American
DRUG INDEX

42nd Edition

American DRUG INDEX

1998

42nd Edition

NORMAN F. BILLUPS, R.Ph., M.S., Ph.D.

Dean and Professor of Pharmacy
College of Pharmacy
The University of Toledo

Associate Editor

SHIRLEY M. BILLUPS, R.N., L.P.C., M.Ed.

Oncology Nurse
Licensed Professional Counselor

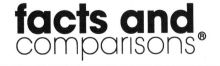

A **Wolters Kluwer** Company

Facts and Comparisons® Staff

Vin Parker
president

Cathy Reilly
coordinating editor

Steven K. Hebel, BS Pharm
director, editorial/production

Noël A. Shamleffer
special projects editor

Bernie R. Olin, PharmD
director of drug information

Julie A. Scott
quality control editor

Heidi L. Meredith
business development

Linda Jones
Bridget Sinclair
Orlando Thomas
assistant editors

ISBN 1-57439-029-5
ISSN 0065-8111

Library of Congress Catalog Card Number 55-6286

Printed in the United States of America

Published by
Facts and Comparisons®
A **Wolters Kluwer** Company
111 West Port Plaza, Suite 300
St. Louis, Missouri 63146-3098

Preface

The 42nd Edition of the *American Drug Index (ADI)* has been prepared for the identification, explanation and correlation of the many pharmaceuticals available to the medical, pharmaceutical and allied health professions. The need for this index has become even more acute as the variety and number of drugs and drug products have continued to multiply. Hence, *ADI* should be useful to pharmacists, nurses, healthcare administrators, physicians, medical transcriptionists, dentists, sales personnel, students and teachers in the fields incorporating pharmaceuticals.

Special note to medical transcriptionists: All generic names are in lowercase and all trade names are in upper/lowercase as appropriate to facilitate transcription. (Tradenames which happen to start with a lowercase letter have been set in uppercase for consistency.) The names for officially designated products (eg, United States Pharmacopeia or U.S.P.) are preceded by a bullet (•) and should appear in lowercase in transcription.

The organization of *ADI* falls into 18 major sections:
Monographs of Drug Products
Common Abbreviations Used in Medical Orders
Common Systems of Weights and Measures
Approximate Practical Equivalents
International System of Units
Normal Laboratory Values
Trademark Glossary
Medical Terminology Glossary
Container Requirements for U.S.P. 23 Drugs
Container and Storage Requirements for Sterile U.S.P. 23 Drugs
Oral Dosage Forms that Should Not Be Crushed or Chewed
Drug Names that Look Alike and Sound Alike
Recommended Childhood Immunization Schedule
Radio-Contrast Media
Radio-Isotopes
Agents for Imaging
Pharmaceutical Company Labeler Code Index
Pharmaceutical Manufacturer and Drug Distributor Listing

MONOGRAPHS: The organization of the monograph section of *ADI* is alphabetical with extensive cross-indexing. Names listed are generic (also called nonproprietary, public name or common name); brand (also called trademark, proprietary or specialty); and chemical. Synonyms that are in general use also are included. All names used for a pharmaceutical appear in alphabetical order with the pertinent data given under the brand name by which it is made available.

The monograph for a typical brand name product appears in upper/lowercase as appropriate, and consists of the manufacturer, generic name, composition and strength, pharmaceutical dosage forms available, package size and use; and appropriate legend designation (eg, *Rx, otc, c-v*).

Generic names appear in lowercase in alphabetical order, followed by the pronunciation and the corresponding recognition of the drug to the U.S.P. (United States Pharmacopeia), N.F. (National Formulary) and USAN (USP Dictionary of United States Adopted Names and International Drug Names). Each of these official generic names is preceded by a bullet (•) at the beginning of each entry. The information is in accord with the U.S.P. 23 and N.F. 18 which became official on January 1, 1995; Supplement 1 which became official on January 1, 1995; the USAN-1996 which became official July 1, 1995; and the 1997 Edition of the USP Dictionary.

Pronunciations have been included for many of the generic drugs. However, not every drug will have a corresponding pronunciation. Some of the most common names are not listed for every drug. The following list is included as a guide to very common names.

Acetate	ASS-eh-tate	Lactobionate	LACK-toe-BYE-oh-nate
Besylate	BESS-ih-late	Maleate	MAL-ee-ate
Borate	BOE-rate	Mesylate	MEH-sih-LATE
Bromide	BROE-mide	Monosodium	MAHN-oh-SO-dee-uhm
Butyrate	BYOO-tih-rate	Nitrate	NYE-trate
Calcium	KAL-see-uhmn	Pendetide	PEN-deh-TIDE
Chloride	KLOR-ide	Pentetate	PEN-teh-tate
Citrate	SIH-trate	Phosphate	FOSS-fate
Dipotassium	die-poe-TASS-ee-uhm	Potassium	poe-TASS-ee-uhm
Disodium	die-SO-dee-uhm	Propionate	PRO-pee-oh-nate
Edetate	eh-deh-TATE	Sodium	SO-dee-uhm
Fosfatex	foss-FAH-tex	Succinate	SUCK-sih-nate
Fumarate	FEW-mah-rate	Sulfate	SULL-fate
Hydrobromide	HIGH-droe-BROE-mide	Tartrate	TAR-trate
Hydrochloride	HIGH-droe-KLOR-ide	Trisodium	try-SO-dee-uhm
Iodide	EYE-oh-dide		

Because of the multiplicity of brand names used for the same therapeutic agent or the same combination of therapeutic agents, it was apparent that some correlation could be done. As an example of this, please turn to tetracycline HCl. Here under the generic name are listed the various brand names. Following are combinations of tetracycline HCl organized in a manner to point out relationships among the many products. Reference then is made to the brand name or names having the indicated composition. Under the brand name are given manufacturer, composition, available forms, sizes, dosage and use.

The multiplicity of generic names for the same therapeutic agent has complicated the nomenclature of these agents. Examples of multiple generic names for the same chemical substance are: (1) parabromdylamine, brompheniramine; (2) acetaminophen, p-hydroxy acetanilid, N-acetyl-p-aminophenol; (3) guaifenesin, glyceryl guaiacolate, glyceryl guaiacol ether, guaianesin, guaifylline, guaiphenesin, guayanesin, methphenoxydiol; (4) pyrilamine, pyranisamine, pyranilamine, pyraminyl, anisopyradamine.

The cross-indexing feature of *ADI* permits the finding of drugs or drug combinations when only one major ingredient is known. For example, a combination of aluminum hydroxide gel and magnesium trisilicate is available. This combination can be found by looking under the name of either of the two ingredients, and in each case the brand names are given. A second form of cross-indexing lists drugs under various therapeutic and pharmaceutical classes (ie, antacids, antihistamines, diuretics, laxatives, etc.).

ABBREVIATIONS: The listing of Common Abbreviations used in Medical Orders is included as an aid in interpreting medical orders. The Latin or Greek word and abbreviation are given with the meaning.

WEIGHTS AND MEASURES: Tables containing the Common Systems of Weights and Measures are included to aid the practitioner in calculating dosages in the metric, apothecary and avoirdupois systems, as well as the International System of Units.

CONVERSION FACTORS: A listing of Approximate Practical Equivalents is added as an aid in calculating and converting dosages among the metric, apothecary and avoirdupois systems.

INTERNATIONAL SYSTEM OF UNITS: A modernized version of the metric system listed in tables for rapid reference.

NORMAL LABORATORY VALUES: Tables containing normal reference values for commonly requested laboratory tests are included as a guideline for the healthcare practitioner.

TRADEMARK GLOSSARY: An alphabetical listing of trademarked dosage forms and package types is included to aid in the identification of drug products listed in *ADI*.

MEDICAL TERMINOLOGY GLOSSARY: Commonly used terms are listed and defined as an aid in interpreting the use given for drug monographs included in *ADI.*

CONTAINER AND STORAGE REQUIREMENTS FOR U.S.P. 23 DRUGS AND STERILE DRUGS: These sections on container and storage requirements specified by the U.S.P. 23 for compendial drugs have been added to aid the practitioner in storing and dispensing.

ORAL DOSAGE FORMS THAT SHOULD NOT BE CRUSHED OR CHEWED: This section has been added to alert the healthcare practitioner about oral dosage forms that should not be crushed, and to serve as an aid in consulting with patients. Examples of products falling into the "non-crush" category are extended-release, enteric-coated, encapsulated beads, wax matrix, sublingual dosage forms and encapsulated liquid formulations.

DRUG NAMES THAT LOOK ALIKE AND SOUND ALIKE: A listing of common drugs that look alike and sound alike. Familiarity with this list may save the prescriber from making a dispensing error.

RECOMMENDED CHILDHOOD IMMUNIZATION SCHEDULE: This section contains dosing and scheduling information for routine childhood vaccines.

RADIO-CONTRAST MEDIA AND ISOTOPES: These tables provide the generic and trade names, dose form and packaging, and manufacturer information as an aid to the healthcare provider.

AGENTS FOR IMAGING: This table provides the generic and trade names, dose form and packaging, and manufacturer information as an aid to the healthcare provider.

LABELER CODE INDEX: The Pharmaceutical Labeler Code Index is presented to aid in the identification of drug products. The codes are listed in numerical order followed by the name of the manufacturer.

MANUFACTURER ADDRESSES: The name, address and zip code of virtually every American pharmaceutical manufacturer and drug distributor are listed in alphabetical order in this section. Additionally, a pharmaceutical labeler code number appears before the address of each company as a further aid in identifying drug products.

Special appreciation and acknowledgment are given to my wife, Shirley, who served again this year as my Associate Editor – and to Dr. Bernie R. Olin, Director of Drug Information of Facts and Comparisons, for compiling the monograph section of this volume. Special thanks are also extended to the manufacturers who supplied product information, to Dr. Kenneth S. Alexander for organizing the Container and Storage Requirements information, to Dr. John F. Mitchell for the table on Oral Dosage Forms that Should Not Be Crushed or Chewed, and to Drs. Charles O. Wilson and Tony E. Jones for their earlier contributions to *ADI*.

Correspondence or communication with reference to a drug or drug products listed in *ADI* should be directed to Editorial/Production, Attn: ADI, Facts and Comparisons, 111 West Port Plaza, Suite 300, St. Louis, Missouri 63146, or call 1-800-223-0554.

Norman F. Billups, RPh, MS, PhD

Contents

[•] Denotes official name: Generic name or chemical name recognized by the U.S.P., N.F., or USAN.

Monographs

A

AA-HC Otic. (Schein) Hydrocortisone 1%, acetic acid glacial 2%, propylene glycol diacetate 3%, benzethonium Cl 0.02%, sodium acetate 0.015%, citric acid 0.2%. Soln. Bot. 10 ml. *Rx.*
Use: Otic preparation.

A and D Ointment. (Schering-Plough) Fish liver oil, cholecalciferol. Tube 1.5 oz, 4 oz. Jar lb. *otc.*
Use: Emollient.

A & D Tablets. (Barth's) Vitamins A 10,000 IU, D 400 IU/Tab. Bot. 100s, 500s. *otc.*
Use: Vitamin supplement.

•**abacavir succinate.** USAN.
Use: Antiviral.

•**abafilcon a.** (ab-ah-FILL-kahn) USAN.
Use: Contact lens material (hydrophilic).

•**abamectin.** (abe-ah-MEK-tin) USAN.
Use: Antiparasitic.

Abbokinase. (Abbott) Urokinase 250,000 IU/5 ml. Lyophilized pow. Vial 5 ml. *Rx.*
Use: Thrombolytic enzyme.

Abbokinase Open-Cath. (Abbott) Urokinase for catheter clearance 5000 IU/ml. Univial 1 ml. *Rx.*
Use: Thrombolytic enzyme.

Abbott AFP-EIA. (Abbott Diagnostics) Enzyme immunoassay for the quantitative measurement of alpha-fetoprotein (AFP) in human serum and amniotic fluid. Test kits 100s.
Use: Diagnostic aid.

Abbott AFP-EIA Monoclonal. (Abbott Diagnostics) Enzyme immunoassay for the quantitative measurement of alpha-fetoprotein (AFP) in human serum and amniotic fluid.
Use: Diagnostic aid.

Abbott Anti-Delta. (Abbott Diagnostics) Radioimmunoassay for the detection of antibody to delta antigen (HDAg) in human serum or plasma. For research only. Not for use in diagnostic procedures.
Use: Research.

Abbott Anti-Delta EIA. (Abbott Diagnostics) Enzyme immunoassay for the detection of antibody to hepatitis delta antigen in human serum or plasma. For research only. Not for use in diagnostic procedures.
Use: Research.

Abbott β-HCG 15/15. (Abbott Diagnostics) Enzyme immunoassay for the quantitative determination of human chorionic gonadotropin in human serum.
Use: Diagnostic aid.

Abbott CA125-EIA. (Abbott Diagnostics) Enzyme immunoassay for the quantitative measurement of cancer antigen (CA) 125 in human serum. For research only. Not for use in diagnostic procedures.
Use: Research.

Abbott CEA-EIA Monoclonal. (Abbott Diagnostics) Enzyme immunoassay for the quantitative measurement of carcinoembryonic antigen (CEA) in human serum or plasma to aid in the management of cancer patients and assessing prognosis.
Use: Diagnostic aid.

Abbott CEA-RIA. (Abbott Diagnostics) Solid phase radioimmunoassay for the quantitative measurement of carcinoembryonic antigen (CEA) in human serum or plasma to aid in the management of cancer patients and assessing prognosis.
Use: Diagnostic aid.

Abbott CMV Total AB EIA. (Abbott Diagnostics) Enzyme immunoassay for the detection of antibody to cytomegalovirus in human serum, plasma, and whole blood. Test kits 100s.
Use: Diagnostic aid.

Abbott Diagnostic Reagents. (Abbott Diagnostics) A series of diagnostic tests for cancer, cardiovascular, hepatitis, infectious disease and immunology, metabolic and digestive disease, OB/GYN, rubella and thyroid.
Use: Diagnostic aid.

Abbott ER-EIA Monoclonal. (Abbott Diagnostics) Enzyme immunoassay for the quantitative measurement of human estrogen receptor in tissue cytosol. For research only. Not for use in diagnostic procedures.
Use: Research.

Abbott ER-ICA Monoclonal. (Abbott Diagnostics) Immunoassay for the detection of estrogen receptor. For research only. Not for use in diagnostic procedures.
Use: Research.

Abbott-HB EIA. (Abbott Diagnostics) Enzyme immunoassay for the detection of hepatitis Be antigen or antibody to hepatitis Be antigen.
Use: Diagnostic aid.

Abbott-HBe Test. (Abbott Diagnostics) Radioimmunoassay or enzyme immunoassay for detection of hepatitis Be

antigen or antibody to hepatitis Be antigen. Test kits 100s.
Use: Diagnostic aid.

Abbott HIVAB HIV-1 EIA. (Abbott Diagnostics) Enzyme immunoassay for the antibody to human immunodeficiency virus type 1 (HIV-1) in serum or plasma. Test kits 100s, 1000s.
Use: Diagnostic aid.

Abbott HIVAG-1. (Abbott Diagnostics) Enzyme immunoassay for the human immunodeficiency virus type 1 (HIV-1) antigens in serum or plasma. Test kits 100s, 1000s.
Use: Diagnostic aid.

Abbott HTLV I EIA. (Abbott Diagnostics) To detect antibody to Human T-Lymphotropic Virus Type I in serum or plasma. Test kits 100s.
Use: Diagnostic aid.

Abbott HTLV III Antigen EIA. (Abbott Diagnostics) Enzyme immunoassay for the detection of Human T-Lymphotropic Virus Type III (HIV) antigens. For research only. Not for use in diagnostic procedures.
Use: Research.

Abbott HTLV III Confirmatory EIA. (Abbott Diagnostics) Enzyme immunoassay for confirmation of specimens found to be positive to antibody to HTLV III. Test kits 100s.
Use: Diagnostic aid.

Abbott HTLV III EIA. (Abbott Diagnostics) Enzyme immunoassay for the detection of antibody to Human T-Lymphotropic Virus Type III (HIV) in human serum or plasma. Test kits 1s.
Use: Diagnostic aid.

Abbott IGE EIA. (Abbott Diagnostics) Enzyme immunoassay for quantitative determination of IgE in human serum and plasma. Test kits 100s.
Use: Diagnostic aid.

Abbott PAP-EIA. (Abbott Diagnostics) Enzyme immunoassay for the measurement of prostatic acid phosphatase (PAP) in serum or plasma.
Use: Diagnostic aid.

Abbott RSV-EIA. (Abbott Diagnostics) Enzyme immunoassay for the detection of respiratory syncytial virus (RSV) in nasopharyngeal washes and aspirates.
Use: Diagnostic aid.

Abbott SCC-RIA. (Abbott Diagnostics) Radioimmunoassay for the quantitative measurement of squamous cell carcinoma associated antigen in human serum. For research only. Not for use in

diagnostic procedures.
Use: Research.

Abbott TdT EIA. (Abbott Diagnostics) Enzyme immunoassay for the quantitative measurement of terminal deoxynucleotidyl transferase (TdT), in extracts of human whole blood or isolated mononuclear cells.
Use: Diagnostic aid.

Abbott Testpack hCG-Serum. (Abbott Diagnostics) Monoclonal antibody, enzyme immunoassay for the qualitative determination of human chorionic gonadotropin (hCG) in serum. No instrumentation required.
Use: Diagnostic aid.

Abbott Testpak hCG-Urine. (Abbott Diagnostics) Monoclonal antibody, enzyme immunoassay for the qualitative determination of human chorionic gonadotropin (hCG) in urine. No instrumentation required.
Use: Diagnostic aid.

Abbott Testpack-Strep A. (Abbott Diagnostics) A rapid screening and confirmatory test for the detection of Group A beta-hemolytic streptococci from throat swabs. No instrumentation required.
Use: Diagnostic aid.

Abbott Toxo-G EIA. (Abbott Diagnostics) Enzyme immunoassay for the qualitative and quantitative determination of IgG antibody to toxoplasma gondii in human serum and plasma.
Use: Diagnostic aid.

Abbott Toxo-M EIA. (Abbott Diagnostics) Enzyme immunoassay for the qualitative determination of IgM antibody to toxoplasma gondii in human serum.
Use: Diagnostic aid.

ABC to Z. (NTBY) Iron 18 mg, Vitamins A 5000 IU, D 400 IU, E 30 IU, B_1 1.5 mg, B_2 1.7 mg, B_3 20 mg, B_5 10 mg, B_6 2 mg, B_{12} 6 mcg, C 60 mg, folic acid 0.4 mg, biotin 30 mcg, Ca, P, I, Mg, Cu, Mn, K, Cl, Cr, Mo, Se, Ni, Si, Sn, V, B, vitamin K, Zn 15 mg/Tab. Bot. 100s. *otc.*
Use: Vitamin/mineral supplement.

•**abciximab.** (ab-SICK-sih-mab) USAN.
Use: Monoclonal antibody (antithrombotic).
See: ReoPro (Lilly).

Abelcet. (Liposome) Amphotericin B 5 mg, 1.5 mg per ml/inj. Vial 20 mg. *Rx.*
Use: Antibiotic.

Abitrexate. (International Pharm. Products) Methotrexate sodium 25 mg/ml. Vial 2 ml, 4 ml, 8 ml. *Rx.*

Use: Antineoplastic.

●**ablukast.** (ab-LOO-kast) USAN.
Use: Antiasthmatic (leukotriene antagonist).

●**ablukast sodium.** (ab-LOO-kast) USAN.
Use: Antiasthmatic (leukotriene antagonist).
See: Ulpax (Hoffman-LaRoche).

abortifacients.
See: Hemabate, Inj. (Pharmacia & Upjohn).
Prostin E_2, Supp. (Pharmacia & Upjohn).

absorbable cellulose cotton or gauze.
See: Oxidized Cellulose (Various Mfr.).

●**absorbable dusting powder,** U.S.P. 23.
Use: Surgical glove lubricant.

●**absorbable gelatin film,** U.S.P. 23.
Use: Hemostatic.
See: Gelfilm (Pharmacia & Upjohn).
Gelfilm Ophthalmic (Pharmacia & Upjohn).

absorbable gelatin powder.
Use: Hemstatic, topical.
See: Gelfoam, Pow. (Pharmacia & Upjohn).

●**absorbable gelatin sponge,** U.S.P. 23.
Use: Local hemostatic.
See: Gelfoam (Pharmacia & Upjohn).

●**absorbable surgical suture,** U.S.P. 23.
Use: Surgical aid.

Absorbase. (Carolina Medical) Petrolatum, mineral oil, ceresin wax, wool wax, alcohol. Oint. Tube 114 g, 454 g. *otc.*
Use: Ointment and lotion base.

●**absorbent gauze,** U.S.P. 23.
Use: Surgical aid.

Absorbent Rub Relief Formula. (De-Witt) Green soap 11.64%, camphor 1.63%, menthol 1.63%, pine tar soap 0.87%, wintergreen oil 0.71%, sassafras oil 0.54%, benzocaine 0.48%, capsicum 0.03%, wormwood oil 0.6%, isopropyl alcohol 75%. Bot. 2 oz. *otc.*
Use: Analgesic, topical.

Absorbine Antifungal. (W.F. Young) Tolnaftate 1%. **Pow.:** Jar 56.7 g. **Cream:** Glyceryl monosterate, propylene glycol, diazolidinyl urea, parabens. Tube 21.3 g. *otc.*
Use: Antifungal, topical.

Absorbine Antifungal Foot Powder. (W.F. Young) Miconazole nitrate 2%, alcohol 10%. Aerosol 85 g. *otc.*
Use: Antifungal, topical.

Absorbine Athlete's Foot Care. (W.F. Young) Tolnaftate 1%, menthol. Liq. Bot. 59.2 ml. *otc.*
Use: Antifungal, topical.

Absorbine Foot Powder. (W.F. Young) Zinc stearate, parachloroxylenol, aluminum chlorhydroxy, allantonate, benzethonium Cl, menthol. Plastic bot. 3 oz w/shaker top. *otc.*
Use: Antifungal, topical.

Absorbine Jock Itch. (W.F. Young) Tolnaftate 1%. Pow. Jar 56.7 g. *otc.*
Use: Antifungal, topical.

Absorbine, Jr. (W.F. Young) Wormwood, thymol, chloroxylenol, menthol, acetone, zinc stearate, parachloroxylenol, aluminum chlorhydroxy, allantonate, benzethonium Cl, menthol. Liq. Bot. 1 oz, 2 oz, 4 oz, 12 oz w/applicator. *otc.*
Use: Analgesic, antifungal, topical.

Absorbine Jr. Antifungal. (W.F. Young) Tolnaftate 1%. Spray Liq. Bot. 59.2 ml, 118.3 ml. *otc.*
Use: Antifungal, topical.

Absorbine Jr. Extra Strength Liniment. (W.F. Young) Natural menthol 4%, plant extracts of calendula, echinacea and wormwood, acetone, chloroxylenol iodine, potassium iodide, thymol, wormwood oil. Lot. Bot. 59 ml, 118 ml. *otc.*
Use: Rub or liniment.

Absorbine Jr. Extra Strength Liquid. (W.F. Young) Menthol 4%. Liq. Bot. 59 ml, 118 ml. *otc.*
Use: Rub or liniment.

Absorbine Jr. Liniment. (W.F. Young) Menthol 1.27%, plant extracts of calendula, echinacea and wormwood, iodine, potassium iodide, thymol, acetone, chloroxylenol. Lot. Bot. 60 ml, 120 ml. *otc.*
Use: Rub or liniment.

Absorbine Power Gel. (W.F. Young) Menthol 4%. Tube 88 g. *otc.*
Use: Rub or liniment.

Abuscreen. (Roche Diagnostics) An immunological and radiochemical assay for morphine and morphine glucuronide in nanogram levels. Utilizes I-125 labeled morphine requiring gamma scintillation equipment. Tests 100s.
Use: Diagnostic aid.

●**acacia,** N.F. 18.
Use: Pharmaceutic aid (suspending or viscosity agent).

●**acadesine.** (ack-AH-dess-een) USAN.
Use: Platelet aggregation inhibitor.

●**acarbose.** (A-car-bose) USAN.
Use: Antidiabetic.
See: Precose, Tab. (Bayer).

Accolate. Zafirlukast 20 mg/Tab. Bot. 60s, 100s. *Rx.*

Use: Treatment of asthma.

Accupep HPF. (Sherwood) Hydrolyzed lactalbumin, maltodextrin, MCT oil, corn oil, mono- and diglycerides, vitamins A, B_1, B_2, B_3, B_5, B_6, B_{12}, C, D, E, K, Ca, Cl, Cu, Fe, I, Mg, Mn, P, Zn, biotin and choline. Pks. 128 g. *otc.*
Use: Nutritional supplement.

Accupril. (Parke-Davis) Quinapril 5 mg, 10 mg, 20 mg, 40 mg/Tab. Bot. Lactose. 90s and UD 100s. *Rx.*
Use: Antihypertensive.

Accurbron. (Hoechst Marion Roussel) Theophylline, anhydrous 10 mg/ml. Bot. Pt. *Rx.*
Use: Bronchodilator.

Accusens T Taste Function Kit. (Westport) Test for ability to distinguish among salty, sweet, sour and bitter tastants. Kit contains 15 bottles (60 ml) tastants and 30 taste record forms.
Use: Diagnostic aid.

Accutane. (Roche) Isotretinoin 10 mg, 20 mg, or 40 mg/Cap. Bot. UD 100s. *Rx.*
Use: Antiacne, oral.

A-C-D Solution. Sodium citrate, citric acid and dextrose in sterile pyrogen-free solution. (Baxter) 600 ml bot. with 70 ml, 120 ml, 300 ml Soln.; 1000 ml Bot. with 500 ml Soln. (Cutter) 500 ml Bot. with 75 ml, 120 ml Soln.; 650 ml bot. with 80 ml, 130 ml Soln. (Diamond) (Abbo-Vac) 250 ml, 500 ml. *Rx.*
Use: Anticoagulant for preparation of plasma or whole blood.

A-C-D Solution Modified. (Squibb) Acid citrate dextrose anticoagulant solution modified. *Rx.*
Use: Anticoagulant for use in radiolabeling red blood cells.

•**acebutolol.** (ass-cee-BYOO-toe-lahl) USAN. (Mylan) 200 mg or 400 mg/Cap. Bot. 100s.
Use: Antihypertensive (β-receptor).
See: Sectral, Cap. (Wyeth-Ayerst).

•**acebutolol hydrochloride,** U.S.P. 23.
Use: Antiadrenergic (β-receptor).
See: Sectral, Cap. (Wyeth-Ayerst).

•**acecainide hydrochloride.** (ASS-eh-CANE-ide) USAN.
Use: Cardiac depressant (antiarrhythmic).
See: Napa (Medco Research/Parke-Davis).

•**aceclidine.** (ass-ECK-lih-DEEN) USAN. 3-Quinuclidinol acetate (ester). Glaucostat.
Use: Cholinergic.

See: Glaucostat (Kingshill Pharmaceuticals Inc., Switzerland).

•**acedapsone.** (ASS-eh-DAP-sone) USAN. 4′,4″-Sulfonylbis (acetanilide).
Use: Antimalarial; antibacterial (leprostatic).

Acedoval. (Pal-Pak) Dover's powder 15 mg, ipecac 1.5 mg, aspirin 162 mg, caffeine anhydrous 8.1 mg/Tab. Bot. 1000s, 5000s. *otc.*
Use: Analgesic, antispasmodic, antiperistaltic.

•**aceglutamide aluminum.** (AH-see-GLUE-tah-mide ah-LOO-min-uhm) USAN.
Use: Antiulcerative.

Acel-Imune. (Lederle) Diphtheria toxoid 7.5 Lf units, tetanus toxoid 5 Lf units, acellular pertussis vaccine 300 hemagglutinating units and aluminum ≤ 0.85 mg/0.5 ml. With formaldehyde ≤ 0.02%, thimerosal final concentration of 1:10,000. Aluminum hydroxide and phosphate, thimerosal, gelatin, glycine, polysorbate 80. 5 ml/vial for inj. *Rx.*
Use: Agent for immunization.

•**acemannan.** (ah-see-MAN-an) USAN.
Use: Antiviral; immunomodulator.
See: Carrisyn (Carrington).

Aceon. (Ortho) Perindopril erbumine 2 mg, 4 mg or 8 mg. Tab. Bot. 100s and UD blister packs. *Rx.*
Use: Antihypertensive.

Acephen. (G & W) **Adult:** Acetaminophen 650 mg/Supp. Box 12s, 100s. **Pediatric:** Acetaminophen 120 mg/Supp. Box 12s, 100s. *otc.*
Use: Analgesic.

acepromazine. (ASS-ee-PRO-mah-zeen) (Wyeth-Ayerst) *Rx.*
Use: Tranquilizer.

Acerola-C. (Barth's) Vitamin C 300 mg/Wafer. Bot. 30s, 90s, 180s, 360s. *otc.*
Use: Vitamin C supplement.

Acerola-Plex. (Barth's) Vitamin C 100 mg, bioflavonoids 50 mg/Tab. Bot. 100s, 500s. *otc.*
Use: Vitamin supplement.

Aceta. (Century) Acetaminophen 325 mg or 500 mg/Tab. Bot. 100s, 1000s. *otc.*
Use: Analgesic.

Aceta w/Codeine. (Century) Acetaminophen 300 mg, codeine phosphate 30 mg/Tab. Bot. 100s. *c-III.*
Use: Narcotic analgesic combination.

Aceta Elixir. (Century) Acetaminophen 160 mg/5 ml, alcohol 7%. Elix. Bot. 120 ml, 1 gal. *otc.*
Use: Analgesic.

Aceta-Gesic. (Rugby) Acetaminophen 325 mg, phenyltoloxamine citrate 30 mg/Tab. Bot. 100s, 1000s. *otc.*
Use: Analgesic, antihistamine.
•**acetaminophen,** (ass-cet-ah-MEE-noe-fen) U.S.P. 23. APAP.
Use: Analgesic, antipyretic.
See: Acephen, Supp. (G & W).
Aceta, Tab., Elix., Supp. (Century).
Acetaminophen Uniserts, Supp. (Upsher-Smith).
Actamin, Tab. (Buffington).
Actamin Extra, Tab. (Buffington).
Aminodyne, Elix. (Jones Medical).
Anacin-3, Chew. tab., Tab., Elix., Drops (Whitehall Robins).
Anapap, Tab. (Forest).
Apap, Cap., Tab. (Various Mfr.).
Aspirin Free Anacin, Capl., Gel Capl., Tab. (Whitehall Robins).
Dapa, Tab. (Ferndale).
Datril 500, Tab. (Bristol-Myers).
Dorcol, Prods. (Sandoz Consumer).
Fendon, Tab. (APC).
G-1 (Roberts).
Genapap, Chew. tab. (Goldline).
Genebs, Tab., Cap. (Goldline).
Halenol, Tab., Elix. (Halsey).
Lestemp, Elix. (Solvay).
Liquiprin, Soln. (SK-Beecham).
Meda Cap, Cap. (Circle).
Meda Tab, Tab. (Circle).
Neopap, Supp. (PolyMedica).
Panadol, Cap., Chew. tab., Tab., Liq. Drops (Bayer).
Panex, Tab. (Roberts).
Parten, Tab. (Parmed).
Phenaphen, Cap., Tab. (Robins).
Proval, Cap., Elix., Drops, Tab. (Solvay).
Suppap-120, 325, 650, Supp. (Raway).
Tapanol Extra Strength, Tab. (Republic).
Temetan, Elix., Tab. (Nevin).
Tempra, Drops, Syr., (Bristol-Myers).
Ty-Caplets, Tab. (Major).
Ty-Caps, Cap. (Major).
Tylenol, Drops, Elix., Liq., Tab., Chew. tab. (McNeil).
Tylenol Extra-Strength, Tab., Cap. (McNeil).
Ty-Pap, Supp., Elix. (Major).
Ty-Tabs, Tab. (Major).
acetaminophen w/combinations.
See: Aceta w/Codeine, Tab. (Century).
Actifed Plus, Tab. (Glaxo Wellcome).
Actifed Sinus Daytime/Nightime, Capl., (Glaxo Wellcome).
Allerest Headache Strength, Tab. (Novartis).

Allergy-Sinus Comtrex, Capl., Tab. (Bristol-Myers).
Alumadrine, Tab. (Fleming).
Anexsia, Tab. (Mallinckrodt).
Anodynos Forte, Tab. (Buffington).
Apap w/Codeine, Tab. (Schwarz Pharma).
Aspirin Free Anacin P.M., Tab. (Robins).
Axocet, Cap. (Savage).
Bayer Select Flu Relief, Capl. (Bayer).
Bayer Select Head Cold, Capl. (Bayer).
Bayer Select Night Time Cold, Capl. (Bayer).
BQ Cold, Tab. (Bristol-Myers).
Bromo-Seltzer, Gran. (Warner-Lambert).
Capital and Codeine, Susp. (Carnrick).
Codimal, Tab. (Schwarz Pharma).
Comtrex Caplets (Bristol-Myers).
Comtrex Liquid (Bristol-Myers).
Comtrex Liqui-Gels (Bristol-Myers).
Comtrex Tablets (Bristol-Myers).
Contac Day & Night Allergy/Sinus Caplets (SK-Beecham).
Contac Day & Night Colds & Flu Caplets (SK-Beecham).
Coricidin, Tab. (Schering-Plough).
Coricidin D, Tab. (Schering-Plough).
Coricidin Sinus Headache, Tab. (Schering-Plough).
Darvocet-N 100, Tab. (Lilly).
DHC Plus, Cap. (Purdue Frederick).
Dristan Cold Multi-Symptom Formula, Tab. (Whitehall Robins).
Drixoral Cold & Flu, Tab. (Schering-Plough).
Drixoral Cough & Sore Throat, Liquid caps. (Schering-Plough).
Esgic, Tab. (Gilbert).
Excedrin Aspirin Free, Cap. (Bristol-Myers).
Excedrin Sinus, Capl., Tab. (Bristol-Myers).
Histosal #2, Tab. (Ferndale).
Hycomine Compound, Tab. (DuPont Merck).
Hy-Phen, Tab. (Ascher).
Hydrocet, Cap. (Carnrick).
Liquiprin, Soln. (Menley & James)
Mapap CF, Tab. (Major).
Midol Maximum Strength, Tab. (Bayer).
Midol Teen, Cap. (Bayer).
Midrin, Cap. (Carnrick).
Naldegesic, Tab. (Bristol-Myers Squibb).
N-D Gesic, Tab. (Hyrex).
Nyquil, Liq. (Procter & Gamble).

Ornex, (Menley & James).
Ornex Maximum Strength, Cap. (Menley & James).
Pamprin Prods. (Chattem Labs.).
Percocet, Tab. (Dupont).
Percogesic, Tab. (DuPont Merck).
Phenaphen #2, #3, #4 (Robins).
Phrenilin, Tab. (Carnrick).
Phrenilin Forte, Cap. (Carnrick).
Propacet 100, Tab. (Lemmon).
Proval No. 3, Tab. (Solvay).
Quiet World, Tab. (Whitehall Robins).
Renpap, Tab. (Wren).
Repan, Tab. (Everett).
Robitussin Night Relief, (Whitehall Robins).
Saleto, Tab. (Roberts).
Saleto-D, Tab. (Roberts).
Sinarest, Tab. (Novartis).
Sine-Aid Maximum Strength, Cap., Tab. (McNeil-CPC).
Sine-Off Maximum Strength No Drowsiness Formula, Capl. (SK-Beecham).
Sine-Off Sinus Medicine, Capl. (SK-Beecham).
Sinulin, Tab. (Carnrick).
Sinutab, Prods. (Warner-Lambert).
St. Joseph Cold Tablets for Children, Tab. (Schering-Plough).
Sudafed Cold & Cough, Liq. Cap. (Glaxo Wellcome).
Sudafed Severe Cold, Tab. (Glaxo Wellcome).
Supac, Tab. (Mission).
Talacen, Cap. (Sanofi Winthrop).
Triaminic Sore Throat Formula, Liq. (Sandoz).
Triaprin, Cap. (Dunhall).
Two-Dyne, Tab. (Hyrex).
Tylenol Children's Chewable Tablets (McNeil).
Tylenol Children's Cold Tablets (McNeil).
Tylenol Children's Suspension (McNeil).
Tylenol Cold, Liq., Cap., Tab. (McNeil).
Tylenol Cold & Flu No Drowsiness, Pow. (McNeil).
Tylenol Cold, Liq., Cap., Tab. (McNeil).
Tylenol Cold Night Time, Liq. (McNeil).
Tylenol Cold No Drowsiness, Capl., Gelcap. (McNeil).
Tylenol Cough, Liq. (McNeil).
Tylenol Cough w/ Decongestant, Liq. (McNeil).
Tylenol Extended Relief, Capl. (McNeil).

Tylenol w/ Codeine, Tab. (McNeil).
Tylenol, Preps. (McNeil).
Tylox, Cap. (McNeil).
Vanquish, Tab. (Bayer).
Vicodin, Tab. (Knoll).
Viro-Med, Tab. (Whitehall Robins).
Wygesic, Tab. (Wyeth-Ayerst).
Zydone, Cap. (DuPont Merck).

acetaminophen and aspirin tablets.
Use: Analgesic.

acetaminophen and caffeine capsules.
Cap., Tab.
Use: Analgesic.

acetaminophen, aspirin and caffeine.
Cap., Tab.
Use: Analgesic.

Acetaminophen Buffered. *otc.*
Use: Analgesic.
See: Bromo-Seltzer (Warner Lambert Consumer Health Products).

Acetaminophen w/Codeine. (ass-cet-ah-MEE-noe-fen) (Various Mfr.) **Tab.:** Codeine phosphate 15 mg, acetaminophen 300 mg/Tab. Bot. 100s, 500s, 1000s. Codeine phosphate 30 mg, acetaminophen 300 mg/Tab. Bot. 100s, 500s, 1000s, UD 100s, RN 100s. Codeine phosphate 60 mg, acetaminophen 300 mg/Tab. Bot. 100s, 500s, 1000s. *c-III.* **Soln.:** Codeine phosphate 12 mg, acetaminophen 120 mg/5 ml. Bot. 120 ml, 500 ml, pt, gal, UD 5 ml, 12.5 ml, 15 ml. *c-v.*
Use: Narcotic analgesic combination.

acetaminophen and codeine phosphate oral solution.
Use: Analgesic.

acetaminophen and diphenhydramine citrate tablets.
Use: Analgesic, antihistamine.

acetaminophen and pseudoephedrine hydrochloride tablets.
Use: Analgesic, decongestant.

acetaminophen oral solution.
Use: Analgesic.

acetaminophen oral suspension.
Use: Analgesic.

acetaminophen suppositories.
Use: Analgesic.

acetaminophen uniserts. (Upsher-Smith) Acetaminophen **120 mg or 325 mg/Supp.:** Ctn. 12s, 50s; **650 mg/Supp.:** Ctn. 12s, 50s, 500s. *otc.*
Use: Analgesic.

acetaminophenol.
See: Acetaminophen.

acetanilid. (Various Mfr.) (Acetylaminobenzene, acetylaniline, antifebrin) N-phenylacetamide cry.

Use: Analgesic (former use).

Acetasol.
See: Acetarsone.

acetarsone. 3-Acetamido-4-hydroxy-phenylarsonic acid. Acetarsol, Acet-phenarsine, Amarsan, Dynarsan, Ehrlich 594, Limarsol, Orarsan, Osar-sal, Osvarsan, Paroxyl, Stovarsol.

acetarsone salt of arecoline.
See: Drocarbil.

Acetasol HC Otic. (Goldline) Hydrocortisone 1%, acetic acid 2%. Bot. 10 ml. *Rx.*
Use: Otic corticosteroid, anti-infective.

Acetasol Otic. (Goldline) Acetic acid (non-aqueous) 2%. Bot. 5 ml. *Rx.*
Use: Anti-infective, otic.

•**acetazolamide,** (uh-seet-uh-ZOLE-uh-mide) U.S.P. 23. (Various Mfr.) **Tab.:** 125 mg, Bot. 100s; 250 mg, Bot. 100s, 1000s, UD 100s. **Pow.:** 500 mg/vial.
Use: Carbonic anhydrase inhibitor.
See: Diamox (Lederle)

•**acetazolamide sodium, sterile,** U.S.P. 23.
Use: Carbonic anhydrase inhibitor.

acet-dia-mer-sulfonamide. Sulf-acetamide, sulfadiazine and sulfamera-zine, Susp. *Rx.*
Use: Antibacterial, sulfonamide.

Acetest Reagent Tablets. (Bayer) Sodium nitroprusside, disodium phosphate, aminoacetic acid, lactose. Tab. Bot. 100s, 250s.
Use: Diagnostic aid.

•**acetic acid,** N.F. 18.
Use: Pharmaceutic aid (acidifying agent).
See: Otic Domeboro, Soln. (Bayer). Vosol Otic Solution, (Wallace).

•**acetic acid, glacial.** U.S.P. 23.
Use: Pharmaceutic aid (acidifying agent).
See: Aci-Jel (Ortho).

acetic acid irrigation. 0.25% soln. (Abbott) 250 ml glass cont.; 250 ml, 1000 ml.
Use: Irrigating solution.

Acetic Acid Otic. (Various Mfr.) Acetic acid 2% with propylene glycol diacetate 3%, benzethonium chloride 0.02% and sodium acetate 0.015%. Soln. Bot. 15 ml, 30 ml, 60 ml. *Rx.*
Use: Otic preparation.

acetic acid, potassium salt. Potassium Acetate, U.S.P. 23.

•**acetohexamide,** (uh-seet-toe-HEX-uh-mide) U.S.P. 23.
Use: Antidiabetic.

acetohexamide. (Various Mfr.) 250 or 500 mg/Tab. 100s. *Rx.*
Use: Antidiabetic.
See: Dymelor, Tab. (Lilly).

•**acetohydroxamic acid,** (ass-EE-toe-high-drox-AM-ik) U.S.P. 23.
Use: Enzyme inhibitor (urease).
See: Lithostat (Mission Pharmacal).

acetomeroctol.
Use: Antiseptic, topical.

•**acetone,** N.F. 18.
Use: Pharmaceutic aid (solvent).

acetone or diacetic acid test.
See: Acetest, Tab. (Bayer).

•**acetophenazine maleate.** (ASS-ee-toe-FEN-ah-zeen) U.S.P. XXII.
Use: Antipsychotic.

acetophenetidin. Phenacetin, Ethoxyacetanilide.
Use: Analgesic, antipyretic.

•**acetosulfone sodium.** USAN.
Use: Antibacterial (leprostatic).

acetoxyphenylmercury.
See: Phenylmercuric acetate.

n-acetyl-p-aminophenol. Acetaminophen.

acetylaniline.
See: Acetanilid (Various Mfr.).

acetyl-bromo-diethylacetyl-carbamide.
See: Acetylcarbromal (Various Mfr.).

acetylcarbromal. Acetyladalin, acetyl-bromodiethylacetylcarbamide. Pow. for manufacturing.
Use: Sedative.
See: Paxarel, Tab. (Circle).
W/Bromisovalum, scopolamine aminoxide HBr.

•**acetylcholine chloride,** U.S.P. 23.
Use: Cardiac depressant; cholinergic; mitotic; vasodilator (peripheral).
See: Miochol Ophthalmic (Ciba Vision). Miochol-E (Ciba Vision).

acetylcholine-like therapeutic agents.
See: Cholinergic agents.

•**acetylcysteine,** (ASS-cee-till-SIS-teen) U.S.P. 23.
Use: Mucolytic [Orphan drug].
See: Acetylcysteine (Various Mfr.).
Mucosil (Dey Labs).
Mucomyst, Soln. (Bristol).

acetylcysteine. (Various Mfr.) Soln: 10%, in 4, 10, and 30 ml vials; 20%, in 4, 10, 30 and 100 ml vials. *Rx.*
Use: Mucolytic.

acetylcysteine and isoproterenol hydrochloride inhalation solution.
Use: Mucolytic.

acetylcysteine (Flumucil). (Zambon). Phase I HIV, ARC, AIDS.

Use: Immunomodulator.

acetylin.
See: Acetylsalicylic Acid (Various Mfr.).

acetylphenylisatin. *Rx.*
See: Oxyphenisatin Acetate.

acetylprocainamide-n.
Use: Cardiac depressant.
See: acecainide, NAPA.

acetylsalicylic acid. Aspirin.
Use: Analgesic; antipyretic; antirheumatic.
See: Aspirin Preps. (Various Mfr.).

acetyl sulfamethoxypyridazine. 3-(N-Acetylsulfanilamido)-6-methoxypyridazine.

n¹-acetylsulfanilamide. (Albucid; p-Aminobenzenesulfonacetamide; Sulfacet; Sulfacetamide, N-Sulfanilylacetamide). *Rx.*
Use: Sulfonamide therapy.

acetyl sulfisoxazole. Sulfisoxazole Acetyl, U.S.P. 23.

acetyltannic acid. Tannic acid acetate.
Use: Antiperistaltic.

AC Eye Drops. (Walgreen) Tetrahydrozoline HCl 0.05%, zinc sulfate 0.25%. Bot. 0.75 oz. *otc.*
Use: Decongestant combination, ophthalmic.

achlorhydria determination.
See: Diagnex Blue, Preps. (Squibb).

achlorhydria therapy.
See: Glutamic Acid HCl (Various Mfr.).

Achol. (Enzyme Process) Vitamin A 4000 units, ketocholanic acids 62 mg/Tab. Bot. 100s, 250s. *otc.*
Use: Vitamin A supplement.

acid acriflavine.
See: Acriflavine HCl (Various Mfr.).

acid citrate dextrose anticoagulant solution modified.
See: A-C-D Solution Modified (Squibb).

acid citrate dextrose solution.
See: A.C.D. Soln. (Various Mfr.).

acidifiers.
See: Ammonium Cl (Various Mfr.).
K-Phos M.F. (Beach).

Acid Mantle. (Sandoz Consumer) Aluminum sulfate, calcium acetate, cetearyl alcohol, glycerin, light mineral oil, methylparaben, sodium lauryl sulfate, synthetic beeswax, white petrolatum, ammonium hydroxide, citric acid. Cream. Jar 120 g. *otc.*
Use: Ointment and lotion base.

Acid Mantle Creme. (Sandoz Consumer) Aluminum acetate in specially prepared water-soluble hydrophilic cream at pH 4.2. Tube 1 oz, Jar 4 oz, lb. *otc.*

Use: Prophylactic agent, topical.

acidophilus.
See: Bacid (Medeva).
Lactinex (Becton Dickinson).
More-Dophilus (Freeda).

acidophilus w/pectin. (Barth's) *Lactobacillus acidophilus* w/natural citrus pectin 100 mg/Cap. Bot. 100s. *otc.*
Use: Antidiarrheal.

acid trypaflavine.
See: Acriflavine HCl. (Various Mfr.).

Acidulated Phosphate Fluoride. (Scherer) Fluoride ion 0.31% in 0.1 molar phosphate. Soln. Bot. 64 oz. (Office Product).
Use: Dental caries preventative.

•**acifran.** (ACE-ih-FRAN) USAN.
Use: Antihyperlipoproteinemic.

Aci-Jel. (Ortho) Glacial acetic acid 0.92%, ricinoleic acid 0.7%, oxyquinoline sulfate 0.025%, glycerin 5%. Propylparaben, tube 85 g w/dose applicator. *Rx.*
Use: Vaginal preparation.

•**acitretin.** (ASS-ih-TREH-tin) USAN.
Use: Antipsoriatic.
See: Soriatane (Hoffman-LaRoche).

•**acivicin.** (ace-ih-VIH-sin) USAN.
Use: Antineoplastic.

•**aclarubicin.** (ack-lah-ROO-bih-sin) USAN.
Use: Antineoplastic.

Aclophen. (Nutripharm) Phenylephrine HCl 40 mg, chlorpheniramine maleate 8 mg, acetaminophen 500 mg/S.R. tab. Dye free. Bot. 100s. *Rx.*
Use: Decongestant, antihistamine, analgesic.

Aclovate. (Glaxo Wellcome) Alclometasone dipropionate 0.05%. Cream or Oint. Tube 15 g, 45 g. *Rx.*
Use: Anti-inflammatory, topical.

A.C.N. (Person & Covey) Vitamin A 25,000 IU, ascorbic acid 250 mg, niacinamide 25 mg/Tab. Bot. 100s. *otc.*
Use: Vitamin supplement.

Acnaveen. (Rydelle)
See: Aveenobar Medicated (Rydelle).

Acna-Vite. (Cenci) Vitamins A 10,000 IU, C 250 mg, hesperidin 50 mg, niacinamide 25 mg/Cap. Bot. 75s. *otc.*
Use: Antiacne, vitamin supplement.

Acne-5. (Various Mfr.) Benzoyl peroxide 5%. Mask 30 ml. *otc.*
Use: Antiacne.

Acne-10. (Various Mfr.) Benzoyl peroxide 10%. Bot. 30 ml. *otc.*
Use: Antiacne.

Acne Lotion 10. (C & M) Benzoyl peroxide 10% in odorless, greaseless, vanishing lotion. Bot. 60 ml. *otc.*
Use: Antiacne.

Acno Cleanser. (Baker/Cummins) Isopropyl alcohol 60%, laureth-23, tetrasodium EDTA. Bot. 240 ml. *otc.*
Use: Antiacne.

Acno Lotion. (Baker/Cummins) Micronized sulfur 3%. Bot. 120 ml. *otc.*
Use: Antiacne.

Acnomel. (Menley & James) Resorcinol 2%, sulfur 8%, alcohol 11%. Cream Tube 28 g. *otc.*
Use: Antiacne.

Acnotex. (C & M) Sulfur 8%, resorcinol 2%, isopropyl alcohol 20%, acetone. In lotion base. Bot. 60 ml. *otc.*
Use: Antiacne.

•**acodazole hydrochloride.** (ah-KOE-dah-ZOLE)
Use: Antineoplastic.

aconiazide.
Use: Antituberculous agent. [Orphan drug]

Acotus. (Whorton) Phenylephrine HCl 5 mg, guaiacol glyceryl ether 100 mg, menthol 1 mg, alcohol by volume 10%/5 ml. Bot. 4 oz, 12 oz, gal. *otc.*
Use: Decongestant, antitussive.

ACR. (Western Research) Ammonium Cl 7.5 gr/Tab. Handicount 28s (36 bags of 28 tab.). *Rx.*
Use: Diuretic.

acriflavine. (Lilly) Tab. 1.5 gr. Bot. 100s.
Use: Antiseptic.

acriflavine hydrochloride. (Various Mfr.) Hydrochloride form of acriflavine. Acid acriflavine, acid trypaflavine, flavine, trypaflavine. National Aniline-Pow., Bot. (1 g, 5 g, 10 g, 25 g, 50 g). Tab. (1.5 gr). Bot. 50s, 100s. *Rx.*
Use: Antibacterial.

•**acrisorcin.** (ACK-rih-sahr-sin) USAN, U.S.P. XXII.
Use: Antifungal.
See: Akrinol (Schering-Plough).

•**acrivastine.** (ACK-rih-VASS-teen) USAN.
Use: Antihistaminic.
See: Semprex-D, Cap. (Glaxo Wellcome)

•**acronine.** (ACK-row-neen) USAN. Under study.
Use: Antineoplastic.

ACT. Dactinomycin, U.S.P. 23.
Use: Antineoplastic.
See: Actinomycin D.

ACT. (J & J) **Rinse:** 0.02% (from 0.05% sodium fluoride). **Mint:** Tartrazine, alcohol 8%. **Cinnamon:** Alcohol 7%. Bot. 360 ml, 480 ml. *otc.*
Use: Dental Rinse.

A-C Tablet. (Century) Aspirin 6 gr, caffeine 0.5 gr/Tab. Bot. 100s, 1000s. *otc.*
Use: Salicylate analgesic.

Actacin-C Syrup. (Vangard) Codeine phosphate 10 mg, triprolidine HCl 2 mg, pseudoephedrine HCl 20 mg, guaifenesin 100 mg/5 ml. Bot. pt, gal. *c-v.*
Use: Antitussive, antihistamine, decongestant, expectorant.

Actacin Tablets. (Vangard) Triprolidine HCl 2.5 mg, pseudoephedrine HCl 60 mg/Tab. Bot. 100s, 1000s. *otc, Rx.*
Use: Antihistamine, decongestant.

Actagen Syrup. (Goldline) Triprolidine HCl 1.25 mg, pseudoephedrine HCl 30 mg/5 ml. Bot. 118 ml. *otc.*
Use: Antihistamine, decongestant.

Actagen Tablets. (Goldline) Triprolidine HCl 2.5 mg, pseudoephedrine HCl 60 mg/Tab. Bot. 100s, 1000s. *otc.*
Use: Antihistamine, decongestant.

Actagen-C Cough Syrup. (Goldline) Triprolidine HCl 1.25 mg, pseudoephedrine HCl 30 mg, codeine phosphate 10 mg/5 ml, alcohol 4.3%. Bot. 120 ml, pt, gal. *c-v.*
Use: Antihistamine, decongestant, antitussive.

Actal Plus Tablets. (Sanofi Winthrop) Aluminum hydroxide, magnesium hydroxide. *otc.*
Use: Antacid.

Actal Suspension. (Sanofi Winthrop) Aluminum hydroxide. *otc.*
Use: Antacid.

Actal Tablets. (Sanofi Winthrop) Aluminum hydroxide. *otc.*
Use: Antacid.

Actamin. (Buffington) Acetaminophen 325 mg/Tab. Dispens-A-Kit 100s, 200s, 500s. *otc.*
Use: Analgesic.

Actamin Extra. (Buffington) Acetaminophen 500 mg/Tab. Bot. 100s, 200s, 500s. *otc.*
Use: Analgesic.

Actamin Super. (Buffington) Acetaminophen 500 mg, caffeine. Sugar, salt, and lactose free. Tab. Dispens-A-Kit 500s, Medipak 200s. *otc.*
Use: Analgesic.

Actamine. (H. L. Moore) **Tab.:** Pseudoephedrine HCl 60 mg, triprolidine HCl 2.5 mg. Bot. 100s, 1000s. **Syr.:** Pseudoephedrine HCl 30 mg, triprolidine HCl 1.25 mg/5 ml. Bot. 120 ml, pt, gal. *otc, Rx.*

Use: Decongestant, antihistamine.

ACTH-Actest Gel. (Forest) Repository corticotropin 40 units or 80 units/ml. Vial 5 ml. *Rx.*
Use: Corticosteroid.

ACTH. Adrenocorticotropic hormone. Adrenocorticotropin. *Rx.*
Use: Corticosteroid.
See: Corticotropin, U.S.P.
(Hauck) (40 units/ml, 5 ml).
(Forest) 40 units or 80 units/ml, 5 ml.
(Parke-Davis) 25 units/vial; 40 units/vial.
(Pharmex) 40 units or 80 units/ml, 5 ml.

ACTH Gel, Purified. (Arcum) 40 or 80 units/ml, vial 5 ml. (Conal) 40 or 80 units/ml, vial 5 ml. (Hart Labs.) 40 units/ml, vial 5 ml. (Jones Medical) Adrenocorticotropic hormone 40 units, aqueous gelatin 16%, phenol 0.5%/ml. Vial 5 ml. *Rx.*
Use: Repository corticotropin.
See: (Arcum) 40 or 80 units/ml, 5 ml.
(Bell) 40 or 80 units/ml, 5 ml.
(Jones Medical) 40 units/ml, 5 ml.
(Hyrex) 40 or 80 units/ml, 5 ml.
(Jenkins) 40 or 80 units/ml, 5 ml.
(Wesley Pharm.) 40 or 80 units/ml, vial 5 ml.
(Wyeth-Ayerst) 40 or 80 units/ml or Tubex.

Acthar. (Centeon) Corticotropin for inj. Vial 25 units, 40 units/vial. (Lyophilized w/gelatin). *Rx.*
Use: Corticosteroid.

ActHIB. (Pasteur-Merieux-Connaught) Inactivated tetanus toxoid 24 mcg, diphtheria toxoid 6.7 Lf, tetanus toxoid 5 Lf, pertussis vaccine ≈ 4 protective units/0.5 ml. Vials. *Rx.*
Use: Agent for immunization.

ActHIB. (Pasteur-Merieux-Connaught) Purified capsular polysaccharide of *Haemophilus influenzae* type b 10 mcg, tetanus toxoid 24 mcg/0.5 ml, sucrose 8.5%. Pow. for inj. Equivalent to OmniHIB. *Rx.*
Use: Typhoid vaccine.

ActHIB/DTP. (Pasteur-Merieux-Connaught) Diphtheria and tetanus toxoids and pertussis and *Haemophilus influenzae* type b vaccines. One package consists of one 7.5 ml vial of Connaught's DTwP and 10 single-dose vials of ActHIB vaccine. *Rx.*
Use: Agent for immunization.

ActiBath. (Jergens) Colloidal oatmeal 20%. Tab. Effervescent. Pkg. 4s. *otc.*
Use: Emollient.

Acticort 100 Lotion. (Baker/Cummins) Hydrocortisone 1%. Bot. 60 ml. *Rx.*
Use: Corticosteroid, topical.

Actidose. (Paddock) Activated charcoal. Soln. 25 g/120 ml or 50 g/240 ml. *otc.*
Use: Antidote.

Actidose-Aqua. (Paddock) Activated charcoal. Aqueous susp. 25 g/120 ml or 50 g/240 ml. *otc.*
Use: Antidote.

Actidose w/Sorbitol. (Paddock) Activated charcoal. Liq: 25 g in 120 ml susp. w/sorbitol, 50 g in 240 ml susp. w/sorbitol. *otc.*
Use: Antidote.

Actifed. (Warner Lambert Consumer Health Products) **Tab.:** Triprolidine HCl 2.5 mg, pseudoephedrine HCl 60 mg/Tab. Pkg. 12s. Bot. 24s, 48s, 100s. *otc.* **Cap.:** Triprolidine HCl 2.5 mg, pseudoephedrine HCl 60 mg/Cap. Box 10s, 20s. *otc.*
Use: Antihistamine, decongestant.

Actifed Allergy. (Warner Lambert Consumer Health Products) **Daytime:** Pseudoephedrine 30 mg; **Nighttime:** Pseudoephedrine 30 mg, diphenhydramine HCl 25 mg/ Capl. Pkg. 24 daytime, 8 nighttime. *otc.*
Use: Decongestant, antihistamine.

Actifed 12-Hour Capsules. (Glaxo Wellcome) Triprolidine HCl 5 mg, pseudoephedrine HCl 120 mg/Cap. Box 10s, 20s. *otc.*
Use: Antihistamine, decongestant.

Actifed Plus. (Warner Lambert Consumer Health Products) Pseudoephedrine HCl 30 mg, triprolidine HCl 1.25 mg, acetaminophen 500 mg/Tab. or Cap. Bot. 20s, 40s. *otc.*
Use: Decongestant, antihistamine, analgesic.

Actifed Sinus Daytime/Nightime. (Warner Lambert Consumer Health Products) **Daytime:** Pseudoephedrine HCl 30 mg, acetaminophen 500 mg/ Capl. pk. 18s. **Nighttime:** Pseudoephedrine HCl 30 mg, diphenhydramine HCl 25 mg, acetaminophen 500 mg/ Capl. pk. 6s. *otc.*
Use: Decongestant, antihistamine, analgesic.

Actifed with Codeine Cough Syrup. (Glaxo Wellcome) Codeine phosphate 10 mg, triprolidine HCl 1.25 mg, pseudoephedrine HCl 30 mg/5 ml, alcohol 4.3%. Bot. pt, gal. *c-v.*
Use: Antitussive, antihistamine, decongestant.

Actigall. (Novartis) Ursodiol (Ursodeoxycholic acid) 300 mg/Cap. Bot. 100s. *Rx.*
Use: Gallstone solubilizing agent.

Actimmune. (Genentech) Inteferon gamma-1b 100 mcg (3 million units)/vial. *Rx.*
Use: Treatment of infections associated with chronic granulomatous disease.

Actinex. (Schwarz Pharma) Masoprocol 10%, isostearyl and stearyl alcohol, light mineral oil, parabens, polyethylene glycol 400, propylene glycol and sodium metabisulfite. Cream, Tube 30 g. *Rx.*
Use: Antineoplastic.

actinomycin c. Name previously used for Cactinomycin.

actinomycin d. Dactinomycin, U.S.P. 23. *Rx.*
Use: Antineoplastic.
See: Cosmegen (Merck & Co.).

•**actinoquinol sodium.** USAN.
Use: Ultraviolet screen.

actinospectocin. Name previously used for Spectinomycin.

Actisite. (Alza) Tetracycline HCl 12.7 mg/23 cm. Fiber. In 10s. *Rx.*
Use: Mouth and throat product.

•**actisomide.** (ackt-EYE-so-MIDE) USAN.
Use: Cardiac depressant (antiarrhythmic).

Activase. (Genentech) Alteplase recombinant. Inj. Vial 20 mg, 50 mg, 100 mg. *Rx.*
Use: Thrombolytic enzyme.

activated attapulgite.
W/Aluminum hydroxide, magnesium carbonate coprecipitate, compressed gel.
See: Hykasil, Cream (Philips Roxane).
W/Polysorbate 80, colloidal sulfur, salicylic acid, propylene glycol. *otc.*
Use: Antiacne.
See: Sebasorb Lotion (Summers Labs.).

activated charcoal tablets. (Cowley) 5 gr/Tab. Bot. 1000s. *otc.*
Use: Antidote.

activated charcoal powder. (Various Mfr.) 15, 30, 40, 120 and 140 g. *otc.*
Use: Antidote.

activated charcoal liquid. (Various Mfr.) 12.5 g or 25 g with propylene glycol. 60 ml (12.5 g), 120 ml (25 g). *otc.*
Use: Antidote.

activated 7-dehydrocholesterol.
See: Vitamin D-3 (Various Mfr.).

activated ergosterol.

See: Calciferol.

•**actodigin.** (ACK-toe-dihj-in) USAN.
Use: Cardiotonic.

actoquinol sodium.
Use: Ultraviolet screen.

Actron. (Bayer) Ketoprofen 12.5 mg/Capl.; lactose. *otc.*
Use: Analgesic.

Acucron. (Seatrace) Acetaminophen 300 mg, salicylamide 200 mg, phenyltoloxamine 20 mg/Tab. Bot. 100s, 1000s, 5000s. *otc.*
Use: Analgesic, antihistamine.

Acu-Dyne. (Acme-United) **Douche:** Povidone-iodine. Pkt. 240 ml. **Oint.:** Povidone-iodine. Jar. lb. Pkt. 1.2, 2.7 (100s). **Perineal wash conc.:** Available iodine 1%. Bot. 40 ml. **Prep. Soln.:** Povidone-iodine. Bot. 240 ml, pt, qt, gal. Pkt. 30 ml, 60 ml. **Skin Cleanser:** Povidone-iodine. Bot. 60 ml, 240 ml, pt, qt, gal. **Soln, prep. swabs:** Available iodine 1%. Bot. 100s. **Soln, swabsticks:** Povidone-iodine. Pkt. 1 or 3 in 25s. **Whirlpool conc.:** Available iodine 1%. Bot. gal. *otc.*
Use: Antiseptic, germicide.

Acular. (Allergan) Ketorolac tromethamine 0.5% Ophth. Soln. Drop. Bot. 5 ml. *Rx.*
Use: Nonsteroidal anti-inflammatory agent, ophthalmic.

Acutrim Late Day. (Novartis Consumer Health) Phenylpropanolamine HCl 75 mg./Tab., precision release Bot. 20s. *otc.*
Use: Nonprescription diet aid.

Acutrim Maximum Strength. (Novartis Consumer Health) Phenylpropanolamine HCl 75 mg./Tab., precision release Bot. 20s, 40s. *otc.*
Use: Nonprescription diet aid.

Acutrim II Maximum Strength. (Novartis Consumer Health) Phenylpropanolamine HCl 75 mg/Tab. precision release, Bot. 20s, 40s. *otc.*
Use: Nonprescription diet aid.

Acutrim 16 Hour. (Novartis Consumer Health) Phenylpropanolamine HCl 75 mg/Tab., precision release. Bot. 20s, 40s. *otc.*
Use: Nonprescription diet aid.

•**acyclovir,** (A-SIKE-low-vir) U.S.P. 23.
Use: Antiviral.
See: Zovirax Cap., Oint., Tab., Susp. (Glaxo Wellcome).

•**acyclovir sodium.** (A-SIKE-low-vir) USAN.
Use: Antiviral.

See: Zovirax Sterile Powder (Glaxo Wellcome).

Adagen. (Enzon) Pegademase bovine 250 units/ml. Vial 1.5 ml. *Rx.*
Use: Enzyme (ADA) replacement therapy.

Adalat. (Bayer) Nifedipine 10 mg or 20 mg/Cap. Bot. 100s, 300s. UD 100s. *Rx.*
Use: Calcium channel blocking agent.

Adalat CC. (Bayer) Nifedipine 30 mg, 60 mg or 90 mg. ER Tab. Bot. 100s, 1000s. *Rx.*
Use: Calcium channel blocking agent.

adamantanamine hydrochloride.
See: Amantadine HCl.
Symmetrel, Cap., Syr. (DuPont Merck).

•**adapalene.** (ADE-ah-PALE-een) USAN.
Use: Antiacne.
See: Differin (Galderma).

Adapettes. (Alcon) Povidone and other water-soluble polymers, sorbic acid, EDTA. Soln. Bot. 15 ml. *otc.*
Use: Contact lens care.

Adapettes for Sensitive Eyes. (Alcon) Povidone and other water-soluble polymers, EDTA, sorbic acid. Pkg. 15 ml. *otc.*
Use: Contact lens care.

Adapin. (Lotus) Doxepin HCl **10 mg, 75 mg, 100 mg:** Cap. Bot. 100s, 1000s, UD 100s; **25 mg, 50 mg:** Cap. Bot. 100s, 1000s, 5000s, UD 100s; **150 mg:** Cap. Bot. 50s, 100s. *Rx.*
Use: Antidepressant.

•**adaprolol maleate.** (ad-AH-prole-ole) USAN.
Use: Antihypertensive (β-blocker, ophthalmic).

Adapt. (Alcon) Povidone, EDTA 0.1%, thimerosal 0.004%. Bot. 15 ml. *otc.*
Use: Contact lens care.

Adapt Wetting Solution. (Alcon) Adsorbobase with thimerosol 0.004%, EDTA 0.1%. Soln. Bot. 15 ml. *otc.*
Use: Hard contact lens care.

•**adatanserin hydrochloride.** (ahd-at-AN-ser-in) USAN.
Use: Antianxiety agent, antidepressant.

AdatoSil 5000. (Escalon Ophthalmics) Polydimethylsiloxane oil. Inj. Vial 10 ml, 15 ml. *Rx.*
Use: Ophthalmic.

Adavite. (Hudson) Vitamins A 5000 IU, D 400 IU, E 30 mg, B_1 3 mg, B_2 3.4 mg, B_3 30 mg, B_5 10 mg, B_6 3 mg, B_{12} 9 mcg, C 90 mg, folic acid 0.4 mg, biotin 35 mcg, beta carotene 1250 IU/Tab. Bot. 130s. *otc.*

Use: Vitamin/mineral supplement.

Adavite. (NTBY) Vitamins A 5500 IU, D 400 IU, E 30 mg, B_1 3 mg, B_2 3.4 mg, B_3 30 mg, B_5 10 mg, B_6 3 mg, B_{12} 9 mcg, C 120 mg, folic acid 0.4 mg, biotin 15 mcg. Tab. Bot. 100s. *otc.*
Use: Vitamin supplement.

Adavite-M. (Hudson) Iron 27 mg, Vitamins A 5000 IU, D 400 IU, E 30 mg, B_1 3 mg, B_2 3.4 mg, B_3 20 mg, B_5 10 mg, B_6 3 mg, B_{12} 9 mcg, C 190 mg, folic acid 0.4 mg, Ca, Cl, Cr, Cu, I, K, Mg, Mn, Mo, P, Se, Zinc 15 mg, biotin 30 mcg/Tab. Bot. 130s. *otc.*
Use: Vitamin/mineral supplement.

ADC with Fluoride. (Various Mfr.) Drops: Flouride 0.5 mg, vitamins A 1500 IU, D 400 IU, C 35 mg, methylparaben/ml. Bot. 50 ml. *Rx.*
Use: Vitamin/mineral supplement.

Adderall. (Richwood) **10 mg:** Dextroamphetamine sulfate 2.5 mg, dextroamphetamine saccharate 2.5 mg, amphetamine aspartate 2.5 mg, amphetamine sulfate 2.5 mg/Tab. Bot. 100s. **20 mg:** dextroamphetamine sulfate 5 mg, dextroamphetamine saccharide 5 mg, amphetamine aspartate 5 mg, amphetamine sulfate 5 mg/Tab. Bot. 100s. *c-ii.*
Use: Amphetamine combination.

Adeecon. (CMC) Vitamins A 5000 IU, D 1000 IU/Cap. Bot. 1000s. *otc.*
Use: Vitamin supplement.

Adeflor M Tablets. (Kenwood/Bradley) Vitamins A 6000 IU, D 400 IU, B_1 1.5 mg, B_2 2.5 mg, C 100 mg, B_3 20 mg, B_5 10 mg, B_6 10 mg, B_{12} 2 mcg, fluoride 1 mg, calcium 250 mg, iron 30 mg, sorbitol, sucrose/Tab. Bot. 100s, 500s. *Rx.*
Use: Vitamin supplement, dental caries preventative.

•**adefovir.** (ah-DEF-fah-vihr) USAN.
Use: Antiviral.

•**adefovir dipivoxil.** USAN.
Use: Antiviral (treatment of HIV and HBV infections.

ADEKs. (Scandipharm) Vitamins A 4000 IU, D 400 IU, E 150 IU, vitamin K, C 60 mg, B_1 1.2 mg, B_2 1.3 mg, B_3 10 mg, B_6 1.5 mg, B_{12} 12 mcg, B_5 10 mg, folic acid 0.2 mg, biotin 50 mcg, beta carotene 3 mg, Zn 1.1 mg, fructose. Tab. Bot. 60s. *otc.*
Use: Vitamin/mineral supplement.

ADEKs Pediatric Drops. (Scandipharm) Vitamin A 1500 IU, D 400 IU, E 40 IU, K_1 0.1 mg, C 45 mg, B_1 0.5 mg, B_2 0.6 mg, B_3 6 mg, B_5 3 mg, B_6 0.6 mg, B_{12} 4 mcg, biotin 15 mcg, Zn 5 mg,

betacarotene 1 mg per ml/drop. 60 ml. *otc.*
Use: Multivitamin.

•**adenine,** U.S.P. 23.
Use: Vitamin.

adeno-associated viral-based vector cystic fibrosis gene therapy. (Targeted Genetics)
Use: Treatment for cystic fibrosis. [Orphan Drug]

Adeno Twelve Gel Injection. (Forest Pharm) Adenosine-5-monophosphate 25 mg, methionine 25 mg, niacin 10 mg/ml. Vial 10 ml. *Rx.*
Use: Arthritis, bursitis, tendinitis and other degenerative diseases.

Adenocard. (Fujisawa) Adenosine 6 mg/2 ml. NaCl 9 mg/ml. Preservative free. Inj. Vial 2 ml, 5 ml. *Rx.*
Use: Antiarrhythmic.

Adenolin Forte. (Lincoln) Adenosine-5-monophosphate 25 mg, methionine 25 mg, niacin 10 mg/ml. Vial 15 ml. *Rx.*
Use: Arthritis, bursitis, tendinitis and other degenerative diseases.

Adenoscan. (Fujisawa) Inj.: Adenosine 3 mg/ml. Vial 30 ml. *Rx.*
Use: In vivo diagnostic aid.

•**adenosine.** (ah-DEN-oh-seen) USAN.
Use: Cardiac depressant (antiarrhythmic).
See: Adenocard, Inj. (Fujisawa).
Adenoscan, Inj. (Fujisawa).

adenosine. (ah-DEN-oh-seen) (Medco Research) *Rx.*
Use: Treatment of brain tumors. [Orphan drug]

adenosine in gelatin. (Forest Pharm) **Forte:** Adenosine-5-monophosphate 50 mg/ml. **Super:** Adenosine-5-monophosphate 100 mg/ml. *Rx.*
Use: Treatment of caricaose vein complications.

•**adenosine phosphate.** (ah-DEN-oh-seen) USAN. Adenosine monophosphate, AMP.
Use: Nutrient.
See: Cobalasine, Inj. (Keene).

adenosine phosphate. (Various Mfr.) 25 mg/ml. May contain benzyl alcohol. 10 ml, 30 ml/Inj. *Rx.*
Use: Treatment of statis dermatitis.

adenovirus vaccine type 4. (Wyeth Lederle) Adenovirus vaccine live type 4. At least 32,000 TCID$_{50}$ per Tab. Bot. 100s. *Rx.*
Use: Agent for immunization.

adenovirus vaccine type 7. (Wyeth Lederle) Adenovirus vaccine live type 7. At least 32,000 TCID$_{50}$ per Tab. Bot. 100s. *Rx.*
Use: Agent for immunization.

adepsine oil.
See: Petrolatum Liquid (Various Mfr.).

•**adinazolam.** (AHD-in-AZE-oh-lam) USAN.
Use: Antidepressant, sedative-hypnotic.

•**adinazolam mesylate.** (AHD-in-AZE-oh-lam) USAN.
Use: Antidepressant.
See: Deracyn (Pharmacia & Upjohn).

Adipex-P. (Lemmon) **Cap.:** Phentermine HCl 37.5 mg. Bot. 100s, 400s. **Tab.:** Phentermine HCl 37.5 mg. Bot. 100s, 400s, 1000s. *c-iv.*
Use: Anorexiant.

•**adiphenine hydrochloride.** (ah-DIH-fehneen) USAN.
Use: Relaxant (smooth muscle).

Adipost. (Jones) Phendimetrazine tartrate 105 mg/S.R. Cap. 100s. *c-iii.*
Use: Anorexiant.

Adisol Tab. (Major) Disulfiram **250 mg/Tab:** Bot. 100s. **500 mg/Tab:** Bot. 50s. *Rx.*
Use: Antialcoholic.

Adlerika. (Last) Magnesium sulfate 4 g/15 ml. Bot. 12 oz. *otc.*
Use: Laxative.

Adlone. (UAD) Methylprednisolone acetate 40 mg, 80 mg/Inj. Vial 5 ml. *Rx.*
Use: Glucocorticoid.

Adolph's Salt Substitute. (Adolph's) Potassium Cl 2480 mg/5 g, silicon dioxide, tartaric acid. Gran. Bot. 99.2 g. *otc.*
Use: Salt substitute.

Adolph's Seasoned Salt Substitute. (Adolph's) Potassium Cl 1360 mg/5 g, silicon dioxide, tartaric acid. Gran. Bot. 92.1 g. *otc.*
Use: Salt substitute.

Adonidine. (City Chem.) Bot. g. *Rx.*
Use: Cardiac stimulant.

•**adozelesin.** (ADE-oh-ZELL-eh-sin) USAN.
Use: Antineoplastic.

Adprin-B. (Pfeiffer) Aspirin 325 mg w/calcium carbonate, magnesium carbonate, magnesium/Chew. tab. Bot. 130s. *otc.*
Use: Analgesic.

Adprin-B, Extra Strength. (Pfeiffer) Aspirin 500 mg w/calcium carbonate, magnesium carbonate, magnesium oxide/Tab. Bot. 130s. *otc.*
Use: Analgesic.

ADR.
Use: Antineoplastic.

See: Doxorubicin HCl.

adrenalin(e).
See: Epinephrine. (Various Mfr.).

Adrenalin Chloride Solution. (Parke-Davis) Epinephrine HCl. Principle of the medullary portion of suprarenal glands. **Amp:** 1:1000-1 ml Epinephrine 1 mg/ml with not more than 0.1% sodium bisulfite as antioxidant. Amp. 10s. **Steri-Vial 1:1000:** Epinephrine 100 mg/ml in isotonic sodium Cl solution with 0.5% chlorobutanol as preservative and not more than 0.15% sodium bisulfite as antioxidant. Vial 30 ml. **Soln. 1:1000:** Bot. 30 ml. (Same as Steri-Vial). **Soln. 1:100:** Each 100 ml contains 1 g epinephrine HCl dissolved in sodium Cl citrate buffer soln w/ phemerol Cl 0.2 mg/ml as preservative, sodium bisulfite 0.2% as antioxidant. Bot. 0.25 oz. *Rx.*
Use: Sympathomimetic.

adrenaline hydrochloride.
See: Epinephrine Hydrochloride. (Various Mfr.)

•**adrenalone.** (ah-DREN-ah-lone) USAN.
Use: Adrenergic (ophthalmic).

adrenamine.
See: Epinephrine (Various Mfr.).

adrenergic agents.
See: Sympathomimetic agents.

adrenergic-blocking agents.
See: Sympatholytic agents.

adrenine.
See: Epinephrine (Various Mfr.).

adrenocorticotropic hormone. ACTH acts by stimulating the endogenous production of cortisone. *Rx.*
See: ACTH.
Corticotropin, U.S.P.

Adrenomist Inhalant and Nebulizers. (Nephron) Epinephrine 1%, Bot. 0.5 oz, 1.25 oz. *otc, Rx.*
Use: Bronchodilator.

Adrenucleo. (Enzyme Process) Vitamin C 250 mg, d-calcium pantothenate 12.5 mg, bioflavonoids 62.5 mg/Tab. Bot. 100s, 250s. *otc.*
Use: Vitamin C supplement.

Adriamycin. (Pharmacia & Upjohn) Doxorubicin HCl 20 mg/vial. *Rx.*
Use: Antineoplastic.

Adriamycin PFS. (Pharmacia & Upjohn) Doxorubicin HCl 2 mg/ml. Inj. Vial: 5 ml, 10 ml, 25 ml. *Rx.*
Use: Antineoplastic.

Adriamycin RDF. (Pharmacia & Upjohn) Doxorubicin HCl. **10 mg:** Methylparaben 1 mg, lactose 50 mg/Vial. Pkg. 10s.

20 mg: Methylparaben 2 mg, lactose 100 mg/Vial. Pkg. 5s. **50 mg:** Methylparaben 5 mg, lactose 250 mg/Vial. Ctn. 1s. **150 mg:** Methylparaben 15 mg, lactose 750 mg/multi-dose vial. Rapid dissolution formula. *Rx.*
Use: Antineoplastic.

Adrucil. (Pharmacia & Upjohn) Fluorouracil 50 mg/10 ml. Amp. 10 ml. *Rx.*
Use: Antineoplastic.

Adsorbocarpine. (Alcon) Pilocarpine HCl 1%, 2% or 4%. Bot. 15 ml. *Rx.*
Use: Miotic.

Adsorbonac Ophth. Solution. (Alcon) Sodium Cl 2% or 5%. Vial 15 ml. *otc.*
Use: Hyperosmolar preparation.

Adsorbotear. (Alcon) Hydroxyethylcellulose 0.4%, povidone 1.67%, water-soluble polymers, thimerosal 0.004%, EDTA 0.1%. Soln. Bot. dropper 15 ml. *otc.*
Use: Artificial tears solution.

Advance. (Ross) **Ready-to-Feed infant formula:** (16 cal/fl oz.) Can 13 fl oz. **Conc. liq:** 32 fl oz. *otc.*
Use: Nutritional supplement.

Advance Pregnancy Test. (Advanced Care) Can be used as early as 3 days after a missed period. Gives results in 30 min. Test kit 1s.
Use: Diagnostic aid.

Advanced Care Cholesterol Test. (Johnson & Johnson)
Use: At home cholesterol test.

Advanced Formula Centrum Liquid. (Lederle) Vitamins A 2500 IU, E 30 IU, C 60 mg, B_1 1.5 mg, B_2 1.7 mg, B_3 20 mg, B_5 10 mg, B_6 2 mg, B_{12} 6 mcg, D 400 IU, iron 9 mg, biotin 300 mcg, I, Zn 3 mg, Mn, Cr, Mo, alcohol 6.7%, sucrose. Bot. 236 ml. *otc.*
Use: Vitamin/mineral supplement.

Advanced Formula Centrum Tablets. (Lederle) Iron 18 mg, vitamins A 5000 IU, D 400 IU, E 30 IU, B_1 1.5 mg, B_2 1.7 mg, B_3 20 mg, B_5 10 mg, B_6 2 mg, B_{12} 6 mcg, C 60 mg, folic acid 0.4 mg, biotin 30 mcg, B, Ca, Cl, Cr, Cu, I, K, Mg, Mn, Mo, Ni, P, Se, Si, Sn, V, Zn 15 mg, vitamin K/Tab. Bot. 60s, 130s, 200s. *otc.*
Use: Vitamin/mineral supplement.

Advanced Formula Oxy Sensitive. (SK-Beecham) Benzoyl peroxide 2.5%, diazolidinyl urea, EDTA. Gel. 30 g. *otc.*
Use: Antiacne.

Advanced Formula Plax. (Pfizer) Tetrasodium pyrophosphate, alcohol, saccharin. Mouthwash. In 120 ml, 240 ml,

473 ml, 720 ml, 1740 ml. *otc.*
Use: Antibacterial.

Advanced Formula Tegrin. (Block) Coal tar solution USP 7%, alcohol 7%, hydroxypropyl methylcellulose, parabens. Shampoo. Bot. 207 ml. *otc.*
Use: Antiseborrheic.

Advanced Formula Zenate. (Solvay) Vitamins A 4000 IU, D 400 IU, E 10 IU, C 70 mg, folic acid 1 mg, B_1 1.5 mg, B_2 1.6 mg, B_3 17 mg, B_6 2.2 mg, B_{12} 2.2 mcg, Ca, I, iron 65 mg, Mg, Se, Zn 15 mg. Tab. Bot. 100s. *Rx.*
Use: Vitamin/mineral supplement.

Advantage 24. (Women's Health Institute) Nonoxynol-9 3.5%. Gel. 1.5 g (3s, 6s). *otc.*
Use: Spermicide.

Advera. (Ross) Protein 60 g (soy protein hydrolysate, sodium caseinate, carnitine 127 mg and taurine 212 mg per L), carbohydrates 215.8 g (hydrolyzed cornstarch, sucrose), fat 22.8 g (canola oil, medium-chain triglycerides, refined deodorized sardine oil), dietary fiber 8.9 g (soy fiber), vitamins A 10,778 IU, D 338 IU, E 38.1 IU, K 67.6 mcg, C 381 mg, folic acid 507 mcg, B_1 3.17 mg, B_2 2.88 mg, B_6 3.38 mg, B_{12} 50.68 mcg, B_3 25.4 mg, biotin, B_5 12.7 mg, Na 1046 mg, K 2827 mg, Cl 1536 mg, Ca 845 mg, P, Mg, I, Mn, Cu, Zn 15.9 mg, Fe 19.1 mg, Se, Cr, Mo, choline, 1280 calories/L. Liq. 240 ml. *otc.*
Use: Dietary management in HIV infection or AIDS.

Advil. (Whitehall Robins) Ibuprofen 200 mg, sucrose (Tab.), parabens (Capl.). In 8s, 24s, 50s, 100s, 165s, 250s (Tab.). *otc.*
Use: Nonsteroidal anti-inflammatory drug; analgesic.

Advil, Children's. (Whitehall Robins) Ibuprofen Susp. 100 mg per 5 ml. Fruit flavor, sorbitol, sucrose, EDTA. Liq. Bot. 199 ml, 473 ml. *Rx.*
Use: Nonsteroidal anti-inflammatory drug; analgesic.

Advil Cold & Sinus. (Whitehall Robins) Pseudoephedrine HCl 30 mg, ibuprofen 200 mg/Tab. Pkg. 20s. Bot. 40s, 75s. *otc.*
Use: Decongestant, analgesic.

A.E.R. (Birchwood) Hamamelis water (witch hazel) 50%, glycerin 12.5%, methylparaben, benzalkonium chloride. Pads. Jar 40s. *otc.*
Use: Topical drug, miscellaneous.

Aerdil. (Econo Med) Triprolidine HCl 1.25 mg, pseudoephedrine HCl 30 mg/5 ml. Bot. pt, gal. *otc.*

Use: Antihistamine, decongestant.

Aeroaid. (Graham-Field) Thimerosal 1:1000, alcohol 72%. Spray bot 90 ml.
Use: Antiseptic.

Aeroaid merthiolate. (Health & Medical Techniques) Merthiolate (Lilly) 1:1000, alcohol 72%. Spray bot. 3 oz.
Use: Antiseptic.

Aerobid. (Forest) Flunisolide in an inhaler system. Canister 7 g, 100 metered inhalations. *Rx.*
Use: Corticosteroid.

Aerobid M. (Forest) Flunisolide in an inhaler system. Canister 7 g, 100 metered inhalations. Menthol flavor. *Rx.*
Use: Corticosteroid.

Aerocaine. (Health & Medical Techniques) Benzocaine 13.6%, benzethonium Cl 0.5%. Spray bot. 0.5 oz, 2.5 oz. *otc.*
Use: Local anesthetic, topical.

Aerocell. (Health & Medical Techniques) Exfoliative cytology fixative spray. Bot. 3.5 oz.
Use: Exfoliative cytology fixative spray.

Aerodine. (Health & Medical Techniques) Povidone-iodine. Bot. 3 oz.
Use: Antiseptic.

Aerofreeze. (Graham-Field) Trichloromonofluoromethane and dichlorodifluoromethane. 240 ml/Aerosol spray. Cont. 8 oz. (12s). *otc.*
Use: Local anesthetic.

Aerolate-III. (Fleming) Theophylline 65 mg/T.D. Cap. Bot. 100s, 1000s. *Rx.*
Use: Bronchodilator.

Aerolate Sr. & Jr. (Fleming) **Cap.:** Theophylline 4 gr for Sr., 2 gr for Jr./Cap. Bot. 100s, 1000s. **Syr.:** 160 mg/15 ml. Bot. pt, gal. *Rx.*
Use: Bronchodilator.

Aeropin.
Use: Cystic fibrosis.
See: Heparin, 2-0-desulfated.

Aeropure. (Health & Medical Techniques) Isopropanol 7.8%, triethylene glycol 3.9%, essential oils 3%, methyldodecyl benzyl trimethyl ammonium Cl 0.12%, methyldodecylxylene bis (trimethyl ammonium Cl) 0.03%, inert ingredients, 85.15%. Bot. 0.8 oz, 4.5 oz.
Use: Air sanitizer, deodorizer.

Aerosan. (Ulmer) Aerosol 16.6 oz.
Use: Air sanitizer, deodorizer.

Aeroseb-Dex. (Allergan Herbert) Dexamethasone 0.01%, alcohol 65.1%. Aerosol 58 g. *Rx.*
Use: Corticosteroid, topical.

Aerosil. (Health & Medical Techniques)

Dimethylpolysiloxane. Bot. 4.5 oz.
Use: Silicone lubricant, protectant.

aerosol ot.
See: Docusate Sodium, U.S.P.

Aerosolv. (Health & Medical Techniques) Isopropyl alcohol, methylene Cl, silicone. Aerosol 5.5 oz.
Use: Adhesive tape remover.

Aerosporin Sterile Powder. (Glaxo Wellcome) Polymyxin B sulfate 500,000 units/vial. Multidose vial 20 ml. *Rx.*
Use: Antibacterial.

Aerotherm. (Health & Medical Techniques) Benzethonium Cl 0.5%, benzocaine 13.6%. Spray bot. 5 oz. *otc.*
Use: Local anesthetic, topical.

AeroZoin. (Health & Medical Techniques) Comp. tr. of benzoin 30%, isopropyl alcohol 44.8%. Spray bot. 3.5 oz. *otc.*
Use: Skin protectant.

Afaxin Capsules. (Sanofi Winthrop) Vitamin A Palmitate 10,000 IU or 50,000 IU/Cap. *otc, Rx.*
Use: Vitamin A supplement.

A-Fil. (GenDerm) Methyl anthranilate 5%, titanium dioxide 5% in vanishing cream base. Tube 45 g. Neutral or dark. *otc.*
Use: Sunscreen.

Afko-Lube. (APC) Docusate sodium 100 mg/Cap. Bot. 100s. *otc.*
Use: Laxative.

Afko-Lube Lax. (APC) Docusate sodium 100 mg, casanthranol 30 mg/Cap. Bot. 100s. *otc.*
Use: Laxative.

Afrikol. (Citroleum) Bot. 4 oz.
Use: Sunscreen.

Afrin. (Schering-Plough) Oxymetazoline HCl 0.05%. **Nose Drops:** Drop. Bot. 20 ml. **Nasal Spray:** Reg.: Bot. 15 ml, 30 ml; Menthol: Bot. 15 ml. **Children's Nose Drops:** Oxymetazoline HCl 0.025%. Drop. Bot. 20 ml. *otc.*
Use: Decongestant.

Afrin Moisturizing Saline Mist. (Schering-Plough) 0.64% sodium chloride, benzalkonium chloride, EDTA/Soln. Bot. 30 ml. *otc.*
Use: Decongestant.

Afrin Sinus. (Schering-Plough) Oxymetazoline HCl 0.05%, benzyl alcohol. Spray. 15 ml. *otc.*
Use: Decongestant.

Afrinol Repetabs. (Schering-Plough) Pseudoephedrine sulfate 120 mg/Repeat Action Tab. Box 12s. Bot. 100s, dispensary pack 48s. *otc.*
Use: Decongestant.

Aftate for Athlete's Foot. (Schering-Plough) Tolnaftate 1%. **Gel:** Tube 15 g **Pump Spray Liq.:** 45 ml (with alcohol 83%). **Pow.:** 67.5 g, 45 g squeeze bot. **Aerosol pow.:** 105 g (with alcohol 14% and talc). **Aerosol liq.:** 120 ml (with alcohol 36%). *otc.*
Use: Antifungal, topical.

Aftate for Jock Itch. (Schering-Plough) **Aerosol powder:** Tolnaftate 1% (with alcohol 14% and talc). 75 ml. **Gel:** Tolnaftate 1%. Tube 15 g. **Powder:** Tolnaftate 1%. Can 56.7 g. *otc.*
Use: Antifungal, topical.

After Bite. (Tender) Ammonium hydroxide 3.5% in aqueous solution. Pen-like dispenser. *otc.*
Use: Antipruritic, analgesic, topical.

After Burn. (Tender) Lidocaine 0.5% in aloe vera 98% solution. *otc.*
Use: Local anesthetic, topical.

•**agar,** N.F. 18.
Use: Pharmaceutical aid (suspending agent).
W/Mineral oil.
See: Agoral, Emulsion (Parke-Davis Prods).
Petrogalar (Wyeth-Ayerst).

aglucerase injection. (Genzyme Corp.)
Use: Treatment of Type II and III Gaucher's disease. [Orphan drug]

Agoral. (Parke-Davis) Phenolphthalein 0.2 g, mineral oil 4.2 g/15 ml in an emulsion containing agar, tragacanth, egg-albumin, acacia, glycerin. Marshmallow and raspberry flavor. Bot. 240 ml, 480 ml. *otc.*
Use: Laxative.

Agrylin. (Roberts) Anagrelide HCl 0.5 mg and 1 mg/cap. Bot. 100s. *Rx.*
Use: Treatment of essential thrombocythemia.

A/G-Pro. (Miller) Protein hydrolysate 50 gr w/essential and nonessential amino acids 45%, l-lysine 300 mg, methionine 75 mg, Vitamins C, B_6, Fe, Cu, I, Mn, K, Zn, Mg/6 Tab. Bot. 180s. *otc.*
Use: Nutritional supplement.

agurin.
See: Theobromine Sodium Acetate (Various Mfr.).

AH-Chew. (WE Pharm) Chlorpheniramine maleate 2 mg, phenylephrine HCl 10 mg, methscopolamine nitrate 1.25 mg. Chew. tab. 100s. *Rx.*
Use: Decongestant, antihistamine.

AH-Chew D. (WE Pharm) Phenylephrine 10 mg/Tab. Chewable. Bot. 100s. *Rx.*
Use: Decongestant.

AHF.

See: Antihemophilic factor.

A-Hydrocort. (Abbott Hospital Prods) Hydrocortisone sodium succinate. 100 mg or 250 mg/2 ml Univial, with benzyl alcohol; 500 mg/4 ml Univial with benzyl alcohol; 1000 mg/8 ml Univial with benzyl alcohol. *Rx.*
Use: Corticosteroid.

AIDS vaccine. (MicroGeneSys/Genentech/Immuno AG/NIH/Wyeth-Ayerst) Phase I-III AIDS, HIV prophylaxis and treatment. *Rx.*
Use: Antiviral.

Airet. (Adams) Albuterol sulfate 0.083%. Soln. for inhalation. Vial. *Rx.*
Use: Bronchodilator.

•**air, medical,** U.S.P. 23.
Use: Gas, medicinal.

Al-RSA. (Autoimmune, Inc.)
Use: Autoimmune uveitis. [Orphan drug]

air & surface disinfectant. (Health & Medical Techniques) Aerosol 16 oz.
Use: Air sanitizer, deodorizer.

Akarpine. (Akorn) Pilocarpine HCl 1%, 2% or 4%. Soln. Bot. 15 ml. *Rx.*
Use: Miotic.

AKBeta. (Akorn) Levobunolol HCl 0.25%. Ophthalmic Soln. 5 ml, 10 ml. Levobunolol HCl 0.5%. Soln. Bot. 5 ml, 10 ml, 15 ml. *Rx.*
Use: Glaucoma agent.

AK-Chlor. (Akorn) **Oint.:** Chloramphenicol 10 mg/g. Tube 3.5 g. **Soln.:** Chloramphenicol 5 mg/ml. Bot. 7.5 ml, 15 ml. *Rx.*
Use: Anti-infective, ophthalmic.

AK-Cide. (Akorn) **Susp.:** Prednisolone acetate 0.5%, sulfacetamide sodium 10%. Dropper bot. 5 ml. **Oint.:** Prednisolone acetate 0.5%, sodium sulfacetamide 10%. Tube 3.5 g. *Rx.*
Use: Ophthalmic corticosteroid, anti-infective.

AK-Con. (Akorn) Naphazoline HCl 0.1%. Soln. Bot. 15 ml. *Rx.*
Use: Vasoconstrictor/mydriatic.

AK-Con-A. (Akorn) Naphazoline HCl 0.025%, pheniramine maleate 0.3%, benzalkonium Cl 0.01%, EDTA. Soln. Bot. 15 ml. *Rx.*
Use: Ophthalmic antihistamine, decongestant.

AK-Dex. (Akorn) Dexamethasone phosphate (as sodium phosphate). **Oint.:** 0.05%. Tube 3.5 g. **Soln.:** 0.1%. Bot 5 ml. *Rx.*
Use: Corticosteroid, ophthalmic.

AK-Dilate. (Akorn) Phenylephrine HCl 2.5% or 10%. Bot. 2 ml, 5 ml (10%), 15 ml (2.5%). *Rx.*

Use: Vasoconstrictor/mydriatic.

AK-Fluor. (Akorn) Fluorescein sodium. **10%:** Amp. 5 ml, Vial 5 ml; **25%:** Amp. 2 ml, Vial 2 ml.
Use: Ophthalmic diagnostic.

AK-Homatropine. (Akorn) Homatropine HBr 5%, benzalkonium Cl 0.01%, hydroxyethyl cellulose, EDTA. Soln. Bot. 5 ml. *Rx.*
Use: Cycloplegic mydriatic.

Akineton. (Knoll) Biperiden HCl 2 mg/ Tab. Bot. 100s, 1000s. *Rx.*
Use: Antiparkinsonian.

Akineton Lactate. (Knoll) Biperiden lactate 5 mg in aqueous 1.4% sodium lactate soln/ml. Amp 1 ml, Box 10s. *Rx.*
Use: Antiparkinsonian.

AK-Homatropine. (Akorn) Homatropine HBr 5%. In 5 ml/Soln. *Rx.*
Use: Cycloplegic mydriatic.

AK-Mycin. (Akorn) Erythromycin 5 mg/g with white petrolatum, mineral oil. Oint. Tube 3.75 g. *Rx.*
Use: Anti-infective, ophthalmic.

AK-NaCl. (Akorn) **Oint.:** Sodium Cl hypertonic 5%. Tube 3.5 g. **Soln.:** Sodium Cl, hypertonic 5%. Bot. 15 ml. *otc.*
Use: Ophthalmic hyperosmolar preparation.

Akne Drying Lotion. (Alto) Zinc oxide 12%, urea 10%, sulfur 6%, salicylic acid 2%, benzalkonium Cl 0.2%, isopropyl alcohol 70%, in a base containing menthol, silicon dioxide, iron oxide, perfume. Bot. ¾ oz, 2.25 oz. *otc.*
Use: Antiacne.

AK-Nefrin. (Akorn) Phenylephrine HCl. Soln. Bot. 15 ml. *otc.*
Use: Vasoconstrictor/mydriatic.

Akne-Mycin. (Hermal) Erythromycin. **Oint.:** 2%. Tube 25 g. **Soln.:** 2%. Bot. 60 ml. *Rx.*
Use: Antiacne.

AK-Neo-Dex. (Akorn) Dexamethasone sodium phosphate 0.1% and neomycin sulfate 0.35%. Ophth. Soln. 5 ml. *Rx.*
Use: Corticosteroid/anti-infective, ophthalmic.

Akne Scrub. (Alto) Povidone iodine with polyethylene granules. Bot. ¾ oz. *otc.*
Use: Antiacne.

AK-Pentolate. (Akorn) Cyclopentolate HCl 1%, benzalkonium Cl 0.01%, EDTA. Soln. Bot. 2 ml, 15 ml. *Rx.*
Use: Cycloplegic mydriatic.

AK-Poly-Bac. (Akorn) Polymyxin B sulfate 10,000 units, bacitracin zinc 500 units/g. Oint. Tube 3.5 g. *Rx.*

Use: Anti-infective, ophthalmic.

AK-Pred. (Akorn) Prednisolone sodium phosphate 0.125% or 1%. **0.125%:** Soln. Bot. 5 ml. **0.1%:** Soln. Bot. 5 ml, 15 ml. *Rx.*
Use: Corticosteroid, ophthalmic.

AKPro. (Akorn) Dipivefrin HCl 0.1%. 2, 5, 10, 15 ml/Liq. *Rx.*
Use: Glaucoma agent.

AK-Ramycin. (Akorn) Doxycycline hyclate 100 mg/Cap. Bot. 50s, 100s, 200s, 250s, 500s, UD 100s. *Rx.*
Use: Anti-infective, tetracycline.

AK-Ratabs. (Akorn) Doxycycline hyclate 100 mg/Tab. Bot. 50s. *Rx.*
Use: Anti-infective, tetracycline.

Akrinol. (Schering-Plough) Acrisorcin.
Use: Antifungal.

AK-Rinse. (Akorn) Sodium carbonate, potassium Cl, boric acid, EDTA, benzalkonium Cl 0.01%. Soln. Bot. 30 ml, 118 ml. *otc.*
Use: Ophthalmic irrigation solution.

AK-Spore. (Akorn) **Oint.:** Polymyxin B sulfate 10,000 units, neomycin (as sulfate) 3.5 mg, bacitracin zinc 400 units/g. Tube 3.5 g. **Soln.:** Polymyxin B sulfate 10,000 units, neomycin sulfate 1.75 mg, gramicidin 0.025 mg/ml. Soln. Dropper bot. 2 ml, 10 ml. *Rx.*
Use: Anti-infective, ophthalmic.

AK-Spore H.C. ophthalmic. (Akorn) **Susp.:** Hydrocortisone 1%, neomycin sulfate 0.35%, polymyxin B sulfate 10,000 units. Soln. Bot. 7.5 ml. **Oint.:** Hydrocortisone 1%, neomycin sulfate 0.35%, bacitracin zinc 400 units, polymyxin B sulfate 10,000 units. Tube 3.5 g. *Rx.*
Use: Corticosteroid, anti-infective.

AK-Spore H.C. Otic. (Akorn) **Susp.:** Hydrocortisone 1%, neomycin sulfate 5 mg, polymyxin B sulfate 10,000 units/ml. Bot. w/dropper 10 ml. **Soln.:** Hydrocortisone 1%, neomycin sulfate 5 mg, polymyxin B sulfate 10,000 units/ml. Bot. w/dropper 10 ml. *Rx.*
Use: Corticosteroid, anti-infective.

AK-Sulf. (Akorn) **Soln.:** Sodium sulfacetamide 10%. Dropper Bot. 2 ml, 5 ml, 15 ml; **Oint.:** Sodium sulfacetamide 10%. Tube 3.5 g. *Rx.*
Use: Anti-infective, ophthalmic.

AK-Taine. (Akorn) Proparacaine HCl 0.5%, glycerin, chlorobutanol, benzalkonium Cl. Dropper bot. 2 ml, 15 ml. *Rx.*
Use: Local anesthetic, ophthalmic.

AK-Tate. (Akorn) Prednisolone acetate 1%, benzalkonium Cl, EDTA, polysor-

bate 80, polyvinyl alcohol, hydroxyethyl cellulose. Susp. Dropper bot. 5 ml, 10 ml, 15 ml. *Rx.*
Use: Corticosteroid, ophthalmic.

AKTob. (Akorn)Tobramycin 0.3%. Soln. Bot. 5 ml. *Rx.*
Use: Anti-infective, ophthalmic.

AK-Tracin. (Akorn) Bacitracin 500 units/g. Oint. Tube 3.5 g. *Rx.*
Use: Anti-infective, ophthalmic.

AK-Trol. (Akorn) **Susp.:** Dexamethasone 0.1%, neomycin sulfate equivalent to 0.35% neomycin base, polymyxin B sulfate 10,000 units. Bot. 5 ml. **Oint.:** Dexamethasone 0.1%, neomycin sulfate equivalent to 0.35% neomycin base, polymyxin B sulfate 10,000 units. Tube 3.5 g. *Rx.*
Use: Ophthalmic corticosteroid, anti-infective.

Akwa Tears. (Akorn) **Soln.:** Polyvinyl alcohol 1.4%, sodium Cl, sodium phosphate, benzalkonium Cl 0.01%, EDTA. Bot. 15 ml. **Oint.:** White petrolatum, mineral oil, lanolin. Tube 3.5 g. *otc.*
Use: Artificial tears.

al-721. (Matrix Laboratories) Phase I/II AIDS, ARC, HIV positive.
Use: Antiviral.

Ala-Bath. (Del-Ray) Bath oil. Bot. 8 oz. *otc.*
Use: Emollient.

Ala-Cort. (Del-Ray) Hydrocortisone 1%. **Cream:** Tube 1 oz, 3 oz. **Lot.:** Bot. 4 oz. *Rx.*
Use: Corticosteroid, topical.

Ala-Derm. (Del-Ray) Lot. Bot 8 oz, 12 oz.
Use: Emollient.

Aladrine. (Scherer) Ephedrine sulfate 8.1 mg, secobarbital sodium 16.2 mg/Tab. Bot. 100s. *c-II.*
Use: Decongestant, sedative/hypnotic.

Alamag. (Barre) Magnesium-aluminum hydroxide gel. Susp. Bot. Pt. *otc.*
Use: Antacid.
W/Belladonna alkaloid. Susp. Bot. 8 oz.

Alamag Suspension. (Goldline) Aluminum hydroxide 225 mg, magnesium hydroxide 200 mg, sorbitol, sucrose, parabens. Bot. 355 ml. *otc.*
Use: Antacid.

Alamag Plus Antacid. (Goldline) Magnesium hydroxide 200 mg, aluminum hydroxide 225 mg, simethicone 25 mg/5 ml. Bot. 355 ml. *otc.*
Use: Antacid.

•**alamecin.** (al-ah-MEE-sin) USAN.
Use: Antibacterial.

•**alanine,** (AL-ah-NEEN) U.S.P. 23. $C_3H_7NO_2$. L-Alanine.
Use: Amino acid.

•**alaproclate.** (AL-ah-PRO-klate) USAN.
Use: Antidepressant.

Ala-Quin 0.5%. (Del-Ray) Hydrocortisone, iodochlorhydroxyquin cream. Tube 1 oz. *otc, Rx.*
Use: Corticosteroid, topical.

Ala-Scalp HP 2%. (Del-Ray) Hydrocortisone lotion. Bot. 1 oz. *Rx.*
Use: Corticosteroid, topical.

Ala-Seb Shampoo. (Del-Ray) Bot. 4 oz, 12 oz. *otc.*
Use: Antiseborrheic.

Ala-Seb T Shampoo. (Del-Ray) Bot. 4 oz, 12 oz. *otc.*
Use: Antiseborrheic.

Alasulf. (Major) Sulfanilamide 15%, aminacrine HCl 0.2%, allantoin 2%. Vaginal Cream Tube w/applicator 120 g. *Rx.*
Use: Anti-infective, vaginal.

Alatone. (Major) Spironolactone 25 mg/Tab. Bot. 100s, 250s, 500s, 1000s, UD 100s. *Rx.*
Use: Antihypertensive.

•**alatrofloxacin mesylate.** (al-at-row-FLOX-ah-sin) USAN.
Use: Antibacterial.

Alaxin. (Delta) Oxyethlene oxypropylene polymer 240 mg/Cap. Bot. 100s. *otc.*
Use: Laxative.

Al-Ay. (Jones Medical) *otc.* **Green Oblong Tube:** Phenylephrine HCl 5 mg, chlorpheniramine maleate 2 mg, aspirin 162 mg, caffeine 15 mg, aminoacetic acid 162 mg/Tab. Bot. 100s, 1000s. **Dark Green S.C:** Phenylephrine HCl 5 mg, chlorpheniramine maleate 2 mg, acetaminophen 160 mg, caffeine 15 mg/Tab. Bot. 100s, 1000s. *otc.*
Use: Decongestant, antihistamine, analgesic.

alazanine trichlorphate. *Rx.*
Use: Anthelmintic.

Alazide Tabs. (Major) Spironolactone w/ hydrochlorothiazide. Bot. 250s, 1000s. *Rx.*
Use: Antihypertensive, diuretic.

Alazine Tabs. (Major) Hydralazine 10 mg, 25 mg or 50 mg/Cap. Bot. 100s, 1000s. *Rx.*
Use: Antihypertensive.

Albalon. (Allergan) Naphazoline HCl 0.1%. Bot. 15 ml. *Rx.*
Use: Vasoconstrictor, ophthalmic.

Albamycin. (Pharmacia & Upjohn) Novobiocin sodium 250 mg/Cap. Bot. 100s. *Rx.*

Use: Anti-infective.

Albay. (Bayer) Freeze-dried venom and venom protein. Vials of 550 mcg for each of honey bee, white-faced hornet, yellow hornet, yellow jacket or wasp. Vials of 1,650 mcg for mixed vespids (white-faced hornet, yellow hornet, yellow jacket). 10 ml/Inj. *Rx.*
Use: Hymenoptera venom.

•**albendazole,** (AL-BEND-ah-zole) U.S.P. 23.
Use: Anthelmintic.
See: Zentel (SK-Beecham).

albendazole. (SK-Beecham) 200 mg/Tab. Bot. 112s. *Rx.*
Use: Anthelmintic.
See: Albenza.

Albenza. (SK-Beecham) Albendazole 200 mg/Tab. Bot. 112s. *Rx.*
Use: Anthelmintic.

Albolene Cream. (SK-Beecham) Unscented or scented. Jar 6 oz, 12 oz.

Albuconn 25% Solution. (Cryosan) Normal serum albumin (human) 12.5 g in 50 ml solution for IV administration. Vial 50 ml. *Rx.*
Use: Treatment of plasma or blood volume deficit, acute hypoproteinemia, oncotic deficit.

•**albumin, aggregated.** (al-BYOO-min AGG-reh-GAY-tuhd) USAN.
Use: Diagnostic aid (lung-imaging).
See: Technescan MAA.

•**albumin, aggregated iodinated I 131,** U.S.P. 23.
Use: Radioactive agent.

•**albumin, aggregated iodinated I 131 serum.** USAN. Blood serum aggregates of albumin labeled with iodine-131.
Use: Radioactive agent.

•**albumin, chromated cr 51 serum.** USAN. Blood serum albumin labeled with chromium-51.
Use: Radioactive agent.
See: Chromalbin (Squibb).

•**albumin human,** (al-BYOO-MIN human) U.S.P. 23. Normal Human Serum Albumin.
Use: Plasma protein fraction; blood volume supporter.
See: Albutein 5%, Inj. (Alpha Therapeutic).
Albutein 25%, Inj. (Alpha Therapeutic).
Buminate, Soln. (Baxter).
Plasbumin-5, (Bayer).
Plasbumin-25, (Bayer). Proserum 5, Inj. (Hoechst Marion Roussel).

albumin human, 5%. (al-BYOO-MIN human) (Immuno-US) Normal serum albumin 5%. Inj. Vial 250 ml. *Rx.*
Use: Plasma protein fraction.
See: Albuminar-5, Inj. (Centeon).
　Albutein 5%, Inj. (Alpha Therapeutic).
　Buminate 5%, Inj. (Baxter).
　Plasbumin-5, Inj. (Bayer).
albumin human, 25%. (al-BYOO-MIN human) (Immuno-US) Normal serum albumin 25%. Inj. Vial 10 ml, 50 ml. *Rx.*
Use: Plasma protein fraction.
See: Albuminar-25, Inj. (Centeon).
　Albutein 25%, Inj. (Alpha Therapeutics).
　Buminate 25%, Inj. (Baxter).
　Plasbumin-25, Inj. (Bayer).
•**albumin, iodinated I 125,** U.S.P. 23, injection. Albumin labeled with iodine-125.
Use: Diagnostic aid (blood volume determination); radioactive agent.
•**albumin, iodinated I 131 serum,** U.S.P. XIX.
•**albumin, iodinated I 125 serum,** U.S.P. XIX.
Use: Diagnostic aid (blood volume determination); radioactive agent.
Use: Diagnostic aid (blood volume determination; intrathecal imaging); radioactive agent.
See: Albumotope-LS (Squibb).
•**albumin, iodinated I 131,** U.S.P. 23. Albumin labeled with iodine-131. Inj.
Use: Diagnostic aid (blood volume determination; intrathecal imaging); radioactive agent.
albumin, normal serum 5%. (Immuno-US) Albumin human 5%. Inj. vial 120 ml. *Rx.*
Use: Plasma protein fraction.
albumin, normal serum 25%. (Immuno-US) Albumin human 25%. Inj. vial 10 ml, 50 ml. *Rx.*
Use: Plasma protein fraction.
albumin-saline diluent. (Bayer) Dilute allergenic extracts and venom products for patient testing and treating. Premeasured vials 1.8 ml, 4 ml, 4.5 ml, 9 ml, 30 ml. Vial 2 ml, 5 ml, 10 ml, 30 ml.
Use: Diagnostic aid, treatment.
Albuminar-5 and Albuminar-25. (Centeon) Albumin, (human) U.S.P. 5%: solution with administration set. Bot. 50 ml, 250 ml, 500 ml, 1000 ml. 25%: solution. Vial 20 ml, 50 ml, 100 ml with administration set. *Rx.*
Use: Plasma protein fraction.
Albumotope I-131. (Squibb) Albumin, Iodinated I-131 Serum (50 uCi).

Use: Diagnostic aid.
Albunex. (Mallinkrodt) Albumin (human) 5%, sonicated. Sodium acetyl tryptophanate 0.08 mmol, sodium caprylate 0.08 mmol/g albumin. Vial. 5 ml, 10 ml, 20 ml. *Rx.*
Use: Plasma protein fractions.
Albustix Reagent Strips. (Bayer) Firm paper reagent strips impregnated with tetrabromphenol blue, citrate buffer and a protein-adsorbing agent. Bot. 50s, 100s.
Use: Diagnostic aid.
Albutein 5%. (Alpha Therapeutic) Normal serum albumin 5%. Inj. Vial w/IV set: 250 ml, 500 ml. *Rx.*
Use: Plasma protein fraction.
Albutein 25%. (Alpha Therapeutic) Normal serum albumin 25%. Inj. Vial w/IV set: 50 ml. *Rx.*
Use: Plasma protein fraction.
•**albuterol,** (al-BYOO-ter-ahl) U.S.P 23. USAN.
Use: Bronchodilator.
See: Proventil Inhaler (Schering-Plough).
　Ventolin, Inh. Aerosol (Glaxo Wellcome).
albuterol aerosol. (Various Mfr.) 90 mcg per activation. 17 g. *Rx.*
Use: Bronchodilator.
•**albuterol sulfate,** (al-BYOO-teh-rahl) U.S.P. 23. USAN.
Use: Bronchodilator.
See: Airet, Inhalation soln. (Adams).
　Proventil, Repetabs, Tab., Soln., Syr. (Schering-Plough).
　Ventolin, Inhalation Soln., Syr., Tab., Nebules (Glaxo Wellcome).
　Ventolin Rotacaps (Glaxo Wellcome).
　Volmax, ER Tab. (Muro).
albuterol tablets.
Use: Bronchodilator.
•**albutoin.** (al-BYOO-toe-in) USAN.
Use: Anticonvulsant.
Alcaine. (Alcon) Proparacaine HCl 0.5%, glycerin, sodium Cl, benzalkonium Cl. Bot. 15 ml. *Rx.*
Use: Local anesthetic, ophthalmic.
Alcare. (SK-Beecham) Ethyl alcohol 62%. Foam Bot. 210 ml, 300 ml, 600 ml. *otc.*
Use: Antiseptic.
Alclear Eye Lotion. (Walgreen) Sterile isotonic fluid. Bot. 8 oz. *otc.*
Use: Eye irritation relief.
•**alclofenac.** (al-KLOE-feh-nak) USAN.
Use: Analgesic, anti-inflammatory.
See: Mervan (Continental Pharma, Belgium).

•**alclometasone dipropionate,** (al-kloe-MEH-tah-zone die-PRO-pee-oh-nate) U.S.P. 23.
Use: Anti-inflammatory (topical).
See: Aclovate, Cream, Oint. (Glaxo Wellcome).

•**alcloxa.** (al-KLOX-ah) USAN.
Use: Astringent, keratolytic.

Alco-Gel. (Tweezerman) Ethyl alcohol 60%. Tube 60 g, 480 g. *otc.*
Use: Skin cleanser.

•**alcohol,** U.S.P. 23. Ethanol, ethyl alcohol.
Use: Anti-infective, topical; pharmaceutic aid (solvent).
See: Anbesol, Gel, Liq. (Whitehall Robins)
Anbesol Maximum Strength, Gel. Liq. (Whitehall Robins).
Ru-Tuss Expectorant (Knoll). Ru-Tuss w/ Hydrocodone (Knoll).
Ru-Tuss Liquid (Knoll).

alcohol, dehydrated.
Use: Solvent, vehicle.

•**alcohol, diluted,** N.F. 18.
Use: Pharmaceutic aid (solvent).

•**alcohol, rubbing,** U.S.P. 23.
Use: Rubefacient.
See: Lavacol (Parke-Davis).

Alcohol 5% and Dextrose 5%. (Abbott Hospital Prods) Alcohol 5 ml, dextrose 5 g/100 ml. Bot. 1000 ml. *Rx.*
Use: Parenteral nutritional supplement.

Alcojet. (Alconox) Biodegradable machine washing detergent and wetting agent. Ctn. 9 × 4 lb, 25 lb, 50 lb, 100 lb, 300 lb. *otc.*
Use: Detergent, wetting agent.

Alcolec. (American Lecithin) Lecithin w/ choline base, cephalin, lipositol. Cap. 100s. Gran. 8 oz, lb. *otc.*
Use: Nutritional supplement.

Alconefrin 12 and 50. (PolyMedica) Phenylephrine HCl 0.16% w/benzalkonium Cl. Dropper bot. 30 ml. *otc.*
Use: Decongestant.

Alconefrin 25. (PolyMedica) Phenylephrine HCl 0.25% w/benzalkonium Cl. Dropper bot. 30 ml. Spray Pkg. 30 ml. *otc.*
Use: Decongestant.

Alcon Enzymatic Cleaning Tablets for Extended Wear. (Alcon Lenscare) Pancreatin tablets. Pkg. 12s. *otc.*
Use: Contact lens care.

Alcon Lens Case. (Alcon Lenscare) Two lens cases. Ctn. 12s. *otc.*
Use: Contact lens care.

Alcon Opti-Pure Sterile Saline Solu-tion. (Alcon Lenscare) Sterile unpreserved saline solution. Aerosol 8 oz. *otc.*
Use: Soft contact lens care.

Alcon Saline Solution for Sensitive Eyes. (Alcon Lenscare) Sodium Cl, edetate disodium, borate buffer system, sorbic acid. Bot. 360 ml. *otc.*
Use: Soft contact lens care.

Alconox. (Alconox) Biodegradable detergent and wetting agent. Box 4 lb, Container 25 lb, 50 lb, 100 lb, 300 lb. *otc.*
Use: Anionic detergent, wetting agent.

Alcotabs. (Alconox) Tab. Box 6s, 100s.
Use: Test tube cleaner.

•**alcuronium chloride.** (al-cure-OH-nee-uhm) USAN. Diallyldinortoxiferin dichloride.
Use: Muscle relaxant.
See: Alloferin (Roche).
Toxiferene (Roche).

Aldactazide Tablets. (Searle) Spironolactone and hydrochlorothiazide. **25 mg/25 mg:** Bot. 100s, 500s, 1000s, 2500s, UD 100s. **50 mg/50 mg:** Bot. 100s, UD 32s, UD 100s. *Rx.*
Use: Antihypertensive, diuretic.

Aldactone Tablets. (Searle) Spironolactone. **25 mg/Tab.:** Bot. 100s, 500s, 1000s, UD 100s. **50 mg/Tab.:** Bot. 100s, UD 100s. **100 mg/Tab.:** Bot. 100s, UD 100s. *Rx.*
Use: Antihypertensive.

Aldara. (3M Pharm) Imiquimod 5%/ Cream Box. 12s. (In 250 mg single-use packets.) *Rx.*
Use: Treatment of external gential and perianal warts/condyloma.

•**aldesleukin.** (al-dess-LOO-kin) USAN.
Use: Biological response modifier; antineoplastic; immunostimulant. [Orphan drug]
See: Proleukin, Pow for Inj. (Chiron).

aldinamide.

•**aldioxa.** (al-DIE-ox-ah) USAN. Aluminum dihydroxy allantoinate.
Use: Astringent, keratolytic.

Aldoclor 150. (Merck) Methyldopa 250 mg, chlorothiazide 150 mg/Tab. Bot. 100s. *Rx.*
Use: Antihypertensive.

Aldoclor 250. (Merck) Methyldopa 250 mg, chlorothiazide 250 mg/Tab. Bot. 100s. *Rx.*
Use: Antihypertensive.

Aldomet. (Merck) Methyldopa. **125 mg/ Tab.:** Bot. 100s. **250 mg/Tab.:** Bot. 100s, 1000s, UD 100s, Unit-of-use 100s. **500 mg/Tab.:** Bot. 100s, 500s, UD 100s, Unit-of-use 60s, 100s. *Rx.*

Use: Antihypertensive.

W/Chlorothiazide.
See: Aldoclor, Tab. (Merck).

W/Hydrochlorothiazide.
See: Aldoril, Tab. (Merck).

Aldomet Ester Hydrochloride. (Merck)
Methyldopate HCl 250 mg/5 ml, citric
acid anhydrous 25 mg, sodium bisulfite
16 mg, disodium edetate 2.5 mg, monothioglycerol 10 mg, sodium hydroxide
to adjust pH, methylparaben 0.15%,
propylparaben 0.02% w/water for inj.
q.s. to 5 ml. Vial 5 ml. *Rx.*
Use: Antihypertensive.

Aldomet Oral Suspension. (Merck)
Methyldopa 250 mg/5 ml, alcohol 1%,
benzoic acid 0.1%, sodium bisulfite
0.2%. Bot. 473 ml. *Rx.*
Use: Antihypertensive.

Aldoril-15. (Merck) Methyldopa 250 mg,
hydrochlorothiazide 15 mg/Tab. Bot.
100s, 1000s. *Rx.*
Use: Antihypertensive.

Aldoril-25. (Merck) Methyldopa 250 mg,
hydrochlorothiazide 25 mg/Tab. Bot.
100s, 1000s, UD 100s. *Rx.*
Use: Antihypertensive.

Aldoril D30 & D50. (Merck) Methyldopa
500 mg, hydrochlorothiazide 30 mg or
50 mg. Tab. Bot. 100s. *Rx.*
Use: Antihypertensive.

Aldosterone RIA Diagnostic Kit. (Abbott Diagnostics) Test kits 50s.
Use: Diagnostic aid.

•**alendronate sodium.** (al-LEN-droe-nate)
USAN.
Use: Bone resorption inhibitor.
See: Fosamax, Tab. (Merck).

Alenic Alka Liquid. (Rugby) Aluminum
hydroxide 31.7 mg, magnesium carbonate 137.3 mg, sodium alginate, EDTA,
sodium 13 mg. Bot. 355 ml. *otc.*
Use: Antacid.

Alenic Alka Tablets. (Rugby) Aluminum
Hydroxide 80 mg, magnesium trisilicate 20 mg, sodium bicarbonate, calcium stearate, sugar. Chew Tab. Bot.
100s. *otc.*
Use: Antacid.

Alenic Alka Tablets, Extra Strength.
(Rugby) Aluminum hydroxide 160 mg,
magnesium carbonate 105 mg, sodium
29.9 mg. Chew. tab. Bot. 100s. *otc.*
Use: Antacid.

•**alentemol hydrobromide.** (al-EN-teh-
mole) USAN
Use: Antipsychotic; dopamine agonist.

Alersule Capsules. (Misemer) Chlorpheniramine maleate 8 mg, phenyleph-

rine HCl 20 mg/Cap. Bot. 100s. *otc, Rx.*
Use: Antihistamine, decongestant.

Alert-Pep. (Approved) Caffeine 200 mg/
Cap. Bot. 16s. *otc.*
Use: CNS stimulant.

•**aletamine hydrochloride.** (al-ETT-ah-
meen) USAN.
Use: Antidepressant.

Aleve. (Procter & Gamble) Naproxen sodium 220 mg (naproxen base 200 mg
with sodium 20 mg) Tab. Bot. 24s, 50s,
100s. *otc.*
Use: Nonsteroidal anti-inflammatory
agent.

•**alexidine.** (ah-LEX-ih-DEEN) USAN.
Use: Antibacterial.

alfa interferon-2a.
See: Roferon A (Roche).

alfa interferon-2b.
See: Intron A (Schering-Plough).

alfa interferon-n3.
See: Alferon N (Purdue Frederick).

Alfenta. (Janssen) Alfentanil 0.5 mg/ml.
Amp. 2 ml, 5 ml, 10 ml, 20 ml. *c-ii.*
Use: Narcotic analgesic, anesthetic,
monitored anesthesia care.

•**alfentanil hydrochloride.** (al-FEN-tuh-
NILL) USAN.
Use: Narcotic analgesic, anesthetic,
monitored anesthesia care.
See: Alfenta, Inj. (Janssen).

Alferon N. (Purdue Frederick) Interferon
alfa-n3 5 mIU/vial. Vial 1 ml. *Rx.*
Use: Condylomata acuminata (genital
warts).

•**alfuzosin hydrochloride.** (al-FEW-zoe-
sin) USAN.
Use: Antihypertensive (α-blocker.

Algel. (Faraday) Magnesium trisilicate
0.5 g, aluminum hydroxide 0.25 g/Tab.
Bot. 100s. Susp. Bot. gal. *otc.*
Use: Antacid.

•**algeldrate.** (AL-jell-drate) USAN.
Use: Antacid.

Algemin. (Thurston) Macrocystis pyrifera
alga. Pow. Jar 8 oz. Tab. Bot. 300s. *otc.*
Use: Dietary aid.

Algenic Alka Improved Tablets. (Rugby)
Aluminum hydroxide 240 mg, magnesium hydroxide 100 mg/Chew. tab. Bot.
100s, 500s. *otc.*
Use: Antacid.

Algenic Alka Liquid. (Rugby) Aluminum
hydroxide 31.7 mg/ml, magnesium
carbonate 137 mg/ml, sodium alginate,
sorbitol. Bot. 355 ml. *otc.*
Use: Antacid.

•**algestone acetonide.** USAN.
Use: Anti-inflammatory.

•**algestone acetophenide.** (al-JESS-tone ah-SEE-toe-FEN-ide) USAN.
Use: Progestin.

Algex liniment. (Approved) Menthol, camphor, methylsalicylate, eucalyptus. Bot. 4 oz. *otc.*
Use: Analgesic, topical.

algin.
See: Sodium Alginate, N.F. 18.

Algin-All. (Barth's) Sodium alginate from kelp. Tab. Bot. 100s, 500s.

•**alginic acid,** N.F. 18.
Use: Pharmaceutic aid (tablet binder, emulsifying agent).

alginic acid. W/Aluminum hydroxide dried gel, magnesium trisilicate, sodium bicarbonate. *otc.*
Use: Antacid.
See: Gaviscon Foamtabs (Hoechst Marion Roussel).

•**alglucerase.** (al-GLUE-ser-ACE) USAN.
Use: Enzyme replacement therapy (glucocerebrosidase). [Orphan drug]
See: Ceredase, Inj. (Genzyme).

algreldrate.
Use: Antacid.

alidine dihydrochloride or phosphate.
Anileridine, N.F.

•**aliflurane.** (al-IH-flew-rane) USAN.
Use: Anesthetic (inhalation).

Alikal Powder. (Sanofi Winthrop) Sodium bicarbonate, tartaric acid powder. *otc.*
Use: Antacid.

Alimentum. (Ross) Casein hydrolysate, sucrose, tapioca starch, MCT (fractionated coconut oil), safflower oil, soy oil. Qt ready-to-use. *otc.*
Use: Enteral nutritional supplement.

•**alipamide.** (al-IH-pam-ide) USAN.
Use: Diuretic, antihypertensive.

alisobumal.
See: Butalbital, U.S.P. 23.

•**alitame.** (AL-ih-TAME) USAN.
Use: Sweetener.

alkalinizers, minerals and electrolytes.
See: Polycitra (Baker Norton).
Oracit (Carolina Medical Products).
Bicitra (Baker Norton).

alkalinizers urinary tract products.
See: Sodium Bicarbonate (Various Mfr.).
Urocit-K (Mission).
Citrolith (Beach Pharm.).
Polycitra (Baker Norton).
Bicitra (Baker Norton).

Alkalol. (Alkalol Co.) Thymol, eucalyptol, menthol, camphor, benzoin, potassium alum, potassium chlorate, sodium bi-carbonate, sodium Cl, sweet birch oil, spearmint oil, pine and cassia oil, alcohol 0.05%. Bot. Pt. Nasal douche cup pkg. 1s. *otc.*
Use: Eyes, nose, throat and all inflamed mucous membranes.

Alka-Med Liquid. (Halsey) Aluminum hydroxide 200 mg, magnesium hydroxide 200 mg/ 5 ml. Bot. 8 oz. *otc.*
Use: Antacid.

Alka-Med Tablets. (Halsey) Magnesium hydroxide, aluminum hydroxide. Bot. 60s. *otc.*
Use: Antacid.

Alka-Mints. (Bayer) Calcium carbonate 850 mg/Chew. tab. Carton 30s. *otc.*
Use: Antacid.

Alka-Seltzer. (Bayer) Heat treated sodium bicarbonate 1916 mg, citric acid 1000 mg, aspirin 325 mg, sodium 567 mg/Tab. Bot. 36s. *otc.*
Use: Effervescent antacid, analgesic.

Alka-Seltzer, Advanced Formula.
(Bayer) Heat treated sodium bicarbonate 465 mg, citric acid 900 mg, acetaminophen 325 mg, potassium bicarbonate 300 mg, calcium carbonate 280 mg/Tab. Foil pack 36s. *otc.*
Use: Effervescent antacid, analgesic.

Alka-Seltzer Effervescent, Gold Tablets. (Bayer) Heat treated sodium bicarbonate 958 mg, citric acid 832 mg, potassium bicarbonate 312 mg, sodium 311 mg/Tab. Bot. 20s, 36s. *otc.*
Use: Effervescent antacid, analgesic.

Alka-Seltzer, Extra Strength. (Bayer) Aspirin 500 mg, heat treated sodium bicarbonate 1985 mg, citric acid 1000 mg, sodium 588 mg/Tab. Bot. 12s, 24s. *otc.*
Use: Effervescent antacid, analgesic.

Alka-Seltzer Flavored Effervescent Antacid-Analgesic. (Bayer) Aspirin 325 mg, sodium bicarbonate 1700 mg, citric acid 1000 mg, phenylalanine 9 mg, sodium 506 mg, aspartame, lemon-lime flavor. Tab. Bot. 24s. *otc.*
Use: Effervescent antacid, analgesic.

Alka-Seltzer Plus. (Bayer) Chlorpheniramine maleate 2 mg, phenylpropanolamine bitartrate 24 mg, aspirin 324 mg, sodium 506 mg/Tab. Foil pack 20s, 36s. *otc.*
Use: Antihistamine, decongestant, analgesic.

Alka-Seltzer Plus Allergy Liqui-Gels.
(Bayer) Pseudoephedrine HCl 30 mg, brompheniramine maleate 2 mg, acetaminophen 500 mg/Tab. Pkg. 12s. *otc.*
Use: Decongestant, antihistamine, analgesic.

Alka-Seltzer Plus Cold and Cough Liqui-Gels. (Bayer) Dextromethorphan HBr 10 mg, pseudoephedrine HCl 30 mg, chlorpheniramine maleate 2 mg, acetaminophen 250 mg/Cap. Pkg. 12s, 20s. *otc.*
Use: Antitussive, decongestant, antihistamine, analgesic.

Alka-Seltzer Plus Cold & Cough Tablets. (Bayer) Phenylpropanolamine bitartrate 20 mg, chlorpheniramine maleate 2 mg, dextromethorphan HBr 10 mg, aspirin 325 mg, phenylalanine 11.2 mg/Tab. 12s, 20s, 36s. *otc.*
Use: Decongestant, antihistamine, antitussive, analgesic.

Alka-Seltzer Plus Cold Liqui-Gels. (Bayer) Chlorpheniramine maleate 2 mg, pseudoephedrine HCl 30 mg, acetaminophen 250 mg/Cap. Pkg. 12s, 20s. *otc.*
Use: Antihistamine, decongestant, analgesic.

Alka-Seltzer Plus Cold Medicine. (Bayer) Phenylpropanolamine bitartrate 20 mg, chlorpheniramine maleate 2 mg, aspirin 325 mg/Tab. 12s, 20s, 36s, 48s. *otc.*
Use: Decongestant, antihistamine, analgesic.

Alka-Seltzer Plus Cold Tablets. (Bayer) Phenylpropanolamine bitartrate 24.08 mg, chlorpheniramine maleate 2 mg, aspirin 325 mg/Tab. Pkg. 12s, 20s. Bot. 36s, 48s. *otc.*
Use: Decongestant, antihistamine, analgesic.

Alka-Seltzer Plus Flu & Body Aches Non-Drowsy Liqui-Gels. (Bayer) Pseudoephedrine HCl 30 mg, dextromethorphan HBr 10 mg, acetaminophen 250 mg/Tab. Pkg. 12s. *otc.*
Use: Decongestant, antitussive, analgesic.

Alka-Seltzer Plus Nighttime Cold Liqui-Gels. (Bayer) Pseudoephedrine HCl 30 mg, dextromethorphan HBr 10 mg, doxylamine succinate 6.25 mg, acetaminophen 250 mg/Cap. Pkg. 20s. *otc.*
Use: Decongestant, antitussive, antihistamine.

Alka-Seltzer Plus Night-Time Cold Tablets. (Bayer) Phenylpropanolamine bitartrate 20 mg, doxylamine succinate 6.25 mg, dextromethorphan HBr 15 mg, aspirin 500 mg, phenylalanine 16.2 mg/Tab. Bot. 12s, 20s, 36s. *otc.*
Use: Decongestant, antihistamine, analgesic.

Alka-Seltzer Plus Sinus. (Bayer) Phenylpropanolamine bitartrate 20 mg, aspirin 325 mg, aspartame, phenylalanine 8.98 mg/Tab. Pkg. 20s. *otc.*
Use: Decongestant, analgesic.

Alka-Seltzer Plus Sinus Allergy. (Bayer) Phenylpropanolamine bitartrate 24.08 mg, brompheniramine maleate 2 mg, aspirin 500 mg, aspartame, phenylalanine 9 mg/Tab. Bot. 16s, 32s. *otc.*
Use: Decongestant, antihistamine, analgesic.

Alka-Seltzer Special Effervescent Antacid. (Bayer) Heat treated sodium bicarbonate 958 mg, citric acid 832 mg, potassium bicarbonate 312 mg, sodium 284 mg/Tab. Foil pack 12s, 20s, 36s. *otc.*
Use: Effervescent antacid.

Alka-Seltzer Tablets. (Bayer) Aspirin 325 mg, citric acid 1000 mg, phenylalanine 9 mg, sodium 506 mg/Tab. Bot. 24s. *otc.*
Use: Effervescent antacid, analgesic.

Alka-Seltzer w/Aspirin. (Bayer) Sodium bicarbonate 1916 mg, citric acid 1000 mg, aspirin 325 mg and sodium 567 mg. 17.2 mEq acid neutralizing capacity. Foil pack 8s, 12s, 24s, 26s and 36s. *otc.*
Use: Effervescent antacid, analgesic.

Alkeran. (Glaxo Wellcome) Melphalan 2 mg/Tab. Bot. 50s. *Rx.*
Use: Antineoplastic.

Alkets. (Roberts Hauck) Calcium carbonate 500 mg, dextrose, peppermint flavor. Chew. tab. Bot. 36s, 96s, 150s. *otc.*
Use: Antacid.

alkylbenzyldimethylammonium chloride. Benzalkonium Cl, N.F. 18.
W/Methylrosaniline Cl, polyoxyethylene-nonylphenol, polyethylene glycol tert-dodecylthioether.
See: Hyva, Tab. (Holland-Rantos).

•**allantoin.** (al-AN-toe-in) USAN.
Use: Vulnerary (topical).
See: Cutemol (Summers).
W/Aminacrine, sulfanilamide.
See: Par Cream (Parmed).
Vagidine, Cream (Zeneca).
Vagitrol, Cream (Syntex).
W/Balsam, Lano-sil, silicone.
See: Balmex Med. Lot. (Macsil).
W/p-Chloro-m-xylenol.
See: Cebum, Shampoo (Dermik).
W/Coal tar extract, hexachlorophene, glycerin, lanolin.
See: Pso-Rite, Cream (DePree).
W/Coal tar in cream base.
See: Tegrin Cream (Block Drug).

W/Coal tar solution, isopropyl myristate, psorilan.
See: Psorelief, Soln. (Quality Generics).

W/Dienestrol, sulfanilamide, aminacrine HCl.
See: AVC/Dienestrol Cream, Supp. (Hoechst Marion Roussel).

W/Hydrocortisone.
See: Tarcortin, Cream (Schwarz Pharma).

W/Nitrofurazone.
See: Eldezol, Oint. (Zeneca).

W/Pramoxine HCl, benzalkonium Cl.
See: Perifoam, Aerosol (Solvay).

W/Resorcinol, hexachlorophene, menthol.
See: Tackle, Gel. (Colgate Oral).

W/Salicylic acid, sulfur.
See: Neutrogena Disposables (Neutrogena).

W/Sulfanilamide, 9-aminoacridine HCl.
Nil Vaginal Cream (Century).
Vagisan, Creme (Sandia).
Vagisul, Creme (Sheryl).

W/Sulfisoxazole, Aminoacridine.
Use: Topically, aid in the promotion of granulation.
See: Vagilia, Cream, Supp. (Lemmon).

W/Tarbonis.
See: Sebical, Shampoo (Schwarz Pharma).

W/Vitamins A, D.
See: A-D Dressing (LaCrosse).

Allay. (LuChem) Acetaminophen 650 mg, hydrocodone bitartrate 7.5 mg/ Cap. Bot. 100s. *c-III.*
Use: Narcotic analgesic combination.

Allbee C-800. (Robins) Vitamins E 45 IU, C 800 mg, B$_1$ 15 mg, B$_2$ 17 mg, B$_3$ 100 mg, B$_5$ 25 mg, B$_{12}$ 12 mcg/Tab. Bot. 60s. *otc.*
Use: Vitamin supplement.

Allbee C-800 Plus Iron. (Robins) Vitamins E 45 IU, C 800 mg, B$_1$ 15 mg, B$_2$ 17 mg, niacin 100 mg, B$_6$ 25 mg, B$_{12}$ 12 mcg, pantothenic acid 25 mg, iron 27 mg, folic acid 0.4 mg/Tab. Bot. 60s. *otc.*
Use: Vitamin/mineral supplement.

Allbee w/C. (Robins) Vitamins B$_1$ 15 mg, B$_6$ 5 mg, B$_2$ 10.2 mg, B$_3$ 50 mg, B$_5$ 10 mg, C 300 mg/Cap. Bot. 30s. *otc.*
Use: Vitamin supplement.

Allbee-T. (Robins) Vitamins B$_1$ 15.5 mg, B$_2$ 10 mg, B$_6$ 8.2 mg, B$_5$ 23 mg, B$_3$ 100 mg, C 500 mg, B$_{12}$ 5 mcg/Tab. Bot. 100s, 500s. *otc.*
Use: Vitamin supplement.

Allbex. (Approved) Vitamins B$_1$ 5 mg, B$_2$ 2 mg, B$_6$ 0.25 mg, calcium pantothe-

nate 3 mg, niacinamide 20 mg, ferrous sulfate 194.4 mg, inositol 10 mg, choline 10 mg, B$_{12}$ (concentrate) 3 mcg/ Cap. Bot. 100s, 1000s. *otc.*
Use: Vitamin/mineral supplement.

All-Day-C. (Barth's) Vitamin C 200 mg/ Cap. or 500 mg/Tab. with rose hip extract. Bot. 30s, 90s, 180s, 360s. *otc.*
Use: Vitamin supplement.

All-Day Iron Yeast. (Barth's) Iron 20 mg, Vitamins B$_1$ 2 mg, B$_2$ 4 mg, niacin 0.57 mg/Cap. Bot. 30s, 90s, 180s. *otc.*
Use: Vitamin/mineral supplement.

All-Day-Vites. (Barth's) Vitamins A 10,000 IU, D 400 IU, B$_1$ 3 mg, B$_2$ 6 mg, niacin 1 mg, C 120 mg, B$_{12}$ 10 mcg, E 30 IU/Cap. Bot. 30s, 90s, 180s, 360s. *otc.*
Use: Vitamin supplement.

Allegra. (Hoechst Marion Roussel) Fexofenadine HCl 60 mg/Cap. Bot. 60s, 100s, 500s, UD 100s. *Rx.*
Use: Antihistamine.

allegron. Nortriptyline.
Use: Antidepressant.

Allent. (Ascher) Pseudoephedrine HCl 120 mg, brompheniramine maleate 12 mg. Slow-release cap. Bot. 100s. *Rx.*
Use: Decongestant, antihistamine.

Allerben Injection. (Forest) Diphenhydramine 10 mg/ml. Vial 30 ml. *Rx.*
Use: Antihistamine.

Allerchlor injection. (Forest) Chlorpheniramine maleate 10 mg/ml. Vial 30 ml. *Rx.*
Use: Antihistamine.

Aller-Chlor. (Rugby) Chlorpheniramine maleate. **Tab.:** 4 mg. Bot. 24s, 100s, 1000s. **Syr.:** 2 mg/5 ml. Bot. 4 oz, pt, gal. *otc.*
Use: Antihistamine.

Allercon. (Parmed) Pseudoephedrine HCl 60 mg, triprolidine HCl 2.5 mg/Tab. Bot. 24s, 100s and 1000s. *otc.*
Use: Decongestant, antihistamine.

Allercreme Skin Lotion. (Galderma) Mineral oil, petrolatum, lanolin, lanolin oil, lanolin alcohols, glycerin, triethanolamine, cetyl alcohol, stearic acid, parabens. Lot. Bot. 240 ml. *otc.*
Use: Emollient.

Allercreme Ultra Emollient. (Galderma) Mineral oil, petrolatum, lanolin, lanolin alcohol, lanolin oil, glycerin, glyceryl stearate, PEG-100 stearate, squalane, cetyl alcohol, sorbitan laurate, quaternium-15, parabens. Cream Bot. 60 g. *otc.*
Use: Emollient.

Allerdec Capsules. (Towne) Phenyl-propanolamine HCl 25 mg, chlorphenir-amine maleate 1 mg, pyrilamine male-ate 5 mg/Cap. Bot. 25s, 50s. *otc.*
Use: Decongestant, antihistamine.

Allerest. (Novartis Consumer Health) **Tab.:** Phenylpropanolamine HCl 18.7 mg, chlorpheniramine maleate 2 mg/Tab. Sleeve Pack 24s, 48s. Bot. 72s. **Chew. tab. for Children:** Phenyl-propanolamine HCl 9.4 mg, chlor-pheniramine maleate 1 mg/Tab. Sleeve Pack 24s. **Eye Drops:** Naphazoline HCl 0.012%. Bot. 0.5 oz. **Headache Strength Tab.:** Acetaminophen 325 mg, pseudoephedrine HCl 30 mg, chlor-pheniramine maleate 2 mg/Tab. Pkg. 24s. **Nasal Spray:** Oxymetazoline HCl 0.05%. Bot. 0.5 oz. *otc.*
Use: Decongestant, antihistamine; anal-gesic (Headache strength Tab only).

Allerest 12-Hour. (Ciba Consumer) Phenylpropanolamine HCl 75 mg, chlorpheniramine maleate 8 mg/Cap. Sleeve pak 10s. Nasal spray: Oxymeta-zoline HCl 0.05%, benzalkonium Cl, EDTA. 15 ml. *otc.*
Use: Decongestant, antihistamine.

Allerest, Children's. (Novartis) Phenyl-propanolamine HCl 94 mg, chlorphenir-amine maleate 6 mg. Chew. tab. Bot. 24s. *otc.*
Use: Pediatric decongestant, antihista-mine.

Allerest Maximum Strength. (Medeva) Pseudoephedrine 30 mg, chlorphenir-amine maleate 2 mg/Tab. Bot. 24s, 48s, 72s. *otc.*
Use: Decongestant, antihistamine.

Allerest Maximum Strength 12-Hour Caplets. (Novartis) Phenylpropanol-amine HCl 75 mg, chlorpheniramine maleate 12 mg/Capl. Pkg. 10s. *otc.*
Use: Decongestant, antihistamine.

Allerest No Drowsiness. (Novartis) Pseudoephedrine 30 mg, acetamino-phen 325 mg/Tab. Bot. 20s. *otc.*
Use: Decongestant, analgesic.

Allerest Sinus Pain Formula. (Novartis) Acetaminophen 500 mg, pseudoephed-rine HCl 30 mg, chlorpheniramine ma-leate 2 mg/Tab. Pkg. 20s. *otc.*
Use: Analgesic, decongestant, antihis-tamine.

Allerfrim. (Rugby) **Tab.:** Pseudoephed-rine HCl 60 mg, triprolidine HCl 2.5 mg. Bot. 24s, 100s, 1000s. **Syr.:** Pseudoephedrine HCl 30 mg, triproli-dine HCl 1.25 mg. Bot. 118 ml, 473 ml. *otc.*

Use: Decongestant, antihistamine.

Allerfrin OTC Syrup. (Rugby) Pseudo-ephedrine 30 mg, triprolidine 1.25 mg. Syr. Bot. Pt. *otc.*
Use: Decongestant, antihistamine.

Allerfrin w/Codeine. (Rugby) Pseudo-ephedrine HCl 30 mg, triprolidine HCl 1.25 mg, codeine phosphate 10 mg, al-cohol 4.3%. Syr. Bot. 120 ml, pt, gal. *c-v.*
Use: Decongestant, antihistamine, anti-tussive.

Allergan Enzymatic. (Allergan) Papain, sodium Cl, sodium carbonate, sodium borate, edetate disodium. Kits 12s, 24s, 36s, 48s. *otc.*
Use: Soft contact lens care.

Allergan Hydrocare Cleaning & Disin-fecting Solution. (Allergan) tris(2-hy-droxyethyl)tallow ammonium Cl 0.013%, thimerosal 0.002%, bis(2-hy-droxyethyl)tallow ammonium Cl, sodium bicarbonate, dibasic, monobasic and anhydrous sodium phosphate, hydro-chloric acid, propylene glycol, polysor-bate 80, special soluble polyhema. Bot. 4 oz, 8 oz, 12 oz. *otc.*
Use: Soft contact lens care.

Allergan Hydrocare Preserved Saline Solution. (Allergan) Sodium Cl, so-dium hexametaphosphate, sodium hydroxide, boric acid, sodium borate, EDTA 0.01%, thimerosal 0.001%. Bot. 8 oz, 12 oz. *otc.*
Use: Soft contact lens care.

Allergen Ear Drops. (Goldline) Benzo-caine 1.4%, antipyrine 5.4%, glycerin, oxyquinoline sulfate. Bot. 0.5 oz. *Rx.*
Use: Otic preparation.

allergen patch test kit. (Hermal) Box of tubes of semi-solid pastes or solutions. Allergens are either suspended in 4.5 g petrolatum, USP, or dissolved in 5.5 g water. Kit includes 20 reclosable sy-ringes for topical use only (not for injec-tion), each exuding sufficient allergen to test 150 patients, housed in a plastic case with two drawers. Allergens in-clude benzocaine, mercaptobenzothia-zole, colophony, p-phenylenediamine, imidazolidinyl urea (Germall 115), cin-namin aldyhyde, lanolin alcohol (wool wax alcohols), carba rubber mix, neo-mycin sulfate, thiuram rubber mix, formaldehyde, ethylenediamine dihydrochloride, epoxy resin, quater-nium 15, p-tert-butylphenol formalde-hyde resin, mercapto rubber mix, black rubber p-phenylenediamine mix, po-tassium dichromate, balsam of Peru and nickel sulfate.

allergen test patches.
Use: For diagnosis of allergic contact dermatitis.
See: T.R.U.E. Test (Glaxo Wellcome).
Allergenic Extracts. (Various Mfr.) Allergenic extracts of pollen, mold, house dust, inhalants, epidermals, insects in saline 0.9% and phenol 0.4% up to 1:10 w/v or 40,000 PNU/ml in sets or vials up to 30 ml.
Use: Diagnosis of specific allergies, relief of allergic symptoms.
Allergenic Extracts. (Bayer) Allergenic extracts of pollens, foods, inhalants, epidermals, fungi, insects, miscellaneous antigens.
Use: Diagnosis of specific allergies, relief of allergic symptoms.
allergenic extracts, alum-precipitated.
See: Allpyral (Bayer).
Certer-Al (Center).
Allergex. (Bayer) Silicones, polyethylene and triethylene glycol, antioxidants, mineral oil concentrate. Bot. Pt. Aerosol pt.
Use: Control of house dust allergens.
Allergy. (Parmed) Chlorpheniramine maleate 4 mg/Tab. Bot. 24s, 100s. *otc.*
Use: Antihistamine.
Allergy Drops. (Bausch & Lomb) Naphazoline HCl 0.012%. Bot. 15 ml. *otc.*
Use: Mydriatic/vasoconstrictor.
allergy preparations.
See: Antihistamine Preparations.
allergy relief medicine.
Use: Decongestant, antihistamine.
See: A.R.M. Caplets (SK-Beecham).
Allergy-Sinus Comtrex. (Bristol-Myers) Pseudoephedrine HCl 30 mg, chlorpheniramine maleate 2 mg, acetaminophen 500 mg/Capl. or Tab. Bot. 50s, UD 24s. *otc.*
Use: Decongestant, antihistamine, analgesic.
Allergy Tablets. (Weeks & Leo) Phenylpropanolamine HCl 37.5 mg, chlorpheniramine 4 mg/Tab. Bot. 30s. *otc.*
Use: Decongestant, antihistamine.
AllerMax. (Pfeiffer) Diphenhydramine HCl 50 mg/Cap. Pkg. 20s. 12.5 mg/5ml/Syr. Bot. 118 ml. *otc.*
Use: Antihistamine.
Allerphed Syrup. (Great Southern) Pseudoephedrine HCl 30 mg, triprolidine HCl 1.25 mg/5 ml. Syr. Bot. 118 ml. *otc.*
Use: Decongestant, antihistamine.
Allersone. (Roberts) Hydrocortisone 0.5%, diperodon HCl 0.5%, zinc oxide 5%, sodium lauryl sulfate, propylene glycol, cetyl alcohol, petrolatum, methyl and propyl parabens. Oint. Tube 15 g. *otc, Rx.*
Use: Corticosteroid, topical.
Allersule Forte. (Misemer) Phenylephrine HCl 20 mg, chlorpheniramine maleate 8 mg, methscopolamine nitrate 2.5 mg/Cap. Bot. 100s. *otc, Rx.*
Use: Decongestant, antihistamine, anticholinergic.
All-Nite Cold Formula. (Major) Pseudoephedrine HCl 10 mg, doxylamine succinate 1.25 mg, dextromethorphan HBr 5 mg, acetaminophen 167 mg/5 ml. Liq. Bot. 177 ml. *otc.*
Use: Decongestant, antihistamine, antitussive, analgesic.
•**allobarbital.** (AL-low-BAR-bih-tal) USAN.
Use: Sedative, hypnotic.
W/Acetaminophen, salicylamide, caffeine.
See: Allylvon, Cap. (Zeneca).
W/Aspirin, acetaminophen, aluminum aspirin.
See: Allylgesic, Tab. (Zeneca).
W/Ergotamine tartrate.
See: Allylgesic w/Ergotamine, Cap. (Zeneca).
allobarbitone.
See: Diallylbarbituric Acid (Various Mfr.).
•**allopurinol,** (AL-oh-PURE-ee-nahl) U.S.P. 23.
Use: Antigout, xanthine oxidase inhibitor.
See: Lopurin, Tab. (Knoll).
Zyloprim, Tab. (Glaxo Wellcome).
allopurinol riboside.
Use: Antiprotozoal.
allopurinol sodium.
Use: Ex vivo preservation of cadaveric kidneys for transplantation; antineoplastic. [Orphan drug]
Allpyral. (Bayer) Allergenic extracts, alum-precipitated. For subcutaneous inj. pollens, molds, epithelia, house dust, other inhalants, stinging insects.
Use: Diagnosis of specific allergies, relief of allergic symptoms.
allylbarbituric acid. Allylisobutyl-barbituric acid, butalbital. Tab. (Various Mfr.).
Use: Sedative.
W/A.P.C.
See: Anti-Ten, Tab. (Century).
Fiorinal, Cap., Tab. (Sandoz).
Tenstan (Standex).
W/Acetaminophen, homatropine methylbromide.
See: Panitol H.M.B., Tab. (Wesley).
W/Acetaminophen, salicylamide, caffeine.
See: Renpap, Tab. (Wren).

allylestrenol.

allyl-isobutylbarbituric acid.
See: Allylbarbituric Acid.

allylisopropylmalonylurea.
See: Aprobarbital.

•**allyl isothiocyanate,** U.S.P. 23.
Use: Counterirritant in neuralgia.

4-allyl-2-methoxyphenol, U.S.P. 23.

n-allylnoroxymorphone hcl, U.S.P. 23.

5-allyl-sec-butylbarbituric acid.
See: Talbutal.

Almacone. (Rugby) **Chew tab.:** Aluminum hydroxide 200 mg, magnesium hydroxide 200 mg, simethicone 20 mg/ Bot. 100s, 1000s. **Liq.:** Aluminum hydroxide 200 mg, magnesium hydroxide 200 mg, simethicone 20 mg, sodium 0.75 mg/5 ml. Bot. 360 ml, gal. *otc.*
Use: Antacid.

Almacone II Double Strength Liquid. (Rugby) Aluminum hydroxide 400 mg, magnesium hydroxide 400 mg, simethicone 40 mg/5 ml. Bot. 360 ml, gal. *otc.*
Use: Antacid.

•**almadrate sulfate.** (AL-ma-drate) USAN. Aluminum magnesium hydroxide-oxide-sulfate-hydrate.
Use: Antacid.

•**almagate.** (AL-mah-gate) USAN.
Use: Antacid.

almagucin. Gastric mucin, dried aluminum hydroxide gel, magnesium trisilicate. *otc.*
Use: Antacid.

Almebex Plus B$_{12}$. (Dayton) Vitamins B$_1$ 1 mg, B$_2$ 2 mg, B$_3$ 5 mg, B$_6$ 0.4 mg, B$_{12}$ 5 mcg, choline 33 mg/5 ml. 473 ml (with B$_{12}$ in separate container). *otc.*
Use: Vitamin supplement.

•**almond oil,** N.F. 18.
Use: Pharmaceutic aid (emollient, perfume, vehicle; oleaginous).

Almora. (Forest) Magnesium gluconate 0.5 g/Tab. Pkg. 100s. *otc.*
Use: Mineral supplement.

Alnyte. (Mayer) Scopolamine aminoxide HBr 0.2 mg, salicylamide 250 mg/Tab. Pkg. 16s. *Rx.*
Use: Anticholinergic, analgesic.

Alocass Laxative. (Western Research) Aloin 0.25 gr, cascara sagrada 0.5 gr, rhubarb 0.5 gr, ginger 1/32 gr, powdered extract of belladonna gr/Tab. Bot. 1000s. Pak 28s. *otc.*
Use: Laxative.

Alodopa-15 Tablets. (Major) Hydrochlorothiazide 15 mg, methyldopa 250 mg. Bot. 100s. *Rx.*
Use: Antihypertensive.

Alodopa-25 Tablets. (Major) Hydrochlorothiazide 25 mg, methyldopa 250 mg. Bot. 100s. *Rx.*
Use: Antihypertensive.

•**aloe,** U.S.P. 23.
Use: See Compound Benzoin Tincture.

Aloe Grande Creme. (Gordon) Aloe, vitamins E 1500 IU, A 100,000 units/oz in cream base. Jar 2.5 oz. *otc.*
Use: Emollient.

aloe vera active principle.
See: Alvagel, Oint. (Kenyon).

Aloe Vesta Perineal. (SK-Beecham) Solution of sodium C14-16 olefin sulfonate, propylene glycol, aloe vera gel, hydrolyzed collagen. Bot. 118 ml, 236 ml, gal. *otc.*
Use: Perianal hygiene.

•**alofilcon a.** (AL-oh-FILL-kahn) USAN.
Use: Contact lens material (hydrophilic).

aloin. (Baker, J.T.) A mixture of crystalline pentosides from various aloes. Bot. oz. *otc.*
Use: Laxative.
W/Ox bile (desiccated), phenolphthalein, cascara sagrada extract, podophyllin.
See: Bilgon (Solvay).

Alomide. (Alcon) Lodoxamide tromethamine 0.1%. Soln. Drop-tainers 10 ml. *Rx.*
Use: Antiallergy agent, ophthalmic.

•**alonimid.** (ah-LAHN-ih-mid) USAN.
Use: Sedative-hypnotic.

Alophen Pills. (Warner-Lambert Consumer) Phenolphthalein 60 mg/Tab. Bot. 100s. *otc.*
Use: Laxative.

Alor 5/500. (Atley) Hydrocodone bitartrate 5 mg, aspirin 500 mg/Tab. Bot. 100s. *Rx.*
Use: Narcotic analgesic.

Alora. (Procter & Gamble) Estradiol 1.5 mg, 2.3 mg and 3 mg/Patch. Calendar packs, 48 and 24 systems. *Rx.*
Use: Estrogen replacement.

•**alosetron hydrochloride.** (al-OH-seh-trahn) USAN.
Use: Antiemetic.

Alotone. (Major) Triamcinolone 4 mg/ Tab. Bot. 100s. *Rx.*
Use: Corticosteroid.

•**alovudine.** (al-OHV-you-deen) USAN.
Use: Antiviral.

•**alpertine.** (al-PURR-teen) USAN.
Use: Antipsychotic.

l-alpha-acetyl-methadol (LAAM). (Biodevelopment) *Rx.*
Use: Treatment of heroin addicts.

•**alpha amylase.** (AL-fah AM-ih-lace)
USAN. A concentrated form of alpha
amylase produced by a strain of non-
pathogenic bacteria.
Use: Digestive aid; anti-inflammatory.
See: Kutrase, Cap. (Schwarz Pharma
Kremers-Urban).
Ku-Zyme, Cap. (Schwarz Pharma
Kremers-Urban).

alpha-amylase w-100. W/Proteinase W-
300, cellase W-100, lipase, estrone,
testosterone, vitamins, minerals. *Rx.*
Use: Digestive aid.
See: Geramine, Tab. (Zeneca).

alpha-1-adrenergic blockers.
Use: Antihypertensive.
See: Cardura (Roerig).

**alpha-1-antitrypsin (recombinant DNA
origin).**
Use: Supplementation therapy for al-
pha$_1$-antitrypsin deficiency in the ZZ
phenotype population. [Orphan drug]

alpha/beta-adrenergic blocker.
See: Normodyne (Schering-Plough).
Trandate (Allen & Hanburys).

alpha-chymotrypsin.
See: Alpha Chymar, Vial (Centeon).
Zolyse, Vial (Alcon).

Alphaderm. (Lemmon) Hydrocortisone
1%. Cream 30 g, 100 g. *otc, Rx.*
Use: Corticosteroid, topical.

alpha-d-galactosidase.
Use: Antiflatulent.

Alpha-E. (Barth's) d-Alpha tocopherol.
50 IU or 100 IU: Cap. Bot. 100s, 500s,
1000s. **200 IU:** Cap. Bot. 100s, 250s.
400 IU: Cap. Bot. 100s, 250s, 500s. *otc.*
Use: Vitamin E Supplement.

alpha-estradiol. Known to be beta-estradiol.
See: Estradiol (Various Mfr.).

alpha-estradiol benzoate.
See: Estradiol benzoate (Various Mfr.).

Alpha Fast. (Eastwood) Bath oil. Bot. 16
oz. *otc.*
Use: Emollient.

alpha-fetoprotein w/tc-99m. USAN.
Use: Diagnostic aid.

alpha-galactosidase.
See: Aspergillus niger enzyme.

alpha-galactosidase a. *Rx.*
Use: Fabry's disease. [Orphan drug]

alpha-galactoside a. USAN.
Use: Treatment of Fabry's disease.

Alphagan. (Allergan) Brimonidine tartrate 0.2%, polyvinyl alcohol/Soln. Dropper Bot. 5 ml, 10 ml. *Rx.*
Use: Agent for glaucoma.

alpha-hypophamine.
See: Oxytocin Inj.

alpha interferon-2a.
See: Roferon-A (Roche).

alpha interferon-2b.
See: Intron A (Schering-Plough).

alpha interferon-N3.
See: Alferon-N (Purdue-Frederick).

Alpha-Keri. (Westwood Squibb) **Therapeutic Bath:** Mineral oil, lanolin oil,
PEG-4-dilaurate, benzophenone-3, D &
C green #6, fragrance. Bot. 4 oz, 8 oz,
16 oz. **Spray:** 5 oz. **Cleansing Bar:** Bar
containing sodium tallowate, sodium
cocoate, water, mineral oil, fragrance,
PEG-75, glycerin, titanium dioxide,
lanolin oil, sodium Cl, BHT, EDTA, D &
C green #5, D & C yellow # 10. 120 g.
otc.
Use: Emollient.

alpha-methyldopa. Name previously
used for Methyldopa.

Alphanate. (Alpha Therapeutics) ≥ 10 IU
FVIII: C/mg total protein. 0.05 to 1 g
albumin (human), ≤ 10 mmol Ca/ml, ≤
750 mcg glycine/IU FVIII: C, ≤ 2 IU
heparin/ml, ≤ 300 mmol arginine/L, ≤
2.5 mg PEG, 80/IU FVIII: C, ≤ 10 mEq
Na/vial after reconstitution. Pow. Lyphi-
lized. Single-dose vials with diluent.
Rx.
Use: Antihemophilic.

AlphaNine. (Alpha Therapeutic) Purified
heat-treated/solvent preparation of
coagulation Factor IX from human
plasma. With ≥ 50 units Factor IX per
mg protein, < 5 units each Factor II (prothrombin) and Factor VII (proconvertin) per 100 IU Factor IX and < 20 units
Factor X (Stuart-Power Factor) per 100
IU Factor IX. In single-dose vials with
diluent, double-ended needle and microaggregated filter. Pow. for inj. *Rx.*
Use: Prevention and control of bleeding in Factor IX deficiency.

AlphaNine SD. (Alpha Therapeutic) Purified, solvent detergent treated preparation of Factor IX derived from human
plasma, ≥ 50 units Factor IX per mg protein, < 5 units each Factor II (prothrombin) and Factor VII (proconvertin)
per 100 IU Factor IX, < 20 units Factor X (Stuart-Power factor) per 100 IU
Factor IX. Heparin, dextrose. Inj. In a
single-dose vial with 10 ml diluent,
double-ended needle and microaggre-
gate filter. *Rx.*
Use: Prevention and control of bleeding in Factor IX deficiency due to hemophilia B.

alpha-phenoxyethyl penicillin, potassium.
See: Phenethicillin Potassium.

alpha-1-proteinase inhibitor.
Use: Treatment of Alpha-1-antitrypsin deficiency. [Orphan drug]
See: Prolastin (Bayer).

alphasone acetophenide. Name previously used for Algestone acetonide.

alpha-tocopherol.
See: Dalfatol, Cap. (Solvay).
Tocopherol, Alpha (Various Mfr.).

dl-alpha-tocopherol succinate.
See: DAlpha-E, Cap. (Alto).

Alphatrex. (Savage) **Cream and Oint.:**
Betamethasone dipropionate 0.05%.
Tube 15 g, 45 g. **Lot.:** Betamethasone dipropionate 0.05%. Bot. 60 ml. *Rx.*
Use: Corticosteroid, topical.

Alpha Vee-12. (Schlicksup) Hydroxocobalamin 1000 mcg/ml. Vial 10 ml. *Rx.*
Use: Vitamin B_{12} supplement.

Alphosyl. (Schwarz Pharma) Allantoin 1.7%, special crude coal tar extracts 5%. **Lot.:** Bot. 8 fl oz. **Cream:** 2 oz. *otc.*
Use: Antipruritic.

•**alpidem.** (AL-PIH-dem) USAN.
Use: Antianxiety (anxiolytic).

•**alprazolam,** (al-PRAY-zoe-lam) U.S.P. 23.
Use: Sedative, hypnotic.
See: Xanax, Tab. (Pharmacia & Upjohn).

alprazolam. (Various Mfr.) Alprazolam **0.25 mg, 0.5 mg, 1 mg:** Tab. Bot. 30s, 100s, 500s, 1000s, UD 100s; **2 mg:** Tab. Bot. 100s, 500s. *c-ɪv.*
Use: Management of anxiety disorders.

alprazolam. (Roxane) **Oral soln.:** Alprazolam 0.5 mg/ml, sorbitol, saccharin. Bot. 500 ml, UD 2.5 ml, UD 5 ml, UD 10 ml. **Intensol soln.:** Alprazolam 1 mg/ml. Bot. 30 ml with dropper. *c-ɪv.*
Use: Management of anxiety disorders.

•**alprenolol hydrochloride.** (al-PREH-no-lole) USAN.
Use: Antiadrenergic (β-receptor).

•**alprenoxime hydrochloride.** (al-PREN-ox-eem) USAN.
Use: Antiglaucoma agent.

•**alprostadil,** (al-PRAHST-uh-dill) U.S.P. 23.
Use: Vasodilator; agent for impotence; agent for patient ductus arteriosus.
See: Caverject (Pharmacia & Upjohn).
Muse (Vivus).
Prostin VR, Inj. (Pharmacia & Upjohn).
Prostin VR Pediatric, Inj. (Pharmacia & Upjohn).

Alramucil. (Alra) Psyllium hydrophilic mucoloid 3.6 g, citric acid, sucrose, saccharin, potassium bicarbonate, sodium bicarbonate, 4 calories and < 0.01 g sodium per packet. Pow. effervescent Pkg. 30s. *otc.*
Use: Laxative.

Alredase. (Wyeth-Ayerst). Tolrestat. *Rx.*
Use: Aldose reductase inhibitor.

•**alrestatin sodium.** (AHL-reh-STAT-in) USAN.
Use: Enzyme inhibitor (aldose reductase).

Alsorb Gel. (Standex) Magnesium and aluminum hydroxide. Colloidal Susp. *otc.*
Use: Antacid.

Alsorb Gel, C.T. (Standex) Calcium carbonate 2 gr, glycine 3 gr, magnesium trisilicate 3 gr/Tab. *otc.*
Use: Antacid.

Altace. (Hoechst Marion Roussel/Pharmacia & Upjohn) Ramipril 1.25 mg, 2.5 mg, 5 mg or 10 mg/Cap. Bot. 100s, UD 100s. *Rx.*
Use: Antihypertensive; congestive heart failure.

•**altanserin tartrate.** (AL-TAN-ser-in) USAN.
Use: Serotonin antagonist.

•**alteplase,** (AL-teh-PLACE) U.S.P. 23
Use: Plasminogen activator.
See: Activase, Inj. (Genentech).

ALternaGEL. (J & J-Merck) Aluminum hydroxide 600 mg/5 ml. Liq. Bot. 150 ml, 360 ml. *otc.*
Use: Antacid.

•**althiazide.** (al-THIGH-azz-ide) USAN.
Use: Antihypertensive; diuretic.

•**altretamine.** (ahl-TRETT-uh-meen) USAN.
Use: Antineoplastic. [Orphan drug]
See: Hexalen (US Bioscience).

Alu-Cap. (3M Pharm) Aluminum hydroxide gel 400 mg/Cap. Bot. 100s. *otc.*
Use: Antacid.

Al-U-Creme. (MacAllister) Aluminum hydroxide equivalent to 4% aluminum oxide. Susp. Bot. pt, gal. *otc.*
Use: Antacid.

Aludrox. (Wyeth-Ayerst) Aluminum hydroxide gel 307 mg, magnesium hydroxide 103 mg/5 ml. Susp. Bot. 355 ml. *otc.*
Use: Antacid.

alukalin. Activated kaolin.
Use: Antidiarrheal.
See: Lusyn, Tab. (Medeva).

Alulex. (Lexington) Magnesium trisilicate

3.25 gr, aluminum hydroxide gel 3.5 gr, phenobarbital ⅛ gr, homatropine methylbromide gr/Tab. Bot. 100s. *Rx.*
Use: Agent for peptic ulcer.

alum. Sulfuric acid, aluminum ammonium salt (2:1:1), dodecahydrate. Sulfuric acid, aluminum potassium salt (2:1:1), dodecahydrate.
Use: Astringent.

•**alum, ammonium,** U.S.P. 23.
Use: Astringent, topical.

•**alum, potassium,** U.S.P. 23.
Use: Astringent, topical.

alum-precipitated allergenic extracts.
See: Allpyral (Bayer).
Center-Al (Center).

Alumadrine. (Fleming) Acetaminophen 500 mg, phenylpropanolamine HCl 25 mg, chlorpheniramine maleate 4 mg/Tab. Bot. 100s, 1000s. *Rx.*
Use: Analgesic, decongestant, antihistamine.

Alumate-HC. (Dermco) Hydrocortisone 0.125%, 0.25%, 0.5% or 1%/Cream. Pkg. 0.5 oz, 1 oz, 4 oz. *otc.*
Use: Corticosteroid, topical.

Alumate Mixture. (Schlicksup) Aluminum hydroxide gel, milk of magnesia/5 ml. Bot. 12 oz, gal. *otc.*
Use: Antacid.

alumina hydrated powder.
W/Activated attapulgite, pectin. *otc.*
Use: Antidiarrheal.
See: Polymagma, Plain, Tab. (Wyeth-Ayerst).

alumina, magnesia and calcium carbonate tablets.
Use: Antacid.

alumina, magnesia, calcium carbonate and simethicone tablets.
Use: Antacid.

alumina, magnesia and calcium chloride oral suspension.
Use: Antacid.

alumina and magnesia oral suspension.
Use: Antacid.

alumina and magnesia tablets.
Use: Antacid.

alumina, magnesia and simethicone.
Use: Antacid, antiflatulent.

alumina, magnesia and simethicone suspension. (Roxane) Aluminum hydroxide 213 mg, magnesium hydroxide 200 mg, simethicone 20 mg, parabens, sorbitol/5 ml. Susp. Bot. UD 15, 30 ml. *otc.*
Use: Antacid.

alumina and magnesium carbonate oral suspension.
Use: Antacid.

alumina, magnesium carbonate and magnesium oxide tablets.
Use: Antacid.

alumina and magnesium trisilicate oral suspension.
Use: Antacid.

alumina and magnesium trisilicate tablets.
Use: Antacid.

Aluminostomy. (Richards Pharm.) Aluminum pow. 18%, zinc oxide, zinc stearate in a bland water repellent ointment. Jar 2 oz, 6 oz, lb.
Use: Skin protectant.

aluminum. (uh-LOO-min-uhm)
See: Aluminostomy (Richards Pharm.).

aluminum acetate.
Use: Astringent.
See: Acid Mantle Creme (Sandoz Consumer).
Buro-Sol pow. (Doak).
W/Salicylic acid, boric acid.

•**aluminum acetate,** U.S.P. 23.
Use: Astringent.
See: Bluboro Powder (Allergan Herbert).
Buro-Sol Antiseptic Powder Conc. (Doak).
Burotor, Emul. (Torch).
Domeboro, Pow., Tab. (Bayer).
Domeboro Otic, Soln. (Bayer).

aluminum aminoacetate, dihydroxy.
See: Dihydroxy aluminum aminoacetate (Various Mfr.)

aluminum carbonate basic.
Use: Antacid.
See: Basaljel, Susp. (Wyeth-Ayerst).

aluminum carbonate, dried basic, gel.
Cap., Tab.
Use: Antacid.

•**aluminum carbonate, basic,** U.S.P. XXII.
Use: Antacid.
See: Basaljel, Susp., Cap., Tab. (Wyeth-Ayerst).

aluminum chlorhydroxy allantoinate.
See: Alcloxa (Schuylkill).

•**aluminum chloride,** U.S.P. 23. Aluminum Cl hexahydrate.
Use: Astringent, topical.
Drysol (Person & Covey).
Xerac AC (Person & Covey).
W/Oxyquinoline sulfate, benzalkonium Cl.
See: Alochor Stypic (Gordon Labs.).

aluminum chloride hexahydrate.

Use: Astringent.
See: Drysol (Person & Covey).
• **aluminum chlorohydrate,** (ah-LOO-min-uhm) U.S.P. 23.
Use: Anhidrotic.
See: Ostiderm, Lot., Roll-On (Pedinol).
• **aluminum chlorohydrex.** (ah-LOO-min-uhm) USAN.
Use: Astringent, topical.
• **aluminum chlorohydrex propylene glycol,** U.S.P. 23.
Use: Anhidrotic.
aluminum dihydroxyaminoacetate.
See: Dihydroxy Aluminum Aminoacetate, U.S.P. 23. (Various Mfr.).
aluminum glycinate, basic.
See: Dihydroxy Aluminum Aminoacetate, U.S.P. 23.
W/Aspirin, Magnesium carbonate.
See: Bufferin, Tab. (Bristol-Myers).
• **aluminum hydroxide gel,** U.S.P. 23.
Use: Antacid.
See: Alterna GEL, Liq. (J & J-Merck).
Alu-Cap, Cap. (3M Pharm).
Al-U-Creme, Susp. (MacAllister).
Alu-Tab, Tab. (3M Pharm).
Amphojel, Susp., Tab. (Wyeth-Ayerst).
Dialume, Cap. (Rhone-Poulenc Rorer).
Gelusil, Chew. tab. (Parke-Davis).
Maalox HRF, Liq. (Rhone-Poulenc Rorer).
Maalox Plus, Tab. (Rhone-Poulenc Rorer).
Nutrajel (Cenci).
W/Aminoacetic acid, magnesium trisilicate.
See: Maracid-2, Tab. (Marin).
W/Belladonna extract, magnesium hydroxide.
See: Trialka, Liq., Tab. (Del Pharm.).
W/Calcium carbonate.
See: Alkalade, Susp., Tab. (DePree).
W/Calcium carbonate, magnesium carbonate, magnesium trisilicate.
See: Marblen, Susp., Tab. (Fleming).
W/Clioquinol, methylcellulose, atropine sulfate, hyoscine HBr, hyoscyamine sulfate.
See: Enterex, Tab. (Person & Covey).
W/Dicyclomine HCl, magnesium hydroxide, methylcellulose.
See: Triactin Liq., Tab. (Procter & Gamble).
W/Gastric mucin, magnesium glycinate.
See: Mucogel, Liq., Tab. (Inwood).
W/Kaolin, pectin.
See: Metropectin, Liq. (Medeva).
W/Magnesium carbonate.
See: Algicon, Tab. (Rhone-Poulenc Rorer).

Estomul-M Liq., Tab. (3M Pharm).
W/Magnesium carbonate, calcium carbonate, amino-acetic acid.
See: Glycogel Tab., Susp. (Schwarz Pharma).
W/Magnesium hydroxide.
See: Alsorb Gel (Standex).
Aludrox, Susp., Tab. (Wyeth-Ayerst).
Delcid, Liq. (Hoechst Marion Roussel).
Kolantyl, Gel, Wafer (Hoechst Marion Roussel).
Maalox, Susp. (Rhone-Poulenc Rorer).
Mylanta, Tab. (Stuart).
Mylanta II, Tab. (Stuart).
Neutralox, Susp. (Lemmon).
WinGel, Liq., Tab. (Sanofi Winthrop Consumer Products).
W/Magnesium hydroxide, aspirin.
See: Ascriptin, Tab. (Rhone-Poulenc Rorer).
Ascriptin Extra Strength, Tab. (Rhone-Poulenc Rorer).
Calciphen, Tab. (Westerfield).
Cama, Tab. (Sandoz).
Cama Inlay-Tab. (Sandoz Consumer).
W/Magnesium hydroxide, belladonna extract
W/Magnesium hydroxide, calcium carbonate.
See: Camalox, Susp. (Rhone-Poulenc Rorer).
W/Magnesium hydroxide, glycine, magnesium trisilicate, belladonna extract.
W/Magnesium hydroxide and simethicone.
See: DI-GEL, Liq. (Schering-Plough).
Maalox Plus, Susp. (Rhone-Poulenc Rorer).
Mylanta, Liq. (Stuart).
Mylanta-II, Liq. (Stuart).
Silain-Gel, Liq., Tab. (Robins).
Simeco, Liq. (Wyeth-Ayerst).
W/Magnesium trisilicate.
See: Antacid G, Tab. (Walgreen).
Antacid Tablets, Tab. (Panray).
Arcodex Antiacid, Tab. (Arcum).
Gacid, Tab. (Arcum).
Malcogel, Susp. (Pharmacia & Upjohn).
Malcotabs (Pharmacia & Upjohn).
Manalum, Tab. (Paddock).
Trisogel, Pulv., Susp. (Lilly).
W/Phenindamine tartrate, phenylephrine HCl, aspirin, caffeine, magnesium carbonate.
See: Dristan, Tab. (Whitehall Robins).
W/Phenol, zinc oxide, camphor, eucalyptol, ichthammol.
See: Almophen, Oint. (Jones Medical).

W/Prednisolone.
See: Fernisolone-B (Ferndale).
Predoxine, Tab. (Roberts).
W/Sodium salicylate, acetaminophen, vitamin C.
See: Gaysal-S., Tab. (Geriatric).
aluminum hydroxide gel. (Various Mfr.)
320 mg/5 ml. Susp. Bot. 360 ml, 480 ml, UD 15 and 30 ml. *otc.*
Use: Antacid.
aluminum hydroxide gel, concentrated. (Various Mfr.) 600 mg/5 ml. Liq. Bot. 30 ml, 180 ml, 480 ml. *otc.*
Use: Antacid.
aluminum hydroxide gel, concentrated. (Roxane) Susp. **450 mg/5 ml:** Bot. 500 ml, UD 30 ml; **675 mg/5 ml:** Bot. 180 ml, 500 ml, UD 20 ml and 30 ml. *otc.*
Use: Antacid.
•**aluminum hydroxide gel, dried,** U.S.P. 23.
Use: Antacid.
See: ALterna GEL, Liq. (J & J-Merck)
Alu-Cap, Cap. (3M Pharm)
Amphojel, Tab. (Wyeth-Ayerst)
Ascriptin, Tab. (Rhone-Poulenc Rorer)
Di-Gel, Liq. (Schering-Plough)
Mylanta, Liq., Tab. (J & J-Merck).
aluminum hydroxide gel, dried w/combinations.
Use: Antacid.
See: Aludrox, Susp., Tab. (Wyeth-Ayerst).
Alurex, Tab. (Rexall).
Banacid, Tab. (Buffington).
Camalox, Tab. (Rhone-Poulenc Rorer).
Delcid, Liq. (Hoechst Marion Roussel).
Eulcin, Tab. (Leeds).
Fermalox, Tab. (Rhone-Poulenc Rorer).
Gaviscon, Foamtab (Hoechst Marion Roussel).
Gelusil, Preps. (Parke-Davis).
Kolantyl, Wafers (Hoechst Marion Roussel).
Maalox, Tab. (Rhone-Poulenc Rorer).
Maalox Plus, Tab. (Rhone-Poulenc Rorer).
Malcotabs, Tab. (Pharmacia & Upjohn).
Mylanta, Tab., Liq. (Stuart).
Mylanta II, Tab., Liq. (Stuart).
Phencaset Improved, Tab. (Zeneca).
Presalin, Tab. (Roberts).
Spasmosorb, Tab. (Roberts).
aluminum hydroxide glycine.
See: Dihydroxy aluminum aminoacetate.

aluminum hydroxide magnesium carbonate.
Use: Antacid.
See: Aloxine (Forest).
DI-GEL, Tab. (Schering-Plough).
Magnagel, Susp., Tab. (Roberts).
W/Aminoacetic acid, calcium carbonate.
See: Eugel, Tab., Liq. (Solvay).
W/Dicyclomine HCl, magnesium trisilicate, methylcellulose.
See: Triactin, Liq., Tab. (Procter & Gamble).
W/Magnesium trisilicate.
See: Escot, Cap. (Solvay).
W/Magnesium trisilicate, bismuth alum.
See: Escot, Cap. (Solvay).
•**aluminum monostearate,** N.F. 18.
Use: Pharmaceutic necessity for preparation of penicillin G procaine w/aluminum stearate suspension.
See: Penicillin G procaine w/aluminum stearate suspension.
aluminum oxide.
See: Epi-Clear Scrub Cleanser (Squibb).
Aluminum Paste. (Paddock) Metallic aluminum 10%. Oint. Jar lb. *otc.*
Use: Topical combination, miscellaneous.
aluminum phenosulfonate.
See: AR-EX Cream Deodorant (Ar-Ex).
•**aluminum phosphate gel,** U.S.P. 23.
Use: Antacid.
See: Phosphaljel, Susp. (Wyeth-Ayerst).
•**aluminum sesquichlorohydrate.** (ah-LOO-min-uhm sess-kwih-KLOR-oh-HIGH-drate) USAN.
Use: Anhidrotic.
aluminum sodium carbonate hydroxide.
See: Dihydroxyaluminum Sodium Carbonate.
•**aluminum subacetate topical solution,** U.S.P. 23.
Use: Astringent.
•**aluminum sulfate,** U.S.P. 23.
Use: Pharmaceutic necessity for preparation of aluminum subacetate solution.
See: Aluminum Subacetate, Soln.
Bluboro, Pow. (Allergan Herbert).
•**aluminum zirconium octachlorohydrate,** U.S.P. 23.
Use: Anhidrotic.
•**aluminum zirconium octachlorohydrex gly,** U.S.P. 23.
Use: Anhidrotic.
•**aluminum zirconium pentachlorohy-**

drate, U.S.P. 23.
Use: Anhidrotic.

•**aluminum zirconium pentachlorohydrex gly,** U.S.P. 23.
Use: Anhidrotic.

•**aluminum zirconium tetrachlorohydrate,** U.S.P. 23.
Use: Anhidrotic.

•**aluminum zirconium tetrachlorohydrex gly,** (ah-LOO-min-uhm zihr-KOE-nee-uhm teh-trah-KLOR-oh-HIGH-drex Gly) U.S.P. 23.
Use: Anhidrotic.

•**aluminum zirconium trichlorohydrate,** U.S.P. 23.
Use: Anhidrotic.

•**aluminum zirconium trichlorohydrex gly,** (ah-LOO-min-uhm zihr-KOE-nee-uhm try-KLOR-oh-HIGH-drex Gly) U.S.P. 23.
Use: Anhidrotic.

Alupent. (Boehringer Ingelheim) Metaproterenol sulfate. **Metered dose inhaler:** 225 mg in 15 ml. **Tab.:** 10 mg or 20 mg. Bot. 100s. **Syr.:** 10 mg/5 ml. Bot. Pt. **Inhalant Soln.: 0.4%:** 2.5 ml UD vial. **0.6%:** 2.5 ml UD vial. **5%:** Bot. 10 ml, 30 ml UD. *Rx.*
Use: Bronchodilator.

Alurate. (Roche) Aprobarbital 40 mg/5 ml. Alcohol 20%. Elix. Bot. Pt. *c-III.*
Use: Sedative, hypnotic.

Alurex. (Rexall) Magnesium-aluminum hydroxide. **Susp.:** (200 mg-150 mg/5 ml) Bot. 12 oz. **Tab:** (400 mg-300 mg) Box 50s. *otc.*
Use: Antacid.

Alu-Tab. (3M Pharm) Aluminum hydroxide gel 500 mg/Tab. Bot. 250s. *otc.*
Use: Antacid.

Alvedil Caps. (Luly-Thomas) Theophylline 4 gr, pseudoephedrine HCl 50 mg, butabarbital 15 mg/Cap. Bot. 100s. *Rx.*
Use: Bronchodilator, decongestant, sedative, hypnotic.

•**alverine citrate.** (AL-ver-een) N.F. XIII.
Use: Anticholinergic.
See: Spacolin, Tab. (Philips Roxane).

•**alvircept sudotox.** (AL-vihr-sept SOOD-ah-tox) USAN.
Use: Antiviral.

Alzapam. (Major) Lorazepam 0.5 mg, 1 mg or 2 mg/Tab. Bot. 100s, 500s. *c-IV.*
Use: Antianxiety.

Ama. (Wampole-Zeus) Antimitochondrial antibodies test by IFA. Test 48s.
Use: Diagnostic aid.

amacetam sulfate,
Use: Cognition adjuvant.

•**amadinone acetate.** (aim-AD-ih-nohn) USAN.
Use: Progestin.

amanozine hydrochloride.

amantadine hydrochloride, (uh-MAN-tuh-deen) U.S.P. 23.
Use: Antiviral.

amantadine hydrochloride, (uh-MAN-tuh-deen) (Various Mfr.) **Cap.:** 100 mg. Bot. 100s, 250s, 500s, UD 100s. **Syrup:** 50 mg/5 ml Bot. pint.
Use: Antiviral agent, treatment of Parkinson's disease.
See: Symmetrel, Cap., Syr. (DuPont Merck).

amaranth.
Use: Color (Not for internal use).

Amaryl. (Hoechst Marion Roussel) Glimepiride 1, 2 or 4 mg, lactose/Tab. 100s, UD 100s. *Rx.*
Use: Antidiabetic.

amazone.

ambenonium chloride.
Use: Cholinergic for treatment of myasthenia gravis.
See: Mytelase, Cap. (Sanofi-Winthrop).

Ambenyl Cough Syrup. (Forest) Codeine phosphate 10 mg, bromodiphenhydramine HCl 12.5 mg/5 ml, alcohol 5%. Bot. 4 oz, pt, gal. *c-v.*
Use: Antitussive, antihistamine.

Ambenyl-D Liquid. (Forest) Guaifenesin 100 mg, pseudoephedrine HCl 30 mg, dextromethorphan HBr 15 mg/10 ml, alcohol 9.5%. Bot. 4 oz. *otc.*
Use: Expectorant, decongestant, antitussive.

Amberlite, I.R.P.-64. (Rohm and Haas). Polacrilin.

Amberlite, I.R.P.-88. (Rohm and Haas). Polacrilin potassium.

Ambi 10 Cream. (Kiwi Brands) Benzoyl peroxide 10%, parabens. Cream. Tube 28.3 g. *otc.*
Use: Antiacne.

Ambi 10 Soap. (Kiwi Brands) Triclosan, sodium tallouate, PEG-20, titanium dioxide. Soap, Bar 99 g. *otc.*
Use: Antiacne.

Ambien. (Searle) Zolpidem tartrate 5 mg, 10 mg/Tab. Bot. 100s, 500s, UD 100s. *c-IV.*
Use: Sedative, hypnotic.

Ambi Skin Tone. (Kiwi Brands) Hydroquinone, padimate O, sodium metabisulfite, parabens, EDTA, vitamin E. Cream. Tube 57 g, 28.4 g. *otc.*
Use: Topical drug, miscellaneous.

•**ambomycin.** (AM-boe-MY-sin) USAN.
Isolated from filtrates of *Streptomyces ambofaciens*.
Use: Antineoplastic.

•**ambruticin.** (am-brew-TIE-sin) USAN.
Use: Antifungal.

ambucaine. Ambutoxate HCl.

ambucetamide.

•**ambuphylline.** (AM-byoo-fill-in) USAN.
Use: Diuretic, smooth muscle relaxant.

•**ambuside.** (AM-buh-SIDE) USAN.
Use: Diuretic.
See: Novohydrin.

ambutonium bromide.
Use: Antispasmodic.

ambutoxate hydrochloride.

AMC. (Schlicksup) Ammonium Cl 7.5 gr/
Tab. Bot. 1000s. *Rx.*
Use: Diuretic, expectorant.

Amcill. (Parke-Davis) **Cap.:** Ampicillin trihydrate 250 mg or 500 mg/Cap. Bot.
100s, 500s, UD pkg 100s. **Oral Susp.:**
125 mg or 250 mg/5 ml. Bot. 100 ml,
200 ml.
Use: Anti-infective, penicillin.

•**amcinafal.** (am-SIN-ah-fal) USAN.
Use: Anti-inflammatory.

•**amcinafide.** (am-SIN-ah-fide) USAN.
Use: Anti-inflammatory.

•**amcinonide,** (am-SIN-oh-nide) U.S.P. 23.
Use: Glucocorticoid.
See: Cyclocort, Cream, Oint. (Lederle).

Amcort. (Keene) Triamcinolone diacetate 40 mg/ml. Vial 5 ml. *Rx.*
Use: Corticosteroid.

•**amdinocillin,** (am-DEE-no-SILL-in)
U.S.P. 23.
Use: Antibacterial.

•**amdinocillin pivoxil.** (am-DEE-no-SILL-
in pihv-OX-ill) USAN.
Use: Antibacterial.

ameban.
See: Carbarsone.

amebicides.
See: Acetarsone (Various Mfr.).
Aralen HCl, Inj. (Sanofi Winthrop).
Aralen Phosphate, Tab. (Sanofi Winthrop).
Carbarsone, Pulv., Tab. (Lilly).
Chiniofon, Tab. (Various Mfr.).
Chloroquine Phosphate, Tab. (Various Mfr.).
Diiodohydroxyquin (Various Mfr.).
Diodoquin, Tab. (Searle).
Emetine HCl (Various Mfr.).
Flagyl, Tab. (Searle).
Humatin, Kapseal, Syr. (Parke-Davis).
Yodoxin, Tab. (Glenwood).

Amechol.
Use: Diagnostic aid.
See: Methacholine Cl.

•**amedalin hydrochloride.** (ah-MEH-dah-
lin) USAN.
Use: Antidepressant.

•**ameltolide.** (AH-mell-TOE-lide) USAN.
Use: Anticonvulsant.

Amen. (Carnrick) Medroxyprogesterone
acetate 10 mg/Tab. Bot. 50s, 100s,
1000s. *Rx.*
Use: Progestin.

Americaine Aerosol. (Novartis) Benzocaine 20% in a water-soluble vehicle.
In 60 ml Bot. 0.67 oz, 2 oz, 4 oz. *otc.*
Use: Local anesthetic, topical.

Americaine Anesthetic Lubricant.
(Medeva) Benzocaine 20%, benzethonium Cl 0.1%. 30 g, UD 2.5 g. Gel.
Rx.
Use: Local anesthetic, topical.

Americaine First Aid Burn Ointment.
(Novartis) Benzocaine 20%, benzethonium Cl 0.1% in a water-soluble polyethylene glycol base. Tube 0.75 oz. *otc.*
Use: Anesthetic, topical.

Americaine Hemorrhoidal Ointment.
(Novartis) Benzocaine 20%. Tube 22.5
g w/rectal applicator. *otc.*
Use: Local anesthetic.

Americaine Otic. (Novartis) Benzethonium Cl 0.1%, benzocaine 20% in a
water-soluble base of 1% (w/w) glycerin, polyethylene glycol 300. Bot. 0.5
oz. *Rx.*
Use: Otic preparation.

Ames Dextro System Lancets. (Bayer)
Sterile disposable lancet. Box 100s.
Use: Diagnostic aid.

•**amesergide.** (am-eh-SIR-jide) USAN.
Use: Serotonin antagonist.

•**ametantrone acetate.** (am-ETT-an-
TRONE) USAN.
Use: Antineoplastic.

A-Methapred Univial. (Abbott Hospital
Prods) Methylprednisolone sodium
succinate. **40 mg/ml:** Pkg. 1s, 25s, 50s,
100s; 125 mg/2 ml Pkg. 1s, 5s, 25s,
50s, 100s; **500 mg/4 ml:** Pkg. 1s, 5s,
25s, 100s; **1000 mg/8 ml:** Pkg. 1s, 5s,
25s, 100s. *Rx.*
Use: Corticosteroid.

amethocaine hydrochloride.
Use: Local anesthetic.
See: Tetracaine HCl.

amethopterin.
Use: Antineoplastic.
See: Methotrexate (Lederle).

•**amfenac sodium.** (AM-fen-ack SO-dee-
uhm) USAN.

Use: Anti-inflammatory.

● **amfilcon a.** (AM-FILL-kahn A) USAN.
Use: Contact lens material (hydrophilic).

● **amflutizole.** (am-FLEW-tih-zole) USAN.
Use: Treatment of gout.

amfodyne.
See: Imidecyl iodine.

● **amfonelic acid.** (am-fah-NEH-lick Acid) USAN.
Use: Central nervous system stimulant.

Amgenal Cough Syrup. (Goldline) Bromodiphenhydramine HCl 12.5 mg, codeine phosphate 10 mg/5 ml, alcohol 5%. Bot. 120 ml, pt, gal. *c-v.*
Use: Antihistamine, antitussive.

amibiarson.
See: Carbarsone (Various Mfr.).

Amicar. (Immunex) Tab.: Aminocaproic acid 500 mg. In 100s. Syrup: Aminocaproic acid 250 mg/ml, sorbitol, saccharin. In 480 ml. Inj.: Aminocaproic acid 250 mg/ml, benzyl alcohol 0.9%. In 20 or 96 ml. *Rx.*
Use: Systemic hemostatic.

● **amicycline.** (AM-ee-SIGH-kleen) USAN.
Use: Antibacterial.

Amidate. (Abbott Hospital Prods) Etomidate 2 mg/ml, propylene glycol 35%. Single dose Amp 20 mg/10 ml or 40 mg/20 ml; Abboject syringe 40 mg/20 ml. *Rx.*
Use: General anesthetic.

● **amidephrine mesylate.** (AM-ee-DEH-frin MEH-sih-LATE) USAN.
Use: Adrenergic.

amidofebrin.
See: Aminopyrine (Various Mfr.).

amidone hydrochloride.
Use: Narcotic agonist analgesic.
See: Methadone HCl (Various Mfr.).

amidopyrazoline.
See: Aminopyrine (Various Mfr.).

amidotrizoate, sodium.
See: Diatrizoate sodium.

● **amifloxacin.** (am-ih-FLOX-ah-SIN) USAN.
Use: Antibacterial.

● **amifloxacin mesylate.** (am-ih-FLOX-ah-SIN MEH-sih-LATE) USAN.
Use: Antibacterial.

● **amifostine.** (am-ih-FOSS-teen) USAN.
Use: Protectant (topical); radioprotector.
See: Ethyol (Alza/US Bioscience).

Amigen. (Baxter) Protein hydrolysate. *Rx.* 5%: Bot. 500 ml, 1000 ml; **10%:** Bot. 500 ml, 1000 ml. **5% w/dextrose 5%:** Bot. 500 ml, 1000 ml. **5% w/dextrose 5%, alcohol 5%:** Bot. 1000 ml.

5% w/fructose 10%: Bot. 1000 ml. **5% w/fructose 12.5%, alcohol 2.4%:** Bot. 1000 ml.
Use: Nutritional supplement.

Amigesic. (Amide) Salsalate 500 mg/Cap or Tab. Salsalate 75 mg/capl. Bot. 100s, 500s. *Rx.*
Use: Salicylate analgesic.

● **amikacin,** (am-ih-KAE-sin) U.S.P. 23.
Use: Antibacterial.

amikacin. (Bedford Labs) Amikacin sulfate 250 mg, sodium metabisulfite 0.66%, sodium citrate dihydrate 2.5%/ml. Inj. Vial 2 ml, 4 ml. *Rx.*
Use: Antibacterial.

amikacin. (Gensia) 50 mg (as sulfate) per ml. sodium metabisulfite 0.13%, sodium citrate dihydrate 0.5%. Inj. Vial 2, 4 ml. *Rx.*
Use: Antibacterial.

● **amikacin sulfate,** (am-ih-KAE-sin) U.S.P. 23.
Use: Antibacterial.

amikacin sulfate injection. (Various Mfr.) Amikacin sulfate 50 mg/ml. Vial 2 ml, 4 ml (10s).
Use: Antibacterial.
See: Amikin, Inj. (Bristol).

Amikin. (Bristol) Amikacin sulfate. Inj. Vial 100 mg, 500 mg, 1 g, disposable syringes 500 mg. *Rx.*
Use: Antibacterial, aminoglycoside.

● **amiloride hydrochloride,** (uh-MILL-oh-ride) U.S.P. 23.
Use: Diuretic.
See: Midamor, Tab. (Merck).

amiloride hydrochloride solution for inhalation. (Glaxo)
Use: Cystic fibrosis. [Orphan drug]

amiloride hydrochloride and hydrochlorthiazide tablets.
Use: Diuretic, antihypertensive.
See: Moduretic, Tab. (Merck).

Amin-Aid. (McGaw) Instant drinks, puddings. *otc.*
Use: Nutritional supplement.

Amin-Aid Instant Drink Powder. (McGaw) Essential amino acids, maltodextrin, sucrose, partially hydrogenated soybean oil, lecithin, mono and diglycerides. Packet 162 g. *otc.*
Use: Nutritional supplement.

Amina-21. (Miller) L-form amino acids 600 mg/Cap. Bot. 100s, 300s.
Use: Tissue repair.

aminacrine. F.D.A. 9-Aminoacridine.
Use: Anti-infective, topical.

● **aminacrine hydrochloride.** (ah-MEE-nah-kreen) USAN. 9-Aminoacridine hydrochloride.

Use: Anti-infective, topical.
W/Dienestrol, sulfanilamide, allantoin.
See: AVC/Dienestrol Cream, Supp.
(Hoechst Marion Roussel).
Use: Bacteriostatic agent.
W/Oxyquinoline benzoate.
See: Triva, Vaginal Jelly (Boyle).
W/Sulfanilamide, allantoin.
See: AVC, Cream, Supp. (Hoechst
Marion Roussel).
Femguard Vaginal Cream (Solvay).
Sulfem Vaginal Cream (Federal
Pharm.).
Vagidine, Cream (Zeneca).
Vagitrol, Cream, Supp. (Lemmon).

aminarsone.
See: Carbarsone (Various Mfr.).

amine resin.
See: Polyamine Methylene Resin.

Aminess. (Clintec) Essential amino ac-
ids. 10 Tab. = adult amino acid MDR.
Jar 300s. *Rx.*
Use: Parenteral nutritional supplement.

Aminess 5.2%. (Clintec) Amino acids
and electrolytes, Inj. *Rx.*
Use: Parenteral nutritional supplement.

Aminicotin.
Use: Vitamin supplement.
See: Nicotinamide (Various Mfr.).

aminoacetic acid. Glycerine, U.S.P. 23.
(Various Mfr.) (Glycine, glycocoll) avail-
able as elix., pow., tab.
Use: Myasthenia gravis, irrigating solu-
tion.
W/Aluminum hydroxide, magnesium
hydroxide, calcium carbonate.
See: Eugel, Tab., Liq. (Solvay).
W/Calcium carbonate.
See: Antacid pH, Tab. (Towne).
Eldamint, Tab. (Zeneca).
W/Calcium carbonate, aluminum hydrox-
ide, magnesium carbonate.
See: Glytabs, Tab. (Pharmics).
W/Calcium carbonate, magnesium carbo-
nate, bismuth subcarbonate, dried alu-
minum hydroxide gel.
See: Buffer-Tabs (Forest).
W/Magnesium trisilicate, aluminum
hydroxide.
See: Maracid-2, Tab. (Marin).
W/Phenylephrine HCl, pyrilamine male-
ate, acetylsalicylic acid, caffeine.
See: Al-Ay, Tab. (Jones Medical).
W/Phenylephrine HCl, chlorpheniramine
maleate, acetaminophen, caffeine.
See: Codimal, Tab. (Schwarz Pharma).

aminoacetic acid & calcium carbonate.
W/Lysine.
See: Lycolan, Elix. (Lannett).

amino acid & protein prep.
See: Aminoacetic Acid, U.S.P. 23.
Glutamic Acid.
Histidine HCl.
Lysine.
Phenylalanine.
Thyroxine.

amino acids.
Use: Amino acid supplement.
See: Aminosol, Soln. (Abbott).
Aminosyn, Soln. (Abbott).
W/Estrone, testosterone, vitamins, miner-
als.
See: Geramine, Tab., Inj. (ICN Pharm).
W/Vitamin B_{12}.
See: Stuart Amino Acids and B_{12}, Tab.
(Stuart).

amino acid combinations.
See: Dequasine (Miller).
NeuRecover-LT (NeuroGenesis).
NeuroSlim (NeuroGenesis/Matrix).
NeuRecover-DA (NeuroGenesis/Ma-
trix).
NeuRecover-SA (NeuroGenesis/Ma-
trix).
Herpetrol (Alva).
A/G-Pro (Miller).
Jets (Freeda).
PDP Liquid Protein (Wesley Pharm.).

Amino-Min-D Capsules. (Tyson) Ca 250
mg, D 100 IU, Fe 7.5 mg, Zn 5.6 mg,
Mg, I, Mn, Cu, K, Cr, Se, betaine HCl,
glutamic acid HCl. Cap. Bot. 100s. *otc.*
Use: Vitamin/mineral supplement.

aminoacridine. (ah-MEE-no-ACK-rih-
deen)
Use: Bacteriostatic agent.
See: 9-aminoacridine.

9-aminoacridine hydrochloride. (9-ah-
MEE-no-ACK-rih-deen) (Various Mfr.)
Aminacrine HCl.
Use: Anti-infective, vaginal.
See: Vagisec Plus (Schmid).
W/Hydrocortisone acetate, tyrothricin,
phenylmercuric acetate, polysorbate-
80, urea, lactose.
See: Aquacort, Vaginal Supp. (Poly-
Medica).
W/Iodoquinol.
See: Vagitric, Oint. (Zeneca).
W/Phenylmercuric acetate, tyrothricin,
urea, lactose.
See: Trinalis, Vaginal Supp. (Poly-
Medica).
W/Polyoxyethylene nonyl phenol, sodium
edetate, docusate sodium.
See: Vagisec Plus, Supp. (Schmid).
W/Pramoxine HCl, acetic acid, parachlo-
rometa-xylenol, methyl-dodecylbenz-
yltrimethyl ammonium Cl.

See: Drotic No. 2, Drops (Ascher).
W/Sulfanilamide, allantoin.
See: AVC Cream, Supp. (Hoechst
Marion Roussel).
Nil Vaginal Cream (Century).
Par Cream (Parmed).
Vagisan, Creme (Sandia).
Vagisul, Creme (Sheryl).
W/Sulfisoxazole, allantoin.
See: Vagilia, Cream (Lemmon).
p-aminobenzene-sulfonylacetylimide.
See: Sulfacetamide.
•**aminobenzoate potassium,** U.S.P. 23.
Use: Analgesic.
See: Potaba, Pow., Tab. (Glenwood).
W/Hydrocortisone, ammonium salicylate,
ascorbic acid.
See: Neocylate sodium free, Tab.
(Schwarz Pharma).
W/Potassium salicylate.
See: Pabalate-SF, Tab. (Robins).
•**aminobenzoate sodium,** U.S.P. 23.
Use: Analgesic.
See: PABA sodium, Tab. (Various Mfr.).
W/Phenobarbital, colchicine salicylate, Vi-
tamin B_1, aspirin.
See: Doloral, Tab. (Alamed).
W/Salicylamide, ascorbic acid.
See: Sylapar, Tab. (Forest).
W/Salicylamide, sodium salicylate, ascor-
bic acid, butabarbital sodium.
See: Bisalate, Tab. (Allison Lab).
W/Sodium salicylate.
See: Pabalate, Tab. (Robins).
Salpara, Tab. (Solvay).
•**aminobenzoic acid,** U.S.P. 23.
Use: Ultraviolet screen.
See: Pabafilm (Galderma).
Pabanol, Lot. (Zeneca).
W/Mephenesin, salicylamide.
See: Sal-Phenesin, Tab. (Hoechst
Marion Roussel).
W/Sodium salicylate, ascorbic acid.
See: Nucorsal, Tab. (Westerfield).
p-aminobenzoic acid, salts.
See: p-Aminobenzoate potassium and
p-Aminobenzoate sodium.
•**aminocaproic acid,** (uh-mee-no-kuh-
PRO-ik) U.S.P. 23.
Use: Hemostatic.
See: Amicar, Syr., Tab., Vial (Immu-
nex).
aminocaproic acid. (Various Mfr.)
250mg/ml. 20 ml/Inj. *Rx.*
Use: Inhibitor of fibrinolytic activity.
aminocardol.
Use: Bronchodilator.
See: Aminophylline (Various Mfr.).
Amino-Cerv pH 5.5. (Milex) Urea 8.34%,
sodium propionate 0.5%, methionine

0.83%, cystine 0.35%, inositol 0.83%,
benzalkonium Cl 0.000004%, buffered
to pH 5.5. Tube with applicator 82.5 g,
82.5 g refill. *Rx.*
Use: Vaginal preparation.
Aminodyne Compound. (Jones Medical) Acetaminophen 2.5 gr, aspirin 3.5
gr, caffeine 0.5 gr/Tab. Bot. 100s,
1000s. *otc.*
Use: Analgesic combination.
2-aminoethanethiol. USAN.
Use: Nephropathic cystinosis.
amino-ethyl-propanol.
See: Aminoisobutanol.
W/Bromotheophyllin.
See: Pamabrom (Various Mfr.).
Aminofen. (Dover) Acetaminophen 325
mg/Tab. Sugar, lactose and salt free.
UD Box 500s. *otc.*
Use: Analgesic.
Aminofen Max. (Dover) Acetaminophen
500 mg/Tab. Sugar, lactose and salt
free. UD Box 500s. *otc.*
Use: Analgesic.
aminoform.
Use: Anti-infective, urinary.
See: Methenamine (Various Mfr.).
Aminogen. (Christina) Vitamin B complex, folic acid. Amp. 2 ml Box 12s,
24s, 100s. Vial 10 ml. *Rx.*
Use: Vitamin B supplement.
•**aminoglutethimide,** U.S.P. 23.
Use: Treatment of Cushing's syndrome;
adrenocortical suppressant; antineoplastic.
See: Cytadren, Tab. (Novartis).
•**aminohippurate sodium,** U.S.P. 23.
Use: Diagnostic aid (renal function determination).
aminohippurate sodium. (Merck) 0.2g/
10 ml. Amp 10 ml, 50 ml.
Use: I.V., diagnostic aid for renal
plasma flow and function determination.
•**aminohippuric acid,** U.S.P. 23.
Use: Component of aminohippurate sodium (Inj.); diagnostic aid (renal function determination).
aminoisobutanol.
See: Butaphyllamine.
Pamabrom for combinations
aminoisometradine.
See: Methionine.
Aminonat. Protein hydrolysates (oral).
aminonitrozole. N-(5-Nitro-2-thiazolyl)
acetamide.
Use: Antitrichomonal.
Amino-Optic-C. (Tyson) Lemon bioflavonoids 250 mg, rutin, hesperidin, vitamin

C and rose hips powder 1000 mg/SR Tab. Bot. 100s. *otc.*
Use: Vitamin supplement.

Amino-Opti-E. (Tyson) 165 mg/Cap. Bot. 100s. *otc.*
Use: Vitamin E supplement.

aminopentamide sulfate.
Use: Anticholinergic.

Aminophyllin. (Searle) Trademark for Aminophylline. **100 mg/Tab.** Bot. 100s, 1000s, UD 100s. **200 mg/Tab.** Bot. 100s, 1000s, UD 100s. *Rx.*
Use: Bronchodilator.

Aminophyllin Injection. (Searle) Trademark for Aminophylline. Amp. **250 mg:** 10 ml; 25s, 100s; **500 mg:** 20 ml; 25s, 100s. *Rx.*
Use: Bronchodilator.

•**aminophylline,** (am-in-AHF-ih-lin) U.S.P. 23.
Use: Smooth muscle relaxant.
See: Aminodur, Dura-Tab. (Berlex).
Lixaminol, Elix. (Ferndale).
Phyllocontin, Tab. (Purdue Frederick).
Rectalad-Aminophylline (Wallace).
Somophyllin Oral Liq. (Medeva).
Somophyllin Rectal Soln. (Medeva).

aminophylline combinations.
Amesec, Cap. (Glaxo).
Amphedrine Compound, Cap. (Lannett).
Asminorel, Tab. (Solvay).
B.M.E., Elix. (Brothers).
Lixaminol AT/5 ml (Ferndale).
Mudrane GG-2, Tab. (ECR Pharm.).
Orthoxine and Aminophylline, Cap. (Pharmacia & Upjohn).
Quinamm, Tab. (Hoechst Marion Roussel).
Quinite, Tab. (Solvay).
Strema, Cap. (Foy).

aminophylline injection. (Abbott) Amp. 250 mg/10 ml, 500 mg/20 ml; Fliptop vial 10 mg/20 ml, 20 mg/50 ml.
Use: Bronchodilator.

aminophylline injection. Theophylline ethylenediamine. Amp. 3¾ gr, 7.5 gr (Various Mfr.).
Use: Smooth muscle relaxant.

aminophylline suppositories. 3⅜ gr, 7.5 gr (Various Mfr.).
Use: Smooth muscle relaxant.

aminophylline tablets. Plain or enteric coated 1.5 gr, 3 gr (Various Mfr.).
Use: Smooth muscle relaxant.

aminophylline with phenobarbital combinations.
Amodrine, Tab. (Searle).

Mudrane, Tab. (ECR Pharm.).
Mudrane GG, Tab. (ECR Pharm.).

Aminoprel. (Taylor Pharmaceuticals) L-lysine 60 mg, dl-methionine 15 mg, hydrolyzed protein 750 mg, iron 2 mg, Cu, I, K, Mg, Mn, Zn. Cap. Bot. 180s.
Use: Nutritional supplement.

aminopromazine. (I.N.N.). Proquamezine.

4-aminopyridine.
Use: Relief of symptoms of multiple sclerosis. [Orphan drug]

aminopyrine. Amidofebrin, Amidopyrazoline, Anafebrina, Novamidon, Pyradone.
Use: Antipyretic, analgesic.
See: Dipyrone, Vial (Maurry).

aminoquin naphthoate.
See: Pamaquine Naphthoate.

4-aminoquinoline derivatives.
Use: Antimalarial.
See: Aralen HCl (Sanofi Winthrop).
Chloroquine Phosphate (Various Mfr.).
Plaquenil Sulfate (Sanofi Winthrop).

8-aminoquinoline derivatives.
Use: Antimalarial.
See: Primaquine Phosphate, U.S.P.
Primaquine Phosphate (Sanofi Winthrop).

•**aminorex.** (am-EE-no-rex) USAN.
Use: Anorexic.
See: Apiquel fumarate.

aminosalicylate calcium, U.S.P. XXI. (Dumas-Wilson) 7.5 gr, Bot. 1000s.
Use: Tuberculosis therapy.
W/Isoniazid, pyridoxine HCl.
See: Calpas-Inah-6, Tab. (Amer. Chem. & Drug).

aminosalicylate potassium. Monopotassium 4-aminosalicylate.
Use: Antibacterial (tuberculostatic).
See: Paskalium, Tab., Pow. (Glenwood).

•**aminosalicylate sodium,** (uh-MEE-no-suh-LIS-ih-LATE) U.S.P. 23.
Use: Antibacterial (tuberculostatic) Crohn's disease. [Orphan drug]
See: Neopasalate, tAb. (Mallinckrodt).
Pasara Sodium, Pow., Tab. (Sandoz).
Pasdium, Tab. (Kasar).
Sodium P.A.S. (Lannett).

•**aminosalicylic acid,** U.S.P. 23.
Use: Antibacterial (tuberculostatic).

4-aminosalicylic acid.
Use: Treatment of ulcerative colitis in patients intolerant to sulfasalazine. [Orphan drug]

5-aminosalicylic acid.
See: Mesalamine.

p-aminosalicylic acid salts.
See: Aminosalicylate Calcium.

Aminosalicylate Potassium.
Aminosalicylate Sodium.

aminosidine.
Use: Mycobacterium avium complex.
[Orphan drug]
See: Gabbromicina.

Aminosyn. (Abbott Hospital Prods) Crystalline amino acid solution. **3.5%:** 1000 ml; **5%:** Container 250 ml, 500 ml, 1000 ml; **7%:** 500 ml; 7% kit (cs/3); **8.5%:** Single dose container 500 ml, 1000 ml. **10%:** 500 ml, 1000 ml. Rx.
W/Dextrose.
W/Electrolytes.
   7%: 500 ml; **8.5%:** 500 ml.
Use: Parenteral nutritional supplement.

Aminosyn (pH6). (Abbott) Crystalline amino acid infusion. **10%:** 500 ml, 1000 ml. Rx.
Use: Parenteral nutritional supplement.

Aminosyn-HBC 7%. (Abbott) Crystalline amino acid infusion for high metabolic stress. 500 ml, 1000 ml. Rx.
Use: Parenteral nutritional supplement.

Aminosyn M 3.5%. (Abbott) Crystalline amino acid infusion with electrolytes. 1000 ml. Rx.
Use: Parenteral nutritional supplement.

Aminosyn-PF. (Abbott) Crystalline amino acid infusions for pediatric use. **7%:** 250 ml, 500 ml; **10%:** 1000 ml. Rx.
Use: Parenteral nutritional supplement.

Aminosyn-RF. (Abbott) Crystalline amino acid infusion for renal failure patients. **5.2%:** 300 ml. Rx.
Use: Parenteral nutritional supplement.

Aminosyn II. (Abbott) Crystalline amino acid infusion. **3.5%:** 1000 ml; **5%:** 1000 ml; **7%:** 500 ml; **8.5%:** 500 ml, 1000 ml; **10%:** 500 ml, 1000 ml. Rx.
W/Dextrose.
   3.5% in 5% dextrose: 1000 ml; **3.5% in 25% dextrose:** 1000 ml; **5% in 25% dextrose:** 1000 ml. Rx.
W/Dextrose and electrolytes.
   3.5% in 5% dextrose: 1000 ml; **3.5% in 25% dextrose:** 1000 ml; **4.25% in 10% dextrose:** 1000 ml; **4.25% in 25% dextrose:** 1000 ml. Rx.
W/Electrolytes.
   7%: 1000 ml; **8.5%:** 1000 ml; **10%:** 1000 ml. Rx.
Use: Parenteral nutritional supplement.

Aminosyn II M. (Abbott) Crystalline amino acid infusion with maintenance electrolytes, 10% dextrose. Soln. 1000 ml. Rx.
Use: Parenteral nutritional supplement.

Amino-Thiol. (Marcen) Sulfur 10 mg, casein 50 mg, sodium citrate 5 mg, phe-

nol 5 mg, benzyl alcohol 5 mg/ml. Vial 10 ml, 30 ml. Rx.
Use: Treatment of arthritis, neuritis.

aminotrate phosphate. Trolnitrate phosphate.
See: Triethanolamine, Preps.

aminoxytropine tropate hydrochloride. Atropine-N-oxide HCl.

•**amiodarone.** (A-MEE-oh-duh-rone) USAN.
Use: Cardiac depressant (antiarrhythmic agent). [Orphan drug]

amiodarone hydrochloride.
Use: Antiarrhythmic.
See: Cordarone, Tab., Inj. (Wyeth-Ayerst).

Ampaque. (Sanofi Winthrop) Metrizamide 18.75%/20 ml Vial.
Use: Radiopaque agent.

amiphenazole hydrochloride.

•**amiprilose hydrochloride.** (ah-MIH-prih-LOHS) USAN.
Use: Antibacterial, antifungal, anti-inflammatory, antineoplastic, antiviral, immunomodulator.

•**amiquinsin hydrochloride.** (AM-ih-KWIN-sin) USAN. Under study.
Use: Antihypertensive.

Ami-Tex LA. (Amide) Phenylpropanolamine HCl 75 mg, guaifenesin 400 mg/tab. Bot. 100s, 500s, 1000s. Rx.
Use: Decongestant, expectorant.

Amitin. (Thurston) Vitamin C 200 mg, lemon bioflavonoid 100 mg, niacinamide 60 mg, methionine 100 mg/Tab. Bot. 100s, 500s. Rx.
Use: Vitamin supplement.

Amitone. (Menley & James) Calcium carbonate 350 mg/Chew. tab. Bot. 100s. otc.
Use: Antacid.

•**amitriptyline hydrochloride,** (am-ee-TRIP-tih-leen) U.S.P. 23.
Use: Antidepressant.
See: Amitril, Tab. (Parke-Davis).
   Elavil HCl, Tab., Inj. (Merck).
   Emitrip, Tab. (Major).
   Endep, Tab. (Roche).
W/Chlordiazepoxide.
   See: Limbitrol, Tab. (Roche).
W/Perphenazine.
   See: Etrafon, Prods. (Schering-Plough).
   Triavil, Tab. (Merck).

•**amlexanox.** (am-LEX-an-ox) USAN.
Use: Treatment of mouth ulcers.
See: Aphthasol.

•**amlinitide.** USAN.
Use: Treatment of insulin-dependent diabetes mellitus.

amlodipine. (am-LOW-dih-PEEN)
Use: Calcium channel blocking agent.
See: Norvasc (Pfizer).

•**amlodipine besylate.** (am-LOW-dih-PEEN) USAN.
Use: Antianginal; antihypertensive.
See: Norvasc (Pfizer).

•**amlodipine maleate.** (am-LOW-dih-PEEN) USAN.
Use: Antianginal, antihypertensive.

Ammens Medicated Powder. (Bristol-Myers) Boric acid 4.55%, zinc oxide 9.10%, talc, starch. Can 6.25 oz, 11 oz. *otc.*
Use: Skin protectant.

ammoidin. Methoxsalen.
Use: Psoralen.

•**ammonia n 13,** (ah-MOE-nee-ah N13) U.S.P. 23.
Use: Diagnostic aid (cardiac imaging, liver imaging); radioactive agent.

•**ammonia solution, strong,** N.F. 18.
Use: Pharmaceutic aid (source and solvent of ammonia).

•**ammonia spirit, aromatic,** U.S.P. 23.
Use: Stimulant (respiratory).

ammoniated mercury. (Various Mfr.)
Use: Anti-infective, topical.
See: Mercuronate 5% Oint. (Jones Medical).
W/Salicylic acid.
See: Emersal, Lot. (Medco).

•**ammonio methacrylate copolymer,** N.F. 18.
Use: Pharmaceutic aid (coating agent).

ammonium benzoate.
Use: Urinary antiseptic.

ammonium biphosphate, sodium biphosphate and sodium acid pyrophosphate.
Use: Urinary tract product.
See: pHos-pHaid (Guardian).

•**ammonium carbonate,** N.F. 18.
Use: Pharmaceutic aid (source of ammonia).

•**ammonium chloride,** U.S.P. 23.
Use: Acidifier; diuretic.
See: Nodema, Tab. (Towne).

ammonium chloride. (Various Mfr.) **Delayed Release Tab.:** Plain or E.C. 5 gr, 7.5 gr. (Bayer) **Inj.:**120 mEq/30 ml. Vial.
Use: Acidifier; diuretic; expectorant; alkalosis.

Ammonium Chloride, Enseals. (Lilly) Ammonium Cl. Tab. Enseal 7.5 gr. Bot. 100s. *Rx.*
Use: Urinary acidifier.

•**ammonium lactate.** (ah-MOE-nee-uhm LACK-tate) USAN.
Use: Antipruritic (topical).

ammonium mandelate. Ammonium salt of mandelic acid. Syr. 8 g/fl oz. Bot. pt, gal.
Use: Urinary antiseptic, oral.

•**ammonium molybdate,** U.S.P. 23.

ammonium nitrate.
See: Reditemp-C, Cold Pack (Wyeth-Ayerst).

•**ammonium phosphate,** N.F. 18. Phosphoric acid diammonium salt. Diammonium phosphate.
Use: Pharmaceutic aid.

ammonium tetrathiomolybdate. *Rx.*
Use: Treatment of Wilson's disease. [Orphan drug]

ammonium valerate.
Use: Sedative.

ammophyllin.
Use: Bronchodilator.
See: Aminophylline, U.S.P. 23. (Various Mfr.).

amobarbital. (am-oh-BAR-bih-tahl) (Various Mfr.) Tab. Elix.
Use: Hypnotic of intermediate duration.
See: Amytal, Elix., Pulv. (Lilly).

amobarbital w/combinations.
See: Amodex, Cap. (Forest).
Ectasule, Cap. (Fleming). (Lannett).

•**amobarbital sodium,** (am-oh-BAR-bih-tahl) U.S.P. 23.
Use: Sedative, hypnotic.

amobarbital sodium. (Various Mfr.) Cap. **1 gr:** Bot. 100s, 500s; **3 gr:** Bot. 100s, 500s, 1000s (Various Mfr.). Tab. **30 mg:** Bot. 100s; **50 mg:** Bot. 100s; **100 mg:** Bot. 100s. (Lilly). Vial 250 mg, 500 mg. (Lilly).
Use: Hypnotic of intermediate duration, sedative.
See: Amytal sodium (Lilly).
W/Ephedrine HCl, theophylline, chlorpheniramine maleate.
See: Theo-Span, Cap. (Scrip).
W/Secobarbital sodium.
See: Compobarb, Cap. (Eon Labs).
Dusotal, Cap. (Harvey).
Tuinal, Cap. (Lilly).

AMO Endosol. (Allergan) Sodium chloride 0.64%, potassium chloride 0.075%, calcium chloride dihydrate 0.048%, magnesium chloride hexahydrate 0.03%, sodium acetate trihydrate 0.39%, sodium citrate dihydrate 0.17%. Preservative free. Soln. 18,500 ml. *Rx.*
Use: Physiological irrigating solution.

AMO Endosol Extra. (Allergan) **Part I:**

water for injection with sodium chloride 7.14 mg, potassium chloride 0.38 mg, calcium chloride dihydrate 0.154 mg, magnesium chloride hexahydrate 0.2 mg, dextrose 0.92 mg, sodium hydroxide or hydrochloric acid/ml. Soln. Bot. 515 ml. **Part II:** Sodium bicarbonate 1081 mg, dibasic sodium phosphate anhydrous 216 mg, glutathione disulfide 95 mg. Soln. Bot. 60 ml. *Rx.*
Use: Ophthalmic irrigation solution.

•**amodiaquine,** U.S.P. 23.
Use: Antiprotozoal.

•**amodiaquine hydrochloride,** U.S.P. 23.
Use: Antimalarial.

Amodopa. (Major) Methyldopa 125 mg, 250 mg or 500 mg. **125 mg:** 100s, UD 100s. **250 mg:** 100s, 1000s, UD 100s. **500 mg:** 100s, 500s, UD 100s. *Rx.*
Use: Antihypertensive.

Amol. Mono-n-amyl-hydroquinone ether.
See: B-F-I, Pow. (SK-Beecham).

Amoline. (Major) Aminophylline 100 mg or 200 mg/Tab. Bot. 100s, 1000s, UD 100s. *otc, Rx.*
Use: Bronchodilator.

amopyroquin hydrochloride.
See: Propoquin.

•**amorolfine.** (am-OH-role-feen) USAN.
Use: Antimycotic.

Amosan. (Oral-B) Sodium perborate, saccharin. 1.76 g single-dose packet box. 20s, 40s. *otc.*
Use: Mouth and gum product.

Amotriphene. *Rx.*
Use: Coronary vasodilator.

AMO Vitrax. (Allergan) Sodium hyaluronate 30 mg/ml. Inj. Disp. syringe 0.65 ml. *Rx.*
Use: Viscoelastic agent, ophthalmic.

•**amoxapine,** (am-OX-uh-peen) U.S.P. 23.
Use: Antidepressant.
See: Asendin, Tab. (Lederle).

amoxapine tablets.
Use: Antidepressant.

•**amoxicillin,** (a-MOX-ih-sil-in) U.S.P. 23.
Use: Antibacterial.
See: Amoxil, Preps. (SK-Beecham).
Polymox, Preps. (Bristol).
Sumox, Preps. (Solvay).

amoxicillin. (Various Mfr.) Chew. tab. 250 mg. Lactose, sucrose. 100s, 500s. *Rx.*
Use: Anti-infective.

amoxicillin and clavulanate potassium for oral suspension. (a-MOX-ih-sil-in and CLAV-you-lon-ate poe-TASS-ee-uhm)
Use: Anti-infective, inhibitor (β-*lactamase*).

See: Augmentin (SK-Beecham).

amoxicillin and clavulanate potassium tablets. (a-MOX-ih-sil-in and CLAV-you-lon-ate poe-TASS-ee-uhm)
Use: Anti-infective, inhibitor (β-*lactamase*).
See: Augmentin, Tab., Chew Tab., Pow for Susp. (SK-Beecham).

amoxicillin intramammary infusion.
Use: Anti-infective, penicillin.

amoxicillin trihydrate.
Use: Anti-infective, penicilliln.
See: Amoxil Chew. tab. (SK-Beecham).
Polymox, Cap., Susp. (Bristol).
Trimox, Preps. (Squibb Mark).
Utimox, Cap, Susp. (Parke-Davis).
Wymox, Cap, Liq. (Wyeth-Ayerst).
W/Clavulanate Potassium.
See: Augmentin, Tab., Chew. tab., Pow. for susp. (SK-Beecham).

Amoxil. (SK-Beecham) Amoxicillin. **Cap.:** 250 mg. Bot. 100s, 500s, UD 10 × 10; 500 mg Bot. 50s. 100s. UD 10 × 10; **Pow. for Oral Susp.:** 125 mg or 250 mg/5 ml. Bot. 80 ml, 100 ml, 150 ml, UD 5 ml. *Rx.*
Use: Anti-infective, penicillin.

Amoxil Chewable Tablets. (SK-Beecham) Amoxicillin trihydrate. 125 mg or 250 mg/Tab. Bot. 60s. *Rx.*
Use: Anti-infective, penicillin.

Amoxil Pediatric Drops. (SK-Beecham) Amoxicillin 50 mg/ml. Bot. 15 ml, 30 ml. *Rx.*
Use: Anti-infective, penicillin.

d-AMP. (Dunhall) Ampicillin trihydrate 500 mg. Cap. Bot. 100s. *Rx.*
Use: Anti-infective, penicillin.

amp. Adenosine Phosphate, USAN.
Use: Nutrient.

amperil. (Armenpharm, Ltd.) Ampicillin trihydrate 250 mg or 500 mg/Cap. Bot. 100s, 500s. *Rx.*
Use: Anti-infective, penicillin.

•**amphecloral.** (AM-feh-klahr-ahl) USAN.
Use: Sympathomimetic; anorexic.

amphenidone.
Use: CNS stimulant.

amphetamine hydrochloride. (am-FET-uh-meen) **Amp:** 20 mg/ml, 1 ml (Various Mfr.). **Cap:** (Various Mfr.) *Rx.*
Use: Vasoconstrictor, CNS stimulant.

amphetamine, levo.
Use: CNS stimulant.
See: Levamphetamine.

amphetamine phosphate.
Use: CNS stimulant.

amphetamine phosphate, dextro. Tab. Dextroamphetamine phosphate. (Various Mfr.).

Use: CNS stimulant.

amphetamine phosphate, dibasic,
(Various Mfr.) Racemic amphetamine phosphate. **Cap:** 5 mg or 10 mg. **Tab:** 5 mg or 10 mg. *Rx.*
Use: CNS stimulant.

amphetamines.
See: Amphetamine Sulfate, Tab. (Lannett).
Biphetamine, Cap. (Medeva).
Desoxyn, Tab. (Abbott).
Desoxyn Gradumets, Long-acting tab. (Abbott).
Dexampex, Cap., Tab. (Lemmon).
Dexedrine, Elix., Tab., S.R. Cap. (SK-Beecham).
Dextroamphetamine Sulfate, Tab., S.R. Cap. (Various Mfr.).
Ferndex, Tab. (Ferndale).
Methampex, Tab. (Lemmon).

•**amphetamine sulfate,** U.S.P. 23.
Use: CNS stimulant.

amphetamine sulfate. (Various Mfr.) 5 mg, 10 mg/Cap. Tab; 20 mg/ml Vial
Use: CNS stimulant.

amphetamine sulfate, dextro.
Use: CNS stimulant.
See: Dextroamphetamine Sulfate, U.S.P. 23.

amphetamine with dextroamphetamine as resin complexes.
Use: Appetite depressant.
See: Biphetamine, Cap. (Medeva).

Amphocaps. (Halsey) Ampicillin 250 mg or 500 mg/Cap. Bot. 100s. *Rx.*
Use: Anti-infective, penicillin.

Amphojel. (Wyeth-Ayerst) Aluminum hydroxide gel. **Susp.:** 320 mg/5 ml. Bot. 355 ml; **Tab.:** 300 mg or 600 mg. Bot. 100s. *otc.*
Use: Antacid.

•**amphomycin.** (AM-foe-MY-sin) USAN. An antibiotic produced by *Streptomyces canus.*
Use: Antibacterial.
See: Ecomytrin.

Amphotec. (Sequus Pharmaceuticals) Amphotericin B (as cholesteryl) 50 mg and 100 mg/Pow. for Inj. Vial 20 ml, 50 ml. *Rx.*
Use: For treatment of certain fungal infections.

amphotericin.
Use: Antifungal.
See: Fungizone, Preps. (Squibb).

•**amphotericin b,** (am-foe-TER-ih-sin B) U.S.P. 23.
Use: Antifungal.
See: Abelcet, Susp. for Inj. (Liposome Co.).

Amphotec (Sequus Pharmaceuticals).
Amphotericin B (Fujisawa).
Fungizone, Preps. (Squibb).
W/Tetracycline and K metaphosphate.
See: Mysteclin-F, Preps. (Squibb).

amphotericin B. (Pharmatek) 50mg w/ sodium desoxycholate 41 mg/Inj. *Rx.*
Use: Antifungal.

amphotericin B lipid complex. (B-M Squibb) *Rx.*
Use: Treatment of cryptococcal meningitis. [Orphan drug]

•**ampicillin,** (am-pih-SILL-in) U.S.P. 23.
Use: Antibacterial.
See: Omnipen, Preps. (Wyeth-Ayerst).
Polycillin, Preps. (Bristol).
Principen, Preps. (Squibb Mark).
Totacillin, Preps. (SK-Beecham).
W/Probenecid.
See: Polycillin-PRB, UD (Bristol).
Principen W/Probenecid Cap. (Squibb).

ampicillin and probenecid, Cap., Oral Susp.
Use: Anti-infective, penicillin.
See: Principen w/Probenecid (Squibb).
Polycillin PRB (Bristol).
Probanpacin (Various Mfr.).

•**ampicillin sodium,** U.S.P. 23.
Use: Antibacterial.
See: Omnipen-N, Inj. (Wyeth-Ayerst).
Polycillin-N (Bristol-Myers).
Totacillin-N, Vial (SK-Beecham).

ampicillin sodium/sulbactam sodium. (am-pih-SILL-in/sull-BAK-tam)
Use: Anti-infective, penicillin.
See: Unasyn (Roerig).

ampicillin trihydrate. (Various Mfr.) Cap., Oral Susp. *Rx.*
Use: Anti-infective, penicillin.
See: Amcil, Cap., Susp. (Parke-Davis).
D-Amp, Cap., Susp. (Dunhall).
Marcillin, Cap., Susp. (Marnel).
Omnipen, Cap., Susp. (Wyeth-Ayerst).
Polycillin Preps. (Bristol).
Principen, Cap., Susp. (Squibb).
Totacillin, Cap., Susp. (SK-Beecham).

Amplicor. (Roche)
Use: For endocervical and male urethral and urine specimens for *Chlamydia trachomatis* test. Kits 10s, 96s, 100s. *Rx.*

Amplicor HIV-1 Monitor. (Roche) Kit. 24 tests.
Use: Test kit for plasma HIV-1 tests.

Ampligen. (HEM Pharmaceutical) Poly I: Poly C12U. Phase II/III HIV.
Use: Immunomodulator.

amprotropine phosphate.
●**ampyzine sulfate.** (AM-pih-zeen) USAN.
Use: Central nervous system stimulant.
●**amquinate.** (am-KWIN-ate) USAN.
Use: Antimalarial.
●**amrinone.** (AM-rih-nohn) USAN.
Use: Cardiotonic.
See: Inocor Lactate Inj. (Sanofi Winthrop).
amrinone lactate. (AM-rih-nohn LAKtate)
See: Inocor (Sanofi Winthrop).
●**amsacrine.** (AM-sah-KREEN) USAN.
Use: Antineoplastic. [Orphan drug]
Am-Tuss Elixir. (T.E. Williams) Codeine phosphate 10 mg, phenylephrine HCl 10 mg, phenylpropanolamine HCl 5 mg, prophenpyridamine maleate 12.5 mg, guaifenesin 44 mg, fluid extract of ipecac 0.17 min., citric acid 60 mg, sodium citrate 197 mg/5 ml, alcohol 5%. Bot. pt, gal. *c-v.*
Use: Antitussive, decongestant, antihistamine, expectorant.
Amvisc. (Chiron) **Inj.:** Sodium hyaluronate 12 mg/ml. Disp. syringe 0.5 ml, 0.8 ml. *Rx.*
Use: Viscoelastic agent.
Amvisc Plus. (Chiron) **Inj.:** Sodium hyaluronate 16 mg/ml. Disp. syringe: 0.5 ml, 0.8 ml. *Rx.*
Use: Viscoelastic agent.
Am-Wax. (Amlab) Urea, benzocaine, propylene glycol, glycerin. Bot. 10 ml. *otc.*
Use: Otic preparation.
amyl. Phenyl phenol, phenyl mercuric nitrate.
See: Lubraseptic Jelly (Guardian).
●**amyl nitrite,** (A-mill NYE-trite) U.S.P. 23.
Use: Vasodilator.
amyl nitrite. Isoamyl nitrite. Isopentyl nitrite. (Glaxo Wellcome). Vaporole 0.18 ml or 0.3 ml. Box 12s. (Lilly). Aspirols 0.3 ml. Box 12s.
Use: Inhalation, coronary vasodilator in angina pectoris.
W/Sodium nitrite, sodium thiosulfate.
See: Cyanide Antidote Pkg. (Lilly).
α**amylase.**
W/Calcium carbonate, glycine, belladonna extract.
See: Trialka, Tab. (Del Pharm.).
W/Pancreatin, protease, lipase.
See: Dizymes, Cap. (Recsei).
W/Pepsin, homatropine methyl bromide, lipase, protease, bile salts.
See: Digesplen, Tab., Elix. (Med. Prod. Panamericana).
W/Pepsin, pancreatin, ox bile extract.

See: Gourmase, Cap. (Solvay).
W/Phenobarbital, belladonna, pepsin, amylase, pancreatin, ox bile extract.
See: Gourmase-PB, Cap. (Solvay).
●**amylene hydrate,** N.F. 18.
Use: Pharmaceutic aid (solvent).
amylolytic enzyme.
W/Butabarbital sodium, belladonna extract, cellulolytic enzyme, proteolytic enzyme, lipolytic enzyme, iron ox bile.
See: Butibel-Zyme, Tab. (McNeil).
W/Calcium carbonate, glycine, proteolytic and cellulolytic enzymes.
See: Co-Gel, Tab. (Arco).
W/Cellulolytic, proteolytic and lipolytic enzymes, hyoscyamine sulfate.
See: Converspaz, Tab. (Ascher).
W/Lipase, proteolytic, cellulolytic enzymes, phenobarbital, hyoscyamine sulfate, atropine sulfate.
See: Arco-Lipase Plus, Tab. (Arco).
W/Proteolytic, cellulolytic, lipolytic enzymes, iron, ox bile.
See: Spaszyme, Tab. (Dooner).
W/Proteolytic enzyme, d-sorbitol.
See: Kuzyme, Cap. (Schwarz Pharma Kremers-Urban).
W/Proteolytic, cellulolytic, lipolytic enzymes.
See: Arco-Lase, Tab. (Arco).
Zymme, Tab. (Scrip).
W/Proteolytic enzyme (Papain), homatropine methylbromide, d-sorbitol.
See: Converzyme, Liq. (Ascher).
W/Proteolytic enzyme, lipolytic enzyme, cellulolytic enzyme, belladonna extract.
See: Mallenzyme Improved, Tab. (Roberts).
Amytal Sodium. (Lilly) Amobarbital sodium. Pow. for Inj.: 15 g, 30 g. Vial: 250 mg/vial or 500 mg/vial. Traypak 10s, 25s. *c-II.*
Use: Sedative, hypnotic.
Ana. (Wampole-Zeus) Antinuclear antibodies test by IFA. Test 54s.
Use: Diagnostic aid.
Ana Hep-2. (Wampole-Zeus) Antinuclear antibodies test by IFA. Tests 60s.
Use: Diagnostic aid.
anabolic agents. These agents stimulate constructive processes leading to retention of nitrogen and increasing the body protein.
See: Adroyd, Tab. (Parke-Davis).
Anabolin-IM, Vial (Alto).
Anadrol, Tab. (Syntex).
Anavar, Tab. (Searle).
Android, Tab. (Zeneca).
Androlone, Vial (Keene).
Crestabolic, Vial (Nutrition).

Deca-Durabolin, Amp., Vial (Organon).
Dianabol, Tab. (Novartis).
Di Genik, Vial (Savage).
Drolban, Vial (Lilly).
Durabolin, Amp., Vial (Organon).
Halotestin, Tab. (Pharmacia & Upjohn).
Hybolin, Vial (Hyrex).
Maxibolin, Elix., Tab. (Organon).
Nandrobolic, Vial (Forest Pharm).
Ora-Testryl, Tab. (Squibb).
Os-Cal-Mone, Tab. (Hoechst Marion Roussel).
Winstrol, Tab. (Sanofi Winthrop).
W/Vitamins and minerals.
See: Dumogran, Tab. (Squibb).
Anabolin. (Alto) Nandrolone phenpropionate 50 mg, benzyl alcohol 2%, sesame oil q.s./ml. Vial 2 ml. *Rx.*
Use: Anabolic steroid.
Anabolin-IM. (Alto) Nandrolone phenpropionate 50 mg, benzyl alcohol 2%, sesame oil q.s./ml. Vial 2 ml. *Rx.*
Use: Anabolic steroid.
Anabolin LA-100. (Alto) Nandrolone decanoate 100 mg/ml. Vial 2 ml. *Rx.*
Use: Anabolic steroid.
Anacaine. (Gordon) Benzocaine 10%. Jar oz, lb. *otc.*
Use: Local anesthetic, topical.
Anacin Tablets. (Whitehall Robins) Aspirin 400 mg, caffeine 32 mg. **Tab.:** Tin 12s, bot. 30s, 50s, 100s, 200s. **Cap.:** Bot. 30s, 50s, 100s. *otc.*
Use: Analgesic.
Anacin Maximum Strength. (Whitehall Robins) Aspirin 500 mg, caffeine 32 mg/ Tab. Bot. 12s, 20s, 24s, 40s, 72s, 75s, 150s. *otc.*
Use: Analgesic.
Anadrol-50. (Syntex) Oxymetholone 50 mg/Tab. Bot. 100s. *c-III.*
Use: Anabolic steroid.
anafebrina.
See: Aminopyrine (Various Mfr.).
Anafranil. (Novartis) Clomipramine HCl 25 mg, 50 mg or 75 mg/Cap. Bot. 100s, UD 100s. *Rx.*
Use: Antidepressant.
• **anagestone acetate.** (AN-ah-JEST-ohn) USAN.
Use: Progestin.
See: Anatropin (Ortho).
• **anagrelide hydrochloride.** (AN-AGG-reh-lide) USAN.
Use: Antithrombotic.
See: Agrylin (Roberts).
Ana-Guard Epinephrine. (Bayer) Epi-

nephrine 1:1000, chlorobutanol < 5 mg and sodium bisulfite 1.5 mg per ml. In 1 ml syringes designed to deliver 2 doses of 0.3 ml each. *Rx.*
Use: Anaphylaxis or severe allergy treatment.
• **anakinra.** USAN.
Use: Anti-inflammatory (nonsteroidal); suppressant (inflammatory bowel disease).
Ana-Kit. (Bayer) Syringe, epinephrine 1:1000 in 1 ml; four (each 2 mg) chlorpheniramine maleate; two sterilized swabs, tourniquet, instructions/kit. *Rx.*
Use: Anaphylaxis reaction.
Analbalm Improved Formula. (Schwarz Pharma) Methyl salicylate 10%, menthol 1.25%, camphor 3%. Liq. Bot.
Green: 4 oz, gal. **Pink:** 4 oz, pt, gal. *otc.*
Use: Counterirritant.
analeptics. Usually a term applied to agents with stimulant action, particularly on the central nervous system. See also central nervous system stimulants.
See: Amphetamine salts (Various Mfr.).
Caffeine (Various Mfr.).
Cylert, Tab. (Abbott).
Dextroamphetamine salts (Various Mfr.).
Dopram, Vial (Robins).
Ephedrine Salts (Various Mfr.).
Methamphetamine salts (Various Mfr.).
Ritalin HCl, Tab. (Novartis).
Sodium Succinate (Various Mfr.).
Analgesia Creme. (Rugby) Trolamine sulfate 10%. Cream, Tube 85 g. *otc.*
Use: Rubs and liniment.
analgesic balm. (Various Mfr.) Menthol w/methyl salicylate in a suitable base. *otc.*
Use: Counterirritant.
See: A.P.C., 1.5 oz, lb.
Fougera, oz.
Horton & Converse, oz, lb.
Lilly, oz.
Musterole (Schering-Plough).
Stanlabs, oz, pt.
Wisconsin, 1 lb, 5 lb.
Analgesic Liquid. (Weeks & Leo) Triethanolamine salicylate 20% in an alcohol base. Bot. 4 oz. *otc.*
Use: Analgesic, topical.
Analgesic Lotion. (Weeks & Leo) Methyl nicotinate 1%, methyl salicylate 10%, camphor 0.1%, menthol 0.1%. Bot. 4 oz. *otc.*
Use: Analgesic, topical.

Analpram-HC. (Ferndale) Hydrocortisone acetate 1% or 2%, pramoxine HCl 1%. Cream Tube 30 g. *Rx.*
Use: Corticosteroid, local anesthetic (topical).

Analval Tablets. (Pal-Pak) Aspirin 227 mg, acetaminophen 162 mg, caffeine 32 mg/Tab. Bot. 1000s. *otc.*
Use: Analgesic combination.

Anamine. (Mayrand) Pseudoephedrine HCl 30 mg, chlorpheniramine maleate 2 mg/5 ml. Syr. Bot. 473 ml. *Rx.*
Use: Decongestant, antihistamine.

Anamine HD Syrup. (Mayrand) Phenylephrine HCl 5 mg, chlorpheniramine maleate 2 mg, hydrocodone bitartrate 1.67 mg. 10 ml tid or qid. *c-III.*
Use: Decongestant, antihistamine, antitussive.

Anamine T.D. Capsules. (Mayrand) Chlorpheniramine maleate 8 mg, pseudoephedrine HCl 120 mg/T.D. Cap. Bot. 100s. *Rx.*
Use: Antihistamine, decongestant.

Ananain, Comosain.
Use: Burn treatment. [Orphan drug]
See: Vianain (Genzyme).

Anaplex. (ECR Pharm.) Pseudoephedrine HCl 30 mg, chlorpheniramine maleate 2 mg/5 ml. Syr. Bot. 473 ml. *Rx.*
Use: Decongestant, antihistamine.

Anaplex HD Syrup. (ECR Pharm.) Hydrocodone bitartrate 1.7 mg, phenylephrine HCl 5 mg, chlopheniramine maleate 2 mg. Bot. 120 ml, 480 ml. *c-III.*
Use: Antitussive, decongestant, antihistamine.

Anaprox. (Syntex) Naproxen sodium 275 mg (naproxen base 250 mg with sodium 25 mg), lactose/Tab. Bot. 100s, 500s. UD 100s. *Rx.*
Use: Nonsteroidal anti-inflammatory agent.

Anaprox DS. (Syntex) Naproxen sodium 550 mg (naproxen base 500 mg with sodium 50 mg)/Tab. Bot. 100s, 500s, UD 100s. *Rx.*
Use: Nonsteroidal anti-inflammatory agent.

anarel. Guanadrel sulfate.

•**anaritide acetate.** (an-NAR-ih-TIDE) USAN.
Use: Antihypertensive, diuretic. [Orphan drug]

Anaspaz. (Ascher) l-Hyoscyamine sulfate 0.125 mg/Tab. Bot. 100s, 500s. *Rx.*
Use: Anticholinergic, antispasmodic.

•**anastrozole.** (an-ASS-troe-zole) USAN.
Use: Antineoplastic.
See: Arimidex, Tab. (Zeneca).

Anatrast. (Lafayette Pharm.) GI contrast agent, 100% paste. Tube 500 g.

Anatuss DM. (Mayrand) **Syrup:** Guaifenesin 100 mg, pseudoephedrine HCl 30 mg, dextromethorphan HBr 10 mg/5 ml. Bot. 480 ml; **Tab.:** Guaifenesin 400 mg, pseudoephedrine HCl 60 mg, dextromethorphan HBr 20 mg. Bot. 100s. *otc.*
Use: Antitussive, expectorant, decongestant.

Anatuss LA. (Mayrand) Guaifenesin 400 mg, pseudoephedrine HCl 120 mg. Tab. Bot. 100s. *Rx.*
Use: Expectorant, decongestant.

Anatuss Syrup. (Mayrand) Dextromethorphan HBr 15 mg, phenylpropanolamine HCl 25 mg, guaifenesin 100 mg/10 ml. Bot. 120 ml, 480 ml. *otc.*
Use: Antitussive, decongestant, expectorant.

Anatuss Tabs. (Mayrand) Guaifenesin 100 mg, acetaminophen 325 mg, dextromethorphan HBr 15 mg, phenylpropanolamine HCl 25 mg/Tab. Bot. 100s, 500s. *Rx.*
Use: Expectorant, analgesic, antitussive, decongestant.

Anatuss w/Codeine. (Mayrand) **Syr.:** Phenylpropanolamine HCl 25 mg, codeine phosphate 10 mg, guaifenesin 100 mg/5 ml. Bot. 120 ml, 480 ml. *c-v.* **Tab.:** Phenylpropanolamine HCl 25 mg, codeine phosphate 10 mg, guaifenesin 100 mg, acetaminophen 300 mg. Bot. 100s. *c-III.*
Use: Decongestant, antitussive, expectorant, analgesic (Tab. only).

Anavar. (Searle) Oxandrolone 2.5 mg/Tab. Bot. 100s. *Rx.*
Use: Anabolic steroid.

anayodin.
See: Chiniofon.

•**anazolene sodium.** USAN. Sodium Anoxynaphthonate.
Use: Diagnostic aid (blood volume and cardiac output determination).
See: Coomassie Blue (Wyeth-Ayerst).

Anbesol Baby Gel. (Whitehall Robins) Benzocaine 7.5%. Tube 0.25 oz. *otc.*
Use: Local anesthetic, topical.

Anbesol Gel. (Whitehall Robins) Benzocaine 6.3%, phenol 0.5%, alcohol 70%. Tube 7.5 g. *otc.*
Use: Anesthetic, topical combination.

Anbesol Liquid. (Whitehall Robins)

Benzocaine 6.3%, phenol 0.5%, povidone-iodine 0.04%, alcohol 70%. Bot. 9 ml, 22 ml. *otc.*
Use: Local anesthetic, topical combination.

Anbesol Maximum Strength. (Whitehall Robins) **Gel:** Benzocaine 20%, alcohol 60%, carbomer 934P, polyethylene glycol, saccharin. Tube 7.2 g. **Liq.:** Benzocaine 20%, alcohol 60%, saccharin, polyethylene glycol. Bot. 9 ml. *otc.*
Use: Local anesthetic, topical.

Ancef. (SK-Beecham) Cefazolin sodium. **Vial:** Equivalent to 250 mg, 500 mg or 1 g of cefazolin. **Multi Pack:** 500 mg or 1 g/Pack. 25s. **Bulk Vial:** 5 g, 10 g. **Piggyback Vial:** 500 mg or 1 g/100 ml. **Minibag:** 1 g/50 ml w/5% dextrose inj. (D5W). 500 mg/50 ml D5W. *Rx.*
Use: Anti-infective, cephalosporin.

Ancet. (C & M Pharm) Sodium lauryl sulfate, lauramide DEA, propylene glycol, hydroxyethyl ethylcellulose, PCMX. Liq. Bot. 240 ml. *otc.*
Use: Therapeutic skin cleanser.

Ancid Tablet and Suspension. (Sheryl) Calcium aluminum carbonate, di-amino acetate complex. Tab. 100s. Susp. pt. *otc.*
Use: Antacid.

Ancobon. (Roche) Flucytosine 250 mg or 500 mg/Cap. Bot. 100s. *Rx.*
Use: Anti-infective.

•**ancrod.** (AN-krahd) USAN. An active principle obtained from the venom of the Malayan pit viper *Agkistrodon rhodostoma.*
Use: Anticoagulant. [Orphan drug]
See: Arvin.

Andesterone Suspension. (Lincoln) Estrone 2 mg, testosterone 6 mg/ml. Vial 15 ml. **Forte:** Estrone 1 mg, testosterone 20 mg/ml. Inj. Vial 15 ml. *Rx.*
Use: Estrogen, androgen combination.

Andrest 90-4. (Seatrace) Testosterone enanthate 90 mg, estradiol valerate 4 mg/ml. Vial 10 ml. *Rx.*
Use: Androgen, estrogen combination.

Andro 100. (Forest) Testosterone 100 mg/ml. Vial 10 ml. *c-III.*
Use: Androgen.

Androcur. Cyproterone acetate. *Rx.*
Use: Hirsutism, severe. [Orphan Drug] Sponsor: Berlex.

Andro-Cyp 100. (Keene) Testosterone cypionate 100 mg/ml. Vial 10 ml. *c-III.*
Use: Androgen.

Andro-Cyp 200. (Keene) Testosterone

cypionate 200 mg/ml. Vial 10 ml. *c-III.*
Use: Androgen.

Androderm. (SmithKline-Beecham) 12.2 mg testosterone USP. 37 cm². Transdermal patch, releases 2.5 mg/day. 30s, 60s. *c-III.*
Use: Treatment of endogenous testosterone deficiency/absence.

Andro-Estro 90-4. (Rugby) Estradiol valerate 4 mg, testosterone enanthate 90 mg/ml with chlorobutanol in sesame oil. Inj. Vial. 10 ml. *Rx.*
Use: Estrogen, androgen combination.

androgens. Substances which possess masculinizing activities.
See: Methyltestosterone.
Testosterone.
Testosterone cyclopentylpropionate.
Testosterone enanthate.
Testosterone heptanoate.
Testosterone phenylacetate.
Testosterone propionate.

androgen-estrogen therapy.
See: Dienestrol with Methyltestosterone.
Estradiol Esters with Methyltestosterone.
Estradiol Esters with Testosterone.
Estrogenic Substance, Conjugated with Methyltestosterone.
Estrogenic Substance Mixed with Methyltestosterone.
Estrogenic Substance Mixed with Testosterone.
Estrone with Testosterone.
Gynetone, Tab. (Schering-Plough).

androgen hormone inhibitor.
See: Proscar (Merck).

Android-10 and 25. (Zeneca) Methyltestosterone 5 mg/Buccal Tab., 10 mg/Tab. or 25 mg/Tab. Bot. 60s. *c-III.*
Use: Androgen.

Andro L.A. 200. (Forest) Testosterone enanthate 200 mg/ml. Inj. vial 10 ml. *c-III.*
Use: Androgen.

Androlin. (Lincoln) Testosterone 100 mg/ml. Vial 10 ml. *c-III.*
Use: Androgen.

Androlone. (Keene) Nandrolone phenpropionate 25 mg/ml in sesame oil. Vial 5 ml. *c-III.*
Use: Anabolic steroid.

Androlone-D 200. (Keene) Nandrolone decanoate w/benzyl alcohol, 200 mg/ml. Inj. Vial 1 ml. *c-III.*
Use: Anabolic steroid.

Andronaq-50. (Schwarz Pharma) Testosterone 50 mg/ml, sodium carboxy-

methylcellulose, methylcellulose, povidone, DSS, thimerosal. Inj. Vial. 10 ml. *c-III*.
Use: Androgen.

Andronaq LA. (Schwarz Pharma) Testosterone cypionate 100 mg, benzyl alcohol 0.9% in cottonseed oil. Vial 10 ml. Bot. 12s. *c-III*.
Use: Androgen.

Andronate 100. (Taylor Pharmaceuticals) Testosterone cypionate 100 mg/ml with benzyl alcohol in cottonseed oil. Vial 10 ml. *c-III*.
Use: Androgen.

Andronate 200. (Taylor Pharmaceuticals) Testosterone cypionate 200 mg/ml with benzyl alcohol, benzyl benzoate in cottonseed oil. Vial 10 ml. *c-III*.
Use: Androgen.

Andropository 200. (Rugby) Testosterone enanthate 200 mg/ml in sesame oil with chlorobutanol. Inj. Vial 10 ml. *c-III*.
Use: Androgen.

androstanazole.
See: Stanozolol.

androstane-17-(beta)-ol-3-one.
See: Stanolone.

androstanolone. (I.N.N.) Stanolone.

androstenopyrazole. Anabolic steroid; pending release.

Androtest P.
See: Testosterone propionate.

Androvite. (Optimax) Tab.: Iron 3 mg, vitamins A 4167 IU, D 67 IU, E 67 IU, B_1 8.3 mg, B_2 8.3 mg, B_3 8.3 mg, B_5 16.7 mg, B_6 16.7 mg, B_{12} 20.8 mcg, C 167 mg, folic acid 0.06 mg, PABA, inositol, biotin, betaine, B, Cr, Cu, I, Mg, Mn, Se, Zn 8.3 mg, pancreatin, hesperidin, rutin. Bot. 180s. *otc*.
Use: Vitamin/mineral supplement.

Andryl 200. (Keene) Testosterone enanthate 200 mg/ml. Vial 10 ml. *c-III*.
Use: Androgen.

Andylate Forte. (Vita Elixir) Acetaminophen 3 gr, salicylamide 3 gr, caffeine 0.25 gr/Tab. *otc*.
Use: Analgesic combination.

Andylate Rub. (Vita Elixir) Methylnicotinate, methylsalicylate, camphor, dipropyleneglycol salicylate, oil of cassia, oleoresin of capsicum, oleoresin of ginger. *otc*.
Use: Analgesic, topical.

Andylate Tablets. (Vita Elixir) Sodium salicylate 10 gr/Tab. *otc*.
Use: Salicylate analgesic.

Anectine. (Glaxo Wellcome) Succinyl-choline Cl. Soln. 20 mg/ml. Multidose Vial 10 ml. Sterile Pow. Flo-Pak 500 mg or 1000 mg. Box 12s. *Rx*.
Use: Muscle relaxant.

Anefrin Nasal Spray, Long Acting. (Walgreen) Oxymetazoline HCl 0.05%. Bot. 0.5 oz. *otc*.
Use: Decongestant.

Anergan 50. (Forest) Promethazine HCl 50 mg/ml. Vial 10 ml. *Rx*.
Use: Antihistamine.

anertan.
See: Testosterone propionate.

Anestacon. (PolyMedica) Lidocaine HCl 20 mg/ml. Jelly, 15 ml, 240 ml. *Rx*.
Use: Local anesthetic.

Anesthesin. Ethyl-p-aminobenzoate.
Use: Local anesthetic.
See: Benzocaine, U.S.P. 23.

anethaine.
See: Tetracaine HCl.

•**anethole.** N.F. 18.
Use: Pharmaceutic aid (flavor).

aneurine hydrochloride.
See: Thiamine HCl, Preps. (Various Mfr.).

Anexsia 5/500 tablets. (Mallinckrodt) Hydrocodone bitartrate 5 mg, acetaminophen 500 mg/Tab. Bot. 100s. *c-III*.
Use: Narcotic analgesic combination.

Anexsia 7.5/650. (Mallinckrodt) Hydrocodone bitartrate 7.5 mg, acetaminophen 650 mg/Tab. Bot. 100s. *c-III*.
Use: Narcotic analgesic combination.

Anexsia 10/660. (Mallinckrodt) Hydrocodone bitartrate 10 mg, acetaminophen 660 mg/Tab. Bot. 100s and 1000s. *c-III*.
Use: Narcotic analgesic combination.

Angel Sweet. (Garrett) Vitamins A and D_2. Cream 90 g. *otc*.
Use: Skin protectant.

Angen. (Davis & Sly) Estrone 2 mg, testosterone 25 mg/ml Aqueous susp. Vial 10 ml. *Rx*.
Use: Estrogen, androgen combination.

Angerin. (Kingsbay) Nitroglycerin 1 mg/Cap. Bot. 60s. *Rx*.
Use: Coronary vasodilator.

Angex. (Janssen) Lidoflazine. *Rx*.
Use: Coronary vasodilator.

Angio-Conray. (Mallinckrodt) Iothalamate sodium 80% (48% iodine), EDTA. Inj. Vial 50 ml.
Use: Radiopaque agent.

•**angiotensin amide.** (an-JEE-oh-TEN-sin AH-mid) USAN. N.F. XIII.
Use: Vasoconstrictor.
See: Hypertensin (Novartis).

angiotensin-converting enzyme inhibitors.
Use: Antihypertensive; congestive heart failure.
See: Accupril, Tab. (Parke-Davis).
Altace, Cap. (Hoechst Marion Roussel).
Capoten, Tab. (Squibb).
Lotensin, Tab. (Novartis).
Monopril, Tab. (Bristol-Myers).
Prinivil, Tab. (Merck).
Univasc, Tab. (Schwarz Pharma Kremers Urban).
Vasotec, Tab. (Merck).
Vasotec I.V., Inj. (Merck).
Zestril, Tab. (Stuart).

Angiovist 282. (Berlex) Diatrizoate meglumine 60% (iodine 28%). Vial 50 ml, 100 ml or 150 ml. Box 10s.
Use: Radiopaque agent.

Angiovist 292. (Berlex) Diatrizoate meglumine 52%, diatrizoate sodium 8% (iodine 29.2%). Vial 30 ml, 50 ml or 100 ml. Box 10s.
Use: Radiopaque agent.

Angiovist 370. (Berlex) Diatrizoate meglumine 66%, diatrizoate sodium 10%, (iodine 37%). Vial 50 ml, 100 ml, 150 ml or 200 ml. Box 10s.
Use: Radiopaque agent.

anhydrohydroxyprogesterone. Ethisterone.

•**anidoxime.** (AN-ih-DOX-eem) USAN.
Use: Analgesic.
See: Bamoxine (U.S.V. Pharm.).

A-Nil. (Vangard) Codeine phosphate 10 mg, bromodiphenhydramine HCl 3.75 mg, diphenhydramine HCl 8.75 mg, ammonium Cl 80 mg, potassium guaiacolsulfonate 80 mg, menthol 0.5 mg/5 ml, alcohol 5%. Bot. Pt. gal. *c-v.*
Use: Antitussive, expectorant.

•**anilerdine,** U.S.P. 23.
Use: Analgesic (narcotic).

•**anileridine hydrochloride,** U.S.P. 23.
Use: Analgesic (narcotic).
See: Leritine HCl, Tab. (Merck).

•**anilopam hydrochloride.** (AN-ih-low-pam) USAN.
Use: Analgesic.

Animal Shapes. (Major) Vitamin A 2500 IU, D 400 IU, E 15 IU, C 60 mg, B_1 1.05 mg, B_2 1.2 mg, B_3 13.5 mg, B_6 1.05 mg, B_{12} 4.5 mcg, folic acid 0.3 mg. Chew. tab. Bot. 100s, 250s. *otc.*
Use: Vitamin supplement.

Animal Shapes + Iron. (Major) Vitamin A 2500 IU, D 400 IU, E 15 IU, C 60 mg, B_1 1.05 mg, B_2 1.2 mg, B_3 13.5 mg,

B_6 1.05 mg, B_{12} 4.5 mcg, folic acid 0.3 mg, iron 15 mg. Chew. tab. Bot. 100s, 250s. *otc.*
Use: Vitamin/mineral supplement.

anion exchange resins.
See: Polyamine-Methylene Resin.

•**aniracetam.** (AN-ih-RASS-eh-tam) USAN.
Use: Mental performance enhancer.

•**anirolac.** (ah-NIH-role-ACK) USAN.
Use: Anti-inflammatory, analgesic.

anise oil, N.F. XVI.
Use: Flavor.

anisindione.
See: Miradon (Schering-Plough).

anisopyradamine.
See: Pyrilamine Maleate.

anisotropine. F.D.A. Tropine 2-propylvalerate.

•**anisotropine methylbromide.** (ah-NIH-so-TROE-peen meth-ill-BROE-mide) USAN.
Use: Anticholinergic.
See: Valpin 50, Tab. (DuPont).

•**anistreplase.** (uh-NISS-truh-place) USAN.
Use: Fibrinolytic, thrombolytic.
See: Eminase (SK-Beecham).

•**anitrazafen.** (AN-ih-TRAY-zaff-en) USAN.
Use: Anti-inflammatory, topical.

anodynon.
See: Ethyl Cl.

Anodynos. (Buffington) Aspirin 420.6 mg, salicylamide 34.4 mg caffeine 34.4 mg/Tab. Sugar, lactose and salt free. Dispens-A-Kit 500s, Bot. 100s, 500s, Medipak 200s. *otc.*
Use: Analgesic combination.

Anodynos-DHC Tablets. (Forest) Hydrocodone bitartrate 5 mg, acetaminophen 500 mg/Tab. Bot. 100s. *c-III.*
Use: Narcotic analgesic combination.

Anodynos Forte. (Buffington) Chlorpheniramine maleate, phenylephrine HCl, salicylamide, acetaminophen, caffeine/Tab. Sugar, lactose and salt free. Dispens-A-Kit 500s, Bot. 100s. *Rx.*
Use: Antihistamine, decongestant, analgesic.

Anoquan. (Roberts Med) Butalbital 50 mg, caffeine 40 mg, acetaminophen 325 mg/Cap. Bot. 100s, 1000s. *Rx.*
Use: Sedative, hypnotic, analgesic.

Anorex. (Dunhall) Phendimetrazine 35 mg/Tab. Bot. 100s. *c-III.*
Use: Anorexiant.

anorexigenic agents. Appetite depressants.

See: Amphetamine Preps.
Didrex, Tab. (Pharmacia & Upjohn).
Plegine, Tab. (Wyeth-Ayerst).
Preludin HCl (Boehringer Ingelheim).
Sanorex, Tab. (Sandoz).
Tenuate (Hoechst Marion Roussel).
Tepanil, Tab. (3M Pharm).
Wilpo, Tab. (Sandoz).

anovlar. Norethindrone plus ethinyl estradiol. *Rx.*
Use: Oral contraceptive.

•**anoxomer.** (an-OX-ah-MER) USAN.
Use: Pharmaceutic aid (antioxidant); food additive.

anoxynaphthonate sodium. Anazolene Sodium.

Ansaid. (Pharmacia & Upjohn) Flurbiprofen 50 mg or 100 mg. Tab. 100s, 500s, UD 100s. *Rx.*
Use: Nonsteroidal anti-inflammatory agent.

Anspor. (SK-Beecham) Cephradine (a semisynthetic cephalosporin) **Cap.:** 250 mg. Bot. 100s, UD 100s; 500 mg. Bot. 20s, 100s, UD 100s. **Oral Susp.:** 125 mg or 250 mg/5 ml. Bot. 100 ml.
Use: Anti-infective, cephalosporin.

Answer. (Carter Products) Reagent in-home pregnancy test kit for urine testing. Test kit box 1s.
Use: Diagnostic aid.

Answer 2. (Carter Products) Reagent in-home pregnancy test kit for urine testing. Test kit box 2s.
Use: Diagnostic aid.

Answer Ovulation. (Carter Products) Home test to predict time of ovulation. In 6 day test kits.
Use: Ovulation prediction.

Answer Plus. (Carter Products) Reagent in-home pregnancy test kit for urine testing. Test kit box 1s.
Use: Diagnostic aid.

Answer Plus 2. (Carter Products) Reagent in-home pregnancy test kit for urine testing. Test kit box 2s.
Use: Diagnostic aid.

Answer Quick & Simple. (Carter Products) Reagent in-home kit for urine testing. Test kit box 1s.

Antabuse. (Wyeth-Ayerst) Disulfiram. **250 mg/Tab.** Bot. 100s; **500 mg/Tab.** Bot. 50s, 1000s. *Rx.*
Use: Antialcoholic agent.

Antacid. (Walgreen) Calcium carbonate 500 mg/Tab. Bot. 75s. *otc.*
Use: Antacid.

Antacid #2. (Global Pharms) Calcium carbonate 5.5 gr, magnesium carbonate

2.5 gr/Tab. Bot. 100s. *otc.*
Use: Antacid.

Antacid M Liquid. (Walgreen) Aluminum oxide 225 mg, magnesium hydroxide 200 mg/5 ml. Bot. 12 oz, 26 oz. *otc.*
Use: Antacid.

Antacid No. 6. (Jones Medical) Calcium carbonate 0.42 g, glycine 0.18 g/Tab. Bot. 100s. *otc.*
Use: Antacid.

Antacid Relief Tablets. (Walgreen) Dihydroxyaluminum sodium carbonate 334 mg/Tab. Bot. 75s. *otc.*
Use: Antacid.

antacids. Drugs that neutralize excess gastric acid.
See: Alka-Seltzer, Tab. (Bayer).
Alka-Seltzer Plus, Tab. (Bayer).
Alka-Seltzer Special Effervescent Antacid, Tab. (Bayer).
Alka-2 Chewable Antacid, Tab. (Bayer).
Aluminum Hydroxide Gel (Various Mfr.).
Aluminum Hydroxide Gel w/Combinations (Various Mfr.).
Aluminum Hydroxide Gel Dried (Various Mfr.).
Aluminum Hydroxide Gel Dried w/ Combinations (Various Mfr.).
Aluminum Hydroxide Magnesium Carbonate, Tab. (Various Mfr.).
Aluminum Phosphate Gel (Wyeth-Ayerst).
Aluminum Proteinate, Tab. (Solvay).
Amitone, Tab. (SmithKline-Beecham).
Calcium Carbonate, Precipitated (Various Mfr.).
Calcium Carbonate Tab. (Various Mfr.).
Carbamine (Key Pharm.).
Ceo-Two, Supp. (Beutlich).
Chooz, Gum Tab. (Schering-Plough).
Citrocarbonate, Liq. (Pharmacia & Upjohn).
Dicarbosil, Tab. (Arch).
Di-Gel, Liq., Tab. (Schering-Plough).
Dihydroxyaluminum Aminoacetate (Various Mfr.).
Dihydroxyaluminum Sodium Carbonate Tab. (Warner-Lambert).
Magaldrate, Tab., Susp. (Wyeth-Ayerst).
Magnesium Carbonate (Various Mfr.).
Magnesium Glycinate, Tab. (Various Mfr.).
Magnesium Hydroxide (Various Mfr.).
Magnesium Oxide, Tab., Cap. (Various Mfr.).
Magnesium Trisilicate (Various Mfr.).

Neutralox, Susp. (Lemmon).
Oxaine, Susp. (Wyeth-Ayerst).
Ratio, Tab. (Pharmacia & Upjohn).
Rolaids, Tab. (Warner-Lambert).
Romach, Tab. (ROR Pharmacal).
Sodium Bicarbonate, Inj., Tab. (Various Mfr.).
Tums, Tab. (SmithKline-Beeecham).

Antacid Suspension. (Geneva Pharm.) Aluminum hydroxide 225 mg, magnesium hydroxide 200 mg/5 ml. Bot. 360 ml. *otc.*
Use: Antacid.

Antacid Tablets. (Goldline) Calcium carbonate 500 mg/Chew. tab. Bot. 150s. *otc.*
Use: Antacid.

Antacid Extra Strength. (Various Mfr.) Calcium carbonate 750 mg/Tab. Bot. 96s. *otc.*
Use: Antacid.

Anta-Gel. (Halsey) Aluminum hydroxide 200 mg, magnesium hydroxide 200 mg, simethicone 20 mg/5 ml. Bot. 12 oz. *otc.*
Use: Antacid, antiflatulent.

antagonists of curariform drugs.
See: Neostigmine Methylsulfate.
Tensilon Cl (Roche).

antastan.
See: Antazoline Hydrochloride, U.S.P. 23.

antazoline hydrochloride. Antastan.
See: Arithmin, Tab. (Lannett).

•**antazoline phosphate,** U.S.P. 23.
Use: Antihistamine.
W/Naphazoline, boric acid, phenylmercuric acetate, sodium Cl, sodium carbonate anhydrous.
See: Vasocon-A Ophthalmic, Soln. (Smith, Miller & Patch).
W/Naphazoline HCl, polyvinyl alcohol.
See: Albalon-A Liquifilm, Ophth. Soln. (Allergan).

Antazoline-V. (Rugby) Naphazoline HCl 0.05%, antazoline phosphate 0.5%, PEG 8000, polyvinyl alcohol, EDTA, benzalkonium chloride 0.01%. Soln. Drop. Bot. 5 ml, 15 ml. *Rx.*
Use: Ophthalmic decongestant combination.

anterior pituitary.
See: Pituitary, anterior.

anthelmintic. A remedy for worms.
See: Antiminth, Susp. (Roerig).
Atabrine, Tab. (Sanofi Winthrop).
Betanaphthol Benzoate (Various Mfr.).
Biltricide, Tab. (Bayer).
Carbon Tetrachloride (Various Mfr.).

Gentian Violet (Various Mfr.).
Jayne's PW Vermifuge (Bayer).
Jayne's RW, Tab. (Bayer).
Mintezol, Tab., Susp. (Merck).
Niclocide, Chew. tab. (Bayer).
Piperazine Preps. (Various Mfr.).
Povan, Tab., Susp. (Parke-Davis).
Terramycin (Various Mfr.).
Tetrachloroethylene.
Vansil, Cap. (Pfipharmecs).
Vermox, Chew tab., Oral Susp. (Merck).

•**anthelmycin.** (AN-thell-MY-sin) USAN.
Use: Anthelmintic.

Anthelvet. Tetramisole HCl.

Anthra-Derm. (Dermik) Anthralin 0.1%, 0.25%, 0.5% or 1% in petrolatum ointment base. Tube 1.5 oz. *Rx.*
Use: Antipsoriatic.

•**anthralin,** U.S.P. 23.
Use: Antipsoriatic.
See: Anthra-Derm Oint. (Dermik) .
Drithocreme, Cream (Dermik).
Dritho-Scalp, Cream (Dermik).
Lasan, Cream, Oint. (Stiefel).
W/Mineral oil.
See: Lasan Pomade (Stiefel).

•**anthramycin.** (an-THRAH-MY-sin) USAN.
Use: Antineoplastic.

anthraquinone of cascara.
See: Cascara Sagrada, Prods.

anthrax vaccine. (Michigan Department of Public Health) Vial 5 ml. *Rx.*
Use: Agent for immunization.

anti-a blood grouping serum.
Use: Diagnostic aid (blood in vitro).

anti-b blood grouping serum.
Use: Diagnostic aid (blood in vitro).

Antiacid. (Hillcrest North) Aluminum hydroxide, magnesium trisilicate, calcium carbonate/Tab. Bot. 100s. *otc.*
Use: Antacid.

Antialcoholic.
See: Disulfiram (Various Mfr.).
Antabuse (Wyeth-Ayerst).

Anti-Allergy tablet. (Walgreen) Phenylpropanolamine HCl 18.7 mg, chlorpheniramine maleate 2 mg/Tab. Bot. 24s. *otc.*
Use: Decongestant, antihistamine.

antiandrogen.
See: Eulexin (Schering-Plough).

antiasthmatic combinations.
See: Cromolyn Sodium, Cap. (Various Mfr.).
Decadron Respihaler, Aerosol. (Merck).
Ephedrine HCl (Various Mfr.).

Ephedrine Sulfate (Various Mfr.).
Isoephedrine HCl (Various Mfr.).
Isoetharine (Sanofi Winthrop).
Isoetharine HCl (Sanofi Winthrop).
Isoetharine Mesylate (Sanofi Winthrop).
Isoproterenol HCl (Various Mfr.).
Isoproterenol Sulfate (Various Mfr.).
Methoxyphenamine HCl (Various Mfr.).
Phenylephrine HCl (Various Mfr.).
Phenylpropanolamine HCl (Various Mfr.).
Pseudoephedrine HCl (Various Mfr.).
Racephedrine HCl (Various Mfr.).
antiasthmatic inhalant.
See: AsthmaHaler (SmithKline-Beecham Beecham).
AsthmaNefrin, Soln. (SmithKline-Beecham).
antibacterial antibodies.
See: Botulinum antitoxin.
Diphtheria antitioxin.
Immune globulin IM.
Immune globulin IV.
Tetanus immune globulin.
antibason.
See: Methylthiouracil (Various Mfr.).
Antibiotic. (Parnell) **Otic susp.:** Polymyxin B sulfate 10,000 units, neomycin (as sulfate) 3.5 mg, hydrocortisone 10 mg/ml, thimerosal 0.01%. Bot. 10 ml w/dropper. **Otic soln.:** Polymyxin B sulfate 10,000 units, neomycin (as sulfate) 3.5 mg, hydrocortisone 10 mg/ml. Bot. 10 ml w/dropper. *Rx.*
Use: Anti-infective, anti-inflammatory.
antibiotics/anti-infectives.
See: Amebicides, general.
Amikacin Sulfate, vial (Various Mfr.).
Amoxicillin (Various Mfr.).
Amoxicillin and Potassium Clavulanate (SK-Beecham).
Amoxicillin w/Comb. (Various Mfr.).
Ampicillin (Various Mfr.).
Ampicillin w/Comb. (Various Mfr.).
Anthelmintic agents, general.
Antimalarial agents, general.
Antiprotozoan agents, general.
Antituberculosis agents, general.
Antiviral agents, general.
Azithromycin, Caps. (Pfizer).
Aztreonam, Vial (Squibb).
Bacampicillin HCl (Roerig).
Bacitracin (Various Mfr.).
Carbenicillin (Various Mfr.).
Cefaclor (Various Mfr.).
Cefadroxil (Various Mfr.).
Cefamandole Nafate (Lilly).
Cefazolin Sodium, Vial (Various Mfr.).

Cefixime (Lederle).
Cefmetazole Sodium (Pharmacia & Upjohn).
Cefonicid Sodium, Vial (SK-Beecham).
Cefoperazone Sodium, Vial (Roerig).
Cefotaxime Sodium, Vial (Hoechst Marion Roussel).
Cefotetan Disodium, Vial (Stuart).
Cefoxitin Sodium, Vial (Merck).
Cefpodoxime Proxetil (Pharmacia & Upjohn).
Cefprozil (Bristol-Myers).
Ceftazidime, Vial (Various Mfr.).
Ceftizoxime Sodium, Vial (Fujisawa).
Ceftriaxone Sodium, Vial (Roche).
Cefuroxime (Various Mfr.).
Cephalexin (Various Mfr.).
Cephalexin Monohydrate, Pulv., Susp. (Various Mfr.).
Cephalothin, Sodium, Vial (Various Mfr.).
Cephradine (Various Mfr.).
Chloramphenicol (Various Mfr.).
Cinoxacin, Cap. (Various Mfr.).
Ciprofloxacin (Bayer).
Clarithromycin (Abbott).
Clindamycin (Various Mfr.).
Clofazimine, Cap. (Novartis).
Cloxacillin Sodium (Various Mfr.).
Colistimethate Sodium, Inj. (Parke-Davis).
Colistin Sulfate (Various Mfr.).
Dapsone, Tab. (Jacobus).
Demeclocycline (Lederle).
Dicloxacillin, Cap., Susp. (Various Mfr.).
Doxycycline (Various Mfr.).
Enoxacin, Tab. (Rhone-Poulenc Rorer).
Erythromycin (Various Mfr.).
Erythromycin w/Comb. (Various Mfr.).
Fungicides, general.
Furazolidone (Procter & Gamble).
Gentamicin Sulfate (Various Mfr.).
Imipenem-Cilastatin, Vial (Merck).
Kanamycin Sulfate (Various Mfr.).
Lincomycin (Various Mfr.).
Lomefloxacin HCl, Tab. (Searle).
Loracarbef (Lilly).
Methacycline HCl, Cap., Syr. (Wallace).
Methenamine (Various Mfr.).
Methenamine w/Comb. (Various Mfr.).
Methicillin Sodium, Vial, Pow. (Various Mfr.).
Methylene Blue, Tab. (Various Mfr.).
Metronidazole (Various Mfr.).
Mezclocillin Sodium, Vial (Bayer).
Minocycline (Lederle).
Nafcillin Sodium, Vial, Cap., Pow. (Wyeth-Ayerst).

Nalidixic Acid (Sanofi Winthrop).
Netilmicin Sulfate, Vial (Schering-Plough).
Neomycin Sulfate (Various Mfr.).
Nitrofurantion (Various Mfr.).
Norfloxacin, Tab. (Roberts).
Novobiocin (Various Mfr.).
Ofloxacin (Ortho).
Oxacillin, Sodium (Various Mfr.).
Oxytetracycline (Various Mfr.).
Paromomycin, Cap., Syr. (Parke-Davis).
Penicillin G Benzathine (Various Mfr.).
Penicillin G Benzathine w/ Comb. (Various Mfr.).
Penicillin G, Potassium (Various Mfr.).
Penicillin G Potassium w/Comb. (Various Mfr.).
Penicillin G Procaine (Various Mfr.).
Penicillin G Procaine w/Comb. (Various Mfr.).
Penicillin G Sodium (Various Mfr.).
Penicillin V Potassium (Various Mfr.).
Pentamidine Isethionate (Fujisawa).
Phenoxymethyl Penicillin (Various Mfr.).
Piperacillin Sodium, Vial (Lederle)
Piperacillin Sodium w/Comb. (Various Mfr.).
Polymyxin B Sulfate (Various Mfr.).
Spectinomycin, Vial (Pharmacia & Upjohn).
Streptomycin Sulfate (Various Mfr.).
Sulfadiazine (Various Mfr.).
Sulfamethizole, Tab. (Wyeth-Ayerst).
Sulfamethoxazole (Various Mfr.).
Sulfamethoxazole w/Comb. (Various Mfr.).
Sulfasalazine (Various Mfr.).
Sulfasalazine w/Comb. (Various Mfr.).
Sulfisoxazole (Various Mfr.).
Tetracycline HCl (Various Mfr.).
Ticarcillin w/Comb. (Various Mfr.).
Ticarcillin Disodium, Vial (SK-Beecham).
Tobramycin Sulfate (Various Mfr.).
Triacetyloleandomycin (Various Mfr.).
Trimethoprim (Various Mfr.).
Trimethoprim w/Comb. (Various Mfr.).
Trimetrexate Glucuronate, Vial (US Bioscience).
Troleandomycin, Cap. (Roerig).
Vancomycin HCl (Lilly).
anticholinergic agents. Parasympatholytic agents.
See: Akineton (Knoll).
Antrenyl Bromide (Novartis).
Artane HCl (Lederle).
Atropine Preps.
Atrovent, Spray (Boehringer Ingelheim).

Banthine Bromide (Searle).
Belladonna Preps.
Cantil Preps. (Hoechst Marion Roussel).
Cogentin (Merck).
Daricon, Tab. (SK-Beecham).
Dicyclomine HCl (Various Mfr.).
Disipal (3M Pharm).
Donabarb Sr., Cap. (Zeneca).
Homatropine methylbromide.
Hybephen, Prods. (SK-Beecham).
Kemadrin, Tab. (Glaxo Wellcome).
Kinesed, Tab. (Stuart).
L-Hyoscyamine, Tab. (Schwarz Pharma Kremers-Urban).
Murel, Amp. (Wyeth-Ayerst).
Norflex, Inj., Tab. (3M Pharm).
Oxyphencyclimine HCl (Various Mfr.).
Pagitane HCl, Tab. (Lilly).
Pamine Bromide, Tab., Soln. (Pharmacia & Upjohn).
Panparnit HCl.
Parsidol HCl, Tab. (Parke-Davis).
Pathilon (Lederle).
Phenoxene HCl (Hoechst Marion Roussel).
Prantal Methylsulfate, Tab. (Schering-Plough).
Pro-Banthine Bromide, Preps. (Searle).
Robinul, Tab., Inj. (Robins).
Scopolamine methylbromide.
Scopolamine methylbromide HBr.
Tral, Preps. (Abbott).
Trihexyphenidyl HCl (Various Mfr.).
Trocinate, Tab. (ECR Pharm.).
Valpin 50, Tab. (DuPont Merck).
Valpin 50-PB, Tab. (DuPont Merck).
•**anticoagulant citrate dextrose solution,** U.S.P. 23.
Use: Anticoagulant (for storage of whole blood).
See: A.C.D. Solution. (Various Mfr.).
•**anticoagulant citrate phosphate dextrose adenine solution,** U.S.P. 23.
Use: Anticoagulant (for storage of whole blood).
•**anticoagulant citrate phosphate dextrose solution,** U.S.P. 23.
Use: Anticoagulant (for storage of whole blood).
•**anticoagulant heparin solution,** U.S.P. 23.
Use: Anticoagulant (for storage of whole blood).
anticoagulants.
See: Acenocoumarin.
Anisindione.
Calciparine, Inj. (DuPont Merck).
Coumadin, Amp., Tab. (DuPont Merck).

Dalteparin Sodium.
Depo-Heparin, Sodium (Pharmacia & Upjohn).
Dipaxin, Tab. (Pharmacia & Upjohn).
Diphenadione.
Eridione, Tab. (Eric, Kirk & Gary).
Enoxaparin Sodium.
Ethyl Biscoumacetate, Tab.
Fragmin (Pharmacia & Upjohn).
Hedulin, Tab. (Hoechst Marion Roussel).
Heparin Calcium.
Heparin, Sodium (Various Mfr.).
Liquaemin Sodium, Vial (Organon).
Liquamar, Tab. (Organon).
Lovenox (Rhone-Poulenc Rorer).
Miradon, Tab. (Schering-Plough).
Panheprin, Amp., Vial (Abbott).
Panwarfin, Tab. (Abbott).
Phenindione, Tab. (Various Mfr.).
ReoPro (Lilly).
Sofarin (Lemmon).
Warfarin (Various Mfr.).
•**anticoagulant sodium citrate solution,** U.S.P. 23.
Use: Anticoagulant (for plasma and blood fractionation).
anticonvulsants.
See: Acetazolamide, Tab. (Various Mfr.).
Amytal Sodium, Amp. (Lilly).
Carbamazepine, Tab. (Various Mfr.).
Celontin Kapseals (Parke-Davis).
Clorazepate, Tab. (Various Mfr.).
Depakene (Abbott).
Diamox, Tab., Inj. (Lederle).
Diazepam, Tab., Soln. (Various Mfr.).
Diazepam Intensol, Soln. (Roxane).
Dilantin, Preps. (Parke-Davis).
Epitol, Tab. (Lemmon).
Felbatol, Tab., Susp. (Wallace Labs).
Gen-Xene, Tab. (Alra).
Klonopin, Tab. (Roche).
Lamictal, Tab. (Glaxo Wellcome).
Magnesium sulfate (Various Mfr.).
Mephobarbital, Tab. (Sanofi Winthrop).
Mesantoin, Tab. (Sandoz).
Milontin, Kapseals (Parke-Davis).
Mysoline, Tab., Susp. (Wyeth-Ayerst).
Neurontin, Cap. (Parke-Davis).
Peganone, Tab. (Abbott).
Phenobarbital (Various Mfr.).
Phenurone, Tab. (Abbott).
Phenytoin, Susp., Tab. (Various Mfr.).
Phenytoin Sodium, Cap. (Various Mfr.).
Primidone, Tab. (Various Mfr.).
Tegretol, Tab. (Novartis).
Tranxene, Tab. (Abbott).
Tranxene-SD, Tab. (Abbott).

Tranxene-T, Tab. (Abbott).
Tridione (Abbott).
Valium, Tab. (Roche).
Valrelease, Cap. (Roche).
Zarontin, Cap., Syr. (Parke-Davis).
anti-cytomegalovirus monoclonal antibodies.
Use: Treatment of cytomegalovirus.
antidepressants.
See: Adapin, Cap. (Lotus).
Amitriptyline HCl (Various Mfr.).
Amoxapine, Tab. (Various Mfr.).
Anafranil, Cap. (Novartis).
Asendin, Tab. (Lederle).
Aventyl HCl, Pulv., Liq. (Lilly).
Deprol, Tab. (Wallace).
Desipramine HCl, Cap., Tab. (Various Mfr.).
Desyrel, Tab. (Bristol-Myers).
Effexor, Tab. (Wyeth-Ayerst).
Elavil Tab., Inj. (Merck).
Endep, Tab. (Roche).
Imipramine HCl, Amp., Tab. (Various Mfr.).
Imipramine Pamoate, Cap. (Novartis).
Janimine, Tab. (Abbott).
Ludiomil, Tab. (Novartis).
Luvox, Tab. (Solvay).
Maprotiline HCl, Tab. (Various Mfr.).
Monoamine oxidase inhibitors.
Nardil, Tab. (Parke-Davis).
Norpramin, Preps. (Hoechst Marion Roussel).
Pamelor, Cap., Liq. (Sandoz).
Parnate Sulfate, Tab. (SK-Beecham).
Paxil, Tab. (SK-Beecham).
Pertofrane, Cap. (Rhone-Poulenc Rorer).
Protriptyline HCl (Merck).
Prozac, Liq., Pulv. (Dista).
Serzone, Tab. (Bristol-Myers Squibb).
Sinequan, Cap. (Pfizer).
Surmontil, Cap. (Wyeth-Ayerst).
Tofranil, Amp., Tab. (Novartis).
Tofranil-PM, Cap. (Novartis).
Trazodone HCl, Tab. (Various Mfr.).
Triavil, Tab. (Merck).
Vivactil, Tab. (Merck).
Wellbutrin, Tab. (Glaxo Wellcome).
Zoloft, Tab. (Roerig).
antidiarrheals.
See: Attapulgite, Activated (Various Mfr.).
Bismatrol, Tab. (Major).
Cantil, Liq., Tab. (Hoechst Marion Roussel).
Coly-Mycin S, Oral Susp., (Parke-Davis).
DIA-Quel Liq. (Inter. Pharm. Corp.).

Diasorb, Liq., Tab. (Columbia).
Diphenoxylate HCl w/atropine sulfate, Tab., Liq. (Various Mfr.).
Donnagel, Chew. tab., Liq., Susp. (Wyeth-Ayerst).
Furoxone Liq., Tab. (Eaton).
Imodium, Cap. (Janssen).
Imodium A-D, Tab., Liq. (McNeil-CPC).
Kaodene Non-Narcotic, Liq. (Pfeiffer).
Kaolin (Various Mfr.)
Kaolin Colloidal (Various Mfr.).
Kaopectate, Prods. (Pharmacia & Upjohn).
Kao-Spen, Susp. (Century).
Kapectolin (Various Mfr.).
K-C, Susp. (Century).
K-Pek, Susp. (Rugby).
Lactinex, Tab., Gran. (Becton Dickinson).
Lactobacillus acidophilus & bulgaricus mixed culture, Tab. (Becton Dickinson).
Lactobacillus acidophilus, viable culture (Various Mfr.).
Logen, Tab. (Goldline).
Lomanate, Liq. (Various Mfr.).
Lomotil, Liq., Tab., (Searle).
Lonox, Liq. (Geneva Pharm.).
Loperamide, Cap., Liq. (Various Mfr.).
Maalox Antidiarrheal, Capl. (Rhone-Poulenc Rorer).
Milk of Bismuth (Various Mfr.).
Motofen, Tab. (Carnrick).
Mycifradin Sulfate, Soln., Tab. (Pharmacia & Upjohn).
Parepectolin, Susp. (Rhone-Poulenc Rorer).
Pepto-Bismol, Liq., Tab. (Procter & Gamble).
Pepto Diarrhea Control, Liq. (Procter & Gamble).
Pink Bismuth, Liq. (Various Mfr.).
Rheaban Maximum Strength, Capl. (Pfizer).
antidiuretics.
  See: Pitressin, Amp. (Parke-Davis).
  Pitressin Tannate In Oil, Amp. (Parke-Davis).
  Pituitary Post. Inj. (Various Mfr.).
antiemetic/antivertigo agents.
  See: Antivert, Tab. (Roerig).
  Antrizine, Tab. (Major).
  Arrestin, Inj. (Vortech).
  Atarax, Tab., Syr. (Roerig).
  Bonine, Tab. (Pfizer).
  Bucladin-S, Softab Tab. (Stuart).
  Calm-X, Tab. (Republic Drug).
  Compazine, Preps. (SK-Beecham).
  Dimenhydrinate, Tab., Inj., Liq. (Various Mfr.).

Dimetabs, Tab. (Jones Medical).
Dinate, Inj. (Seatrace).
Dizmiss, Tab. (Jones Medical).
Dramamine, Preps. (Searle).
Dramanate, Inj. (Taylor Pharmaceuticals).
Dramilin, Inj. (Kay Pharm.).
Dramoject, Inj. (Mayrand).
Dymenate, Inj. (Keene).
Emecheck, Liq. (Savage).
Emetrol, Liq. (Rhone-Poulenc Rorer).
Hydrate, Inj. (Hyrex).
Kytril, Tab., Inj. (SK-Beecham).
Marezine, Tab. (Glaxo Wellcome).
Marinol, Cap. (Roxane).
Maxolon, Tab. (SK-Beecham).
Meclizine HCl, Tab. (Various Mfr.).
Meni-D, Cap. (Seatrace).
Mepergan, Inj. (Wyeth-Ayerst).
Metoclopramide, Tab. (Various Mfr.).
Naus-A-Tories, Supp. (Table Rock).
Naus-A-Way, Soln. (Roberts).
Nausetrol, Syr. (Medical Chemicals).
Octamide, Tab. (Pharmacia & Upjohn).
Phenergan, Preps. (Wyeth-Ayerst).
Prochlorperazine, Supp. (Various Mfr.).
Reclomide, Tab. (Major).
Reglan, Inj., Syr., Tab. (Robins).
Ru-Vert-M, Tab. (Solvay).
Tebamide, Supp. (G & W Labs).
T-Gen, Supp. (Goldline).
Thorazine, Preps. (SK-Beecham).
Ticon, Inj. (Roberts).
Tigan, Preps. (SK-Beecham).
Torecan Amp., Supp., Tab. (Sandoz).
Transderm-Scop, Transdermal Therapeutic System (Novartis).
Trilafon, Preps. (Schering-Plough).
Trimazide, Cap., Supp. (Major).
Trimethobenzamide HCl, Cap., Inj., Supp. (Various Mfr.).
Triptone, Capl. (Del Pharm.)
Vesprin, Inj. (Bristol-Myers).
Vistaril, Cap., Susp., Soln. (Pfizer).
Vontrol, Tab. (SK-Beecham).
Zofran, Inj., Tab. (Glaxo).
antiepilepsirine.
  Use: Anticonvulsant. [Orphan drug]
antiepileptic agents.
  See: Anticonvulsants.
antiestrogen. Tamoxifen citrate.
  Use: Hormone for cancer therapy.
  See: Nolvadex (Zeneca).
  Tamoxifen (Barr).
antifebrin.
  See: Acetanilid (Various Mfr.).
antiflatulents.
  See: Di-Gel, Prods. (Schering-Plough).

Silain, Tab., Gel (Robins).
Simethicone Prods.

Antifoam A Compound. (Hoechst Marion Roussel).
Use: Antiflatulent.
See: Simethicone, U.S.P. 23.

antifolic acid.
See: Methotrexate, Tab. (Lederle).

Antiformin. Sodium hypochlorite in sodium hydroxide 7.5%, available chlorine 5.2%; may be colored with meta cresol purple.
Use: Antiseptic, germicide.

antifungal agents.
See: Fungicides.

•**antihemophilic factor,** U.S.P. 23.
Use: Antihemophilic.

antihemophilic factor. (Baxter & Alpha Therapeutics) Antihemophilic Factor, human. Method for Syringe Administration 10 ml 450 A.H.F. or 300 A.H.F. units/Pkg. W/Syringe 30 ml or 900 A.H.F. units/Pkg.
Use: Antihemophilic.
See: Alphanate, Inj. (Alpha Therapeutic).
Bioclate, Inj. (Centeon).
Helixate, Inj. (Centeon).
Hemofil, Vial (Baxter).
Humate-P, Inj. (Centeon).
Koate HP, Inj. (Bayer).
KoGENate, Inj. (Bayer).
Monoclate-P, Inj. (Centeon).
Profilate HP. Inj. (Alpha Therapeutic).
Recombinate, Inj. (Baxter).

antihemophilic factor, human.
Use: Treatment of Von Willebrand's disease. [Orphan drug]
See: Humate P.

Antihemophilic Factor (Porcine) Hyate: C. (Speywood) Freeze-dried concentrate of Antihemophilic Factor, 400 to 700 porcine units of Factor VIII:C. Pow. for inj. Vials. *Rx.*
Use: Antihemophilic.

antihemophilic factor (recombinant).
Use: Prophylaxis/treatment of bleeding in hemophilia A. [Orphan drug]
See: Kogenate.

antiheparin.
See: Protamine Sulfate.

Antihist-1. (Various Mfr.) Clemastine fumarate 1.34 mg. Pkg. 16s. *otc.*
Use: Antihistamine.

Antihistamine Cream. (Towne) Methapyrilene HCl 10 mg, pyrilamine maleate 5 mg, allantoin 2 mg, diperodon HCl 2.5 mg, benzocaine 10 mg, menthol 2 mg/g. Cream Jar 2 oz. *otc.*

Use: Antihistamine, topical.

antihistamines.
See: Aller-Chlor, Syr., Tab. (Rugby).
AllerMax, Capl. (Pfeiffer).
Anergan, Inj. (Forest).
Banophen, Cap., Capl. (Major).
Belix, Elix. (Halsey).
Benadryl, Preps. (Parke-Davis).
Bena-D, Inj. (Seatrace).
Benahist, Inj. (Keene).
Ben-Allergin-50, Inj. (Dunhall).
Benoject, Inj. (Mayrand).
Benylin Cough, Syr. (Parke-Davis).
Brompheniramine, Tab., Elix. (Various Mfr.).
Bromphen, Elix. (Various Mfr.).
Bydramine, Syr. (Major).
Chlo-Amine, Tab. (Bayer).
Chlorate, Tab. (Major).
Chlorpheniramine Maleate (Various Mfr.).
Chlor-Pro, Inj. (Schein).
Chlortab, Tab. (Vortech).
Chlor-Trimeton, Inj., Syr., Tab. (Schering-Plough).
Claritin, Tab. (Schering-Plough).
Cophene-B, Inj. (Dunhall).
Co-Pyronil 2, Pulv., Susp. (Lilly).
Cyproheptadine HCl, Syr., Tab. (Various Mfr.).
Dexchlor, Tab. (Schein).
Dexchlorpheniramine Maleate, Tab. (Various Mfr.).
Dimetane, Preps. (Robins).
Diphen Cough, Syr. (Rosemont).
Diphenhydramine HCl (Various Mfr.).
Diphenylpyraline HCl (Various Mfr.).
Disophrol, Prods. (Schering-Plough).
Doxylamine Succinate (Various Mfr.).
Drixoral, Prods. (Schering-Plough).
Diphen Cough, Syr. (Rosemont).
Genahist, Cap., Tab., Elix. (Goldline).
Hismanal, Tab. (Janssen).
Histaject, Inj. (Mayrand).
Hydramyn, Syr. (HN Norton).
Hyrexin-50, Inj. (Hyrex).
Myidyl, Syr. (Rosemont).
Nasahist B, Inj. (Keene).
ND Stat, Inj. (Hyrex).
Nidryl, Elix. (Geneva Pharm.).
Nolahist, Tab. (Carnrick).
Optimine, Tab. (Schering-Plough).
Oraminic, Inj. (Vortech).
PBZ, Tab. (Novartis).
PBZ-SR, Tab. (Novartis).
Pelamine, Tab. (Major).
Pentazine, Inj. (Century Pharm.).
Periactin, Syr., Tab. (Merck).
Pfeiffer's Allergy, Tab. (Pfieffer).
Phenameth, Tab. (Major).
Phenazine, Inj. (Keene).

Phendry, Prods. (HN Norton).
Phenergan, Prods .(Wyeth-Ayerst).
Phenoject-50, Inj. (Mayrand).
Poladex, Tab. (Major).
Polaramine, Syr., Tab. (Schering-
Plough).
Poly-Histine, Elix. (Bock).
Pro-50, Inj. (Dunhall).
Prometh-50, Inj. (Seatrace).
Promethazine HCl (Various Mfr.).
Prophenpyridamine Maleate (Various
Mfr.).
Prorex, Inj. (Hyrex).
Prothazine, Prods. (Vortech).
Pyrilamine Maleate (Various Mfr.).
Seldane, Tab. (Hoechst Marion Rous-
sel).
Tacaryl, Tab., Syr. (Westwood
Squibb).
Tavist, Tab. Syr. (Sandoz).
Telachlor, Cap. (Major).
Teldrin, Cap. (SK-Beecham).
Temaril, Tab., Span., Syr. (Allergan
Herbert).
Tripelennamine HCl (Various Mfr.).
Triprolidine HCl (Various Mfr.).
Tusstat, Syr. (Century Pharm.).
V-Gan, Inj. (Roberts).
Wehdryl, Inj. (Roberts).
antihyperlipidemics.
See: Atromid-S, Cap. (Wyeth-Ayerst).
Choloxin, Tab. (Knoll Pharm.).
Clofibrate, Cap. (Various Mfr.).
Mevacor, Tab. (Merck).
Niacin, Prods. (Various Mfr.).
Pravachol, Tab. (Bristol-Myers
Squibb).
Questran, Prods. (Bristol-Myers).
Zocor, Tab. (Merck).
antihypertensives.
See: Accupril, Tab. (Parke-Davis).
Acebutolol hydrochloride.
Aceon, Tab. (Ortho).
Adaprolol maleate.
Alazide, Tab. (Major).
Alazine, Tab. (Major).
Aldactazide, Tab. (Searle).
Aldactone, Tab. (Searle).
Aldoclor 250, Tab. (Merck).
Aldomet, Tab. (Merck).
Aldoril, Tab. (Merck).
Alfuzosin hydrochloride.
Aldopa, Tab. (Major).
Alpha 1-adrenergic blockers.
Altace, Cap. (Hoechst Marion Rous-
sel, Pharmacia & Upjohn).
Althiazide.
Amiquinsin hydrochloride.
Amlodipine besylate.
Amlodipine maleate.
Amodopa (Major).

Anaritide acetate.
ACE inhibitors.
Apresazide, Cap. (Novartis).
Apresodex, Tab. (Rugby).
Apresoline, Amp., Tab. (Novartis).
Aprozide, Cap. (Major).
Arcum R-S, Tab. (Arcum).
Arlix (Hoechst Marion Roussel).
Artarau, Tab. (Archer-Taylor).
Atenolol/chlorthalidone, Tab. (Various
Mfr.).
Atiprosin maleate.
Belfosdil.
Bendacalol mesylate.
Bendroflumethiazide.
Benzthiazide.
Betaxolol hydrochloride.
Bethanidine sulfate.
Bevantolol hydrochloride.
Biclodil hydrochloride.
Bosoprolol.
Bisoprolol fumarate.
Bucindolol hydrochloride.
Cam-Ap-Es, Tab. (Camall).
Candoxatril.
Candoxatrilat.
Capoten, Tab. (Bristol-Myers Squibb).
Capozide, Tab. (Bristol-Myers
Squibb).
Captopril.
Cardura, Tab. (Roerig).
Carvedilol.
Catapres, Tab. (Boehringer Ingel-
heim).
Ceronapril.
Chlorothiazide sodium.
Chlorthalidone, Tab. (Various Mfr.).
Cicletanine.
Cilazapril.
Cithal, Cap. (Table Rock).
Citrin, Cap. (Table Rock).
Clentiazem maleate.
Clonidine.
Clonidine hydrochloride.
Clonidine hydrochloride and Chlor-
thalidone, Tab. (Various Mfr.).
Clopamide.
Combipres, Tab. (Boehringer Ingel-
heim).
Coreg, Tab., (SK-Beecham).
Cyclothiazide.
Debrisoquin sulfate.
Delapril hydrochloride.
Demser, Cap. (Merck).
De Serpa, Tab. (de Leon).
Diaserp, Tab. (Major).
Diazoxide.
Diazoxide parenteral.
Dibenzyline, Cap. (SK-Beecham).
Dilevalol hydrochloride.
Diovan, Cap. (Novartis).

Ditekiren.
Diucardin, Tab. (Wyeth-Ayerst).
Diulo, Tab. (Searle).
Diurigen w/Reserpine, Tab. (Gold-
line).
Diuril, Tab., Susp. (Merck).
Diuril sodium, I.V., (Merck).
Diutensen-R, Tab. (Wallace).
Doxazosin mesylate.
Elserpine, Tab. (Canright).
Enalapril maleate.
Enalaprilat.
Enalkiren.
Endralazine mesylate.
Enduronyl, Tab. (Abbott).
Enduronyl forte, Tab. (Abbott).
Eprosartan.
Eprosartan mesylate.
Eserdine, Tab. (Major).
Eserdine forte, Tab. (Major).
Esidrix, Tab. (Novartis).
Esimil, Tab. (Novartis).
Exna, Tab. (Robins).
Fenoldopam mesylate.
Flavodilol maleate.
Flolan, Pow. for Inj. (Glaxo Wellcome).
Flordipine.
Flosequinan.
Forasartan.
Fosinopril.
Fosinopril sodium.
Fosinoprilat.
Guanabenz.
Guanabenz acetate.
Guanacline sulfate.
Guanadrel sulfate.
Guancydine.
Guanethidine monosulfate.
Guanethidine sulfate.
Guanfacine hydrochloride.
Guanisoquin.
Guanisoquin sulfate.
Guanoclor sulfate.
Guanocitine hydrochloride.
Guanoxabenz.
Guanoxan sulfate.
Guanoxyfen sulfate.
Harbolin, Tab. (Arcum).
H.H.R., Tab. (Geneva Pharm.).
Hiwolfia, Tab. (Jones Medical).
Hydralazine, Inj. (Solopak).
Hydralazine hydrochloride, Tab. (Vari-
ous Mfr.).
Hydralazine polistirex.
Hydrap-ES, Tab. (Parmed).
Hydraserp, Tab. (Geneva Pharm).
Hydrazide, Cap. (Goldline).
Hydra-Zide, Cap. (Par Pharm).
Hydrochloroserpine, Tab. (Freeport).
Hydrochlorothiazide/hydralazine, Cap.
(Various Mfr.).

Hydroflumethiazide.
Hydromox-R, Tab. (Lederle).
Hydropine, Tab. (Rugby).
Hydropine H.P., Tab. (Rugby).
Hydropres-50, Tab. (Merck).
Hydroserp, Tab. (Zenith).
Hydroserp-50, Tab. (Freeport).
Hydroserpine #1, #2 (Various Mfr.).
Hydrosine 25, 50, Tab. (Major).
Hydrotensin-50, Tab. (Mayrand).
Hydroxyisoindolin.
Hylorel, Tab. (Hyrex).
Hyperstat, I.V. Inj. (Schering-Plough).
Hytrin, Tab., Cap. (Abbott).
Hyzaar, Tab. (Merck).
Indacrinone.
Indapamide.
Inderide, Tab. (Wyeth-Ayerst).
Inderide LA, Cap. (Wyeth-Ayerst).
Indolapril hydrochloride.
Indoramin.
Indoramin hydrochloride.
Indorenate hydrochloride.
Ingadine, Tab. (Major).
Inhibace (Roche/Glaxo Wellcome).
Inversine, Tab. (Merck).
Irbesartan.
Ismelin, Tab. (Novartis).
Labetalol hydrochloride.
Leniquinsin.
Levcromakalim.
Lexxel, ER Tab. (Astra Merck).
Lofexidine hydrochloride.
Loniten, Tab. (Pharmacia & Upjohn).
Lopressor HCT, Tab. (Novartis).
Losartan potassium.
Losulazine hydrochloride.
Lotensin, Tab. (Novartis).
Lotrel, Cap. (Novartis).
Lozol, Tab. (Rhone-Poulenc Rorer).
Marapres, Tab. (Marnel).
Mavik, Tab. (Knoll).
Maxzide, Tab. (Lederle).
Mebutamate.
Mecamylamine hydrochloride.
Medroxalol.
Medroxalol hydrochloride.
Metatensin, Tab. (Hoechst Marion
Roussel).
Methalthiazide.
Methyclodine, Tab. (Rugby).
Methyclothiazide.
Methyldopa.
Methyldopa and Chlorothiazide, Tab.
Methyldopa and Hydrochlorothiazide,
Tab. (Various Mfr.).
Methyldopate hydrochloride, Inj. (Fu-
jisawa).
Metipranolol.
Metipranolol hydrochloride.
Metolazone.

Metoprolol fumarate.
Metoprolol succinate.
Metoprolol tartrate and Hydrochloro-
thiazide.
Metryosine.
Midamor, Tab. (Merck).
Minipress, Cap. (Pfizer).
Minizide, Cap. (Pfizer).
Minoxidil, Tab. (Rugby).
Moduretic, Tab. (Merck).
Moexipril hydrochloride.
Monopril, Tab. (Bristol-Myers).
Muzolimine.
Nadolol, Tab. (Various Mfr.).
Nadolol and Bendroflumethiazide.
Natrico, Pulvoid (Drug Products).
Nebivolol.
Nitrendipine.
Nitropress, Vial (Abbott).
Nitroprusside sodium.
Normodyne, Inj., Tab. (Schering-
Plough).
Normotensin, Inj. (Marcen).
Pargyline hydrochloride.
Pelanserin hydrochloride.
Pentina, Tab. (Freeport).
Pentolinium tartrate.
Perindopril erbumine.
Pheniprazine hydrochloride.
Phenoxybenzamine hydrochloride.
Phentolamine hydrochloride.
Pinacidil.
Pivopril.
Prazosin hydrochloride, Cap. (Vari-
ous Mfr.).
Prinivil, Tab. (Merck).
Prinzide, Tab. (Merck).
Priscoline, Vial (Novartis).
Prizidilol hydrochloride.
Propranolol hydrochloride and Hydro-
chlorothiazide, Tab. (Various Mfr.).
Quinapril hydrochloride.
Quinaprilat.
Quinazosin hydrochloride.
Quinelorane hydrochloride.
Quiniprole hydrochloride.
Quinuclium bromide.
Ramipril.
Rauneed, Tab. (Hanlon).
Raunescine (Penick).
Raurine, Tab., Cap. (New Eng. Phr.
Co.).
Rautina, Tab. (Fellows).
Rauval, Tab. (Pal-Pak).
Rauwolfia/bendroflumethiazide, Tab.
(Various Mfr.).
Rauwolfia serpentina.
Rauwolscine.
Rauzide, Tab. (B-M Squibb).
Rawfola, Tab. (Foy).
Regroton, Tab. (Rhone-Poulenc
Rorer).

Regroton Demi, Tab. (Rhone-Poulenc
Rorer).
Renese, Tab. (Pfizer).
Renese-R, Tab. (Pfizer).
Reserpaneed, Tab. (Hanlon).
Reserpine.
Reserpine and Chlorothiazide, Tab.
Reserpine and Hydrochlorothiazide,
Tab. (Various Mfr.).
Reserpine, hydralazine hydrochloride
and Hydrochlorothiazide, Tab. (Vari-
ous Mfr.).
R-HCTZ-H, Tab. (Lederle).
Salazide, Tab. (Major).
Salazide-Demi, Tab. (Major).
Salutensin, Tab. (Roberts).
Salutensin-Demi, Tab. (Bristol-My-
ers).
Saprisartan potassium.
Saralasin acetate.
Sectral, Cap. (Wyeth-Ayerst).
Ser-A-Gen, Tab. (Goldline).
Ser-Ap-Es, Tab. (Novartis).
Serpasil-Apresoline, Tab. (Novartis).
Serpasil-Esidrix, Tab. (Novartis).
Serpazide, Tab. (Major).
Sertabs, Tab. (Table Rock).
Sertina, Tab. (Fellows).
Sodium nitroprusside, Pow. for Inj. (El-
kins-Sinn).
Sulfinalol hydrochloride.
Tarka, Tab. (Knoll).
Teludipine hydrochloride.
Temocapril hydrochloride.
Tenex, Tab. (Robins).
Tenoretic, Tab. (Zeneca).
Tenormin, Amp, Tab. (Zeneca).
Terazosin hydrochloride.
Tiamenidine hydrochloride.
Ticrynafen.
Timolide 10-25, Tab. (Merck).
Timolol maleate
Timolol maleate and Hydrochloride,
Tab.
Tinabinol.
Tipentosin hydrochloride.
Tolazoline hydrochloride.
Toprol XL, Tab. (Astra).
Trandate, Tab., Inj. (Allen & Han-
burys).
Trandate hydrochlorothiazide, Tab.
(Allen & Hanburys).
Tri-Hydroserpine, Tab. (Rugby).
Trimazosin hydrochloride.
Trimethamide.
Trimethaphan camsylate.
Trimoxamine hydrochloride.
T-Sert, Tab. (Tennessee).
Tryosine hydroxylase inhibitor.
Univasc, Tab. (Schwarz Pharma).
Valsartan.

Vaseretic, Tab. (Merck).
Vasotec, Tab., Inj. (Merck).
Visken, Tab. (Sandoz).
Xipamide.
Zankiren hydrochloride.
Zepine, Tab. (Foy).
Zestoretic, Tab. (Zeneca).
Zestril, Tab. (Zeneca).
Ziac, Tab. (Lederle).
Zofenoprilat arginine.

anti-infectives.
See: antibiotics/anti-infectives.

anti-inhibitor coagulant complex.
Use: Antihemophilic.
See: Autoplex T. (Baxter).
Feiba VH. (Immuno-U.S.).

Anti-Itch Cream. (Rugby) Burow's solution 5%, phenol 0.5%, menthol 0.5%, camphor 1% in washable base. Tube oz. *otc.*
Use: Antipruritic, counterirritant.

Antilerge. (Metz) Chlorpheniramine maleate 8 mg, phenylephrine HCl 12 mg/ Tab. Bot. 30s. *otc.*
Use: Antihistamine, decongestant.

antileukemia.
See: Antineoplastic agents.

Antilirium. (Forest) Physostigmine salicylate 1 mg/ml, benzyl alcohol 2%, sodium bisufite 0.1%. 2 ml. *Rx.*
Use: Antidote.

antimalarial agents.
See: Amodiaquin HCl.
Aralen HCl, Inj. (Sanofi Winthrop).
Aralen Phosphate (Sanofi Winthrop).
Aralen Phosphate w/Primaquine (Sanofi Winthrop).
Atabrine HCl, Tab. (Sanofi Winthrop).
Chloroguanide HCl.
Daraprim Tab. (Glaxo Wellcome).
Hydroxychloroquine Sulfate.
Paludrine HCl, Tab. (Wyeth-Ayerst).
Pamaquine Naphthoate.
Plaquenil Sulfate, Tab. (Sanofi Winthrop).
Plasmochin Naphthoate.
Primaquine Phosphate, Tab. (Sanofi Winthrop).
Pyrimethamine.
Quinacrine HCl, Tab.
Quinine Salts (Various Mfr.).
Quinine Sulfate (Various Mfr.).
Totaquine, Pow.

Antiminth. (Pfizer Laboratories) Pyrantel pamoate 250 mg/5 ml. Oral susp. Bot. 60 ml. *otc.*
Use: Anthelmintic.

•**antimony potassium tartrate,** U.S.P. 23. (Various Mfr.).
Use: Antischistosomal, leishmaniasis,

expectorant, emetic.
W/Cocillana, euphorbia pilulifera, squill, senega.
See: Cylana, Syr. (Jones Medical).
W/Guaifenesin, codeine phosphate.
See: Cheracol, Syr. (Pharmacia & Upjohn).
W/Guaifenesin, dextromethorphan HBr.
See: Cheracol-D, Syr. (Pharmacia & Upjohn).
W/Paregoric, glycyrrhiza fluid extract.
See: Brown Mixture (Lilly).
W/Thenylpyramine HCl, ammonium Cl, sodium citrate, menthol, aromatics.
See: Histacomp, Syr., Tab. (Approved Pharm.).

antimony preparations.
See: Antimony Potassium Tartrate (Various Mfr.).
Antimony Sodium Thioglycollate (Various Mfr.).
Tartar Emetic (Various Mfr.).

•**antimony sodium tartrate,** U.S.P. 23.
Use: Antischistosomal.

antimony sodium thioglycollate. (Various Mfr.) *Rx.*
Use: Schistosomiasis, leishmaniasis, filariasis.

•**antimony trisulfide colloid.** USAN.
Use: Pharmaceutic aid.

antimonyl potassium tartrate.
See: Antimony Potassium Tartrate, U.S.P. 23.

anti-my9-blocked ricin. USAN.
Use: Leukemia treatment.

antinauseants.
See: Antiemetic/antivertigo agents.

antineoplastic agents.
See: Adriamycin, Vial (Pharmacia & Upjohn & Pharmacia & Upjohn).
Alkeran, Tab. (Glaxo Wellcome).
Amsacrine.
Azacitidine
Blenoxane, Amp. (Bristol).
Cosmegen, Inj. (Merck).
Elspar, Inj. (Merck).
Emcyt, Cap. (Pharmacia & Upjohn).
Estinyl, Tab. (Schering-Plough).
5-Fluorouracil, Amp. (Roche).
FUDR, Vial (Roche).
Hexalen (US Bioscience).
Hydrea, Cap. (Squibb).
Idamycin (Pharmacia & Upjohn).
Leukeran, Tab. (Glaxo Wellcome).
Lysodren, Tab. (Bristol-Myers Oncology).
Matulane, Cap. (Roche).
Medroxyprogesterone Acetate Tab., Vial (Various Mfr.).
Megace, Tab. (Bristol-Myers).

Mercaptopurine, Tab.
Methotrexate, Tab. (Lederle).
Methotrexate Sodium, Vial (Lederle).
Mithracin, Vial (Pfizer).
Mustargen, Inj. (Merck).
Myleran, Tab. (Glaxo Wellcome).
Nolvadex, Tab. (Zeneca).
Oncovin, Amp. (Lilly).
Purinethol, Tab. (Glaxo Wellcome).
TACE, Cap. (Hoechst Marion Roussel).
Tamoxifen, Tab. (Barr).
Thioguanine, Tab. (Glaxo Wellcome).
Thio Tepa, Vial (Lederle).
Uracil Mustard, Cap. (Pharmacia & Upjohn).
Velban, Amp. (Lilly).

antiobesity agents.
See: Acutrim, Prods. (Novartis).
Adderall (Richwood).
Adipex-P, Tab., Cap. (Lemmon).
Amphetamine Preps. (Various Mfr.).
Anorex, Cap. (Dunhall).
Bontril, Prods. (Carnrick).
Control, Cap. (Thompson).
Dexatrim Pre-Meal, Cap. (Thompson).
Dextroamphetamine Preps. (Various Mfr.).
Didrex, Tab. (Pharmacia & Upjohn).
Diethylpropion HCl.
Dieutrim T.D., Cap. (Legere).
Fastin, Cap. (SK-Beecham).
Ionamin, Cap. (Medeva).
Levo-Amphetamine.
Maximum Strength Dexatrim, Cap. (Thompson).
Mazanor, Tab. (Wyeth-Ayerst).
Melfiat-105 Unicelles, Cap. (Solvay)
Methamphetamine Preps. (Various Mfr.).
Obe-Nix 30, Cap. (Holloway).
Obephen, Cap. (Roberts).
Obestin-30, Cap. (Ferndale).
Phendimetrazine Tartrate, Cap., Tab. (Various Mfr.).
Phentermine HCl, Tab., Cap. (Various Mfr.)
Phentermine Resin, Cap. (Various Mfr.).
Phenyldrine, Tab. (Rugby).
Pondimin, Tab. (Robins).
Prelu-2, Cap. (Boehringer Ingelheim).
Sanorex, Tab. (Sandoz).
Slim-Mint, Gum (Thompson).
Tenuate, Tab. (Hoechst Marion Roussel).
Tenuate Dospan, Tab. (SK-Beecham).
Tepanil, Tab. (3M Pharm).
Trimstat, Tab. (Laser).
Wehless Timecelles, Cap. (Roberts).

Antiox. (Mayrand) Vitamin C 120 mg, vitamin E 100 IU, beta carotene 25 mg. Cap. Bot. 60s. *otc.*
Use: Vitamin supplement.

Anti-Pak Compound. (Lowitt) Phenylephrine HCl 5 mg, salicylamide 0.23 g, acetophenetidin 0.15 gr, caffeine 0.03 g, ascorbic acid 50 mg, hesperidin complex 50 mg, chlorprophen-pyridamine maleate 2 mg/Tab. Bot. 30s, 100s. *otc.*
Use: Decongestant, analgesic, antihistamine combination.

antiparasympathomimetics.
See: Parasympatholytic agents.

anti-pellagra vitamin.
See: Nicotinic acid.

anti-pernicious anemia principle.
See: Vitamin B_{12}.

Antiphlogistine. (Denver) Medicated poultice. Jar 5 oz, lb. Tube 8 oz. Can 5 lb.

antiplatelet antibodies.
See: ReoPro (Lilly).

antiprotozoan agents.
See: Antimony Preps.
Arsenic Preps.
Bismuth Preps.
Chiniofon (Various Mfr.).
Diiodohydroxyquinoline.
Emetine HCl (Various Mfr.).
Furazolidone.
Iodocholohydroxyquinoline.
Iodohydroxyquinoline Sulfonate Sodium.
Levofuraltadone.
Ornidyl (Hoechst Marion Roussel).
Quinoxyl.
Suramin Sodium.

•**antipyrine,** U.S.P. 23.
Use: Analgesic, antipyretic.
W/Benzocaine, chlorobutanol.
See: G.B.A., Drops (Scrip).
W/Carbamide, benzocaine, cetyldimethylbenzylammonium HCl.
See: Auralgesic, Liq. (ICN Pharm).
W/Phenylephrine HCl, benzocaine.
See: Tympagesic, Liq. (Pharmacia & Upjohn).
W/Pyrilamine maleate, phenylephrine, benzalkonium.
See: Prefrin-A Ophthalmic (Allergan).

antipyrine and benzocaine otic solution.
Use: Local anesthetic.
See: Auro Ear Drops (Del Pharm).
Lanaurine, Drops (Lannett).
Pyrocaine Eardrop, Liq. (Med. Chem.).

antipyrine, benzocaine and phenylephrine hydrochloride otic solution.
Use: Local anesthetic, decongestant eardrop.

•**antirabies serum,** U.S.P. 23.
Use: Immunizing agent (passive).

antirickettsial agents.
See: p-Aminobenzoic Acid (Various Mfr.).
p-Aminobenzoate Sodium (Various Mfr.).
Aureomycin, Preps. (Lederle).
Chloromycetin, Preps. (Parke-Davis).
Terramycin, Preps. (Pfizer).

antiscorbutic vitamin.
See: Ascorbic Acid.

antiseptic, chlorine, active.
See: Antiseptic, N-Chloro Compounds, Hypochlorite Preps.

antiseptic, dyes.
See: Acriflavine (Various Mfr.).
Aminoacridine HCl.
Bismuth Violet, Preps. (Table Rock).
Brilliant Green.
Crystal Violet.
Fuchsin.
Gentian Violet (Various Mfr.).
Methylrosaniline Cl (Various Mfr.).
Methyl Violet.
Pyridium, Tab. (Parke-Davis).
Serenium, Tab. (Squibb).

antiseptic, mercurials.
See: Mercresin (Pharmacia & Upjohn).
Merthiolate, Preps. (Lilly).
Phenylmercuric Acetate (Various Mfr.).
Phenylmercuric Borate (Various Mfr.).
Phenylmercuric Nitrate (Various Mfr.).
Phenylmercuric Picrate (Various Mfr.).
Thimerosal.

antiseptic, n-chloro compounds.
See: Chloramine-T (Various Mfr.).
Chlorazene, Pow., Tab. (Badger).
Dichloramine-T (Various Mfr.).
Halazone, Tab. (Abbott).

antiseptic, phenols.
See: Anthralin (Various Mfr.).
Bithionol.
Coal Tar Products (Various Mfr.).
Creosote (Various Mfr.).
Cresols (Various Mfr.).
Guaiacol (Various Mfr.).
Hexachlorophene (Various Mfr.).
Hexylresorcinol (Various Mfr.).
Methylparaben (Various Mfr.).
o-Phenylphenol (Various Mfr.).
Oxyquinoline Salts (Various Mfr.).
Parachlorometaxylenol (Various Mfr.).
Phenol (Various Mfr.).

Picric Acid (Various Mfr.).
Propylparaben (Various Mfr.).
Pyrogallol (Various Mfr.).
Resorcinol (Various Mfr.).
Resorcinol Monoacetate (Various Mfr.).
Thymol (Various Mfr.).
Trinitrophenol (Various Mfr.).

antiseptics.
See: Furacin, Preps. (Eaton).
Iodine Products.
Mercurials.
N-Chloro Compounds.
Phenols.
Surface-Active Agents.

antiseptic, surface-active agents.
See: Bactine, Preps. (Bayer).
Benzalkonium Cl (Various Mfr.).
Benzethonium Cl (Various Mfr.).
Ceepryn (Hoechst Marion Roussel).
Cēpacol Preps. (Hoechst Marion Roussel).
Cetylpyridinium Cl (Various Mfr.).
Diaparene Cl, Preps. (Bayer).
Methylbenzethonium Cl (Various Mfr.).
Zephiran Cl, Preps. (Sanofi Winthrop).

Antispas. (Keene) Dicyclomine HCl 10 mg/ml. Vial 10 ml. *Rx.*
Use: Antispasmodic.

antispasmodics. Parasympatholytic agents.
See: Anticholinergic Agents.
Spasmolytic Agents.

Antispasmodic Capsules. (Lemmon) Phenobarbital 16.2 mg, hyoscyamine sulfate 0.1037 mg, atropine sulfate 0.0194 mg, scopolamine HBr 0.0065 mg/Cap. Bot. 1000s. *Rx.*
Use: Sedative, hypnotic, anticholinergic/antispasmodic.

Antispasmodic Elixir. (Various Mfr.) Atropine sulfate 0.0194 mg, scopolamine HBr 0.0065 mg, hyoscyamine HBr or SO$_4$ 0.1037 mg, phenobarbital 16.2 mg/ml w/alcohol 23%. Elix. Bot. 120 ml, pt, gal and UD 5 ml. *Rx.*
Use: Anticholinergic/antispasmodic, sedative, hypnotic.

antistreptolysin-O. Titration procedure.
See: Also (Wampole Labs).

antisterility vitamin.
See: Vitamin E.

anti-t lymphocyte immunotoxin xmmly-h65-rta. (Xoma)
See: Anti Pan T Lymphocyte Monoclonal Antibody.

Anti-Tac, Humanized. (Roche) *Rx.*
Use: Prevention of acute renal allograft rejection. [Orphan drug]

Anti-Ten. (Century) Allylisobutylbarbituric acid ¾ gr, aspirin 3 gr, phenacetin 2 gr, caffeine gr/Tab. Bot. 100s, 1000s. *Rx.*
Use: Sedative, analgesic, CNS stimulant.

Antithrombin III Concentrate IV. *Rx.*
Use: Prophylaxis/treatment of thromboembolic episodes in AT-III deficiency. [Orphan drug]

antithrombin III human. *Rx.*
Use: Thromboembolic agent. [Orphan drug]
See: ATnativ (Baxter).

antithymocyte globulin. *Rx.*
Use: Prevention of allograft rejection. [Orphan drug]
See: Atgam (Pharmacia & Upjohn).

antithyroid agents.
See: Iothiouracil Sodium.
Methimazole.
Methylthiouracil (Various Mfr.).
Propylthiouracil (Various Mfr.).
Tapazole, Tab. (Lilly).

antitoxins.
See: Botulism Antitoxin.
Diphtheria Antitoxin.
Tetanus Immune Globulin.

antitrypsin, alpha 1.
See: alpha-1-antitrypsin.

antituberculosis agents.
See: Aminosalicylates (Na, Ca, K) (Various Mfr.).
Benzoylpas Calcium (Various Mfr.).
Capastat Sulfate, Amp. (Lilly).
Cycloserine.
Dihydrosteptomycin (Various Mfr.).
Isoniazid (Various Mfr.).
Myambutol, Tab. (Lederle).
Niconyl, Tab. (Parke-Davis).
P.A.S. Acid, Tab. (Kasar).
Pasdium, Tab. (Kasar).
Pyrazinamide, Tab. (Lederle).
Rifadin, Cap., Inj. (Hoechst Marion Roussel).
Rimactane, Cap. (Novartis).
Rimactane/INH (Novartis).
Seromycin, Pulv. (Lilly).
Streptomycin (Various Mfr.).
Trecator-SC, Tab. (Wyeth-Ayerst).
Triniad, Tab. (Kasar).
Triniad Plus 30 (Kasar).
Uniad, Tab. (Kasar).
Uniad-Plus 5,10, Tab. (Kasar).

Anti-Tuss. (Century) Guaifenesin 100 mg/5 ml. Bot. 4 oz, gal. *otc.*
Use: Expectorant.

Anti-Tuss D.M. (Century) Guaifenesin 100 mg, dextromethorphan HBr 15 mg/5 ml. Bot. 4 oz, pt, gal. *otc.*
Use: Expectorant, antitussive.

Anti-Tussive. (Canright) Dextromethorphan HBr 10 mg, potassium guaiacol sulfonate 125 mg, terpin hydrate 100 mg, phenylpropanolamine HCl 12.5 mg, pyrilamine maleate 12.5 mg/Tab. Bot. 60s. *otc.*
Use: Antitussive, expectorant, decongestant, antihistamine.

Antitussive Cough Syrup. (Weeks & Leo) Chlorpheniramine 2 mg, phenylephrine HCl 5 mg, dextromethorphan 15 mg, ammonium Cl 50 mg/5 ml. *otc.*
Use: Antihistamine, decongestant, antitussive, expectorant.

Antitussive Cough Syrup with Codeine. (Weeks & Leo) Chlorpheniramine maleate 2 mg, phenylephrine HCl 5 mg, codeine phosphate 10 mg, ammonium Cl 50 mg/5 ml. Bot. 4 oz. *c-v.*
Use: Antihistamine, decongestant, antitussive, expectorant.

antitussive-decongestant.
See: St. Joseph Cough Syrup for Children (Schering-Plough).
Tussend, Tab., Liq. (Hoechst Marion Roussel).

•**antivenin (latrodectus mactans),** U.S.P. 23.
Use: Immunizing agent (passive).

antivenin (latrodectus mactans). Black widow spider antivenin. Each vial contains not less than 6000 antivenin units. Thimerosal (mercury derivative) 1:10,000 added as preservative. Vial 2.5 ml of Sterile Water for Injection and a 1 ml vial of normal horse serum for sensitivity testing.
Use: Treatment of black widow spider bites.

•**antivenin (micrurus fulvius),** U.S.P. 23.
Use: Immunizing agent (passive).

antivenin (micrurus fulvius). North American coral snake antivenin. Lyophilized antivenin of animal origin (*Micrurus fulvius*) with phenol 0.25% and thimerosal 0.005% as preservatives. Bacteriostatic water w/phenylmercuric nitrate 1:100,000 as preservative. Combination package. Vial 10 ml.
Use: Bites of North American coral snake and Texas coral snake.

antivenin Centruroides sculpturatus. (Arizone State University) Available in Arizona only. 5 ml vials.
Use: Neutralizes the venom of the bark scorpion.

•**antivenin (crotalidae) polyvalent,** U.S.P. 23.

Use: Immunizing agent (passive).

antivenin (crotalidae) polyvalent. (Wyeth-Ayerst) Rattlesnake, copperhead and cottonmouth moccasin antitoxic serum. One vial lyophilized serum with 0.25% phenol and 0.005% thimerosal. One vial, 10 ml of bacteriostatic water for inj. w/phenyl mercuric nitrate 0.001%; one vial normal horse serum 1:10, as sensitivity testing material w/ thimerosal 0.005% and phenol 0.35%.
Use: Bites of crotalid snakes of North, Central and South America.

antivenin, polyvalent crotalid (ovine) fab. *Rx.*
Use: Bites of North American crotalid snakes. [Orphan drug]
See: Crotab (Therapeutic Antibodies).

Antivenom (Crotalidae) Purified (Avian). (Ophidian)
Use: Bites of snakes of the crotalidae family. [Orphan drug]

Antivert. (Roerig) Meclizine HCl 12.5 mg, 25 mg or 50 mg/Tab., 25 mg/Chew. tab. **12.5 mg:** Bot. 100s, 1000s, UD 100s; **25 mg:** Bot. 100s, 1000s, UD 100s. **50 mg:** Bot. 100s. *Rx.*
Use: Antiemetic, antivertigo.

antiviral agents.
See: Cytovene, Inj. (Syntex).
Famvir, Tab. (SK-Beecham).
Foscavir, Inj. (Astra).
Hivid, Tab. (Roche).
Retrovir, Preps. (Glaxo Wellcome).
Symmetrel, Cap., Syr. (DuPont Merck).
Videx, Pow., Tab. (Bristol-Myers Squibb).
Vira-A, Inj. (Parke-Davis).
Virazole, Pow. for Reconstitution for aerosol (ICN).
Zerit, Cap. (B-M Squibb).
Zovirax, Cap, Inj. (Glaxo Wellcome).

antiviral antibodies.
See: Cytomegalovirus immune globulin.
Immune globulin IM.
Immune globulin IV.
Hepatitis B immune globulin.
Rabies immune globulin.
Vaccinia immune globulin.
Varicella-zoster immune globulin.

antixerophthalmic vitamin.
See: Vitamin A.

Antrizine Tabs. (Major) Meclizine 12.5 mg, 25 mg or 50 mg/Tab. **12.5 mg:** 100s, 500s, 1000s. **25 mg:** 100s, 500s, 1000s, UD 100s. **50 mg:** 100s. *Rx.*
Use: Antiemetic, antivertigo.

Antrocol Elixir. (ECR) Atropine sulfate 0.195 mg, phenobarbital 16 mg, alcohol 20%/5 ml. Sugar free. Bot. Pt. *Rx.*
Use: Anticholinergic/antispasmodic, sedative/hypnotic.

Antrypol. Suramin. *Rx.*
Use: CDC anti-infective agent.

Anturane. (Novartis) Sulfinpyrazone, U.S.P. **100 mg/Tab.:** Bot 100s. **200 mg/Cap.:** Bot. 100s. *Rx.*
Use: Agent for gout.

Anucaine. (Calvin) Procaine 50 mg, butyl-p-aminobenzoate 200 mg, benzyl alcohol 265 mg in sweet almond oil/5 ml. Amp. 5 ml. Box 6s, 24s, 100s. *otc.*
Use: Anorectal preparation.

Anucort-HC. (G & W) Hydrocortisone acetate 25 mg in a hydrogenated vegetable oil base. Supp. Box 12s, 24s, 100s. *Rx.*
Use: Anorectal preparation.

Anuject. (Roberts) Procaine. Soln. Vial 5 ml or 10 ml. *Rx.*
Use: Anorectal preparation.

Anumed. (Major) Bismuth subgallate 2.25%, bismuth resorcin compound 1.75%, benzyl benzoate 1.2%, zinc oxide 11%, balsam Peru 1.8% in a hydrogenated vegetable oil base. Supp. Box 12s. *otc.*
Use: Anorectal preparation.

Anumed HC. (Major) Hydrocortisone acetate 10 mg. Supp. Box 12s. *Rx.*
Use: Anorectal preparation.

Anuprep HC. (Great Southern) Hydrocortisone acetate 25 mg. Supp. Box 12s.
Use: Anorectal preparation.

Anuprep Hemorrhoidal. (Great Southern) Bismuth subgallate 2.25%, bismuth resorcin compound 1.75%, benzyl benzoate 1.2%, peruvian balsam 1.8% and zinc oxide 11% in a hydrogenated vegetable oil base. Supp. Box 12s, 24s. *Rx.*
Use: Anorectal prepration.

Anusol. (Glaxo Wellcome) Topical starch 51%, benzyl alcohol, soybean oil, tocopheryl acetate. Supp. 12s. *otc.*
Use: Anorectal preparation.

Anusol-HC 2.5%. (Parke-Davis) Hydrocortisone 2.5%. Cream Tube 30 g. *Rx.*
Use: Corticosteroid, topical.

Anusol HC 1. (Parke-Davis) Hydrocortisone 1%, diazolidinyl urea, parabens, mineral oil, sorbitan sesquioleate, white petrolatum. Oint. Tube 21 g. *otc.*
Use: Corticosteroid, topical.

Anusol Ointment. (Parke-Davis Prods)

Pramoxine HCl 1%, zinc oxide 12.5%/g, benzyl benzoate 1.2%, pramoxine HCl 1% in a mineral oil and cocoa butter. Tube. 30 g. *otc.*
Use: Anorectal preparation.

Anxanil. (Econo Med) Hydroxyzine HCl 25 mg/Tab. Bot. 100s. *Rx.*
Use: Antianxiety agent.

Aosept. (Ciba Vision) Hydrogen peroxide 3%, sodium Cl 0.85%, phosphonic acid, phosphate buffer. Soln. Bot. 120 ml, 240 ml, 360 ml. *otc.*
Use: Contact lens care.

Apacet. (Parmed) Acetaminophen 80 mg/Chew. tab. Bot. 100s. *otc.*
Use: Analgesic.

•**apalcillin sodium.** (APE-al-SIH-lin) USAN.
Use: Antibacterial.

APAP.
See: Acetaminophen.

Apatate w/Fluoride. (Kenwood/Bradley) Vitamins B_1 15 mg, B_6 0.5 mg, B_{12} 25 mcg, F 0.5 mg/5 ml. Liq. Bot. 120 ml. *Rx.*
Use: Vitamin/mineral supplement.

Apatate Liquid. (Kenwood/Bradley) Vitamins B_1 15 mg, B_{12} 25 mcg, B_6 0.5 mg/5 ml. Liq. Bot. 120 ml, 240 ml. *otc.*
Use: Vitamin supplement.

Apatate Tablets. (Kenwood/Bradley) Vitamins B_1 15 mg, B_{12} 25 mcg, B_6 0.5 mg/Tab. Bot. 50s. *otc.*
Use: Vitamin supplement.

•**apaxifylline.** (A-pock-SIH-fih-leen) USAN.
Use: Selective adenosine A_1 antagonist.

•**apazone.** (APP-ah-zone) USAN.
Use: Anti-inflammatory.

A.P.C. (Various Mfr.) Aspirin, phenacetin, caffeine. Cap., Tab.
Use: Analgesic combination.
See: A.S.A. Compound, Preps. (Lilly).
P.A.C. Compound, Cap., Tab. (Pharmacia & Upjohn).
Pan-APC, Tab. (Panray).
Phensal, Tab. (Hoechst Marion Roussel).
W/Codeine phosphate. (Various Mfr.).
See: Anexsia w/Codeine, Tab. (SK-Beecham).
Anexsia D, Tab. (SK-Beecham).

A.P.C. w/gelsemium combinations.
See: Aidant, Tab. (Noyes).
Ansemco, No. 2, Tab. (Zeneca).
Asphac-G, Tab. (Schwarz Pharma).
Valacet, Tab. (Pal-Pak).

Apcogesic. (Apco) Sodium salicylate 5 gr, colchicine 1/320 gr, calcium carbonate 65 mg, dried aluminum hydroxide gel 130 mg, phenobarbital ⅛ gr/Tab. Bot. 100s. *Rx.*
Use: Agent for gout, sedative/hypnotic.

Apcohist. (APC) Phenylpropanolamine HCl 25 mg, chlorpheniramine maleate 1 mg/Tab. Bot. 100s. *otc.*
Use: Decongestant, antihistamine.

Apcoretic. (APC) Caffeine anhydrous 100 mg, ammonium Cl 325 mg/Tab. Bot. 90s. *Rx.*
Use: Diuretic.

Ap Creme. (T.E. Williams) Hydrocortisone 0.5%, iodochlorhydroxyquin 3%. Tube oz. *otc, Rx.*
Use: Corticosteroid, antifungal (topical).

Apetil. (Kenwood/Bradley) B_1 1.7 mg, B_2 0.3 mg, B_3 6.7 mg, B_6 2.5 mg, B_{12} 5 mcg, Zn 14.6 mg, Mg, Mn, I-lysine. Liq. Bot. 237 ml. *otc.*
Use: Vitamin/mineral supplement.

APF. (Whitehall Robins).
Use: Salicylate analgesic.
See: Arthritis Pain Formula. (Whitehall Robins).

Aphco Hemorrhoidal Combination. (APC) Combination package of Aphco Hemorrhoidal Ointment 1.5 oz tube, Aphco Hemorrhoidal Supp. Box 12s, 1000s. *otc.*
Use: Anorectal preparation.

Aphen Tabs. (Major) Trihexyphenidyl 2 mg or 5 mg/Tab. Bot. 250s, 1000s. *Rx.*
Use: Antiparkinson agent.

Aphrodyne. (Star) Yohimbine HCl 5.4 mg/Tab. Bot. 100s, 1000s. *Rx.*
Use: Alpha-adrenergic blocking agent.

Aphthasol. (Block) Amlexanox 5%, benzyl alcohol, glyceryl monostearate, mineral oil, petrolatum/Paste. Tube. 5 g. *Rx.*
Use: Treatment of mouth ulcers.

Apicillin. D-(-)-α-Aminobenzyl penicillin.
See: Ampicillin.

A.P.L. (Wyeth-Ayerst) Chorionic Gonadotropin for Injection. 5000 units, 10,000 units or 20,000 units, sterile diluent, w/ benzyl alcohol, phenol, lactose. *Rx.*
Use: Chorionic gonadotropin therapy.

APL 400-200. (Apollon)
Use: Treatment of cutaneous t-cell lymphoma. [Orphan drug]

Aplisol. (Parke-Davis) Tuberculin purified protein derivative diluted 5 units/0.1 ml, polysorbate 80, potassium and sodium phosphates, phenol. Vial 1 ml (10 tests), 5 ml (50 tests).
Use: Diagnostic aid.

Aplitest. (Parke-Davis) Purified tuberculin protein derivative buffered with potassium and sodium phosphates, phenol 0.5%/single-use, multipuncture unit. 25s.
Use: Diagnostic aid.

•**apomorphine hydrochloride,** U.S.P. 23.
Use: Treatment of Parkinson's disease; emetic.

aporphine-10, 11-diol hydrochloride.
See: Apomorphine HCl.

Appedrine. (Thompson Medical) Phenylpropanolamine HCl 25 mg, multivitamins, caffeine 100 mg/Tab. *otc.*
Use: Diet aid.

appetite-depressants.
See: Anorexiants.

APPG.
See: Penicillin G, Procaine, Aqueous.

apraclonidine hydrochloride, (app-rah-KLOE-nih-deen) U.S.P. 23.
Use: Adrenergic (α_2-agonist).
See: Iopidine (Alcon).

•**apramycin.** (APP-rah-MY-sin) USAN.
Use: Antibacterial.

Aprazone. (Major) Sulfinpyrazone. **Cap.:** 200 mg. Bot. 100s, 500s, 1000s. **Tab.:** 100 mg. Bot. 100s. *Rx.*
Use: Agent for gout.

Apresazide. (Novartis) **25/25:** Hydralazine HCl 25 mg, hydrochlorothiazide 25 mg/Cap. **50/50:** Hydralazine HCl 50 mg, hydrochlorothiazide 50 mg/Cap. **100/50:** Hydralazine 100 mg, hydrochlorothiazide 50 mg/Cap. Bot. 100s. *Rx.*
Use: Antihypertensive.

Apresodex. (Rugby) Hydrochlorothiazide 15 mg, hydralazine HCl 25 mg. Tab. Bot. 100s, 1000s. *Rx.*
Use: Antihypertensive.

Apresoline. (Novartis) Hydralazine HCl. **Amp.:** 20 mg w/propylene glycol, methyl and propyl parabens/ml. Pkg. 5s. **Tab.:** 10 mg Bot. 100s, 1200s; 25 mg or 50 mg Bot. 100s, 1000s; 100 mg Bot. 100s. Consumer pack 100s. *Rx.*
Use: Antihypertensive.
W/Serpasil.
See: Serpasil Prods., Preps. (Novartis).

Apresoline-Esidrix. (Novartis) Hydralazine HCl 25 mg, hydrochlorothiazide 15 mg/Tab. Bot. 100s. *Rx.*
Use: Antihypertensive.

•**aprindine.** (APE-rin-deen) USAN.
Use: Cardiac depressant (antiarrhythmic).

•**aprindine hydrochloride.** (APE-rin-deen) USAN.

Use: Cardiac depressant (antiarrhythmic).

aprobarbital. Pow. *c-iii.*
Use: Sedative/hypnotic.
See: Alurate, Elix. (Roche).

Aprobee w/C. (Approved) Vitamins B_1 15 mg, B_2 10 mg, B_6 5 mg, niacinamide 50 mg, calcium pantothenate 10 mg, C 250 mg/Cap. or Tab. **Cap.:** Bot. 100s, 1000s. **Tab.:** Bot. 50s, 100s, 1000s. *otc.*
Use: Vitamin/mineral supplement.

Aprodine. (Major) **Tab.:** Pseudoephedrine HCl 60 mg, triprolidine HCl 2.5 mg. Bot. 24s, 100s, 1000s, UD 100s. **Syr.:** Pseudoephedrine HCl 30 mg, triprolidine HCl 1.25 mg/5 ml. Bot. 120 ml, pt. *otc.*
Use: Decongestant, antihistamine.

Aprodine w/C. (Major) Pseudoephedrine HCl 30 mg, triprolidine HCl 1.25 mg, codeine phosphate 10 mg. Syr. Bot. pt, gal. *c-v.*
Use: Decongestant, antihistamine.

•**aprotinin.** (app-row-TIE-nin) USAN. A polypeptide proteinase inhibitor.
Use: Enzyme inhibitor (proteinase). [Orphan drug]
See: Trasylol, Inj. (Bayer).

Aprozide 25/25 capsules. (Major) Hydralazine 25 mg, hydrochlorothiazide 25 mg/Cap. Bot. 100s, 250s. *Rx.*
Use: Antihypertensive.

Aprozide 50/50 capsules. (Major) Hydrochlorothiazide 50 mg, hydralazine 50 mg/Cap. Bot. 100s, 250s. *Rx.*
Use: Antihypertensive.

A.P.S. Aspirin, phenacetin and salicylamide.

•**aptazapine maleate.** USAN.
Use: Antidepressant.

•**aptiganel hydrochloride.** (app-tih-GAN-ehl) USAN.
Use: Stroke and brain injury treatment (NMDA ion channel blocker).

APSAC. Thrombolytic enzyme.
See: Eminase (SK-Beecham).

apyron.
See: Magnesium acetylsalicylate.

AQ-4B. (Western Research) Trichlormethiazide 4 mg/Tab. Bot. 1000s. *Rx.*
Use: Diuretic.

Aqua-Ban. (Thompson Medical) Caffeine 100 mg, ammonium Cl 325 mg/Tab. Bot. 60s. *otc.*
Use: Diuretic.

Aqua-Ban Plus. (Thompson Medical) Ammonium Cl 650 mg, caffeine 200 mg, iron 6 mg/Tab. Bot. 30s. *otc.*

Use: Diuretic, mineral supplement.

Aquabase. (Pal-Pak) Cetyl alcohol, propylene glycol, sodium lauryl sulfate, white wax, purified water. Jar lb. *otc.*
Use: Hydrophilic ointment base.

Aquacare Cream. (Allergan Herbert) Urea 2%, benzyl alcohol, carbomer 934, cetyl esters wax, fragrance, glycerin, oleth-3 phosphate, petrolatum, phenyl dimethicone, water, sodium hydroxide. Tube 2.5 oz. *otc.*
Use: Emollient.

Aquacare/HP. (Allergan Herbert) Urea 10%, benzyl alcohol. **Cream:** Tube 2.5 oz. **Lot.:** Bot. 8 oz, 16 oz. *otc.*
Use: Emollient.

Aquacare Lotion. (Allergan Herbert) Benzyl alcohol, oleth-3 phosphate, phenyl dimethicone, fragrance. Bot. 8 oz. *otc.*
Use: Emollient.

Aquachloral. (PolyMedica) Chloral hydrate, polyethylene glycol, spreading agent. Supp. 5 gr, 10 gr. Strip 12s. *c-iv.*
Use: Sedative, hypnotic (rectal).

Aquacillin G. (Armenpharm Ltd.) Penicillin G. *Rx.*
Use: Anti-infective, penicillin.

Aquacycline. (Armenpharm, Ltd.) Tetracycline HCl. *Rx.*
Use: Anti-infective, tetracycline.

Aquaderm. (C & M Pharmacal) Purified water, glycerin 25%, salicylic acid 0.1%, octoxynol-9 0.03%, FD & C; Red #40 0.0001%. Bot. 2 oz. *otc.*
Use: Emollient.

Aquaderm. (Baker Cummins). Octyl methoxycinnamate 7.5%, oxybenzone 6%. SPF 15. Cream 105 g. *otc.*
Use: Sunscreen.

Aquaflex Ultrasound Gel Pad. (Parker) Clear, solid, flexible, moist, standoff gel pad for use where transducer movement is impeded by bony or irregular body surfaces. 2 cm × 9 cm.
Use: Ultrasound agent.

Aquafuren. (Armenpharm Ltd.) Nitrofurantoin. *Rx.*
Use: Anti-infective, urinary.

Aquagen. (ALK Laboratories) Allergenic extracts. Vials.

aquakay.
See: Menadione (Various Mfr.).

Aqua Lacten Lotion. (Herald Pharmacal) Demineralized water, urea, petrolatum, propylene glycol monostearate, sorbitan monostearate, lactic acid. Bot. 8 oz. *otc.*
Use: Emollient.

Aquamephyton Injection. (Merck) Phytonadione 2 mg/ml or 10 mg/ml, vitamin K-1, w/polyoxyethylated fatty acid derivative 70 mg, dextrose 37.5 mg, benzyl alcohol 0.9%, water for injection q.s. to 1 ml. Inj. Amp. 1 mg/0.5 ml Box 25s; 10 mg/1 ml Box 6s, 25s. Vial 10 mg/ml 2.5 ml, 5 ml. *Rx.*
Use: Prothrombogenic.

Aqua Mist. (Faraday) Nasal spray. Squeeze Bot. 20 ml.

Aquamycin. (Armenpharm, Ltd.) Erythromycin. *Rx.*
Use: Anti-infective, erythromycin.

Aquanil. (Sig) Mersalyl 100 mg, theophylline (hydrate) 50 mg, methylparaben 0.18%, propylparaben 0.02%. Vial 10 ml. *otc.*
Use: Diuretic, bronchodilator.

Aquanil Cleanser. (Person & Covey) Glycerin, cetyl, stearyl and benzyl alcohol, sodium laureth sulfate, xanthan gum. Lipid free. Lot. Bot. 240 ml, 480 ml. *otc.*
Use: Therapeutic skin cleanser.

Aquanine. (Armenpharm Ltd.) Quinine HCl. *Rx.*
Use: Antimalarial.

Aquaoxy. (Armenpharm, Ltd.) Oxytetracycline HCl. *Rx.*
Use: Anti-infective, tetracycline.

Aquaphenicol. (Armenpharm, Ltd.) Chloramphenicol. *Rx.*
Use: Anti-infective.

Aquaphilic Ointment. (Medco Lab) Hydrated hydrophilic oint. Jar 16 oz. *otc.*
Use: Emollient, ointment base.

Aquaphilic Ointment with Carbamide 10% and 20%. (Medco Lab) Stearyl alcohol, white petrolatum, sorbitol, propylene glycol, sodium lauryl sulfate, lactic acid, methylparaben, propylparaben.
Use: Prescription compounding, emollient.

Aquaphor Natural Healing. (Beiersdorf) Petrolatum, mineral oil, mineral wax, woolwax alcohol, panthenol, glycerin, chamomile essense. Oint. Tube 52.5 g. *otc.*
Use: Emollient.

Aquaphor. (Beiersdorf) Cholesterolized anhydrous petrolatum ointment base. Tube 1.75 oz, 3.25 oz, 16 oz, Jar 5 lb, Bar 3 oz. *otc.*
Use: Water-miscible ointment base.
See: Eucerin, Emulsion (Duke).

Aquaphor Antibiotic. (Beiersdorf) 10,000 units polymyxin B sulfate and

500 units bacitracin zinc/g in a cholesterolized ointment base. Oint. Tube 15 g. *otc.*
Use: Anti-infective, topical.

Aquaphyllin Syrup. (Ferndale) Theophylline anhydrous 80 mg/15 ml UD pk. 15 ml, 30 ml. Bot. 16 oz, gal. *Rx.*
Use: Bronchodilator.

Aquapool Concentrate. (Parker) Color additive for hydrotherapy to control foaming. Bot. pt, gal.

AquaSite. (Ciba Vision) PEG-400 0.2%, dextran 70, polycarbophil, NaCl, EDTA, sodium hydroxide. Preservative free. Soln. Single-use vials 0.6 ml, 15 ml. *otc.*
Use: Artificial tears.

Aquasol A. (Astra) Water-miscible Vitamin A. Chlorobutanol 0.5%, polysorbate 80, butylated hydroxyanisole, butylated hydroxytoluene. **Inj.:** 50,000 U.S.P. units/ml. Vial 2 ml Box 10s. **Cap.:** 25,000 U.S.P. units/Cap. Bot. 100s. 50,000 U.S.P. units/Cap. Bot. 100s, 500s. **Drops:** 5000 U.S.P. units/0.1 ml. Bot. 30 ml w/dropper. *otc, Rx.*
Use: Vitamin A supplement.

Aquasol E. (Astra) Vitamin E. **Cap.:** 73.5 mg Bot. 100s; 400 IU Bot. 30s. **Drops:** 50 mg/ml Bot. 12 ml, 30 ml w/dropper. *otc.*
Use: Vitamin E supplement.

Aquasonic 100. (Parker) Water-soluble, viscous, contact medium gel for ultrasonic transmission. Bot. 250 ml, 1 L, 5 L.
Use: Ultrasound agent.

Aquasonic 100 sterile. (Parker) Water-soluble, sterile gel for ultrasonic transmission. Overwrapped Foil Pouches 15 g, 50 g.
Use: Ultrasound agent.

Aquasulf. (Armenpharm, Ltd.) Triple sulfa tablet. *Rx.*
Use: Anti-infective.

Aquatar Therapeutic Tar Gel. (Allergan Herbert) Coal tar extract (BioTar) 2.5% w/DEA oleth-3 phosphate, glycerin, imidurea, methylparaben, mineral oil, oleth-3, oleth-10, oleth-20, poloxamer 407, polysorbate 80, propylparaben, purified water. Tube 3 oz. *otc.*
Use: Antipruritic, keratoplastic, antipsoriatic.

Aquatensen. (Wallace) Methyclothiazide 5 mg/Tab. Bot. 100s, 500s. *Rx.*
Use: Diuretic, antihypertensive.

Aquavite. (Armenpharm, Ltd.) Soluble multivitamin.
Use: Vitamin supplement.

Aquazide. (Western Research) Trichlormethiazide 4 mg/Tab. Bot. 100s. *Rx.*
Use: Antihypertensive, diuretic.

Aquazide H. (Western Research) Hydrochlorothiazide 50 mg/Tab. Bot. 1000s. *Rx.*
Use: Diuretic.

Aquazol. (Armenpharm, Ltd.) Sulfisoxazole.
Use: Anti-infective.

Aqueous Allergens. (Bayer).
Use: Allergenic extracts.

Aquest. (Dunhall) Estrone 2 mg/ml. Sodium carboxymethylcellulose, povidone, benzyl alcohol, parabens. Vial 10 ml. *Rx.*
Use: Estrogen.

aquinone.
See: Menadione, U.S.P. 23.

Aquol Bath Oil. (Lamond) Vegetable oil, olive oil. Bot. 4 oz, 6 oz, 16 oz, qt, gal. *otc.*
Use: Emollient, antipruritic.

ar-121. (Argus) Phase I/II HIV. *Rx.*
Use: Antiviral.

ARA-A.
See: Vidarabine.

ARA-C.
See: Cytarabine.

Aralen Hydrochloride. (Sanofi Winthrop) Chloroquine HCl 50 mg/ml. Amp 5 ml. *Rx.*
Use: Antimalarial, amebicide.

Aralen Phosphate. (Sanofi Winthrop) Chloroquine phosphate 500 mg/Tab. Bot. 25s. *Rx.*
Use: Antimalarial, amebicide.

Aralis Tablets. (Sanofi Winthrop) Glycobiarsol, chloroquine phosphate. *Rx.*
Use: Amebicide.

Aramine. (Merck) Metaraminol bitartrate (equivalent to metaraminol) 10 mg/ml, sodium Cl 4.4 mg, water for injection q.s. ad. 1 ml, methylparaben 0.15%, propylparaben 0.02%, sodium bisulfite 0.2%. Vial 10 ml. *Rx.*
Use: Treatment of acute hypotension.

•**aranotin.** (AR-ah-NO-tin) USAN.
Use: Antiviral.

•**arbaprostil.** USAN.
Use: Antisecretory (gastric).

Arbolic. (Burgin-Arden) Methandriol dipropionate 50 mg/ml. Vial 10 ml. *Rx.*
Use: Anabolic steroid.

Arbutal. (Arcum) Butalbital ¾ gr, phenacetin 2 gr, aspirin 3 gr, caffeine gr/Tab. Bot. 100s, 1000s. *Rx.*
Use: Sedative, hypnotic, analgesic.

•**arbutamine hydrochloride.** (ahr-BYOO-tah-meen) USAN.
Use: Cardiac stimulant.

Arcet. (EconoMed) Butalbital 50 mg, acetaminophen 325 mg, caffeine 40 mg/Tab. Bot. 100s. *Rx.*
Use: Analgesic, sedative, hypnotic.

•**arcitumomab.** (ahr-sigh-TOO-moe-mab) USAN.
Use: Monoclonal antibody.
See: CEA-Scan (Immunomedics, Mallinckrodt).

•**arclofenin.** (AHR-kloe-FEN-in) USAN.
Use: Diagnostic aid for hepatic function determination.

Arcoban Tablets. (Arcum) Meprobamate 400 mg/Tab. Bot. 50s, 1000s. *Rx.*
Use: Antianxiety agent.

Arcobee w/C. (NTBY) Vitamins B_1 15 mg, B_2 10.2 mg, B_3 50 mg, B_5 10 mg, B_6 5 mg, C 300 mg, tartrazine. Cap. Box 100s. *otc.*
Use: Vitamin supplement.

Arcobex Extra Strength Caps. (Arcum) Vitamins B_1 100 mg, B_2 2 mg, B_6 5 mg, niacinamide 125 mg, panthenol 10 mg, B_{12} 30 mcg, benzyl alcohol 1%, genistic acid ethanolamine 2.5%/ml. Vial 30 ml. *Rx.*
Use: Vitamin B supplement.

Arcodex Antacid Tablets. (Arcum) Magnesium trisilicate 500 mg, aluminum hydroxide 250 mg/Tab. Bot. 100s, 1000s. *otc.*
Use: Antacid.

Arco-Lase. (Arco) Trizyme 38 mg (amylase 30 mg, protease 6 mg, cellulase 2 mg), lipase 25 mg/Tab. Bot. 50s. *Rx.*
Use: Digestive aid.

Arco-Lase Plus. (Arco) Phenobarbital 8 mg, hyoscyamine sulfate 0.1 mg, atropine sulfate 0.02 mg, trizyme 38 mg, lipase 25 mg/Tab. Bot. 50s. *Rx.*
Use: Sedative, hypnotic, digestive aid.

Arcosterone. (Arcum) Methyltestosterone. **Oral:** 10 mg or 25 mg/Tab. Bot. 100s, 1000s. **Sublingual:** 10 mg/Tab. Bot. 100s, 1000s. *Rx.*
Use: Androgen.

Arco-Thyroid. (Arco) Thyroid 1.5 gr/Tab. Bot. 1000s. *Rx.*
Use: Thyroid hormone.

Arcotrate. (Arcum) Pentaerythritol tetranitrate 10 mg/Tab. **No. 2:** Pentaerythritol tetranitrate 20 mg/Tab. **No. 3:** Pentaerythritol tetranitrate 20 mg, phenobarbital ⅛ gr/Tab. Bot. 100s, 1000s. *Rx.*
Use: Antianginal.

Arcoval Improved. (Arcum) Vitamin A palmitate 10,000 IU, D 400 IU, thiamine mononitrate 15 mg, B_2 10 mg, nicotinamide 150 mg, B_6 5 mg, calcium pantothenate 10 mg, B_{12} 5 mcg, C 150 mg, E 5 IU/Cap. Bot. 100s, 1000s. *otc.*
Use: Vitamin/mineral supplement.

Arcum R-S. (Arcum) Reserpine 0.25 mg/Tab. Bot. 100s, 1000s. *Rx.*
Use: Antihypertensive.

Arcum V-M. (Arcum) Vitamin A palmitate 5000 IU, D 400 IU, B_1 2.5 mg, B_2 2.5 mg, B_6 0.5 mg, B_{12} 2 mcg, C 50 mg, niacinamide 20 mg, calcium pantothenate 5 mg, iron 18 mg/Cap. Bot. 100s, 1000s. *otc.*
Use: Vitamin/mineral supplement.

A-R-D. (Birchwood) Anatomically shaped dressing. Dispenser 24s.
Use: Rectal counterirritant, antipruritic.

Ardeben. (Burgin-Arden) Diphenhydramine HCl 10 mg, chlorobutanol 0.5%. Inj. Vial 30 ml. *Rx.*
Use: Antihistamine.

Ardecaine 1%. (Burgin-Arden) Lidocaine HCl 1%. Inj. Vial 30 ml. *Rx.*
Use: Anesthetic, topical.

Ardecaine 2%. (Burgin-Arden) Lidocaine HCl 2%. Inj. Vial 30 ml. *Rx.*
Use: Anesthetic, topical.

Ardecaine 1% w/Epinephrine. (Burgin-Arden) Lidocaine HCl 1%, epinephrine. Inj. Vial 30 ml. *Rx.*
Use: Anesthetic, topical.

Ardecaine 2% w/Epinephrine. (Burgin-Arden) Lidocaine HCl 2%, epinephrine. Inj. Vial 30 ml. *Rx.*
Use: Anesthetic, topical.

Ardefem 10. (Burgin-Arden) Estradiol valerate 10 mg/ml. Vial 10 ml. *Rx.*
Use: Estrogen.

Ardefem 20. (Burgin-Arden) Estradiol valerate 20 mg/ml. Vial 10 ml. *Rx.*
Use: Estrogen.

Ardefem 40. (Burgin-Arden) Estradiol valerate 40 mg/ml. Vial 10 ml. *Rx.*
Use: Estrogen.

•**ardeparin sodium.** USAN.
Use: Anticoagulant.

Ardepred Soluble. (Burgin-Arden) Prednisolone 20 mg, niacinamide 25 mg, disodium edetate 0.5 mg, sodium bisulfite 1 mg, phenol 5 mg/ml. Vial 10 ml. *Rx.*
Use: Corticosteroid combination.

Arderone 100. (Burgin-Arden) Testosterone enanthate 100 mg/ml. Vial 10 ml. *c-III.*
Use: Androgen.

Arderone 200. (Burgin-Arden) Testosterone enanthate 200 mg/ml. Vial 10 ml. *c-III.*
Use: Androgen.

Ardevila tablets. (Sanofi Winthrop) Inositol hexanicotinate. *Rx.*
Use: Vasodilator.

Ardiol 90/4. (Burgin-Arden) Testosterone enanthate 90 mg, estradiol valerate 4 mg/ml. Vial 10 ml. *Rx.*
Use: Androgen/estrogen combination.

Arduan. (Organon) Pipecuronium Br 10 mg/10 ml. Vial. *Rx.*
Use: Neuromuscular blocking agent.

arecoline acetarsone salt.
See: Drocarbil.

Aredia. (Novartis) Pamidronate disodium 30 mg, 60 mg, 90 mg. Lyophilized inj. Vial. *Rx.*
Use: Treatment of hypercalcemia.

Ar-EX products. (Ar-Ex) A series of hypo-allergenic products for sensitive skin including: *otc.*
Skin Care Products:
Body Lotion.
Chap Cream.
Cleansing Cream.
Cold Cream.
Cream For Dry Skin.
Enriched Night Cream.
Eye Cream.
Moisture Cream.
Moisture Lotion.
Personal Care Products:
Bath Oil.
Bath Soap.
Cream Deodorant.
Roll-On Deodorant.
Safe Suds (liquid detergent).
Shampoo.
Soap.
Cosmetics and Eye Make-up:
Brush-On.
Disappear (blemish stick).
Eye Make-Up Remover Pads.
Eye Pencil.
Face and Compact Powder.
Foundation Lotion.
Lip Gloss.
Lipstick.
Mascara.

Argesic. (Econo Med) Methyl salicylate and triethanolamine in a nongreasy vanishing cream base. Jar 60 g. *otc.*
Use: Analgesic, topical.

Argesic-SA. (Econo Med) Disalicylic acid 500 mg/Tab. Bot. 100s. *Rx.*
Use: Analgesic, topical.

•**arginine,** (AHR-jih-neen) U.S.P. 23.
Use: Ammonia detoxicant; diagnostic aid (pituitary function determination).

arginine butyrate. (AHR-jih-neen) *Rx.*
Use: Treatment of sickle cell disease and beta-thalassemia. [Orphan drug]

•**arginine glutamate.** (AHR-jih-neen GLUE-tah-mate) USAN.
Use: Ammonia detoxicant.
See: Modumate (Abbott).

arginine hydrochloride. (AHR-jih-neen)
Use: Diagnostic aid.
See: R-Gene 10, Inj. (Pharmacia & Upjohn).

•**arginine hydrochloride,** U.S.P. 23.
Use: Ammonia detoxicant.

8-arginine-vasopressin.
See: Vasopressin.

•**argipressin tannate.** (AHR-JIH-press-in TAN-ate) USAN.
Use: Antidiuretic.

argyn.
See: Mild Silver Protein (Various Mfr.).

Aricept. (Eisai/Pfizer) Donepezil HCl 5 mg and 10 mg/Tab. Blister pack. 30s and 100s. *Rx.*
Use: Treatment of mild to moderate dementia associated with Alzheimer's disease.

Aridol. (MPL) Pamabrom 52 mg, pyrilamine maleate 30 mg, homatropine methylbromide 1.2 mg, hyoscyamine sulfate 0.10 mg, scopolamine HBr 0.02 mg, methamphetamine HCl 1.5 mg/Tab. Bot. 100s. *Rx.*
Use: Diuretic, anticholinergic, antispasmodic, CNS stimulant.

•**arildone.** (AR-ill-dohn) USAN.
Use: Antiviral.

Armidex. (Zeneca) Anastrozole 1 mg, lactose/Tab. 30s *Rx.*
Use: Aromatase inhibitor.

Aris Phenobarbital Reagent Strips. (Bayer) Box 25s.
Use: Diagnostic aid.

Aris Phenytoin Reagent Strips. (Bayer) Box 25s.
Use: Diagnostic aid.

Aristocort. (Lederle) Triamcinolone.
Tab.: 1 mg Bot. 50s; 2 mg Bot. 100s; 4 mg Bot. 30s, 100s; 8 mg Bot. 50s.
Syr.: Diacetate (w/methylparaben 0.08%, propylparaben 0.02%) 2 mg/5 ml. Bot. 4 oz. *Rx.*
Use: Corticosteroid.

Aristocort A Cream. (Fujisawa) Triamcinolone acetonide w/emulsifying wax, isopropyl palmitate, glycerin, sorbitol, lactic acid, benzyl alcohol.
0.025% w/Aquatain: Tube 15 g, 60 g.
0.1%: Tube 15 g, 60 g, Jar 240 g.

0.5%: Tube 15 g. *Rx.*
Use: Corticosteroid, topical.
Aristocort Acetonide, Sodium Phosphate Salt. (Lederle)
Use: Corticosteroid, topical.
See: Aristocort Preps.
Sodium Phosphate Triamcinolone Acetonide.
Aristocort A Ointment. (Fujisawa) Triamcinolone acetonide 0.1%. Tube 15 g, 60 g. *Rx.*
Use: Corticosteroid, topical.
Aristocort Cream. (Fujisawa) Triamcinolone acetonide w/emulsifying wax, polysorbate 60, mono and diglycerides, squalane, sorbitol soln., sorbic acid, potassium sorbate. **LP: 0.025%:** Tube 15 g, 60 g, Jar 240 g, 480 g; **R: 0.1%:** Tube 15 g, 60 g, Jar 240 g, 480 g; **HP: 0.5%:** Tube 15 g, Jar 240 g. *Rx.*
Use: Corticosteroid, topical.
Aristocort Forte. (Lederle) Triamcinolone diacetate 40 mg/ml. Vial 1 ml, 5 ml. *Rx.*
Use: Corticosteroid.
Aristocort Intralesional. (Lederle) Triamcinolone diacetate 25 mg/ml. Vial 5 ml. *Rx.*
Use: Corticosteroid.
Aristocort Ointment. (Fujisawa) Triamcinolone acetonide. **R: 0.1%:** Tube 15 g, 60 g, Jar 240 g. **HP: 0.5%:** Tube 15 g, Jar 240 g. *Rx.*
Use: Corticosteroid, topical.
Aristo-Pak. (Lederle) Triamcinolone 4 mg/Tab. 16s. *Rx.*
Use: Corticosteroid.
Aristospan Intra-Articular. (Lederle) Triamcinolone hexacetonide 20 mg/ml micronized susp., polysorbate 80 0.4% w/v, sorbitol soln. 64% w/v, water q.s., benzyl alcohol 0.9% w/v. Vial 1 ml, 5 ml. *Rx.*
Use: Corticosteroid.
Aristospan Intralesional. (Lederle) Triamcinolone hexacetonide 5 mg/ml, polysorbate 80 0.2% w/v, sorbitol soln. 64% w/v, water q.s., benzyl alcohol 0.9% w/v. Vial 5 ml. *Rx.*
Use: Corticosteroid.
Arlacel 83. (Zeneca) Sorbitan Sesquioleate.
Use: Surface-active agent.
Arlacel 165. (Zeneca) Glyceryl monostearate, PEG-100 stearate nonionic self-emulsifying.
Use: Surface-active agent.
Arlacel C. (Zeneca) Sorbitan Sesquioleate. Mixture of oleate esters of sorbitol and its anhydrides.

Use: Surface-active agent.
Arlamol E. (Zeneca) Polyoxypropylene (15), stearyl ether, BHT 0.1%.
Use: Emollient.
Arlatone 507. (Zeneca) Padimate O. *otc.*
Use: Sunscreen.
Arlix. (Hoechst Marion Roussel) Piretanide HCl. *Rx.*
Use: Diuretic, antihypertensive.
Arm-a-Med Isoetharine Hydrochloride. (Astra) Isoetharine 0.125%, sodium metabisulfite, glycerin. Soln. for nebulization. Bot. UD 4 ml. *Rx.*
Use: Bronchodilator.
Arm-a-Med Metaproterenol Sulfate. (Centeon) Soln. for nebulization: Metaproterenol sulfate 0.4% or 0.6% with sodium Cl, EDTA. Vial UD 2.5 ml for use with IPPB device. *Rx.*
Use: Bronchodilator.
Arm-a-Vial. (Centeon) Sterile water, sodium Cl 0.45% or 0.9%. Box 100s. Plastic vial 3 ml, 5 ml.
Use: Electrolyte.
A.R.M. Caplets. (Menley & James) Chlorpheniramine maleate 4 mg, phenylpropanolamine HCl 25 mg/Capl. Pkg. 20s, 40s. *otc.*
Use: Antihistamine, decongestant.
Aromatic Ammonia Vaporole. (Glaxo Wellcome) Inhalant. Vial 5 min. Box 10s, 12s, 100s. *Rx.*
Use: Respiratory/CNS stimulant.
•**aromatic elixir.** N.F. 18.
Use: Pharmaceutic aid (vehicle; flavored, sweetened).
aromatic elixir. (Lilly) Alcohol 22%. Bot. 16 fl. oz.
Use: Flavored vehicle.
Arnica Tincture. (Lilly) Arnica 20% in alcohol 66%. Bot. 120 ml, 480 ml. *otc.*
Use: Analgesic, topical.
•**arprinocid.** (ahr-PRIN-oh-sid) USAN.
Use: Coccidiostat.
arseclor.
See: Dichlorophenarsine HCl (Various Mfr.).
arsenic compounds.
Use: Rarely employed in modern medicine; there are no longer any official compounds.
See: Acetarson.
Arsphenamine.
Carbarsone (Various Mfr.).
Dichlorophenarsine HCl.
Ferric Cacodylate.
Glycobiarsol.
Neoarsphenamine.
Oxophenarsine HCl.

Sodium Cacodylate (Various Mfr.). Tryparsamide.

arsenobenzene.
See: Arsphenamine.

arsenphenolamine.
See: Arsphenamine.

Arsobal. Melarsoprol (Mel B).
Use: CDC anti-infective agent.

arsphenamine. Arsenobenzene, arseno-benzol, arsenphenolamine, Ehrlich 606, salvarsan.
Use: Formerly used as antisyphilitic.

arsthinol. Cyclic.
Use: Antiprotozoal.

Artane. (Lederle) Trihexyphenidyl HCl. **Elix.:** 2 mg/5 ml w/methylparaben 0.08%, propylparaben 0.02%, Bot. Pt. **Tab.:** 2 mg or 5 mg, Bot. 100s, 1000s, UD 10×10 in 10s. **Sequel:** 5 mg Bot. 60s, 500s. *Rx.*
Use: Antiparkinsonian.

Artarau. (Archer-Taylor) Rauwolfia serpentina 50 mg or 100 mg/Tab. Bot. 100s, 1000s. *Rx.*
Use: Antihypertensive.

Arta-Vi-C. (Archer-Taylor) Multivitamins with Vitamin C 100 mg/Tab. Bot. 100s. *otc.*
Use: Vitamin supplement.

Artazyme. (Archer-Taylor) Bot. 13 ml.
Use: Autolyzed proteolytic enzyme.

•**arteflene.** (AHR-teh-fleen) USAN.
Use: Antimalarial.

•**artegraft.** (AHR-teh-graft) USAN. Arterial graft composed of a section of bovine carotid artery that has been subjected to enzymatic digestion with ficin and tanned with dialdehyde starch.
Use: Prosthetic aid (arterial).

arterenol.
See: Norepinephrine bitartrate.

Artha-G. (T.E. Williams) Salsalate 750 mg/Tab. Bot. 120s. *Rx.*
Use: Salicylate analgesic.

Arthralgen. (Robins) Salicylamide 250 mg, acetaminophen 250 mg/Tab. Bot. 30s, 100s, 500s. *otc.*
Use: Analgesic combination.

Arthricare Daytime Formula. (Del Pharm.) Menthol 1.25%, methyl nico-tinate 0.25%, capsaicin 0.025%, with aloe vera gel, carbomer 940, DMDM hydantoin, glyceryl stearate SE, myristyl propionate, propylparaben, triethanol-amine. Cream. Jar 90 g. *otc.*
Use: Analgesic for arthritis, topical.

Arthricare Double Ice. (Del Pharm.) Menthol 4%, camphor 3.1%, with aloe vera gel, carbomer 940, dioctyl sodium sulfosuccinate, propylene glycol, tri-ethanolamine. Gel. Jar 90 g. *otc.*
Use: Analgesic for arthritis, topical.

Arthricare Odor Free Rub. (Del Pharm.) Menthol 1.25%, methyl nicotinate 0.25%, capsaicin 0.025%, aloe vera gel, carbomer 940, DMDM hydantoin, emulsifying wax, glyceryl stearate SE, isopropyl alcohol, myristyl propionate, propylparaben, triethanolamine. Oint. Jar 90 g. *otc.*
Use: Rub and liniment.

Arthricare Triple Medicated. (Del Pharm.) Methylsalicylate 30%, menthol 1.25%, methyl nicotinate 0.7%, dioc-tyl sodium sulfosuccinate, hydroxypro-pylmethylcellulose, isopropyl alcohol, propylene glycol. Gel. Tube 3 oz. *otc.*
Use: Analgesic, topical.

Arthritic Pain Lotion. (Walgreen) Tri-ethanolamine salicylate 10%. Bot. 6 oz. *otc.*
Use: Analgesic, topical.

Arthritis Bayer Timed Release Aspirin. (Bayer) Aspirin 650 mg/TR Tab. Bot. 30s, 72s, 125s. *otc.*
Use: Salicylate analgesic.

Arthritis Foundation Pain Reliever. (McNeil-PPC) Aspirin 500 mg/Tab. Bot. 50s. *otc.*
Use: Analgesic.

Arthritis Hot Creme. (Thompson) Methyl salicylate 15%, menthol 10%, glyceryl stearate, carbomer 934, lanolin, PEG-100 stearate, propylene glycol, trola-mine, parabens. Cream Jar 90 g. *otc.*
Use: Rub and liniment.

Arthritis Pain Formula. (Whitehall Rob-ins) Aspirin 486 mg, aluminum hydrox-ide gel 20 mg, magnesium hydroxide 60 mg/Tab. Bot. 40s, 100s, 175s. *otc.*
Use: Analgesic combination.

Arthritis Pain Formula, Aspirin Free. (Whitehall Robins) Acetaminophen 500 mg/Tab. Bot. 30s, 75s. *otc.*
Use: Analgesic.

Arthropan Liquid. (Purdue Frederick) Choline salicylate 870 mg/5 ml. Bot. 8 oz, 16 oz. *Rx.*
Use: Analgesic.

Arthrotrin Tablets. (Whiteworth Towne) Enteric coated aspirin 325 mg/Tab. Bot. 100s.
Use: Salicylate analgesic.

Articulose-50. (Seatrace) Prednisolone acetate 50 mg/ml. Vial 10 ml, 30 ml.
Use: Corticosteroid.

Articulose L. A. (Seatrace) Triamcino-lone diacetate 40 mg/ml. Vial 5 ml. *Rx.*

Use: Corticosteroid.

artificial tanning agent.
See: QT, Prods. (Schering-Plough).
Sudden Tan, Prods. (Schering-
Plough).

artificial tear insert.
See: Lacrisert (Merck).

artificial tears. (Various Mfr.) Benzalkonium Cl 0.01%. May also contain
EDTA, NaCl, polyvinyl alcohol. Sol. Bot.
15 ml or 30 ml. *otc.*
Use: Lubricant, ophthalmic.

Artificial Tears Ointment. (Rugby) White
petrolatum, anhydrous liquid lanolin,
mineral oil. Ophth. Oint. Tube 3.5 g. *otc.*
Use: Ocular lubricant.

Artificial Tears Plus. (Various Mfr.) Polyvinyl alcohol 1.4%, povidone 0.6%,
chlorobutanol 0.5%, NaCl. Soln. Bot.
15 ml. *otc.*
Use: Lubricant, ophthalmic.

•**artilide fumarate.** (AHR-tih-lide) USAN.
Use: Cardiac depressant (antiarrhythmic).

Artra Beauty Bar. (Schering-Plough) Triclocarban 1% in soap base. Cake 3.6
oz. *otc.*
Use: Skin cleanser.

Artra Skin Tone Cream. (Schering-
Plough) Hydroquinone 2%. Oint. Tube
1 oz. (normal only), 2 oz, 4 oz.
Use: Skin bleaching agent.

AS-101. (Wyeth-Ayerst) Phase I/II ARC,
AIDS. *Rx.*
Use: Immunomodulator.

5-asa. Mesalamine.
See: Asacol (Procter & Gamble
Pharm.).
Rowasa (Solvay).

ASA. (Wampole-Zeus) Anti-skin antibodies test by IFA. Test 48s.
Use: Diagnostic aid.

A.S.A. (Lilly) Aspirin. Acetylsalicylic acid.
Enseal: 5 gr or 10 gr. Bot. 100s, 1000s.
Supp.: 5 gr or 10 gr. Pkg. 6s, 144s.
otc.
Use: Salicylate analgesic.

Asacol. (Procter & Gamble Pharm.)
Mesalamine 400 mg/Tab. DR Bot. 100s.
Rx.
Use: Anti-inflammatory.

asafetida, emulsion of. Milk of Asafetida.

Asaped Tablets. (Sanofi Winthrop)
Acetylsalicylic acid. *otc.*
Use: Analgesic.

Asawin Tablets. (Sanofi Winthrop)
Acetylsalicylic acid. *otc.*
Use: Analgesic.

A.S.B. (Femco) Calcium carbonate, magnesium carbonate, bismuth subcarbonate, sodium bicarbonate, kaolin. Pow.,
Can 3 oz. Tabs. 50s. *otc.*
Use: Antacid.

Asclerol. (Spanner) Liver injection crude
(2 mcg/ml) 50%, Vitamins B_1 20 mg,
B_2 3 mg, B_6 1 mg, B_{12} 30 mcg, niacinamide 100 mg, panthenol 2.8 mg, choline Cl 20 mg, inositol 10 mg/ml. Multiple dose vial 10 ml. *Rx.*
Use: Vitamin supplement.

ascorbate sodium. Antiscorbutic vitamin.

•**ascorbic acid,** U.S.P. 23.
Use: Vitamin (antiscorbutic); aicidifier
(urinary).

ascorbic acid, (ASS-kor-bik) Antiscorbic
vitamin; Vitamin C. **Cap.:** (Various Mfr.)
25 mg, 100 mg, 250 mg, 500 mg. **Inj.:**
(Various Mfr.) Amp. (100 mg/ml) 1 ml, 2
ml, 5 ml; (200 mg/ml) 5 ml, (500 mg)
2 ml, 5 ml, 10 ml, 30 ml, (250 mg/ml) 10
ml; (1000 mg/ml) 10 ml. **Tab.:** (Vari-
ous Mfr.) 50 mg, 100 mg, 250 mg, 500
mg. **Chew. tab.:** (Various Mfr.) 100 mg,
250 mg, 500 mg. **SR Tab.:** (Various
Mfr.) 500 mg, 1500 mg. **SR Cap.:** 500
mg. **Pow.:** (Various Mfr.) 4 g/5 ml.
Soln.: (Various Mfr.) 35 mg/0.6 ml or
100 mg/ml.
Use: Vitamin C supplement.
See: Ascorbicap, Cap. (ICN).
Ascorbineed, Cap. (Hanlon).
C-Caps 500 (Drug Industries).
Cecon, Soln. (Abbott).
Cenolate, Amp. (Abbott).
Cetane, Cap., Vial (Forest).
Cevalin, Tab., Amp. (Lilly).
Cevi-Bid, Cap. (Geriatric).
Ce-Vi-Sol, Drops (Bristol-Myers).
Neo-Vadrin, Preps. (Scherer).
Solucap C, Cap. (Jamieson-McK-
ames).
Sunkist Vitamin C, Capl., Chew. tab.
(Novartis).

ascorbic acid injection.
Use: Vitamin C supplement.
See: Cevalin, Amp. (Lilly).

ascorbic acid salts.
See: Bismuth Ascorbate.
Calcium Ascorbate.
Sodium Ascorbate.

Ascorbicap. (ICN) Ascorbic acid 500 mg/
S.R. Cap. Bot. 50s. *otc.*
Use: Vitamin C supplement.

Ascorbin/11. (Taylor Pharmaceuticals)
Lemon bioflavonoids 110 mg, Vitamin
C 1 g, rose hips powder 50 mg, rutin 25
mg/S.R. Tab. Bot. 100s. *otc.*

Use: Vitamin supplement.

Ascorbineed. (Hanlon) Vitamin C 500 mg/T-Cap. Bot. 100s. *otc.*
Use: Vitamin C supplement.

Ascorbocin Powder. (Paddock) Vitamin C 500 mg, niacin 500 mg, B_1 50 mg, B_6 50 mg, d-α-tocopheryl, polyethylene glycol 1000 succinate 50 IU, lactose/ 3 g. Bot. lb. *otc.*
Use: Vitamin supplement.

•**ascorbyl palmitate,** N.F. 18. L-Ascorbic acid 6-palmitate.
Use: Preservative; pharmaceutic aid (antioxidant).

Ascorvite S.R. (Eon Labs) Vitamin C 500 mg/S.R. Cap. *otc.*
Use: Vitamin C supplement.

Ascriptin. (Rhone-Poulenc Rorer) Aspirin 325 mg, magnesium hydroxide 50 mg, aluminum hydroxide 50 mg/Tab. Bot. 50s, 100s, 225s, 500s. *otc.*
Use: Analgesic, antacid.

Ascriptin A/D. (Rhone-Poulenc Rorer) Acetylsalicylic acid 325 mg with magnesium hydroxide 75 mg, aluminum hydroxide and calcium carbonate 75 mg/Capsule shape coated tabs. Bot. 225s. *otc.*
Use: Analgesic, antacid.

Ascriptin Extra Strength. (Rhone-Poulenc Rorer) Aspirin 500 mg with magnesium hydroxide 80 mg, aluminum hydroxide and calcium carbonate 80 mg. Capsule shape coated tabs. Bot. 50s. *otc.*
Use: Analgesic, antacid.

Asendin. (Lederle) Amoxapine. **25 mg/ Tab.:** Bot. 100s; **50 mg/Tab.:** Bot. 100s, 500s, UD 100s; **100 mg/Tab.:** Bot. 100s, UD 100s; **150 mg/Tab.:** Bot. 30s. *Rx.*
Use: Antidepressant.

aseptichrome.
See: Merbromin (Various Mfr.).

Aslum. (Drug Products) Carbolic acid 1%, aluminum acetate, ichthammol, zinc oxide, aromatic oils in a petrolatum-stearin base. Tube oz. Jar lb.
Use: Astringent, dressing.

Asma. (Wampole-Zeus) Anti-smooth muscle antibody test by IFA. Test 48.
Use: Diagnostic aid.

Asmalix. (Century) Theophylline 80 mg, alcohol 20%/15 ml. Bot. qt, gal. *Rx.*
Use: Bronchodilator.

Asma-Tuss. (Halsey) Phenobarbital 4 mg, theophylline 15 mg, ephedrine sulfate 12 mg, guaifenesin 50 mg/5 ml. Bot. 4 oz. *Rx.*

Use: Bronchodilator.

Asolectin. (Associated Conc.) Chemical lecithin 25%, chemical cephalin 22%, inositol phosphatides 16%, soybean oil 2.5%, other miscellaneous sterols and lipids 34.5%. *otc.*
Use: Diet supplement.

•**asparaginase.** (ass-PAR-uh-jin-aze) USAN. L-asparagine amidohydrolase.
Use: Antineoplastic.
See: Elspar, Inj. (Merck).

•**aspartame,** (ass-PAR-tame) N.F. 18.
Use: Sweetener.

•**aspartic acid.** (ass-PAR-tick Acid) USAN. Aspartic acid; aminosuccinic acid.
Use: Management of fatigue; amino acid.

•**aspartocin.** (ass-PAR-toe-sin) USAN.
Use: Antibacterial.

A-Spas. (Hyrex) Dicyclomine HCl 10 mg/ ml. Vial 10 ml. *Rx.*
Use: Antispasmodic.

A-Spas S/L. (Hyrex) Hyoscyamine sulfate 0.125 mg/Tab., sublingual. 100s. *Rx.*
Use: Antispasmodic.

Aspercreme. (Thompson Medical) Triethanolamine salicylate 10% in cream base. *otc.*
Use: Analgesic, topical.

aspergillus niger enzyme. Alpha-galactosidase. *otc.*
See: Beano, Tab. (AK-Pharma).

aspergillus oryzae enzyme. Diastase.
See: Taka-Diastase, Preps. (Parke-Davis).

Aspergum. (Schering-Plough) Aspirin 227.5 mg/1 Gum. Tab. Orange or Cherry flavor. Box 16s, 40s. *otc.*
Use: Salicylate analgesic.

asperkinase. Proteolytic enzyme mixture derived from aspergillus oryzae.

•**asperlin.** (ASS-per-lin) USAN.
Use: Antibacterial, antineoplastic.

Aspermin. (Buffington) Aspirin 325 mg/ Tab. Sugar, caffeine, lactose, and salt free. Dispens-A-Kit 500s. *otc.*
Use: Salicylate analgesic.

Aspermin Extra. (Buffington) Aspirin 500 mg/Tab. Sugar, caffeine, lactose, and salt free. Dispens-A-Kit 500s. *otc.*
Use: Salicylate analgesic.

•**aspirin,** (ASS-pihr-in) U.S.P. 23. Acetophen, Acetol, Acetosal, Acetosalin, Aceticyl, Acetylin, Acetylsal, Empirin, Saletin. Acetylsalicylic acid, Benzoic acid, 2-(acetyloxy)-., Salicylic acid acetate.
Use: Analgesic, antipyretic, antirheu-

matic. Prophylactic to reduce risk of death or non-fatal MI in patients with a previous infarction or unstable angina pectoris.
See: A.S.A., Preps. (Lilly).
Aspergum, Gum, Tab. (Schering-Plough).
Bayer Children's Aspirin, Tab. (Bayer).
Bayer, 8-Hour Timed-Release, Tab. (Bayer).
Easprin, Tab. (Parke-Davis).
Ecotrin, Tab. (SK-Beecham).
Ecotrin Maximum Strength, Capl., Tab. (SK-Beecham).
Empirin, Tab. (Glaxo Wellcome).
Genprin, Tab. (Goldline).
Genuine Bayer Aspirin, Tab., Capl. (Bayer).
Halfprin 81, EC Tab. (Kramer).
Maximum Bayer Aspirin, Tab., Capl. (Bayer).
Norwich Aspirin, Tab. (Procter & Gamble).
St. Joseph, Prods. (Schering-Plough).
ZORprin, Tab. (Knoll Pharm.).

aspirin, alumina, and magnesia tablets.
Use: Analgesic, antacid.

aspirin, alumina, and magnesium oxide tablets.
Use: Analgesic, antacid.

aspirin-barbiturate combinations.
Use: Analgesic, sedative, hypnotic.
See: Axotal, Tab. (Warren-Teed).
BA-C, Tab. (Mayrand).
Butalbital, Tab., Cap. (Various Mfr.).
Fiorgen, Tab. (Goldline).
Fiorinal, Cap., Tab. (Sandoz).
Isollyl, Tab. (Rugby).
Marnal, Tab., Cap. (Vortech).

aspirin, caffeine and dihydrocodeine bitartrate capsules.
Use: Analgesic.

aspirin w/codeine no. 3. (Various Mfr.)
Codeine phosphate 30 mg, aspirin 325 mg Tab. Bot. 100s, 1000s. *c-III.*
Use: Narcotic analgesic, combination.

aspirin w/codeine no. 4. (Various Mfr.)
Codeine phosphate 60 mg, aspirin 325 mg Tab. Bot. 100s, 500s, 1000s. *c-III.*
Use: Narcotic analgesic, combination.

aspirin, codeine, phosphate alumina, and magnesia tablets.
Use: Analgesic.

aspirin and codeine phosphate tablets.
Use: Analgesic.

aspirin delayed-release capsules.
Use: Analgesic.

aspirin delayed-release tablets.
Use: Analgesic.
See: Bayer Low Adult Strength (Bayer).

aspirin, enteric coated.
Use: Analgesic.
See: A.S.A., Preps. (Lilly).
Ecotrin, Tab. (SK-Beecham).

Aspirin Free Anacin Maximum Strength. (Whitehall Robins) Acetaminophen 500 mg. **Capl., Gel Capl.:** Bot. 100s; **Tab.:** Bot. 60s. *otc.*
Use: Analgesic.

Aspirin Free Anacin P.M. (Robins) Diphenhydramine HCl 25 mg, acetaminophen 500 mg/Tab. Bot. 20s. *otc.*
Use: Nonprescription sleep aid.

Aspirin-Free Bayer Select Allergy Sinus. (Bayer) Pseudoephedrine HCl 30 mg, chlorpheniramine maleate 2 mg, acetaminophen 500 mg/Cap. Pkg. 16s. *otc.*
Use: Decongestant, antihistamine, analgesic.

Aspirin-Free Bayer Select Head & Chest Cold. (Bayer) Pseudoephedrine HCl 30 mg, dextromethorphan HBr 10 mg, guaifenesin 100 mg, acetaminophen 325 mg. Cap. Bot. 16s. *otc.*
Use: Expectorant, analgesic, decongestant.

Aspirin-Free Bayer Select Headache. (Bayer) Acetaminophen 500 mg, caffeine 65 mg. Cap. Bot. 50s. *otc.*
Use: Analgesic combination.

Aspirin-Free Bayer Select Excedrin. (Bristol-Myers) Acetaminophen 500 mg, caffeine 65 mg/Tab., Capl. Bot. 20s, 40s, 80s. *otc.*
Use: Analgesic combination.

Aspirin-Free Bayer Select Excedrin Dual. (B-M Squibb) Acetaminophen 500 mg, calcium carbonate 111 mg, magnesium carbonate 64 mg, magnesium oxide 30 mg/Capl. Bot. 100s. *otc.*
Use: Analgesic combination.

Aspirin Free Pain Relief. (Hudson) Acetaminophen 325 mg/Tab. Bot. 100s. *otc.*
Use: Analgesic.

aspirin w/o.t.c. combinations.
See: Alka Seltzer, Tab. (Bayer).
Alka Seltzer Plus, Tab. (Bayer).
Anacin, Cap., Tab. (Whitehall Robins).
A.P.C., Tab., Cap. (Various Mfr.).
Arthritis Strength BC Powder (Block).
Ascriptin, Tab. (Rhone-Poulenc Rorer Consumer).
Ascriptin A/D, Tab. (Rhone-Poulenc Rorer Consumer).
Ascriptin, Extra Strength, Tab.

(Rhone-Poulenc Rorer Consumer).
Bayer Aspirin Preps. (Bayer).
BC, Powder, Tab. (Block Drug).
Buffaprin, Tab. (Buffington).
Buffets, Tab. (JMI).
Cama, Tab. (Sandoz Consumer).
Cope, Tab. (Mentholatum).
Excedrin, Cap., Tab. (Bristol-Myers).
4-Way, Tab., Spray (Bristol-Myers).
Gelpirin, Tab. (Alra).
Gensan, Tab. (Goldline).
Goody's Headache Powders (Goody).
Midol, Cap., Spray (Bayer).
Momentum, Cap. (Whitehall Robins).
Night-Time Effervescent, Tab. (Goldline).
Pain Reliever, Tab. (Rugby).
Presalin, Tab. (Roberts).
Saleto, Preps. (Roberts).
Salocol, Tab. (Roberts).
Sine-Off Tablets (Menley & James).
Stanback, Pow., Tab. (Stanback).
St. Joseph Cold Tablets For Children (Schering-Plough).
Supac, Tab. (Mission).
Vanquish, Cap. (Bayer).

aspirin & oxycodone. (Various Mfr.) Oxycodone HCl 4.5 mg, oxycodone terephthalate 0.38 mg, aspirin 325 mg/Tab. Bot. 100s, 500s, 1000s, UD 25s. *c-II.*
Use: Narcotic analagesic combination.

Aspirin Plus. (Walgreen) Aspirin 400 mg, caffeine 32 mg/Tab. Bot. 100s. *otc.*
Use: Analgesic combination.

aspirin salts.
See: Calcium Acetylsalicylate.

aspirin tablets, buffered.
Use: Salicylate analgesic.

Aspirin Uniserts. (Upsher-Smith) Aspirin 125 mg, 300 mg or 650 mg/supp. Ctn. 12s, 50s. *otc.*
Use: Salicylate analgesic.

Aspirtab. (Dover) Aspirin 325 mg/Tab. Sugar, lactose and salt free. UD Box 500s. *otc.*
Use: Salicylate analgesic.

Aspirtab Max. (Dover) Aspirin 500 mg/Tab. Sugar, lactose and salt free. UD Box 500s. *otc.*
Use: Analgesic.

Aspogen. Dihydroxyaluminum aminoacetate.

Asprimox. (Invamed) Capl.: aspirin (buffered) 325 mg. Bot. 100s, 500s. Tab.: aspirin 325 mg, aluminum hydroxide gel (dried) 50 mg, magnesium hydroxide 50 mg, calcium carbonate. 100s, 500s. *otc.*
Use: Analgesic.

Asprimox Extra Protection for Arthritis Pain. (Invamed) Aspirin (buffered) 325 mg/Capl. Bot. 100s, 500s. *otc.*
Use: Analgesic.

Astaril tablets. (Sanofi Winthrop) Theophylline anhydrous, ephedrine sulphate. *Rx.*
Use: Bronchodilator.

Astelin. (Wallace) Azelatine HCl 137 mcg, benzalkonium chloride, EDTA/Spray. Bot. 17 mg per bottle. 2s. *Rx.*
Use: Antihistamine.

•**astemizole.** (ASS-TEM-ih-zole) USAN.
Use: Antihistamine; antiallergic
See: Hismanal, Tab. (Janssen).

asterol.
Use: Antifungal.

Asthmahaler. (SK-Beecham) Epinephrine bitartrate 0.3 mg/ml in an inert propellant. Oral inhaler, 15 ml with mouthpiece; 15 ml refills. *otc.*
Use: Bronchodilator.

Asthmalixir. (Reese Pharmaceutical Inc.) Theophylline 45 mg, ephedrine sulfate 36 mg, guaifenesin 150 mg, phenobarbital 12 mg/ 15 ml. Alcohol 19%. Bot. *Rx.*
Use: Bronchodilator, expectorant, sedative/hypnotic.

AsthmaNefrin. (Menley & James) Racepinephrine HCl 2.25%. Soln. Nebulizer 15 ml, 30 ml. *otc.*
Use: Sympathomimetic.

AsthmaNefrin Solution & Nebulizer. (SK-Beecham) Racepin (racemic epinephrine) as HCl equivalent to epinephrine base 2.25%, chlorobutanol 0.5%. Bot. 0.5 fl oz. With sodium bisulfite. Bot. 1 fl oz. *otc.*
Use: Bronchodilator.

•**astifilcon a.** (ASS-tih-FILL-kahn) USAN.
Use: Contact lens material (hydrophilic).

Astramorph PF. (Astra) Morphine sulfate 0.5 mg/ml or 1 mg/ml preservative free. Amp. 10 ml, Vial 10 ml. *c-II.*
Use: Narcotic analgesic.

Astroglide. (BioFilm) Purified water, glycerin, propylene glycol and parabens. Vaginal gel. Bot 70.5 ml. Travel pks. 5 ml. *otc.*
Use: Vaginal lubricant.

•**astromicin sulfate.** (ASS-troe-MY-sin) USAN.
Use: Antibacterial.

Astro-Vites. (Faraday) Vitamins A 3500 IU, D 400 IU, C 60 mg, B_1 0.8 mg, B_2 1.3 mg, niacinamide 14 mg, B_6 1 mg, B_{12} 2.5 mcg, folic acid 0.05 mg, panto-

thenic acid 5 mg, iron 12 mg/Tab. Bot. 100s, 250s. *otc.*
Use: Vitamin/mineral supplement.

AST/SGOT Reagent Strips. (Bayer) Seralyzer reagent strip. A quantitative strip test for asparate transaminase/ serum glutamic oxaloacetic transaminase in serum or plasma. Bot. Strip 25s.
Use: Diagnostic aid.

Asupirin. (Suppositoria) Aspirin 60 mg, 120 mg, 200 mg, 300 mg, 600 mg or 1.2 g/Supp. Box 12s, 100s, 1000s. *otc.*
Use: Salicylate analgesic.

A.T. 10.
See: Dihydrotachysterol.

Atabee TD. (Defco) Vitamins C 500 mg, B_1 15 mg, B_2 10 mg, B_6 2 mg, nicotinamide 50 mg, calcium pantothenate 10 mg/Cap. Bot. 30s, 1000s. *otc.*
Use: Vitamin supplement.

Atarax. (Roerig) Hydroxyzine HCl. **Tab.:** 10 mg or 25 mg Bot. 100s, 500s, UD 10 × 10s, Unit-of-use 40s; 50 mg Bot. 100s, 500s, UD 10 10s; 100 mg Bot. 100s, UD 10 × 10s. **Syr.:** 10 mg/5 ml, alcohol 0.5%. Bot. Pt. *Rx.*
Use: Antianxiety agent.
W/Ephedrine sulfate, theophylline.
See: Marax, Tab., Syr. (Roerig).
W/Penta-erythrityltetranitrate.
See: Cartrax, Tab. (Roerig).

atarvet. Acepromazine.

●**atenolol.** (ah-TEN-oh-lahl) U.S.P. 23.
Use: Beta-adrenergic blocking agent.
See: Tenormin, Tab. (Stuart).

atenolol/chlorthalidone. (ah-TEN-oh-lahl/klor-THAL-ih-dohn) (Various Mfr.) Atenolol 50 mg or 100 mg, chlorthalidone 25 mg/Tab. Bot. 50s, 100s, 250s, 500s, 1000s. *Rx.*
Use: Antihypertensive.

●**atevirdine mesylate.** (at-TEH-vihr-DEEN) USAN.
Use: Antiviral.

Atgam. (Pharmacia & Upjohn) Lymphocyte immune globulin, antithymocyte globulin 250 mg protein (50 mg/ml). Amp. 5 ml. *Rx.*
Use: Management of allograft rejection in renal transplant patients.

Athlete's Foot Ointment. (Walgreen) Zinc undecylenate 20%, undecylenic acid 5%. Tube 1.5 oz. *otc.*
Use: Antifungal, topical.

●**atipamezole.** (AT-ih-pam-EH-zole) USAN.
Use: Antagonist (α_2-receptor).

●**atiprimod dihydrochloride.** (at-TIH-prih-mahd) USAN.

Use: Anti-inflammatory, antiarthritic (immunomodulator, suppressor cell inducing agent), antirheumatic (disease modifying).

●**atiprosin maleate.** (ah-TIH-pro-SIN) USAN.
Use: Antihypertensive.

Ativan Injection. (Wyeth-Ayerst) Lorazepam in 2 mg/ml or 4 mg/ml. Vial 1 ml, 10 ml/2 ml Tubex (w/1 ml fill). Pkg. 10s. *c-IV.*
Use: Antianxiety agent.

Ativan Tablets. (Wyeth-Ayerst) Lorazepam 0.5 mg, 1 mg or 2 mg/Tab. Bot. 100s, 500s, 1000s, Redipak 25s. *c-IV.*
Use: Antianxiety agent.

●**atlafilcon a.** (at-LAH-FILL-kahn A) USAN.
Use: Contact lens material (hydrophilic).

ATnativ. (Baxter) Antithrombin III (human), lyophilized powder/500 IU. Inj. Bot. 50 ml w/10 l sterile water. *Rx.*
Use: Thromboembolic agent.

●**atolide.** (ATE-oh-lide) USAN. Under study.
Use: Anticonvulsant.

Atolone. (Major) Triamcinolone 4 mg/ Tab. Bot. 100s, Uni-Pak 16s. *Rx.*
Use: Corticosteroid.

●**atorvastatin calcium.** USAN.
Use: HMG-CoA reductase inhibitor; antihyperlipidemic.
See: Lipitor, Tab. (Parke-Davis).

●**atosiban.** (at-OH-sih-ban) USAN.
Use: Antagonist, oxytocin.

●**atovaquone.** (uh-TOE-vuh-KWONE) USAN.
Use: Antpneumocystic; antiprotozoal. [Orphan drug]
See: Mepron (Glaxo Wellcome).

Atozine Tabs. (Major) Hydroxyzine HCl 10 mg, 25 mg or 50 mg/Tab; **10 and 25 mg:** Bot. 100s, 250s, 1000s, UD 100s; **50 mg:** Bot. 100s, 250s, 500s, UD 100s. *Rx.*
Use: Antianxiety agent.

Atpeg. (Zeneca) Polyethylene glycol available as 300, 400, 600 or 4000.
Use: Surfactant, humectant.

●**atracurium besylate.** (AT-rah-CUE-ree-uhm BESS-ih-late) USAN.
Use: Neuromuscular blocking agent; skeletal muscle relaxant.
See: Tracrium (Glaxo Wellcome).

Atretol. (Athena Neurosciences) Carbamazepine 200 mg, lactose/Tab. 100s. *Rx.*
Use: Antiepileptic.

Atridine. (Interstate) Triprolidine 2.5 mg,

pseudoephedrine HCl 60 mg/Tab. Bot. 100s, 1000s. *otc.*
Use: Antihistamine, decongestant.

Atrocap. (Freeport) Atropine sulfate 0.06 mg, hyoscyamine sulfate 0.3 mg, hyoscine hydrobromide 0.02 mg, phenobarbital 50 mg/T.R. Cap. Bot. 1000s. *Rx.*
Use: Sedative, hypnotic, anticholinergic, antispasmodic.

Atrocholin Tablets. (Glaxo) Dehydrocholic acid 130 mg/Tab. Bot. 100s. *otc.*
Use: Laxative.

Atrofed. (Genetco) Pseudoephedrine HCl 60 mg, triprolidine HCl 2.5 mg. Tab. Bot. 24s, 100s, 1000s. *otc.*
Use: Antihistamine, decongestant.

Atrohist LA. (Adams) Pseudoephedrine HCl 120 mg, brompheniramine maleate 4 mg, phenyltoloxamine citrate 50 mg/SR Tab with atropine sulfate 0.0242 mg available for immediate release. Bot. 100s. *Rx.*
Use: Decongestant, antihistamine.

Atrohist Pediatric Capsules. (Adams) Chlorpheniramine maleate 4 mg, pseudoephedrine HCl 60 mg/SR Cap. Bot. 100s. *Rx.*
Use: Antihistamine, decongestant.

Atrohist Pediatric Suspension. (Adams) Phenylephrine tannate 5 mg, chlorpheniramine tannate 2 mg, pyrilamine tannate 12.5 mg. Susp. Bot. 473 ml. Unit-of-use 118 ml. *Rx.*
Use: Decongestant, antihistamine.

Atrohist Plus Tablets. (Adams) Phenylephrine HCl 25 mg, phenylpropanolamine HCl 50 mg, chlorpheniramine maleate 8 mg, hyoscyamine sulfate 0.19 mg, atropine sulfate 0.04 mg, scopolamine HBr 0.01 mg/SR Tab. Bot. 100s. *Rx.*
Use: Decongestant, antihistamine, anticholinergic.

Atrohist Sprinkle. (Adams) Pseudoephedrine HCl 120 mg, brompheniramine maleate 2 mg, phenytoloxamine citrate 25 mg/SR Cap. Bot. 100s. *Rx.*
Use: Decongestant, antihistamine.

Atromid-S. (Wyeth-Ayerst) Clofibrate 500 mg/Cap. Bot. 100s. *Rx.*
Use: Antihyperlipidemic.

Atropen Auto-Injecter. (Survival Technology) Atropine sulfate, phenol 2 mg. In prefilled automatic injection device. *Rx.*
Use: For toxic exposure to organophosphorus or carbamate insecticides.

•**atropine,** (AT-troe-peen) U.S.P. 23.

Use: Anticholinergic.

Atropine-1. (Optopics) Atropine sulfate 1% soln. Bot. 2, 5, 15 ml. *Rx.*
Use: Cycloplegic mydriatic.

Atropine Care. (Akorn) Atropine sulfate 1%. Soln. Bot. 2 ml, 5 ml, 15 ml. *Rx.*
Use: Cycloplegic mydriatic.

atropine and demerol injection. (Sanofi Winthrop) Atropine sulfate 0.4 mg, meperidine HCl 50 mg or 75 mg/Carpuject. *c-ii.*
Use: Preoperative sedative.

atropine-hyoscine-hyoscyamine combinations. (See also Belladonna Products)
See: Barbella, Tab., Elix. (Forest).
Barbeloid, Tab. (Pal-Pak).
Bar-Don, Tab., Elix. (Warren-Teed).
Belakoids TT, Tab. (Philips Roxane).
Belbutal No. 2 Kaptabs. (Churchill).
Brobella-P.B., Tab. (Brothers).
Buren, Tab. (Ascher).
Donnagel, Susp. (Robins).
Donnamine, Elix., Tab. (Tennessee Pharm.).
Donnatal, Cap., Elix., Tab. (Robins).
Donnatal #2, Tab. (Robins).
Donnatal Extentabs, Tab. (Robins).
Donnazyme, Tab. (Robins).
Eldonal, Preps. (Canright).
Hyatal, Elix. (Winsale).
Hybephen, Preps. (SK-Beecham).
Hyonal, Preps. (Paddock).
Hyonatol B, Preps. (Jones Medical).
Hytrona, Tab. (PolyMedica).
Kinesed, Tab. (Stuart).
Koryza, Tab. (Forest).
Maso-Donna, Elix., Tab. (Mason).
Nilspasm, Tab. (Parmed).
Sedamine, Tab. (Dunhall).
Sedapar, Tab. (Parmed).
Seds, Tab. (Taylor Pharmaceuticals).
Spabelin, Elix. (Arcum).
Spasdel, Cap. (Marlop).
Spasloids, Tab. (G.F. Harvey).
Spasmolin, Tab. (Bell).
Spasquid, Elix. (Geneva Pharm.).
Uriseptin, Tab. (Blaine).
Urogesic, Tab. (Edwards).

atropine methylnitrate. (Various Mfr.) dl-Hyoscyamine methylnitrate.
See: Harvatrate, Tab. (Forest Pharm.).
Thitrate W.P., Tab. (Blaine).
W/Hyoscine HBr, hyoscyamine sulfate, amobarbital sodium.
See: Amocine, Tab. (Roberts).
W/Methenamine mandelate and phenylazodiaminopyridine HCl.
See: Uritral, Cap. (Schwarz Pharma).
W/Phenobarbital and dihydroxyaluminum aminoacetate.

See: Atromal, Tab. (Blaine).
Harvatrate A, Tab. (Forest Pharm.).
atropine-n-oxide hydrochloride.
See: Atropine Oxide HCl.
•**atropine oxide hydrochloride.** (AT-row-peen OX-ide) USAN. Atropine N-oxide HCl.
Use: Anticholinergic.
See: X-Tro (Xttrium).
•**atropine sulfate, U.S.P. 23.**
Use: Anticholinergic (ophthalmic).
atropine sulfate. (Various Mfr.) **Pediatric Inj.:** 0.05 mg/ml 5 ml Abboject.
Tab, Hypodermic: 0.3 mg, 0.4 mg and 0.6 mg/Tab. Bot. 100s. **Tab, Oral:** 0.4 mg/Tab. Bot. 100s. **Inj.:** 0.1 mg/ml 5 ml and 10 ml Abboject 0.3 mg/ml. Vial 1 ml; 0.4 mg/ml. Amp. 1 ml, vial 20 ml; 0.8 mg/ml. Amp. 1 ml, dosette 0.5 ml; 1 mg/ml. Amp., vial 1 ml, syringe 10 ml; 1.2 mg/ml. Vial 1 ml syringe. **Lyophilized:** Lyopine (Hyrex). **Ophth. Oint:** 1%. Tube 3.5 g., UD 1 g. **Ophth. Soln:** 1%. Bot. UD 1 ml, 2 ml, 5 ml, 15 ml; 2%. Bot. 2 ml.
Use: Anticholinergic (ophthalmic).
See: Atropine-1, Soln., (Optopics).
Atropine Care, Soln., (Akorn).
Atropine Sulfate S.O.P., Oint., (Allergan).
Atropisol, Soln., (Ciba Vision).
Isopto-Atropine (Alcon).
Lyopine, Inj. (Hyrex).
Parasympatholytic and antispasmodic.
Sal-Tropine (Hope Pharm.).
W/Ephedrine sulfate.
See: Enuretrol, Tab. (Berlex).
atropine sulfate/edrophonium chloride. Anticholinesterase muscle stimulant.
See: Enlon-Plus (Ohmeda Pharmaceuticals).
atropine sulfate and meperidine hcl.
See: Atropine and Demerol. (Sanofi Winthrop.).
atropine sulfate and morphine sulfate.
See: Morphine and Atropine Sulfates. (SK-Beecham).
atropine sulfate S.O.P. (Allergan) 0.5%, 1%. Oint. Tube 3.5 g. *Rx.*
Use: Cycloplegic mydriatic.
atropine sulfate w/phenobarbital.
See: Antrocol, Tab., Cap. (ECR Pharm.).
Arco-Lase Plus, Tab. (Arco).
Barbeloid, Tab. (Pal-Pak).
Briabell, Tab. (Briar).
Brobella-P.B., Tab. (Brothers).
Donnatal, Cap., Extentab, Tab., Elix. (Robins).

Donnatal #2, Tab. (Robins).
Hyatal Elix. (Winsale).
Palbar No. 2, Tab. (Roberts).
Seds, Tab. (Taylor Pharmaceuticals).
Spabelin, Elix. (Arcum).
Spasdel, Cap. (Marlop).
Stannitol (Standex).
Atropisol. (Ciba Vision) Atropine sulfate 1%. Soln. Dropperette 1 ml. *Rx.*
Use: Cycloplegic mydriatic.
Atrosed. (Freeport) Atropine sulfate 0.0195 mg, hyoscine HBr 0.0065 mg, hyoscyamine sulfate 0.104 mg, phenobarbital 0.25 gr/Tab. Bot. 1000s, 5000s. *Rx.*
Use: Anticholinergic, antispasmodic, sedative, hypnotic.
Atrosept. (Geneva Pharm.) Methenamine 40.8 mg, phenyl salicylate 18.1 mg, atropine sulfate 0.03 mg, hyoscyamine 0.03 mg, benzoic acid 4.5 mg, methylene blue 5.4 mg/Tab. Bot. 100s, 1000s. *Rx.*
Use: Urinary anti-infective.
Atrovent. (Boehringer Ingelheim) Ipratropium bromide. **Aerosol:** 18 mcg/dose. 14 g; **Soln.:** 0.02% (500 mg/vial) 25s. **Spray:** 0.03% in 30 ml vials; 0.06% in 15 ml vials. *Rx.*
Use: Bronchodilator.
A/T/S. (Hoechst Marion Roussel) Erythromycin 2%. Gel. Tube 30 g. *Rx.*
Use: Antiacne.
A/T/S Topical Solution. (Hoechst Marion Roussel) Erythromycin 2% topical soln. Bot. 60 ml. *Rx.*
Use: Antiacne.
AT-Solution. (Sanofi Winthrop) Dihydrotachysterol solution.
Use: Hypocalcemic tetany.
Attain Liquid. (Sherwood). Sodium caseinate, calcium caseinate, maltodextrin, corn oil, soy lecithin. Can 250 ml and 1000 ml closed system. *otc.*
Use: Nutritional supplement.
•**attapulgite, activated,** U.S.P. 23.
Use: Antidiarrheal; pharmaceutic aid (suspending agent).
See: Quintess, Susp. (Lilly).
W/Pectin, hydrated alumina powder.
See: Polymagma Plain Tab. (Wyeth-Ayerst).
W/Polysorbate 80, salicylic acid, propylene glycol.
See: Sebasorb Lot. (Summer).
Attenuvax. (Merck) Measles virus vaccine, live, attenuated w/neomycin 25 mcg/Vial. Single-dose vial w/diluent. Pkg. 1s, 10s. *Rx.*
Use: Agent for immunization.

W/Meruvax.
See: M-R-Vax-II, Vial (Merck).
W/Mumpsvax, Meruvax.
See: M-M-R II, Vial (Merck).
Atuss DM. (Atley) Dextromethorphan 15 mg, phenylephrine HCl 5 mg, chlorpheniramine maleate 2 mg, sucrose, saccharin Syr. Bot. 480 ml. *Rx.*
Use: Decongestant, antitussive, antihistamine.
Atuss EX. (Atley) Hydrocodone bitartrate 5 mg, guaifenesin 100 mg/Syrup Bot. 480 ml. *c-iii.*
Use: Narcotic expectorant.
Atuss G. (Atley) Hydrocodone bitartrate 2 mg, phenylephrine HCl 10 mg, guaifenesin 100 mg, sucrose/Syr. Bot. 480 ml. *c-iii.*
Use: Narcotic decongestant expectorant.
Atuss HD. (Atley) Hydrocodone bitartrate 2.5 mg, phenylephrine HCl 5 mg, chlorpheniramine maleate 2mg/5ml. Menthol, sucrose. Liq. Bot. 480 ml. *c-iii.*
Use: Antitussive, decongestant, antihistamine.
Augmented Betamethasone Dipropionate.
Use: Corticosteroid, topical.
See: Diprolene (Schering-Plough).
Augmentin Chewable Tablets. (SK-Beecham) **125:** Amoxicillin 125 mg, clavulanic acid 31.25 mg, saccharin/Tab. Ctn. 30s. **250:** Amoxicillin 250 mg, clavulanic acid 62.5 mg, saccharin/Tab. Ctn. 30s. *Rx.*
Use: Anti-infective, penicillin.
Augmentin Oral Suspension. (SK-Beecham) **125:** Amoxicillin 125 mg, clavulanic acid (as potassium salt) 31.25 mg/5 ml. Bot. 75 ml, 150 ml. **200:** Amoxicillin 200 mg, clavulanic acid/5ml. Mannitol, aspartame/Pow. Bot. 50 ml, 75 ml, 100 ml. **250:** Amoxicillin 250 mg, clavulanic acid (as potassium salt) 62.5 mg/5 ml. Bot. 75 ml, 150 ml. **400:** Amoxicillin 400 mg, clavulanic acid 28.5 mg/5ml. Mannitol, aspartame/Pow. Bot. 50 ml, 75 ml, and 100 ml. *Rx.*
Use: Anti-infective, penicillin.
Augmentin Tablets. (SK-Beecham) Amoxicillin trihydrate 250 mg, 500 mg or 850 mg, clavulanic acid (as potassium salt) 125 mg/Tab. **250:** Bot. 30s, UD 100s. **500:** Bot. 30s, 100s. **850:** 20s, UD 100s. *Rx.*
Use: Anti-infective, penicillin.
Auralgan Otic Solution. (Wyeth-Ayerst) Antipyrine 54 mg, benzocaine 14 mg/ml w/oxyquinoline sulfate in dehydrated glycerin (contains not more than 0.6% moisture). Bot. w/dropper 15 ml. *Rx.*
Use: Otic preparation.
Auralgesic. (Wesley) Carbamide 10%, antipyrine 5%, benzocaine 2.5%, cetyldimethylbenzylammonium HCl 0.2%. Bot. 0.5 oz. *Rx.*
Use: Otic preparation.
•**auranofin.** (or-RAIN-oh-fin) USAN.
Use: Antirheumatic.
See: Ridaura, Cap. (SK-Beecham).
aureomycin preparations. (Storz Lederle) Chlortetracycline HCl. **Ophth. Oint.:** 1% (10 mg/g) Tube 0.125 oz. **Topical Oint.:** 3% (30 mg/g) in white petrolatum, anhydrous lanolin base. Tube 0.5 oz, 1 oz. *Rx.*
Use: Anti-infective.
Aureoquin Diamate. Name previously used for Quinetolate.
Aurinol Ear Drops. (Various Mfr.) Chloroxylenol and acetic acid, w/benzalkonium chloride and glycerin. Soln. Bot. 15 ml. *Rx.*
Use: Otic preparation.
Aurocein. (Christina) Gold naphthyl sulfhydryl derivative. 5% or 12.5% Amp. 10 ml. *Rx.*
Use: Antirheumatic agent.
Auro-Dri. (Del Pharm.) Boric acid 2.75% in isopropyl alcohol. Bot. oz. *otc.*
Use: Otic preparation.
Auro Ear Drops. (Del Pharm.) Carbamide peroxide 6.5% in a specially prepared base. Bot. 15 ml. *otc.*
Use: Otic preparation.
Aurolate. (Taylor Pharmaceuticals) Gold sodium thiomalate 50 mg, benzyl alcohol 0.5%/ml. Inj. Vial 2 ml, 10 ml. *Rx.*
Use: Antirheumatic agent.
aurolin.
See: Gold sodium thiosulfate.
auropin.
See: Gold sodium thiosulfate.
aurosan.
See: Gold sodium thiosulfate.
aurothioblycanide.
Use: Antirheumatic agent.
•**aurothioglucose, U.S.P. 23.**
Use: Antirheumatic.
aurothioglucose injection.
See: Sterile aurothioglucose suspension.
aurothiomalate, sodium.
See: Gold Sodium Thiomalate, U.S.P. 23.
Auroto Otic. (Barre) Benzocaine 1.4%, antipyrine 5.4%, glycerin and oxyquinoline sulfate/Soln. Bot. 15 ml w/dropper. *Rx.*

Use: Otic preparation.

Ausab. (Abbott Diagnostics) Radioimmunoassay or enzyme immunoassay for detection of antibody to hepatitis B surface antigen. Test kit 100s.
Use: Diagnostic aid.

Ausab EIA. (Abbott Diagnostics) Enzyme immunoassay for the detection of antibody to hepatitis B surface antigen.
Use: Diagnostic aid.

Auscell. (Abbott Diagnostics) Reverse passive hemagglutination test for hepatitis B surface antigen. Test kit 110s, 450s, 1800s.
Use: Diagnostic aid.

Ausria II-125. (Abbott Diagnostics) Radioimmunoassay for detection of hepatitis B surface antigen. Test kit 100s, 500s, 600s, 700s, 800s, 900s, 1000s.
Use: Diagnostic aid.

Auszyme II. (Abbott Diagnostics) Enzyme immunoassay for detection of hepatitis B surface antigen (HBsAg) in human serum or plasma. Test kit 100s, 500s.
Use: Diagnostic aid.

Auszyme Monoclonal. (Abbott Diagnostics) Qualitative third generation enzyme immunoassay for the detection of hepatitis B surface antigen (HBsAg) in human serum or plasma.
Use: Diagnostic aid.

Autoantibody Screen. (Wampole-Zeus) Autoantibody screening system. To screen serum for the presence of a variety of autoantibodies. Test 48s.
Use: Diagnostic aid.

Autolet Kit. (Bayer) Automatic blood letting spring-loaded device to obtain capillary blood samples from fingertips, earlobes or heels.
Use: Diagnostic aid.

Autolymphocyte Therapy; ALT. (Callcor) *Rx.*
Use: Treatment of renal cancer. [Orphan drug]

Autoplex. (Baxter) Anti-inhibitor coagulant complex prepared from pooled human plasma. Vial 30 ml.
Use: Diagnostic aid.

Autoplex T. (Baxter) Dried anti-inhibitor coagulant complex. With a maximum of heparin 2 units and polyethylene glycol 2 mg per ml reconstituted material. Inj. Vial with diluent and needles. *Rx.*
Use: Diagnostic aid.

Autrinic. Intrinsic factor concentrate. *Rx.*
Use: To increase absorption of Vitamin B_{12}.

Auxotab Enteric 1 & 2. (Colab) Rapid identification of enteric bacteria and *pseudomonas.* Test contains capillary units with selective biochemical reagents.
Use: Diagnostic aid.

Avail. (Menley & James) Iron 18 mg, vitamin A 5000 IU, D 400 IU, E 30 mg, B_1 2.25 mg, B_2 2.55 mg, B_3 20 mg, B_6 3 mg, B_{12} 9 mcg, C 90 mg, folic acid 0.4 mg, Ca, Cr, I, Mg, Se and zinc 22.5 mg/Tab. Bot. 60s. *otc.*
Use: Vitamin/mineral supplement.

Avalgesic Lotion. (Various Mfr.) Methyl salicylate, menthol, camphor, methyl nicotinate, dipropylene glycol salicylate, oil of cassia, oleoresins capsicum and ginger. Bot. 120 ml, pt, gal. *otc.*
Use: Analgesic, topical.

A-Van. (Stewart-Jackson) Dimenhydrinate 50 mg/Cap. Bot. 100s.
Use: Antivertigo agent.

AVC Cream. (Hoechst Marion Roussel) Sulfanilamide 15% in a water-miscible base of propylene glycol, stearic acid, diglycol stearate to acid pH. Tube 4 oz. w/applicator. *Rx.*
Use: Anti-infective, vaginal.

AVC Suppositories. (Hoechst Marion Roussel) Sulfanilamide 1.05 g in a base made from polyethylene glycol 400, polysorbate 80, polyethylene glycol 3350, glycerin, inert glycerin-gelatin covering. Box 16s w/inserter. *Rx.*
Use: Anti-infective, vaginal.

Aveeno Anti-Itch. (Rydelle) Calamine 3%, pramoxine HCl, camphor 0.3% in a base of glycerin, distearyldimonium chloride, petrolatum, oatmeal flour, isopropyl palmitate, cetyl alcohol, dimethicone and sodium chloride. Cream 30 g, Lotion 120 ml. *otc.*
Use: Antipruritic.

Aveenobar Medicated. (Rydelle) Aveeno colloidal oatmeal 50%, sulfur 2%, salicylic acid 2%, in soap-free cleansing bar. Formerly Acnaveen. Bar 3.5 oz. *otc.*
Use: Antipruritic.

Aveenobar Oilated. (Rydelle) Vegetable oils, lanolin derivative, glycerine 29%, aveeno colloidal oatmeal 30% in soap-free base. Formerly Emulave. Bar. 3 oz. *otc.*
Use: Emollient.

Aveenobar Regular. (Rydelle) Colloidal oatmeal 50%, anionic sulfonate, hypoallergenic lanolin. Formerly Aveeno Bar. Bar 3.2 oz, 4.4 oz. *otc.*
Use: Skin cleanser.

Aveeno Bath. (Rydelle) Colloidal oatmeal. Box 1 lb, 4 lb. *otc.*
Use: Emollient.

Aveeno Cleansing for Acne Prone Skin. (Rydelle) Sulfur 2%, salicylic acid 2%, colloidal oatmeal 50%, glycerin, titanium dioxide. Soap Bar 90 g. *otc.*
Use: Antiacne.

Aveeno Cleansing Bar. (Rydelle) **Combination Skin:** Soap free. Colloidal oatmeal 51%, sodium cocoyl isethionate, glycerin, lactic acid, sodium lactate, petrolatum, magnesium aluminum silicate, potassium sorbate, titanium dioxide, PEG 14M. Bar 90 g. **Dry Skin:** Soap free. Colloidal oatmeal 51%, sodium cocoyl isethionate, vegetable oil and shortening, glycerin, PEG-75, lauramide DEA, lactic acid, sodium lactate, sorbic acid, titanium dioxide. Bar 90 g. *otc.*
Use: Therapeutic skin cleanser.

Aveeno Colloidal Oatmeal. (Rydelle) Colloidal oatmeal. Box 1 lb, 4 lb. *otc.*
Use: Emollient.

Aveeno Dry. (Rydelle) Dry skin formula, soap free, emollient colloidal oatmeal, vegetable oils, lanolin derivative and glycerin 29% in mild surfactant base. Cleansing bar 90 g. *otc.*
Use: Skin cleansers.

Aveeno Lotion. (Rydelle) Colloidal oatmeal in aqueous lotion base. Glycerin, petrolatum, dimethicone, phenylcarbinol. Bot. 6 oz. *otc.*
Use: Emollient.

Aveeno Moisturizing Cream. (Rydelle) Colloidal oatmeal, glycerin, petrolatum, dimethicone, phenylcarbinol. Cream Tube 120 g. *otc.*
Use: Emollient.

Aveeno Normal. (Rydelle) Normal to oily skin formula, soap free. Colloidal oatmeal 50%, lanolin derivative and mild surfactant. Cleansing bar 96 g, 132 g. *otc.*
Use: Skin cleanser.

Aveeno Oilated. (Rydelle) Aveeno colloidal oatmeal impregnated with 35% liquid petrolatum, refined olive oil. Box 8 oz, 2 lb. *otc.*
Use: Emollient.

Aveeno Shave. (Rydelle) Oatmeal flour. Gel. Can 210 g. *otc.*
Use: Emollient.

Aveeno Shower & Bath. (Rydelle) Colloidal oatmeal, 5% mineral oil, glyceryl stearate, PEG 100 stearate, laureth-4, benzyl alcohol, silica benzaldehyde. Oil. Bot. 240 ml. *otc.*
Use: Emollient.

Aventyl Hydrochloride. (Lilly) Nortriptyline HCl. **Liq.:** Equivalent to 10 mg base/5 ml in alcohol 4%. Bot. 16 fl. oz. **Pulv.:** Equivalent to 10 mg base or 25 mg base/Cap. Bot. 100s, 500s, Blisterpak 10 × 10s. *Rx.*
Use: Antidepressant.

Avertin. Tribromoethanol (Various Mfr.).

•**avilamycin.** (ah-VILL-ah-MY-sin) USAN.
Use: Antibacterial.

Avinar. Uredepa.
Use: Antineoplastic.

Avitene Hemostat. (Med Chem) Hydrochloric acid salt of purified bovine corium collagen. **Fibrous Form:** Jar 1 g, 5 g. **Web Form:** Blister Pak. Sheets of 70 mm × 70 mm, 70 mm × 35 mm, 35 mm × 35 mm. *Rx.*
Use: Hemostat, topical.

•**avobenzone.** (AV-ah-BENZ-ohn) USAN.
Use: Sunscreen.

Avonex. (Biogen) Interferon Beta-1a 33 mcg (6.6 million IU) albumin human 15 mg, sodium chloride and sodium phosphates. Pow. for inj. Vials. Single-use vial w/ 10 ml vial of diluent, swabs, syringe, access pin, needle and bandage. *Rx.*
Use: Relapsing multiple sclerosis.

Avonique. (Armenpharm, Ltd.) Vitamins A 4000 IU, D 400 IU, B_1 1 mg, B_2 1.2 mg, B_6 2 mg, B_{12} 2 mcg, calcium pantothenate 5 mg, B_3 10 mg, C 30 mg, calcium 100 mg, phosphorous 76 mg, iron 10 mg, manganese 1 mg, magnesium 1 mg, zinc 1 mg. *otc.*
Use: Vitamin/mineral supplement.

•**avoparcin.** (AVE-oh-PAR-sin) USAN.
Use: Antibacterial.

•**avridine.** (AV-rih-deen) USAN.
Use: Antiviral.

Awake. (Walgreen) Caffeine 100 mg/ Tab. Bot. 36s. *otc.*
Use: CNS stimulant.

axerophthol.
See: Vitamin A.

Axid. (Lilly) Nizatidine 150 mg or 300 mg/ Cap. Bot. 30s, 60s. *Rx.*
Use: H_2 antagonist.

Axid AR. (Whitehall-Robins) Nizatidine 75 mg/Tab. Bot. 6s, 12s, 18s, 30s. *otc.*
Use: Prevention of heartburn.

Axocet. (Savage) Butalbital 50 mg, acetaminophen 650 mg/Cap. Bot. 100s. *Rx.*
Use: Sedative, hypnotic, analgesic.

Axsain.
See: Zostrix (GenDerm).

Ayds Appetite Suppressant Candy.
(DEP Corp.) Benzocaine 5 mg in chewy candy base w/25 cal./Cube. Ctn. 12s, 48s, 96s. *otc.*
Use: Nonprescription diet aid.

Aygestin. (Wyeth-Ayerst) Norethindrone acetate 5 mg/Tab. Bot. 50s, Cycle pack 10s. *Rx.*
Use: Progestin.

Ayr Saline Nasal Drops. (Ascher) Sodium Cl 0.65% adjusted with phosphate buffers to proper tonicity and pH to prevent nasal irritation. **Drops:** Bot. 20 ml. **Mist:** Bot. 50 ml. *otc.*
Use: Moisture replenisher.

•**azabon.** (AZE-ah-bahn) USAN.
Use: Central nervous system stimulant.

•**azacitidine.** (AZE-ah-SIGH-tih-deen) USAN.
Use: Antineoplastic.

•**azaclorzine hydrochloride.** (AZE-ah-KLOR-zeen) USAN.
Use: Coronary vasodilator.

•**azaconazole.** (AZE-ah-CONE-ah-zole) USAN.
Use: Antifungal.

AZA-CR. NCI Investigational agent.
See: Azacitadine.

Azactam for Injection. (Squibb) L-arginine 780 mg/g aztreonam. **Single dose 15 ml vial:** 500 mg/Vial Pkg. 10s, 25s. 1 g/Vial Pkg. 10s, 25s. 2 g/vial Pkg. 10s, 25s. **Single dose 100 ml IV infusion bottle w/ball bands:** 500 mg/ Bot. Pkg. 10s. 1 g/vial Pkg. 10s. 2 g/ vial Pkg. 10s. *Rx.*
Use: Antibacterial.

azacyclonol hydrochloride.

5-aza-2 deoxycytidine.
Use: Treatment of acute leukemia.

•**azalanstat dihydrochloride.** USAN.
Use: Hypolipidemic.

Azaline Tabs. (Major) Sulfasalazine 500 mg/Tab. Bot. 100s, 500s, 1000s.
Use: Agent for ulcerative colitis.

•**azaloxan fumarate.** (aze-ah-LOX-ahn) USAN.
Use: Antidepressant.

azamethonium bromide. (Novartis) *Rx.*
Use: Ganglionic blocking agent.

•**azanator maleate.** (AZE-an-nay-tore) USAN.
Use: Bronchodilator.

•**azanidazole.** (AZE-ah-NIH-dah-zole) USAN.
Use: Antiprotozoal.

•**azaperone,** (AZE-app-eh-RONE) U.S.P. 23.
Use: Antipsychotic.

azapetine phosphate.

•**azaribine.** (aze-ah-RYE-bean) USAN.
Use: Treatment of psoriasis.

•**azarole.** (AZE-ah-role) USAN.
Use: Immunoregulator.

•**azaserine.** (AZE-ah-SER-een) USAN.
Use: Antifungal.

•**azatadine maleate,** (aze-AT-ad-EEN) U.S.P. 23.
Use: Antihistamine.
See: Optimine, Tab. (Schering-Plough). Trinalin, Tab. (Schering-Plough).

•**azathioprine,** (AZE-uh-THIGH-oh-preen) U.S.P. 23.
Use: Immunosuppressant.
See: Imuran, Inj., Tab. (Glaxo Wellcome).

•**azathioprine sodium,** U.S.P. 23.
Use: Immunosuppressant.

Azathioprine Sodium. (Bedford) Powd. for inj. 100 mg. Vial. 20 ml. *Rx.*
Use: Anti-leukemic.

5-azc.
See: Azacitidine.

Azdone. (Schwarz Pharma) Hydrocodone bitartrate 5 mg, aspirin 500 mg/Tab. Bot. 100s, 1000s. *c-III.*
Use: Narcotic analgesic combination.

•**azelaic acid.** (aze-eh-LAY-ik) USAN.
Use: Antiacne agent.
See: Azelex, cream. (Allergan Herbert).

•**azelastine hydrochloride.** (ah-ZELL-ass-teen) USAN.
Use: Antiallergic, antiasthmatic.
See: Astelin (Wallace).

Azelex. (Allergan Herbert) Azelaic acid 20%, glycerin, cetearyl, alcohol, benzoic acid. Cream 30 g. *Rx.*
Use: Agent for acne vulgaris.

•**azepindole.** (AZE-eh-PIN-dole) USAN.
Use: Antidepressant.

•**azetepa.** (AZE-eh-teh-pah) USAN.
Use: Antineoplastic.

•**3-azido-2, 3 dideoxyuridine.** USAN.
Use: Treatment of AIDS.

azidothymidine.
See: Zidovudine.

Azidouridine. (Berlex) Phase I HIV positive symptomatic, ARC, AIDS. *Rx.*
Use: Antiviral.

•**azimilide dihydrochloride.** (azz-IM-ih-lide die-HIGH-droe-KLOR-ide) USAN.
Use: Cardiac depressant (antiarrhythmic).

•**azipramine hydrochloride.** (aze-IPP-RAH-meen) USAN.
Use: Antidepressant.

•**azithromycin,** (UHZ-ith-row-MY-sin) U.S.P. 23.

Use: Antibacterial.
See: Zithromax, Cap., Susp.(Pfizer).

Azlin. (Bayer) Azlocillin sodium. Vial 2 g, 3 g, 4 g.
Use: Anti-infective; penicillin.

•**azlocillin.** (AZZ-low-SILL-in) USAN.
Use: Antibacterial.
See: Azlin, Inj. (Bayer).

•**azlocillin sodium, sterile,** U.S.P. 23.
Use: Antibacterial.

Azma-Aid. (Purepac) Theophylline 118 mg, ephedrine 24 mg, phenobarbital 8 mg/Tab. Bot. 100s, 250s, 1000s. *Rx.*
Use: Bronchodilator.

Azmacort Inhaler. (Rhone-Poulenc Rorer) Triamcinolone acetonide ≈ 100 mcg delivered from the collapsible expansion chamber activator. Canister 20 g, contains triamcinolone acetonide 60 mg w/oral adapter. *Rx.*
Use: Corticosteroid.

AZO-100. (Scruggs) Phenylazodiaminopyridine HCl 100 mg/Tab. Bot. 100s, 1000s. *otc.*
Use: Urinary tract analgesic.

azoconazole.
Use: Antifungal.

Azodyne.
W/Sulfadiazine, sulfamethizole.
See: Suladyne, Tab. (Stuart).

Azodyne Hydrochloride.
See: Pyridium, Tab. (Parke-Davis).

•**azolimine.** (aze-OLE-ih-meen) USAN.
Use: Diuretic.

AZO Negacide Tablets. (Sanofi Winthrop) Nalidixic acid, phenazopyridine HCl. *Rx.*
Use: Urinary anti-infective.

•**azosemide.** (AZE-oh-SEH-mide) USAN.
Use: Diuretic.

AZO-Standard. (PolyMedica) Phenazopyridine HCl 100 mg/Tab. Bot. 360s. *otc.*
Use: Urinary analgesic.

Azostix Reagent Strips. (Bayer) Bromthymol blue, urease, buffers. Colorimetric test for blood urea nitrogen level. Bot 25 strips.
Use: Diagnostic aid.

azo-sulfisoxazole. (Various Mfr.) Sulfisoxazole 500 mg, phenazopyridine HCl 50 mg/Tab. Bot. 100s, 1000s. *Rx.*
Use: Urinary anti-infective.

•**azotomycin.** (aze-OH-toe-MY-sin) USAN. Antibiotic isolated from broth filtrates of *Streptomyces ambofaciens.*
Use: Antineoplastic.

Azovan Blue.
See: Evans Blue Dye, Amp. (City Chemical; Harvey).

AZO Wintomylon. (Sanofi Winthrop) Nalidixic acid, phenazopyridine HCl. *Rx.*
Use: Urinary anti-infective.

AZT.
See: Zidovudine.

AZT-P-DDI. (Baker Norton) Phase I AIDS.
Use: Antiviral.

•**aztreonam,** (AZZ-TREE-oh-nam) U.S.P. 23.
Use: Antimicrobial.
See: Azactam, Vial (Squibb).

Azulfidine Tablets and En-Tabs. (Pharmacia & Upjohn) Sulfasalazine (salicylazosulfapyridine) 500 mg/Tab or En-tab. Bot. 100s, 500s, UD 100s, 1000s. *Rx.*
Use: Agent for ulcerative colitis.

•**azumolene sodium.** (AH-ZUH-moe-leen) USAN.
Use: Relaxant (skeletal muscle).

B

B₁. Thiamine HCl.

B₂. Riboflavin.

B₃. Niacin, nicotinamide.

B₅. Calcium pantothenate.

B₆. Pyridoxine HCl.

B₆ 50. (Western Research) Vitamin B₆ 50 mg/Tab. Bot. 1000s. *otc.*
Use: Vitamin B₆ supplement.

B₁₂. Cyanocobalamin. *otc.*

B-50. (NBTY) Vitamins B₁ 50 mg, B₂ 50 mg, B₃ 50 mg, B₅ 50 mg, B₆ 50 mg, B₁₂ 50 mcg, folic acid 0.1 mg, d-biotin 50 mcg, PABA, choline bitartrate, inositol/Tab. Bot. 50s, 100s. *otc.*
Use: Vitamin/mineral supplement.

B-50 Time Release. (NBTY) Vitamins B₁ 50 mg, B₂ 50 mg, B₃ 50 mg, B₅ 50 mg, B₆ 50 mg, B₁₂ 50 mcg, folic acid 0.1 mg, d-biotin 50 mcg, PABA 50 mg, choline bitartrate 50 mg, inositol 50 mg, lecithin/Tab. Bot. 100s. *otc.*
Use: Vitamin/mineral supplement.

B 100. (Fibertone) B₁ 100 mg, B₂ 100 mg, B₃ 100 mg, B₅ 100 mg, B₆ 100 mg, B₁₂ 100 mcg, FA 0.4 mg, biotin 50 mcg, PABA 100 mg, choline bitartrate 100 mg, inositol 100 mg/ SR Tab. Bot. 100s. *otc.*
Use: Vitamin supplement.

B-100. (NBTY) Vitamins B₁ 100 mg, B₂ 100 mg, B₃ 100 mg, B₅ 100 mg, B₆ 100 mg, B₁₂ 100 mcg, folic acid 0.1 mg, d-biotin 100 mcg, PABA 100 mg, choline bitartrate, inositol, lecithin. Tab. Bot. 50s, 100s. *otc.*
Use: Vitamin/mineral supplement.

B125. (NBTY) Vitamins B₁ 125 mg, B₂ 125 mg, B₃ 125 mg, B₅ 125 mg, B₆ 125 mg, B₁₂ 125 mcg, folic acid 0.1 mg, d-biotin 125 mcg, PABA 125 mg, choline bitartrate 125 mg, inositol 125 mg, lecithin. Tab. Bot. 100s. *otc.*
Use: Vitamin/mineral supplement.

B150. (NBTY) Vitamins B₁ 150 mg, B₂ 150 mg, B₃ 150 mg, B₅ 150 mg, B₆ 150 mg, B₁₂ 150 mcg, folic acid 0.1 mg, d-biotin 150 mcg, PABA 150 mg, choline bitartrate 150 mg, inositol 150 mg, lecithin. Tab. Bot. 100s. *otc.*
Use: Vitamin/mineral supplement.

B & A. (Eastern Research) Sodium bicarbonate, potassium, aluminum, borax. Hygenic pow. Jar. 8 oz, 5 lb. *Rx.*
Use: Vaginal preparation.

B.A. Gradual. (Federal) Theophylline 260 mg, pseudoephedrine HCl 50 mg, butabarbital 15 mg/Gradual. Bot. 50s, 1000s. *Rx.*

Use: Bronchodilator, decongestant, sedative/hypnotic.

Babee Teething. (Pfeiffer) Benzocaine 2.5%, cetalkonium Cl 0.02%, alcohol, eucolyptol, menthol, camphor. Soln. Bot. 15 ml. *otc.*
Use: Local anesthetic, topical.

Baby Anbesol. (Whitehall Robins) Benzocaine 7.5%, saccharin. Gel Tube 7.2 g. *otc.*
Use: Mouth and throat product.

Baby Cough Syrup. (Towne) Ammonium Cl 300 mg, sodium citrate 600 mg/ oz w/citric acid. Bot. 4 oz.
Use: Antitussive.

Baby Orajel. (Del Pharm) Benzocaine 7.5%, saccharin, sorbitol, alchol free. Gel. Tube 9.45 g. *otc.*
Use: Mouth and throat product.

Baby Orajel Nighttime Formula. (Del Pharm) Benzocaine 10%, saccharin, sorbitol, alcohol free. Gel. Tube 6 g. *otc.*
Use: Mouth and throat product.

Baby Oragel Teeth & Gum Cleanser. (Del Pharm) Poloxamer 407 2%, simethicone 0.12%, parabens, saccharin, sorbitol. Gel Tube 14.2 g. *otc.*
Use: Mouth and throat product.

Baby Vitamin Drops. (Goldline) Vitamins A 1500 IU, D 400 IU, E 5 IU, B₁ 0.5 mg, B₂ 0.6 mg, B₃ 8 mg, B₆ 0.4 mg, B₁₂ 2 mcg, C 35 mg/ml/ Drop. Bot. 50 ml. *otc.*
Use: Vitamin supplement.

Baby Vitamin Drops with Iron. (Goldline) Iron 10 mg, vitamins A 1500 IU, D 400 IU, E 5 IU, B₁ 0.5 mg, B₂ 0.6 mg, B₃ 8 mg, B₆ 0.4 mg, C 35 mg/ml/ Bot. 50 ml. *otc.*
Use: Vitamin/mineral supplement.

BAC. Benzalkonium Cl.

•**bacampicillin HCl,** (BACK-am-PIH-sill-in) U.S.P. 23.
Use: Antibacterial.
See: Spectrobid (Roerig). [NAME]ô[/ NAME](Roberts) Vitamins C 300 mg, B₁ 15 mg, B₂ 10.2 mg, B₃ 50 mg, B₆ 5 mg, B[SUB]5[/Sub] 10 mg/Caplets. Bot. 100s.*otc.*
Use: Vitamin supplement.

Bacco-Resist. (Vita Elixir) Lobeline sulfate 1/64 gr.
Use: Antismoking lozenge.

Bacid. (Novartis) A specially cultured strain of human *Lactobacillus acidophilus*, sodium carboxymethylcellulose 100 mg, sodium 0.5 mEq/Cap. Bot. 50s, 100s. *otc.*
Use: Antidiarrheal/nutritional supplement.

Baciguent Antibiotic Ointment. (Pharmacia & Upjohn) Bacitracin 500 units/g. Oint. Tube 0.5 oz, 1 oz, 4 oz. *otc.*
Use: Anti-infective, external.

bacitracin. (Various Mfr.). An antibiotic produced by a strain of *Bacillus subtilis.*
Diagnostic Tabs. Oint., Ophthalmic Oint. 500 units/Gm. Tube 3.5 g, 3.75 g. *Rx.*
Soluble Tab., Systemic Use, Vial., Topical Use, Vial., Troche. Vaginal Tab.
Use: Antibacterial. [Orphan drug]

•**bacitracin, U.S.P. 23.**
Use: Antibacterial.
See: AK-Tracin, Oint. (Akorn).
Baciquent, Oint. (Pharmacia & Upjohn).
W/Neomycin sulfate.
See: Bacimycin, Oint. (Hoechst Marion Roussel).
Bacitracin-Neomycin, Oint., Ophth. Oint. (Various Mfr.).
W/Neomycin, polymyxin B sulfate.
See: Baximin, Oint. (Quality Generics).
BPN Ointment (Procter & Gamble).
Mycitracin, Oint., Ophth. Oint. (Pharmacia & Upjohn).
Neosporin, Oint., Ophth. Oint., Aerosol, Pow. (Glaxo Wellcome).
Neo-Thrycex, Oint. (Del Pharm.).
Tigo, Oint. (Burlington).
Tri-Biotic Oint. (Burgin-Arden).
Tri-Biotic, Oint. (Standex).
Tri-Bow Oint. (Jones Medical).
Triple Antibiotic Oint. (Towne).
W/Neomycin sulfate, polymyxin B sulfate, diperodon HCl.
See: Epimycin A, Oint. (Delta).
Mity-Mycin, Oint. (Solvay).
W/Neomycin sulfate, polymyxin B sulfate, hydrocortisone acetate.
See: Neopolycin-HC, Oint., Ophth. Oint. (Hoechst Marion Roussel).
W/Polymyxin B sulfate.
See: Polysporin, Oint., Ophth. Oint. (Glaxo Wellcome).
W/Polymyxin B sulfate and neomycin sulfate.
See: Trimixin, Oint. (Hance).
W/Polymyxin B sulfate, neomycin sulfate and hydrocortisone-free alcohol.
See: Biotic-Ophth. W/HC, Oint. (Scrip).
Cortisporin, Preps. (Glaxo Wellcome).

bacitracin-neomycin ointment. (Various Mfr.) Neomycin sulfate equivalent to 3.5 mg base, bacitracin 500 units/Gm. Topical Oint. Tube 0.5 oz, 1 oz, Ophth. Oint. ⅛ oz. *otc.*

Use: Anti-infective, topical.

bacitracin/neomycin/polymyxin B ointment. (Various Mfr.) Polymyxin B sulfate 10,000 units/g, neomycin sulfate 3.5 mg/g, bacitracin zinc 400 units/g. Tube 3.5 g. *Rx.*
Use: Anti-infective, ophthalmic.

bacitracin and polymyxin b sulfate.
Topical Aerosol.
Use: Anti-infective, topical.
See: Polysporin Oint., Pow. (Glaxo Wellcome).

bacitracin zinc. (Pharmacia & Upjohn) Sterile pow. 10,000 units, 50,000 units/Vial.
Use: Anti-infective.

•**bacitracin zinc, U.S.P. 23.**
Use: Antibacterial.
W/Neomycin sulfate, polymyxin B sulfate
See: AK-Spore Ophth. Oint. (Akorn).
Neomixin, Oint. (Roberts)
Neosporin, Prods. (Glaxo Wellcome).
Neotal, Oint. (Roberts)
Ocutricin Ophth. Oint. (Bausch & Lomb)
Triple Antibiotic Ophth. Oint. (Various Mfr.).
W/Neomycin sulfate, polymyxin B, benzalkonium Cl.
See: Biotres, Oint. (Schwarz Pharma)
W/Neomycin sulfate, polymyxin B sulfate, hydrocortisone acetate
See: Biotres HC, Cream (Schwarz Pharma).
Coracin, Oint. (Roberts).
W/Polymyxin B sulfate, neomycin sulfate.
See: Ophthel, Ophth. Oint. (ICN Pharm.).

bacitracin zinc/neomycin sulfate/polymixin B sulfate/hydrocortisone. (Various Mfr.) Hydrocortisone 1%, neomycin sulfate 0.35%, bacitracin zinc 400 units, polymyxin B sulfate 10,000 units. Tube 3.5 g. *Rx.*
Use: Anti-infective, corticosteroid, ophthalmic.

bacitracin zinc ointment. Bacitracin zinc is an anhydrous ointment base.
(Bausch & Lomb) Polymyxin B sulfate 10,000 units, bacitracin zinc 500 units. Tube 3.5 g
Use: Antibacterial, topical.

bacitracin zinc and polymyxin b sulfate ointment. Ophth. Oint.,
Use: Anti-infective, ophthalmic. *Rx.*
See: Polysporin (Glaxo Wellcome).

Bacit White. (Whiteworth Towne) Bacitracin. Oint. Tube 0.5 oz, 1 oz. *otc.*
Use: Anti-infective, topical.

Backache Maximum Strength Relief.
(B-M Squibb) Magnesium salicylate anhydrous (as tetrahydrate) 467 mg. Capl. Bot. 24s, 50s.*otc.*
Use: Salicylate analgesic.

baclofen. (BACK-low-fen) **Tab.** Bot. 10 mg, 20 mg. 100s, UD 100s; **Intrathecal.** 10 mg/20 ml, 10 mg/5 ml. Single use amps 1 amp refill kit (10 mg/20 ml), 2 or 4 amp refill kit (10 mg/5 ml).
Use: Muscle relaxant.

•**baclofen,** U.S.P. 23.
Use: Muscle relaxant.
See: Baclofen, Tab. (Eon Labs).
Lioresal, Tab. (Novartis).

baclofen, l-baclofen. *Rx.*
Use: Treatment of muscle spasticity.
[Orphn Drug]
See: Neuralgon.

Bacmin. (Marnel) Iron 27 mg, Vitamin A 5000 IU, E 30 IU, C 500 mg, B_1 20 mg, B_2 20 mg, B_3 100 mg, B_5 25 mg, B_6 25 mg, B_{12} 50 mcg, biotin 0.15 mg, folic acid 0.8 mg, Cr, Cu Mg, Mn, Zn 22.5 mg/Tab. Bot. 100s*Rx.*
Use: Vitamin/mineral supplement.

Bac-Neo-Poly Ointment. (Burgin-Arden) Bacitracin 400 units, neomycin sulfate 5 mg, polymyxin B sulfate 5000 units/ Gm. Tube 5 oz.*otc.*
Use: Anti-infective, topical.

Bactal Soap. (Whittaker General) Triclosan 0.5% and anhydrous soap 10%. Liq. 240 ml, 1/2 gal.*otc.*
Use: Antiseptic soap.

bacteriostatic sodium chloride. (Various Mfr.) Sodium Cl 0.9%. Also contains benzyl alcohol or parabens. Inj. Bot. 10 ml, 20 ml, 30 ml. *Rx.*
Use: Parenteral diluent.

bacteriostatic water for injection.
U.S.P. 23. (Abbott) 30 ml. Multiple-dose Fliptop vial (plastic).
Use: Pharmaceutic aid for diluting and dissolving drugs for injection.

bacteriuria tests. In vitro diagnostic aids.
See: Isocult for bacteriuria (SmithKline Diagnostics)
Microstix-3 strips (Bayer)
Uricult (Orion Diagnostica).

Bacti-Cleanse. (Pedinol) Benzylkonium Cl, mineral oil, isopropyl palmitate, cetyl alcohol, glycerine, glyceryl stearate, PEG-100 stearate, dimethicone, diazolidinyl urea, parabens, DMDM hydantion, EDTA. Liq. Bot. 453.6 ml. *otc.*
Use: Therapeutic skin cleanser.

Bacticort. (Rugby) Hydrocortisone 1%, neomycin sulfate equivalent to 0.35%

neomycin base, polymyxin B sulfate 10,000 units/ml, benzalkonium Cl, cetyl alcohol, glyceryl monostearate, mineral oil, polyoxyl 40 stearate, propylene glycol. Ophth. Soln. Bot. 7.5 ml.*Rx.*
Use: Corticosteroid; anti-infective, ophthalmic.

Bactigen Group A Streptococcus.
(Wampole) Latex agglutination slide test for the qualitative detection of group A streptococcal antigen directly from throat swabs. Test kit 60s.
Use: Diagnostic aid.

Bactigen Group A Streptococcus with Gast Trak Slides. (Wampole) Latex agglutination slide test for qualitative detection of group A streptococcal antigen directly from throat swabs. Test 24s. Test kit 48s.
Use: Diagnostic aid.

Bactigen Group B Streptococcus.
(Wampole) Latex agglutination slide test for the qualitative detection of group B streptococcus antigen in urine, cerebrospinal fluid and serum. Test kit 15s.
Use: Diagnostic aid.

Bactigen H. Influenzae. (Wampole) Rapid latex agglutination slide test for the qualitative detection of *Haemophilus influenzae*, type b antigen in cerebrospinal fluid, serum and urine. Test kit 15s, 30s.
Use: Diagnostic aid.

Bactigen Meningitis Panel. (Wampole) Rapid latex agglutination slide test for the qualitative detection of *Haemophilus influenzae* type b, *Neisseria meningitidis* A/B/C/Y/W135 and Streptococcus pneumoniae antigens in cerebrospinal fluid, serum and urine. Test kit 18.
Use: Diagnostic aid.

Bactigen N. Meningitidis. (Wampole) Rapid latex agglutination slide test for the qualitative detection of *Neisseria meningitidis*, serogroups A/B/C/Y/W135 antigens in cerebrospinal fluid, serum and urine. Test kit 15s, 30s.
Use: Diagnostic aid.

Bactigen Salmonella-Shigella. (Wampole) Latex agglutination slide test for the qualitative detection of *Salmonella* or *Shigella* from cultures. 96s.
Use: Diagnostic aid.

Bactine Antiseptic/Anesthetic First Aid Spray. (Bayer) Benzalkonium Cl 0.13%, lidocaine 2.5%. **Squeeze Bot.:** 2 oz, 4 oz. **Liq.:** 16 oz. **Aerosol:** 3 oz. *otc.*
Use: Antiseptic, anesthetic, topical.

Bactine First Aid Antibiotic. (Bayer) Polymyxin B sulfate 5,000 units, baci-

tracin 500 units, neomycin sulfate 5 mg/ g in mineral oil, white petrolatum. Oint. Tube 15 g. *otc.*
Use: Anti-infective, topical.

Bactine First Aid Antibiotic Plus Anesthetic. (Bayer) Polymyxin B sulfate 5,000 units, neomycin 3.5 mg/g, bacitracin 400 units, diperodon HCl 10 mg, in mineral oil and white petrolatum. Oint. Tube 15 g. *otc.*
Use: Anti-infective, topical.

Bactine Hydrocortisone Skin Cream. (Bayer) Hydrocortisone 0.5%. Tube 0.5 oz. *otc.*
Use: Corticosteroid, topical.

Bactine Maximum Strength. (Bayer) Hydrocortisone 1%, glycerin, mineral oil, methylparaben, white petrolatum. Cream tube 30 g. *otc.*
Use: Corticosteroid, topical.

Bactocill. (SK-Beecham) Oxacillin sodium. **Cap.:** 250 mg or 500 mg Bot. 100s. **Vial:** (w/dibasic sodium phosphate 40 mg, methylparaben 3.6 mg, propylparaben 0.4 mg, sodium 3.1 mEq/ Gm) 500 mg, 1 g, 2 g or 4 g/Vial; 10s. Piggyback vial 1 g, 2 g; 25s. Bulk pharm pkg 10 g; Box 25s. *Rx.*
Use: Anti-infective; penicillin.

Bactoshield Foam. (Amsco) Chlorhexidine gluconate 4%, isopropyl alcohol 4%/Foam. Bot. 180 ml. *otc.*
Use: Surgical hand scrub and hand wash.

Bactoshield Solution. (Amsco) Chlorhexidine gluconate 4%/Soln. Bot. 960 ml. *otc.*
Use: Surgical scrub, hand wash, preoperative skin preparation, skin wound and general skin cleanser.

Bactoshield 2. (Amsco) Chlorhexidine glyconate 2%, isorpropyl alcohol 4%. Soln. Bot. 960 ml. *otc.*
Use: Pre-operative skin preparation/ cleanser.

Bactrim. (Roche) Sulfamethoxazole 400 mg, trimethoprim 80 mg/Tab. Bot. 100s. *Rx.*
Use: Anti-infective.

Bactrim DS. (Roche) Trimethoprim 160 mg, sulfamethoxazole 800 mg/Tab. Bot. 100s, 200s, 500s. *Rx.*
Use: Anti-infective.

Bactrim IV Infusion. (Roche) Sulfamethoxazole 400 mg, trimethoprim 80 mg/5 ml. Multidose vials. 10ml, 30ml. *Rx.*
Use: Anti-infective.

Bactrim Pediatric Suspension. (Roche) Trimethoprim 40 mg, sulfamethoxazole

200 mg/5 ml. Bot. 480 ml. *Rx.*
Use: Anti-infective combination.

Bactrim Suspension. (Roche) Sulfamethoxazole 200 mg, trimethoprim 40 mg/5 ml. Bot. 16 oz. *Rx.*
Use: Anti-infective.

Bactroban. (SK-Beecham) Mupirocin 2% in a polyethylene glycol base/Oint (Topical). Tube 15 g. Mupirocin calcium 2%/ Oint (Intranasal). Tube 1 g. *Rx.*
Use: Anti-infective, topical; anti-infective used in adult patients and healthcare workers during institutional outbreaks (intranasal).

Bacturcult. (Wampole) A urinary bacteria culture medium diagnostic urine culture system for urine collection, bacteriuria screening and presumptive bacterial identification. Test kit 10s, 100s.
Use: Diagnostic aid.

Bain de Soleil All Day For Kids SPF 30. (Procter & Gamble) Ethylhexyl p-methoxycinnamate, 2-ethylhexyl 2-cyano-3, 3 diphenyl acrylate, oxybenzone, titanium dioxide, stearyl alcohol, tocopheryl acetate, EDTA. PABA free. Waterproof. Lot. Bot. 120 ml. *otc.*
Use: Sunscreen.

Bain de Soleil All Day Waterproof Sunblock. (Procter & Gamble) SPF 15, 30. Ethylhexyl p-methoxycinnamate, 2-ethylhexyl 2-cyano-3, 3-diphenyl acrylate, oxybenzone, titanium dioxide, stearyl alcohol, vitamin E, EDTA. Lot. Bot. 120 m/g. *otc.*
Use: Sunscreen.

Bain de Soleil All Day Waterproof Sunfilter. (Procter & Gamble) SPF 4, 8. 2-ethylhexyl 2-cyano-3, 3 diphenyl acrylate, ethylhexyl p-methoxycinnamate, titanium dioxide, stearyl alcohol, vitamin E, EDTA. Lot. Bot. 120 ml. *otc.*
Use: Sunscreen.

Bain de Soleil Body Silkening Creme. (Procter & Gamble) Padimate O, ethylhexyl p-methoxycinnamate, oxybenzone, benzyl alcohol. Waterproof cream. Bot. 94 g. *otc.*
Use: Sunscreen.

Bain de Soleil Body Silkening Spray. (Procter & Gamble) Padimate O, oxybenzone, ethylhexyl p-methoxycinnamate. Waterproof lotion. Bot. 240 ml. *otc.*
Use: Sunscreen.

Bain de Soleil Body Silkening Stick. (Procter & Gamble) Padimate O, ethylhexyl p-methoxycinnamate, oxybenzone, dioxybenzone. Stick 53 g. *otc.*
Use: Sunscreen.

Bain de Soleil Face Creme. (Procter & Gamble) Padimate O, ethylhexyl p-methoxycinnamate, oxybenzone. Waterproof cream. Bot. 60 g. *otc.*
Use: Sunscreen.

Bain de Soleil Kids Sport. (Procter & Gamble) SPF 25. Ethylhexyl-p-methoxycinnamate, 2-ethylhexyl 2-cyano-3, 3-diphenyl acrylate, titanium dioxide, PVP/eicosene copolymer, dimethicone, cyclomethicone, triethanolamine, glyceryl tribehenate, tocopheryl acetate, carbomer, EDTA, DMDM hydantoin. PABA free. Waterproof, all day protection. Lot. Bot. 120 ml. *otc.*
Use: Sunscreen.

Bain de Soleil Lip Protecteur. (Procter & Gamble) Ethylhexyl p-methoxycinnamate, oxybenzone, 2-ethylhexyl salicylate, oleyl alcohol, petrolatum. PABA free lip balm, 3 g. *otc.*
Use: Sunscreen.

Bain de Soleil Megatan. (Procter & Gamble) Ethylhexyl p-methoxycinnamate, 2-ethylhexyl salicylate, lanolin, cocoa butter, palm oil, aloe, DMDM hydantoin, xanthan gum, shea butter, EDTA. Lot. Bot. 120 ml. *otc.*
Use: Sunscreen.

Bain de Soleil Orange Gelee SPF 4. (Procter & Gamble) Ethylhexyl p-methoxycinnamate, 2-ethylhexyl salicylate. PABA free. Gel Tube 93.75 g. *otc.*
Use: Sunscreen.

Bain de Soleil SPF 8 + Color. (Procter & Gamble) Octyl methoxycinnamate, octocrylene, mineral oil, cetyl alcohol, EDTA. Lot. Bot. 118 ml. *otc.*
Use: Sunscreen.

Bain de Soleil SPF 15 + Color. (Procter & Gamble) Octyl methoxycinnamate, octocrylene, oxybenzone, mineral oil, cetyl alcohol, EDTA. Lot. Bot. 118 ml. *otc.*
Use: Sunscreen.

Bain de Soleil SPF 30 + Color. (Procter & Gamble). Octocrylene, octyl methoxycinnamate, oxybenzone, mineral oil, cetyl alcohol, EDTA. Lot. Bot. 118 ml. *otc.*
Use: Sunscreen.

Bain de Soleil Sport. (Procter & Gamble). SPF 15. 2-ethylhexyl 2-cyan-3, 3 diphenyl acrylate, ethylhexyl-p-methoxycinnamate, titanium dioxide, dimethicone, cyclomethicone, panthenol, tocopheryl acetate, carbomer, EDTA, DMDM hydantoin. PABA free. Waterproof, sweatproof, all day protection. Lot. Bot. 180 ml. *otc.*
Use: Sunscreen.

Bain de Soleil Tropical Deluxe SPF 4. (Procter & Gamble) Ethylhexyl p-methoxycinnamate, 2-ethylhexyl salicylate, cetyl alcohol, EDTA. PABA free. Waterproof. Lot. Bot. 240 ml. *otc.*
Use: Sunscreen.

Bain de Soleil Under Eye. (Procter & Gamble) Ethylhexyl p-methoxycinnamate, oxybenzone, 2-ethylhexyl salicylate. Stick 1.5 g. *otc.*
Use: Sunscreen.

Bakers Best. (Scherer) Water, alcohol 38%, propylene glycol, extract of capsicum, glycerin, boric acid, Tween 80, diethylphthalate, rose oil, pyrilamine maleate, glacial acetic acid, Uvinul MS 40, hexetidine, benzalkonium Cl 50%, sodium hydroxide 76%. Bot. 8 oz. *otc.*
Use: Antipruritic, antiseborrheic, topical.

•**balafilcon A.** (ba-lah-FILL-kahn A) USAN.
Use: Contact lens material (hydrophilic).

Balanced B$_{100}$. (Fibertone) Vitamins B$_1$ 100 mg, B$_2$ 100 mg, B$_3$ 100 mg, B$_5$ 100 mg, B$_6$ 100 mg, B$_{12}$ 100 mcg, folic acid 0.1 mg, PABA 100 mg, inositol 100 mg, d-biotin 100 mcg/SR Tab. Bot. 50s.
Use: Vitamin/mineral supplement.

Balanced Salt Solution. (Various Mfr.) Sodium Cl 0.64%, potassium Cl, 0.075%, calcium Cl 0.048%, magnesium Cl 0.03%, sodium acetate 0.39%, sodium citrate 0.17%, sodium hydroxide or hydrochloric acid. Soln. Droptainer 18 ml, 500 ml.
Use: Intraocular irrigant.

Baldex Ophthalmic Ointment. (Bausch & Lomb) Dexamethasone phosphate 0.05%. 3.75 g. *Rx.*
Use: Corticosteroid, ophthalmic.

Baldex Ophthalmic Solution. (Bausch & Lomb) Dexamethasone phosphate 0.01%. Dropper Bot. 5 ml. *Rx.*
Use: Corticosteroid, ophthalmic.

BAL in Oil. (Becton Dickinson) 2,3-dimercaptopropanol 100 mg, benzyl benzoate 210 mg, peanut oil 680 mg/ml. Amp. 3 ml Box 10s. *Rx.*
Use: Antidote.

Balmex Baby Powder. (Macsil) Specially purified balsam Peru, zinc oxide, starch, calcium carbonate. Shaker top can. 4 oz. *otc.*
Use: Adsorbent, emollient.

Balmex Emollient Lotion. (Macsil) Fraction of lanolin, allantoin, specially purified balsam Peru, silicone in a non-mineral oil base. Bot. 6 fl. oz. *otc.*
Use: Emollient.

Balmex Ointment. (Macsil) Specially purified balsam Peru, Vitamins A and D, zinc oxide, bismuth subnitrate in a base w/silicone. Tube 1 oz, 2 oz, 4 oz. Jar lb. *otc.*
Use: Emollient.

Balneol Perianal Cleansing. (Solvay) Mineral oil, lanolin oil, methylparaben. Bot. 120 ml. *otc.*
Use: Anorectal preparation.

Balnetar. (Westwood Squibb) Tar equivalent to 2.5% coal tar, U.S.P. Bot. 8 oz. *otc.*
Use: Bath dermatological.

•**balsalazide disodium.** (bahl-SAL-ah-zide) USAN.
Use: Anti-inflammatory (gastrointestinal).

Balsan. Specially purified balsam Peru.
See: Balmex Prods. (Macsil).

•**bambermycins.** (BAM-ber-MY-sinz) USAN.
Use: Anti-bacterial.

•**bamethan sulfate.** USAN.
Use: Vasodilator.

•**bamifylline hydrochloride.** (BAM-ih-FILL-in) USAN.
Use: Bronchodilator.

•**bamnidazole.** (bam-NIH-DAH-zole) USAN.
Use: Antiprotozoal (trichomonas).

Banacid Tablets. (Buffington) Magnesium trisilicate 220 mg. Bot. 100s, 200s, 500s. *otc.*
Use: Antacid.

Banadyne-3. (Norstar) Lidocaine 4%, menthol 1%, alcohol 45%. Soln. Bot. 7.5 ml. *otc.*
Use: Relief of cold sores, fever blisters.

Banalg. (Forest) Methyl salicylate 4.9%, camphor 2%, menthol 1%. Lot. Bot. 60 ml and 480 ml. *otc.*
Use: Analgesic, topical.

Banalg Hospital Strength Liniment. (Forest) Methyl salicylate 14%, menthol 3%. Bot. 60 ml. *otc.*
Use: Analgesic, topical.

Bancap HC. (Forest) Acetaminophen 500 mg, hydrocodone bitartrate 5 mg/Cap. Bot. 100s, 500s. *c-III.*
Use: Narcotic analgesic combination.

•**bandage, adhesive,** U.S.P. 23.
Use: Surgical aid.

•**bandage, gauze,** U.S.P. 23.
Use: Surgical aid.

Banex Capsules. (LuChem) Phenylpropanolamine HCl 45 mg, phenylephrine HCl 5 mg, guaifenesin 200 mg. Bot. 100s, 500s. *otc.*

Use: Decongestant, expectorant.

Banex-LA Tablets. (LuChem) Phenylpropanolamine HCl 75 mg, guaifenesin 400 mg. Bot. 100s, 500s. *otc.*
Use: Decongestant, expectorant.

Banflex. (Forest) Orphenadrine citrate 30 mg/ml. Inj. Vial 10 ml. *Rx.*
Use: Skeletal muscle relaxant.

Bangesic. (H.L. Moore) Menthol, camphor, methyl salicylate, eucalyptus oil in non-greasy base. Bot. 2 oz, gal. *otc.*
Use: Analgesic, topical.

Banocide.
See: Diethylcarbamazine Citrate, U.S.P.

Banophen. (Major) **Cap.** Pseudoephedrine HCl 60 mg, diphenhydramine HCl 25 mg. **Elixir.** Diphenhydramine HCl 12.5 mg/ 5ml, alcohol 5.6%, EDTA, saccharin, sugar. In 118 ml and 240 ml. *otc.*
Use: Decongestant, antihistamine.

Bansmoke. (Thompson) Benzocaine 6 mg, corn syrup, dextrose, lecithin, sucrose. Gum Pack 24s. *otc.*
Use: Smoking deterrent.

Banthine. (Schiapparelli Searle) Methantheline bromide 50 mg/Tab. Bot. 100s. *Rx.*
Use: Anticholinergic.

Bantron Smoking Deterrent Tablets. (DEP Corp.) Magnesium carbonate 129.6 mg, lobeline sulfate 2 mg, tribasic calcium phosphate 129.6 mg/Tab. Carton 18s, 36s. *otc.*
Use: Smoking deterrent.

Barbased. (Major) **Tab.:** Butabarbital 0.25 gr or 0.5 gr/Tab. Bot. 1000s. **Elix.:** Butabarbital- 30 mg/5 ml, alcohol 7%. Bot. 480 ml. *Rx.*
Use: Sedative, hypnotic.

Barbatose No. 2 Tablets. (Pal-Pak) Barbital 64.8 mg/Tab. w/hyoscyamus sulfate, passiflora, valarian. Bot. 1000s. *Rx.*
Use: Sedative.

Barbella Elixir. (Forest) Phenobarbital 0.25 gr, hyoscyamine sulfate 0.1037 mg, atropine sulfate 0.0194 mg, scopolamine HBr 0.0065 mg, alcohol 23%/5 ml. Bot. 4 oz, gal. *Rx.*
Use: Sedative, hypnotic, anticholinergic, antispasmodic.

Barbella Tablets. (Forest) Phenobarbital 16.2 mg, atropine sulfate 0.0194 mg, hyoscyamine sulfate 0.1037 mg, hyoscine HBr 0.0065 mg/Tab. Bot. 100s, 1000s, 5000s. *Rx.*
Use: Sedative, hypnotic, anticholinergic, antispasmodic.

Barbeloid. (Pal-Pak) Phenobarbital 16.2

mg, hyoscyamine sulfate 0.1037 mg, atropine sulfate 0.0194 mg, scopolamine HBr 0.0065 mg/Tab. Bot. 100s, 1000s. *Rx.*
Use: Sedative, hypnotic, anticholinergic, antispasmodic.

Barbenyl.
See: Phenobarbital.

Barbidonna. (Wallace) Phenobarbital 16 mg, hyoscyamine sulfate 0.1286 mg, atropine sulfate 0.025 mg, scopolamine HBr 0.0074 mg, lactose. Tab. Bot. 100s, 500s. *Rx.*
Use: Sedative, hypnotic, anticholinergic, antispasmodic.

Barbidonna No. 2. (Wallace) Phenobarbital 32 mg, hyoscyamine sulfate 0.1286 mg, atropine sulfate 0.025 mg, scopolamine HBr 0.0074 mg, lactose. Tab. Bot. 100s. *Rx.*
Use: Sedative, hypnotic, anticholinergic, antispamodic.

Barbiphenyl.
See: Phenobarbital.

barbital. Barbitone, Deba, Dormonal, Hypnogene, Malonal, Sedeval, Uronal, Veronal, Vesperal, diethylbarbituric acid, diethylmalonylurea.
Use: Sedative, hypnotic.
W/Aspirin, caffeine, niacinamide.
See: Mentran, Tab. (Pasadena Research).

barbital sodium. Barbitone Sodium, diethylbarbiturate monosodium, diethylmalonylurea sodium, Embinal, Medinal, Veronal Sodium.
Use: Sedative, hypnotic.

barbitone.
See: Barbital.

barbitone sodium.
See: Barbital Sodium.

barbiturate-aspirin combinations.
See: Aspirin-Barbiturate Combination.

barbiturates, intermediate duration.
See: Butabarbital (Various Mfr.).
Butethal (Various Mfr.).
Diallylbarbituric Acid (Various Mfr.).
Lotusate, Cap. (Sanofi Winthrop).
Vinbarbital. (Various Mfr.).

barbiturates, long duration.
See: Barbital (Various Mfr.).
Mebaral, Tab. (Sanofi Winthrop).
Mephobarbital (Various Mfr.).
Phenobarbital (Various Mfr.).
Phenobarbital Sodium (Various Mfr.).

barbiturates, short duration.
See: Amobarbital (Various Mfr.).
Amobarbital Sodium (Various Mfr.).
Butalbital (Various Mfr.).

Butallylonal (Various Mfr.).
Cyclobarbital (Various Mfr.).
Cyclopal.
Pentobarbital Salts (Various Mfr.).
Sandoptal.
Secobarbital (Various Mfr.).

barbiturates, triple.
See: Butseco, S.C.T., Tab. (Jones Medical).
Ethobral, Cap. (Wyeth-Ayerst).

barbiturates, ultrashort duration.
See: Hexobarbital.
Neraval.
Pentothal Sodium, Amp. (Abbott).
Surital Sodium, Amp., Vial (Parke-Davis).
Thiopental Sodium (Various Mfr.).

Barc Gel. (Del Pharm.) Pyrethrins 0.18%, piperonyl butoxide technical 2.2%, petroleum distillate 4.8% in gel base. Tube oz. *otc.*
Use: Pediculicide.

Barc Liquid. (Del Pharm.) Pyrethrins 0.18%, piperonyl butoxide technical 2.2%, petroleum distillate 5.52%. Bot. 2 oz. *otc.*
Use: Pediculicide.

Barc Non-Body Lice Control Spray. (Del Pharm.) Spray can 5 oz. *otc.*
Use: Pediculicide.

Baricon. (Lafayette) Barium sulfate 95% pow. for susp. In UD 340 g. *Rx.*
Use: Gastrointestinal contrast agent.

Baridium. (Pfeiffer) Phenazopyridine HCl 100 mg/Tab. Bot.32s. *otc.*
Use: Urinary analgesic.

Bari-Stress M. (Barre) Vitamins B_1 10 mg, B_2 10 mg, niacinamide 100 mg, C 300 mg, B_6 2 mg, B_{12} 4 mcg, folic acid 1.5 mg, calcium pantothenate 20 mg/ Cap or Tab. **Cap.:** Bot. 30s, 100s, 1000s. **Tab.:** Bot. 100s, 1000s. *Rx.*
Use: Vitamin/mineral supplement.

•**barium hydroxide lime,** U.S.P. 23.
Use: Carbon dioxide absorbant.

•**barium sulfate,** U.S.P. 23.
Use: Diagnostic aid (radiopaque medium).

barium sulfate preparation.
See: Barotrast, Pow., Cream (Pilkington Barnes Hind).
Fleet.
Raybar, Susp. (Fleet).
Redi-Flow, Susp. (Berlex).
Rugar, Susp. (McKesson).

Barlevite. (Barth's) Vitamins B_6 0.6 mg, B_{12} 3 mcg, pantothenic acid 0.6 mg, D 3 IU, l-lysine 20 mg/0.6 ml. 100-Day Supply. *otc.*

Use: Vitamin/mineral supplement.

●**barmastine.** (BAR-mast-een) USAN.
Use: Antihistamine.

Barnes-Hind Cleaning and Soaking Solution. (Pilkington Barnes Hind) Cleaning and buffering agents, benzalkonium Cl 0.01%, disodium edetate 0.2%. Bot. 1.2 oz, 4 oz. *otc.*
Use: Hard contact lens care.

Barnes-Hind Saline for Sensitive Eyes. (Pilkington Barnes Hind) Potassium sorbate 0.13%, EDTA 0.025%. Soln. Bot. 360 ml (2s). *otc.*
Use: Contact lens care.

Barnes-Hind Wetting & Soaking Solution. (Pilkington Barnes Hind) Polyvinyl alcohol, povidone, hydroxyethyl cellulose, octylphenoxy (oxyethylene) ethanol, benzalkonium Cl, edetate disodium. Bot. 4 oz. *otc.*
Use: Hard contact lens care.

Barnes-Hind Wetting Solution. (Pilkington Barnes Hind) Polyvinyl alcohol, edetate disodium 0.02%, benzalkonium Cl 0.004%. Bot. 35 ml, 60 ml. *otc.*
Use: Hard contact lens care.

Baro-Cat. (Lafayette) Barium sulfate 1.5% susp. 300 ml, 900 ml.
Use: Gastrointestinal contrast agent.

Baros. (Lafayette) Sodium bicarbonate 460 mg (sodium 126 mg) and tartaric acid 420 mg/g with simethicone. Granules, effervescent. Plastic amp. 3 g.
Use: Diagnostic aid.

Baroset. (Lafayette) Air contrast stomach. Unit-of-use kit. Case 12s.
Use: Radiopaque agent.

barosmin.
See: Diosmin.

Barosperse. (Lafayette) Barium sulfate 95%, suspending agent. Susp. 25 lb.
Use: Radiopaque agent.

Barosperse 110. (Lafayette) Barium sulfate 95%. Susp. 900 g.
Use: Radiopaque agent.

W/Iron. Ferric pyrophosphate 250 mg/5 ml plus Barovite liquid formula.

Basa. (Freeport) Acetylsalicylic acid 324 mg/Tab. Bot. 1000s. *otc.*
Use: Salicylate analgesic.

Basaljel. (Wyeth-Ayerst) Aluminum carbonate gel. **Susp.:** Equivalent to aluminum hydroxide 400 mg/5 ml. Bot. 355 ml. **Cap.:** Equivalent to 608 mg dried aluminum hydroxide gel or 500 mg aluminum hydroxide. Bot. 100s, 500s. **Tab.:** Equivalent to 608 mg dried aluminum hydroxide gel or 500 mg aluminum hydroxide. Bot. 100s. *otc.*

Use: Antacid.

basic aluminum aminoacetate.
See: Dihydroxyaluminum Aminoacetate.

basic aluminum carbonate.
See: Basaljel, Susp. (Wyeth-Ayerst).

basic aluminum glycinate.
See: Dihydroxyaluminum aminoacetate.

basic bismuth carbonate.
See: Bismuth Subcarbonate.

basic bismuth gallate.
See: Bismuth Subgallate (Various Mfr.).

basic bismuth nitrate.
See: Bismuth Subnitrate (Various Mfr.).

basic bismuth salicylate.
See: Bismuth Subsalicylate.

basic fuchsin.
See: Carbol-Fuchsin Topical Soln., U.S.P. 23.

●**basifungin.** (bass-ih-FUN-jin) USAN.
Use: Antifungal.

Basis, Glycerin Soap. (Beiersdorf) **Bar:** Tallow, coconut oil, glycerin. **Sensitive:** Bar 90 g, 150 g. **Normal to dry:** Bar 90 g, 150 g. *otc.*
Use: Therapeutic skin cleanser.

Basis, Superfatted Soap. (Beiersdorf) **Bar:** Sodium tallowate, sodium cocoate, petrolatum, glycerin, zinc oxide, sodium Cl, titanium dioxide, lanolin, alcohol, beeswax, BHT, EDTA. Bar 99 g, 225 g. *otc.*
Use: Therapeutic skin cleanser.

●**batanopride hydrochloride.** (bah-TAN-oh-pride) USAN.
Use: Antiemetic.

●**batelapine maleate.** (bat-EH-lap-EEN) USAN.
Use: Antipsychotic.

●**batimastat.** (bat-IM-ah-stat) USAN.
Use: Antineoplastic.

Bayer 8-Hour Timed-Release Aspirin. (Bayer) Aspirin 10 gr (650 mg)/T.R. Tab. Bot. 30s, 72s, 125s. *otc.*
Use: Salicylate analgesic.

Bayer 205.
See: Suramin Sodium. (No Mfr. currently listed.).

Bayer 2502.
See: Nifurtimox. (No Mfr. currently listed.).

Bayer Aspirin, Genuine. (Bayer) Aspirin 325 mg/Tab. Bot. 50s, 100s, 200s, 300s. Pkg. 12s, 24s. *otc.*
Use: Salicylate analgesic.

Bayer Aspirin, Maximum. (Bayer) Aspirin 500 mg/Tab. Bot. 30s, 60s, 100s. *otc.*

Use: Salicylate analgesic.

Bayer Buffered Aspirin. (Bayer) Buffered aspirin 325 mg. Tab. Bot. 100s. *otc.*
Use: Salicylate analgesic.

Bayer Children's Chewable Aspirin. (Bayer) Aspirin 1.25 gr (81 mg)/Tab. Bot. 30s. *otc.*
Use: Salicylate analgesic.

Bayer Children's Cold Tablets. (Bayer) Phenylpropanolamine HCl 3.125 mg, aspirin 1.25 gr (81 mg)/Tab. Bot. 30s. *otc.*
Use: Decongestant, salicylate analgesic.

Bayer Cough Syrup for Children. (Bayer) Phenylpropanolamine HCl 9 mg, dextromethorphan HBr 7.5 mg/5 ml w/alcohol 5%. Bot. 3 oz. *otc.*
Use: Decongestant, antitussive.

Bayer Low Adult Strength. (Bayer) Aspirin 81 mg, lactose. DR Tab. Bot. 120s. *otc.*
Use: Salicylate analgesic.

Bayer Plus Extra Strength. (Bayer) Aspirin 500 mg buffered with calcium carbonate, magnesium carbonate, magnesium oxide. Cap. Bot. 30s, 60s. *otc.*
Use: Salicylate analgesic with antacid buffers.

Bayer Select Chest Cold. (Bayer) Dextromethorphan HBr 15 mg, acetaminophen 500 mg. Caplets in Pkg. 16s. *otc.*
Use: Antitussive, analgesic.

Bayer Select Flu Relief. (Bayer) Acetaminophen 500 mg, pseudoephedrine HCl 30 mg, dextromethorphan HBr 15 mg, chlorpheniramine maleate 2 mg. Capl. Blister-pack 16s. *otc.*
Use: Decongestant, antitussive, antihistamine, analgesic.

Bayer Select Head Cold. (Bayer) Pseudoephedrine HCl 30 mg, acetaminophen 500 mg. Capl. Pkg. 16s. *otc.*
Use: Decongestant, analgesic, expectorant.

Bayer Select Maximum Strength Backache. (Bayer) Magnesium salicylate tetrahydrate 580 mg. Capl. bot. 24s, 50s. *otc.*
Use: Analgesic.

Bayer Select Maximum Strength Headache. (Bayer) Acetaminophen 500 mg, caffeine 65 mg/Cap. Bot. 36s. *otc.*
Use: Analgesic combination.

Bayer Select Maximum Strength Menstrual. (Bayer) Acetaminophen 500 mg, pamabrom 25 mg/Capl. Bot. 24s, 50s. *otc.*
Use: Analgesic, diuretic.

Bayer Select Maximum Strength Night Time Pain Relief. (Bayer) Acetaminophen 500 mg, diphenhydramine HCl/Tab. Bot. 24s, 50s. *otc.*
Use: Antihistamine.

Bayer Select Maximum Strength Sinus Pain Relief. (Bayer) Acetaminophen 500 mg, pseudoephedrine HCl 30 mg/Tab. Bot. 50s. *otc.*
Use: Analgesic, decongestant.

Bayer Select Night Time Cold. (Bayer) Acetaminophen 500 mg, pseudoephedrine HCl 30 mg, dextromethorphan HBr 15 mg, triprolidine HCl 1.25 mg. Capl. Blister-pack 16s. *otc.*
Use: Analgesic, decongestant, antitussive, antihistamine.

Bayer Select Pain Relief Formula. (Bayer) Ibuprofen 200 mg/Cap. Bot. 50s. *otc.*
Use: Nonsteroidal anti-inflammatory agent, analgesic.

Bayer Therapy Caplets. (Bayer) Aspirin, 325 mg, enteric coated. Tab. Bot. 50s, 100s. *otc.*
Use: Analgesic.

BayHep B. (Bayer) Hepatitis B immune globulin (Human). Vial 250 unit, prefilled syringe 250 unit. Vial 1 ml. *Rx.*
Use: Agent for immunization.

Baylocaine 2% Viscous. (Bay Labs) Lidocaine 2% w/sodium carboxymethylcellulose. Soln. Bot. 100 ml. *otc.*
Use: Local anesthetic, topical.

Baylocaine 4%. (Bay Labs) Lidocaine 4% w/methylparaben. Soln. Bot. 50 ml, 100 ml.
Use: Local anesthetic, topical.

Baypress. Type II calcium channel blocking agent. *Rx.*
See: Nitrendipine.

Bayrab. (Bayer) Rabies immune globulin (Human) 150 IU/ml. Vial 2 ml, 10 ml. *Rx.*
Use: Agent for immunization.

BayRho D. (Bayer) Rh_o (D) immune globulin (Human). Prefilled single dose syringe. Single dose syringe. Single dose vial. Pkg. *Rx.*
Use: Immune serum.

Baytet. (Bayer) Tetanus immune globulin (Human). Vial 250 units, Disp. Syringe 250 units. *Rx.*
Use: Immune serum.

BC-1000. (Solvay) Vitamins B_1 50 mg, B_2 5 mg, B_{12} 1000 mcg, B_6 5 mg, d-panthenol 6 mg, niacinamide 125 mg,

ascorbic acid 50 mg, benzyl alcohol 1%/ml. Vial 10 ml. *otc.*
Use: Vitamin supplement.

BC Arthritis Strength. (Block) Aspirin 742 mg, salicylamide 222 mg, caffeine 36 mg/Pow. Bot. 6s, 24s, 50s. *otc.*
Use: Nonnarcotic analgesic combination.

B-C-Bid. (Roberts) Vitamins B_1 15 mg, B_2 10 mg, B_3 50 mg, B_5 10 mg, B_6 5 mg, vitamin C 300 mg, B_{12} 5 mcg /Cap. Bot. 30s, 100s, 500s. *otc.*
Use: Vitamin/mineral supplement.

B-C Bid Caplets. (Roberts) Vitamin C 300 mg, B_1 15 mg, B_2 10.2 mg, B_3 50 mg, B_5 10 mg B_6 5 mg/Cap. Bot. 100s. *otc.*
Use: Vitamin supplement.

BC Cold-Sinus-Allergy Powder. (Block) Phenylpropanolamine HCl 25 mg, chlorpheniramine maleate 4 mg, aspirin 650 mg, lactose. Pow. Pck. 6s, 24s. *otc.*
Use: Decongestant, antihistamine, analgesic.

BC Cold-Sinus Powder. (Block) Phenylpropanolamine HCl 25 mg, aspirin 650 mg, lactose. Pkg. 6s.*otc.*
Use: Decongestant combination.

B-Complex-50. (Nion) Vitamins B_1 50 mg, B_2 50 mg, B_3 50 mg, B_5 50 mg, B_6 50 mg, B_{12} 50 mcg, FA 0.4 mg, biotin 50 mcg, PABA 50 mg, choline bitartrate 50 mg, inositol 50 mg/SR Tab. Bot. 100s. *otc.*
Use: Vitamin/mineral supplement.

B-Complex-150. (Nion) Vitamins B_1 150 mg, B_2 150 mg, B_3 150 mg, B_5 150 mg, B_6 150 mg, B_{12} 1 mcg, FA 0.4 mg, biotin 150 mcg, PABEA 100 mg, choline bitartrate 150 mg, inositol 150 mg. SR Tab. Bot. 30s. *otc.*
Use: Vitamin/mineral supplement.

B-Complex Elixir. (Nion) B_1 2.3 mg, B_2 1 mg, B_3 6.7 mg, B_6 0.3 mg, alcohol 10%. Elix. Bot. 240 ml, 480 ml.*otc.*
Use: Vitamin/mineral supplement.

•**bcg vaccine,** U.S.P. 23.
Use: Immunizing agent (active).

bcg vaccine. (Various Mfr.) Prepared from a Glaxo culture of a Danish strain of BCG bacillus. Amp. 2 ml. *Rx.*
Use: Immunization against tuberculosis, active.
See: Theracys (Pasteur-Merieux-Connaught)

BCNU.
Use: Antineoplastic.
See: BiCNU, Inj. (Bristol).

BCO. (Western Research) Vitamins B_1

10 mg, B_2 2 mg, B_6 1.5 mg, B_{12} 25 mcg, niacinamide 50 mg/Tab. Bot. 1000s. *otc.*
Use: Vitamin supplement.

B-Com. (Century) Vitamins B_1 3 mg, B_2 3 mg, B_6 0.5 mg, niacinamide 20 mg, calcium pantothenate 5 mg, B_{12} 1 mcg, desiccated liver (undefatted) 60 mg, debittered brewer's dried yeast 60 mg/Cap. Bot. 100s, 1000s. *otc.*
Use: Vitamin/mineral supplement.

B-Complex 25-25 Inj. (Forest) Niacinamide 100 mg, Vitamins B_1 25 mg, B_2 1 mg, B_6 2 mg, pantothenic acid 2 mg/ml. Vial 30 ml. *Rx.*
Use: Vitamin supplement.

B-Complex "50". (Vitaline) Vitamins B_1 50 mg, B_2 50 mg, B_3 50 mg, B_4 50 mg, B_5 50 mg, B_6 50 mg, B_{12} 50 mcg, FA 0.1 mg, PABA 30 mg, inositol 50 mg, biotin 50 mcg, choline bitartrate 50 mg. Reg. or TR tabs. Bot. 90s, 1000s. *otc.*
Use: Vitamin supplement.

B-Complex #100. (Medical Chem) Vitamins B_1 100 mg, B_2 2 mg, B_6 4 mg, d-panthenol 4 mg, niacinamide 100 mg/ml. Vial 30 ml. *Rx.*
Use: Vitamin supplement.

B-Complex 100. (Rabin-Winters) Vitamins B_1 100 mg, B_2 2 mg, B_6 2 mg, niacinamide 125 mg, panthenol 10 mg/ml. Vial 30 ml. *Rx.*
Use: Vitamin supplement.

B-Complex 100/100. (Sandia) Vitamins B_1 100 mg, B_2 2 mg, B_6 2 mg, niacinamide 100 mg/ml. Inj. Vial 30 ml. *Rx.*
Use: Vitamin supplement.

B-Complex and B_{12}. (NBTY) Vitamins B_1 7 mg, B_2 14 mg, B_3 4.5 mg, B_{12} 25 mcg, protease 10 mg/Tab. Bot. 90s. *otc.*
Use: Vitamin supplement.

B-Complex with B-12. (Goldline) B_1 1.5 mg, B_2 1.7 mg, B_3 20 mg, B_5 10 mg, B_6 2 mg, B_{12} 6 mcg, FA 0.4 mg/Tab. Bot. 100s *otc.*
Use: Vitamin/mineral supplement.

B-Complex Capsules. (Arcum) Vitamins B_1 1.5 mg, B_2 2 mg, niacinamide 10 mg, B_6 0.1 mg, calcium pantothenate 1 mg, desiccated liver 70 mg, dried yeast 100 mg/Cap. Bot. 100s, 1000s. *otc.*
Use: Vitamin/mineral supplement.

B-Complex Capsules J.F. (Bryant) Vitamins B_1 1 mg, B_2 0.3 mg, nicotinic acid 0.3 mg, B_6 0.25 mg, desiccated liver 0.15 g, yeast powder, dried 0.15 g/Cap. Bot. 100s, 1000s. *otc.*
Use: Vitamin/mineral supplement.

B-Complex Injection with Vitamin C.

Use: Vitamin supplement.
See: Cplex Cap. (Arcum).

B Complex with B$_{12}$ Capsules. (Bryant) Vitamins B$_1$ 2 mg, B$_2$ 2 mg, B$_6$ 0.5 mg, niacinamide 10 mg, B$_{12}$ 2 mcg, biotin 10 mcg, calcium pantothenate 1.5 mg, choline dihydrogen citrate 40 mg, inositol 30 mg, desiccated liver 1 gr, brewer's yeast 3 gr/Cap. Bot. 100s, 1000s. *otc.*
Use: Vitamin/mineral supplement.

B-Complex/Vitamin C Caplets. (Geneva) Vitamins B$_1$ 15 mg, B$_2$ 10.2 mg, B$_3$ 50 mg, B$_5$ 10 mg, B$_6$ 5 mg, C 300 mg/Capl. Bot. 100s. *otc.*
Use: Vitamin supplement.

B-Complex with Vitamin C and B$_{12}$-10,000. (Fujisawa) Vitamins B$_1$ 20 mg, B$_2$ 3 mg, B$_3$ 75 mg, B$_5$ 5 mg, B$_6$ 5 mg, B$_{12}$ 1000 mcg, C 100 mg. Covial. 10 ml multiple dose. *Rx.*
Use: Vitamin supplement.

B Complex + C. (Various Mfr.) Vitamins B$_1$ 15 mg, B$_2$ 10 mg, B$_3$ 100 mg, B$_5$ 20 mg, B$_6$ 5 mg, B$_{12}$ 10 mcg, C 500 mg/Tab. Bot. 100s. *otc.*
Use: Vitamin supplement

B-Complex + C. (NBTY) C 200 mg, B$_1$ 10 mg, B$_2$ 10 mg, B$_3$ 50 mg, B$_5$ 10 mg, B$_6$ 5 mg/Tab. Bot. 100s. *otc.*
Use: Vitamin supplement.

B Complex with C and B-12 Injection. (Goldline) B$_1$ 50 mg, B$_2$ 5 mg, B$_3$ 125 mg, B$_5$ 6 mg, B$_6$ 5 mg, B$_{12}$ 1000 mcg, C 50 mg/Inj. 10 ml. *Rx.*
Use: Vitamin supplement.

BC Powder. (Block) Aspirin 650 mg, salicylamide 145 mg, caffeine 32 mg/Pow. Pkg. 2s, 6s, 24s, 50s. *otc.*
Use: Salicylate analgesic combination.

BC Powder, Arthritis Strength. (Block) Aspirin 742 mg, salicylamide 222 mg, caffeine 36 mg/Powder. Pkg. 6s, 24s, 50s. *otc.*
Use: Salicylate analgesic combination.

BC Tablets. (Block) Aspirin 325 mg, salicylamide 95 mg, caffeine 16 mg/Tab. Pkg 4s. Bot. 50s, 100s. *otc.*
Use: Salicylate analgesic combination.

B-C with Folic Acid. (Geneva) Vitamins B$_1$ 15 mg, B$_2$ 15 mg, B$_3$ 100 mg, B$_5$ 18 mg, B$_6$ 4 mg, B$_{12}$ 5 mcg, C 500 mg, folic acid 0.5 mg/Tab. Bot. 100s. *Rx.*
Use: Vitamin/mineral supplement.

B-C w/Folic Acid Plus. (Geneva Pharm.) Fe 27 mg, vitamins A 5000 IU, E 30 IU, B$_1$ 20 mg, B$_2$ 20 mg, B$_3$ 100 mg, B$_5$ 25 mg, B$_6$ 25 mg, B$_{12}$ 50 mcg, C 500 mg, FA 0.8 mg, biotin 0.15 mg, Cr, Cu, Mg,

Mn, Zn 22.5 mg. Tab. Bot. 100s. *Rx.*
Use: Vitamin/mineral supplement.

B-Day Tablets. (Barth's) Vitamins B$_1$ 7 mg, B$_2$ 14 mg, niacin 4.67 mg, B$_{12}$ 5 mcg/Tab. Bot. 100s, 500s. *otc.*
Use: Vitamin B supplement.

B-D Glucose. (Becton Dickinson) Glucose 5 g. Chew. Tab. Bot. 36s. *otc.*
Use: Glucose elevating agent.

bdep.
See: Benzathine Penicillin G.

B Dozen. (Standex) Vitamin B$_{12}$ 25 mcg Tab. Bot. 1000s. *otc.*
Use: Vitamin B supplement.

B-Dram w/C Computabs. (Dram) Vitamins B$_1$ 5mg, B$_2$ 10 mg, B$_6$ 5 mg, nicotinamide 50 mg, calcium pantothenate 20 mg/Tab. Bot. 100s. *otc.*
Use: Vitamin/mineral supplement.

Beano. (AK Pharma) alpha-D-galactosidase derived from *Aspergillus niger*, a fungal source in carrier of water and glycerol. Liq. Bot. 75 serving size at 5 drops per dose. Tab. Pkg. 12s. Bot. 30s, 100s. *otc.*
Use: Antiflatulent.

Bebatab No. 2. (Freeport) Belladonna ⅛ gr, phenobarbital 0.25 gr/Tab. Bot. 1000s. *Rx.*
Use: Anticholinergic, antispasmodic, sedative, hypnotic.

•**becanthone hydrochloride.** (BEE-kanthone) USAN.
Use: Antischistosomal.

Because. (Schering Plough) Nonoxynol 9 8%. Vaginal foam. Bot. 10 g (6 dose contraceptor unit). *otc.*
Use: Spermicide.

•**becaplermin.** (beh-kah-PLER-min) USAN.
Use: Chronic dermal ulcers treatment.

Beceevite Capsules. (Halsey) Vitamins C 300 mg, B$_1$ 15 mg, B$_2$ 10 mg, niacin 50 mg, B$_6$ 5 mg, pantothenic acid 10 mg/Tab. Bot. 100s. *otc.*
Use: Vitamin supplement.

•**beclomethasone dipropionate,** (BEK-low-METH-uh-zone die-PRO-peo-uh-NATE) U.S.P. 23.
Use: Glucocorticoid.
See: Beclovent Inhalation Aerosol (Allen & Hanburys).
Beconase Nasal Inhaler (Allen & Hanburys).
Beconase AQ Nasal Spray (Allen & Hanburys).
Vancenase Nasal Inhaler (Schering Plough).
Vanceril Inhaler (Schering Plough).

beclomycin dipropionate.
Use: Corticosteroid.

Beclovent Inhalation Aerosol. (Glaxo Wellcome) Beclomethasone dipropionate 42 mcg/actuation. Aerosol canister (16.8 g) containing 200 metered inhalations. Canister 16.8 g w/oral adapter. Refill canister 16.8 g. *Rx.*
Use: Corticosteroid.

Becomp-C. (Cenci) Vitamins C 250 mg, B_1 25 mg, B_2 10 mg, nicotinamide 50 mg, B_6 2 mg, calcium pantothenate 10 mg, hesperidin complex 50 mg/Cap. Bot. 100s, 500s. *otc.*
Use: Vitamin/mineral supplement.

Beconase AQ Nasal Spray. (Glaxo Wellcome) Beclomethasone dipropionate 42 mcg/metered spray. Pump aerosol bot. 25 g (200 metered inhalations). *Rx.*
Use: Corticosteroid.

Beconase Inhalation Aerosol. (Glaxo Wellcome) Beclomethasone dipropionate 42 mcg/actuation. Aerosol canister (16.8 g) containing 200 metered inhalations. Canister 16.8 g. *Rx.*
Use: Corticosteroid.

Becotin-T. (Dista) Vitamins B_1 15 mg, B_2 10 mg, B_6 5 mg, niacinamide 100 mg, pantothenic acid 20 mg, B_{12} 4 mcg, C 300 mg/Tab. Bot. 100s, 1000s, Blister pkg. 10 × 10s. *otc.*
Use: Vitamin supplement.

•**bectumomab.** (beck-TYOO-moe-mab) USAN.
Use: Monoclonal antibody (diagnosis of non-Hodgkin's lymphoma and detection of AIDS-related lymphoma).

Bedoce. (Lincoln) Crystalline anhydrous vitamin B_{12} 1000 mcg/ml. Vial 10 ml. *Rx.*
Use: Vitamin B_{12} supplement.

Bedoce-Gel. (Lincoln) Vitamin B_{12} 1000 mcg/ml in 17% gelatin soln. Vial 10 ml. *Rx.*
Use: Vitamin B_{12} supplement.

Bedside Care. (Sween) Bot. 8 oz, gal.
Use: Non-rinsing shampoo, body wash.

Beeceevites Capsules. (Halsey)
Use: Vitamin supplement.

beechwood creosote.
See: Creosote, N.F.

Bee-Forte w/C. (Rugby) Vitamins B_1 25 mg, B_2 12.5 mg, B_3 50 mg, B_5 10 mg, B_6 3 mg, B_{12} 2.5 mcg, C 250 mg/Cap. Bot. 100s. *otc.*
Use: Vitamin supplement.

beef peptones. (Sandia) Water soluble peptones derived from beef 20 mg/2 ml. Inj. Vial 30 ml. *Rx.*

Use: Parenteral nutritional supplement.

Beelith. (Beach) Pyridoxine HCl 20 mg, magnesium oxide 600 mg/Tab. Bot. 100s. *otc.*
Use: Vitamin/mineral supplement.

Beepen-VK. (SK-Beecham) Penicillin VK. **Tab.:** 250 mg. Bot. 1000s; 500 mg. Bot. 500s. **Oral Susp.:** 125 mg/5 ml Bot. 100 ml, 200 ml; 250 mg/5 ml Bot. 100 ml, 200 ml. *Rx.*
Use: Anti-infective; penicillin.

Bee-Thi. (Burgin-Arden) Cyanocobalamin 1000 mcg, thiamine HCl 100 mg in isotonic soln. of sodium Cl/ml. Vial 10 ml, 20 ml. *Rx.*
Use: Vitamin B supplement.

Bee-Twelve 1000. (Burgin-Arden) Cyanocobalamin 1000 mcg /ml. Vial 10 ml, 30 ml. *Rx.*
Use: Vitamin B supplement.

Bee-Zee. (Rugby) Vitamins E 45 mg, B_1 15 mg, B_2 10.2 mg, B_3 100 mg, B_5 25 mg, B_6 10 mg, B_{12} 6 mcg, C 600 mg, zinc 5.2 mg/Tab. Bot. 60s. *otc.*
Use: Vitamin/mineral supplement.

Behepan.
See: Vitamin B_{12}.

Belatol No. 1; No. 2. (Cenci) **No. 1:** Belladonna leaf extract ⅛ gr, phenobarbital 0.25 gr/Tab. 100s, 1000s. **No. 2:** Belladonna leaf extract gr, phenobarbital 0.5 gr/Tab. Bot. 100s, 1000s. *Rx.*
Use: Anticholinergic, antispasmodic, sedative, hypnotic.

Belatol Elixir. (Cenci) Phenobarbital 20 mg, belladonna 6.75 min./5 ml w/ alcohol 45%. Elix. Bot. pt, gal. *Rx.*
Use: Sedative, hypnotic, anticholinergic, antispasmodic.

Belbutal No. 2 Kaptabs. (Churchill) Phenobarbital 32.4 mg, hyoscyamine sulfate 0.1092 mg, atropine sulfate 0.0215 mg, hyoscine HBr 0.0065 mg/Tab. Bot. 100s. *Rx.*
Use: Sedative, hypnotic, anticholinergic, antispasmodic.

Beldin. (Halsey) Diphenhydramine HCl 12.5 mg/5 ml w/alcohol 5%. Bot. gal. *otc.*
Use: Antihistamine.

Belexal. (Pal-Pak) Vitamins B_1 1.5 mg, B_2 2 mg, B_6 0.167 mg, calcium pantothenate 1 mg, niacinamide 10 mg/Tab. w/brewer's yeast. Bot. 1000s, 5000s. *otc.*
Use: Vitamin/mineral supplement.

Belexon Fortified Improved. (APC) Liver fraction No. 2, 3 gr, yeast extract 3 gr, vitamins B_1 5 mg, B_2 6 mg, niac-

inamide 10 mg, calcium pantothenate 2 mg, cyanocobalamin 1 mcg, iron 10 mg/Cap. Bot. 100s. *otc.*
Use: Vitamin/mineral supplement.

Belfer. (Forest) Vitamins B₁ 2 mg, B₂ 2 mg, B₁₂ 10 mcg, B₆ 2 mg, C 50 mg, iron 17 mg/Tab. Bot. 100s. *otc.*
Use: Vitamin/mineral supplement.

•**belfosdil.** (bell-FOSE-dill) USAN.
Use: Antihypertensive (calcium channel blocker).

Belganyl. CDC anti-infective agent. *Rx.*
See: Suramin.

Belix Elixir. (Halsey) Diphenhydramine HCl 12.5 mg/5 ml. Bot. 118 ml. *otc.*
Use: Antihistamine.

belladonna alkaloids.
Use: Anticholinergic, antispasmodic.
W/Combinations.
See: Accelerase-PB, Cap. (Organon).
Belphen Timed Cap. (Robinson).
Coryztime, Cap. (ICN Pharm.).
Fitacol Stankap (Standex).
Nilspasm, Tab. (Parmed).
Ultabs, Tab. (Burlington).
Urised, Tab. (PolyMedica).
U-Tract, Tab. (Jones Medical).
Wigraine, Tab., Supp. (Organon).
Wyanoids, Supp. (Wyeth-Ayerst).

belladonna alkaloids w/phenobarbital.
(Various Mfr.) Atropine sulfate 0.0194 mg, scopolamine HBr 0.0065 mg, hyoscyamine HBr or SO₄ 0.1037 mg, phenobarbital 16.2 mg/Tab. Bot. 20s, 1000s, UD 100s. *Rx.*
Use: Anticholinergic, antispasmodic, sedative, hypnotic.

•**belladonna extract,** U.S.P.23.
Use: Anticholinergic.

belladonna extract. (Lilly) 15 mg (0.187 mg belladonna)/Tab.
Use: Intestinal antispasmodic.

belladonna extract combinations.
Use: Anticholinergic, antispasmodic.
See: Amobell, Cap. (Bock).
Amsodyne, Tab. (ICN Pharm.).
B & O Supprettes (PolyMedica).
Belap, Tab. (Lemmon).
Bellkatal, Tab. (Ferndale).
Butibel, Tab., Elix. (McNeil).
Gelcomul, Liq. (Del Pharm.).
Hycoff Cold, Cap. (Saron).
Phebe (Western Research).
Rectacort, Supp. (Century).

belladonna leaf.
Use: Intestinal antispasmodic.
W/Phenobarbital and benzocaine.
Use: Anticholinergic.
See: Gastrolic, Tab. (Roberts).

belladonna products and phenobarbital combinations.
Use: Anticholinergic, antispasmodic, sedative, hypnotic.
See: Accelerase-PB, Cap. (Organon).
Alised, Tab. (ICN Pharm.).
Atrocap, Cap. (Freeport).
Atrosed, Tab. (Freeport).
Bebatab, Tab. (Freeport).
Belap, Tab., Elix. (Lemmon).
Belatol, Tab., Elix. (Cenci).
Bellergal, Tab., Spacetab. (Sandoz).
Bellkatal, Tab. (Ferndale).
Bellophen, Tab. (Richlyn).
B-Sed, Tab. (Scrip).
Chardonna, Tab. (Rhone-Poulenc Rorer).
Donabarb, Tab., Elix. (ICN Pharm.).
Donnafed Jr., Tab. (Jenkins).
Donnatal, Tab., Extentab, Cap., Elix. (Robins).
Donnatal #2, Tab. (Robins).
Donnazyme, Tab. (Robins).
Gastrolic, Tab. (Roberts).
Hypnaldyne, Tab. (Vortech).
Kinesed, Tab. (Stuart).
Mallenzyme, Tab. (Roberts).
Medi-Spas, Elix. (Medical Chemicals).
Phenobarbital and Belladonna, Tab. (Lilly).
Sedapar, Tab. (Parmed).
Spabelin, Tab. (Arcum).
Spabelin No. 2, Tab. (Arcum).
Spasnil, Tab. (Rhode).

belladonna tincture. (Lilly) Bot. 4 oz, 16 oz.
Use: Intestinal antispasmodic.

Bellafoline. (Sandoz) Levorotatory alkaloids of belladonna. **0.25 mg/Tab.**: Bot. 100s. **0.5 mg/ml.**: Amp 1 ml. *Rx.*
Use: Anticholinergic, antispasmodic.

Bellaneed. (Hanlon) Belladonna, phenobarbital 16 mg/Cap. Bot. 100s. *Rx.*
Use: Anticholinergic, antispasmodic, sedative, hypnotic.

Bell/ans. (C.S. Dent) Sodium bicarbonate 520 mg, sodium content 144 mg/Tab. Bot. 30s, 60s. *otc.*
Use: Antacid.

Bellastal. (Wharton) Atropine sulfate 0.0194 mg, scopolamine HBr 0.0065 mg, hyoscyamine HBr or SO₄ 0.1037 mg, phenobarbital 16.2 mg Cap. Bot. 1000s. *Rx.*
Use: Anticholinergic, antispasmodic.

Bellatal. (Richwood) Phenobarbital 16.2 mg (hyoscyamine sulfate 0.1037 mg, atropine sulfate 0.0194 mg, scopolamine HBr 0.0065 mg), Lactose/Tab. Bot. 100s, 500s. *Rx.*

Use: Sedative, hypnotic.

Bellergal-S. (Sandoz) Ergotamine tartrate 0.6 mg, bellafoline 0.2 mg, phenobarbital 40 mg, tartrazine, lactose, sucrose. SR Tab. Bot. 100s. *Rx.*
Use: Anticholingergic, antispasmodic, sedative, hypnotic.

•**beloxamide.** (bell-OX-ah-mid) USAN.
Use: Antihyperlipoproteinemic.

Bel-Phen-Ergot S. (Goldline) Phenobarbital 40 mg, ergotamine tartrate 0.6 mg, l-alkaloids of belladonna 0.2 mg. Tab. Bot. 100s. *Rx.*
Use: Anticholingergic, antispasmodic, sedative, hypnotic.

Bel-Phen-Ergot SR. (Goldline) l-alkaloids of belladonna 0.2 mg, phenobarbital 40 mg, ergotamine tartrate 0.6 mg, lactose/SR Tabs. Bot. 100s. *Rx.*
Use: Anticholinergic.

•**bemarinone hydrochloride.** (BEH-mahrih-NOHN) USAN.
Use: Cardiotonic (positive inotropic, vasodilator).

•**bemesetron.** (beh-meh-SET-rone) USAN.
Use: Antiemetic.

Beminal 500. (Whitehall) Vitamins B_1 25 mg, B_2 12.5 mg, B_3 100 mg, B_6 10 mg, B_5 20 mg, C 500 mg, B_{12} 5 mcg/Tab. Bot. 100s. *otc.*
Use: Vitamin supplement.

Beminal Forte w/Vit. C. (Wyeth-Ayerst) Vitamins B_1 25 mg, B_2 12.5 mg, niacinamide 50 mg, B_6 3 mg, calcium pantothenate 10 mg, C 250 mg, B_{12} 2.5 mcg/Cap. Bot. 100s. *otc.*
Use: Vitamin/mineral supplement.

Beminal Stress Plus Iron. (Wyeth-Ayerst) Vitamins B_1 25 mg, B_2 12.5 mg, B_3 100 mg, B_6 20 mg, B_6 10 mg, B_{12} 25 mcg, folic acid 400 mcg, C 700 mg, E 45 IU, iron 27 mg. Dye-free. Tab. Bot. 60s. *otc.*
Use: Vitamin/mineral supplement.

Beminal Stress Plus Zinc. (Wyeth-Ayerst) Vitamins B_1 25 mg, B_2 12.5 mg, B_3 100 mg, B_5 20 mg, B_6 10 mg, B_{12} 25 mcg, C 700 mg, E 45 IU, zinc 45 mg/Tab. Bot. 60s, 250s. *otc.*
Use: Vitamin/mineral supplement.

•**bemitradine.** (beh-MIH-trah-DEEN) USAN.
Use: Antihypertensive, diuretic.

•**bemoradan.** (beh-MOE-rah-DAN) USAN.
Use: Cardiotonic.

Benacen. (Cenci) Probenecid 0.5 g/Tab. Bot. 100s, 1000s. *Rx.*
Use: Agent for gout.

Benacol. (Cenci) Dicyclomine HCl 20 mg/Tab. Bot. 100s, 1000s. *Rx.*
Use: Anticholinergic, antispasmodic.

benactyzine hydrochloride. 2-Diethylaminoethyl benzilate HCl.
Use: Tranquilizer.
W/Meprobamate.
See: Deprol, Tab. (Wallace).

benactyzine/meprobamate. Psychotherapeutic combination.
See: Deprol (Wallace).

Benadryl. (Parke-Davis) Diphenhydramine HCl. *otc, Rx.* **Cap.:** 25 mg. Bot. 100s, 1000s, UD 100s. **Cream:** 1%. Tube 1 oz. **Elix. (w/alcohol 14%):** 12.5 mg/5 ml. Bot. 4 oz, pt, gal, UD 5 ml 100s. **Spray:** 1%. Bot. 2 oz. **Tab.:** 25 mg. Bot. 100s.
Use: Antihistamine.

Benadryl-25 Capsules. (Parke-Davis) Diphenhydramine HCl 25 mg/Cap. Box 24s. *otc.*
Use: Antihistamine.

Benadryl Allergy. (Warner Lambert Consumer Health Products) Diphenhydramine HCl, phenylalanine 4.2 mg. **Kapseal:** 25 mg/Cap. Bot. 24s, 48s. **Chew. Tab.:** 12.5 mg/Tab. Pkg. 24s. **Tab.:** 25 mg/Tab. Bot. 24s, 100s. **Liq.:** 12.5 mg/5 ml. Liq. Bot. 120 ml, 480 ml. *otc.*
Use: Antihistamine.

Benadryl Allergy Decongestant Liquid. (Warner Lambert Consumer Health Products) Pseudoephedrine HCl 30mg, diphenhydramine HCl 12.5 mg/5ml. Liq. Bot. 118 ml. *otc.*
Use: Decongestant, antihistamine.

Benadryl Allergy/Sinus Headache Caplets. (Warner Lambert Consumer Health Products) Pseudoephedrine HCl 30 mg, diphenhydramine HCl 12.5 mg, acetaminophen 500 mg/Capl. Bot. 24s. *otc.*
Use: Decongestant, antihistamine, analgesic.

Benadryl Cold Liquid. (Parke-Davis) Pseudoephedrine HCl 10 mg, diphenhydramine HCl 8.3 mg, acetaminophen 167 mg, alcohol 10%, saccharin. Liq. Bot. 180 ml. *otc.*
Use: Decongestant, antihistamine.

Benadryl Cough Preparation.
See: Benylin Cough Syrup (Parke-Davis).

Benadryl Decongestant Allergy Capsules. (Warner Lambert Consumer Health Products) Diphenhydramine HCl 25 mg, pseudoephedrine HCl 60 mg/Cap. Box 24s. *otc.*

Use: Antihistamine, decongestant.

Benadryl Dye Free. (Warner Lambert Consumer Health Products) Diphenhydramine HCl 6.25 mg/5 ml. Liq. 236 ml. *otc.*
Use: Antihistamine.

Benadryl Dye-Free Allergy Liqui Gels. (Parke-Davis) Diphenhydramine HCl 25 mg, sorbitol/Softgel Cap/Bot. 24s. *otc.*
Use: Antihistamine.

Benadryl Dye Free LiquiGels. (Warner Lambert Consumer Health Products) Diphenhydramine HCl 2.5 mg/Cap. Pkg. 24s. *otc.*
Use: Antihistamine.

Benadryl Elixir. (Parke-Davis) Diphenhydramine HCl 12.5 mg/5 ml w/alcohol 14%. Bot. 4 oz, pt, gal, UD (5 ml) 100s. *otc.*
Use: Antihistamine.

Benadryl Injection. (Parke-Davis) Diphenhydramine HCl. *Rx.* **Amp:** 50 mg/ml. Amp. 1 ml. Box 10s. **Steri-Dose:** 50 mg/ml, pH adjusted w/HCl or sodium hydroxide. Amp. 1 ml. Box 10s. Disposable syringe 1 ml. **Steri-Vial:** 10 mg/ml. Phemerol benzethonium Cl as germicidal agent. pH adjusted w/sodium hydroxide or HCl 10 ml, 30 ml. (50 mg/ml) 10 ml.
Use: Antihistamine.

Benadryl Itch Relief. (Warner Lambert Consumer Health Products) Diphenhydramine HCl 2%, zinc acetate 0.1%, alcohol 73.6%, aloe vera. Spray. 59 ml. *otc.*
Use: Antihistamine.

Benadryl Itch Stopping Gel Children's Formula. (Warner Lambert Consumer Health Products) Diphenhydramine HCl 1%, zinc acetate 1%. Tube 118 ml. *otc.*
Use: Antihistamine.

Benadryl Itch Stopping Gel Maximum Strength. (Warner Lambert Consumer Health Products) Diphenhydramine HCl 2%, zinc acetate 1%. Tube 118 g. *otc.*
Use: Antihistamine.

Benadryl Itch Relief Children's. (Warner Lambert Consumer Health Products) **Cream:** Diphenhydramine HCl 1%, zinc acetate 0.1%, aloe vera, cetyl alcohol, parabens. Jar 14.2 g. **Spray:** Diphenhydramine HCl 1%, zinc acetate 0.1%, alcohol 73.6%, aloe vera, povidone. Can. 59 ml. *otc.*
Use: Antihistamine.

Benadryl Maximum Strength. (Parke-Davis) **Cream:** Diphenhydramine HCl 2% and parabens in a greaseless base in 15 g. **Non-aerosol spray:** Diphenhydramine HCl 2%, alcohol 85% in 60 ml. *otc.*
Use: Antipruritic, topical.

Benadryl Maximum Strength 2%. (Parke-Davis) **Cream:** Diphenhydramine HCl 2%, parabens. 15 g. **Spray, non-aerosol:** Diphenhydramine HCl 2%, alcohol 85%. 60 ml. *otc.*
Use: Antipruritic, topical.

Benadryl Plus. (Parke-Davis) Pseudoephedrine 30 mg, diphenhydramine 12.5 mg, acetaminophen 500 mg/Tab. 24s. *otc.*
Use: Decongestant, antihistamine, analgesic.

Benadryl Plus Nighttime. (Parke-Davis). Pseudoephedrine 30 mg, diphenhydramine 25 mg, acetaminophen 500 mg/5 ml. 180 ml, 300 ml. *otc.*
Use: Decongestant, antihistamine, analgesic.

Benahist 10. (Keene) Diphenhydramine 10 mg/ml. Vial 30 ml. *Rx.*
Use: Antihistamine.

Benahist 50. (Keene) Diphenhydramine 50 mg/ml. Vial 10 ml. *Rx.*
Use: Antihistamine.

Ben-Allergin-50. (Mayrand) Diphenhydramine HCl 50 mg/ml w/chlorobutanol. Inj. Vial 10 ml. *Rx.*
Use: Antihistamine.

benaneerin hydrochloride.
benanserin hydrochloride.
Use: Serotonin antagonist.

Benapen.
See: Benethamine.

Benaphen Caps. (Major) Diphenhydramine 25 mg or 50 mg/Cap. Bot. 100s, 1000s. *otc, Rx.*
Use: Antihistamine.

•**benapryzine hydrochloride.** (BEN-ah-PRY-zeen) USAN.
Use: Anticholinergic.

Ben-Aqua. (Syosset) **Gel:** Benzoyl peroxide 5% or 10% w/polyoxyethylene laurylether. Tube 45 g, 120 g. *otc.*
Use: Antiacne.

Benase. (Ferndale) Proteolytic enzymes extracted from Carica papaya 20,000 units enzyme activity. Tab. Bot. 1000s. *Rx.*
Use: Reduction of edema, relief of episiotomy.

Benat-12. (Roberts) Cyanocobalamin 30 mcg, liver injection 0.5 ml, vitamins B_1 10 mg, B_2 2 mg, niacinamide 50 mg, d-panthenol 1 mg, B_6 1 mg/ml, benzyl alcohol 4%, phenol 0.5%. Vial 10 ml. *Rx.*
Use: Vitamin/mineral supplement.

•**benazepril hydrochloride.** (BEN-AZE-
eh-prill) USAN.
Use: ACE inhibitor.
See: Lotensin (Novartis).

•**benazeprilat.** (BEN-AZE-eh-prill-at)
USAN.
Use: ACE inhibitor.

•**bendacalol mesylate.** (ben-DACK-ah-
LOLE) USAN.
Use: Antihypertensive.

•**bendazac.** (BEN-dah-ZAK) USAN.
Use: Anti-inflammatory.

•**bendroflumethiazide,** U.S.P. 23.
Use: Diuretic, antihypertensive.
See: Naturetin, Tab. (Squibb).
W/Potassium Cl.
See: Naturetin W-K, Tab. (Squibb).
W/Rauwolfia serpentina.
See: Rauzide, Tab. (B-M Squibb)
W/Rauwolfia serpentina, potassium Cl.
See: Rautrax-N, Tab. (Squibb).
Rautrax-N Modified, Tab. (Squibb).

Benefix. (Genetics Inst.) Non-pyrogenic
lyophilized powder preparation. Purified protein produced by recombinant
DNA. Single dose vial with diluent
needle, filter, infusion set and alcohol
swabs. 250, 500 and 1000 IU. *Rx.*
Use: For use in therapy of Factor IX deficiency.

Benemid. (Merck) Probenecid 0.5 g/Tab.
Bot. 100s, 1000s, UD 100s. *Rx.*
Use: Agent for gout.
W/Colchicine.
See: Colbenemid, Tab. (Merck).

**Benephen Antiseptic Medicated Pow-
der.** (Halsted) Methylbenzethonium Cl
1:1800, magnesium carbonate in cornstarch base. Shaker can 3.56 oz. *otc.*
Use: Deodorant, antiseptic.

**Benephen Antiseptic Ointment w/Cod
Liver Oil.** (Halsted) Methylbenzethonium Cl 1:1000, water-repellent base
of zinc oxide, cornstarch. Tube 1.5 oz,
jar lb. *otc.*
Use: Antiseptic.

**Benephen Antiseptic Vitamin A & D
Cream.** (Halsted) Methylbenzethonium
Cl 1:1000, cod liver oil w/vitamins A
and D in petrolatum and glycerin base.
Tube 2 oz, jar lb. *otc.*
Use: Antiseptic.

Benepro Tabs. (Major) Probenecid 500
mg/Tab. Bot. 100s, 1000s. *Rx.*
Use: Agent for gout.

bengal gelatin.
See: Agar.

Ben-Gay Children's Vaporizing Rub.
(Pfizer) Camphor, menthol, w/oils of
turpentine, eucalyptus, cedar leaf, nut-
meg, thyme in stainless white base.
Jar 1.125 oz. *otc.*
Use: Analgesic, topical.

Ben-Gay Extra Strength Balm. (Pfizer)
Methylsalicylate 30%, menthol 8%. Jar
3.75 oz. *otc.*
Use: Analgesic, topical.

Ben-Gay Extra Strength Sports Balm.
(Pfizer) Methylsalicylate 28%, menthol
10%. Tube 1.25 oz, 3 oz. *otc.*
Use: Analgesic, topical.

Ben-Gay Gel. (Pfizer) Methylsalicylate
15%, menthol 7%, alcohol 40%. Tube
1.25 oz, 3 oz. *otc.*
Use: Analgesic, topical.

Ben-Gay Greaseless Ointment. (Pfizer)
Methylsalicylate 18.3%, menthol 16%.
Tube 1.25 oz, 3 oz, 5 oz. *otc.*
Use: Analgesic, topical.

Ben-Gay Lotion. (Pfizer) Methylsalicy-
late 15%, menthol 7% in lotion base.
Bot. 2 oz, 4 oz. *otc.*
Use: Analgesic, topical.

Ben-Gay Original. (Pfizer) Methyl salicy-
late 18.3% and menthol 16%. Oint.
Tube. 37.5 g, 90 g, 150 g. *otc.*
Use: Analgesic, topical.

Ben-Gay Ointment. (Pfizer) Methylsalicylate 15%, menthol 10% in ointment
base. Tube 1.25 oz, 3 oz, 5 oz. *otc.*
Use: Analgesic, topical.

Ben-Gay Sportsgel. (Pfizer) Methylsalicylate, menthol, alcohol 40%. Tube
1.25 oz, 3 oz. *otc.*
Use: Analgesic, topical.

Benoquin. (ICN Pharm.) Monobenzone
20% in cream base. Tube 35 g, 453.6
g. *Rx.*
Use: Treatment of vitiligo.

•**benorterone.** (bee-NAHR-ter-ohn)
USAN.
Use: Antiandrogen.

•**benoxaprofen.** (ben-OX-ah-PRO-fen)
USAN.
Use: Anti-inflammatory, analgesic.

•**benoxinate hydrochloride,** U.S.P. 23.
Use: Anesthetic (topical).
See: Fluress (Pilkington Barnes Hind).

Benoxyl Lotion. (Stiefel) Benzoyl peroxide 5% or 10% in mild lotion base. Bot.
30 ml, 60 ml. *otc.*
Use: Antiacne.

•**benperidol.** (BEN-peh-rih-dahl) USAN.
Use: Antipsychotic.
See: Anquil.

•**bensalan.** (BEN-sal-an) USAN. Under
study.
Use: Disinfectant.

•**benserazide.** (ben-SER-ah-zide) USAN.
Use: Inhibitor (decarboxylase); treatment of Parkinson's disease.

Bensulfoid Cream. (ECR Pharm) Sulfur 8%, resorcinol 2%, alcohol 12%. 15 g. *otc.*
Use: Antiacne.

•**bentazepam.** (BEN-tay-zeh-pam) USAN.
Use: Sedative, hypnotic.

Bentical. (Lamond) Bentonite, zinc oxide, zinc carbonate, titanium dioxide. Bot. 4 oz, 6 oz, 8 oz, 16 oz, 32 oz, 0.5 gal, gal.
Use: Bland lotion.

•**bentiromide.** (ben-TIRE-oh-mide) USAN.
Use: Diagnostic aid (pancreas function determination).
See: Chymex, Soln. (Pharmacia & Upjohn).

•**bentonite, N.F. 18.**
Use: Pharmaceutic aid (suspending agent).

bentonite magma.
Use: Pharmaceutic aid (suspending agent).

bentonite, purified.
Use: Pharmaceutic aid.

•**bentoquatam.** (BEN-toe-KWAH-tam) USAN.
Use: Barrier for prevention of allergic contact dermatitis.

Bentyl. (SK-Beecham) Dicyclomine HCl. **Cap.:** 10 mg. Bot. 100s, 500s, UD 100s. **Tab.:** 20 mg. Bot. 100s, 500s, 1000s, UD 100s. **Syr.:** 10 mg/5 ml. Bot. pt. **Inj.:** 10 mg/ml. Amp. 2 ml, syringe 2 ml. Vial 10 ml (also contains chlorobutanol). *Rx.*
Use: Anticholinergic, antispasmodic.

•**benurestat.** (BEN-YOU-reh-stat) USAN.
Use: Enzyme inhibitor (urease).

Benylin Adult. (Warner Lambert Consumer Health Products) Dextromethorphan HBr 15 mg. Liq. Bot. 118 ml. *otc.*
Use: Antitussive.

Benylin DM Cough Syrup. (Parke-Davis) Dextromethorphan HBr 10 mg/5 ml, alcohol 5%. Bot. 4 oz, 8 oz. *otc.*
Use: Antitussive.

Benylin DME. (Parke-Davis) **Liq.:** Dextromethorphan HBr 5 mg, guaifenesin 100 mg, alcohol 5%, saccharin, menthol. Bot. 240 ml. *otc.*
Use: Antitussive, expectorant.

Benylin Expectorant Liquid. (Warner Lambert Consumer Health Products) Dextromethorphan HBr 5 mg, guaifenesin 100 mg, saccharin, menthol, sucrose. Bot. Liq. 118, 236 ml. *otc.*

Use: Antitussive, expectorant.

Benylin Multi-Symptom. (Warner Lambert Consumer Health Products) Dextromethorphan HBr 5 mg, pseudoephedrine HCl 15 mg, guaifenesin 100 mg/5 ml. Liq. Bot. 118 ml. *otc.*
Use: Antitussive, decongestant, expectorant.

Benylin Pediatric. (Warner Lambert Consumer Health Products) Dextromethorphan HBr 5 ml. Liq. Bot. 118 ml. *otc.*
Use: Antitussive.

Benza. (Century) Benzalkonium Cl 1:5000 and 1:750. Bot. 2 oz, 4 oz.
Use: Antiseptic, germicide.

Benzac 5 & 10. (Galderma) Benzoyl peroxide 5% or 10%, alcohol 12%. Tube 60 g, 90 g. *Rx.*
Use: Antiacne.

Benzac w/ 2.5, 5 & 10. (Galderma) Benzoyl peroxide 2.5%, 5%, 10%. Tube 60 g, 90 g. *Rx.*
Use: Antiacne.

Benzac AC 2.5, 5, & 10. (Galderma) Benzoyl peroxide 2.5%, 5% or 10%, glycerine and EDTA in water base. Gel. Tube. 60 g, 90 g. *Rx.*
Use: Antiacne.

Benzac AC Wash 2.5, 5, & 10. (Galderma) Benzoyl peroxide 2.5%, 5%, 10%, glycerin. Liq. Bot. 240 ml. *Rx.*
Use: Antiacne.

Benzac w Wash 5, & 10. (Galderma) Benzoyl peroxide 5% or 10%. **5%:** Bot. 120 ml, 240 ml. **10%:** Bot. 240 ml. *Rx.*
Use: Antiacne.

5- & 10-Benzagel. (Dermik) Benzoyl peroxide 5% or 10% in gel base of water, alcohol 14%, laureth-4 6% (10% only). Tube 42.5 g, 85 g. *Rx.*
Use: Antiacne.

•**benzaldehyde, N.F. 18.**
Use: Pharmaceutic aid (flavor).

benzalkonium chloride, N.F. 18.
Use: Surface antiseptic, antimicrobial preservative.
See: Benz-All, Liq. (Xttrium).
Econopred, Susp. (Alcon).
Eye-Stream, Liq. (Alcon).
Germicin, Soln. (Consolidated Mid.).
Hyamine 3500 (Rohm & Haas).
Otrivin Spray (Novartis).
Ultra Tears (Alcon).
Zalkon Conc., Liq. (Gordon).
Zephiran Chloride Preps. (Sanofi Winthrop).
W/Aluminum Cl, oxyquinoline sulfate.
See: Alochor Styptic, Liq. (Gordon).

W/Bacitracin zinc, polymyxin B, neomycin sulfate.
See: Biotres, Oint. (Schwarz Pharma).
W/Benzocaine, benzyl alcohol.
See: Aerocain, Oint. (Aeroceuticals).
W/Benzocaine, orthohydroxyphenyl-mercuric Cl, parachlorometaxylenol.
See: Unguentine, Aerosol (Procter & Gamble).
W/Berberine HCl, sodium borate, phenylephrine HCl, sodium Cl, boric acid.
See: Ocusol, Eye Lotion, Drops (Procter & Gamble).
W/Boric acid, potassium Cl, sodium carbonate anhydrous, disodium edetate.
See: Swim-Eye, Drops (Savage).
W/Chlorophyll.
See: Mycomist, Spray Liq. (Gordon).
W/Hydrocortisone.
See: Barseb Thera-Spray, Soln. (Pilkington Barnes Hind).
W/Diperodon HCl, carbolic acid, ichthammol, thymol, camphor, juniper tar.
See: Boro Oint. (Scrip).
W/Disodium edetate, potassium Cl, isotonic boric acid.
See: Dacriose (Smith, Miller & Patch).
W/Epinephrine.
See: Epinal, Soln. (Alcon).
W/Epinephrine bitartrate, pilocarpine HCl, mannitol.
See: E-Pilo Ophth., Preps. (Smith, Miller & Patch).
W/Ethoxylated lanolin, methylparaben, hamamelis water, glycerin.
See: Mediconet, clothwipes. (Medicone).
W/Gentamicin sulfate disodium phosphate, monosodium, phosphate, sodium Cl.
See: Garamycin Ophth. Soln., Preps. (Schering Plough).
W/Hydroxypropyl methylcellulose.
See: Isopto Plain & Tears (Alcon).
W/Hydroxypropyl methylcellulose, disodium edetate.
See: Goniosol (Smith, Miller & Patch).
W/Isopropyl alcohol, methyl salicylate.
See: Cydonol Massage Lotion (Gordon).
W/Lidocaine, phenol.
See: Unguentine, spray (Procter & Gamble).
W/Methylcellulose.
See: Tearisol (Smith, Miller & Patch).
W/Methylcellulose, phenylephrine HCl.
See: Efricel % (Professional Pharmacal).
W/Oxyquinolin sulfate, distilled water.
See: Oxyzal Wet Dressing, Soln. (Gordon).

W/Phenylephrine, pyrilamine maleate, antipyrine.
See: Prefrin-A, Ophth. (Allergan).
W/Pilocarpine HCl, epinephrine bitartrate, mannitol.
See: E-Pilo Ophth., Preps. (Smith, Miller & Patch).
W/Polymyxin B, neomycin sulfate, zinc bacitracin.
See: Biotres, Oint. (Schwarz Pharma).
W/Polyoxyethylene ethers.
See: Ionax, Aerosol Can (Galderma).
W/Polyvinyl alcohol.
See: Contique Artificial Tears (Alcon).
W/Pramoxin.

• **benzbromarone.** USAN.
  Use: Uricosuric.
• **benzethonium chloride,** U.S.P. 23.
  Use: Anti-infective (topical), pharmaceutic aid (preservative).
• **benzetimide hydrochloride.** USAN.
  Use: Anticholinergic.
• **benzilonium bromide.** USAN.
  Use: Anticholinergic.
• **benzindopyrine hydrochloride.** USAN.
  Use: Antipsychotic.
  benzoate and pheylacetate.
  Use: Treatment of hyperammonemia. [Orphan drug]
  Benzo-C. (Freeport) Benzocaine 5 mg, cetalkonium Cl 5 mg, ascorbic acid 50 mg/Troche. Bot. 1000s, cello-packed boxes 1000s. *otc.*
  Use: Local anesthetic, topical.
• **benzocaine,** U.S.P. 23. Ethyl-p-aminobenzoate. Anesthesin, orthesin, parathesin.
  Use: Anesthetic (topical).
  See: BanSmoke, Gum (Thompson).
  W/Combinations.
  See: Aerocaine, Oint. (Aeroceuticals).
  Aerotherm, Oint. (Aeroceuticals).
  Americaine, Oint., Aerosol (DuPont Merck).
  Americaine Anesthetic Lubricant Gel. (Novartis).
  Anacaine, Oint. (Gordon).
  Auralgan, Otic Drops (Wyeth-Ayerst).
  Auralgesic, Liq. (ICN Pharm.).
  Benadex, Oint. (Fuller).
  Benzo-C, Troche (Freeport).
  Benzocol, Oint. (Roberts).
  Benzodent, Oint. (Richardson-Vicks).
  Bicozene, Cream. (Sandoz).
  Boil-Ease Anesthetic, Oint (Del Pharm.).
  Bowman Drawing Paste, Oint. (Jones Medical).
  20-Cain Burn Relief, (Alto).
  Calamatum, Preps. (Blair).

Cetacaine, Preps. (Cetylite).
Chiggerex, Oint. (Scherer).
Chiggertox, Liq. (Scherer).
Chloraseptic Children's Lozenges (Procter & Gamble).
Cepacol, Troches (Hoechst Marion Roussel).
CPI Hemorrhoidal, Supp. (Century).
Culminal, Cream (Culminal).
D.D.D. Cream (Campana).
Dent's Dental Poultice (C.S. Dent).
Dent's Lotion, Jel (C.S. Dent).
Dent's Toothache Gum (C.S. Dent).
Derma Medicone (Medicone).
Derma Medicone-HC (Medicone).
Dermoplast, Lot (Wyeth-Ayerst).
Detane, Gel (Del).
Diplan, Cap. (Solvay).
Dulzit, Cream (Del Pharm.).
Epinephricaine, Oint. (Pharmacia & Upjohn).
Erase, Supp. (LaCrosse).
E.R.O. Forte, Liq. (Scherer).
Foille, Preps. (Carbisulphoil).
Foille, Spray (Blistex).
Foille Medicated First Aid, Oint, Spray. (Blistex).
Foille Plus, Spray (Blistex)
Formula 44 Cough Control Discs, Loz. (Richardson-Vicks).
Fung-O-Spray (Scrip).
G.B.A. Drops (Scrip).
Hemocaine, Oint. (Roberts).
Hurricane, Liq, Spray or Gel (Beutlich).
Isodettes Loz. (SK-Beecham).
Jiffy, Drops (Block Drug).
Lanaiane, Spray, Cream (Whitehall-Robins).
Listerine Cough Control Lozenges (Warner-Lambert).
Maximum Strength Anbesol, Liq, Gel (Whitehall).
Medicone Dressing (Medicone).
Meditrating Throat Lozenge, Loz. (Richardson-Vicks).
My-Cort Drops (Scrip).
Myringacaine, Liq. (Pharmacia & Upjohn).
Nilatus, Loz. (Jones Medical).
Off-Ezy Corn Remover, Liq. (Del Pharm.).
Oracin, Loz. (Richardson-Vicks).
Orabase (Colgate-Palmolive).
Oradex-C, Troche (Del Pharm.).
Orajel Mouth-Aid, Liq, Gel (Del).
Ora-Jel, Gel. (Del Pharm.).
Pazo, Oint., Supp. (Bristol-Myers).
Pyrogallic Acid Oint. (Gordon).
Rectal Medicone (Medicone).
Rectal Medicone-HC, Supp. (Medicone).

Rectal Medicone Unguent (Medicone).
Ridupois Capsule (ICN Pharm.).
Robitussets, Troche (Robins).
Salicide, Oint. (Gordon).
Scrip, Preps. (Scrip).
Solarcaine, Lot, Spray (Schering Plough).
Spec-T Sore Throat-Cough Suppressant Loz. (Squibb).
Spec-T Sore Throat-Decongestant Loz. (Squibb).
Sucrets Cold Decongestant Lozenge (SK-Beecham).
Sucrets Cough Control Lozenge (SK-Beecham).
Tanac, Liq. (Del Pharm.).
Tympagesic, Liq. (Pharmacia & Upjohn).
Unguentine Aerosol (Procter & Gamble).
Vicks Cough Silencers, Loz. (Richardson-Vicks).
Vicks Formula 44 Cough Control Discs, Loz. (Richardson-Vicks).
Vicks Medi-Trating Throat Lozenges, Loz. (Richardson-Vicks).
Vicks Oracin, Loz. (Richardson-Vicks).

benzochlorophene sodium. The sodium salt of ortho-benzyl-para-chlorophenol.

•**benzoctamine hydrochloride.** USAN.
Use: Muscle relaxant, sedative, hypnotic.

Benzodent. (Procter & Gamble) Benzocaine 20%. Tube 30 g. *otc.*
Use: Local anesthetic, topical.

•**benzodepa.** (BEN-zoe-DEH-pah) USAN.
Use: Antineoplastic.

benzoic acid. (Various Mfr.) Pkg. 0.25 lb, 1 lb. *otc.*
Use: Fungistatic, fungicidal.

benzoic acid, U.S.P. 23.
Use: Pharmaceutic aid (antifungal).
W/Boric acid, zinc oxide, zinc stearate.
See: Ting, Cream, Pow. (Novartis).
W/Salicylic acid.
See: Whitfield's Oint. (Various Mfr.).

benzoic acid, 2-hydroxy. Salicylic Acid.

benzoic and salicylic acids ointment.
Use: Antifungal (topical).
See: Whitfield's Oint. (Various Mfr.).

•**benzoin,** U.S.P. 23.
Use: Topical protectant, expectorant.
See: Arcum–Bot. 2 oz, 4 oz, pt, gal.
Lilly–Bot. 4 fl oz, pt.
Rals–Aerosol 12 oz.
Stanlabs–Bot. 2 oz, 4 oz, pt, Compound. Bot. 1 oz, 4 oz, pt.

W/Methyl salicylate, guaiacol.
See: Methagul, Oint. (Gordon).
W/Podophyllum resin.
See: Podoben, Liq. (Maurry).
W/Polyoxyethylene dodecanol, aromatics.
See: Vicks Vaposteam, Liq. (Richardson-Vicks).

Benzoin Spray. (Morton) Benzoin, tolu balsam, styrax, alcohol w/propellant. Aerosol can 7 oz. *otc.*
Use: Skin protectant.

benzol. Usually refers to benzene.

Benzo-Menth Tablets. (Pal-Pak) Benzocaine 2.2 mg/Tab. Bot. 1000s. *otc.*
Use: Anesthetic, topical.

•**benzonatate,** U.S.P. 23.
Use: Antitussive.
See: Tessalon, Perles (DuPont Merck).

Benzonatate Softgels. (Various Mfr.) Benzonatate 100 mg. Cap. Bot. 100s, 1000s. *Rx.*
Use: Antitussive.

benzophenone.
See: Pan Ultra, Lot., Lipstick (Cummins).
W/Oxybenzone, dioxybenzone.
See: Solbar Lotion (Person & Covey).

benzopyrrolate.
See: Benzopyrronium.

benzoquinolimine.
See: Emete-Con (Pfizer).

benzoquinonium chloride. (Various Mfr.) *Rx.*
Use: Skeletal muscle relaxant.

benzosulfimide.
See: Saccharin, U.S.P. 23.

benzosulphinide sodium. Name previously used for Saccharin Sodium.

•**benzoxiquine.** (benz-OX-ee-kwine) USAN.
Use: Disinfectant.

benzoyl p-aminosalicylic. (BEN-zoyl)
See: Benzapas, Pow., Tab. (Sandoz).

•**benzoylpas calcium.** USAN.
Use: Antibacterial (tuberculostatic).
See: Benzapas, Tab., Pow. (Sandoz).

benzoyl peroxide, hydrous, (BEN-zoyl per-OX-ide) Peroxide, dibenzoyl. (Various) **Mask:** 5%. In 30 ml. **Lotion:** 5%, 10%. Bot. 30 ml. **Gel:** 5%, 10%. 45 g, 90 g (10% only).
Use: Keratolytic.

benzoyl peroxide, hydrous, (BEN-zoyl per-OX-ide) U.S.P. 23.
Use: Keratolytic.
See: Benoxyl, Lot. (Stiefel)
Benzac AC, Gel, Liq. (Galderma).
Benzagel-5 & 10, Oint. (Dermik).

Brevoxyl, Gel (Stiefel).
Clearasil Acne Treatment, Cream (Richardson-Vicks).
Clearasil Antibacterial Acne Lotion (Richardson-Vicks).
Dermoxyl, Gel (Zeneca).
Epi-Clear Antiseptic Lotion, Scrub (Squibb).
Exact, Cream (Advanced Polymer Systems).
Oxy-5 Acne Pimple Medication (SK-Beecham).
Oxy-10 Maximum Strength Acne-Pimple Medication (SK-Beecham).
Oxy Wash Antibacterial Skin Wash (SK-Beecham).
Panoxyl, Bar (Stiefel).
Peroxin A5, A10, Gel (Dermol).
Persadox, Cream, Lot. (Ortho).
Persadox HP, Cream, Lot. (Galderma).
Persa-Gel, Gel (Ortho).
Theroxide, Liq., Lot. (Medicis).
Topex, Lot. (Richardson-Vicks).
W/Chlorhydroxyquinoline, hydrocortisone.
See: Loroxide-HC, Lot. (Dermik).
Vanoxide-HC, Lot. (Dermik).
W/Polyoxyethylene lauryl ether.
See: Benzac 5 & 10, Gel (Galderma).
Desquam-X, Gel (Westwood Squibb).
W/Sulfur.
See: Sulfoxyl Lotion (Stiefel).

Benzoyl Peroxide Wash, 5% & 10%. (Glades) Benzoyl peroxide 5%. Liq. Bot. 120 ml, 150 ml, 240 ml. 10%. Liq. Bot. 150 ml, 240 ml. *Rx.*
Use: Keratolytic.

n'-benzoylsulfanilamide.
See: Sulfabenzamide.
W/Sulfacetamide, sulfathiazole, urea.
See: Sultrin, Tab, Cream (Ortho).

benzphetamine hydrochloride. (benz-FET-uh-meen) N-Benzyl-N-α-dimethylphenethylamine HCl, dextro. *c-iii.*
Use: Anorexiant.
See: Didrex, Tab. (Pharmacia & Upjohn).

benzpyrinium bromide.

•**benzquinamide.** (benz-KWIN-ah-mid) USAN.
Use: Antiemetic.
See: Emete-Con, Vial (Roerig).
Quantril (Roerig).

benzquinamide hydrochloride.
See: Emete-Con. (Roerig).

benzthianide.

•**benzthiazide,** U.S.P. 23.
Use: Diuretic, antihypertensive.
See: Aquatag, Tab. (Solvay).

Exna, Tab. (Robins).
Hydrex, Tab. (Trimen).
Proaqua, Tab. (Solvay).
Urazide, Tab. (Roberts).
W/Reserpine.
See: Exna-R, Tab. (Robins).
•benztropine mesylate, (BENZ-troe-peen) U.S.P. 23.
Use: Parasympatholytic, antiparkinso-nian.
W/sodium Cl.
See: Cogentin, Tab., Amp. (Merck).
benztropine methanesulfonate.
See: Benztropine mesylate.
•benzydamine hydrochloride. (ben-ZIH-dah-meen) USAN.
Use: Analgesic, anti-inflammatory, anti-pyretic.
benzydroflumethiazide.
See: Bendroflumethiazide.
benzyhydryl-n-methylpiperazine hy-drochloride.
See: n-benzyhydryl-n-methylpiperazine HCl.
•benzyl alcohol, N.F. 18. Phenylcarbinol.
Use: Antiseptic, local anesthetic, phar-maceutic aid (antimicrobial).
See: Topic, Gel (Ingram).
Vicks Blue Mint, Regular & Wild Cherry Medicated Cough Drops (Richardson-Vicks).
•benzyl benzoate,
Use: Pharmaceutical necessity for Dimercaprol Inj.
benzyl benzoate saponated. Triethanol-amine 20 g, oleic acid 80 g, benzyl ben-zoate q.s. 1000 ml.
benzyl carbinol.
See: Phenylethyl Alcohol, U.S.P. 23.
benzylpenicillin, benzylpenicilloic, benzylpenilloic acid. (Kremers-Urban) Rx.
Use: Assessment of penicillin sensitiv-ity. [Orphan drug]
See: Pre-Pen/MDM.
benzyl penicillin-C-14. (Nuclear-Chi-cago) Carbon-14 labelled penicillin. Vacuum-sealed glass vial 50 microcu-ries, 0.5 millicuries.
Use: Radioisotope.
benzyl penicillin G, potassium.
See: Penicillin G Potassium.
benzyl penicillin G, sodium.
See: Penicillin G Sodium.
•benzylpenicilloyl polylysine concen-trate, U.S.P. 23.
Use: Diagnostic aid (penicillin sensitiv-ity).
See: Pre-Pen (Kremers-Urban).

bepanthen.
See: Panthenol.
bephedin. Benzyl ephedrine.
bephenium bromide.
bephenium hydroxynaphthoate, U.S.P. XXI.
Use: Anthelmintic (hookworms).
•bepridil hydrochloride. USAN.
Use: Vasodilator.
See: Vascor (McNeil).
•beractant. (ber-ACT-ant) USAN.
Use: Lung surfactant. [Orphan drug]
See: Survanta (Ross).
beractant intrathecal suspension. Rx.
Use: Lung surfactant. [Orphan drug]
See: Survanta.
•beraprost. USAN.
Use: Platelet aggregation inhibitor, im-proves ischemic syndromes.
•beraprost sodium. (BEH-reh-prahst) USAN.
Use: Platelet aggregation inhibitor, im-proves ischemic action.
berberine.
W/Hydrastine, glycerin.
See: Murine, Ophth. Soln.
berberine hydrochloride.
W/Borax, sodium Cl, boric acid, camphor water, cherry laurel water, rose water, thimerosol.
See: Lauro, eye irrigator and drops (Otis Clapp).
•berefrine. (BEH-reh-FREEN) USAN.
Use: Mydriatic.
Ber-Ex. (Dolcin) Calcium succinate 2.8 gr, acetylsalicylic acid 3.7 gr/Tab. Bot. 100s, 500s. otc.
Use: Anti-arthritic, antirheumatic.
Berocca Plus Tablets. (Roche) Vitamins A 5000 IU, E 30 IU, C 500 mg, B₁ 20 mg, B₂ 20 mg, B₃.
•berythromycin. USAN.
Use: Antiamebic, antibacterial.
Beserol Tablets. (Sanofi Winthrop) Acetaminophen, chlormezanone. Rx.
Use: Analgesic, tranquilizer, muscle re-laxant.
•besipirdine hydrochloride. (beh-SIH-pihr-deen) USAN.
Use: Cognition enhancer (Alzheimer's disease).
Besta Capsules. (Roberts) Vitamins B₁ 20 mg, B₂ 15 mg, niacinamide 100 mg, calcium pantothenate 20 mg, E 50 IU, magnesium sulfate 70 mg, zinc 18.4 mg, B₁₂ 4 mcg, B₆ 25 mg, C 300 mg/Cap. Bot. 100s. otc.
Use: Vitamin/mineral supplement.

Best C Caps. (Roberts) Ascorbic acid 500 mg/TR Cap. Bot. 100s. *otc.*
Use: Vitamin C supplement.
Bestrone Injection. (Bluco) Estrone in aqueous susp. 2 mg or 5 mg/ml. Vial 10 ml. *Rx.*
Use: Estrogen.
Beta-2. (Nephron) Isoetharine HCl 1% with glycerin, sodium bisulfite, parabens. Bot. 10 ml, 30 ml. *Rx.*
Use: Respiratory therapy, oral inhalant.
beta-adrenergic blockers.
See: Blocadren, Tab. (Merck).
  Brevibloc, Inj. (DuPont Merck).
  Cartrol, Tab. (Abbott).
  Corgard, Tab. (Bristol-Myers).
  Inderal, Tab., Inj. (Wyeth-Ayerst).
  Inderal LA, Sustained Release Cap. (Wyeth-Ayerst).
  Kerlone, Tab. (Searle).
  Levatol, Tab. (Schwarz Pharma).
  Lopressor, Tab., Inj. (Novartis).
  Nadolol, Tab. (Various Mfr.)
  Propranolol HCl, Tab. (Various Mfr.).
  Propranolol HCl, Inj. (SoloPak).
  Sectral, Cap. (Wyeth-Ayerst).
  Tenormin, Tab. (ICI Pharm.).
  Timolol, Tab. (Various Mfr.).
  Visken, Tab. (Sandoz).
beta-adrenergic blockers, ophthalmic.
See: Betagan Liquifilm, Soln. (Allergan).
  Betoptic, Soln. (Alcon).
  Ocupress, Soln. (Otsuka).
  OptiPranolol, Soln. (Bausch & Lomb).
  Timoptic in Ocudose, Soln. (Merck).
  Timoptic, Soln. (Merck).
• **beta carotene,** (BAY-tah CARE-oh-teen) U.S.P. 23.
Use: Ultraviolet screen.
See: Max-Caro (Marlyn).
  Provatene (Solgar).
  Solatene (Roche).
Betachron E-R. (Inwood) Propranolol HCl 60 mg, 80 mg, 120 mg, 160 mg. ER Cap. **60 mg, 120mg, 160 mg:** Bot. 100s. **80 mg:** Bot. 100s, 250s (80 mg only). *Rx.*
Use: Beta-adrenergic blockers.
• **beta cyclodextrin.** N.F. 18.
Use: Pharmaceutic aid (sequestering agent).
Betadine. (Purdue Frederick) Povidone-iodine. *otc.*
  Aerosol Spray, Bot. 3 oz.
  Antiseptic Gz. Pads 3"×9". Box 12s.
  Antiseptic Lubricating Gel, Tube 5 g.
  Disposable Medicated Douche, concentrated packette w/cannula and 6 oz water.

Douche, Bot. 1 oz, 4 oz, 8 oz.
Douche Packette, 0.5 oz (6 per carton).
Helafoam Solution Canister 250 g.
Mouthwash/Gargle, Bot. 6 oz.
Oint., Tube 1 oz, Jar 1 lb, 5 lb.
Oint., packette oz, oz.
Perineal Wash Conc. Kit, Bot. 8 oz w/ dispenser.
Skin Cleanser, Bot. 1 oz, 4 oz.
Skin Cleanser Foam, Canister 6 oz.
Solution, 0.5 oz, 8 oz, 16 oz, 32 oz, gal.
Solution Packette, oz.
Solution Swab Aid, 100s.
Solution Swabsticks, 1s Box 200s; 3s Box 50s.
Surgical Scrub, Bot. pt, pt w/dispenser, qt, gal, packette 0.5 oz.
Surgi-prep Sponge-Brush 36s.
Vaginal Suppositories, Box 7s w/vaginal applicator.
Viscous Formula Antiseptic Gauze Pads: 3"×9", 5"×9". Box 12s.
Whirlpool Concentrate, Bot. gal.
Use: Antiseptic for uses indicated in product labeling.
Betadine Antiseptic. (Purdue Frederick) Povidone-iodine 10%. Vaginal gel. 18 g with applicator. *otc.*
Use: Vaginal preparation.
Betadine Cream. (Purdue-Frederick) Povidone-iodine 5% mineral oil, polyoxyethylene stearate, polysorbate, sorbitan monostearate, white petrolatum. Cream Tube 14 g. *otc.*
Use: Antiseptic/germicide, topical.
Betadine First Aid Antibiotics & Moisturizer. (Purdue Frederick) Polymyxin B sulfate 10,000 IU, bacitracin zinc 500 IU. Oint. 14 g. *otc.*
Use: Antibiotic, topical.
Betadine 5% Sterile Ophthalmic Prep Solution. (Akorn) Povidone iodine 5%. Soln. Bot. 50 ml. *Rx.*
Use: Antiseptic, ophthalmic.
Betadine Medicated Disposable Douche. (Purdue Frederick) Povidone-iodine 10% Soln (0.3% when diluted). Vial 5.4 ml with 180 ml bot. Sanitized water. 1 and 2 packs. *otc.*
Use: Vaginal preparation.
Betadine Medicated Douche. (Purdue Frederick) Povidone-iodine 10% (0.3% when diluted). Soln. In 15 ml (6s) packettes and 240 ml. *otc.*
Use: Vaginal preparation.
Betadine Medicated Premixed Disposable Douche. (Purdue Frederick) Povidone-iodine 10% soln (0.3% when di-

luted). Bot. 180 ml. 1s, 2s. *otc.*
Use: Vaginal preparation.

Betadine Medicated Vaginal Gel and Suppositories. (Purdue Frederick) **Gel:** Povidone-iodine 10%. Tube 18 g, 85 g w/applicator. **Supp:** Povidone-iodine 10%. In 7s w/applicator. *otc.*
Use: Vaginal preparation.

Betadine Shampoo. (Purdue-Frederick) Povidone-iodine 7.5%. Shampoo Bot. 118 ml. *otc.*
Use: Antiseborrheic.

beta-estradiol.
See: Estradiol, U.S.P. 23.

betaeucaine hydrochloride. Name previously used for Eucaine HCl.

Betagan Liquiflim. (Allergan) Levobunolol HCl 0.25% or 0.5%. Bot. 2 ml (0.5%), 5 ml, 10 ml (0.25%) w/ B.I.D. C Cap and Q.D. C Cap (0.5%). *Rx.*
Use: Beta-adrenergic blocking agent, ophthalmic.

Betagen. (Enzyme Process) Vitamins B_1 1 mg, B_2 1.2 mg, niacin 15 mg, B_6 18 mg, pantothenic acid 18 mg, choline 1.8 g, betaine 96 mg/6 Tab. Bot. 100s, 250s. *otc.*
Use: Vitamin/mineral supplement.

Betagen Ointment. (Goldline) Povidone iodine. Oint. Tube oz. Jar lb. *otc.*
Use: Antiseptic.

Betagen Solution. (Goldline) Povidone iodine. Bot. pt, gal. *otc.*
Use: Antiseptic.

Betagen Surgical Scrub. (Goldline) Povidone iodine. Bot. pt, gal. *otc.*
Use: Antiseptic.

•**betahistine hydrochloride.** (BEE-tah-HISS-teen) USAN.
Use: Vasodilator. Meniere's disease. A diamine oxidase inhibitor. Increase microcirculation.

beta-hypophamine.
See: Vasopressin.

betaine anhydrous. (Orphan Medical) *Rx.*
Use: Treatment of hemocystinuria.
See: Cystadane (Orphan Medical).

•**betaine hydrochloride,** U.S.P. 23. Acidol HCl, lycine HCl.
Use: Replenisher adjunct (electrolyte).
W/Ferrous fumarate, docusate sodium, desiccated liver, vitamins, minerals.
See: Hemaferrin, Tab. (Western Research).
W/Pancreatin, pepsin, ammonium Cl.
See: Zypan, Tab. (Standard Process).
W/Pepsin.
See: Normacid, Tab. (Stuart).

Betalin S. (Lilly) Thiamine HCl 50 mg or 100 mg. Tab. Bot. 100s. *otc.*
Use: Vitamin B_1 supplement.

•**betamethasone,** (BAY-tuh-METH-uh-zone) U.S.P. 23.
Use: Glucocorticoid.
See: Celestone, Inj., Syr., Tab. (Schering Plough).

•**betamethasone acetate,** (BAY-tuh-METH-uh-zone) U.S.P. 23.
Use: Glucocorticoid.

•**betamethasone benzoate,** U.S.P. 23.
Use: Glucocorticoid.

•**betamethasone dipropionate,** (BAY-tah-METH-ah-zone die-PRO-pee-oh-nate) U.S.P. 23.
Use: Glucocorticoid.
See: Alphatrex Prods. (Savage).
Diprolene Prods. (Schering Plough).
Diprosone Prods. (Schering Plough).
Psorion Cream (Zeneca).

•**betamethasone sodium phosphate,** (BEE-tah-METH-ah-zone) U.S.P. 23.
Use: Glucocorticoid.
See: Celestone Phosphate Inj. (Schering Plough).

betamethasone sodium phosphate and betamethasone acetate suspension, sterile,
See: Celestone Soluspan (Schering Plough).

•**betamethasone valerate,** (BAY-tah-METH-ah-zone VAL-eh-rate) U.S.P. 23.
Use: Glucocorticoid.
See: Betatrex Prods. (Savage).
Beta-Val Prods. (Lemmon).
Valisone Prods. (Schering Plough).
Valnac Prods. (Schering Plough).

•**betamicin sulfate.** (bay-tah-MY-sin) USAN.
Use: Antibacterial.

betanaphthol. 2-Naphthol.
Use: Parasiticide.

Betapace. (Berlex) Sotalol HCl 80 mg, 120 mg, 160 mg, 240 mg/Tab. Bot. 100s, UD 100s. *Rx.*
Use: Beta-adrenergic blocking agent.

Betapen-VK. (Bristol) Penicillin V potassium. **Oral Soln.:** 125 mg/ml Bot. 100 ml. 250 mg/5 ml Bot. 100 ml, 200 ml. **Tab.:** 250 mg/Tab. Bot. 100s, 1000s; 500 mg/Tab. Bot. 100s. *Rx.*
Use: Anti-infective; penicillin.

beta-phenyl-ethyl-hydrazine. Phenelzine dihydrogen sulfate.
See: Nardil, Tab. (Parke-Davis).

beta-propiolactone.
See: Betaprone, Vial (Forest).

beta-pyridyl-carbinol. Nicotinyl alcohol.

Alcohol corresponding to nicotinic acid.
See: Roniacol, Elix., Tab. (Roche Lab.).

Betasept. (Purdue-Frederick) Chlorhexidine gluconate 4%, isopropyl 4%, alcohol/Liq. Bot. 946 ml. *otc.*
Use: Skin cleanser.

Betaseron. (Berlex) Interferon beta 1b 0.3 mg, (9.6 million IU per vial, albumin human 15 mg, dextrose 15 mg. Pow. for Inj. Single-use Vial w/2 ml vial of diluent. *Rx.*
Use: Relapsing-remitting multiple sclerosis.

Betatrex. (Savage) Betamethasone valerate 0.1%. Cream, Oint. Tube 15 g, 45 g; Lot. Bot. 60 ml. *Rx.*
Use: Corticosteroid, topical.

Beta-Val Cream. (Lemmon) Betamethasone valerate equivalent to 0.1% betamethasone base in cream base. Tube 15 g, 45 g. *Rx.*
Use: Corticosteroid, topical.

•**betaxolol hydrochloride,** (BAY-TAX-oh-lahl) U.S.P. 23.
Use: Antianginal, antihypertensive.
See: Betoptic, Ophth. (Alcon).
Kerlone (Searle).

betaxolol ophthalmic solution,
Use: Beta-adrenergic blocking agent.

•**bethanechol chloride,** (beth-AN-ih-kole) U.S.P. 23.
Use: Cholinergic.
See: Duvoid, Tab. (Procter & Gamble).
Myotonachol, Tab., Amp. (Glenwood).
Urabeth, Tab. (Major).
Urecholine, Tab., Amp. (Merck).
Vesicholine, Tab. (Star).

bethanidine.
Use: Hypotensive.

•**bethanidine sulfate.** (beth-AN-ih-deen) USAN.
Use: Antihypertensive.

Bethaprim. (Major) Trimethoprim 40 mg, sulfamethoxazole 200 mg/5 ml, alcohol 0.26%, saccharin and sorbitol. Susp. *Rx.*
Use: Anti-infective.

Bethaprim DS Tabs. (Major) Trimethoprim 160 mg, sulfamethoxazole 800 mg/Tab. Bot. 100s, 500s, UD 100s. *Rx.*
Use: Anti-infective.

Bethaprim SS Tabs. (Major) Trimethoprim 80 mg, sulfamethoxazole 400 mg/Tab. Bot. 100s, 500s. *Rx.*
Use: Anti-infective.

•**betiatide.** (BEH-tie-ah-tide) USAN.
Use: Pharmaceutic aid.

Betimol. (Ciba Vision) Timolol 0.25% or 0.5%, benzalkonium Cl 0.01%/Soln. Bot. 2.5 ml, 5 ml, 10 ml, 15 ml. *Rx.*
Use: Agent for glaucoma.

Betoptic. (Alcon) Betaxolol HCl 0.5%. Bot. 2.5 ml, 5 ml, 10 ml, 15 ml. *Rx.*
Use: Beta-adrenergic blocking agent, ophthalmic.

Betoptic S. (Alcon) Betaxalol HCl 0.25%. Bot. 2.5 ml, 5 ml, 10 ml, 15 ml. *Rx.*
Use: Beta-adrenergic blocking agent, ophthalmic.

Betuline. (Ferndale) Methyl salicylate, camphor, menthol, peppermint oil in a water soluble base. Lot. Bot. 60 ml, pt. *otc.*
Use: Analgesic, topical.

•**bevantolol hydrochloride.** (beh-VAN-toe-LOLE) USAN.
Use: Antianginal, antihypertensive, cardiac depressant (antiarrhythmic).

Bexomal-C. (Roberts) Vitamins B_1 6 mg, B_2 7 mg, B_3 80 mg, B_5 10 mg, B_6 5 mg, B_{12} 6 mcg, C 250 mg/Tab. Bot. 50s. *otc.*
Use: Vitamin supplement.

•**bezafibrate.** (BEH-zah-FIE-brate) USAN.
Use: Antihyperlipoproteinemic.
See: Bezalip (Procter & Gamble).

Bezon. (Whittier) Vitamins B_1 5 mg, B_2 3 mg, niacinamide 20 mg, pantothenic acid 3 mg, B_6 0.5 mg, C 50 mg, B_{12} 1 mcg/Cap. Bot. 30s, 100s. *otc.*
Use: Vitamin supplement.

Bezon Forte. (Whittier) Vitamins B_1 25 mg, B_2 12.5 mg, niacinamide 50 mg, pantothenic acid 10 mg, B_6 5 mg, C 250 mg/Cap. Bot. 30s, 100s. *otc.*
Use: Vitamin supplement.

B-F-I Powder. (SK-Beecham) Bismuth-formic-iodide, zinc phenolsulfonate, bismuth subgallate, amol, potassium alum, boric acid, menthol, eucalyptol, thymol and inert diluents. Can 0.25 oz, 1.25 oz, 8 oz. *otc.*
Use: Antiseptic, topical.

B.G.O. (Calotabs) Iodoform, salicylic acid, sulfur, zinc oxide, phenol (liquefied) 1%, calamine, menthol, petrolatum, lanolin, mineral oil, undecylenic acid 1%. Jar ⅞ oz, Tube 1 oz. *otc.*
Use: Antiseptic, antifungal, topical.

•**bialamicol hydrochloride.** (bye-AH-lam-IH-KAHL) USAN.
Use: Antiamebic.

•**biapenem.** USAN.
Use: Antibacterial.

biaphasic insulin injection. A suspension of insulin crystals in a solution of insulin buffered at pH 7. Insulin Novo Rapitard.

Biavax-II. (Merck) Rubella and mumps virus vaccine, live. See details under Meruvax-II and Mumpsvax. Single-dose vial w/diluent. Pkg. 1s, 10s. *Rx.*
Use: Agent for immunization.

Biaxin. (Abbott) Clarithromycin 250 mg, 500 mg/Tab. Bot. 60s, UD 100s. Clarithromycin 125 mg/5 ml and 250 mg/5 ml/Gran for oral susp. Bot. 50 ml, 100 ml. *Rx.*
Use: Anti-infective, erythromycin.

• **bicalutamide.** (bye-kah-LOO-tah-mide) USAN.
Use: Antineoplastic.
See: Casodex, Tab (Zeneca).

• **bicifadine hydrochloride.** (bye-SIGH-fah-deen) USAN.
Use: Analgesic.

Bicillin. (Wyeth-Ayerst) Penicillin G benzathine 200,000 units/Tab. Bot. 36s. *Rx.*
Use: Anti-infective; penicillin.

Bicillin C-R. (Wyeth-Ayerst) Penicillin G benzathine 150,000 units, penicillin G procaine 150,000 units/ml w/lecithin, povidone, methyl and propylparabens. Vial 10 ml. Bicillin 300,000 units, penicillin G procaine 300,000 units/1 ml w/lecithin, povidone, methyl and propylparaben. Tubex cartridge 1 ml. Pkg. 10s. Bicillin 600,000 units, penicillin G procaine 600,000 units with parabens, lecithin and povidone/2 ml Tubex cartridge. Pkg. 10s. Bicillin 1,200,000 units, penicillin G procaine 1,200,000 units with parabens, lecithin and povidone/4 single-dose disposable syringe, 10s, 4 ml. *Rx.*
Use: Anti-infective; penicillin.

Bicillin C-R 900/300 Injection. (Wyeth-Ayerst) Penicillin G benzathine 900,000 units, penicillin G procaine 300,000 units with parabens, lecithin and povidone/2 ml. Tubex. Pkg. 10s. *Rx.*
Use: Anti-infective; penicillin.

Bicillin Long-Acting. (Wyeth-Ayerst) Penicillin G benzathine 300,000 units/ml w/lecithin, povidone, methyl and propylparabens. 300,000 units/ml. Vial 10 ml 600,000 units/Tubex. 1,200,000 units/2 ml Tubex 10s. 2,400,000 units/4 ml single dose disposable syringe, 10s. *Rx.*
Use: Anti-infective; penicillin.

• **biciromab.** (bye-SIH-rah-mab) USAN
Use: Monoclonal antibody (antifibrin).

Bicitra. (Baker Norton) Sodium citrate dihydrate 500 mg, citric acid monohydrate 334 mg, 5 mEq sodium ion/5 ml.

Shohl's Solution. Bot. 4 oz, pt, gal, Unit-dose 15 ml, 30 ml. *Rx.*
Use: Systemic alkalinizer.

• **biclodil hydrochloride.** (BYE-kloe-DILL) USAN.
Use: Antihypertensive (vasodilator).

BiCNU. (Bristol-Myers/Bristol Oncology) Carmustine (BCNU) 100 mg, sterile diluent (dehydrated alcohol USP inj.) 3 ml/Vial. *Rx.*
Use: Antineoplastic agent.

Bicozene Cream. (Sandoz) Benzocaine 6%, resorcinol 1.66% in cream base/Cream. Tube 30 g. *otc.*
Use: Anesthetic, topical.

Bicycline. (Knight) Tetracycline HCl 250 mg/Cap. Bot. 100s.
Use: Anti-infective.

• **bidisomide.** USAN.
Use: Cardiac depressant (antiarrhythmic).

• **bifonazole.** (BYE-FONE-ah-zole) USAN.
Use: Antifungal.

bile acids, oxidized. Note also dehydrocholic acid.
W/Atropine methyl nitrate, ox and hog bile extract, phenobarbital.
See: G.B.S., Tab. (Forest).
W/Bile whole (desiccated), dessicated whole pancreas, homatropine methylbromide.
See: Pancobile, Tab. (Solvay).
W/Ox bile, steapsin, phenobarbital, homatropine methylbromide.
See: Oxacholin, Tab. (Roxane).

bile acid suquestrants. *Rx.*
See: Cholybar (Parke-Davis)
Questran (Bristol-Myers)
Questran Light (Bristol-Myers)
Colestid (Pharmacia & Upjohn)

bile extract. (Various Mfr.) Pow. 0.25 lb, 1 lb.
W/Cascara sagrada, dandelion root, podophyllin, nux vomica.
See: Oxachol, Liq. (Roxane).
W/Dehydrocholic acid, homatropine methylbromide, phenobarbital.
See: Neocholan, Tab. (Hoechst Marion Roussel).
W/Pancreatic substance, dl-methionine, choline bitartrate.
See: Licoplex, Tab. (Mills).

bile extract, ox. Purified ox gall. (Lilly) Enseal 5 gr, Bot. 100s, 500s, 1000s.
C. D. Smith–Tab. 5 gr, Bot. 1000s. Stoddard–Tab. 3 gr, Bot. 100s, 500s, 1000s.
W/Cellulase, pepsin, glutamic acid HCl, pancreatin.
See: Kanulase, Tab. (Sandoz).

W/Cellulase, pepsin, glutamic acid HCl, pancreatin, methscopolamine nitrate, pentobarbital.
See: Kanumodic, Tab. (Sandoz).
W/Colcynth compound extract, cascara sagrada extract, podophyllin, hyoscyamus extract.
See: Bileo-Secrin Compound Tablets (First Texas).
W/Dehydrocholic acid, homatropine methylbromide, phenobarbital.
See: Bilamide, Tab. (Norgine).
W/Dehydrocholic acid, pepsin, homatropine methylbromide.
See: Biloric, Cap. (Arcum).
W/Desoxycholic acid, oxidized bile acids, pancreatin.
See: Bilogen, Tab. (Organon).
W/Enzyme concentrate, pepsin, dehydrocholic acid, belladonna extract.
See: Ro-Bile, Tab. (Solvay).
W/Oxidized bile acids, steapsin, phenobarbital, homatropine methylbromide.
See: Oxacholin, Tab. (Philips).
W/Pepsin, pancreatic enzyme concentrate.
See: Konzyme, Tab. (Brunswick).
Nu'Leven, Tab. (Lemmon).
Nu'Leven Plus, Tab. (Lemmon).
W/Sodium salicylate, phenolphthalein, chionanthus extract, cascara sagrada extract, sodium glycocholate, sodium taurocholate.
See: Glycols, Tab. (Jones Medical).
bilein. Bile salts obtained from ox bile.
bile-like products.
See: Zanchol, Tab. (Searle).
bile products.
See: Bile Salts.
Dehydrocholic Acid.
Desoxycholic Acid.
Ketocholanic Acid.
bile salts. Sodium glycocholate and taurocholate. Note also Bile Extract, Ox and oxidized bile acids. (Lilly) Enseal 5 gr, Bot. 100s.
See: Bilein.
Bisol, Tab. (Paddock).
Ox Bile Extract.
Oxidized Bile Acids.
W/Belladonna, nux vomica compound Bile salts 60 mg, belladonna leaf extract 5 mg, nux vomica extract 2 mg, phenolphthalein 30 mg, sodium salicylate 15 mg, aloin 15 mg/Tab. Bot. 1000s.
Use: Laxative, antispasmodic.
W/Cascara sagrada, phenolphthalein, capsicum oleoresin, peppermint oil.
See: Torocol, Tab. (Plessner).
W/Cellulase, calcium carbonate, pancrelipase.

See: Accelerase, Cap. (Organon).
W/Cellulase, pancrelipase, calcium carbonate, belladonna alkaloids, phenobarbital.
See: Accelerase-PB, Cap. (Organon).
W/Dehydrocholic acid, pancreatic substance.
See: Depancol, Tab. (Parke-Davis).
W/Dehydrocholic acid, pepsin, pancreatin.
See: Progestive, Tab. (NCP).
W/Pancrelipase, cellulase.
See: Cotazym-B, Tab. (Organon).
W/Papain, cascara sagrada extract, phenolphthalein, capsicum oleoresin.
See: Torocol Compound, Tab. (Plessner).
W/Pepsin, homatropine, methylbromide, amylase, lipase, protease.
See: Digesplen, Tab., Elix., Drops (Med. Prod.).
W/Phenolphthalein, chionanthus extract.
See: Bile Anthus Compound, Cap. (Scrip).
W/Sodium salicylate, phenolphthalein, chionanthus extract, bile extract, cascara sagrada extract.
See: Glycols, Tab. (Jones Medical).
bile, whole desiccated.
W/Pancreatin, mycozyme diastase, pepsin, nux vomica extract.
See: Enzobile, Tab. (Roberts).
Bili-Labstix Reagent Strips. (Bayer) Reagent strips. Bot. 100s. Test for pH, protein, glucose, ketones, bilirubin and blood in urine.
Use: Diagnostic aid.
Bili-Labstix SG Reagent Strips. (Bayer) Bot. 100s. Urinalysis reagent strip test for specific gravity, pH, protein, glucose, ketone, bilirubin, and blood.
Use: Diagnostic aid.
Bilirubin Reagent Strips. (Bayer) Seralyzer reagent strip. Bot. 25s. Quantitative strip test for total bilirubin in serum or plasma.
Use: Diagnostic aid.
Bilirubin Test.
See: Ictotest. (Bayer).
Bilivist. (Berlex) Ipodate sodium 500 mg/Cap. Bot. 120s. *Rx.*
Use: Radiopaque agent.
Bilopaque. (Sanofi Winthrop) Tyropanoate sodium 750 mg/Cap. Catchcovers of 4 cap. Box 20s, Bot. 100s, 500s. *Rx.*
Use: Radiopaque agent.
Biloric. (Arcum) Pepsin 9 mg, ox bile 160 mg/Cap. Bot. 100s, 1000s. *otc, Rx.*
Use: Antispasmodic.

Bilstan. (Standex) Bile salts 0.5 gr, cascara sagrada powder extract 0.5 gr, phenolphthalein 0.5 gr, aloin ⅛ gr, podophyllin gr/Tab. Bot. 100s. *otc.*
Use: Laxative.

Biltricide. (Bayer) Praziquantel 600 mg/Tab. Bot. 6s. *Rx.*
Use: Anthelmintic.

bimethoxycaine lactate.

•**bindarit.** (BIN-dah-rit) USAN.
Use: Antirheumatic.

•**biniramycin.** (bih-NEER-ah-MY-sin) USAN.
Use: Antibacterial.

•**binospirone mesylate.** (bih-NO-spy-rone) USAN.
Use: Antianxiety agent.

Bintron Tablets. (Madland) Liver fraction 4.6 gr, ferrous sulfate 5 gr, vitamins B_1 3 mg, B_2 0.5 mg, B_6 0.15 mg, C 20 mg, calcium pantothenate 0.3 mg, niacinamide 10 mg/Tab. Bot. 100s, 1000s. *otc.*
Use: Vitamin/mineral supplement.

Bio-Acerola C Complex. (Solgar) Vitamin C 500 mg, citrus bioflavonoids 10 mg, rutin 5 mg in a natural base of acerola, rose hips, buckwheat, black currant and green pepper concentrate powders, cherry flavored. Wafers. Bot. 50s, 100s. *otc.*
Use: Vitamin supplement.

Biobrane. (Sanofi Winthrop) A temporary skin substitute available in various sizes. *otc.*
Use: Temporary skin substitute.

Biocal 250. (Bayer) Calcium 250 mg/Chew. Tab. Bot. 75s. *otc.*
Use: Calcium supplement.

Biocal 500. (Bayer) Calcium 500 mg/Tab. Bot. 75s. *otc.*
Use: Calcium supplement.

Biocef. (Inter. Ethical Labs) Cephalexin monohydrate 500 mg/Cap. Bot. 100s. Cephalexin monohydrate 125 mg/ml and 250 mg/ml/Pow. for susp. Bot. 100 ml. *Rx.*
Use: Anti-infective, cephalosporin.

Bioclate. (Centeon) Concentrated recombinant hemophilic factor. After reconstitution, also contains albumin (human) 12.5 mg/ml, PEG-3350 1.5 mg/ml, sodium 180 mEq/L, histidine 55 mM, polysorbate 80 1.5 mcg/AHF IU, calcium 0.2 mg/ml. Bot. IU 250, 500, 1000. *Rx.*
Use: Antihemophilic.

Biocult-GC. (Orion Diagnostica) Swab Test for gonorrhea. For endocervical, urethral, rectal and pharyngeal cultures. Box 1 test per kit.
Use: Diagnostic aid.

biodegradable polymer implant containing carmustine.
Use: Treatment of recurrent malignant glioma. [Orphan drug]
See: Biodel Implant/BCNU.

Biodel Implant/BCNU. (Scios Nova) Biodegradable polymer implant containing carmustine. *Rx.*
Use: Treatment of recurrent malignant glioma.

Biodine. (Major) Iodine 1%. Soln. Bot. pt, gal. *otc.*
Use: Antiseptic, germicide, topical.

bio-flavonoid compounds. Vitamin P.

bio-flavonoid compound, citrus. W/Vitamin C.
See: C.V.P. Syr., Cap. (Rhone-Poulenc Rorer).
  Mevanin-C, Cap. (Beutlich).
  Mevatinic-C, Tab. (Beutlich).
  Peridin-C, Tab. (Beutlich).
  Pregent, Tab. (Beutlich).

Biogastrone.
See: Carbenoxolone.

Biohist-LA. (Wakefield) Carbinoxamine maleate 8 mg, pseudoephedrine HCl 120 mg/TR Tab. Bot. 100s. *Rx.*
Use: Antihistamine, decongestant.

•**biological indicator for dry-heat sterilization, paper strip,** U.S.P. 23.
Use: Biological indicator, sterilization.

•**biological indicator for ethylene oxide sterilization, paper strip,** U.S.P. 23.
Use: Biological indicator, sterilization.

•**biological indicator for steam sterilization, paper strip,** U.S.P. 23.
Use: Biological indicator, sterilization.

Biomox. (Inter. Ethical Labs) Amoxicillin 250 mg/Cap. Bot. 100s. *Rx.*
Use: Anti-infective.

Bion Tears. (Alcon) Dextran 70 0.1%, hydroxypropyl methylcellulose 2910 0.3%, NaCl, KCl, sodium bicarbonate. Preservative free. Soln. In single-use 0.45 ml containers (28s). *otc.*
Use: Artificial tears.

Bionate 50-2. (Seatrace) Testosterone cypionate 50 mg, estradiol cypionate 2 mg/ml. Vial 10 ml. *Rx.*
Use: Androgen, estrogen combination.

Bioral.
See: Carbenoxolone.

Bios I.
See: Inositol.

Bio-Tab. (Inter. Ethical Labs) Doxycycline hyclate 100 mg, film coated. Tab.

Bot. 50s, 100s, 500s. *Rx.*
Use: Anti-infective, tetracycline.

Biotel Diabetes. (Biotel) In vitro diagnostic test for diabetes and other metabolic disorders by screening for glucose in the urine. Test Kit 12s.
Use: In vitro diagnostic aid.

Biotel Kidney. (Biotel) In vitro diagnostic test for early detection of diseases of the kidneys, bladder and urinary tract by screening for hemoglobin, red blood cells and albumin in the urine. Test Kit 12s.
Use: In vitro diagnostic aid.

Biotel U.T.I. (Biotel) In vitro diagnostic home test to detect urinary tract infections by screening for nitrate in urine. Test Kit 12s.
Use: In vitro diagnostic aid.

Biotexin.
See: Novobiocin.

Biothesin. (Pal-Pak). Phosphorated carbohydrate solution cerium oxalate 120 mg, bismuth subnitrate 120 mg, benzocaine 15 mg, aromatics/Tab. 1000s.
otc.
Use: Antiemetic/antivertigo combination.

•**biotin,** U.S.P. 23.
Use: Vitamin.

Biotin Forte 3 mg. (Vitaline) B_1 10 mg, B_2 10 mg, B_3 40 mg, B_5 10 mg, B_6 25 mg, B_{12} 10 mc/g, C 200 mg, biotin 3 mg, FA 800 mcg, Zn 30 mg. *Rx.*
Use: Vitamin/mineral supplement.

Biotin Forte 5 mg Extra Strength. (Vitaline) B_1 10 mg, B_2 10 mg, B_3 40 mg, B_5 10 mg, B_6 25 mg, B_{12} 10 mcg, C 100 mg, biotin 5 mg, FA 800 mcg/Tab. Bot. 60s. *Rx.*
Use: Vitamin supplement.

Bio-Tytra. (Approved) Neomycin sulfate 2.5 mg, gramicidin 0.25 mg, benzocaine 10 mg/Troche. Box 10s. *Rx.*
Use: Anti-infective.

•**bipenamol hydrochloride.** (bye-PEN-ah-MAHL) USAN.
Use: Antidepressant.

•**biperiden,** (by-PURR-ih-den) U.S.P. 23.
Use: Anticholinergic; antiparkinsonian.

•**biperiden hydrochloride,** U.S.P. 23.
Use: Anticholinergic; antiparkinsonian.

biperiden hydrochloride and lactate.
Use: Anticholinergic, antiparkinson agent.
See: Akineton, Amp., Tab. (Knoll Pharm).

•**biperiden lactate, injection,** U.S.P. 23.
Use: Anticholinergic, antiparkinsonian.

•**biphenamine hydrochloride.** (bye-FEN-ah-meen) USAN.
Use: Topical anesthetic, antibacterial; antifungal.

biphosphonates.
See: Didronel (Procter & Gamble).
Didronel IV (MGI Pharma).
Aredia (Novartis).

Bipole-S. (Spanner) Testosterone 25 mg, estrone 2 mg/ml/Inj. Vial. 10 ml. *Rx.*
Use: Androgen, estrogen combination.

bis (acetoxphenyl0 oxindol.
See: Oxyphenisatin.

•**bisacodyl,** (BISS-uh-koe-dill) U.S.P. 23.
Use: Laxative.
See: Bisacodyl Uniserts, Supp. (Upsher-Smith).
Bisco-Lax, Supp (Raway).
Dacodyl, Tab. Supp. (Major).
Deficol, Tab., Supp. (Vangard).
Delco-Lax, Tab. (Delco).
Dulcagen, Tab., Supp. (Goldline).
Dulcolax, Tab. Supp. (Novartis Self-Medication)
Fleet Bisacodyl, Tab. Supp. (Fleet).
Theralax, Tab., Supp. (SK-Beecham).

•**bisacodyl tannex.** USAN. Water-soluble complex of bisacodyl and tannic acid.
Use: Laxative.
See: Clysodrast, packet (Pilkington Barnes Hind).

Bisacodyl Uniserts. (Upsher-Smith) Bisacodyl 5 mg and 10 mg/Supp. Pack. 12, 50s, 500s. *otc.*
Use: Laxative.

Bisalate. (Allison) Sodium salicylate 5 gr, salicylamide 2.5 gr, sodium paraminobenzoate 5 gr, ascorbic acid 50 mg, butabarbital sodium 1/8 gr/Tab. Bot. 100s and 1000s. *Rx.*
Use: Antirrheumatic.

•**bisantrene hydrochloride.** USAN.
Use: Antineoplastic.

bisatin.
See: Oxyphenisatin.

Bisco-Lax. (Raway) Bisacodyl 10 mg/Supp. Box of foil UD 12s, 50s, 100s, 500s, 1000s. *otc.*
Use: Laxative.

bishydroxycoumarin.
See: Dicumarol, U.S.P. 23.

Bismapec Tablets. (Pal-Pak) Bismuth hydroxide 137.7 mg, colloidal kaolin 648 mg, citrus pectin 129.6 mg/Tab. Bot. 1000s. *otc.*
Use: Antidiarrheal.

Bismu-Kino. (Denver) Bismuth oxycarbonate 10 gr, eucalyptus gum 6 gr, phenyl salicylate, camphor, menthol,

carminative oils of nutmeg and clove in soothing, demulcent base w/alcohol 2%/fl oz. Bot. 4 oz, pt. *otc.*
Use: Stomach and intestinal upset.

•**bismuth aluminate.** USAN. Aluminum bismuth oxide.
See: Escot, Cap. (Solvay).

•**bismuth carbonate.** (BISS-muth) USAN.
Use: Protectant (topical).

bismuth glycolylarsanilate. (BISS-muth)
Use: Antiamebic.
See: Glycobiarsol, N.F. 18.

bismuth hydroxide.
See: Milk of Bismuth, U.S.P. 23.

bismuth, insoluble products.
See: Bismuth Subgallate (Various Mfr.).
Bismuth Subsalicylate (Various Mfr.).
Bismuth Tribromophenate (N.Y. Quinine).

bismuth, magma. Name previously used for Milk of Bismuth.

•**bismuth, milk of,** (BISS-muth) U.S.P. 23.
Use: Astringent, antacid.

bismuth oxycarbonate.
See: Bismuth Subcarbonate.

bismuth potassium tartrate. Basic bismuth potassium bismuthotartrate. (Brewer) 25 mg/ml Amp. 2 ml. (Miller) 0.016 g/ml Amp. 2 ml, Box 12s, 100s; Bot. 30 ml, 60 ml. (Raymer) 2.5% Amp. 2 ml, Box 12s, 100s. *Rx.*
Use: Agent for syphilis.

bismuth resorcin compound.
W/Bismuth subgallate, balsam Peru, benzocaine, zinc oxide, boric acid.
See: Bonate, Supp. (Suppositoria).
W/Bismuth subgallate, balsam Peru, zinc oxide, boric acid.
See: Versal, Supp. (Suppositoria).
W/Bismuth subgallate, zinc oxide, boric acid, balsam Peru.
See: Anulan, Supp. (Lannett).

bismuth sodium tartrate. (BISS-muth)
Use: I.M., syphilis.

bismuth subbenzoate. (BISS-muth)
Use: Dusting powder for wounds.

•**bismuth subcarbonate,** (BISS-muth) U.S.P. 23.
Use: Protectant (topical).

bismuth subcarbonate. (BISS-muth)
Use: Gastroenteritis, diarrhea.
W/Benzocaine, zinc oxide, boric acid.
See: Aracain Rectal Supp. (Del Pharm.).
W/Calcium carbonate, magnesium carbonate, aminoacetic acid, dried aluminum hydroxide gel.
See: Buffertabs, Tab. (Forest).

W/Charcoal and ginger.
See: Harv-a-carbs, Tab. (Forest).
W/Hydrocortisone acetate, belladonna extract, ephedrine sulfate, zinc oxide, boric acid, balsam Peru, cocoa butter.
See: Rectacort, Supp. (Century).
W/Kaolin, pectin.
See: K-C, Liq. (Century).
W/Pectin, kaolin, opium powder.
See: KBP/O, Cap. (Cole).
W/Phenyl salicylate, zinc phenolsulfonate, pepsin.
See: Bismuth, salol, zinc compound (Jones Medical).
W/Phenyl salicylate, chloroform, eucalyptus gum, camphor.
See: Bismu-Kino, Liq. (Denver Chem.).
W/Ephedrine sulfate, belladonna extract, zinc oxide, boric acid, bismuth oxyiodide, balsam Peru.
See: Wyanoids, Preps. (Wyeth-Ayerst).

•**bismuth subgallate,** U.S.P. 23.
Use: Topically for skin conditions; orally as an antidiarrheal.

bismuth subgallate, (BISS-muth) (Various Mfr.) Dermatol.
Use: Topically for skin conditions; orally as an antidiarrheal.
See: Devrom, Tab (Parthenon).
W/Benzocaine, resorcin, cod liver oil, lanolin, zinc oxide.
See: Biscolan, Supp. (Lannett).
W/Benzocaine, zinc oxide, boric acid, balsam Peru.
See: Anocaine, Supp. (Roberts).
W/Bismuth oxyiodide, bismuth resorcin compound, benzocaine, boric acid.
See: Bonate, Supp. (Suppositoria).
W/Bismuth resorcin compound, balsam Peru, benzocaine, zinc oxide, boric acid.
See: Bonate, Supp. (Suppositoria).
W/Bismuth resorcin compound, zinc oxide, boric acid, balsam Peru.
See: Anulan, Supp. (Lannett).
Versal, Supp. (Suppositoria).
W/Cod liver oil, benzocaine, lanolin, zinc oxide, resorcin, balsam Peru, hydrocortisone.
See: Doctient HC, Supp. (Suppositoria).
W/Hydrocortisone acetate, bismuth resorcin compound, zinc oxide, balsam Peru, benzyl benzoate.
See: Anusol-HC, Supp. (Parke-Davis).
W/Diethylaminoacet-2,6-xylidide, zinc oxide, aluminum subacetate, balsam Peru.
See: Xylocaine Suppositories (Astra).
W/Kaolin, colloidal.
See: Diastop, Liq. (ICN Pharm.).

W/Kaolin colloidal, calcium carbonate, magnesium trisilicate, papain, atropine sulphate.
See: Kaocasil, Tab. (Jenkins).
W/Kaolin, opium, zinc phenolsulfonate, pectin.
See: Cholactabs, Tab. (Roxane).
W/Kaolin, pectin, zinc phenolsulfonate, opium powder.
See: Diastay, Tab. (ICN Pharm.).
W/Opium powder, pectin, kaolin, zinc phenolsulfonate.
See: Bismuth, Pectin, Paregoric (Lemmon).
W/Zinc oxide, bismuth resorcin compound, balsam Peru, benzyl benzoate.
See: Anugesic, Supp., Oint. (Parke-Davis).
Anusol, Supp., Oint. (Parke-Davis).
bismuth subiodide.
See: Bismuth oxyiodide.
•**bismuth subnitrate,** (BISS-muth) U.S.P. 23.
Use: Pharmaceutic necessity, gastroenteritis, amebic dysentery, locally for wounds.
W/Calcium carbonate, magnesium carbonate.
See: Antacid No. 2, Tab. (Jones Medical).
Maygel, Tab. (Century).
W/Sodium bicarbonate, magnesium carbonate, diastase, papain.
Panacarb, Tab. (Lannett).
•**bismuth subsalicylate.** (BISS-muth) USAN. Basic bismuth salicylate.
Use: Agent for syphilis. Used in combination with metronidazole and tetracycline HCl to treat active duodenal ulcer associated with H. pylori infection.
W/Calcium carbonate, glycocoll.
See: Pepto-Bismol, Tab. (Procter & Gamble).
W/Pectin, salol, kaolin, zinc sulfocarbolate, aluminum hydroxide.
See: Wescola Antidiarrheal-Stomach Upset (Western Research).
W/Phenylsalicylate, zinc phenolsulfonate, methylcellulose, magnesium aluminum silicate.
See: Pepto-Bismol, Liq. (Procter & Gamble).
bismuth tannate. (BISS-muth) (Various Mfr.) Tanbismuth. otc.
Use: Astringent and protective in GI disorders.
bismuth tribromophenate. (BISS-muth)
Use: Intestinal antiseptic.
bismuth violet. (BISS-muth) (Table Rock) Bismuth Violet. **Oint.** 1%. Jar oz,

lb. **Soln.** 0.5%. Bot. 0.5 oz, 6 oz, pt, gal. **Tr.** 0.5%. Bot. 6 oz, pt, also 1% w/ benzoic and salicylic acid. Bot. 0.5 oz, 6 oz, pt. otc.
Use: Anti-infective, topical.
bismuth, water-soluble products.
See: Bismuth Potassium Tartrate (Various Mfr.).
•**bisnafide dimesylate.** (BISS-nah-fide die-MEH-sih-late) USAN.
Use: Antineoplastic.
•**bisobrin lactate.** (BISS-oh-brin LACK-tate) USAN.
Use: Fibrinolytic.
•**bisoprolol.** (bih-SO-pro-lahl) USAN.
Use: Antihypertensive (beta blocker).
•**bisoprolol fumarate.** USAN.
Use: Antihypertensive (beta blocker).
See: Zebeta (Lederle).
Ziac, Tab. (Lederle).
•**bisoxatin acetate.** (biss-OX-at-in) USAN.
Use: Laxative.
bispecific antibody 520C9x22. (Medarex) Rx.
Use: Serotherapy of ovarian cancer. [Orphan drug]
bisphosphonates.
Use: Treatment of hypercalcemia; bone resorption inhibitor.
See: Didronel (Procter & Gamble).
Didronel IV (MGI Pharma).
Aredia, Inj (Novartis).
Fosamax, Tab (Merck).
•**bispyrithione magsulfex.** (BISS-PIHR-ih-thigh-ohn mag-sull-fex) USAN.
Use: Antidandruff, antibacterial, antifungal.
bisquadine. (Sterwin) Alexidine.
bis-tropamide. Tropicamide.
See: Mydriacyl, Soln. (Alcon).
Bite & Itch Lotion. (Weeks & Leo) Pramoxine HCl 1%, pyrilamine maleate 2%, pheniramine maleate 0.2%, chlorpheniramine maleate 0.2%. Bot. 4 oz. otc.
Use: Antipruritic, topical.
•**bithionolate, sodium.** USAN.
Use: Topical anti-infective.
Bitin. CDC Anti-infective agent.
See: Bithionol.
•**bitolterol mesylate.** (by-TOLE-tor-ole) USAN.
Use: Bronchodilator.
See: Tornalate, Inhalation soln. (Dura).
Bitrate. (Arco) Phenobarbital 15 mg, pentaerythritol tetranitrate 20 mg/Tab. Bot. 100s. Rx.
Use: Sedative, hypnotic, antianginal.

•**bivalirudin.** (bye-VAL-ih-ruh-din) USAN.
Use: Anticoagulant, antithrombotic.

•**bizelesin.** (bye-ZELL-eh-sin) USAN.
Use: Antineoplastic.

B-Ject-100. (Hyrex) Vitamins B$_1$ 100 mg,
B$_2$ 2 mg, B$_3$ 100 mg, B$_5$ 2 mg, B$_6$ 2 mg/
ml. Inj. Vial 10 ml, 30 ml. *Rx.*
Use: Vitamin B supplement.

Black and White Bleaching Cream.
(Schering Plough) Hydroquinone 2%.
Tube 0.75 oz, 1.5 oz. *Rx.*
Use: Skin bleaching agent.

Black and White Ointment. (Schering
Plough) Resorcinol 3%. Tube 0.62 oz,
2.25 oz.
Use: Antiseptic, antipruritic, topical.

Black Draught. (Chattem) Powdered
senna extract. **Tab.:** 600 mg. Bot. 30s.
Gran.: 1.65 g/0.5 tsp. Jar 22.5 g. *otc.*
Use: Laxative.

Black Draught Syrup. (Chattem) Casanthranol 90 mg w/senna, rhubarb, anise,
methyl salicylate, ginger, peppermint
oil, spearmint oil, menthol, alcohol 5%,
tartrazine/Tbsp. Bot. 2 oz, 5 oz. *otc.*
Use: Laxative.

black widow spider, antivenin.
See: Antivenin (Lactrodectus mactens),
Inj. (Merck).

Blairex Hard Contact Lens Cleaner.
(Blairex) Anionic detergent. Liq. Bot. 60
ml. *otc.*
Use: Hard contact lens care.

Blairex Lens Lubricant. (Blairex) Isotonic. Sorbic acid 0.25%, EDTA 0.1%,
borate buffer, NaCl, hydroxypropylmethylcellulose, glycerin. Soln. Bot. 15 ml.
otc.
Use: Soft contact lens care.

Blairex Sterile Saline Solution. (Blairex)
Sodium Cl, boric acid, sodium borate.
Aerosol. 90 ml, 240 ml, 360 ml. *otc.*
Use: Soft contact lens care.

Blairex System. (Blairex Labs) Sodium
Cl 135 mg/Tab. 200s, 365s w/15 ml
bot. *otc.*
Use: Soft contact lens care.

Blairex System II. (Blairex Labs) Sodium Cl 250 mg/Tab. 90s, 180s w/27.7
ml bot. *otc.*
Use: Soft contact lens care.

Blaud Strubel. (Strubel) Ferrous sulfate
5 gr/Cap. Bot. 100s. *otc.*
Use: Iron supplement.

Blefcon. (Madland) Sodium sulfacetamide 30%. Oint. Tube ⅛ oz. *Rx.*
Use: Anti-infective, ophthalmic.

BlemErase. (Young) Benzoyl peroxide
10%. Lot. Bot. 12 ml. *otc.*

Use: Antiacne.

Blenoxane. (Bristol-Myers/B-M Squibb
Oncology) Bleomycin sulfate 15 units/
Vial. 1s, 10s. *Rx.*
Use: Antineoplastic.

•**bleomycin sulfate, sterile,** (BLEE-oh-
MY-sin) U.S.P. 23. Antibiotic obtained
from cultures of *Streptomyces verticil-
lus.*
Use: Antineoplastic.
See: Blenoxane, Inj. (Bristol).

Bleph-10. (Allergan) Sulfacetamide sodium 10%. Dropper Bot. 2.5 ml, 5 ml,
15 ml. *Rx.*
Use: Anti-infective, ophthalmic.

Bleph-10 Sterile Ophthalmic Ointment.
(Allergan) Sulfacetamide sodium 10%.
Tube 3.5 g. *Rx.*
Use: Anti-infective, ophthalmic.

Blephamide. (Allergan) Sulfacetamide
sodium 10%, prednisolone acetate
0.2%. Bot. 2.5 ml, 5 ml, 10 ml. *Rx.*
Use: Anti-inflammatory, anti-infective,
ophthalmic.

Blephamide Ophthalmic Ointment. (Allergan) Prednisolone acetate 0.2%, sulfacetamide sodium 10%. Tube 3.5 g.
Rx.
Use: Anti-inflammatory, anti-infective,
ophthalmic.

Blinx. (Akorn) Sodium Cl, potassium Cl,
sodium phosphate, benzalkonium Cl
0.005%, EDTA 0.02%. Soln. Bot. 120
ml. *otc.*
Use: Extraocular irrigation solution.

Blis. (Del Pharm.) Boric acid 47.5%, salicylic acid 17%. Bot. 7 oz. *otc.*
Use: Antifungal, topical.

Blistergard. (Medtech) Alcohol 6.7%, pyroxylin solution, oil of cloves, B-hydroxy-
quinolone. Liq. Bot. 30 ml. *otc.*
Use: Skin protectant.

Blistex. (Blistex) Camphor 0.5%, phenol
0.5%, allantoin 1%, lanolin, mineral oil.
Tube 4.2 g, 10.5 g. *otc.*
Use: Lip balm.

Blistex Lip Balm. (Blistex) SPF 10. Camphor 0.5%, phenol 0.5%, allantoin 1%,
dimethicone 2%, pamidate 0.25%, oxybenzone, parabens, petrolatum. Tube.
4.5 g. *otc.*
Use: Lip balm.

Blistex Ultra Protection. (Blistex) Octyl
methoxycinnamate, oxybenzone, octyl
salicylate, menthyl anthranilate, homosalate, dimethicone. Tube 4.2 g. *otc.*
Use: Lip balm.

Blistik. (Blistex) Padimate O 6.6%, oxybenzone 2.5%, dimethicone 2%. Lip

balm stick 4.5 g. *otc.*
Use: Lip protectant.
Blis-To-Sol. (Chattem) **Liq.:** Tolnaftate 1%. Bot. 30 ml, 55.5 ml. **Pow.:** Zinc undecylenate 12%. Bot. 60 g. **Soln:** Tolnaftate 1% Bot. 30 ml and 55.5 ml. *otc.*
Use: Antifungal, topical.
BLM.
See: Bleomycin sulfate.
Blocadren. (Merck) Timolol maleate 5 mg, 10 mg or 20 mg/Tab. **5 mg:** Bot. 100s; **10 mg:** Bot. 100s, UD 100s; **20 mg:** Bot. 100s. *Rx.*
Use: Beta-adrenergic blocking agent.
Block Out By Sea & Ski. (Carter) Padimate O, octyl methoxycinnamate, oxybenzone. Cream. Tube 120 g. *otc.*
Use: Sunscreen.
Block Out Clear By Sea & Ski. (Carter) Padimate O, octyl methoxycinnamate, octyl salicylate, SD alcohol 40. Lot. Bot. 120 ml. *otc.*
Use: Sunscreen.
blood, anticoagulants.
See: Anticoagulants.
•**blood cells, red.** U.S.P. 23.
Use: Blood replenisher.
blood coagulation.
See: Hemostatics.
blood fractions.
See: Albumin (Human) Salt-Poor (Armour; Baxter).
blood glucose concentrator.
See: Glucagon (Lilly).
blood glucose test.
See: Chemstrip bG Strips. (Boehringer Mannheim).
Dextrostix Reagent Strips. (Bayer).
First Choice, Strips (Polymer Technology, Int.).
Glucostix Strips. (Bayer).
Visidex II Reagent Strips. (Bayer).
•**blood grouping serum, anti-a.** U.S.P. 23.
Use: Diagnostic aid (in vitro, blood).
•**blood grouping serum, anti-b,** U.S.P. 23.
Use: Diagnostic aid (in vitro, blood).
•**blood grouping serums anti-d, anti-C, anti-E, anti-C, anti-E,** U.S.P. 23.
Use: Diagnostic aid (in vitro, blood).
•**blood group specific substances a, b and ab,** U.S.P. 23.
Use: Blood neutralizer.
•**blood, whole,** U.S.P. 23.
Use: Blood replenisher.
•**Blu-12 100.** (Bluco) Cyanocobalamin 100 mcg /ml. Vial 30 ml. *Rx.*
Use: Vitamin B$_{12}$ supplement.

Blu-12 1000. (Bluco) Cyanocobalamin 1000 mcg /ml. Vial 30 ml. *Rx.*
Use: Vitamin B$_{12}$ supplement.
Bluboro Powder. (Allergan Herbert) Aluminum sulfate 53.9%, calcium acetate 43% w/boric acid, FD&C; Blue 1. Packet 1.9 g. Box 12s. *otc.*
Use: Astringent, topical.
Bludex. (Burlington) Methenamine 40.8 mg, methylene blue 5.4 mg, phenyl salicylate 18.1 mg, atropine sulfate 0.03 mg, hyoscyamine 0.03 mg, benzoic acid 4.5 mg/Tab. Bot. 100s, 1000s. *Rx.*
Use: Urinary antiseptic, antispasmodic.
Blue. (Various Mfr.) Pyrethrins 0.3%, piperonyl butoxide 3%, petroleum distillate 1.2%. Gel Bot. 30 g, 480 g. *otc.*
Use: Pediculicide.
Blue Gel Muscular Pain Reliever. (Rugby) Menthol in a specially formulated base. Gel. Tube 240 g. *otc.*
Use: Rubs & liniments.
Blue Star Ointment. (McCue Labs.) Salicylic acid, benzoic acid, methyl salicylate, camphor, lanolin, petrolatum. Jar 2 oz. *otc.*
Use: Minor skin irritations, ringworm, corn or callus removal.
blutene chloride.
B-Major. (Barth's) Vitamins B$_1$ 7 mg, B$_2$ 14 mg, niacin 2.35 mg, B$_{12}$ 7.5 mcg, B$_6$ 0.15 mg, pantothenic acid 0.37 mg, choline 85 mg, inositol 6 mg, biotin, folic acid, aminobenzoic acid/Cap. Bot. 1s, 3s, 6s, 12s. *otc, Rx.*
Use: Vitamin/mineral supplement.
B.M.E. (Brothers) Aminophylline 32 mg, ephedrine sulfate 8 mg, phenobarbital 8 mg, chlorpheniramine maleate 2 mg, alcohol 15%/5 ml. Bot. pt. *Rx.*
Use: Bronchodilator, decongestant, sedative, hypnotic, antihistamine.
B-N. (Eric, Kirk & Gary). Bacitracin 500 units, neomycin sulfate 5 mg. Oint. Tube 0.5 oz. *otc.*
Use: Anti-infective, external.
b-naphthyl salicylate. Betol, Naphthosalol, Salinaphthol.
Use: G.I. & G.U., antiseptic.
B-Nutron Tablets. (Nion) Vitamins B$_1$ 2 mg, niacinamide 18 mg, B$_2$ 3 mg, B$_6$ 2.2 mg, cyanocobalamin 3 mcg, folic acid 0.4 mg, iron 6 mg, pantothenic acid 3.3 mg, B complex as provided by 150 mg Brewer's yeast/Tab. Bot. 100s, 500s. *otc.*
Use: Vitamin/mineral supplement.
B and O Supprettes No. 15A & No. 16A. (PolyMedica) Opium 30 mg or 60 mg,

belladonna extract 16.2 mg/Supp. Jar 12s. c-II.
Use: Narcotic analgesic, antispasmodic.

Bobid. (Boyd) Phenylpropanolamine HCl 50 mg, chlorpheniramine maleate 8 mg, methscopolamine bromide 2.5 mg/Cap. Bot. 100s. *otc.*
Use: Decongestant, antihistamine, anticholinergic.

Bo-Cal. (Fibertone) Calcium 250 mg, magnesium 125 mg, vitamin D$_3$ 100 IU, boron 0.75 mg/Tab. Bot. 120s. *otc.*
Use: Vitamin/mineral supplement.

Boil-Ease Salve. (Del) Benzocaine 20%, camphor, eucalyptus oil, menthol, petrolatum, phenol. Oint. 30 g. *otc.*
Use: Anesthetic drawing salve.

BoilnSoak. (Alcon) Sodium Cl 0.7%, boric acid, sodium borate, thimerosal 0.001%, disodium edetate 0.1%. Bot. 8 oz, 12 oz. *otc.*
Use: Soft contact lens care.

•**bolandiol dipropionate.** (bole-AN-die-ole die-PRO-pee-oh-nate) USAN.
Use: Anabolic.

•**bolasterone.** (BOLE-ah-STEE-rone) USAN.
Use: Anabolic.

Bolax. (Boyd) Docusate sodium 240 mg, phenolphthalein 30 mg, dihydrocholic acid ¾ gr/Cap. Bot. 100s. *otc.*
Use: Laxative.

•**boldenone undecylenate.** (BOLE-deen-ohn uhn-deh-sih-LEN-ate) USAN. Parenabol. Under study.
Use: Anabolic.

•**bolenol.** (BOLE-ee-nahl) USAN.
Use: Anabolic.

•**bolmantalate.** (BOLE-MAN-tah-late) USAN.
Use: Anabolic.

Bonacal Plus Tablets. (Kenwood) Vitamins A 5000 IU, D 400 IU, C 100 mg, B$_1$ 3 mg, B$_2$ 3 mg, B$_6$ 10 mg, B$_{12}$ 4 mcg, niacinamide 20 mg, d-calcium pantothenate 3.3 mg, iron 42 mg, calcium 350 mg, manganese 0.33 mg, zinc 0.1 mg, magnesium 1.67 mg, potassium 1.67 mg/Tab. Bot. 100s. *otc.*
Use: Vitamin/mineral supplement.

Bonamil Infant Formula with Iron. (Wyeth-Ayerst) Protein 2.3 g (from nonfat milk, taurine), fat 5.4 g (from soybean and coconut oils, soy lecithin), carbohydrase 10.7 g (from lactose), linoleic acid 1300 mg, vitamin A 300 IU, D 60 IU, E 2.85 IU, K 8 mcg, B$_1$ 100 mcg, B$_2$ 150 mcg, B$_6$ 63 mcg, B$_{12}$ 0.2 mcg, B$_3$ 750 mcg, folic acid 7.5 mcg, B$_5$ 315

mcg, biotin 2.2 mcg, vitamin C 8.3 mg, choline 15 mg, Ca 69 mg, P 54 mg, Mg 6 mg, Fe 1.8 mg, Zn 0.75 mg, Mn 15 mcg, Cu 70 mcg, I 5 mcg, Na 27 mg, K 93 mg, Cl 63 mg/100 cal (5.3 cal/g). Powd. Bot. 453 g. *otc.*
Use: Enteral nutritional therapy, infant foods with iron.

Bonate. (Suppositoria) Bismuth subgallate, balsam Peru, benzocaine, zinc oxide/Supp. Box 12s, 100s, 1000s. *otc.*
Use: Anorectal preparation.

Bone Meal w/ Vitamin D. (Natures Bounty) Calcium 220 mg, vitamin D 100 IU, phosphorus 100 mg, iron 0.45 mg, copper 3.25 mg, zinc 20 mcg, manganese 2.75 mcg, magnesium 0.925 mg. Tab. Bot. 100s, 250s. *otc.*
Use: Vitamin/mineral supplement.

Bonine. (Leeming) Meclizine HCl 25 mg/Chew. tab. Pkg. 8s, 48s. *otc.*
Use: Antiemetic, antivertigo.

Bontril PDM. (Schwarz Pharma) Phendimetrazine tartrate 35 mg/3 layer Tab. Bot. 100s, 1000s. c-III.
Use: Anorexiant.

Bontril Slow Release Capsules. (Schwarz Pharma) Phendimetrazine tartrate 105 mg/Cap. Bot. 100s, 1000s c-III.
Use: Anorexiant.

Boost. (B-M Squibb) Protein 10 mg, fat 7 g, carbohydrate 35 g, sodium 130 mg, potassium 400 mg, vitamins A, C, D, E, B$_1$, B$_2$, B$_3$, B$_5$, B$_6$, B$_9$, B$_{12}$, biotin, Ca, P, I, Mg, Zn, Cu, sugar, corn syrup. Liq. Bot. 237 ml. *otc.*
Use: Enteral nutritional supplement.

Bopen-VK. (Boyd) Potassium phenoxymethyl penicillin 400,000 units/Tab. Bot. 100s.
Use: Anti-infective; penicillin.

borax. Sodium Borate, N.F. 18.

•**boric acid,** N.F. 18.
Use: Mild antiseptic, pharmaceutic necessity.
See: Borofax, Oint. (Glaxo Wellcome). W/Combinations.
See: Saratoga Ointment (Blair).

boric acid ointment. (Various Mfr.) Topical ointment 5% or 10%. Tube, Jar 30 g, 52.5 g, 60 g, 120 g, 454 g. Ophth. oint. 0.5% or 10%. Tube, Jar. 3.5 g, 3.75 g, 30 g, 60 g, 480 g. *otc, Rx.*
Use: Minor skin irritations.

2-bornanone. Camphor, U.S.P. 23.

•**bornelone.** (BORE-neh-LONE) USAN.
Use: Ultraviolet screen.

•**bornyl acetate.** USAN.

•**borocaptate sodium B 10.** (bore-oh-CAP-tate) USAN.
Use: Antineoplastic, radioactive agent.

Borofair. (Major) Acetic acid 2% in aluminum acetate soln. Bot. 60 ml. *Rx.*
Use: Otic preparation.

Borofax Skin Protectant. (Warner Lambert Consumer Health Products) Zinc oxide 15%, petrolatum 68.6%, lanolin, mineral oil. Oint. Tube 50 g. *otc.*
Use: Minor skin irritations.

Boroglycerin. Glycerol borate. (Emerson) Bot. pt.

boroglycerin glycerite. Boric acid 31 parts, glycerin 96 parts.
Use: Agent for dermatitis.

Boropak Powder. (Glenwood) Aluminum sulfate and calcium acetate. One packet dissolved in a pint of water yields a 1:40 dilution. Pcks 2.4 g. 100s. *otc.*
Use: Anti-inflammatory, topical.

borotannic complex. Boric acid 31 mg, tannic acid 50 mg.
W/salicylic acid, ethyl alcohol.
See: Onycho-Phytex, Liq. (Unimed).

•**bosentan.** (boe-SEN-tan) USAN.
Use: Antagonist (endothelin receptor).

Boston Advance Cleaner. (Polymer Tech) Concentrated homogenous surfactant with friction-enhancing agents. Soln. Bot. 30 ml. *otc.*
Use: Contact lens care.

Boston Advance Comfort Formula. (Polymer Tech) Buffered, slightly hypertonic. Polyaminopropyl biguanide 0.00015%, EDTA 0.05%, cationic cellulose derivative polymer. Soln. Bot. 120 ml. *otc.*
Use: Contact lens care.

Boston Advance Conditioning Solution. (Polymer Tech) Sterile, buffered, slightly hypertonic. Polyaminopropyl biguanide 0.0015%, EDTA 0.05%. Bot. 120 ml or with cleaner in a convenience pack. *otc.*
Use: Contact lens care.

Boston Advance Rewetting Drops. (Polymer Tech) Buffered, slightly hypertonic. Polyaminopropyl biguanide 0.0015%, EDTA 0.05%. Bot. 10 ml. *otc.*
Use: Contact lens care.

Boston Cleaner. (Polymer Tech) Concentrated homogenons surfactant with friction-enhancing agents, sodium Cl. Soln. Bot. 30 ml. *otc.*
Use: Contact lens care.

Boston Conditioning Solution. (Polymer Tech) Sterile, buffered, slightly hypertonic, low viscosity. EDTA 0.05%,

chlorhexidine gluconate 0.006%. Bot. 120 ml. *otc.*
Use: Contact lens care.

Boston Reconditioning Drops. (Polymer Tech) Hydrophilic polyelectrolyte, polyvinyl alcohol, hydroxyethylcellulose, chlorhexidine gluconate, EDTA. Soln. Bot. 120 ml. *otc.*
Use: Contact lens care.

Boston Rewetting Drops. (Polymer Tech) Buffered, slightly hypertonic. Chlorhexidine gluconate 0.006%, EDTA 0.05%, cationic cellulose derivative polymer. Soln. Bot. 10 ml. *otc.*
Use: Contact lens care.

Botox. (Allergan) Botulinum toxin type A 100 units, albumin 0.05 mg, sodium chloride 0.9mg. Pow. for inj. (lyophilized). Vials. *Rx.*
Use: Treatment of strabismus or blepharospasm.

BottomBetter. (Inno Visions) Petrolatum 49%, lanolin 15.5%, beeswax, sodium borate, lanolin alcohols, methylsalicylate, sorbitan sesquioleate, parabens, oxyquinolone, EDTA. Oint. Pkg. 18s. *otc.*
Use: Diaper rash product.

botulinum toxin type A.
Use: Treatment of strabismus and blepharospasm. [Orphan drug]
See: Botox (Allergan).

botulinum toxin type B. *Rx.*
Use: Cervical dystonia [Orphan drug]

botulinum toxin type F. *Rx.*
Use: Cervical dystonia; essential blepharospasm. [Orphan drug]

•**botulism antitoxin,** U.S.P. 23.
Use: Prophylaxis and treatment of the toxins of C. botulinum, Types A or B; passive immunizing agent.

botulism immune globulin.
Use: Infant botulism. [Orphan drug]

Bounty Bears. (NBTY) Vitamins A 2500 IU, D 400 IU, E 15 IU, C 60 mg, B_1 1.05 mg, B_2 1.2 mg, B_3 13.5 mg, B_6 1.05 mg, B_{12} 4.5 mcg, folic acid 0.3 mg/Tab. Bot. 100s. *otc.*
Use: Vitamin/mineral supplement.

Bounty Bears Plus Iron. (NBTY) Vitamins A 2500 IU, D 400 IU, E 15 IU, C 60 mg, B_1 1.05 mg, B_2 1.2 mg, B_3 13.5 mg, B_6 1.05 mg, B_{12} 4.5 mcg, folic acid 0.3 mg, iron 15 mg/Tab. Bot. 100s. *otc.*
Use: Vitamin/mineral supplement.

bourbonal.
See: Ethyl Vanillin, N.F. 18.

bovine colostrum. *Rx.*
Use: AIDS-related diarrhea. [Orphan drug]

bovine whey protein concentrate. *Rx.*
Use: Treatment of cryptosporidiosis.
[Orphan drug]
See: Immuno-C.

Bowman Cold Tabs. (Jones Medical)
Acetaminophen 324 mg, phenylpropanolamine HCl 24.3 mg, caffeine 16.2
mg/Tab. Bot. 1000s, 5000s. *otc.*
Use: Analgesic, decongestant.

Bowman's Poison Antidote Kit. (Jones
Medical) Syrup of ipecac 1 oz, 1 bottle;
activated charcoal liquid 2 oz, 3
bottles. *otc.*
Use: Antidote.

Bowsteral. (Jones Medical) Isopropanol
60%. Bot. pt, gal.
Use: Antirust disinfectant for surgical instruments.

●**boxidine.** USAN.
Use: Adrenal steroid blocker, antihyperlipoproteinemic.

Boylex. (Approved) Diperodon, hexachlorophene, rosin cerate, ichthammol,
carbolic acid, thymol, camphor, juniper tar. Tube oz. *otc.*
Use: Drawing salve.

Boyol. (Pfeiffer) Ichthammol 10%, benzocaine, lanolin and petrolatum base.
Salve Tube 30 g. *otc.*
Use: Antiseptic, local anesthetic, topical.

B-Pap. (Wren) Acetaminophen 120 mg,
sodium butabarbital 15 mg/5 ml. Bot.
pt, gal. *Rx.*
Use: Analgesic, sedative.

b-pas.
See: Calcium Benzoyl PAS.

B-Plex. (Goldline) Vitamins B₁ 15 mg, B₂
15 mg, B₃ 100 mg, B₅ 18 mg, B₆ 4 mg,
B₁₂ 5 mcg, C 500 mg, folic acid 0.5
mg/Tab. Bot. 100s. *Rx.*
Use: Vitamin/mineral supplement.

BP-Papaverine. (Burlington) Papaverine
HCl 150 mg/S.R. Cap. Bot. 50s. *Rx.*
Use: Vasodilator.

BP Cold Tablets. (Bristol-Myers) Acetaminophen 325 mg, phenylpropanolamine HCl 12.5 mg, chlorpheniramine
maleate 2 mg/Tab. Card 16s, Bot. 16s,
30s, 50s. *otc.*
Use: Analgesic, decongestant, antihistamine.

Brace. (SK-Beecham) Denture adhesive.
Tube 1.4 oz, 2.4 oz.

Bradosol Bromide. (Novartis) Domiphen
bromide.

Branchamin 4%. (Baxter) Isoleucine
1.38 g, leucine 1.38 g, valine 1.25 g,
phosphate 31.6 mOsm/100 ml. Bot. 500
ml. *Rx.*

Use: Adjunct to regular TPN therapy
for highly stressed or traumatized patients.

branched chain amino acids. *Rx.*
Use: Nutritional supplement; amyotrophic lateral sclerosis. [Orphan drug]

Brasivol Fine, Medium and Rough.
(Stiefel) Aluminum oxide scrub particles
in a surfactant cleansing base. **Fine:**
Jar 153 g. **Medium:** Jar 180 g. **Rough:**
Jar 195 g. *otc.*
Use: Scrub cleanser.

Breacol Decongestant Cough Medication. (Bayer) Dextromethorphan HBr
10 mg, phenylpropanolamine HCl 37.5
mg, alcohol 10%, chlorpheniramine
maleate 4 mg/5 ml. Bot. 3 oz, 6 oz. *otc.*
Use: Antitussive, decongestant, antihistamine.

Breatheasy. (Pascal) Racemic epinephrine HCl soln. 2.2% inhaled by use of
nebulizer. Bot. 0.25 oz, 0.5 oz, 1 oz. *otc.*
Use: Bronchodilator.

Breezee Mist. (Pedinol) Aluminum chlorhydrate, undecylenic acid, menthol.
Aerosol Bot. 4 oz. *otc.*
Use: Antifungal, deodorant, antiperspirant, foot powder.

Breezee Mist Antifungal. (Pedinol) Tolnaftate 1%, talc, menthol. Pow. Bot.
113 g. *otc.*
Use: Antifungal, topical.

Breonesin. (Sanofi Winthrop-Breon)
Guaifenesin 200 mg/Cap. Bot. 100s.
otc.
Use: Expectorant.

●**brequinar sodium.** (BREh-kwih-NAHR)
USAN.
Use: Antineoplastic.

●**bretazenil.** (bret-AZZ-eh-nill) USAN
Use: Antianxiety agent.

Brethaire. (Novartis) Terbutaline sulfate
inhaler 7.5 ml. (10.5 g) w/mouthpiece.
Rx.
Use: Bronchodilator.

Brethancer. (Novartis) Inhaler (complete
unit to be used with Brethaire).

Brethine. (Novartis) Terbutaline sulfate.
Tab.: 2.5 mg. Bot. 100s, 1000s, UD
100s, Gy-Pak 90s, 100s. 5 mg. Bot.
100s, 1000s, UD 100s, Gy-Pak 90s,
100s. **Amp.:** 1 mg/ml. Box 10s, 100s.
Rx.
Use: Bronchodilator.

●**bretylium tosylate,** (bre-TILL-ee-uhm
TAH-sill-ate) U.S.P. 23.
Use: Hypotensive, antiadrenergic, cardiac depressant (antiarrhythmic).
See: Bretylol, Inj. (DuPont Merck).

bretylium tosylate in 5% dextrose. (Various Mfr.) 500 mg or 1000 mg/vial. Inj. vial 250 ml. *Rx.*
Use: Antiarrhythmic.

Bretylol. (DuPont Merck) Bretylium tosylate 50 mg/ml. Amp. 10 ml. *Rx.*
Use: Antiarrhythmic.

Brevibloc. (Ohmeda) Esmolol HCl 10 mg/ml or 250 mg/ml, propylene glycol 25%. **10 mg/ml:** Vial 10 ml. **250 mg/ml:** Amp 10 ml. *Rx.*
Use: Beta-adrenergic blocking agent.

Brevicon. (Syntex) Norethindrone 0.5 mg, ethinyl estradiol 0.035 mg/Tab. 21 and 28 day (7 inert tabs) Wallette. *Rx.*
Use: Oral contraceptive.

Brevital Sodium. (Lilly) Methohexital sodium. **Vial:** 500 mg/50 ml, 500 mg/50 ml w/diluent. 2.5 g/250 ml, 5 g/500 ml. **Amp.:** 2.5 g, 5 g. *Rx.*
Use: General anesthetic.

Brevoxyl. (Stiefel) Benzyol peroxide 4%, cetyl and stearyl alcohol. Gel. Tube 42.5 g, 90 g. *Rx.*
Use: Antiacne product.

brewer's yeast. (NTBY) Vitamins B$_1$ 0.06 mg, B$_2$ 0.02 mg, B$_3$ 0.2 mg/Tab. Bot 250s. *otc.*
Use: Vitamin supplement.

Brexin EX Liquid. (Savage) Pseudoephedrine HCl 30 mg, guaifenesin 200 mg/5 ml. *otc.*
Use: Decongestant, expectorant.

Brexin EX Tablet. (Savage) Pseudoephedrine HCl 60 mg, guaifenesin 400 mg/Tab. Bot. 100s. *otc.*
Use: Decongestant, expectorant.

Brexin L.A. (Savage) Chlorpheniramine maleate 8 mg, pseudoephedrine HCl 120 mg/L.A. Cap. Bot. 100s. *otc.*
Use: Antihistamine, decongestant.

Bricanyl Injection. (SK-Beecham) Terbutaline sulfate 1 mg/Amp. 1 ml. 10s. *Rx.*
Use: Bronchodilator.

Bricanyl Tablets. (SK-Beecham) Terbutaline sulfate 2.5 mg or 5 mg/Tab. Bot. 100s, 1000s, UD 100s. *Rx.*
Use: Bronchodilator.

•**brifentanil hydrochloride.** (brih-FEN-tah-NILL) USAN.
Use: Analgesic (narcotic).

Brigen-G. (Grafton) Chlordiazepoxide 5 mg, 10 mg or 25 mg/Tab. Bot. 500s. *c-iv.*
Use: Antianxiety agent.

Brij 96 and 97. (ICI Americas) Polyoxyl 10 oleyl ether available as 96 and 97.
Use: Surface-active agent.

Brij-721. (ICI Americas) Polyoxyethylene 21 stearyl ether (100% active).
Use: Surface-active agent.

•**brimonidine tartrate.** (brih-MOE-nih-DEEN) USAN.
Use: Adrenergic (ophthalmic).
See: Alphagan (Allergan).

•**brinolase.** (BRIN-oh-laze) USAN. Fibrinolytic enzyme produced by *Aspergillus oryzae.*
Use: Fibrinolytic.

Brirel w/Superinone. (Sanofi Winthrop) Hexahydropyrazine, hexahydrate. *Rx.*
Use: Anthelmintic.

Bristoject. (Bristol) Prefilled disposable syringes w/needle.
Aminophylline: 250 mg/10 ml.
Atropine Sulfate: 5 mg/5 ml or 1 mg/ml. 10s.
Calcium Cl: 10%. 10 ml. 10s.
Dexamethasone: 20 mg/5 ml.
Dextrose: 50%. 50 ml. 10s.
Diphenhydramine: 50 mg/5 ml.
Dopamine HCl: 200 mg/5 ml, 400 mg/10 ml.
Ephedrine: 50 mg/10 ml.
Epinephrine: 1:10,000. 10 ml. 10s.
Lidocaine HCl.: 1%: 5 ml, 10 ml; 2%: 5 ml; 4%: 25 ml, 50 ml; 20%: 5 ml, 10 ml.
Magnesium Sulfate: 5 g/10 ml. 10s.
Metaraminol: 1%. 10 ml.
Sodium Bicarbonate: 7.5%: 50 ml; 8.4%: 50 ml. 10s.

british anti-lewisite. Dimercaprol.
See: BAL.

Brobella-P.B. (Brothers) Atropine sulfate 0.0195 mg, hyoscine HBr 0.0065 mg, hyoscyamine sulfate 0.1040 mg, phenobarbital 0.25 gr/Tab. Bot. 100s, 1000s. *Rx.*
Use: Anticholinergic, antispasmodic, sedative, hypnotic.

•**brocresine.** (broe-KREE-seen) USAN.
Use: Histidine decarboxylase inhibitor.
See: Contramine phosphate.

•**brocrinat.** (BROE-krih-NAT) USAN.
Use: Diuretic.

Brocycline. (Brothers) Tetracycline HCl 250 mg/Cap. Bot. 100s, 1000s. *Rx.*
Use: Anti-infective; tetracycline.

Brofed. (Marnel) Pseudoephedrine HCl 30 mg, brompheniramine maleate 4 mg/5 ml. Elix. Bot. 473 ml. *otc.*
Use: Decongestant, antihistamine.

•**brofoxine.** (BROE-fox-een) USAN.
Use: Antipsychotic.

Brolade. (Brothers) Chlorpheniramine

maleate 8 mg, phenylephrine HCl 20 mg, methscopolamine nitrate 2.5 mg/Cap. Bot. 50s, 500s. *Rx.*
Use: Antihistamine, decongestant, anticholinergic.

bromacrylide.

•**bromadoline maleate.** (BROE-mah-DOE-leen) USAN.
Use: Analgesic.

bromaleate.
See: Pamabrom.

Bromaline Elixir. (Rugby) Phenylpropanolamine HCl 12.5 mg, brompheniramine maleate 2 mg, alcohol 2.3%. Elix. Bot. 118 ml, 473 ml and gal. *otc.*
Use: Decongestant, antihistamine.

Bromaline Plus. (Rugby) Phenylpropanolamine HCl 12.5 mg, brompheniramine maleate 2 mg, acetaminophen 500 mg. Captabs. Bot. 24s. *otc.*
Use: Decongestant, antihistamine, analgesic.

Bromalix. (Century) Bromphenramine maleate 4 mg, phenylephrine HCl 5 mg, phenylpropanolamine HCl 5 mg, alcohol 2.3%/5 ml. Bot. 4 oz, pt, gal. *otc.*
Use: Antihistamine, decongestant.

Bromanate DC Cough Syrup. (Various Mfr.) Phenylpropanolamine HCl 12.5 mg, brompheniramine maleate 2 mg, codeine phosphate 10 mg, alcohol 0.95%. Syr. Bot. 120 ml, pt, gal. *c-v.*
Use: Decongestant, antihistamine, antitussive.

Bromanate Elixir. (Barre-National) Phenylpropanolomine HCl 12.5 mg, brompheniramine maleate 2 mg/5 ml. Elix. Bot. 118 ml, 237 ml, 473 ml, gal. *otc.*
Use: Decongestant, antihistamine.

Bromanyl. (Various Mfr.) Bromodiphenhydramine HCl 12.5 mg, codeine phosphate 10 mg, alcohol 5%. Syr. Bot. pt, gal. *c-v.*
Use: Antihistamine, antitussive.

Bromarest DX. (Warner Chilcott) Pseudoephedrine HCl 30 mg, brompheniramine maleate 2 mg, dextromethorphan HBr 10 mg, alcohol 0.95%. Butterscotch favor. Syr. Bot. 480 ml. *Rx.*
Use: Antitussive, decongestant, antihistamine.

Bromatane D.C. Cough Syrup. (Goldline) Brompheniramine maleate, phenylpropanolamine HCl, codeine phosphate. Bot. gal. *c-v.*
Use: Antihistamine, decongestant, antitussive.

Bromatane DX Cough Syrup. (Goldline) Pseudoephedrine HCl 30 mg, brompheniramine maleate 2 mg, dextromethorphan HBr 10 mg. Bot. 480 ml. *Rx.*
Use: Decongestant, antihistamine, antitussive.

Bromatap Elixir. (Goldline) Brompheniramine maleate 2 mg, phenylephrine HCl 12.5 mg, alcohol 2.3%/5 ml. Bot. 4 oz, 8 oz, pt, gal. *otc.*
Use: Antihistamine, decongestant.

Bromatapp Tablets. (Copley) Brompheniramine maleate 12 mg, phenylpropanolamine HCl 75 mg/Tab. Bot. 100s. *otc.*
Use: Antihistamine, decongestant.

bromauric acid. Hydrogen tetrabromoaurate.

•**bromazepam.** (broe-MAY-zeh-pam) USAN.
Use: Tranquilizer (minor).

bromazine.
See: Ambodryl HCl, Elix., Kapseal (Parke-Davis).

Brombay Elixir. (Rosemont) Brompheniramine maleate 2 mg/5 ml, alcohol 3%. Bot. 4 oz, pt, gal. *otc.*
Use: Antihistamine.

•**bromchlorenone.** (brome-KLOR-ee-nohn) USAN. (Maumee) Vinyzene.
Use: Anti-infective (topical).

•**bromelains.** (BROE-meh-lanes) USAN.
Use: Anti-inflammatory.
See: Dayto-Anase, Tab. (Dayton).

Bromenzyme. (Barth's) Bromelain 40 mg/Tab. Bot. 100s, 250s, 500s. *otc, Rx.*
Use: Digestive aid.

Bromezyme. (Barth's) Bromelain 40 mg, papaya fruit, papain enzyme/Tab. Bot. 100s, 250s, 500s. *otc, Rx.*
Use: Digestive aid.

bromethol.
See: Avertin.

Bromfed Capsules. (Muro) Brompheniramine maleate 12 mg, pseudoephedrine HCl 120 mg/TR Cap. Bot. 100s, 500s. *Rx.*
Use: Antihistamine, decongestant.

Bromfed-DM Syrup. (Muro) Brompheniramine maleate 2 mg, pseudoephedrine HCl 30 mg, dextromethorphan HBr 10 mg/5 ml. Bot. 120 ml, 240 ml, 480 ml. *Rx.*
Use: Antihistamine, decongestant, antitussive.

Bromfed-PD Capsules. (Muro) Brompheniramine maleate 6 mg, pseudoephedrine HCl 60 mg/TR Cap. Bot. 100s, 500s. *Rx.*

Use: Antihistamine, decongestant.

Bromfed Syrup. (Muro) Brompheniramine maleate 2 mg, pseudoephedrine HCl 30 mg/5 ml. Bot. 120 ml, 473 ml. *otc.*
Use: Antihistamine, decongestant.

Bromfed Tablets. (Muro) Brompheniramine maleate 4 mg, pseudoephedrine HCl 60 mg/Tab. Bot. 100s. *Rx.*
Use: Antihistamine, decongestant.

•**bromfenac sodium.** (BROME-fen-ACK) USAN.
Use: Analgesic.

Bromfenex. (Ethex) Brompheniramine maleate 12 mg, pseudoephedrine HCl 120 mg/ER Cap. Bot. 100s, 500s. *Rx.*
Use: Decongestant, antihistamine.

Bromfenex PD. (Ethex) Brompheniramine maleate 6 mg, pseudoephedrine HCl 60 mg, sucrose/ER Cap. Bot. 100s, 500s. *Rx.*
Use: Decongestant, antihistamine.

•**bromhexine hydrochloride.** (brome-HEX-een) USAN.
Use: Expectorant, mucolytic.
See: Bisolvon (Boehringer Ingelheim).

bromhexine. *Rx.*
Use: Mild/moderate keratoconjunctivitis sicca. [Orphan drug]

bromides.
See: Lanabrom, Elix. (Lannett).
Peacocks Bromides, Liq. (Natcon).

bromide salts.
See: Calcium Bromide.
Ferrous Bromide.
Potassium Bromide.
Sodium Bromide.
Strontium Bromide.

Bromi-Lotion. (Gordon) Aluminum hydroxychloride 20%, emollient base. Bot. 1.5 oz, 4 oz. *otc.*
Use: Antiperspirant.

•**bromindione.** (BROME-in-die-ohn) USAN.
Use: Anticoagulant.
See: Circladin.

Bromi-Talc. (Gordon) Potassium alum, bentonite, talc. Shaker can 3.5 oz, 1 lb, 5 lb. *otc.*
Use: Bromidrosis, hyperhidrosis.

•**bromocriptine.** (BROE-moe-KRIP-teen) USAN.
Use: Prolactin inhibitor.

•**bromocriptine mesylate.** (BROE-moe-KRIP-teen) U.S.P. 23.
Use: Prolactin inhibitor.
See: Parlodel, Tab. (Sandoz).

bromodiethylacetylurea.
See: Carbromal.

•**bromodiphenhydramine hydrochloride.** U.S.P. 23.
Use: Antihistamine.

Bromodiphenhydramine HCl/Codeine Cough Syrup. (Rosemont) Bromodiphenhydramine HCl 12.5 mg, codeine phsophate 10 mg. Syr. Bot. 480 ml. *c-v.*
Use: Antitussive combination.

bromofrom. Tribromomethane.

bromoisovaleryl urea. Alpha, bromoisovaleryl urea.
See: Bromisovalum.

Bromophen T.D. (Rugby) Phenylpropanolamine HCl 15 mg, phenylephrine HCl 15 mg, brompheniramine maleate 12 mg/Tab. Bot. 100s, 1000s. *Rx.*
Use: Decongestant, antihistamine.

Bromophin.
See: Apomorphine HCl (Various Mfr.).

Bromo Quinine Cold Tablets.
See: BQ Cold Tablets (Bristol-Myers).

Bromo-Seltzer. (Warner-Lambert) Acetaminophen 325 mg, sodium bicarbonate 2.78 g, citric acid 2.22 g (when dissolved, forms sodium citrate 2.85 g)/Dose. Large (2⅝ oz), King (4.25 oz), Giant (9 oz), Foil pack, single dose 48s. *otc.*
Use: Antacid, analgesic.

Bromo-Seltzer Effervescent Granules. (Warner-Lambert) Sodium bicarbonate 2781 mg, acetaminophen 325 mg, citric acid 2224 mg, sodium 761 mg, sugar. Bot. 127.5 g. *otc.*
Use: Antacid, analgesic.

8-bromotheophylline.
See: Pamabrom.

bromotheophyllinate aminoisobutanol.
See: Pamabrom.

bromotheophyllinate pyranisamine.
See: Pyrabrom.

bromotheophyllinate pyrilamine.
See: Pyrabrom.

Bromotuss W/ Codeine. (Rugby) Bromodiphenhydramine HCl 12.5 mg, codeine phosphate 10 mg, alcohol 5 %. Syr. Bot. 120 ml, pt, gal. *c-v.*
Use: Antihistamine, antitussive.

•**bromoxanide.** (broe-MOX-ah-nide) USAN.
Use: Anthelmintic.

•**bromperidol.** (brome-PURR-ih-dahl) USAN.
Use: Antipsychotic.

•**bromperidol decanoate.** (brome-PURR-ih-dole deh-KAN-oh-ate) USAN.
Use: Antipsychotic.

Bromphen DC w/ Codeine Cough Syrup. (Various Mfr.) Phenylpropanolamine HCl 12.5 mg, brompheniramine maleate 2 mg, codeine phosphate 10 mg, alcohol 0.95%. Syr. Bot. 120 ml, pt, gal. *c-v.*
Use: Decongestant, antihistamine, antitussive.

Bromphen DX. (Rugby) Pseudoephedrine HCl 30 mg, brompheniramine maleate 2 mg, dextromethorphan HBr 10 mg, alcohol 0.95%. Syr. Bot. 480 ml. *Rx.*
Use: Decongestant, antihistamine, antitussive.

Bromphen Expectorant. (Various Mfr.) Phenylpropanolamine HCl 5 mg, phenylephrine HCl 5 mg, brompheniramine maleate 2 mg, guaifenesin 100 mg, alcohol 3.5%. Liq. Bot. 120 ml, pt, gal. *otc.*
Use: Decongestant, antihistamine, expectorant.

Brompheniramine Cough Syrup. (Geneva Pharm.) Pseudoephedrine HCl 30 mg, brompheniramine maleate 2 mg, dextromethorphan HBr 10 mg, alcohol 0.95%. Bot. 480 ml. *Rx.*
Use: Decongestant, antihistamine, antitussive.

Brompheniramine DC. (Geneva Pharm.) Phenylpropanolamine HCl 12.5 mg, brompheniramine maleate 2 mg, codeine phosphate 10 mg, alcohol 0.95%. Syr. Bot. 120 ml. *c-v.*
Use: Decongestant, antihistamine, antitussive.

•**brompheniramine maleate,** (brome-fen-AIR-uh-meen) U.S.P. 23.
Use: Antihistamine.
See: Dimetane, Tab., Elix., Inj. (Robins). Symptom 3, Liq. (Parke-Davis). Veltane (Lannett).

brompheniramine maleate w/combinations.
See: Bro-Expectorant W/Codeine, Liq. (Solvay).
Bromepaph, Preps. (Quality Generics).
Cortane, Preps. (Standex).
Cortapp, Elix. (Standex).
Dimetane Decongestant, Tab., Elix. (Robins).
Dimetane Expectorant, Liq. (Robins).
Dimetane Expectorant-DC, Liq. (Robins).
Dimetapp Extentabs, Elix. (Robins).
Eldatapp, Tab., Liq. (ICN Pharm.).

Brompton's Cocktail. Heroin or morphine 10 mg, cocaine 10 mg, alcohol, chloroform water, syrup. *c-ii.*
Use: Narcotic agonist analgesic.

Bromtapp. (Halsey) Brompheniramine maleate 4 mg, phenylephrine HCl 5 mg, phenylpropanolamine HCl 5 mg/5 ml. Bot. 16 oz, gal. *otc.*
Use: Antihistamine, decongestant.

Bronchial Capsules. (Various Mfr.) Theophylline 150 mg, guaifenesin 90 mg. Cap. Bot. 100s, 1000s. *Rx.*
Use: Antiasthmatic, expectorant.

Broncholate Capsules. (Bock) Ephedrine HCl 12.5 mg, guaifenesin 200 mg/Cap. Bot. 100s, 1000s. *Rx.*
Use: Bronchodilator, expectorant.

Broncholate Softgels. (Bock) Ephedrine HCl 12.5 mg, guaifenesin 200 mg. Cap. Bot. 100s. *Rx.*
Use: Bronchodilator, expectorant.

Broncholate Syrup. (Bock) Ephedrine HCl 6.25 mg, guaifenesin 100 mg/5 ml. Bot. pt. *Rx.*
Use: Bronchodilator, expectorant.

Broncho Saline. (Blairex) 0.9% sodium Cl for diluting bronchodilator solutions for inhalation. Soln. 90 ml, 240 ml w/metered dispensing valve. *otc.*
Use: Inhalation diluent.

Brondecon. (Parke-Davis) **Tab.:** Oxtriphylline 200 mg, guaifenesin 100 mg/Tab. Bot. 100s. **Elix.:** Oxtriphylline 100 mg, guaifenesin 50 mg/5 ml w/alcohol 20%. Bot. 8 oz, 16 oz. *Rx.*
Use: Bronchodilator, expectorant.

Brondelate. (Various Mfr.) Oxtriphylline 300 mg, guaifenesin 150 mg/5 ml. Elix. Bot. 480 ml, gal. *Rx.*
Use: Bronchodilator, expectorant.

Bronitin. (Whitehall Robins) Theophylline hydrous 120 mg, guaifenesin 100 mg, ephedrine HCl 24.3 mg, pyrilamine maleate 16.6 mg/Tab. Bot. 24s, 60s. *otc.*
Use: Bronchodilator.

Bronitin Mist. (Whitehall Robins) Epinephrine bitartrate in inhalation aerosol. Each spray releases 0.3 mg epinephrine bitartrate equivalent to 0.16 mg epinephrine base. Bot 15 ml or 15 ml refills. *otc.*
Use: Bronchodilator.

Bronkaid Dual Action. (Bayer) Ephedrine sulfate 25 mg, guaifenesin 400 mg. Capl. Bot. 24s. *otc.*
Use: Bronchodilator, expectorant.

Bronkaid Mist. (Sanofi Winthrop) Epinephrine 0.5% in inhalation aerosol. Each spray releases 0.25 mg epinephrine. Aerosol 10 g or 16.7 g w/adapter; 15 g, 25 g refills. *otc.*
Use: Bronchodilator.

Bronkaid Mist Suspension. (Sanofi Winthrop) Epinephrine bitartrate 0.7%. Each spray releases 0.3 mg epinephrine bitartrate equivalent to 0.16 mg epinephrine base. Bot. 10 ml, 15 ml with and without adapter. *otc.*
Use: Bronchodilator.

Bronkodyl. (Sanofi Winthrop) Theophylline 100 mg or 200 mg/Cap. Bot. 100s. Theophylline 300 mg/SR Cap. Bot. 100s. *Rx.*
Use: Bronchodilator.

Bronkometer. (Sanofi Winthrop) Isoetharine mesylate 0.61%, saccharin, menthol, alcohol 30%. Metered dose of 340 mcg isoetharine in fluoro hydrocarbon propellant. Bot. w/nebulizer 10 ml, 15 ml. Refill 10 ml, 15 ml. *Rx.*
Use: Bronchodilator.

Bronkosol. (Sanofi Winthrop) Isoetharine HCl 1% w/glycerin, sodium bisulfite, parabens for oral inhalation. Bot. 10 ml, 30 ml. *Rx.*
Use: Bronchodilator.

Bronkotuss. (Hyrex) Chlorpheniramine maleate 4 mg, guaifenesin 100 mg, ephedrine sulfate 8.216 mg, hydriodic acid syrup 1.67 mg/5 ml w/alcohol 5%. Bot. pt, gal. *Rx.*
Use: Antihistamine, expectorant, decongestant.

Brontex Liquid. (Proctor & Gamble) Codeine phosphate 2.5 mg, guaifenesin 75 mg per 5 ml, methylparaben, saccharin, sucrose/Liq. Bot. 473 ml. *c-iv.*
Use: Narcotic antitussive w/expectorant.

Brontex Tablets. (Procter & Gamble) **Tab:** Codeine phosphate 10 mg, guaifenesin 300 mg/Tab. 100s. *c-iii.*
Use: Narcotic antitussive w/expecotrant.

•**broperamole.** (BROE-PURR-ah-mole) USAN.
Use: Anti-inflammatory.

•**bropirimine.** (broe-PIE-rih-MEEN) USAN.
Use: Antineoplastic, antiviral.

Broserpine. (Brothers) Reserpine 0.25 mg/Tab. Bot. 250s, 100s.
Use: Antihypertensive.

Brotane Expectorant. (Halsey) Guaifenesin 100 mg, brompheniramine maleate 2 mg, phenylephrine HCl 5 mg, phenylpropanolamine HCl 5 mg/5 ml, alcohol 3.5%. Bot. 16 oz. *otc.*
Use: Expectorant, antihistamine, decongestant.

•**brotizolam.** (broe-TIE-zoe-LAM) USAN.

Use: Hypnotic, sedative.

Bro-T's. (Brothers) Bromisovalum 0.12 g, carbromal 0.2 g/Tab. Bot. 100s, 1000s. *Rx.*
Use: Sedative, tranquilizer.

Bro-Tuss. (Brothers) Dextromethorphan HBr 15 mg, chlorpheniramine maleate 2 mg, phenylephrine HCl 5 mg, ammonium Cl 100 mg, sodium citrate 150 mg, vitamin C 30 mg/10 ml. Bot. 4 oz, pt, gal. *otc.*
Use: Antitussive, antihistamine, decongestant, expectorant.

Bro-Tuss A.C. (Brothers) Acetaminophen 120 mg, codeine phosphate 10 mg, phenylephrine HCl 5 mg, chlorpheniramine maleate 2 mg, menthol 1 mg, alcohol 10%/5 ml. Bot. pt, gal. *c-v.*
Use: Analgesic, antitussive, decongestant, antihistamine.

Bryrel Syrup. (Sanofi Winthrop) Piperazine citrate anhydrous 110 mg/ml. Bot. oz. *Rx.*
Use: Anthelmintic.

B-Salt Forte. (Akorn) **Part I:** Sodium Cl 7.14 mg, potassium Cl 0.38 mg, calcium chloride dihydrate 0.154 mg, magnesium chloride hexahydrate 0.2 mg, dextrose 0.92 mg, hydrochloric acid or sodium hydroxide/ml. Soln. Bot. 515 ml. **Part II:** Sodium bicarbonate 1081 mg, dibasic sodium phosphate (anhydrous) 216 mg, glutathione disulfide 95 mg/vial. Soln. Bot. 60 ml. *Rx.*
Use: Intraocular irrigating solution.

B-Scorbic. (Pharmics) Vitamins C 300 mg, B_1 25 mg, B_2 10 mg, calcium pantothenate 10 mg, niacinamide 50 mg, lemon flavored complex 200 mg/Tab. Bot. 100s, 1000s. *otc.*
Use: Vitamin/mineral supplement.

BSS. (Alcon) Sodium Cl 0.64%, potassium Cl 0.075%, magnesium Cl 0.03%, calcium Cl 0.048%, sodium acetate 0.39%, sodium citrate 0.17%, sodium hydroxide or hydrochloric acid. Bot. 15 ml, 30 ml, 250 ml, 500 ml. *Rx.*
Use: Intraocular irrigating solution.

BSS Plus. (Alcon) **Part I:** Sodium Cl 7.44 mg, potassium Cl 0.395 mg, dibasic sodium phosphate 0.433 mg, sodium bicarbonate 2.19 mg, hydrochloric acid or sodium hydroxide/ml. Soln. Bot. 240 ml. **Part II:** Calcium chloride dihydrate 3.85 mg, magnesium chloride hexahydrate 5 mg, dextrose 23 mg, glutathione disulfide 4.5 mg/ml. Soln. Bot. 10 ml. *Rx.*
Use: Intraocular irrigating solution.

BTA Rapid Urine Test. (Bard) Reagent kit for detection of bladder tumor associated analytes in urine to aid in management of bladder cancer. In kits of 15 and 30 tests. *Rx.*
Use: Diagnostic tests.

•**bucainide maleate.** (byoo-CANE-ide) USAN.
Use: Cardiac depressant (antiarrhythmic).

Bucet. (UAD) Butalbital 50 mg, acetaminophen 650 mg. Cap. Bot. 100s. *Rx.*
Use: Analgesic.

buchu.
See: Barosmin.

•**bucindolol hydrochloride.** (BYOO-SIN-doe-lole) USAN. A B-M Squibb investigational drug.
Use: Investigative, antihypertensive.

Bucladin-S. (Zeneca) Buclizine HCl 50 mg. Softab. Tab. Bot. 100s. *Rx.*
Use: Antiemetic, antivertigo.

•**buclizine hydrochloride.** (BYOO-klih-zeen) USAN.
Use: Antiemetic, antinauseant.
See: Bucladin-S, Tab. (Stuart).

•**bucromarone.** (byoo-KROE-mah-rone) USAN.
Use: Cardiac depressant (antiarrhythmic).

•**bucrylate.** (BYOO-krih-late) USAN.
Use: Surgical aid (tissue adhesive).

•**budesonide.** (BYOO-DESS-oh-nide) USAN.
Use: Anti-inflammatory.

Buf Acne Cleansing Bar. (3M Products) Salicylic acid 1%, sulfur 1% in detergent cleansing bar. 3.5 oz. *otc.*
Use: Antiacne.

Buf-Bar. (3M Products) Sulpher 3% and titanium dioxide. Bar 105 g. *otc.*
Use: Antiacne.

Buf Body Scrub. (3M Products) Round cleansing sponge on plastic handles. *otc.*
Use: Cleansing sponge.

Buff-A. (Mayrand) Aspirin acid 5 gr. buffered w/magnesium hydroxide, aluminum hydroxide dried gel. Tab. Bot. 100s, 1000s. *otc.*
Use: Analgesic, antacid.

Buffaprin. (Buffington) Aspirin 325 mg. buffered with magnesium oxide. Sugar, caffeine, lactose, salt free. Tab. Dispens-A-Kit 500s. *otc.*
Use: Salicylate analgesic.

Buffasal. (Dover) Aspirin 325 mg/Tab. w/magnesium oxide. Sugar, lactose, salt free. UD Box 500s. *otc.*

Use: Salicylate analgesic.

Buffasal Max. (Dover) Aspirin 500 mg/Tab w/magnesium oxide. Sugar, lactose, salt free. *otc.*
Use: Salicylate analgesic.

Bufferin AF Nite Time. (B-M Squibb) Acetaminophen 500 mg, diphenhydramine citrate 38 mg, simethicone. Cap shaped tab. Bot. 24s and 50s. *otc.*
Use: Nonprescription sleep aid, analgesic.

Buffered Aspirin. (Various Mfr.) Aspirin 325 mg with buffers. Tab. Bot. 100s, 500s, 1000s and UD 100s and 200s. *otc.*
Use: Analgesic.

Buffets II. (JMI) Aspirin 227 mg, acetaminophen 162 mg, caffeine 32.4 mg, aluminum hydroxide 50 mg/Tab. Bot. 1000s. *otc.*
Use: Analgesic combination.

Buffex. (Roberts Med) Aspirin 325 mg w/ dihydroxyaluminum aminoacetate. Tab. Bot. 1000s, Sanipack 1000s. *otc.*
Use: Salicylate analgesic.

Buf Foot Care Kit. (3M Products) Cleansing system for the feet. *otc.*
Use: Foot preparation.

Buf Foot Care Lotion. (3M Products) Moisturizing lotion for feet. *otc.*
Use: Foot preparation.

Buf Foot Care Soap. (3M Products) Bar 3.5 oz. *otc.*
Use: Foot preparation.

•**bufilcon a.** (BYOO-fill-kahn A) USAN.
Use: Contact lens material (hydrophilic).

Buf Kit for Acne. (3M Products) Cleansing sponge, cleansing bar. 3.5 oz w/ booklet, holding tray. *otc.*
Use: Antiacne.

Buf Lotion. (3M Products) Moisturizing lotion. *otc.*
Use: Emollient.

•**buformin.** (BYOO-FORE-min) USAN.
Use: Antidiabetic.

Bufosal. (Table Rock) Sodium salicylate 15 gr/dram w/calcium carbonate, sodium bicarbonate as granulated effervescent powder. Bot. 4 oz. *otc.*
Use: Salicylate analgesic, antacid.

Buf-Ped Non Medicated Cleansing Sponge. (3M Products) Abrasive cleansing sponge. *otc.*
Use: Cleansing skin on feet.

Buf-Puf Acne Cleansing. (3M Products) Salicyclic acid 2%, vitamin E acetate, EDTA. Cake. 99 g. *otc.*
Use: Antiacne.

Buf Puf Bodymate. (3M Products) Oval two-sided cleansing sponge. Abrasive/gentle. *otc.*
Use: Cleansing all areas of the body.

Buf-Puf Medicated. (3M Products) Water-activated. Salicylic acid 0.5% (reg. strength), alcohols benzoate, EDTA, triethanolamine and vitamin E acetate. Salicylic acid 2% (max. strength). Pads. Jar 30s. *otc.*
Use: Antiacne.

Buf-Puf Non-Medicated cleansing sponge. (3M Products) Abrasive cleansing sponge. *otc.*
Use: Skin cleansing.

Buf-Sul Tablets and Suspension. (Sheryl) Sulfacetamide 167 mg, sulfadiazine 167 mg, sulfamerazine 167 mg. Tab. 100s. Susp. pt. *Rx.*
Use: Anti-infective, sulfonamide.

Buf-Tabs. (Halsey) Aspirin 5 gr/Tab. w/ aluminum hydroxide, glycine magnesium carbonate. Bot. 100s. *otc.*
Use: Salicylate analgesic, antacid.

Bug-Pruf. (Scherer) n, n diethyl-m-toluamide (DEET) 94.525%, other isomers 4.975%, fragrance 0.5%. Bot. 2 oz.
Use: Insect repellent.

Bugs Bunny Chewable Vitamins and Minerals. (Bayer) Vitamins A 5000 IU, D 400 IU, E 30 IU, C 60 mg, folic acid 0.4 mg, B_1 1.5 mg, B_2 1.7 mg, niacin 20 mg, B_6 2 mg, B_{12} 6 mcg, biotin 40 mcg, pantothenic acid 10 mg, iron 18 mg, calcium 100 mg, phosphorus 100 mg, iodine 150 mcg, magnesium 20 mg, copper 2 mg, zinc 15 mg/Tab. Bot 60s. *otc.*
Use: Vitamin/mineral supplement.

Bugs Bunny Complete. (Bayer) Ca 100 mg, iron 18 mg, vitamins A 5000 IU, D 400 IU, E 30 mg, B_1 1.5 mg, B_2 1.7mg, B_3 20 mg, B_5 10 mg, B_6 mcg, C 60 mg, folic acid 0.4 mg, biotin 40 mcg, Cu, I, Mg, P, aspartame, phenylalanine, Zn 15 mg/Tab. Bot 60s. *otc.*
Use: Vitamin/mineral supplement.

Bugs Bunny Plus Iron. (Bayer) Vitamins A 2500 IU, E 15 IU, C 60 mg, folic acid 0.3 mg, B_1 1.05 mg, B_2 1.2 mg, niacin 13.5 mg, B_6 1.05 mg, B_{12} 4.5 mcg, D 400 IU, iron 15 mg/Chew. tab. Bot. 60s. *otc.*
Use: Vitamin/mineral supplement.

Bugs Bunny With Extra C. (Bayer) Vitamins A 2500 IU, D 400 IU, E 15 IU, C 250 mg, folic acid 0.3 mg, B_1 1.05 mg, B_2 1.2 mg, niacin 13.5 mg, B_6 1.05 mg, B_{12} 4.5 mcg/Tab. Bot. 60s. *otc.*
Use: Vitamin/mineral supplement.

bulkogen. A mucin extracted from the seeds of *Cyanopsis tetragonaloba.*

Bullfrog. (Chattem) Benzophenone-3, octyl methoxycinnamate, isostearyl alcohol, aloe, hydrogenated vegetable oil, vitamin E. Waterproof. Stick 16.5 g. *otc.*
Use: Sunscreen.

Bullfrog Extra Moisturizing Gel. (Chattem) Benzophenone-3, octocrylene, octyl methoxycinnamate, vitamin E, aloe. SPF 18. Tube 90 g. *otc.*
Use: Sunscreen.

Bullfrog for Kids. (Chattem). SPF 18. Octocrylene, octyl methoxycinnamate, octyl salicylate, vitamin E, aloe, alcohols benzoate. Gel Tube 60 g. *otc.*
Use: Sunscreen.

Bullfrog Sport Lotion. (Chattem) SPF 18. Benzophenone-3, octocrylene, octyl methoxycinnamate, octyl salicylate, titanium dioxide, diazolidinyl urea, EDTA, parabens, vitamin E, aloe. Bot. 120 ml. *otc.*
Use: Sunscreen.

Bullfrog Sunblock. (Chattem) SPF 18, 36. Benzophenone-3, octocrylene, octyl methoxycinnamate, aloe, vitamin E, isostearyl alcohol. PABA free. Waterproof. Gel Tube 120 g. *otc.*
Use: Sunscreen.

• **bumetanide,** U.S.P. 23.
Use: Diuretic.
See: Bumex, Inj., Tab. (Roche).

bumetanide, (BYOO-MET-uh-nide) U.S.P. 23, Tab., Inj., (Mylan) **Tab:** 0.5 mg, 1 mg, 2 mg/Tab. Bot. 100s. (Various Mfr.) **Inj.:** 0.25 mg/ml. In 4 ml fill in 5 ml.
Use: Diuretic.

• **bumetrizole.** (BYOO-meh-TRY-zole) USAN.
Use: Ultraviolet screen.

Bumex. (Roche) Bumetanide 0.5 mg, 1 mg or 2 mg/Tab. 0.5 mg and 1 mg Bot. 100s, 500s, UD 100s. 2 mg Bot. 100s, UD 100s. Inj. Amp 2 ml, 0.25 mg/ml. Box 10s. Vial 2 ml, 4 ml or 10 ml, 0.25 mg/ml. Box 10s. *Rx.*
Use: Loop diuretic.

Buminate. (Baxter) Normal serum albumin (human) **25%** soln. in 20 ml w/o administration set; 50 ml and 100 ml w/ administration set. **5%** soln. in 250 ml and 500 ml w/administration set. *Rx.*
Use: Albumin replacement.

• **bunamide hydrochloride.** (BYOO-NAM-ih-deen) USAN.
Use: Anthelmintic.

bunamiodyl sodium.
Use: Diagnostic aid (radiopaque medium).

•**bunaprolast.** (BYOO-nah-PROLE-ast) USAN.
Use: Antiasthmatic.

•**bunolol hydrochloride.** (BYOO-no-lole) USAN.
Use: Antiadrenergic (β-receptors).

Bun Reagent Strips. (Bayer) Seralyzer reagent strips. A quantitative strip test for BUN in serum or plasma. Bot 25s.
Use: Diagnostic aid.

Buphenyl. (Ucyclyd Pharma) Sodium phenylbutyrate 500 mg/Tab. Bot. 250s, 500s. 3.2 g (3 g sodium phenylbutyrate)/tsp. and 9.1 g (8.6 g sodium phenylbutyrate)/tsp/Pow. for inj. Bot. 500 ml and 950 ml. *Rx.*
Use: Antihyperammonemic.

•**bupicomide.** (byoo-PIH-koe-mide) USAN.
Use: Antihypertensive.

•**bupivacaine hydrochloride,** (byoo-PIH-vah-cane) U.S.P. 23.
Use: Anesthetic (local).

Bupivacaine HCl. (Abbott) Bupivacaine 0.25%/Inj. Vial. 20 ml, 50 ml. Bupivacaine HCl 0.5%/Inj. Vial. 20 ml, 30 ml. Bupivacaine HCl 0.75%/Inj. Vial. 20 ml. *Rx.*
Use: Local anesthetic.

bupivacaine in dextrose injection.
Use: Local anesthetic.

bupivacaine and epinephrine injection.
Use: Local anesthetic.
See: Marcaine w/Epinephrine, Inj. (Sanofi Winthrop).

bupivacaine hydrochloride.
Use: Local anesthetic.
See: Marcaine, Inj (Astra).
Marcaine w/Epinephrine, Inj. (Cook-Waite).
Marcaine Spinal, Inj (Astra).
Sensorcaine MPF, Inj (Astra).
Sensorcaine MPF Spinal, Inj (Astra).
Bupivacaine HCl, Inj (Abbott).
Sensorcaine, Inj. (Astra).

Buprenex Injection. (Reckitt & Colman) Buprenorphine HCl 0.3 mg/ml w/50 mg anhydrous dextrose. Amp. 1 ml. [c-v] c-v.
Use: Narcotic analgesic.

•**buprenorphine hydrochloride,** (BYOO-preh-NAHR-feen) U.S.P. 23.
Use: Analgesic; treatment of opiate addiction. [Orphan drug]

•**bupropion hydrochloride.** (byoo-PRO-pee-ahn) USAN.

Use: Antidepressant.
See: Wellbutrin (Glaxo Wellcome).

•**buramate.** (BYOO-rah-mate) USAN.
Use: Anticonvulsant, tranquilizer, antipsychotic.
See: Hyamate (Xttrium).

Burdeo. (Hill) Aluminum subacetate 100 mg, boric acid 300 mg/oz. Bot. 3 oz. Roll-on 8 oz. *otc.*
Use: Deodorant.

Burn-a-Lay. (Ken-Gate) Chlorobutanol 0.75%, oxyquinoline benzoate 0.025%, zinc oxide 2%, thymol 0.5%. Cream. Tube oz. *otc.*
Use: Burn remedy.

Burnate. (Burlington) Vitamins A 4000 IU, D-2 400 IU, thiamine HCl 3 mg, riboflavin 2 mg, niacinamide 10 mg, pyridine HCl 2 mg, cyanocobalamin 5 mcg, calcium pantothenate 0.5 mg, folic acid 0.4 mg, ascorbic acid 50 mg, ferrous fumarate 300 mg, calcium 200 mg, iodine 0.15 mg, copper 1 mg, magnesium 5 mg, zinc 1.5 mg/Tab. Bot. 100s. *otc.*
Use: Vitamin/mineral supplement.

burn therapy.
See: Americaine, Preps. (DuPont Merck).
Amertan, Jelly (Lilly).
Burn-A-Lay, Cream (Ken-Gate).
Burnicin, Oint. (Quality Generics).
Burn-Quel, Aerosol (Halperin).
Butesin Picrate Oint. (Abbott).
Foille, Preps. (Carbisulphoil).
Kip, Preps. (Youngs Drug Prod.).
Nupercainal, Oint. (Novartis).
Silvadene, Cream (Hoechst Marion Roussel).
Solarcaine, Preps. (Schering Plough).
Sulfamylon, Cream (Sanofi Winthrop).
Unguentine, Preps. (Procter & Gamble).

Burn-Quel. Halperin aerosol dispenser. 1 oz, 2 oz.
Use: Burn remedy.

Buro-Sol Antiseptic Powder. (Doak) Contents make a diluted Burow's Solution. Aluminum acetate topical soln. plus benzethonium Cl. Pkg. (2.36 g) 12s, 100s. Bot. Pow. 4 oz, 1 lb, 5 lb. *otc.*
Use: Astringent wet dressing.

Buro-Sol Solution. (Doak) Aluminum acetate 0.23%. Soln. Pkt. 12s.
Use: Astringent wet dressing.

Burow's Solution. Aluminum Acetate Topical Solution, U.S.P. 23.
See: Buro-Sol Pow. (Doak).
Domeboro, Pow., Tab. (Bayer).

W/Boric acid, acetic acid.
See: Star-Otic, Drops (Star).
Bursul. (Burlington) Sulfamethiazole 500 mg/Tab. Bot. 100s. *Rx.*
Use: Anti-infective; sulfonamide.
Bur-Tuss. (Burlington) Chlorpheniramine maleate 2 mg, phenylephrine HCl 5 mg, phenylpropanolamine HCl 5 mg, guaifenesin 100 mg, alcohol 2.5%/5 ml. Bot. pt, gal. *otc.*
Use: Antihistamine, decongestant, expectorant.
Bur-Zin. (Lamond) Aluminum acetate solution 2%, zinc oxide 10%. Bot. 4 oz, 8 oz, pt, qt, gal. Also w/o lanolin. *otc.*
Use: Antipruritic, counterirritant.
•**buserelin acetate.** (BYOO-seh-REH-lin ASS-eh-tate) USAN.
Use: Gonad-stimulating principle.
BuSpar Tablets. (Bristol-Myers) Buspirone HCl 5 mg or 10 mg/Tab. *Rx.*
Use: Antianxiety agent.
•**buspirone hydrochloride.** (byoo-SPY-rone) U.S.P. 23.
Use: Antianxiety agent; tranquilizer (minor).
See: BuSpar, Tab. (Bristol-Myers).
•**busulfan.** (byoo-SULL-fate) U.S.P. 23. Tabs, U.S.P. 23.
Use: Antineoplastic, chronic myeloid leukemia. [Orphan drug]
See: Myleran, Tab. (Glaxo Wellcome).
•**butabarbital,** (byoo-tah-BAR-bih-tahl) U.S.P. 23
Use: Sedative, hypnotic.
See: BBS, Tab. (Solvay).
   Butisol, Prods. (Wallace).
   Da-Sed, Tab. (Sheryl).
   Expansatol, Cap. (Merit).
   Medarsed, Elix., Tab. (Medar).
W/Acetaminophen.
See: G-3, Tab. (Roberts).
   Sedapap, Elix. (Mayrand).
   Sedapap-10, Tab. (Mayrand).
W/Acetaminophen, codeine phosphate.
See: G-3, Cap. (Roberts).
W/Acetaminophen, mephenesin.
See: See:T-Caps, Cap. (Burlington).
W/Acetaminophen, phenacetin, caffeine.
See: Windolor, Tab. (Winston).
W/Acetaminophen, salicylamide, phenyltoloxamine citrate.
See: Dengesic, Tab. (Scott-Alison).
   Scotgesic, Cap., Elix. (Scott/Cord).
W/Ambutonium bromide, aluminum hydroxide, magnesium hydroxide.
See: Aludrox, Susp., Tab. (Wyeth-Ayerst).
W/Aminophylline, phenylpropanolamine HCl, chlorpheniramine maleate, aluminum hydroxide, magnesium trisilicate.
See: Asmacol, Tab. (Pal-Pak).
W/Carboxyphen.
See: Bontril Timed No. 2, Tab. (G. W. Carnrick).
W/Chlorpheniramine maleate, hyoscine HBr.
See: Pedo-Sol, Tab., Elix. (Warren Pharmacal).
W/Dihydroxypropyl theophylline, ephedrine HCl.
See: Airet R, Tab. (Baylor).
W/Ephedrine sulfate, theophylline.
See: Airet Y, Tab., Elix. (Baylor).
W/Ephedrine HCl, theophylline, guaifenesin.
See: Quibron Plus, Cap., Elix. (Bristol).
W/Ephedrine HCl, theophylline, isoproterenol.
W/Ephedrine sulfate, theophylline, guaifenesin.
See: Broncholate, Cap., Elix. (Bock).
W/l-Hyoscyamine.
See: Cystospaz-SR, Cap. (PolyMedica).
W/Hyoscyamine sulfate, atropine sulfate, hyoscine HBr, homatropine methylbromide.
See: Butabell HMB, Tab., Elix. (Saron).
W/Hyoscyamine sulfate, scopolamine methylnitrate, atropine sulfate.
See: Banatil, Cap., Elix. (Trimen).
W/Nitroglycerin.
See: Nitrodyl-B, Cap. (Bock).
W/Pentaerythritol tetranitrate.
See: Petn Plus (Saron).
W/Pentobarbital, phenobarbital.
See: Quiess, Tab. (Forest).
W/Phenazopyridine, hyoscyamine HBr.
See: Pyridium Plus, Tab. (Parke-Davis).
W/Phenazopyridine, scopolamine HBr, atropine sulfate, hyoscyamine sulfate.
See: Buren, Tab. (Ascher).
W/Phenobarbital, pentobarbital, hyoscyamine sulfate, hyoscine HBr, atropine sulfate.
See: Neoquess, Tab. (Forest).
W/Salicylamide.
See: Dapco, Tab. (Mericon).
W/Secobarbital.
See: Monosyl, Tab. (Arcum).
W/Secobarbital, pentobarbital, phenobarbital.
See: Quad-Set, Tab. (Kenyon).
W/Theophylline.
See: Theobid, Cap. (Meyer).
W/Theophylline, pseudoephedrine HCl.
See: Asmadil, Cap. (Solvay).
   Ayr, Liq. (Ascher).
   Ayrcap, Cap. (Ascher).
   Az-Kap, Cap. (Keene).

B. A., Prods. (Federal).
Bronchobid, Duracap (Meyer).
●**butabarbital sodium,** U.S.P. 23.
  Use: Sedative, hypnotic.
  See: BBS, Tab. (Solvay).
    Butalan, Elix. (Lannett).
    Butisol Sodium, Elix., Tab. (Wallace).
    Expansatol, Cap. (Merit).
    Quiebar, Spantab, Tab (Nevin).
    Renbu, Tab. (Wren).
    Soduben Tab., Elix. (Arcum).
  W/Acetaminophen.
    See: Amino-Bar, Tab. (Jones Medical).
    Minotal, Tab. (Schwarz Pharma).
  W/Acetaminophen, aspirin, caffeine.
    See: Dolor Plus, Tab. (Geriatric).
  W/Acetaminophen, caffeine.
    See: Dularin-TH, Tab. (Donner).
    Phrenilin, Tab. (Schwarz Pharma).
  W/Acetaminophen, mephenesin, codeine
  phosphate.
    See: Bancaps-C, Cap. (Westerfield).
  W/Acetaminophen, salicylamide.
    See: Banesin Forte, Tab. (Westerfield).
    Indogesic, Tab. (Century).
  W/Acetaminophen, salicylamide, d-
  amphetamine sulfate, hexobarbital,
  secobarbital sodium, phenobarbital.
    See: Sedragesic, Tab. (Lannett).
  W/d-Amphetamine sulfate.
    See: Bontril, Tab. (Schwarz Pharma).
  W/Ascorbic acid, sodium p-aminobenzo-
  ate, salicylamide, sodium salicylate.
    See: Bisalate, Tab. (Allison).
  W/Atropine sulfate, hyoscyamine HBr, al-
  cohol, hyoscine HBr.
    See: Hyonatol Tab., Hyonatol B Elix.,
    Hexett, Tab. (Jones Medical).
  W/Belladonna extract
    See: Butibel, Tab., Elix. (McNeil).
    Quiebel, Elix., Cap. (Nevin).
  W/Dehydrocholic acid, belladonna ex-
  tract.
    See: Decholin-BB, Tab. (Bayer).
  W/Methscopolamine bromide, aluminum
  hydroxide gel, dried, magnesium trisili-
  cate.
    See: Eulcin, Tab. (Leeds).
  W/Pentobarbital sodium, phenobarbital
  sodium.
    See: Trio-Bar, Tab. (Jenkins).
  W/Salicylamide, mephenesin.
    See: Metrogesic, Tab. (Lexis).
  W/Secobarbital sodium.
    See: Monosyl, Tab. (Arcum).
  W/Secobarbital sodium, pentobarbital so-
  dium, phenobarbital.
    See: Nidar, Tab. (Centeon).
  W/Secobarbital sodium, phenobarbital.
    See: S.B.P., Tab. (Lemmon).
  W/Simethicone, hyoscyamine sulfate,

atropine sulfate, hyoscine HBr.
  See: Sidonna, Tab. (Schwarz Pharma).
W/Theophylline, pseudoephedrine HCl.
  See: Dilorbron, Cap. (Roberts).
butabarbital sodium, (Various Mfr.)
  Tab.: 15 mg. Bot. 1000s; 30 mg Bot.
  100s, 1000s. **Elixir:** 30 mg/5ml Bot. pt.
  Use: Sedative, hypnotic.
butacaine.
  Use: Local anesthetic.
  See: Butyn Dental Oint. (Abbott).
●**butacetin.** (byoot-ASS-ih-tin) USAN.
  Use: Analgesic, antidepressant.
●**butaclamol hydrochloride.** USAN.
  Use: Antipsychotic.
Butagen Caps. (Goldline) Phenylbuta-
  zone 100 mg/Cap. Bot. 100s, 500s.
  Rx.
  Use: Antirheumatic.
  Use: Sedative, hypnotic.
●**butalbital,** (BYOO-TAL-bih-tuhl) U.S.P.
  23.
  Use: Sedative, hypnotic.
  See: Buff-A-Comp #3 (Mayrand).
    Lotusate, Cap. (Sanofi Winthrop).
    Sandoptal, Preps. (Sandoz).
  W/Acetaminophen.
    See: Phrenilin, Tab. (Schwarz Pharma).
    Phrenilin Forte, Cap. (Schwarz
    Pharma).
  W/Acetaminophen, codeine.
    See: Phrenilin w/Codeine, Cap.
    (Schwarz Pharma).
  W/Acetaminophen, caffeine.
    See: Arbutal, Tab. (Arcum).
    Buff-A-Comp, Tab., Cap. (Mayrand).
    Esgic, Tab. (Gilbert).
    Cefinal, Tab. (Alto).
    Protension, Tab. (Blaine).
    Repan, Tab. (Everett).
  W/Aspirin, caffeine.
    See: Duogesic, Cap. (Western Re-
    search).
    Fiorinal, Cap., Tab. (Sandoz).
  W/Aspirin, caffeine, codeine phosphate.
    See: Buff-A-Comp, Tab w/Codeine.
    (Mayrand).
    Fiorinal With Codeine, Cap. (San-
    doz).
  W/Caffeine, aspirin, acetaminophen.
    See: Anaphen, Cap. (Roberts).
**butalbital, acetaminophen and caffeine
  tablets.** (BYOO-TAL-bih-tuhl, us-seet-
  uh-min-oh-fen and kaff-EEN)
  Use: Analgesic.
butalbital, aspirin & caffeine. (Various
  Mfr.) (BYOO-TAL-bih-tuhl, ass-pihr-in
  and kaff-EEN) **Tab.:** Aspirin 325 mg,
  caffeine 40 mg, butalbital 50 mg. Bot.
  20s, 100s, 1000s, UD 100s. **Cap.:** Aspi-

rin 325 mg, caffeine 40 mg, butalbital 50 mg. Bot. 100s, 1000s. *c-III.*
Use: Nonnarcotic analgesic combination.

•**butalbital and aspirin tablets,**
Use: Analgesic, sedative.

butalbital compound. (Various Mfr.) Tab., Cap. Bot. 100s, 500s, 1000s.
Use: Nonnarcotic analgesic.

W/Acetaminophen, butalbital.
See: Phrenilin (Schwarz Pharma).
Bancap (Forest).
Bucet, Cap. (UAD).
Sedapap-10 (Mayrand).
Tencon, Cap. (Inter. Ethical Labs).
Triaprin (Dunhall).

W/Acetaminophen, caffeine, butalbital.
See: Arcet, Tab. (EconoMed).
Amaphen (Trimen).
Endolor (Keene).
Esgic (Forest).
Esgic-Plus, Tab. (Forest).
Fioricet (Sandoz).
G-1 (Roberts).
Isocet, Tab. (Rugby).
Margesic, Cap. (Marnel).
Medigesic Plus (U.S. Pharm. Corp.).
Phrenilin Forte (Schwarz Pharma).
Repan (Everett).
Sedapap-10 (Mayrand).
Triad, Cap. (UAD).

W/Aspirin, butalbital.
See: Axotal (Pharmacia & Upjohn).

W/Aspirin, caffeine, butalbital.
See: Fiorgen PF (Goldline).
Fiorinal (Sandoz).
Isollyl Improved (Rugby).
Lanorinal (Lannett).
Lorprn (Whitby).
B-A-C (Mayrand).

Butalan Elixir. (Lannett) Sodium butabarbital 0.2 g/30 ml. Bot. pt, gal.
Use: Sedative, hypnotic.

butalgin.
See: Methadone HCl (Various Mfr.).

butallylonal. (Pernocton).
Use: Hypnotic.

•**butamben,** (BYOO-tam-ben) U.S.P. 23.
Use: Anesthetic (topical).

•**butamben picrate.** (BYOO-tam-ben PIC-rate) USAN.
Use: Anesthetic (topical).
See: Butesin Picrate, Oint. (Abbott).

•**butamirate citrate.** (byoo-tah-MY-rate SIH-trate) USAN.
Use: Antitussive.

•**butane,** N.F. 18.
Use: Aerosol propellant.

butanisamide.

•**butaperazine.** USAN.
Use: Antipsychotic.

•**butaperazine maleate.** (BYOO-tah-PURR-ah-zeen) USAN.
Use: Antipsychotic.

butaphyllamine. Ambuphylline. Theophylline aminoisobutanol. Theophylline with 2-amino-2-methyl-1-propanol.

Butapro Elixir. (Approved) Butabarbital sodium 0.2 g/30 ml. Bot. pt, gal. *c-v.*
Use: Sedative, hypnotic.

•**butaprost.** (BYOO-tah-PRAHST) USAN.
Use: Bronchodilator.

Butazone. (Major) Phenylbutazone. **Cap.:** 100 mg. Bot. 100s, 500s. **Tab.:** 100 mg. Bot. 500s. *Rx.*
Use: Antirheumatic.

•**butedronate tetrasodium.** (BYOO-teh-DROE-nate TET-rah-SO-dee-uhm) USAN.
Use: Diagnostic aid (bone imaging).

butelline.
See: Butacaine Sulfate (Various Mfr.).

butenafine hydrochloride. (Penederm).
Use: Treatment of interdigital tinea pedis (athlete's foot).
See: Mentax (Penederm).

•**buterizine.** (byoo-TER-ih-ZEEN) USAN.
Use: Vasodilator (peripheral).

Butesin Picrate. (Abbott) n-Butyl-p-aminobenzoate. Lidocaine 1%, lanolin, parabens, mineral oil/Oint. Jar. 28.4 g. *otc.*
Use: Topical anesthetic. *otc.*

Butesin Picrate Ointment. (Abbott) Butamben picrate 1%. Tube oz. *otc.*
Use: Local anesthetic, topical.

butethal. (Various Mfr.) *Rx.*
Use: Sedative, hypnotic.

butethamine formate.

butethamine hydrochloride.
See: Dentocaine (Amer. Chem. & Drug).

butethanol.
See: Tetracaine.

•**buthiazide.** (byoo-THIGH-azz-IDE) USAN.
Use: Diuretic, antihypertensive.

Butibel. (Wallace) Butabarbital sodium 15 mg, belladonna extract 15 mg/Tab or 5 ml. **Tab.** Bot. 100s. **Elix.:** (w/alcohol 7%) Bot. pt. *Rx.*
Use: Sedative, hypnotic, anticholinergic, antispasmodic.

•**butikacin.** (BYOO-tih-KAY-sin) USAN.
Use: Antibacterial.

•**butilfenin.** (BYOO-till-FEN-in) USAN.
Use: Diagnostic aid (hepatic function determination).

•**butirosin sulfate.** (byoo-TIHR-oh-sin) USAN. A mixture of the sulfates of the A and B forms of an antibiotic produced by *Bacillus circularis.*
Use: Antibacterial.

Butisol Sodium. (Wallace) Butabarbital sodium. **Elix.:** 30 mg/5 ml. Bot pt, gal. **Tab.:** 15 mg, 30 mg. Bot. 100s, 1000s. 50 mg or 100 mg. Bot. 100s. *c-III.*
Use: Sedative, hypnotic.
See: Buticaps, Cap. (Wallace).
W/Belladonna extract.
See: Butibel, (Wallace).

•**butixirate.** (BYOO-TIX-ih-rate) USAN.
Use: Analgesic, antirheumatic.

•**butoconazole nitrate,** (BYOO-toe-KOE-nuh-zole) U.S.P. 23.
Use: Antifungal.
See: Femstat, Cream (Procter-Syntex). Femstat 3 (Procter-Syntex).

butolan. Benzylphenyl carbamate.

•**butonate.** (BYOO-tahn-ate) USAN.
Use: Anthelmintic.

•**butopamine.** (BYOO-TOE-pah-meen) USAN.
Use: Cardiotonic.

•**butoprozone hydrochloride.** (byoo-TOE-pro-ZEEN) USAN.
Use: Cardiac depressant (antiarrhythmic), antianginal.

butopyronoxyl. (Indalone) Butylmesityl oxide.
Use: Insect repellant.

•**butorphanol.** (BYOO-TAR-fan-ahl) USAN.
Use: Analgesic, antitussive.

•**butorphanol tartrate,** U.S.P. 23.
Use: Analgesic, antitussive.
See: Stadol, Inj. (Bristol).

•**butoxamine hydrochloride.** (byoo-TOX-ah-meen) USAN.
Use: Antidiabetic, antihyperlipoproteinemic.

•**butriptyline hydrochloride.** (BYOO-TRIP-till-een) USAN.
Use: Antidepressant.

•**butyl alcohol,** N.F. 18. Butyl alcohol is n-butyl alcohol.
Use: Pharmaceutic aid (solvent).

butyl aminobenzoate. n-Butyl p-Amino-benzoate. Scuroforme.
Use: Local anesthetic.
W/Benzocaine, tetracaine HCl.
See: Cetacaine, Preps. (Cetylite).
W/Benzyl alcohol, phenylmercuric borate, benzocaine.
See: Dermathyn, Oint. (Davis & Sly).

W/Procaine, benzyl alcohol, in sweet almond oil.
See: Anucaine, Amp. (Calvin).
W/Tetracaine.
See: Pontocaine, Oint. (Sanofi Winthrop).

•**butylated hydroxyanisole,** N.F. 18.
Use: Pharmaceutic aid (antioxidant).

•**buylated hydroxytoluene.** N.F. 18.
Use: Pharmaceutic aid (antioxidant).

•**butylparaben,** N.F. 18.
Use: Pharmaceutic aid (antifungal).

butylphenamide.

butylphenylsalicylamide.
See: Butylphenamide.

butyrophenone. Class of antipsychotic agents. *Rx.*
See: Haloperidol.

butyrylcholinesterase. *Rx.*
Use: Treat cocaine overdose; post-surgical apnea. [Orphan drug]

B vitamins, parenteral.
See: B-Ject-100 (Hyrex) Becomject-100 (Mayrand)

B vitamins with vitamin C, parenteral.
See: Key-Plex Injection (Hyrex) Neurodep Injection (Medical Products) Vicam Injection (Keene)

B-Vite Injection. (Bluco) Vitamins B_1 50 mg, B_2 5 mg, B_6 5 mg, niacinamide 125 mg, B_{12} 1000 mcg, dexpanthenol 6 mg, C 50 mg/10 ml. Mono vial w/benzyl alcohol 1% in water for injection. *Rx.*
Use: Vitamin supplement.

BVU.
See: Bromisovalum.

Byclomine. (Major) Dicyclomine. **Cap.:** 10 mg. Bot. 100s, 250s, 1000s. **Tab.:** 20 mg. Bot. 100s, 250s, 1000s. *Rx.*
Use: Antispasmodic.

Byclomine w/Phenobarbital. (Major) **Cap.:** Dicyclomine HCl 10 mg, phenobarbital 15 mg. Bot. 250s, 1000s. **Tab.:** Dicyclomine HCl 20 mg, phenobarbital 15 mg. Bot. 100s, 250s, 1000s. *Rx.*
Use: Antispasmodic, sedative, hypnotic.

Bydramine. (Major) Diphenhydramine HCl 12.5 mg/5 ml, alcohol 5%. Syr. Bot. 118 ml, pt, gal. *otc.*
Use: Antihistamine.

Bydramine Cough. (Major) Diphenhydramine HCl 12.5 mg/5 ml, alcohol 5%. Syr. Bot. 118 ml, pt, gal. *otc.*
Use: Antitussive.

C

c1-esterase-inhibitor, human, pasteurized. *Rx.*
Use: Prevention/treatment of angioedema. [Orphan Drug]

c1 inhibitor. *Rx.*
Use: Treatment of angioedema. [Orphan drug]

c vitamin.
See: Ascorbic Acid, Prep.

●**cabergoline.** (cab-ERR-go-leen) USAN.
Use: Antiparkinsonian; hyperolactinemic disorders treatment.
See: Dostinex, Tab. (Pharmacia & Upjohn).

●**cabufocan a.** USAN.
Use: Contact lens material (hydrophobic).

●**cabufocon b.** (cab-YOU-FOE-kahn B) USAN.
Use: Contact lens material (hydrophobic).

Cachexon. (Telluride Pharm)
See: L-Glutathione.

cacodylic acid salts.
Ferric Salt.
Iron Salt.
Sodium Salt.

●**cactinomycin.** (KACK-tih-no-MY-sin) USAN.
Use: Antineoplastic.
See: Sanamycin (FBA Pharm).

cade oil.
See: Juniper Tar.

●**cadexomer iodine.** (kad-EX-oh-mer) USAN.
Use: Antiseptic, antiulcerative.

C & E Softgels. (NBTY) E 400 mg, C 500 mg/Cap. Bot. 50s. *otc.*
Use: Vitamin supplement.

Cafatine Supps. (Major) Ergotamine tartrate 2 mg, caffeine 100 mg. Supp. Box 12s. *Rx.*
Use: Agent for migraine.

Cafatine-PB. (Major) Ergotamine tartrate 2 mg, caffeine 100 mg, belladonna alkaloids 0.25 mg, pentobarbital 60 mg/Supp. Box foil 10s. *Rx.*
Use: Agent for migraine.

Cafenol. (Sanofi Winthrop) Aspirin, caffeine. *otc.*
Use: Analgesic combination.

Cafergot P-B Suppositories. (Sandoz) Ergotamine tartrate 2 mg, caffeine 100 mg, bellafoline 0.25 mg, pentobarbital 60 mg/Supp. Box 12s. *Rx.*
Use: Agent for migraine.

Cafergot P-B Tablets. (Sandoz) Ergotamine tartrate 1 mg, caffeine 100 mg, bellafoline 0.125 mg, pentobarbital sodium 30 mg/Tab. SigPak dispensing pkg. of 90s, 250s. *c-iv.*
Use: Agent for migraine.

Cafergot Suppositories. (Sandoz) Ergotamine tartrate 2 mg, caffeine 100 mg in cocoa butter base. Supp. Box 12s. *Rx.*
Use: Agent for migraine.

Cafergot Tablets. (Sandoz) Ergotamine tartrate 1 mg, caffeine 100 mg/S.C. Tab. Bot. 250s. SigPak dispensing pkg. of 90s. *Rx.*
Use: Agent for migraine.

Cafetrate Supps. (Schein) Ergotamine tartrate 2 mg, caffeine 100 mg/Supp. Box 12s. *Rx.*
Use: Agent for migraine.

Caffedrine. (Thompson) Caffeine 200 mg/T.R. Cap. Bot. 20s. *otc.*
Use: CNS stimulant.

●**caffeine,** U.S.P. 23.
Use: CNS stimulant; apnea of prematurity. [Orphan drug]
See: Enerjets, Loz. (Chilton).
Femicin, Tab. (SK-Beecham).
Nodoz, Tab. (Bristol-Myers).
Stim 250, Cap. (Scrip).
Tirend (SK-Beecham).
Vivarin, Tab. (J.B. Williams).

caffeine citrated.
Use: CNS stimulant.

caffeine sodio-benzoate.
See: Caffeine sodium benzoate.

caffeine sodium benzoate injection.
Approximately equal parts of caffeine and sodium benzoate. (Various Mfr.) Amp. (3 ¾ gr and 7.5 gr) 2 ml. Box 12s, 100s. Hypo Tab. (1 gr) Tube 20s, 100s and Pow.
Use: Orally, I.M. central nervous system stimulant.

caffeine sodium salicylate. (Various Mfr.) Bot. 1 oz; Pkg. 0.25 lb, 1 lb. *otc.*
Use: See caffeine.

caffeine-theophylline compound.
W/Nux Vomica Ext.
See: Xanthinux, Tab. (Cole).

Cagol. (Harvey) Guaiacol 0.1 g, eucalyptol 0.08 g, iodoform 0.2 g, camphor 0.05 g/2 ml in olive oil. Vial 30 ml. *Rx.*
Use: Expectorant.

Caladryl. (Parke-Davis) Calamine 8%, pramoxine HCl 1%, alcohol 2.2%, camphor, diazolidinyl urea, parabens. Lot. Bot. 180 ml. *otc.*
Use: Antipruritic, topical.

Caladryl Clear. (Parke-Davis) Pramoxine HCl 1%, zinc acetate 0.1%, alcohol 2%, camphor, diazolidinyl urea, parabens. Lot. Bot. 180 ml. *otc.*
Use: Antipruritic, topical.

Caladryl for Kids. (Parke-Davis) Calamine 8%, pramoxine HCl 1%, camphor, cetyl alcohol, diazolidinyl urea, parabens. Cream. Tube 45 g. *otc.*
Use: Antipruritic, topical.

Calaformula. (Eric, Kirk & Gary) Ferrous gluconate 130 mg, calcium lactate 130 mg, vitamins A 1000 IU, D 400 IU, B_1 2 mg, B_2 2 mg, niacinamide 5 mg, ascorbic acid 20 mg, folic acid 0.13 mg, magnesium 0.25 mg, copper 0.25 mg, zinc 0.25 mg, manganese 0.25 mg, potassium 0.075 mg/Cap. Bot. 50s, 100s, 500s, 1000s, 5000s. *otc.*
Use: Vitamin/mineral supplement.

Calaformula F. (Eric, Kirk & Gary) Calaformula plus fluorine 0.333 mg/Tab. Bot. 100s. *Rx.*
Use: Vitamin/mineral supplement, dental caries preventative.

Cala-Gen. (Goldline) Diphenhydramine HCl 1%, camphor, alcohol 2%. Lot. Bot. 178 ml. *otc.*
Use: Antipruritic, topical.

Calahist Lotion. (Walgreen) Diphenhydramine HCl 1%, calamine 8.1%, camphor 0.1%. Lot. Bot. 6 oz. *otc.*
Use: Antipruritic, topical.

Calamatum. (Blair) **Lot.:** Calamine, zinc oxide, phenol, camphor, benzocaine 3%, nongreasy base. Bot. 1125 ml. **Oint:** Calamine, zinc oxide, phenol, camphor, benzocaine. Tube 45 g. *otc.*
Use: Minor skin irritations.

Calamatum Aerosol Spray. (Blair) Benzocaine 3%, zinc oxide, calamine, phenol, camphor. Spray can 3 oz. *otc.*
Use: Local anesthetic, topical.

•**calamine,** U.S.P. 23.
Use: Protectant (topical).

calamine. (Various Mfr.) Calamine 8%, zinc oxide 8%, glycerin 2%, bentonite maga, calcium hydroxide soln. Lot. Bot. 120 ml, 240 ml, pt, gal.
Use: Astringent, mild antiseptic

Calamine, Phenolated. (Humco) Calamine 8%, zinc oxide 8%, glycerin 2%, bentonite maga and phenol 1% in calcium hydroxide solution. Lot. Bot. 120, 240 ml. *otc.*
Use: Astringent, mild antiseptic.

Calamox. (Roberts) Prepared calamine 0.17 g. Oint. Tube 60 g. *otc.*
Use: Astringent, mild antiseptic.

Calamycin. (Pfeiffer) Pyrilamine maleate, zinc oxide 10%, calamine 10%, benzocaine, chloroxylenol, zirconium oxide, isopropyl alcohol 10%. Lot. Bot. 120 ml. *otc.*
Use: Antipruritic, topical.

Calan. (Searle) Verapamil HCl 40 mg, 80 mg or 120 mg/Tab. Bot. 100s, 500s, 1000s, UD 100s. *Rx.*
Use: Calcium channel blocking agent.

Calan SR. (Searle) Verapamil HCl **120 mg, 180 mg/SR Tab.** Bot. 100s, UD 100s. **240 mg/SR Tab:** Bot. 100s, 500s, UD 100s. *Rx.*
Use: Calcium channel blocker.

Cal-Bid. (Geriatric) Elemental calcium 250 mg, ascorbic acid 100 mg, vitamin D 125 IU/Tab. Bot. 100s. *otc.*
Use: Vitamin/mineral supplement.

Cal Carb-HD. (Konsyl Pharm) Calcium 6.5 g per packet, simethicone. Pow. 7 g packets, Bot. 210 g. *otc.*
Use: Antacid.

Calcet. (Mission) Elemental calcium 153 mg, vitamin D 100 units/Tab. Bot. 100s. *otc.*
Use: Vitamin/mineral supplement.

Calcet Plus. (Mission) Elemental calcium 152.8 mg, elemental iron 18 mg, vitamins A 5000 IU, D 400 IU, E 30 mg, B_1 2.25 mg, B_2 2.55 mg, B_3 30 mg, B_5 15 mg, B_6 3 mg, B_{12} 9 mcg, C 500 mg, folic acid 0.8 mg, zinc 15 mg, sugar/Tab. Bot 60s. *otc.*
Use: Vitamin/mineral supplement.

Calcibind. (Mission) Inorganic phosphate content 34%, sodium content 11%. Packets: Cellulose sodium phosphate 25 g. Single dose 90 packets, 300 g bulk pack. *Rx.*
Use: Urinary tract product.

CalciCaps. (Nion) Calcium (dibasic calcium phosphate, calcium gluconate, calcium carbonate) 125 mg, vitamin D 67 IU, phosphorus 60 mg/Tab. Bot. 100s, 500s. *otc.*
Use: Vitamin/mineral supplement.

CalciCaps with Iron. (Nion) Calcium 125 mg, phosphorus 60 mg, vitamin D 67 IU, ferrous gluconate 7 mg, tartrazine/Tab. Bot. 100s, 500s. *otc.*
Use: Vitamin/mineral supplement.

CalciCaps M-Z. (Nion) Ca 400 mg, Mg 133 mg, Zn 5 mg, vitamin A 1667 mg, D 133 IU, Se. Tab. Bot. 90s. *otc.*
Use: Vitamin/mineral supplement.

CalciCaps, Super. (Nion) Calcium 400 mg, phosphorus 41.7 mg, vitamin D 100 IU/Tab. Bot. 90s. *otc.*

Use: Vitamin/mineral supplement.

Calci-Chew. (R & D) Calcium carbonate 1.25 g (500 mg calcium)/Chew. Tab. Bot. 100s. *otc.*
Use: Calcium supplement.

Calciday-667. (NBTY) Calcium carbonate 667 mg (266.8 mg calcium)/Tab. Bot. 60s. *otc.*
Use: Calcium supplement.

Calcidrine syrup. (Abbott) Codeine 8.4 mg, calcium iodide anhydrous 152 mg, alcohol 6%/5 ml. Bot. 120 ml, 480 ml. *c-v.*
Use: Antitussive, expectorant.

•**calcifediol,** (KAL-sih-feh-DIE-ahl) U.S.P. 23.
Use: Calcium regulator.
See: Calderol (Organon).

calciferol. Ergosterol. (D_2) **Liq:** 8000 IU/ml. Bot. 60 ml. **Tab:** 50,000 IU. Bot. 100s. **Inj:** 500,000 IU/ml. Amp. 1 ml.
Use: Refractory rickets, familial hypophosphatemia, hypoparathyroidism.

Calcijex. (Abbott) Calcitriol injection 1 mcg or 2 mcg/ml. Amp. 1 ml. *Rx.*
Use: Hypocalcemia and hypoparathyroidism.

Calcimar Injection, Synthetic. (Rhone-Poulenc Rorer) Calcitonin solution (Salmon origin), phenol/200 IU/ml. Vial 2 ml. *Rx.*
Use: Treatment of Paget's disease.

Calci-Mix. (R & D) Calcium carbonate 1250 mg. Cap. Bot. 100s. *otc.*
Use: Calcium supplement.

•**calcipotriene.** (kal-sih-POE-try-een) USAN.
Use: Antipsoriatic.
See: Dovonex, Oint. (Westwood Squibb).

•**calcitonin.** (kal-sih-TOE-nin) USAN.
Use: Treatment of Paget's disease, calcium regulator.
See: Calcimar (Rhone-Poulenc Rorer).
Cibacalcin (Novartis).
Miacalcin (Sandoz).

calcitonin human. (kal-sih-TOE-nin human) Hormone from thyroid gland.
Use: Plasma hypocalcemic hormone; symptomatic Paget's disease of bone [Orphan drug]
See: Cibacalcin (Novartis).

calcitonin salmon. (kal-sih-TOE-nin salmon)
Use: Antihypercalcemic.
See: Calcimar (Rhone-Poulenc Rorer).
Miacalcin (Sandoz).
Osteocalcin, Inj. (Arcola).

calcitonin salmon nasal spray. *Rx.*

Use: Symptomatic Paget's disease of bone. [Orphan drug]
See: Miacalcin (Sandoz).

•**calcitriol.** (KAL-sih-TRY-ole) USAN.
Use: Management of hypocalcemia in chronic renal dialysis patients; calcium regulator.
See: Calcijex, Inj. (Abbott).
Rocaltrol, Cap. (Roche).

Calcium-600. (Schein) Calcium 600 mg. Tab. Bot. 60s. *otc.*
Use: Calcium supplement.

Calcium 600/Vitamin D. (Schein) Ca 600 mg, D 125 IU. Tab. Bot. 60s. *otc.*
Use: Vitamin/mineral supplement.

•**calcium acetate,** (KAL-see-uhm) U.S.P. 23.
Use: Pharmaceutic aid (buffering agent). Hyperphosphatemia [Orphan drug].

calcium acetate mineral/electrolytes.
See: Phos-Ex 62.5 Mini-Tabs (Vitaline).
Phos-Ex 167 (Braintree).
Phos-Ex 250 (Vitaline).
Phos-Ex 125 (Vitaline).
PhosLo (Braintree).

calcium acetylsalicylate. Kalmopyrin, kalsetal, soluble aspirin, tylcalsin.
Use: Salicylate analgesic.

calcium aluminum carbonate. W/Dl-Amino acetate complex.
See: Ancid Tab., Susp. (Sheryl).

calcium aminosalicylate. Aminosalicylate calcium, N.F. 18.

calcium amphomycin.
See: Amphomycin.

calcium and magnesium carbonates tablets.
Use: Antacid.

•**calcium ascorbate,** U.S.P. 23.
Use: Nutritional supplement.

calcium ascorbate. (Freeda) **Tab.:** Calcium ascorbate 610 mg (equivalent to 500 mg ascorbic acid). Bot. 100s, 250s, 500s. **Pow.:** Calcium ascorbate 1 g (equivalent to 826 mg ascorbic acid) per ¼ tsp. Bot. 120 g, 448 g. *otc.*
Use: Calcium/nutritional supplement.

calcium 4-benzamidosalicylate. Calcium Aminacyl B-PAS. Benzoylpas Calcium.
See: Benzapas, Pow., Tab. (Sandoz).

calcium benzoyl-p-aminosalicylate.
See: Benzoylpas calcium.

calcium benzoylpas.
See: Benzoylpas calcium.

calcium bis-dioctyl sulfosuccinate.
See: Dioctyl calcium.

calcium carbimide. Calcium cyanamide. Sulfosuccinate.
See: Alka-Mints (Bayer).
Amitone, Tab. (Menley & James).
Antacid Tablets (Goldline).
Chooz (Schering-Plough).
Dicarbosil, Tab. (SK-Beecham).
Equilet (Mission).
Extra Strength Antacid (Various Mfr.).
Maalox Antacid (RPR).
Mallamint, Tab. (Roberts).
Mylanta (J & J-Merck).
Tums (SK-Beecham).
•**calcium carbonate,** U.S.P. 23.
Use: Antacid.
calcium carbonate. (Various Mfr.) Precipitated chalk; carbonic acid, calcium salt (1:1).
Use: Antacid.
calcium carbonate. *Rx.*
Use: Hyperphosphatemia. [Orphan drug]
calcium carbonate. (Various Mfr.) 500 mg/Tab. 100s, 120s, UD 100s; 600 mg/Tab. 60s, 72s, 150s, UD 100s; 650 mg/Tab. 100s, 1000s. *otc.*
Use: Antacid/calcium supplement.
calcium carbonate. (Roxane) **Tab.:** 1250 mg. Bot. 100s, UD 100s. **Susp.:** 1250 mg/5 ml. Bot. 500 ml, UD 5 ml. *otc.*
Use: Antacid/calcium supplement.
calcium carbonate, aromatic. (Lilly) Calcium carbonate 10 gr/Tab. Bot. 100s, 1000s. *otc.*
Use: Antacid.
calcium carbonate w/combinations.
See: Accelerase, Cap. (Organon).
Alkets, Tab. (Pharmacia & Upjohn).
Camalox, Tab., Susp. (Rhone-Poulenc Rorer Consumer).
Ca-Plus, Tab. (Miller).
Co-Gel, Tab. (Arco).
Lactocal, Tab. (Laser).
Natabec, Prep. (Parke-Davis).
Titralac, Liq., Tab. (3M).
calcium carbonate 600/vitamin d. (Major) Ca 600 mg, D 125 IU. Tab. Bot. 60s. *otc.*
Use: Vitamin/mineral supplement.
calcium caseinate.
See: Casec, Pow. (Bristol-Myers).
calcium channel blockers.
Use: Angina pectoris, vasospastic and unstable angina.
See: Adalat, Cap. (Bayer).
Calan, Inj., Tab. (Searle).
Calan SR, SR Cap. (Searle).
Cardene, Cap. (Syntex).
Cardene SR, SR Cap. (Syntex).
Cardene IV, Inj. (DuPont Merck).

Cardizem, Tab. (Hoechst Marion Roussel).
Diltiazem HCl, ER Cap. (Various Mfr.).
DynaCirc, Cap. (Sandoz).
Isoptin, Inj., Tab. (Knoll).
Isoptin SR, SR Cap. (Knoll).
Nimotop, Cap. (Bayer).
Plendil, SR Tab. (Merck & Co.).
Procardia, Cap. (Pfizer).
Vascor, Tab. (McNeil).
Verapamil HCl, Inj., Tab. (Various Mfr.).
Calcium Chel 330. (Novartis).
Use: Heavy metal antagonist.
See: Calcium Trisodium Pentetate.
•**calcium chloride,** U.S.P. 23.
Use: Electrolyte, calcium replenisher.
•**calcium chloride Ca 45.** USAN.
Use: Radioactive agent.
•**calcium chloride Ca 47.** USAN.
Use: Radioactive agent.
calcium chloride injection. (Pharmacia & Upjohn) 1 g Amp. 10 ml, 25s. (Torigian) 1 g Amp. 10 ml 12s, 25s, 100s. (Trent) 10% Amp. 10 ml (Bayer) 13.6 mEq./10 ml Vial.
Use: IV, hypocalcemic tetany.
•**calcium citrate,** U.S.P. 23.
Use: Calcium supplement.
calcium cyclamate. Calcium cyclohexanesulfamate.
calcium cyclobarbital.
Use: Central depressant.
calcium cyclohexanesulfamate.
See: Calcium Cyclamate.
Calcium 600 + D. (NBTY) Calcium 600 mg, vitamin D 125 IU. Film coat. Tab. Bot. 60s. *otc.*
Use: Vitamin/mineral supplement.
calcium dl-pantothenate. Calcium Pantothenate, Racemic, U.S.P. 23.
calcium dioctyl sulfosuccinate. Docusate Calcium, U.S.P. 23.
See: Surfak (Hoechst Marion Roussel).
calcium disodium edathamil.
See: Edetate Calcium Disodium, U.S.P. 23.
calcium disodium edetate. (KAL-see-uhm die-SO-dee-uhm ed-deh-TATE) Edetate Calcium Disodium, U.S.P. 23.
Use: Antidote for acute and chronic lead poisoning, lead encephalopathy.
See: Calcium Disodium Versenate (3M).
calcium disodium versenate. (3M) Calcium Disodium Edetate U.S.P. Inj.: 200 mg/ml. Amp 5 ml. *Rx.*
Use: IV or IM for lead poisoning and lead encephalopathy.

calcium edetate sodium.
See: calcium disodium edetate.

calcium EDTA.
See: Calcium Disodium Versenate, Amp. (3M).

•**calcium glubionate,** (KAL-see uhm glue-BYE-oh-nate) U.S.P. 23.
Use: Calcium replenisher.
See: Neo-Calglucon (Sandoz).

•**calcium gluceptate,** U.S.P. 23.
Use: Calcium replenisher.
See: Calcium Gluceptate (Abbott).
Calcium Gluceptate (I.M.S.).
Calcium Gluceptate (Lilly).

•**calcium gluceptate.** (Various Mfr.) 1.1 g (5 ml) contains 90 mg (4.5 mEq) calcium. Inj.: 1.1 g/5 ml. Amp. 5 ml. Vial 50 ml.
Use: Calcium electrolyte replacement.

calcium glucoheptonate. (Various Mfr.)
Cal. D-glucoheptonate O. otc.
Use: Nutritional supplement.

•**calcium gluconate,** U.S.P. 23.
Use: Calcium replenisher.

calcium gluconate gel. Rx.
Use: Topical treatment of hydrogen fluoride burns. [Orphan drug]

calcium glycerophosphate. Neurosin. (Various Mfr.).

•**calcium hydroxide,** U.S.P. 23.
Use: Astringent; pharmaceutic necessity for calamine lotion.

calcium hydroxide powder. (Lilly) Powder 4 oz/Bot.
Use: Preparation of lime water solution.

calcium hypophosphite. (N.Y. Quinine & Chem. Works).

calcium iodide.
W/Codeine phosphate.
See: Calcidrine Syr. (Abbott).
W/Chloral hydrate, ephedrine HCl.
See: Iophed, Syr. (Marsh Labs).

calcium iodized.
See: Cal-Lime-1, Tab. (Scrip).
W/Calcium creosotate.
See: Niocrese, Tab. (Noyes).
W/Ipecac, hyoscyamus extract, licorice extract.
See: Kaldifane, Tab. (Noyes).

calcium iodobehenate. Calioben. (Various Mfr.).

calcium ipodate. Ipodate Calcium, U.S.P. 23.
See: Oragrafin Calcium, Granules (Squibb).

calcium kinate gluconate. Kinate is hexahydrotetrahydroxybenzoate. Calcium Quinate.

•**calcium lactate,** U.S.P. 23.
Use: Calcium replenisher.
W/Calcium glycerophosphate.
See: Calphosan, Amp., Vial (Carlton).
W/Calcium glycerophosphate, phenol, sodium Cl solution.
See: Calpholac, Vial (Century).
Calphosan, Inj. (Zeneca).
W/Niacinamide, folic acid, ferrous gluconate, vitamins.
See: Pergrava No. 2, Cap. (Arcum).
W/Phenobarbital, extract hyoscyamus, terpin hydrate, guaifenesin.
W/Theobromine sodium salicylate, phenobarbital.
See: Theolaphen, Tab. (Zeneca).
W/Zinc sulfate.
See: Zinc-220, Cap. (Alto).

•**calcium lactobionate,** U.S.P. 23.
Use: Calcium supplement.

calcium lactophosphate. Lactic acid hydrogen phosphate calcium salt.

calcium leucovorin. Leucovorin Calcium, U.S.P. 23. Inj. Tab. Powder for Oral. Powder for Inj. Rx.
Use: For overdosage of folic acid antagonists; megalobastic anemias.
See: Leucovorin Calcium (Lederle).
Wellcovorin (Glaxo Wellcome).

•**calcium levulinate,** U.S.P. 23.
Use: Calcium replenisher.

Calcium Magnesium Chelated. (NBTY) Ca 500 mg, Mg 250 mg/Tab. Bot. 50s, 100s. otc.
Use: Mineral supplement.

Calcium Magnesium Zinc. (NBTY) Ca 333 mg, Mg 133 mg, Zn 8.3 mg/Tab. Bot. 100. otc.
Use: Mineral supplement.

calcium novobiocin. Calcium salt of an antibacterial substance produced by Streptomyces niveus.
Use: Anti-infective.

calcium orotate.
See: Calora, Tab. (Miller).

calcium oxytetracycline. Oxytetracycline Calcium, N.F. XIV.

•**calcium pantothenate,** U.S.P. 23.
Use: Pantothenic acid (B_5) deficiency, coenzyme A precursor, vitamin (enzyme co-factor).
See: Calcium Pantothenate (Freeda).
Calcium Pantothenate (Fibertone).
W/Ascorbic acid, niacinamide, vitamins B_1, B_2, B_6, B_{12}, A, D, E.
See: Tota-Vi-Caps Gelatin Capsule, Cap. (Zeneca).
W/Calcium carbonate.
See: Ilomel, Pow. (Warren-Teed).
W/Calcium carbonate, ferrous fumarate, niacinamide.

See: Prenatag, Tab. (Solvay).
W/Danthron.
See: Modane, Tab., Liq. (Warren-Teed).
Parlax, Tab. (Parmed).
W/Docusate sodium.
See: Pantyl, Tab. (McGregor).
W/Docusate sodium, acetphenolisatin.
See: Android-Plus, Tab. (Zeneca).
Peri-Pantyl, Tab. (McGregor).
W/Methoscopolamine nitrate, mephobarbital.
See: Ilocalm, Tabs. (Warren-Teed).
W/Niacinamide and vitamins.
See: Allbee C-800, Prods. (Robins).
Allbee T, Cap. (Robins).
Allbee with C, Cap. (Robins).
Ferrovite, Tab. (Laser).
Fumatinic, Tab. (Laser).
Maintenance Vitamin Formula, Tab. (Burgin-Arden).
Mulvidren, Tab. (Stuart).
OB-Tabs, Tab. (Laser).
Probec, Tab. (Stuart).
Probec-T, Tab. (Stuart).
Stuart Hematinic, Tab. (Stuart).
Stuart Therapeutic Multivitamin, Tab. (Stuart).
W/Niacinamide, vitamins B_1, B_2, B_6.
See: Noviplex Capsules, Cap. (Zeneca).
W/Vitamins B_1, B_2, B_6, B_{12}, niacinamide, choline Cl, inositol, dl-methionine, testosterone, estrone, procaine.
See: Gerihorm, Inj. (Burgin-Arden).
W/Vitamin complex, ferrous fumarate, folic acid, calcium lactate, niacinamide.
See: Vitanate, Tab. (Century).
W/Vitamins A, D, B_1, B_2, C, niacinamide, calcium phosphorus, iron, B_6, B_{12}, E, magnesium, manganese, potassium, zinc, choline bitartrate, inositol.
See: Geriatric Vitamin Formula, Tab. (Burgin-Arden).
W/Vitamins A, E, C, zinc sulfate, magnesium sulfate, niacinamide, B_1, B_2, manganese Cl, B_6, folic acid, B_{12}.
See: Vicon Forte, Cap. (Glaxo).
W/Vitamin C, niacin, zinc sulfate, vitamins E, B_1, B_2, B_6, B_{12}.
See: Z-Bec, Tab. (Robins).
W/Vitamin complex, iron.
See: Vita-iron, Tab. (Century).
W/Vitamins, minerals, niacinamide.
See: Arcum-VM, Cap. (Arcum).
Capre, Tab. (Hoechst Marion Roussel).
Orovimin, Tab. (Solvay).
Os-Cal Forte, Tab. (Hoechst Marion Roussel).
Os-Vim, Tab. (Hoechst Marion Roussel).

Stuartinic, Tab. (Stuart).
Theramin, Tab. (Arcum).
Theron, Tab. (Stuart).
Uplex, Cap. (Arcum).
W/Vitamins, minerals, methyl testosterone, ethinyl estradiol, niacinamide.
See: Geritag, Cap. (Solvay).
W/Vitamin C, niacinamide, zinc sulfate, magnesium sulfate, vitamins B_1, B_2, B_6.
See: Vicon-C, Cap. (Glaxo).
W/Zinc sulfate, niacinamide, magnesium sulfate, manganese sulfate, vitamin complex.
See: Vicon Plus, Cap. (Glaxo).
●**calcium pantothenate, racemic,** U.S.P. 23. β-Alanine, N-(2,4-dihydroxy-3,3-dimethyl-1-oxo-butyl-, calcium salt (2:1), (±-Calcium DL-pantothenate (1:2).
Use: Vitamin B (enzyme cofactor).
See: Pantholin (Lilly).
●**calcium phosphate, dibasic,** U.S.P. 23.
Use: Calcium replenisher, pharmaceutic aid (tablet base).
See: Dicalcium Phosphate.
Diostate D, Tab. (Pharmacia & Upjohn).
calcium phosphate, monocalcium.
See: Dicalcium Phosphate.
●**calcium phosphate, tribasic,** N.F. 18.
Use: Calcium replenisher.
See: Posture (Wyeth-Ayerst).
calcium-phosphorus-free.
See: Fosfree, Tab. (Mission).
●**calcium polycarbophil,** (KAL-see-uhm PAHL-ee-CAR-boe-fill) U.S.P. 23.
Use: Laxative.
See: Fibercon, Tab. (Lederle).
calcium polysulfide.
Use: Wet dressing, soak.
See: Vlemasque, Cream. (Dormik).
Vleminckx, Soln. (Ulmer).
calcium propionate.
See: Propionate-caprylate mixtures.
calcium quinate.
See: Calcium Kinate Gluconate.
●**calcium saccharate,** U.S.P. 23.
Use: Sweetening agent, pharmaceutic aid (stabilizer).
calcium saccharin. Saccharin Calcium, U.S.P. 23.
Use: Sweetening agent.
calcium salicylate, theobromine.
See: Theocalcin, Tab., Pow. (Knoll).
calcium salts of sennosides a & b.
Use: Laxative.
See: Gentle Nature, Tab. (Sandoz).
Nytilax, Tab. (Mentholatum).
●**calcium silicate,** N.F. 18. A compound

of calcium oxide and silicon dioxide.
Use: Pharmaceutic aid (tablet excipient).

•**calcium stearate,** N.F. 18.
Use: Pharmaceutic aid (tablet and capsule lubricant).

calcium succinate.
W/Aspirin.
See: Ber-Ex, Tab. (Dolcin).
Dolcin, Tab. (Dolcin).

•**calcium sulfate,** N.F. 18.
Use: Pharmaceutic aid (tablet and capsule diluent).

calcium thiosulfate.
Use: Wet dressing, soak.
See: Vlemasque Cream (Dermik).
Vleminckx, Soln. (Ulmer).

calcium trisodium pentetate. (KAL-see-uhm try-SO-dee-uhm PEN-teh-tate)
Use: Heavy metal antagonist.
See: Calcium Chel 330 (Novartis).

•**calcium undecylenate,** U.S.P. 23.
Use: Antifungal.

calcium undecylenate. 10% calcium undecylenate Pow.
Use: Antifungal, topical.
See: Caldesene, Pow. (Novartis).
Cruex Squeeze Pow. (Novartis).

calcium with vitamin D tablets.
Use: Vitamin/mineral supplement.

Calcium with Vitamin D. (Schein) Calcium 600 mg, vitamin D 125 IU Bot. 60s. *otc.*
Use: Vitamin/mineral supplement.

Caldecort Spray. (Novartis) Hydrocortisone 0.5%. Aerosol can 1.5 oz. *otc.*
Use: Corticosteroid, topical.

Calderol. (Organon) Calcifediol 20 mcg or 50 mcg/Tab. Bot. 60s. *Rx.*
Use: Metabolic bone disease or hypocalcemia in renal dialysis patients.

Caldesene. (Novartis) **Oint.:** Cod liver oil (vitamins A, D) zinc oxide 15%, lanolin, petroleum 54%, talc. Tube 37.5 g. **Pow.:** Calcium undecylenate 10%. Bot. 60 g, 120 g. *otc.*
Use: Antifungal, topical.

•**caldiamide sodium.** (KAL-DIE-ah-MIDE) USAN.
Use: Pharmaceutic aid.

Cal-D-Mint. (Enzyme Process) Calcium 800 mg, magnesium 150 mg, iron 18 mg, iodine 0.1 mg, copper 2 mg, vitamin D 200 IU/2 Tab. Bot. 100s, 250s. *otc.*
Use: Vitamin/mineral supplement.

Cal-D-Phos. (Archer-Taylor) Dicalcium phosphate 4.5 gr, calcium gluconate 3 gr, vitamin D/Tab. Bot. 1000s. *otc.*

Use: Vitamin/mineral supplement.

Calel-D Tablets. (Rhone-Poulenc Rorer) Calcium 500 mg, vitamin D 200 IU/Tab. Bot. 60s, 75s. *otc.*
Use: Vitamin/mineral supplement.

Calglycine Antacid. (Rugby) Calcium carbonate 420 mg, glycine 150 mg. Sugar free. Chew Tab. Bot. 250s, 1000s. *otc.*
Use: Antacid.

Cal-Guard. (Rugby) Calcium carbonate 50 mg. Softgel Cap. Bot. 60s. *otc.*
Use: Calcium supplement.

Calicylic Creme. (Gordon) Salicylic acid 10%, mineral oil, cetyl alcohol, propylene glycol, white wax, sodium lauryl sulfate, oleic acid, methyl and propyl parabens, triethanolamine. 60 g. *otc.*
Use: Keratolytic.

Cal-Im. (Standex) Calcium glycerophosphate 1%, calcium levulinate 1.5%. Vial 30 ml. *Rx.*
Use: Calcium supplement.

Calinate-FA. (Solvay) Calcium 250 mg, vitamins A 4000 IU, D 400 IU, B_1 3 mg, B_2 3 mg, B_6 5 mg, B_{12} 1 mcg, folic acid 1 mg, C 50 mg, B_3 (niacinamide) 20 mg, B_5 (d-panthenol 1 mg), iron 60 mg, iodine 0.02 mg, manganese 0.2 mg, magnesium 0.2 mg, zinc 0.1 mg, copper 0.15 mg/Tab. Bot. 100s. *Rx.*
Use: Vitamin/mineral supplement.

calioben.
See: Calcium Iodobehenate.

Calivite. (Apco) Calcium carbonate 885 mg, ferrous sulfate 199 mg, vitamins A 3600 IU, D 400 IU, C 75 mg, B_1 1.5 mg, B_2 1.95 mg, B_6 0.75 mg, nicotinic acid 15 mg, B_{12} activity 0.025 mcg, choline 1500 mcg, inositol 2500 mcg, pantothenic acid 75 mcg, folic acid 25 mcg, p-aminobenzoic acid 12 mcg, potassium 10 mg, magnesium 1 mg, zinc 0.075 mg, manganese 0.02 mg, copper 0.01 mg, cobalt 0.02 mcg/Tab. Bot. 100s. *otc.*
Use: Vitamin/mineral supplement.

Cal-Lime-1. (Scrip) Calcium iodized 1 gr/Tab. Bot. 1000s.

Calmol 4. (Mentholatum) **Supp.:** Cocoa butter 80%, zinc oxide 10%, parabens. Box 12s, 24s. *otc.*
Use: Anorectal preparation.

Calmosin. (Spanner) Calcium gluconate, strontium bromide. Amp. 10 ml. 100s.

Cal-Nor. (Vortech) Calcium glycerophosphate 100 mg, calcium levulinate 150 mg/10 ml. Inj. Vial 100 ml. *Rx.*
Use: Calcium supplement.

Calocarb Tablets. (Pal-Pak) Calcium carbonate 648 mg/Tab. w/cinnamon flavor. Bot. 1000s. *otc.*
Use: Antacid.

calomel. Mercurous Cl.
Use: Cathartic.

Calotabs. Reformulated. (Calotabs) Docusate sodium 100 mg, casanthranol 30 mg/Tab. Box 10s. *otc.*
Use: Laxative.

caloxidine (iodized calcium).
See: Calcium Iodized.

Calphosan. (Glenwood) Calcium glycerophosphate 50 mg, calcium lactate 50 mg/10 ml sodium Cl solution. Contains calcium 0.08 mEq/ml. Inj. Amp. 10 ml, Vial 60 ml. *Rx.*
Use: Calcium supplement.

Calphron. (Nephro-Tech) Calcium acetate 667 mg/Tab. Bot. 200s. *Rx.*
Use: Calcium supplement.

Cal-Plus. (Geriatric) Calcium carbonate 1500 mg/Tab. Bot. 100s. *otc.*
Use: Calcium supplement.

Calsan. (Burgin-Arden) Calcium glycerophosphate 10 mg, calcium levulinate 15 mg, chlorobutanol 0.5%/ml. Inj. Vial 100 ml. *Rx.*
Use: Calcium supplement.

Cal Sup Instant 1000. (3M Personal Care Products) Elemental calcium 1000 mg, vitamins D 400 IU, C 60 mg. Pow. Packet 12s. *otc.*
Use: Vitamin/mineral supplement.

Cal Sup 600 Plus. (3M Personal Care Products) Elemental calcium 600 mg, vitamins D 200 IU, C 30 mg/Tab. Bot. 60s. *otc.*
Use: Vitamin/mineral supplement.

•**calteridol calcium.** (KAL-TER-ih-dahl KAL-see-uhm) USAN.
Use: Pharmaceutic aid.

Caltrate 600. (Lederle) Calcium carbonate 1.5 g (calcium 600 mg). Bot. 60s, 120s. *otc.*
Use: Calcium supplement.

Caltrate 600 + D. (Lederle) D 200 IU, Ca 600 mg. Sugar free. Tab. Bot. 60s. *otc.*
Use: Vitamin/mineral supplement.

Caltrate 600 + Iron. (Lederle) Calcium carbonate 600 mg, iron 18 mg, vitamin D 125 IU/Tab. Bot. 60s. *otc.*
Use: Vitamin/mineral supplement.

Caltrate Jr. (Lederle) Calcium carbonate 750 mg (300 mg calcium)/Chew. Tab. Bot. 60s. *otc.*
Use: Calcium supplement.

Caltrate Plus. (Lederle) D 200 IU, Ca 600 mg, Zn 7.5 mg, Mg, Cu, Mn, B.

Sugar free. Tab. Bot. 60s. *otc.*
Use: Vitamin/mineral supplement.

Caltro. (Geneva Pharm.) Elemental calcium 250 mg, vitamin D 125 IU/Tab. Bot. 100s, 1000s. *otc.*
Use: Vitamin/mineral supplement.

•**calusterone.** USAN.
Use: Antineoplastic.

Cama Arthritis Pain Reliever. (Sandoz Consumer) Aspirin 500 mg, magnesium oxide 150 mg, aluminum hydroxide 125 mg, methylparaben. Tab. Bot. 100s. *otc.*
Use: Salicylate analgesic; antacid.

Cam-Ap-Es. (Camall) Hydrochlorothiazide 15 mg, reserpine 0.1 mg, hydralazine HCl 25 mg/Tab. Bot. 100s. *Rx.*
Use: Antihypertensive.

•**cambendazole.** (kam-BEND-ah-zole) USAN.
Use: Anthelmintic.

Camellia Lotion. (O'Leary) Moisturizer lotion for face, hands and body. For normal to oily skin. Bot. 4 oz. *otc.*
Use: Emollient.

Cameo Oil. (Medco Lab) Mineral oil, isopropyl myristate, lanolin oil, PEG-8-Dioleate. Plastic Bot. 8 oz, 16 oz, 32 oz. *otc.*
Use: Emollient.

•**camiglibose.** (kah-mih-GLIE-bose) USAN.
Use: Antidiabetic (Glucohydrolase inhibitor).

Camouflage Crayon. (O'Leary) Coverup for minor skin discolorations, under eye concealer, lipstick fixer. Available in 6 shades. Crayon 0.05 oz. *otc.*
Use: Skin coverup.

Campho-Phenique. (Sanofi Winthrop) Camphor 10.8%, phenol 4.7%. **Liq.:** 22.5 ml, 45 ml, 120 ml. **Gel:** 6.9 g, 15 g. *otc.*
Use: Analgesic; antiseptic, topical.

Campho-Phenique Antibiotic Plus Pain Reliever. (Sanofi Winthrop) Bacitracin 500 units, neomycin 3.5 mg, polymyxin B 5000 units/g, lidocaine 40 mg. Oint. Tube 5 g. *otc.*
Use: Anti-infective, topical.

•**camphor,** U.S.P. 23.
Use: Topical antipruritic; anti-infective; pharmaceutic necessity for camphorated phenol, paregoric and flexible collodion, antitussive, expectorant, local counterirritant, nasal decongestant.
See: Vicks Inhaler (Procter & Gamble). Vicks Regular and Wild Cherry Medi-

cated Cough Drops (Procter & Gamble).

Vicks Medi-Trating Throat Lozenges (Procter & Gamble).

Vicks Sinex, Nasal Spray (Procter & Gamble).

Vicks Vaporub, Oint. (Procter & Gamble).

Vicks Vaposteam, Liq. (Procter & Gamble).

Vicks Va-Tro-Nol, Nose Drops (Procter & Gamble).

camphor, monobromated.

•**camphorated, parachlorophenol.**
Use: Anti-infective (dental).

camphoric acid.

camphoric acid ester. Ester of p-Tolyl-methylcarbinal as Diethanolamine Salt.

Camptosar. (Pharmacia & Upjohn) Irinotecan HCl 20 mg/ml, sorbitol/Inj. Vial. 5 ml. *Rx.*
Use: Treatment of metastatic carcinoma of the colon or rectum.

•**candicidin,** (KAN-dih-SIDE-in) U.S.P. 23. An antifungal antibiotic derived from *Strep. griseus.*
Use: Antifungal.
See: Candeptin, Vaginal Tab., Oint. (Julius Schmid).
Vanobid, Oint., Vaginal Tab. (Merrell Dow).

candida albicans skin test antigen.
Use: In vivo diagnostic.
See: Candin, Inj. (Allermed, ALK Laboratories).

candida test. (SmithKline Diagnostics) Culture test for candida. 4s.
Use: Diagnostic aid.

Candin. (Allermed, ALK Laboratories) Candida albicans skin test antigen prepared from the culture filtrate and cells of two strains of *Candida albicans*. Vial 1 ml. *Rx.*
Use: Evaluation of cell-mediated immunity; in vivo diagnostic.

•**candoxatril.** (kan-DOXE-at-trill) USAN.
Use: Antihypertensive.

•**candoxatrilat.** (kan-DOXE-at-trill-at) USAN.
Use: Antihypertensive.

Candycon. (Allison) Chlorprophenpyridamine maleate 2 mg, phenylephrine HCl 5 mg/Tab. Bot. 50s. *otc.*
Use: Antihistamine, decongestant.

cannabinoids. Antiemetic/Antivertigo agent.
See: Dronabinol.

cannabis. Antiemetic, antivertigo.
See: Dronabinol.

Canopar. (Glaxo Wellcome).
See: Thenium closylate.

•**canrenoate potassium.** USAN.
Use: Aldosterone antagonist.

•**canrenone.** USAN.
Use: Aldosterone antagonist.

cantharidin.
Use: Keratolytic.

Cantil. (Hoechst Marion Roussel) Mepenzolate bromide 25 mg/Tab. Bot. 100s. *Rx.*
Use: Anticholinergic, antispasmodic.

Ca-Orotate. (Miller) Calcium (as calcium orotate) 50 mg/Tab. Bot. 100s. *otc.*
Use: Calcium supplement.

C-A-P. (Eastman Kodak) Cellulose acetate phthalate.

Capahist-DMH. (Freeport) Chlorpheniramine maleate 8 mg, phenylpropanolamine HCl 50 mg, atropine sulfate $\frac{1}{180}$ gr, dextromethorphan HBr 20 mg/T.R. Cap. *Rx.*
Use: Antihistamine, decongestant, anticholinergic, antispasmodic, antitussive.

Capastat Sulfate. (Dura) Capreomycin sulfate 1 g/5 ml. Vial 5 ml. *Rx.*
Use: Antituberculous agent.

•**capecitabine.** USAN.
Use: Antineoplastic.

Capital with Codeine. (Carnrick) **Susp.:** Acetaminophen 120 mg, codeine phosphate 12 mg/5 ml. Bot. 473 ml. *c-v.* **Tab.:** Codeine phosphate 30 mg, acetaminophen 325 mg/Tab. scored. Bot. 100s. *c-III.*
Use: Narcotic analgesic combination.

Capitrol Cream Shampoo. (Westwood Squibb) Tube 85 g. *Rx.*
Use: Antiseborrheic.

Ca-Plus-Protein. (Miller) Calcium (as contained in a calcium-protein complex made with specially isolated soy protein) 280 mg/Tab. Bot. 100s. *otc.*
Use: Calcium supplement.

Capnitro. (Freeport) Nitroglycerin 6.5 mg/TR Cap. Bot. 100s. *Rx.*
Use: Antianginal agent.

•**capobenate sodium.** (CAP-oh-BEN-ate) USAN.
Use: Cardiac depressant (antiarrhythmic).

•**capobenic acid.** (CAP-oh-BEN-ik) USAN.
Use: Cardiac depressant (antiarrhythmic).

Capoten. (Bristol-Myers Squibb) Captopril 12.5 mg, 25 mg, 50 mg or 100 mg, lactose. Tab. Bot 100s, 1000s (except

100 mg), UD 100s. *Rx.*
Use: Antihypertensive.

Capozide. (Bristol-Myers Squibb) Captopril/hydrochlorothiazide 25/15 mg, 25/25 mg, 50/15 mg or 50/25 mg/Tab. Bot. 100s. *Rx.*
Use: Antihypertensive.

•**capreomycin sulfate, sterile,** (CAP-ree-oh-MY-sin) U.S.P. 23. An antibiotic derived from *Streptomyces capreolus.* Caprocin.
Use: Antibiotic (tuberculostatic).
See: Capastat Sulfate, Amp. (Lilly).

caprochlorone.

•**capromab pendetide.** (CAP-row-mab PEN-deh-TIDE) USAN.
Use: Monoclonal antibody.
See: Prostascint (Cytogen).

caprylate-propionate mixtures.
See: Sopronol, Preps. (Wyeth-Ayerst).

caprylate, salts.
See: Sodium Caprylate.
Zinc Caprylate.

caprylate sodium, injection. (Ingram) Amp. 33%, 1 ml Pkg. 12s, 25s, 100s.
Use: Antifungal.
See: Sodium Caprylate Preps.

capsaicin. (kap-SAY-uh-sin)
Use: Analgesic, topical.
See: R-Gel (Healthline Labs).
Zostrix Cream (GenDerm).

•**capsicum,** U.S.P. 23.
Use: Carminative, counterirritant (external), stomachic.

•**capsicum oleoresin,** U.S.P. 23.
Use: Carminative; counterirritant (external); stomachic.

Capsin. (Flemming) Capsaicin 0.025% or 0.075%, benzyl alcohol, propylene glycol, denatured alcohol. Lot. Bot. 59 ml. *otc.*
Use: External analgesic.

capsules, empty gelatin. (Lilly) Lilly markets clear empty gelatin capsules in sizes 000,00,0,1,2,3,4,5.

•**captamine hydrochloride.** (CAP-tam-een) USAN.
Use: Depigmentor.

captodiame hydrochloride.

•**captopril,** (KAP-toe-prill) U.S.P. 23.
Use: Antihypertensive, enzyme inhibitor (angiotensin-converting).
See: Capoten, Tab. (Squibb).

•**capuride.** (CAP-you-ride) USAN.
Use: Hypnotic, sedative.

Capzasin-P. (Thompson Medical) Capsaicin 0.025%, benzyl and cetyl alcohol. Cream. 42.5 g. *otc.*
Use: External analgesic.

Caquin. (Forest) Hydrocortisone 1%, iodochlorhydroxyquin 3%, hydrophilic base. Cream. Tube 20 g. *otc, Rx.*
Use: Corticosteroid, topical.

•**caracemide.** (car-ASS-eh-MIDE) USAN.
Use: Antineoplastic.

Carafate. (Hoechst Marion Roussel)
Tab.: Sucralfate 1 g. Bot. 100s, 120s, 500s, UD 100s. **Susp.:** Sucralfate 1 g/10 ml. Bot. 420 ml. *Rx.*
Use: Antiulcer agent.

•**caramel,** N.F. 18.
Use: Pharmaceutic aid (color).

caramiphen edisylate.
W/Phenylpropanolamine.
See: Tuss-Ornade, Prods. (SK-Beecham).

caramiphen ethanedisulfonate.
W/Phenylephrine HCl, phenindamine tartrate.
See: Dondril, Tab. (Whitehall Robbins).

caramiphen hydrochloride.
Use: Proposed antiparkinson agent.

caraway, N.F. XVI.
Use: Flavor.

•**carbachol,** U.S.P. 23.
Use: Parasympathomimetic, cholinergic (ophthalmic).
See: Miostat Intraocular, Soln. (Alcon).
Murocarb, Soln. (Muro).
W/Methylcellulose.
See: Carbuptic, Soln. (Optopic).
Isopto Carbachol, Soln. (Alcon).

carbacrylamine resins.
Use: Cation-exchange resin.

•**carbadox.** (CAR-bah-dox) USAN.
Use: Antibacterial.

carbamate.
See: Valmid, Tab. (Lilly).

•**carbamazepine,** (KAR-bam-AZE-uh-peen) U.S.P. 23.
Use: Analgesic, anticonvulsant.
See: Atretol, Tab. (Athena Neurosciences).
Carbamazepine (Rugby).
Epitol, Tab. (Lemmon).
Tegretol, Tab. (Novartis).

carbamazepine. (KAR-bam-AZE-uh-peen) (Various Mfr.) **Chew. Tab.:** 100 mg. Bot. 100s. **Tab.:** 200 mg. Bot. 100s, 500s, 1000s, UD 100s.
Use: Treatment of epilepsy and trigeminal neuralgia.

carbamide. (Various Mfr.) Urea. Cream, Lot.
Use: Emollient.
See: Aquacare (Allergan Herbert).
Carmol 20 (Syntex).
Elaqua XX (Zeneca).

Nutraplus (Galderma).
Rea-Lo (Whorton).
Ultra Mide Moisturizer (Baker/Cummins).
Ureacin-20 (Pedinol).
Ureacin-40 (Pedinol).

carbamide compounds.
See: Acetylcarbromal (Various Mfr.).
Bromisovalum (Various Mfr.).
Bromural, Tab. (Knoll).
Carbrital, Elix., Kap. (Parke-Davis).
Carbromal (Various Mfr.).
Sedamyl, Tab. (3M).

•**carbamide peroxide,** U.S.P. 23. Urea compound w/hydrogen peroxide (1:1).
Use: Anti-infective, topical (dental); anti-inflammatory; analgesic.
See: Gly-Oxide (Hoechst Marion Roussel).
Orajel Brace-aid Rinse (Del Pharm.).
Orajel Perioseptic, Liq. (Del Pharm.).
Proxigel (Schwarz Pharma).

carbamide peroxide 6.5% in glycerin.
Use: Otic preparation.
See: Murine Ear Drops (Abbott).
Murine Ear Wax Removal System (Abbott).

carbamylcholine chloride.
See: Carbachol.

carbamylmethylcholine chloride.
See: Urecholine, Tab., Inj. (Merck & Co.).

•**carbantel lauryl sulfate.** (CAR-ban-tell LAH-ruhl) USAN.
Use: Anthelmintic.

carbapenem.
See: Imipenem-Cilastatin.

carbarsone, U.S.P. 21. Caps., U.S.P. 21. (Various Mfr.) N-carbamoylarsanilic acid. Amabevan, ameban, amibiarson, arsambide, fenarsone, leucarsone, aminarsone, amebarsone. p-Ureidobenzenearsonic acid.
Use: Acute and chronic amebiasis and trichomoniasis.

•**carbaspirin calcium.** USAN.
Use: Analgesic.

Carbastat. (Ciba Vision) Carbachol 0.1%, sodium Cl 0.064%, potassium Cl 0.075%, calcium Cl dihydrate 0.048%, magnesium Cl hexahydrate 0.03%, sodium acetate trihydrate 0.39%, sodium citrate dihydrate 0.17%. Soln. Vial 1.5 ml. Rx.
Use: Agent for glaucoma.

•**carbazeran.** (CAR-BAY-zeh-ran) USAN.
Use: Cardiotonic.

•**carbenicillin disodium, sterile,** (CAR-ben-ih-SILL-in die-SO-dee-uhm) U.S.P. 23.

Use: Antibacterial.
See: Geopen, Vial (Roerig).
Pyopen, Inj. (SK-Beecham).

•**carbenicillin indanyl sodium,** (car-BEN-ih-SILL-in IN-duh-nil) U.S.P. 23.
Use: Antibacterial.
See: Geocillin, Tab. (Roerig).

•**carbenicillin phenyl sodium.** (CAR-ben-ih-SILL-in FEN-ill) USAN.
Use: Antibacterial.

•**carbenicillin potassium.** (CAR-ben-ih-SILL-in) USAN.
Use: Antibacterial.

•**carbenoxolone sodium.** (CAR-ben-ox-ah-lone) USAN.
Use: Glucocorticoid.

carbetapentane citrate.
Use: Antitussive.
W/Codeine phosphate, chlorpheniramine maleate, guaifenesin.
See: Tussar-2, Syr. (Rhone-Poulenc Rorer).
Tussar SF, Liq. (Rhone-Poulenc Rorer).

carbethoxysyringoyl methylreserpate.
See: Singoserp, Tab. (Novartis).

carbethyl salicylate.
See: Sal-Ethyl Carbonate, Tab. (Parke-Davis).

•**carbetimer.** (car-BEH-tih-MER) USAN.
Use: Antineoplastic.

Carbex. (Dupont Pharma) Selegiline HCl 5 mg, lactose/Tab. Bot. 60s. Rx.
Use: Used in combination with levodopa/carbidopa for treatment of Parkinson's disease.

•**carbidopa,** (CAR-bih-doe-puh) U.S.P. 23.
Use: Decarboxylase inhibitor.
See: Lodosyn, Tab. (Merck & Co.).
W/Levodopa.
See: Sinemet, Tab. (DuPont Pharma).

carbidopa and levodopa tablets.
Use: Treatment of Parkinson's disease.
See: Sinemet, Tab. (DuPont Pharma).

carbidopa & levodopa. (Various) Carbidopa 10 mg, levodopa 100 mg; carbidopa 25 mg, levodopa 100 mg; carbidopa 25 mg, levodopa 250 mg. Tab. Bot. 100s, 1000s. Rx.
Use: Antiparkinsonian.

carbimazole.

Carbinoxamine Compound Drops. (Rosemont) Pseudoephedrine HCl 25 mg, carbinoxamine maleate 2 mg, dextromethorphan HBr 4 mg. Grape flavor. Drop. Bot. 30 ml. Rx.
Use: Decongestant, antitussive, antihistamine.

Carbinoxamine Compound Syrup.

(Rosemont) Pseudoephedrine HCl 60 mg, dextromethorphan HBr 15 mg, carbinoxamine maleate 4 mg. Grape flavor. Syr. Bot. 120 ml, pt, gal. *Rx.*
Use: Decongestant, antitussive, antihistamine.

•**carbinoxamine maleate,** U.S.P. 23.
Use: Antihistamine.

•**carbiphene hydrochloride.** (CAR-bih-FEEN) USAN.
Use: Analgesic.

Carbiset Tablets. (Nutripharm) Pseudoephedrine 60 mg, carbinoxamine maleate 4 mg/Tab. Bot. 100s, 500s. *Rx.*
Use: Decongestant, antihistamine.

Carbiset-TR. (Nutripharm) Pseudoephedrine HCl 120 mg, carbinoxamine maleate 8 mg/Tab. Bot. 100s. *Rx.*
Use: Decongestant, antihistamine.

Carbocaine. (Cook-Waite) Mepivacaine HCl 3%. Inj. Dental cartridge 1.8 ml. *Rx.*
Use: Local anesthetic.

Carbocaine. (Sanofi Winthrop) Mepivacaine HCl. **1%:** Vial 30 ml, 50 ml. **1.5%:** Vial 30 ml. **2%:** Vial 20 ml, 50 ml. *Rx.*
Use: Local anesthetic.

Carbocaine with Neo-Cobefrin. (Cook-Waite) Mepivacaine HCl 2% with levonorefrin 1:20,000. Inj. Dental cartridge 1.8 ml. *Rx.*
Use: Local anesthetic.

•**carbocloral.** (CAR-boe-KLOR-uhl) USAN.
Use: Hypnotic, sedative.
See: Chloralurethane.
Prodorm (Parke-Davis).

•**carbocysteine.** (car-boe-SIS-teen) USAN.
Use: Mucolytic.

Carbodec. (Rugby) Pseudoephedrine HCl 60 mg, carbinoxamine maleate 4 mg/5 ml. Syr. Bot. 473 ml. *Rx.*
Use: Decongestant, antihistamine.

Carbodec DM Products. (Rugby) **Syr.:** Pseudoephedrine HCl 60 mg, carbinoxamine maleate 4 mg, dextromethorphan HBr 15 mg, alcohol < 0.6%/5 ml. Bot. 30 ml, 120 ml, pt, gal. **Drops (Pediatric):** Pseudoephedrine HCl 25 mg, carbinoxamine maleate 2 mg, dextromethorphan HBr 4 mg, alcohol 0.6%/ml. Bot. 30 ml. *Rx.*
Use: Decongestant, antihistamine, antitussive.

Carbodec Tablets. (Rugby) Pseudoephedrine HCl 60 mg, carbinoxamine maleate 4 mg/Tab. Bot. 100s. *Rx.*

Use: Decongestant, antihistamine.

Carbodec TR. (Rugby) Pseudoephedrine HCl 120 mg, carbinoxamine maleate 8 mg/Tab. Bot. 100s. *Rx.*
Use: Decongestant, antihistamine.

carbol-fuchsin paint. Original fuchsin formula known as Castellani's Paint. Basic Fuchsin 0.3%, phenol 4.5%, resorcinol 10%, acetone 5%, alcohol 10%. Bot. 30 ml, 120 ml, 480 ml.
Use: Antifungal, topical.
See: Carfusin, Soln. (Rhone-Poulenc Rorer).
Castellani's Paint (Various Mfr.).

•**carbol-fuchsin, topical solution.** U.S.P. 23.
Use: Antifungal.

carbomer, (CAR-boe-mer) N.F. 18. A polymer of acrylic acid, crosslinked with a polyfunctional agent.
Use: Pharmaceutic aid (emulsifying, suspending agent).
See: Carbopol 934 P (Goodrich).

•**carbomer 910,** (CAR-boe-mer 910) N.F. 18.
Use: Pharmaceutic aid, (emulsifying, suspending agent).

•**carbomer 934,** (CAR-boe-mer 934) N.F. 18.
Use: Pharmaceutic aid (emulsifying, suspending agent).

•**carbomer 934p,** (CAR-boe-mer 934) N.F. 18.
Use: Pharmaceutic aid (emulsifying, suspending viscosity, thickening agent).

•**carbomer 940,** (CAR-boe-mer 940) N.F. 18.
Use: Pharmaceutic aid (emulsifying, suspending agent).

•**carbomer 941,** (CAR-boe-mer 941) N.F. 18.
Use: Pharmaceutic aid (emulsifying, suspending agent).

•**carbomer 1342,** (CAR-boe-mer 1342) N.F. 18.
Use: Pharmaceutic aid (emulsifying, suspending agent).

carbomycin. An antibiotic from *Streptomyces halstedii.*
Use: Anti-infective.

•**carbon dioxide,** U.S.P. 23.
Use: Inhalation, respiratory stimulant.
See: Ceo-Two, Supp. (Beutlich).

•**carbon monoxide c 11,** (CAR-bahn moe-NOX-ide C11) U.S.P. 23.
Use: Diagnostic aid (blood volume determination), radioactive agent.

carbonic acid, dilithium salt. Lithium

Carbonate, U.S.P. 23.

carbonic acid, disodium salt. Sodium Carbonate, N.F. 18.

carbonic acid, monosodium salt. Sodium Bicarbonate, U.S.P. 23.

carbonic anhydrase inhibitors.
See: Acetazolamide, Tab. (Various Mfr.).
AK-ZOL, Tab. (Akorn).
Daranide, Tab. (Merck & Co.).
Dazamide, Tab. (Major).
Diamox, Tab., Sequel, Vial (Lederle).
Neptazane, Tab. (Lederle).

Carbonis Detergens, Liquor.
See: Coal Tar Solution.

carbonyl diamide.
See: Chap Cream (Ar-Ex).

carbon tetrachloride. N.F. XVII. Benzinoform. (Various Mfr.).
Use: Pharmaceutic aid (solvent).

•**carboplatin,** (car-boe-PLATT-in) U.S.P. 23.
Use: Antineoplastic.

•**carboprost.** (CAR-boe-prahst) USAN.
Use: Oxytocic.

•**carboprost methyl.** (CAR-boe-prahst METH-ill) USAN.
Use: Oxytocic

•**carboprost tromethamine,** (CAR-boe-prahst troe-METH-ah-meen) U.S.P. 23.
Use: Oxytocic.
See: Prostin, Amp. (Pharmacia & Upjohn).

Carboptic. (Optopics) Carbachol 3%. Soln. Bot. 15 ml. *Rx.*
Use: Ophthalmic, topical.

carbose d.
See: Carboxymethylcellulose sodium, Prep.

Carbovir. *Rx.*
Use: AIDS treatment. [Orphan drug]

carbowax. 300, 400, 1540, 4000. Polyethylene glycol 300, 400, 1540, 4000.

•**carboxymethylcellulose calcium,** N.F. 18.
Use: Pharmaceutic aid (tablet disintegrant).

carboxymethylcellulose salt of dextroamphetamine. Carboxyphen.
See: Bontril Timed Tab. (Carnrick).

•**carboxymethylcellulose sodium,** U.S.P. 23.
Use: Pharmaceutic aid (suspending agent, tablet excipient), and viscosity-increasing agent; cathartic.
W/Acetphenolisatin, docusate sodium.
See: Scrip-Lax, Tab. (Scrip).
W/Alginic acid, sodium bicarbonate.
See: Pretts, Tabs. (Hoechst Marion Roussel).

W/Belladonna extract, kaolin, pectin, zinc phenosulfonate.
See: Gelcomul, Liq. (Del Pharm.).
W/Digitoxin.
See: Foxalin, Cap. (Standex).
Thegitoxin (Standex).
W/Docusate sodium.
See: Dialose, Cap. (Stuart).
W/Docusate sodium, casanthranol.
See: Dialose Plus, Cap. (Stuart).
Tri-Vac, Cap. (Rhode).
W/Docusate sodium, oxyphenisatin acetate.
See: Dialose Plus, Cap. (Stuart).
W/Methylcellulose.
See: Ex-Caloric, Wafer (Eastern Research).
W/Testosterone, estrone, sodium Cl.
See: Tostestro, Inj. (Jones Medical).

•**carboxymethylcellulose sodium 12,** N.F. 18.
Use: Pharmaceutic aid (suspending, viscosity-increasing agent).
Use: Mucolytic agent.

carboxyphen.
W/Butabarbital.
See: Bontril, Timed Tab. (Carnrick).

Carbromal. (Various Mfr.) Bromodiethylacetylurea, bromadel, nyctal, planadalin, uradal. *Rx.*
Use: Sedative, hypnotic.
W/Bromisovalum (Bromural).
See: Bro-T's, Tab. (Brothers).

carbutamide.
Use: Hypoglycemic.

•**carbuterol hydrochloride.** (car-BYOO-ter-ole) USAN.
Use: Bronchodilator.

cardamon. Oil, seed, Cpd. Tincture.
Use: Flavor.

Cardec DM Drops. (Various Mfr.) Carbinoxamine maleate 2 mg, pseudoephedrine HCl 25 mg, dextromethorphan HBr 4 mg, alcohol < 0.6%/ml. Drop. Bot. 30 ml. *Rx.*
Use: Antihistamine, decongestant, antitussive.

Cardec DM Pediatric Syrup. (Schein) Pseudoephedrine HCl 60 mg, dextromethorphan HBr 15 mg, carbinoxamine maleate 4 mg, < 0.6% alcohol. Bot. pt. *Rx.*
Use: Decongestant, antitussive, antihistamine.

Cardec DM Syrup. (Various Mfr.) Carbinoxamine maleate 4 mg, pseudoephedrine HCl 60 mg, dextromethorphan HBr 15 mg, alcohol > 0.6%/5 ml. Bot. 30 ml, 120 ml, pt, gal. *Rx.*
Use: Antihistamine, decongestant, antitussive.

Cardec-S. (Barre-National) Pseudo-ephedrine HCl 60 mg, carbinoxamine maleate 4 mg/5 ml. Syr. Bot. 473 ml. *Rx.*
Use: Decongestant, antihistamine.

Cardene. (Syntex) Nicardipine 20 mg or 30 mg/Cap. Bot. 100s, 500s, UD 100s. *Rx.*
Use: Calcium channel blocking agent.

Cardene IV. (Wyeth-Ayerst) Nicardipine HCl 2.5 ml, sorbitol 48 mg/ml. Inj. 10 ml amps. *Rx.*
Use: Calcium channel blocking agent.

Cardene SR. (Syntex) Nicardipine HCl 30 mg, 45 mg, 60 mg/Cap. SR Bot. 60s, 200s, UD 100s. *Rx.*
Use: Calcium channel blocking agent.

Cardenz. (Miller) Vitamins C 25 mg, E 5 mg, inositol 30 mg, p-aminobenzoic acid 9 mg, A 2000 IU, B_6 1.5 mg, B_{12} 1 mcg, D 100 IU, niacinamide 20 mg, magnesium 23 mg, iodine 0.05 mg, potassium 8 mg/Tab. Bot. 100s. *otc.*
Use: Vitamin/mineral supplement.

cardiamid.
See: Nikethamide. (Various Mfr.).

cardiazol.
See: Metrazol, Preps. (Knoll).

Cardilate. (Glaxo Wellcome) Erythrityl tetranitrate 10 mg/Tab. Bot. 100s.
Use: Antianginal.

Cardio-Green (CG). (Becton-Dickinson) Indocyanine Green 25 mg or 50 mg. Inj. Amps 10 ml (2s).
Use: Diagnostic aid.

Cardio-Green Disposable Unit. (Becton Dickinson) Vial Cardio-Green, ampule aqueous solvent and calibrated syringe. 10 mg.
Use: Diagnostic aid.

Cardi-Omega 3. (Thompson Medical) EPA 180 mg, DHA 120 mg, cholesterol 5 mg, less than 2% RDA of vitamins A, B_1, B_2, B_3, C, D, Fe, Ca/Cap. Bot. 60s. *otc.*
Use: Vitamin/mineral supplement.

cardioplegic solution.
Use: During open heart surgery.
See: Plegisol, Soln. (Abbott).

Cardioquin Tablets. (Purdue Frederick) Quinidine polygalacturonate 275 mg equivalent to quinidine sulfate 200 mg/Tab. Bot. 100s, 500s. *Rx.*
Use: Antiarrhythmic.

Cardiotrol-CK. (Roche Diagnostics) Lyophilized human serum containing three CK isoenzymes from human tissue source. 10 × 2 ml.
Use: Suitable for use as a quality control for immunochemical or electrophoretic assays.

Cardiotrol-LD. (Roche Diagnostics) Lyophilized human serum containing all LD isoenzymes from human tissue source. 10 × 1 ml.
Use: Suitable for use as a quality control for immunochemical or electrophoretic assays.

Cardizem. (Hoechst Marion Roussel) Diltiazem HCl **30 mg/Tab:** Bot. 100s, 500s, UD 100s. **60 mg/Tab:** Bot. 90s, 100s, 500s, UD 100s. **90 mg/Tab:** Bot 90s, 100s, UD 100s. **120 mg/Tab:** Bot. 100s and UD 100s. *Rx.*
Use: Calcium channel blocking agent.

Cardizem CD. (Hoechst Marion Roussel) Diltiazem HCl 120 mg, 180 mg, 240 mg, 300 mg/Ext. Rel. Cap. Bot. 30s, 90s, 5000s and UD 100s. *Rx.*
Use: Calcium channel blocking agent.

Cardizem Injection. (Hoechst Marion Roussel) **25 mg (5 mg/ml)/Inj:** Diltiazem HCl, 3.75 mg citric acid, 3.25 mg sodium citrate dihydrate and 357 mg sorbitol solution. 5 ml vials. **50 mg (5 mg/ml)/Inj:** Diltiazem HCl, 7.5 mg citric acid, 6.5 mg sodium citrate dihydrate and 714 mg sorbitol solution. 10 ml vials. *Rx.*
Use: Calcium channel blocking agent.

Cardizem SR. (Hoechst Marion Roussel) Diltiazem HCl 60 mg, 90 mg or 120 mg/S.R. Cap. Bot. 100s, UD 100s. *Rx.*
Use: Calcium channel blocking agent.

Cardophyllin.
See: Aminophylline. (Various Mfr.).

Cardoxin. (Vita Elixir) Digoxin 0.25 mg/Tab. *Rx.*
Use: Cardiac glycoside.

Cardura. (Roerig) Doxazosin mesylate 1 mg, 2 mg, 4 mg, 8 mg/Tab. Bot. 100s. *Rx.*
Use: Antihypertensive.

carena.
See: Aminophylline (Various Mfr.).

•**carfentanil citrate.** (car-FEN-tah-NILL SIH-trate) USAN.
Use: Narcotic analgesic.

Cargentos.
See: Silver Protein, Mild.

•**carisoprodol,** (car-eye-so-PRO-dole) U.S.P. 23.
Use: Skeletal muscle relaxant.
See: Rela, Tab. (Schering-Plough). Soma, Tab. (Wallace).

carisoprodol. (Various Mfr.) 350 mg. Tab. Bot. 30s, 60s, 100, 500s, 1000s, UD 100s.
Use: Skeletal muscle relaxant.

carisoprodol and aspirin tablets.
Use: Analgesic, muscle relaxant.
See: Soma Compound Tab. (Wallace).

carisoprodol, aspirin, and codeine phosphate tablets.
Use: Analgesic, muscle relaxant.
See: Soma Compound w/Codeine Tab. (Wallace).

Carisoprodol Compound. (Various Mfr.) Carisoprodol 200 mg, aspirin 325 mg/Tab. Bot. 15s, 30s, 40s, 100s, 500s, 1000s. *Rx.*
Use: Skeletal muscle relaxant, salicylate analgesic.

Cari-Tab. (Jones Medical) Fluoride 0.5 mg, vitamins A 2000 IU, D 200 IU, C 75 mg/Softab. Bot. 100s. *Rx.*
Use: Vitamin supplement, dental caries preventative.

•**carmantadine.** (car-MAN-tah-deen) USAN.
Use: Treatment of Parkinson's disease.

Carmol 10. (Doak Dermatologics) Urea (carbamide) 10% in hypoallergenic water-washable lotion base. Bot. 6 fl oz. *otc.*
Use: Emollient.

Carmol 20. (Doak Dermatologics) Urea (carbamide) 20% in hypoallergenic vanishing cream base. Tube 3 oz, Jar lb. *otc.*
Use: Emollient.

Carmol-HC Cream 1%. (Doak Dermatologics) Micronized hydrocortisone acetate 1%, urea 10% in water-washable base. Tube 1 oz, Jar 4 oz. *Rx.*
Use: Corticosteroid, topical.

•**carmustine.** (CAR-muss-teen) USAN.
Use: Antineoplastic.
See: Bicnu, Inj. (Bristol).

Carnation Follow-Up. (Carnation) Protein (from non-fat milk) 18 g, carbohydrate (from lactose and corn syrup) 89.2 g, fat 27.7 g, vitamins A, D, E, K, C, B$_1$, B$_2$, B$_3$, B$_6$, B$_{12}$, B$_5$, biotin, choline, Ca, P, Cl, Mg, I, Mn, Cu, Zn, Fe 13 mg, inositol, cholesterol 11.4 mg, taurine, sodium 264 mg, potassium 913 mg. Pow. 360 g Con. 390 ml. *otc.*
Use: Nutritional supplement.

Carnation Good-Start. (Carnation) Protein 16 g, carbohydrate 74.4 g, fat 34.5 g, vitamins A, D, E, K, B$_1$, B$_2$, B$_3$, B$_5$, B$_6$, B$_{12}$, C, biotin, choline, inositol, cholesterol 68 mg, taurine, Ca, P, Mg, Fe 10 mg, Zn, Mn, Cu, I, Cl, sodium 162 mg, potassium 663 mg. Pow 360 g Con. 390 ml. *otc.*
Use: Nutritional supplement.

Carnation Instant Breakfast. (Carnation) Non-fat instant breakfast containing 280 K calories w/15 g protein and 8 oz whole milk. Pkt. 35 g, Ctn. 6s. Six flavors. *otc.*
Use: Nutritional supplement.

•**carnidazole.** (car-NIH-dah-zole) USAN. Methyl-nitro-imidazole.
Use: Antiparasitic, antiprotozoal.

Carnitor. (Siga-Tau) Levocarnitine. **Liq.:** 100 mg/ml. Bot. 10 ml. **Tab.:** 330 mg. Bot. 90s. **Inj.:** 1 g/5 ml. Single-dose amps 5 ml. *Rx.*
Use: Vitamin supplement.

•**caroxazone.** (car-OX-ah-zone) USAN.
Use: Antidepressant.

•**carphenazine maleate.** (car-FEN-azz-een) USAN.
Use: Antipsychotic.

•**carprofen.** USAN.
Use: Nonsteroidal anti-inflammatory drug; analgesic.
See: Rimadyl. (Roche).

•**carrageenan,** N.F. 18.
Use: Pharmaceutic aid (suspending, viscosity-increasing agent).

Carrisyn. (Carrington Labs) Phase I AIDS, ARC. *Rx.*
Use: Antiviral, immunomodulator.

•**carsatrin succinate.** (car-SAT-rin) USAN.
Use: Cardiotonic.

•**cartazolate.** (car-TAZZ-oh-late) USAN.
Use: Antidepressant.

•**carteolol hydrochloride,** (CAR-tee-oh-lahl) U.S.P. 23.
Use: Antiadrenergic (β-receptor).
See: Ocupress, Ophth. Soln. (Otuska America).

Carter's Little Pills. (Carter Products) Bisacodyl 5 mg/Pill. Pills 30s, 85s. *otc.*
Use: Laxative.

Cartrol. (Abbott) Carteolol 2.5 mg or 5 mg/Tab. Bot. 100s. *Rx.*
Use: Beta-adrenergic blocking agent.

Cartucho Cook with Ravocaine. (Sanofi Winthrop) Ravocaine, novocaine, levophed or neo-cobefrin. *Rx.*
Use: Dental anesthetic.

•**carubicin hydrochloride.** (kah-ROO-bih-sin) USAN.
Use: Antineoplastic.

•**carumonam sodium.** (kah-roo-MOE-nam) USAN.
Use: Antibacterial.

•**carvedilol.** (CAR-veh-DILL-ole) USAN.
Use: Antianginal, antihypertensive.
See: Coreg, Tab. (SmithKline Beecham).

Car-Vit. (Mericon) Ascorbic acid 60 mg, vitamins A acetate 4000 IU, D-2 400 IU, ferrous fumarate 90 mg (elemental iron 30 mg), oyster shell 600 mg (calcium 230 mg)/Cap. Bot. 90s, 1000s. *otc.*
Use: Vitamin/mineral supplement.

•**carvotroline hydrochloride.** (car-VAH-trah-leen) USAN.
Use: Antipsychotic.

•**carzelesin.** (car-ZELL-eh-sin) USAN.
Use: Antineoplastic (site-selective DNA binding).

carzenide.
Use: Carbonic anhydrase inhibitor.

casa-dicole. (Halsey) Docusate sodium 100 mg, casanthrol 30 mg/Cap. Bot. 100s. *otc.*
Use: Laxative.

•**casanthranol,** (kass-AN-thrah-nole) U.S.P. 23. A purified mixture of the anthranol glycosides derived from Cascara sagrada.
Use: Laxative.
See: Black Draught, Prods. (Chattem Labs.).
W/Docusate sodium.
See: Bu-Lax-Plus, Cap. (Ulmer).
Calotabs, Tab. (Calotabs).
Comfolax-Plus, Cap. (Rhone-Poulenc Rorer).
Comfolax-Plus, Cap. (Searle).
Comfula-Plus (Searle).
Constiban, Cap. (Quality Generics).
Diolax, Cap. (Century).
Dio-Soft (Standex).
Disulans, Cap. (Noyes).
Easy-Lax Plus, Cap. (Walgreen).
Genericace, Cap. (Forest Pharm.).
Neo-Vardin D-S-S-C, Cap. (Scherer).
Nuvac, Cap. (LaCrosse).
Peri-Colace, Cap., Syr. (Bristol-Myers).
Sodex, Cap. (Roberts).
Stimulax, Cap. (Geriatric).
Tonelax Plus, Cap. (A.V.P.).
W/Docusate sodium, sodium carboxymethylcellulose.
See: Dialose Plus, Cap. (Stuart).
Tri-Vac, Cap. (Rhode).
W/Mineral oil, irish moss.
See: Neo-Kondremul, Liq. (Medeva).

Cascara. (Lilly) Cascara 150 mg/Tab. Bot. 100s. *otc.*
Use: Laxative.

cascara fluid extract, aromatic.
Use: Laxative.
W/Psyllium husk powder, prune powder.
See: Casyllium, Pow. (Pharmacia & Upjohn).

Cascara Glycosides.
Use: Laxative.

•**cascara sagrada,** U.S.P. 23.
Use: Cathartic.
W/Bile salts, papain, phenolphthalein, capsicum oleoresin.
See: Torocol Compound, Tab. (Plessner).
W/Bile salts, phenolphthalein, capsicum oleoresin, peppermint oil.
See: Torocol, Tab. (Plessner).
W/Ox bile (desiccated), phenolphthalein, aloin, podophyllin.
See: Bilgon, Tab. (Solvay).
W/Oxgall, dandelion root, podophyllin, tincture nux vomica.
See: Oxachol, Liq. (Philips Roxane).
W/Pancreatin, pepsin, sodium salicylate.
See: Bocresin, Liq. (Scrip).
W/Phenolphthalein, sodium glycocholate, sodium taurocholate, aloin.
See: Bicholax, Tab. (Zeneca).
Oxiphen, Tab. (PolyMedica).
W/Sodium salicylate, phenolphthalein, chionanthus extract, bile extract, sodium glycocholate, sodium taurocholate.
See: Glycols, Tab. (Jones Medical).

cascara sagrada. (Various Mfr.) 325 mg/Tab. Bot. 100s, 1000s.
Use: Cathartic.

cascara sagrada fluid extract. (Parke-Davis) Alcohol 18%. Bot. pt, gal, UD 5 ml.
Use: Laxative. [Orphan drug]
See: Cas-Evac, Liq. (Parke-Davis).
Bilstan (Standex).

cascara sagrada fluid extract aromatic. Aromatic Cascara Fluid extract. Liq. Alcohol ≈ 18%/5 ml. Bot. 60 ml, 120 ml, pt, gal, UD 5 ml.
Use: Laxative.
W/Psyllium husk powder, prune powder.
See: Casyllium, Granules (Pharmacia & Upjohn).

cascarin.
See: Casanthranol (Various Mfr.).

Casec. (Bristol-Myers) Calcium caseinate (derived from skim milk curd and calcium carbonate). Pow. Can 2.5 oz. *otc.*
Use: Calcium supplement.

Casodex. (Zeneca) Bicalutamide 50 mg, lactose/Tab. In 100s and UD 30s. *Rx.*
Use: Prostate cancer treatment.

CAST. (Biomerica) Color Allergy Screening Test: A visual ELISA test for quantitative determination of Human Immunoglobulin E in serum.
Use: Diagnostic aid.

CAST. (Biomerica) Reagent test for immunoglobulin E in serum. Tube Kit 25s.
Use: In vitro diagnostic aid.

Castel Minus. (Syosset) Resorcinol 10%, acetone, basic fuchsin, hydroxyethyl cellulose, alcohol 10%. Non-staining. Liq. Bot. 30 ml. *otc.*
Use: Antifungal, topical.

Castel Plus. (Syosset) Resorcinol 10%, acetone, basic fuchsin, hydroxyethyl cellulose, alcohol 10%. Liq. Bot. 30 ml. *otc.*
Use: Antifungal, topical.

Castellani Paint Modified. (Pedinol) Basic fuchsin, phenol resorcinol, acetone, alcohol. Bot. 30 ml, 120 ml, 480 ml. Also available as colorless solution without basic fuchsin. Bot. 30 ml, 120 ml, 480 ml. *Rx.*
Use: Antifungal, topical.

Castellani's Paint. (Archer-Taylor) Bot. 4 oz, 16 oz. *Rx.*
Use: Antifungal, topical.

Castellani's Paint. (Penta) Carbol-fuchsin solution. Fuchsin 0.3%, phenol 4.5%, resorcinol 10%, acetone 1.5%, alcohol 13%. Bot. 1 oz, 4 oz, pt. *Rx.*
Use: Antifungal, topical.

• **castor oil,** (KASS-ter oil) U.S.P. 23.
Use: Laxative, pharmaceutic aid (plasticizer).
See: Neoloid (Lederle).
Purge (Fleming).

castor oil. (KASS-ter oil) Aromatic Caps. Liq. emulsion. Liq. Bot. 60 ml, 120 ml, pt.
Use: Laxative, pharmaceutic aid (plasticizer).

castor oil emulsion.
Use: Cathartic.
See: Emulsoil (Paddock).
Fleet Flavored (Fleet).

castor oil, hydrogenated.
Use: Laxative.

Cataflam. (Novartis) Diclofenac 50 mg (as potassium) Tab. Bot. 100s, UD 100s. *Rx.*
Use: Nonsteroidal anti-inflammatory drug; analgesic.

Catapres. (Boehringer Ingelheim) Clonidine HCl 0.1 mg, 0.2 mg or 0.3 mg/Tab. Bot. 100s. 0.1 mg, 0.2 mg: Bot. 1000s, UD 100s. *Rx.*
Use: Antihypertensive.

Catapres-TTS. (Boehringer Ingelheim) Clonidine 2.5 mg, 5 mg or 7.5 mg/Transdermal patch. Pkg. 4s, 12s. *Rx.*
Use: Antihypertensive.

Catarase 1:5000. (Ciba Vision) Chymotrypsin 300 units in a 2-chamber vial with 2 ml sodium Cl. *Rx.*
Use: Ophthalmic enzyme.

Catatrol. (Zeneca) Viloxazine.
Use: Antidepressant.

cathomycin calcium. Calcium novobiocin.
Use: Anti-infective.

cathomycin sodium. Novobiocin sodium.
Use: Anti-infective.

cationic resins.
See: Resins, Sodium-Removing.

Catrix Correction. (Donell DerMedex) SPF 15. Octyl methoxycinnamate, menthyl anthranilate, benzophenone 3, titanium dioxide, sesame oil, cetearyl alcohol, urea, EDTA, imidazolidinyl urea, parabens. Cream Tube 39 g. *otc.*
Use: Sunscreen.

Caverject. (Pharmacia & Upjohn) Alprostadil 11.9 mcg (10 mcg/ml) or 23.2 mcg (20 mcg/ml). Lyophilized powd. for inj. In vials with diluent syringes. *Rx.*
Use: Agent for impotence.

Cav-X Fluoride Treatment. (Palisades) Stannous fluoride 0.4% gel. Bot. 121.9 g. *Rx.*
Use: Dental caries preventative.

C-Bio. (Barth's) Vitamin C 150 mg, citrus bioflavonoid complex 100 mg, rutin 50 mg/Tab. Bot. 100s, 500s, 1000s. *otc.*
Use: Vitamin supplement.

C-B Time Liquid. (Arco) Vitamins C 300 mg, B$_1$ 15 mg, B$_2$ 10 mg, B$_3$ 100 mg, B$_5$ 20 mg, B$_6$ 5 mg, B$_{12}$ 5 mcg. Liq. Bot. 120 ml. *otc.*
Use: Vitamin supplement.

CCD 1042. (Cocensys) *Rx.*
Use: Treatment of infantile spasms. [Orphan drug]

ccnu. Lomustine.
Use: Antineoplastic.
See: CeeNu, Tab. (Bristol).

C-Crystals. (NBTY) Vitamin C 5,000 mg/tsp. Crystals. Bot. 180 g. *otc.*
Use: Vitamin C supplement.

CD4 human truncated 369 AA polypeptide. *Rx.*
Use: AIDS treatment.

CD4 immunoglobulin G, recombinant human. *Rx.*
Use: AIDS treatment. [Orphan drug]

CD4, recombinant soluble human (rCD4). *Rx.*
Use: AIDS treatment. [Orphan drug]

CD5-t lymphocyte immunotoxin. *Rx.*
Use: Rejection in bone marrow transplants. [Orphan drug]

CD-45 monoclonal antibodies. *Rx.*
Use: Prevent graft rejection in organ transplants. [Orphan drug]

cddp.
Use: Antineoplastic.
See: Cisplatin.

C.D.P. Caps. (Goldline) Chlordiazepoxide HCl 5 mg, 10 mg or 25 mg/Cap. Bot. 100s, 500s, 1000s. *c-iv.*
Use: Antianxiety.

Cea. (Abbott Diagnostics) Radioimmunoassay or enzyme immunoassay for quantitative measurement of carcinoembryonic antigen in human serum or plasma. Test kit 100s.
Use: Diagnostic aid.

Cea-Roche. (Roche Diagnostics) Radioimmunoassay capable of detecting and measuring plasma levels of CEA in the nanogram range. Sensitivity-0.5 ng./ml of CEA.
Use: Diagnostic aid.

Cea-Roche Test Kit. (Roche Diagnostics) Carcinoembryonic antigen, a glycoprotein which is a constituent of the glycocalyx of embryonic entodermal epithelium. Test kit.
Use: Diagnostic aid.

CEA-Scan. (Immunomedics, Mallinckrodt) Arcitumomab 1.25 mg for conjugation in indium-111. Kit. *Rx.*
Use: For detection of recurrent or metastatic colorectal carcinoma of the liver, extrahepatic abdomen and pelvis; radioimmunoscintigraphy.

Cebid Timecelles. (Roberts) Ascorbic acid 500 mg/Cap. Bot. 100s. *otc.*
Use: Vitamin C supplement.

Ceb Nuggets. (Scott/Cord) Vitamins B_1 15 mg, B_2 15 mg, B_6 5 mg, B_{12} 5 mcg, C 600 mg, niacinamide 100 mg, E 40 IU, calcium pantothenate 20 mg, folic acid 0.1 mg/Nugget. Bot. 60s. *otc.*
Use: Vitamin/mineral supplement.

Cebo-Caps. (Forest) Placebo capsules. *otc.*

C & E Capsules. (NBTY) Vitamins C 500 mg, E 400 mg/Cap. Bot. 50s, 100s. *otc.*
Use: Vitamin supplement.

Ceclor. (Lilly) **Pulv.:** Cefaclor 250 mg or 500 mg. Bot. 15s, 100s, UD 100s. **Oral Susp.:** Cefaclor 125 mg, 250 mg/5ml. Bot. 75 ml, 150 ml; 187 mg, 375 mg/5 ml. Bot. 50 ml, 100 ml. *Rx.*
Use: Anti-infective, cephalosporin.

Ceclor CD. (Eli Lilly) Cefaclor (as monohydrate) 375 mg or 500 mg, mannitol/ER Tab. Bot. 60s. *Rx.*
Use: Antibiotic.

Cecon Solution. (Abbott) Ascorbic acid 10% in propylene glycol. Each drop from enclosed dropper supplies 2.5 mg ascorbic acid; each ml contains 100 mg Bot. w/dropper 50 ml. *otc.*
Use: Vitamin C supplement.

Cedax. (Schering-Plough) Cap.: Ceftibuten 400 mg, parabens/Bot 20s, 100s, UD 100s. Susp.: Ceftibuten 90 or 180 mg/5 ml, sucrose/Bot 30, 60, 120 ml. *Rx.*
Use: Cephalosporin.

•**cedefingol.** (seh-deh-FIN-gole) USAN.
Use: Antineoplastic adjunct, antipsoriatic.

•**cedelizumab.** USAN.
Use: Monoclonal antibody, immunosuppressant.

Ceebevim. (NBTY) Vitamins B_1 15 mg, B_2 10.2 mg, B_3 50 mg, B_5 10 mg, B_6 5 mg, C 300 mg/Cap. Bot. 100s, 300s. *otc.*
Use: Vitamin supplement.

CeeNu. (Bristol-Myers/Bristol Oncology) Lomustine (CCNU) 10 mg, 40 mg or 100 mg/Cap. Dose pk. of two cap. each of all three strengths. *Rx.*
Use: Antineoplastic.

Ceepa. (Geneva Pharm.) Theophylline 130 mg, ephedrine HCl 24 mg, phenobarbital 8 mg/Tab. Bot. 100s, 1000s. *Rx.*
Use: Bronchodilator, decongestant, sedative, hypnotic.

Ceepryn. Cetylpyridinium Cl. *otc.*
Use: Antiseptic.
See: Cēpacol Lozenges, Soln., Troches (J.B. Williams).

Cee with Bee. (Wesley) Vitamins B_1 15 mg, B_2 10.2 mg, B_3 50 mg, B_5 10 mg, B_6 5 mg, C 300 mg, tartrazine. Bot. 100s, 1000s. *otc.*
Use: Vitamin supplement.

•**cefaclor,** (SEFF-uh-klor) U.S.P. 23.
Use: Antibacterial, cephalosporin.
See: Ceclor, Cap. (Lilly).

•**cefadroxil,** (SEFF-uh-DROX-ill) U.S.P. 23.
Use: Antibacterial, cephalosporin.
See: Duricef, Cap., Tab., Susp. (Bristol-Myers).

cefadroxil. (Various Mfr.) Cefadroxil Cap.: 500 mg/Bot 100s. **Tab.:** 1 g/Bot 24s. **Oral Susp.:** 125 mg/5ml, 250 mg/5ml, 500 mg/5 ml. Bot 50 and 100 ml (125 and 250 mg only). *Rx.*

Use: Anti-infective, cephalosporin.

Cefadyl. (Apothecon) Cephapirin sodium 500 mg, 1 g or 2 g/Vial.; Piggyback vial 1 g, 2 g or 4 g; Bulk vial 20 g. *Rx.*
Use: Anti-infective, cephalosporin.

•**cefamandole.** (SEFF-ah-MAN-dole) USAN.
Use: Antibacterial.

•**cefamandole nafate for injection,** (SEFF-uh-MAN-dahl NA-fate) U.S.P. 23.
Use: Antibacterial, cephalosporin.
See: Mandol, Amp. (Lilly).

•**cefamandole sodium,** U.S.P. 23.
Use: Antibacterial, cephalosporin.

Cefanex. (Apothecon) Cephalexin monohydrate 250 mg or 500 mg/Cap. Bot. 100s. *Rx.*
Use: Anti-infective, cephalosporin.

•**cefaparole.** (SEFF-ah-pah-ROLE) USAN.
Use: Antibacterial.

•**cefatrizine.** (SEFF-ah-TRY-zeen) USAN.
Use: Antibacterial, cephalosporin.

•**cefazaflur sodium.** (seff-AZE-ah-flure) USAN.
Use: Antibacterial, cephalosporin.

•**cefazolin,** U.S.P. 23.
Use: Antibacterial (systemic), cephalosporin.

•**cefazolin sodium, injection,** (seff-uh-zoe-lin) U.S.P. 23.
Use: Antibacterial (systemic), cephalosporin.
See: Ancef, Vial (SK-Beecham).
  Kefzol, Amp. (Lilly).

cefazolin sodium. (Apothecon). 250 mg/Vial; 500 mg, 1 g/Vial, piggyback vial; 5 g, 10 g, 20 g,/bulk pkg.
Use: Antibacterial (systemic), cephalosporin.

•**cefbuperazone.** (SEFF-byoo-PURR-ah-zone) USAN.
Use: Antibacterial, cephalosporin.

•**cefdinir.** (SEFF-dih-ner) USAN.
Use: Antibacterial, cephalosporin.

•**cefepime.** (SEFF-eh-pim) USAN.
Use: Antibacterial.

•**cefepime hydrochloride.** (SEFF-eh-pim) USAN.
Use: Antibacterial.
See: Maxipime, Pow. for Inj. (B-M Squibb).

•**cefetecol.** (seff-EH-teh-kahl) USAN.
Use: Antibacterial, cephalosporin.

Cefinal II. (Alto) Salicymide 150 mg, acetaminophen 250 mg, doxylamine succinate 25 mg/Tab. Bot. 100s. *otc.*
Use: Analgesic combination.

•**cefixime.** (SEFF-IKS-eem) U.S.P. 23.
Use: Antibacterial, cephalosporin.
See: Suprax (Lederle).

Cefizox. (SK-Beecham) Semisynthetic cephalosporin equivalent to: **Vials:** 1 g, 2 g, 10 g of ceftizoxime/Vial. **Piggyback Vials:** 1 g, 2 g/100 ml. **Minibags:** 1 g, 2 g/50 ml w/dextrose injection (D5W). *Rx.*
Use: Anti-infective, cephalosporin.

•**cefmenoxine hydrochloride, sterile,** U.S.P. 23.
Use: Antibacterial, cephalosporin.
See: Takeda (Abbott).

•**cefmetazole,** (seff-MET-ah-zole) U.S.P. 23.
Use: Antibacterial, cephalosporin.

•**cefmetazole sodium, sterile,** (seff-MET-ah-zole) U.S.P. 23.
Use: Antibacterial, cephalosporin.
See: Zefazone (Pharmacia & Upjohn).

Cefobid. (Roerig) Cefoperazone sodium 1 g or 2 g/Vial. 1 g, 2 g PBU 10 pack. *Rx.*
Use: Anti-infective, cephalosporin.

Cefol Filmtab. (Abbott) Vitamins B_1 15 mg, B_2 10 mg, B_6 5 mg, B_{12} 6 mcg, C 750 mg, E 30 mg, B_5 20 mg, B_3 100 mg, folic acid 0.5 mg/Tab. Bot. 100s. *otc.*
Use: Vitamin/mineral supplement.

•**cefonicid monosodium.** (seh-FAHN-ih-SID MAHN-oh-SO-dee-uhm) USAN.
Use: Antibacterial, cephalosporin.

•**cefonicid sodium, sterile,** (seh-FAHN-ih-SID) U.S.P. 23.
Use: Antibacterial, cephalosporin.

•**cefoperazone sodium,** (SEFF-oh-PUR-uh-zone) U.S.P. 23.
Use: Antibacterial, cephalosporin.
See: Cefobid, Inj. (Roerig).

•**ceforanide for injection,** (seh-FAR-ah-NIDE) U.S.P. 23.
Use: Antibacterial, cephalosporin.

Cefotan. (Zeneca) Cefotetan disodium 1 g/10 ml, 1 g/100 ml or 2 g/100 ml. Vial. *Rx.*
Use: Anti-infective, cephalosporin.

•**cefotaxime sodium,** (seff-oh-TAX-eem) U.S.P. 23.
Use: Antibacterial, cephalosporin.
See: Claforan, Inj. (Hoechst Marion Roussel).

•**cefotetan,** (SEFF-oh-tee-tan) U.S.P. 23.
Use: Antibacterial, cephalosporin.

•**cefotetan disodium sterile,** (SEFF-oh-tee-tan die-SO-dee-uhm) U.S.P. 23.
Use: Antibacterial
See: Cefotan (Zeneca).

•**cefotiam hydrochloride sterile,** (SEFF-

oh-TIE-am) U.S.P. 23.
Use: Antibacterial, cephalosporin.

•**cefoxitin.** (seff-OX-ih-tin) USAN.
Use: Antibacterial, cephalosporin.
See: Mefoxin, Inj. (Merck).

•**cefoxitin sodium,** (seff-OX-ih-tin) U.S.P. 23.
Use: Antibacterial, cephalosporin.

•**cefpimizole.** (seff-PIH-mih-zole) USAN.
Use: Antibacterial, cephalosporin.

•**cefpimizole sodium.** (seff-PIH-mih-zole) USAN.
Use: Antibacterial, cephalosporin.
See: Mefoxin, Inj., Pow. for Inj. (Merck).

•**cefpiramide,** (SEFF-PIHR-am-ide) U.S.P. 23.
Use: Antibacterial, cephalosporin.

•**cefpiramide sodium.** (SEFF-PIHR-am ide) USAN.
Use: Antibacterial, cephalosporin.

•**cefpirome sulfate.** (SEFF-pihr-ome) USAN.
Use: Antibacterial, cephalosporin.

cefpodoxime proxetil. (SEFF-pode-OX-eem PROX-uh-til) USAN.
Use: Antibacterial, cephalosporin.
See: Vantin Gran. for Susp., Tab. (Pharmacia & Upjohn).

•**cefprozil,** (SEFF-pro-zill) U.S.P. 23.
Use: Antibacterial, cephalosporin.
See: Cefzil Pow. for Susp., Tab. (Bristol Labs.)

•**cefroxadine.** (SEFF-ROX-ah-deen) USAN.
Use: Antibacterial, cephalosporin.

•**cefsulodin sodium,** (SEFF-SULL-ohdin) USAN.
Use: Antibacterial, cephalosporin.

•**ceftazidime,** (seff-TAZE-ih-deem) U.S.P. 23.
Use: Antibacterial, cephalosporin.
See: Ceptaz, Inj. (Glaxo).
Fortaz, Inj. (Glaxo).
Tazicef, Inj. (Abbott)
Tazidime, Inj. (Lilly).

•**ceftibuten.** (seff-TIE-byoo-ten) USAN.
Use: Antibacterial.
See: Cedax, Cap., Susp. (Schering-Plough).

Ceftin. (Glaxo Wellcome) Cefuroxime axetil **Tab:** 125 mg, 250 mg or 500 mg/ Tab. Bot. 20s, 60s, UD 50s, 100s. *Rx.*
Susp.: 125 mg/5 ml, sucrose/Bot. 50 ml, 100 ml, 200 ml. *Rx.*
Use: Anti-infective, cephalosporin.

•**ceftizoxime sodium,** (SEFF-tih-ZOX-eem) U.S.P. 23.
Use: Antibacterial, cephalosporin.

•**ceftriaxone sodium,** (SEFF-TRY-AXE-own) U.S.P. 23.
Use: Antibacterial, cephalosporin.
See: Rocephin, Inj. (Roche).

•**cefuroxime,** (SEFF-yur-OX-eem) U.S.P. 23
Use: Antibacterial, cephalosporin.
See: Ceftin, Tab. (Glaxo Wellcome).

•**cefuroxime axetil.** (SEFF-your-OX-eem ACK-seh-TILL) USAN. U.S.P. 23.
Use: Antibacterial, cephalosporin.
See: Ceftin, Tab. (Allen & Hanburys).

•**cefuroxime pivoxetil.** (SEFF-your-OX-eem pih-VOX-eh-till) USAN.
Use: Antibacterial, cephalosporin.

•**cefuroxime sodium,** U.S.P. 23.
Use: Antibacterial, cephalosporin.
See: Kefurox, Pow. for Inj. (Lilly).
Zinacef, Inj., Pow. for Inj. (Glaxo Wellcome).

cefuroxime sodium. (Various) Pow. for Inj.: 750, 1.5 g in 10 ml (750 mg only), 20 ml (1.5 g only), 100 ml piggyback vials; 7.5 g/vial pharmacy bulk package. *Rx.*
Use: Anti-infective, cephalosporin.

cefuroxime sodium, sterile.
Use: Anti-infective, cephalosporin.
See: Kefurox, Inj. (Lilly).
Zinacef, Inj. (Glaxo).

Cefzil. (Bristol-Myers) Cefprozil. **Tab:** 250 mg, 500 mg. Bot. 100s and UD 100s.
Pow. Susp.: 125 mg/5 ml, 250 mg/5 ml. Sucrose, aspartame, phenylalanine 28 mg/5 ml. Bot. 50 and 100 ml. *Rx.*
Use: Anti-infective, cephalosporin.

•**celgosivir hydrochloride.** USAN.
Use: Antiviral.

Celestone. (Schering-Plough) **Tab.:** Betamethasone 0.6 mg. Bot. 100s, 500s, UD 21s. **Syr.:** Betamethasone 0.6 mg/5 ml, alcohol < 1%. Bot. 120 ml. *Rx.*
Use: Corticosteroid.

Celestone Phosphate Injection. (Schering-Plough) Betamethasone sodium phosphate 4 mg/ml equivalent to betamethasone alcohol 3 mg/ml. Vial 5 ml. *Rx.*
Use: Corticosteroid.

Celestone Soluspan. (Schering-Plough) Betamethasone sodium phosphate 3 mg, betamethasone acetate 3 mg, dibasic sodium phosphate 7.1 mg, monobasic sodium phosphate 3.4 mg, edetate disodium 0.1 mg, benzalkonium Cl 0.2 mg/ml. Vial 5 ml. *Rx.*
Use: Corticosteroid.

•**celiprolol hydrochloride.** (SEE-lih-PRO-lahl) USAN.

Use: Anti-adrenergic (β-receptor).

Cellaburate. (Eastman Kodak) Cellulose acetate butyrate.
Use: Pharmaceutic aid (plastic filming agent).

Cellase W-100.
W/Alpha-amylase W-100, proteinase W-300, lipase, estrone, testosterone, vitamins, minerals.
See: Geramine, Tab. (Zeneca).

CellCept. (Roche) Mycophenolate mofetil 250 mg/Cap. Bot. 100s, 500s, UD 100s. *Rx.*
Use: Immunosuppressive drug.

Cellepacbin. (Arthrins) Vitamins A 1200 IU, B_1 1.5 mg, B_2 1.5 mg, B_6 0.75 mg, niacinamide 7.5 mg, panthenol 3 mg, C 20 mg, B_{12} 2 mcg, E 1 IU/Cap. Bot. 180s. *otc.*
Use: Vitamin supplement.

Cellothyl. (Numark) Methylcellulose 0.5 g/Tab. Bot. 100s, 1000s. *otc.*
Use: Laxative.

Cellufresh. (Allergan) Carboxymethylcellulose sodium 0.5%, NaCl. In 0.3 ml single-use containers (4s, 30s). *otc.*
Use: Ocular lubricant.

•**cellulase.** (SELL-you-lace) USAN. A concentrate of cellulose-splitting enzymes derived from *Aspergillus niger* and other sources.
Use: Enzyme (digestive adjunct).
W/Bile salts, mixed conjugated, pancrelipase.
See: Cotazym-B, Tab. (Organon).
W/Mylase, prolase, calcium carbonate, magnesium glycinate.
See: Zylase, Tab. (Eon Labs).
W/Mylase, prolase, lipase.
See: Ku-Zyme, Cap. (Kremers-Urban).
W/Pepsin, glutamic acid, pancreatin, ox bile extract.
See: Kanulase, Tab. (Sandoz Consumer).
W/Pepsin, pancreatin, dehydrocholic acid.
See: Gastroenterase, Tab. (Wallace).

cellulose. (SELL-you-lohs)
W/Hexachlorophene.
See: ZeaSorb, Pow. (Stiefel).

•**cellulose acetate,** (SELL-you-lohs) N.F. 18.
Use: Pharmaceutic aid (coating agent), polymer membrane (insoluble).

•**cellulose acetate phthalate,** (SELL-you-lohs) N.F. 18. Cellulose, acetate, 1,2-benzenedicarboxylate.
Use: Pharmaceutic aid (tablet coating agent).

cellulose, carboxymethyl, sodium salt. (SELL-you-lohs) Carboxymethylcellulose Sodium, U.S.P. 23.

cellulose, hydroxypropyl methyl ether. Hydroxypropyl Methylcellulose, U.S.P. 23.

cellulose methyl ether. (SELL-you-lohs)
See: Methylcellulose, Prep. (Various Mfr.).

•**cellulose microcrystalline,** (SELL-you-lohs) N.F. 18.
Use: Pharmaceutic aid (tablet and capsule diluent).

cellulose, nitrate. Pyroxylin.

•**cellulose, oxidized,** (SELL-you-lohs) U.S.P. 23.
Use: Local hemostatic.

•**cellulose, oxidized regenerated,** (SELL-you-lohs) U.S.P. 23.
Use: Local hemostatic.

cellulose, powdered. (SELL-you-lohs)
Use: Tablet and capsule diluent.

•**cellulose sodium phosphate,** (SELL-you-lohs) U.S.P. 23.
Use: Antiurolithic.
See: Calcibind (Mission).

cellulosic acid.
See: Oxidized Cellulose. (Various Mfr.).

cellulolytic.
W/Amylolytic, proteolytic.
See: Trienzyme, Tab. (Forest Pharm.).

cellulolytic enzyme.
See: Cellulase (Various Mfr.).
W/Amylolytic, proteolytic enzymes, lipase, phenobarbital, hyoscyamine sulfate, atropine sulfate.
See: Arco-Lipase Plus, Tab. (Arco).
W/Amylolytic enzyme, proteolytic enzyme, lipolytic enzyme, butisol sodium, belladonna.
See: Butibel-zyme, Tab. (McNeil).
W/Calcium carbonate, glycine, amylolytic and proteolytic enzymes.
See: Co-Gel, Tab. (Arco).
W/Proteolytic enzyme, amylolytic enzyme, lipolytic enzyme.
See: Ku-Zyme, Cap. (Kremers-Urban). Zymme, Cap. (Scrip).
W/Proteolytic, amylolytic, lipolytic enzymes, iron, ox bile.
See: Spaszyme, Tab. (Dooner).

Celluvisc. (Allergan) Carboxymethylcellulose 1%, NaCl, KCl, sodium lactate. Ophthalmic soln. Single use containers 0.3 ml (UD 30s). *otc.*
Use: Artificial tear solution.

Celontin. (Parke-Davis) Methsuximide 150 mg or 300 mg/Kapseal. Bot. 100s. *Rx.*

Use: Anticonvulsant.

Cel-U-Jec. (Roberts) Betamethasone sodium phosphate 4 mg (equivalent to betamethasone alcohol 3 mg)/ml. Soln. Inj. Vial 5 ml. *Rx.*
Use: Corticosteroid.

Cenafed. (Century) **Tab.:** Pseudoephedrine HCl 30 mg or 60 mg. Bot. 100s, 1000s. **Syr.:** Pseudoephedrine HCl 30 mg/5 ml. Bot. 120 ml, pt, gal. *otc.*
Use: Decongestant.

Cenafed Plus. (Century) Pseudoephedrine HCl 60 mg, triprolidine HCl 2.5 mg/Tab. Bot. 100s. *otc.*
Use: Decongestant, antihistamine.

Cena-K. (Century) Potassium and Cl 20 mEq/15 ml (10% KCl), saccharin. Bot. pt, gal. *Rx.*
Use: Potassium supplement.

Cenalax. (Century) Bisacodyl. **Tab.:** 5 mg. Bot. 100s, 1000s. **Supp.:** 10 mg. Pkg. 12s, 1000s. *otc.*
Use: Laxative.

Cenolate. (Abbott Hospital Prods) Sodium ascorbate 562.5 mg/ml (equivalent to 500 mg/ml ascorbic acid), sodium hydrosulfate 0.5%. Inj. Amp. 1 ml, 2 ml. *Rx.*
Use: Vitamin C supplement.

Centeon Thyroid. (Rhone-Poulenc Rorer) Dessicated animal thyroid glands (active thyroid hormones) T-4 thyroxine, T-3 thyronine 0.25 gr, 0.5 gr, 1 gr, 1.5 gr, 2 gr, 3 gr, 4 gr or 5 gr/Tab. Bot. 100s, 1000s. Handy Hundreds, Carton Strip 100s. *Rx.*
Use: Thyroid hormone.

Center-Al. (Center) Allergenic extracts, alum precipitated 10,000 PNU/ml or 20,000 PNU/ml. Vial 10 ml, 30 ml. *Rx.*
Use: Treatment of allergy due to pollens or house dust.

Centrafree. (NBTY) Iron 27 mg, vitamins A 5000 IU, D 400 IU, E 30 IU, B_1 2.25 mg, B_2 2.6 mg, B_3 20 mg, B_5 10 mg, B_6 3 mg, B_{12} 9 mcg, C 90 mg, folic acid 0.4 mg, biotin 45 mcg, Ca, Cl, Cr, Cu, I, K, Mg, Mn, Mo, P, Se, Zn/Tab. Bot. 100s. *otc.*
Use: Vitamin/mineral supplement.

central nervous system depressants.
See: Sedatives.

central nervous system stimulants.
See: Amphetamine (Various Mfr.).
D-Amphetamine (Various Mfr.).
Anorexigenic agents.
Caffeine (Various Mfr.).
Coramine, Liq., Inj. (Novartis).

Desoxyephedrine HCl, Tab. (Various Mfr.).
Desoxyn HCl, Tab. Gradumet. (Abbott).
Dexedrine, Preps. (SK-Beecham).
Methamphetamine HCl (Various Mfr.).
Ritalin HCl, Tab., Inj. (Novartis).

Centrovite Advanced Formula. (Rugby) Fe 18 mg, A 5000 IU, D 400 IU, E 30 IU, B_1 1.5 mg, B_2 1.7 mg, B_3 20 mg, B_5 10 mg, B_6 2 mg, B_{12} 6 mcg, C 60 mg, Fa 0.4 mg, biotin 30 mcg, Ca, Cl, Cr, Cu, I, vitamin K, Mg, Mn, Mo, Ni, P, Se, Si, Sn, V, Zn, K. Tab. Bot. 100s. *otc.*
Use: Vitamin/mineral supplement.

Centrovite Jr. (Rugby) Iron 18 mg, vitamins A 5000 IU, D 400 IU, E 15 IU, B_1 1.5 mg, B_2 1.7 mg, B_3 20 mg, B_5 10 mg, B_6 2 mg, B_{12} 6 mcg, C 60 mg, folic acid 0.4 mg, biotin 45 mcg, Cr, Cu, I, Mg, Mn, Mo, Zn/Chew. Tab. Bot. 60s. *otc.*
Use: Vitamin/mineral supplement.

Centrum. (Lederle) Vitamins A 5000 IU, E 30 IU, C 90 mg, folic acid 400 mcg, B_1 2.25 mg, B_2 2.6 mg, B_6 3 mg, niacinamide 20 mg, B_{12} 9 mcg, D 400 IU, biotin 45 mcg, pantothenic acid 10 mg, calcium 162 mg, phosphorus 125 mg, iodine 150 mcg, iron 27 mg, magnesium 100 mg, potassium 30 mg, manganese 5 mg, chromium 25 mcg, selenium 25 mcg, molybdenum 25 mcg, zinc 15 mg, copper 2 mg, K 25 mcg, Cl 27.2 mg/Tab. *otc.*
Use: Vitamin/mineral supplement.

Centrum, Advanced Formula. (Lederle) Vitamins A 2500 IU, E 30 IU, C 60 mg, B_1 1.5 mg, B_2 1.7 mg, B_3 20 mg, B_5 10 mg, B_6 2 mg, B_{12} 6 mcg, D_2 400 IU, iron 9 mg, biotin 300 mcg per 15 ml. With I, Zn, Mn, Cr, Mo, alcohol. 6.6%. Liq. Bot. 236 ml. *otc.*
Use: Vitamin/mineral supplement.

Centrum Jr. (Lederle) Vitamins A 5000 IU, D 400 IU, E 30 IU, C 60 mg, folic acid 400 mcg, B_1 1.5 mg, B_6 2 mg, B_{12} 6 mcg, riboflavin 1.7 mg, niacinamide 20 mg, iron 18 mg, magnesium 25 mg, copper 2 mg, zinc 15 mg, biotin 45 mcg, panthothenic acid 10 mg, molybdenum 20 mcg, chromium 20 mcg, iodine 150 mcg, manganese 1 mg/Chew. Tab. Bot. 60s. *otc.*
Use: Vitamin/mineral supplement.

Centrum Jr. + Extra C. (Lederle) Vitamins A 5000 IU D 400 IU, E 30 IU, C 300 mg, folic acid 400 mcg, biotin 45 mcg, B_1 1.5 mg, B_5 10 mg, B_2 1.7 mg, B_3 20 mg, B_6 2 mg, B_{12} 6 mcg, K, iron

18 mg, Mg, I, Cu, P, calcium 108 mg, zinc 15 mg, Mn, Mo, Cr, biotin 45 mcg, sugar, lactose/Chew. Tab. Bot. 60s. *otc.*
Use: Vitamin/mineral supplement.

Centrum, Jr. + Extra Calcium. (Lederle) Calcium 160 mg, iron 18 mg, vitamins A 5000 IU, D 400 IU, E 30 mg, B_1 1.5 mg, B_2 1.7 mg, B_3 20 mg, B_5 10 mg, B_6 2 mg, B_{12} 6 mcg, C 60 mg, folic acid 400 mcg, Cr, Cu, I, Mn, Mg, Mo, P, Zn 15 mg, vitamin K, biotin 45 mcg, sugar/Chew. Tab. Bot. 60s. *otc.*
Use: Vitamin/mineral supplement.

Centrum, Jr. + Iron. (Lederle) Iron 18 mg, vitamins A 5000 IU, D 400 IU, E 30 IU, B_1 1.5 mg, B_2 1.7 mg, B_3 20 mg, B_5 10 mg, B_6 2 mg, B_{12} 6 mcg, C 60 mg, folic acid 0.4 mg, Ca, Cr, Cu, I, Mg, Mn, Mo, P, zinc 15 mg, biotin 45 mcg, vitamin K/Chew. Tab. Bot. 60s. *otc.*
Use: Vitamin/mineral supplement.

Centrum Silver. (Lederle) Tab.: Vitamin A 5000 IU, D 400 IU, E 45 IU, B_1 1.5 mg, B_2 1.7 mg, B_3 20 mg, B_5 10 mg, B_6 3 mg, B_{12} 25 mcg, C 60 mg, iron 4 mg, folic acid 0.4 mg, Ca 200 mg, Zn 15 mg, biotin 30 mcg, vitamin K, Cu, I, Mg, P, Cl, Cr, Mn, Mo, Ni, Se, Si, V. Bot. 60s, 100s, 180s, *otc.*
Use: Vitamin/mineral supplement.

Centrum Silver Gel-Tabs. (Lederle) Vitamins A 6000 IU, D 400 IU, E 45 IU, B_1 1.5 mg, B_2 1.7 mg, B_3 20 mg, B_5 10 mg, B_6 3 mg, B_{12} 25 mcg, C 60 mg, K 10 mcg, biotin 30 mcg, folic acid 200 mcg, Fe 9 mg. With Ca 200 mg, Cu, I, Mg, P, Zn, Cl, Cr, Mn, Mo, Ni, K, Se, Si and V. Tab. Bot. 60s. *otc.*
Use: Vitamin/mineral supplement.

Centurion A-Z. (Mission) Fe 27 mg, A 5000 IU, D 400 IU, E 30 IU, B_1 2.25 mg, B_2 2.6 mg, B_3 20 mg, B_5 10 mg, B_6 3 mg, B_{12} 9 mcg, C 90 mg, Fa 0.4 mg, biotin 0.45 mg, Ca, Cl, Cr, Cu, I, K, Mg, Mn, Mo, P, Se, Zn, vitamin K. Tab. Bot. 130s. *otc.*
Use: Vitamin/mineral supplement.

Ceo-Two. (Beutlich) Potassium bitartrate, sodium bicarbonate in polyethylene glycol base/Supp. 10s. *otc.*
Use: Laxative.

Cēpacol. (J.B. Williams) Cetylpyridinium Cl 0.05%, alcohol 14%, tartrazine, saccharin. Liq. Bot. 360 ml, 540 ml, 720 ml, 960 ml. *otc.*
Use: Antiseptic.

Cēpacol Anesthetic Lozenges. (J.B. Williams) Benzocaine 10 mg, cetylpyridinium Cl 0.07%, tartrazine. Pkg. 18s, 24s. *otc.*

Use: Anesthetic, antiseptic.

Cēpacol Throat Lozenges. (J.B. Williams) Cetylpyridinium Cl 0.07%, benzyl alcohol 0.3%, tartrazine. Pkg. 27s, 40s. *otc.*
Use: Antiseptic.

Cēpastat Cherry Lozenges. (SK-Beecham) Phenol 14.5 mg, menthol, sorbitol, saccharin. Sugar free. Box 18s. *otc.*
Use: Anesthetic.

Cēpastat Extra Strength. (SK-Beecham) Phenol 29 mg, menthol, sorbitol, eucalyptus oil. Sugar free. Loz. Pkg. 18s. *otc.*
Use: Anesthetic.

cephacetrile sodium. (SEFF-ah-seh-TRILE) USAN.
Use: Antibacterial, cephalosporin.

•**cephalexin,** (SEFF-ah-LEX-in) U.S.P. 23.
Use: Antibacterial, cephalosporin.
See: Biocef, Cap., Pow. (Inter. Ehtical Labs).
  Keflex, Cap., Susp. (Dista).

•**cephalexin hydrochloride,** (SEFF-ah-LEX-in) U.S.P. 23.
Use: Antibacterial, cephalosporin.
See: Keftab, Tab. (Dista).

cephalexin monohydrate. (SEFF-ah-LEX-in)
Use: Anti-infective, cephalosporin.
See: Biocef, Cap., Pow.. (Inter. Ethical Labs).
  Cefalexin, Cap., Tab., Susp. (Various).
  Keflex, Cap., Susp. (Dista).

cephalin.
W/Lecithin with choline base, lipositol.
See: Alcolec, Cap., Granules (American Lecithin).

•**cephaloglycin.** (SEFF-ah-low-GLIE-sin) USAN. U.S.P. XX.
Use: Antibacterial.

•**cephaloridine.** (SEFF-ah-lor-ih-deen) USAN. U.S.P. XX.
Use: Antibacterial, cephalosporin.

•**cephalothin sodium,** (seff-AY-low-thin) U.S.P. 23.
Use: Antibacterial, cephalosporin.
See: Keflin, Vial (Lilly).

•**cephapirin benzathine,** U.S.P. 23.
Use: Antibacterial.

•**cephapirin sodium, sterile,** (SEFF-uh-PIE-rin) U.S.P. 23.
Use: Antibacterial, cephalosporin.
See: Cefadyl, Vial (Bristol).

cephazolin sodium.
See: Cefazolin.

•**cephradine,** (SEFF-ruh-deen) U.S.P. 23.

Cap., Inj., Oral Susp., Sterile U.S.P. 23.
Use: Antibacterial, cephalosporin.
See: Velosef, Cap., Inj., Susp. (Squibb).

Cephulac. (Hoechst Marion Roussel) Lactulose syrup 10 g/15 ml (less than galactose 2.2 g, lactose 1.2 g, other sugars 1.2 g). Bot. 473 ml, 1890 ml, UD 15 ml, 30 ml. Box 100s. *Rx.*
Use: Laxative.

Ceptaz. (Glaxo Wellcome) Ceftazidime pentahydrate with L-arginine at a concentration of 349 mg/g ceftazidime activity equivalent to anhydrous ceftazidime. Vial. 1 and 2 g, Infusion packs 1 and 2 g, Pharmacy bulk packages 10 g. *Rx.*
Use: Anti-infective, cephalosporin.

ceramide trihexosidase/alpha- galactosidase a.
Use: Fabry's disease. [Orphan drug]

Cerapon. Triethanolamine Polypeptide Oleate-Condensate. (Purdue Frederick).
See: Cerumenex, Drops (Purdue Frederick).

Cerebyx. (Parke-Davis) Fosphenytoin 150 mg (100 mg phenytoin sodium) in 2 ml vials and 750 mg (500 mg phenytoin sodium) in 10 ml vials. *Rx.*
Use: Treatment of certain types of seizures.

Ceredase. (Genzyme) Alglucerase. Inj. 10 U/ml or 80 U/ml. Bot. 5 ml. *Rx.*
Use: Enzyme replacement for Gaucher's disease.

cerelose.
See: Glucose (Various Mfr.).

Ceretex. (Enzyme Process) Iron 15 mg, vitamins B_{12} 10 mcg, B_1 2 mg, B_6 1 mg, niacinamide 1 mg, pantothenic acid 0.15 mg, B_2 2 mg, iodine 15 mg/2 ml. Bot. 60 ml, 8 oz. *otc.*
Use: Vitamin/mineral supplement.

Cerezyme. (Genzyme) Imiglucerase 212 units (equiv. to a withdrawal dose of 200 units). Pow. for Inj. Vials. *Rx.*
Use: Treatment for Gaucher's disease.

•cerivastatin sodium. (seh-RIHV-ah-statin) USAN.
Use: Antihyperlipidemic; inhibitor.

•ceronapril. (seh-ROW-nap-rill) USAN.
Use: Antihypertensive.

Cerose. (Wyeth-Ayerst) Dextromethorphan HBr 15 mg, chlorpheniramine maleate 4 mg, phenylephrine HCl 10 mg/5 ml, alcohol 2.4%, saccharin. Sugar free. Liq. Bot. 120 ml, 480 ml. *otc.*
Use: Antitussive, antihistamine, decongestant.

Cerovite. (Rugby) Iron 18 mg, vitamins A 5000 IU, D 400 IU, E 30 IU, B_1 1.5 mg, B_2 1.7 mg, B_3 20 mg, B_5 10 mg, B_6 2 mg, B_{12} 6 mcg, C 60 mg, folic acid 0.4 mg, Ca, Cl, Cr, Cu, I, Mg, Mn, Mo, Ni, P, Se, Si, SN, V, biotin 30 mcg, vitamin K, Zn 15 mg/Tab. Bot. 130s. *otc.*
Use: Vitamin/mineral supplement.

Cerovite Advanced Formula. (Rugby) Iron 18 mg, vitamins A 5000 IU, D 400 IU, E 30 IU, B_1 1.5 mg, B_2 1.7 mg, B_3 20 mg, B_5 10 mg, B_6 2 mg, B_{12} 6 mcg, C 60 mg, folic acid 0.4 mg, biotin 30 mcg, Ca, P, I, Mg, Cu, Mn, K, Cl, Cr, Mo, Se, Ni, Si, Sn, V, vitamin K, Zn 15 mg/Tab. Bot. 130s, 200s. *otc.*
Use: Iron with vitamin supplement.

Cerovite Jr.. (Rugby) Iron 18 mg, vitamins A 5000 IU, D 400 IU, E 15 IU, B_1 1.5 mg, B_2 1.7 mg, B_3 20 mg, B_5 10 mg, B_6 2 mg, B_{12} 6 mcg, C 60 mg, folic acid 0.4 mg, Cu, I, Mg, Zn, Mn, Mo, biotin 45 mcg, Cr, sugar/Tab. Bot. 60s. *otc.*
Use: Vitamin/mineral supplement.

Cerovite Senior. (Rugby) Vitamins A 6000 IU, D 400 IU, E 45 IU, B_1 1.5 mg, B_2 1.7 mg, B_3 20 mg, B_5 10 mg, B_6 3 mg, B_{12} 25 mcg, C 60 mg, iron 9 mg, folic acid 0.2 mg, Ca 200 mg, Zn 15 mg, biotin 30 mcg, Cu, I, Mg, P, Cl, Cr, Mn, Mo, Ni, Se, Si, V, vitamin K. Tab. Bot. 60s. *otc.*
Use: Vitamin/mineral supplement.

Certagen. (Goldline) Iron 18 mg, A 5000 IU, D 400 IU, E 30 IU, B_1 1.5 mg, B_2 1.7 mg, B_3 20 mg, B_5 10 mg, B_6 2 mg, B_{12} 6 mcg, C 60 mg, folic acid 0.4 mg, biotin 30 mcg, Ca, P, I, Mg, Cu, Mn, K, Cl, Cr, Mo, Se, Ni, Si, Sn, V, vitamin K, Zn 15 mg/Tab. Bot. 130s, 1000s. *otc.*
Use: Vitamin/mineral supplement.

Certagen Liquid. (Goldline) Vitamins A 2500 IU, B_1 1.5 mg, B_2 1.7 mg, B_3 20 mg, B_5 10 mg, B_6 2 mg, B_{12} 6 mcg, C 60 mg, D_3 400 IU, E 30 IU, biotin 300 mcg, iron 9 mg, Zn 3 mg, Cr, I, Mn, Mo/15 ml. Alcohol 6.6%. Liq. Bot. 237 ml. *otc.*
Use: Vitamin/mineral supplement.

Certagen Senior. (Goldline) Vitamin A 6000 IU, B_1 1.5 mg, B_2 1.7 mg, B_6 3 mg, B_{12} 25 mcg, C 60 mg, D 400 IU, E 45 IU, vitamin K, biotin 30 mcg, folic acid 200 mcg, B_3 20 mg, B_5 10 mg, Ca 80 mg, Cl, Cr, Cu, I, Fe 3 mg, Mg, Mn, Mo, Ni, P, K, Se, Si, V, Zn 15 mg/Tab. Bot. 60s. *otc.*
Use: Vitamin and mineral supplement.

CertaVite. (Major) Vitamin A 5000 IU, D

400 IU, E 30 IU, K$_1$, C 60 mg, B$_1$ 1.5 mg, B$_2$ 1.7 mg, B$_3$ 20 mg, B$_6$ 2 mg, B$_{12}$ 6 mcg, B$_5$ 10 mg, folic acid 0.4 mg, biotin 30 mcg, iron 18 mg, Ca, P, I, Mg, Cu, Zn, Mn, K, Cl, Cr, Mo, Se, Ni, Si, V, B. Tab. Bot. 130s, 300s. *otc.*
Use: Vitamin/mineral supplement.

Certa-Vite Golden. (Major) Vitamin A 6000 IU, D 400 IU, E 45 IU, B$_1$ 1.5 mg, B$_2$ 1.7 mg, B$_3$ 20 mg, B$_5$ 10 mg, B$_6$ 3 mg, B$_{12}$ 25 mcg, C 60 mg, vitamin K, calcium 200 mg, zinc 15 mg, biotin 30 mcg, Cl, Cr, Cu, I, K, Mg, Mn, Mo, Ni, P, Se, Si, V. Tab. Bot. 60s. *otc.*
Use: Vitamin/mineral supplement.

cervical ripening agent.
See: Cervidil, Insert. (Forest).
Prepidil, Gel. (Pharmacia & Upjohn).

Cervidil. (Forest) Dinoprostone 10 mg/ Insert. 1 each. *Rx.*
Use: Agent for cervical ripening.

•**ceruletide.** (seh-ROO-leh-tide) USAN.
Use: Stimulant (gastric secretory).

•**ceruletide diethylamine.** (seh-ROO-leh-tide die-ETH-ill-ah-meen) USAN.
Use: Stimulant (gastric secretory).

Cerumenex Drops. (Purdue Frederick) Triethanolamine polypeptide oleate-condensate 10%, chlorobutanol in propylene glycol 0.5%. Liq. Dropper bot. 6 ml, 12 ml. *Rx.*
Use: Otic preparation.

cervical ripening agents.
See: Prepidil (Pharmacia & Upjohn).

Cervidil. (Forest) Dinoprostone 10 mg. Insert. 1s. *Rx.*
Use: Agent for cervical ripening.

Ces. (I.C.N.) Conjugated estrogens 0.625 mg, 1.25 mg or 2.5 mg/Tab. *Rx.*
Use: Estrogen.

•**cesium chloride Cs 131.** (SEE-zee-uhm KLOR-ide) USAN.
Use: Radioactive agent.

Ceta. (C & M Pharm) Soap Free. Propylene glycol, hydroxyethylcellulose, cetyl and cetearyl alcohols, sodium lauryl sulfate, parabens. Liq. Bot. 240 ml. *otc.*
Use: Therapeutic skin cleanser.

Ceta-Plus. (Seatrace) Hydrocodone bitartrate 5 mg, acetaminophen 500 mg/ Cap. Bot. 100s. *c-III.*
Use: Narcotic analgesic combination.

•**cetaben sodium.** (SEE-tah-ben) USAN.
Use: Antihyperlipoproteinemic.

Cetacaine. (Cetylite) Benzocaine 14%, butyl aminobenzoate 2%, tetracaine HCl 2%, benzalkonium Cl 0.5%, cetyl dimethyl ethyl ammonium bromide 0.005%. **Aerosol Spray:** 56 g. **Liq.:** 56

g. **Oint.:** Jar 37 g, flavored. **Hosp. Gel:** 29 g. *Rx.*
Use: Local anesthetic, topical.

Cetacort. (Galderma) Hydrocortisone in concentrations of 0.25%, 0.5%, 1% w/ cetyl alcohol, propylene glycol, stearyl alcohol, sodium lauryl sulfate, butylparaben, methylparaben, propylparaben, purified water. Bot. 120 ml (0.25% only), 60 ml (0.5%, 1%). *Rx.*
Use: Corticosteroid, topical.

cetalkonium. (SEET-al-KOE-nee-uhm) F.D.A. Benzylhexadecyldimethylammonium ion.

•**cetalkonium chloride.** (SEET-al-KOE-nee-uhm) USAN.
Use: Anti-infective (topical).
W/Phenylephrine, pyrilamine maleate, thimerosal.
See: Anti-B Mist (DePree).

Cetamide. (Alcon) Sulfacetamide sodium 10%. Sterile ophthalmic oint. Tube 3.5 g. *Rx.*
Use: Anti-infective, ophthalmic.

•**cetamolol hydrochloride.** (SEET-AM-oh-lahl) USAN.
Use: Anti-adrenergic (β-recptor).

Cetaphil. (Galderma) Cetyl alcohol, stearyl alcohol, propylene glycol (cream only), sodium lauryl sulfate, methylparaben, propylparaben, butylparaben, purified water. Cream, Lot. Bot. 480 g (cream), 120 ml, 240 ml, 480 ml (lotion). *otc.*
Use: Skin cleanser.

Cetapred. (Alcon) Sulfacetamide sodium 10%, prednisolone acetate 0.25%. Ophth. Oint. Tube 3.5 g. *Rx.*
Use: Anti-infective, ophthalmic.

Cetazol. (Professional Pharmacal) Acetazolamide 250 mg/Tab. Bot. 100s. *Rx.*
Use: Anticonvulsant, diuretic.

•**cetiedil citrate.** (see-TIE-eh-DILL SIH-trate) USAN.
Use: Vasodilator (peripheral).

•**cetirizine hydrochloride.** USAN.
Use: Antihistamine.
See: Zyrtec, Tab. (Pfizer).

•**cetocycline hydrochloride.** (SEE-toe-SIGH-kleen) USAN.
Use: Antibacterial.

•**cetophenicol.** USAN.
Use: Antibacterial.

•**cetostearyl alcohol,** N.F. 18.
Use: Pharmaceutic aid (emulsifying agent).

•**cetraxate hydrochloride.** (seh-TRAX-ate) USAN.
Use: Antiulcerative (gastrointestinal).

•**cetyl alcohol,** N.F. 18. 1-Hexadecanol.
Use: Pharmaceutic aid (emulsifying and stiffening agent).

Cetylcide Solution. (Cetylite) Cetyldimethylethyl ammonium bromide 6.5%, benzalkonium Cl 6.5%, isopropyl alcohol 13%. Inert ingredients 74%, including sodium nitrite. Bot. 16 oz, 32 oz.
Use: Disinfectant.

cetyldimethyl benzyl ammonium chloride.
W/Benzocaine, ascorbic acid.
See: Locane, Troches (Solvay).
W/Phenylephrine HCl, pyrilamine maleate.
See: Dalihist, Nasal Spray (Dalin).

•**cetyl esters wax,** N.F. 18.
Use: Pharmaceutic aid (stiffening agent).

•**cetylpyridinium chloride,** U.S.P. 23.
Use: Anti-infective (topical), pharmaceutic aid (preservative).
See: Bactalin (LaCrosse).
W/Benzocaine.
See: Axon Throat Loz. (McKesson).
Cēpacol, Throat Loz., (J.B. Williams).
Coirex, Preps. (Solvay).
Oradex-C, Troches (Del Pharm.).
Semets, Troches (SK-Beecham).
Spec-T Sore Throat Loz. (Squibb).
Vicks Medi-Trating Throat Lozenges (Procter & Gamble).
W/Benzocaine.
See: Cēpacol Antiseptic Lozenges (J.B. Williams).
W/Benzocaine, menthol, camphor, eucalyptus oil.
See: Vicks Medi-Trating Throat Lozenges (Procter & Gamble).
W/Dextromethorphan HBr, benzocaine.
See: Thorzettes (Towne).
W/d-Methorphan HBr, phenyltoloxamine dihydrogen citrate, sodium citrate.
See: Exo-Kol, Cough Syrup, Spray, Tab. (Inwood).
W/Phenylephrine HCl, methapyrilene HCl, menthol, eucalyptol, camphor, methyl salicylate.
See: Vicks Sinex Nasal Spray (Procter & Gamble).
W/Phenylpropanolamide HCl, benzocaine, terpin hydrate.
See: S.A.C. Throat Lozenges (Towne).

cetyltrimethyl ammonium bromide.
(Bio Labs.) Cetrimide B.P., Cetavlon, CTAB.
Use: Antiseptic.
W/Lidocaine, hexachlorophene.
See: Aerosept, Aerosol (Dalin).

Cevalin. (Lilly) Ascorbic acid 100 mg or 500 mg/ml. Inj. Amp. 10 ml (100 mg), 1 ml (500 mg). *Rx.*
Use: Vitamin C supplement.

Cevi-Bid. (Geriatric) Ascorbic acid 500 mg/TR Caps. Bot. 30s, 100s, 500s. *otc.*
Use: Vitamin C supplement.

Cevi-Fer. (Geriatric) Ascorbic acid 300 mg, ferrous fumarate 20 mg, folic acid 1 mg/Cap. Bot. 30s, 100s. *Rx.*
Use: Vitamin/mineral supplement.

•**cevimeline hydrochloride.** USAN.
Use: Treatment of Alzheimer's disease.

Ce-Vi-Sol. (Bristol-Myers) Ascorbic acid 35 mg/0.6 ml, alcohol 5%. Bot. w/dropper 50 ml. *otc.*
Use: Vitamin C supplement.

cevitamic acid.
See: Ascorbic acid.

cevitan.
See: Ascorbic acid.

Cewin Tablets. (Sanofi Winthrop) Ascorbic acid. *otc.*
Use: Vitamin C supplement.

ceylon gelatin.
See: Agar.

Cezin. (UAD) Vitamins B_1 20 mg, B_2 10 mg, B_3 100 mg, B_5 20 mg, B_6 5 mg, C 300 mg, magnesium sulfate 70 mg, zinc sulfate 80 mg. Cap. Bot. 100s. *otc.*
Use: Vitamin supplement.

Cezin-S. (UAD) Vitamins A 10,000 IU, D 50 IU, E 50 IU, B_1 10 mg, B_2 5 mg, B_3 50 mg, B_5 10 mg, B_6 2 mg, C 200 mg, folic acid 0.5 mg, zinc 18 mg, Mg, Mn/ Cap. Bot. 100s. *Rx.*
Use: Vitamin supplement.

C Factors "1000" Plus. (Solgar) Vitamins C with rosehips 1000 mg, citrus bioflavonoids 250 mg, rutin 50 mg, hesperidin complex 25 mg. Tab. Bot. 50s, 100s, 250s. *otc.*
Use: Vitamin supplement. *otc.*

C.G. (Sig) Chorionic gonadotropin (lyophilized) 10,000 units, mannitol 100 mg, supplied with diluent. Univial 10 ml. *Rx.*
Use: Chorionic gonadotropin.

CG Disposable Unit.
See: Cardio Green, Vial (Becton Dickinson).

CG Ria. (Abbott Diagnostics) Radioimmunoassay for the quantitative measurement of total circulating serum cholylglycine.
Use: Diagnostic aid.

Chap Cream. (Ar-Ex) Carbonyl diamide. Tube 1.5 oz, 3.25 oz. Jar 4 oz, 9 oz, 18 oz. *otc.*

Use: Emollient.

Chapoline Cream Lotion. (Wade) Glycerine, boric acid, chlorobutanol 0.5%, alcohol 10%. Bot. 4 oz, pt, gal. *otc.*
Use: Emollient.

Chapstick Medicated Lip Balm. (Robins) **Jar:** Petrolatum 60%, camphor 1%, menthol 0.6%, phenol 0.5%, microcrystalline wax, mineral oil, cocoa butter, lanolin, paraffin wax, parabens 7 g. **Squeezable tube:** Petrolatum 67%, camphor 1%, menthol 0.6%, phenol 0.5%, microcrystalline wax, mineral oil, cocoa butter, lanolin, parabens 10 g. **Stick:** Petrolatum 41%, camphor 1%, menthol 0.6%, phenol 0.5%, paraffin wax, mineral oil, cocoa butter, 2-octyl dodecanol, arachidyl propionate, polyphenyl methylsiloxane 556, white wax, oleyl alcohol, isopropyl lanolate, carnauba wax, isopropyl myristate, lanolin, cetyl alcohol, parabens 4.2 g. *otc.*
Use: Mouth/throat product.

Chapstick Sunblock 15. (Robins) Padimate O 0.7%, oxybenzone 3%. Stick 4.25 g. *otc.*
Use: Lip protectant, sunscreen.

Chapstick Sunblock 15 Petroleum Jelly Plus. (Robins) White petrolatum 89%, padimate O 7%, oxybenzone 3%, aloe, lanolin. Stick 10 g. *otc.*
Use: Lip protectant, sunscreen.

CharcoAid. (Requa) Activated charcoal 15 g/120 ml, 30 g/150 ml, sorbitol/ Susp. Bot. *otc.*
Use: Antidote.

CharcoAid 2000. (Requa) Activated charcoal 15 g/120 ml, 50 g/240 ml with and without sorbitol/Liq. 15 g/240 ml. Granules. Bot. *otc.*
Use: Antidote.

charcoal. (CHAR-kole) (Various Mfr.) Cap., Tab. *otc.*
Use: Antiflatulent.
See: Charcoal (Paddock).
　Charcoal (Rugby).

•**charcoal, activated,** (CHAR-kole) U.S.P. 23.
Use: Antidote (general purpose), pharmaceutic aid (adsorbant).
See: Actidose-Aqua, Liq. (Paddock).
　CharcoAid, Susp. (Requa).
　Liqui-Char, Liq. (Jones Medical).
W/Nux vomica, bismuth subgallate, pepsin, berberis, diastase, pancreatin, hydrastis, papain.
See: Charcocaps, Cap. (Requa).
　Charcotabs, Tab. (Requa).

Charcoal Plus. (Kramer) Activated charcoal 250 mg, simethicone 40 mg. Tab. Bot. 120s. *otc.*

Use: Antiflatulent.

charcoal and simethicone. Antiflatulent.
See: Charcoal Plus (Kramer).
　Flatulex (Dayton).

CharcoCaps. (Requa) Activated charcoal 260 mg/Cap. Bot. 36s. *otc.*
Use: Antiflatulent.

Chardonna-2. (Kremers-Urban) Belladonna extract 15 mg, phenobarbital 15 mg/Tab. Bot. 100s. *Rx.*
Use: Anticholinergic, antispasmodic, sedative, hypnotic.

Charo Scatter-Paks. (Requa) Activated charcoal 5 g/Packet.
Use: Odor absorber.

Chaz Scalp Treatment Dandruff Shampoo. (Revlon) Zinc pyrithione 1% in liquid shampoo. *otc.*
Use: Antiseborrheic.

Chealamide Injection. (Vortech) Disodium edetate 150 mg/ml. Vial 20 ml. *Rx.*
Use: Chelating agent.

Checkmate. (Oral-B) Acidulated phosphate fluoride 1.23%. Bot. 2 oz, 16 oz. *Rx.*
Use: Dental caries preventative.

Chek-Stix Urinalysis Control Strips. (Bayer) Bot. 25s.
Use: Diagnostic aid.

chelafrin.
See: Epinephrine.

Chelated Calcium Magnesium. (NBTY) Calcium^{++} 500 mg, magnesium 250 mg/ Tab. Protein coated. Bot. 50s. *otc.*
Use: Mineral supplement.

chelated calcium magnesium zinc. (NBTY) Calcium^{++} 333 mg, magnesium 133 mg, zinc 8.3 mg/Tab. Bot. 100s. *otc.*
Use: Mineral supplement.

Chelated Magnesium. (Freeda) Magnesium amino acids chelate 500 mg (magnesium 100 mg)/Tab. Bot. 100s, 250s, 500s. *otc.*
Use: Magnesium supplement.

Chelated Manganese. (Freeda) Manganese 20 mg or 50 mg/Tab. Bot. 100s, 250s, 500s. *otc.*
Use: Manganese supplement.

chelating agent.
See: BAL, Amp. (Becton Dickinson).
　Calcium Disodium Versenate, Amp., Tab. (3M).
　Desferal, Amp. (Novartis).
　Endrate Disodium, Amp. (Abbott).
　Magora, Tab. (Miller).

chelen.

See: Ethyl Chloride.

Chemet. (Bock) Succimer 100 mg. Cap. Bot. 100s. *Rx.*
Use: Chelating agent.

Chemipen. Potassium phenethicillin.
Use: Anti-infective, penicillin.

Chemovag Supps. (Forest Pharm.) Sulfisoxazole 0.5 g/Supp. Bot. 12s w/applicators. *Rx.*
Use: Anti-infective, sulfonamide.

Chemozine. (Tennessee Pharm.) Sulfadiazine, 0.167 g, sulfamerazine 0.167 g, sulfamethazine 0.167 g/Tab. Bot. 100s, 1000s. Susp. Bot. pt, gal. *Rx.*
Use: Anti-infective, sulfonamide.

Chemstrip 6. (Boehringer Mannheim) Broad range test for glucose, protein, pH, blood, ketones and leukocytes. Bot. strip 100s.
Use: Diagnostic aid.

Chemstrip 7. (Boehringer Mannheim) Broad range test for glucose, protein, pH, blood, ketones, bilirubin and leukocytes. Bot. strip 100s.
Use: Diagnostic aid.

Chemstrip 8. (Boehringer Mannheim) Broad range urine test for glucose, protein, pH, blood, ketones, bilirubin, urobilinogen and leukocytes. Bot. Strip 100s.
Use: Diagnostic aid.

Chemstrip 9. (Boehringer Mannheim) Broad range test for glucose, protein, pH, blood, ketones, bilirubin, urobilinogen, nitrite and leukocytes in urine. Bot. strip 100s.
Use: Diagnostic aid.

Chemstrip 10 SG. (Boehringer Mannheim) Broad range test for glucose, protein, pH, blood, ketones, bilirubin, urobilinogen, nitrite and leukocytes in urine. Bot. Strip 100s.
Use: Diagnostic aid.

Chemstrip 4 the OB. (Boehringer Mannheim) Broad range test for glucose, protein, blood and leukocytes in urine. Bot. Strip 100s.
Use: Diagnostic aid.

Chemstrip BG. (Boehringer Mannheim) For measuring glucose in blood. Bot. strip 25s, 50s.
Use: Diagnostic aid.

Chemstrip 2 GP. (Boehringer Mannheim) Broad range test for glucose and protein. Bot. strip 100s.
Use: Diagnostic aid.

Chemstrip-K. (Boehringer Mannheim) Reagent papers for ketones in urine. Bot. paper 25s, 100s.

Use: Diagnostic aid.

Chemstrip 2 LN. (Boehringer Mannheim) Broad range test for nitrite and leukocytes. Bot. strip 100s.
Use: Diagnostic aid.

Chemstrip Micral. (Boehringer Mannheim) In vitro reagent strips to detect albumin in urine. In 5s, 30s.
Use: Diagnostic aid.

Chemstrip Mineral. (Boehringer Mannheim) In vitro reagent strips used to detect albumin in urine. Strips. 5s, 30s.
Use: In vitro diagnostic aid.

Chemstrip UG. (Boehringer Mannheim) Test for glucose in urine using the glucose oxidase method. Bot. Strip 100s.
Use: Diagnostic aid.

Chemstrip uGK. (Boehringer Mannheim) Broad range test for glucose and ketones. Bot. strip 50s, 100s.
Use: Diagnostic aid.

Chenatal. (Miller) Calcium 580 mg, magnesium 200 mg, vitamins C 100 mg, folic acid 0.4 mg, A 5000 IU, D 400 IU, B_1 3 mg, B_2 3 mg, B_6 5 mg, B_{12} 9 mcg, niacinamide 30 mg, pantothenic acid 5 mg, tocopherols (mixed) 10 mg, iron 20 mg, copper 1 mg, manganese 2 mg, potassium 10 mg, zinc 25 mg, iodine 0.1 mg/2 Tabs. Bot. 100s. *otc.*
Use: Vitamin/mineral supplement.

chenodeoxycholic acid.
Use: Gallstone solubilizing agent.
See: Chenodiol.

•**chenodiol.** (KEEN-oh-DIE-ahl) USAN.
Use: Anticholelithogenic. [Orphan drug]

Cheracol. (Roberts) Codeine phosphate 10 mg, guaifenesin 100 mg/5 ml, alcohol 4.75%. Bot. 2 oz, 4 oz, pt. *c-v.*
Use: Antitussive, expectorant.

Cheracol D. (Roberts) Dextromethorphan HBr 10 mg, guaifenesin 100 mg/ 5 ml, alcohol 4.75%. Bot. 2 oz, 4 oz, 6 oz. *otc.*
Use: Antitussive, expectorant.

Cheracol Nasal. (Roberts) Oxymetazoline HCl 0.05%, phenylmercuric acetate 0.02 mg/ml, benzalkonium chloride, glycine, sorbitol. Soln. Spray 30 ml. *otc.*
Use: Decongestant.

Cheracol Plus. (Roberts) Phenylpropanolamine HCl 8.3 mg, dextromethorphan HBr 6.7 mg, chlorpheniramine maleate 1.3 mg/5 ml. Bot. 4 oz. *otc.*
Use: Decongestant, antitussive, antihistamine.

Cheracol Sore Throat. (Roberts) Phe-

nol 1.4%, saccharin, sorbitol, alcohol 12.5%. Spray Bot. 180 ml. *otc.*
Use: Mouth and throat product.

Cheratussin Cough Syrup. (Towne) Dextromethorphan HBr 45 mg, ammonium Cl 575 mg, citrate sodium 280 mg/Fl oz. Bot. 4 oz. *otc.*
Use: Antitussive, expectorant.

Chero-Trisulfa-V. (Vita Elixir) Sulfadiazine 0.166 g, sulfacetamide 0.166 g, sulfamerazine 0.166 g, sodium citrate 0.5 g/5 ml. Susp. Bot. pt.
Use: Anti-infective, sulfonamide.

cherry juice, N.F. XVI.
Use: Flavor.

cherry syrup.
Use: Pharmaceutic aid (Vehicle).

Chestamine. (Leeds) Chlorpheniramine maleate 8 mg or 12 mg/Cap. Bot. 50s. *Rx.*
Use: Antihistamine.

Chest Throat Lozenges. (Lane) Eucalyptol, anise, horehound, tolu balsam, benzoin tincture, sugar, corn syrup. Pkg. 30s. *otc.*
Use: Antiseptic.

Chewable C. (Approved Pharm.) Vitamin C 100 mg, 250 mg, 300 mg and 500 mg/Tab. Bot. 100s. *otc.*
Use: Vitamin C supplement.

Chewable Multivitamins w/Fluoride. (Moore) Tab.: Fluoride 1 mg, vitamins A 2500 IU, D 400 IU, E 15 IU, B_1 1.05 mg, B_2 1.2 mg, B_3 13.5 mg, B_6 1.05 mg, B_{12} 4.5 mcg, C 60 mg, folic acid 0.3 mg, sucrose/ Bot. 100s. *Rx.*
Use: Vitamin/mineral supplement; dental caries preventative.

Chew-Vims. (Barth's) Vitamins A 5000 IU, D 400 IU, B_1 3 mg, B_2 6 mg, niacin 1.71 mg, C 100 mg, B_{12} 5 mcg, E 5 IU/Tab. Bot. 30s, 90s, 180s, 360s. *otc.*
Use: Vitamin supplement.

Chew-Vi-Tab. (Halsey) Vitamins A 2500 IU, D 400 IU, E 15 IU, C 60 mg, folic acid 0.3 mg, B_1 1.05 mg, B_2 1.2 mg, niacin 13.5 mg, B_6 1.05 mg, B_{12} 4.5 mcg/ Tab. Bot. 100s. *otc.*
Use: Vitamin supplement.

Chew-Vi-Tab with Iron. (Halsey) Vitamins A 5000 IU, C 60 mg, E 15 IU, folic acid 0.4 mg, B_1 1.5 mg, B_2 1.7 mg, niacin 20 mg, B_6 2 mg, B_{12} 6 mcg, D 400 IU, iron 18 mg/Tab. Bot. 100s. *otc.*
Use: Vitamin/mineral supplement.

Chibroxin. (Merck) Norfloxacin 3 mg/ml. Soln. Drop. Bot. 5 ml Ocumeters. *Rx.*
Use: Antibiotic, ophthalmic.

chicken pox vaccine.

See: Varivax (Merck).

Chiggerex. (Scherer) Benzocaine 0.02%, camphor, menthol, peppermint oil, olive oil, clove oils, pegosperse, methylparaben, distilled water. Oint. Jar 50 g. *otc.*
Use: Local anesthetic, counterirritant.

Chigger-Tox. (Scherer) Benzocaine 2.1%, benzyl benzoate 21.4%, soft soap, isopropyl alcohol. Liq. Bot. 30 ml. *otc.*
Use: Local anesthetic, topical.

Children's Advil. (Wyeth-Ayerst) Ibuprofen 100 mg/5 ml. Susp. Bot. 119 ml, 473 ml. *Rx.*
Use: Nonsteroidal anti-inflammatory drug; analgesic.

Children's Allerest. (Novartis) Phenylpropanolamine HCl 9.4 mg, chlorpheniramine maleate 1 mg. Chew. Tab. Bot. 24s. *otc.*
Use: Pediatric decongestant, antihistamine.

Children's Dramamine. (Pharmacia & Upjohn) Dimenhydrinate 12.5 mg/5 ml, alcohol 5%, sucrose/Bot. 120 ml. *otc.*
Use: Antiemetic/antivertigo agent.

Children's Feverall. (Upsher-Smith) Acetaminophen 120 mg or 325 mg/ Supp. Pkg. 6s. *otc.*
Use: Analgesic.

Children's Formula Cough Syrup. (Pharmakon) Guaifenesin 50 mg, dextromethorphan HBr 5 mg, sucrose, corn syrup. Alcohol free. Grape flavor. Syr. Bot. 118 ml, 236 ml. *otc.*
Use: Expectorant, antitussive.

Children's Hold 4-Hour Cough Suppressant & Decongestant. (Beecham Products) Dextromethorphan HBr 3.75 mg, phenylpropanolamine HCl 6.25 mg/ Loz. Pkg. 10s. *otc.*
Use: Antitussive, decongestant.

Children's Kaopectate. (Pharmacia & Upjohn) Attapulgite 600 mg. Liq. Bot. 180 ml. *otc.*
Use: Antidiarrheal.

Children's Mapap. (Major) Acetaminophen 160 mg/5ml, alcohol free/Elixir. Bot. 120 ml. *otc.*
Use: Analgesic.

Children's Motrin. (McNeil) Ibuprofen 100 mg/5 ml, alcohol free/Susp. Bot. 120 ml, 480 ml. *otc, Rx.*
Use: Nonsteroidal anti-inflammatory drug, analgesic.

Children's No Aspirin Elixir. (Walgreen) Acetaminophen 80 mg/2.5 ml. Nonalcoholic. Bot. 4 oz. *otc.*
Use: Analgesic.

Children's No-Aspirin Tablets. (Walgreen) Acetaminophen 80 mg/Tab. Bot. 30s. *otc.*
Use: Analgesic.

Children's Nyquil. (Procter & Gamble) Pseudoephedrine HCl 10 mg, chlorpheniramine maleate 0.6 mg, dextromethorphan HBr 5 mg/5 ml. Bot. 120 ml, 240 ml. *otc.*
Use: Decongestant, antihistamine, antitussive.

Children's Nyquil Nightime Head Cold, Allergy Formula. (Procter & Gamble) Pseudoephedrine HCl 10 mg, chlorpheniramine maleate 0.67 mg/5 ml. Alcohol free. Sorbitol, sucrose. Grape flavor. Liq. Bot. 120 ml. *otc.*
Use: Decongestant, antihistamine.

Children's Silapap. (Silarx) Acetaminophen 80 mg/2.5 ml, sugar free, alcohol free/Liq. Bot. 237 ml. *otc.*
Use: Analgesic.

Children's Silfedrine. (Silarx) Pseudoephedrine HCl 30 mg/5 ml. Liq. Bot. 118 ml. *otc.*
Use: Nasal decongestant.

Children's SunKist Multivitamins Complete. (Novartis) Iron 18 mg, vitamin A 5000 IU, D_3 400 IU, E 30 IU, B_1 1.5 mg, B_2 1.7 mg, B_3 20 mg, B_5 10 mg, B_6 2 mg, B_{12} 6 mcg, C 60 mg, folic acid 0.4 mg, Ca, Cu, I, K, Mg, Mn, P, zinc 10 mg, biotin 40 mcg, vitamin K, sorbitol, aspartame, phenylalanine, tartrazine/Chew. Tab. Bot. 60s. *otc.*
Use: Vitamin/mineral supplement.

Children's SunKist Multivitamins + Extra C. (Novartis) Vitamin A 2500 IU, E 15 IU, D_3 400 IU, B_1 1.05 mg, B_2 1.2 mg, B_3 13.5 mg, B_6 1.05 mg, B_{12} 4.5 mcg, C 250 mg, folic acid 0.3 mg, vitamin K_1 5 mcg, sorbitol, aspartame, phenylalanine, tartrazine. Chew. Tab. Bot. 60s. *otc.*
Use: Vitamin/mineral supplement.

Children's SunKist Multivitaminins + Iron. (Novartis) Iron 15 mg, vitamin A 2500 IU, E 15 IU, D_3 400 IU, B_1 1.05 mg, B_2 1.2 mg, B_3 13.5 mg, B_6 1.05 mg, B_{12} 4.5 mcg, C 60 mg, folic acid 0.3 mg, vitamin K_1 5 mcg, sorbitol, aspartame, phenylalanine, tartrazine. Chew. Tab. Bot. 60s. *otc.*
Use: Vitamin with Iron supplement.

Children's Tylenol Cold Tablets. (McNeil-CPC) Pseudoephedrine HCl 7.5 mg, chlorpheniramine maleate 0.5 mg, acetaminophen 80 mg, aspartame, sucrose, phenylalanine 4 mg. Chewable. Grape flavor. Tab. Bot. 24s. *otc.*
Use: Decongestant, antihistamine, analgesic.

Children's Tylenol Cold Liquid. (McNeil-CPC) Pseudoephedrine HCl 15 mg, chlorpheniramine maleate 1 mg, acetaminophen 160 mg, sorbitol, sucrose. Alcohol free. Grape flavor. Liq. Bot. 120 ml. *otc.*
Use: Decongestant, antihistamine, analgesic.

Children's Tylenol Cold Multi Symptom Plus Cough. (McNeil-CPC) Acetaminophen 160 mg, dextromethorphan HBr 5 mg, chlorpheniramine maleate 1 mg, pseudoephedrine HCl 15 mg/5 ml. Liq. Bot. 120 ml. *otc.*
Use: Decongestant, antihistamine, antitussive.

Children's Tylenol Cold Plus Cough. (McNeil) Acetaminophen 80 mg, pseudoephedrine HCl 7.5 mg, dextromethorphan HBr 2.5 mg, chlorpheniramine maleate 0.5 mg/Tab. Chewable. Pkg. 24s. *otc.*
Use: Analgesic, decongestant, antitussive, antihistamine.

Children's Tylenol Elixir. (McNeil-CPC) Acetaminophen 160 mg/5 ml. Elix. Bot. 60 ml, 120 ml. *otc.*
Use: Analgesic.

Children's Ty-Tabs. (Major) Acetaminophen 80 mg. Tab. Bot. 100s, 1000s. *otc.*
Use: Analgesic.

chimeric m-t412 (human-murine) igg monoclonal anti-cd4. *Rx.*
Use: Multiple sclerosis. [Orphan drug]

chimeric (murine variable, human constant) mab to cd20. (Idec Pharm) *Rx.*
Use: Treatment of non-Hodgkin's B-cell lymphoma. [Orphan drug]

chinese gelatin.
See: Agar.

chinese isinglass.
Use: Amebicide.

chiniofon.
Use: Amebicide.

Chinosol. (Vernon) 8-Hydroxyquinoline sulfate 7.5 gr/Tab. Vial 6s. Trit. Tab. (⅜ gr) Bot. 50s. Pow. 1 oz.
Use: Antiseptic.

chlamydia trachomatis test.
Use: Diagnostic aid.
See: MicroTrak (Syva).

Chlamydiazyme. (Abbott Diagnostics) Enzyme immunoassay for detection of *Chlamydia trachomatis* from urethral or urogenital swabs. Test kit 100s.
Use: Diagnostic aid.

Chlo-Amine. (Bayer) Chlorpheniramine maleate 2 mg/Chew. Tab. Box 24x4 mg Tab. Packages. *otc.*
Use: Antihistamine.

chlophedianol. (KLOE-fee-DIE-ah-nole) F.D.A.

•**chlophedianol hydrochloride.** (KLOE-fee-DIE-ah-nole) USAN.
Use: Antitussive.

Chloracol 0.5%. (Horizon) Chloramphenicol 5 mg/ml with chlorobutanol, hydroxypropyl methylcellulose. Dropper bot. 7.5 ml. *Rx.*
Use: Anti-infective, ophthalmic.

Chlorafed. (Roberts) Chlorpheniramine maleate 2 mg, pseudoephedrine HCl 30 mg/5 ml, alcohol, dye, sugar and corn free. Liq. Bot. 120 ml, 480 ml. *otc.*
Use: Antihistamine, decongestant.

Chlorafed H.S. Timecelles. (Roberts Hauck) Chlorpheniramine maleate 4 mg, pseudoephedrine HCl 60 mg/SR Cap. Bot. 100s. *Rx.*
Use: Antihistamine, decongestant.

Chlorafed Timecelles. (Roberts Hauck) Chlorpheniramine maleate 8 mg, pseudoephedrine HCl 120 mg/SA timecelles. Bot. 100s. *Rx.*
Use: Antihistamine, decongestant.

Chlorahist. (Evron) Chlorpheniramine maleate **4 mg/Tab.:** Bot. 100s, 1000s. **8 mg or 12 mg/Cap.:** Bot. 250s, 1000s. **Syr. 2 mg/4 ml.:** Bot. qt. *otc, Rx.*
Use: Antihistamine.

•**chloral betaine.** (KLOR-uhl BEE-taheen) USAN. N.F. XIV.
Use: Sedative, hypnotic.

chloralformamide.

•**chloral hydrate,** (KLOR-uhl HIGH-drate) U.S.P. 23.
Use: Hypnotic, sedative.
See: Aquachloral Supprettes, Supp. (PolyMedica).
Noctec, Cap., Syr. (Squibb).
Generic Products:
Quality Generics (7.5 gr) Bot. 100s.
G.F. Harvey-Cap. (3 gr) Bot. 100s; (7.5 gr) Bot. 100s.
Lederle-Cap. (500 mg) 100s.
Pacific Pharm. Corp. Cap. (7.5 gr) Bot. 100s, 1000s.
Parke, Davis-Cap. (500 mg) Bot. 100s, UD 100s.
Stayner-Cap. (250 mg or 500 mg) Bot. 100s, (500 mg) Bot. 1000s, Crystals Bot. 1 lb. and 5 lbs.
West-Ward-Cap. (3 gr, 7.5 gr) Bot. 100s.

chloral hydrate betaine (1:1) compound. Chloral Betaine.

chloralpyrine dichloralpyrine.
See: Dichloralantipyrine.

chloralurethane. Name used for Carbochloral.

Chloraman. (Rasman) Chlorpheniramine maleate 12 mg/Tab. Bot. 100s, 500s, 1000s. *Rx.*
Use: Antihistamine.

•**chlorambucil,** (klor-AM-byoo-sill) U.S.P. 23.
Use: Antineoplastic.
See: Leukeran, Tab. (Glaxo Wellcome).

Chloramine-T. Sodium paratoluenesulfan chloramide, chloramine, chlorozone.
Lilly-Tab. (0.3 g), Bot. 100s, 1000s.
Robinson, Pow., 1 oz.
Use: Antiseptic, deodorant.
See: Chlorazene (Badger).

chloramphenicol. (KLOR-am-FEN-ihkahl) (Various Mfr.) **Soln.:** 5 mg/ml Bot. 7.5 ml, 15 ml; **Oint.:** 10 mg/g Tube 3.5 g; **Cap.:** 250 mg Bot. 100s.
Use: Antibacterial, antirickettsial.

•**chloramphenicol,** (KLOR-am-FEN-ihkahl) U.S.P. 23.
Use: Antibacterial, antirickettsial.
See: AK-Chlor, Preps. (Akorn).
Chloromycetin, Preps. (Parke-Davis).
Chloroptic Ophth. Oint. (Allergan).
Chloroptic S.O.P. Ophth. Oint. (Allergan).
Econochlor, Soln., Oint. (Alcon).
Mychel, Cap. (Houba).
Ophthochlor, Soln. (Parke-Davis).
W/Polymixin B.
Use: Treatment of superficial ocular infections involving the conjunctiva and/or cornea caused by susceptible organisms.
See: Chloromyxin Ophthalmic Oint. (Parke-Davis).
W/Polymixin B, Hydrocortisone.
See: Ophthocort, Oint. (Parke-Davis).

chloramphenicol and hydrocortisone acetate for ophthalmic suspension.
Use: Anti-infective, anti-inflammatory.
See: Chloromycetin, Prods. (Parke-Davis).

chloramphenicol, polymyxin b sulfate, and hydrocortisone acetate ophthalmic ointment.
Use: Anti-infective, anti-inflammatory.
See: Chloromycetin, Prods. (Parke-Davis).

chloramphenicol and polymyxin b sulfate ophthalmic ointment.
Use: Anti-infective.

●**chloramphenicol palmitate,** U.S.P. 23.
Use: Antibacterial, antirickettsial.
See: Chloromycetin Palmitate, Oral
Susp. (Parke-Davis).

●**chloramphenicol pantothenate complex.** (KLOR-am-FEN-ih-kahl PAN-toe-
THEH-nate) USAN. A complex consisting of 4 parts of chloramphenicol to
one part of calcium pantothenate. Pan-
tofenicol.
Use: Antibacterial, antirickettsial.

**chloramphenicol and prednisolone
ophthalmic ointment.**
Use: Antibiotic, steroid combination.
See: Chloromycetin, Prods. (Parke-
Davis).

●**chloramphenicol sodium succinate,
sterile,** U.S.P. 23.
Use: Antibacterial, antirickettsial.
See: Chloromycetin Succinate, Inj.,
(Parke-Davis).
Mychel-S, IV. (Houba).

chloramphenicol sodium succinate.
(Various Mfr.) 100 mg/ml. Inj. Vial. 1 g
in 15 ml.
Use: Antibacterial, antirickettsial.

chloranil.

Chloraseptic Children's Lozenges.
(Procter & Gamble) Benzocaine 5 mg/
Loz. Pkg. 18s. *otc.*
Use: Local anesthetic.

Chloraseptic Liquid. (Procter & Gamble)
Total phenol 1.4% as phenol and sodium phenolate, saccharin. Menthol and
cherry flavors. Bot. 180 ml, 360 ml
(mouthwash/gargle); 45 ml, 240 ml, 360
ml (throat spray). *otc.*
Use: Antiseptic, local anesthetic.

Chloraseptic Lozenge. (Procter &
Gamble) Total phenol 32.5 mg/lozenge
as phenol and sodium phenolate. Menthol and cherry flavors. Pkg. 18s, 36s.
otc.
Use: Local anesthetic, antiseptic.

Chlorate. (Major) Chlorpheniramine maleate 4 mg/Tab. Bot. 24s, 100s, 1000s.
otc.
Use: Antihistamine.

chlorazanil hydrochloride.

Chlorazene. (Badger) Chloramine-T, so-
dium p-toluene-sulfonchloramide.
Pow.: UD Pkg. 20 g, 38 g, 50 g, 88 g,
200 g, 240 g, 320 g, Bot. 1 lb, 5 lb.
Aromatic Pow. (5%): Bot. 1 lb, 5 lb.
Tab. (0.3 g): Bot. 20s, 100s, 1000s,
5000s. *otc.*
Use: Antiseptic, deodorant.

chlorazepate dipotassium.
Use: Antianxiety agent, anticonvulsant.

See: Clorazepate dipotassium.

chlorazepate monopotassium.
See: Clorazepate monopotassium.

Chlorazine Tabs. (Major) Prochlorperazine 5 mg or 10 mg/Tab. Bot. 100s.
Use: Antiemetic, antivertigo, antipsychotic.

chlorazone.
See: Chloramine-T.

Chlor Benzo Mor, A and D Ointment.
(Wade) Vitamins A and D fortified,
chlorobutanol 3%, benzocaine 2%,
benzyl alcohol 3%, actamer 1%, in
lanolin and petrolatum base. Tube 1 oz,
Jar 1 oz, lb. *otc.*
Use: Antiseptic, local anesthetic.

Chlor Benzo Mor Spray. (Wade) Vitamin A and D fortified, chlorobutanol
3%, benzocaine 2%, benzyl alcohol 3%,
and actamer 1%, in lanolin and mineral oil base. Bot. 2 oz, 11 oz. *otc.*
Use: Antiseptic, local anesthetic.

chlorbutanol.
See: Chlorobutanol, N.F. 18.

chlorbutol.
See: Chlorobutanol, N.F. 18.

chlorcyclizine hydrochloride, N.F. XVI.
Use: Antihistamine.
W/Hydrocortisone acetate.
See: Mantadil, Cream (Glaxo Well-
come).
W/Pseudoephedrine HCl.
See: Fedrazil, Tab. (Glaxo Wellcome).

●**chlordantoin.** (CLOR-dan-toe-in) USAN.
Use: Antifungal.
See: Sporostacin Cream (Ortho).

●**chlordiazepoxide,** (klor-DIE-aze-ee-
POX-side) U.S.P. 23.
Use: Tranquilizer (minor).
See: A-poxide, Cap. (Abbott).
Brigen-G, Tab. (Grafton).
Libritabs, Tab. (Roche).
Menrium, Tab. (Roche).
W/Amitriptyline.
See: Limbitrol, Tab. (Roche).

**chlordiazepoxide and amitriptyline HCl
tablets.** (klor-DIE-aze-ee-POX-ide and
am-ee-TRIP-tih-leen)
Use: Antianxiety agent.
See: Limbitrol, Tab. (Roche).

●**chlordiazepoxide hydrochloride,** (klor-
DIE-aze-ee-POX-ide) U.S.P. 23.
Use: Sedative, hypnotic.
See: A-poxide, Cap. (Abbott).
Chlordiazachel, Cap. (Houba).
Librium, Cap., Inj. (Roche).
Screen, Cap. (Foy).
Zetran, Cap. (Roberts).
W/Clidinium bromide.

See: Librax, Cap. (Roche).

chlordiazepoxide w/clindinium bromide. (Various Mfr.) Clindinium 2.5 mg, chlordiazepoxide HCl 5 mg/Cap. Bot. 30s, 100s, 500s, 1000s, UD 100s. *c-iv.*
Use: Gastrointestinal anticholinergic combination.

Chlordrine S.R. (Rugby) Pseudoephedrine HCl 120 mg, chlorpheniramine maleate 8 mg/Cap. Bot. 100s.
Rx.
Use: Decongestant, antihistamine.

Chloren 4. (Wren) Chlorpheniramine maleate 4 mg/Tab. Bot. 100s, 1000s. *otc.*
Use: Antihistamine.

Chloren 8 T.D. (Wren) Chlorpheniramine maleate 8 mg/Tab. Bot. 100s, 1000s. *otc.*
Use: Antihistamine.

Chloren 12 T.D. (Wren) Chlorpheniramine maleate 12 mg/Tab. Bot. 100s, 1000s. *otc, Rx.*
Use: Antihistamine.

Chloresium. (Rystan) **Oint.:** Chlorophyllin copper complex 0.5% in hydrophilic base. Tube 1 oz, 4 oz, Jar lb. **Soln.:** Chlorophyllin copper complex 0.2% in isotonic saline soln. Bot. 60 ml, 240 ml, qt. *otc.*
Use: Healing agent, deodorizer.

Chloresium Tablets. (Rystan) Chlorophyllin copper complex 14 mg/Tab. Bot. 100s, 1000s. *otc.*
Use: Oral deodorant.

Chloresium Tooth Paste. (Rystan) Chlorophyllin copper complex. Tube 3.25 oz. *otc.*
Use: Oral deodorant.

chlorethyl.
See: Ethyl Chloride.

Chlorgest-HD. (Great Southern) Phenylephrine HCl 5 mg, chlorpheniramine maleate 4 mg, hydrocodone bitartrate 1.67 mg. Alcohol free. Liq. Bot. pt, gal. *c-iii.*
Use: Decongestant, antihistamine, antitussive.

chlorguanide hydrochloride.
See: Chloroguanide HCl (Various Mfr.).

chlorhexadol.

chlorhexidine. (klor-HEX-ih-deen) F.D.A. *otc.*
Use: Antiseptic.
See: BactoShield, Foam, Soln. (Amsco).
BactoShield 2, Soln. (Amsco).
Hibiclens.
Hibiscrub.
Hibitane.

Lisium.
Rotersept.

•**chlorhexidine gluconate.** (klor-HEX-ih-deen GLUE-koe-nate) USAN. Oral rinse or topical skin cleanser.
Use: Antimicrobial. [Orphan drug]
See: BactoShield, Foam, Soln. (Amsco).
BactoShield 2, Soln. (Amsco).
Hibiclens, Liq. (Stuart).
Hibistat, Liq. (Stuart).
Peridex (Procter & Gamble).

•**chlorhexidine hydrochloride.** (klor-HEX-ih-deen) USAN.
Use: Anti-infective, topical.

•**chlorhexidine phosphanilate.** (klor-HEX-ih-deen FOSS-fah-nih-LATE) USAN.
Use: Antibacterial.

chlorhydroxyquinolin.
See: Quinolor Compound, Oint. (Squibb).

chlorinated and iodized peanut oil. Chloriodized Oil.

•**chlorindanol.** (klor-IN-dah-nahl) USAN. 7-Chloro-4-indanol.
Use: Antiseptic, spermaticide.

chlorine compound, antiseptic. Antiseptics, Chlorine.

chloriodized oil. Chlorinated and iodized peanut oil.

chlorisondamine chloride.

•**chlormadinone acetate.** (klor-MAD-ih-nohn) USAN. NF XIII.
Use: Progestin.

Chlor Mal w/Sal + APAP S.C. (Global Pharms) Chlorpheniramine maleate 2 mg, acetaminophen 150 mg, salicylamide 175 mg/Tab. Bot. 1000s. *otc.*
Use: Antihistamine, analgesic.

chlormerodrin. Mercloran. *Rx.*
Use: Diuretic.

•**chlormerodrin hg 197.** USAN. U.S.P. XX.
Use: Diagnostic aid (renal function determination), radioactive agent.

•**chlormerodrin hg 203.** USAN. U.S.P. XX.
Use: Diagnostic aid (renal function determination), radioactive agent.

chlormezanone. Chlormethazanone. *Rx.*
Use: Antianxiety agent.
See: Trancopal, Cap. (Sanofi Winthrop).

Chlor-Niramine Allergy Tabs. (Whiteworth Towne) Chlorpheniramine maleate 4 mg/Tab. Bot. 24s, 100s. *otc.*
Use: Antihistamine.

chloroazodin. Alpha, alpha, Azobis-(chloroformamidine).

•**chlorobutanol,** N.F. 18.
Use: Anesthetic, antiseptic, hypnotic; pharmaceutic aid (antimicrobial).
See: Cerumenex, Drops (Purdue-Frederick).
Pre-Sert (Allergan).
W/Atropine sulfate, chlorpheniramine maleate, phenylpropanolamine HCl.
See: Decongestant, Inj. (Century).
W/Calcium glycerophosphate, calcium levulinate.
See: Cal San, Inj. (Burgin-Arden).
W/Cetyltrimethylammonium Br, methapyrilene HCl, phenylephrine HCl, hydrocortisone.
See: T-Spray, Liq. (Saron).
W/Diphenhydramine HCl.
See: Ardeben, Inj. (Burgin-Arden).
W/Ephedrine HCl, sodium Cl.
See: Efedron HCl Nasal Jelly (Hart).
W/Estradiol cypionate, testosterone cypionate.
See: Depo-Testadiol, Vial (Pharmacia & Upjohn).
Depotestogen, Vial (Hyrex).
W/Glycerin, anhydrous.
See: Ophthalgan, Liq. (Wyeth-Ayerst).
W/Liquifilm.
See: Liquifilm Tears (Allergan).
W/Methylcellulose.
See: Lacril (Allergan).
W/Myristyl-gamma-picolinium Cl.
See: Wet Tone, Soln. (3M).
W/Nonionic lanolin derivative.
See: Lacri-Lube, Ophthalmic Ointment (Allergan).
W/Polyethylene glycol, polyoxyl 40 stearate.
See: Blink-N-Clean (Allergan).
W/Sodium Cl.
See: Ocean, Liq. (Fleming).
W/Tannic acid, isopropyl alcohol.
See: Outgro, Soln. (Whitehall Robbins).
W/Vitamins B_1, B_2, B_6, niacinamide, calcium pantothenate, benzyl alcohol.

•**chlorocresol,** (KLOR-oh-KREE-sole) N.F. 18.
Use: Antiseptic, disinfectant.

chloroethane.
See: Ethyl Chloride. anticholinergic, antispasmodic.

Chlorofair. (Pharmafair) **Soln.:** Chloramphenicol 5 mg/ml. Bot. 7.5 ml **Oint.:** Chloramphenicol 10 mg/g in white petrolatum base with mineral oil, polysorbate 60. Tube 3.5 g. *Rx.*
Use: Anti-infective, ophthalmic.

chloroguanide hydrochloride. (Various Mfr.) (Proguanil HCl) *Rx.*
Use: Antimalarial.

Chlorohist-LA. (Roberts) Xylometazoline HCl 0.1%. Soln. Spray 15 ml. *otc.*
Use: Decongestant.

chloro-iodohydroxyquinoline.
See: Clioquinol, U.S.P. 23.

chloromethapyrilene citrate.
See: Chlorothen Citrate.

Chloromycetin. (Parke-Davis) Chloramphenicol. **Ophth. Oint.:** (1%) in base of petrolatum, polyethylene. Tube 3.5 g. **Inj.:** 100 mg/ml (as sodium succinate) when reconstituted. In 1 g in 15 ml vials. **Ophth. Soln.:** (25 mg) Bot. w/dropper 15 ml (dry). Soln. Plastic dropper Bot. 15 ml. **Oral:** 150 mg/5 ml (palmitate), alcohol, sucrose, sodium benzoate 0.5%. Custard flavor. Bot. 60 ml. **Otic Drops:** (0.5%) 5 mg/ml w/propylene glycol. Bot. 15 ml. *Rx.*
Use: Anti-infective.

Chloromycetin/Hydrocortisone. (Parke-Davis) Hydrocortisone acetate 0.5% (2.5% as powder), chloramphenicol 0.25% (1.25% as powder). Pow. Bot. with dropper 5 ml. *Rx.*
Use: Anti-infective, ophthalmic.

Chloromycetin Sodium Succinate I.V. (Parke-Davis) Chloramphenicol sodium succinate dried powder which when reconstituted contains chloromycetin 100 mg/ml. Steri-vial 1 g, 10s. *Rx.*
Use: Anti-infective.

chlorophenothane.
Use: Pediculocide.

chlorophyll. (Freeda Vitamins) Chlorophyll 20 mg, sugar free/Tab. Bot. 100s, 250s, 500s. *otc.*
Use: Oral deodorizer.

Chlorophyll "A" Ointment.
See: Chloresium Oint. (Rystan).

Chlorophyll "A" Solution. (Chlorophyllin).
See: Chloresium Soln. (Rystan).

chlorophyll derivatives, systemic.
See: chlorophyll (Freeda).
Derifil (Rystan).
Chloresium (Rystan).

chlorophyll derivatives, topical.
See: Chloresium (Rystan).

chlorophyll tablets. *otc.*
See: Derifil, Tab. (Rystan).
Nullo, Tab. (Depree).

chlorophyll, water-soluble. (Various Mfr.) Chlorophyllin.
See: Chloresium Prep. (Rystan).
Derifil, Pow. (Rystan).

chlorophyllin. (KLOR-oh-FILL-in)
Use: Healing agent, deodorizer.

•**chlorophyllin copper complex.** (KLOR-

oh-FILL-in KAHP-uhr) USAN.
Use: Deodorant.
See: Nullo, Tab. (Chattem).
PALS, Tab. (Palisades).
•**chlorophyllin copper complex sodium,** U.S.P. 23.
•**chloroprocaine hydrochloride,** U.S.P. 23.
Use: Anesthetic (local).
See: Nesacaine, Inj. (Astra).
Nescaine-MPF, Inj. (Astra).
Chloroptic. (Allergan) Chloramphenicol 0.5%. **Soln.:** Dropper bot. 2.5 ml, 7.5 ml. *Rx.*
Use: Anti-infective, ophthalmic.
Chloroptic S.O.P. (Allergan) Chloramphenicol 10 mg/g. Oint. Tube 3.5 g. *Rx.*
Use: Anti-infective, ophthalmic.
•**chloroquine,** (KLOR-oh-kwin) U.S.P. 23.
Use: Antiamebic, antimalarial.
See: Aralen HCl Prods. (Sanofi Winthrop).
•**chloroquine hydrochloride inj.,** U.S.P. 23.
Use: Antiamebic, antimalarial.
See: Aralen HCl (Sanofi Winthrop).
•**chloroquine phosphate,** U.S.P. 23. Tab. U.S.P. 23. Nivaquine.
Use: Antiamebic, antimalarial, lupus erythematosus suppressant.
See: Aralen Phosphate, Tab. (Sanofi Winthrop).
chlorothen.
Use: Antihistamine.
chlorothen citrate. (Whittier) Tab., Bot. 100s.
Use: Antihistamine.
W/Pyrilamine, thenylpyramine.
See: Derma-Pax, Liq. (Recsei).
chlorothenylpyramine. Chlorothen, Prep.
Chlorotheophyllinate w/Benadryl.
See: Dramamine, Prep. (Searle).
•**chlorothiazide,** U.S.P. 23.
Use: Diuretic.
See: Diuril, Tab., Susp. (Merck & Co.).
W/Methyldopa.
See: Aldoclor, Tab. (Merck & Co.).
W/Reserpine. Tab.: Chlorothiazide 250 mg or 500 mg, reserpine 0.125 mg. Bot. 100s.
See: Diupres, Tab. (Merck & Co.).
Use: Diuretic.
•**chlorothiazide sodium for injection,** U.S.P. 23.
Use: Diuretic, antihypertensive.
See: Sodium Diuril, Vial (Merck & Co.).
chlorothymol. 6-Chlorothymol.

Use: Antibacterial.
•**chlorotrianisene,** (klor-oh-try-AN-ih-seen) U.S.P. 23.
Use: Estrogen.
chlorotrianisene capsules.
Use: Estrogen.
See: Tace, Cap. (Hoechst Marion Roussel).
β **chlorovinyl ethynyl carbinol.**
See: Placidyl, Cap. (Abbott).
•**chloroxine.** (KLOR-ox-een) USAN.
Use: Antiseborrheic.
•**chloroxylenol,** (KLOR-oh-ZIE-len-ole) U.S.P. 23.
Use: Antibacterial.
W/Benzocaine, menthol, lanolin.
See: Unburn, Spray, Cream, Lot. (Leeming-Pacquin).
W/Hexachlorophene.
See: Desitin, Preps. (Leeming-Pacquin).
W/Methyl salicylate, menthol, camphor, thymol, eucalyptus oil, isopropyl alcohol.
See: Gordobalm, Balm (Gordon).
Chlorpazine. (Major) Prochlorperazine maleate 5 mg, 10 mg or 25 mg/Tab. Bot. 100s, UD 100s (5 mg, 10 mg only). *Rx.*
Use: Antipsychotic.
Chlorphed Injection. (Roberts) Brompheniramine maleate 10 mg/ml. Vial 10 ml. *Rx.*
Use: Antihistamine.
Chlorphed-LA. (Roberts) Oxymetazoline 0.05%. Soln. Spray 15 ml. *otc.*
Use: Decongestant.
Chlorphedrine SR. (Goldline) Chlorpheniramine maleate 8 mg, pseudoephedrine HCl 120 mg/Cap. Bot. 100s. *Rx.*
Use: Antihistamine, decongestant.
chlorphenesin. (KLOR-fen-ss-sin) F.D.A.
•**chlorphenesin carbamate.** (KLOR-fen-ee-sin CAR-bah-mate) USAN.
Use: Muscle relaxant (skeletal).
See: Maolate, Tab. (Pharmacia & Upjohn).
•**chlorpheniramine maleate,** (klor-fen-IHR-ah-meen) U.S.P. 23.
Use: Antihistamine.
See: Alermine, Tab. (Solvay).
Chestamine, Cap. (Leeds).
Chlo-Amine, Tab. (Bayer).
Chloraman, Tab. (Rasman).
Chloren, Preps. (Wren).
Chlor-4, Tab. (Mills).
Chlor-Niramine, Tab. (Whiteworth Towne).
Chlorophen, Vial (Medical Chem.).

Chlor-pen, Tab., Vial (American Chemical & Drug).
Chlor-Span, Cap. (Burlington).
Chlortab, Tab., Cap., Inj. (Vortech).
Chlor-Trimeton Maleate, Preps. (Schering-Plough).
Cosea, Preps. (Center).
Histacon, Tab., Syr. (Marsh Labs).
Histaspan, Cap. (Rhone-Poulenc Rorer).
Histex, Cap. (Roberts).
Nasahist (Keene).
Polaramine, Tab., Syr. (Schering-Plough).
Pyranistan, Tab. (Standex).
Rhinihist, Elix. (Schwarz Pharma).
Teldrin, Spansule (SK-Beecham).
Trymegen (Medco).
chlorpheniramine maleate w/combinations.
See: Al-Ay, Preps. (Jones Medical).
Alka-Seltzer Plus, Tab. (Bayer).
Allerdec, Cap. (Towne).
Allerest, Prods. (Novartis).
Alumadrine, Tab. (Fleming).
A.R.M., Tab. (SK-Beecham).
Atussin-D.M. Expectorant, Liq. (Federal).
B.M.E., Liq. (Brothers).
Bobid, Cap. (Boyd).
Breacol Cough Medication, Liq. (Bayer).
Brolade, Cap. (Brothers).
Bur-Tuss Expectorant (Burlington).
Cenahist, Cap. (Century).
Cenaid, Tab. (Century).
Centuss, Tab. (Century).
Chlorpel, Cap. (Santa).
Chlor-Trimeton, Preps. (Schering-Plough).
Codimal, Tab. (Schwarz Pharma).
Col-Decon, Tab. (Quality Generics).
Colrex Compound, Preps. (Solvay).
Comtrex, Tab., Cap., Liq. (Bristol-Myers).
Conalsyn Croncap, Cap. (Cenci).
Contac, Cap. (SK-Beecham).
Cophene No. 2, Cap. (Dunhall).
Cophene-S, Syr. (Dunhall).
Coricidin, Preps. (Schering-Plough).
Corilin, Liq. (Schering-Plough).
Corizahist, Preps. (Mason).
Coryban-D, Cap. (Pfizer).
Co-Tylenol, Preps. (McNeil).
Dallergy, Tab., Cap., Syr. (Laser).
Deconamine, Tab., Cap., Syr. (Berlex).
Dehist, Cap. (Forest).
Demazin, Tab., Syr. (Schering-Plough).
Derma-Pax, Lot. (Recsei).

Dezest, Cap. (Geneva Pharm.).
Donatussin, Liq., Syr. (Laser).
Dristan, Preps. (Whitehall Robbins).
Drucon, Elix. (Standard Drug).
Efricon Expectorant (Lannett).
Extendryl, Tab., Cap., Syr. (Fleming).
F.C.A.H., Cap. (Scherer).
Fedahist, Prods. (Donner).
Fitacol (Standex).
Histabid, Cap. (Glaxo).
Histacon, Tab., Syr. (Marsh Labs).
Histapco, Tab. (Apco).
Histaspan-D, Cap. (Rhone-Poulenc Rorer).
Histaspan Plus, Cap. (Rhone-Poulenc Rorer).
Hista-Vadrin, Tab., Cap., Syr. (Scherer).
Histine Prods. (Freeport).
Histogesic, Tab. (Century).
Hycomine Compound, Tab. (DuPont Merck).
Infantuss, Liq. (Scott/Cord).
Koryza, Tab. (Forest Pharm.).
Kronofed-A, Cap. (Ferndale).
Mapap CF, Tab. (Major).
Marhist (Marlop).
Neo-Pyranistan, Tab. (Standex).
Nilcol, Tab., Elix. (Parke-Davis).
Nolamine, Tab. (Carnrick).
Novafed A, Cap., Liq. (Hoechst Marion Roussel).
Novahistine, Preps. (Hoechst Marion Roussel).
Partuss, Liq. (Parmed).
Partuss T.D., Tab. (Parmed).
Phenahist, Preps. (T.E. Williams).
Phenchlor, Prods. (Freeport).
Polytuss-DM, Liq. (Rhode).
Pyma, Cap., Vial (Forest Pharm.).
Pyristan, Cap., Elix. (Arcum).
Pyranistan (Standex).
Quelidrine, Syr. (Abbott).
Rentuss, Cap., Syr. (Wren).
Rhinex D M, Tab., Syr. (Lemmon).
Rhinogesic, Tab. (Pal-Pak).
Rohist-D, Cap. (Rocky Mtn.).
Ryna, Liq. (Wallace).
Ryna-tussadine, Tab., Liq. (Wallace).
Salphenyl, Cap. (Roberts).
Scotcof, Liq. (Scott/Cord).
Scotnord (Scott/Cord).
Scotuss Liq. (Scott/Cord).
Shertus, Liq. (Sheryl).
Sialco, Tab. (Foy).
Sinarest, Tab. (Novartis).
Sine-Off, Prods. (SK-Beecham).
Sino-Compound, Tab. (Bio-Factor).
Sinovan Timed, Cap. (Drug Ind.).
Sinucol, Cap., Vial (Tennessee).
Sinulin, Tab. (Carnrick).

Sinutab Extra Strength, Cap. (Warner-Lambert).
Spantuss, Tab., Liq. (Arco).
Statomin Maleate CC, Tab. (Jones Medical).
Sudafed Plus, Tab., Syr. (Glaxo Wellcome).
Symptrol, Cap. (Saron).
T.A.C., Cap. (Towne).
Tonecol, Tab., Syr. (A.V.P.).
Triamininc, Prods. (Sandoz Consumer).
Triamincin Chewables (Sandoz Consumer).
Turbilixir, Liq. (Burlington).
Turbispan Leisurecaps, Cap. (Burlington).
Tusquelin, Syr. (Circle).
Tussar, Prods. (Rhone-Poulenc Rorer).
Valihist, Cap. (Otis Clapp).

d-chlorpheniramine maleate.
See: Polarmine Expectorant, Tab., Syr. (Schering-Plough).

chlorpheniramine maleate w/pseudoephedrine hydrochloride. (Eon) Pseudoephedrine HCl 120 mg, chlorpheniramine maleate 8 mg/Cap. Bot. 100s, 250s, 1000s. *otc.*
Use: Decongestant, antihistamine.

•**chlorpheniramine polistirex.** (klor-fen-IHR-ah-meen pahl-ee-STIE-rex) USAN.
Use: Antihistamine.

chlorpheniramine resin w/combinations.
See: Omni-Tuss, Liq. (Medeva).

chlorpheniramine tannate.
W/Carbetapentane tannate, ephedrine tannate, phenylephrine tannate.
See: Rynatuss Tab., Susp. (Wallace).
W/Phenylephrine tannate, pyrilamine tannate.
See: Rynatan, Tab., Susp. (Wallace).

•**chlorphentermine hydrochloride.** (klor-FEN-ter-meen) USAN.
Use: Anorexic.

chlorphthalidone.
See: Chlorthalidone.

Chlor-Pro 10. (Schein) Chlorpheniramine maleate 10 mg/ml, benzyl alcohol. Inj. Vial 30 ml. *Rx.*
Use: Antihistamine.

•**chlorpromazine,** (klor-PRO-muh-zeen) U.S.P. 23.
Use: Antiemetic, antipsychotic.
See: Chloractil.
Largactil.

•**chlorpromazine hydrochloride,** U.S.P. 23.
Use: Antiemetic, antipsychotic.

See: Chlorzine, Inj. (Roberts).
Promachlor, Tab. (Geneva Pharm.).
Promapar, Tab. (Parke-Davis).
Promaz, Inj. (Keene).
Sonazine, Tab. (Solvay).
Terpium, Tab. (Scrip).
Thorazine, Tab., Cap., Liq., Syr., Supp., Amp. (SK-Beecham).

Chlorpromazine Hydrochloride Intensol Oral Solution. (Roxane) Chlorpromazine HCl concentrated oral soln. **30 mg/ml:** Bot. 120 ml. **100 mg/ml:** Bot. 240 ml. *Rx.*
Use: Antiemetic, antipsychotic.

•**chlorpropamide,** (klor-PRO-puh-mide) U.S.P. 23.
Use: Antidiabetic.
See: Diabinese, Tab. (Pfizer Laboratories).

chlorprophenpyridamine maleate.
See: Chlorpheniramine Maleate, U.S.P. 23.

chlorquinaldol. 5,7-Dichloro-8-hydroxyquinal-dine.

chlorquinol. A mixture of the chlorinated products of 8-hydroxyquinoline containing about 65% of 5,7-dichloro-8-hydroxyquinoline. Quixalin.

Chlor-Rest. (Rugby) Phenylpropanolamine HCl 18.7 mg, chlorpheniramine maleate 2 mg/Tab. Bot. 100s. *otc.*
Use: Decongestant, antihistamine.

chlor-span. (Burlington) Chlorpheniramine maleate 8 mg/S.R. Cap. Bot. 60s. *otc.*
Use: Antihistamine.

chlortetracycline and sulfamethazine bisulfates soluble powder.
Use: Anti-infective.

•**chlortetracycline bisulfate,** U.S.P. 23.
Use: Antibacterial.

•**chlortetracycline hydrochloride,** U.S.P. 23.
Use: Antiprotozoal.
See: Aureomycin, Oint. (Storz/Lederle)

•**chlorthalidone,** (klor-THAL-ih-dohn) U.S.P. 23.
Use: Diuretic, antihypertensive.
See: Hygroton, Tab. (Rhone-Poulenc Rorer).
Thaliton, Tab. (Horus Therapeutics).
W/Reserpine.
See: Demi-Regroton, Tab. (Rhone-Poulenc Rorer).
Regroton, Tab. (Rhone-Poulenc Rorer).

chlorthalidone. (Various). Tab.: 25, 50, or 100 mg. Bot. 100s (25 mg); 100s, 250s, 1000s, (50 mg); 100s, 500s,

1000s (100 mg). *Rx.*
Use: Diuretic, antihypertensive.
Chlor-Trimeton. (Schering-Plough)
Chlorpheniramine maleate. **Tab.:** 4 mg.
Box 24s. Bot. 100s, 1000s. **Repetabs:**
8 mg. Box 24s, 48s. Bot. 100s, 1000s.
12 mg. Bot. 100s, 1000s. Blister packs
12s, 24s. **Syr.:** 2 mg/5 ml. Bot. 4 oz, pt,
gal. *otc, Rx.*
Use: Antihistamine.
Chlor-Trimeton Allergy. (Schering-
Plough) Chlorpheniramine maleate 4
mg, lactose/Tab. Pkg. 24s. *otc.*
Use: Antihistamine.
Chlor-Trimeton Allergy-Sinus. (Scher-
ing-Plough) Phenylpropanolamine HCl
12.5 mg, chlorpheniramine maleate 2
mg, acetaminophen 500 mg/Capl. Box
24s. *otc.*
Use: Decongestant, antihistamine, anal-
gesic.
Chlor-Trimeton w/Combinations. (Sch-
ering-Plough) Chlorpheniramine male-
ate.
W/Acetaminophen.
See: Coricidin, Tab. (Schering-Plough).
W/Acetaminophen, phenylpropanol-
amine.
See: Coricidin "D", Prods. (Schering-
Plough).
W/Phenylephrine HCl.
See: Demazin, Prods. (Schering-
Plough).
W/Pseudoephedrine sulfate.
See: Chlor-Trimeton Decongestant Tab.
(Schering-Plough).
Chlor-Trimeton 12 Hour Allergy (Sch-
ering-Plough).
W/Salicylamide, phenacetin, caffeine, vi-
tamin C.
See: Coriforte, Cap. (Schering-Plough).
W/Sodium salicylate, amino acetic acid.
See: Corilin, Liq. (Schering-Plough).
Chlor-Trimeton 4-Hour Relief Tablets.
(Schering-Plough) Chlorpheniramine
maleate 4 mg, pseudoephedrine sulfate
60 mg/Tab. Box 24s, 48s. *otc.*
Use: Antihistamine, decongestant.
Chlor-Trimeton 12 Hour Allergy. (Scher-
ing-Plough) Chlorpheniramine maleate
8 mg, pseudoephedrine sulfate 120
mg/SR Tab. Box 24s, 48s. UD 96s. *otc.*
Use: Antihistamine, decongestant.
Chlor-Trimeton 12-Hour Relief Tablets.
(Schering-Plough) Chlorpheniramine 8
mg, pseudoephedrine sulfate 120 mg/
Tab. Box 12s. Bot. 36s. *otc.*
Use: Decongestant, antihistamine.
Chlorzide. (Foy) Hydrochlorothiazide 50
mg/Tab. Bot. 1000s. *Rx.*

Use: Diuretic.
•**chlorzoxazone,** (klor-ZOX-uh-zone)
U.S.P. 23.
Use: Muscle relaxant (skeletal).
See: Paraflex, Tab. (McNeil).
Parafon Forte DSC, Capl. (McNeil).
Remular-S (Inter. Ethical).
W/Acetaminophen.
See: Blanex, Cap. (Edwards).
chlorzoxazone. (Various Mfr.) 250 mg,
500 mg/Tab. Bot. 100s, 500s (500 mg
only), 1000s.
Use: Muscle relaxant (skeletal).
**chlorzoxazone and acetaminophen
capsules.**
Use: Muscle relaxant, analgesic.
**chlorzoxazone and acetaminophen
tablets.**
Use: Muscle relaxant, analgesic.
Choice 10. (Whiteworth Towne) Potassium Cl 10% soln., unflavored. Bot.
gal. *Rx.*
Use: Potassium supplement.
Choice 20. (Whiteworth Towne) Potassium Cl 20% soln., unflavored. Bot.
gal. *Rx.*
Use: Potassium supplement.
Choice dm. (B-M Squibb) Protein 10.6
g, fat 12 g, carbohydrate 25 g, vita-
mins A, D, E, K, C, FA, B_1, B_2, B_3, B_5,
B_6, B_{12}, biotin, Ca, P, I, Fe, Mg, Cu,
Zn, Mn, Cl, Na, Se, Cr, Mo, sucrose,,
250 calories/240 ml. Lactose free/Liq.
240 ml. *otc.*
Use: For abnormal glucose tolerance.
Cholac. (Alra) Lactulose 10 g/15 ml. Bot.
240 ml, pt, UD 30 ml. *Rx.*
Use: Laxative.
cholacrylamine resin. An anion exchange resin consisting of a water
soluble polymer having a molecular
weight equivalent between 350 and 360
in which aliphatic quaternary amine
groups are attached to an acrylic back-
bone by ester linkages.
cholalic acid.
See: Cholic Acid.
Cholan-DH. (Medeva) Dehydrocholic
acid 250 mg/Tab. Bot. 100s.
Use: Laxative.
Cholan-HMB. (Novartis Consumer
Health) Dehydrocholic acid 250 mg/Tab.
Bot. 100s. *otc.*
Use: Laxative.
cholanic acid. Dehydrodesoxycholic
acid.
Cholebrine. (Mallinckrodt) Iocetamic acid
(62% iodine) 750 mg/Tab. Bot. 100s,
150s.

Use: Radiopaque agent.

•**cholecalciferol,** U.S.P. 23.
Use: Vitamin (antirachitic).
See: Decavitamin Cap., Tab.

cholecystography agents.
See: Bilopaque, Cap. (Sanofi Winthrop).
Iodized Oil (Various Mfr.).
Iophendylate Inj.
Pantopaque, Amp. (Lafayette).
Telepaque, Tab. (Sanofi Winthrop).

Choledyl SA. (Parke-Davis) Oxtriphyl-
line 400 mg or 600 mg/Tab. Bot. 100s,
UD 100s. *Rx.*
Use: Bronchodilator.

•**cholera vaccine,** U.S.P. 23.
Use: Active immunizing agent.

cholera vaccine. (Wyeth Lederle) 8 units
each of Ogawa and Inaba strains per
ml. Vial, 1.5 ml, 20 ml.
Use: Active immunizing agent.

choleretic. Bile salts.
See: Bile Preps. and Forms.
Dehydrocholic Acid.
Desoxycholic Acid.
Tocamphyl, Tab. (Various Mfr.).

cholesterin.
See: Cholesterol.

•**cholesterol,** N.F. 18. (Various Mfr.).
Use: Pharmaceutic aid (emulsifying
agent).

cholesterol reagent strips. (Bayer) A
quantitative strip test for cholesterol
in serum. Seralyzer reagent strips. Bot.
25s.
Use: Diagnostic aid.

cholestyramine. (koe-less-TIE-ruh-
meen) An antihyperlipidemic agent used
to lower cholesterol. Consists of anhydrous cholestyramine 4 g/dose.
See: Cholybar, Bar (Parke-Davis).
Questran, Pow. (Bristol Labs.).
Questran Light, Pow. (Bristol Labs.).

cholestyramine. (koe-less-TIE-ruh-
meen) U.S.P. 23.
Use: Ion-exchange resin (bile salts), antihyperlipoproteinemic.

•**cholestyramine powder.** (Goldline) 4 g
(as anhydrous resin), phenylalanine
14.1 mg/5.5 g powder, aspartame/Pow.
Packets. 42 and 60 single dose 5.5 g
Packets. *Rx.*
Use: Bile acid sequestrant.

•**cholestyramine resin,** U.S.P. 23. A sty-
ryl-divinyl-benzene copolymer (about
2% divinylbenzene) containing quaternary ammonium groups.
Use: Antihyperlipidemic, ion-exchange
resin (bile salts).
See: Questran, Pow. (Bristol).

cholic acid.

Cholidase. (Freeda) Choline 450 mg,
inositol 150 mg, vitamins B_6 2.5 mg, B_{12}
5 mcg, E 7.5 mg/Tab. Bot. 100s, 250s,
500s. *otc.*
Use: Lipotropic/vitamin supplement.

choline. (Various Mfr.) Choline. Tab.: **250
mg:** Bot. 100s, 250s, 500s, 1000s. **500
mg:** Bot. 100s. **650 mg:** Bot. 90s,
100s, 250s, 500s. *otc.*
Use: Lipotropic.

choline bitartrate.
W/Bile extract, pancreatic substance, dl-
methionine.
See: Licoplex, Tab. (Mills).
W/Methionine, inositol, desiccated liver,
vitamin B_{12}.
See: Limvic, Tab. (Briar).
W/Mucopolysaccharide, epinephrine neu-
tralizing factor, pancreatic lipotropic
fraction, dl-methionine, inositol, bile ex-
tract.
See: Lipo-K, Cap. (Marcen).
W/d-Pantothenyl alcohol.
See: Ilopan-Choline, Tab. (Pharmacia
& Upjohn).
W/Safflower oil, whole liver, soybean, leci-
thin, inositol, methionine, natural to-
copherols, vitamins B_6, B_{12}, panthenol.
See: Nutricol, Cap., Vial (Nutrition Con-
trol).

choline chloride. (Various Mfr.).
Use: Liver supplement. [Orphan drug]
W/Inositol, methionine, vitamin B_{12}.
See: Lychol-B, Inj. (Burgin-Arden).
W/Methionine, vitamins, niacinamide,
panthenol.
See: Minoplex, Vial (Savage).
W/Panthenol, inositol, vitamins, minerals,
estrone, testosterone.
See: Geramine, Inj. (Zeneca).
W/Panthenol, inositol, vitamins, minerals,
estrone, testosterone, polydigestase.
See: Geramine, Tab. (Zeneca).
W/Vitamin B_1, niacinamide, B_2, B_6, cal-
cium pantothenate, cyanocobalamin,
B_{12}, inositol, dl-methionine, testoster-
one, estrone, procaine.
See: Gerihorm, Inj. (Burgin-Arden).

choline chloride, carbamate. Carbachol, U.S.P. 23.

choline chloride succinate.
See: Succinylcholine Chloride, U.S.P.
23.

choline citrate, tricholine citrate.
W/Inositol, methionine, vitamin B_{12}.
See: Cholimeth Tab. (Schwarz
Pharma).

choline dihydrogen citrate. 2-Hydroxy-
ethyl trimethylammonium citrate-U.S.

vitamin 0.5 g. Bot. 100s, 500s.
Use: Lipotropic.
See: Cholinate, Liq. (Cenci).
choline magnesium trisalicylate. (Sidmak) 500 mg, 750 mg or 1000 mg. Tab. Bot. 100s, 500s. *Rx.*
Use: Salicylate analgesic.
See: Trilisate, Tab. (Purdue Frederick).
cholinergic agents.
(Parasympathomimetic Agents).
See: Mecholyl Cl, Inj. (Baker).
Mestinon, Tab., Syr., Amp. (Roche).
Mytelase, Cap. (Sanofi Winthrop).
Pilocarpine Nitrate (Various Mfr.).
Prostigin Bromide, Tab. (Roche).
Prostigin Methylsulfate, Inj. (Roche).
Tensilon, Inj. (Roche).
Urecholine, Inj., Tab. (Merck & Co.).
cholinergic blocking agents.
See: Parasympatholytic agents.
•**choline salicylate.** USAN.
Use: Analgesic (salicylate).
cholinesterase inhibitors. Agents that inhibit the enzyme cholinesterase and enhance the effects of endogenous acetylcholine.
Use: Glaucoma therapy.
See: Eserine Sulfate, Oint., (Various, eg, Harber, Iolab, Pharmaderm).
Isopto Eserine, Soln., (Alcon).
Eserine Salicylate, Soln., (Alcon).
Use: Muscle stimulants.
See: Prostigin, Tab., (Roche).
Neostigine Methylsulfate, Inj., (Various Mfr.).
Prostigin, Inj., (Roche).
choline theophyllinate.
See: Oxtriphylline.
Cholinoid. (Goldline) Choline 111 mg, inositol 111 mg, vitamins B_1 0.33 mg, B_2 0.33 mg, B_3 3.33 mg, B_5 1.7 mg, B_6 0.33 mg, B_{12} 1.7 mcg, C 100 mg, lemon bioflavonoid complex 100 mg/ Cap. Bot. 100s. *otc.*
Use: Lipotropic/vitamin supplement.
Chol Meth in B. (Esco) Choline bitartrate 235 mg, inositol 112 mg, methionine 70 mg, betaine anhydrous 50 mg, vitamins B_{12} 6 mcg, B_1 6 mg, B_6 3 mg, niacin 10 mg/Cap. Bot. 500s, 1000s. *otc.*
Use: Vitamin supplement.
Cholografin Meglumine. (Squibb) Iodipamide meglumine **10.3%** (iodine 5.1%)/ 100 ml, Vial 100 ml. **52%** (26% iodine)/ 20 ml, Vial 20 ml.
Use: Cholangiography, cholecystography.
Cholografin Sodium.

Choloxin. (Knoll Pharm.) Sodium dextrothyroxine 1 mg, 2 mg or 4 mg/Tab. Tartrazine (2 mg, 4 mg only). Bot. 100s, Bot. 250s (2 mg, 4 mg only). *Rx.*
Use: Antihyperlipidemic.
cholyglycine.
See: CG RIA, Kit (Abbott).
chondodendron tomentosum.
See: Curare.
Chondroitinase. (Storz).
Use: For patients undergoing vitrectomy. [Orphan Drug]
chondrotin sulfate and sodium hyaluronate. A surgical aid in anterior segent procedures including cataract extraction and intraocular lens implantation. *Rx.*
See: Viscoat, Soln., (Cilco).
chondrus. Irish Moss.
W/Petrolatum, Liq.
See: Kondremul, Liq. (Medeva).
Chooz. (Schering-Plough) Calcium carbonate 500 mg/Gum tab. Pkg. 16s. *otc.*
Use: Antacid.
Chorex 5. (Hyrex) Chorionic gonadotropin 5000 units, mannitol, benzyl alcohol 0.9%/Vial 10 ml. *Rx.*
Use: Chorionic gonadotropin.
Chorex 10. (Hyrex) Chorionic gonadotropin 10,000 units. Mannitol, benzyl alcohol 0.9%/Vial 10 ml. *Rx.*
Use: Chorionic gonadotropin.
chorionic gonadotropin. 5000 units/ Vial w/diluent 10 ml, 10,000 units/Vial w/ diluent 10 ml, 20,000 units/vial w/diluent 10 ml (Various) mannitol, benzyl alcohol 0.9%/Vial 10 ml. Vial.
Use: Prepubertal cryptorchidism or induction of ovulation and pregnancy in anovulatory women.
See: Antuitrin-S (Parke-Davis).
A.P.L., Inj. (Wyeth-Ayerst).
C-G-10, Vial (Scrip).
Chorex 5, Vial (Hyrex).
Chorex 10, Vial (Hyrex).
Choron 10, Vial (Forest).
Gonadex (Continental Dist.).
Gonic, Vial (Hauck).
Khorion (Hickam).
Neovital-Diluent, Inj. (Taylor).
Pregnyl, Vial (Organon).
Profasi, Vial (Serono).
Rochoric, Inj. (Rocky Mtn.).
Choron 10. (Forest) Chorionic gonadotropin 10,000 units/vial with diluent 10 ml, mannitol, benzyl alcohol 0.9%/Inj. Vial 10 ml. *Rx.*
Use: Chorionic gonadotropin.

Chromagen. (Savage) **Cap.:** Ferrous fumarate 66 mg, vitamins C 250 mg, B$_{12}$ activity 10 mcg, desiccated stomach substances 100 mg/soft gelatin cap. Bot. 100s, 500s. *Rx.*
Use: Vitamin/mineral supplement.

Chromalbin. (Squibb) 100 uCi containing chromium Cr^{51} and human albumin. *Rx.*

Chroma-Pak. (SoloPak) Chromium **4 mcg/ml:** Vial 10 ml, 30 ml. **20 mcg/ml:** Vial 5 ml. *Rx.*
Use: Parenteral nutritional supplement.

chromargyre.
See: Merbromin (Various Mfr.).

chromated. Solution (Cr^{51}).
See: Chromitope sodium (Squibb).

Chromelin Complexion Blender. (Summers) Dihydroxyacetone 5%, alcohol 50%. Bot. oz. *otc.*
Use: Agent for vitiligo.

chromic acid, disodium salt. Sodium Chromate Cr^{51} Inj., U.S.P. 23.

•**chromic chloride,** U.S.P. 23.
Use: Supplement (trace mineral).
See: Chrometrace, Inj. (Centeon).

•**chromic chloride Cr^{51}.** USAN.
Use: Radioactive agent.
See: Chromitope Cl (Squibb).

•**chromic phosphate Cr^{51}.** USAN.
Use: Radioactive agent.

•**chromic phosphate P^{32} suspension,** U.S.P. 23.
Use: Radioactive agent.

Chromitope Sodium. (Squibb) Chromate Cr^{51}, Sodium for Inj. 0.25 mCi.
Use: Radioactive agent.

chromium. A trace metal used in IV nutritional therapy that helps maintain normal glucose metabolism and peripheral nerve function.
See: Chromium, Inj. (Various Mfr.).
  Chromic Chloride, Inj. (Various Mfr.).
  Chromium Chloride, Inj. (Various Mfr.).
  Chroma-Pak, Inj. (Solopak).
  Chromium Trace Metal Additive, Inj. (IMS).
  Concentrated Chrmic Chloride, Inj. (American Regent).

•**chromonar hydrochloride.** (KROE-moe-nahr) USAN.
Use: Coronary vasodilator.

Chronulac. (Hoechst Marion Roussel) Lactulose 10 g/15 ml (< 2.2 g galactose, 1.2 g lactose, 1.2 g other sugars). Bot. 473 ml, 1890 ml, UD 15 ml, 30 ml. Box 100s. *Rx.*
Use: Laxative.

chrysazin.
See: Danthron, N.F. 18.

Chur-Hist. (Churchill) Chlorpheniramine 4 mg/Kaptab. Bot. 100s.
Use: Antihistamine.

Chymex. (Pharmacia & Upjohn) Bentiromide 500 mg/7.5 ml w/propylene glycol 40%. Screening test for pancreatic exocrine insufficiency.
Use: Diagnostic aid.

Chymodiactin. (Smith) 4 nKat units, 1.4 mg sodium L-cysteinate HCl with diluent. Pow. for Inj. Vial 2 ml. *Rx.*
Use: Proteolytic enzyme.

•**chymopapain.** (KIE-moe-pap-ANE) USAN. Proteolytic enzyme isolated from papaya latex, differing from papain in electrophoretic mobility, solubility and substrate specificity.
Use: Proteolytic enzyme.

•**chymotrypsin,** U.S.P. 23. An enzyme, α-Chymotrypsin obtained in crystalline form from mammalian pancreas by aqueous acid extraction of its proenzyme, chymotrypsinogen, and subsequent conversion with trypsin to chymotrypsin.
Use: Proteolytic enzyme.
See: Catarase, Soln. (Ciba Vision).
W/Trypsin.
  See: Orenzyme, Tab. (Hoechst Marion Roussel).
W/Trypsin, neomycin palmitate.
  See: Biozyme, Oint. (Centeon).

C.I. Basic Violet 3. Gentian Violet, U.S.P. 23.

Ciba Vision Cleaner. (Ciba Vision) Cocoamphocarboxyglycinate, sodium lauryl sulfate, sorbic acid 0.1%, hexylene glycol, EDTA 0.2%. Soln. 5 ml or 15 ml. *otc.*
Use: Soft contact lens care.

Ciba Vision Saline. (Ciba Vision) Buffered, isotonic with NaCl, boric acid. Soln. Bot. 90 ml, 240 ml, 360 ml. *otc.*
Use: Solution for rinsing/storage of soft contact lens.

cibenzoline. (SIGH-BEN-zoe-leen)
See: Cifenline Succinate. USAN.

•**ciclafrine hydrochloride.** (SICK-lah-freen) USAN.
Use: Antihypotensive.

•**ciclazindol.** (sigh-CLAY-zin-dole) USAN.
Use: Antidepressant.

•**cicletanine.** (sick-LET-ah-neen) USAN.
Use: Antihypertensive.

•**ciclopirox.** (sigh-kloe-PEER-ox) USAN.
Use: Antifungal.

•**ciclopirox olamine,** (sigh-kloe-PEER-ox

OLE-ah-meen) U.S.P. 23.
Use: Antifungal.
See: Loprox, Cream (Hoechst Marion Roussel).

•**cicloprofen.** (SICK-low-pro-fen) USAN.
Use: Anti-inflammatory.

•**cicloprolol hydrochloride.** (SIGH-kloe-PRO-lahl) USAN.
Use: Anti-adrenergic (beta receptor).

Cidex. (Johnson & Johnson) Activated dialdehyde soln. Bot. qt, gal, 2.5 gal.
Use: Sterilizing, disinfecting agent.

Cidex-7. (Johnson & Johnson) Glutaraldehyde 2% and vial of activator with aqueous potassium salt as buffer and sodium nitrite as a corrosive inhibitor. Soln. Bot. qt, 1 gal, 5 gal.
Use: Sterilizing, disinfecting agent.

Cidex Plus. (Johnson & Johnson) 3.2% glutaraldehyde. Soln. Gal.
Use: Sterilizing, disinfecting agent.

C.I. Direct Blue 53 Tetrasodium Salt. Evans Blue, U.S.P. 23. *Rx.*

•**cidofovir.** (sigh-DAH-fah-vihr) USAN
Use: Antiviral.
See: Vistide (Gilead Sciences).

•**cidoxepin hydrochoride.** (sih-DOX-eh-PIN) USAN.
Use: Antidepressant.

•**cifenline.** (sigh-FEN-leen) USAN. *Formerly cibenzoline.*
Use: Cardiac depressant (antiarrhythmic).

•**cifenline succinate.** (sigh-FEN-leen) USAN.
Use: Cardiac depressant (antiarrhythmic).

•**ciglitazone.** (sigh-GLIE-tah-ZONE) USAN.
Use: Antidiabetic.

cignolin.
See: Anthralin (Various Mfr.).

•**ciladopa hydrochloride.** (SIGH-lah-doe-pah) USAN.
Use: Treatment of Parkinson's disease, dopaminergic.

cilastatin-imipenem. A formulation of imipenem, a thienamycin antibiotic, and cilastatin sodium, the inhibitor of the renal dipeptidase, dehydropeptidase-1.
Use: Anti-infective.
See: Primaxin I.V., Pow. (Merck). Primaxin I.M., Pow. (Merck).

•**cilastatin sodium,** (SIGH-lah-STAT-in) U.S.P. 23.
Use: Enzyme inhibitor.
W/Imipenem.
See: Primaxin, Inj. (Merck).

•**cilazapril.** (sile-AZE-ah-PRILL) USAN.
Use: Antihypertensive.

•**cilexetil.** (sigh-LEX-eh-till) USAN.
Use: Antibacterial.
Sanfetrinem Cilexetil.

Cilfomide Tablets. (Sanofi Winthrop) Inositol hexanicotinate. *Rx.*
Use: Hypolipidimic, peripheral vasodilator.

ciliary neurotrophic factor. (Regeneron Pharm) *Rx.*
Use: Treatment of amyotrophic lateral sclerosis. [Orphan drug]

ciliary neurotrophic factor (recombinant human). *Rx.*
Use: Treatment of motor neuron disease. [Orphan drug]

Cillium. (Whiteworth Towne) Psyllium seed husk pow. 4.94 g, 14 calories/rounded tsp. Bot. 420 g, 630 g. *otc.*
Use: Laxative.

•**cilmostim.** USAN.
Use: Hematopoietic (macrophage colony-stimulating factor).

•**cilobamine mesylate.** (SIGH-low-BAM-een) USAN. *Formerly clobamine mesylate.*
Use: Antidepressant.

•**cilofungin.** (SIGH-low-FUN-jin) USAN.
Use: Antifungal.

Ciloxan. (Alcon) Ciprofloxacin HCl 3.5 mg (equivalent to 3 mg base)/ml. Soln., Drop-Tainer dispensers. 2.5 ml, 5 ml. *Rx.*
Use: Anti-infective.

•**cimaterol.** (sigh-MAH-teh-role) USAN.
Use: Repartitioning agent.

•**cimetidine,** (sigh-MET-ih-deen) U.S.P. 23.
Use: H_2 histamine antagonist.
See: Tagamet, Tab., Inj. (SK-Beecham).

cimetidine. (Various Mfr.) 200 mg, 300 mg, 400 mg, 800 mg/Tab. Bot. 100s, 500s, 1000s, UD 100s.
Use: HB_2 histamine antagonist.

•**cimetidine hydrochloride.** (sigh-MET-ih-deen) USAN.
Use: H_2 histamine antagonist.

cimetidine hydrochloride. (sigh-MET-ih-deen) (Endo) Cimetidine HCl 150 mg, phenol 5 mg/ml. Inj. In 2 ml vials and 8 ml multiple dose vials. *Rx.*
Use: Histamine H_2 antagonist.

cimetidine oral solution. (sigh-MET-ih-deen) (Barre-National) 300 mg (as HCl)/5 ml. Bot. 240 ml, 470 ml. *Rx.*
Use: Histamine H_2 antagonist.

Cinacort Span. (Foy) Triamcinolone acetonide 40 mg/ml. Vial 5 ml. *Rx.*

Use: Corticosteroid.

•**cinalukast.** USAN.
Use: Antiasthmatic (leukotriene antagonist).

•**cinanserin hydrochloride.** (sin-AN-ser-in) USAN.
Use: Serotonin inhibitor.

cinchona bark. (Various Mfr.).
Use: Antimalarial, tonic.
W/Anhydrous quinine, cinchonidine, cinchonine, quinidine, quinine.
See: Totaquine, Pow. (Various Mfr.).
W/Iron oxide, nux vomica, vitamin B_1, alcohol.
See: Briatonic, Liq. (Briar).

cinchonidine sulfate.

cinchonine salts. (Various Mfr.).
Use: Quinine dihydrochloride.

cinchophen.
Use: Analgesic.

•**cinepazet maleate.** (SIN-eh-PAZZ-ett) USAN.
Use: Antianginal.

•**cinflumide.** (SIN-flew-mide) USAN.
Use: Muscle relaxant.

•**cingestol.** (sin-JESS-tole) USAN.
Use: Progestin.

cinnamaldehyde. N.F. IX.

•**cinnamedrine.** (sin-am-ED-reen) USAN.
Use: Smooth muscle relaxant.
See: Midol, Tab. (Bayer).

cinnamic aldehyde. Name previously used for Cinnamaldehyde.

cinnamon, N.F. XVI.
Use: Flavoring agent.

cinnamon oil, N.F. XVI. (Various Mfr.).
Use: Pharmaceutic aid.

cinnamyl ephedrine hydrochloride.
W/Acetaminophen, homatropine methylbromide.
See: Periodic, Cap. (Towne).

•**cinnarizine.** (sin-NAHR-ih-zeen) USAN.
Use: Antihistamine.

cinnopentazone. INN for Cintazone.

Cinobac. (Oclassen) Cinoxacin **250 mg/ Cap.:** Bot. 40s. **500 mg/Cap.:** Bot. 50s. *Rx.*
Use: Urinary anti-infective.

•**cinoxacin,** (sin-OX-ah-sin) U.S.P. 23.
Use: Antibacterial.
See: Cinobac, Cap. (Dista).

cinoxacin. (sin-OX-ah-sin) (Various Mfr.)
250 mg/Cap. Bot. 40s, 100s. 500 mg/ Cap. Bot. 50s, 100s. *Rx.*
Use: Urinary anti-infective.

•**cinoxate,** (sin-OX-ate) U.S.P. 23.
Use: Ultraviolet screen.
See: Sundare Prods. (Rydelle).

W/Methyl anthranilate.
See: Maxafil Cream (Rydelle).

•**cinperene.** (SIN-peh-reen) USAN.
Use: Antipsychotic.

Cin-Quin. (Solvay) Quinidine sulfate. (Contains 83% anhydrous quinidine alkaloid.) **Tab.:** 100 mg, 200 mg or 300 mg. Bot. 100s, 1000s, UD 100s. **Cap.:** 200 mg. Bot. 100s. 300 mg. Bot. 100s, 1000s, UD 100s. *Rx.*
Use: Antiarrhythmic.

•**cinromide.** (SIN-row-mide) USAN.
Use: Anticonvulsant.

•**cintazone.** (SIN-tah-zone) USAN.
Use: Anti-inflammatory.

•**cintriamide.** (sin-TRY-ah-mid) USAN.
Use: Antipsychotic.

•**cioteronel.** (SIGH-oh-TEH-row-nell) USAN.
Use: Treatment of acne, adrogenic alopecia and keloid (antiandrogen).

•**cipamfylline.** (sigh-PAM-fih-lin) USAN.
Use: Antiviral.

Cipralan. (Roche) Cifenline succinate, formerly cibenzoline. *Rx.*
Use: Antiarrhythmic.

•**ciprefadol succinate.** (sih-PREH-fah-dahl) USAN.
Use: Analgesic.

Cipro. (Bayer) Ciprofloxacin HCl 100 mg, 250 mg, 500 mg or 750 mg/Tab. Bot. 50s (750 mg only), 100s (except 750 mg), UD 100s, 100 mg in *Cipro Cystitis Packs* 6s. *Rx.*
Use: Anti-infective, fluoroquinolone.

Cipro I.V.. (Bayer) Ciprofloxacin 200 mg and 400 mg (with lactic acid). Inj. Vial: 20 ml (1%), 40 ml (1%). Flex Bot.: 100 ml (in 5% dextrose) and 200 ml (in 5% dextrose). *Rx.*
Use: Anti-infective, fluoroquinolone.

•**ciprocinonide.** (sih-PRO-SIN-oh-nide) USAN.
Use: Adrenocortical steroid.

•**ciprofibrate.** (sip-ROW-FIE-brate) USAN.
Use: Antihyperlipoproteinemic.

•**ciprofloxacin,** (sip-ROW-FLOX-ah-sin) U.S.P. 23.
Use: Antibacterial.

•**ciprofloxacin hydrochloride,** (sip-ROW-FLOX-ah-sin) U.S.P. 23.
Use: Antibacterial.
See: Ciloxan, Soln. (Alcon).
Cipro (Bayer).

•**ciprostene calcium.** (sigh-PRAHS-teen) USAN.
Use: Platelet aggregation inhibitor.

•**ciramadol.** (sihr-AM-ah-dole) USAN.
Use: Analgesic.

•**ciramadol hydrochloride.** (sihr-AM-ah-dole) USAN.
Use: Analgesic.

Cirbed. (Boyd) Papaverine HCl 150 mg/Cap. Bot. 100s. *Rx.*
Use: Antispasmodic.

Circavite-T. (Circle) Iron 12 mg, vitamins A 10,000 IU, D 400 IU, E 15 mg, B$_1$ 10.3 mg, B$_2$ 10 mg, B$_3$ 100 mg, B$_5$ 18.4 mg, B$_6$ 4.1 mg, B$_{12}$ 5 mcg, C 200 mg, Cu, I, Mg, Mn, zinc 1.5 mg. Bot. 100s. *otc.*
Use: Vitamin/mineral supplement.

•**cirolemycin.** (sih-ROW-leh-MY-sin) USAN.
Use: Antibacterial, antineoplastic.

•**cisapride.** (SIS-uh-PRIDE) USAN.
Use: Treatment of heartburn, stimulant (peristaltic).
See: Propulsid, Tab. (Janssen).

•**cisatracurium besylate.** (sis-ah-trah-CURE-ee-uhm BESS-ih-late) USAN.
Use: Nondepolarizing neuromuscular blocking agent; muscle relaxant; adjunct to anesthesia.
See: Nimbex, Inj. (Glaxo Wellcome).

•**cisconazole.** (SIS-KOE-nah-zahl) USAN.
Use: Antifungal.

•**cisplatin.** (SIS-plat-in) U.S.P. 23.
Use: Antineoplastic.
See: Platinol, Inj. (Bristol).

cis-retinoic acid. (13-cis-Retinoic Acid). *Rx.*
Use: Antiacne.
See: Isotretinoin.
   Accutane (Roche).

citanest hydrochloride. (Astra) **Plain:** Prilocaine HCl 4%/1.8 ml dental cartridge. *Rx.*
Use: Local anesthetic.

Citanest Hydrochloride Forte. (Astra) Prilocaine HCl 4% with epinephrine 1:200,000. Contains sodium metabisulfite. Dental cartridge 1.8 ml. Inj. *Rx.*
Use: Local anesthetic.

•**citenamide.** (sigh-TEN-ah-MIDE) USAN.
Use: Anticonvulsant.

Cithal Capsules. (Table Rock) Watermelon seed extract 2 gr, theobromine 4 gr, phenobarbital 0.25 gr/Cap. Bot. 100s, 500s. *Rx.*
Use: Antihypertensive.

•**citicoline sodium.** (SIGH-tih-koe-leen) USAN.
Use: Post-stroke and post-head trauma treatment.

Citracal. (Mission) Calcium citrate 950 mg/Tab. Bot. 100s. *otc.*

Use: Calcium supplement.

Citracal 1500 + D. (Mission) Calcium citrate 1500 mg, vitamin D 200 IU/Tab. Bot. 60s. *otc.*
Use: Vitamin/mineral supplement.

Citracal Liquitab. (Mission) Calcium citrate 2376 mg/Effervescent tab. Box. 30s. *otc.*
Use: Calcium supplement.

Citra Forte. (Boyle) Hydrocodone bitartrate 5 mg, ascorbic acid 30 mg, pheniramine maleate 2.5 mg, pyrilamine maleate 3.33 mg, potassium citrate 150 mg/5 ml. Bot. pt, gal. *c-III.*
Use: Antitussive, vitamin C supplement, antihistamine.

Citramin-500. (Thurston) Vitamin C 500 mg, rose hips, acerola with mixed bioflavonoids/Loz. Bot. 100s, 250s, 1000s. *otc.*
Use: Vitamin/mineral supplement.

Citranox. (Alconox)
Use: Liquid acid detergent for manual and ultrasonic washers.

Citra pH. (Val Med) Sodium citrate dihydrate 450 mg/30 ml. Soln. 30 ml. *otc.*
Use: Antacid.

Citrasan B. (Sandia) Lemon bioflavonoid complex 300 mg, vitamins C 300 mg, B$_1$ 30 mg, B$_2$ 10 mg, B$_6$ 5 mg, B$_{12}$ 4 mcg, calcium pantothenate 10 mg, niacinamide 50 mg/Tab. Bot. 100s, 1000s. *otc.*
Use: Vitamin/mineral supplement.

Citrasan K-250. (Sandia) Vitamins C 250 mg, K 1 mg, lemon bioflavonoid 250 mg/Tab. Bot. 100s, 1000s. *otc.*
Use: Vitamin supplement.

Citrasan K Liquid. (Sandia) Vitamins C 125 mg, K 0.66 mg, lemon bioflavonoid complex 125 mg/5 ml. Bot. pt, gal. *otc.*
Use: Vitamin supplement.

citrate acid.
See: Bicitra Soln. (Baker Norton).

citrate and citric acid solution.
Use: Alkalinizer.
See: Polycitra (Baker Norton).
   Polycitra-LC (Baker Norton).
   Polycitra-K (Baker Norton).
   Oracit (Carolina Medical Products.).
   Bicitra (Baker Norton).

Citrate of Magnesia. (Various Mfr.) Magnesium citrate. Soln. Bot. 300 ml. *otc.*
Use: Laxative.

citrated normal human plasma.
See: Plasma, Normal Human.

Citresco-K. (Esco) Vitamins C 100 mg, K 0.7 mg, citrus bioflavonoid complex

100 mg/Cap. Bot. 100s, 500s, 1000s. *otc.*

Use: Vitamin supplement.

•**citric acid,** U.S.P. 23.

Use: Component of anticoagulant solutions and drug products.

citric acid and d-gluconic acid irrigant. *Rx.*

Use: Genitourinary irrigant. [Orphan drug]

See: Renacidin (Guardian).

citric acid, magnesium oxide, and sodium carbonate irrigation.

Use: Irrigating solution.

citrin.

See: Vitamin P.

Citrin Capsules. (Table Rock) Watermelon seed extract 4 gr/Cap. Bot. 100s, 500s. *Rx.*

Use: Antihypertensive.

Citrocarbonate. (Pharmacia & Upjohn) Sodium bicarbonate 0.78 g, sodium citrate anhydrous 1.82 g/3.9 g. Bot. 4 oz, 8 oz. *otc.*

Use: Antacid.

Citrocarbonate Effervescent Granules. (Roberts-Hauck) Sodium bicarbonate 780 mg, sodium citrate anhydrous 1820 mg, sodium 700.6 mg/5 ml. Bot. 150 g. *otc.*

Use: Antacid, analgesic.

Citro Cee, Super. (Marlyn) Bioflavonoids 500 mg, rutin 50 mg, vitamin C 500 mg, rose hips powder 500 mg/Tab. Bot. 50s, 100s. *otc.*

Use: Vitamin supplement.

Citro-Flav 200. (Goldline) Citrus bioflavonoid compound 200 mg/Cap. Bot. 100s, 1000s. *otc.*

Use: Vitamin supplement.

Citroleum Sunburn Creme. (Citroleum) Bot. 4 oz.

Citrolith. (Beach) Potassium citrate 50 mg, sodium citrate 950 mg/Tab. Bot. 100s, 500s. *Rx.*

Use: Urinary alkalinizer.

Citroma. (Century) Magnesium citrate. Oral soln. Bot. 10 oz. *otc.*

Use: Laxative.

Citroma Low Sodium. (National Magnesia) Magnesium citrate. Oral soln w/lemon or cherry flavor in sugar-free vehicle. Bot. 10 oz. *otc.*

Use: Laxative.

Citrotein. (Sandoz Nutrition) Sucrose, pasteurized egg white solids, amino acids, maltodextrin, citric acid, natural and artificial flavors, mono and diglycerides, partially hydrogenated soybean oil, 0.66 cal/ml, protein 40.7 g, carbohydrate 120.7 g, fat 1.55 g, sodium 698 mg, potassium 698 mg/L. Tartrazine (orange flavor only). Pow. 1.57 oz/packet, Can 14.16 oz. Orange, grape and punch flavors. *otc.*

Use: Enteral nutritional supplement.

citrovorum factor. Leucovorin Calcium, U.S.P. 23.

See: Leucovorin Calcium (Lederle) Folinic Acid.

Citrucel. (SK-Beecham) Methylcellulose 2 g/heaping tbsp. dose w/citric acid. Bot. 16 oz, 30 oz. *otc.*

Use: Laxative.

Citrucel Sugar Free. (SK-Beecham) Methylcellulose 2 g, aspartame, phenylalanine 52 mg. Pow. Can. 479 g. *otc.*

Use: Laxative.

citrus bioflavonoid compound.

See: Bioflavonoid Compounds (Various Mfr.).

C.V.P., Syr. (Rhone-Poulenc Rorer). Vitamin P.

W/Ascorbic acid, phenyltoloxamine dihydrogen citrate, salicylamide, acetyl p-aminophenol, caffeine, racemic amphetamine sulfate.

See: Euphenex, Tab. (Westerfield).

Citrus-Flav C 500. (Fibertone) Citrus bioflavonoids complex 200 mg, vitamin C 200 mg, hesperidin complex 40 mg, acerola 50 mg, rutin 10 mg, in citrus base of orange and lemon powder, grapefruit concentrate powder and citrus pectin. Tabs. Bot. 100s, 250s. *otc.*

Use: Nutritional supplement.

C-Ject. (Lincoln) Ascorbic acid 2000 mg, sodium bisulfite 0.1%, disodium sequestrene 0.01%/10 ml. Amp. 10 ml, "Score-Break" Box 25s. *Rx.*

Use: Nutritional supplement.

C-Ject with B. (Lincoln) When mixed with 10 ml of diluent, each vial contains: Vitamins C 2000 mg, B$_1$ 50 mg, B$_2$ 5 mg, B$_6$ 10 mg, nicotinamide 100 mg, methylparaben 0.89 mg, propylparaben 0.22 mg, sodium bisulfite 10 mg, disodium sequestrene 1 mg. Box of 6 lyophilized plugs and 6 10 ml vials of Sterile Diluent. *Rx.*

Use: Nutritional supplement.

CKA Canker Aid. (Pannett Prod.) Benzocaine, aluminum hydrate, magnesium trisilicate, sodium acid carbonate. Pow. *otc.*

Use: Cold-canker sore.

CK(CPK) Reagent Strips. (Bayer) Seralyzer reagent strips for creatinine phosphokinase in serum or plasma. Bot. 25s.

Use: Diagnostic aid.

●**cladribine.** (KLAD-rih-BEAN) USAN.
Use: Antineoplastic. [Orphan drug]
See: Leustatin (Ortho Biotech).

Claforan. (Hoechst Marion Roussel)
Cefotaxime sodium 1 g, 2 g or 10 g/Vial.
Infusion Bot.: 1 g, 2 g. Viaflex (pre-
mixed frozen) Bag: 1 g, 2 g. Add-Van-
tage System: Vial 1 g, 2 g. Pow. for
Inj. 500 mg/Vial. 10s. *Rx.*
Use: Anti-infective, cephalosporin.

●**clamoxyquin hydrochloride.** (KLAM-
OX-ee-kwin) USAN.
Use: Amebicide.

Claretin-12.
See: Vitamin B$_{12}$.

●**clarithromycin,** (kluh-RITH-row-MY-sin)
U.S.P. 23.
Use: Antibacterial.

clarithromycin. A semi-synthetic macrolide antibiotic. *Rx.*
Use: Anti-infectant, erythromycin, used
in combination with omeprazole for
the treatment of duodenal ulcer associated with *H. pylori*
See: Biaxin Tabs., Gran. for Oral Susp.
(Abbott).

Claritin. (Schering-Plough) Loratadine
10 mg, lactose/Tab. Bot. 100s, unit-
of-use 14s, 30s and UD 100s. Loratadine 1 mg/ml/Syr. Bot. 480 ml. Loratadine 10 mg, mannitol/Reditabs. Blister
pack. 30s. *Rx.*
Use: Antihistamine.

Claritin-D. (Schering-Plough) Loratadine
5 mg, pseudoephedrine sulfate 120 mg/
SR Tab. Bot. 100s, unit-of-use 10s,
30s, UD 100s. *Rx.*
Use: Antihistamine, decongestant.

Claritin-D 24-Hour. (Schering-Plough)
Loratadine 10 mg, pseudoephedrine
sulfate 240 mg/ER Tab. Bot. 100s, UD
100s. *Rx.*
Use: Antihistamine, decongestant.

●**clavulanate potassium,** (CLAV-you-lah-
nate) U.S.P. 23.
Use: Inhibitor (β-*lactamase*).

clavulanate potassium, sterile. (CLAV-
you-lah-nate)
Use: Inhibitor (β-*lactamase*).

clavulanate potassium and ticarcillin.
Use: Anti-infective, pencillin.
See: Timentin, Pow. for Inj. (SK-
Beecham).
Timentin, Soln. (SK-Beecham).

clavulanic acid/amoxicillin.
Use: Anti-infective, penicillin.
See: Augentin Tab. (SK-Beecham).

clavulanic acid/ticarcillin.

Use: Anti-infective, penicillin.
See: Timentin Pow. for Inj. (SK-
Beecham).

●**clazolam.** (CLAY-zoe-lam) USAN.
Use: Tranquilizer (minor).

●**clazolimine.** (clay-ZOLE-ih-meen)
USAN.
Use: Diuretic.

Clean-n-Soak. (Allergan) Cleaning agent
with phenylmercuric nitrate 0.004%.
Bot. 120 ml. *otc.*
Use: Hard contact lens care.

Clearasil 10%. (Proter & Gamble) Benzoyl peroxide 10%. Bot. oz. *otc.*
Use: Antiacne.

Clearasil Adult Care Cream. (Procter &
Gamble) Sulfur, resorcinol, alcohol
10%, parabens. Cream. Tube. 17 g. *otc.*
Use: Antiacne.

**Clearasil Adult Care Medicated Blem-
ish Stick.** (Procter & Gamble) Sulfur
8%, resorcinol 1%, bentonite 4%,
laureth-4, titanium dioxide. Stick ⅛ oz.
otc.
Use: Antiacne.

Clearasil Antibacterial Soap. (Procter &
Gamble) Triclosan 0.75%, 92 g. *otc.*
Use: Antiacne.

**Clearasil Clearstick, Maximum
Strength.** (Procter & Gamble) Salicylic
acid 2%, alcohol 39%, menthol, EDTA.
Liq. 35 ml. *otc.*
Use: Antiacne.

Clearasil Clearstick, Regular Strength.
(Procter & Gamble) Salicylic acid
1.25%, alcohol 39%, aloe vera gel,
menthol, EDTA. Liq. 35 ml. *otc.*
Use: Antiacne.

**Clearasil Clearstick for Sensitive Skin,
Maximum Strength.** (Procter &
Gamble) Salicylic acid 2%, alcohol
39%, aloe vera gel, menthol, EDTA. Liq.
35 ml. *otc.*
Use: Antiacne.

Clearasil Daily Face Wash. (Procter &
Gamble) Triclosan 0.3%, glycerin, aloe
vera gel, EDTA. Liq. Bot. 135 ml. *otc.*
Use: Antiacne.

Clearasil Double Clear. (Procter &
Gamble) **Pads, maximum strength:**
Salicylic acid 2%, alcohol 40%, witch
hazel distillate, menthol, Jar 32s. **Pads,
regular strength:** Salicylic acid 1.25%,
alcohol 40%, witch hazel distillate,
menthol. Jar 32s. *otc.*
Use: Antiacne.

Clearasil Double Textured Pads. (Procter & Gamble) **Pads, regular strength:**
Salicylic acid 2%, alcohol 40%, gly-

cerin, aloe vera gel, EDTA. In 32s, 40s.

Pads, maximum strength: Salicylic acid 2%, alcohol 40%, menthol, aloe vera gel, EDTA. In 32s, 40s. *otc.*
Use: Antiacne.

Clearasil Maximum Strength Cream. (Procter & Gamble) Benzoyl peroxide 10%, parabens in tinted or vanishing base. Tube 18 g, 28 g. *otc.*
Use: Antiacne.

Clearasil Maximum Strength Lotion. (Procter & Gamble) Benzoyl peroxide 10%, cetyl alcohol, parabens in vanishing base. Bot. 29 ml. *otc.*
Use: Antiacne.

Clearasil Medicated Deep Cleanser. (Procter & Gamble) Salicylic acid 0.5%, alcohol 42%, menthol, EDTA, aloe vera gel, hydrogenated castor oil. Liq. Bot. 229 ml. *otc.*
Use: Antiacne.

Clear Away. (Schering-Plough) Salicyclic acid 40%. Disc Pck. 18s. *otc.*
Use: Antiacne.

Clear Away Plantar. (Schering-Plough) Salicyclic acid 40%. Disc (for feet) Pck. 24s. *otc.*
Use: Antiacne.

Clearblue Easy. (Whitehall Robbins) Dip stick for in-home pregnancy test. Kit 1, 2s.
Use: Diagnostic aid.

Clearblue Pregnancy Test. (VLI) Dip stick for pregnancy test. Kit 2s.
Use: Diagnostic aid.

Clear by Design. (SK-Beecham) Benzoyl peroxide 2.5% in an invisible, greaseless gel base. Tube 45 g. *otc.*
Use: Antiacne.

Clearex Acne Cream. (Approved) Allantoin, sulfur, resorcinol, d-panthenol, isopropanol. Tube 1.5 oz. *otc.*
Use: Antiacne.

Clear Eyes ACR Eye Drops. (Ross) Naphazoline HCl 0.012%. Bot. 15 ml, 30 ml. *otc.*
Use: Ophthalmic vasoconstrictor, mydriatic.

Clear Eyes Eye Drops. (Ross) Naphazoline HCl 0.012%. Bot. 15 ml, 30 ml. *otc.*
Use: Ophthalmic vasoconstrictor, mydriatic.

Clearly Cala-Gel. (TecLabs) Diphenhydramine HCl, zinc acetate, menthol, EDTA. Gel In 180 g. *otc.*
Use: Antipruritis, topical.

Clearplan. (VLI) Ovulation prediction test. Box 10s.

Use: Diagnostic aid.

Clear Total Lice Elimination System. (Care Technologies) **Shampoo:** Pyrethium extract 0.3%, piperonyl butoxide 3%. 2 ml, 4 ml. **Lice egg remover:** Enzymes including oxidoreductase, tranferase, lyase, hydrolase, isomerase, ligase and hydroxyethyl cellulose, sodium benzoate. *otc.*
Use: Lice removal system.

Clear Tussin 30. (Goldline) Dextromethorphan HBr 15 mg, guaifenesin 100 mg/5 ml, alcohol, dye, sugar free/ Liq. Bot. 118 ml. *otc.*
Use: Decongestant, expectorant.

•**clebopride.** (KLEH-boe-PRIDE) USAN.
Use: Antiemetic.

•**clemastine.** (KLEM-ass-teen) USAN.
Use: Antihistamine.
See: Tavist, Tab., Syr. (Sandoz).

•**clemastine fumarate,** (KLEM-ass-teen) U.S.P. 23.
Use: Antihistamine.

clemastine fumarate. (Various Mfr.) 0.5 mg/5 ml. Syr. Bot. 118 ml. 1.34 mg, 2.68 mg/Tab. Bot. 100s.
Use: Antihistamine.

clemizole hydrochloride.

Clens. (Alcon) Cleansing agent with benzalkonium Cl 0.02%, EDTA 0.1%. Soln. Bot. 60 ml. *otc.*
Use: Hard contact lens care.

•**clentiazem maleate.** (klen-TIE-ah-zem) USAN.
Use: Antianginal, antihypertensive, antagonist (calcium channel).

Cleocin Hydrochloride. (Pharmacia & Upjohn) Clindamycin HCl 75 mg, 150 mg or 300 mg/Cap. Tartrazine. Bot. 100s. (75 mg); 16s, 100s, UD 100s (150 mg, 300 mg). *Rx.*
Use: Anti-infective.

Cleocin Pediatric. (Pharmacia & Upjohn) Clindamycin palmitate HCl equivalent to clindamycin 75 mg/5 ml when reconstituted as directed. Bot. 100 ml. *Rx.*
Use: Anti-infective.

Cleocin Phosphate. (Pharmacia & Upjohn) Clindamycin phosphate equivalent to clindamycin 150 mg/ml. **300 mg:** Vial 2 ml w/disodium edetate 1 mg, benzyl alcohol 18.9 mg. Pack 25s, 100s. **600 mg:** Vial 4 ml w/disodium edetate 2 mg, benzyl alcohol 37.8 mg. Pack 25s, 100s. **900 mg:** Vial 6 ml. Pack 25s, 100s. **9000 mg:** Bulk Vial 60 ml. Pack 5s. *Rx.*
Use: Anti-infective.

Cleocin T. (Pharmacia & Upjohn) Clindamycin phosphate 10 mg/ml. Topical soln., gel, lot. Bot. 30 ml, 60 ml, pt. (topical soln.). Bot. 7.5 g, 30 g (gel). Lot. Bot. 60 ml (lotion). *Rx.*
Use: Anti-infective.

Cleocin Vaginal. (Pharmacia & Upjohn) Clindamycin phosphate 2%, mineral oil, benzyl alcohol, propylene glycol, polysorbate 60, sorbitan, monostearate. Cream. Tube with 7 disposable applicators 40 g. *Rx.*
Use: Anti-infective, vaginal.

Clerz Drops for Hard Lenses. (Ciba Vision) Hypertonic solution with hydroxyethylcellulose, sorbic acid, poloxamer 407, EDTA 0.1%, thimerosal 0.001%. Soln. Bot. 25 ml. *otc.*
Use: Hard contact lens care.

Clerz Drops for Soft Lenses. (Ciba Vision) Hypertonic solution with hydroxyethylcellulose, sodium borate, poloxamer 407, sorbic acid, thimerosal 0.001%, EDTA 0.1%. Soln. Bot. 25 ml. *otc.*
Use: Soft contact lens care.

Clerz 2 for Hard Lenses. (Ciba Vision) Isotonic solution with hydroxyethylcellulose, poloxamer 407, sodium Cl, potassium Cl, sodium borate, boric acid, sorbic acid, EDTA. Soln. Bot. 5 ml, 15 ml, 30 ml. *otc.*
Use: Hard contact lens care.

Clerz 2 for Soft Lenses. (Ciba Vision) Isotonic solution with sodium Cl, potassium Cl, hydroxyethylcellulose, poloxamer 407, sodium borate, boric acid, sorbic acid, EDTA. Soln. Bot. 5 ml (2s), 15 ml, 30. *otc.*
Use: Soft contact lens care.

•**clidinium bromide,** (KLIH-dih-nee-uhm BROE-mide) U.S.P. 23.
Use: Anticholinergic.
See: Quarzan, Cap. (Roche).
W/Chlordiazepoxide.
See: Librax, Cap. (Roche).

Climara. (Berlex) Estradiol 3.9 mg or 7.8 mg/Transdermal Patch. In 4s. *Rx.*
Use: Estrogen.

•**clinafloxacin hydrochloride.** (klin-ah-FLOX-ah-sin) USAN.
Use: Antibacterial.

Clinda-Derm. (Paddock) Clindamycin phosphate 10 mg/ml, isopropyl alcohol 51.5%, propylene glycol. Soln. Bot. 60 ml. *Rx.*
Use: Antiacne.

•**clindamycin.** (KLIN-dah-MY-sin) USAN.
Use: Antibacterial. Topical antibiotic for acne. Oral as antibiotic. Vaginal as anti-infective. AIDS associated pneumonia [Orphan drug]
See: Cleocin T (Pharmacia & Upjohn).
Cleocin (Pharmacia & Upjohn).
Cleocin Vaginal Cream (Pharmacia & Upjohn).

•**clindamycin hydrochloride,** (KLIN-dah-MY-sin) U.S.P. 23.
Use: Antibacterial.
See: Cleocin HCl A.D.T., Cap. (Pharmacia & Upjohn).

•**clindamycin palmitate hydrochloride,** (KLIN-dah-MY-sin PAL-mih-tate) U.S.P. 23.
Use: Antibacterial.
See: Cleocin Pediatric (Pharmacia & Upjohn).
Cleocin T, Liq. (Pharmacia & Upjohn).

•**clindamycin phosphate,** (KLIN-dah-MY-sin) U.S.P. 23.
Use: Antibacterial.
See: Cleocin phosphate, Inj. (Pharmacia & Upjohn).
Clinda-Derm, Soln. (Paddock).

clindamycin phosphate. (KLIN-dah-MY-sin) (Various Mfr.) Clindamycin phosphate 10 mg/ml. Topical Soln., gel, lotion. Bot. 30 ml, 60 ml (Topical Soln.). Tube 30 g (gel). Bot. 60 ml (lot.). *Rx.*
Use: Antiacne.

Clindex. (Rugby) Clidinium bromide 2.5 mg, chlordiazepoxide HCl 5 mg/Cap. Bot. 100s, 500s, 1000s. *c-iv.*
Use: Anticholinergic, antispasmodic.

Clinistix Reagent Strips. (Bayer) Glucose oxidase, peroxidase and orthotolidine. Diagnostic test for glucose in urine. Bot. 50s.
Use: Diagnostic aid.

Clinitest. (Bayer) 2-drop and 5-drop combination packages w/color charts for both 2-drop and 5-drop use. Reagent tablets containing copper sulfate, sodium hydroxide, heat-producing agents. Patient's plastic set; Tab. refills. **Box:** 100s, 500s, sealed in foil. **Child-resistant bot.:** 36s, 100s.
Use: Diagnostic aid.

Clinocaine Hydrochloride.
See: Procaine HCl.

Clinoril. (Merck & Co.) Sulindac 150 mg or 200 mg/Tab. Bot. 100s, UD 100s. Unit-of-use 60s, 100s. *Rx.*
Use: Nonsteroidal anti-inflammatory drug; analgesic.

Clinoxide Capsules. (Geneva Pharm.) Clidinium 2.5 mg, chlordiazepoxide HCl, 5 mg. Cap. Bot. 100s, 500s. *c-iv.*
Use: Gastrointestinal anticholinergic combination.

•**clioquinol,** U.S.P. 23. *Formerly Iodo-chlorhydroxyquin.*
Use: Antiamebic, anti-infective (topical).
See: HCV Creame (Saron).
Quin III, Cream (Lemmon).
Quinoform, Oint., Cream, Lot. (C & M Pharmacal).
Torofor, Cream, Oint. (Torch).
Vioform, Prep. (Novartis).
W/Aluminum acetate solution, hydrocortisone.
See: Hydrelt, Cream, Oint. (Zeneca).
W/Hydrocortisone acetate.
See: Viotag Cream (Solvay).
W/Hydrocortisone acetate, lidocaine.
See: Lidaform-HC, Creme, Lot. (Bayer).
W/Hydrocortisone, lidocaine.
See: Bafil Lotion (Scruggs).
HIL-20 Lotion (Solvay).
W/Hydrocortisone, chlorobutanol.
See: Hc-Form, Jelly (Recsei).
W/Hydrocortisone, coal tar extract.
See: Racet LCD, Cream (Lemmon).
W/Hydrocortisone and pramoxine HCl.
See: Dermarex Cream (Hyrex).
Sherform-HC, Oint. (Sheryl).
Stera-Form Creme (Mayrand).
V-Cort, Cream (Scrip).
W/Methylcellulose, aluminum hydroxide, atropine sulfate, hyoscine HBr, hyoscyamine sulfate.
See: Enterex, Tab. (Person & Covey).
W/Nystatin.
See: Nystaform, Oint. (Bayer).
clioquinol and hydrocortisone cream.
Use: Topical antifungal.
See: Bafil, Cream (Skruggs).
Caquin Cream (Forest).
Coidocort Cream (Coast).
Domeform-HC, Cream (Bayer).
Hi-Form Cream (Blaine).
Hydrelt, Cream (Zeneca).
Hysone, Cream (Roberts).
Ido-Cortistan Oint. (Standex).
Iodocort, Cream (Ulmer).
Iohydro, Cream (Freeport).
Maso-Form, Cream (Mason).
Mity-Quin Cream (Solvay).
Racet, Cream (Lemmon).
Racet Forte, Cream (Lemmon).
Vioform-Hydrocortisone, Cream, Oint., Lot. (Novartis).
Vio-Hydrocort, Cream, Oint. (Quality Generics).
clioquinol and hydrocortisone ointment.
Use: Topical antifungal.
See: Hysone, Cream (Roberts).
Vioform-Hydrocortisone, Cream, Oint., Lot. (Novartis).

Vio-Hydrocort, Cream, Oint. (Quality Generics).
•**clioxanide.** (klie-OX-ah-nide) USAN.
Use: Anthelmintic.
Clipoxide. (Schein) Clidinium bromide 2.5 mg, chlordiazepoxide HCl 5 mg/Cap. Bot. 100s, 500s. *c-v.*
Use: Anticholinergic, antispasmodic.
•**cliprofen.** (klih-PRO-fen) USAN.
Use: Anti-inflammatory.
clobamine mesylate. (KLOE-bah-meen)
Name previously used. See cilobamine mesylate.
Use: Antidepressant.
•**clobazam.** (KLOE-bazz-am) USAN.
Use: Tranquilizer (minor).
clobenztropine.
•**clobetasol propionate,** (kloe-BEE-tah-sahl PRO-pee-oh-nate) U.S.P. 23.
Use: Anit-inflammatory.
See: Cormax, Oint. (Oclassen).
Temovate, Cream, Oint., Scalp application (Glaxo Dermatology).
clobetasol propionate. (Various Mfr.)
Cream: 0.05%. Tube 15 g, 30 g, 45 g. **Ointment:** 0.05%, white petrolatum. 15 g, 30 g, 45 g.
Use: Corticosteroid (topical).
•**clobetasone butyrate.** (kloe-BEE-tih-sone BYOO-tah-rate) USAN.
Use: Corticosteroid, anti-inflammatory.
•**clocortolone acetate.** (kloe-CORE-toe-lone) USAN.
Use: Glucocorticoid.
•**clocortolone pivalate,** (kloe-CORE-toe-lone PIH-vah-late) U.S.P. 23.
Use: Glucocorticoid.
Clocream. (Pharmacia & Upjohn) Vitamins A and D in vanishing base. Tube oz. *otc.*
Use: Emollient.
•**clodanolene.** USAN.
Use: Relaxant (skeletal muscle).
•**clodazon hydrochloride.** (KLOE-dah-zone) USAN.
Use: Antidepressant.
Cloderm. (Hermal) Clocortolone pivalate cream 0.1%. Tube 15 g, 45 g. *Rx.*
Use: Corticosteroid, topical.
•**clodronic acid.** (kloe-DRAHN-ik acid) USAN.
Use: Calcium regulator.
•**clofazimine,** U.S.P. 23.
Use: Antibacterial (tuberculostatic, leprostatic). [Orphan drug]
See: Lamprene, Cap. (Novartis).
•**clofibrate,** (kloe-FIH-brate) U.S.P. 23.
Use: Antihyperlipidemic.
See: Atromid S, Cap. (Wyeth-Ayerst).

•**clofilium phosphate.** (KLOE-FILL-ee-uhm) USAN.
Use: Cardiac depressant (antiarrythmic).

•**cloflucarban.** (KLOE-flew-CAR-ban) USAN.
Use: Antiseptic, disinfectant.

•**clogestone acetate.** USAN. Under study.
Use: Progestin.

•**clomacran phosphate.** (KLOE-mah-KRAN) USAN. Under study.
Use: Antipsychotic.

•**clomegestone acetate.** (KLOE-meh-JESS-tone) USAN. Under study.
Use: Progestin.

•**clometherone.** (kloe-METH-ehr-OHN) USAN.
Use: Antiestrogen.

Clomid. (Hoechst Marion Roussel) Clomiphene citrate 50 mg/Tab. Carton 30s. *Rx.*
Use: Ovulation stimulant.

•**clominorex.** (kloe-MEE-no-rex) USAN.
Use: Anorexic.

•**clomiphene citrate,** (KLOE-mih-feen SIH-trate) U.S.P. 23.
Use: Antiestrogen.
See: Clomid, Tab. (Hoechst Marion Roussel).
Milophene, Tab. (Milex).
Serophene, Tab. (Serono).

clomiphene citrate. (Various Mfr.) 50 mg/Tab. Pkg. 10s, 30s.
Use: Ovulation stimulant.

•**clomipramine hydrochloride.** (kloe-MIH-pruh-meen) USAN.
Use: Antidepressant.
See: Anafranil (Novartis).

Clomycin. (Roberts) Bacitracin 500 U, neomycin sulfate equivalent to 3.5 mg neomycin base, polymyxin B sulfate 5000 U, lidocaine 40 mg, yellow petrolatum, anhydrous, lanolin, light mineral oil/g. Oint. Tube 28.35 g. *otc.*
Use: Antibiotic, topical.

•**clonazepam,** (kloe-NAY-ze-pam) U.S.P. 23.
Use: Anticonvulsant.
See: Klonopin, Tab. (Roche).

clonazepam. 0.5 mg, 1 mg, 2 mg/Tab. Bot. 100s. *c-iv.*
Use: Anticonvulsant.

•**clonidine.** (KLOE-nih-DEEN) USAN.
Use: Antihypertensive.
See: Catapres (Boehringer Ingelheim).

•**clonidine hydrochloride,** (KLOE-nih-DEEN) U.S.P. 23.
Use: Antihypertensive. Epidural use for pain in cancer patients [Orphan drug]

See: Catapres, Tab. (Boehringer Ingelheim).
Duraclon, Inj. (Fujisawa).

clonidine hydrochloride and chlorthalidone tablets. (Various Mfr.) Clonidine HCl 0.1 mg, 0.2 mg or 0.3 mg, chlorthalidone 15 mg/Tab. Bot. 100s, 500s, 1000s.
Use: Antihypertensive, diuretic.
See: Combipres, Tab. (Boehringer Ingelheim).

•**clonitrate.** (KLOE-nye-trate) USAN.
Use: Coronary vasodilator.

•**clonixeril.** (kloe-NIX-ehr-ill) USAN.
Use: Analgesic.

•**clonixin.** (kloe-NIX-in) USAN.
Use: Analgesic.

•**clopamide.** (kloe-PAM-id) USAN.
Use: Antihypertensive, diuretic.
See: Aquex, Tab. (Lannett).

•**clopenthixol.** (KLOE-pen-THIX-ole) USAN.
Use: Antipsychotic.
See: Sordinol (Wyeth-Ayerst).

•**cloperidone hydrochloride.** (KLOE-per-ih-dohn) USAN.
Use: Sedative, hypnotic.

clophedianol hydrochloride.
See: Acutuss, Tab., Expect. (Philips Roxane).

clophenoxate hydrochloride.
Use: Cerebral stimulant.

•**clopimozide.** (KLOE-PIM-oh-zide) USAN.
Use: Antipsychotic.

•**clopipazan mesylate.** (KLOE-pip-ah-ZAN) USAN.
Use: Antipsychotic.

•**clopirac.** (KLOE-pih-rack) USAN.
Use: Anti-inflammatory.

•**cloprednol.** (kloe-PRED-nahl) USAN.
Use: Glucocorticoid.

•**cloprostenol sodium.** (kloe-PROSTE-een-ole) USAN.
Use: Prostaglandin.

•**clorazepate dipotassium,** (klor-AZE-eh-PATE DIE-poe-TASS-ee-uhm) U.S.P. 23.
Use: Antianxiety, anticonvulsant, minor tranquilizer.
See: Tranxene, Cap. (Abbott).

clorazepate dipotassium. (Various Mfr.) 3.75 mg, 7.5 mg, 15 mg/Tab. Bot. 100s, 500s.
Use: Antianxiety, anticonvulsant, minor tranquilizer.

•**clorazepate monopotassium.** (clor-AZE-eh-PATE MAHN-oh-poe-TASS-ee-uhm) USAN.

Use: Minor tranquilizer.
●**clorethate.** (klahr-ETH-ate) USAN.
Use: Sedative, hypnotic.
●**clorexolone.** (KLOR-ex-oh-LONE)
USAN.
Use: Diuretic.
See: Nefrolan.
Clorfed II. (Stewart-Jackson) Chlor-
pheniramine 4 mg, pseudoephedrine 60
mg/Tab. Bot. 100s. *otc.*
Use: Antihistamine, decongestant.
Clorfed Capsules. (Stewart-Jackson)
Chlorpheniramine 8 mg, pseudoephed-
rine 120 mg/Cap. Bot. 100s. *otc, Rx.*
Use: Antihistamine, decongestant.
Clorfed Expectorant. (Stewart-Jackson)
Pseudoephedrine 30 mg, guaifensen
100 mg, codeine 10 mg. Bot. pt. *c-v.*
Use: Decongestant, expectorant, anti-
tussive.
●**cloroperone hydrochloride.** (KLOR-oh-
PURR-ohn) USAN.
Use: Antipsychotic.
●**clorophene.** (KLOR-oh-feen) USAN.
Use: Disinfectant.
See: Santophen 1 (Monsanto).
Clorpactin WCS-90. (Guardian) Sodium
oxychlorosene. Bot. 2 g, 5s.
Use: Antiseptic.
●**clorprenaline hydrochloride.** (klor-
PREN-ah-leen) USAN. *Formerly Iso-*
prophenamine HCl.
Use: Bronchodilator.
●**clorsulon,** (KLOR-sull-ahn) U.S.P. 23.
Use: Antiparasitic, fasciolicide.
●**clortermine hydrochloride.** (klor-TER-
meen) USAN.
Use: Anorexic.
●**closantel.** (KLOSE-an-tell) USAN.
Use: Anthelmintic.
●**closiramine aceturate.** (kloe-SIH-rah-
meen ah-SEE-tur-ate) USAN.
Use: Antihistamine.
●**clothiapine.** (KLOE-THIGH-ah-peen)
USAN.
Use: Antipsychotic.
●**clothixamide maleate.** (kloe-THIX-ah-
mid) USAN.
Use: Antipsychotic.
●**cloticasone propionate.** (kloe-TICK-ah-
SONE PRO-pee-oh-nate) USAN.
Use: Anti-inflammatory.
●**clotrimazole,** (kloe-TRIM-uh-zole) U.S.P.
23.
Use: Antifungal.
See: FemCare, Vaginal Tab., Cream.
(Schering-Plough).
Gyne-Lotrimin, Cream, Vaginal Tab.
(Schering-Plough).

Gyne-Lotrimin Combination Pack.
(Schering-Plough).
Lotrimin, Cream, Soln. (Schering-
Plough).
Mycelex, Cream, Soln., Tab. (Bayer).
Mycelex-7, Vaginal Cream, Tab.
(Bayer).
Mycelex-G, Vaginal Supp. (Bayer).
clotrimazole. (Various Mfr.) **Vaginal**
Tab.: 100 mg, in 7s with applicator.
Vaginal cream: 1% Tube 45 g with ap-
plicator.
Use: Antifungal, candida infections.
clotrimazole. (NMC) Clotrimazole 1%,
benzyl alcohol. Vaginal cream. In 45
g with 7 disposable applicators. *otc.*
Use: Antifungal, vaginal.
clotrimazole. (Taro) Clotrimazole 1% in
a vanishing cream base, benzyl alco-
hol 1%, cetostearyl alcohol. Cream.
Tube 15 g, 30 g, 45 g, 2 × 45 g. *otc.*
Use: Antifungal, topical.
clotrimazole and betamethasone di-
propionate cream.
Use: Antifungal, anti-inflammatory.
clotrimidazole. (Fujisawa)
Use: Sickle cell disease. [Orphan Drug]
clove oil.
Use: Pharmaceutic aid (flavor).
Cloverine. (Medtech) White salve. Tin
oz. *otc.*
Use: Minor skin irritations.
Clovocain. (Vita Elixir) Benzocaine, oil
of cloves. *otc.*
Use: Local anesthetic, topical.
●**cloxacillin benzathine,** (KLOX-ah-SILL-
in BENZ-ah-theen) U.S.P. 23.
Use: Antibacterial.
●**cloxacillin sodium,** (KLOX-ah-SILL-in)
U.S.P. 23.
Use: Antibiotic for resistant staph infec-
tions; antibacterial.
See: Cloxapen, Cap. (SK-Beecham).
Tegopen, Cap., Granules (Bristol).
Cloxapen. (SK-Beecham) Cloxacillin so-
dium 250 mg or 500 mg/Cap. Bot. 100s.
Rx.
Use: Anti-infective, penicillin.
●**cloxyquin.** (KLOX-ee-kwin) USAN.
Use: Antibacterial.
●**clozapine.** (KLOE-zuh-PEEN) USAN.
Rx.
Use: Antipsychotic.
See: Clozaril (Sandoz).
Clozaril. (Sandoz) Clozapine 25 mg or
100 mg/Tab. UD 100s, total daily dose
packages of 150 mg, 200 mg, 250 mg,
300 mg, 400 mg, 500 mg, 600 mg/
day. *Rx.*

Use: Antipsychotic.

Clusivol Syrup. (Whitehall Robbins) Vitamins A 2500 U.S.P. units, D-2 400 U.S.P. units, C 15 mg, B_{12} 2 mcg, B_1 1 mg, B_2 1 mg, niacinamide 5 mg, d-panthenol 3 mg, B_6 0.6 mg, manganese, 0.5 mg, zinc 0.5 mg, magnesium 3 mg/5 ml. Bot. 8 fl oz, 16 fl oz. *otc.*
Use: Vitamin/mineral supplement.

Clysodrast. (Rhone-Poulenc Rhone) Tannic acid, 2.5 g, bisacodyl 1.5 mg per packet. Pow. Box 25s, 50s. *Rx.*
Use: Laxative.

C-Max. (Bio-Tech) Vitamin C 1000 mg, magnesium 40 mg, zinc 5 mg, potassium 10 mg, manganese 1 mg, pectin 10 mg in a base of rose hips. Tabs. Bot. 100s. *otc.*
Use: Vitamin/mineral supplement.

C.M.C. Cellulose Gum.
See: Carboxymethylcellulose Sodium, Preps.

CMV. (Wampole-Zeus) Cytomegalovirus antibody test system for the qualitative and semi-quantitative detection of CMV antibody in human serum. Test 100s.
Use: Diagnostic aid.

CMV-IGIV.
Use: Immune serum.
See: Cytogam, Vial (Med Immune).
Cytomegalovirus Immune Globulin Intravenous, (Human).
Soln. (Massachusetts Public Health Biologic Laboratories)

Coadvil. (Whitehall Robins) Ibuprofen 200 mg, pseudoephedrine HCl 30 mg/ Tab. Bot. 100s. *otc.*
Use: Analgesic, decongestant.

coagulation factor ix.
Use: Treatment of hemophilia B. [Orphan drug]
See: Mononine.

coagulation factor ix (human).
Use: Treatment of hemophilia B. [Orphan drug]
See: AlphaNine.

coagulation factor ix (recombinant). (Genetics Institute)
Use: Treament of hemophilia B. [Orphan Drug]

coagulants.
See: Hemostatics.

•**coal tar,** U.S.P. 23.
Use: Topical antieczematic; antipsoriatic.
See: Balnetar, Liq. (Westwood Squibb).
Estar, Gel (Westwood Squibb).
L.C.D. Compound, Oint., Soln. (Almay).

Polytar Bath, Liq. (Stiefel).
Protar Protein, Shampoo (Dermol).
Tarbonis, Cream (Schwarz Pharma).
Zetar, Preps. (Dermik).
W/Allantoin, hydrocortisone.
See: Alphosyl-HC, Lot., Cream (Schwarz Pharma).
W/Hydrocortisone.
See: Doak Oil Forte, Liq. (Doak).
Tarcortin, Cream (Schwarz Pharma).
W/Iodoquinol, hydrocortisone.
See: Ze Tar-Quin, Cream (Dermik).
W/Zinc oxide.
See: Tarpaste, Paste (Doak).

coal tar, distillate.
Use: Tar-containing preparation, topical.
See: Lavatar, Liq. (Doak).
Syntar, Cream (Zeneca).
W/Sulfur, salicylic acid.
See: Pragatar, Oint. (Menley & James).

coal tar extract.
Use: Tar-containing preparation, topical.
W/Allantoin, hexachlorophene.
See: Sebical Cream (Schwarz Pharma).
W/Allantoin, hexachlorophene, glycerin, lanolin.
See: Pso-Rite, Cream (DePree).
W/Allantoin, salicylic acid, perhydrosqualine.
See: Skaylos Cream (Ambix).
Skaylos Lotion (Ambix).
W/Salicylic acid, resorcinol, benzoic acid.
See: Mazon Cream (SK-Beecham).

coal tar paste.
Use: Tar-containing preparation, topical.
W/Zinc paste.
See: Tarpaste, Paste (Doak).

coal tar topical solution. Liquor Carbonis Detergens. L.C.D.
Use: Anti-eczematic, topical.
See: Advanced Formula Tegrin, Shampoo (Block).
Balnetar, Liq. (Westwood Squibb).
Estar, Gel (Westwood Squibb).
L.C.D. Compound Oint., Soln. (Almay).
MG217 Medicated, Shampoo, Cond. (Triton).
Psorigel, Gel (Galderma).
PsoriNail, Liq. (Summers).
Wright's Soln. (Fougera).
Zetar, Emulsion, Shampoo (Dermik).
W/Allantoin, psorilan, myristate.
See: Iocon, Shampoo (Galderma).
Psorelief, Cream (Quality Generics).
W/Hydrocortisone, iodoquinol.
See: Cor-Tar-Quin, Cream, Lot. (Bayer).

W/Hydrocortisone alcohol, clioquinololine, diperodon HCl, vitamins A, D.
See: Pentacort, Cream (Dalin).
W/Robane (perhydrosqualene).
See: Skaylos Shampoo (Ambix).
W/Salicylic acid.
See: Epidol, Soln. (Spirt).
Ionil T, Shampoo (Galderma).
W/Salicylic acid, sulfur, protein.
See: Vanseb-T Tar Shampoo (Allergan Herbert).

Co-APAP. (Various Mfr.) Pseudoephedrine HCl 30 mg, chlorpheniramine maleate 2 mg, dextromethorphan HBr 15 mg, acetaminophen 325 mg/Tab. Bot. 24s, 50s, 1000s. *otc.*
Use: Decongestant, antihistamine, antitussive, analgesic.

cobalamine concentrate, U.S.P. 21.
Use: Hematopoietic vitamin.
See: Vitamin B_{12} (Various Mfr.).

cobalt chloride.
W/Ferrous gluconate, vitamin B_{12}, duodenum whole desiccated.
See: Bitrinsic-E, Cap. (Zeneca).

cobalt gluconate.
W/Ferrous gluconate, vitamin B_{12} activity, desiccated stomach substance, folic acid.
See: Chromagen, Cap., Inj. (Savage).

cobalt-labeled vitamin B_{12}.
See: Rubratope-57 (Squibb).

cobalt standards for vitamin B_{12}.
See: Cobatope-57, and Cobatope-60 (Squibb).

•**cobaltous chloride Co 57.** USAN.
Use: Radioactive agent.

•**cobaltous chloride Co 60.** USAN.
Use: Radioactive agent.

cobatope-57. (Squibb) Cobaltous Cl Co 57.

cobex 1000. (Standex) Vitamin B_{12} 1000 mcg/10 ml. Vial 30 ml. *Rx.*
Use: Vitamin B_{12} supplement.

Co-Bile. (Western Research) Hog bile 64.8 mg, pancreas substance 64.8 mg, papain-pepsin complex 97.2 mg, diatase malt 16.2 mg, papain 48.6 mg, pepsin 48.6 mg/Tab. Bot. 1000s. *otc, Rx.*
Use: Digestive enzyme.

•**cocaine,** U.S.P. 23.
Use: Anesthetic (topical).

•**cocaine hydrochloride,** U.S.P. 23.
Use: Anesthetic (topical).

cocaine HCl. Top. Soln.: Cocaine HCl 4%, 10%/Bot. 10 ml, UD 4 ml. (Various). **Pow.:** 5 g, 25 g. (Mallinckrodt). *c-II.*

Use: Mucosal anesthetic.

cocaine viscous. (Various) Cocaine viscous 4%, 10%/Soln. Top. Bot. 10 ml, UD 4 ml. *c-II.*
Use: Local anesthetic, topical.

•**coccidioidin,** U.S.P. 23.
Use: Diagnostic aid (dermal reactive indicator).
See: BioCox, Vial (Iatric).
Spherulin (ALK Laboratories).

cocculin.
See: Picrotoxin, Inj. (Various Mfr.).

Cocilan Syrup. (Approved) Euphorbia, wild lettuce, cocillana, squill, senega, cascarin (bitterless). Bot. gal. Available w/codeine. Bot. gal.

cocillana.
W/Euphorbia pilulifera, squill, antimony potassium tartrate, senega.
See: Cylana Syr. (Jones Medical).

cocoa, N.F. XVI.
Use: Pharmaceutic aid (flavor; flavored vehicle).

•**cocoa butter,** N.F. 18.
Use: Pharmaceutic aid (suppository base).

Codamine Pediatric Syrup. (Barre-National) Hydrocodone bitartrate 2.5 mg, phenylpropanolamine HCl 12.5 mg. Bot. pt. *c-III.*
Use: Antitussive, decongestant.

Codamine Syrup. (Goldline) Hydrocodone bitartrate 5 mg, phenylpropanolamine HCl 25 mg/5 ml. Bot. pt, gal. *c-III.*
Use: Antitussive, decongestant.

Codanol Ointment. (A.P.C.) Vitamins A, D, hexachlorophene, zinc oxide. Tube 1.5 oz, 4 oz, Jar lb. *otc.*
Use: Minor skin irritations.

Codap. (Solvay) Codeine phosphate 32 mg, acetaminophen 325 mg/Tab. Bot. 250s. *c-III.*
Use: Narcotic analgesic combination.

Codegest Expectorant. (Great Southern) Guaifenesin 100 mg, phenylpropanolamine HCl 12.5 mg, codeine phosphate 10 mg. Alcohol, dye free. Liq. Bot. pt, gal. *c-v.*
Use: Antitussive, decongestant, expectorant.

Codehist DH Elixir. (Geneva Pharm.) Pseudoephedrine 30 mg, chlorpheniramine maleate 2 mg, codeine phosphate 10 mg, alcohol 5.7%. Bot. 120 ml, 480 ml. *c-v.*
Use: Decongestant, antihistamine, antitussive.

•**codeine,** (KOE-deen) U.S.P. 23.

Use: Analgesic (narcotic); antitussive.

codeine combinations.
See: Actifed-C, Expectorant, Syr. (Glaxo Wellcome).
Anexsia w/Codeine, Tab. (SK-Beecham).
APAP w/Codeine, Tab. (Schwarz Pharma).
A.P.C. w/Codeine, Tab. (Various Mfr.).
Ascriptin W/Codeine No. 2, Tab. (Rhone-Poulenc Rorer).
Ascriptin W/Codeine No. 3, Tab. (Rhone-Poulenc Rorer).
Buff-A-Compound, Tab. (Mayrand).
Calcidrine Syr. (Abbott).
Capital w/Codeine, Susp. (Carnrick).
Cheracol, Syr. (Pharmacia & Upjohn).
Chlor-Trimeton Expectorant (Schering-Plough).
Codasa I and II, Cap. (Stayner).
Colrex Compound, Cap., Elix. (Solvay).
Cosanyl Cough Syrup (Health Care Ind.).
Drucon w/Codeine, Liq. (Standard Drug).
Empirin No. 1, No. 2, No. 3, No. 4, Tab. (Glaxo Wellcome).
Fiorinal w/Codeine, Cap. (Sandoz).
G-3, Cap. (Roberts).
Golacol, Syr. (Arcum).
Novahistine, Expectorant (Hoechst Marion Roussel).
Nucofed, Liq. (Beecham).
Partuss AC (Parmed).
Pediacof, Syr. (Sanofi Winthrop).
Phenaphen #2, #3, #4, Cap. (Robins).
Phenaphen-650, Cap. (Robins).
Phenergan Expectorant w/Codeine, Troches (Wyeth-Ayerst).
Proval No. 3, Tab. (Solvay).
Prunicodeine, Syr. (Lilly).
Robitussin A-C, DAC (Robins).
Tolu-Sed, Elix. (Scherer).
Tussar-2, Syr. (Rhone-Poulenc Rorer).
Tussar SF, Liq. (Rhone-Poulenc Rorer).
Tussi-Organidin, Liq. (Wallace).
Tylenol w/Codeine No. 1, No. 2, No. 3, No. 4 Tab. (McNeil).
Tylenol w/Codeine, Elix. (McNeil).
Vasotus, Liq. (Sheryl).

codeine methylbromide. Eucodin.
Use: Antitussive.

•**codeine phosphate,** (KOE-deen FOSS-fate) U.S.P. 23.
Use: Narcotic analgesic, antitussive.

codeine phosphate. (Various Mfr.) Pow. Bot. ⅛ oz, 0.25 oz, 0.5 oz, 1 oz.
Use: Narcotic analgesic, antitussive.

codeine phosphate and guaifenesin. (Goldline) Codeine phospate 10 mg, guaifenesin 300 mg/Tab. Bot. 100s. *Rx.*
Use: Narcotic antitussive, expectorant.

•**codeine polistirex.** (KOE-deen pahl-ee-STIE-rex) USAN.
Use: Antitussive.

codeine resin complex combinations.
See: Omni-Tuss, Liq. (Medeva).

•**codeine sulfate,** (KOE-deen) U.S.P. 23.
Use: Antitussive, analgesic (narcotic).

codelcortone.
See: Prednisolone.

Codiclear DH Syrup. (Schwarz Pharma) Hydrocodone bitartrate 5 mg, guaifenesin 100 mg/5 ml. Bot. 4 oz, pt. *c-III.*
Use: Antitussive, expectorant.

Codimal. (Schwarz Pharma) Chlorpheniramine maleate 2 mg, pseudoephedrine HCl 30 mg, acetaminophen 325 mg/Cap. or Tab. Bot. 24s, 100s, 1000s. *otc.*
Use: Antihistamine, decongestant, analgesic.

Codimal DH Syrup. (Schwarz Pharma) Hydrocodone bitartrate 1.66 mg, phenylephrine HCl 5 mg, pyrilamine maleate 8.33 mg/5 ml. Bot. 4 oz, pt, gal. *c-III.*
Use: Antitussive, decongestant, antihistamine.

Codimal DM. (Schwarz Pharma) Dextromethorphan HBr 10 mg, phenylephrine HCl 5 mg, pyrilamine maleate 8.33 mg/5 ml, alcohol 4%, saccharin, sorbitol. Sugar free. Bot. 4 oz, pt, gal. *otc.*
Use: Antitussive, decongestant, antihistamine.

Codimal-L.A. (Schwarz Pharma) Chlorpheniramine maleate 8 mg, pseudoephedrine HCl 120 mg/SR Cap. Bot. 100s, 1000s. *Rx.*
Use: Antihistamine, decongestant.

Codimal-L.A. Half Capsules. (Schwarz Pharma) Pseudoephedrine HCl 60 mg, chlorpheniramine maleate 4 mg, sucrose. Cap. Bot. 100s. *Rx.*
Use: Decongestant, antihistamine.

Codimal pH Syrup. (Schwarz Pharma) Codeine phosphate 10 mg, phenylephrine HCl 5 mg, pyrilamine maleate 8.33 mg/5 ml. Bot. 4 oz, pt, gal. *c-v.*
Use: Antitussive, decongestant, antihistamine.

Codimal Tablets. (Schwarz Pharma) Chlorpheniramine maleate 2 mg, pseudoephedrine HCl 30 mg, acetaminophen 325 mg/Tab. Bot. 24s, 100s, 1000s.

Use: Antihistamine, decongestant, analgesic.

•**cod liver oil,** U.S.P. 23. Emulsion.
Use: Vitamin A and D therapy.
See: Cod Liver Oil Concentrate Cap. (Schering-Plough).
W/Anesthesin, zinc oxide, hydroxyquinoline.
See: Medicone Dressing. (Medicone).
W/Benzocaine.
See: Morusan, Oint. (SK-Beecham).
W/Creosote.
(Bryant) Cod liver oil 9 min, creosote 1 min/Cap. Bot. 100s.
W/Malt extract.
(Glaxo Wellcome) Vitamins A 6450 IU, D 645 IU. Bot. 10 fl oz, 20 fl oz.
W/Methylbenzethonium Cl.
See: Benephen, Prods. (Halsted).
W/Viosterol.
(Abbott) Vitamins A 2800 IU, D 255 IU/g. Bot. 12 fl oz.
(Squibb) Vitamins A 2000 IU, D 440 IU/g. Bot. 4 fl oz, 12 fl oz.
W/Zinc oxide.
See: Desitin, Preps. (Pfizer).
cod liver oil concentrate. (Schering-Plough) Concentrate of cod liver oil with vitamins A and D added. **Cap.:** Bot. 40s, 100s. **Tab.:** Bot. 100s, 240s. Also W/Vitamin C. Bot. 100s. *otc.*
Use: Vitamin supplement.
cod liver oil ointment. *otc.*
See: Moruguent, Oint. (SK-Beecham).
codorphone hydrochloride. (KOE-dahr-fone) Name previously used.
Use: Analgesic.
See: Conorphone HCl.
•**codoxime.** (CODE-ox-eem) USAN.
Use: Antitussive.
codoxy. (Halsey) Oxycodone HCl 4.5 mg, oxycodone terephthalate 0.38 mg, aspirin 325 mg/Tab. Bot. 100s.
Use: Narcotic analgesic combination.
Cogentin. (Merck & Co.) Benztropine Mesylate **Tab.:** 0.5 mg Bot. 100s; 1 mg Bot. 100s, UD 100s; 2 mg Bot. 100s, 1000s, UD 100s. **Inj.:** Benztropine mesylate 1 mg/ml w/sodium Cl 9 mg and water for injection q.s. to 1 ml Amp. 2 ml, Box 6s. *Rx.*
Use: Antiparkinsonian.
Co-Gesic. (Schwarz Pharma) Hydrocodone bitartrate 5 mg, acetaminophen 500 mg/Tab. Bot. 100s, 500s. *c-III.*
Use: Narcotic analgesic combination.
Cognex. (Parke-Davis) Tacrine HCl 10 mg, 20 mg, 30 mg, 40 mg/Cap. Bot. 120s, UD 100s. *Rx.*

Use: Psychotherapeutic.
Co-Hep-Tral. (Davis & Sly) Folic acid 10 mg, vitamin B₁₂ 100 mcg, liver injection q.s./ml. Vial 10 ml. *Rx.*
Use: Vitamin/mineral supplement.
Co-Hist. (Roberts Med.) Pseudoephedrine HCl 30 mg, chlorpheniramine 2 mg, acetaminophen 325 mg/Tab. Bot. 500s, 1000s. *otc.*
Use: Decongestant, antihistamine, analgesic.
Colabid Tabs. (Major) Probenecid 500 mg, colchicine 0.5 mg/Tab. Bot. 100s, 1000s. *Rx.*
Use: Agent for gout.
Colace. (Bristol-Myers) Docusate sodium. **Cap.:** 50 mg or 100 mg. Bot. 30s, 60s, 250s, 1000s, UD 100s. **Syr.:** 60 mg/15 ml with alcohol < 1%. Bot. 240 ml, 480 ml. **Liq.:** 150 mg/15 ml. Bot. 30 ml, 480 ml with calibrated droppers. *otc.*
Use: Laxative.
Colagyn. (Smith) Zinc sulfocarbolate, potassium, oxyquinoline sulfate, lactic acid, boric acid. Jelly. Tube w/applicator and refill 6 oz. Douche Pow. 3 oz, 7 oz, 14 oz. *otc.*
Colana Syrup. (Hance) Euphorbia pilulifera tincture 8 ml, wild lettuce syrup 8 ml, cocillana tincture 2.5 ml, squill compound syrup 1.5 ml, cascara 0.25 g, menthol 4.8 mg/fl oz. Bot. 4 fl oz, gal. Also w/Dionin 15 mg/fl oz. Bot. gal.
Co-Lav. (Copley) Polyethylene glycol 3350 60g, sodium chloride 1.46 g, potassium chloride 0.745 g, sodium bicarbonate 1.68 g, sodium sulfate 5.68 g per L/Pow. for Soln. Jug 4 L. *Rx.*
Use: Bowel evacuant.
Colax. (Rugby) Docusate sodium 100 mg, phenolphthalein 65 mg/Tab. Bot. 30s. *otc.*
Use: Laxative.
•**colchicine,** (KOHL-chih-seen) U.S.P. 23.
Use: Gout suppressant. Treat multiple sclerosis [Orphan drug]
W/Benemid.
See: Colbenemid, Tab. (Merck & Co.).
W/Methyl salicylate. (Parke-Davis) Colchicine gr, methyl salicylate 3 min/Cap. Bot. 100s, 500s, 1000s.
Use: Orally, gout therapy.
W/Probenecid.
See: Benn-C, Tab. (Scrip).
Colbenemid, Tab. (Merck & Co.).
Robenecid with colchicine, Tab. (Robinson).
W/Sodium salicylate.
See: Salcoce, Tab. (Cole).

W/Sodium salicylate, calcium carbonate, dried aluminum hydroxide gel, phenobarbital.
See: Apcogesic, Tabs. (Apco).

W/Sodium salicylate, potassium iodide.
See: Bricolide, Tab. (Briar).

colchicine. (Various Mfr.) 0.5 mg/Tab. Bot. 100s.
Use: Gout suppressant. Treat multiple sclerosis [Orphan drug].

colchicine salicylate.
W/Phenobarbital, sodium p-aminobenzoate, vitamin B₁, aspirin.
See: Doloral, Tab. (Alamed).

Cold & Allergy Elixir. (Goldline) Phenylpropanolamine HCl 12.5 mg, brompheniramine maleate 2 mg/5 ml. Liq. Bot. 118 ml, 237 ml, 473 ml, gal. *otc.*
Use: Decongestant, antihistamine.

cold cream, U.S.P. 21.
Use: Emollient; water in oil emulsion ointment base.

Cold-Gest Cold Capsules. (Major) Chlorpheniramine maleate 8 mg, pseudoephedrine HCl 75 mg/Cap. Pkg. 10s, 20s. *otc.*
Use: Antihistamine, decongestant.

Coldloc. (Flemming) Phenylpropanolamine HCl 20 mg, phenylephrine 5 mg, guaifenesin 100 mg/5 ml, sorbitol. Alcohol, sugar, dye free/Elixir. Bot. Pt. *Rx.*
Use: Decongestant, expectorant.

Coldloc-LA. (Flemming) Phenylpropanolamine HCl 75 mg, guaifenesin 600 mg/SR Cap. Bot. 50s, 100s. *Rx.*
Use: Decongestant, expectorant.

Coldonyl. (Dover) Acetaminophen, phenylephrine HCl/Tab. Sugar, lactose and salt free. UD Box 500s. *otc.*
Use: Analgesic, decongestant.

Coldran. (Halsey) Phenylephrine HCl 5 mg, chlorpheniramine maleate 2 mg, salicylamide 1.5 gr, acetaminophen 0.5 gr, caffeine/Tab. Bot. 30s. *otc.*
Use: Decongestant, antihistamine, analgesic.

Cold Relief. (Rugby) Phenylpropanolamine HCl 12.5 mg, chlorpheniramine maleate 2 mg, dextromethorphan HBr 10 mg, acetaminophen 325 mg/Tab. Bot. 50s. *otc.*
Use: Decongestant, antihistamine, antitussive, analgesic.

Coldrine. (Roberts) Acetaminophen 325 mg, pseudoephedrine HCl 30 mg, sodium metabisulfite/Tab. Bot. 1000s, 500s (packets), 4-dose boxes. *otc.*
Use: Analgesic, decongestant.

Cold Sore Lotion. (Purepac) Camphor, benzoin, aluminum Cl. Bot. 0.5 oz.
Use: Cold sores.

Cold Symptoms Relief. (Major) Pseudoephedrine HCl 30 mg, chlorpheniramine maleate 2 mg, dextromethorphan HBr 10 mg, acetaminophen 325 mg/Tab. Bot. 50s. *otc.*
Use: Decongestant, antihistamine, antitussive, analgesic.

Cold Tablets. (Walgreen) Phenylephrine HCl 5 mg, chlorpheniramine maleate 2 mg, acetaminophen 325 mg/Tab. Bot. 50s. *otc.*
Use: Decongestant, antihistamine, analgesic.

Cold Tablets Multiple Symptom. (Walgreen) Acetaminophen 500 mg, pseudoephedrine HCl 30 mg, chlorpheniramine maleate 2 mg, dextromethorphan HBr 10 mg/Tab. Bot. 50s. *otc.*
Use: Analgesic, decongestant, antihistamine, antitussive.

Colestid. (Pharmacia & Upjohn) Colestipol HCl. **Unflavored:** Bot. 300 g, 500 g. Pkt. 5 g. **Flavored:** Bot. 450 g. Pkt. 7.5 g (5 g colestipol HCl). *Rx.*
Use: Antihyperlipidemic.

Colestid Tablets. (Pharmacia & Upjohn) Colestipol HCl 1 g/Tab. 120s and 250s. *Rx.*
Use: Antihyperlipidemic.

•**colestipol hydrochloride,** (koe-LESS-tih-pole) U.S.P. 23.
Use: Antihyperlipidemic.
See: Colestid (Pharmacia & Upjohn).

•**colestolone.** (koe-LESS-toe-LONE) USAN.
Use: Hypolipidemic.

Col-Evac. (Forest) Potassium bitartrate, bicarbonate of soda and a blended base of polyethylene glycols. Supp. 2s, 12s.

Colfed-A Capsules. (Parmed) Pseudoephedrine HCl 120 mg, chlorpheniramine maleate 8 mg. Bot 100s. *Rx.*
Use: Decongestant, antihistamine.

•**colforsin.** (kole-FAR-sin) USAN.
Use: Antiglaucoma agent.

•**colfosceril palmitate.** (kahl-FOSE-uhr-ILL PAL-mih-TATE) USAN.
Use: Pulmonary surfactant, antiatelectic; prevention/treatment of hyaline membrane disease. [Orphan drug]
See: Exosurf (Glaxo Wellcome).

colimycin sodium methanesulfonate. (Parke-Davis).
See: Colistimethate Sodium.

colimycin sulfate. (Parke-Davis).
See: Coly-Mycin, Preps. (Parke-Davis).

•**colistimethate sodium, sterile,** (koe-LISS-tih-METH-ate) U.S.P. 23. Sodium Colistin Methanesulfonate. Colistin methane sulfonic acid, pentasodium salt. Pentasodium colistin methanesulfonate.
Use: Antibacterial.
See: Coly-Mycin-M, Injectable (Parke-Davis).

colistin base.
W/Neomycin base, hydrocortisone acetate, thonzonium bromide, polysorbate 80, acetic acid, sodium acetate.
See: Coly-Mycin Otic W/Neomycin and Hydrocortisone, Liq. (Parke-Davis).

colistin methanesulfonate.
See: Colistimethate Sodium.

colistin and neomycin sulfates and hydrocortisone acetate otic suspension.
Use: Anti-infective, anti-inflammatory.

•**colistin sulfate,** U.S.P. 23.
Use: Antibacterial.

Co-Liver. (Standex) Folic acid 1 mg, vitamin B_{12} 100 mcg, liver 10 mcg/ml. Vial 10 ml. *Rx.*
Use: Vitamin/mineral supplement.

Colladerm. (C & M Pharmacal) Purified water, glycerin, soluble collagen, hydrolysed elastin, allantoin, ethylhydroxycellulose, sorbic, octoxynol-9. Bot. 2.3 oz. *otc.*
Use: Emollient.

collagenase.
See: Santyl (Knoll).

collagenase abc ointment. (Advance Biofactures) Collagenase 250 units/g in white petrolatum. 25 g, 50 g. *otc.*
Use: Topical enzyme preparation.

collagen implant. (Lacrimedics) In 0.2 mm, 0.3 mm, 0.4 mm, 0.5 mm. 0.6 mm. Box 12s. *Rx.*
Use: Collagen implant, ophthalmic.

collagen implant.
See: Zyderm I. (Collagen Corp.).
Zyderm II. (Collagen Corp.).

Collastin Oil Free Moisturizer. (Dermol) Soluble collagen, hydrolyzed elastin. Lot. Bot. 60 ml. *otc.*
Use: Emollient.

•**collodion,** U.S.P. 23.
Use: Topical protectant.

colloidal aluminum hydroxide.
See: Aluminum Hydroxide Gel, U.S.P. 23.

colloidal gold.
See: Aureotope (Squibb).

colloidal silver iodide.
See: Neo-Silvol, Soln. (Parke-Davis).

Collyrium for Fresh Eyes. (Wyeth-Ayerst) Boric acid, sodium borate, benzalkonium Cl. Bot. 120 ml. *otc.*
Use: Extraocular irrigating solution.

Collyrium Fresh Eye Drops. (Wyeth-Ayerst) Tetrahydrozoline HCl 0.05%. Drop. Bot. 15 ml. *otc.*
Use: Ophthalmic vasoconstrictor, mydriatic.

Colocare. (Helena Labs) In-home fecal test. Kit. 3s.
Use: Diagnostic aid.

Coloctyl. (Eon Labs) Docusate sodium 100 mg/Cap. Bot. 100s, 1000s, UD 1000s. *otc.*
Use: Laxative.

Cologel. (Lilly) Methylcellulose 450 mg/5 ml, alcohol 5%, saccharin. Bot. 16 fl oz. *otc.*
Use: Laxative.

colony stimulating factor.
Use: Adjunct during antineoplastic therapy.
See: Leukine (Immunex)
Neupogen (Amgen).

color allergy screening test.
See: CAST (Biomerica).

Color Ovulation Test. (Biomerica) Monoclonal antibody-based enzyme immunoassay test for hLH in urine. Kit. 9-day test kit.
Use: To predict ovulation.

Coloscreen. (Helena Labs) Occult blood screening test. Kit 12s, 25s, 50s. 3 tests per kit.
Use: Diagnostic aid.

Coloscreen/VPI. (Helena Labs) Occult blood screening test. Box 100s, 1000s.
Use: Diagnostic aid.

Colovage. (Dyna Pharm) Powder for reconstitution to produce 1 gal soln. Containing sodium Cl 5.53 g, potassium Cl 2.82 g, sodium bicarbonate 6.36 g, sodium sulfate anhydrous 21.5 g, polyethylene glycol 3350. Pkg. 1s. *Rx.*
Use: Laxative.

Col-Probenecid. (Various Mfr.) Probenecid 500 mg, colchicine 0.5 mg/Tab. Bot. 100s, 1000s, UD 100s. *Rx.*
Use: Agent for gout.

Coltab Children's. (Roberts) Phenylephrine HCl 2.5 mg, chlorpheniramine maleate 1 mg/Chew. tab. Bot. 30s. *otc.*
Use: Decongestant, antihistamine.

•**colterol mesylate.** (KOLE-ter-ole) USAN.
Use: Bronchodilator.

Coly-Mycin M Parenteral. (Parke-Davis) Colistimethate sodium equivalent 150

mg colistin base per vial. *Rx.*
Use: Anti-infective.

Coly-Mycin S Otic Drops w/ Neomycin and Hydrocortisone. (Parke-Davis) Colistin base as the sulfate 3 mg, neomycin base as the sulfate 3.3 mg, hydrocortisone acetate 10 mg, thonzonium bromide 0.5 mg/ml, polysorbate 80, acetic acid, sodium acetate, thimerosal. Dropper bot. 5 ml, 10 ml. *Rx.*
Use: Anti-infective.

CoLyte. (Schwarz Pharma) **2L:** PEG (Polyethylene glycol-electrolyte solution) 3350 120 g, sodium sulfate 11.36 g, sodium bicarbonate 3.36 g, sodium Cl 2.92 g, potassium Cl 1.49 g. **1 gal:** PEG 3350 227.1 g, sodium sulfate 21.5 g, sodium bicarbonate 6.36 g, sodium Cl 5.53 g, potassium Cl 2.82 g. **6 L:** PEG 3350 360 g, sodium sulfate 34.08 g, sodium bicarbonate 10.08 g, sodium Cl 8.76 g, potassium Cl 4.47 g. Pack 5. Bot. 2 L, gal, 4L, 6L. *Rx.*
Use: Bowel evacuant for GI exams.

Combichole. (Trout) Dehydrocholic acid 2 gr, desoxycholic acid 1 gr/Tab. Bot. 100s, 1000s. *Rx.*
Use: Hydrocholeretic.

Combipres Tablets. (Boehringer Ingelheim) **0.1 mg:** Clonidine HCl 0.1 mg, chlorthalidone 15 mg/Tab. Bot. 100s, 1000s. **0.2 mg:** Clonidine HCl 0.2 mg, chlorthalidone 15 mg/Tab. Bot. 100s, 1000s. **0.3 mg:** Clonidine HCl 0.3 mg, chlorthalidone 15 mg/Tab. Bot. 100s. *Rx.*
Use: Antihypertensive.

Combistix. (Bayer) Urine test for glucose, protein and blood/Test. In 100s.
Use: Diagnostic aid.

Combistix Reagent Strips. (Bayer) Protein test-tetrabromphenol blue, citrate buffer, protein-absorbing agent; glucose test area-glucose oxidase, orthotolidin and a catalyst; pH test area methyl red and bromthymol blue. Box, strips, 100s.
Use: Diagnostic aid.

Combivent. (Boehringer Ingelheim) Per actuation - ipratropium bromide 18 mg, albuterol sulfate 103 mcg (90 mcg base)/Aerosol Can 14.7 g (200 inhalations). *Rx.*
Use: Secondary treatment of chronic obstructive pulmonary disease (COPD).

ComfortCare GP Wetting & Soaking. (Pilkington Barnes Hind) Buffered, isotonic. Chlorhexidine gluconate 0.005%, EDTA 0.02%, octylphenoxy (oxyethylene) ethanol, povidone, polyvinyl alcohol, propylene glycol, hydroxyethylcellulose, NaCl. Soln. Bot. 120 ml or 240 ml. *otc.*
Use: Contact lens care.

Comfort Drops. (Pilkington Barnes Hind) Isotonic solution containing naphazoline 0.03%, benzalkonium Cl 0.005%, edetate disodium 0.02%. Bot. 15 ml. *otc.*
Use: Hard contact lens care.

Comfort Eye Drops. (Pilkington Barnes Hind) Naphazoline HCl 0.03%. Bot. 15 ml. *otc.*
Use: Ophthalmic decongestant.

Comfort Gel Liquid. (Walgreen) Aluminum hydroxide compressed gel 200 mg, magnesium hydroxide 200 mg, simethicone 20 mg/5 ml. Bot. 12 oz. *otc.*
Use: Antacid, antiflatulent.

Comfort Gel Tablets. (Walgreen) Magnesium hydroxide 85 mg, simethicone 25 mg, aluminum hydroxide-magnesium carbonate codried gel 282 mg/Tab. Bot. 100s. *otc.*
Use: Antacid, antiflatulent.

Comfortine. (Dermik) Zinc oxide 12%, vitamins A and D, lanolin in protective base. Oint. Tube 1.5 oz, 4 oz. *otc.*
Use: Emollient.

Comfort Tears. (Pilkington Barnes Hind) Hydroxyethyl cellulose, benzalkonium Cl 0.005%, edetate disodium 0.02%. Bot. 15 ml. *otc.*
Use: Soft contact lens care.

Comhist L.A. Capsules. (Roberts) Phenylephrine HCl 20 mg, chlorpheniramine maleate 4 mg, phenyltoloxamine citrate 50 mg/Cap. Bot. 100s. *Rx.*
Use: Decongestant, antihistamine.

Comhist Tablets. (Roberts) Phenylephrine HCl 10 mg, chlorpheniramine maleate 2 mg, phenyltoloxamine citrate 25 mg/Tab. Bot. 100s. *Rx.*
Use: Decongestant, antihistamine.

Compal. (Solvay) Dihydrocodeine 16 mg, acetaminophen 356.4 mg, caffeine 30 mg/Cap. Bot. 100s. *c-III.*
Use: Analgesic combination.

Compat Nutrition Enteral Delivery System. (Sandoz Nutrition) Top fill feeding containers 600 ml, 1400 ml. Gravity delivery set. Pump delivery set. Compat enteral feeding pump.
Use: Nutritional supplement.

Compazine. (SK-Beecham) Prochlorperazine as the maleate. **Tab.:** 5 mg, 10 mg or 25 mg. Bot. 100s, 1000s, UD 100s (except for 25 mg). **Inj.:** Edisylate

salt 5 mg/ml. Amp. 2 ml, vial 10 ml, disposable syringe 2 ml. **SR Spansule:** Maleate salt 10 mg, 15 mg or 30 mg. Bot. 50s, 500s, UD 100s. **Supp.:** 2.5 mg, 5 mg or 25 mg. Box 12s. **Syr.:** Edisylate salt 5 mg/5 ml. Bot. 4 fl oz. *Rx.*
Use: Antiemetic, antipsychotic.

Compete. (Mission) Iron 27 mg, vitamins A 5000 IU, D 400 IU, E 45 IU, B_1 2 mg, B_2 2.6 mg, B_3 30 mg, B_6 20.6 mg, B_{12} 9 mcg, C 90 mg, folic acid 0.4 mg, Zn 22.5/Tab. Bot. 100s. *otc.*
Use: Vitamin/mineral supplement.

Compleat-B Meat Base Formula. (Sandoz Nutrition) Beef, nonfat milk, hydrolyzed cereal solids, maltodextrin, pureed fruits and vegetables, corn oil, mono and diglycerides. Bot. 250 ml, Can 250 ml. *otc.*
Use: Enteral nutritional supplement.

Compleat-Modified Formula Meat Base. (Sandoz Nutrition) Hydrolyzed cereal solids, calcium caseinate, pureed fruits and vegetables, corn oil, beef puree, mono and diglycerides. Can 250 ml. *otc.*
Use: Enteral nutritional supplement.

Compleat-Regular Formula. (Sandoz Nutrition) Deionized water, beef puree, hydrolyzed cereal solids, green bean puree, pea puree, nonfat milk, corn oil, maltodextrin, peach puree, orange juice, mono and diglycerides, carrageenan, vitamins, minerals. Bot. 250 ml, Can 250 ml. *otc.*
Use: Enteral nutritional supplement.

Complete. (Mission) Vitamins A 5000 IU, D 400 IU, E 45 IU, C 90 mg, B_1 2.25 mg, folic acid 0.4 mg, B_2 2.6 mg, B_3 30 mg, B_6 25 mg, B_{12} 9 mcg, ferrous gluconate 233 mg, zinc 22.5 mg/Tab. Bot. 100s, 1000s. *otc.*
Use: Vitamin/mineral supplement.

Complete. (Allergan) Buffered, isotonic. Sodium Cl, polyhexamethylene biguanide 0.0001%, tromethamine, tyloxapol, EDTA. Soln. Bot. 15 ml. *otc.*
Use: Contact lens care.

Complete All-In-One. (Allergan) Buffered, isotonic. Sodium Cl, polyhexamethylone biguanide, EDTA. Soln. Bot. 60, 120, 360 ml. *otc.*
Use: Contact lens care.

Complete Weekly Enzymatic Cleaner. (Allergan) Effervescing, buffering and tableting agents. Sublitisin A. Tab. Pkg. 8s. *otc.*
Use: Contact lens care.

Completone Elixir Fort. (Sanofi Winthrop) Ferrous gluconate.
Use: Iron supplement.

Complex 15 Cream. (Baker/Cummins) Jar 4 oz. *otc.*
Use: Emollient.

Complex 15 Lotion. (Baker/Cummins) Bot. 8 oz. *otc.*
Use: Emollient.

Complex Zinc Carbonates.
See: Zinc (Sublingual Products).

Comply Liquid. (Sherwood) Sodium caseinate, calcium caseinate, hydrolyzed cornstarch, sucrose, corn oil, soy lecithin, vitamins A, B_1, B_2, B_3, B_5, B_6, B_{12}, C, D, E, K, folic acid, biotin, choline, Ca, Cl, Cu, Fe, I, Mg, Mn, P, Zn. Can 250 ml, Bot. 200 ml. *otc.*
Use: Enteral nutritional supplement.

compound 42.
See: Warfarin (Various Mfr.).

compound b.
See: Corticosterone (Various Mfr.).

compound cb3025.
See: Alkeran, Tab. (Glaxo Wellcome).

compound e. (McGaw).
See: Cortisone Acetate. (Various Mfr.).

compound f.
See: Hydrocortisone (Various Mfr.).

compound q.
Use: Antiviral.
See: Trichosanthine (Genelabs).

compound s.
Use: Antiviral.
See: Retrovir (Glaxo Wellcome). Zidovudine.

Compound W. (Whitehall Robbins) Salicylic acid 17% w/w in flexible collodion vehicle w/ether 63.5%. Bot. 0.31 oz. *otc.*
Use: Keratolytic.

Compoz. (Medtech) **Tab.:** Diphenhydramine HCl 50 mg Pkg. 12s, 24s. **Cap.:** Diphenhydramine HCl 25 mg Pkg. 16s. *otc.*
Use: Nonprescription sleep aid.

comprecin.
See: Penetrex (Warner-Lambert).

Comtrex. (Bristol-Myers) Acetaminophen 325 mg, pseudoephedrine HCl 30 mg, chlorpheniramine maleate 2 mg, dextromethorphan HBr 10 mg/Tab. Bot. 24s, 50s. *otc.*
Use: Analgesic, decongestant, antihistamine, antitussive.

Comtrex Allergy-Sinus. (Bristol-Myers) Pseudoephedrine HCl 30 mg, chlorpheniramine maleate 2 mg, acetaminophen 500 mg/Tab. or Capl. Bot. 24s, 50s. *otc.*

Use: Decongestant, antihistamine, analgesic.

Comtrex Caplets. (Bristol-Myers) Acetaminophen 325 mg, pseudoephedrine HCl 30 mg, chlorpheniramine maleate 2 mg, dextromethorphan HBr 10 mg/ Capl. Bot. 24s, 50s. *otc.*
Use: Analgesic, decongestant, antihistamine, antitussive.

Comtrex Cough Formula. (Bristol-Myers) Pseudoephedrine HCl 15 mg, dextromethorphan 7.5 mg, guaifenesin 50 mg, acetaminophen 125 mg/5 ml, alcohol 20%. Bot. 120 ml, 240 ml. *otc.*
Use: Decongestant, antitussive, expectorant, analgesic.

Comtrex Day-Night. (Bristol-Myers) **Night:** Pseudoephedrine HCl 30 mg, chlorpheniramine maleate 2 mg, dextromethorphan HBr 10 mg, acetaminophen 325 mg/Tab. Pkg. 6s. **Day:** Pseudoephedrine HCl 30 mg, dextromethorphan HBr 10 mg, acetaminophen 500 mg/Tab. Pkg. 18s. *otc.*
Use: Antitussive, decongestant, antihistamine.

Comtrex Liquid. (Bristol-Myers) Pseudoephedrine HCl 10 mg, dextromethorphan HBr 3.3 mg, chlorpheniramine maleate 0.67 mg, acetaminophen 108.3 mg, alcohol 20%, sucrose. Bot. 180 ml. *otc.*
Use: Decongestant, antitussive, antihistamine.

Comtrex Liquid Multi-Symptom Cold Reliever. (Bristol-Myers) Acetaminophen 650 mg, phenylpropanolamine HCl 25 mg, chlorpheniramine maleate 4 mg, dextromethorphan HBr 20 mg/30 ml, alcohol 20%. Bot. 6 oz, 10 oz. *otc.*
Use: Analgesic, decongestant, antihistamine, antitussive.

Comtrex Liqui-Gels. (Bristol-Myers) Acetaminophen 325 mg, phenylpropanolamine HCl 12.5 mg, chlorpheniramine maleate 2 mg, dextromethorphan HBr 10 mg/Tab. Blister pkg. 24s, 50s. *otc.*
Use: Analgesic, decongestant, antihistamine, antitussive.

Comtrex, Maximum Strength. (Bristol-Myers) Phenylpropanolamine HCl 12.5 mg, dextromethorphan HBr 15 mg, chlorpheniramine maleate 2 mg, acetaminophen 500 mg. Cap. 24s, 50s. *otc.*
Use: Decongestant, antihistamine, antitussive.

Comtrex Maximum Strength Multi-Symptom Cold & Flu Relief. (Bristol-Myers) Phenylpropanolamine HCl 12.5 mg, chlorpheniramine maleate 2 mg, dextromethorphan HBr 15 mg, acetaminophen 500 mg/Capl. or Tab. Pkg. 24s. *otc.*
Use: Decongestant, antihistamine, antitussive, analgesic.

Comtrex Maximum Strength Non-Drowsy. (Bristol-Myers) Pseudoephedrine HCl 30 mg, dextromethorphan HBr 15 mg, acetaminophen 500 mg/Capl. Pkg. 24s. *otc.*
Use: Decongestant, antitussive, analgesic.

Comax. (Merck) *Haemophilus influenzae* type b and hepatitis b vaccines, combined 7.5 mcg Hib polysaccharide and 5 mcg hepatitis B surface antigen per 0.5 ml. Single-dose vial. *Rx.*
Use: Vaccine.

Conceive Ovulation Predictor. (Quidel) In vitro diagnostic test for luteinizing hormone in urine.
Use: Pregnancy test.

Concentraid. (Ferring Labs) Desmopressin acetate 0.1 mg/ml (0.1 mg equals 400 IU arginine vasopressin). Soln. Disposable intranasal pipettes containing 20 mcg/2 ml. *Rx.*
Use: Posterior pituitary hormones.

Concentrated Cleaner. (Bausch & Lomb) Anionic sulfate surfactant with friction-enhancing agents and sodium chlorine. Soln. Bot. 30 ml. *otc.*
Use: Contact lens care.

Concentrated Milk of Magnesia-Cascara. (Roxane) Magnesium hydroxide 2.34 g, aromatic cascara fluid extract U.S.P. 5 ml, alcohol 7%/Susp. UD 15 ml. *otc.*
Use: Laxative.

Concentrated Multiple Trace Element. (American Regent) Zinc (as sulfate) 5 mg, copper (as sulfate) 1 mg, manganese (as sulfate) 0.5 mg, chromium (as chloride) 10 mcg. Vial. 10 ml. *Rx.*
Use: Therapeutic supplement.

concentrated oleovitamin a & d.
See: Oleovitamin A & D, Concentrated, Cap. (Various Mfr.).

Concentrated Phillips' Milk of Magnesia. (Phillips) Magnesium hydroxide 800 mg/5 ml, sorbitol and sugar. Strawberry and orange vanilla creme flavors. Liq. 8 fl. oz. *otc.*
Use: Antacid, laxative.

Concentrin Caps. (Parke-Davis) Dextromethorphan HBr 15 mg, pseudoephedrine HCl 30 mg, guaifenesin 100 mg/ Cap. Bot. 12s. *otc.*
Use: Antitussive, decongestant, expectorant.

Conceptrol Contraceptive Inserts. (Advanced Care) Nonoxynol-9 150 mg. Supp. 10s. *otc.*
Use: Spermicide.

Conceptrol Disposable Contraceptive. (Advanced Care) Nonoxynol-9 4%. Vaginal gel. Tube. 2.7 g (6s, 10s). *otc.*
Use: Spermicide.

Condol Suspension. (Sanofi Winthrop) Dipyrone, chlormezanone. *Rx.*
Use: Analgesic, muscle relaxant.

Condol Tablets. (Sanofi Winthrop) Dipyrone, chlormezanone. *Rx.*
Use: Analgesic, muscle relaxant.

Condrin-LA. (Roberts) Phenylpropanolamine HCl 75 mg, chlorpheniramine maleate 12 mg. Bot. 1000s. *otc.*
Use: Decongestant, antihistamine.

condylox. (Oclassen) Podofilox 0.5%, alcohol 95%. Soln. Bot. 3.5 ml. *Rx.*
Use: Keratolytic.

Conest. (Grafton) Conjugated estrogens 0.625 mg, 1.25 mg or 2.5 mg/Tab. Bot. 100s, 1000s. *Rx.*
Use: Estrogen.

Conex-DA. (Forest) Phenylpropanolamine HCl 37.5 mg, chlorpheniramine maleate 4 mg/Tab. Bot. 100s, 1000s. *otc.*
Use: Decongestant, antihistamine.

Conex Plus. (Forest) Phenylpropanolamine HCl 25 mg, chlorpheniramine maleate 4 mg, acetaminophen 325 mg/Tab. Bot. 1000s. *otc.*
Use: Decongestant, antihistamine, analgesic.

Conex Syrup. (Forest) Phenylpropanolamine HCl 12.5 mg, guaifenesin 100 mg/5 ml. Bot. 4 oz. *otc.*
Use: Decongestant, expectorant.

Conex with Codeine. (Forest) Codeine phosphate 10 mg, guaifenesin 100 mg, phenylpropanolamine HCl 12.5 mg/5 ml. Bot. 4 oz. *c-v.*
Use: Antitussive, expectorant, decongestant.

Confide. (Direct Access Diagnostics) Reagent kit for HIV blood tests. Kit contains materials to draw a blood sample, a test card and a protective mailer for 1 test. *otc.*
Use: Diagnostic aid.

Confident. (Block) Carboxymethylcellulose gum, ethylene oxide polymer, petrolatum/mineral oil base. Tube 0.7 oz, 1.4 oz, 2.4 oz. *otc.*
Use: Denture adhesive.

Congess. (Fleming) **Sr.:** Guaifenesin 250 mg, pseudoephedrine HCl 120 mg/SR Cap. **Jr.:** Guaifenesin 125 mg, pseudoephedrine HCl 60 mg/TR Cap. Bot. 100s, 1000s. *otc, Rx.*
Use: Expectorant, decongestant.

Congess Jr. (Fleming) Pseudoephedrine HCl 60 mg, guaifenesin 125 mg/Cap. Bot. 100s, 1000s. *Rx.*
Use: Decongestant, expectorant.

Congess Sr. (Fleming) Pseudoephedrine HCl 120 mg, guaifenesin 250 mg/Cap. Bot. 100s, 1000s. *Rx.*
Use: Decongestant, expectorant.

Congestac. (Menley & James) Pseudoephedrine HCl 60 mg, guaifenesin 400 mg/Tab. Bot. 24s. *otc.*
Use: Decongestant, expectorant.

Congestant D. (Rugby) Phenylpropanolamine HCl 12.5 mg, chlorpheniramine maleate 2 mg, acetaminophen 325 mg, sucrose. Tab. Bot. 100s, 1000s. *otc.*
Use: Decongestant, antihistamine.

congo red. Injection.
Use: Hemostatic in hemorrhagic disorders.

conjugated estrogens.
See: Estrogens, Conjugated (Various Mfr.).
Use: Estrogen.

Conjunctamide. (Horizon) Prednisolone acetate 0.5%, sodium sulfacetamide 10%, hydroxypropyl methylcellulose, polysorbate 80, sodium thiosulfate, benzalkonium Cl 0.01%. Susp. Dropper bot. 5 ml, 15 ml. *Rx.*
Use: Corticosteroid, anti-infective, ophthalmic.

•**conorphone hydrochloride.** (KOE-nahr-fone) USAN. *Formerly Codorphone.*
Use: Analgesic.

Conray. (Mallinckrodt) Iothalamate meglumine 60% (28.2% iodine), EDTA. Inj. Vial 20 ml, 30 ml, 50 ml, 100 ml, 150 ml. *Rx.*
Use: Radiopaque agent.

Conray-30. (Mallinckrodt) Iothalamate meglumine 30% (14.1% iodine), EDTA. Inj. Vial 300 ml. *Rx.*
Use: Radiopaque agent.

Conray-43. (Mallinckrodt) Iothalamate meglumine 43% (20.2% iodine), EDTA. Inj. Vial 50 ml, 100 ml, 250 ml. *Rx.*
Use: Radiopaque agent.

Conray-325. (Mallinckrodt) Iothalamate sodium 54.3% (32.5% iodine), EDTA. Inj. Vial 30 ml, 50 ml. *Rx.*
Use: Radiopaque agent.

Conray-400. (Mallinckrodt) Iothalamate sodium 66.8% (40% iodine), EDTA. Inj. Vial 25 ml, 50 ml. *Rx.*

Use: Radiopaque agent.

Consin Compound Salve. (Wisconsin) Carbolic acid ointment. Jar 2 oz, lb. *otc.*
Use: Minor skin irritations.

Constilac. (Alra) Lactulose syrup 10 g/15 ml. Bot. 8 oz, 16 oz, UD 30 ml. *Rx.*
Use: Laxative.

Constonate 60. Docusate sodium 100 mg, 250 mg/Cap. Bot. 100s, 1000s. *otc.*
Use: Laxative.

Constulose. (Barre-National) Lactulose 10 g, galactose < 2.2 g, lactose 1.2 g, other sugars ≤ 1.2 g/15 ml. Syr. Bot. 237 ml, 946 ml. *Rx.*
Use: Laxative, analgesic.

Contac-12 Hour Capsules. (SK-Beecham) Phenylpropanolamine HCl 75 mg, chlorpheniramine maleate 8 mg/CA Cap. Pkg. 10s, 20s. *otc.*
Use: Decongestant, antihistamine.

Contac Cough & Chest Cold Liquid. (SK-Beecham) Pseudoephedrine HCl 15 mg, dextromethorpan HBr 5 mg, guaifenesin 50 mg, acetaminophen 125 mg, alcohol 10%, saccharin, sorbitol. Liq. Bot. 4 fl. oz. *otc.*
Use: Decongestant, antitussive, expectorant, analgesic.

Contac Cough and Sore Throat Formula. (SK-Beecham) Dextromethorphan HBr 5 mg, acetaminophen 125 mg, alcohol 10%. Bot. 120 ml. *otc.*
Use: Antitussive, analgesic.

Contac Day & Night Allergy/Sinus Caplets. (SK-Beecham) **Day:** Pseudoephedrine HCl 60 mg, acetaminophen 650 mg/Capl. **Night:** Pseudoephedrine HCl 60 mg, diphenhydramine HCl 50 mg, acetaminophen 650 mg/Capl. Pkg. 20 (15 day; 5 night). *otc.*
Use: Decongestant, antihistamine, analgesic.

Contac Day & Night Cold & Flu Caplets. (SK-Beecham) **Night:** Pseudoephedrine HCl 60 mg, diphenhydramine HCl 50 mg, acetaminophen 650 mg/Cap. Pkg. 5s. **Day:** Pseudoephedrine HCl 60 mg, dextromethorphan HRr 30 mg, acetaminophen 650 mg/Cap. Pkg. 15s. *otc.*
Use: Decongestant, antihistamine, antitussive, analgesic.

Contac Jr. (SK-Beecham) Pseudoephedrine HCl 15 mg, acetaminophen 160 mg, dextromethorphan HBr 5 mg, saccharin, sorbitol/5 ml. Bot. 4 oz. *otc.*
Use: Decongestant, analgesic, antitussive.

Contac Maximum Strength 12-hour Caplets. (SK-Beecham) Phenylpropanolamine HCl 75 mg, chlorpheniramine maleate 12 mg/Capl. Pkg. 10, 20s. *otc.*
Use: Decongestant, antihistamine.

Contac Nighttime Cold. (SK-Beecham) Acetaminophen 167 mg, dextromethorphan HBr 5 mg, pseudoephedrine HCl 10 mg, doxylamine succinate 1.25 mg/5 ml, alcohol 25%. Bot. 177 ml. *otc.*
Use: Analgesic, antitussive, decongestant, antihistamine.

Contac Non-Drowsy Formula Sinus. (SK-Beecham) Pseudoephedrine HCl 30 mg, acetaminophen 500 mg/Capl. or Tab. Pkg. 24s. *otc.*
Use: Decongestant, analgesic.

Contac Severe Cold Formula. (SK-Beecham) Phenylpropanolamine HCl 12.5 mg, acetaminophen 500 mg, chlorpheniramine maleate 2 mg, dextromethorphan HBr 15 mg/Capl. Pkg. 10s, 20s. *otc.*
Use: Decongestant, analgesic, antihistamine, antitussive.

Contac Severe Cold & Flu Nighttime Liquid. (SK-Beecham) Pseudoephedrine HCl 10 mg, chlorpheniramine maleate 0.67 mg, dextromethorphan HBr 5 mg, acetaminophen 167 mg, alcohol 18.5%, saccharin, sorbitol, glucose. Liq. Bot. 180 ml. *otc.*
Use: Decongestant, antihistamine, antitussive.

contact lens products, soft. (Hydrogel). *otc.*
Use: Rinsing/storage solutions.
See: Allergan Hydrocare Preserved Saline (Allergan).
Boil n Soak (Alcon).
Lensrins (Allergan).
Opti-Soft (Alcon).
ReNu Saline (Bausch & Lomb).
Saline Solution, Sterile Preserved (Bausch & Lomb).
Murine Preserved All-Purpose Saline Solution (Ross).
Sensitive Eyes Plus (Bausch & Lomb).
Sensitive Eyes Saline (Bausch & Lomb).
Soft Mate Saline for Sensitive Eyes (Pilkington Barnes Hind).
Allergan Sorbi-Care Saline (Allergan).
Sterile Saline (Bausch & Lomb).
Blairex Sterile Saline (Blairex).
Hypo-Clear (Bausch & Lomb).
Lens Plus Preservative Free (Allergan).

Ciba Vision Saline (Ciba Vision).
Hypo-Clear (Bausch & Lomb).
Purisol 4 (Amcon).
Unisol (Wesley-Jessen).
Unisol 4 (Wesley-Jessen).
Soft Mate Saline Preservative-Free
(Pilkington Barnes Hind).
Use: Salt tablets for normal saline.
See: Soft Rinse 135 (Professional Supplies).
Amcon 250 (Amcon).
Easy Eyes (Eaton Medicals).
Marlin Salt System II (Marlin).
Soft Rinse 250 (Professional Supplies).
Use: Surfactant cleaning solutions.
See: Ciba Vision Cleaner (Ciba Vision).
Daily Cleaner (Bausch & Lomb).
Preflex for Sensitive Eyes (Alcon).
DURAcare II (Blairex).
LC-65 (Allergan).
Lens Clear (Allergan).
Lens Plus Daily Cleaner (Allergan).
Mira Flow Extra Strength (Ciba Vision).
Murine Contact Lens Cleaner (Ross).
Opti-Clean II (Alcon).
Pliagel (Wesley-Jessen).
Sensitive Eyes Saline/Cleaning Solution (Bausch & Lomb).
Sof/Pro-Clean (Sherman).
Sof/Pro-Clean (s.a.) (Sherman).
Soft Mate Hands Off Daily Cleaner
(Pilkington Barnes Hind).
Soft Mate Protein Remover (Pilkington Barnes Hind).
Soft Mate Daily Cleaning for Sensitive Eyes (Pilkington Barnes Hind).
Use: Enzymatic cleaners.
See: Allergan Enzymatic (Allergan).
Extenzyme Protein Cleaner (Allergan).
Opti-zyme Enzymatic Cleaner (Alcon).
ReNu Effervescent Enzymatic
Cleaner (Bausch & Lomb).
ReNu Thermal Enzymatic Cleaner
(Bausch & Lomb).
Ultrazyme Enzymatic Cleaner (Allergan).
Use: Re-wetting solutions.
See: Adapettes for Sensitive Eyes (Alcon).
Clerz Drops (Wesley-Jessen).
Clerz 2 (Wesley-Jessen).
Comfort Tears (Pilkington Barnes
Hind).
Lens Drops (Ciba Vision).
Lens Fresh (Allergan).
Lens Lubricant (Bausch & Lomb).
Lens Plus Rewetting Drops (Allergan).

Lens-Wet (Allergan).
Murine Sterile Lubricating and Rewetting Drops (Ross).
Opti-Tears (Alcon).
Sensitive Eye Drops (Bausch &
Lomb).
Soft Mate Comfort Drops (Pilkington
Barnes Hind).
Soft Mate Lens Drops (Pilkington Barnes Hind).
Sterile Lens Lubricant (Blairex).
Use: Chemical disinfection systems.
See: Allergan Hydrocare Cleaning and
Disinfecting (Allergan).
Aosept (Ciba Vision).
Disinfecting Solution (Bausch &
Lomb).
Flex-Care (Alcon).
Lens Plus Oxysept System (Allergan).
Lensept (Ciba Vision).
MiraSept System (Wesley-Jessen).
Opti-Free (Alcon).
Pure Sept (Ross).
Quik-Sept System (Bausch & Lomb).
ReNu Multi-Action (Bausch & Lomb).
Soft Mate (Pilkington Barnes Hind).
Soft Mate Consept (Pilkington Barnes
Hind).
ConTE-PAK-4. (SoloPak) Zinc 5 mg, copper 1 mg, manganese 0.5 mg, chromium 10 mcg/ml. Soln. Vial 1 ml, 10 ml.
Rx.
Use: Parenteral nutritional supplement.
contraceptives.
See: Oral Contraceptives (Various Mfr.).
Foams, Vaginal.
See: Delfen, Vaginal Foam (Ortho).
Emko, Vaginal Foam (Schering-Plough).
Intrauterine System.
See: Progestasert, (Alza).
Jellies & Creams, Vaginal.
See: Colagyn, Jel (Smith).
Colagyn, Jel (Smith).
Conceptrol, Cream, Gel (Ortho).
Gynol II, Gel (Ortho).
Immolin, Cream-Jel (Schmid).
Koromex-A, Jelly (Holland-Rantos).
Koromex, Cream or Jelly (Holland-Rantos).
Ortho-Creme (Ortho).
Ortho-Gynol, Jelly (Ortho).
Miscellaneous.
See: Norplant (Wyeth-Ayerst).
VCF, Film (Apothecus).
Suppositories, Vaginal.
See: Intercept, Inserts (Ortho).
Lorophyn, Supp., Jelly (Eaton).
Contrin. (Geneva Pharm.) Iron (from fer-

rous fumarate) 110 mg, B_{12} 15 mcg, IFC (intrinisic factor as concentrate or from stomach preparations) 240 mg, C 75 mg, folic acid 0.5 mg/Cap. Bot. 100s. *Rx.*
Use: Vitamin/mineral supplement.

Control. (Thompson) Phenylpropanolamine HCl 75 mg/TR Cap. Bot. 14s, 28s, 56s. *otc.*
Use: Nonprescription diet aid.

Contuss Liquid. (Parmed) Phenylpropanolamine HCl 20 mg, phenylephrine HCl 5 mg, guaifenesin 100 mg, alcohol 5%, saccharin, sorbitol, sucrose. Liq. Bot. 16 fl. oz. *Rx.*
Use: Antihistamine, decongestant, antitussive.
Use: Digestive enzymes.

Converspaz. (Ascher) Cellulase 5 mg, protease 10 mg, amylase 30 mg, lipase 13 mg, l-hyoscamine sulfate 0.0625 mg/Cap. Bot. 100s. *Rx.*
Use: Digestive enzymes.

Cool-Mint Listerine. (Warner-Lambert) Thymol, eucalyptol, methyl salicylate, menthol, alcohol 21.6%. Liq. Bot. 90 ml, 180 ml, 360 ml, 540 ml, 720 ml, 960 ml. *otc.*
Use: Mouthwash.

Coopervision Balanced Salt Solution. (Ciba Vision) Sterile intraocular irrigation soln. Bot. 15 ml, 500 ml.
Use: Intraocular irrigating solution.

Copavin Pulvules. (Lilly) Codeine sulfate 15 mg, papaverine HCl 15 mg/Cap. Bot. 100s. *c-v.*
Use: Antitussive.

Copaxone. Glatiramer acetate, mannitol 40 mg/Vial, 2 ml. 32s. *Rx.*
Use: Treatment of relapsing-remitting multiple sclerosis.

Cope. (Mentholatum) Aspirin 421 mg, magnesium hydroxide 50 mg, aluminum hydroxide 25 mg, caffeine 32 mg/Tab. Bot. 36s, 60s. *otc.*
Use: Salicylate analgesic, antacid.

Cophene-B. (Dunhall) Brompheniramine maleate 10 mg/ml/Inj. Vial 10 ml with methyl and propyl parabens. *Rx.*
Use: Antihistamine.

Cophene #2. (Dunhall) Chlorpheniramine maleate 12 mg, pseudoephedrine HCl 120 mg/Time Cap. Bot. 100s, 500s. *Rx.*
Use: Antihistamine, decongestant.

Cophene Injectable. (Dunhall) Atropine sulfate 0.2 mg, phenylpropanolamine HCl 12.5 mg, chlorpheniramine maleate 5 mg/ml. Pkg. 10 ml. *Rx.*

Use: Anticholinergic, antispasmodic, decongestant, antihistamine.

Cophene-PL. (Dunhall) Phenylephrine HCl 20 mg, phenylpropanolamine HCl 20 mg, chlorpheniramine maleate 5 mg/5 ml. Bot. 16 oz. *otc, Rx.*
Use: Decongestant, antihistamine.

Cophene-S. (Dunhall) Dihydrocodone bitartrate 3 mg, phenylephrine HCl 20 mg, phenylpropanolamine HCl 20 mg, chlorpheniramine maleate 5 mg/5 ml. Bot. pt. *c-iii.*
Use: Antitussive, decongestant, antihistamine.

Cophene-X. (Dunhall) Carbetapentane citrate 20 mg, phenylephrine HCl 10 mg, phenylpropanolamine HCl 10 mg, chlorpheniramine maleate 2.5 mg, potassium guaiacolsulfonate 45 mg/Cap. Bot. 100s. *Rx.*
Use: Antitussive, decongestant, antihistamine, expectorant.

Cophene-XP Syrup. (Dunhall) Carbetapentane citrate 20 mg, phenylephrine HCl 10 mg, phenylpropanolamine HCl 20 mg, chlorpheniramine maleate 2.5 mg, potassium guaiacolsulfonate 45 mg/5 ml. Bot. pt. *Rx.*
Use: Antitussive, decongestant, antihistamine, expectorant.

copolymer 1, (cop 1). *Rx.*
Use: Treat multiple sclerosis. [Orphan drug]

copper. (Abbott) Copper 0.4 mg/ml (as 0.85 mg cupric Cl.) Inj. Vial 10 ml, 30 ml. *Rx.*
Use: Parenteral nutritional supplement.

•**copper gluconate,** U.S.P. 23.
Use: Supplement (trace mineral).

copperhead bite therapy.
See: Antivenin, Snake Polyvalent Inj. (Wyeth-Ayerst).

Copperin. (Vernon) Iron ammonium citrate, copper (6 gr). "A" adult dose, "B" children dose. Bot. 30s, 100s, 500s.
Use: Mineral supplement.

Coppertone. (Schering-Plough) A series of sun-care products marketed under the Coppertone name including Waterproof Lotions SPF 4, 6, 8, 15 and 25. Bot. 4 fl oz, 8 fl oz. Oil SPF 2: Bot. 4 fl oz, 8 fl oz; Lite Formula Oil SPF 2: Bot. 4 fl oz; Lite Lotion SPF 4: Bot. 4 fl oz; Dark Tanning Body Mousse SPF 4: Tube 4 oz; Suntanning Gel SPF 4: Tube 3 oz; Noskote SPF 8: Tube 0.44 oz, Jar 1 oz; Noskote SPF-15: Jar 1 oz. Contain one or more of the following ingredients: Padimate O, oxybenzone, homosalate, ethylhexyl p-methocinnamate. *otc.*

Use: Sunscreen.

Coppertone Dark Tanning Spray. (Schering-Plough) Padimate O in spray base (SPF 2). Bot. 8 fl oz. *otc.*
Use: Sunscreen.

Coppertone Face. (Schering-Plough) A series of sunscreen lotions with SPF 2, 4, 6 and 15 in a non-greasy base with Padimate O, oxybenzone (SPF 15 only). *otc.*
Use: Sunscreen.

Coppertone Kids Sunblock. (Schering-Plough) **SPF 15:** Ethylhexyl p-methoxycinnamate, oxybenzone, 2-ethylhexyl salicylate, homosalate. Lot. Bot. 120 ml, 240 ml. **SPF 30:** Octocrylene, ethylhexyl p-methoxycinnamate, oxybenzone, 2-ethylhexyl salicylate. Lot. Bot. 120 ml, 240 ml. *otc.*
Use: Sunscreen.

Coppertone Lipkote. (Schering-Plough) Ethylhexyl p-methoxycinnamate, oxybenzone. SPF 15. Stick 4.5 g. *otc.*
Use: Sunscreen.

Coppertone Moisturizing Sunblock. (Schering-Plough) **SPF 45:** Ethylhexyl p-methoxycinnamate, 2-ethylhexyl salicylate, octocrylene, oxybenzone. Lot. Bot. 120 ml, 300 ml. **SPF 30, 25:** Ethylhexyl p-methoxycinnamate, oxybenzone, 2-ethylhexyl salicylate, homosalate. Lot. Bot. SPF 30: 120 ml, 240 ml; SPF 25: 120 ml. **SPF 15:** Ethylhexyl p-methoxycinnamate, oxybenzone. Lot. Bot. 120 ml, 240 ml, 300 ml. *otc.*
Use: Sunscreen.

Coppertone Moisturizing Sunscreen. (Schering-Plough) Ethylhexyl p-methoxycinnamate, oxybenzone, benzyl alcohol, vitamin E, aloe. PABA free. SPF 6, 8. Waterproof. Lot. Bot. 120 ml, 240 ml. *otc.*
Use: Sunscreen.

Coppertone Moisturizing Suntan. (Schering-Plough) **SPF 4:** ethylhexyl p-methoxycinnamate, oxybenzone, benzyl alcohol, vitamin E, aloe. PABA free. Waterproof. Lot. Bot. 120 ml, 240 ml. **SPF 2:** homosalate, vitamin E, aloe. PABA free. Waterproof. Oil. Bot. 120 ml. *otc.*
Use: Sunscreen.

Coppertone Noskote. (Schering-Plough) Homosalate 8%, oxybenzone 3%. (SPF 8) Oint. Jar 13.2 g, 30 g. *otc.*
Use: Sunscreen.

Coppertone SPF-25 Sunblock Lotion. (Schering-Plough) Ethylhexyl p-methoxycinnamate, oxybenzone, Padimate O in lotion base (SPF-25). Bot. 4 fl oz. *otc.*

Use: Sunscreen.

Coppertone Sport. (Schering-Plough) Ethylhexyl p-methoxycinnamate, oxybenzone. SPF 4, 8, 15, 30. Lot. Bot. 120 ml. *otc.*
Use: Sunscreen.

Coppertone Tan Magnifier Suntan. (Schering-Plough). **SPF 2:** Triethanolamine salicylate. Oil Bot. 120 ml. **SPF 4: Lotion:** Ethylhexyl p-methoxycinnamate. Bot. 120 ml. **Gel:** 2-phenylbenzimidazole-5-sulfonic acid. Tube 120 g. *otc.*
Use: Sunscreen

copper trace metal additive. (IMS) Copper 1 mg. Inj. Vial 10 ml. *Rx.*
Use: Copper supplement.

•**copper undecylenate.** USAN.
W/Sodium propionate, sodium caprylate, propionic acid, undecylenic acid, salicylic acid.

Co-Pyronil 2. (Dista) Chlorpheniramine maleate 4 mg, pseudoephedrine HCl 60 mg/Pulvule. Bot. 100s. *otc.*
Use: Antihistamine, decongestant.

Corab. (Abbott Diagnostics) Radioimmunoassay for detection of antibody to hepatitis B core antigen. Test kit 100s.
Use: Diagnostic aid.

Corab-M. (Abbott Diagnostics) Radioimmunoassay for the qualitative determination of specific Ig antibody to hepatitis B virus core antigen (Anti-HBc Ig) in human serum or plasma and may be used as an aid in the diagnosis of acute or recent hepatitis B infection.
Use: Diagnostic aid.

Corace Injection. (Forest Pharm.) Cortisone acetate 50 mg/ml. Vial 10 ml. *Rx.*
Use: Glucocorticoid.

Coracin. (Roberts Hauck) Hydrocortisone acetate 1%, neomycin sulfate 0.5%, bacitracin zinc 400 units, polymyxin B sulfate 10,000 units/g in white petrolatum and mineral oil base. Oint. Tube 3.5 g. *Rx.*
Use: Corticosteroid, anti-infective, ophthalmic.

Coral. (Young Dental Mfr.) Fluoride ion 1.23%, 0.1 molar phosphate. Jar 250 g, Coral II: 180 disposable cup units/carton. *Rx.*
Use: Phosphate/fluoride prophylaxis paste.

Coral/Plus. (Young Dental Mfr.) Free fluoride ion 2.2%, recrystallized kaolinite. Tube 250 g. *Rx.*

coral snake (North American) antivenin.

See: Antivenin (Micrurus fulvius). (Wyeth-Ayerst).

Corane Capsules. (Forest Pharm.) Pyrilamine maleate 25 mg, pheniramine maleate 10 mg, phenylpropanolamine HCl 25 mg, phenylephrine HCl 10 mg/Cap. Bot. 100s, 500s, 1000s. *otc.*
Use: Antihistamine, decongestant.

Corbicin-125. (Arthrins) Vitamin C 125 mg/Cap. Bot. 100s. *otc.*
Use: Vitamin C supplement.

Cordarone. (Wyeth-Ayerst) Tab.: Amiodarone HCl 200 mg, lactose. Bot. 60s, UD 100s. Inj.: Amiodarone 50 mg/ml, benzyl alcohol 20.2 mg/ml. Amps. 3 ml. *Rx.*
Use: Antiarrhythmic.

Cordran. (Dista) Flurandrenolide 0.025%, 0.05% in emulsified petrolatum base/g. **0.025%:** Tube 30 g, 60 g, Jar 225 g. **0.05%:** Tube 15 g, 30 g, 60 g, Jar 225 g. *Rx.*
Use: Corticosteroid, topical.

Cordran Lotion. (Dista) Flurandrenolide 0.05%, cetyl alcohol, benzyl alcohol, stearic acid, glyceryl monostearate, polyoxyl 40 stearate, glycerin, mineral oil, menthol, purified water. Squeeze bot. 15 ml, 60 ml. *Rx.*
Use: Corticosteroid, topical.

Cordran-N Cream & Ointment. (Dista) Flurandrenolide 0.5 mg, neomycin sulfate 5 mg/g. Tube 15 g, 30 g, 60 g. *Rx.*
Use: Corticosteroid, topical.

Cordran SP. (Dista) Flurandrenolide 0.025%, 0.05% in emulsified base w/ cetyl alcohol, stearic acid, polyoxyl 40 stearate, mineral oil, propylene glycol, sodium citrate, citric acid, purified water. **0.025%:** Tube 30 g, 60 g, Jar 225 g. **0.05%:** Tube 15 g, 30 g, 60 g, Jar 225 g. *Rx.*
Use: Corticosteroid, topical.

Cordran Tape. (Dista) Flurandrenolide 4 mcg/sq. cm. Roll 7.5 cm × 60 cm, 7.5 cm 200 cm. *Rx.*
Use: Corticosteroid, topical.

Cordrol. (Vita Elixir) Prednisolone 5 mg, 10 mg or 20 mg/Tab. Bot. 100s. *Rx.*
Use: Corticosteroid.

Coreg. (SmithKline Beecham) Carvedilol, lactose, sucrose/Tab. 6.25, 12.5 or 25 mg. In 30s, 100s or UD 100s. Film-coated *Rx.*
Use: Antihypertensive.

Corega Powder. (Block) Denture adhesive containing polyethyleneoxide polymer w/peppermint oil, karaya gum.

Pkg.: pocket 0.7 oz; medium 1.15 oz; economy 3.55 oz. *otc.*
Use: Denture adhesive.

Corgard. (Bristol Myers Squibb) Nadolol 20 mg, 40 mg, 80 mg, 120 mg or 160 mg/Tab. Bot. 100s, 1000s, UD 100s. *Rx.*
Use: Beta-adrenergic blocker.

•**coriander oil,** N.F. XVI.
Use: Pharmaceutic aid (flavor).

Coricidin. (Schering-Plough) Chlorpheniramine maleate 2 mg, acetaminophen 325 mg/Tab. Bot. 100s. *otc.*
Use: Antihistamine, analgesic.

Coricidin D Tablets. (Schering-Plough) Chlorpheniramine maleate 2 mg, acetaminophen 325 mg, phenylpropanolamine HCl 12.5 mg/Tab. Bot. 12s, 24s, 48s, 100s. *otc.*
Use: Antihistamine, analgesic, decongestant,

Coricidin Demilets. (Schering-Plough) Phenylpropanolamine HCl 6.25 mg, chlorpheniramine maleate 1 mg, acetaminophen 80 mg, saccharin, lactose. Tab. Bot. 24s, 36s. *otc.*
Use: Pediatric decongestant, antihistamine, analgesic.

Coricidin Extra Strength Sinus Headache Tablets. (Schering-Plough) Acetaminophen 500 mg, phenylpropanolamine HCl 12.5 mg, chlorpheniramine maleate 2 mg/Tab. Box 24s. *otc.*
Use: Analgesic, decongestant, antihistamine.

Coricidin Maximum Strength Sinus Headache. (Schering-Plough) Phenylpropanolamine HCl 12.5 mg, chlorpheniramine maleate 2 mg, acetaminophen 500 mg/Tab. Box 24s. *otc.*
Use: Decongestant, antihistamine, analgesic.

Corilin Infant Liquid. (Schering-Plough) Chlorpheniramine maleate 0.75 mg, sodium salicylate 80 mg/ml, alcohol < 1%. Bot. 30 ml. *otc.*
Use: Antihistamine, salicylate analgesic.

Cormax. (Oclassen) Clobetasol propionate 0.05%, white petrolatum, sorbitan sesquioleate/Oint. Tube. 15 g and 45 g. *Rx.*
Use: Topical corticosteroid.

Cormed.
See: Nikethamide (Various Mfr.).

•**cormethasone acetate.** (core-METH-ah-sone) USAN.
Use: Anti-inflammatory (topical).

Corn Huskers Lotion. (Warner-Lambert Prods.) Glycerin 6.7%, SD alcohol, al-

gin, TEA-oleoyl sarcosinate, guar gum, methylparaben, calcium sulfate, calcium Cl, TEA-fumarate, TEA-borate. Bot. 4 oz, 7 oz. *otc.*
Use: Emollient.

•**corn oil, N.F.** 18.
Use: Pharmaceutic aid (solvent, oleaginous vehicle).
See: G. B. Prep Emulsion (Gray).
Lipomul-Oral, Liq. (Pharmacia & Upjohn).

Corns-O-Poppin. (Ries-Hamly) Salicylic acid 6.5%, benzoic acid 12%. *otc.*
Use: Cauterizing agent.

Corotrope. (Winthop Pharm.) Milrinone for IV use. *Rx.*
Use: Cardiotonic agent.

corpus luteum, extract (water soluble).
See: Progesterone, Preps. (Various Mfr.).

Corque. (Geneva Pharm.) Hydrocortisone 1%, iodochlorhydroxyquin 3%. Cream. Tube 20 g. *Rx.*
Use: Corticosteroid, topical.

Correctol Extra Gentle. (Schering-Plough) Docusate sodium 100 mg. Cap. Bot. 30s. *otc.*
Use: Laxative.

Correctol Tablets. (Schering-Plough) Docusate sodium 100 mg, yellow phenolphthalein 65 mg/Tab. Box 15s, 30s, 60s, 90s. *otc.*
Use: Laxative.

Cortaid, Maximum Strength. (Pharmacia & Upjohn) **Cream:** Hydrocortisone in parabens 1%, cetyl and stearyl alcohols, glycerin and white petrolatum. Tube 15 g, 30 g. *otc.*
Use: Corticosteroids, topical.

Cortaid Maximum Strength Spray. (Pharmacia & Upjohn) Hydrocortisone 1%, alcohol 55%, glycerin, methylparaben. Pump spray. Bot. 45 ml. *otc.*
Use: Corticosteroid, topical.

Cortan. (Halsey) Prednisone 5 mg/Tab. Bot. 1000s. *Rx.*
Use: Corticosteroid.

Cortane D.C. Expectorant. (Standex) Brompheniramine maleate 2 mg, guaifenesin 100 mg, phenylephrine HCl 5 mg, phenylpropanolamine HCl 5 mg, codeine phosphate 10 mg, alcohol 3.5%/5 ml. Bot. pt. *c-v.*
Use: Antihistamine, expectorant, decongestant, antitussive.

Cortane Expectorant. (Standex) Brompheniramine maleate 2 mg, guaifenesin 100 mg, phenylephrine 5 mg, phenylpropanolamine HCl 5 mg, alcohol

3.5%/5 ml. Bot. pt. *otc.*
Use: Antihistamine, expectorant, decongestant.

Cortapp Elixir. (Standex) Brompheniramine maleate 5 mg, phenylephrine HCl 5 mg, phenylpropanolamine HCl 5 mg, alcohol 2.3%/5 ml. Bot. pt. *otc.*
Use: Antihistamine, decongestant.

Cortatrigen Ear Suspension. (Goldline) Hydrocortisone 1%, neomycin sulfate 5 mg, polymyxin B sulfate 10,000 units/ml. Bot. 10 ml. *Rx.*
Use: Corticosteroid, anti-infective, otic.

Cortatrigen Modified Ear Drops. (Goldline) Bot. 10 ml. *Rx.*
Use: Corticosteroid, anti-infective, otic.

Cort-Dome. (Bayer) Hydrocortisone alcohol. **Cream:** 0.25%: 1 oz, 4 oz; 0.5%: 1 oz; 1%: 1 oz. **Lot.:** 0.25%: 4 oz; 0.5%: 4 oz; 1%: 1 oz. *Rx.*
Use: Corticosteroid, topical.

Cort-Dome High Potency. (Bayer) Hydrocortisone acetate 25 mg in a monoglyceride base. Supp. Box 12s. *Rx.*
Use: Corticosteroid, topical.

Cortef Acetate Ointment. (Pharmacia & Upjohn) Hydrocortisone acetate 10 mg/g, lanolin (anhydrous), white petrolatum, mineral oil. Tube 20 g (10 mg/g). *Rx.*
Use: Corticosteroid, topical.

Cortef Feminine Itch Cream. (Pharmacia & Upjohn) Hydrocortisone acetate equivalent to hydrocortisone 5 mg/g. Tube 0.5 oz. *Rx.*
Use: Corticosteroid, topical.

Cortef Oral Suspension. (Pharmacia & Upjohn) Hydrocortisone 10 mg/5 ml (as 13.4 mg hydrocortisone cypionate). Oral susp. Bot. 4 oz. *Rx.*
Use: Corticosteroid.

Cortef Tablets. (Pharmacia & Upjohn) Hydrocortisone. **5 mg/Tab.:** Bot. 50s; **10 mg or 20 mg/Tab.:** Bot. 100s. *Rx.*
Use: Corticosteroid.

Cortenema. (Solvay) Hydrocortisone 100 mg in aqueous solution w/carboxypolymethylene, polysorbate 80, methylparaben 0.18%/60 ml. Bot. w/applicator. UD 1s. *Rx.*
Use: Corticosteroid, topical.

cortenil.
See: Desoxycorticosterone Acetate, Preps. (Various Mfr.).

cortical hormone products.
See: Adrenal Cortex Extract (Various Mfr.).
Aristocort, Preps. (Lederle).

Corticotropin, Preps. (Various Mfr.).
Hydrocortisone, Preps. (Various Mfr.).
Cortisone Acetate, Preps. (Various Mfr.).
Decadron LA, Inj. (Merck & Co.).
Decadron, Tab., Elix., Inj. (Merck & Co.).
Desoxycorticosterone Acetate, Preps. (Various Mfr.).
Dexamethasone, Tab. (Various Mfr.).
Fludrocortisone (Various Mfr.).
Hydeltrasol, Inj. (Merck & Co.).
Hydrocortone Acetate, Inj. (Merck & Co.).
Hydrocortone Phosphate, Inj. (Merck & Co.).
Kenacort, Prep. (Squibb).
Lipo-Adrenal Cortex, Inj. (Pharmacia & Upjohn).
Medrol, Preps. (Pharmacia & Upjohn).
Methylprednisolone, Tab. (Various Mfr.).
Prednisolone, Tab. (Various Mfr.).
Prednisone, Tab. (Various Mfr.).
Triamcinolone, Tab. (Various Mfr.).

Cortic Ear Drops. (Everett) Hydrocortisone 10 mg, pramoxine HCl 10 mg, chloroxylenol 1 mg/ml, propylene glycol diacetate 3%/Drops. Bot. 10 ml. *Rx.*
Use: Otic preparation.

•**corticorelin ovine triflutate.** (core-tih-kah-REH-lin OH-vine TRY-flew-TATE) USAN.
Use: Hormone (corticotropin-releasing); diagnostic aid for adrenal cortical function and Cushing's syndrome. [Orphan drug]

corticosteroid/mydriatic combo, ophthalmics. Prednisolone acetate 0.25%, atropine sulfate 1%. *Rx.*
Use: Treatment of anterior uveitis.
See: Mydrapred, Susp. (Alcon).

corticotropin highly purified.
See: H. P. Acthar Gel. Vial. (Centeon).

•**corticotropin injection,** (core-tih-koe-TROE-pin) U.S.P. 23. ACTH, Adrenocorticotropic hormone or adrenocorticotrop(h)in or corticotropin.
Use: Adrenal corticotropic hormone; glucocorticoid; diagnostic aid (adrenocortical insufficiency).
See: ACTH.
Acthar (Centeon).
Cortrophin Gel, Vial, Amp. (Organon).

•**corticotropin injection, repository,** (core-tih-koe-TROE-pin) U.S.P. 23.
Use: Hormone (adrenocorticotropic); glucocorticoid; diagnostic aid (adrenocortical insufficiency).
See: Acthar Gel Vial (Centeon).

ACTH Gel Purified (Various Mfr.).
Cortrophin Gel Amp., Vial (Organon).
H.P. Acthar Gel, Vial (Centeon).

Cortifoam. (Schwarz Pharma) Hydrocortisone acetate 10% in an aerosol foam w/propylene glycol, emulsifying wax, steareth 10, cetyl alcohol, methylparaben, propylparaben, trolamine, water, inert propellants. Container 20 g w/rectal applicator for 14 applicatorfuls. *Rx.*
Use: Corticosteroid, topical.

cortisol.
See: Hydrocortisone, U.S.P. 23.
Note: Cortisol was the official published name for hydrocortisone in U.S.P. 23. The name was changed back to Hydrocortisone, U.S.P. in Supplement 1 to the U.S.P. 23.

cortisol cyclopentylpropionate.
See: Cortef Fluid, Susp., Tab. (Pharmacia & Upjohn).

•**cortisone acetate,** (CORE-tih-sone) U.S.P. 23.
Use: Glucocorticoid.
See: Cortistan (Standex).
Cortone Acetate, Tab. (Merck & Co.).

cortisone acetate. (Kendall's Compund E, Pharmacia & Upjohn) 5 mg, 10 mg, 25 mg/Tab. Bot. 50s, 100s, 500s.
Use: Adrenocortical steroid (anti-inflammatory).

Cortisporin Cream. (Glaxo Wellcome) Polymyxin B sulfate 10,000 units, neomycin sulfate 5 mg, hydrocortisone acetate 5 mg/g, methylparaben 0.25%. Tube 7.5 g. *Rx.*
Use: Anti-infective; corticosteroid, topical.

Cortisporin Ointment. (Glaxo Wellcome) Polymyxin B sulfate 5000 units, bacitracin zinc 400 units, neomycin sulfate 5 mg, hydrocortisone (1%) 10 mg/g in petrolatum base. Tube 30 g. *Rx.*
Use: Anti-infective; corticosteroid, topical.

Cortisporin Ophthalmic Ointment. (Glaxo Wellcome) Polymyxin B sulfate 10,000 units, bacitracin 400 units, neomycin sulfate 0.35%, hydrocortisone 0.1%. Tube 3.5 g. *Rx.*
Use: Anti-infective; corticosteroid, ophthalmic.

Cortisporin Ophthalmic Suspension. (Glaxo Wellcome) Polymyxin B sulfate 10,000 units, neomycin sulfate 0.35%, hydrocortisone 1%. Dropper bot. 7.5 ml Sterile. *Rx.*
Use: Anti-infective; corticosteroid, ophthalmic.

Cortisporin Otic Solution Sterile. (Glaxo Wellcome) Polymyxin B sulfate 10,000 units, neomycin sulfate 5 mg, hydrocortisone 10 mg/ml, glycerin, propylene glycol, vitamin K metabisulfite 0.1%. Dropper bot. 10 ml Sterile. *Rx.*
Use: Anti-infective, corticosteroid, otic.

Cortisporin Otic Suspension. (Glaxo Wellcome) Polymyxin B sulfate 10,000 units, neomycin sulfate 5 mg, hydrocortisone free alcohol 10 mg/ml, cetyl alcohol, propylene glycol, polysorbate 80, thimerosal. Dropper bot. 10 ml Sterile. *Rx.*
Use: Anti-infective; corticosteroid, otic.

Cortistan. (Standex) Cortisone 25 mg/10 ml. *Rx.*
Use: Corticosteroid.

●**cortivazol.** (core-TIH-vah-zole) USAN.
Use: Glucocorticoid.

Cortizone-5. (Thompson Med.) Hydrocortisone 0.5%, glycerin, mineral oil, white petrolatum. Tube 30 g. *otc.*
Use: Corticosteroid, topical.

Cortizone-S, Maximum Strength. (Thompson Medical) Hydrocortisone 0.5%. Tube. *otc.*
Use: Corticosteroid, topical.

●**cortodoxone.** (CORE-toe-dox-OHN) USAN.
Use: Anti-inflammatory.

Cortogen Acetate. Cortisone acetate.

Cortone Acetate. (Merck & Co.) Cortisone acetate. **5 mg/Tab.:** Bot. 50s. **10 mg/Tab.:** Bot. 100s. **25 mg/Tab.:** Bot. 100s, 500s, 1000s, UD 100s. **Inj.:** 50 mg/ml. Vial 10 ml. *Rx.*
Use: Corticosteroid.

Cortril Topical Ointment 1%. (Pfizer Laboratories) Hydrocortisone 1%, cetyl and stearyl alcohol, propylene glycol, sodium lauryl sulfate, petrolatum, cholesterol, mineral oil, methyl and propyl parabens in ointment base. Tube 0.5 oz.
Use: Corticosteroid, topical.

Cortrosyn Injection. (Organon) Cosyntropin 0.25 mg, mannitol 10 mg, lyophilized powder/ml. Vial. Pkg. w/1 ml amp. diluent. Box 10s. Vial. *Rx.*
Use: Corticosteroid.

Corubeen. (Spanner) Vitamin B_{12} crystalline 1000 mcg/ml. Vial 10 ml. *Rx.*
Use: Vitamin B_{12} supplement.

Corvert. (Pharmacia & Upjohn) Ibutilide fumarate 0.1 mg/ml/Soln. Vial. 10 ml. *Rx.*
Use: Antiarrhythmatic.

Coryza Brengle. (Roberts) Pseudo-ephedrine HCl 30 mg, acetaminophen 200 mg/Cap. Bot. 1000s. *otc.*
Use: Decongestant, analgesic.

Corzide. (Bristol-Myers) Nadolol 40 mg, bendroflumethiazide 5 mg/Tab or Nadolol 80 mg, bendroflumethiazide 5 mg/Tab. Bot. 100s. *Rx.*
Use: Antihypertensive.

Corzyme. (Abbott Diagnostics) Enzyme immunoassay for detection of antibody to hepatitis B core antigen in serum or plasma. Test kit 100s.
Use: Diagnostic aid.

Corzyme-M. (Abbott Diagnostics) Enzyme immunoassay for the detection of Ig antibody to hepatitis B core antigen. (Anti-HBc Ig) In human serum or plasma. Test kit 100s.
Use: Diagnostic aid.

Cosmegen. (Merck & Co.) Actinomycin D (dactinomycin) 0.5 mg (lyophilized powder)/3 ml. *Rx.*
Use: Antineoplastic.

Cosmoline.
See: Petrolatum.

Cosulid. (Novartis) Sulfachloropyridazine.

●**cosyntropin.** (koe-sin-TROE-pin) USAN.
Use: Hormone (adrenocorticotropic).
See: Cortrosyn, Vial (Organon).

Cotaphylline Tabs. (Major) Oxtriphylline 100 mg or 200 mg/Tab. Bot. 100s, 500s. *Rx.*
Use: Bronchodilator.

cotarnine chloride. Cotarnine hydrochloride.

cotarnine hydrochloride.
See: Cotarnine Chloride.

Cotazym. (Organon) Pancrelipase, lipase 8000 units, protease 30,000 units, amylase 30,000 units, calcium carbonate 25 mg/Cap. Bot. 100s, 500s. *Rx.*
Use: Digestive enzymes.

Cotazym-S. (Organon) Pancrelipase spheres, lipase 5,000 units, protease 20,000 units, amylase 20,000 units/Cap. Bot. 100s, 500s. *Rx.*
Use: Digestive enzyme.

●**cotinine fumarate.** (koe-TIH-neen) USAN.
Use: Antidepressant, psychomotor stimulant.

Cotolate Tabs. (Major) Benztropine 1 mg or 2 mg/Tab. Bot. 100s, 1000s. *Rx.*
Use: Antiparkinsonian.

Cotrim. (Lemmon) Sulfamethoxazole 400 mg, trimethoprim 80 mg/Tab. Bot. 100s, 500s. *Rx.*
Use: Anti-infective.

Cotrim D.S. (Lemmon) Sulfamethoxazole 800 mg, trimethoprim 160 mg/Tab. Bot. 100s, 500s. *Rx.*
Use: Anti-infective.

Cotrim Pediatric. (Lemmon) Sulfamethoxazole 200 mg, trimethoprim 40 mg/5 ml. Bot. 473 ml. *Rx.*
Use: Anti-infective.

•**cotton, purified,** U.S.P. 23.
Use: Surgical aid.

•**cottonseed oil,** N.F. 18.
Use: Pharmaceutic aid, solvent, oleaginous vehicle.

Co-Tuss V Liquid. (Rugby) Hydrocodone bitartrate 5 mg, guaifenesin 100 mg. Bot. 480 ml. *c-III.*
Use: Antitussive, expectorant.

Cotylenol Chewable Cold Tablet. (McNeil Prods.) Acetaminophen 80 mg, phenylpropanolamine HCl 3.125 mg, chlorpheniramine maleate 0.5 mg/Tab. Bot. 24s. *otc.*
Use: Analgesic, decongestant, antihistamine.

Cotylenol Children's Chewable Cold Tablet. (McNeil Prods.) Acetaminophen 80 mg, chlorpheniramine maleate 0.5 mg, pseudoephedrine HCl 7.5 mg/Tab. Bot. 24s. *otc.*
Use: Analgesic, antihistamine, decongestant.

Cotylenol Children's Liquid Cold Formula. (McNeil Prods.) Acetaminophen 160 mg, chlorpheniramine maleate 1 mg, pseudoephedrine HCl 15 mg, sorbitol/5 ml. Bot. 4 oz. *otc.*
Use: Analgesic, antihistamine, decongestant.

Cotylenol Cold Formula. (McNeil Prods.) Chlorpheniramine maleate 2 mg, dextromethorphan HBr 15 mg, pseudoephedrine HCl 30 mg, acetaminophen 325 mg/Tab. or Capl. **Tab.:** Box 24s, Bot. 50s, 100s. **Capl.:** Bot. 24s, 50s. *otc.*
Use: Antihistamine, antitussive, decongestant, analgesic.

Cotylenol Liquid Cold Formula. (McNeil Prods.) Acetaminophen 650 mg, chlorpheniramine maleate 4 mg, pseudoephedrine HCl 60 mg, dextromethorphan HCl 30 mg/30 ml, alcohol 7.5%, sorbitol. Bot. 5 oz. *otc.*
Use: Analgesic, antihistamine, decongestant, antitussive.

Cough Formula Comtrex. (Bristol-Myers) Pseudoephedrine HCl 15 mg, dextromethorphan HBr 7.5 mg, guaifenesin, saccharin, sucrose. Liq. Bot. 120 ml, 240 ml. *otc.*
Use: Antitussive, expectorant.

Cough Syrup. (Goldline) Phenylephrine HCl 5 mg, dextromethorphan HBr 10 mg, guaifenesin 100 mg, alcohol free. Bot. 120 ml. *otc.*
Use: Decongestant, antitussive, expectorant.

Cough-X. (Ascher) Dextromethorphan 5 mg, benzocaine 2 mg, dye free/Loz. Pkg. 9s. *otc.*
Use: Local anesthetic, antitussive.

Coumadin. (DuPont) Warfarin sodium crystalline. **Tab.:** 1 mg, 2 mg, 2.5 mg, 4 mg, 5 mg, 7.5 mg or 10 mg. Bot. 100s, 1000s, UD 100s. **Powd. for Inj., lyophilized:** Warfarin sodium 2 mg, sodium phosphate 4.98 mg, dibasic,, heptahydrate, sodium phosphate 0.194 mg, monobasic, monohydrate, NaCl 0.1 mg, mannitol 38 mg/ml when reconstituted. Vial. 5 mg. *Rx.*
Use: Anticoagulant.

coumarin.
Use: Anticoagulant; treat renal cell carcinoma. [Orphan Drug]

coumarin and indandione derivatives.
Use: Anticoagulant.
See: Coumadin, Tab. (DuPont Merck).
Warfarin Sodium, Tab. (Various Mfr.).
Panwarfin, Tab. (Abbott).
Sofarin, Tab. (Lemmon).
Miradon, Tab. (Schering-Plough).

•**coumermycin.** (KOO-mer-MY-sin) USAN. Antibiotic derived from *Streptomyces rishiriensis.*
Use: Antibacterial.

•**coumermycin sodium.** (KOO-mer-MY-sin) USAN.
Use: Antibacterial.

Counterpain Rub. (Squibb Mark) Methyl salicylate, eugenol, menthol. Oint. Tube 1 oz. *otc.*
Use: Analgesic, topical.

Covangesic. (Wallace) Phenylpropanolamine HCl 12.5 mg, phenylephrine HCl 7.5 mg, chlorpheniramine maleate 2 mg, pyrilamine maleate 12.5 mg, acetaminophen 275 mg, tartrazine/Tab. Bot. 24s. *otc.*
Use: Decongestant, antihistamine, analgesic.

Covera-HS. (Searle) Verapamil HCl 180 or 240 mg/ER Tab. Bot. 30s, 100, UD 100s. *Rx.*
Use: Calcium channel blocker.

Covermark. (O'Leary) Neutral cream, hypoallergenic, opaque, greaseless. Jars 1 oz, 3 oz, available in eleven shades. *otc.*

Use: Conceals birthmarks and skin discolorations.

Covermark Stick. (O'Leary) For normal to oily skin, available in 7 shades. *otc.*
Use: Conceals birthmarks and skin discolorations.

Co-Xan Syrup. (Schwarz Pharma) Theophylline anhydrous 150 mg, ephedrine HCl 25 mg, guaifenesin 100 mg, codeine phosphate 15 mg, alcohol 10%/ 15 ml. Bot. 1 pt. *Rx.*
Use: Bronchodilator, decongestant, expectorant, antitussive.

Cozaar. (Merck) Losartan potassium 25 mg, 50 mg/Tab. Bot. 30s (50 mg only), 90s, 100s, UD 100s. *Rx.*
Use: Antihypertensive.

CPA TR. (Schein) Phenylpropanolamine HCl 75 mg, chlorpheniramine maleate 12 mg/Cap. Bot. 100s, 1000s. *otc.*
Use: Decongestant, antihistamine.

Cplex. (Arcum) Vitamins B_1 10 mg, B_2 10 mg, B_6 5 mg, B_{12} 10 mcg, niacinamide 100 mg, calcium pantothenate 25 mg, C 150 mg, liver 50 mg, dried yeast 50 mg/Cap. Bot. 100s, 1000s. *otc.*
Use: Vitamin/mineral supplement.

C.P.M. Tablets. (Goldline) Chlorpheniramine 4 mg/Tab. Bot. 1000s. *otc.*
Use: Antihistamine.

c-reactive protein test.
See: LA test-CRP kit. (Fisher).

Cream Camellia. (O'Leary) Jar 2 oz. *otc.*
Use: Emollient.

Creamy Tar. (C & M) Coal tar topical solution 6.65%, crude coal tar 0.67%. Shampoo. Bot. 240 ml. *otc.*
Use: Antiseborrheic.

•**creatinine,** N.F. 18.
Use: Bulking agent for freeze drying.

creatinine reagent strips. (Bayer) Seralyzer reagent strips. A quantitative strip test for creatinine in serum or plasma. Bot. 25s.
Use: Diagnostic aid.

Cremagol. (Cremagol) Emulsion of liquid petrolatum, agar agar, acacia, glycerin. Bot. 14 oz.
W/cascara 11 gr/oz, Bot. 14 oz.
W/phenolphthalein 2 gr/oz, Bot. 14 oz. *otc.*
Use: Laxative.

Creomulsion Cough Medicine. (Creomulsion) Beechwood creosote, cascara, ipecac, menthol, white pine, wild cherry w/alcohol. For adults. Bot. 4 fl oz, 8 fl oz. *otc.*
Use: Coughs and bronchial irritations due to colds.

Creomulsion for Children. (Creomulsion) Beechwood creosote, cascara, ipecac, menthol, white pine, wild cherry w/alcohol. For children. Bot. 4 fl oz, 8 fl oz. *otc.*
Use: Coughs and bronchial irritations due to colds.

Creon. (Solvay) Lipase 8000 units, amylase 30,000 units, protease 13,000 units, pancreatin 300 mg/Cap. Bot. 100s, 250s. *Rx.*
Use: Digestive enzyme.

Creon 10. (Solvay) Lipase 10,000 USP units, amylase 33,200 USP units, protease 37,500 USP units. DR Cap. Bot. 100s, 250s. *Rx.*
Use: Digestive enzyme.

Creon 20. (Solvay) Lipase 20,000 USP units, amylase 66,400 USP units, protease 75,000 USP units. DR Cap. Bot. 100s, 250s. *Rx.*
Use: Digestive enzyme.

Creon 25. (Solvay) Lipase 25,000 units, amylase 74,700 units, protease 62,500 units, pancreatin 300 mg. Cap. Bot. 100s. *Rx.*
Use: Digestive enzyme.

creosote. Wood creosote, creosote, beechwood creosote.
W/Ipecac, menthol, licorice, white pine, wild cherry, cascara, vitamin C.
See: Creozets, Loz. (Creomulsion).

Creo-Terpin. (Lee) Dextromethorphan HBr 10 mg/15 ml, tartrazine, alcohol 25%, terpin hydrate, creosote, saccharin, corn syrup. Liq. Bot. 120 ml. *otc.*
Use: Antitussive.

Crescormon. (Pharmacia & Upjohn) Somatotropin 4 IU/Vial. IM administration. *Rx.*
Use: Growth hormone.
   Note: Crescormon will be available only for patients who qualify for treatment. Apply to Kabi Group Inc. for approval.

•**cresol,** N.F. 18. Mixture of 3 isomeric cresols. Phenol, methyl cresol.
Use: Antiseptic, disinfectant.

cresol preparations.
Use: Antiseptic, disinfectant.
See: Cresol, Soln. (Various Mfr.).
   Cresylone, Liq. (Parke-Davis).
   Saponated Cresol Soln.

m-cresyl-acetate.
See: Cresylate, Liq. (Recsei).

Cresylate. (Recsei) M-cresyl-acetate 25%, isopropanol 25%, chlorobutanol 1%, benzyl alcohol 1%, castor oil 5%, propylene glycol/15 ml. Bot. 15 ml, pt. *Rx.*

Use: Otic preparation.

cresylic acid. Same as Cresol.

•**crilvastatin.** (krill-vah-STAT-in) USAN.
Use: Antihyperlipidemic.

•**crisnatol mesylate.** (KRISS-nah-tole) USAN.
Use: Antineoplastic.

Criticare HN. (Bristol-Myers) High nitrogen elemental diet. Protein 14%, fat 4.3%, carbohydrate 81.5%. Bot. 8 oz. *otc.*
Use: Enteral nutritional supplement.

Crixivan. (Merck) Indinavir sulfate 200 mg, 400 mg, lactose/Cap. Bot. 270s and 360s (200 mg only), 180s (400 mg only). *Rx.*
Use: Antiviral.

Croferrin. (Forest Pharm.) Iron peptonate 50 mg, liver injection 2.5 mcg, vitamin B_{12} 12.5 mcg, lidocaine HCl 1%, phenol 0.5%, sodium citrate 0.125%, sodium bisulfite 0.009%/ml. Vial 10 ml, 30 ml. *Rx.*
Use: Vitamin/mineral supplement.

•**crofilcon A.** (kroe-FILL-kahn A) USAN.
Use: Contact lens material (hydrophilic).

Crolom. (Bausch & Lomb) Cromolyn sodium 4%. Soln. Bot. 2.5 ml, 10 ml w/ controlled drop tip. *Rx.*
Use: For vernal keratoconjunctivitis, vernal conjunctivitis and vernal keratitis.

Cro-Man-Zin. (Freeda) Cr 200 mcg, Mn 5 mg, Zn 25 mg, kosher, sugar free/ Tab. Bot. 100s, 250s. *otc.*
Use: Mineral/electrolyte supplement.

•**cromitrile sodium.** (KROE-mih-TRILE) USAN.
Use: Antiasthmatic.

cromolyn sodium. *Rx.*
Use: Treatment of mastocytosis. [Orphan drug]
See: Gastrocrom (Medeva).

•**cromolyn sodium,** (KROE-moe-lin) U.S.P. 23.
Use: Antiasthmatic (prophylactic).
See: Gastrocrom (Medeva).
   Intal (Medeva).
   Nasalcrom (Medeva).
   Opticrom (Medeva).

cromolyn sodium. (Dey) **Inhalation:** 20 mg/2 ml. In unit-dose vials. **Soln. for nebulization:** 20 mg/2 ml. Vial. 2 ml. *Rx.*
Use: Respiratory inhalant.

cromolyn sodium 4% ophthalmic solution. *Rx.*
Use: Vernal keratoconjunctivitis. [Orphan drug]

See: Crolom, Ophth. Soln. (Bausch & Lomb)

Cronetal.
See: Disulfiram.

•**croscarmellose sodium,** (KRAHS-CAR-mell-ose) N.F. 18. *Formerly crosslinked Carboxymethylcellulose Sodium and Modified Cellulose Gum.*
Use: Pharmaceutic aid (tablet disintegrant).

•**crospovidone,** N.F. 18.
Use: Pharmaceutic aid (tablet excipient).

Cross Aspirin. (Cross) Aspirin 325 mg/ Tab. Sugar, salt and lactose free. Bot. 100s, 1000s. *otc.*
Use: Salicylate analgesic.

Crotab. (Therapeutic Antibodies) *Rx.*
See: Antivenin, Polyvalent Crotalic (Ovine) Fab.

Crotalidae Antivenin Polyvalent. (Wyeth-Ayerst) 1 vial of lyophilized serum, 1 vial of bacteriostatic water 10 ml, USP, 1 vial normal horse serum. Inj. Vials combination Pkg. *Rx.*
Use: Antivenin.

crotaline antivenin, polyvalent. Antivenin Crotalidae Polyvalent, U.S.P. 23. North and South American Antisnakebite serum. *Rx.*
Use: Passive immunizing agent.

•**crotamiton,** U.S.P. 23.
Use: Scabicide.
See: Eurax, Cream, Lot. (Novartis).
   Component of Eurax (Westwood-Squibb).

CRPA, CRPA Latex Test. (Laboratory Diagnostics) Rapid latex agglutination test for the qualitative determination of C reactive protein. CRPA, 1 ml–CRP Positest Control, 0.5 ml CRPA Latex Test Kit.
Use: Diagnostic aid.

Cruex Cream. (Novartis Consumer Health) Total undecylenate 20% as undecylenic acid and zinc undecylenate. Tube 0.5 oz. *otc.*
Use: Antifungal, topical.

Cruex Spray Powder. (Novartis) Undecylenic acid 2% and zinc undecylenate 20%. Aeros.ol can 1.8 oz, 3.5 oz, 5.5 oz. *otc.*
Use: Antifungal, topical.

Cruex Squeeze Powder. (Novartis) Calcium undecylenate 10%. Plastic squeeze bot. 1.5 oz. *otc.*
Use: Antifungal, topical.

Cryptolin. (Hoechst Marion Roussel) Gonadorelin in nasal spray. *Rx.*

Use: Cryptorchism treatment.

cryptosporidium hyperimmune bovine colostrum IgG concentrate. *Rx.*
Use: Treat diarrhea in AIDS patients.
[Orphan drug]

cryptosporidium parvum bovine immunoglobulin concentrate. *Rx.*
Use: Treat infection of GI tract in immunocompromised patients. [Orphan drug]

crystalline trypsin. Highly purified preparation of enzyme as derived from mammalian pancreas glands.
See: Tryptar, Inj. (Centeon).

crystal violet.
See: Methylrosaniline Chloride, U.S.P.

Crystamine. (Dunhall) Cyanocobalamin 100 mcg or 1000 mcg/ml, benzyl alcohol. Vial 10 ml, 30 ml. *Rx.*
Use: Vitamin B_{12} supplement.

Crysti-1000. (Roberts Hauck) Cyanocobalamine crystalline 1000 mcg/ml. Inj. Vial 10 ml, 30 ml. *Rx.*
Use: Vitamin B_{12}.

Crysticillin 300 A.S. (Apothecon) Sterile procaine penicillin G suspension U.S.P. 300,000 units/ml, povidone, lecithin, sodium citrate, sodium formaldehyde sulfoxylate, sodium carboxymethylcellulose, methylparaben, propylparaben. Vial 10 ml. *Rx.*
Use: Anti-infective, penicillin.

Crysticillin 600 A.S. (Apothecon) Sterile procaine penicillin G suspension 600,000 units/1.2 ml, lecithin, phenol, povidone, sodium citrate, sodium carboxymethylcellulose, sodium formaldehyde sulfoxylate, methylparaben, propylparaben. Vial 12 ml. *Rx.*
Use: Anti-infective, penicillin.

Crysti-Liver. (Roberts) Liver injection (equivalent to B_{12} 10 mcg), crystalline B_{12} 100 mcg, folic acid 0.4 mg. Vial 10 ml. *Rx.*
Use: Vitamin/mineral supplement.

Crystodigin. (Lilly) Digitoxin 0.05 mg and 0.1 mg/Tab. Bot. 100s. *Rx.*
Use: Cardiac glycoside.

Crystografin. Meglumine diatrizoate.
Use: Contrast medium.

C-Solve. (Syosset) Alcohol 36%, glycerin, polysorbate 20, laureth-4, water soluble cellulose gum, PVA, collagen, gelatin hydrolysate, midazolidinyl urea, sorbic acid. Lot. Bot. 50 ml. *otc.*
Use: Lotion base.

C Speridin. (Marlyn) Hesperidin 100 mg, lemon bioflavonoids 100 mg, vitamin C 500 mg/SR Tab. Bot. 100s. *otc.*

Use: Vitamin supplement.

CTab.
See: Cetyl Trimethyl Ammonium Bromide.

C/T/S. (Hoescht-Roussel) Clindamycin phosphate 10 mg/ml. Top. Soln. 30 ml, 60 ml. *Rx.*
Use: Antiacne.

C-Tussin. (Century) Codeine phosphate 10 mg, pseudoephedrine HCl 30 mg, guaifenesin 100 mg/5 ml, alcohol 7.5%. Bot. 120 ml, gal. *c-v.*
Use: Antitussive, decongestant, expectorant.

Culminal. (Culminal) Benzocaine 3% in water miscible cream base. Tube oz. *otc.*
Use: Local anesthetic.

Culturette 10 Minute Group A Step ID. (Hoechst Marion Roussel) Latex slide agglutination test for group A streptococcal antigen on throat swabs. Kit 55 determinations.
Use: Diagnostic aid.

•**cupric acetate Cu 64.** USAN.
Use: Radioactive agent.

•**cupric chloride,** U.S.P. 23.
Use: Supplement (trace mineral).
See: Coppertrace, Inj. (Centeon).

•**cupric sulfate,** U.S.P. 23.
Use: Antidote to phosphorus.
W/Zinc sulfate, camphor.
See: Dalibour, Pow. (Doak).

Cuprid. (Merck & Co.) Trientine HCl 250 mg/Cap. Bot. 100s. *Rx.*
Use: Chelating agent.

Cuprimine. (Merck & Co.) Penicillamine 125 mg or 250 mg/Cap. Bot. 100s. *Rx.*
Use: Metal chelating agent.

•**cuprimyxin.** (KUH-prih-mix-in) USAN.
Use: Antifungal.

Cupri-Pak. (SoloPak) Copper **0.4 mg/ml:** Vial 10 ml, 30 ml. **2 mg/ml:** Vial 5 ml. *Rx.*
Use: Parenteral nutritional supplement.

curare.
Use: Muscle relaxant.
See: d-Tubocurarine Salts (Various Mfr.).

curare antagonist.
See: Neostigine Methylsulfate Inj. (Various Mfr.).
Tensilon, Amp. (Roche).

Curel. (Bausch & Lomb) Glycerin, petrolatum, dimethicone, parabens. Lot. 180, 300, 390 ml. Cream 90 g. *otc. Rx.*
Use: Emollient.

Curosurf. (Chiesi Pharm)
See: Pulmonary Surfactant Replacement.

curral.
See: Diallyl Barbituric Acid, Tab. (Various Mfr.).

Curretab. (Solvay) Medroxyprogesterone acetate 10 mg/Tab. Bot. 50s. Rx.
Use: Progestin.

Cutar Bath Oil. (Summers) Liquor carbonis detergens 7.5% in liquid petrolatum, isopropyl myristate, acetylated lanolin, lanolin alcohols extract. Bot. 180 ml. otc.
Use: Emollient.

Cutemol Emollient Cream. (Summers) Allantoin 0.2%, liquid petrolatum, acetylated lanolin, lanolin alcohols extract, isopropyl myristate, water. Jar 2 oz. otc.
Use: Emollient.

Cuticura Medicated Shampoo. (DEP Corp.) Sodium lauryl sulfate, sodium stearate, salicylic acid, protein, sulfur. Tube 3 oz. otc.
Use: Antidandruff shampoo.

Cuticura Medicated Soap. (DEP Corp.) Triclocarban 1%, petrolatum, sodium tallowate, sodium cocoate, glycerin, mineral oil, sodium Cl, tetrasodium EDTA, sodium bicarbonate, magnesium silicate, iron oxides. Bar 3.5 oz, 5.5 oz. otc.
Use: Antibacterial, topical.

Cutivate. (Glaxo Wellcome) Fluticasone propionate. **Cream:** 0.05%. Jar 15,30,60 g. **Oint.:** 0.005%. Jar 15, 30, 60 g. Rx.
Use: Corticosteroid, topical.

Cutter Insect Repellent. (Bayer) N,N-Diethyl-meta-toluamide 28.5%, other isomers 1.5%. Vial 1 oz; Foam, Can 2 oz; Spray 2 oz, 14 oz aerosol can; Assortment Pack; First Aid Kits, Trial Pack, 6s; Marine Pack 3s; Camp Pack 4s; Pocket Pack, Travel Pack.
Use: Insect repellent.

CY-1503. (Cytel) Rx.
Use: Anti-thromboembolic. [Orphan drug]

CY-1899. (Cytel) Rx.
Use: Treatment of hepatitis B. [Orphan drug]

Cyanide Antidote Package. (Lilly) 2 Amp. (300 mg/10 ml) sodium nitrite; 2 Amp. (12.5 g/50 ml), sodium thiosulfate; 12 aspirols amyl nitrite (0.3 ml), syringes, stomach tube, tourniquet/Pkg. Check exact dosage before administration. Rx.
Use: Antidote, cyanide poisoning.

Cyanocob. (Paddock) Vitamin B_{12} 1000 mcg/ml. Bot. 1000 ml, Vial 10 ml. Rx.
Use: Vitamin B_{12} supplement.

•**cyanocobalamin,** (sigh-an-oh-koe-BAL-uh-min) U.S.P. 23.
Use: Vitamin (hematopoietic).
See: Redisol, Inj., Tab. (Merck & Co.).

•**cyanocobalamin Co 57,** U.S.P. 23.
Use: Diagnostic aid (pernicious anemia).

•**cyanocobalamin Co 60.** USAN. U.S.P. XXII.
Use: Diagnostic aid (pernicious anemia), radioactive agent.

cyanocobalamin crystalline. otc, Rx.
Use: Vitamin B_{12} supplement.
See: Vitamin B_{12}, Inj., Tab. (Various Mfr.).
Cobex, Inj. (Pasadena).
Crystamine, Inj. (Dunhall).
Rubcamin PC, Inj. (Apothecon).
Berubigen, Inj. (Pharmacia & Upjohn).
Betalin 12, Inj. (Lilly).
Crysti-12, Inj. (Roberts).
Crysti 1000, Inj. (Roberts Hauck).
Cyanoject, Inj. (Mayrand).
Cyomin, Inj. (Forest).
Kaybovite-1000, Inj. (Kay).
Redisol, Inj. (Merck & Co.).
Rubesol-1000, Inj. (Schwarz Pharma).
Sytobex, Inj. (Park-Davis).

Cyanoject. (Mayrand) Vitamin B_{12} 1000 mcg/ml, benzyl alcohol. Vial 10 ml, 30 ml. Rx.
Use: Vitamin B_{12} supplement.

Cyanover. (Research Supplies) Cyanocobalamin 100 mcg, liver injection 10 mcg, folic acid 10 mg/ml. Lyo-layer vial 10 ml with vial of diluent 10 ml. Rx.
Use: Vitamin/mineral supplement.

•**cyclacillin,** (SIGH-klah-SILL-in) U.S.P. 23.
Use: Antibacterial.

cyclamate sodium. Cyclohexanesulfamate dihydrate salt.

•**cyclamic acid.** (sigh-KLAM-ik) USAN. N-Cyclohexylsulfamic acid. Hexamic Acid. Cyclohexanesulfamic acid. Currently banned in U.S.
Use: Sweetener (non-nutritive).

Cyclan Caps. (Major) Cyclandelate 200 mg or 400 mg/Tab. Bot. 100s, 1000s, UD 100s. 400 mg: Bot. 250s also. Rx.
Use: Vasodilator.

cyclandelate.
Use: Vasodilator.
See: Cyclan, Cap. (Major).
Cyclospasmol, Tab., Cap. (Wyeth-Ayerst).

•**cyclazocine.** (SIGH-CLAY-zoe-seen)

USAN. Under study.
Use: Analgesic.

•**cyclindole.** (sigh-KLIN-dole) USAN.
Use: Antidepressant.

Cyclinex-1. (Ross) Protein 7.5 g (from carnitine, cystine, histidine, isoleucine, leucine, lysine, methionine, phenylalanine, taurine, threonine, tryptophan, tyrosine, valine), fat 27 g (from palm oil, hydrogenated coconut oil, soy oil), carbohydrate 52 g (from hydrolyzed corn starch), linoleic acid 2000 mg, Fe 10 mg, Na 215 mg, Ca, vitamins A, B_1, B_2, B_3, B_5, B_6, B_{12}, C, D, E, K, biotin, choline, folic acid, inositol, Cl, Cu, I, Mg, Mn, P, Se, Zn and 515 Cal per 100 g. Nonessential amino acid free. Pow. Can 350 g. *otc.*
Use: Nutritional/mineral supplement.

Cyclinex-2. (Ross) Protein 15 g (from carnitine, cystine, histidine, isoleucine, leucine, lysine, methionine, phenylalanine, taurine, threonine, tryptophan, tyrosine, valine), fat 20.7 g (from palm oil, hydrogenated coconut oil, soy oil), carbohydrate 40 g (from hydrolyzed cornstarch), Fe 17 mg, Na 1175 mg, K 1830 mg, Ca, vitamins A, B_1, B_2, B_3, B_5, B_6, B_{12}, C, D, E, K, biotin, choline, folic acid, inositol, Cl, Cu, I, Mg, Mn, P, Se, Zn and 480 Cal per 100 g. Nonessential amino acid free. Pow. Can 325 g. *otc.*
Use: Nutritional/mineral supplement.

•**cycliramine maleate.** (SIGH-klih-rah-meen) USAN.
Use: Antihistamine.

•**cyclizine,** U.S.P. 23.
Use: Antihistamine.
See: Marzine (hydrochloride).
Valoid (hydrochloride or lactate).

•**cyclizine hydrochloride,** U.S.P. 23.
Use: Antiemetic.
See: Marezine HCl and lactate, Preps. (Glaxo Wellcome).
W/Ergotamine tartrate, caffeine.
See: Migral, Tab. (Glaxo Wellcome).

•**cyclizine lactate injection,** U.S.P. 23. A sterile soln. of cyclizine lactate in water for injection.
Use: Antihistamine, antinauseant.

cyclobarbital.
Use: Central depressant.

cyclobarbital calcium.
Use: Sedative, hypnotic.

•**cyclobendazole.** (SIGH-kloe-BEN-dah-zole) USAN.
Use: Anthelmintic.

•**cyclobenzaprine hydrochloride,** (SIGH-

kloe-BEN-zuh-preen) U.S.P. 23.
See: Flexeril, Tab. (Merck & Co.).
Use: Muscle relaxant.

cyclobenzaprine hydrochloride. (Various Mfr.) 10 mg/Tab. Bot. 30s, 100s, 1000s.
Use: Muscle relaxant.

Cyclocort Cream. (Lederle) Amcinonide 0.1% in Aquatain hydrophilic base. Tubes 15 g, 30 g, 60 g. *Rx.*
Use: Corticosteroid, topical.

Cyclocort Ointment. (Lederle) Amcinonide 0.1% in ointment base. Tube 15 g, 30 g, 60 g. *Rx.*
Use: Corticosteroid, topical.

cyclocumarol.
Use: Anticoagulant.

•**cyclofilcon a.** (SIGH-kloe-FILL-kahn A) USAN.
Use: Contact lens material (hydrophilic).

Cyclogen. (Schwarz Pharma) Dicyclomine HCl 10 mg, sodium Cl 0.9%, chlorobutanol hydrate 0.5%. Vial 10 ml, Box 12s. *Rx.*
Use: Antispasmodic.

•**cycloguanil pamoate.** (SIGH-kloe-GWAHN-ill PAM-oh-ate) USAN.
Use: Antimalarial.

Cyclogyl. (Alcon) Cyclopentolate HCl Soln. 0.5%, 1% or 2%. Droptainer 2 ml, 5 ml, 15 ml. *Rx.*
Use: Cycloplegic, mydriatic.

•**cycloheximide.** (sigh-KLOE-HEX-ih-mid) USAN.
Use: Antipsoriatic.

•**cyclomethicone,** N.F. 18.
Use: Pharmaceutic aid (wetting agent).

cyclomethycaine and methapyrilene.
Use: Anesthetic, topical.
See: Surfadil Cream, Lot. (Lilly).

cyclomethycaine sulfate, U.S.P. XXI.
Use: Topical anesthetic.
See: Surfacaine, Prep. (Lilly).
W/Methapyrilene.
See: Surfadil, Cream, Lot. (Lilly).

cyclomethycaine and thenylpyramine.
See: Surfadil Cream, Lot. (Lilly).

Cyclomydril. (Alcon) Phenylephrine HCl 1%, cyclopentolate HCl 0.2%. Droptainer 2 ml, 5 ml. *Rx.*
Use: Mydriatic.

Cyclonil. (Seatrace) Dicyclomine HCl 10 mg/ml. Vial 10 ml. *Rx.*
Use: Anticholinergic/antispasmodic.

Cyclopal.

Cyclopar. (Parke-Davis) Tetracycline HCl 250 mg or 500 mg/Cap. **250 mg:** Bot. 100s, 1000s. **500 mg:** Bot. 100s, UD 100s. *Rx.*

Use: Anti-infective, tetracycline.

cyclopentamine hydrochloride, U.S.P. XXI.
Use: Adrenergic (vasoconstrictor).
See: Clopane Hydrochloride, Nasal Soln. (Dista).
W/Aludrine.
See: Aerolone Compound, Soln. (Lilly).
W/Chlorpheniramine.
See: Hista-Clopane, Pulvule (Lilly).

cyclopentenyl-allyl-barbituric acid.
See: Cyclopal.

•**cyclopenthiazide.** (SIHG-kloe-pen-THIGH-ah-zide) USAN.
Use: Diuretic, antihypertensive.
See: Navidrex.

•**cyclopentolate hydrochloride,** U.S.P. 23.
Use: Anticholinergic (ophthalmic).
See: AK-Pentolate, Soln. (Akorn).
Cyclogyl, Soln. (Alcon).
W/Phenylephrine HCl.
See: Cyclomydril, Soln. (Alcon).

cyclopentolate hydrochloride. (Various Mfr.) 1% Soln. Bot. 2 ml, 15 ml.
Use: Anticholinergic (ophthalmic).

cyclopentylpropionate.
See: Depo-Testosterone, Vial (Pharmacia & Upjohn).

•**cyclophenazine hydrochloride.** (SIGH-kloe-FEH-nazz-een) USAN.
Use: Antipsychotic.

•**cyclophosphamide,** (sigh-kloe-FOSS-fuh-mide) U.S.P. 23.
Use: Antineoplastic, immunosuppressant.
See: Cytoxan, Tab., Vial (Bristol Oncology).

•**cyclopropane,** U.S.P. 23. Trimethylene.
Use: Inhalation anesthetic.

•**cycloserine,** (sigh-kloe-SER-een) U.S.P. 23.
Use: Antibacterial (tuberculostatic).
See: Seromycin, Cap. (Lilly).

l-cycloserine.
Use: Treat Gaucher's disease. [Orphan drug].

Cyclospasmol Tablets. (Wyeth-Ayerst) Cyclandelate 100 mg/Tab. Bot. 100s, 500s. *Rx.*
Use: Vasodilator.

cyclosporin a.
Use: Immunosuppressant.
See: Cyclosporine, U.S.P. 23.

•**cyclosporine,** (SIGH-kloe-spore-EEN) U.S.P. 23.
Use: Immunosuppressant.
See: Sandimmune, Inj., Oral Soln. (Sandoz).

Neoral, Cap., Oral Soln. (Sandoz).

cyclosporine ophthalmic. (SIGH-kloe-spore-EEN) *Rx.*
Use: Severe keratoconjunctivitis sicca; graft rejection following keratoplasty. [Orphan drug]

cyclosporine 2% ophthalmic ointment. (Allergan)
Use: Treatment of graft rejection after keratoplasty and corneal melting syndromes. [Orphan Drug]

•**cyclothiazide.** (SIGH-kloe-thigh-AZZ-ide) USAN.
Use: Diuretic; antihypertensive.

Cycofed Pediatric. (Cypress) Codeine phosphate 10 mg, pseudoephedrine HCl 30 mg, guaifenesin 100 mg, alcohol 6%/Syr. Bot. 1 pt. *c-v.*
Use: Antitussive, expectorant.

Cycrin. (ESI Pharma) Medroxyprogesterone acetate 2.5 mg, 5 mg, 10 mg/Tab. Bot. 100s. *Rx.*
Use: Progestin.

Cydonol Massage Lotion. (Gordon) Isopropyl alcohol 14%, methyl salicylate, benzalkonium Cl. Bot. 4 oz, gal. *otc.*
Use: Counterirritant.

•**cyheptamide.** (sigh-HEP-tah-mid) USAN.
Use: Anticonvulsant.

Cyklokapron. (Pharmacia & Upjohn) **Tab.:** Tranexamic acid 500 mg. Bot. 100s. **Inj.:** 100 mg/ml. Amp. 10 ml. *Rx.*
Use: Hemostatic.

Cylert Chewable Tablets. (Abbott) Pemoline 37.5 mg/Tab. Bot. 100s. *c-iv.*
Use: Psychotherapeutic.

Cylert Tablets. (Abbott) Pemoline 18.75, 37.5 or 75 mg/Tab. Bot. 100s. *c-iv.*
Use: Psychotherapeutic.

Cylex Sugar Free. (PharmaKon) Benzocaine 15 mg, cetylpyridinium Cl 5 mg, sorbitol. Loz. Pkg. 12s. *otc.*
Use: Antiseptic; analgesic, topical.

Cylex Throat. (PharmaKon) Benzocaine 15 mg, cetylpyridinium Cl 5 mg, sorbitol. Loz. Pkg. 12s. *otc.*
Use: Antiseptic; analgesic, topical.

Cynobal. (Arcum) Cyanocobalamin 100 mcg or 1000 mcg/ml. Inj. **100 mcg:** Vial 30 ml. **1000/mcg/ml.:** Inj. Vial 10 ml, 30 ml. *Rx.*
Use: Vitamin B_{12} supplement.

Cyomin. (Forest) Cyanocobalamin 1000 mcg/ml. Vial 10 ml, 30 ml. *Rx.*
Use: Vitamin B_{12} supplement.

•**cypenamine hydrochloride.** (sigh-PEN-ah-meen) USAN. 2-Phenylcyclopentylamine HCl.

Use: Antidepressant.
- **cyprazepam.** (sigh-PRAY-zeh-pam) USAN.
  Use: Sedative, hypnotic.
- **cyproheptadine hydrochloride,** (sip-row-HEP-tuh-deen) U.S.P. 23.
  Use: Antihistamine, antipruritic.
  See: Periactin, Tab., Syr. (Merck & Co.).
- **cyprolidol hydrochloride.** (sigh-PRO-lih-dahl) USAN.
  Use: Antidepressant.
- **cyproterone acetate.** (sigh-PRO-ter-ohn) USAN.
  Use: Antiandrogen.
- **cyproximide.** (sigh-PROX-ih-MIDE) USAN.
  Use: Antipsychotic, antidepressant.
  cyren a.
  See: Diethylstilbestrol Prep. (Various Mfr.).
  cyrimine hydrochloride.
  See: Pagitane HCl, Tab. (Lilly).
  Cyronine. (Major) Liothyronine sodium 25 mcg/Tab. Bot. 100s. *Rx.*
  Use: Thyroid hormone.
  Cystadine. (Orphan Medical) Betaine anhydrous 1 g/1.7 ml/Pow. Bot. 180 g. *Rx.*
  Use: Treatment of homocystinuria.
  Cystagon. (Mylan) Cysteamine bitartrate 50 mg, 150 mg/Cap. Bot. 100s, 500s. *Rx.*
  Use: Treatment of nephropathic cystinosis.
  Cystamin.
  See: Methenamine, Tab. (Various Mfr.).
  Cystamine. (Tennessee) Methenamine 2 gr, phenyl salicylate 0.5 gr, phenazopyridine HCl 10 mg, benzoic acid ⅛ gr, hyoscyamine sulfate gr, atropine sulfate gr/SC Tab. Bot. 100s, 1000s. *Rx.*
  Use: Urinary anti-infective.
- **cysteamine.** (sis-TEE-ah-MEEN) USAN.
  Use: Antiurolithic (cysteine calculi), nephropathic cystinosis. [Orphan Drug]
- **cysteamine hydrochloride.** (sis-TEE-ah-MEEN) USAN.
  Use: Antiurolithic treatment of nephropathic cystinosis.
  See: Cystagon.
- **cysteine hydrochloride,** U.S.P. 23. L-Cysteine hydrochloride monohydrate.
  Use: Amino acid for replacement therapy, treatment of photosensitivity in erythropoietic protoporphyria. [Orphan Drug]
  See: Cysteine HCl (Abbott).
  Cystex. (Numark) Methenamine 162 mg, sodium salicylate 162.5 mg, benzoic acid 32 mg/Tab. Bot. 40s, 100s. *otc.*

Use: Urinary anti-infective.
cystic fibrosis gene therapy. *Rx.*
  Use: Cystic fibrosis. [Orphan Drug]
cystic fibrosis transmembrane conductance regulator gene. (Genetic Therapy) *Rx.*
  Use: Treatment of cystic fibrosis. [Orphan Drug]
cystic fibrosis TR gene therapy (recombinant adenovirus). (Gerac)
  Use: Treament of cystic fibrosis. [Orphan Drug]
- **cystine.** (SIS-TEEN) USAN. An essential amino acid.
  Use: Amino acid replacement therapy, an additive for infants on TPN.
  Cysto. (Freeport) Methenamine 40.8 mg, methylene blue 5.4 mg, phenyl salicylate 18.1 mg, atropine sulfate 0.03 mg, hyoscyamine 0.03 mg, benzoic acid 4.5 mg/Tab. Bot. 1000s. *Rx.*
  Use: Urinary anti-infective.
  Cysto-Conray. (Mallinckrodt) Iothalamate meglumine 43% (iodine 20.2%) with EDTA. Soln. Vial 50 ml, 100 ml. Bot. 250 ml.
  Use: Radiopaque agent.
  Cysto-Conray II. (Mallinckrodt) Iothalamate meglumine 17.2% (iodine 8.1%) with EDTA. Soln. Bot. 250 ml, 500 ml.
  Use: Radiopaque agent.
  Cystografin. (Squibb) Meglumine diatrizoate 30% (bound iodine 14%), EDTA 0.04%. Bot. 100 ml, 300 ml.
  Use: Radiopaque agent.
  Cystografin Dilute. (Squibb) Diatrizoate meglumine 18% (organically-bound iodine 85 mg)/ml. Vial 300 ml, 500 ml.
  Use: Radiopaque agent.
  CystoSpaz. (Polymedica) l-Hyoscyamine 0.15 mg/Tab. Bot. 100s. *Rx.*
  Use: Anticholinergic, antispasmodic.
  CystoSpazM. (Polymedica) Hyoscyamine sulfate 375 mcg/Cap. Bot. 100s. *Rx.*
  Use: Anticholinergic, antispasmodic.
  Cytadren. (Novartis) Aminoglutethimide 250 mg/Tab. Bot. 100s. *Rx.*
  Use: Adrenal steroid inhibitor; treatment of Cushing's syndrome.
- **cytarabine,** (SIGH-tar-ah-bean) U.S.P. 23.
  Use: Antineoplastic, antiviral.
  See: Cytosar, Inj. (Pharmacia & Upjohn).
  cytarabine. (Various Mfr.) 100 mg, 500 mg/Pow. for Inj. Vials.
  Use: Antineoplastic, antiviral.
  cytarabine, depofoam encapsulated.

Rx.
Use: Neoplastic meningitis. [Orphan Drug]

•**cytarabine hydrochloride.** USAN. *Formerly Cytsosine Arabinosde Hydrochloride* 1-Arabinoluranosylcytosine hydrochloride.
Use: Antiviral management of acute leukemias.
See: Cytosar-U, Vial (Pharmacia & Upjohn).

CytoGam. (MedImmune) Cytomegalovirus immune globulin IV (human) 2500 mg ±500 mg/Inj. Solvent/detergent treated. Vial 2.5 g. *Formerly called cytomegalovirus immune globulin (human) IV. Rx.*
Use: Cytomegalovirus disease associated with kidney transplantation.

cytomegalovirus immune globulin (human). *Rx.*
Use: Cytomegalovirus disease associated with organ transplant. [Orphan drug]
See: CytoGam, Vial (MedImmune).

cytomegalovirus immune globulin (human) iv. Now named CytoGam (MedImmune).
Use: CMV pneumonia in bone marrow transplants. [Orphan Drug]
See: CytoGam, Inj., (MedImmune).

cytomegalovirus monoclonal antibody (human).
Use: Cytomegalovirus disease associated with organ transplant; treatment of cytomegalovirus retinitis in AIDS patients. [Orphan Drug]

Cytomel. (SK-Beecham) Liothyronine sodium 5 mcg, 25 mcg or 50 mcg/Tab. Bot. 100s. 25 mcg: Bot. 100s. *Rx.*
Use: Thyroid hormone.

Cytosar-U. (Pharmacia & Upjohn) Cytarabine 20 mg/ml in powder, 50 mg/ml reconstituted. Vial 100 mg, 500 mg. *Rx.*
Use: Antineoplastic agent.

cytosine arabinoside hydrochloride. Cytarabine HCl.
See: Cytosar-U (Pharmacia & Upjohn).

Cytosol. (Cytosol Ophthalmics) Calcium chloride 48 mg, magnesium chloride 30 mg, potassium chloride 75 mg, sodium acetate 390 mg, sodium chloride 640 mg, sodium citrate 170 mg/100 ml. Soln. Bot. 200 ml, 500 ml. *Rx.*
Use: Sterile irrigating solution.

Cytotec. (Searle) Misoprostol 200 mcg/Tab. Bot. 100s, UD 100s. *Rx.*
Use: Prostaglandins.

Cytovene. (Roche) Ganciclovir (as sodium) . **Cap.:** 250 mg/Tab. Bot. 180s. **Inj.:** 500 mg/Pow. Vial. 10 ml. *Rx.*
Use: Antiviral.

Cytox. (MPL) Cyanocobalamin 500 mcg, vitamins B_6 20 mg, B_1 100 mg, benzyl alcohol 2% in isotonic solution of sodium Cl/ml. Inj. Vial 10 ml. *Rx.*
Use: Vitamin supplement.

Cytoxan Lyophilized. (Bristol-Myers Squibb Oncology) Cyclophosphamide. Vial 500 mg. *Rx.*
Use: Antineoplastic.

Cytoxan Powder. (Bristol-Myers Squibb Oncology) Cyclophosphamide powder 100 mg, 200 mg, 500 mg, 1 g or 2 g/Vial. *Rx.*
Use: Antineoplastic.

Cytoxan Tablets. (Bristol-Myers Squibb Oncology) Cyclophosphamide 25 mg or 50 mg/Tab. **25 mg/Tab.:** Bot. 100s; **50 mg/Tab.:** Bot. 100s, 1000s, UD 100s. *Rx.*
Use: Antineoplastic.

Cytra-20. (Cypress) Sodium citrate dihydrate 500 mg, citric acid monohydrate 334 mg/5 ml/Soln. Bot. 16 oz. *Rx.*
Use: Systemic alkalinizers.

Cytra-30. (Cypress) Potassium citrate monohydrate 550 mg, sodium citrate dihydrate 500 mg, citric acid monohydrate 334 mg/5 ml/Syr. Bot. 16 oz. *Rx.*
Use: Systemic alkalinizers.

Cytra-K. (Cypress) Potassium citrate monohydrate 1100 mg, citric acid monohydrate 334 mg/5 ml/Soln. Bot. 473 ml. *Rx.*
Use: Systemic alkalinizer.

Cytra-LC. (Cypress) Potassium citrate monohydrate 550 mg, sodium citrate dihydrate 500 mg, citric acid monohydrate 334 mg/5 ml/Soln. Bot. 16 oz. *Rx.*
Use: Systemic alkalinizer.

D

D-2. One of the D vitamins.
See: Ergocalciferol.

D-3. One of the D vitamins.
See: Cholecalciferol.

daa.
See: Dihydroxy Aluminum Aminoacetate.

•**dacarbazine,** (da-CAR-buh-zeen) U.S.P. 23.
Use: Antineoplastic.
See: Dtic-Dome, Inj. (Bayer).

D.A. Chew Tabs. (Dura) Phenylephrine HCl 10 mg, chlorpheniramine 2 mg, methscopolamine nitrate 1.25 mg/Tab. Bot. 100s. *Rx.*
Use: Decongestant, antihistamine, anticholinergic.

D.A. II. (Dura) Chlorpheniramine maleate 4 mg, phenylephrine HCl 10 mg, methscopolamine nitrate 1.25 mg/Tab. Bot. 100s. *Rx.*
Use: Decongestant, antihistamine, anticholinergic.

•**dacliximab.** (dak-LICK-sih-mab) USAN.
Use: Monoclonal antibody (immunosuppressant).
See: Zenapax (Hoffmann-LaRoche).

Dacodyl. (Major) **Tab.:** Bisacodyl 5 mg/Tab. 100s, 250s, 1000s. UD 100s. **Supp.:** Bisacodyl 10 mg. Box 12s, 100s. *otc.*
Use: Laxative.

Dacriose. (Ciba Vision) Sodium Cl, potassium Cl, sodium hydroxide, sodium phosphate, benzalkonium Cl 0.01%, edetate disodium. Bot. 15 ml, 120 ml. *otc.*
Use: Irrigating solution, ophthalmic.

•**dactinomycin,** (DAK-tih-no-MY-sin) U.S.P. 23.
Use: Antineoplastic.
See: Cosmegen, Vial (Merck).

Daily Care. (Pfizer) Zinc oxide 10%, mineral oil, white petrolatum, parabens. Oint. Tube 57 g. *otc.*
Use: Diaper rash product.

Daily Cleaner. (Bausch & Lomb) Isotonic solution with sodium Cl, sodium phosphate, tyloxapol, hydroxyethylcellulose, polyvinyl alcohol with thimerosal 0.004%, EDTA 0.2%. Soln. Bot. 45 ml. *otc.*
Use: Soft contact lens care.

Daily Conditioning Treatment. (Blistex) Padimate O 7.5%, oxybenzone 3.5%, petrolatum. Stick 11.4 g. SPF 15. *otc.*
Use: Lip protectant, sunscreen.

Daily Vitamins Liquid. (Rugby) Vitamins A 2500 IU, D 400 IU, E 15 IU, C 60 mg, B_1 1.2 mg, B_2 1.2 mg, B_6 1.05 mg, B_{12} 4.5 mcg, niacinamide 13.5 mg/5 ml. Bot. 273 ml, 473 ml. *otc.*
Use: Vitamin supplement.

Daily Vitamins Tablets. (Kirkman Sales) Vitamins A 5000 IU, D 400 IU, C 50 mg, B_1 3 mg, B_2 2.5 mg, B_6 1 mg, B_{12} 1 mcg, niacinamide 20 mg, d-calcium pantothenate 1 mg/Tab. Bot. 100s. *otc.*
Use: Vitamin supplement.

Daily Vitamins w/Iron. (Kirkman Sales) Vitamins A 5000 IU, D 400 IU, B_1 2 mg, B_2 2.5 mg, B_6 1 mg, B_{12} 1 mcg, niacinamide 20 mg, d-calcium pantothenate 1 mg, iron 18 mg/Tab. Bot. 100s. *otc.*
Use: Vitamin supplement.

Daily-Vite w/Iron & Minerals. (Rugby) Iron 18 mg, vitamins A 18 mg, D 400 IU, E 30 mg, B_1 1.5 mg, B_2 1.7 mg, B_3 20 mg, B_5 10 mg, B_6 2 mg, B_{12} 6 mcg, C 60 mg, folic acid 0.4 mg, Ca, Cl, Cr, Cu, I, K, Mg, Mn, Mo, P, Se, zinc 15 mg, biotin, vitamin K/Tab. Bot. 100s. *otc.*
Use: Vitamin/mineral supplement.

Dairy Ease. (Sanofi Winthrop) Lactase 3300 FCC units, mannitol. Tab. Bot. 60s. *otc.*
Use: Lactase enzyme.

Daisy 2 Pregnancy Test. (Advanced Care) Home pregnancy test. Test kit 2s.
Use: Diagnostic aid.

Dakin's Solution.
See: Sodium Hypochlorite Solution Diluted.

Dakin's Solution-Full Strength. (Century) Sodium hypochlorite 0.5%. Soln. Bot. pt, gal. *otc.*
Use: Anti-infective, topical.

Dakin's Solution-Half Strength. (Century) Sodium hypochlorite 0.25%. Soln. Bot. pt. *otc.*
Use: Anti-infective, topical.

Dalalone. (Forest) Dexamethasone sodium phosphate 4 mg/ml, methyl and propyl parabens, sodium bisulfite. Vial 5 ml. *Rx.*
Use: Corticosteroid.

Dalalone D.P. (Forest) Dexamethasone acetate 16 mg/ml, polysorbate 80, carboxymethylcellulose, sodium bisulfite, EDTA, benzyl alcohol. Vial 1 ml, 5 ml. *Rx.*
Use: Corticosteroid.

Dalalone L.A. (Forest) Dexamethasone 8 mg/ml, polysorbate 80, carboxymethylcellulose, sodium bisulfite, EDTA, benzyl alcohol. Vial 5 ml. *Rx.*

Use: Corticosteroid.

d-ala-peptide t.
Use: Antiviral.
See: Peptide T (Carl Biotech/National Institute of Mental Health).

•**daledalin tosylate.** (dah-LEH-dah-lin TAH-sill-ate) USAN.
Use: Antidepressant.

•**dalfopristin.** (dal-FOE-priss-tin) USAN.
Use: Antibacterial.

Dalgan. (Wyeth-Ayerst) Dezocine 5 mg, 10 mg or 15 mg/ml. **5 mg/ml:** Vial (SD) 1 ml. **10 mg/ml:** Vial (SD) 1 ml, Vial (MD) 10 ml, syringes (prefilled) 1 ml. **15 mg/ml:** Vial (SD) 1 ml, syringes (prefilled) 1 ml. *Rx.*
Use: Narcotic analgesic.

Dallergy. (Laser) Chlorpheniramine maleate 8 mg, phenylephrine HCl 20 mg, methscopolamine nitrate 2.5 mg/ER Capl. Bot. 100s. *Rx.*
Use: Antihistamine, decongestant, anticholinergic.

Dallergy-D Syrup. (Laser) Chlorpheniramine maleate 2 mg, phenylephrine HCl 5 mg/5 ml. Bot. 118 ml. *otc.*
Use: Antihistamine, decongestant.

Dallergy-Jr Capsules. (Laser) Brompheniramine maleate 6 mg, pseudoephedrine HCl 60 mg/Cap. Bot. 100s. *Rx.*
Use: Antihistamine, decongestant.

Dallergy Syrup. (Laser) Chlorpheniramine maleate 2 mg, phenylephrine HCl 10 mg, methscopolamine nitrate 0.625 mg/5 ml. Bot. 473 ml. *Rx.*
Use: Antihistamine, decongestant, anticholinergic, antispasmodic.

Dallergy Tablets. (Laser) Chlorpheniramine maleate 4 mg, phenylephrine HCl 10 mg, methscopolamine nitrate 1.25 mg/Tab. Bot. 100s. *Rx.*
Use: Antihistamine, decongestant, anticholinergic, antispasmodic.

Dalmane. (Roche) Flurazepam HCl 15 mg or 30 mg/Cap. Bot. 100s, 500s, Prescription Pak 300s. RNP (Reverse Numbered Packages) 4 rolls × 25 cap. or 4 cards × 25 cap. UD 100s. *c-IV.*
Use: Sedative, hypnotic.

•**dalteparin sodium.** (dal-TEH-puh-rin) USAN.
Use: Anticoagulant; antithrombotic.
See: Fragmin, Soln. (Pharmacia & Upjohn).

•**daltroban.** (DAL-troe-ban) USAN.
Use: Platelet aggregation inhibitor, immunosuppressant.

•**dalvastatin.** (DAL-vah-STAT-in) USAN.

Use: Antihyperlipidemic.

Damacet-P. (Mason) Hydrocodone bitartrate 5 mg, acetaminophen 500 mg/Tab. Bot. 100s, 500s. *c-III.*
Use: Narcotic analgesic combination.

Damason-P. (Mason) Hydrocodone bitartrate 5 mg, aspirin 500 mg/Tab. Bot. 100s, 500s, 1000s. *c-III.*
Use: Narcotic analgesic combination.

Dambose.
See: Inositol, Tabs.

D-Amp. (Dunhall) Ampicillin trihydrate 500 mg/Cap. Bot. 100s. *Rx.*
Use: Anti-infective, penicillin.

•**danaparoid sodium.** (dan-AHP-ah-royd) USAN.
Use: Antithrombotic.
See: Orgaran Inj. (Organon).

Danatrol Capsules. (Sanofi Winthrop) Danazol. *Rx.*
Use: Gonadotropin inhibitor.

•**danazol,** (DAN-uh-ZOLE) U.S.P. 23.
Use: Anterior pituitary suppressant.
See: Danocrine, Cap. (Sanofi Winthrop) Chronogyn (Sterling Winthrop).

danazol. (Various Mfr.) 200 mg/Cap. Bot. 50s, 100s, 500s.
Use:
Use: Anterior pituitary suppressant.

Dandruff Shampoo. (Walgreen) Zinc pyrithione 2 g/100 ml. Bot. 11 oz. Tube 7 oz. *otc.*
Use: Antiseborrheic.

•**daniplestin.** USAN.
Use: Treatment of chemotherapy-induced bone marrow suppression.

Danocrine. (Sanofi Winthrop) Danazol 50 mg, 100 mg or 200 mg/Cap. Bot. 100s. *Rx.*
Use: Gonadotropin inhibitor.

Danogar Tablets. (Sanofi Winthrop) Danazol. *Rx.*
Use: Gonadotropin inhibitor.

Danol Capsules. (Sanofi Winthrop) Danazol. *Rx.*
Use: Gonadotropin inhibitor.

Dantrium. (Procter & Gamble) Dantrolene sodium. **25 mg/Cap.:** Bot. 100s, 500s, UD 100s; **50 mg/Cap.:** Bot. 100s; **100 mg/Cap.:** Bot. 100s, UD 100s. *Rx.*
Use: Skeletal muscle relaxant.

Dantrium I.V. (Procter & Gamble) Dantrolene sodium 20 mg/Vial. Vial 70 ml. *Rx.*
Use: Skeletal muscle relaxant.

•**dantrolene.** (dan-troe-LEEN) USAN.
Use: Skeletal muscle relaxant.

•**dantrolene sodium.** (dan-troe-LEEN) USAN.
Use: Skeletal muscle relaxant.

See: Dantrium, Cap., I.V. (Procter & Gamble).

Dapacin Cold Capsules. (Ferndale) Phenylpropanolamine 12.5 mg, chlorpheniramine maleate 2 mg, acetaminophen 325 mg. Bot. 100s. *otc.*
Use: Decongestant, antihistamine, analgesic.

Dapa Extra Strength Tablets. (Ferndale) Acetaminophen 500 mg/Cap. Bot. 50s, 100s, 1000s, UD 100s. *otc.*
Use: Analgesic.

Dapa Tablets. (Ferndale) Acetaminophen 324 mg/Tab. Bot. 100s, 1000s, UD 100s. *otc.*
Use: Analgesic.

Dapco. (Schlicksup) Salicylamide 300 mg, butabarbital 15 mg/Tab. Bot. 100s, 1000s. *c-III.*
Use: Salicylate analgesic, sedative, hypnotic.

•**dapiprazole hydrochloride.** (DAP-ih-PRAY-zole) USAN.
Use: Alpha-adrenergic blocking agent, neuroleptic, psychotropic, antiglaucoma agent.
See: Rēv-Eyes, Pow. (Storz/Lederle).

•**dapoxetine hydrochloride.** (dap-OX-eh-teen) USAN.
Use: Antidepressant.

•**dapsone,** (DAP-sone) U.S.P. 23. *Formerly Diaminodiphenylsulfone.*
Use: Antibacterial (leprostatic); dermitis herpetiformis suppressant; prevention/treatment of *Pneumocystis carinii* pneumonia. [Orphan drug]

dapsone. (Jacobus) 25 mg or 100 mg/Tab. Bot. 100s.
Use: Antibacterial (leprostatic), dermitis herpetiformis suppressant, prevention/treatment of *Pneumocystis carinii* pneumonia. [Orphan drug]

•**daptomycin.** (DAP-toe-MY-sin) USAN.
Use: Antibacterial.

Daragen. (Galderma) Collagen polypeptide, benzalkonium Cl in a mild amphoteric base. Shampoo. Bot. 8 oz. *otc.*
Use: Shampoo.

Dara Soapless Shampoo. (Galderma) Purified water, potassium coco hydrolyzed protein, sulfated castor oil, pentasodium triphosphate, sodium benzoate, sodium lauryl sulfate, fragrance. Shampoo. Bot. 8 oz, 16 oz. *otc.*
Use: Scalp protectant.

Daranide. (Merck) Dichlorphenamide 50 mg/Tab. Bot. 100s. *Rx.*
Use: Agent for glaucoma.

Daraprim. (Glaxo Wellcome) Pyrimethamine 25 mg/Tab. Bot. 100s. *Rx.*
Use: Antimalarial.

Darco G-60. (Zeneca) Activated carbon from lignite.
Use: Purifier.

•**darglitazone sodium.** (dahr-GLIH-tah-zone) USAN.
Use: Oral hypoglycemic.

Daricon. (SK-Beecham) Oxyphencyclimine HCl 10 mg/Tab. Bot. 60s, 500s. *Rx.*
Use: Antispasmodic.

•**darodipine.** (DA-row-dih-PEEN) USAN.
Use: Antihypertensive, bronchodilator, vasodilator.

Darvocet-N 100. (Lilly) Propoxyphene napsylate 100 mg, acetaminophen 650 mg/Tab. Bot. 100s (Rx Pak) 500s, UD 100s, 500s, RN 500s. *c-IV.*
Use: Narcotic analgesic combination.

Darvon. (Lilly) Propoxyphene HCl 65 mg/Pulv. Bot. 100s. Rx Pak 500s; Blister pkg. 10 × 10s; UD 20 rolls 25s. *c-IV.*
Use: Narcotic analgesic.

Darvon Compound-65. (Lilly) Propoxyphene HCl 65 mg, aspirin 389 mg, caffeine 32.4 mg/Pulv. Bot. 100s (Rx Pak) 500s. *c-IV.*
Use: Narcotic analgesic combination.

Darvon-N. (Lilly) Propoxyphene napsylate. **Tab.:** 100 mg. Bot. 100s (Rx Pak), 500s; Blister pkg. 10 × 10s; Rx Pak 20 × 50s. *c-IV.*
Use: Narcotic analgesic.

Da-Sed Tablet. (Sheryl) Butabarbital 0.5 gr/Tab. Bot. 100s. *c-III.*
Use: Sedative, hypnotic.

Dasin. (SK-Beecham) Ipecac 3 mg, acetylsalicylic acid 130 mg, camphor 15 mg, caffeine 8 mg, atropine sulfate 0.13 mg/Cap. Bot. 100s, 500s. *Rx.*
Use: Analgesic, anticholinergic, antispasmodic.

Daturine Hydrobromide.
See: Hyoscyamine Salts (Various Mfr.)

•**daunorubicin hydrochloride,** (DAW-no-RUE-bih-sin) U.S.P. 23.
Use: Antineoplastic.
See: Cerubidine, Inj. (Wyeth-Ayerst).

daunorubicin, liposomal. (DAW-no-RUE-bih-sin) (Vestar)
Use: Treatment of advanced HIV-associated Kaposi's sarcoma.
See: DaunoXome (NeXstar).

DaunoXome. (NeXstar) Daunorubicin citrate liposomal 2 mg/ml (equivalent to 50 mg daunorubicin base). Inj. Vials. 1, 4, 10 unit packs. *Rx.*
Use: Treatment of advanced HIV-asso-

ciated Kaposi's sarcoma.

Davitamon K.
See: Menadione Inj., Tab. (Various Mfr.)

Davosil. (Colgate Oral) Silicon carbide in glycerin base. Jar 8 oz, 10 oz. *otc.*
Use: Agent for oral hygiene.

Dayalets. (Abbott) Vitamins B_1 1.5 mg, B_2 1.7 mg, A 5000 IU, C 60 mg, D 400 IU, niacinamide 20 mg, B_6 2 mg, B_{12} 6 mcg, E 30 IU, folic acid 0.4 mg/Filmtab. Bot. 100s. *otc.*
Use: Vitamin supplement.

Dayalets Plus Iron. (Abbott) Vitamins B_1 1.5 mg, B_2 1.7 mg, niacinamide 20 mg, B_6 2 mg, C 60 mg, A 5000 IU, D 400 IU, E 30 IU, B_{12} 6 mcg, iron 18 mg, folic acid 0.4 mg/Filmtab. Bot. 100s. *otc.*
Use: Vitamin/mineral supplement.

Day Caps. (Towne) Vitamins A 5500 IU, D 400 IU, B_1 3 mg, B_2 3 mg, B_6 0.5 mg, B_{12} 4 mcg, C 50 mg, calcium pantothenate 5 mg, niacinamide 20 mg/Cap. Bot. 120s, 300s.
Use: Vitamin supplement.

Day Cap Tabs-M. (Towne) Vitamins A 5500 IU, D 400 IU, B_1 3 mg, B_2 3 mg, B_6 0.5 mg, B_{12} 4 mcg, C 50 mg, niacinamide 20 mg, calcium pantothenate 5 mg, l-Lysine HCl 15 mg, iron 10 mg, zinc 1.5 mg, manganese 1 mg, iodine 0.1 mg, copper 1 mg, potassium 5 mg, magnesium 6 mg/Cap. or Tab. Bot. 100s, 250s.
Use: Vitamin/mineral supplement.

Daycare. (Procter & Gamble) Pseudoephedrine HCl 10 mg, dextromethorphan HBr 3.3 mg, guaifenesin 33.3 mg, acetaminophen 108 mg, alcohol 10% and saccharin. Expectorant Liq. Bot. 180 ml, 300 ml. *otc.*
Use: Decongestant, antitussive, expectorant, analgesic.

Day-Night Comtrex. (Bristol-Myers) Pseudoephedrine HCl 30 mg, chlorpheniramine maleate 2 mg, dextromethorphan HBr 10 mg, acetaminophen 325 mg/Tab. Pkg. 6s. *otc.*
Use: Decongestant, antihistamine, antitussive, analgesic.

Daypro. (Searle) Oxaprozin 600 mg/Tab. Bot. 100s, UD 100s. *Rx.*
Use: Nonsteroidal anti-inflammatory, analgesic.

Day Tab. (Towne) Vitamins A 5000 IU, D 400 IU, B_1 15 mg, B_2 10 mg, C 600 mg, niacinamide 20 mg, B_6 5 mg, folic acid 400 mcg, pantothenic acid 10 mg, zinc 15 mg, copper 2 mg, B_{12} 5 mcg/Tab. Bot. 100s, 200s. *otc.*

Use: Vitamin/mineral supplement.

Day Tab Essential. (Towne) Vitamins A 5000 IU, D 400 IU, E 15 IU, C 60 mg, folic acid 0.4 mg, B_1 1.5 mg, B_2 1.7 mg, niacin 20 mg, B_6 2 mg, B_{12} 6 mcg/Tab. Bot. 200s. *otc.*
Use: Vitamin supplement.

Day Tabs, New. (Towne) Vitamins A 5000 IU, E 15 IU, D 400 IU, C 60 mg, folic acid 0.4 mg, B_1 1.5 mg, B_2 1.7 mg, niacin 20 mg, B_6 20 mg, B_{12} 6 mcg/Tab. Bot 100s, 250s. *otc.*
Use: Vitamin supplement.

Day Tab Plus Iron. (Towne) Iron 18 mg, vitamins A 5000 IU, D 400 IU, B_1 1.5 mg, B_2 1.7 mg, niacinamide 20 mg, C 60 mg, B_6 2 mg, pantothenic acid 10 mg, B_{12} 6 mcg, folic acid 0.1 mg/Tab. Bot. 100s. *otc.*
Use: Vitamin/mineral supplement.

Day Tabs Plus Iron, New. (Towne) Vitamins A 5000 IU, E 15 IU, D 400 IU, C 60 mg, folic acid 0.4 mg, B_1 1.5 mg, B_2 1.7 mg, niacin 20 mg, B_6 20 mg, B_{12} 6 mcg, iron 18 mcg/Tab. Bot. 250s. *otc.*
Use: Vitamin/mineral supplement.

Day Tab Stress Complex. (Towne) Vitamins A 5000 IU, C 600 mg, B_1 15 mg, B_2 10 mg, niacin 100 mg, D 400 IU, E 30 IU, B_6 5 mg, folic acid 400 mcg, B_{12} 6 mcg, pantothenic acid 20 mg, iron 18 mg, zinc 15 mg, copper 2 mg/Tab. Bot. 60s. *otc.*
Use: Vitamin/mineral supplement.

Day Tab with Iron. (Towne) Vitamins A 5000 IU, D 400 IU, E 15 IU, C 60 mg, folic acid 1.5 mg, B_1 15 mg, B_2 1.7 mg, niacin 20 mg, B_6 2 mg, B_{12} 6 mcg, iron 18 mg/Tab. Bot. 200s. *Rx.*
Use: Vitamin/mineral supplement.

Dayto-Anase. (Dayton) Bromelains 50,000 IU (protease activity). Tab. Bot. 60s. *otc.*
Use: Enzyme.

Dayto Himbin. (Dayton) Yohimbine 5.4 mg/Tab. Bot. 60s. *Rx.*
Use: Alpha-adrenergic blocker.

Dayto Sulf. (Dayton) Sulfathiazole 3.42%, sulfacetamide 2.86%, sulfabenzamide 3.7%, urea 0.64%. Cream. Tube 78 g with 8 disposable applicators. *Rx.*
Use: Anti-infective, vaginal.

•**dazadrol maleate.** (DAY-zah-drole) USAN.
Use: Antidepressant.

Dazamide Tabs. (Major) Acetazolamide 250 mg/Tab. Bot. 100s, 250s, 1000s, UD 100s. *Rx.*

Use: Diuretic.

•**dazepinil hydrochloride.** (dahz-EH-pih-NILL) USAN.
Use: Antidepressant.

•**dazmegrel.** (DAZE-meh-grell) USAN.
Use: Inhibitor (thromboxane synthetase).

•**dazopride fumarate.** (DAY-zoe-PRIDE) USAN.
Use: Peristaltic stimulant.

•**dazoxiben hydrochloride.** (DAZE-OX-ih-ben) USAN.
Use: Antithrombotic.

DB Electrode Paste. (Day-Baldwin) Tube 5%.

Dbed. Dibenzylethylenediamine dipenicillin G.
Use: Anti-infective, penicillin.
See: Benzathine penicillin G, Susp.

DCA.
See: Desoxycorticosterone acetate preps. (Various Mfr.)

DCF. Pentostatin (2'-deoxycoformycin).
Rx.
Use: Anti-infective.
See: Nipent, Pow. (Parke-Davis).

DCP. (Towne) Calcium 180 mg, phosphorus 105 mg, vitamins D 66.7 IU/Tab.
Bot. 100s. *otc.*
Use: Vitamin/mineral supplement.

DC Softgels. (Goldline) Docusate calcium 240 mg/Cap. Bot. 100s, 500s. *otc.*
Use: Laxative.

DC 240. (Goldline) Docusate calcium 240 mg/Cap. Bot. 100s, 500s. *otc.*
Use: Laxative.

DDAVP Injection. (Rorer). Desmopressin acetate 4 mcg, chlorobutanol 5 mg/ml. Amp. 1 ml. Vials. 10 ml. *Rx.*
Use: Antidiuretic.

DDAVP Spray. (Rorer) Desmopressin acetate 0.1 mg, chlorobutanol 5 mg/ml. Bot. 5 ml. Vial 2.5 ml w/applicator tubes for nasal administration. *Rx.*
Use: Antidiuretic.

DDAVP Tablets. (Rhone-Poulenc Rorer) Desmopressin acetate 0.1 or 0.2 mg/Tab. Bot 100s. *Rx.*
Use: Antidiuretic.

ddC. Dideoxycytidine.
Use: Antiviral.
See: HIVID (Roche).

ddl. Didanosine.
Use: Antiviral.
See: Videx, Tab., Pow. (Bristol-Myers Squibb).

D-Diol. (Burgin-Arden) Testosterone cypionate 50 mg, estradiol cypionate 2 mg/ml. Vial 10 ml. *Rx.*
Use: Androgen, estrogen.

DDS.
See: Dapsone Tab., U.S.P. 23.

DDT.
See: Chlorophenothane.

Deacetyllanatoside C.
See: Deslanoside, U.S.P. 23.

deadly nightshade leaf.
See: Belladonna Leaf, U.S.P. 23.

1-deamino-8-d-arginine vasopressin.
Desmopressin acetate.
Use: Posterior pituitary hormone.
See: Concentraid, Soln. (Ferring Labs.).
DDAVP, Inj., Soln. (Rhone-Poulenc Rorer).

deba.
See: Barbital (Various Mfr.)

Debrisan. (Johnson & Johnson) Dextranomer. **Beads:** Spherical hydrophilic 0.1-0.3 mm diameter. Bot. 25 g, 60 g, 120 g. Pk. 7 × 4 g, 14 × 14 g. U.S. distributor Johnson & Johnson Products. **Paste:** 10 g. Foil packets 6s. *otc.*
Use: Wound and ulcer cleansing.

•**debrisoquin sulfate.** (deb-RICE-oh-kwin) USAN. *Formerly Isocaramidine Sulfate.*
Use: Antihypertensive.

Debrox. (Hoechst Marion Roussel) Carbamide peroxide 6.5% in anhydrous glycerol. Plastic squeeze bot. 0.5 oz, 1 oz. *otc.*
Use: Otic preparation.

Decabid. (Lilly) Indecainide HCl 50 mg, 75 mg or 100 mg/SR tab. Bot. 100s, UD 100s. [Approved but not marketed].
Use: Antiarrhythmic.

Deca-Bon. (Barrows) Vitamins A 3000 IU, D 400 IU, C 60 mg, B_1 1 mg, B_2 1.2 mg, niacinamide 8 mg, B_6 1 mg, panthenol 3 mg, B_{12} 1 mcg, biotin 30 mcg/0.6 ml. Drops Bot. 50 ml. *otc.*
Use: Vitamin supplement.

Decaderm. (Merck) Dexamethasone 0.1% w/isopropyl myristate gel, wood alcohols, refined lanolin alcohol, microcrystalline wax, anhydrous citric acid, anhydrous sodium phosphate dibasic. Tube 30 g. *Rx.*
Use: Corticosteroid.

Decadrol. (Paddock) Dexamethasone sodium phosphate 4 mg/ml. Vial 5 ml. *Rx.*
Use: Corticosteroid.

Decadron. (Merck) Dexamethasone. **Tab.:** 0.5 mg: Bot. 100s, UD 100s; 0.75 mg: 100s, UD 100s; 1.5 mg: Bot. 50s, UD 100s; 4 mg: Bot. 50s, UD 100s.

Elix.: 0.5 mg/5 ml, benzoic acid 0.1%, alcohol 5% Bot. w/dropper 100 ml, Bot. w/out dropper 237 ml. *Rx.*
Use: Corticosteroid.
W/Neomycin sulfate.
See: NeoDecadron, Ophth. Soln., Ophth. Oint., Topical, Cream (Merck).

Decadron-LA Suspension. (Merck) Dexamethasone acetate equivalent to dexamethasone 8 mg/ml w/sodium Cl 6.67 mg, creatinine 5 mg, disodium edetate 0.5 mg, sodium carboxymethylcellulose 5 mg, polysorbate 80 0.75 mg, sodium hydroxide to adjust pH, benzyl alcohol 9 mg, sodium bisulfite 1 mg, water for injection q.s. 1 ml. Vial 1 ml, 5 ml. *Rx.*
Use: Corticosteroid.

Decadron Phosphate. (Merck) Dexamethasone sodium phosphate equivalent in various forms: **Ophth. Soln.:** 0.1%. Ocumeter dispenser 5 ml. *Rx.* **Ophth. Oint.:** 0.05%. Tube 3.5 g. *Rx.* **Cream:** 0.1% w/stearyl alcohol, cetyl alcohol, mineral oil, polyoxyl 40 stearate, sorbitol solution, methyl polysilicone emulsion, creatinine, purified water, sodium citrate, disodium edetate, sodium hydroxide to adjust pH, methylparaben 0.15%, sorbic acid 0.1%. Tube 15 g, 30 g.
Use: Corticosteroid, ophthalmic.
W/Neomycin.
Use: Corticosteroid, anti-infective.
See: NeoDecadron, Ophth. Soln., Ophth. Oint., Topical Cream (Merck)
W/Xylocaine.
Dexamethasone sodium phosphate equivalent to dexamethasone phosphate 4 mg, lidocaine HCl 10 mg, citric acid 10 mg, creatinine 8 mg, sodium bisulfite 0.5 mg, disodium edetate 0.5 mg, sodium hydroxide to adjust pH, water for injection, methylparaben 1.5 mg, propylparaben 0.2 mg/ml. Inj. Vial 5 ml.
Use: Corticosteroid.

Decadron Phosphate Injection. (Merck) Dexamethasone sodium phosphate 4 mg or 24 mg/ml, creatinine 8 mg, sodium citrate 10 mg, disodium edetate 0.5 mg (24 mg/ml only), sodium hydroxide to adjust pH, sodium bisulfite 1 mg, methylparaben 1.5 mg, propylparaben 0.2 mg/ml. **4 mg/ml:** Vial 1 ml, 5 ml, 25 ml. **24 mg/ml** (for I.V. use only): Vial 5 ml, 10 ml. *Rx.*
Use: Corticosteroid.

Decadron w/Xylocaine. (Merck) Dexamethasone sodium phosphate 4 mg,

lidocaine HCl 10 mg/ml. Soln. Vial 15 ml. *Rx.*
Use: Corticosteroid.

Deca-Durabolin. (Organon) Nandrolone decanoate injection w/benzyl alcohol 10%. **50 mg/ml:** Multidose vial 2 ml. **100 mg/ml:** Multidose vial 2 ml, syringe 1 ml. **200 mg/ml:** Multidose vial 1 ml, syringe 1 ml. *c-III.*
Use: Anabolic steroid.

Deca-Durabolin Rediject Syringes. (Organon) Nandrolone decanoate 50 mg, 100 mg or 200 mg/ml. Syringe 1 ml Box 25s. *c-III.*
Use: Anabolic steroid.

Decagen. (Goldline) Iron 18 mg, vitamins A 5000 IU, D 400 IU, E 30 IU, B_1 1.7 mg, B_2 2 mg, B_3 20 mg, B_5 10 mg, B_6 3 mg, B_{12} 6 mcg, C 60 mg, folic acid 0.4 mg, Ca, Cl, Cr, Cu, B, I, K, Mg, Mn, Mo, Ni, P, Se, Si, Sn, V, Zn 15 mg, vitamin K, biotin 30 mcg/Tab. Bot. 130s. *otc.*
Use: Vitamin/mineral supplement.

Decaject. (Mayrand) Dexamethasone sodium phosphate 4 mg/ml. Vial 5 ml, 10 ml. *Rx.*
Use: Corticosteroid.

Decaject-L.A. (Mayrand) Dexamethasone acetate 8 mg/ml suspension, polysorbate 80, carboxymethylcellulose, sodium bisulfite, EDTA, benzyl alcohol. Inj. vial 5 ml. *Rx.*
Use: Corticosteroid.

Decajest LA. (Mayrand) Dexamethasone acetate 8 mg/ml. Vial 5 ml. *Rx.*
Use: Corticosteroid.

Decalix. (Pharmed) Dexamethasone 0.5 mg/5 ml. Bot. 100 ml. *Rx.*
Use: Corticosteroid.

Decameth. (Foy) Dexamethasone sodium phosphate injection 4 mg/5 cc vial. *Rx.*
Use: Corticosteroid.

Decameth L.A. (Foy) Dexamethasone sodium phosphate injection 8 mg/ml. Vial/5 ml. *Rx.*
Use: Corticosteroid.

Decameth Tablets. (Foy) Dexamethasone 0.75 mg/Tab. Bot. 1000s. *Rx.*
Use: Corticosteroid.

Decapryn. (Hoechst Marion Roussel) Doxylamine succinate 12.5 mg/Tab. Bot. 100s. *otc.*
Use: Antihistamine.
W/Pyridoxine HCl.
See: Bendectin, Tab. (Hoechst Marion Roussel).

Decasone Injection. (Forest Pharm.)

Dexamethasone sodium phosphate equivalent to dexamethasone phosphate 4 mg/ml. Vial 5 ml. *Rx.*
Use: Corticosteroid.

decavitamin. U.S.P. XXI. Vitamins A 4000 IU, D 400 IU, C 70 mg, calcium pantothenate 10 mg, B$_{12}$ 5 mcg, folic acid 100 mcg, nicotinamide 20 mg, B$_6$ 2 mg, B$_2$ 2 mg, B$_1$ 2 mg/Cap. or Tab. *otc.*
Use: Vitamin therapy.

Decholin. (Bayer) Dehydrocholic acid 250 mg/Tab. Bot. 100s, 500s. *otc.*
Use: Hydrocholeric.

Decicain. Tetracaine HCl.

•**decitabine.** (deh-SIGH-tah-BEAN) USAN.
Use: Antineoplastic.

declaben. (DEH-klah-BEN) (previously used name) see lodelaben.
Use: Antiarthritic, emphysema therapy adjunct.

Declomycin Hydrochloride. (Lederle) Demeclocycline HCl. **Cap.:** 150 mg. Bot. 100s. **Tab.:** 150 mg. Bot. 100s; 300 mg. Bot. 48s. *Rx.*
Use: Anti-infective, tetracycline.

Decofed. (Various Mfr.) Pseudoephedrine HCl 30 mg/5 ml. Syr. Bot. 120 ml, 240 ml, pt, gal. *otc.*
Use: Decongestant.

Decohist Capsules. (Towne) Chlorpheniramine maleate 1 mg, phenylpropanolamine HCl 12.5 mg, salicylamide 180 mg, caffeine 15 mg/Cap. Bot. 18s. *otc.*
Use: Antihistamine, decongestant, analgesic.

Decohistine DH Liquid. (Morton Grove) Pseudoephedrine HCl 30 mg, chlorpheniramine maleate 2 mg, codeine phosphate 10 mg, alcohol. Liq. Bot. 120 ml, pt and gal. *c-v.*
Use: Decongestant, antihistamine, antitussive.

Decohistine Elixir. (Rosemont) Phenylephrine HCl 5 mg, chlorpheniramine maleate 2 mg, alcohol 5%. Elix. Bot. 120 ml, pt. and gal. *otc.*
Use: Decongestant, antihistamine.

Deconade. (H.L. Moore) Phenylpropanolamine HCl 75 mg, chlorpheniramine maleate 12 mg/Cap. Bot. 100s, 1000s. *otc.*
Use: Decongestant, antihistamine.

Deconamine CX Liquid. (Bradley) Hydrocodone bitartrate 5 mg, pseudoephedrine HCl 60 mg, guaifenesin 200 mg/5 ml. Bot. 480 ml. *Rx.*
Use: Antitussive, expectorant.

Deconamine CX Tablets. (Kenwood/Bradley) Hydrocodone bitartrate 5 mg, pseudoephedrine HCl 30 mg, guaifenesin 300 mg/Tab. Bot. 100s. *Rx.*
Use: Antitussive, expectorant.

Deconamine SR Capsules. (Kenwood/Bradley) Chlorpheniramine maleate 8 mg, d-pseudoephedrine HCl 120 mg/Cap. Bot. 100s, 500s. *Rx.*
Use: Antihistamine, decongestant.

Deconamine Syrup. (Kenwood/Bradley) Chlorpheniramine maleate 2 mg, d-pseudoephedrine HCl 30 mg/5 ml, sorbitol. Bot. 473 ml. *Rx.*
Use: Antihistamine, decongestant.

Deconamine Tablets. (Kenwood/Bradley) Chlorpheniramine maleate 4 mg, d-pseudoephedrine HCl 60 mg/Tab. Bot. 100s. *Rx.*
Use: Antihistamine, decongestant.

Decongestabs. (Various Mfr.) Phenylpropanolamine HCl 40 mg, phenylephrine HCl 10 mg, chlorpheniramine maleate 5 mg, phenyltoloxamine citrate 15 mg/Tab. Bot. 100s, 1000s. *Rx.*
Use: Decongestant, antihistamine.

Decongestant Expectorant Liquid. (Schein) Pseudoephedrine HCl 30 mg, codeine phosphate 10 mg, guaifenesin 100 mg, alcohol 7.5%. Bot. 480 ml. *c-v.*
Use: Decongestant, antitussive, expectorant.

Decongestant Formula Mediquell. (Parke-Davis Prods) Dextromethorphan HBr 30 mg, pseudoephedrine HCl 60 mg/Square.
Use: Antitussive, decongestant.

Decongestant Tablets, Extended Release. (Various Mfr.) Phenylpropanolamine HCl 40 mg, phenylephrine HCl 10 mg, chlorpheniramine maleate 5 mg, phenyltoloxamine citrate 15 mg/Tab. Bot. 50s, 100s, 1000s. *Rx.*
Use: Decongestant, antihistamine.

Deconhist L.A. (Goldline) Phenylephrine HCl 25 mg, phenylpropanolamine HCl, chlorpheniramine maleate 8 mg, hyoscyamine sulfate 0.19 mg, atropine sulfate 0.04 mg, scopolamine hydrobromide 0.01 mg/SR Tab. Bot. 100s.
Use: Decongestant, antihistamine, anticholinergic.

Deconomed. (Iomed) Chlorpheniramine maleate 8 mg, pseudoephedrine HCl 120 mg/Cap. Bot. 100s, 500s. *Rx.*
Use: Antihistamine, decongestant.

Deconsal II Capsules. (Adams) Pseudoephedrine 60 mg, guaifenesin 600 mg/Cap. Bot. 100s. *Rx.*

Use: Decongestant, expectorant.

Deconsal Pediatric. (Adams) Codeine phosphate 10 mg, pseudoephedrine HCl 30 mg, guaifenesin 100 mg/5 ml, alcohol 6%. Syr. Bot. 480 ml. *c-v.*
Use: Decongestant, expectorant.

Deconsal Sprinkle Capsule. (Adams) Phenylephrine HCl 10 mg, guaifenesin 300 mg/S.R. Cap. Bot. 100s. *Rx.*
Use: Decongestant, expectorant.

•**dectaflur.** (DECK-tah-flure) USAN.
Use: Dental caries prophylactic.

Decubitex. (I.C.P) **Oint.:** Biebrich scarlet red sulfonated 0.1%, balsam Peru, castor oil, zinc oxide, starch, sodium propionate, parabens. Jar 15 g, 60 g, 120 g, lb. **Pow.:** Biebrich scarlet red sulfonated 0.1%, starch, zinc oxide, sodium propionate, parabens. Bot. 30 g, UD 1 g. *otc.*
Use: Wound-healing agent, emollient, antipruritic.

Decylenes. (Rugby) Undecylenic acid, zinc undecylenate. Oint. Tube 30 g, lb. *otc.*
Use: Antifungal, topical.

Deep Down Pain Relief Rub. (SK-Beecham) Methyl salicylate 15%, menthol 5%, camphor 0.5%. Tube 1.25 oz, 3 oz. *otc.*
Use: Analgesic, topical.

Deep Strength Musterole. (Schering-Plough) Methyl salicylate 30%, menthol 3%, methyl nicotinate 0.5%. Tube 1.25 oz, 3 oz. *otc.*
Use: Analgesic, topical.

Defed-60. (Ferndale) Pseudoephedrine 60 mg/Tab. Bot 1000s. *otc.*
Use: Decongestant.

Defen-LA. (Horizon) Pseudoephedrine HCl 60 mg, guaifenesin 600 mg/SR Tab. Bot. 100s. *Rx.*
Use: Decongestant, expectorant.

•**deferoxamine.** (DEE-fer-OX-ah-meen) USAN.
Use: Chelating agent for iron.

•**deferoxamine hydrochloride.** USAN.
Use: Chelating agent for iron.

•**deferoxamine mesylate,** (DEE-fer-OX-ah-meen) U.S.P. 23.
Use: Iron depleter, antidote to iron poisoning, chelating agent.
See: Desferal Mesylate, Pow. for Inj. (Novartis).

defibrotide.
Use: Thrombotic thrombocytopenic purpura. [Orphan drug]

Deficol. (Vangard) Bisacodyl 5 mg/Tab. Bot. 100s, 1000s. *otc.*

Use: Laxative.

•**deflazacort.** (deh-FLAZE-ah-cart) USAN.
Use: Anti-inflammatory.

d4T.
Use: Antiviral.
See: Stavudine (B-M Squibb).

Degas. (Invamed) Simethicone 80 mg/Tab. Chewable. Bot. 100s. *otc.*
Use: Antiflatulent.

Degest-2. (Akorn) Naphazoline HCl 0.012%. Bot. 15 ml. *otc.*
Use: Ophthalmic decongestant.

Dehydrex.
Use: Recurrent corneal erosion. [Orphan drug]

dehydrocholate sodium inj., U.S.P. XXI.
Use: Relief of liver congestion; diagnosis of cardiac failure.
See: Decholine Sodium, Inj. (Bayer).

7-dehydrocholesterol, activated. (Various Mfr.) Vitamin D-3.
Use: Vitamin D supplement.

•**dehydrocholic acid, U.S.P. 23.**
Use: Orally, hydrocholeretic and choleretic.
See: Atrocholin,Tab. (Glaxo).
  Cholan-DH, Tab. (Medeva).
  Decholin (Bayer).
  Dilabil (Sterling Winthrop).
  Ketocholanic acid.
  Neocholan, Tab. (Hoechst Marion Roussel).
  Procholon (Bristol-Myers Squibb).
W/Amyloytic and proteolytic enzymes, desoxycholic acid.
See: Bilezyme, Tab. (Geriatric).
W/Bile, homatropine methylbromide, pepsin.
See: Biloric, Caps. (Arcum).
W/Bile, homatropine methylbromide, phenobarbital.
See: Bilamide, Tab. (Norgine).
W/Bile extract, pepsin, pancreatin.
See: Progestive, Tab. (NCP).
W/Desoxycholic acid.
See: Combichole, Tab. (F. Trout).
  Ketosox, Tab. (Ascher).
W/Docusate sodium.
See: Dubbalax-B, Cap. (Redford).
  Dubbalax-N, Cap. (Redford).
  Neolax, Tab. (Schwarz Pharma).
W/Docusate sodium, phenolphthalein.
See: Bolax, Cap. (Boyd).
  Sarolax (Saron).
  Tripalax, Cap. (Redford).
W/Homatropine methylbromide.
See: Cholan V, Tab. (Medeva).
  Dranochol, Tab. (Marin).
W/Homatropine methylbromide, sodium pentobarbital.

See: Homachol, Tab. (Lemmon).
W/Methscopolamine, ox bile, amobarbital.
See: Hydrochol Plus, Tab. (Zeneca)
W/Ox bile, homatropine methylbromide, phenobarbital.
See: Bilamide, Tab. (Norgine).
W/Pancreatin, pepsin, ox bile, belladonna extract.
See: Ro-Bile, Tab. (Solvay).
W/Pepsin, pancreatin, ox bile extract, papain.
See: Canz, Tab. (Cole).
W/Pepsin, pancreatin enzyme concentrate, cellulase.
See: Gastroenterase, Tab (Wallace).
W/Phenobarbital, homatropine methylbromide.
See: Cholan-HMB, Tab. (Medeva).
W/Phenobarbital, homatropine methylbromide, gerilase, geriprotase, desoxycholic acid.
See: Bilezyme Plus, Tabs. (Geriatric).
W/Phenolphthalein, docusate sodium.
See: Sarolax, Cap. (Saron).
dehydrocholin.
Use: Hydrocholeretic.
See: Dehydrocholic acid.
dehydroepiandrosterone. (Genelabs)
Use: Treatment of systemic lupus erythematosus (SLE). [Orphan drug].
dehydrodesoxycholic acid.
See: Cholanic acid.
Dekasol. (Seatrace) Dexamethasone phosphate 4 mg/ml. Vial 5 ml, 10 ml. *Rx.*
Use: Corticosteroid.
Dekasol L.A. (Seatrace) Dexamethasone acetate 8 mg/ml. Vial 5 ml. *Rx.*
Use: Corticosteroid.
De-Koff. (Whiteworth Towne) Terpin hydrate w/dextromethorphan. Elix. Bot. 4 oz. *otc.*
Use: Antitussive, expectorant.
Delacort Lotion. (Mericon) Hydrocortisone 0.5%. Bot. 4 oz. *otc.*
Use: Corticosteroid, topical.
•**delapril hydrochloride.** (DELL-ah-prill) USAN.
Use: Antihypertensive; angiotensin-converting enzyme inhibitor.
Delaqua-5. (Del-Ray) Benzoyl peroxide 5%. Tube 42.5 g. *Rx.*
Use: Antiacne.
Delaqua-10. (Del-Ray) Benzoyl peroxide 10%. 42.5 g. *Rx.*
Use: Antiacne.
Delaquin Lotion. (Schlicksup) Hydrocortisone 0.5%, iodoquin 3%. Bot. 3 oz. *Rx.*

Use: Corticosteroid, antifungal.
Delatest. (Dunhall) Testosterone enanthate 100 mg/ml, chlorobutanol in sesame oil. Amp. 10 ml. *c-III.*
Use: Androgen.
Delatestadiol. (Dunhall) Testosterone enanthate 90 mg, estradiol valerate 4 mg/ml, chlorobutanol in sesame oil. Amp. 10 ml. *Rx.*
Use: Androgen, estrogen combination.
Delatestryl. (Bio-Technology General) Testosterone enanthate 200 mg/ml in sesame oil, chlorobutanol 0.5%. Vial 5 ml. *c-III.*
Use: Androgen.
•**delavirdine mesylate.** USAN.
Use: Antiviral.
Delcid. (SK-Beecham) Aluminum hydroxide 600 mg, magnesium hydroxide 665 mg/5 ml, alcohol 0.3%, saccharin. Bot. 8 oz. *otc.*
Use: Antacid.
Del-Clens. (Del-Ray) Soapless cleanser. Bot. 8 oz. *otc.*
Use: Skin cleanser.
Delcort. (Roberts) Hydrocortisone 0.5% or 1%. Cream. Pack. 1 g, 20 g, 1 lb. (1% only). *otc.*
Use: Corticosteroid, topical.
Delco-Lax. (Delco) Bisacodyl 5 mg/Tab. Bot. 1000s. *otc.*
Use: Laxative.
Delcozine. (Delco) Phendimetrazine tartrate 70 mg/Tab. Bot. 1000s, 5000s. *c-III.*
Use: Anorexiant.
•**delequamine hydrochloride.** (deh-LEH-kwah-meen) USAN.
Use: Impotence therapy adjunct.
Delestrec. Estradiol 17-undecanoate. *Rx.*
Use: Estrogen.
Delestrogen. (Bristol-Myers) Estradiol valerate **10 mg/ml:** In sesame oil, chlorobutanol 0.5%. Vial 5 ml. **20 mg/ml:** In castor oil, benzyl benzoate 20%, benzyl alcohol 2%. Vial 5 ml or 1 ml unimatic single dose syringe. **40 mg/ml:** In castor oil, benzyl benzoate 40%, benzyl alcohol 2%. Vial 5 ml. *Rx.*
Use: Estrogen.
Delfen Contraceptive Foam. (Advanced Care) Nonoxynol-9 12.5% in an oil-in-water emulsion at pH 4.5 to 5.0. Starter can with applicator 20 g. Refill 20 g, 42 g. *otc.*
Use: Spermicide.
delinal. Propenzolate HCl.
•**delmadinone acetate.** USAN.
Use: Progestin, antiandrogen, antiestrogen.

See: Delmate (Syntex).

Del-Mycin. (Del-Ray) Erythromycin 2%, ethyl alcohol 66%. Topical soln. Bot. 60 ml. *Rx.*
Use: Antiacne.

Del-Stat. (Del-Ray) Abradent cleaner. Jar 2 oz. *otc.*
Use: Antiacne.

Delsym Cough Suppressant Liquid. (McNeil Prods) Dextromethorphan HBr 30 mg/5 ml. Bot. 3 oz. *otc.*
Use: Antitussive.

delta-1-cortisone.
Use: Corticosteroid.
See: Deltasone, Tab. (Pharmacia & Upjohn).

delta-1-hydrocortisone.
Use: Corticosteroid.
See: Prednisolone (Various Mfr.)

Delta-Cortef. (Pharmacia & Upjohn) Prednisolone 5 mg/Tab. Bot. 100s, 500s. *Rx.*
Use: Corticosteroid.

Deltacortone. Prednisone.
Use: Corticosteroid.

Delta-Cortril. Prednisolone.
Use: Corticosteroid.

Delta-D. (Freeda) Vitamin D$_3$ 400 IU/ Tab. Bot. 250s, 500s. *otc.*
Use: Vitamin D supplement.

•**deltafilcon a.** (DELL-tah-FILL-kahn A) USAN.
Use: Contact lens material, hydrophilic.

•**deltafilcon b.** (DELL-tah-FILL-kahn B) USAN.
Use: Contact lens material (hydrophilic).
See: Amsof (Lombart).
Amsof-Thin (Lombart).

Deltasone. (Pharmacia & Upjohn) Prednisone. **2.5 mg:** Tab. Bot. 100s. **5 mg:** Tab. Bot. 100s, 500s, UD 100s, Dosepak 21s. **10 mg, 20 mg:** Tab. Bot. 100s, 500s, UD 100s. **50 mg:** Tab. Bot. 100s, UD 100s. *Rx.*
Use: Corticosteroid.

Delta-Tritex. (Dermol) Triamcinolone acetonide. **Cream:** 0.1% Tube 30 and 80 g. **Oint.:** 0.1% Tube 30 g. *Rx.*
Use: Corticosteroid, topical.

Del-Trac. (Del-Ray) Acne lotion. Bot. 2 oz. *otc.*
Use: Antiacne.

Deltastab.
Use: Corticosteroid.
See: Prednisolone (Various Mfr.)

•**deltibant.** USAN.
Use: Antagonist (bradykinin).

Del-Vi-A. (Del-Ray) Vitamin A 50,000 IU/ Cap. Bot. 100s. *Rx.*

Use: Vitamin A supplement.

Delysid. Lysergic acid diethylamide.
Use: Potent psychotogenic.

Demadex. (Boehringer Mannheim) **Tab.:** Torsemide 5 mg, 10 mg, 20 mg, 100 mg. Bot. UD 100s. **Inj.:** Torsemide 10 mg/ml. Amps. 2 ml or 5 ml. *Rx.*
Use: Diuretics, loop.

Demazin. (Schering-Plough) **Syr.:** Chlorpheniramine maleate 2 mg, phenylpropanolamine HCl 12.5 mg/5 ml, alcohol 7.5%, menthol. Bot. 118 ml. **Tab.:** Chlorpheniramine maleate 4 mg, phenylpropanolamine HCl 25 mg. Box 24s. Bot. 100s. *otc.*
Use: Antihistamine, decongestant.

•**demecarium bromide,** U.S.P. 23.
Use: Cholinergic, (ophthalmic).
See: Humorsol, Soln. (Merck).

•**demeclocycline,** U.S.P. 23. *Formerly Demethylchlortetracycline.*
Use: Antibacterial.
See: Declomycin Prods. (Lederle).
Ledermycin Prods. (Lederle).

•**demeclocycline hydrochloride,** (DEH-meh-kloe-SIGH-kleen) U.S.P. 23.
Use: Antibacterial.
See: Declomycin HCl, Preps. (Lederle).

•**demeclocycline hydrochloride and nystatin capsules,** U.S.P. 23.
Use: Anti-infective.
See: Declostatin, Cap. (Lederle).

demeclocycline hydrochloride and nystatin tablets.
Use: Anti-infective.
See: Declostatin, Tab. (Lederle).

•**demecycline.** (DEH-meh-SIGH-kleen) USAN.
Use: Antibacterial.

Demerol Hydrochloride. (Sanofi Winthrop) Meperidine HCl. **Syr.:** 50 mg/ 5 ml, saccharin. Bot. 16 fl oz. **Inj.:** Detecto-Seal, Carpuject, Sterile Cartridge-Needle Unit. **2.5%** (25 mg/ml), **5%** (50 mg/ml), **7.5%** (75 mg/ml), **10%** (100 mg/ ml), Box 10s. **Uni-Amp 5%:** 0.5 ml (25 mg)/Amp., 1 ml (50 mg)/Amp., 1.5 ml (75 mg)/Amp., 2 ml (100 mg)/Amp. Box 25s; **10%:** 1 ml (100 mg)/Amp. Box 25s. **Uni-Nest 5%:** 0.5 ml (25 mg)/ Amp., 1 ml (50 mg)/Amp., 1.5 ml (75 mg)/Amp., 2 ml (100 mg)/Amp. Box 25s; **10%:** 1 ml/Amp. Box 25s. **Vial:** 5% multiple-dose vial/30 ml Box 1s. **Tab.:** 50 mg or 100 mg. Bot. 100s, 500s. *c-II.*
Use: Narcotic analgesic.

demethylchlortetracycline hydrochloride.
Use: Anti-infective, tetracycline.

See: Demeclocycline HCl, U.S.P. 23.

Demi-Regroton. (Rhone-Poulenc Rorer) Chlorthalidone 25 mg, reserpine 0.125 mg/Tab. Bot. 100s. *Rx.*
Use: Antihypertensive, diuretic.

•**demoxepam.** (dem-OX-eh-pam) USAN.
Use: Minor tranquilizer.

Demser. (Merck) Metyrosine 250 mg/Cap. Bot. 100s. *Rx.*
Use: Antihypertensive.

Demulen 1/35-21. (Searle) Ethynodiol diacetate 1 mg, ethinyl estradiol 35 mcg/Tab. Compack disp. 21s, 6 × 21, 2421. Refill 21s, 1221. *Rx.*
Use: Oral contraceptive.

Demulen 1/35-28. (Searle) Ethynodiol diacetate 1 mg, ethinyl estradiol 35 mcg/Tab. Compack 28s: 21 active tabs, 7 placebo tabs. Compack 6 × 28, 2428. Refill 28s, 1228. *Rx.*
Use: Oral contraceptive.

Demulen 1/50-21. (Searle) Ethynodiol diacetate 1 mg, ethinyl estradiol 50 mcg/Tab. Compack Disp. 21s, 6 × 21, 2421. Refill 21s, 1221. *Rx.*
Use: Oral contraceptive.

Demulen 1/50-28. (Searle) Ethynodiol diacetate 1 mg, ethinyl estradiol 50 mcg/Tab. Compack 28s: 21 active tabs, 7 placebo tabs. Compack Disp. of 28, 6 × 28, 2428. Refill 28s, 1228. *Rx.*
Use: Oral contraceptive.

Denalan Denture Cleanser. (Whitehall Robins) Sodium percarbonate 30%. Bot. 7 oz., 13 oz. *otc.*
Use: Agent for oral hygiene.

•**denatonium benzoate,** (DEE-nah-TOE-nee-uhm BEN-zoh-ate) N.F. 18.
Use: Pharmaceutic aid (flavor, alcohol denaturant).
See: Bitrex.

Denavir. (SmithKline Beecham) Penciclovir 10 mg/g/Cream. Tube 2 g. *Rx.*
Use: Treatment of recurrent herpes labialis (cold sores).

Dencorub. (Last) Methyl salicylate 20%, menthol 0.75%, camphor 1%, eucalyptus oil 0.5%. Tube 1.25 oz, 2.75 oz. *otc.*
Use: Analgesic, topical.

Dencorub Analgesic Liquid. (Last) Oleoresin capsicum suspension in aqueous vehicle. Bot. 6 oz. *otc.*
Use: Analgesic, topical.

•**denofungin.** (DEE-no-FUN-jin) USAN.
Use: Antifungal, antibacterial.

Denorex. (Whitehall Robins) Coal tar solution 9%, menthol 1.5%. Shampoo Bot. 4 oz, 8 oz. *otc.*

Use: Antiseborrheic.

Denorex Extra Strength. (Whitehall Robins) Coal tar solution 12.5%, menthol 1.5%, alcohol 10.4%. Shampoo. Bot. 120, 240, 360 ml. *otc.*
Use: Antiseborrheic.

Denorex Mountain Fresh. (Whitehall Robins) Coal tar solution 9%, menthol 1.5%. Bot. 4 oz, 8 oz. *otc.*
Use: Antiseborrheic.

Denorex with Conditioners. (Whitehall Robins) Coal tar solution 9%, menthol 1.5%. Bot 4 oz, 8 oz. *otc.*
Use: Antiseborrheic.

Denquel. (Procter & Gamble) Potassium nitrate 5%, calcium carbonate, glycerin, flavors. Tube 1.6 oz, 3 oz, 4.5 oz. *otc.*
Use: Agent for oral hygiene, preparation for sensitive teeth.

Dental Caries Preventive. (Colgate Oral) Fluoride ion 1.2%, alumina abrasive. 2 g Box 200s, Jar 9 oz. *Rx.*
Use: Dental caries preventative.

Dentipatch. (Noven) Lidocaine 23 mg or 46.1 mg/2 cm^2 patch, aspartame/Patch. Box 50s, 100s. *Rx.*
Use: Topical anesthesia.

Dentrol. (Block) Carboxymethylcellulose, polyethelyne oxide homopolymer, peppermint and spearmint in mineral oil base. Bot. 0.9 oz, 1.8 oz. *otc.*
Use: Denture adhesive.

Dent's Dental Poultice. (C.S. Dent) Glycerin, mineral oil, polyoxyethylene sorbitan monooleate. Bot. 0.125 oz, 0.25 oz. *otc.*
Use: Dental poultice.

Dent's Ear Wax Drops. (C.S. Dent) Glycerin, mineral oil, polyoxyethylene sorbitan monooleate. Bot. 0.125 oz, 0.25 oz. *otc.*
Use: Otic preparation.

Dent's Extra Strength Toothache Gum. (C.S. Dent) Benzocaine. Box. 1 g. *otc.*
Use: Local anesthetic, oral.

Dent's Lotion-Jel. (C.S. Dent) Benzocaine in special base. Tube 0-2 oz. *otc.*
Use: Local anesthetic, oral.

Dent's Maximum Strength Toothache Drops. (C.S. Dent) Benzocaine, alcohol 74%, chlorobutanol anhydrous 0.09%. Liq. 3.7 ml. *otc.*
Use: Local anesthetic, oral.

Dent's Toothache Drops Treatment. (C.S. Dent) Alcohol 60%, chlorobutanol anhydrous (chloroform derivative) 0.09%, propylene glycol, eugenol. Bot. 0.125 oz. *otc.*

Use: Local anesthetic, oral.

Dent's Toothache Gum. (C.S. Dent) Benzocaine, eugenol, petrolatum in base of cotton and wax. Box 0.035 oz. *otc.*
Use: Local anesthetic, oral.

Denture Orajel. (Del Pharm) Benzocaine 10%, saccharin. Gel. Tube. 9.45 g. *otc.*
Use: Local anesthetic, oral.

Dent-Zel-Ite. (Last) **Oral Mucosal Analgesic:** Benzocaine 5%, alcohol, glycerin. Bot. ¹⁄₁₆ oz. **Temporary Dental Filling:** Sandarac gum, alcohol. Bot. oz. **Toothache Drops:** Eugenol 85% in alcohol. Bot. oz. *otc.*
Use: Local anesthetic, oral.

denyl sodium.
Use: Anticonvulsant.
See: Diphenylhydantoin Sodium, Cap. (Various Mfr.)

deodorizers, systemic. Chlorophyll derivatives (chlorophyllin). *otc.*
Use: **Oral:** Control of fecal and urinary odors in colostomy, ileostomy or incontinence. **Topical:** Reduce pain and inflammation (wounds, burns, surface ulcers, skin irritation).
See: Chlorophyll, Tab. (Freeda).
  Derifil, Tab. (Rystan).
  Chloresium, Tab., Soln., Oint. (Rystan).

deoxyadenosine, 2-chloro-2¹. (St. Jude Children's Hospital) *Rx.*
Use: Antineoplastic. [Orphan drug]

deoxycholic acid.
See: Desoxycholic Acid, Tab. (Various Mfr.)

2'deoxycoformycin. Pentostatin.
Use: Antibiotic, antineoplastic.
See: Nipent, Pow. (Parke-Davis).

deoxycytidine, 5-AZA-2'. (Pharmachemie U.S.A.) *Rx.*
Use: Antineoplastic. [Orphan drug]

deoxynojirmycin. (Searle) Butyl-DNJ. *Rx.*
Use: Antiviral.

Dep Gynogen. (Forest) Estradiol cypionate in cottonseed oil 5 mg/ml, cottonseed oil, chlorobutanol. Vial 10 ml. *Rx.*
Use: Estrogen.

Dep Medalone 40. (Forest) Methylprednisolone acetate in aqueous suspension 40 mg/ml, polyethylene glycol, myristyl-gamma-picolinium Cl. Vial 5 ml. *Rx.*
Use: Corticosteroid.

Dep Medalone 80. (Forest) Methylprednisolone acetate 80 mg/ml, polyethylene glycol, myristyl-gamma-pico-

linium Cl. Vial 5 ml. *Rx.*
Use: Corticosteroid.

Depacon. (Abbott) Valproic acid 5 ml (as valproic sodium)/Inj. Vial 10s. *Rx.*
Use: Anticonvulsant.

Depakene. (Abbott) Valproic acid. **Cap.:** 250 mg. Bot. 100s, UD 100s. **Syr.:** 250 mg/5 ml, sorbitol. Bot. 480 ml. *Rx.*
Use: Anticonvulsant.

Depakote. (Abbott) Divalproex sodium 125 mg, 250 mg or 500 mg/Delayed Release Tab and 125 mg/sprinkle cap. **DR Tab.:** Bot. 100s, 500s, UD 100s. **Sprinkle Cap.:** Bot. 100s, UD 100s. *Rx.*
Use: Anticonvulsant.

DepAndro 100. (Forest) Testosterone cypionate in cottonseed oil 100 mg/ml, benzyl alcohol. Vial 10 ml. *c-III.*
Use: Androgen.

DepAndro 200. (Forest) Testosterone cypionate in cottonseed oil 200 mg/ml, benzyl benzoate, benzyl alcohol. Vial 10 ml. *c-III.*
Use: Androgen.

DepAndrogyn. (Forest) Testosterone cypionate 50 mg, estradiol cypionate 2 mg/ml. Vial 10 ml. *Rx.*
Use: Androgen, estrogen combination.

Depa-Syrup. (Alra) Valproic acid syrup 250 mg/5 ml. Bot. 4 oz, 16 oz. *Rx.*
Use: Anticonvulsant.

Depen Tablets. (Wallace) Penicillamine 250 mg/Tab. Bot. 100s. *Rx.*
Use: Chelating agent.

depepsen. Amylosulfate sodium.
Use: Digestive aid.

Depoestra. (Tennessee Pharm.) Estradiol cypionate 5 mg/ml. Vial 10 ml. *Rx.*
Use: Estrogen.

Depo-Estradiol. (Pharmacia & Upjohn) Estradiol cypionate 1 mg or 5 mg/ml, chlorobutanol anhydrous 5.4 mg/ml, cottonseed oil. **1 mg/ml:** Vial 10 ml. **5 mg/ml:** Vial 5 ml. *Rx.*
Use: Estrogen.

Depogen. (Hyrex) Estradiol cypionate 5 mg/ml, cottonseed oil, chlorobutanol. Vial 10 ml. *Rx.*
Use: Estrogen.

Depoject. (Mayrand) Methylprednisolone acetate 40 mg or 80 mg/ml suspension with polyethylene glycol and myristyl-gamma-picolinium Cl. Inj. Vial 5 ml. *Rx.*
Use: Corticosteroid.

Depo-Medrol. (Pharmacia & Upjohn) Methylprednisolone acetate, 20 mg/Inj. Vial. 5 ml, 10 ml. Methylprednisolone acetate, 40 mg/Inj. Vial. 5 ml, 10 ml. Methylprednisolone acetate 80 mg/Inj.

Vial. 1 ml, 5 ml. *Rx.*
Use: Corticosteroid.

Deponit. (Schwarz Pharma Kremers Urban) Nitroglycerin transdermal delivery system containing 16 mg or 32 mg. Box 30s, 100s. *Rx.*
Use: Vasodilator, antianginal.

Depopred 40. (Hyrex) Methylprednisolone acetate suspension 40 mg/ml, polyethylene glycol, myristyl-gamma-picolinum Cl. Vial 5 ml, 10 ml. *Rx.*
Use: Corticosteroid.

Depopred 80. (Hyrex) Methylprednisolone acetate 80 mg/Inj. Vial. 5 ml. *Rx.*
Use: Corticosteroid.

Depo-Provera. (Pharmacia & Upjohn) Medroxyprogesterone acetate 400 mg/ml. Suspended in polyethylene glycol 3350 20.3 mg, sodium sulfate (anhydrous) 11 mg, myristyl-gamma-picolinium Cl 1.69 mg. Vial 2.5 ml, 10 ml, 1 ml U-Ject. *Rx.*
Use: Progestin.

Depo-Provera Contraceptive Injection. (Pharmacia & Upjohn) Medroxyprogesterone acetate 150 mg/ml, with PEG-3350 28.9 mg, polysorbate 80 2.41 mg, sodium Cl 8.68 mg, methylparaben 1.37 mg, propylparaben 0.15 mg/Inj. Vial. 1 ml. *Rx.*
Use: Contraceptive.

Depotest. (Hyrex) Testosterone cypionate. **100 mg:** With cottonseed oil, benzyl alcohol. **200 mg:** With cottonseed oil, benzyl benzoate, benzyl alcohol. Vial 10 ml. *c-III.*
Use: Androgen.

Depo-Testadiol. (Roberts) Testosterone cypionate 50 mg, estradiol cypionate 2 mg/ml. Vial 10 ml. *Rx.*
Use: Androgen estrogen combination.

Depotestogen. (Hyrex) Testosterone cypionate 50 mg, estradiol cypionate 2 mg/ml. Vial 10 ml. *Rx.*
Use: Androgen, estrogen combination.

Depo-Testosterone. (Pharmacia & Upjohn) Testosterone cypionate. **100 mg/ml:** In benzyl alcohol 9.45 mg, cottonseed oil 736 mg/ml. Vial 1 ml. **200 mg/ml:** In benzyl benzoate 0.2 ml, benzyl alcohol 9.45 mg, cottonseed oil 560 mg/ml. Vial 1 ml, 10 ml. *c-III.*
Use: Androgen.

deprenyl. Selegiline HCl.
See: Eldepryl (Somerset).

Deproist Expectorant with Codeine. (Geneva Pharm.) Pseudoephedrine HCl 30 mg, codeine phosphate 10 mg, guaifenesin 100 mg/5 ml. Bot. 120 ml, 480 ml. *c-v.*

Use: Decongestant, antitussive, expectorant.

•deprostil. (deh-PRAHST-ill) USAN.
Use: Antisecretory, gastric.

Dep-Test. (Sig) Testosterone cypionate 100 mg/ml. Vial 10 ml. *c-III.*
Use: Androgen.

Dequasine. (Miller) L-lysine 20 mg, l-cysteine 100 mg, dl-methionine 50 mg, vitamin C 200 mg, iron 5 mg, Cu, I, Mg, Mn, Zn. Tab. Bot. 100s. *otc.*
Use: Vitamin/mineral supplement.

Derifil. (Rystan) Chlorophyllin copper complex 100 mg/Tab. Bot. 30s, 100s, 1000s. *otc.*
Use: Oral deodorant.

Dermabase. (Paddock) Mineral oil, petrolatum, cetostearyl alcohol, propylene glycol, sodium lauryl sulfate, isopropyl palmitate, imidazolidinyl urea, methyl and propylparabens. Cream. Jar 1 lb. *otc.*
Use: Emollient.

Dermacoat Aerosol Spray. (Century) Benzocaine 4.5%. Bot. 7 oz. *otc.*
Use: Local anesthetic, topical.

Dermacort Cream. (Solvay) Hydrocortisone 0.5% or 1% in a water soluble cream of stearyl alcohol, cetyl alcohol, isopropyl palmitate, citric acid, polyoxyethylene 40 stearate, sodium phosphate, propylene glycol, water, benzyl alcohol, buffered to pH 5.0. 0.5% in 30 g, 1% in 1 lb. *Rx.*
Use: Corticosteroid, topical.

Dermacort Lotion. (Solvay) Hydrocortisone 1% in lotion base, buffered to pH 5.0. Paraben free. Bot. 120 ml. *Rx.*
Use: Corticosteroid, topical.

Derma-Cover. (Scrip) Sulfur, salicylic acid, hyamine 10x, isopropyl alcohol 22%, in powder film forming base. Bot. 2 oz. *otc.*
Use: Keratolytic.

Dermaflex. (Zila) Lidocaine 2.5%, alcohol 79%. Gel. Tube 15 g. *otc.*
Use: Local anesthetic, topical.

Derma-Guard. (Greer) Protective adhesive pow. Can w/sifter top, 4 oz. Spray top Bot. 4 oz, pkg. 1 lb. Rings. Pkg. 5s, 10s. *otc.*
Use: Skin protectant.

Dermal-Rub Balm. (Roberts) Menthol racemic 7%, camphor 1%, methyl salicylate 1%, cajuput oil 1%. Cream. Jar 1 oz, 1 lb. *otc.*
Use: Analgesic, topical.

Dermamycin. (Pfeiffer) Diphenhydramine HCl 2% in a base of parabens, polyeth-

ylene glycol monostearate and propylene glycol. Cream 28.35 g. *otc.*
Use: Antihistamine, topical.

Dermaneed. (Hanlon) Zirconium oxide 4.5%, calamine 6%, zinc oxide 4%, actamer 0.1% in bland lotionized base. Bot. 4 oz. *otc.*
Use: Antipruritic, topical.

Derma-Pax. (Recsei) Methapyrilene HCl 0.22%, chlorothenylpyramine maleate 0.06%, pyrilamine maleate 0.22%, benzyl alcohol 1%, chlorobutanol 1%, isopropyl alcohol 40%. Liq. 4 oz, pt. *otc.*
Use: Topical antipruritic; antihistamine, topical.

Derma-Pax HC. (Recsei) Hydrocortisone 0.5%, pyrilamine maleate 0.2%, pheniramine maleate 0.2%, chlorpheniramine 0.06%, benzyl alcohol 1%. Liq. Bot. 60 ml, 120 ml, 480 ml.
Use: Topical corticosteroid; antihistamine, topical.

Dermarest. (Del) Diphenhydramine HCl 2%, resorcinol 2%, aloe vera gel, benzalkonium chloride, EDTA, menthol, methylparaben, propylene glycol. Gel Tube 29.25 g, 56.25 g. *otc.*
Use: Antihistamine, topical.

Dermarest Dricort. (Del) Hydrocortisone 1%, white petrolatum cream. Bot. 14 g. *otc.*
Use: Corticosteroid, topical.

Dermarest Plus. (Del) **Gel:** Diphenhydramine HCl 2%, menthol 1%, aloe vera gel, benzalkonium chloride, isopropyl alcohol, methylparaben; propylene glycol. Tube 15 g, 30 g. **Spray:** Diphenhydramine HCl 2%, menthol 1%, aloe vera gel, benzalkonium chloride, methylparaben propylene glycol, SDA 40 alcohol, EDTA. Bot. 60 ml. *otc.*
Use: Antihistamine, topical.

Dermasept Antifungal. (PharmaKon) Tannic acid 6.098%, zinc Cl 5.081%, benzocaine 2.032%, methylbenzethonium HCl, tolnaftate 1.017%, undecylenic acid 5.081%, ethanol 38B 58.539%, phenol, benzyl alcohol, benzoic acid, coal tar, camphor, menthol. Liq. Bot. 30 ml. *otc.*
Use: Antifungal (topical).

Dermasil. (Chesebrough-Ponds) Glycerin and dimethicone in a base containing cyclomethicone, sunflower seed oil, petrolatum, borage seed oil, lecithin, vitamin E acetate, vitamin A palmitate, vitamin D_3, corn oil, EDTA, methylparaben. Lot. Bot. 120 ml, 240 ml. *otc.*
Use: Emollient.

Derma-Smoothe/FS Oil. (Hill) Fluocinolone acetonide 0.01%. Oil. Bot. 4 oz. *Rx.*
Use: Antipsoriatic; antiseborrheic, topical.

Derma-Smoothe Oil. (Hill) Refined peanut oil, mineral oil in lipophilic base. *otc.*
Use: Antipruritic, skin protectant.

Derma Soap. (Ferndale) Dowicil 0.1%. 4 oz w/dispenser. *otc.*
Use: Antiseptic.

Derma-Soft. (Vogarell) Medicated cream. Salicylic acid, castor oil, triethanolamine. Tube ¾ oz. *otc.*
Use: Keratolytic.

Derma-Sone 1%. (Hill) Hydrocortisone 1%, pramoxine HCl 1%, cetyl alcohol, glyceryl monosterate, isopropyl myristate, potassium sorbate, furcelleran. *otc, Rx.*
Use: Corticosteroid, local anesthetic.

Dermasorcin. (Lamond) Resorcin 2%, sulfur 5%. Bot. 1 oz, 2 oz, 4 oz, 8 oz, pt, 32 oz, 0.5 gal. *otc.*
Use: Antiacne; antiseborrheic, topical.

Dermastringe. (Lamond) Bot. 4 oz, 6 oz, 8 oz, pt, 32 oz, gal. *otc.*
Use: Skin cleanser.

Dermasul. (Lamond) Sulfur 5%. Bot. 1 oz, 2 oz, 4 oz, 8 oz, pt, 32 oz, 0.5 gal, gal. *otc.*
Use: Antiacne; antiseborrheic, topical.

Dermathyn. (Davis & Sly) Benzyl alcohol 3%, benzocaine 3.5%, butyl-p-aminobenzoate 1%, phenylmercuric borate. Tube 1 oz. *otc.*
Use: Local anesthetic, topical.

Dermatic Base. (Whorton) Compounding cream base. Bot. 16 oz.
Use: Cream and lotion base.

Dermatol.
See: Bismuth subgallate, Preps. (Various Mfr.)

Dermatop. (Hoechst Marion Roussel) Prednicarbate 0.1%, white petrolatum, lanolin alcohols, mineral oil, cetostearyl alcohol, EDTA, lactic acid. Cream 15 g, 60 g. *Rx.*
Use: Corticosteroids, topical.

Dermatophytin (trichophytin). (Bayer) Prepared from the filtrates of mixtures of 21-day maltose broth cultures of *Trichophyton mentagrophytes, T rubrum* and *T tonsurans.* Vial 5 ml (undiluted) and 5 ml (diluted 1:30).
Use: Diagnostic aid.

Dermatophytin "O" (oidiomycin). (Bayer) Prepared from the filtrate of a 21-day maltose broth culture of *Candida*

albicans (Monillia). Vials 5 ml (undiluted) and 5 ml (diluted 1:100).
Use: Diagnostic aid.

Derma Viva. (Rugby) Mineral oil, glyceryl stearate, laureth-4, lanolin oil, PEG-100 stearate, PEG-40 stearate, PEG-4 dilaurate, trolamine, diocetyl sodium sulfosuccinate, parabens. Lot. Bot. 237 ml. *otc.*
Use: Emollient.

Dermed. (Holloway) Vitamins A and D with hydrogenated vegetable oil. Cream. Tube 60 g, 120 g. *otc.*
Use: Emollient.

Dermeze. (Premo) Thenylpyramine HCl 2%, benzocaine 2%, tyrothricin 0.25 mg/g. Massage Lot. Bot. 5¾ oz. *otc.*
Use: Topical antihistamine, antibiotic, anesthetic.

Dermol HC. (Dermol) **Cream:** Hydrocortisone 1% or 2.5%. Tube 30 g. **Oint.:** Hydrocortisone 1%. Tube 30 g. *Rx.*
Use: Anorectal preparation.

Dermolate Anti-Itch. (Schering-Plough) Hydrocortisone 0.5% petrolatum, mineral oil, chlorocresol. Cream Tube 15 g, 30 g. *otc.*
Use: Corticosteroid, topical.

Dermolin. (Roberts) Menthol racemic, methyl salicylate, camphor, mustard oil, isopropyl alcohol 8%. Bot. 3 oz, pt, gal. *otc.*
Use: Liniment, topical.

Dermoplast. (Whitehall-Robins) **Spray:** Benzocaine 20%, menthol, methylparaben, aloe, lanolin. Bot. 82.5 ml. **Lot.:** Benzocaine 8%, menthol, aloe, glycerin, parabens, lanolin. Bot. 90 ml. *otc.*
Use: Topical anesthetic.

Dermovan. (Galderma) Glyceryl stearate, spermaceti, mineral oil, glycerin, cetyl alcohol, butylparaben, methylparaben, propylparaben, purified water. Vanishing-type base, Jar 1 lb. *otc.*
Use: Skin protectant.

Dermtex HC. (Pfeiffer) Hydrocortisone 0.5% in a glycerin base. Tube 15 g. *otc.*
Use: Corticosteroid, topical.

Dermuspray. (Warner-Chilcott) Trypsin 0.1 mg, Balsam Peru 72.5 mg, castor oil 650 mg/0.82 ml. Aer. Bot. 120 g. *Rx.*
Use: Topical enzyme combination.

D.E.S.
See: Diethylstilbestrol.

desacchromin. A nonprotein bacterial colloidal dispersion of polysaccharide.

•**desciclovir.** (DESS-sigh-kloe-veer) USAN.
Use: Antiviral.

•**descinolone acetonide.** (DESS-SIN-oleohn ah-SEE-toe-nide) USAN.
Use: Glucocorticoid.

Desenex. (Novartis) **Cream:** Undecylenic acid, zinc undecylenate 25%, lanolin, parabens, white petrolatum. Tube 0.5 oz, 1 oz. **Oint.:** Undecylenic acid 5%, zinc undecylenate 20%, lanolin, parabens, white petrolatum. Tube 0.9 oz, 1.8 oz, Can 1 lb. **Pow.:** Undecylenic acid 5%, zinc undecylenate 20%, talc. Can 1.5 oz, 3 oz, Carton 1 lb. **Liq.:** Undecylenic acid 10%, isopropyl alcohol 47.1%. Pump spray bot. 1.5 oz. **Spray Pow.:** Undecylenic acid 5%, zinc undecylenate 20%, menthol, talc. Aerosol can 2.7 oz, 5.5 oz. **Penetrating Foam:** Undecylenic acid 10%, isopropyl alcohol 29.2%. Can 1.5 oz. *otc.*
Use: Antifungal, topical.

Desenex Foot & Sneaker Spray. (Novartis) Aluminum chlorohydrex w/alcohol 89.3%. Aerosol can 2.7 oz. *otc.*
Use: Foot deodorant, antiperspirant.

Desenex Maximum Strength. (Medeva) Total undecylenate 25%, lanolin, parabens, white petrolatum. Oint. Tube 15 g. *otc.*
Use: Antifungal, topical.

De Serpa. (de Leon) Reserpine 0.25 mg or 0.5 mg/Tab. Bot. 100s, 500s, 1000s (0.25 mg only).
Use: Antihypertensive.

Desert Pure Calcium. (Cal-White Mineral Co.) Calcium (from calcium carbonate) 500 mg, vitamin D 125 IU. Tab. Bot. 200s. *otc.*
Use: Vitamin/mineral supplement.

Desferal. (Novartis) Deferoxamine mesylate 500 mg/5 ml. Amp. 4s. *Rx.*
Use: Antidote.

•**desflurane,** (dess-FLEW-rane) U.S.P. 23.
Use: Anesthetic.
See: Suprane (Ohmeda).

•**desipramine hydrochloride,** (dess-IPP-ruh-meen) U.S.P. 23.
Use: Antidepressant.
See: Norpramin, Tab. (Hoechst Marion Roussel).
Pertofrane, Cap. (Rhone-Poulenc Rorer).

•**desirudin.** (deh-SIHR-uh-din) USAN.
Use: Anticoagulant.

Desitin. (Pfizer) **Pow.:** Talc. Can 3 oz, 7 oz, 10 oz. **Oint.:** Cod liver oil, zinc oxide 40%, talc, petrolatum, lanolin. Tube 1 oz, 2 oz, 4 oz, 8 oz, Jar 1 lb. *otc.*
Use: Astringent, skin protectant.

Desitin with Zinc Oxide. (Pfizer) Cornstarch 88.2%, zinc oxide 10%. Pow. 28 g, 397 g. *otc.*
Use: Diaper rash product.
•**deslanoside,** U.S.P. 23.
Use: Cardiotonic.
See: Cedilanid-D (Sandoz Consumer).
•**deslorelin.** (DESS-low-REH-lin) USAN.
Use: Gonadotropin inhibitor. [Orphan drug], LHRH agonist.
See: Somagard [as acetate] (Roberts Pharmaceutical).
Desma. (Tablicaps) Diethylstilbesterol 25 mg/Tab. Patient dispenser 10s. *Rx.*
Use: Estrogen.
•**desmopressin acetate.** (DESS-moe-PRESS-in) USAN.
Use: Treatment of diabetes insipidus, mild hemophilia A and von Willebrand's disease [Orphan drug], antidiuretic.
See: Stimate (Centeon).
DDAVP, Liq. (Rhone-Poulenc Rorer).
desmopressin acetate. (Various Mfr.) Desmopressin acetate 4 mcg/ml. Inj. 1 ml, 10 ml. *Rx.*
Use: Treatment of diabetes insipidus, mild hemophilia A and von Willebrand's disease [Orphan drug].
Desogen. (Organon) Desogestrel 0.15 mg, ethinyl estradiol 0.03 mg/Tab. Pck. 28s. *Rx.*
Use: Oral contraceptive.
•**desogestrel.** (DESS-oh-JESS-trell) USAN.
Use: Progestin.
W/ Ethinyl estradiol.
See: Desogen, Tab. (Organon).
Ortho-Cept, Tab. (Ortho).
•**desonide.** (DESS-oh-nide) USAN. (Various Mfr.) Desonide 0.05%. Oint. 15 g, 60 g.
Use: Anti-inflammatory; corticosteroid, topical.
See: Tridesilon, Cream (Bayer).
desonide. (Various Mfr.) Desonide 0.05%. Oint. 15 g, 60 g.
Use: Anti-inflammatory, corticosteroid (topical).
Desonide Cream. (Galderma) Desonide 0.05% in cream base. Tube 15 g, 60 g. *Rx.*
Use: Corticosteroid, topical.
Desowen. (Galderma) Desonide 0.05%. Cream. Tube 15 g, 60 g. *Rx.*
Use: Corticosteroid, topical.
•**desoximetasone,** (dess-OX-ee-MET-ah-sone) U.S.P. 23.
Use: Corticosteroid (topical), anti-inflammatory.

See: Topicort (Hoechst Marion Roussel).
•**desoxycorticosterone acetate,** U.S.P. 23.
Use: Adrenocortical steroid (salt-regulating).
•**desoxycorticosterone pivalate,** U.S.P. 23.
Use: Adrenocortical steroid (salt-regulating).
desoxycorticosterone pivalate injectable suspension.
Use: Adrenocortical steroid (salt-regulating).
desoxycorticosterone trimethylacetate, U.S.P. XVI.
Use: Adrenocortical steroid (salt-regulating).
desoxyephedrine hydrochloride. (Various Mfr.) *c-ii.*
Use: CNS stimulant.
See: Methamphetamine HCl, Prep.
Desoxyn. (Abbott) Methamphetamine HCl. **Tab.:** 5 mg. Bot. 100s. **Gradumets:** 5 mg. Bot. 100s; 10 mg. Bot. 100s; 15 mg. Bot. 100s. *c-ii.*
Use: CNS stimulant.
desoxy norephedrine.
Use: CNS stimulant.
See: Amphetamine HCl, Preps. (Various Mfr.)
desoxyribonuclease.
W/Fibrinolysin.
Use: Topical enzyme preparation.
See: Elase, prep. (Parke-Davis).
Desquam-E 2, 5, & 10. (Westwood Squibb) Benzoyl peroxide 2.5%, 5% or 10%. Gel. Tube 42.5 g. *Rx.*
Use: Antiacne.
Desquam-X 5% or 10% Gel. (Westwood Squibb) Benzoyl peroxide 5% or 10%, water base with EDTA. Tube 42.5 ml; 85 g (5% only). *Rx.*
Use: Antiacne.
Desquam-X 5% or 10% Wash. (Westwood Squibb) Benzoyl peroxide 5% or 10%, EDTA. Bot. 150 ml. *Rx.*
Use: Antiacne.
D-Est. (Burgin-Arden) Estradiol cypionate 5 mg/ml. Vial 10 ml. *Rx.*
Use: Estrogen.
De-Stat. (Sherman) Surfactant cleaner, benzalkonium Cl 0.01%, EDTA 0.25%. Soln. Bot. 118 ml. *otc.*
Use: Hard contact lens care.
De-Stat 3. (Sherman) Octylphenoxypolyethoxyethanol, benzyl alcohol 0.1%, EDTA 0.5%, lauryl sulfate salt of imidazoline. Soln. Bot. 118 ml. *otc.*

Use: Hard contact lens care.

De-Stat 4. (Sherman) Benzyl alcohol 0.3%, EDTA 0.5%, lauryl sulfate, salt of imidazole, octylphenoxypolyethoxyethanol. Thimerosol free. Soln. Bot. 118 ml. *otc.*
Use: Rigid gas permeable contact lens care.

Desyrel. (Bristol-Myers) Trazodone HCl 50 mg or 100 mg. **50 mg:** Bot. 100s, 1000s, UD 100s. **100 mg:** Bot. 500s. *Rx.*
Use: Antidepressant.

Desyrel Dividose. (Bristol-Myers) Trazodone HCl 150 mg or 300 mg/Dividose tab. Dividose design breakable into fragments for dosing convenience. Bot. 100s, 500s (150 mg). *Rx.*
Use: Antidepressant.

Detachol. (Ferndale) Bland, nonirritating liquid for removing adhesive tape. Pkg. 4 oz.
Use: Adhesive remover.

De Tal. (de Leon) Phenobarbital 0.25 gr, hyoscyamine sulfate 0.1037 mg, atropine sulfate 0.0194 mg, hyoscine HBr 0.0065 mg/Tab. or 5 ml. **Tab.:** Bot. 100s. **Elix.:** With alcohol 20%. Bot. pt. *Rx.*
Use: Sedative, hypnotic, anticholinergic, antispasmodic.

Detane. (Del Pharmaceuticals) Benzocaine 7.5%. Tube 0.5 oz. *otc.*
Use: Local anesthetic, topical.

●**deterenol hydrochloride.** (dee-TEER-eh-nahl) USAN.
Use: Adrenergic (ophthalmic).

detergents, surface-active.
See: pHisoDerm, Liq. (Sanofi Winthrop).
pHisoHex, Liq. (Sanofi Winthrop).
Zephiran, Prods. (Sanofi Winthrop).

detigon hydrochloride.
See: Chlophedianol HCl (Various Mfr.)

●**detirelix acetate.** (DEH-tih-RELL-ix)
Use: Antagonist (LHRH).

●**detomidine hydrochloride.** USAN.
Use: Sedative, hypnotic.

Detuss. (Various Mfr.) Phenylpropanolamine HCl 75 mg and caramiphen edisylate 40 mg/TR Cap. Bot. 100s, 500s, 1000s. *otc.*
Use: Decongestant, antitussive.

Detussin Expectorant Liquid. (Various Mfr.) Pseudoephedrine HCl 60 mg, hydrocodone bitartrate 5 mg, guaifenesin 200 mg, alcohol. Liq. Bot. 480 ml. *c-III.*
Use: Decongestant, antitussive, expectorant.

Detussin Liquid. (Various Mfr.) Pseudoephedrine HCl 60 mg, hydrocodone bitartrate 5 mg. Liq. Bot. Pt, Gal. *c-III.*
Use: Decongestant, antitussive.

●**deuterium oxide.** USAN.
Use: Radioactive agent.

●**devazepide.** (dev-AZE-eh-PIDE) USAN.
Use: Antispasmodic, gastrointestinal; antagonist (cholecystokinin).

Devrom. (Parthenon). Bismuth subgallate 200 mg, lactose, sugar/chew. tab. Bot. 100s. *otc.*
Use: Systemic deodorizer.

Dex 4 Glucose. (Can-Am Care) Glucose. Tab. Bot. 10s, 50s. *otc.*
Use: Glucose-elevating agent.

Dexacidin Ointment. (Ciba Vision) Neomycin sulfate 0.35%, dexamethasone 0.1% polymyxin B sulfate 10,000 units. Tube 3.5 g. *Rx.*
Use: Anti-infective, corticosteroid, ophthalmic.

Dexacidin Ophthalmic Suspension. (Ciba Vision) Neomycin 0.35%, polymyxin B sulfate 10,000 units, dexamethasone 1%. Bot. 5 ml. *Rx.*
Use: Anti-infective, corticosteroid, ophthalmic.

Dexacort Phosphate in Turbinaire. (Adams) Dexamethasone sodium phosphate 0.1 mg equivalent to dexamethasone 0.084 mg w/fluorochlorohydrocarbons as propellants and alcohol 2%. Aerosol w/nasal applicator. Container 170 sprays; refill package without nasal applicator.
Use: Nasal corticosteroid.

Dexacort Phosphate Respihaler. (Adams) Dexamethasone sodium phosphate equivalent to 0.1 mg dexamethasone phosphate (approximately 0.084 mg dexamethasone) w/fluorochlorohydrocarbons as propellants, alcohol 2%. Aerosol for oral inhalation, 170 sprays in 12.6 g pressurized container.
Use: Bronchodilator.

Dex-a-Diet Caffeine Free. (Columbia) Phenylpropanolamine HCl 75 mg/Cap. or Capl. Pkg. 3s, 6s, 20s, 40s.
Use: Diet aid.

Dex-a-Diet Original Formula. (Columbia) Phenylpropanolamine HCl 75 mg, ascorbic acid 200 mg/Cap. Pkg. 3s, 6s, 10s, 24s, 48s.
Use: Diet aid.

Dexafed. (Mallard) Phenylephrine HCl 5 mg, dextromethorphan HBr 10 mg, guaifenesin 100 mg/5 ml. Syr. Bot. 120 ml. *otc.*

Use: Decongestant, antitussive, expectorant.

Dexameth. (Major) **Tab.:** Dexamethasone 0.25 mg, 0.5 mg, 0.75 mg, 1.5 mg or 4 mg. Bot. 100s (0.25 mg, 0.5 mg, 1.5 mg); Bot. 100s, 1000s, Unipak 12s (0.75 mg); Bot. 50s, 100s (4 mg). **Elix.:** 0.5 mg/5 ml, alcohol 5%. Bot. 100 ml, 240 ml. *Rx.*
Use: Corticosteroid.

•**dexamethasone,** (DEX-uh-METH-uh-sone) U.S.P. 23.
Use: Adrenal corticosteroid (anti-inflammatory), glucocorticoid.
See: Aeroseb-Dex, Aerosol (Allergan Herbert).
Decaderm in Estergel (Merck).
Decadron, Tab., Elix. (Merck).
Decameth, Inj. (Foy).
Decameth L.A., Inj. (Foy).
Decaspray, Aerosol (Merck).
Dexaport, Tab. (Freeport).
Dexone TM, Tab. (Solvay).
Dezone, Tab. (Solvay).
Hexadrol, Tab., Elix., Cream (Organon).
Maxidex Ophth. Liq. (Alcon).
W/Neomycin sulfate.
See: NeoDecadron, Prep. (Merck)
NeoDecaspray, Aerosol (Merck).
W/Neomycin sulfate, polymyxin B sulfate.
See: Maxitrol Ophth. Susp., Oint. (Alcon).

dexamethasone. (Steris) 0.1%. Susp. Bot. 5 ml. *Rx.*
Use: Corticosteroid, ophthalmic.

•**dexamethasone acefurate,** (DEX-ah-METH-ah-sone ASS-eh-fer-ate) USAN.
Use: Anti-inflammatory, topical steroid.

•**dexamethasone acetate,** (DEX-ah-METH-ah-sone) U.S.P. 23.
Use: Adrenocortical steroid (anti-inflammatory).
See: Dalalone (Forest).
Decadronal (Merck)
Dexone LA, Ind. (Kay).

•**dexamethasone dipropionate.** (DEX-ah-METH-ah-sone die-PRO-pee-oh-nate) USAN.
Use: Anti-inflammatory, steroid.

Dexamethasone Intensol Oral Solution. (Roxane) Dexamethasone 1 mg/ml concentrated oral soln. Bot. 30 ml w/calibrated dropper. *Rx.*
Use: Corticosteroid.

dexamethasone ophthalmic. (Various Mfr.) Dexamethasone 0.1%. Susp. Bot. 5 ml. *Rx.*
Use: Corticosteroid.

•**dexamethasone sodium phosphate,** U.S.P. 23.
Use: Adrenocortical steroid (anti-inflammatory), glucocorticoid.
See: AK-Dex, Soln., Oint. (Akorn).
Dalalone (Forest).
Decadron Phosphate, Preps. (Merck).
Decadron Phosphate Respihaler (Merck).
Decaject, Vial (Mayrand).
Decameth, Inj. (Foy).
Dexone, Inj. (Keene, Hauck).
Dezone, Inj. (Solvay).
Hexadrol Phosphate, Inj. (Organon).
Maxidex, Oint. (Alcon).
Savacort D, Inj. (Savage).
Solurex, Inj. (Hyrex).
W/Lidocaine (Xylocaine).
See: Decadron Phosphate w/Xylocaine, Inj. (Merck).
W/Neomycin sulfate.
See: NeoDecadron, Prods. (Merck).
W/Neomycin and polymyxin B sulfates.
See: Dexacidin, Prods. (Ciba Vision).

dexamethasone sodium phosphate. (Various Mfr.) **Soln.:** 0.1%. Bot. 5 ml; **Oint.:** 0.05%. Tube 3.5 g.
Use: Adrenocortical steroid (anti-inflammatory), glucocorticoid.

•**dexamisole.** (DEX-AM-ih-sole) USAN.
Use: Antidepressant.

dexamphetamine.
See: Dextroamphetamine (Various Mfr.)

Dexaphen SA Tablets. (Major) Pseudo-ephedrine sulfate 120 mg, dex-brompheniramine maleate 6 mg. In 100s, 500s. *Rx.*
Use: Decongestant, antihistamine.

Dexaport. (Freeport) Dexamethasone 0.75 mg/Tab. Bot. 1000s. *Rx.*
Use: Corticosteroid.

Dexasone. (Various Mfr.) Dexamethasone sodium phosphate 4 mg/ml, methyl and propyl parabens, sodium bisulfite. Vial 5 ml, 10 ml, 30 ml. *Rx.*
Use: Corticosteroid.

Dexasone Injection. (Roberts) Dexamethasone sodium phosphate 4 mg/ml. Vial 5 ml, 30 ml. *Rx.*
Use: Corticosteroid.

Dexasone-L.A. Injection. (Roberts) Dexamethasone acetate 8 mg/ml. Vial 5 ml. *Rx.*
Use: Corticosteroid.

Dexasporin Ointment. (Bausch & Lomb) Dexamethasone 0.1%, neomycin sulfate equivalent to 0.35% neomycin base and 10,000 units polymyxin B sulfate. Ophth. Oint. Tube 3.5 g. *Rx.*
Use: Steroid, antibiotic (ophthalmic).

Dexasporin Suspension. (Various Mfr.) Dexamethasone 0.1%, neomycin sulfate equivalent to 0.35%, neomycin base and 10,000 units polymyxin B sulfate/ml, hydroxypropyl methylcellulose, polysorbate 20, benzalkonium chloride. Drops. Bot. 5 ml. *Rx.*
Use: Corticosteroid, anti-infective, ophthalmic.

Dexatrim-15. (Thompson) Phenylpropanolamine HCl 75 mg/TR Cap. Bot. 20s, 40s. *otc.*
Use: Nonprescription diet aid.

Dexatrim-15 w/Vitamin C. (Thompson) Phenylpropanolamine HCl 75 mg, vitamin C 180 mg/TR Cap. Bot. 20s. *otc.*
Use: Nonprescription diet aid.

Dexatrim Maximum Strength. (Thompson) Phenylpropanolamine HCl 75 mg/Tab. ER Bot. 20s. *otc.*
Use: Nonprescription diet aid.

Dexatrim Plus Vitamins. (Thompson)
TR Caplets: Phenylpropanolamine 75 mg, vitamin C 60 mg, lactose.
Caplets: Vitamin A 5000 IU, E 30 IU, C 60 mg, K_1 25 mg, folic acid 0.4 mg, B_1 1.5 mg, B_2 1.7 mg, B_3 20 mg, B_5 10 mg, B_6 2 mg, B_{12} 6 mcg, D 400 IU, biotin 30 mcg, Ca 162 mg, P, I, Fe 18 mg, Mg, Cu, Zn 15 mg, Mn, K 40 mg, Cl 36.3 mg, Cr, Mo, Se, Ni, Sn, Si, V, B. Pkg. 14s/14s, 28s/28s. *otc.*
Use: Nonprescription diet aid, vitamin/mineral supplement.

Dexatrim Pre-Meal. (Thompson) Phenylpropanolamine HCl 25 mg/TR Cap. Bot. 30s. *otc.*
Use: Nonprescription diet aid.

•**dexbrompheniramine maleate,** U.S.P. 23.
Use: Antihistamine.
W/Pseudoephedrine sulfate.
See: Disophrol Chronotab, Tab. (Schering-Plough).
Drixoral S.A., Tab. (Schering-Plough).

Dexchlor. (Schein) Dexchlorpheniramine maleate 4 mg/RA Tab. Bot. 100s. *Rx.*
Use: Antihistamine.

•**dexchlorpheniramine maleate,** U.S.P. 23.
Use: Antihistamine.
See: Polaramine, Repetabs Tab., Tab., Syr. (Schering-Plough).
W/Pseudoephedrine sulfate, guaifenesin, alcohol.
See: Polaramine Expectorant (Schering-Plough).

•**dexclamol hydrochloride.** (DEX-claymahl) USAN.
Use: Sedative, hypnotic.

Dexedrine. (SK-Beecham) Dextroamphetamine sulfate. **Tab.:** 5 mg Bot. 100s, 1000s. **Spansule:** 5 mg Bot. 50s; 10 mg, 15 mg Bot. 50s, 500s. *c-ii.*
Use: CNS stimulant.

•**dexetimide.** (dex-ETT-ih-mid) USAN.
Use: Treatment of Parkinson's disease, anticholinergic.

•**dexfenfluramine hydrochloride.** (DEX-fen-FLURE-ah-meen) USAN.
Use: Appetite suppressant (systemic).
See: Redux, Cap. (Wyeth-Ayerst).

DexFerrum. (American Regent) Elemental iron 50 mg/ml (as dextran)/Inj. Vial. 2 ml (single dose). *Rx.*
Use: Iron deficiency.

•**dexibuprofen lysine.** (dex-EYE-byoo-PRO-fen LIE-seen) USAN.
Use: Anti-inflammatory, analgesic (cyclooxygenase inhibitor).

•**deximafen.** (dex-IH-mah-fen) USAN.
Use: Antidepressant.

•**dexivacaine.** (dex-IH-vah-CANE) USAN.
Use: Anesthetic.

•**dexmedetomidine.** (DEX-meh-dih-TOE-mih-deen) USAN.
Use: Tranquilizer.

Dexone. (Solvay) Dexamethasone 0.5 mg, 0.75 mg, 1.5 mg or 4 mg/Tab. Bot. 100s, UD 100s. Box 1s, 10s, 150s. *Rx.*
Use: Corticosteroid.

Dexone. (Roberts) Dexamethasone sodium phosphate 4 mg/ml. Amp. 5 ml. *Rx.*
Use: Corticosteroid.

Dexone. (Keene) Dexamethasone sodium phosphate 4 mg/ml, methyl and propyl parabens, sodium bisulfite. Vial 5 ml, 10 ml. *Rx.*
Use: Corticosteroid.

Dexone L.A. (Keene) Dexamethasone acetate suspension equivalent to dexamethasone 8 mg, polysorbate 80, carboxymethylcellulose, sodium bisulfite, EDTA, benzyl alcohol. Vial 5 ml. *Rx.*
Use: Corticosteroid.

•**dexormaplatin.** (DEX-ore-mah-PLAT-in) USAN.
Use: Antineoplastic.

•**dexoxadrol hydrochloride.** (dex-OX-ah-drole) USAN.
Use: Antidepressant; stimulant (central); analgesic.

•**dexpanthenol,** (DEX-PAN-theh-nahl) U.S.P. 23. Preparation, U.S.P. 23.
Use: Treatment of paralytic ileus and postoperative distention, cholinergic.
See: Ilopan, Inj. (Pharmacia & Upjohn).
Panthoderm (Rhone-Poulenc Rorer).

dexpanthenol with choline bitartrate.
See: Ilopan-choline (Pharmacia & Upjohn).

•**dexpemedolac.** USAN.
Use: Analgesic.

•**dexpropanolol hydrochloride.** (DEXpro-PRAN-oh-lole) USAN.
Use: Cardiac depressant (antiarrhythmic); anti-adrenergic (β-receptor).

•**dexrazoxane.** (dex-ray-ZOX-ane) USAN.
Use: Cardioprotectant. [Orphan drug]
See: Zinecard, Pow. for Inj., (Pharmacia & Upjohn).

•**dexsotalol hydrochloride.** (DEX-ah-tahlahl) USAN
Use: Cardiac depressant (antiarrhythmic).

dextran 1.
See: Promit (Pharmacia & Upjohn).

dextran 6%. (Abbott). Rx.
See: Dextran 75, I.V. (Abbott).

•**dextran 40.** USAN. Polysaccharide (m.w. 40,000) produced by the action of Leuconostoc mesenteroides on saccharose.
Use: Blood flow adjuvant, plasma volume extender.
See: Gentran 40 (Baxter Healthcare).
Rheomacrodex (Medisan)
10% LMD, Inj. (Abbott).

dextran 40. (McGaw) Dextran 40 10% with 0.9% sodium chloride or in 5% dextrose. Inj. 500 ml. Rx.
Use: Plasma expander.

dextran 45, 75. Polysaccharide (m.w. 45,000, 75,000) produced by the action of Leuconostoc mesenteroides on saccharose. Rheotran (45). Rx.
Use: Blood volume expander.

•**dextran 70.** (DEX-tran 70) USAN. A polysaccharide.
Use: Plasma volume extender.
See: Aquasite (Ciba Vision).
Dextran 70, Inj. (McGaw).
Gentran 70, Inj. (Baxter).
Hyskon (Kabi Pharmacia & Upjohn).
Macrodex (Medisan).

dextran 70. (DEX-tran 70) (McGaw) Dextran 70 6% in 0.9% sodium chloride. Inj. 500 ml. Rx.
Use: Plasma expander.

•**dextran 75.** USAN. Dextran 75 6% in 0.9% saline. Flask 500 ml; Dextran 75 6% in 5% dextrose. Flask 500 ml.
Use: Plasma volume extender.
See: Dextran 75, Inj. (Abbott).
Macrodex, Inj. (Medisan).

dextran 75. (Abbott) Dextran 75 6% in 0.9% sodium chloride or 5% dextrose. Inj. 500 ml. Rx.

Use: Plasma expander.

dextran adjunct. Rx.
Use: Plasma expander.
See: Promit, Inj. (Pharmacia & Upjohn).

dextran and deferoxamine. Rx.
Use: Acute iron poisoning. [Orphan drug]

dextran sulfate. Rx.
Use: Antiviral. [Orphan drug]
See: Uendex (Ueno Fine Chem Industry Ltd.)

dextran sulfate sodium.
Use: AIDS drug. [Orphan drug]

•**dextrates,** (DEX-traytz) N.F. 18. Mixture of sugars (approximately 92% dextrose monohydrate and 8% higher saccharides; dextrose equivalent is 95 to 97%) resulting from the controlled enzymatic hydrolysis of starch.
Use: Pharmaceutic aid (tablet binder and diluent).

•**dextrin,** N.F. 18.
Use: Pharmaceutic aid (suspending and viscosity-increasing agent, tablet binder, tablet and capsule diluent).

•**dextroamphetamine.** (DEX-troe-am-FET-ah-meen) USAN.
Use: Stimulant (central).

dextroamphetamine with amphetamine as resin complex.
See: Biphetamine 12.5, 20, Cap. (Medeva).

dextroamphetamine phosphate. Monobasic d-a-methylphenethlyamine phosphate. (+)-α-Methylphenethylamine phosphate.
Use: CNS stimulant.
See: d-Amphetamine phosphate combinations.

•**dextroamphetamine sulfate.** (DEX-troe-am-FET-uh-meen) U.S.P. 23.
Use: CNS stimulant.
See: Dexampex, Cap., Tab. (Lemmon).
Dexedrine, Preps. (SK-Beecham).
Diphylets, Granucaps (Solvay).
Tidex Tab. (Allison).

dextroamphetamine sulfate w/combinations.
Use: CNS stimulant.
See: Amphodex, Cap. (Jamieson-McKames).
Delcobese (Delco).
Min-Gera, Tab. (Scrip).
Trimex, Trimex #2, Cap. (Mills).

Dextro-Check Normal Control. (Bayer) Clear liquid containing measured amount of glucose 0.10% w/v.
Use: Perform check of Glucometer re-

fluctance photometer or Dextrometer refluctance photometer using Dextrostix and Glucometer II Blood Glucose Meter using Glucostix.

Dextro-Chek Calibrators. (Bayer) Clear liquid soln. containing measured amounts of glucose. Low calibrator contains 0.05% w/v glucose. High calibrator contains 0.30% w/v glucose. *Use:* Dextrostix to perform calibration procedure for Glucometer reflectance photometer.

Dextro-Chlorpheniramine Maleate.
Use: Antihistamine.
See: Polaramine, Repetab, Tab., Expect., Syr. (Schering-Plough).

•**dextromethorphan,** (DEX-troe-meth-OR-fan) U.S.P. 23.
Use: Cough suppressant, antitussive.

•**dextromethorphan hydrobromide,** (DEX-troe-meth-OR-fan HIGH-droe-BROE-mide) U.S.P. 23.
Use: Antitussive.
See: Benylin DM Cough Syr. (Parke-Davis).
Delsym, Liq. (Medeva).
Mediquell, Tab. (Warner-Lambert).
St. Joseph Cough Syr. (Schering-Plough).
Symptom 1, Liq. (Parke-Davis).
Tus-F, Liq. (Orbit).
Tussade Tab. (Westerfield).
W/Benzocaine, menthol, peppermint oil.
See: Vicks Formula 44 Cough Control Discs, Loz. (Procter & Gamble).

dextromethorphan hydrobromide w/ benzocaine.
Use: Nonnarcotic antitussives.
See: Spec-T, Loz. (Apothecon).
Vicks Formula 44 Cough Control Discs, Loz. (Procter & Gamble)
Vicks Cough Silencers, Loz. (Procter & Gamble)

dextromethorphan hydrobromide w/ combinations.
See: Ambenyl-D, Liq. (Hoechst Marion Roussel).
Anatuss DM, Syr., Tab. (Mayrand).
Anti-Tuss D.M., Liq. (Century).
Anti-Tussive, Tab. (Canright).
Bayer Prods. (Bayer).
Breacol Cough Medication, Liq. (Bayer).
Capahist-DMH, Cap. (Freeport).
Centuss, MLT, Tab. (Century).
Cerose-DM, Liq. (Wyeth-Ayerst).
Cheracol-D, Cough Syr. (Upjohn).
Cheratussin, Cough Syr. (Towne).
Chexit, Tab. (Sandoz Consumer).
Children's Hold 4-Hour Cough Sup-

pressant & Decongestant, Loz. (SK-Beecham).
Codimal DM, Liq. (Schwarz Pharma).
Colrex, Syr. (Solvay).
Comtrex, Cap., Liq. Tab. (Bristol-Myers).
Congespirin Cough Syrup (Bristol-Myers).
Contac Jr., Liq. (SK-Beecham).
Coricidin Children's Cough Syrup (Schering-Plough).
Dimacol, Cap. (Robins).
Donatussin, Syr. (Laser).
Dorcol Ped. Cough Syr. (Sandoz Consumer).
Dristan Cough Formula, Syr. (Whitehall Robins).
End-A-Koff, Jr. Syr. (Quality Generics).
Formula 44 Prods. (Procter & Gamble).
Halls Mentho-Lyptus Decongestant Cough Formula, Liq. (Warner-Lambert).
Histalets, DM, Syr. (Reid Provident).
Infantuss, Liq. (Scott/Cord).
Mapap CF, Tab. (Major).
Maximum Strength Tylenol Flu, Tab. (McNeil-CPC).
Niltuss, Syr. (Minn. Pharm.)
Nyquil, Liq. (Procter & Gamble).
Orthoxicol, Syr. (Pharmacia & Upjohn).
Partuss, Liq. (Parmed).
Phenergan, Pediatric, Liq. (Wyeth-Ayerst).
Polytuss-DM, Liq. (Rhode).
Rentuss, Tab., Syr. (Wren).
Rentuss, Tab. (Wren).
Robitussin-DM, Syr., Loz. (Robins).
Robitussin Cold & Cough, Cap. (Robins).
Robitussin-CF (Robins).
Rondec DM, Drops, Syr. (Ross).
Scotcof Liq. (Scott/Cord).
Scotuss, Pediatric Cough Syr. (Scott/Cord).
Shertus, Liq. (Sheryl).
Sorbase Cough Syr. (Fort David).
Spec-T Sore Throat-Cough Suppressant Loz. (Squibb).
Sudafed Cough Syr. (Glaxo Wellcome).
Synatuss-One, Liq. (Freeport).
Thor, Cough Syr. (Towne).
Tolu-Sed DM, Liq. (Scherer).
Tonecol, Syr., Tab. (A.V.P.).
Triaminic-DM Cough Formula (Sandoz, Consumer).
Triaminicol, Syr. (Sandoz, Consumer).
Trind-DM, Syr. (Bristol-Myers).

Tusquelin, Syr. (Circle).
Tussagesic, Tab., Susp. (Sandoz,
Consumer).
Unproco, Cap. (Solvay).
Vicks Cough Prods. (Procter &
Gamble).
Vicks Daycare, Liq. (Procter &
Gamble).
Vicks Formula 44 Prods. (Procter &
Gamble).
Vicks Nyquil, Liq. (Procter & Gamble).
Wal-Tussin DM, Syr. (Walgreen).
• **dextromethorphan polistirex.** (DEX-
troe-meth-OR-fan pahl-ee-STIE-rex)
USAN.
Use: Antitussive.
dextromoramide tartrate.
Use: Narcotic analgesic.
dextro-pantothenyl alcohol.
See: Panthenol (Various Mfr.)
Ilopan (Pharmacia & Upjohn).
dextropropoxyphene hydrochloride.
c-iv.
Use: Analgesic.
See: Propoxyphene HCl, Cap. (Various
Mfr.)
• **dextrorphan hydrochloride.** (DEX-trore-
fan) USAN.
Use: Treatment of cerebral ischemia.
• **dextrose,** U.S.P. 23.
Use: Fluid and nutrient replenisher.
W/Calcium ascorbate and benzyl alcohol
injection
See: Calscorbate, Amp. (Cole).
W/Psyllium mucilloid.
See: V-lax, Pow. (Century).
Dextrose 5% and Electrolyte #48. (Bax-
ter) Dextrose 50 g, calories 180/L with
Na^+ 25 mEq, K^+ 20 mEq, Mg^{++} 3 mEq,
Cl^- 24 mEq, phosphate 3 mEq, acetate
23 mEq with osmolarity 348 mOsm/
L. Soln. Bot. 250 ml, 500 ml, 1000 ml.
Rx.
Use: Parenteral nutritional supplement.
Dextrose 5% and Electrolyte #75. (Bax-
ter) Dextrose 50 g, calories 180/L with
Na^+ 40 mEq, K^+ 35 mEq, Cl^- 48 mEq,
phosphate 15 mEq and lactate 20 mEq
with osmolarity 402 mOsm/L. Soln.
Bot. 250 ml, 500 ml, 1000 ml. *Rx.*
Use: Parenteral nutritional supplement.
dextrose-alcohol injection. *Rx.*
Use: Parenteral nutritional supplement.
See: 5% alcohol and 5% dextrose in
water (Abbott, Baxter, Kendall Mc-
Gaw)
dextrose-electrolyte solution. *Rx.*
Dextrose 2.5% w/0.45% sodium chloride (Various Mfr.) Soln. 250, 500,
1000 ml.

Dextrose 5% w/0.11% sodium chloride (Kendal McGaw). Soln. 500,
1000 ml.
Dextrose 5% w/0.2% sodium chloride
(Various Mfr.) Soln. 250, 500, 1000
ml.
Dextrose 5% w/0.33% sodium chlor-
ide (Various Mfr.) Soln. 250, 500,
1000 ml.
Dextrose 5% w/0.45% sodium chlor-
ide (Various Mfr.) Soln. 250, 500,
1000 ml.
Dextrose 5% w/0.9% sodium chloride
(Various Mfr.) Soln. 250, 500, 1000
ml.
Dextrose 10% w/0.45% sodium chlor-
ide (McGaw). Soln. 1000 ml.
Dextrose 10% w/0.9% sodium chlor-
ide (Various Mfr.) Soln. 500, 1000
ml.
Potassium chloride 0.075% in D-5-W
(Baxter). Soln. 1000 ml.
Potassium chloride 0.15% in D-5-W
(Various Mfr.) Soln. 1000 ml.
Potassium chloride 0.224% in D-5-W
(Various Mfr.) Soln. 1000 ml.
Potassium chloride 0.3% in D-5-W
(Various Mfr.) Soln. 500, 1000 ml.
0.075% potassium chloride in 5% dextrose and 0.2% sodium chloride
(Various Mfr.) Soln. 1000 ml.
0.15% potassium chloride in 5% dextrose and 0.2% sodium chloride
(Various Mfr.) Soln. 250, 500, 1000
ml.
0.224% potassium chloride in 5% dextrose and 0.2% sodium chloride
(Various Mfr.) Soln. 1000 ml.
0.3% potassium chloride in 5% dextrose and 0.2% sodium chloride
(Various Mfr.) Soln. 1000 ml.
0.15% potassium chloride in 5% dextrose and 0.33% sodium chloride
(Baxter). Soln. 500, 1000 ml.
0.224% potassium chloride in 5% dextrose and 0.33% sodium chloride
(Baxter). Soln. 1000 ml.
0.3% potassium chloride in 5% dextrose and 0.33% sodium chloride
(Various Mfr.) Soln. 1000 ml.
0.075% potassium chloride in 5% dextrose and 0.45% sodium chloride
(Various Mfr.) Soln. 1000 ml.
0.15% potassium chloride in 5% dextrose and 0.45% sodium chloride
(Various Mfr.) Soln. 500, 1000 ml.
0.224% potassium chloride in 5% dextrose and 0.45% sodium chloride
(Various Mfr.) Soln. 1000 ml.
0.3% potassium chloride in 5% dextrose and 0.45% sodium chloride

(Various Mfr.) Soln. 1000 ml.

0.15% potassium chloride in 5% dextrose and 0.9% sodium chloride (Baxter). Soln. 1000 ml.

0.3% potassium chloride in 5% dextrose and 0.9% sodium chloride (Baxter). Soln. 1000 ml.

Isolyte G with 5% dextrose (McGaw) 70 mEq NH_4+. Soln. 1000 ml.

Isolyte G with 10% dextrose (McGaw) 70 mEq NH_4+. Soln. 1000 ml.

5% dextrose and electrolyte #75 (Baxter). Soln. 250, 500, 1000 ml.

Ionosol T and 5% dextrose (Abbott). Soln. 250, 500, 1000 ml.

Isolyte M and 5% dextrose (McGaw). Soln. 1000 ml.

Dextrose 5% in Ringer's (Various Mfr.) Soln. 500, 1000 ml.

Dextrose 2.5% in half-strength lactated Ringer's (Various Mfr.) Soln. 250, 500, 1000 ml.

Dextrose 5% in lactated Ringer's (Various Mfr.) Soln. 250, 500, 1000 ml.

5% dextrose and electrolyte #48 (Baxter). Soln. 250, 500, 1000 ml.

Ionosol MB and 5% dextrose (Abbott). Soln. 250, 500, 1000 ml.

Ionosol B and 5% dextrose (Abbott). Soln. 500, 1000.

Isolyte H with 5% dextrose (McGaw). Soln. 1000 ml.

Normosol-M and 5% dextrose (Abbott). Soln. 500, 1000.

Plasma-Lyte 56 and 5% dextrose (Baxter). Soln. 500, 1000.

Isolyte P with 5% dextrose (McGaw). Soln. 250, 500, 1000.

Isolyte S with 5% dextrose (McGaw). 23 mEq gluconate. Soln. 1000 ml.

Normosol-R and 5% dextrose (Abbott). 23 mEq gluconate. Soln. 500, 1000 ml.

Plasma-Lyte 148 and 5% dextrose (Baxter). 23 mEq gluconate. Soln. 500, 1000 ml.

Ionosol MB and 10% dextrose (Abbott). Soln. 500 ml.

10% dextrose with electrolytes (Abbott). Soln. 21 mEq gluconate. Soln. 500 ml in 1000 ml partial fill container.

10% dextrose and electrolyte no. 48 injection (Baxter). Soln. 250 ml.

Isolyte R with 5% dextrose (McGaw). Soln. 1000 ml.

Plasma-Lyte M and 5% dextrose (Baxter). Soln. 500, 1000 ml.

Plasma-Lyte R and 5% dextrose (Baxter). Soln. 1000 ml.

Isolyte E with 5% dextrose (McGaw). 8 mEq citrate. Soln. 1000 ml. Use: Parenteral nutritional supplement.

•dextrose excipient, N.F. 18. *Use:* Pharmaceutic aid (tablet excipient).

50% Dextrose with Electrolyte Pattern A. (McGaw) Dextrose 500 g/L, calories 1700 cal/L, Na^+ 84 mEq, K^+ 40 mEq, Ca^{++} 10 mEq, Mg^{++} 16 mEq, Cl^- 115 mEq, osmolarity 2,800 mOsm/L, sulfate 16 mEq, gluconate 13 mEq. Soln. 500 ml in 1000 ml partial fill container. *Rx.* Use: Parenteral nutritional supplement.

50% Dextrose with Electrolyte Pattern B. (McGaw) Dextrose 500 g/L, calories 1700 cal/L, Na^+ 32 mEq, Ca^{++} 9 mEq, Mg^{++} 16 mEq, Cl^- 32 mEq, osmolarity 2,615 mOsm/L, sulfate 16 mEq, gluconate 4.2 mEq. Soln. 500 ml in 1000 ml partial fill container. *Rx.* Use: Parenteral nutritional supplement.

50% Dextrose with Electrolyte Pattern N. (McGaw) Dextrose 500 g/L, calories 1,700 cal/L, Na^+ 90 mEq, K^+ 80 mEq, Mg^{++} 16 mEq, Cl^- 150 mEq, phosphate 28 mEq, osmolarity 2,875 mOsm/L, sulfate 16 mEq. 500 ml in 1000 ml partial fill container. *Rx.* Use: Parenteral nutritional supplement.

dextrose large volume parenterals. (Abbott Hospital Prods). *Rx.*

Dextrose 2 0.5% in Water-1000 ml.

Dextrose 2 0.5% in 0.5 Sterile Lactose Ringer's or in 0.5 Sterile Saline-1000 ml.

Dextrose 5% in Water-150 ml, 250 ml, 500 ml, 1000 ml in Abbo-Vac glass or LifeCare flexible plastic container; partial-fill glass: 50 in 200 ml, 50 in 300 ml, 100 in 300 ml, 400 in 500 ml; partial-fill plastic: 50 in 150 ml, 100 in 150 ml.

Dextrose 5% in Lactose Ringer's-250 ml, 500 ml, 1000 ml glass; 500 ml, 1000 ml plastic container.

Dextrose 5% in Ringer's-500 ml, 1000 ml.

Dextrose 5% in Saline 0.9% or in 0.25, 0.33 or 0.5 Sterile Saline-250, 500, 1000 ml glass or plastic container.

Dextrose 10% in Water-250 ml, 500 ml, 1000 ml containers.

Dextrose 20% in Water-500 ml.

Dextrose 50% in Water-500 ml. Dextrose 20%, 30%, 40%, 50%, 60%, 70% Injections, U.S.P. in partial-fill container, 500 ml in 1000 ml.

Dextrose Injection 50%. Bot. 1000 ml.
Dextrose 50% and Injection w/Electrolytes in partial-fill container, 500 ml in 1000 ml.
Dextrose Injection 70%. Bot. 1000 ml.
Use: Parenteral nutritional supplement.

dextrose small volume parenterals.
(Abbott Hospital Prods) **Dextrose 5%:** 50 ml, 100 ml pressurized pintop vial. **Dextrose 10%:** 5 ml amp.; **Dextrose 25%:** 10 ml syringe. **Dextrose 50%:** 50 ml Abboject syringe (18 g × 1.5″), 50 ml Fliptop vial. **Dextrose 70%:** 70 ml pressurized pintop vial. *Rx.*
Use: Parenteral nutritional supplement.

•**dextrose & sodium chloride injection,** U.S.P. 23. (Abbott) 10% Dextrose and 0.225% Sodium Cl. Inj. Single dose container 500 ml.
Use: Parenteral nutritional supplement.

Dextrostat. (Richwood) Dextroamphetamine sulfate 5 mg, sucrose, lactose, tartrazine/Tab. Bot. 100s. *c-II.*
Use: CNS Stimulant.

Dextrostix. (Bayer) A cellulose strip containing glucose oxidase and indicator system. Bot. 25s, 100s. Box 10s.
Use: Blood-glucose test.

•**dextrothyroxine sodium.** USAN. U.S.P. XXI.
Use: Anticholesteremic, antihyperlipidemic.
See: Choloxin, Tab. (Knoll Pharm.)

Dexule. (Approved) Vitamins A 1333 IU, D 133 IU, B₁ 0.33 mg, B₂ 0.4 mg, C 10 mg, niacinamide 3.3 mg, iron 3.3 mg, calcium 29 mg, phosphorous 15 mg, methylcellulose 100 mg, benzocaine 3 mg/Cap. Bot. 21s, 90s. *otc.*
Use: Vitamin/mineral supplement.

Dexyl. (Pinex) Dextromethorphan HBr 15 mg, vitamin C 20 mg/Tab. Box 20s. *otc.*
Use: Antitussive, vitamin C supplement.

Dey-Dose Epinephrine. (Dey Labs) Racemic epinephrine (as HCl) equal to 2.25% epinephrine base, chlorobutanol, sodium metabisulfite. Soln. for nebulization. Vial 0.25 ml. *otc.*
Use: Bronchodilator.

Dey-Dose Isoetharine Hydrochloride. (Dey Labs) Isoetharine HCl 1% with glycerin, sodium metabisulfite and parabens. Soln. for nebulization. Vial 0.25 ml, 0.5 ml. *Rx.*
Use: Brochodilator.

Dey-Dose Isoproterenol Hydrochloride. (Dey Labs) Isoproterenol HCl 0.5% (1:200). Soln. for nebulization. Vial 0.5 ml. *Rx.*

Use: Bronchodilator.

Dey-Dose Metaproterenol Sulfate. (Dey Labs) Metaproterenol sulfate 0.5%. Inhaler 0.3 ml. *Rx.*
Use: Bronchodilator.

Dey-Lute. (Dey Labs) Isoetharine HCl with sodium metabisulfite, glycerin. Soln. **0.08%:** UD 3 ml; **0.1%:** UD 5 ml; **0.17%:** UD 3 ml; **0.25%:** UD 2 ml. *Rx.*
Use: Bronchodilator.

Dey-Lute Metaproterenol Sulfate. (Dey Labs) Metaproterenol sulfate 0.6%. Soln. for inhalation 2.5 ml. *Rx.*
Use: Bronchodilator.

Dey Pak Sodium Chloride 3%. (Dey) Sodium chloride 3%. Soln. Vial 3 ml, 5 ml, 100s and 10 ml, 15 ml, 50s.
Use: To induce sputum production for specimen collection.

Dey-Pak Sodium Chloride 10%. (Dey) Sodium chloride 10%. Soln. Vial 10 ml, 15 ml, 50s.
Use: To induce sputum production for specimen collection.

•**dezaguanine.** (DEH-zah-GWAHN-een) USAN.
Use: Antineoplastic.

•**dezaguanine mesylate.** (DEE-zah-GWAHN-een MEH-sih-late) USAN.
Use: Antineoplastic.

Dezest. (Armenpharm, Ltd.) Atropine sulfate, phenylpropanolamine HCl, chlorpheniramine maleate. Bot. 100s.
Use: Anticholinergic, antispasmodic, decongestant, antihistamine.

•**dezinamide.** (deh-ZIN-ah-mide) USAN.
Use: Anticonvulsant.

•**dezocine.** (DESS-oh-seen) USAN.
Use: Analgesic.
See: Dalgan (Wyeth-Ayerst).

D-Film. (Ciba Vision) Poloxamer 407, EDTA 0.25%, benzalkonium Cl 0.025%. Gel Tube 25 g. *otc.*
Use: Hard contact lens care.

DFMO. Eflornithine HCl. *Rx.*
Use: Anti-infective.
See: Ornidyl, Inj. (Hoechst Marion Roussel).

DFP. Disopropyl fluorophosphate (Various Mfr.)

d-glucose. Dextrose. *Rx.*
Use: Parenteral nutritional supplement.
See: D-2½-W, Soln. (Various Mfr.)
D-5-W, Soln. (Various Mfr.)
D-7.7-W, Soln. (McGaw.)
D-10-W, Soln. (Various Mfr.)
D-20-W, Soln. (Various Mfr.)
D-25-W, Soln. (Various Mfr.)
D-30-W, Soln. (Various Mfr.)

D-38-W, Soln. (McGaw).
D-38.5-W, Soln. (Abbott).
D-40-W, Soln. (Various Mfr.)
D-50-W, Soln. (Various Mfr.)
D-60-W, Soln. (Various Mfr.)
D-70-W, Soln. (Various Mfr.)

DHC Plus. (Purdue Frederick) Dihydrocodeine bitartrate 16 mg, acetaminophen 356.4 mg, caffeine 30 mg. Cap. Bot. 100s. *c-III.*
Use: Narcotic analgesic combination.

DHEA. (Elan Corp) EL10. *Rx.*
Use: Antiviral, immunomodulator.

D.H.E. 45. (Sandoz) Dihydroergotamine mesylate 1 mg/ml, methanesulfonic acid, alcohol 6.1%, glycerin 15%. Inj. in 1 ml amps. *Rx.*
Use: Agent for migraine.

DHPG. Ganciclovir sodium. *Rx.*
Use: Antiviral.
See: Cytovene, Pow. (Syntex).
BW B759U (Glaxo Wellcome).

DHS Conditioning Rinse. (Person & Covey) Conditioning ingredients. Bot. 8 oz. *otc.*
Use: Dermatological hair conditioner.

DHS Shampoo. (Person & Covey) Blend of cleansing surfactants and emulsifiers. Plastic bot. w/dispenser 8 oz, 16 oz. *otc.*
Use: Dermatological hair and scalp shampoo.

DHS Tar Gel Shampoo. (Person & Covey) Coal Tar, U.S.P. 0.5% Bot. 8 oz. *otc.*
Use: Antiseborrheic, antipsoriatic.

DHS Tar Shampoo. (Person & Covey) Coal tar 0.5% in DHS shampoo. Bot. 4 oz, 8 oz, 16 oz. *otc.*
Use: Antiseborrheic, antipsoriatic.

DHS Zinc Shampoo. (Person & Covey) Zinc pyrithione 2% in DHS shampoo. Bot. 6 oz, 12 oz. *otc.*
Use: Antiseborrheic.

DHT. (Roxane) Dihydrotachysterol. **Tab.:** 0.125 mg, 0.2 mg or 0.4 mg/Tab. Bot. 50s, UD 100s (0.125 mg). 100s, UD 100s (0.2 mg). 50s (0.4 mg). **Intensol:** Dihydrotachysterol 0.2 mg/ml, alcohol 20%. Bot. 30 ml w/dropper. *Rx.*
Use: For postoperative tetany; idiopathic tetany; hypoparathyroidism.

DiaBeta Tablets. (Hoechst Marion Roussel) Glyburide. **1.25 mg:** Bot. 50s. **2.5 mg:** Bot. 60s, 100s, 500s, UD 100s. **5 mg:** Bot. 30s, 60s, 90s, 100s, 500s, 1000s, UD 1000s. *Rx.*
Use: Antidiabetic.

Diabetic Tussin. (Roberts) Dextro-

methorphan HBr 10 mg, guaifenesin 100 mg, phenylephrine 5 mg/5 ml. Liq. Bot. 120 ml. *otc.*
Use: Antitussive, expectorant, decongestant.

Diabetic Tussin DM. (Roberts) Dextromethorphan HBr 10 mg, guaifenesin 100 mg, saccharin, methylparaben, menthol, alcohol & dye free. Liq. Bot. 118 ml. *otc.*
Use: Antitussive, expectorant.

Diabetic Tussin EX. (Health Care Products) Guaifenesin 100 mg/5 ml, saccharin, menthol, methylparaben. Liq. Bot. 118 ml. *otc.*
Use: Expectorant.

Diabinese. (Pfizer Laboratories) Chlorpropamide. **100 mg/Tab.:** Bot. 100s, UD 100s; **250 mg/Tab.:** Bot. 100s, 1000s. *Rx.*
Use: Antidiabetic.

diacetic acid test.
See: Acetest, Tab. (Bayer).

Diaceto w/Codeine. (Archer-Taylor) Codeine 0.25 gr, 0.5 gr/Tab. or Cap. Bot. 500s, 1000s. *c-II.*
Use: Narcotic analgesic.

Diaceto w/Gelsemium. (Archer-Taylor) Phenobarbital 0.5 gr, gelsemium 3 min./Tab. Bot. 1000s. *c-IV.*
Use: Sedative, hypnotic.

•**diacetolol hydrochloride.** USAN.
Use: Anti-adrenergic (β-receptor).

diacetrizoate, sodium.
See: Diatrizoate (Various Mfr.)

•**diacetylated monoglycerides,** N.F. 18. Glycerin esterfied with edible fatty acids and acetic acid.
Use: Pharmaceutic aid (plasticizer).

diacetylcholine chloride. Succinylcholine Cl.
See: Anectine Chloride, Inj., Pow. (Burroughs-Wellcome).

diacetyl-dihydroxydiphenylisatin.
See: Oxyphenisatin acetate (Various Mfr.)

diacetyldioxyphenylisatin.
See: Oxyphenisatin acetate (Various Mfr.)

diacetylmorphine salts. Heroin. Illegal in U.S.A. by Federal statute because of its addiction potential.

Di-Ademil.
See: Hydroflumethiazide, Tab. (Various Mfr.)

diagniol.
See: Sodium Acetrizoate.

diagnostic agents.
See: Acholest, Kit (Fougera).

Cardio-Green, Vial (Becton Dickinson).
Cardiografin, Vial (Squibb).
Cea-Roche, Kit (Roche).
Cholografin, Prep. (Squibb).
Coccidioidin, Vial (Cutter).
Dextrostix, Strip (Bayer).
Dey-Pak Sodium Chloride (Dey).
Diptheria Toxin for Schick Test (Various Mfr.)
Evans Blue Dye, Inj. (New World Trading Corp.).
EZ Detect Strep-A Test (Biomerica).
Fertility Tape (Weston Labs.).
First Choice (Polymer Technology Int.).
Fluorescein Sodium Ophth. Soln. (Various Mfr.)
Fluor-I-Strip (Wyeth-Ayerst).
Fluor-I-Strip A.T. (Wyeth-Ayerst).
Fluress, Ophth. Soln. (Pilkington Barnes Hind).
Glucola, Soln. (Bayer).
Hema-Combistix Strips (Bayer).
Hemastix Strips (Bayer).
Histalog, Amp. (Lilly).
Histoplasmin, Vial (Parke-Davis).
Indigo Carmine (Various Mfr.)
HIVAB HIV-1/HIV-2 (rDNA) EIA (Abbot).
Immunex CRP (Wampole).
Mannitol Soln., Inj. (Merck).
Mono-Latex (Wampole).
Mono-Plus (Wampole).
Persantine IV (DuPont Merck).
Phenolsulfonphthalein (Various Mfr.)
Phentolamine Methanesulfonate, Inj. (Various Mfr.)
Regitine, Amp., Tab. (Novartis).
Rheumanosticon Slide Test (Organon).
Rheumatex (Wampole).
Rheumaton (Wampole).
Rocky Mountain Spotted Fever Antigen, Vial (Lederle).
SureCell Chlamydia Test (Kodak).
SureCell Herpes (HSV) Test (Kodak).
SureCell Strep A Test (Kodak).
Sodium Dehydrocholate, Inj. (Various Mfr.)
Tes-Tape (Lilly).
See: See also: Cholecystography Agents.
Kidney Function Agents.
Liver Function Agents.
Urography Agents.

diagnostic agents for urine.
See: Acetest, Tab. (Bayer).
Albustix, Strip (Bayer).
Biotel Diabetes (Biotel).
Biotel Kidney (Biotel).
Biotel U.T.I. (Biotel).
Bumintest, Tab. (Bayer).
Chemstrip Micral, Strips (Boehringer Mannheim).
Clinistix, Strip (Bayer).
Clinitest, Tab. (Bayer).
Fortel Midstream (Biomerica).
Fortel Plus (Biomerica).
Hema-Combistix, Strip (Bayer).
HCG-nostick (Organon Teknika).
Hemastix, Strip (Bayer).
Hematest, Tab. (Bayer).
Icotest, Tab. (Bayer).
Ketostix, Strip (Bayer).
Pheniplate, Preps. (Bayer).
Phenistix, Strip (Bayer).
SureCell hCG-Urine Test (Kodak).
Uristix, Strip (Bayer).
Wampole One-Step hCG (Wampole).

diallybarbituric acid. Allobarbital, Allobarbitone, Curral.

diallylamicol. Diallyl-diethylaminoethyl phenol di HCl.

diallylnortoxiferine.
See: Alloferin (Roche).

dialminate. Mixture of magnesium carbonate and (alminate) dihydroxyaluminum glycinate.
W/Aspirin.
See: Bufferin, Preps. (Bristol-Myers).

Dialose. (J & J-Merck) Docusate sodium 100 mg. Tab. Bot. 36s. *otc.*
Use: Laxative.

Dialose Plus. (J & J-Merck) **Cap.:** Docusate sodium 100 mg, yellow phenolphthalein 65 mg/Cap. Bot. 36s, 100s, 500s. **Tab.:** Docusate sodium 100 mg, yellow phenolphthalein 65 mg, sugar/Tab. Bot 100s. *otc.*
Use: Laxative.

Dialume. (RPR) Aluminum hydroxide gel 500 mg/Cap. Bot. 500s. *otc.*
Use: Antacid.

Dialyte Pattern LM w/1.5% Dextrose. (Gambro) Dextrose 15 g/L, Na$^+$ 131, Ca^{++} 3.5, Mg^{++} 0.5, Cl$^-$ 94 and lactate 40 with osmolarity 345 mOsm/L. Soln. Bot. 1000 ml, 2000 ml, 4000 ml. *Rx.*
Use: Peritoneal dialysis solution.

Dialyte Pattern LM w/2.5% Dextrose. (Gambro) Dextrose 25 g/L, Na$^+$ 131.5, Ca^{++} 3.5, Mg^{++} 0.5, Cl$^-$ 94 and lactate 40 with osmolarity 395 mOsm/L. Soln. Bot. 1000 ml, 2000 ml, 4000 ml. *Rx.*
Use: Peritoneal dialysis solution.

Dialyte Pattern LM w/4.25% Dextrose. (Gambro) Dextrose 42.5 g/L, Na$^+$ 131.5, Ca^{++} 3.5, Mg^{++} 0.5, Cl$^-$ 94 and lactate 40 with osmolarity 485 mOsm/L. Soln. Bot. 1000 ml, 2000 ml, 4000 ml. *Rx.*

Use: Peritoneal dialysis solution.

diamethine.
See: Dimethyl tubocurarine (Various Mfr.)

diaminedipenicillin g.
See: Benzethacil (Various Mfr.)

Diamine T.D. (Major) Brompheniramine maleate 8 mg or 12 mg/TR tab. Bot. 100s, 250s, 1000s.
Use: Antihistamine.

di-amino acetate complex w/calcium aluminum carbonate. Cap. IU.
See: Ancid Tab., Susp. (Sheryl).

diaminodiphenylsulfone. Dapsone, U.S.P. 23.
Use: Treatment of malaria.

diaminopropyl tetramethylene.
See: Spermine.

3,4-diaminopyridine. *Rx.*
Use: Lambert-Eaton myasthenic syndrome. [Orphan drug]

•**diamocaine cyclamate.** (die-AM-oh-CANE SIH-klah-mate) USAN.
Use: Local anesthetic.

Diamox. (Lederle) Acetazolamide. **Tab.:** 125 mg Bot. 100s. 250 mg Bot. 100s, 1000s, UD 10 × 10s. **Inj. Vial:** Sterile sodium salt 500 mg (sodium hydroxide to adjust pH). *Rx.*
Use: Diuretic, anticonvulsant.

Diamox Sequels. (Lederle) Acetazolamide 500 mg/Cap. Bot. 30s, 100s. *Rx.*
Use: Diuretic, anticonvulsant.

diamthazole dihydrochloride. Asterol.

Dianeal w/1.5% Dextrose. (Baxter) Dextrose 15 g/L, Na⁺ 141, Ca⁺⁺ 3.5, Mg⁺⁺ 1.5, Cl⁻ 101, lactate 45 with osmolarity 364 mOsm/L. Soln. Bot. 1000 ml, 2000 ml. *Rx.*
Use: Peritoneal dialysis solution.

Dianeal 137 w/1.5% Dextrose. (Baxter) Dextrose 15 g/L, Na⁺ 132, Ca⁺⁺ 3.5, Mg⁺⁺ 1.5, Cl102, lactate 35 with osmolarity 347 mOsm/L. Soln. Bot. 2000 ml. *Rx.*
Use: Peritoneal dialysis solution.

Dianeal w/4.25% Dextrose. (Baxter) Dextrose 42.5 g/L, Na⁺ 141, Ca⁺⁺ 3.5, Mg⁺⁺ 1.5, Cl⁻ 101, lactate 45 with osmolarity 503 mOsm/L. Soln. Bot. 2000 ml. *Rx.*
Use: Peritoneal dialysis solution.

Dianeal 137 w/4.25% Dextrose. (Baxter) Dextrose 42.5 g/L, Na⁺ 132, Ca⁺⁺ 3.5, Mg⁺⁺ 1.5, Cl⁻ 102, lactate 35 with osmolarity 486 mOsm/L. Soln. Bot. 2000 ml. *Rx.*
Use: Peritoneal dialysis solution.

Dianeal PD-2 Peritoneal Dialysis Soln with 1.1% Amino Acid. *Rx.*
Use: Nutritional supplement for dialysis patients. [Orphan drug]

•**diapamide.** (die-APP-am-ide) USAN.
Use: Diuretic, antihypertensive.

Diapantin. (Janssen) Isopropamide bromide. *Rx.*
Use: Anticholinergic.

Diaparene. (Bayer) Methylbenzethonium Cl. Pow. Bot. 4 oz, 9 oz, 12.5 oz, 14 oz.
Use: Surface-active disinfectant.

Diaparene Medicated. (Reckitt & Coleman) Methylbenzethonium Cl with white petrolatum 0.1%, glycerin, mineral oil, stearyl alcohol. Cream. Tube 30, 60, 120 g. *otc.*
Use: Antimicrobial, topical.

Diaparene Ointment. (Bayer) Methylbenzethonium Cl 0.1% w/petrolatum, glycerin. Tube 1 oz, 2 oz, 4 oz. *otc.*
Use: Antimicrobial, topical.

Diaparene Peri-Anal Cream. (Bayer) Methylbenzethonium Cl 1:1000, zinc oxide, starch, cod liver oil, white petrolatum, lanolin, calcium caseinate. Cream Tube 1 oz, 2 oz, 4 oz. *otc.*
Use: Antimicrobial, astringent.

Diaper Guard. (Del) Dimethicone 1%, white petrolatum 66%, cocoa butter, parabens, vitamins A, D₃, E, zinc oxide. Oint. Tube 49.6 g, 99.2 g. *otc.*
Use: Diaper rash product.

Diaper Rash. (Various Mfr.) Zinc oxide, cod liver oil, lanolin, methylparaben, petrolatum, talc. Oint. Tube 113 g. *otc.*
Use: Diaper rash product.

diaphenylsulfone. Dapsone, U.S.P. 23.
Use: Leprostatic.

Diapid. (Sandoz,) Lypressin synthetic lysine-8-vasopressin. Equiv. to 50 U.S.P. units posterior pituitary/ml (0.185 mg/ml). Nasal spray. Bot. 8 ml. *Rx.*
Use: Pituitary hormone.

Di-Ap-Trol. (Foy) Phendimetrazine tartrate 35 mg/Tab. Bot. 100s, 1000s. *c-III.*
Use: Anorexiant.

Diar-aid. (Thompson) Loperamide HCl 2 mg/Capl. Pkg. 12s. *otc.*
Use: Antidiarrheal.

Diarrest. (Dover) Calcium carbonate, pectin/Tab. Sugar, lactose and salt free. UD box 500s. *otc.*
Use: Antidiarrheal.

diarrhea therapy.
See: Antidiarrheals.

Diaserp Tabs. (Major) Chlorothiazide 250

mg or 500 mg/Tab. w/reserpine. Bot. 100s. *Rx.*
Use: Antihypertensive.

Diasorb. (Columbia) Activated nonfibrous attapulgite. **Liq.:** 750 mg per 5 ml. Bot. 120 ml. **Tab.:** 750 mg. Pkg. 24s. *otc.*
Use: Antidiarrheal.

Diasporal Cream. (Doak) Formerly Sulfur Salicyl Diasporal. Sulfur 3%, salicylic acid 2%, isopropyl alcohol in diasporal base. Cream Jar 3¾ oz. *otc.*
Use: Antiseptic, topical.

Diastase.
See: Aspergillus oryzae enzyme.

Diastix Reagent Strips. (Bayer) Broad range test for glucose in urine. Containing glucose oxidase, peroxidase, potassium iodide/w blue background dye. Tab. Pkg. 50s, 100s.
Use: Diagnostic aid.

diatrizoate.
•**diatrizoate meglumine,** U.S.P. 23.
Use: Diagnostic aid (radiopaque medium).
See: Angiovist 282, Inj. (Berlex).
Cardiografin, Vial (Squibb).
Cystographin, Inj. (Squibb).
Gastrografin, Liq. (Squibb).
Hypaque-Cysto, Liq. (Sanofi Winthrop).
Hypaque Meglumine (Sanofi Winthrop).
Renografin, Inj. (Squibb).
Reno-M-DIP, Inj. (Squibb).
Reno-M-30, Inj. (Squibb).
Reno-M-60, Inj. (Squibb).
Urovist, Prods. (Berlex).
W/Iodipamide methylglucamine.
See: Sinografin, Vial (Squibb).
W/Sodium Diatrizoate.
See: Renovist, Inj. (Squibb).

diatrizoate meglumine and diatrizoate sodium injection.
Use: Diagnostic aid (radiopaque medium).
See: Angiorist 292, Inj. (Berlex).
Angiovist 370, Inj. (Berlex).
Gastrovist, Soln. (Berlex).
Hypaque-M Prods. (Sanofi Winthrop).

diatrizoate meglumine and diatrizoate sodium solution.
Use: Diagnostic aid (radiopaque medium).
See: Gastrografini Soln. (Squibb).
Renografin-60, Soln. (Squibb).
Renografin-76, Soln. (Squibb).
Renovist, Soln. (Squibb).

diatrizoate meglumine 52.7% and iodipamide meglumine 25.8% (38% iodine).
Use: Diagnostic aid (radiopaque agent).
See: Sinografin, Inj. (Bracco DXS).

diatrizoate methylglucamine.
Use: Diagnostic aid (radiopaque medium).
See: Diatrizoate Meglumine, U.S.P. 23.

diatrizoate methylglucamine sodium.
Use: Diagnostic aid (radiopaque medium).

•**diatrizoate sodium,** U.S.P. 23.
Use: Diagnostic aid (radiopaque medium).
See: Hypaque Prods. (Sanofi Winthrop).
Urovist Sodium, Inj. (Berlex).
W/Meglumine diatrizoate.
See: Gastrografin, Liq. (Squibb).
Renografin-60, -76, Vial (Squibb).
Renovist II, Vial (Squibb).
W/Methylglucamine diatrizoate, sodium citrate, disodium ethylenediamine tetraacetate dihydrate, methylparaben, propylparaben.
See: Renovist, Vial (Squibb).

diatrizoate sodium 41.66% (24.9% iodine).
Use: Diagnostic aid (radiopaque agent).
See: Hypaque sodium, Soln. (Sanofi Winthrop.).

diatrizoate sodium (59.87% iodine).
Use: Diagnostic aid (radiopaque agent).
See: Hypaque Sodium, Soln. (Sanofi Winthrop.).

•**diatrizoate sodium I-125.** USAN.
Use: Radioactive agent.

•**diatrizoate sodium I-131.** USAN.
Use: Radioactive agent.

•**diatrizoic acid,** (DIE-at-rih-ZOE-ik) U.S.P. 23.
Use: Diagnostic aid (radiopaque medium).
See: Amidotrizoic Acid.
Hypaque sodium salt.

•**diaveridine.** (DIE-ah-ver-ih-deen) USAN.
Use: Antibacterial.

•**diazepam,** (DIE-aze-uh-pam) U.S.P. 23.
Use: Agent for control of emotional disturbances, sedative, hypnotic, tranquilizer.
See: Valium, Tab. (Roche).
Valrelease, S.R. Cap. (Roche).
Zetran (Roberts).

diazepam. (Various Mfr.) **Tab.:** 2 mg. Bot. 100s, 500s, 1000s; 5 mg or 10 mg. Bot. 100s, 500s, 1000s; **Inj.:** 5 mg/ml Amps 2 ml; vial 1, 2, 5, 10 ml; syringe 1, 2 ml. **Oral Soln.** (Roxane): 5 mg/5 ml. In 500 ml, UD 5 ml, 10 ml patient cups. **Concentrated Oral Soln.** (Roxane): 5

mg/ml In 30 ml w/dropper.
Use: Agent for control of emotional disturbances, sedative, hypnotic, tranquilizer.

Diazepam Intensol. (Roxane) Diazepam 5 mg/ml. Oral Soln. In 30 ml with dropper. *c-iv.*
Use: Antianxiety agent.

diazepam viscous rectal solution. *c-iv.*
Use: To treat acute repetitive seizures. [Orphan drug]

●**diaziquone.** (DIE-azz-ih-kwone) USAN.
Use: Antineoplastic.

diazomycins a, b, & c. Antibiotic obtained from *Streptomyces ambofaciens.* Under study.

●**diazoxide,** (DIE-aze-OX-ide) U.S.P. 23.
Use: Antihypertensive.
See: Proglycem Capsules (Medical Market Specialists).
Proglycem Suspension (Medical Market Specialists).

diazoxide, parenteral. (DIE-aze-OX-ide)
Use: Antihypertensive.
See: Diazoxide Injection USP, Inj. (Various Mfr.)
Hyperstat IV, Inj. (Schering Plough).

dibasic calcium phosphate dihydrate.
Use: Replenisher (calcium); pharmaceutic aid (tablet base).
See: D.C.P. 340, Tab. (Parke-Davis).
Diostate D, Tab. (Pharmacia & Upjohn).

Dibatrol. (Lexis) Chlorpropamide 100 mg or 250 mg/Tab. Bot. 100s, 1000s. *Rx.*
Use: Antidiabetic.

dibencil.
See: Benzathine Penicillin G. (Various Mfr.)

Dibent. (Roberts) Dicyclomine 10 mg/ml with chlorobutanol. Inj. Vial 10 ml. *Rx.*
Use: GI anticholinergic, antispasmodic.

●**dibenzepin hydrochloride.** (die-BEN-zeh-pin) USAN.
Use: Antidepressant.

●**dibenzothiophene.** (die-BEN-zoe-THIGH-oh-feen) USAN.
Use: Keratolytic.

Dibenzyline. (SK-Beecham) Phenoxybenzamine HCl 10 mg/Cap. Bot. 100s. *Rx.*
Use: Antihypertensive.

dibromodulcitol.
Use: Antineoplastic. [Orphan drug]

●**dibromsalan.** (die-BROME-sah-lan) USAN.
Use: Germicide, disinfectant.

●**dibucaine,** U.S.P. 23.
Use: Local anesthetic.

See: D-Caine, Oint. (Century).
Dulzit, Cream (Del).
Nupercainal, Oint., Cream, Supp. (Novartis).
Nupercainal Heavy, Soln. (Novartis).
W/Dextrose.
See: Nupercaine Heavy Soln. (Novartis).
W/Sodium bisulfite.
See: Nupercainal, Cream, Oint. (Novartis).
W/Zinc oxide, bismuth subgallate, acetone sodium bisulfite.
See: Nupercainal, Oint., Supp. (Novartis).

●**dibucaine hydrochloride,** U.S.P. 23.
Use: Local anesthetic.
See: Nupercaine HCl, soln., (Novartis).
W/Antipyrine, hydrocortisone, polymyxin B sulfate, neomycin sulfate.
See: Otocort, Liq. (Lemmon).
W/Colistin sodium methanesulfonate, citric acid, sodium citrate.
See: Coly-Mycin M, Injectable (Warner-Chilcott).

dibutoline sulfate. Ethyl(2-hydroxyethyl)-dimethylammonium sulfate (2:1) bis(dibutyl-carbamate).
Use: Anticholinergic, antispasmodic.

●**dibutyl sebacate.** N.F. 18.
Use: Pharmaceutic aid (plasticizer).

Dical Captabs. (Rugby) Calcium 116 mg, vitamin D 133 IU, phosphorus 90 mg. Bot. 1000s. *otc.*
Use: Calcium, vitamin D supplement.

dicalcium phosphate. (Various Mfr.) Dibasic calcium phosphate, monocalcium phosphate. **Cap.:** 7.5 gr or 10 gr. **Tab.:** 7.5 gr, 10 gr or 15 gr. **Wafer:** 15 gr. *otc.*
Use: Calcium supplement.
W/Calcium gluconate and Vitamin D. (Various Mfr.) Cap., Tab., Wafer.
See: Calcicaps, Tab. (Nion).
W/Iron and Vitamin D. (Various Mfr.)
Lilly–Pulv., Bot. 100s.
W/Vitamin D. (Squibb) Calcium 85 mg, phosphorous 60 mg, vitamin D 41 IU.

Dical D. (Abbott) Calcium 117 mg, vitamin D 133 IU, phosphorus 90 mg. Tab. Bot. 100s, 500s. *otc.*
Use: Calcium, phosphorus, vitamin D supplement.

Dical-D with Vitamin C. (Abbott) Dibasic calcium phosphate containing calcium 116.7 mg, phosphorus 90 mg, vitamin D 133 IU, ascorbic acid 15 mg/Cap. Bot. 100s.
Use: Vitamin/mineral supplement.

Dical-Dee. (Barre) Vitamins D 350 IU, dibasic calcium phosphate 4.5 gr, cal-

cium gluconate 3 gr/Cap. Bot. 100s, 1000s. *otc.*
Use: Vitamin/mineral supplement.

Dicaldel. (Faraday) Dibasic calcium phosphate 300 mg, calcium gluconate 200 mg, vitamin D 33 IU/Cap. Bot. 100s, 250s, 500s, 1000s. *otc.*
Use: Vitamin/mineral supplement.

Dical-D Wafers. (Abbott) Dibasic calcium phosphate containing calcium 232 mg, phosphorus 180 mg, vitamin D 200 IU/Wafer. Box 51s. *otc.*
Use: Vitamin/mineral supplement.

Dicaltabs. (Faraday) Dibasic calcium phosphate 108 mg, calcium gluconate 140 mg, vitamin D 35 IU/Tab. Bot. 100s, 250s, 1000s. *otc.*
Use: Vitamin/mineral supplement.

Dicarbosil. (BIRA) Calcium carbonate 500 mg/Chew. Tab. Roll 12s. *otc.*
Use: Antacid.

Di-Cet. (Sanford & Son) Methylbenzethonium Cl 24.4 g, sodium carbonate monohydrate 48.8 g, sodium nitrite 24.4 g, trisodium ethylenediamine tetra-acetate monohydrate 2.4 g. Pow. Pkg. 2.4 g, Box 24s.
Use: Dental instrument disinfectant.

dichloralantipyrine. Dichloralphenazone. Chloralpyrine. A complex of 2 mol. chloral hydrate with 1 mol. antipyrine. Sominat.
W/Isometheptene mucate, acetaminophen.
See: Midrin, Cap. (Schwarz Pharma).

•**dichloralphenazone.** U.S.P. 23.
Use: Sedative, hypnotic.

Dichloramine T. (Various Mfr.) (1% to 5% in chlorinated paraffin). P-Toluenesulfone-dichloramine.
Use: Antiseptic.

dichloren.
See: Mechlorethamine HCl, Sterile Inj. (Various Mfr.)

dichlorisone acetate.

dichlormethazanone.

dichloroacetate sodium. *Rx.*
Use: Lactic acidosis; hypercholesterolemia. [Orphan drug]

dichloroacetic acid. *Rx.*
Use: Cauterizing agent.
See: Bichloracetic Acid, Liq. (Glenwood).

•**dichlorodifluoromethane,** N.F. 18.
Use: Pharmaceutic aid (aerosol propellant).

dichlorodiphenyl trichloroethane.
See: Chlorophenothane (Various Mfr.)

dichlorophenarsine hydrochloride. (Chlorarsen, Clorarsen, Fontarsol, Halarsol).

dichlorophene. Related to hexachlorophene.
W/Undecylenic acid.
See: Onychomycetin, Liq. (Gordon).
W/Undecylenic acid, salicylicacid, hexachlorophene.
See: Podiaspray, aerosol pow. (Dalin).

•**dichlorotetrafluoroethane,** N.F. 18.
Use: Pharmaceutic aid (aerosol propellant).

•**dichlorphenamide,** U.S.P. 23.
Use: Carbonic anhydrase inhibitor.

dichlorphenamide. *Rx.*
Use: Agent for glaucoma.

•**dichlorvos.** (DIE-klor-vahs) USAN.
Use: Anthelmintic.
See: Atgard (Fermenta).
Equigard (Fermenta).
Task (Fermenta).

•**dicirenone.** (die-sigh-REN-ohn) USAN.
Use: Hypotensive, aldosterone antagonist.

Dickey's Old Reliable Eye Wash. (Dickey Drug) Berberine sulfate, boric acid, propyl parasept, methyl parasept. Plastic dropper bot. 8 ml, 12 ml, 1 oz. *otc.*
Use: Counterirritant, ophthalmic.

•**diclofenac potassium.** (die-KLOE-fen-ak) USAN.
Use: Anti-inflammatory, nonsteroidal analgesic.
See: Cataflam, Tab. (Novartis).

•**diclofenac sodium.** (die-KLOE-fen-ak) USAN.
Use: Anti-inflammatory, nonsteroidal analgesic.
See: Voltaren (Novartis).
Voltaren Ophthalmic (Ciba Vision Ophthalmic).

diclofenac sodium. (Roxane) 25 mg, 50 mg or 75 mg/DR Tab. Bot. 60s, 100s, 1000s, UD 100s.
Use: Anti-inflammatory, nonsteroidal analgesic.

Dicloxacil. (Goldline) Dicloxacillin sodium 250 mg or 500 mg/Cap. Bot. 100s. *Rx.*
Use: Anti-infective, penicillin.

•**dicloxacillin.** (DIE-klox-uh-SILL-in) USAN.
Use: Antibacterial.
See: Dynapen, Cap., Susp. (Bristol).
Pathocil, Cap., Susp. (Wyeth-Ayerst).

•**dicloxacillin sodium.** (DIE-klox-uh-SILL-in) U.S.P. 23.

Use: Antibacterial.
See: Dycill, Cap. (SK-Beecham).
Dynapen, Cap., Soln. (Bristol).
Dicole. (Halsey) Docusate sodium 100 mg/Cap. Bot. 100s. *otc.*
Use: Laxative.
dicophane.
Use: Pediculicide.
See: Chlorophenothane (Various Mfr.), DDT.
dicoumarin.
Use: Anticoagulant.
See: Dicumarol, Preps. (Various Mfr.)
dicoumarol.
Use: Anticoagulant.
See: Dicumarol, U.S.P. 23.
•**dicumarol,** (die-KUME-ah-rahl) USAN. U.S.P. XXII. *Formerly Bishydroxycoumarin.*
Use: Anticoagulant.
dicumarol. (Abbott) 25 mg/Tab. Bot. 100s, 1000s.
Use: Anticoagulant.
•**dicyclomine hydrochloride,** (die-SIGH-kloe-meen) U.S.P. 23.
Use: Antispasmodic, anticholinergic.
See: Antispas, Inj. (Keene).
Bentyl, Amp. Syringe, Cap., Tab., Syr. (Hoechst Marion Roussel).
Dysaps, Tab., Liq., Inj. (Savage).
Nospaz, Vial (Solvay).
Stannitol (Standex).
W/Aluminum hydroxide, magnesium hydroxide, methylcellulose.
See: Triactin Liq., Tab. (Procter & Gamble).
W/Phenobarbital.
See: Bentyl with Phenobarbital, Prods. (Hoechst Marion Roussel).
Dicynene. (Baxter) *Rx.*
Use: Hemostatic.
See: Ethamsylate.
dicysteine.
See: Cystine, Pow. (Various Mfr.)
•**didanosine.** (die-DAN-oh-SEEN) USAN.
Use: Antiviral.
See: Videx, Tab., Pow. (Bristol Myers Squibb).
didehydrodideoxythymidine.
Use: Antiviral.
See: Stavudine (B-M Squibb).
Di-Delamine Gel. (Del Pharm.) Tripelennamine HCl 0.5%, diphenhydramine HCl 1%, benzalkonium Cl 0.12% in clear gel. Tube 1.25 oz. *otc.*
Use: Antipruritic, topical.
Di-Delamine Spray. (Del Pharm.) Tripelennamine HCl 0.5%, diphenhydramine HCl 1%, benzalkonium Cl 0.12%.

Spray pump 4 oz. *otc.*
Use: Antipruritic, topical.
dideoxycytidine. (Roche). *Rx.*
Use: Antiviral.
See: HIVID.
2,3 dideoxycytidine. (Roche; NCI; Bristol-Myers). *Rx.*
Use: Antiviral (AIDS).
dideoxyinisine.
Use: Antiviral.
See: Videx, Tab., Pow. (Bristol-Myers Squibb).
Didrex. (Pharmacia & Upjohn) Benzphetamine HCl. **25 mg/Tab.:** Bot. 100s; **50 mg/Tab.:** Bot. 100s, 500s. *c-III.*
Use: Anorexiant.
Didronel. (Procter & Gamble) Etidronate disodium 200 mg or 400 mg/Tab. Bot. 60s. *Rx.*
Use: Hypercalcemia of malignancy.
Didronel IV. (MGI Pharma) Etidronate disodium 300 mg/6 ml amp. *Rx.*
Use: Hypercalcemia of malignancy.
•**dienestrol,** U.S.P. 23.
Use: Estrogen therapy, atrophic vaginitis.
See: D V, Cream (Hoechst Marion Roussel).
D V, Supp. (Hoechst Marion Roussel).
Ortho Dienestrol Cream (Ortho).
W/Sulfanilamide, aminacrine HCl, allantoin.
See: AVC/Dienestrol Cream, Supp. (Hoechst Marion Roussel).
dienestrol. (Ortho) 0.01%. Tube 78 g w/ applicator.
Use: Estrogen therapy, atrophic vaginitis.
Diet-Aid, Maximum Strength. (Columbia) Phenylpropanolamine HCl 75 mg/ Cap. Pkg. 20s. *otc.*
Use: Nonprescription diet aid.
Diet-Aid Plus Vitamin C, Maximum Strength. (Columbia) Phenylpropanolamine HCl 75 mg, vitamin C 180 mg/ Cap. Pkg. 20s. *otc.*
Use: Nonprescription diet aid.
diet aids, nonprescription.
Use: Diet aid.
See: Appedrine, Tab. (Thompson).
Dex-A-Diet Plus Vitamin C, Cap. (Columbia).
Diet Ayds, Candy (DEP Corp.).
Dieutrim T.D., Cap. (Legere).
Extra Strength Grapefruit Diet Plan w/ Diadax, Cap. (Columbia).
Grapefruit Diet Plan w/Diadax, Cap., Tab. (Columbia).

Maximum Strength Dexatrim Plus Vitamin C, Cap. (Thompsom).
Slim-Mint, Gum (Thompson).

Diet Ayds. (DEP) Benzocaine 6 mg/square. Bot. 48s. *otc.*
Use: Nonprescription diet aid.

•**diethanolamine,** N.F. 18.
Use: Pharmaceutic acid (alkalizing agent).

diethanolamine.
See: Diolamine.

diethazine hydrochloride. 10-(β-Diethylaminoethyl)-pheno-thiazine HCl. Diparcol.
Use: Parkinsonism.

diethoxin. Intracaine HCl.

•**diethyl phthalate,** N.F. 18.
Use: Pharmaceutic aid (plasticizer).

diethyldithiocarbamate.
Use: Trial drug for AIDS. [Orphan drug]
See: Imuthiol.

diethylenediamine citrate. Piperazine Citrate, Piperazine Hexahydrate.
See: Antepar, Syr., Tab., Wafer (Glaxo Wellcome).

diethylmalonylurea.
See: Barbital, Tab. (Various Mfr.)

•**diethylcarbamazine citrate,** U.S.P. 23.
Use: Anthelmintic.
See: Nemacide (Fermenta).

•**diethylpropion hydrochloride,** (die-ETH-uhl-PRO-pee-ahn) U.S.P. 23.
Use: Anorexic.
See: D.E.P.-75
Tenuate, Tab. (Hoechst Marion Roussel).
Tepanil, Tab. (3M).
Tepanil Ten-Tab, Tab. (3M).

diethylpropion. (Various Mfr.) **Tab.:** Diethylpropion 25 mg. Bot. 100s, 500s, 1000s. **SR Tab.:** Diethylpropion 75 mg. Bot. 100s, 250s, 500s, 1000s. *c-iv.*
Use: Anorexiant.

•**diethylstilbestrol.** (die-ETH-uhl-still-BESS-trahl) U.S.P. 23.
Use: Estrogen.
See: Acnestrol, Lot. (Dermik).
Mase-Bestrol, Tab. (Mason).
W/Clioquinol, sulfanilamide.
See: D.I.T.I. Creme (Dunhall).
W/Nitrofurazone, diperodon HCl.
See: Furacin-E Urethral Inserts (Eaton).

diethylstilbestrol. (Lilly) Diethylstilbestrol 1 mg or 5 mg/Tab. Bot. 100s. *Rx.*
Use: Estrogen.

•**diethylstilbestrol diphosphate,** U.S.P. 23.
Use: Estrogen.

See: Stilphostrol, Inj., Tab. (Bayer).

diethylstilbestrol dipropionate, (Various Mfr.) Amp. in oil, 0.5 mg, 1 mg or 5 mg/ml. Tab. 0.5 mg, 1 mg or 5 mg.
Use: Estrogen.

•**diethyltoluamide,** U.S.P. 23.
Use: Repellent (arthropod).
See: RV Pellent, Oint. (Zeneca)

n, n-diethylvanillamide.
See: Ethamivan, Inj. (Various Mfr.)

Diet-Tuss. (Approved) Dextromethorphan 30 mg, thenylpyramine HCl, pyrilamine maleate 80 mg, sodium salicylate 200 mg, sodium citrate 600 mg, ammonium Cl 100 mg/fl oz. Sugar free. Bot. 4 oz. *otc.*
Use: Antitussive, antihistamine, analgesic, expectorant.

Dieutrim T.D. (Legere) Phenylpropanolamine 75 mg, benzocaine 9 mg, sodium carboxymethylcellulose 75 mg/SR Cap. Bot. 100s, 1000s. *otc.*
Use: Nonprescription diet aid.

•**difenoximide hydrochloride.** (DIE-fen-OX-ih-mid) USAN.
Use: Antiperistaltic.

•**difenoxin.** (DIE-fen-OX-in) USAN.
Use: Antidiarrheal, antiperistaltic.
W/Atropine sulfate.
See: Motofen (Schwarz Pharma).

Differin. (Galderma) Adapalene 0.1%, propylene glycol, EDTA, methylparaben/Gel. Tube. 15 g, 45 g. *Rx.*
Use: Topical treatment of acne vulgaris.

•**diflorasone diacetate,** U.S.P. 23.
Use: Anti-inflammatory (topical), antipruritic.
See: Florone, Cream, Oint. (Pharmacia & Upjohn).
Maxiflor, Cream, Oint. (Allergan Herbert).
Psorcon, Cream, Oint. (Dermik).

•**difloxacin hydrochloride.** (die-FLOX-ah-SIN) USAN.
Use: Anti-infective (DNA gyrase inhibitor).

•**difluanine hydrochloride.** (die-FLEW-an-EEN) USAN.
Use: CNS stimulant.

Diflucan. (Roerig) Fluconazole. **Tab.:** 50 mg. Bot. 30s, 100 mg or 200 mg. Bot. 30s, UD 100s; 150 mg. 1s. **Inj.:** 2 mg/ml Vial with sodium chloride 9 mg/ml or *Viaflex Plus* 100 ml, 200 ml. **Pow. for Oral Susp.:** 10 mg/ml in 350 mg or 40 mg/ml in 1400 mg. *Rx.*
Use: Antifungal.

•**diflucortolone.** USAN.
Use: Glucocorticoid.

- **diflucortolone pivalate.** USAN.
  Use: Glucocorticoid.
- **diflumidone sodium.** (die-FLEW-mih-DOHN) USAN.
  Use: Anti-inflammatory.
- **diflunisal,** (die-FLOO-nih-sal) U.S.P. 23.
  Use: Anti-inflammatory, analgesic.
  See: Dolobid, Tab. (Merck).
  diflunisal. (Various Mfr.) Diflunisal 250 mg or 500 mg/Tab. Pkg. UD 60s, 100s, 500s. *Rx.*
  Use: Anti-inflammatory, nonsteroidal analgesic.
- **difluprednate.** (DIE-flew-PRED-nate) USAN.
  Use: Anti-inflammatory.
- **diftalone.** (DIFF-tah-lone) USAN.
  Use: Anti-inflammatory, analgesic.
- **digalloyl trioleate.** USAN.
  Di-Gel Advanced Formula. (Schering-Plough) Magnesium hydroxide 128 mg, calcium carbonate 280 mg, simethicone 20 mg/Tab. Bot. 30s, 60s, 90s. *otc.*
  Use: Antacid, antiflatulent.
  Di-Gel Liquid. (Schering-Plough) Aluminum hydroxide (equivalent to dried gel) 200 mg, magnesium hydroxide 200 mg, simethicone 20 mg/5 ml, saccharin, sorbitol. Bot. 180 ml, 360 ml. *otc.*
  Use: Antacid, antiflatulent.
  Digepepsin. (Kenwood/Bradley) Pepsin 250 mg, pancreatin 300 mg, bile salts 150 mg/Tab. Bot. 60s. *Rx.*
  Use: Digestive enzyme.
  Digestamic. (Lexis) Pancrelipase 300 mg, pepsin 100 mg/Tab. Bot. 50s. *otc, Rx.*
  Use: Digestive aid.
  Digestamic Liquid. (Lexis) Belladonna leaf fluid extract 0.64 min./5 ml. Bot. 8 oz. *otc, Rx.*
  Use: Anticholinergic, antispasmodic.
  Digestant. (Canright) Pancreatin 5.25 gr, ox bile extract 2 gr, pepsin 5 gr, betaine HCl 1 gr/Tab. Bot. 100s, 1000s. *otc, Rx.*
  Use: Digestive aid.
  Digestive Compound. (Thurston) Betaine HCl 3.25 gr, pepsin 1 gr, papain 2 gr, mycozyme 2 gr, ox bile 2 gr/2 Tab. Bot. 100s, 500s. *otc, Rx.*
  Use: Digestive aid.
  digestive enzymes.
  See: Cotazym Capsules (Organon).
  Cotazym-S Capsules (Organon).
  Creon Capsules (Solvay).
  Dizmeys Tablets (Recsei Labs.).
  Festal II Tablets (Hoechst Marion Roussel).

  Hi-Vegi-Lip Tablets (Freeda).
  Ilozyme Tablets (Pharmacia & Upjohn).
  Ku-Zyme HP Capsules (Kremers-Urban).
  Pancrease Capsules (McNeil Pharm.)
  Pancreatin Enseals Tablets (Lilly).
  Pancreatin Tablets (Lilly).
  VioKase Pow., Tab. (Robins).
  digestive products, miscellaneous.
  Use: Digestive enzyme supplement.
  See: Ku-Zyme, Cap. (Kremers-Urban).
  Arco-Lase, Tabs. (Arco).
  Converzyme, Cap. (Ascher).
  Digestozyme, Tab. (Various Mfr.)
  Nu'Leven, Tab. (Lemmon).
  Enzobile Improved (Roberts).
  Sto-Zyme (Misemer).
  Digestozyme Tabs. (Goldline) Pancreatin, pepsin, bile salts. Bot. 1000s. *Rx.*
  Use: Digestive aid.
  Digibind. (Glaxo Wellcome) Digoxin Immune Fab (ovine) fragments 38 mg, sorbitol 75 mg/Vial. Box 1s. *Rx.*
  Use: Antidote.
- **digitalis,** U.S.P. 23.
  Use: Cardiotonic.
  See: Acylanid, Tab. (Sandoz).
  Cedilanid, Tab. (Sandoz).
  Cedilanid-D, Amp. (Sandoz).
  Crystodigin, Tab. Amp., Vial (Lilly).
  Deslanoside, Inj. (Various Mfr.)
  Digiglusin, Tab. (Lilly).
  Digitaline Nativelle, Soln., Tab., Elix. (Savage).
  Digitoxin, Preps. (Various Mfr.)
  Digoxin, Preps. (Various Mfr.)
  Gitaligin, Tab. (Schering).
  Gitalin, Tab. (Various Mfr.)
  Lanatoside C, Inj., Tab. (Various Mfr.)
  Lanoxin, Tab., Inj., Elix. (Glaxo Wellcome).
  Purodigin, Tab. (Wyeth-Ayerst).
  digitalis leaf, powdered.
  Use: Cardiac glycoside.
  See: Pil-Digis, Pill (Key).
  digitalis tincture.
  Use: Cardiac glycoside.
- **digitoxin,** (dih-jih-TOX-in) U.S.P. 23.
  Use: Cardiac glycoside, cardiotonic.
  See: Crystodigin, Tab. (Lilly).
  digitoxin. (Various Mfr.) **Amp.:** (0.2 mg/ml) 1 ml, **Cap. in oil:** 0.1 mg or 0.2 mg. **Tab.:** 0.1 mg, 0.2 mg.
  Use: Cardiac glycoside, cardiotonic.
  digitoxin, acetyl.
  Use: Cardiac glycoside.
  See: Acylanid, Tab. (Sandoz).

α-digitoxin monoacetate.
Use: Cardiac glycoside.
See: Acetyldigitoxin, Tab. (Various Mfr.)
•**digoxin,** (dih-JOX-in) U.S.P. 23.
Use: Cardiac glycoside, cardiotonic.
See: Lanoxicaps (Glaxo Wellcome).
Lanoxin, Preps. (Glaxo Wellcome).
Masoxin, Tab. (Mason).
digoxin. (Roxane) Digoxin 0.05 mg/ml,
alcohol 10%. Bot 60 ml, UD 2.5 ml,
UD 5 ml. *Rx.*
Use: Cardiac glycoside.
digoxin antibody.
See: Digibind (Glaxo Wellcome).
Digoxin Elixir. (Roxane) 0.05 mg/ml. Liq.
Bot. 60 ml, UD 2.5 ml, 5 ml. *Rx.*
Use: Cardiotonic.
digoxin i-125 imusay. (Abbott Diagnos-
tics) Digoxin diagnostic kit for the quan-
titative determination of serum digoxin.
100s, 300s.
Use: Diagnostic aid.
digoxin immune fab (ovine) fragments.
Rx.
Use: Antidote. [Orphan drug]
See: Digibind, Pow. for Inj.(Glaxo Well-
come).
Digoxin Riabead. (Abbott Diagnostics)
Solid-phase radioimmunoassay for
quantitative measurement of serum digoxin. Test kit 100s, 300s.
Use: Diagnostic aid.
dihematoporphyrin ethers.
Use: Photodynamic therapy of transi-
tional cell carcinoma in situ of urinary bladder or primary or recurrent
obstructing esophageal carcinoma.
[Orphan drug]
See: Photofrin (QLT Phototherapeu-
tics).
•**dihexyverine hydrochloride.** (die-HEX-
ih-ver-een) USAN.
Use: Anticholinergic.
Dihistine D.H. (Goldline) Pseudoephedrine HCl 30 mg, chlorpheniramine maleate 2 mg, codeine phosphate 10 mg.
Elix. Bot. 4 oz, pt, gal. *c-v.*
Use: Decongestant, antihistamine, antitussive.
Dihistine Elixir. (Various Mfr.) Phenylephrine HCl 5 mg, chlorpheniramine
maleate 2 mg/5 ml. Bot. pt, gal. *otc.*
Use: Decongestant, antihistamine.
Dihistine Expectorant. (Goldline)
Pseudoephedrine HCl 30 mg, codeine
phosphate 10 mg, guaifenesin 100 mg,
alcohol 7.5%. Bot. 4 oz, pt, gal. *c-v.*
Use: Decongestant, antitussive, expectorant.

dihydan soluble.
See: Phenytoin Sodium (Various Mfr.)
dihydrocodeine. Paracodin. Drocode.
Use: Antitussive, analgesic.
•**dihydrocodeine bitartrate,** U.S.P. 23.
Use: Analgesic.
See: Hydrocodone Bitartrate, U.S.P. 23.
W/Caffeine, phenacetin, aspirin.
See: Drocogesic #3, Tab. (Rand).
Duradyne DHC, Liq. (Forest).
W/Caffeine, aspirin.
See: Synalgos-DC, Cap. (Wyeth-
Ayerst).
W/Caffeine, acetaminophen.
See: DHC Plus, Cap. (Purdue Freder-
ick).
dihydrocodeinone resin complex.
W/Phenyltoloxamine resin complex.
See: Tussionex, Preps. (Medeva).
dihydro-diethylstilbestrol.
See: Hexestrol, Tab., Vial (Various Mfr.)
dihydroergocornine. Ergot alkaline
component of hydergine.
See: Circanol, Tab. (3M).
Deapril-ST, Tab. (Bristol-Myers).
dihydroergocristine. Ergot alkaloid com-
ponent of hydergine.
See: Circanol, Tab. (3M).
Deapril-ST, Tab. (Bristol-Myers).
dihydroergocryptine. Ergot alkaloid
component of hydergine.
See: Circanol, Tab. (3M).
Deapril-ST, Tab. (Bristol-Myers).
dihydroergotamine. (D.H.E. 45) (San-
doz) Dihydroergotamine mesylate.
Amp. *Rx.*
Use: Agent for migraine, antiadrener-
gic.
•**dihydroergotamine mesylate.** (DIE-
high-droe-err-GOT-uh-meen) U.S.P. 23.
Dihydroergotamine methanesulfonate.
Use: Agent for migraine, antiadrenergic.
See: DHE 45, Amp. (Sandoz). *Rx.*
W/Scopolamine HBr, phenobarbital so-
dium, barbital sodium, Sandoptal.
See: Plexonal, Tab. (Sandoz).
dihydroergotoxine. Ergoloid mesylate.
Rx.
Use: Psychotherapeutic.
See: Gerimal, Tab. (Rugby).
Hydergine, Tab. (Sandoz).
Ergoloid Mesylates, Tab. (Various
Mfr.)
Ergoloid Mesylates, Tab. (Various
Mfr.)
Hydergine, Tab. (Sandoz).
Niloric, Tab. (Ascher).
Hydergine LC, Cap. (Sandoz).
Hydergine, Liq. (Sandoz).

dihydrofollicular hormone.
See: Estradiol (Various Mfr.)

dihydrofolliculine.
See: Estradiol (Various Mfr.)

dihydrohydroxycodeinone. Oxycodone.
(Ducodal, Eukodal, Eucodal). *c-II.*
Use: Narcotic analgesic.

dihydrohydroxycodeinone hydrochloride or bitartrate. Oxycodone HCI or
Bitartrate.
W/Combinations.
See: Cophene-S, Syr. (Dunhall).
Corizahist-D, Syr. (Mason).
Damason-P, Tab. (Mason).
Percobarb, Cap. (DuPont Merck).
Percodan, Tab. (DuPont Merck).
Triaprin-DC, Cap. (Dunhall).

dihydromorphinone hydrochloride.
See: Dilaudid, Preps. (Knoll).

•**dihydrostreptomycin sulfate,** U.S.P. 23.
Use: Antibiotic, antibacterial.

•**dihydrotachysterol,** U.S.P. 23. (Roxane)
0.2 mg/Tab. Bot. 100s, UD 100s.
Use: For postoperative tetany, idiopathic tetany, hypoparathyroidism,
calcium regulator.
See: Hytakerol, Cap., Soln. (Sanofi
Winthrop).

dihydrotachysterol. (Roxane) 0.2 mg/
Tab. Bot. 100s, UD 100s.
Use: For postoperative tetany, idiopathic tetany, hypoparathyroidism,
calcium regulator.

dihydrotestosterone.
See: Stanolone.

dihydrotheelin.
See: Estradiol (Various Mfr.)

dihydroxyacetone.
See: Chromelin, Liq. (Summers).
QT, Liq. (Schering-Plough).
Sudden Tan, Liq. (Schering-Plough).

•**dihydroxyaluminum aminoacetate,**
U.S.P. 23.
Use: Antacid.
W/Methscopolamine bromide, sodium
lauryl sulfate, magnesium hydroxide.
See: Alu-Scop, Cap., Susp. (Westerfield).
W/Phenobarbital and atropine methyl nitrate.
See: Harvatrate A, Tab. (O'Neal).
W/Salicylsalicylic acid, aspirin.
See: Salsprin, Tab. (Seatrace).

•**dihydroxyaluminum sodium carbonate,** U.S.P. 23.
Use: Antacid.
See: Rolaids (Parke-Davis).

dihydroxycholecalciferol.
See: Rocaltrol. (Roche).

24,25 dihydroxycholecalciferol. (Lemmon/Tag) *Rx.*
Use: Uremic osteodystrophy. [Orphan
drug]

dihydroxyestrin.
See: Estradiol (Various Mfr.)

dihydroxyfluorane. Fluorescein.

dihydroxyphenylisatin.
See: Oxyphenisatin (Various Mfr.)

dihydroxyphenyloxindol.
See: Oxyphenisatin (Various Mfr.)

dihydroxypropyltheophylline. Dyphylline.
See: Neothylline, Tab., Elix., Inj. (Lemmon).

dihydroxy(stearato)aluminum. Aluminum Monostearate, N.F. 18.

diiodohydroxyquin.
Use: Amebicide.
See: Iodoquinol, U.S.P. 23.

diiodohydroxyquinoline.
See: Iodoquinol, U.S.P. 23.

diisopromine hydrochloride. (Lab. for
Pharmaceutical Development, Inc.).
See: Desquam-X (Westwood Squibb).

diisopropyl phosphorofluoridate.
See: Isofluorophate, U.S.P. 23.
Floropryl, Oint. (Merck).

diisopropyl sebacate.
Use: Moisturizing agent.
See: Delavan, Cream (Bayer).

Dilacor XR. (Rhone-Poulenc Rorer) Diltiazem HCI 120 mg, 180 mg, or 240
mg/Cap. SR 100s, UD 100s. *Rx.*
Use: Calcium channel blocking agent.

dilaminate. Mixture of magnesium carbide and dihydroxy aluminum glycinate. *otc.*
Use: Antacid.

Dilantin. (Parke-Davis) Phenytoin. **30'
Susp.:** 30 mg/5 ml. Bot. 8 oz, UD 5
ml. **125 Susp.:** 125 mg/5 ml. Bot. 8 oz,
UD 5 ml. **Infatab:** 50 mg/Tab. Bot.
100s, UD 100s. *Rx.*
Use: Anticonvulsant.

Dilantin Sodium. (Parke-Davis) Extended phenytoin sodium. **Kapseal:** 30
mg, 100 mg. Bot. 100s, 1000s, UD
100s. **Amp.:** (w/propylene glycol 40%,
alcohol 10%, sodium hydroxide) 100
mg/2 ml. UD 10s; 250 mg/5 ml. Amp.
10s, UD 10s. *Rx.*
Use: Anticonvulsant.

**Dilantin Sodium w/Phenobarbital
Kapseal.** (Parke-Davis) Phenytoin sodium 100 mg, phenobarbital 16 mg or
32 mg/Cap. Bot. 100s, 1000s, UD 100s
(32 mg only). *Rx.*
Use: Anticonvulsant, sedative, hypnotic.

Dilantin-30 Pediatric. (Parke-Davis) Phenytoin 30 mg/5 ml, alcohol 0.6%. Susp. Bot. 240 ml, 5 ml. *Rx.*
Use: Anticonvulsant.

Dilatrate-SR. (Schwarz Pharma) Isosorbide dinitrate 40 mg/SR Cap. Bot. 60s, 100s. *Rx.*
Use: Antianginal.

Dilaudid. (Knoll) Hydromorphone HCl. **Amp.** (w/sodium citrate 0.2%, citric acid soln. 0.2%): 1 mg, 2 mg or 4 mg/ml. Box 10s. 2 mg. Box 25s. **Multiple Dose Vial:** 2 mg/ml. Bot. 20 ml. **Tab.:** 2 mg Bot. 100s, 500s. Strip pack 4 × 25s. 4 mg 100s, 500s. Strip pack 4 × 25s. 8 mg. Bot. 100s. **Pow:** Vial, 15 gr Multiple dose vial 10 ml, 20 ml. 2 mg/ml. **Rectal Supp.:** (in cocoa butter base, w/colloidal silica 1%): 3 mg/Supp. Box 6s. *c-ii.*
Use: Narcotic analgesic.
W/Guaifenesin.
See: Dilaudid Cough Syrup. (Knoll).

Dilaudid Cough Syrup. (Knoll) Hydromorphone HCl 1 mg, guaifenesin 100 mg/ 5ml. Alcohol 5%. Bot. pt. *c-ii.*
Use: Narcotic analgesic, expectorant.

Dilaudid-5. (Knoll) Hydromorphone HCl 5 mg/5 ml. Liq. Bot. Pt. *c-ii.*
Use: Narcotic analgesic.

Dilaudid HP Ampule. (Knoll) Hydromorphone 10 mg/ml. Box 10s; 50 mg/5 ml. Box 1s. *c-ii.*
Use: Narcotic analgesic.

Dilaudid-HP Injection. (Knoll) Hydromorphone HCl 250 mg (10 mg/ml when reconstituted). In vials. *c-ii.*
Use: Narcotic analgesic.

•**dilevalol hydrochloride.** (DIE-LEV-ah-lole) USAN.
Use: Antihypertensive, anti-adrenergic (β-receptor).

dilithium carbonate. Lithium Carbonate, U.S.P. 23.
Use: Antipsychotic.

Dilocaine. (Hauck) Lidocaine HCl 1% or 2%. Bot. 50 ml. *Rx.*
Use: Local anesthetic, topical.

Dilor. (Savage) Dyphylline. **Tab.:** 200 mg. Bot. 100s, 1000s, UD 100s. **Elix.:** 160 mg/15 ml. Bot. pt. *Rx.*
Use: Bronchodilator.

Dilor 400. (Savage) Dyphylline 400 mg. Bot. 100s, 1000s, UD 100s. *Rx.*
Use: Bronchodilator.

Dilor G Liquid. (Savage) Dyphylline 300 mg, guaifenesin 300 mg/15 ml. Bot. pt, gal. *Rx.*
Use: Bronchodilator, expectorant.

Dilor G Tablets. (Savage) Dyphylline 200 mg, guaifenesin 200 mg/Tab. Bot. 100s, 1000s, UD 100s. *Rx.*
Use: Bronchodilator, expectorant.

diloxaride furoate.
Use: Anti-infective.

•**diltiazem hydrochloride,** (dill-TIE-uh-zem) U.S.P. 23.
Use: Vasodilator (coronary).

diltiazem hydrochloride extended-release capsules. (Various Mfr.) Diltiazem HCl 60 mg, 90 mg or 120 mg. Bot. 100s. *Rx.*
Use: Calcium channel blocker.

diltiazem hydrochloride tablets. (Various Mfr.) Diltiazem HCl 30 mg, 60 mg, 90 mg or 120 mg. Bot. 100s, 500s, 1000s and unit of issue 30s, 60s, 90s, 120s. *Rx.*
Use: Calcium channel blocker.

•**diltiazem malate.** (dill-TIE-ah-zem MAL-ate) USAN.
Use: Calcium channel blocker, antihypertensive.

Dimacol. (Robins) Pseudoephedrine HCl 30 mg, dextromethorphan HBr 10 mg, guaifenesin 100 mg/Cap. or 5 ml. **Cap.** Bot. 100s, 500s, Pre-Pack 12s, 24s. **Liq.** (w/alcohol 4.75%) Bot. pt. *otc.*
Use: Decongestant, nonnarcotic antitussive, expectorant.

Dimaphen Elixir. (Major) Phenylpropanolamine HCl 12.5 mg, brompheniramine maleate 2 mg, 237 ml. *otc.*
Use: Decongestant, antihistamine.

Dimaphen Release. (Major) Phenylpropanolamine HCl 75 mg, brompheniramine maleate 12 mg/Tab. Bot. 12s. *otc.*
Use: Decongestant, antihistamine.

Dimaphen Tablets. (Major) Phenylpropanolamine HCl 25 mg, brompheniramine maleate 4 mg. Tab. Bot. 24s. *otc.*
Use: Decongestant, antihistamine.

•**dimefadane.** (DIE-meh-fah-dane) USAN.
Use: Analgesic.

•**dimefilcon a.** (DIE-meh-FILL-kahn A) USAN.
Use: Contact lens material (hydrophilic).

•**dimefline hydrochloride.** (DIE-meh-fleen) USAN.
Use: Respiratory stimulant.

•**dimefocon.** (DIE-meh-FOE-kahn A) USAN.
Use: Contact lens material (hydrophobic).

Dimenest. (Forest Pharm.) Dimenhydrinate 50 mg/ml. Vial 10 ml. *Rx.*

•**dimenhydrinate,** (die-men-HIGH-drih-nate) U.S.P. 23.
Use: Antiemetic, antihistamine.
See: Dimenest, Inj. (Forest Pharm.)
Dimentabs, Tab. (Jones Medical).
Dramamine, Preps. (Pharmacia & Upjohn).
Dramocen, Inj. (Schwarz Pharma).
Dymenate, Inj. (Keene).
Eldadryl, Preps. (Zeneca)
Eldodram, Tab. (Zeneca)
Hydrate, Vial (Hyrex).
Reidamine, Inj. (Solvay).
Signate, Inj. (Sig).
Trav-Arex, Cap. (Quality Generics).
Traveltabs, Tab. (Geneva Pharm.)
Vertab, Cap. (UAD).

Dimentabs. (Jones Medical) Dimenhydrinate 50 mg/Tab. Bot. 100s. *otc.*
Use: Antiemetic, antivertigo.

•**dimepranol acedoben.** (DIE-MEH-prahnahl ah-SEE-doe-BEN) USAN.
Use: Immunomodulator.

•**dimercaprol,** U.S.P. 23. *Formerly BAL.*
Use: Antidote to gold, arsenic and mercury poisoning; metal complexing agent.
See: BAL in oil, Inj. (Becton Dickinson).

Dimetane-DC Cough Syrup. (Robins) Brompheniramine maleate 2 mg, phenylpropanolamine HCl 12.5 mg, codeine phosphate 10 mg/5 ml w/alcohol 0.95%. Bot. pt, gal. *c-v.*
Use: Antihistamine, decongestant, antitussive.

Dimetane Decongestant Caplets. (Robins) Brompheniramine maleate 4 mg, phenylephrine HCl 10 mg/Capl. Bot. 24s, 48s. *otc.*
Use: Antihistamine, decongestant.

Dimetane Decongestant Elixir. (Robins) Brompheniramine maleate 2 mg, phenylephrine HCl 5 mg/5 ml, alcohol 2.3%. Bot. 120 ml. *otc.*
Use: Antihistamine, decongestant.

Dimetane-DX Cough Syrup. (Robins) Pseudoephedrine HCl 30 mg, brompheniramine maleate 2 mg, dextromethorphan HBr 10 mg, alcohol 0.95%, saccharin, sorbitol. Bot. pt. *Rx.*
Use: Decongestant, antihistamine, antitussive.

Dimetane Extabs. (Robins) Brompheniramine maleate 12 mg/Tab. Pkg. 12s. Bot. 100s, 500s. *otc.*
Use: Antihistamine.

Dimetapp Cold & Allergy. (Robins) Brompheniramine maleate 1 mg, phenylpropanolamine HCl 6.25 mg, aspartame, phenylalanine 8 mg, sorbitol. Tab. Chew. Bot. 24s. *otc.*
Use: Decongestant, antihistamine.

Dimetapp Cold & Flu Caplet. (Robins) Phenylpropanolamine HCl 12.5 mg, brompheniramine maleate 2 mg, acetaminophen 500 mg/Capl. Bot. 24s, 48s. *otc.*
Use: Decongestant, antihistamine, analgesic.

Dimetapp DM Elixir. (Robins) Phenylpropanolamine HCl 12.5 mg, brompheniramine maleate 2 mg, dextromethorphan HBr 10 mg, 2.3% alcohol, saccharin, sorbitol. Elix. Bot. 120 ml, 240 ml. *otc.*
Use: Decongestant, antihistamine, antitussive.

Dimetapp Elixir. (Robins) Brompheniramine maleate 2 mg, phenylpropanolamine HCl 12.5 mg/5 ml. Bot. 120 ml, 240 ml, 360 ml, 473 ml, gal, UD 5 ml. *otc.*
Use: Antihistamine, decongestant.

Dimetapp Extentabs. (Robins) Brompheniramine maleate 12 mg, phenylpropanolamine HCl 75 mg/Tab. Bot. 100s, 500s, UD 100s. Blister pack 12s, 24s, 48s. *otc.*
Use: Antihistamine, decongestant.

Dimetapp 4-Hour Liqui-Gels. (Robins) Brompheniramine maleate 4 mg, phenylpropanolamine HCl 25 mg, sorbitol. Cap. Pck. 12s. *otc.*
Use: Decongestant, antihistamine.

Dimetapp Sinus. (Robins) Pseudoephedrine HCl 30 mg, ibuprofen 200 mg/Cap. Bot. 20s, 40s. *otc.*
Use: Decongestant, analgesic.

Dimetapp Tablets. (Robins) Brompheniramine maleate 4 mg, phenylpropanolamine HCl 25 mg/Tab. Blisterpak 24s. *otc.*
Use: Antihistamine, decongestant.

•**dimethadione.** (DIE-meth-ah-DIE-ohn) USAN. (Baxter).
Use: Anticonvulsant.

dimethazan.

•**dimethicone,** N.F. 18. Dimethylsiloxane polymers. Dimethyl polysiloxane.
Use: Prosthetic aid (soft tissue), component of barrier creams; lubricant and hydrophobing agent.
See: Covicone, Cream (Abbott).
Silicone, Oint. (Various Mfr.)

•**dimethicone 350.** (DIE-meth-ih-cone 350) USAN.
Use: Prosthetic aid for soft tissue.

•**dimethindene maleate.** (DIE-METH-in-deen) USAN. U.S.P. XX.
Use: Antihistamine.

•**dimethisoquin hydrochloride.** USAN.

•**dimethisterone.** (DIE-meth-ISS-ter-ohn) USAN. N.F. XIV.
Use: Progestin.

dimetholizine phosphate.

dimethoxyphenyl penicillin sodium.
Use: Anti-infective.
See: Methicillin sodium (Various Mfr.)

dimethpyridene maleate. Dimethindene Maleate, U.S.P. 23.
See: Dimethindene Maleate, U.S.P. 23.

dimethylaminophenazone.
See: Aminopyrine (Various Mfr.)

dimethylamino pyrazine sulfate.
See: Ampyzine Sulfate.

dimethylcarbamate. of 3-Hydroxy-1-Methylpyridinium Bromide.
See: Mestinon, Tab. (Roche).

dimethylhexestrol dipropionate. Promethestrol Dipropionate.
See: Meprane Dipropionate, Tab. (Schwarz Pharma).

dimethyl polysiloxane.
See: Dimethicone (Various Mfr.)
W/Benzocaine, bismuth subcarbonate, carbamide, hexachlorophene, phenylephrine HCl, pyrilamine maleate, zinc oxide.
W/Hexachlorophene, zinc oxide, pyrilamine maleate, tetracaine HCl, methyl salicylate, zirconium oxide.

•**dimethyl sulfoxide,** (die-METH-uhl sull-FOX-ide) U.S.P. 23. Methyl sulfoxide. DMSO.
Use: Anti-inflammatory (topical), increased intracranial pressure. [Orphan drug].
See: Rimso-50 (Research Ind.).

dimethyl-tubocurarine iodide.
Use: Skeletal muscle relaxant.
See: Metocurine Iodide, U.S.P. 23.

dimethylurethimine.
See: Meturedepa (Centeon).

•**dimoxamine hydrochloride.** (die-MOX-AH-meen) USAN.
Use: Memory adjuvant.

Dimycor. (Standard Drug) Pentaerythritol tetranitrate 10 mg, phenobarbital 15 mg/Tab. Bot. 1000s. *Rx.*
Use: Antianginal, sedative, hypnotic.

Dinacrin. (Sanofi Winthrop) Isonicotinic acid, hydrazide. *Rx.*
Use: Antituberculous agent.

Dinate. (Blaine) Dimenhydrinate 50 mg/ml. Vial 10 ml. *Rx.*
Use: Antiemetic, antivertigo.

•**dinoprost.** (DIE-no-proste) USAN.
Use: Oxytocic; prostaglandin.

•**dinoprost tromethamine,** (DIE-no-proste troe-METH-ah-meen) U.S.P. 23.
Use: Oxytocic, prostaglandin.

•**dinoprostone.** (DIE-no-PROSTE-ohn) USAN.
Use: Abortifacient, agent for cervical ripening, oxytocic, prostaglandin.
See: Cervidil, Insert (Forest).
Prepidil, Gel (Pharmacia & Upjohn).
Prostin E₂, Supp. (Pharmacia & Upjohn).

Diocto. (Purepac) Docusate sodium 100 mg or 200 mg/Cap. Bot. 100s. *otc.*
Use: Laxative.

Diocto-C. (Various Mfr.) Docusate sodium 60 mg, casanthranol 30 mg/15 ml. Syr. Bot. 240 ml, pt, gal. *otc.*
Use: Laxative.

Diocto-K. (Rugby) Docusate potassium 100 mg/Cap. Bot. 100s, 1000s. *otc.*
Use: Laxative.

Diocto-K Plus. (Rugby) Docusate sodium 100 mg, casanthranol 30 mg. Cap. Bot. 100s, 1000s. *otc.*
Use: Laxative.

Dioctolose. (Goldline) Docusate potassium 100 mg/Cap. Bot. 100s, 1000s.
Use: Laxative.

Dioctolose Plus Capsules. (Goldline) Docusate 100 mg, casanthranol 30 mg/Cap. Bot. 100s, 1000s. *otc.*
Use: Laxative.

dioctyl calcium sulfosuccinate. (die-OCK-till SULL-foe-SUCK-sih-nate) Docusate Calcium.
Use: Laxative.

dioctyl potassium sulfosuccinate. *otc.*
W/Glycerin, potassium oleate and stearate.
See: Rectalad, Liq. (Wallace).

dioctyl sodium sulfosuccinate.
See: Docusate Sodium, U.S.P. 23.
Use: Non-laxative fecal softener.

diodone injection.
See: Iodopyracet injection.

Dioeze. (Century) Dioctyl sodium sulfosuccinate 250 mg/Cap. Bot. 100s, 1000s. *otc.*
Use: Laxative.

•**diohippuric acid I-125.** USAN.
Use: Radioactive agent.

•**diohippuric acid I-131.** USAN.
Use: Radioactive agent.

Dio-Hist. (Approved) Dextromethorphan 30 mg, thenylpyramine HCl 80 mg, phenylephrine HCl 20 mg, potassium tartrate ¹⁄₂₄ gr/oz. Bot. 4 oz. *otc.*

Use: Antihistamine.

D-Diol. (Burgin-Arden) Testosterone cypionate 50 mg, estradiol cypionate 2 mg/ml. Vial 10 ml. *Rx.*
Use: Androgen, estrogen.

diolamine. Diethanolamine.

diolostene.
See: Methandriol.

Dionex. (Interstate) Docusate sodium 100 mg or 250 mg/Cap. Bot. 100s, 250s, 1000s. *otc.*
Use: Laxative.

dionin. Ethylmorphine HCl.
Use: Orally; cough depressant, ocular lymphagogue.

Dionosil Oily. (Glaxo) Propyliodone 60% in peanut oil. Inj. Vial 20 ml.
Use: Bronchographic contrast medium.

diophyllin.
See: Aminophylline, Preps. (Various Mfr.)

diopterin. Pteroyldiglutamic acid, PDGA, Pteroyl-alpha-glutamylglutamic acid.
Use: Antineoplastic.

Diorapin. (Standex) Estrogenic conjugate 0.625 mg, methyltestosterone 5 mg/Tab. Bot. 100s. Estrone 2 mg, testosterone 25 mg/ml. Inj. Vial 10 ml. *Rx.*
Use: Estrogen, androgen combination.

Diosate D. (Towne) Docusate sodium. Cap. 100 mg or 250 mg/Tab. Bot. 100s. *otc.*
Use: Laxative.

Diosmin. Buchu resin obtained from lvs. of barosma serratifolia and alliedrutaceae.

Dio-Soft. (Standex) Docusate sodium 100 mg, casanthranol 30 mg/Cap. Bot. 100s. *otc.*
Use: Laxative.

Diostate D. (Pharmacia & Upjohn) Vitamin D 400 IU, calcium 343 mg, phosphorus 265 mg/3 Tab. Bot. 100s. *otc.*
Use: Vitamin/mineral supplement.

• **diotyrosine I-125.** USAN.
Use: Radioactive agent.

• **diotyrosine I-131.** USAN.
Use: Radioactive agent.

Dioval XX. (Keene) Estradiol valerate 20 mg/ml. Vial 10 ml. *Rx.*
Use: Estrogen.

Dioval 40. (Keene) Estradiol valerate 40 mg/ml. Vial 10 ml. *Rx.*
Use: Estrogen.

Diovan. (Novartis) Valsartan 80 mg, 160 mg/Cap. Bot. 100s, 4000s, UD blister 100s. *Rx.*
Use: Antihypertensive.

Diovocylin. (Novartis)
See: Estradiol, Preps. (Various Mfr.)

• **dioxadrol hydrochloride.** (die-OX-ah-drole) USAN.
Use: Antidepressant.

dioxindol. Diacetylhydroxyphenylisatin.

dioxyanthranol.
See: Anthralin, N.F. (Various Mfr.)

dioxyanthraquinone.
See: Danthron, U.S.P. 23.

• **dioxybenzone,** U.S.P. 23.
Use: Ultraviolet screen.
W/Oxybenzone, benzophene.
See: Solbar, Lot. (Person & Covey).

dipalmitoylphosphatidylcholine. Colfosceril palmitate.
Use: Synthetic lung surfactant.
See: Exosurf Neonatal, Pow. (Glaxo Wellcome).

dipalmitoylphosphatidylcholine/phosphatidylglycerol.
Use: Neonatal respiratory distress syndrome. [Orphan drug]

diparcol hydrochloride. Diethazine.

Dipegyl.
See: Nicotinamide, Preps. (Various Mfr.)

dipenicillin g.
See: Benzethacil.

Dipentum. (Pharmacia & Upjohn) Osalazine sodium 250 mg/Cap. Bot. 100s, 500s. *Rx.*
Use: Ulcerative colitis.

diperodon hydrochloride.
Use: Anesthetic.
See: Diothane Oint. (Hoechst Marion Roussel).
Proctodon, Cream (Solvay).
W/Bacitracin, neomycin sulfate, polymyxin.
See: Epimycin A, Oint. (Delta).
W/Benzalkonium Cl, ichthammol, thymol, camphor, juniper tar.
See: Boro Oint. (Scrip).
W/Furacin (nitrofurazone).
See: Furacin E Urethral Inserts (Eaton).
Furacin H.C. Urethral Inserts (Eaton).
W/Furacin (nitrofurazone) and Microfur (nituroxime).
See: Furacin Otic, Drops. (Eaton).
W/Hydrocortisone, polymyxin B sulfate, neomycin.
See: My Cort Otic #1, Ear Drops (Scrip).
W/Hydroxyquinoline Benzoate.
See: Diothane, Oint. (Hoechst Marion Roussel).
W/Methapyrilene HCl, pyrilamine maleate, allantoin, benzocaine, menthol.
See: Antihistamine Cream (Towne).

W/Thimerosal, isopropyl alcohol.
See: Earobex, Ear Drops (Roberts).
diphenadione.
Use: Anticoagulant.
See: Dipaxin, Tab. (Pharmacia & Upjohn).
diphenatil.
See: Diphemanil methylsulfate.
Diphenatol. (Rugby) Diphenoxylate HCl 2.5 mg, atropine sulfate 0.025 mg. Tab. Bot. 100s, 500s, 1000s.
Use: Antidiarrheal.
Diphen Cough. (Rosemont) Diphenhydramine HCl 12.5 mg/5 ml. Syr. Bot. 118 ml, pt, gal. *otc.*
Use: Antitussive.
Diphenhist. (Rugby) Diphenhydramine.
Captabs: 25 mg Bot. 100s, UD 24s.
Elix.: 12.5 mg/5 ml. Bot. 120 ml, pt, gal. *otc.*
Use: Antihistamine.
•**diphenhydramine citrate,** U.S.P. 23.
Use: Antihistamine.
diphenhydramine and pseudoephedrine capsules.
Use: Antihistamine, decongestant.
diphenhydramine citrate.
Use: Antihistamine.
•**diphenhydramine hydrochloride,** (die-fen-HIGH-druh-meen) U.S.P. 23.
Use: Antihistamine.
diphenhydramine hydrochloride. (die-fen-HIGH-druh-meen)
Use: Antihistamine.
See: Bax, Cap., Elix., Expectorant (McKesson).
Benadryl Hydrochloride, Preps. (Parke-Davis).
Benahist, Preps. (Keene).
Benylin Cough Syrup (Warner-Lambert).
Clearly Cala-gel (Tec Labs).
Diphen-Ex, Syr. (Quality Generics).
Diphenhydramine HCl (Weeks & Leo).
Fenylhist, Cap. (Roberts).
Histine Prods. (Freeport).
Hyrexin, Inj. (Hyrex).
Mouthkote P/R, Oint., Spray (Parnell).
Span-Lanin, Cap. (Scrip).
Tusstat, Expectorant (Century).
W/Ammonium Cl, menthol.
See: Eldadryl Expectorant, Liq. (Zeneca)
Fenylex, Expectorant (Roberts).
Tusstat Expectorant (Century).
W/Antihistamines.
See: Symptrol, Syr., Cap., Inj. (Saron).
W/Benzethonium Cl.
See: Bendylate, Inj. (Solvay).

W/Chlorobutanol.
See: Ardeben, Inj. (Burgin-Arden).
W/Pheniramine maleate pyrilamine maleate, phenylephrine HCl, phenylpropanolamine HCl.
See: Symptrol, Syr. (Saron).
W/Zinc oxide.
See: Ziradryl, Lot. (Parke-Davis).
•**diphenidol.** (die-FEN-ih-dahl) USAN.
Use: Antiemetic.
See: Vontrol, Preps. (SK-Beecham).
•**diphenidol hydrochloride.** (die-FEN-ih-dahl) USAN.
Use: Antiemetic.
•**diphenidol pamoate.** (die-FEN-ih-dahl) USAN.
Use: Antiemetic.
diphenmethanil methylsulfate.
See: Diphemanil Methylsulfate (Various Mfr.)
•**diphenoxylate hydrochloride,** (die-fen-OX-ih-late) U.S.P. 23.
Use: Antiperistaltic to treat diarrhea.
W/Atropine.
See: Diaction, Tab. (Knoll Pharm.)
Lomotil, Tab., Liq. (Searle).
diphenoxylate hydrochloride and atropine sulfate. (die-fen-OX-ih-late and AT-troe-peen)
Use: Antiperistaltic.
diphenylhydroxycarbinol. Benzhydrol HCl.
diphenylhydantoin. Phenytoin, U.S.P. 23.
Use: Anticonvulsant.
diphenylhydantoin sodium. Phenytoin Sodium, U.S.P. 23.
Use: Anticonvulsant.
diphenylisatin.
See: Oxyphenisatin (Various Mfr.)
diphosphonic acid.
See: Etidronic acid.
diphosphopyridine (dpn).
Use: Antialcoholic. Under study.
diphosphothiamin. Cocarboxylase.
See: Coenzyme-B, Cap., and Inj. (Inwood).
diphoxazide.
diphtheria, acellular pertussis, tetanus vaccine. (diff-THEER-ee-uh, ay-SELL-you-luhr per-TUSS-iss, TET-ah-nus)
Use: Agent for immunization.
See: Acel-Imune (Wyeth Lederle).
Tripedia (Pasteur-Merieux-Connaught).
•**diphtheria antitoxin,** (diff-THEER-ee-uh) U.S.P. 23. (Pasteur-Merieux-Connaught) 20,000 units, tricresol 4%/vial. (Biocine-Sclavo) 20,000 units, m-cre-

sol 0.3%/vial. (not < 500 units/ml).
Use: I.M., slow I.V. infusion; protection, treatment of diphtheria; passive immunizing agent.

diphtheria antitoxin. (Pasteur-Merieux-Connaught) 20,000 units, tricresol 4%/vial. (Biocine-Sclavo) 20,000 units, m-cresol 0.3%/vial. (not < 500 units/ml).
Use: I.M. slow I.V. infusion; protection/treatment of diphtheria; passive immunizing agent.

diphtheria equine antitoxin. *Rx.*
Use: Prophylaxis and treatment of diphtheria.

diphtheria & tetanus toxoids. (diff-THEER-ee-uh & TET-ah-nus)
Use: Agent for immunization.

diphtheria & tetanus toxoids & acellular pertussis vaccine.
See: Acel-Imune, Vial (Wyeth Lederle).
Infanrix, Vial (SK-Beecham).
Tripedia, Vial (Pasteur-Merieux-Connaught).

diphtheria & tetanus toxoids, aluminum phosphate adsorbed. (Wyeth Lederle) Tubex 0.5 ml. Vial 5 ml. Pkg. 10s. Available in pediatric and adult strengths. 10 Lf units diphtheria and 5 Lf units tetanus per 0.5 ml dose. 1.5 Lf units diphtheria, 5 Lf units tetanus per 0.5 ml dose. *Rx.*
Use: Agent for immunization.

diphtheria & tetanus toxoids.
Pediatric: (Pasteur-Merieux-Connaught) 6.6 Lf units diphtheria and 5 Lf units tetanus/0.5 ml dose. Vial 5 ml.
(Wyeth Lederle) 12.5 Lf units diphtheria, 5 Lf units tetanus per 0.5 ml dose. Vial 5 ml.
(Massachusetts Public Health Biologic Labs) 7.5 Lf units diphtheria and 7.5 Lf units tetanus/0.5 ml dose. Vial, multidose. *Rx.*
Adult:
(Pasteur-Merieux-Connaught) 2 Lf units diphtheria and 5 Lf units tetanus/0.5 ml dose. Vial 5 ml, 30 ml.
(Wyeth Lederle) 2 Lf units diphtheria and 5 Lf units tetanus per 0.5 ml dose. Vial 5 ml, disp. syringe 0.5 ml, vial 5 ml.
(Massachusetts Public Health Biologic Labs) 2 Lf units diphtheria and 2 Lf units tetanus/0.5 ml dose. Vial, multidose. *Rx.*
Use: Agent for immunization.

diphtheria & tetanus toxoids & pertussis vaccine. (diff-THEER-ee-uh & TET-ah-nus & per-TUSS-iss)

(Pasteur-Merieux-Connaught) 6.5 Lf units diphtheria, 5 Lf units tetanus, 4 Lf units pertussis/0.5 ml dose. Vial 2.5 ml, 5 ml, 7.5 ml.
(Massachusetts Public Health Biologic Labs) 10 Lf units diphtheria, 5.5 Lf units tetanus and 4 units pertussis/0.5 ml dose. Vial 5 ml.
Use: Prevention against diphtheria, tetanus and pertussis; immunizing agent.
See: Acel-Imune, Vial (Wyeth Lederle)
DTwP (Michigan Dept. of Public Health/SK-Beecham).
Tri-immunol, Vial (Wyeth Lederle).
Tripedia, Vial (Pasteur-Merieux-Connaught).

diphtheria & tetanus toxoids & pertussis vaccine adsorbed. (Wyeth Lederle) Vaccine Vial 7.5 ml. *Rx.*
Use: Agent for immunization.

diphtheria & tetanus toxoids & pertussis vaccine combined, Aluminum Hydroxide Adsorbed.
See: Triogen, Vial (Parke-Davis).

diphtheria & tetanus toxoids & pertussis vaccine combined, aluminum phosphate-adsorbed.
Use: Agent for immunization.
See: Tri-Immunol, Vial (Wyeth Lederle).

•**diphtheria toxin for Schick Test,** U.S.P. 23. *Formerly Diphtheria Toxin, Diagnostic.*
Use: Diagnostic aid (dermal reactivity indicator).

•**diphtheria toxoid,** U.S.P. 23.
Use: Immunization (active).

•**diphtheria toxoid adsorbed,** U.S.P. 23.
Use: Immunization (active).

diphylline.
See: Diazma, Vial (Pharmex).

Dipimol. (Everett) Dipyridamole 25 mg, 50 mg or 75 mg/Tab. Bot. 100s, 500s, 1000s.
Use: Antianginal.

dipivalyl epinephrine.
See: Propine (Allergan).

•**dipivefrin.** (die-PIHV-eh-FRIN) USAN. *Formerly Dipivalyl Epinephrine.*
Use: Adrenergic (ophthalmic).

•**dipivefrin hydrochloride,** U.S.P. 23.
Use: Antiglaucoma agent.
See: Propine, Soln. (Allergan).

dipivefrin hydrochloride. (Various Mfr.) 0.1% Soln. 5 ml, 10 ml, 15 ml. *Rx.*
Use: Antiglaucoma agent.

Dipridamole. (Foy) Dipyridamole 25 mg/Tab. Bot. 1000s. *Rx.*
Use: Antianginal.

Diprivan. (Zeneca) Propofol 10 mg/ml. Inj. Amp. 20 ml, 50 ml or 100 ml infusion vials. *Rx.*
Use: General anesthetic.

Diprolene AF Cream. (Schering Plough) Betamethasone dipropionate cream equivalent to 0.05% betamethasone. 15 g, 45 g. *Rx.*
Use: Topical corticosteroid.

Diprolene Cream 0.05%. (Schering Plough) Betamethasone dipropionate 0.05% in cream base. Tube 15 g. *Rx.*
Use: Anti-inflammatory, antipruritic (topical).

Diprolene Ointment 0.05%. (Schering Plough) Betamethasone dipropionate 0.05%, in ointment base. Tube 15 g, 45 g. *Rx.*
Use: Anti-inflammatory, antipruritic (topical).

dipropylacetic acid.
See: Valproic Acid.

Diprosone Aerosol 0.1%. (Schering Plough) Betamethasone dipropionate 6.4 mg (equiv. to 5 mg bethamethasone) in vehicle of mineral oil, caprylic-capric triglyceride w/isopropyl alcohol 10%, inert hydrocarbon propellants. (propane and isobutane). Can 85 g. *Rx.*
Use: Corticosteroid, topical.

Diprosone Cream 0.05%. (Schering Plough) Betamethasone dipropionate 0.64 mg (equiv. to 0.5 mg betamethasone) w/mineral oil, white petrolatum, polyethylene glycol 1000 monocetyl ether, cetostearyl alcohol, phosphoric acid, monobasic sodium phosphate with 4-chloro-m-cresol as preservative. Tube 15 g, 45 g. *Rx.*
Use: Corticosteroid, topical.

Diprosone Lotion 0.05%. (Schering Plough) Betamethasone dipropionate 0.64 mg (equivalent to 0.5 mg betamethasone) w/isopropyl alcohol (46.8%), purified water. Bot. 20 ml, 60 ml. *Rx.*
Use: Corticosteroid, topical.

Diprosone Ointment 0.05%. (Schering Plough) Betamethasone dipropionate 0.64 mg (equivalent to 0.5 mg betamethasone) in white petrolatum and mineral oil base. Tube 15 g, 45 g. *Rx.*
Use: Corticosteroid, topical.

dipyridamole, (DIE-pih-RID-uh-mole) (Various Mfr.) **25 mg/Tab.:** Bot. 90s, 100s, 500s, 1000s, 5000s, UD 100s. **50 mg, 75 mg/Tab.:** Bot. 100s, 500s, 1000s, UD 100s.
Use: Coronary vasodilator.
See: Persantine (Boehringer Ingelheim).

●**dipyridamole,** (DIE-pih-RID-uh-mole) U.S.P. 23.
Use: Coronary vasodilator.
See: Persantine, Tab. (Boehringer Ingelheim).
Persantine IV (DuPont Merck).

●**dipyrithione.** (DIE-pihr-ih-THIGH-ohn) USAN.
Use: Antibacterial, antifungal.

●**dipyrone.** (DIE-pie-rone) USAN. *Formerly Methampyrone.*
Use: Analgesic, antipyretic.
See: Novaldin (Sterling Winthrop).

●**dirithromycin.** (die-RITH-row-MY-sin) USAN.
Use: Antibacterial.
See: Dynabac, Tab. (Bock).

disaccharide tripeptide glycerol dipalmitoyl. *Rx.*
Use: Antineoplastic. [Orphan drug]

Disalcid. (3M) Salsalate. **Tab.:** 500 mg or 750 mg. Bot. 100s, 500s, UD 100s. **Cap.:** 500 mg. Bot. 100s. *Rx.*
Use: Salicylate analgesic.

Discase. (Omnis Surgical) Chymopapain 5 units/2 ml. Vial 5 ml. *Rx.*
Use: Intradiscal injection for herniated lumbar intervertebral discs.

Disinfecting Solution. (Bausch & Lomb) Sodium Cl, sodium borate, boric acid, chlorhexidine 0.005%, EDTA 0.1%, thimerosal 0.001%. Bot. 355 ml. *otc.*
Use: Soft contact lens care.

●**disiquonium chloride.** (die-SIH-CONE-ee-uhm) USAN.
Use: Antiseptic.

Dismiss Douche. (Schering Plough) Sodium Cl, sodium citrate, citric acid, cetaryl octoate, ceteareth-27, fragrance. Pow. for dilution. Pkg. 2s.
Use: Vaginal preparation.

Disobrom. (Geneva Pharm.) Pseudoephedrine sulfate 120 mg, dexbrompheniramine maleate 6 mg Tab. Bot 100s, 1000s. *Rx.*
Use: Decongestant, antihistamine.

●**disobutamide.** (DIE-so-BYOO-tam-ide) USAN.
Use: Cardiac depressant (antiarrhythmic).

disodium carbonate. Sodium Carbonate, N.F. 18.

disodium chromate. Sodium Chromate Cr 51 Injection, U.S.P. 23.

disodium chromoglycate.
See: Intal (Medeva).
Nasalcrom (Medeva).

disodium clodronate. *Rx.*
Use: Treatment of hypercalcemia of ma-

lignancy. [Orphan drug]

disodium clodronate tetrahydrate. *Rx.*
Use: Increased bone resorption due to malignancy. [Orphan drug]

disodium edathamil.
See: Edathamil Disodium (Various Mfr.)

disodium edetate. Disodium ethylenediaminetetra acetate.
See: Edetate Disodium, U.S.P. 23.

disodium phosphate.
See: Sodium Phosphate, U.S.P. 23.

disodium phosphate heptahydrate. Sodium Phosphate, U.S.P. 23.

disodium silibinin dihemisuccinate. *Rx.*
Use: Antidote for mushroom poisoning. [Orphan drug]

disodium thiosulfate pentahydrate. Sodium Thiosulfate, U.S.P. 23.

di-sodium versenate.
See: Edathamil Disodium (Various Mfr.)

•**disofenin.** (DIE-so-FEN-in) USAN.
Use: Diagnostic aid (carrier agent).

Disophrol. (Schering-Plough) Pseudoephedrine sulfate 60 mg, dexbrompheniramine maleate 2 mg. Tab. Bot. 100s. *otc.*
Use: Decongestant, antihistamine.

Disophrol Chronotabs. (Schering-Plough) Dexbrompheniramine maleate 6 mg, pseudoephedrine sulfate 120 mg/SA Tab. Bot. 100s. *otc.*
Use: Antihistamine, decongestant.

•**disopyramide.** (DIE-so-PIR-uh-mide) USAN.
Use: Cardiac depressant (antiarrhythmic).
See: Rythmodan.

•**disopyramide phosphate,** (DIE-so-PIHR-ah-mid) U.S.P. 23.
Use: Cardiac depressant (antiarrhythmic).
See: Norpace (Searle).

disopyramide phosphate extended-release capsules. (DIE-so-PIHR-ah-mid)
Use: Cardiac depressant (antiarrhythmic).

Disotate. (Forest) Disodium edetate 150 mg/ml. Vial 20 ml. *Rx.*
Use: Treatment of hypercalcemia.

•**disoxaril.** (die-SOX-ar-ILL) USAN.
Use: Antiviral.

Di-Spaz. (Vortech) Dicyclomine HCl.
Cap.: 10 mg. Bot. 1000s. **Inj.:** 10 mg. Vial 10 ml. *Rx.*
Use: Gastrointestinal antispasmodic.

Dispos-A-Med. (Parke-Davis) Isoetharine HCl 0.5% or 1%, isoproterenol HCl

0.25% or 0.5%. Can of prefilled sterile tubes 0.5 ml, 50s. *Rx.*
Use: Bronchodilator.

distaquaine.
See: Penicillin V.

distigmine bromide. Hexamarium bromide.

•**disulfiram,** (die-SULL-fih-ram) U.S.P. 23.
Use: Alcohol deterrent.
See: Antabuse, Tab. (Wyeth-Ayerst).

disulfonamide.
See: Dia-Mer-Sulfonamides (Various Mfr.)

Dital. (UAD) Phendimetrazine tartrate 105 mg/SR Cap. Bot. 100s. *c-III.*
Use: Anorexiant.

Ditate D.S. (Savage) Testosterone enanthate 360 mg, estradiol valerate 16 mg, benzyl alcohol 2% in sesame oil. Syringe 2 ml Box 10s. Vial 2 ml. *Rx.*
Use: Androgen, estrogen combination.

•**ditekiren.** (DIE-teh-KIE-ren) USAN.
Use: Antihypertensive.

dithranol.
See: Anthralin, U.S.P. 23. (Various Mfr.)

D.I.T.I. Creme. (Dunhall) Iodoquinol 100 mg, sulfanilamide 500 mg, diethylstilbestrol 0.1 mg/g Jar. 4 oz. *Rx.*
Use: Anti-infective, vaginal.

D.I.T.I.-2 Creme. (Dunhall) Sulfanilamide 15%, aminacrine HCl 0.2%, allantoin 2%. Tube 142 g. *Rx.*
Use: Anti-infective, vaginal.

Ditropan. (Hoechst Marion Roussel) Oxybutynin Cl 5 mg/Tab. Bot. 100s, 1000s, UD identification pak 100s. *Rx.*
Use: Urinary tract agent.

Ditropan Syrup. (Hoechst Marion Roussel) Oxybutynin Cl. 5 mg/5 ml Bot. 473 ml. *Rx.*
Use: Urinary tract agent.

Diucardin. (Wyeth-Ayerst) Hydroflumethiazide 50 mg/Tab. Bot. 100s. *Rx.*
Use: Diuretic, antihypertensive.

Diulo. (Searle) Metolazone. 2.5 mg, 5 mg or 10 mg/Tab. Bot. 100s. *Rx.*
Use: Diuretic, antihypertensive.

Diurese. (American Urologicals) Trichlormethiazide 4 mg/Tab. Bot. 100s, 1000s. *Rx.*
Use: Diuretic.

diuretic combinations.
See: Moduretic, Tab. (Merck).
Spironolactone w/Hydrochlorothiazide, Tab. (Various Mfr.)
Alazide, Tab. (Major).
Aldactazide, Tab. (Searle).
Dyazide, Cap. (SKB).
Maxzide, Tab. (Lederle).

Maxzide-25 MG, Tab. (Lederle).
Spironazide, Tab. (Schein).
Spirozide, Tab. (Rugby).
Triamterene w/Hydrochlorthiazide,
Cap. (Various Mfr.)
Triamterene w/Hydrochlorothiazide,
Tab. (Various Mfr.)
diuretics, loop.
See: Bumex, Inj., Tab. (Roche).
Edecrin, Tab. (Merck).
Edecrin Sodium, Inj. (Merck).
Fumide, Tab. (Everett).
Furomide M.D., Inj. (Hyrex).
Furosemide, Inj., Tab. (Various Mfr.)
Furosemide, Oral Soln. (Roxane).
Lasix, Inj., Oral Soln., Tab. (Hoechst
Marion Roussel).
Luramide, Tab. (Major).
diuretics, osmotic.
See: Glyrol, Soln. (Ciba Vision).
Ismotic, Soln. (Alcon).
Mannitol, Inj. (Various Mfr.)
Osmitrol, Inj. (Baxter).
Osmoglyn, Soln. (Alcon).
Ureaphil, Inj. (Abbott).
diuretics, potassium-sparing.
See: Alatone, Tab. (Major).
Aldactone, Tab. (Searle).
Amiloride HCl, Tab. (Various Mfr.)
Dyrenium, Cap. (SK-Beecham).
Midamor, Tab. (Merck).
Spironolactone, Tab. (Various Mfr.)
diuretics, thiazides.
See: Anhydron, Tab. (Lilly).
Aquatag, Tab. (Solvay).
Aquatensen, Tab. (Wallace).
Chlorothiazide, Tab. (Various Mfr.)
Chlorthalidone, Tab. (Various Mfr.)
Diachlor, Tab. (Major).
Diaqua, Tab. (Roberts).
Diucardin, Tab. (Wyeth-Ayerst).
Diulo, Tab. (Searle).
Diurese, Tab. (American Urologicals).
Diurigen, Tab. (Goldline).
Diuril, Oral Susp., Tab. (Merck).
Diuril Sodium, Inj. (Merck).
Enduron, Tab. (Abbott).
Esidrix, Tab. (Novartis).
Ethon, Tab. (Major).
Exna, Tab. (Robins).
Hydrex, Tab. (Trimen).
Hydrochlorothiazide, Tab. (Various
Mfr.)
Hydrochlorothiazide, Oral Soln.
(Roxane).
HydroDIURIL, Tab. (Merck).
Hydroflumethiazide, Tab. (Various
Mfr.)
Hydromal, Tab. (Roberts).
Hydromox, Tab. (Lederle).

Hydro-T, Tab. (Major).
Hydro-Z-50, Tab. (Mayrand).
Hydrozide-50, Tab. (T.E. Williams).
Hygroton, Tab. (Rhone-Poulenc
Rorer).
Hylidone, Tab. (Major).
Lozol, Tab. (Rhone-Poulenc Rorer).
Metahydrin, Tab. (Hoechst Marion
Roussel).
Methyclothiazide, Tab. (Various Mfr.)
Mictrin, Tab. (Econo Med).
MyKrox (Medeva).
Naqua, Tab. (Schering Plough).
Naturetin, Tab. (Bristol-Myers).
Niazide, Tab. (Major).
Oretic, Tab. (Abbott).
Proaqua, Tab. (Solvay).
Renese, Tab. (Pfizer).
Saluron, Tab. (Bristol-Myers).
Thalitone, Tab. (Boehringer Ingel-
heim).
Thiuretic, Tab. (Warner-Chilcott).
Trichlormethiazide, Tab. (Various Mfr.)
Zaroxolyn, Tab. (Medeva).
Diuretic Tablets. (Faraday) Buchu
leaves 150 mg, uva ursi leaves 150 mg,
juniper berries 120 mg, bone meal,
parsley, asparagus/Tab. Bot. 100s. Rx.
Use: Diuretic.
Diurigen Tablets. (Goldline) Chloro-
thiazide 500 mg/Tab Bot. 100s, 1000s.
Rx.
Use: Diuretic.
Diurigen w/Reserpine 250 Tablets.
(Goldline). Chlorothiazide 250 mg, re-
serpine 0.125 mg. Tab. Bot. 100s,
1000s. Rx.
Use: Antihypertensive combination.
Diurigen w/Reserpine 500 Tablets.
(Goldline). Chlorothiazide 500 mg, re-
serpine 0.125 mg. Tab. Bot. 100s,
1000s. Rx.
Use: Antihypertensive combination.
Diuril. (Merck) Chlorothiazide, U.S.P.
Tab.: 250 mg Bot. 100s, 1000s; 500 mg
Bot. 100s, 1000s, UD 100s. **Oral
Susp.:** 250 mg/5 ml w/methylparaben
0.12%, propylparaben 0.02%, benzoic
acid 0.1%, alcohol 0.5%. Bot. 237 ml.
Rx.
Use: Diuretic, antihypertensive.
W/Methyldopa.
See: Aldoclor, Tab. (Merck).
W/Reserpine.
See: Diupres, Tab. (Merck).
Diuril Sodium Intravenous. (Merck)
Chlorothiazide sodium equivalent to 0.5
g chlorothiazide w/mannitol 0.25 g so-
dium hydroxide, thimerosal 0.4 mg.
Vial 20 ml. Rx.

Use: Diuretic, antihypertensive.

Diutensen-R. (Wallace) Methyclothiazide 2.5 mg, reserpine 0.1 mg/Tab. Bot. 100s, 500s, 5000s. *Rx.*
Use: Antihypertensive combination.

•**divalproex sodium.** (die-VAL-pro-ex) USAN.
Use: Anticonvulsant.
See: Depakote (Abbott).

divinyl oxide. Vinyl ether, divinyl ether.
Use: Inhalation anesthetic.

Dizac. (Ohmeda) Diazepam 5 mg/ml. Inj. Vial 3 ml. *c-iv.*
Use: Antianxiety agent, anticonvulsant, skeletal muscle relaxant.

Dizmiss. (Jones Medical) Meclizine HCl 25 mg/Tab. Bot. 100s, 1000s. *otc.*
Use: Antiemetic, antivertigo.

•**dizocilpine maleate.** (die-ZOE-sill-PEEN) USAN.
Use: Neuroprotective.

dl-desoxyephedrine hydrochloride.
See: dl-Methamphetamine HCl.

dl-methamphetamine hydrochloride.
dl-Desoxyephedrine HCl.
See: Oxydess, Tab. (Vortech).
W/Pyrilamine maleate, phenyltoloxamine dihydrogen citrate, didesoxyephedrine HCl, codeine phosphate, ammonium Cl, potassium guaiacolsulfonate, chloroform, phenylpropanolamine tartar emetic.
See: Meditussin-X Liquid (Roberts).

dl-norephedrine hydrochloride.
See: Phenylpropanolamine Hydrochloride (Various Mfr.)

DM Cough. (Rosemont) Dextromethorphan HBr 10 mg/5 ml, alcohol 5%. Syr. Bot. 120 ml, pt, gal. *otc.*
Use: Antitussive.

DMCT. (Lederle) Demethylchlortetracycline. *Rx.*
Use: Anti-infective, tetracycline.
See: Declomycin HCl, Preps. (Lederle).

d-methorphan hydrobromide.
See: Dextromethorphan HBr (Various Mfr.).

d-methylphenylamine sulfate.
See: Dextroamphetamine Sulfate, U.S.P. 23. (Various Mfr.).

DML Dermatological Moisturizing Lotion. (Person & Covey) Purified water, petrolatum, glycerin, methyl glucose sesquisterate, dimethicone, methyl gluceth-20 sesquisterate, benzyl alcohol, volatile silicone, glyceryl stearate, stearic acid, palmitic acid, cetyl alcohol, xanthan gum, magnesium aluminum silicate carbomer 941, sodium

hydroxide. Bot. 8 oz. *otc.*
Use: Emollient.

DML Facial Moisturizer. (Person & Covey) Octyl methoxycinnamate 8%, oxybenzone 4%, benzyl alcohol, petrolatum, EDTA. SPF 15. Cream 45 g. *otc.*
Use: Sunscreen.

DML Forte. (Person & Covey) Petrolatum, PPG-2 myristyl ether propionate, glyceryl stearate, glycerin, stearic acid, d-panthenol, DEA-cetyl phosphate, simethicone, PVP eicosene copolymer, benzyl alcohol, cetyl alcohol, silica, disodium EDTA, BHA, magnesium aluminum silicate, sodium carbomer 1342. Tube 113 g. *otc.*
Use: Emollient.

DMSO.
See: Dimethyl sulfoxide.
n-DNA.

DNR.
See: Cerubidine (Wyeth-Ayerst).

Doak Tar Distillate. (Doak) Coal tar distillate 40%. Liq. Bot. 59 ml. *otc.*
Use: Antiseborrheic.

Doak Tar Lotion. (Doak) Tar distillate 5%. Bot. 118 ml. *otc.*
Use: Antiseborrheic.

Doak Tar Oil. (Doak) Tar distillate 2%. Liq. Bot. 237 ml. *otc.*
Use: Antiseborrheic.

Doak Tar Oil Forte. (Doak) Tar distillate 5%. Bot. 4 oz.
Use: Antiseborrheic.

Doak Tar Shampoo. (Doak) Tar distillate 3% in shampoo base. Bot. 237 ml. *otc.*
Use: Antiseborrheic.

Doak Tersaseptic. (Doak) Liquid cleanser, pH 6.8. Bot. 4 oz, pt, gal. *otc.*
Use: Liquid detergent.

Doan's Backache Spray. (DEP Corp.) Methyl salicylate 15%, menthol 8.4%, methyl nicotinate 0.6%. Aerosol can 4 oz. *otc.*
Use: Analgesic, topical.

Doan's Pills. (DEP Corp.) Magnesium salicylate 325 mg/Tab. Ctn. 24s, 48s. *otc.*
Use: Analgesic.

•**dobutamine,** (doe-BYOOT-ah-meen) U.S.P. 23
Use: Cardiotonic.

•**dobutamine hydrochloride.** (doe-BYOOT-ah-meen) U.S.P. 23.
Use: Cardiac stimulant, cardiotonic.
See: Dobutrex, Inj. (Lilly).

dobutamine hydrochloride. (Various Mfr.) 12.5 mg/ml. May contain sulfites. Inj. Vial 20 ml.

Use: Cardiac stimulant, cardiotonic.

• **dobutamine lactobionate.** (doe-BYOOT-ah-meen) USAN.
Use: Cardiac stimulant, cardiotonic.

• **dobutamine tartrate.** (doe-BYOOT-ah-meen) USAN.
Use: Cardiac stimulant, cardiotonic.

Dobutrex Solution. (Lilly) Dobutamine HCl 250 mg. Inj. Vial 20 ml. *Rx.*
Use: Cardiac stimulant.

• **docebenone.** (dah-SEH-beh-nohn) USAN.
Use: Inhibitor (5-lipoxygenase).
See: Antiallergic; antiasthmatic.

• **docetaxel.** USAN.
Use: Antineoplastic.
See: Taxotere (Rhone-Poulenc Rorer).

• **doconazole.** (doe-KOE-nah-zole) USAN.
Use: Antifungal.

Doctar. (Savage) Coal tar 0.5%, conditioner. Shampoo. Bot. 100 ml. *otc.*
Use: Antiseborrheic.

Doctase. (Purepac) Docusate sodium 100 mg, casanthranol 30 mg/Cap. Bot. 100s. *otc.*
Use: Laxative.

Doctyl. (Approved) Docusate sodium 100 mg/Tab. Bot. 40s, 100s, 1000s. *otc.*
Use: Laxative.

Doctylax. (Approved) Docusate sodium 100 mg, acetophenolisatin 2 mg, prune conc. ¾ mg/Tab. Bot. 40s, 100s, 1000s. *otc.*
Use: Laxative.

Docucal-P Softgels. (Parmed) Docusate (as calcium) 60 mg, phenolphthalein 65 mg/Cap. Bot. 100s, 1000s. *otc.*
Use: Laxative.

• **docusate calcium,** (DOCK-you-sate) U.S.P. 23. *Formerly Dioctyl Calcium Sulfosuccinate.*
Use: Laxative; stool softener.
See: Surfak, Cap. (Hoechst Marion Roussel).
  Doxidan, Cap. (Hoechst Marion Roussel).
  Danthron, Tab. (Goldline).

docusate with casanthranol. (DOCK-you-sate) (Various Mfr.) Docusate (as sodium) 100 mg, casanthranol 30 mg/Cap. Bot. 100s, 1000s, UD 100s. *otc.*
Use: Laxative; stool softener.

• **docusate potassium,** U.S.P. 23.
Use: Laxative; stool softener.
See: Dialose, Cap. (Stuart).
  Dialose Plus, Cap. (Stuart).
  Kasof, Cap. (Stuart).

• **docusate sodium,** (DOCK-you-sate) U.S.P. 23. *Formerly Dioctyl Sodium Sulfosuccinate.*

Use: Pharmaceutical aid (surfactant), stool softener.
See: Colace, Cap., Liq., Syr. (Bristol-Myers).
  Coloctyl, Cap. (Eon Labs).
  Comfolax, Cap. (Searle).
  Correctol Extra Gentle, Cap. (Schering-Plough).
  Dialose, Tab. (J & J-Merck).
  Diomedicone, Tab (Medicone).
  Diosate Caps. (Towne).
  Doss, Super Doss, Tab. (Ferndale).
  Doxinate, Cap., Liq. (Hoechst Marion Roussel).
  DSS (Parke-Davis).
  Duosol, Cap. (Kirkman Sales).
  Dynoctol, Cap. (Solvay).
  Easy-Lax, Cap. (Walgreen).
  Konsto, Cap. (Freeport).
  Laxatab, Tab. (Freeport).
  Liqui-Doss, Liq. (Ferndale).
  Modane Soft, Cap. (Pharmacia & Upjohn).
  Peri-Doss, Cap. (Ferndale).
  Regul-Aid, Syr. (Quality Generics).
  Regutol, Tab. (Schering-Plough).
  Revac Supprettes, Supp. (Poly-Medica).
  Stulex, Tab. (Jones Medical).
  Surfak, Cap. (Hoechst Marion Roussel).

W/Ascorbic acid, ferrous fumarate.
See: Hemaspan Cap. (Bock).

W/Betaine HCl, zinc, manganese, molybdenum.
See: Hemaferrin (Western Research).

W/Bisacodyl.
See: Laxadan, Supp. (Lemmon).

W/Brewer's yeast.
See: Doss or Super Doss, Tab. (Ferndale).

W/Casanthranol.
See: Calotabs, Tab. (Calotabs).
  Constiban (Quality Generics).
  Diolax, Cap. (Century).
  Dio-Soft (Standex).
  Di-Sosul Forte, Tab. (Drug).
  Easy-Lax Plus, Cap. (Walgreen).
  Genericace, Cap. (Forest Pharm.)
  Neo-Vadrin D-D-S, Cap. (Scherer).
  Nuvac, Cap. (LaCrosse).
  Peri-Colace, Cap., Syr. (Bristol-Myers).

W/Casanthranol, sodium carboxymethylcellulose.
See: Dialose Plus, Cap. (Stuart).
  Tri-Vac, Cap. (Rhode).

W/Dehydrocholic acid.
See: Dubbalax-B, Cap. (Redford).
  Dubbalax-N, Cap. (Redford).
  Neolax, Tab. (Schwarz Pharma).

W/D-calcium pantothenate and acetphenolisatin.
See: Peri-Pantyl, Tab. (McGregor).
W/Ferrous fumarate, Vitamin C.
See: Hemaspan, Cap. (Bock).
Recoup, Tab. (Lederle).
W/Ferrous fumarate, vitamins.
See: Bevitone, Tab. (Lemmon).
W/Ferrous fumarate, betaine HCl, desiccated liver, vitamins, minerals.
See: Hemaferrin, Tab. (Western Research).
W/Glycerin.
See: Rectalad Enema, Liq. (Wampole).
W/Isobornyl thiocyanoacetate.
See: Barc, Cream, Liq. (Del Pharm.)
W/Petrolatum.
See: Milkinol, Liq., Emulsion (Kremers-Urban).
W/Phenolphthalein.
See: Correctol, Tab. (Schering-Plough).
Ex-Lax Prods. (Sandoz Consumer).
Feen-A-Mint, Pills (Schering-Plough).
W/Phenolphthalein, dehydrocholic acid.
See: Bolax, Cap. (Boyd).
Sarolax, Cap. (Saron).
Tripalax, Cap. (Redford).
W/Polyoxyethylene nonyl phenol, sodium edetate, and 9-aminoacridine HCl.
See: Vagisec Plus Supp. (Schmid).
W/Senna concentrate.
See: Gentlax S, Tab. (Blair).
Sarolax (Saron).
Senokap-DDS, Cap. (Purdue Frederick).
Senokot S, Tab. (Purdue Frederick).
W/Sodium propionate, propionic acid, salicylic acid.
See: Prosal, Liq. (Gordon).
W/Vitamin-mineral combination.
See: Geriplex-FS, Kapseal (Parke-Davis).
Materna 1.60, Tab. (Lederle).
doderlein bacilli.
See: Redoderlein, Vial (Forest Pharm.)
•**dofetilide.** (doe-FEH-till-ide) USAN.
Use: Cardiac depressant (antiarrhythmic).
Dofus. (Miller) Freeze dried *Lactobacillus acidophilus* minimum of 100,000,000 organisms/Cap. w/*Lactobacillus bifidus* organisms added. Bot. 60s. *otc.*
Use: Nutritional supplement, anti-diarrheal.
Dok. (Major) Docusate sodium. **Caps.:** 250 mg. Bot. 100s, 1000s. **Liq.:** 150 mg/15 ml. Bot. pt. **Syrup:** 60 mg/15 ml. Bot. pt, gal. *otc.*
Use: Laxative; stool softener.
Dok-250. (Major) Docusate sodium 250

mg. Cap. Bot. 100s. *otc.*
Use: Laxative; stool softener.
Doktors Spray. (Scherer) Phenylephrine HCl 0.25%, chlorobutanol, sodium bisulfite, benzalkonium chloride. Soln. Bot. 30 ml. *otc.*
Use: Decongestant.
Dolacet. (Roberts Hauck) Hydrocodone bitartrate 5 mg, acetaminophen 500 mg/Cap. Bot. 100s. *c-iii.*
Use: Narcotic analgesic combination.
Dolamide Tabs. (Major) Chlorpropamide 100 mg or 250 mg/Tab. Bot. 100s, 500s, 1000s. *Rx.*
Use: Antidiabetic.
Dolamin. (Harvey) Ammonium sulfate 0.75% with sodium Cl, benzyl alcohol. Amp. 10 ml. In 12s, 25s, 100s. *Rx.*
Use: Antineuralgic.
dolantin.
See: Meperidine HCl, U.S.P. 23.
•**dolasetron mesylate.** (dahl-AH-set-rahn) USAN.
Use: Antiemetic, antimigraine.
See: Anzemet (Hoechst Marion Roussel).
Dolcin. (Dolcin) Aspirin 3.7 gr, calcium succinate 2.8 gr/Tab. Bot. 100s, 200s. *otc.*
Use: Analgesic, salicylate.
Doldram. (Dram) Salicylamide 7.5 gr/Tab. Bot. 100s.
Use: Salicylate analgesic.
Dolene AP-65. (Lederle) Propoxyphene HCl 65 mg, acetaminophen 650 mg/Tab. Bot. 100s, 500s. *c-iv.*
Use: Narcotic analgesic combination.
Dolene Compound-65. (Lederle) Propoxyphene HCl 65 mg, aspirin 389 mg, caffeine 32.4 mg/Cap. Bot. 100s, 500s. *c-iv.*
Use: Narcotic analgesic combination.
Dolene Plain. (Lederle) Propoxyphene HCl 65 mg/Cap. Bot. 100s, 500s. *c-iv.*
Use: Narcotic analgesic.
Dolobid. (Merck) Diflunisal 250 mg or 500 mg/Tab. Unit-of-use 60s, UD 100s. *Rx.*
Use: Salicylate analgesic.
Dolomite. (NBTY) Magnesium 78 mg, calcium 130 mg/Tab. Bot. 100s, 250s. *otc.*
Use: Mineral supplement.
Dolomite. (Halsey) Calcium 426 mg, magnesium 246 mg/3 Tab. w/guar and acacia gum. Bot. 250s. *otc.*
Use: Mineral supplement.
Dolomite Plus Capsules. (Barth's) Magnesium 37 mg, calcium 187 mg, phos-

phorous 50 mg, iodine 0.25 mg/Cap. Bot. 100s, 500s, 1000s. *otc.*
Use: Mineral supplement.

Dolomite Tablets. (Faraday) Calcium 150 mg, magnesium 90 mg/Tab. Bot. 250s. *otc.*
Use: Mineral supplement.

dolonil. (Parke-Davis)
See: Pyridium Plus, Tab. (Parke-Davis).

Dolophine Hydrochloride. (Lilly) Methadone HCl. **Amp.:** (10 mg/ml; sodium Cl 0.9%) 1 ml 12s, 100s. **Vial:** (10 mg/ml) 20 ml (sodium Cl 0.9%, chlorobutanol 0.5%). 1s, 25s. **Tab.:** 5 mg, Bot. 100s. 10 mg, Bot. 100s. *c-II.*
Use: Narcotic analgesic.

Dolopirona Tablets. (Sanofi Winthrop) Dipyrone with chlormezanone. *Rx.*
Use: Analgesic, muscle relaxant, antianxiety agent.

Dolorac. (GenDerm) Capsaicin 0.25%, benzyl alcohol, cetyl alcohol/Cream. Tube 28 g. *otc.*
Use: Topical analgesic.

Doloral. (Progressive Enterprises) Colchicine salicylate 0.1 mg, phenobarbital 8 mg, sodium p-amino-benzoate 15 mg, vitamins B_1 25 mg, aspirin 325 mg/Tab. Bot. 100s, 1000s. *Rx.*
Use: Agent for gout, antiarthritic.

dolosal.
See: Meperidine HCl.

Dolsed. (American Urologicals) Methenamine 40.8 mg, phenylsalicylate 18.1 mg, atropine sulfate 0.03 mg, hyoscyamine 0.03 mg, benzoic acid 4.5 mg, methylene blue 5.4 mg. Tab. Bot. 100s, 1000s. *Rx.*
Use: Urinary anti-infective.

dolvanol.
Use: Narcotic analgesic.
See: Meperidine HCl.

•**domazoline fumarate.** (DOME-AZE-oh-leen) USAN.
Use: Anticholinergic.

Domeboro. (Bayer) Aluminum sulfate and calcium acetate when added to water gives therapeutic effect of Burow's. One pkg. or Tab./pt. water approximately equivalent to 1:40 dilution. **Pkg.:** 2.2 g, 12s, 100s. **Effervescent Tab.:** Box 12s, 100s, 1000s. *otc.*
Use: Anti-inflammatory agent, topical.

Domeboro Otic. (Bayer) Acetic acid 2% (in aluminum acetate solution). Soln. Bot. 60 ml with dropper. *Rx.*
Use: Otic preparation.

Dome-Paste Bandage. (Bayer) Zinc oxide, calamine and gelatin bandage.

Pkg. 4"×10 yd. and 3"×10 yd. impregnated gauze bandage. *otc.*
Use: Treatment of conditions of the extremities.

domestrol.
See: Diethylstilbestrol, Preps. (Various Mfr.)

D.O.M.F.
Use: Germicide.
See: Merbromin (Mercurochrome) (City Chem.).

•**domiodol.** (dome-EYE-oh-DOLE) USAN.
Use: Mucolytic.

•**domiphen bromide.** (DOE-mih-fen) USAN.
Use: Antiseptic; anti-infective (topical).
See: Bradosol.
Domibrom.

Domol Bath and Shower Oil. (Bayer.) D_1-isopropyl sebacate, isopropyl myristate with mineral oil. Bot. 240 ml. *otc.*
Use: Emollient.

•**domperidone.** (dome-PEH-rih-dohn) USAN.
Use: Antiemetic.
See: Motilium (Janssen).

Donatussin DC Syrup. (Laser) Hydrocodone bitartrate 2.5 mg, phenylephrine HCl 7.5 mg, guaifenesin 50 mg/5 ml. Bot. 120 ml, 480 ml. *c-III.*
Use: Antitussive, decongestant, expectorant.

Donatussin Pediatric Drops. (Laser) Guaifenesin 20 mg, chlorpheniramine maleate 1 mg, phenylephrine HCl 2 mg/ml. Drop. Bot. 30 ml. *Rx.*
Use: Expectorant, antihistamine, decongestant.

Donatussin Syrup. (Laser) Phenylephrine 10 mg, chlorpheniramine maleate 2 mg, dextromethorphan HBr 7.5 mg, guaifenesin 100 mg. Bot. pt, gal. *Rx.*
Use: Decongestant, antihistamine, antitussive, expectorant.

Dondril. (Whitehall Robins) Dextromethorphan HBr 10 mg, phenylephrine HCl 5 mg, chlorpheniramine maleate 1 mg/Tab. Bot. 24s. *otc.*
Use: Antitussive, decongestant, antihistamine.

donepezil HCl. (Eisai/Pfizer)
Use: Treatment of mild to moderate dementia of the Alzheimer's type.
See: Aricept, Tab. (Eisai/Pfizer).

•**donetidine.** (doe-NEH-tih-DEEN) USAN.
Use: Antagonist (to Histamine H_2 receptors).

Donna. (Arcum) Menthol, thymol, euca-

lyptol, exsiccated alum, boric acid. 4 oz, 14 oz. *Rx.*
Use: Vaginal preparation.

Donnagel. (Wyeth-Ayerst) Attapulgite 600 mg. Chew. Tab. Pkg. 18s; Liq. Bot. 120 ml, 240 ml. *otc.*
Use: Antidiarrheal.

Donnamar. (H.L. Moore) Atropine sulfate 0.0194 mg, scopolamine HBr 0.0065 mg, hyoscyamine HBr or SO₄ 0.1037 mg, phenobarbital 16.2 mg/5 ml, alcohol 23%. Elix. Bot. 120 ml, pt, gal. *Rx.*
Use: Anticholinergic, antispasmodic.

Donnamar. (Marnel) Hyoscyamine sulfate 0.125 mg. Tab. Bot. 100s. *Rx.*
Use: Anticholinergic, antispasmodic.

Donnaphen Elixir. (Approved) Phenobarbital 16.2 mg, hyoscyamine sulfate 0.1037 mg, atropine sulfate 0.0194 mg, hyoscine HBr 0.0065 mg/5 ml. Bot. pt, gal. *Rx.*
Use: anticholinergic, antispasmodic.

Donnapine Tabs. (Major) Belladonna alkaloids, phenobarbital 16.2 mg. Bot. 100s, 1000s, UD 100s. *Rx.*
Use: Sedative, anticholinergic, antispasmodic.

Donna-Sed Elixir. (Vortech) Atropine sulfate 0.0194 mg, scopolamine HBr 0.0065, hyoscyamine HBr or SO₄ 0.1037 mg, phenobarbital 16.2 mg, alcohol 23%. Liq. Bot. 118 ml, gal. *Rx.*
Use: Gastrointestinal anticholinergic.

Donnatal. (Robins) Hyoscyamine sulfate 0.1037 mg, atropine sulfate 0.0194 mg, scopolamine HBr 0.0065 mg, phenobarbital 16.2 mg. **Cap. & Tab.:** Bot. 100s, 1000s. **Elix.:** w/alcohol 23%. Bot. 4 oz, pt, gal, Dis-Co pack 5 ml, 100s. *Rx.*
Use: Sedative, anticholinergic, antispasmodic.

Donnatal Dis-Co UD Pack. (Robins) Hyoscyamine sulfate 0.1037 mg, atropine sulfate 0.0194 mg, hyoscine HBr 0.0065 mg, phenobarbital 16.2 mg (0.25 gr)/Tab. or 5 ml. **Tab.:** UD 100s. **Elix.:** UD (5 ml) 25s. *Rx.*
Use: Sedative, anticholinergic, antispasmodic.

Donnatal Elixir. (Robins) Atropine sulfate 0.0194 mg, scopolamine HBr 0.0065 mg, hyoscyamine HBr or sulfate 0.1037 mg, phenobarbital 16.2 mg, alcohol 23%, glucose, saccharin/5 ml. Bot. 120 ml, pt., gal, Dis-Co pack 5 ml. *Rx.*
Use: GI anticholinergic.

Donnatal Extentabs. (Robins) Hyoscyamine sulfate 0.3111 mg, atropine sulfate 0.0582 mg, scopolamine HBr 0.0195 mg, phenobarbital 48.6 mg (¾ gr)/Tab. Bot. 100s, 500s, Dis-Co pack 100s. *Rx.*
Use: Sedative, anticholinergic, antispasmodic.

Donnatal #2. (Robins) Phenobarbital 32.4 mg (0.5 gr), hyoscyamine sulfate 0.1037 mg, atropine sulfate 0.0194 mg, scopolamine HBr 0.0065 mg/Tab. Bot. 100s, 1000s. *Rx.*
Use: Sedative, anticholinergic, antispasmodic.

Donnazyme. (Robins) Hyoscyamine sulfate 0.0518 mg, atropine sulfate 0.0097 mg, scopolamine HBr 0.0033 mg, phenobarbital 8.1 mg (⅛ gr), pepsin 150 mg/Tab. in outer layer, pancreatin 300 mg, bile salts 150 mg/Tab. in core. Bot. 100s, 500s. *Rx.*
Use: Anticholinergic, antispasmodic, digestive aid.

Don't. (Del Pharm.) Sucrose octa acetate 5%, isopropyl alcohol 54%. Bot. 0.45 oz. *otc.*
Use: Used to discourage nail biting and thumb sucking.

•**dopamantine.** (DOE-pah-MAN-teen) USAN.
Use: Antiparkinsonian.

dopamine. (DOE-pah-meen) (Astra) Dopamine. **Amp.:** 200 mg/5 ml Amp. Box 10s; 400 mg/10 ml Amp. Box 5s. **Additive Syringe:** 200 mg/5 ml Syr. Box 1s; 400 mg/10 ml Syr. Box 1s. *Rx.*
Use: Inotropic agent.

•**dopamine hydrochloride,** (DOE-puh-meen) U.S.P. 23.
Use: Adrenergic.
See: Intropin, Amp. (DuPont Merck).

dopamine hydrochloride and dextrose injection. (DOE-pah-meen)
Use: Adrenergic, emergency treatment of low blood pressure.

Dopar. (Procter & Gamble) Levodopa 100 mg or 250 mg/Cap. Bot. 100s. 500 mg/Cap. Bot. 100s, 1000s. *Rx.*
Use: Antiparkinsonian.

•**dopexamine.** (doe-PEX-ah-MEEN) USAN.
Use: Cardiovascular agent.

•**dopexamine hydrochloride.** (doe-PEX-ah-MEEN) USAN.
Use: Cardiovascular agent.

Dopram. (Robins) Doxapram HCl 20 mg/ml, 0.9% benzyl alcohol. Vial 20 ml. *Rx.*
Use: Respiratory stimulant.

Doral. (Wallace) Quazepam 7.5 mg or 15 mg/Tab. Bot. 100s, UD 100s. *c-iv.*

Use: Sedative, hypnotic.

•**dorastine hydrochloride.** USAN.
Use: Antihistamine.

Dorcol Children's Cold Formula. (Sandoz Consumer) Pseudoephedrine HCl 15 mg, chlorpheniramine maleate 1 mg/5 ml. Bot. 120 ml. *otc.*
Use: Decongestant, antihistamine.

Dorcol Children's Cough Syrup. (Sandoz Consumer) Dextromethorphan HBr 5 mg, pseudoephedrine HCl 15 mg, guaifenesin 50 mg/5 ml. Bot. 120 ml, 240 ml. *otc.*
Use: Antitussive, decongestant, expectorant.

Dorcol Children's Decongestant Liquid. (Sandoz Consumer) Pseudoephedrine HCl 15 mg/5 ml. Bot. 4 oz. *otc.*
Use: Decongestant.

Dorcol Fever and Pain Reducer. (Sandoz Consumer) Acetaminophen 160 mg/5 ml. Bot. 4 oz. *otc.*
Use: Analgesic.

•**doretinel.** (DOE-REH-tin-ell) USAN.
Use: Antikeratinizing agent.

Doriglute Tabs DEA. (Major) Glutethimide 0.5 g/Tab. Bot. 100s, 250s, 1000s. *c-II.*
Use: Nonbarbiturate hypnotic.

Dormeer. (Taylor Pharmaceuticals) Scopolamine aminoxide HBr 0.2 mg/Cap. Bot. 100s, 1000s. *Rx.*
Use: Sedative, hypnotic.

dormethan.
See: Dextromethorphan HBr. (Various Mfr.)

Dormin. (Randob) Diphenhydramine HCl 25 mg, lactose. Cap. Bot. 32s, 72s *otc.*
Use: Nonprescription sleep aid.

Dormin Sleeping Caplets. (Randob) Diphenhydramine HCl 25 mg/Cap. Bot. 32s. *otc.*
Use: Nonprescription sleep aid.

dormiral.
See: Phenobarbital, Preps. (Various Mfr.).

dormonal.
See: Barbital, Preps. (Various Mfr.).

Dormutol. (Approved) Scopolamine aminoxide HBr 0.2 mg/Cap. Bot. 24s, 60s. *Rx.*
Use: Sedative, hypnotic.

dornase alfa. (DOR-nace AL-fuh)
Use: Treatment of cystic fibrosis. [Orphan drug]
See: Pulmozyme, Soln. (Genentech).

Doryx Pellets. (Parke-Davis) Doxycycline hyclate 100 mg/Cap. Bot. 50s. *Rx.*

Use: Anti-infective, tetracycline.

•**dorzolamide hydrochloride.** (dore-ZOLE-lah-mide) USAN.
Use: Carbonic anhydrase inhibitor.
See: TruSopt, Soln. (Merck).

Dosalax. (Richwood) Extract of senna fruit, parabens, sucrose, alcohol 7%. Syrup. Bot. 237 ml.*Rx.*
Use: Laxative.

D.O.S. Caps. (Goldline) Dioctyl sodium sulfosuccinate SG 100 mg or 250 mg/Cap. Bot. 100s, 1000s. *otc.*
Use: Laxative.

Doss Syrup. (Rosemont) Docusate sodium 20 mg/5 ml. Bot. pt, gal. *otc.*
Use: Laxative; stool softener.

Dostinex. (Pharmacia & Upjohn) Cabergoline 0.5 mg/Tab. Bot. 8s. *Rx.*
Use: Treatment of hyperprolactinemic disorders.

•**dothiepin hydrochloride.** (DOE-THIGH-eh-pin) USAN.
Use: Antidepressant.
See: Prothiaden.

Dotirol. (Sanofi Winthrop) Ampicillin trihydrate available in Cap, Susp., Inj. (IV, IM.). *Rx.*
Use: Anti-infective, penicillin.

Double Action Toothache Kit. (C.S. Dent) **Liquid:** benzocaine, alcohol 74%, chlorobutanol anhydrous 0.09%. Bot. 3.7 ml. **Maronox Pain Relief Tablets:** acetaminophen 325 mg/Tab. Box. 8s. *otc.*
Use: Treatment of toothache.

Double Sal Tablets. (Pal-Pak) Sodium salicylate 648 mg/EC Tab. Bot. 1000s. *otc.*
Use: Salicylate analgesic.

Double Strength Gaviscon-2. (SK-Beecham) Aluminum hydroxide 160 mg, magnesium trisilicate 40 mg, alginic acid, calcium stearate, sodium bicarbonate, sucrose. Tab. Bot. 48s. *otc.*
Use: Antacid.

Dovacet Capsules. (Pal-Pak) Dover's powder 24.3 mg, aspirin 324 mg, caffeine 32.4 mg/Tab. Bot. 1000s.
Use: Analgesic.

Dover's Powder. Ipecac 1 part, opium 1 part, lactose 8 parts.
Use: Analgesic, sedative, diaphoretic.

W/Acetophenetidin, atropine sulfate, aspirin, camphor, caffeine, sodium sulfate, dried.
See: Dovium, Cap. (Hance).

W/Acetophenetidin, camphor, aspirin, caffeine, atropine sulfate.
See: Analgestine, Cap. (Roberts).

W/Acetophenetidin, sodium citrate, potassium guaiacolsulfonate.
See: Doverlyn, Cap., Tab. (Davis & Sly).
W/A.P.C. camphor monobromated.
See: Coldate, Tab. (Zeneca)
W/Aspirin, phenacetin, camphor monobromated, caffeine.
See: Coldate, Tab. (Zeneca)
W/Atropine sulfate, A.P.C., camphor.
See: Dasin, Cap. (SK-Beecham).

Dovonex. (Westwood Squibb) Calcipotriene 0.005%. Oint. Tube 30, 60 or 100 g. *Rx.*
Use: Antipsoriatic, topical.

Dowicil 200.
See: Derma Soap (Ferndale).

Dow-Isoniazid. (Hoechst Marion Roussel) Isoniazid 300 mg/Tab. Bot. 30s. *Rx.*
Use: Antituberculous agent.

•**doxacurium chloride.** (dox-ah-cure-ee-uhm) USAN.
Use: Neuromuscular blocking agent.
See: Nuromax (Glaxo Wellcome).

Doxamin. (Forest) Thiamine HCl 100 mg, vitamin B₆ 100 mg/ml. Vial 10 ml. *Rx.*
Use: Vitamin supplement.

Doxapap-N Tabs. (Major) Propoxyphene napsylate 100 mg, acetaminophen 650 mg Bot. 100s, 500s. *c-iv.*
Use: Narcotic analgesic combination.

Doxaphene Capsules. (Major) Propoxyphene HCl 65 mg/Cap. Bot. 1000s. *c-iv.*
Use: Narcotic analgesic.

Doxaphene Compound 65 Caps. (Major) Propoxyphene HCl, acetaminophen. Bot. 1000s. *c-iv.*
Use: Narcotic analgesic combination.

•**doxapram hydrochloride.** (DOX-uh-pram) U.S.P. 23. (Various Mfr.) 20 mg/ml. Benzyl alcohol. Inj. Vial 20 ml.
Use: Respiratory and CNS stimulant.
See: Dopram, Vial (Robins).

doxapram hydrochloride. (Various Mfr.) 20 mg/ml. Benzyl alcohol. Inj. Vial. 20 ml.
Use: Respiratory and CNS stimulant.

•**doxaprost.** (DOX-ah-proste) USAN.
Use: Bronchodilator.

Doxate. Docusate sodium. *otc.*
Use: Laxative.

•**doxazosin mesylate.** (DOX-uh-ZOE-sin) USAN.
Use: Antihypertensive.
See: Cardura, Tab. (Roerig).

•**doxepin hydrochloride,** (DOX-uh-pin) U.S.P. 23.
Use: Psychotherapeutic drug; antidepressant.

See: Adapin, Cap. (Lotus).
Sinequan, Cap. (Roerig).

Doxidan. (Hoechst Marion Roussel) Yellow phenolphthalein 65 mg, docusate calcium 60 mg/Cap. Bot. 30s, 100s, 1000s, UD 100s, Display Pack 10s. *otc.*
Use: Laxative.

Doxil. (Sequus) Doxorubicin HCl 20 mg/10 ml vial. *Rx.*
Use: Antineoplastic.

•**doxofylline.** (DOX-oh-fill-een) USAN.
Use: Bronchodilator.
See: Maxivent (Roberts).

•**doxorubicin.** (DOX-oh-ROO-bih-sin) USAN.
Use: Antineoplastic.

•**doxorubicin hydrochloride.** (DOX-oh-ROO-bih-sin) U.S.P. 23.
Use: Antineoplastic.
See: Adriamycin, Inj. (Pharmacia & Upjohn).
Rubex, Pow. for Inj. (Bristol-Myers Oncology).

doxorubicin HCl. (Chiron) Doxorubicin HCl. **Pow. for Inj.: 10 mg:** w/lactose 50 mg. **20 mg:** w/lactose 100 mg. **50 mg:** w/lactose 250 mg. **Inj., aqueous:** 2 mg/ml, sodium chloride 0.9%. Vials 5, 10, 25, 100 ml. *Rx.*
Use: Antibiotic.

•**doxpicomine hydrochloride.** (DOX-PIH-koe-meen) USAN. *Formerly Doxpicodin hydrochloride.*
Use: Analgesic.

Doxy 100. (Fujisawa) Doxycycline hyclate for injection. Pow. 100 mg/Vial. *Rx.*
Use: Anti-infective, tetracycline.

Doxy 200. (Fujisawa) Doxycycline hyclate. Pow. 200 mg/Vial. *Rx.*
Use: Anti-infective, tetracycline.

Doxy-Caps. (Edwards) Doxycycline hyclate 100 mg/Cap. Bot. 50s. *Rx.*
Use: Anti-infective, tetracycline.

Doxychel Capsules. (Houba Inc.) Doxycycline hyclate 50 mg or 100 mg/Cap. Bot. 50s, 500s, UD 100s. *Rx.*
Use: Anti-infective, tetracycline.

Doxychel Injectable. (Houba Inc.) Doxycycline hyclate 100 mg or 200 mg/Vial. *Rx.*
Use: Anti-infective, tetracycline.

Doxychel Tablets. (Houba Inc.) Doxycycline hyclate 50 mg or 100 mg/Tab. Bot. 50s, 500s. *Rx.*
Use: Anti-infective, tetracycline.

•**doxycycline,** (DOX-ee-SIGH-kleen) U.S.P. 23.
Use: Antibacterial.

See: Vibramycin for Oral Susp. (Pfizer Laboratories).
Vibramycin IV. (Roerig).

•**doxycycline calcium oral suspension,** (DOX-ee-SIGH-kleen) U.S.P. 23.
Use: Antibacterial, antiprotozoal.

•**doxycycline fosfatex.** USAN. (DOX-ee-SIGH-kleen foss-FAH-tex)
Use: Antibacterial.

•**doxycycline hyclate,** (DOX-ee-SIGH-kleen HIGH-klate) U.S.P. 23.
Use: Antibacterial.
See: Bio-Tab, Tab. (Inter. Ethical Labs).
Doxy-Caps, Cap. (Edwards).
Vibra-Tabs, Tab. (Pfizer Laboratories).
Vibramycin, Cap., Tab., Vial (Pfizer Laboratories).
Vivox, Cap., Tab. (Squibb Mark).

•**doxylamine succinate,** U.S.P. 23.
Use: Antihistamine.
See: Decapryn, Prep. (Hoechst Marion Roussel).
Unisom, Tab. (Pfizer).
W/Acetominophen, ephedrine sulfate, dextromethorphan HBr, alcohol.
See: Nyquil, Liq. (Vick).
W/Dextromethorphan HBr, alcohol.
See: Consotuss Antitussive, Syr. (Hoechst Marion Roussel).
W/Dextromethorphan HBr, sodium citrate, alcohol.
See: Vicks Formula 44 Cough Mixture, Syr. (Procter & Gamble).

Doxy-Lemmon Capsules. (Lemmon) Doxycycline hyclate equivalent to 100 mg of doxycycline base/Cap. Bot. 50s, 500s, UD 100s. *Rx.*
Use: Anti-infective, tetracycline.

Doxy-Lemmon Tablets. (Lemmon) Doxycycline hyclate equivalent to 100 mg of doxycycline base/Tab. Bot. 50s, 500s, UD 100s. *Rx.*
Use: Anti-infective, tetracycline.

Doxy-Tabs. (Houba Inc.) Doxycycline hyclate 100 mg/FC Tab. Bot. 50s, 500s. *Rx.*
Use: Anti-infective, tetracycline.

Doxy-Tabs-50. (Houba Inc.) 50 mg/Tab. Bot. 50s. *Rx.*
Use: Anti-infective, tetracycline.

DPPC. Colfosceril palmitate. *Rx.*
Use: Lung surfactant.
See: Exosurf Neonatal (Glaxo Wellcome).

•**draflazine.** (DRAFF-lah-ZEEN) USAN.
Use: Cardioprotectant.

Dramaject. (Mayrand) Dimenhydrinate 50 mg/ml. Vial 10 ml. *Rx.*
Use: Antiemetic, antivertigo.

Dramamine II. (Pharmacia & Upjohn) Meclizine HCl 25 mg/Tab. Pck. 8s. *otc.*
Use: Antiemetic, antivertigo.

Dramamine Children's. (Pharmacia & Upjohn) Dimenhydrinate 12.5 mg/5 ml, alcohol 5%, sucrose. liq. Bot. 120 ml. *otc.*
Use: Antiemetic, antivertigo.

Dramamine Liquid. (Pharmacia & Upjohn) Dimenhydrinate 12.5 mg/4 ml Bot. 90 ml, pt. *otc.*
Use: Antiemetic, antivertigo.

Dramamine Tablets. (Pharmacia & Upjohn) Dimenhydrinate 50 mg/Tab. Bot. 36s, 100s, 1000s, Blister pkg. 12s, UD 100s. *otc.*
Use: Antiemetic, antivertigo.

Dramanate. (Pasadena) Dimenhydrinate 50 mg/ml. Inj. Vial 10 ml. *Rx.*
Use: Antiemetic, antivertigo.

dramarin.
See: Dramamine, Preps. (Searle).

dramyl.
See: Dramamine, Preps. (Searle).

Drawing Salve. (Whiteworth Towne) Tube oz. *otc.*
Use: Healing agent, topical.

Drawing Salve with Triquinodin. (Towne) Tube 2 oz. *otc.*
Use: Healing agent, topical.

Dr. Berry's Skin Toner. (Last) Hydroquinone 2%. Jar oz. *Rx.*
Use: Skin bleaching agent.

Dr. Caldwell Senna Laxative. (Mentholatum) Senna 7%, alcohol 4.5%. Bot. 130 ml, 360 ml. *otc.*
Use: Laxative.

DRC Peri-Anal Cream. (Xttrium) Lassar's paste 37.5%, anhydrous lanolin, U.S.P. 37.5%, cold cream 25%. Tube 5 oz. *otc.*
Use: Skin protectant, perianal.

Dr. Dermi-Heal. (Quality Formulations) Zinc oxide 25%, allantoin 1%, peruvian balsam, castor oil, white petrolatum. Oint. Tube 75 g. *otc.*
Use: Astringent.

Dr. Drake's Cough Medicine. (Last) Dextromethorphan HBr 10 mg/5 ml Bot. 2 oz. *otc.*
Use: Antitussive.

•**dribendazole.** (dry-BEN-dah-ZOLE) USAN.
Use: Anthelmintic.

Dri-A Caps. (Barth's) Vitamin A 10,000 IU/Cap. Bot. 100s, 500s. *otc.*
Use: Vitamin A supplement.

Dri A & D Caps. (Barth's) Vitamins A 10,000 IU, D 400 IU/Cap. Bot. 100s, 500s. *otc.*

Use: Vitamin A and D supplement.

Dri-E. (Barth's) Vitamin E. **100 IU/Cap.:** Bot. 100s, 500s, 1000s. **200 IU/Cap.:** Bot. 100s, 250s, 500s. **400 IU/Cap.:** Bot. 100s, 250s. *otc.*
Use: Vitamin E supplement.

Dri/Ear. (Pfeiffer) Boric acid 2.75% in isopropyl alcohol. Soln. Dropper Bot. 30 ml. *otc.*
Use: Otic preparation.

dried aluminum hydroxide gel.
Use: Antacid.
See: Aluminum Hydroxide Gel, dried.

dried yeast.
See: Yeast, dried.

Driminate Tabs. (Major) Dimenhydrinate 50 mg/Tab. Bot. 100s, 1000s. *otc.*
Use: Antiemetic, antivertigo.

•**drinidene.** (DRIH-nih-deen) USAN.
Use: Analgesic.

Drisdol. (Sanofi Winthrop) Ergocalciferol (Vitamin D) 8000 IU/ml in propylene glycol. Bot. 60 ml. *Rx.*
Use: Refractory rickets; hypophosphatemia; hypoparathyroidism.

Drisdol 50,000 Unit Capsules. (Sanofi Winthrop) Vitamin D-2, 50,000 IU/Cap. Bot. 50s. *Rx.*
Use: Refractory rickets; hypophosphatemia; hypoparathyroidism.

Dristan 12 Hour. (Whitehall Robins) Chlorpheniramine maleate 4 mg, phenylephrine HCl 20 mg/Cap. Bot. 6s, 10s, 15s. *otc.*
Use: Antihistamine, decongestant.

Dristan Allergy. (Whitehall Robins) Pseudoephedrine HCl 60 mg, brompheniramine maleate 4 mg/Cap. Bot. 20s. *otc.*
Use: Decongestant and antihistamine.

Dristan Capsules. (Whitehall Robins) Phenylephrine HCl 5 mg, chlorpheniramine maleate 2 mg, acetaminophen 325 mg/Cap. Bot. 16s, 36s, 75s. *otc.*
Use: Decongestant, antihistamine, analgesic.

Dristan Cold. (Whitehall Robins) Pseudoephedrine HCl 30 mg, acetaminophen 500 mg/Capl. Bot. 20s, 40s. *otc.*
Use: Decongestant, analgesic.

Dristan Cold & Flu. (Whitehall Robins) Acetaminophen 500 mg, pseudoephedrine HCl 60 mg, chlorpheniramine maleate 4 mg, dextromethorphan HBr 20 mg/Pow. Pkts. 6s. *otc.*
Use: Analgesic, decongestant, antihistamine, antitussive.

Dristan Cold Multi-Symptom Formula. (Whitehall Robins) Phenylephrine HCl 5 mg, chlorpheniramine maleate 2 mg, acetaminophen 325 mg/Tab. Bot. 20s, 40s, 75s. *otc.*
Use: Decongestant, antihistamine, analgesic.

Dristan Juice Mix-In. (Whitehall Robins) Acetaminophen 500 mg, pseudoephedrine HCl 60 mg, dextromethorphan 20 mg/Pow. Pkts. 5s. *otc.*
Use: Analgesic, decongestant, antitussive.

Dristan 12-Hr Nasal. (Whitehall Robins) Oxymetazoline HCl 0.05%, benzalkonium Cl 1:5000, thimerosal 0.002%, hydroxypropylmethylcellulose. Spray. Bot. 15 ml. *otc.*
Use: Nasal decongestant.

Dristan Maximum Strength Caplets. (Whitehall Robins) Pseudoephedrine HCl 30 mg, acetaminophen 500 mg/Capl. Bot. 24s. *otc.*
Use: Decongestant, analgesic.

Dristan Menthol Nasal Mist. (Whitehall Robins) Phenylephrine HCl 0.5%, pheniramine maleate 0.2%. Bot. 0.5 oz, 1 oz. *otc.*
Use: Decongestant, antihistamine.

Dristan Nasal Mist. (Whitehall Robins) Phenylephrine HCl 0.5%, pheniramine maleate 0.2%. Regular: 15 ml, 30 ml. Menthol: 15 ml. *otc.*
Use: Decongestant, antihistamine.

Dristan No Drowsiness Cold. (Whitehall Robins) Pseudoephedrine HCl 30 mg, acetaminophen 500 mg/Cap. Bot. 20s. *otc.*
Use: Decongestant, analgesic.

Dristan Saline Spray. (Whitehall Robins) Sodium chloride. Soln. Bot. 15 ml.
Use: Nasal product.

Dristan Sinus. (Whitehall Robins) Pseudoephedrine HCl 30 mg, ibuprofen 200 mg/Cap. Pkg. 20s. Bot. 24s, 40s. *otc.*
Use: Decongestant; analgesic.

Dritho-Creme. (Dermik) Anthralin 0.1%, 0.25% or 0.5%. Tube 50 g. *Rx.*
Use: Antipsoriatic.

Dritho-Creme HP 1.0%. (Dermik) Anthralin 1%. Tube 50 g. *Rx.*
Use: Antipsoriatic.

Dritho-Scalp. (Dermik) Anthralin 0.25% or 0.5%. Tube 50 g. *Rx.*
Use: Antipsoriatic.

Drixomed. (Iomed) Dexbrompheniramine maleate 6 mg, pseudoephedrine sulfate 120 mg/SR Tab. Bot. 100s, 500s. *Rx.*

Use: Decongestant, antihistamine.

Drixoral. (Schering-Plough) Dexbrompheniramine maleate 6 mg, pseudoephedrine sulfate 120 mg. SA Tab. Box 10s, 20s, 40s. Bot. 48s, 100s. *otc.*
Use: Antihistamine, decongestant.

Drixoral. (Schering-Plough) Pseudoephedrine sulfate 30 mg, brompheniramine maleate 2 mg, sorbitol, sugar. Syrup. Bot. 118 ml. *otc.*
Use: Decongestant, antihistamine.

Drixoral Cold & Allergy. (Schering-Plough) Dexbrompheniramine maleate 6 mg, pseudoephedrine sulfate 120 mg/SR Tab. Pkg. 10s. *otc.*
Use: Antihistamine, decongestant.

Drixoral Cold & Flu. (Schering-Plough) Pseudoephedrine HCl 60 mg, dexbrompheniramine maleate 3 mg, acetaminophen 500 mg/Tab. Bot. 12s, 24s, 48s. *otc.*
Use: Decongestant, antihistamine, analgesic.

Drixoral Cough & Congestion Liquid Caps. (Schering-Plough) Pseudoephedrine HCl 60 mg, dextromethorphan HBr 30 mg/Cap. Pkg. 10s. *otc.*
Use: Decongestant, antihistamine.

Drixoral Cough & Sore Throat Liquid Caps. (Schering-Plough) Dextromethorphan HBr 15 mg, acetaminophen 325 mg, sorbitol. Cap. Pkg. 10s. *otc.*
Use: Antitussive, analgesic.

Drixoral Cough Liquid Caps. (Schering-Plough) Dextromethorphan HBr 30 mg. Cap. Pkg. 10s. *otc.*
Use: Antitussive.

Drixoral Non-Drowsy Formula. (Schering-Plough) Pseudoephedrine sulfate 120 mg, sugar. Tab. Pkg. 10s, 20s. *otc.*
Use: Decongestant.

Drixoral Plus. (Schering-Plough) Pseudoephedrine sulfate 60 mg, dexbrompheniramine maleate 3 mg, acetaminophen 500 mg/TR Tab. Bot. 12s, 24s. *otc.*
Use: Decongestant, antihistamine, analgesic.

Drixoral Sustained-Action Tablets. (Schering-Plough) Pseudoephedrine sulfate 120 mg, dexbrompheniramine maleate 6 mg, sugar, lactose. Tab. Pkg. 10s. Bots. 20s, 40s. *otc.*
Use: Decongestant, antihistamine.

Drize. (Jones Medical) Phenylpropanolamine HCl 75 mg, chlorpheniramine maleate 12 mg/SR Cap. Bot. 100s. *Rx.*
Use: Decongestant, antihistamine.

•**drobuline.** (DROE-byoo-leen) USAN.

Use: Cardiac depressant (antiarrhythmic).

•**drocinonide.** (droe-SIN-oh-nide) USAN.
Use: Anti-inflammatory.

drocode.
See: Dihydrocodeine.

•**droloxifene.** (drole-OX-ih-feen) USAN.
Use: Antineoplastic.

•**droloxifene citrate.** (drole-OX-ih-feen) USAN.
Use: Antineoplastic.

•**drometrizole.** (DROE-meh-TRY-zole) USAN.
Use: Ultraviolet screen.

•**dromostanolone propionate.** (DRAHM-oh-STAN-oh-lone) USAN. U.S.P. XX.
Use: Antineoplastic.

•**dronabinol,** (droe-NAB-ih-nahl) U.S.P. 23.
Use: Antiemetic. [Orphan drug]
See: Marinol, Gel Cap. (Roxane).

drop chalk. (Various Mfr.) Calcium carbonate, prepared. Prepared chalk.

•**droperidol,** (dro-PER-i-dahl) U.S.P. 23.
Use: Tranquilizer; antipsychotic.
See: Inapsine, Inj. (Janssen).
W/Fentanyl citrate.
Use: Tranquilizer.
See: Innovar, Inj. (Janssen).

•**droprenilamine.** (droe-preh-NILL-ah-meen) USAN.
Use: Vasodilator (coronary).

Drotic Sterile Otic Solution. (Ascher) Hydrocortisone 10 mg (1%), polymyxin B sulfate 10,000 units, neomycin 5 mg/ml, preservatives. Dropper bot. 10 ml. *Rx.*
Use: Otic preparation.

•**droxacin sodium.** (DROX-ah-sin) USAN.
Use: Antibacterial.

•**droxifilcon A.** (DROX-ih-fill-kahn A) USAN.
Use: Contact lens material (hydrophilic).

•**droxinavir hydrochloride.** (drox-IN-ah-veer HIGH-droe-KLOR-ide) USAN.
Use: Antiviral.

Dr. Scholl's Advanced Pain Relief Corn Removers. (Schering-Plough) Salicylic acid 40% in a rubber-based vehicle. Disc. 6s. *otc.*
Use: Keratolytic.

Dr. Scholl's Athlete's Foot. (Schering-Plough) Pow.: Tolnaftate 1%. Talc. 63 g. **Spray Liq.:** Tolnaftate 1%, alcohol 36%. 113 ml. **Spray Pow.:** Tolnaftate 1%, SD alcohol 40 14%. 99 g. *otc.*
Use: Antifungal, topical.

Dr. Scholl's Athlete's Foot Cream. (Schering-Plough) Tolnaftate 1%. Tube 0.5 oz. *otc.*

Use: Antifungal, topical.

Dr. Scholl's Callous Removers. (Schering-Plough) Salicylic acid 40% in a rubber-based vehicle. 6 pads, 4 discs. Extra thick in 4 discs. *otc.*
Use: Keratolytic.

Dr. Scholl's Clear Away. (Schering-Plough) Salicylic acid 40% in a rubber-based vehicle. Disc 18s. *otc.*
Use: Keratolytic.

Dr. Scholl's Clear Away Onestep. (Schering-Plough) Salicylic acid 40% in a rubber-based vehicle. Strip 14s. *otc.*
Use: Keratolytic.

Dr. Scholl's Clear Away Plantar. (Schering-Plough) Salicylic acid 40% in a rubber-based vehicle. Disc 24s. *otc.*
Use: Keratolytic.

Dr. Scholl's Corn/Callous Remover. (Schering-Plough) Salicylic acid 12.6% in a flexible collodion, alcohol 18%, ether 55%, hydrogenated vegetable oil. Liq. 10 ml with 3 cushions. *otc.*
Use: Keratolytic.

Dr. Scholl's Corn/Callous Salve. (Schering-Plough) Salicylic acid 15%. Tube 0.4 oz. *otc.*
Use: Keratolytic.

Dr. Scholl's Corn Remover. (Schering-Plough) Salicylic acid 40% in a rubber-based vehicle. Discs: 6s as wraparounds, 9s as ultra thin, small, waterproof, regular, soft and extra-thick. *otc.*
Use: Keratolytic.

Dr. Scholl's Corn Salve. (Schering-Plough) Salicylic acid 15%. Jar 0.4 oz. *otc.*
Use: Keratolytic.

Dr. Scholl's Cracked Heel Relief. (Schering-Plough) Lidocaine 2%, benzalkonium Cl 0.13%. Cream 5.6 g. *otc.*
Use: Local anesthetic, topical.

Dr. Scholl's Ingrown Toenail Reliever. (Schering-Plough) Sodium sulfide 1%. Bot. 0.33 oz. *otc.*
Use: Foot preparation.

Dr. Scholl's Maximum Strength Tritin. (Schering-Plough) **Pow.:** Tolnaftate 1% 56 g. **Spray Pow.:** Tolnaftate 1%, SD alcohol 40 14%, 85 g. *otc.*
Use: Antifungal, topical.

Dr. Scholl's Moisturizing Corn Remover Kit. (Schering-Plough) Salicylic acid 40% in a rubber-based vehicle, moisturizing cream, pain relief cushions. Disc 6s. *otc.*
Use: Keratolytic.

Dr. Scholl's Onestep Corn Removers. (Schering-Plough) Salicylic acid 40% in a rubber-based vehicle. Strips 6s. *otc.*
Use: Keratolytic.

Dr. Scholl's Pro Comfort Jock Itch Spray. (Schering-Plough) Tolnaftate 1%. Aerosol can 3.5 oz. *otc.*
Use: Antifungal, topical.

Dr. Scholl's Wart Remover Kit. (Schering-Plough) Salicylic acid 17% in a flexible collodion, alcohol 17%, ether 52%. Liq. 10 ml with brush and 6 adhesive pads. *otc.*
Use: Keratolytic.

Dr. Scholl's Zino Pads/with Medicated Disks. (Schering-Plough) Salicylic acid 20% or 40%. Protective pads designed for use with and without salicylic acid-impregnated disks. *otc.*
Use: Keratolytic.

Drucon. (Standard Drug) Phenylephrine HCl 5 mg, chlorpheniramine maleate 2 mg, menthol 1 mg, alcohol 5%/5 ml Elix. Bot. pt, gal. *otc.*
Use: Decongestant, antihistamine.

Drucon C R. (Standard Drug) Phenylephrine HCl 25 mg, chlorpheniramine maleate 4 mg/Tab. Bot. 100s. *otc.*
Use: Decongestant, antihistamine.

Drucon with Codeine. (Standard Drug) Codeine phosphate 10 mg, phenylephrine HCl 10 mg, chlorpheniramine maleate 2 mg, menthol 1 mg, alcohol 5%/5 ml. Bot. pt. *c-v.*
Use: Antitussive, decongestant, antihistamine.

Dry Eyes. (Bausch & Lomb) White petrolatum, mineral oil, lanolin. Oint. Tube 3.5 g. *otc.*
Use: Ocular lubricant.

Dry Eyes Solution. (Bausch & Lomb) Polyvinyl alcohol 1.4%, benzalkonium Cl 0.01%, sodium phosphate, EDTA, NaCl. Bot. 15 ml. *otc.*
Use: Lubricant, ophthalmic.

Dry Eye Therapy. (Bausch & Lomb) Glycerin 0.3%, potassium Cl, sodium Cl, sodium citrate, sodium phosphate, zinc Cl. Drop. Single-use Bot. 0.3 ml (UD 32s). *otc.*
Use: Ophthalmic.

Dryox 2.5, 5, 10 & 20. (C & M Pharm.) Benzoyl peroxide 2.5%, 5%, 10%, 20%. Gel. Tube. 30 g, 60 g. *otc.*
Use: Antiacne.

Dryox 10S 5. (C & M Pharm.) Benzoyl peroxide 10%, sulfur 5%, methylparaben. Gel. Tube. 30 g, 60 g. *otc.*
Use: Antiacne.

Dryox 20S 5. (C & M Pharm.) Benzoyl

peroxide 20%, sulfur 10%, methylparaben. Gel. Tube. 30 g, 60 g. *otc.*
Use: Antiacne.

Dryox Wash 5 & 10. (C & M Pharm.) Benzoyl peroxide 5%, 10%. Liq. Bot. 240 ml. *Rx.*
Use: Antiacne.

Dry Skin Creme. (Gordon) Cetyl alcohol, lubricating oils in a water soluble base. Jar 2 oz, 1 lb, 5 lb. *otc.*
Use: Emollient.

Drysol. (Person & Covey) Aluminum Cl hexahydrate 20% in 93% SD alcohol 40. Bot. 37.5 ml. *Rx.*
Use: Astringent.

Drysum Shampoo. (Summers) Alcohol 15%, acetone 6%. Plastic bot. 4 oz. *otc.*
Use: Drying agent for oily hair.

Drytergent. (C & M Pharm.) TEA-dodecylbenzenesulfonate, boric acid, lauramide DEA, propylene glycol, tartrazine, purified water, color, fragrance. Liq. Bot. 240 ml, 480 ml. *otc.*
Use: Antiacne.

Drytex. (C & M Pharm.) Salicylic acid 2%, benzalkonium Cl 0.1%, acetone 10%, isopropyl alcohol 40%, tartrazine. Lot. Bot. 240 ml. *otc.*
Use: Antiacne.

DSMC Plus. (Geneva Pharm.) Docusate potassium 100 mg. Cap. Bot. 100s. *otc.*
Use: Laxative.

DSS. (Dioctyle sodium sulfosuccinate) Docusate sodium. *otc.*
Use: Laxative.
See: Regutol, Tab. (Schering-Plough).
  Colace, Cap. (Bristol-Myers).
  Docusate Sodium, Cap. (Various, eg, Geneva, Marsam, Lederle, Major, Purepac, Rugby, Schein, URL).
  DOK, Cap. (Major).
  DOS, Softgel, Cap. (Goldline).
  D-S-S, Cap. (Warner Chilcott).
  Modane Soft, Cap. (Pharmacia & Upjohn).
  Pro-Sof, Cap. (Vangard).
  Regulax SS, Cap. (Republic).

D-S-S. (Warner-Chilcott) Docusate sodium 100 mg/Cap. Bot. 100s, 1000s and UD 100s. *otc.*
Use: Laxative; stool softener.

DST. Dihydrostreptomycin.
See: Dihydrostreptomycin, Preps. (Various Mfr.)

D-Test 100. (Burgin-Arden) Testosterone cypionate 100 mg/ml. Vial 10 ml. *c-iii.*
Use: Androgen.

D-Test 200. (Burgin-Arden) Testosterone

cypionate 200 mg/ml. Vial 10 ml. *c-iii.*
Use: Androgen.

DTIC. Dacarbazine. *Rx.*
Use: Antineoplastic.
See: Decarbazine, Inj. (Various Mfr.)
  DTIC-Dome, Inj. (Bayer Pharm.).

DTIC-Dome. (Bayer Pharm.) Dacarbazine 100 mg or 200 mg/Vial. Vial 10 ml, 20 ml. *Rx.*
Use: Antineoplastic.

DTP. Diphtheria and tetanus toxoids and pertussis vaccine, adsorbed. *Rx.*
Use: Agent for immunization.
See: Acel-Imune, Vial (Wyeth Lederle).
  Diphtheria and Tetanus Toxoids and Pertussis Vaccine, Inj. (Pasteur-Merieux-Connaught, Massachusetts Public Health Biologic Labs).
  DTwP, Inj. (Michigan Dept of Public Health/SK Beecham).
  Tri-Immunol, Vial, Inj. (Wyeth Lederle).
  Tripedia, Vial (Pasteur-Merieux-Connaught).

DTwP. (Michigan Dept. of Public Health/ SK Beecham) 10 Lf units diphtheria, 5.5 Lf units tetanus and 4 Lf units pertussis/0.5 ml. Vial 5 ml. *Rx.*
Use: Agent for immunization.

Duadacin. (Kenwood/Bradley) Phenylpropanolamine HCl 12.5 mg, chlorpheniramine maleate 2 mg, acetaminophen 325 mg/Cap. Bot. 100s, 1000s. Dispense-A-Pak 1000s. *otc.*
Use: Decongestant, antihistamine, analgesic.

Dual-Wet. (Alcon Lenscare) Polyvinyl alcohol, duasorb water soluble polymeric system, benzalkonium Cl 0.01%, disodium edetate 0.05%. Bot. 2 oz. *otc.*
Use: Hard contact lens care.

•**duazomycin.** (doo-AZE-oh-MY-sin) USAN. Antibiotic isolated from broth filtrates of *Streptomyces ambofaciens*.
Use: Antineoplastic.

Duazomycin A. Name used for Duazomycin.
Use: Antineoplastic.

Duazomycin B. Name used for Azotomycin.
Use: Antineoplastic.

Duazomycin C. Name used for Ambomycin.
Use: Antineoplastic.

Dulcagen Suppositories. (Goldline) Bisacodyl 10 mg/Supp. Box 12s, 100s. *otc.*
Use: Laxative.

Dulcagen Tablets. (Goldline) Bisacodyl

5 mg/Tab. Bot. 100s. *otc.*
Use: Laxative.

Dulcolax. (Novartis Consumer Health) Bisacodyl. **EC Tab.:** 5 mg. Box 10s, 25s, 50s, 100s. Bot. 1000s, UD 100s. **Supp.:** 10 mg. Box 2s, 4s, 8s, 50s, 500s. **Bowel Prep Kit:** 4 tab., 1 supp./ Kit. 5s/box. *otc.*
Use: Laxative.

Dull-C. (Freeda) Ascorbic acid 4 g/tsp. Pow. Bot. 100 g, 500 g, 1000 g. *otc.*
Use: Vitamin C supplement.

•**duloxetine hydrochloride.** (doo-LOX-eh-teen) USAN.
Use: Antidepressant.

Dulphalac. (Solvay) Lactulose 10 g/5 ml. Syr. Bot. 240 ml, 480 ml, 960 ml, UD 30 ml. *Rx.*
Use: Laxative.

Duo. (Norcliff Thayer) Tube 0.5 oz.
Use: Surgical adhesive.

Duo-Cet. (Mason) Hydrocodone bitartrate 5 mg, acetaminophen 500 mg/ Tab. Bot. 100s. *c-III.*
Use: Narcotic analgesic combination.

Duo-Cyp. (Keene) Testosterone cypionate 50 mg, estradiol cypionate 2 mg/ ml. Vial 10 ml. *Rx.*
Use: Androgen, estrogen combination.

duodenal substance.
W/Ox bile extract, pancreatin, papain.
See: Digenzyme, Tab. (Burgin-Arden).

duodenum whole, desiccated & defatted.
W/Ferrous gluconate, Vitamin B_{12}, cobalt Cl.
See: Bitrinsic-E, Cap. (Zeneca).

Duoderm. (Conva Tec) **Sterile dressing:** 10 cm × 10 cm. Pack 5s. 20 cm 20 cm. Pack 3s. **Sterile gran:** Packet 4 g. Pack 5s. *otc.*
Use: Wound-healing agent.

Duoderm Extra Thin. (ConvaTec) Flexible hydroactive sterile dressings. 4" × 4", 6"×6". Pck. 10s. *otc.*
Use: Topical dressing.

Duofilm. (Stiefel) Salicylic acid 16.7%, lactic acid 16.7% in flexible collodion. Bot. 15 ml w/applicator. *otc.*
Use: Keratolytic.

Duo-Flow. (Ciba Vision) Poloxamer 188, benzalkonium Cl 0.013%, EDTA 0.25%. Soln. Bot. 120 ml. *otc.*
Use: Hard contact lens care.

Duo-K. (Various Mfr.) Potassium 20 mEq, chloride 3.4 mEq/15 ml (from potassium gluconate and potassium Cl). Bot. pt, gal. *Rx.*
Use: Mineral supplement.

Duolube. (Bausch & Lomb) White petrolatum, mineral oil. Sterile, preservative and lanolin free. Oint. Tube 3.5 g. *otc.*
Use: Lubricant, ophthalmic.

Duo-Medihaler. (3M) Isoproterenol HCl 0.16 mg, phenylephrine bitartrate 0.24 mg. In 15 ml (300 metered doses) or 22.5 ml (450 metered doses) medihaler. Refill vial 15 ml, 22.5 ml. *Rx.*
Use: Bronchodilator.

duomycin.
See: Aureomycin, Preps. (Lederle).

•**duoperone fumarate.** (DOO-oh-per-OHN) USAN.
Use: Neuroleptic.

Duoplant. (Stiefel). Salicylic acid 27%, alcohol 50%, flexible collodion, hydroxypropylcellulose, lactic acid. Liq. Bot. 14 g. *otc.*
Use: Ketatolytic (wart removal).

Duosol. (Kirkman Sales) Docusate sodium 100 mg or 250 mg/Cap. Bot. 100s, 1000s. *otc.*
Use: Laxative.

Duotal. (Approved) 1.5 gr: Secobarbital sodium ¾ gr, amobarbital gr/Cap. 3 gr: Secobarbital sodium 1.5 gr, amobarbital 1.5 gr/Cap. Bot. 100s, 500s, 1000s. *c-II.*
Use: Sedative, hypnotic.

duotal.
See: Guaiacol Carbonate (Various Mfr.).

Duo-Trach Kit. (Astra) Lidocaine HCl 4%. Inj. 5 ml disp. syringe with laryngotracheal cannula. *Rx.*
Use: Local anesthetic.

Duotrate 30. (Jones Medical) Pentaerythritol tetranitrate 30 mg/SR Cap. Bot. 100s. *Rx.*
Use: Antianginal.

Duotrate 45. (Jones Medical) Pentaerythritol tetranitrate 45 mg/SR Cap. Bot. 100s. *Rx.*
Use: Antianginal.

Duovin-S. (Spanner) Estrone 2.5 mg, progesterone 25 mg/ml. Vial 10 ml. *Rx.*
Use: Estrogen, progestin combination.

Duo-WR, No. 1 & No. 2. (Whorton) **No. 1:** Salicylic acid, compound tincture benzoin. **No. 2:** Compound tincture benzoin, formaldehyde. Bot. 0.25 oz. *otc.*
Use: Keratolytic.

Duphalac. (Solvay) Lactulose 10 g/15 ml (< 2.2 g galactose, 1.2 g lactose, 1.2 g or less of other sugars). Syr. Bot. 240 ml, pt, qt, UD 30 ml. *Rx.*
Use: Laxative.

Duplast. (Beiersdorf) Adhesive coated

elastic cloth. 8" X 4" Strip. Box 10s. 10" X 5"; Strip. Box 8s, 10s.

Duplex. (C & M Pharm.) Sodium lauryl sulfate 15%, lauramide DEA. Liq. Bot. 480 ml. *otc.*
Use: Therapeutic skin cleanser.

Duplex Shampoo. (C & M Pharm.) Sodium lauryl sulfate, lauramide DEA, purified water. Bot. pt, gal. *otc.*
Use: Shampoo.

Duplex T Shampoo. (C & M Pharm.) Sodium lauryl sulfate, purified water, lauramide DEA, solution of coal tar, alcohol 8.3%. Bot. pt, gal. *otc.*
Use: Antiseborrheic.

duponol.
See: Gardinol-type detergents (Sodium Lauryl Sulfate) (Various Mfr.)

Durabolin. (Organon) Nandrolone phenpropionate 25 mg/ml in sesame oil, benzyl alcohol 5%. Inj. Vial 5 ml. *c-III.*
Use: Anabolic steroid.
See: Deca-Durabolin, Inj. (Organon).

Durabolin. (Organon) Nandrolone phenpropionate 50 mg/ml in sterile sesame oil, benzyl alcohol 10%. Inj. Vial 2 ml. *c-III.*
Use: Anabolic steroid.

DURAcare. (Blairex) Buffered hypertonic salt solution, non-ionic detergents with thimerosal 0.004%, EDTA 0.1%. Soln. Bot. 30 ml. *otc.*
Use: Soft contact lens care.

DURAcare II. (Blairex) Buffered hypertonic, ethylene and propylene oxide, octylphenoxypolyethoxyethanol, lauryl sulfate salt of imidazoline, sodium bisulfite 0.1%, sorbic acid 0.1%, EDTA 0.25%. Soln. Bot. 30 ml. *otc.*
Use: Contact lens care.

Duraclon. (Fujisawa) Clonidine HCl 100 mcg/ml/Inj. Vials. 10 ml. *Rx.*
Use: Treatment of severe pain in cancer patients.

Dura-Estrin. (Roberts) Estradiol cypionate in oil 5 mg/ml. Inj. Vial 10 ml. *Rx.*
Use: Estrogen.

Duragen. (Roberts) Estradiol valerate in oil 20 mg or 40 mg/ml. Inj. Vial 10 ml. *Rx.*
Use: Estrogen.

Duragesic. (Janssen) Fentanyl 2.5 mg, 5 mg, 7.5 mg or 10 mg/transdermal patch. Carton 5s. *c-II.*
Use: Narcotic analgesic.

Dura-Gest. (Dura) Phenylpropanolamine HCl 45 mg, phenylephrine HCl 5 mg, guaifenesin 200 mg/Cap. Bot. 100s, 500s. *Rx.*

Use: Decongestant, expectorant.

Duralex. (American Urologicals) Pseudoephedrine HCl 120 mg, chlorpheniramine maleate 8 mg/SR Cap. Bot. 100s, 1000s. *Rx.*
Use: Decongestant, antihistamine.

Duralone Injection. (Roberts) Methylprednisolone acetate 40 mg or 80 mg/ml Susp. for Inj. **40 mg:** Vial 10 ml. **80 mg:** Vial 5 ml. *Rx.*
Use: Corticosteroid.

Duralutin Injection. (Roberts Hauck) Hydroxyprogesterone caproate in oil 250 mg/ml. Vial 5 ml. *Rx.*
Use: Progesterone.

Dura-Meth. (Foy) Methylprednisolone 40 mg/ml. Vial 5 ml, 10 ml. *Rx.*
Use: Corticosteroid.

Duramist Plus. (Pfeiffer) Oxymetazoline HCl 0.05%. Spray. 15 ml. *otc.*
Use: Decongestant.

Duramorph. (Elkins-Sinn) Morphine sulfate. Inj. 0.5 mg/ml or 1 mg/ml. Amp. 10 ml Box 10s. Preservative free. *c-II.*
Use: Narcotic analgesic.

Duranest. (Astra) Etidocaine HCl 1.5%, epinephrine 1:200,000, sodium metabisulfite. Dental cartridges 1.8 ml. *Rx.*
Use: Local anesthetic.

Duranest-MPF. (Astra) Etidocaine. **1%:** w/epinephrine 1:200,000. Vial 30 ml. **1.5%:** w/epinephrine 1:200,000. Amp. 20 ml. *Rx.*
Use: Local anesthetic.

Durapam. (Major) Flurazepam HCl 15 mg or 30 mg/Cap. Bot. 100s, 500s. *c-IV.*
Use: Sedative, hypnotic.

•**durapatite.** (der-APP-ah-tite) USAN.
Use: Prosthetic aid.
See: Alveograf (Sterling Winthrop). Periograf (Sterling Winthrop).

Duraquin. (Parke-Davis) Quinidine gluconate 330 mg/SR Tab. Bot. 100s, UD 100s. *Rx.*
Use: Cardiac depressant.

Durascreen. (Schwarz Pharma) SPF 30. Octyl methoxycinnamate, octyl salicylate, oxybenzone, 2-phenylbenzimidazole-sulfonic acid, titanium dioxide, cetearyl alcohol, diazolidinyl urea, parabens, shea butter. Lot. Bot. 105 ml. *otc.*
Use: Sunscreen.

Durascreen SPF 15. (Schwarz Pharma) SPF 15. Ethylhexyl p-methoxycinnamate, 2-ethylhexyl salicylate, oxybenzone, parabens, titanium dioxide. Lot. Bot. 105 ml. *otc.*

Use: Sunscreen.

Dura-Tap/PD. (Dura) Pseudoephedrine HCl 60 mg, chlorpheniramine maleate 4 mg. Cap. Bot. 100s. *Rx.*
Use: Decongestant, antihistamine.

Duratears Naturale. (Alcon) White petroleum, anhydrous liquid lanolin, mineral oil. Oint. Tube 3.5 g. *otc.*
Use: Ophthalmic lubricant.

Duratest-200/Duratest-100. (Roberts) Testosterone cypionate in oil 100 mg or 200 mg/ml. Inj. Vial 10 ml. *c-III.*
Use: Androgen.

Duratestrin. (Roberts) Estradiol cypionate 2 mg, testosterone cypionate 50 mg/ml. Vial 10 ml. *Rx.*
Use: Estrogen, androgen combination.

Durathate-200 Injection. (Roberts) Testosterone enanthate in oil 200 mg/ml. Vial 10 ml. *c-III.*
Use: Androgen.

Duration Mentholated Vapor Spray. (Schering-Plough) Oxymetazoline HCl 0.05%, aromatics. Squeeze bot. 15 ml. *otc.*
Use: Decongestant.

Duration Mild Nasal Spray. (Schering-Plough) Phenylephrine HCl 0.5%. Bot. 15 ml. *otc.*
Use: Decongestant.

Duration Nasal Spray. (Schering-Plough) Oxymetazoline HCl 0.05%. Aqueous soln. Squeeze bot. 15 ml, 30 ml. *otc.*
Use: Nasal decongestant; androgen, estrogen combination.

Duratuss. (Whitby) Pseudoephedrine HCl 120 mg, guaifenesin 600 mg. LA Tab. Bot. 100s. *Rx.*
Use: Decongestant, expectorant.

Duratuss-G. (UCB Pharma) 1200 mg (UCb/620)/Tab. Bot. 100s. *Rx.*
Use: Expectorant.

Duratuss HD. (Whitby) Hydrocodone bitartrate 2.5 mg, pseudoephedrine HCl 30 mg, guaifenesin 100 mg, alcohol 5%. Elixir Bot. 473 ml. *c-III.*
Use: Antitussive, expectorant, decongestant.

Dura-Vent. (Dura) Phenylpropanolamine HCl 75 mg, guaifenesin 600 mg. SR Tab. Bot. 100s. *Rx.*
Use: Decongestant, expectorant.

Dura-Vent/A. (Dura) Phenylpropanolamine HCl 75 mg, chlorpheniramine maleate 10 mg. SR Cap. Bot. 100s. *Rx.*
Use: Decongestant, antihistamine.

Dura-Vent/DA. (Dura) Phenylephrine HCl 20 mg, chlorpheniramine maleate 8 mg,

methscopolamine nitrate 2.5 mg. SR Tab. Bot. 100s. *Rx.*
Use: Decongestant, antihistamine, anticholinergic.

Durazyme. (Blairex) Nonionic detergent preserved w/thimerosal 0.004%, EDTA 0.1% in sterile buffered hypertonic salt soln. Bot. 30 ml. *otc.*
Use: Contact lens care.

Duricef. (Mead-Johnson) Cefadroxil.
Tab.: 1 g. Bot. 50s, 100s, UD 100s.
Cap.: 500 mg. Bot. 50s, 100s, UD 100s.
Susp.: 125 mg/5 ml, 250 mg/5 ml or 500 mg/5 ml Bot. 50 ml, 75 ml (500 mg/5 ml), 100 ml. *Rx.*
Use: Anti-infective, cephalosporin.

Dusotal. (Harvey) Sodium amobarbital ¾ gr, sodium secobarbital gr/Cap. Bot. 1000s. (3 gr) Bot. 1000s. *c-II.*
Use: Sedative, hypnotic.

•**dusting powder, absorbable,** U.S.P. 23.
Use: Surgical aid (glove lubricant).

dusting powder, surgical.
See: B-F-I Powder (SK-Beecham).

Dutch Drops. Oil of turpentine, sulfurated.

dutch oil. Oil of turpentine, sulfurated.

Duvoid. (Roberts) Bethanechol Cl 10 mg, 25 mg or 50 mg/Tab. Bot. 100s, UD ctn. 100s. *Rx.*
Use: Urinary tract product.

D V Cream. (Hoechst Marion Roussel) Dienestrol 0.01% w/lactose, propylene glycol, stearic acid, diglycol stearate, TEA, benzoic acid, butylated hydroxytoluene, disodium edetate, buffered w/ lactic acid to an acid pH. Tube 3 oz, w/applicator. *Rx.*
Use: Estrogen, vaginal.

D-Vaso-S. (Dunhall) Pentylenetetrazole 50 mg, niacin 50 mg, dimenhydrinate 25 mg, alcohol 18%, sherry wine vehicle. Bot. pt. *Rx.*
Use: Respiratory stimulant.

D-10-W. (Various Mfr.) Dextrose in water injection 10% (amps 3 ml); vials 250 ml, 500 ml, 1000 ml; 17 ml fill in 20 ml, 500 ml fill in 1000 ml, 1000 ml fill in 2000 ml vials. *Rx.*
Use: Carbohydrate.

Dwelle. (Dakryon) EDTA 0.09%, sodium chloride, potassium chloride, boric acid, povidone, NPX 0.001%. Drop. Bot. 15 ml. *otc.*
Use: Artificial tear solution.

d-xylose.
See: Xylo-Pfan. (Pharmacia & Upjohn).

Dyantoin Caps. (Major) Phenytoin sodium 100 mg/Cap. Bot. 100s, 1000s. *Rx.*

Use: Anticonvulsant.

DX 114 Foot Powder. (Amlab) Zinc undecylenate 1%, salicylic acid 1%, benzoic acid 1%, ammonium alum 5%, boric acid 10.5% w/zinc stearate, chlorophyll, talc, kaolin, starch, calcium silicate, oil of wormwood. Cont. 2 oz. *otc.*
Use: Antifungal, topical.

Dyazide. (SK-Beecham) Triamterene 37.5 mg, hydrochlorothiazide 25 mg/Cap. Bot. 1000s, UD 100s, Patient Pack 100s. *Rx.*
Use: Diuretic, antihypertensive.

Dycill. (SK-Beecham) Dicloxacillin sodium 250 mg or 500 mg/Cap. Bot. 100s. *Rx.*
Use: Anti-infective, penicillin.

Dyclone. (Astra) Dyclonine HCl 0.5% or 1%. Soln. Bot. 30 ml. *Rx.*
Use: Local anesthetic, topical.

•**dyclonine hydrochloride,** U.S.P. 23.
Use: Anesthetic (topical).
See: Dyclone, Soln. (Astra).
W/Benzethonium chloride
See: Skin Shield, Liq. (Del).
W/Neomycinsulfate, polymyxin B sulfate, hydrocortisone acetate.
See: Neo-polycin HC, Oint. (Hoechst Marion Roussel).

Dycomene. (Hance) Hydrocodone bitartrate ⅛ gr, pyrilamine maleate 1 gr/fl. oz. Bot. 3 oz, gal. *c-iii.*
Use: Antitussive, sleep aid.

•**dydrogesterone,** (DIE-droe-JESS-ter-ohn) U.S.P. 23.
Use: Progestin.

dyes.
See: Antiseptic, Dyes.

Dyflex-200 Tablets. (Econo Med) Dyphylline 200 mg/Tab. Bot. 100s, 1000s. *Rx.*
Use: Bronchodilator.

Dyflex-G Tablets. (Econo Med) Dyphylline 200 mg, guaifenesin 200 mg/Tab. Bot. 100s, 1000s. *Rx.*
Use: Bronchodilator, expectorant.

dylate. Clonitrate.
Use: Coronary vasodilator.

Dyline-GG Liquid. (Seatrace) Dyphylline 300 mg, guaifenesin 300 mg/15 ml. Bot. pt, gal. *Rx.*
Use: Bronchodilator, expectorant.

Dyline-GG Tablets. (Seatrace) Dyphylline 200 mg, guaifenesin 200 mg/Tab. Bot. 100s, 1000s. *Rx.*
Use: Bronchodilator, expectorant.

•**dymanthine hydrochloride.** (DIE-mantheen) USAN. N,N-dimethyloctadecyl-amine hydrochloride.
Use: Anthelmintic.

Dymelor. (Lilly) Acetohexamide 250 mg or 500 mg/Tab. Bot. 200s. *Rx.*
Use: Antidiabetic.

Dymenate. (Keene) Dimenhydrinate 50 mg/ml. Vial 10 ml. *Rx.*
Use: Antiemetic, antivertigo.

Dynabac. (Bock) Dirithromycin 250 mg/Tab. Enteric coated. Bot. 60s. *Rx.*
Use: Antibiotic.

Dynacin. (Medicis Dermatologics) Minocycline HCl 50 mg, 100 mg. Cap. **50 mg:** Bot. 100s; **100 mg:** Bot. 50s. *Rx.*
Use: Anti-infective, tetracycline.

DynaCirc. (Sandoz Consumer) Isradipine. 2.5 mg or 5 mg/Cap. Bot. 60s, 100s, UD 100s. *Rx.*
Use: Calcium channel blocker.

Dynacoryl.
See: Nikethamide, Preps. (Various Mfr.)

Dynafed Asthma Relief. (BDI) Ephedrine HCl 25 mg, guaifenesin 200 mg/Tab. Bot. 60s. *otc.*
Use: Decongestant, expectorant.

Dynafed Pseudo. (BDI) Pseudoephedrine HCl 60 mg/Tab. Bot. 60s. *otc.*
Use: Decongestant.

Dyna-Hex Skin Cleanser. (Western Medical) Chlorhexidine gluconate 4%, isopropyl alcohol 4%. Liq. Bot. 120 ml, 240 ml, 480 ml, 1 gal. *otc.*
Use: Antiseptic, germicide.

Dyna-Hex 2 Skin Cleanser. (Western Medical) Chlorhexidine gluconate 2%, isopropyl alcohol 4%. Liq. Bot. 120 ml, 2409 ml, 480 ml, 1 gal. *otc.*
Use: Antiseptic, germicide.

dynamine. (Mayo Foundation)
Use: Antispasmodic. Lambert-Eaton myasthenic syndrome; hereditary motor and sensory neuropathy type I (Charcot-Marie-Tooth Disease). [Orphan drug]

Dynapen. (Bristol) Sodium dicloxacillin. **Cap.:** 125 mg, 250 mg or 500 mg. Bot. 24s, 50s, 100s. **Susp.:** 62.5 mg/5 ml. Bot. 80 ml, 100 ml, 200 ml. *Rx.*
Use: Anti-infective, penicillin.

Dynaplex. (Alton) Vitamin B complex. Bot. 100s, 1000s. *otc.*
Use: Vitamin B supplement.

dynarsan.
See: Acetarsone, Tab.

Dy-O-Derm. (Galderma) Purified water, isopropyl alcohol, acetone, dihydroxyacetone, FD&C; yellow No. 6, FD&C; blue No. 1, FD&C; red No. 33. Bot. 4 oz.
Use: Water-soluble vitiligo stain.

Dy-Phyl-Lin. (Foy) Dyphylline 250 mg/ml with benzyl alcohol. Inj. Vial 10 ml. *Rx.*
Use: Bronchodilator.

•**dyphylline,** U.S.P. 23.
Use: Vasodilator, bronchodilator.
See: Brophylline, Inj., Granucaps (Solvay).
Dilor, Preps. (Savage).
Emfabid TD, Tab. (Saron).
Lardet, Inj. (Standex).
Neothylline, Tab. (Lemmon).
Prophyllin, Oint., Pow. (Rystan).
W/Chlorpheniramine maleate, guaifenesin, dextromethorphan HBr, phenylephrine HCl.
See: Hycoff-A, Syr. (Saron).
W/Guaifenesin.
See: Bronkolate-G, Tab. (Parmed).
Dilor-G, Liq., Tab. (Savage).
Embron, Syr., Cap. (T.E. Williams).
Neothylline GG, Liq. (Lemmon).

Dyphylline-GG Elixir. (Various Mfr.) Dyphylline 100 mg, guaifenesin 100 mg/15 ml. Bot. 473 ml. *Rx.*

Use: Bronchodilator.

Dyprotex. (Blistex) Micronized zinc oxide 40%, petrolatum 37.6%, dimethicone 2.5%, cod liver oil, aloe extract, zinc stearate. Pads. Pkgs. 3s (9 applications). *otc.*
Use: Astringent, diaper rash agent.

Dyrenium. (SK-Beecham) Triamterene. **50 mg/Cap.:** Bot. 100s, UD 100s. **100 mg/Cap.:** Bot. 100s, 1000s, UD 100s. *Rx.*
Use: Diuretic.

Dyretic. (Keene) Furosemide 10 mg/ml. Vial 10 ml. *Rx.*
Use: Diuretic.

Dyrexan-OD. (Trimen) Phendimetrazine tartrate 105 mg/SR Cap. Bot. 100s. *c-III.*
Use: Anorexiant.

Dyspel. (Dover) Acetaminophen, ephedrine sulfate, atropine sulfate. Sugar, lactose and salt free. Tab. UD Box 500s. *Rx.*
Use: Analgesic.

E

Eaase. (Neuro Genesis/Matrix) D, L-phenylalanine 500 mg, L-glutamine 15 mg, L-tyrosine 25 mg, L-carnitine 10 mg, L-arginine pyroglutamate 10 mg, L-ornithine/L-aspartate 10 mg, Cr 0.033 mg, Se 0.012 mg, B_1 0.33 mg, B_2 5 mg, B_3 3.3 mg, B_5 0.33 mg, B_6 0.33 mg, B_{12} 1 mcg, E 5 IU, biotin 0.05 mg, FA 0.066 mg, Fe 1 mg, Zn 2.5 mg, Ca 35 mg, I 0.25 mg, Cu 0.33 mg, Mg 25 mg/Cap. Bot. 42s *otc.*
Use: Nutritional supplement.

EACA. (Lederle) Epsilon aminocaproic acid. *Rx.*
Use: Antifibrinolytic.
See: Amicar (Lederle).

Ear Drops. (Weeks & Leo) Carbamide peroxide 6.5% in an anhydrous glycerin base. Bot. oz. *otc.*
Use: Otic preparation.

Ear-Dry. (Scherer) Isopropyl alcohol, boric acid 2.75%. Dropper bot. 30 ml. *otc.*
Use: Otic preparation.

Earex Ear Drops. (Approved) Benzocaine 0.15 g, antipyrine 0.7 g/0.5 oz. Bot. 0.5 oz. *Rx.*
Use: Otic prepartion.

Ear-Eze. (Hyrex) Hydrocortisone 1%, chloroxylenol 0.1%, pramoxine HCl 1%. Dropper bot. 15 ml. *Rx.*
Use: Corticosteroid, antibacterial, local anesthetic (otic), otic preparation.

Earocol Ear Drops. (Roberts) Benzocaine 1.4%, antipyrine 5.4%, glycerin, oxyquinoline sulfate. Soln. Dropper bot. 15 ml. *Rx.*
Use: Otic preparation.

earthnut oil. Peanut Oil.

Easprin. (Parke-Davis) Aspirin 15 gr/EC Tab. Bot. 100s. *Rx.*
Use: Salicylate analgesic.

East-A. (Eastwood) Therapeutic lotion. Bot. 16 oz. *otc.*
Use: Emollient.

Easy-Lax. (Walgreen) Docusate sodium 100 mg/Cap. Bot. 60s. *otc.*
Use: Laxative, stool softener.

Easy-Lax Plus. (Walgreen) Docusate sodium 100 mg, casanthranol 30 mg/Cap. Bot. 60s. *otc.*
Use: Laxative, stool softener.

Eazol. (Roberts) Fructose, dextrose, orthophosphoric acid with controlled hydrogen ion concentration. Bot. 473 ml. *otc.*
Use: Antinauseant.

E-Base. (Barr) Erythromycin. **Cap.:** 333

mg. Bot. 100s, 500s, 1000s. **Tab.:** 500 mg. Bot. 100s, 500s. *Rx.*
Use: Anti-infective, erythromycin.

•**ebastine.** (EBB-ass-teen) USAN.
Use: Antihistamine.

EBV-VCA. (Wampole-Zeus) Epstein-Barr virus, viral capsid antigen antibody test. Qualitative and semi-quantitative detection of EBV antibody in human serum. Test 100s.
Use: Diagnostic aid.

EBV-VCA Ig. (Wampole-Zeus) Epstein-Barr virus, viral capsid antigen Ig antibody. Qualitative and semiqualitative detection of EBV-VCA Ig antibody in human serum. Test 50s.
Use: Diagnostic aid.

•**ecadotril.** (ee-CAD-oh-trill) USAN.
Use: Antihypertensive.

Ecee Plus. (Edwards) Vitamin E 165 mg, ascorbic acid 100 mg, magnesium sulfate 70 mg, zinc sulfate 80 mg/Tab. Bot. 100s. *otc.*
Use: Vitamin/mineral supplement.

•**echothiophate iodide,** U.S.P. 23.
Use: Glaucoma; cholinergic (ophthalmic).
See: Echodide, Ophth. Soln. (Alcon). Phospholine Iodide, Pow. (Wyeth-Ayerst).

•**eclanamine maleate.** (eh-KLAN-ah-MEEN) USAN.
Use: Antidepressant.

•**eclazolast.** (eh-CLAY-zole-AST) USAN.
Use: Antiallergic, inhibitor (mediator release).

Eclipse After Sun. (Sandoz) Petrolatum, glycerin, oleth-3 phosphate, carbomer-934, imidazolidinyl urea, benzyl alcohol, cetyl esters wax. Lot. Bot. 180 ml. *otc.*
Use: Emollient.

Eclipse Lip and Face Protectant. (Sandoz) Padimate O, oxybenzone. Stick 4.5 g. *otc.*
Use: Sunscreen for lips.

Eclipse Original Sunscreen. (Sandoz) Padimate O, glyceryl PABA. Lot. Bot. 120 ml. *otc.*
Use: Sunscreen.

Eclipse Suntan, Partial. (Sandoz) Padimate O. Lot. Bot. 120 ml. *otc.*
Use: Sunscreen.

EC-Naprosyn. (Syntex) Naproxen 375 mg or 500 mg/TR Tab. Bot. 100s. *Rx.*
Use: Nonsteroidal anti-inflammatory drug.

•**econazole.** (ee-CON-uh-zole) USAN.
Use: Antifungal.

econazole nitrate, (ee-CON-uh-zole) U.S.P. 23.
Use: Antifungal.
See: Spectazole (Ortho Pharm).

Econo B & C. (Vanguard) Vitamins B₁ 15 mg, B₂ 10.2 mg, B₃ 50 mg, B₅ 10 mg, B₆ 5 mg, C 300 mg/Capl. Bot. 100s, UD 100s. *otc.*
Use: Vitamin supplement.

Econopred Ophthalmic. (Alcon) Prednisolone acetate 0.125% Susp. Drop-Tainer 5 ml, 10 ml. *Rx.*
Use: Corticosteroid, ophthalmic.

Econopred Plus. (Alcon) Prednisolone acetate 1%. Susp. Drop-Tainer 5 ml, 10 ml. *Rx.*
Use: Corticosteroid, ophthalmic.

Econotrin Adult Low Strength. (SK-Beecham) Aspirin 81 mg., tartrazine/Tab. ent. ctd. Bot. 36s *otc.*
Use: Analgesic.

Ecotrin Maximum Strength. (SK-Beecham) Acetylsalicylic acid 500 mg. **Tab.:** Bot. 60s, 150s. **Cap.:** Bot. 60s. *otc.*
Use: Analgesic.

Ecotrin Regular Strength Tablets. (SK-Beecham) Aspirin 325 mg/EC Tab. Bot. 100s, 250s, 1000s. *otc.*
Use: Salicylate analgesic.

Ed A-Hist. (Edwards) Phenylephrine HCl 10 mg, chlorpheniramine maleate 4 mg/5 ml, alcohol 5%. Liq. Bot. 473 ml. *Rx.*
Use: Decongestant, antihistamine.

Ed A-Hist Tablets. (Edwards) Chlorpheniramine maleate 8 mg, phenylephrine HCl 20 mg/SR Tab. Bot. 100s. *Rx.*
Use: Antihistamine, decongestant.

edathamil. Edetate ethylenediaminetetraacetic acid.
See: Nullapons (General Aniline).

edathamil calcium-disodium. Calcium disodium ethylenediamine tetraacetate.
See: Calcium Disodium Versenate, Amp. & Tab. (3M).

edathamil disodium. Disodium salt of ethylene diamine tetraacetic acid.
See: Endrate, Amp. (Abbott).

edatrexate. (EE-dah-TREX-ate) USAN.
Use: Antineoplastic.

Edecrin. (Merck) Ethacrynic acid 25 mg or 50 mg/Tab. Bot. 100s. *Rx.*
Use: Diuretic.

Edecrin Sodium Intravenous. (Merck) Ethacrynate sodium equivalent to 50 mg ethacrynic acid w/mannitol 62.5 mg, thimerosal 0.1 mg/Vial. Vial 50 ml for reconstitution. *Rx.*
Use: Diuretic.

edetate calcium disodium, (EH-duh-tate) U.S.P. 23. Formerly Edathamil.
Use: Chelating agent (metal).
See: Calcium Disodium Versenate, Amp., Tab. (3M).
Versere CA (dow Chemical).

edetate dipotassium. (EH-deh-tate) USAN.
Use: Pharmaceutic aid (chelating agent).

edetate disodium, (EH-duh-tate) U.S.P. 23.
Use: Chelating agent (metal) pharmaceutic aid (chelating agent).
See: Endrate, Amp. (Abbott).
Sodium Versenate inj. (3M).
W/Benzalkonium Cl, boric acid, potassium Cl, sodium carbonate anhydrous.
See: Swim-Eye Drops (Savage).
W/Phenylephrine HCl, methapyrilene HCl, benzalkonium Cl, sodium bisulfite.
See: Allerest Nasal Spray (Novartis).
W/Phenylephrine HCl, benzalkonium Cl, sodium bisulfate.
See: Sinarest, Aerosol (Novartis).
W/Potassium Cl, benzalkonium Cl, isotonic boric acid.
See: Dacriose (Smith, Miller & Patch).
W/Prednisolone sodium phosphate, niacinamide, sodium bisulfite, phenol.
See: P.S.P. IV. Inj. (Solvay).
W/Sodium thiosulfate, salicylic acid, isopropyl alcohol, propylene glycol, menthol, colloidal alumina.
See: Tinver Lotion (Pilkington Barnes Hind).

edetate disodium. (Various Mfr.) Edetate disodium 150 mg/ml. 20 ml vial. *Rx.*
Use: Treatment of hypercalcemia, control of ventricular arrhythmias associated with digitalis toxicity.

edetate sodium. (EH-deh-tate) USAN. Tetrasodium (ethylenedinitrilo)-tetraacetate, or tetrasodium ethylenediaminetetraacetate.
Use: Chelating agent.
See: Disodium Versenate (3M).
Vagisec, Liq. (Julius Schmid).

edetate trisodium. (EH-deh-tate) USAN. Trisodium hydrogen (ethylenedinitrilo) tetraacetate, or trisodium hydrogen ethylenediaminetetraacetate.
Use: Chelating agent.

edetic acid, N.F. 18. (Ethylenedinitrilo) tetraacetic acid.
Use: Pharmaceutic aid (chelating agent).
See: Versene Acid (Dow Chemical).

edetol. (eh-deh-TOLE) USAN.

Use: Pharmaceutic aid (alkalinizing agent).
See: Neutrol TE (BASF), Quadrol (BASF)

• **edifolone acetate.** (EH-DIH-fah-LONE) USAN.
Use: Cardiac depressant (antiarrhythmic).

edithamil.
See: Edathamil.

• **edobacomab.** (eh-dah-BACK-ah-mab) USAN.
Use: Antiendotoxin monoclonal antibody.

• **edoxudine.** (ee-DOX-you-DEEN) USAN.
Use: Antiviral.

• **edrecolomab.** (edd-reh-KOE-lah-mab) USAN.
Use: Monoclonal antibody (antineoplastic adjuvant).

edrofuradene. Name used for Nifurdazil.

• **edrophonium chloride,** (eh-droe-FOE-nee-uhm) U.S.P. 23.
Use: Antidote to curare principles; diagnostic aid (myasthenia gravis).
See: Enlon, Inj. (Ohmeda Pharmeceuticals).
Reversol (Organon).
Tensilon Chloride, Vial (Roche).

edrophonium chloride/atropine sulfate.
See: atropine sulfate/edrophonium chloride.

ED-SPAZ. (Edwards) Hyoscyamine sulfate 0.125 mg/Tab. Bot. 100s. *Rx.*
Use: Anticholinergic, antispasmodic.

EDTA.
See: Edathamil (Various Mfr.).

Ed-Tlc. (Edwards) Phenylephrine HCl 5 mg, chlorpheniramine maleate 2 mg, hydrocodone bitartrate 1.67 mg/5 ml. Liq. Bot. 473 ml. *c-III.*
Use: Decongestant, antihistamine, antitussive.

Ed-Tuss HC. (Edwards) Phenylephrine HCl 10 mg, chlorpheniramine maleate 4 mg, hydrocodone bitartrate 2.5 mg, alcohol 5%/5 ml. Liq. Bot. 480 ml. *c-III.*
Use: Decongestant, antihistamine, antitussive.

E.E.S. 400 Filmtab. (Abbott) Erythromycin ethylsuccinate representing 400 mg erythromycin activity/Tab. Pkg. 100s, 500s, UD 100s. *Rx.*
Use: Anti-infective, erythromycin.

E.E.S. Drops. (Abbott) Erythromycin ethylsuccinate representing erythromycin activity 100 mg/2.5 ml when re-constituted w/water. Dropper Bot. 50 ml. *Rx.*
Use: Anti-infective, erythromycin.

E.E.S. Granules. (Abbott) Erythromycin ethylsuccinate representing erythromycin activity 200 mg/5 ml oral susp. Gran. Bot. 60 ml, 100 ml, 200 ml, UD 5 ml. *Rx.*
Use: Anti-infective, erythromycin.

E.E.S. Liquid-200 & 400. (Abbott) Erythromycin ethylsuccinate representing erythromycin activity 200 mg/5 ml. Bot. 100 ml, 480 ml; erythromycin activity 400 mg/5 ml. Bot. 100 ml, 480 ml. *Rx.*
Use: Anti-infective, erythromycin.

Efed-II. (Alto) Ephedrine sulfate 25 mg/ Cap. Box 24s. *otc.*
Use: Decongestant.

Efedron Nasal. (Hyrex) Ephedrine HCl 0.6%, chlorobutanol 0.5% w/sodium Cl, menthol and cinnamon oil in a water-soluble jelly base. Tube 20 g. *otc.*
Use: Decongestant.

• **efegatran sulfate.** (EH-feh-GAT-ran) USAN.
Use: Antithrombotic.

E-Ferol Spray. (Forest Pharm.) Alpha tocopherol equivalent to 30 IU Vitamin E/ ml. Can 6 oz. *otc.*
Use: Emollient.

E-Ferol Succinate. (Forest Pharm.) d-alpha Tocopherol acid succinate, equivalent to Vitamin E. *otc.* **100 or 400 IU/Cap.:** Bot. 100s, 500s, 1000s. **200 IU/Cap.:** Bot. 50s, 100s, 500s, 1000s. **50 IU/Tab.:** Bot. 100s, 500s, 1000s.
Use: Vitamin E supplement.

E-Ferol Vanishing Cream. (Forest Pharm.) Alpha tocopherol. Jar 2 oz. *otc.*
Use: Emollient.

Effectin Tablets. (Sanofi Winthrop) Bitolterol mesylate. *Rx.*
Use: Bronchodilator.

Effective Strength Cough Formula. (Barre-National) Chlorpheniramine maleate 2 mg, dextromethorphan HBr 15 mg, alcohol 10%. Liq. Bot. 240 ml. *otc.*
Use: Antihistamine, antitussive.

Effective Strength Cough Formula with Decongestant. (Barre-National) Pseudoephedrine HCl 20 mg, dextromethorhan HBr 10 mg, alcohol 10%. Liq. Bot. 240 ml. *otc.*
Use: Decongestant, antitussive.

Effer-K. (Nomax) Potassium 25 mEq. (as bicarbonate and citrate), saccharin. Effervescent tab. Box foil 30s, 250s. *Rx.*
Use: Mineral supplement.

Effexor. (Wyeth-Ayerst) Venlafaxine 25 mg, 37.5 mg, 50 mg, 75 mg or 100 mg/Tab. Bot. 100s, Redipak 100s. *Rx.*
Use: Antidepressant.

Efficol Cough Whip, Suppressant, Decongestant. (Block) Phenylpropanolamine HCl 6.25 mg, dextromethorphan HBr 2.5 mg/5 ml Bot. 8 oz. *otc.*
Use: Decongestant, antitussive.

Efficol Cough Whip, Suppressant, Decongestant, Antihistamine. (Block) Dextromethorphan HBr 2.5 mg, phenylpropanolamine HCl 6.25 mg, chlorpheniramine maleate 1 mg/5 ml Bot. 8 oz. *otc.*
Use: Antitussive, decongestant, antihistamine.

Efidac/24. (Novartis) Pseudoephedrine HCl 240 mg/Tab. Pkg. 6s, 12s. *otc.*
Use: Decongestant.

Efidac 24 Chlorpheniramine. (Novartis) Chlorpheniramine maleate 16 mg/ER Tab. Pkg. 6s, 12s. *otc.*
Use: Antihistamine.

•**eflornithine hydrochloride.** (ee-FLAHR-nih-THEEN) USAN.
Use: Antineoplastic, antiprotozoal. [Orphan drug]
See: Ornidyl (Hoechst Marion Roussel).

Efo-Dine Ointment. (Fougera) Povidone-iodine oint. Foilpac oz, Tube oz. Jar lb. *otc.*

Efudex. (Roche) Fluorouracil. **Soln:** Fluorouracil 2% or 5%, w/propylene glycol, hydroxypropyl cellulose, parabens, disodium edetate. Drop Dispenser 10 ml. **Cream:** Fluorouracil 5%, in vanishing cream base w/white petrolatum, stearyl alcohol, propylene glycol, polysorbate 60, parabens. Tube 25 g. *Rx.*
Use: Antineoplastic.

egraine. A protein binder from oats.

•**egtazic acid.** (egg-TAY-zik) USAN.
Use: Pharmaceutic aid.

EHDP.
See: Etidronate Disodium.

ehrlich 606.
See: Arspheramine (Various Mfr.).

EL 10. (Elan Corporation) *Rx.*
Use: Antiviral, immunomodulator.

•**elacridar hydrochloride.** USAN.
Use: Potentiation of chemotherapy in cancer (multidrug resistance inhibitor in cancer).

•**elantrine.** (EL-an-treen) USAN.
Use: Anticholinergic.

Elase-Chloromycetin Ointment. (Parke-Davis) Fibrinolysin 10 units, desoxyribonuclease 6666 units, chloramphenicol 100 mg. Tube 10 g. Fibrinolysin 30 units, desoxyribonuclease 20,000 units, chloramphenicol 300 mg and thimerosal. In 30 g. *Rx.*
Use: Enzyme preparation, topical.

Elase Oint. & Pwd. for Sol. (Parke-Davis) **Pow.:** Fibrinolysin 25 units, desoxyribonuclease 15,000 units, thimerosal 0.1 mg/Vial as lyophilized powder. May be reconstituted with 10 ml of isotonic sodium Cl Soln. **Oint.:** Fibrinolysin 30 units, desoxyribonuclease 20,000 units, thimerosal 0.12 mg/30 g Tube. Fibrinolysin 10 units, desoxyribonuclease 6,666 units/10 g w/ thimerosal 0.04 mg as preservative. Ointment base of liquid petrolatum, polyethylene w/sucrose, sodium Cl. Tube 10 g, 30 g. *Rx.*
Use: Enzyme preparation, topical.

•**elastofilcon a.** (ee-LASS-toe-FILL-kahn A) USAN.
Use: Contact lens material, hydrophilic.
See: Silsoft (Bausch & Lomb)

Elavil. (Zeneca) Amitriptyline HCl. **Tab.:** **10 mg:** Bot. 100s, 1000s; **25 mg:** Bot. 100s, 1000s; **50 mg:** Bot. 100s, 1000s; **75 mg, 100 mg:** Bot. 100s; **150 mg:** Bot. 30s, 100s. All strengths in UD 100s. **Inj.:** Vial 10 mg/ml w/dextrose 44 mg, methylparaben 1.5 mg, propylparaben 0.2 mg/ml w/water for injection. q.s. Vial 1 ml, 10 ml. *Rx.*
Use: Antidepressant, tricyclic.

•**eldacimibe.** USAN.
Use: Antiatherosclerotic, antihyperlipidemic.

Eldec Kapseals. (Parke-Davis) Elemental iron 3.3 mg, Vitamins A 1667 IU, E 10 mg, B_1 10 mg, B_2 0.9 mg, B_3 17 mg, B_5 10 mg, B_6 0.7 mg, B_{12} 2 mcg, C 67 mg, folic acid 0.3 mg, calcium iodine/ Cap. Bot. 100s. *otc.*
Use: Vitamin/mineral supplement.

Eldecort. (Zeneca) Hydrocortisone 2.5%, light mineral oil, propylene glycol, allantoin/Cream. Tube 15 g, 30 g. *Rx.*
Use: Corticosteroid, topical.

Eldepryl. (Somerset) Selegiline 5 mg. Cap. Bot. 60s, 300s. *Rx.*
Use: Antiparkinsonian.

Eldercaps. (Mayrand) Vitamins A 4000 IU, D 400 IU, E 25 IU, B, 10mg. B_2 5 mg., B_3 25 mg., B_5 10 mg., B_6 2 mg., C 200 mg, folic acid 1 mg , Zn 15.8 mg. Mg, Mn. /Cap. Bot. 100s. *Rx.*
Use: Vitamin/mineral supplement.

Elder's RVP. Red Vet. Petrolatum.
Use: Dermatoses.

Eldertonic. (Mayrand) Vitamins B₁ 0.17 mg, B₂ 0.19 mg, B₃ 2.22 mg, B₅ 1.11 mg, B₆ 0.22 mg, B₁₂ 0.67 mcg, alcohol 13.5%, Mg, Mn, zinc 1.7 mg/5 ml. Bot. 473 ml. *otc.*
Use: Vitamin/mineral supplement.

Eldisine. (Lilly).
See: Vindesine sulfate.

Eldo-B & C. (Canright) Vitamins C 250 mg, B₁ 25 mg, B₂ 10 mg, niacinamide 150 mg, B₆ 5 mg, d-calcium pantothenate 20 mg/Tab. Bot. 100s, 1000s. *otc.*
Use: Vitamin/mineral supplement.

Eldofe. (Canright) Ferrous fumarate 225 mg/Chew. tab. Bot. 100s, 1000s. *otc.*
Use: Iron supplement.

Eldofe-C. (Canright) Ferrous fumarate 225 mg, ascorbic acid 50 mg/Tab. Bot. 100s. *otc.*
Use: Vitamin/mineral supplement.

Eldopaque. (ICN Pharm.) Hydroquinone 2% in a tinted sunblocking cream base. Tube 15 g, 30 g. *otc.*
Use: Skin bleaching agent.

Eldopaque Forte. (ICN Pharm.) Hydroquinone 4% in a tinted sunblocking cream base. Tube 15 g, 30 g. *Rx.*
Use: Skin bleaching agent.

Eldoquin. (ICN Pharm.) Hydroquinone 2% in a vanishing cream base. Tube 15 g, 30 g. *otc.*
Use: Skin bleaching agent.

Eldoquin Forte. (ICN Pharm.) Hydroquinone 4% in vanishing cream base. Tube 15 g, 30 g. *Rx.*
Use: Skin bleaching agent.

Elecal. (Western Research) Calcium 250 mg, magnesium 15 mg/Tab. Bot. 1000s. *otc.*
Use: Mineral supplement.

Electrolyte #48 Injection. Pediatric maintenance electrolyte solution. Dextrose 5% in electrolyte #48 w/sodium 25 mEq, potassium 20 mEq, magnesium 3 mEq, chloride 22 mEq, lactate 23 mEq, phosphate 3 mEq/L. *Rx.*
Use: Water, caloric, electrolyte supplement.

Electrolyte #75 and 5% Dextrose.
See: 5% Dextrose and Electrolyte #75.

Elegen-G. (Grafton) Amitriptyline 10 mg, 25 mg or 50 mg/Tab. Bot. 100s, 1000s. *Rx.*
Use: Antidepressant, tricyclic.

Elevites. (Barth's) Vitamins A 6000 IU, D 400 IU, B₁ 1.5 mg, B₂ 3 mg, C 60 mg, B₁₂ 10 mcg, niacin 1 mg, E 10 IU, malt diastase 15 mg, iron 15 mg, calcium 381 mg, phosphorus 0.172 mg, citrus bioflavonoid complex 15 mg, rutin 15 mg, nucleic acid 3 mg, red bone marrow 30 mg, peppermint leaves 10 mg, wheat germ 30 mg/Tab. or Cap. Bot. 100s, 500s, 1000s. *Rx.*
Use: Vitamin/mineral supplement.

Elimite. (Allergan Herbert) Permethrin 5%. Cream. Tube 60 g. *Rx.*
Use: Scabicide, pediculicide.

Elixicon. (Berlex) Theophylline 100 mg/ 5 ml with methyl and propyl parabens. Susp. Bot. 237 ml. *Rx.*
Use: Bronchodilator.

Elixiral. (Vita Elixir) Phenobarbital 16.2 mg, hyoscyamine sulfate 0.1037 mg, atropine sulfate 0.194 mg, hyoscine HBr 0.0065 mg/5 ml. Liq. pt, gal. *Rx.*
Use: Sedative, hypnotic, anticholinergic, antispasmodic.

Elixophyllin Capsules, Dye-Free. (Forest) Anhydrous theophylline 100 mg or 200 mg/Cap. **100 mg:** Bot. 100s; **200 mg:** Bot. 100s, 500s, UD 100s. *Rx.*
Use: Bronchodilator.

Elixophyllin Elixir. (Forest) Anhydrous theophylline 80 mg, alcohol 20%/15 ml. Bot. pt, qt, gal. *Rx.*
Use: Bronchodilator.

Elixophyllin-GG Liquid. (Forest) Theophylline 100 mg, guaifenesin 100 mg/ 15 ml. Alcohol free. Bot. 237, 480 ml. *Rx.*
Use: Antiasthmatic combination.

Elixophyllin-KI Elixir. (Forest) Anhydrous theophylline 80 mg, potassium iodide 130 mg/15 ml. Bot. 237 ml. *Rx.*
Use: Antiasthmatic combination.

Ellesdine. (Janssen) Pipenperone. *Rx.*
Use: Tranquilizer.

Elliot's B Solution. (Orphan Medical)
Use: Acute lymphatic leukemias and acute lymphoblastic lymphomas. [Orphan drug] *otc, Rx.*

elm, U.S.P. 23.
Use: Pharmaceutic aid (suspending agent), demulcent.

Elmiron. (Baker Norton) Pentosan polysulfate 100 mg/ Cap. Bot. 100s *Rx.*
Use: Relief of bladder pain associated with interstitial cystitis.

Elocon Cream. (Schering-Plough) Mometasone furoate 0.1%, hexylene glycol, phosphoric acid, propylene glycol stearate, stearyl alcohol, ceteareth-20, titanium dioxide, aluminum starch octenyl succinate, white wax, white petrolatum. 15 g, 45 g. *Rx.*

Use: Corticosteroid, topical.

Elocon Lotion. (Schering-Plough) Mometasone furoate 0.1%. Bot. 30 ml, 60 ml. *Rx.*
Use: Corticosteroid, topical.

Elocon Ointment. (Schering-Plough) Mometasone furoate 0.1%, hexylene glycol, propylene glycol stearate, white wax, white petrolatum. 15 g, 45 g. *Rx.*
Use: Corticosteroid, topical.

Elphemet. (Canright) Phendimetrazine tartrate 35 mg/Tab. Bot. 100s, 1000s. *c-III.*
Use: Anorexiant.

Elprecal. (Canright) Vitamins A 5000 IU, D 400 IU, B_1 3 mg, B_2 2 mg, B_6 0.1 mg, B_{12} 1 mcg, C 50 mg, E 2 IU, calcium pantothenate 2.5 mg, niacinamide 15 mg, inositol 5 mg, choline 5 mg, calcium lactate 500 mg, ferrous sulfate 50 mg, copper 1 mg, manganese 1 mg, magnesium 2 mg, potassium 2 mg, zinc 0.5 mg, sulfur 1 mg/Cap. Bot. 100s. *otc.*
Use: Vitamin/mineral supplement.

•**elsamitrucin.** (els-AM-ih-TRUE-sin) USAN.
Use: Antineoplastic.

Elserpine. (Canright) Reserpine 0.25 mg/Tab. Bot. 100s, 1000s. *Rx.*
Use: Antihypertensive.

Elspar. (Merck) Asparaginase 10,000 IU, mannitol 80 mg/Inj. Vial 10 ml. *Rx.*
Use: Antineoplastic.

•**elucaine.** (eh-LOO-cane) USAN.
Use: Anticholinergic, gastric.

Eltroxin. (Roberts) Levothyroxine sodium 0.05 mg, 0.1 mg, 0.15 mg, 0.2 mg, 0.3 mg/Tab. Bot. 100s, 500s. *Rx.*
Use: Thyroid hormone.

Elvanol. (DuPont Merck) Polyvinyl alcohol.
Use: Pharmaceutical aid.

embechine. Aliphatic chloroethylamine.
Use: Antineoplastic.

Emcodeine Tabs. (Major) Aspirin with codeine as #2, #3 or #4. Bot. 100s, 500s. *c-III.*
Use: Narcotic analgesic combination.

Emcyt. (Pharmacia & Upjohn) Estramustine phosphate sodium equivalent to 140 mg estramustine phosphate sodium 12.5 mg/Cap. Bot. 100s. *Rx.*
Use: Antineoplastic.

Emdol. (Approved) Salicylamide, para-aminobenzoic acid, sodium calcium succinate, vitamin D-1250. Bot. 100s, 1000s. *otc.*
Use: Analgesic combination.

Emecheck. (Savage) Phosphoric acid 21.5 mg, glucose, fructose/5 ml, methylparaben, cherry flavor. Liq. Bot. 120 ml. *otc.*
Use: Antiemetic.

•**emedastine difumarate.** USAN.
Use: Management of allergic conjunctivitis, antiasthmatic, antiallergic, antihistamine.

emergency kits.
See: Ana-Kit (Bayer).
AtroPen Auto-Injector (Survival Technology).
Cyanide Antidote Package (Lilly).
Emergent-Ez Kit (Healthfirst Corp).
EpiPen Auto-Injector (Center Labs).
EpiPen Jr. Auto-Injector (Center Labs).
LidoPen Auto-Injector (Survival Technology).
Poison Antidote Kit (Jones Medical).

Emergent-EZ. (Healthfirst Corp.) Adrenalin 2 amp., aminophylline 1 amp., ammonia inhalants (3), amyl nitrite inhalants (2), atropine 2 amp., diazepam (2 amp.), epinephrine (2 amp), Benadryl 2 amp., nitroglycerin 1 bottle, Solu-Cortef 1 mix-o-vial, Talwin 1 amp., Tigan 1 amp., Valium 2 amp., Wyamine 2 amp., plastic air way (1), disposable syringes, tracheotomy needle (1) and tourniquet (1)/kit. *Rx.*
Use: Emergency kit.

Emeroid. (Delta) Zinc oxide 5%, diperodon HCl 0.25%, bismuth subcarbonate 0.2%, pyrilamine maleate 0.1%, phenylephrine HCl 0.25%, in a petrolatum base containing cod liver oil. Tube 1.25 oz. *otc.*
Use: Anorectal preparation.

Emersal. (Medco Lab) Ammoniated mercury 5%, salicylic acid 2.5%, castor oil 23%, liquid petrolatum, polyoxyl 40 stearate, polysorbate 80, water. Lot. Plastic bot. 120 ml. *Rx.*
Use: Antipsoriatic.

Emerson 1% Sodium Fluoride Dental Gel. (Emerson) Red and plain. Bot. 2 oz. *Rx.*
Use: Dental caries preventative.

emetics.
See: Apomorphine HCl. Cupric Sulfate. Ipecac Syr.

•**emetrine hydrochloride,** U S. P. 23.
Use: Anti-amebic.

Emetrol. (Bock) Oral soln. containing balanced amounts of fructose and dextrose with orthophosphoric acid, with controlled hydrogen ion concentration. Bot. 120 ml, 480 ml. *otc.*
Use: Antiemetic.

Emgel. (Glaxo) Erythromycin 2%. Gel. Tube 27 g. *Rx.*
Use: Anti-acne.

EM-GG. (Econo Med) Guaifenesin 100 mg/5 ml. Bot. pt. *otc.*
Use: Expectorant.

•**emilium tosylate.** (EE-MILL-ee-uhm TAH-sill-ate) USAN.
Use: Cardiac depressant (antiarrhythmic).

Eminase. (Roberts) Anistreplase 30 units/Pow. for Inj. Vials. *Rx.*
Use: Thrombolytic enzyme.

Emitrip Tabs. (Major) Amitriptyline **10 mg or 25 mg/Tab.:** Bot. 100s, 250s, 1000s, UD 100s. **50 mg/Tab.:** Bot. 100s, 250s, 1000s, UD 100s. **75 mg/Tab.:** Bot. 100s, 250s, UD 100s. **100 mg/ Tab.:** Bot. 100s, 250s, 1000s, UD 100s. **150 mg/Tab.:** Bot. 100s, 250s. *Rx.*
Use: Antidepressant, tricyclic.

Emko Because Contraceptor. (Schering-Plough) Nonoxynol-9 (8% concentration). Contraceptor container w/applicator. Tube 10 g. *otc.*
Use: Vaginal contraceptive.

Emko Pre-Fil. (Schering-Plough) Nonoxynol-9 (8% concentration). Aerosol Can 30 g, Refill 60 g. *otc.*
Use: Vaginal contraceptive.

Emko Vaginal Foam. (Schering-Plough) Nonoxynol-9 (8% concentration). Kit Aerosol w/applicator 40 g, Refill 40 g, 90 g. *otc.*
Use: Vaginal contraceptive.

EMLA. (Astra) Lidocaine 2.5%, prilocaine 2.5%/Cream. Tube 5 g, 30 g. *Rx.*
Use: Local anesthetic, topical.

Emollia-Creme. (Gordon) Cetyl alcohol, lubricating oils in water-soluble base. Jar 4 oz, 5 lb. *otc.*
Use: Emollient.

Emollia-Lotion. (Gordon) Water-dispersable waxes, lubricating bland oils in a water-soluble lotion base. Bot. 1 oz, 4 oz, gal. *otc.*
Use: Emollient.

Empirin Aspirin Tablets. (Glaxo Wellcome) Aspirin 325 mg/Tab. Bot. 50s, 100s, 250s. *otc.*
Use: Salicylate analgesic.

Empirin with Codeine. (Glaxo Wellcome) Aspirin 325 mg with codeine phosphate 15 mg, 30 mg or 60 mg/Tab. **No. 2:** Codeine phosphate 15 mg. Bot. 100s. **No. 3:** Codeine phosphate 30 mg. Bot. 100s, 500s, 1000s, Dispenserpak 25s. **No. 4:** Codeine phosphate 60 mg. Bot. 100s, 500s, Dispenserpak 25s. *c-iii.*

Use: Narcotic analgesic combination.

Emulave. (Rydelle)
See: Aveenobar Oilated (Rydelle).

Emul-O-Balm. (Medeva) Menthol, camphor, methyl salicylate. Bot. 2 oz, 8 oz, gal.
Use: Analgesic, topical.

Emulsoil. (Paddock) Castor oil 95%. Bot. 60 ml. *otc.*
Use: Laxative.

E-Mycin. (Pharmacia & Upjohn) Erythromycin. **250 mg**/EC Tab.: Bot. 100s, 500s, UD 100s, Unit-of-Use 40s. **333 mg**/EC Tab.: Bot. 100s, 500s, UD 100s. *Rx.*
Use: Anti-infective, erythromycin.

•**enadoline hydrochloride.** (en-AHD-ole-en) USAN.
Use: Analgesic.

•**enalapril maleate,** (EH-NAL-uh-prill) U.S.P. 23.
Use: Antihypertensive.
See: Vasotec, Tab. (Merck).
W/Hydrochlorothiazide.
See: Vaseretic, Tab. (Merck & Co.).

•**enalaprilat,** (EH-NAL-uh-prill-at) U.S.P. 23.
Use: Antihypertensive.
See: Vasotec Inj(Merck).

•**enalkiren.** (en-al-KIE-ren) USAN.
Use: Antihypertensive.

•**enazadrem phosphate.** (eh-NAZZ-ah-drem FOSS-fate) USAN.
Use: Antipsoriatic inhibitor.

•**encainide hydrochloride.** (EN-CANE-ide) USAN.
Use: Cardiac depressant (antiarrhythmic).
See: Enkaid, Cap. (Bristol).

Encare. (Thompson Medical) Nonoxynol-9 (2.27%). Supp. 12s. *otc.*
Use: Vaginal contraceptive.

•**enciprazine hydrochloride.** (en-SIH-PRAH-zeen) USAN.
Use: Tranquilizer (minor).

•**enclomiphene.** (en-KLOE-mih-FEEN) USAN. Formerly Cisclomiphene.

•**encyprate.** (en-SIGH-prate) USAN.
Use: Antidepressant.

Endafed. (UAD) Pseudoephedrine HCl 120 mg, brompheniramine maleate 12 mg/SR Cap. Bot. 100s. *Rx.*
Use: Decongestant, antihistamine.

Endagen-HD. (Jones Medical) Phenylephrine HCl 5 mg, chlorpheniramine maleate 2 mg, hydrocodone bitartrate 1.67 mg. Bot. 473 ml. *c-iii.*
Use: Decongestant, antihistamine, antitussive.

Endal. (UAD Labs) Phenylephrine HCl 20 mg, guaifenesin 300 mg/TR tab., dye free. Bot. 100s. *Rx.*
Use: Decongestant, expectorant.

Endal Expectorant. (UAD Labs) Codeine phosphate 10 mg, phenylpropanolamine HCl 12.5 mg, guaifenesin 100 mg/5 ml w/alcohol 5%. Bot. pt. *c-iv.*
Use: Antitussive, decongestant, expectorant.

Endal-HD. (UAD Labs) Phenylephrine HCl 5 mg, chlorpheniramine maleate 2 mg, hydrocodone bitartrate 1.67 mg w/menthol, sucrose. Liq. Bot. 480 ml. *c-iii.*
Use: Decongestant, antihistamine, antitussive.

Endal-HD Plus. (UAD) Hydrocodone bitartrate 2 mg, phenylephrine HCl 5 mg, chlorpheniramine maleate 2 mg/5 ml. Liq. Bot. 473 ml. *c-iii.*
Use: Antitussive, decongestant, antihistamine.

Endecon. (DuPont Merck) Phenylpropanolamine HCl 25 mg, acetaminophen 325 mg/Tab. Bot. 60s. *otc.*
Use: Decongestant, analgesic.

Endep. (Roche) Amitriptyline HCl 10 mg, 25 mg, 50 mg, 75 mg, 100 mg or 150 mg/Tab. **10 mg:** Bot. 100s, Tel-E-Dose 100s. **25 mg:** Bot. 100s, 500s, Tel-E-Dose 100s. **50 mg:** Bot. 100s, 500s, Tel-E-Dose 100s. **75 mg:** Bot. 100s, Tel-E-Dose 100s. **100 mg:** Bot. 100s, Tel-E-Dose 100s. **150 mg:** Bot 100s. *Rx.*
Use: Antidepressant, tricyclic.

End Lice. (Thompson) Pyrethrins 0.3%, piperonyl butoxide technical 3%. Liq. Bot. 177 ml. *otc.*
Use: Pediculicide.

endobenziline bromide.
Use: Anticholinergic.

endocaine. Pyrrocaine.
Use: Local anesthetic.

endojodin.
See: Entodon.

Endolor. (Keene) Butalbital 50 mg, caffeine 40 mg, acetaminophen 325 mg/Cap. Bot. 100s. *Rx.*
Use: Sedative, hypnotic, analgesic.

endomycin. A new antibiotic obtained from cultures of *Streptomyces endus.* Under study.

endophenolphthalein. (Roche) Diacetyldioxyphenylisatin-isacen-bisatin. *otc.*
Use: Laxative.
See: Diacetylhydroxphenylisatin, Prep. (Various Mfr.)

•**endralazine mesylate.** (en-DRAL-ahzeen MEH-sih-late) USAN.
Use: Antihypertensive.
See: Migranol (Sandoz).

Endrate. (Abbott Hospital Prods) Edetate disodium 150 mg/ml. Amp. 20 ml. *Rx.*
Use: Treatment of hypercalcemia, control of ventricular arrhythmias associated with digitalis toxicity.

•**endrysone.** (EN-drih-sone) USAN.
Use: Anti-inflammatory (topical, ophthalmic).

Enduron. (Abbott) Methyclothiazide 5 mg/Tab. Bot. 100s, 1000s, UD 100s. *Rx.*
Use: Diuretic.

Enduronyl. (Abbott) Methyclothiazide 5 mg, deserpidine 0.25 mg/Tab. Bot. 100s, 1000s, UD 100s. *Rx.*
Use: Antihypertensive, diuretic.

Enduronyl Forte. (Abbott) Methyclothiazide 5 mg, deserpidine 0.5 mg/Tab. Bot. 100s, 1000s. *Rx.*
Use: Antihypertensive, diuretic.

Enebag 2. (Lafayette) Air contrast barium enema bag. Case 24s.
Use: Radiopaque agent.

Enebag XL. (Lafayette) Air contrast barium enema bag 3000 ml w/lumen tubing, enema tip and side clamp. Case 24s.
Use: Radiopaque agent.

Enecat. (Lafayette) Barium sulfate suspension CT colon exam kit. Case 12s.
Use: Radiopaque agent.

Enemark. (Lafayette) Rectal marker. 85% w/v liquid barium. Case of 12 kits.
Use: Rectal marker during radiation therapy.

Ener-B. (NTBY) Vitamin B_{12} 400 mcg/unit. Nasal gel. Unit 12s. *otc.*
Use: Vitamin supplement.

Enerjets. (Chilton) Caffeine 65 mg/Loz. pkg. 10s. *otc.*
Use: CNS stimulant.

Eneset 1. (Lafayette) Barium sulfate suspension 300 ml/air contrast examination kit. Unit-of-use kit. Case 12s.
Use: Radiopaque agent.

Eneset 2. (Lafayette) Barium sulfate suspension 450 ml/contrast examination kit. Unit-of-use kit. Case 12s.
Use: Radiopaque agent.

Eneset 600. (Lafayette) Barium sulfate suspension 600 ml/air contrast examination kit. Unit-of-use kit. Case 12s.
Use: Radiopaque agent.

Enfamil. (Bristol-Myers) Vitamins A 2000 IU, D 400 IU, E 20 IU, C 52 mg, B_1 0.5

mg, B_2 1 mg, B_6 0.4 mg, B_{12} 1.5 mcg, niacin 8 mg, calcium 440 mg, phosphorus 300 mg, folic acid 100 mcg, pantothenic acid 3 mg, inositol 30 mg, biotin 15 mcg, K-1 55 mcg, choline 100 mg, iron 1.4 mg, potassium 650 mg, chloride 400 mg, copper 0.6 mg, iodine 65 mcg, sodium 175 mg, magnesium 50 mg, zinc 5 mg, manganese 100 mg/Qt. Concentrated Liq. 13 fl oz, Instant Pow. lb. *otc.*
Use: Nutritional supplement.

Enfamil Human Milk Fortifier. (Bristol-Myers) Whey protein, casein, corn syrup solids, lactose, protein 0.7 g, carbohydrate 2.7 g, fat 0.04 g, calories 14. Pow. Packet 0.95 g, Box 100s. *otc.*
Use: Nutritional supplement.

Enfamil with Iron. (Bristol-Myers) Iron 12 mg/Qt. Pkg. Con. Liq. 13 fl oz. 24s. Pow. 1 lb. 6s. *otc.*
Use: Nutritional supplement.

Enfamil with Iron Ready to Use. (Bristol-Myers) Ready-to-use Enfamil with Iron infant formula 20 kcal/fl oz. Can 8 fl oz, 6-can pack; 32 fl oz, 6 cans per case. *otc.*
Use: Nutritional supplement.

Enfamil Next Step. (Bristol-Myers) Protein 17.3 g, carbohydrates 74 g, fat 33.3 g/liter, with appropriate vitamins and minerals. **Liq.:** 390 ml concentrate, 1 qt ready-to-use. **Pow.:** 360 g, 720 g. *otc.*
Use: Nutritional supplement.

Enfamil Nursette. (Bristol-Myers) Ready-to-feed Enfamil 20 kcal/fl oz, 4 fl oz, 6 fl oz and 8 fl oz. 4 bottles/sealed carton. W/Iron. Ready to use. Bot. 6 fl oz 4s, 24s. *otc.*
Use: Nutritional supplement.

Enfamil Premature Formula. (Bristol-Myers) Nonfat milk, whey protein concentrate, corn syrup solids, lactose, coconut oil, corn oil, medium chain triglycerides, soy lecithin. Protein 2.8 g, carbohydrate 10.7 g, fat 4.9 g, calories 96. Pow. Nursettes 120 ml. *otc.*
Use: Nutritional supplement.

Enfamil Ready To Use. (Bristol-Myers) Ready-to-use Enfamil infant formula 20 kcal/fl oz. Can 8 fl oz, 6-can pack; 32 fl oz, 6 cans per case. *otc.*
Use: Nutritional supplement.

•**enflurane,** (EN-flew-rane) U.S.P. 23. Ethrane
Use: Anesthetic (inhalation).
See: Ethrane (Ohio Medical).

enflurane. (Abbott) Enflurane 125 ml and 250 ml/Inhalation. *Rx.*

Use: Anesthetic, inhalation.

Engerix-B. (SK-Beecham) Hepatitis B vaccine (recombinant). **Adult:** 20 mcg 1ml with orange caps: 1 ml single-dose vial, 10 vials, 25 vials; 10 ml multidose vial; 5 1 ml Disp. Single-Dose Syr w/ 23-gauge 1 inch needles/Pkg. **Pediatric/High Risk/Adolescent:** 10 mcg 10.5 ml with blue caps: 0.5 ml single-dose vial; 5 0.5 ml Disp-Single-Dose Syr. with 25-gauge ⅝ inch needle/Pkg.
Use: Vaccine.

•**englitazone sodium.** (EN-GLIH-tah-zone) USAN.
Use: Antidiabetic.

•**enilconazole.** (EE-nill-KOE-nah-zole) USAN.
Use: Antifungal.

•**eniluracil.** USAN.
Use: Potentiator of antineoplastic activity of fluorouracil (uracil reductase inhibitor).

•**enisoprost.** (en-EYE-so-prahst) USAN.
Use: Antiulcerative.

Enisyl. (Person & Covey) L-Lysine monohydrochloride 334 mg or 500 mg/Tab. Bot. 100s, 250s. *otc.*
Use: Dietary supplement.

Enkaid. (Bristol) Encainide HCl 25 mg, 35 mg or 50 mg/Cap. Bot. 100s, UD 100s. *Rx.*
Use: Antiarrhythmic.

•**enlimomab.** (en-LIE-moe-mab) USAN.
Use: Anti-inflammatory, monoclonal antibody.

Enlon Injection. (Ohmeda) Edrophonium Cl 10 mg/ml, phenol 0.45%, sodium sulfite 0.2%. Vial 15 ml. *Rx.*
Use: Cholinergic muscle stimulant.

Enlon-Plus. (Ohmeda) Edrophonium chloride 10 mg, atropine sulfate 0.14 mg. Inj. Amp. 5 ml, Multi-dose Vial 15 ml. *Rx.*
Use: Cholinergic muscle stimulant.

•**enloplatin.** (en-LOW-PLAT-in) USAN.
Use: Antineoplastic.

Ennex Ointment. (Ennex) Aloe vera extract 37.5%. **Skin Oint.:** Zinc oxide 12.5%, coal tar 1.5%, alcohol 4.5%. Tube oz. **Hemorrhoidal Oint.:** Tube oz. *otc.*
Use: Anti-inflammatory, astringent, antipruritic.

•**enofelast.** (EE-no-fell-ast) USAN.
Use: Antiasthmatic.

•**enolicam sodium.** (ee-NO-lih-kam) USAN.
Use: Anti-inflammatory, antirheumatic.

Enomine Capsules. (Major) Phenyl-

propanolamine 45 mg, phenylephrine 5 mg, guaifenesin 200 mg/Cap. Bot. 100s, 500s. *Rx.*
Use: Decongestant, expectorant.

Enovid-E 21. (Searle) Norethynodrel 2.5 mg, mestranol 0.1 mg/Tab. Compack disp. 21s, 6 × 21. Refill 21s, 12 × 21. *Rx.*
Use: Estrogen, progestin combination.

Enovil. (Roberts) Amtriptyline HCl 10 mg/ml. Vial 10 ml. *Rx.*
Use: Antidepressant.

•**enoxacin.** (en-OX-ah-SIN) USAN.
Use: Antibacterial.
See: Penetrex (Rhone-Poulenc Rorer).

•**enoxaparin sodium.** (ee-NOX-ah-PAR-in) USAN.
Use: Antithrombotic.
See: Lovenox (Rhone-Poulenc Rorer).

•**enoximone.** (EN-ox-ih-MONE) USAN.
Use: Cardiotonic.
See: Perfar (Hoechst Marion Roussel).

•**enpiroline phosphate.** (en-PIHR-oh-LEEN) USAN.
Use: Antimalarial.

•**enprofylline.** (en-PRO-fih-lin) USAN.
Use: Bronchodilator.

•**enpromate.** (EN-pro-mate) USAN.
Use: Antineoplastic.

•**enprostil.** (en-PRAHS-till) USAN.
Use: Antisecretory, antiulcerative.
See: Gardrin (Syntex).

Enrich. (Ross) Liquid food with fiber providing complete, balanced nutrition as a full liquid diet, liquid supplement, or tube feeding. One serving provides 5 g dietary fiber. 1100 calories/L. 1530 calories provides 100% US RDA for vitamins and minerals. Can Ready-to-Use 8 fl oz (vanilla, chocolate). *otc.*
Use: Enteral nutritional supplement.

Ensidon. (Novartis) Opipramol HCl. *Rx.*
Use: Antidepressant.

Ensure. (Ross) Liquid food providing 1.06 calories/ml. Can be used as a full liquid diet, liquid supplement or tube feeding. Two quarts (2000 calories) provides 100% US RDA for vitamins and minerals for adults and children over 4 yrs. **Ready-to-Use:** Bot. 8 fl oz (vanilla). Can 8 fl oz (chocolate, black walnut, coffee, strawberry, eggnog, vanilla), 32 fl oz (vanilla, chocolate). **Pow.:** Can 14 oz (400 g) (vanilla). *otc.*
Use: Nutritional supplement.

Ensure HN. (Ross) High nitrogen low residue liquid food providing complete, balanced nutrition as tube feeding or oral supplement with 1.06 calories/ml.

Provides 100% US RDA for vitamins and minerals for adults and children over 4 yrs. 1400 calories (1321 ml). Ready-to-Use: Can 8 fl oz (vanilla). *otc.*
Use: Nutritional supplement.

Ensure High Protein. (Ross) Protein 50.4 g, carbohydrate 129.4 g, fat 25.2 g, < 21 mg cholesterol, Na 1218 mg, K 2100 mg, vitamin A 5250 IU, D 420 IU, E 47.5 IU, K 84 mcg, C 125 mg, folic acid 420 mg, B_1 1.6 mg, B_2 1.8 mg, B_3 21 mg, B_5 10.5 mg, B_6 2.1 mg, B_{12} 6.3 mcg, biotin 315 mcg, Ca 1050 mg, Cl, P, Mg, I, Mn, Cu, Zn 24 mg, Fe 19 mg, Se, Cr, Mo, 945 calories/237 ml. Liq. Bot. 237 ml. *otc.*
Use: Nutritional supplement.

Ensure Osmolite. (Ross).
See: Osmolite (Ross).

Ensure Plus. (Ross) High-calorie liquid food w/caloric density of 1500 calories/L. Six servings (8 oz and 2130 calories each) provides 100% US RDA for vitamins and minerals for adults and children. Ready-to-Use: Bot. 8 fl oz (vanilla). Can 8 fl oz (chocolate, vanilla, eggnog, coffee, strawberry). *otc.*
Use: Nutritional supplement.

Ensure Plus HN. (Ross) High-calorie, high-nitrogen liquid food providing 1.5 calories/ml; 1420 calories provides 100% US RDA for vitamins and minerals for adults and children. Calorie/nitrogen ratio is 150:1. Can 8 fl oz (vanilla). *otc.*
Use: Nutritional supplement.

Ensure Pudding. (Ross) Protein 6.8 g (nonfat milk), carbohydrate 34 g (sucrose, modified food starch), fat 9.7 g (partially hydrogenated soybean oil), vitamin A 850 IU, D 68 IU, E 7.7 IU, K 12 mcg, C 15.4 mg, folic acid 68 mcg, B_1 0.25 mg, B_2 0.29 mg, B_6 0.34 mg, B_{12} 1.1 mcg, B_3 3.4 mg, choline, biotin, B_5 1.7 mg, Na 240 mg, K 330 mg, Cl 220 mg, Ca 200 mg, P, Mg, I, Mn, Cu, Zn 3.83 mg, Fe 3.06 mg, 250 calories/can. Pudding. 150 g. *otc.*
Use: Nutritional supplement.

Entab 650. (Mayrand) Aspirin 650 mg/EC tab. Bot. 100s. *otc.*
Use: Salicylate analgesic.

Entero-Test. (HDC Corp.) Cap. To identify duodenal parasites; to diagnose and locate upper GI bleeding, pH disorders, achlorhydria and esophageal reflux. Bot. 10s, 25s.
Use: Diagnostic aid.

Entero-Test Pediatric. (HDC Corp.) To identify duodenal parasites; to diag-

nose and locate upper GI bleeding, pH disorders, achlorhydria and esophageal reflux. Cap. Bot. 10s, 25s.
Use: Diagnostic aid.

Enterotube. (Roche Diagnostics) Culture-identification method for enterobacteriaceae ACA. Test kit 25s.
Use: Diagnostic aid.

Entertainer's Secret Spray. (KLI Corp.) Sodium carboxymethylcellulose, potassium Cl, dibasic sodium phosphate, aloe vera gel, glycerin, parabens. Soln. 60 ml spray. *otc.*
Use: Saliva substitute.

Entex. (Procter & Gamble) Phenylephrine HCl 5 mg, phenylpropanolamine HCl 45 mg, guaifenesin 200 mg/Cap. Bot. 100s, 500s. *Rx.*
Use: Decongestant, expectorant.

Entex LA. (Procter & Gamble) Phenylpropanolamine HCl 75 mg, guaifenesin 400 mg/T.R. Tab. Bot. 100s, 500s. *Rx.*
Use: Decongestant, expectorant.

Entex Liquid. (Procter & Gamble) Phenylephrine HCl 5 mg, phenylpropanolamine HCl 20 mg, guaifenesin 100 mg/5 ml, alcohol 5%. Elix. Bot. 480 ml. *Rx.*
Use: Decongestant, expectorant.

Entex PSE. (Procter & Gamble) Pseudoephedrine 120 mg, guaifenesin 600 mg. Prolonged action. Tab. Bot. 100s. *Rx.*
Use: Decongestant, expectorant.

entodon.

entoidoin.
See: Entodon.

Entolase HP. (Robins) Lipase 8,000 units, protease 50,000 units, amylase 40,000 units/Cap. (enteric coated microbeads). Bot. 100s, 250s. *Rx.*
Use: Digestive enzymes.

Entrition Half Strength. (Biosearch) Calcium and sodium caseinates, maltodextrin, corn oil, soy lecithin, mono- and diglycerides, protein 17.5 g, carbohydrate 68 g, fat 17.5 g, sodium 350 mg, potassium 600 mg, calories 0.5/ml, osmolarity 120 mOsm/kg, water, vitamins A, B_1, B_2, B_3, B_5, B_6, B_{12}, C, D, E, K, Ca, P, Mg, I, Fe, Zn, Mn, Cu, Cl, biotin, choline, folic acid. Pouch 1 L. *otc.*
Use: Nutritional supplement.

Entrition HN Entri-Pak. (Biosearch). Sodium and calcium caseinates, soy protein isolate, maltodextrin, corn oil, soy lecithin, mono and diglycerides, vitamins A, B_1, B_2, B_3, B_5, B_6, B_{12}, C, D, E, K, folic acid, biotin, choline, Ca, Cl, Cu,

Fe, I, Mg, Mn, P, Zn. Pouch 1 L. *otc.*
Use: Nutritional supplement.

Entrobag Set. (Lafayette) Enteroclysis set. Case 6 sets.
Use: Enteroclysis of the small intestine.

Entrobar. (Lafayette) Barium sulfate 50% w/v susp. Bot. 500 ml, case 12 bot.
Use: Radiopaque agent.

Entrokit. (Lafayette) Barium sulfate susp. (Entrobar), methylcellulose (Entrolcel). Case 4 kits.
Use: Radiopaque agent.

Entrolcel. (Lafayette) Methylcellulose 1.8% w/w concentrate for dilution at time of use. Bot. 500 ml, case 24 Bot.
Use: Diagnostic aid.

•**entsufon sodium.** (ENT-sue-fahn) USAN.
Use: Detergent.

E.N.T. Syrup. (Springbok) Brompheniramine maleate 4 mg, phenylephrine HCl 5 mg, phenylpropanolamine HCl 5 mg/5 ml. Bot. 16 oz. *Rx.*
Use: Antihistamine, decongestant.

Entuss. (Roberts/Hauck) **Tab.:** Hydrocodone bitartrate 5 mg, guaifenesin 300 mg/Tab. Bot. 100s. **Syr.:** 5 mg hydrocodone bitartate, 300 mg potassium guaiacolsulfonate/5 ml. Alcohol free. Bot. 120 ml, 480 ml. *c-III.*
Use: Antitussive, expectorant.

Entuss-D Junior. (Roberts/Hauck) Pseudoepherine HCl 30 mg, hydrocodone bitartrate 2.5 mg, guaifenesin 100 mg w/ alcohol 5%, saccharin, sorbitol, sucrose. Liq. Bot.120 ml, pt. *c-III.*
Use: Antitussive, expectorant combination.

Entuss-D Liquid. (Roberts/Hauck) Hydrocodone bitartrate 5 mg, pseudoephedrine 30 mg/5 ml. 473 ml. *c-III.*
Use: Antitussive, decongestant.

Entuss-D Tablets. (Roberts/Hauck) Pseudoephedrine 30 mg, hydrocodone bitartrate 5 mg, guaifenesin 300 mg/Tab. Bot. 100s. *c-III.*
Use: Decongestant, antitussive, expectorant.

Enuclene. (Alcon) Tyloxapol 0.25%. Soln. Drop-tainer 15 ml. *otc.*
Use: Artificial eye care.

Enulose. (Barre-National) Lactulose 10 g, galactose 2.2 g, lactose 1.2 g, other sugars ≤ 1.2 g. Syr. pt, 2 qt. *Rx.*
Use: Laxative.

•**enviradene.** (en-VIE-rah-DEEN) USAN.
Use: Antiviral.

Enviro-Stress. (Vitaline) Vitamins B_1 50 mg, B_2 50 mg, B_3 100 mg, B_5 50 mg,

B_6 50 mg, B_{12} 25 mcg, C 600 mg, E 30 IU, folic acid 0.4 mg, zinc 30 mg, Mg, Se, PABA. SR Tab. Bot. 90s, 1000s. *otc.*
Use: Vitamin/mineral supplement.

•**enviroxime.** (en-VIE-rox-eem) USAN.
Use: Antiviral.

Envisan Treatment Multipack. (Hoechst Marion Roussel) Dextranomer with PEG 3000 and PEG 600. Paste 10 g packets with nylon net and semi-occlusive film. *otc.*
Use: Wound debridement.

Enzest. (Barth's) Seven natural enzymes, calcium carbonate 250 mg/Tab. Bot. 100s, 250s, 500s. *otc.*
Use: Digestive enzymes, antacid.

Enzobile Improved. (Roberts) Pancreatic enzyme concentrate 100 mg, ox bile extract 100 mg, cellulase 10 mg in inner core and pepsin 150 mg in outer layer. EC tab. Bot. 100s. *otc, Rx.*
Use: Digestive enzymes.

Enzone. (UAD) Hydrocortisone acetate 1%, pramoxine HCl 1% in hydrophilic base w/stearic acid, aquaphor, isopropyl palmitate, polyoxyl-40, stearate, triethanolamine lauryl sulfate. Cream. Tube 30 g w/rectal applicator. *Rx.*
Use: Corticosteroid combination.

Enzymatic Cleaner for Extended Wear. (Alcon) Highly purified pork pancreatin to dilute in saline solution. Tab. Pkg. 12s. *otc.*
Use: Soft contact lens care.

Enzyme Formula #E-2. (Barth's) Amylase 30 mg, lipase 25 mg, bile salts 1 gr, wilzyme 10 mg, pepsin 2 gr, pancreatin 0.5 gr, calcium carbonate 4 gr/Tab. Bot. 100s, 250s. *otc, Rx.*
Use: Digestive aid.

enzymes.
See: Alpha Chymar, Vial (Centeon).
Ananase, Tab. (Rhone-Poulenc Rorer).
Cholinesterase (Various Mfr.).
Chymotrypsin.
Cotazym, Cap. (Organon).
Creon (Solvay).
Diastase (Various Mfr.).
Dornavac, Vial (Merck).
Fibrinolysin. Hyaluronidase (Various Mfr.).
Neutrapen, Vial (3M).
Pancreatin (Various Mfr.).
Papain (Various Mfr.).
Papase, Tab. (Warner-Chilcott).
Penicillinase (Various Mfr.).
Pepsin (Various Mfr.).
Plasmin. Rennin (Various Mfr.).

Taka-Diastase, Prep. (Parke-Davis).
Travase, Oint. (Knoll Pharm.).
Thrombolysin, I.V. Inj. (Merck).
Varidase, Prep. (Lederle).

EPA Capsules. (NTBY) N-3 fat content (mg) EPA 180 mg, DHA 120 mg, vitamin E 1 IU. Bot. 50s, 100s. *otc.*
Use: Nutritional supplement.

•**ephedrine,** (eh-FED-rin) U.S.P. 23. *otc.*
Use: Adrenergic (bronchodilator) Bronchodilator.
See: Bofedrol Inhalant (Jones Medical).
Racephedrine HCl (Various Mfr.).
W/Procaine.
See: Ephedrine and Procaine, Rx "A", Amp. (Lilly).
W/Pyrilamine maleate, guaifenesin, theophylline.
W/Theophylline, guaifenesin, phenobarbital.
See: Duovent, Tab. (3M).

•**ephedrine hydrochloride,** U.S.P. 23.
Use: Bronchodilator

ephedrine hydrochloride. (Various Mfr.) Cryst. Box 0.25 oz, 4 oz.
Use: Bronchodilator.

ephedrine hydrochloride w/combinations.
See: Asma-lief, Tab., Susp. (Quality Generics).
Ceepa, Tab. (Geneva Pharm.).
Co-Xan, Elix. (Schwarz Pharma).
Derma Medicone (Medicone).
Derma Medicone HC, Oint. (Medicone).
Ectasule, Ectasule Minus, Cap. (Fleming).
Golacal, Syr. (Arcum).
Kie, Tab., Syr. (Laser).
Lardet Expectorant, Tab. (Standex).
Lardet, Tab. (Standex).
Mudrane GG, Tab. (ECR Pharm.).
Mudrane, Tab. (ECR Pharm.).
Quadrinal, Tab., Susp. (Knoll).
Quelidrine, Syr. (Abbott).
Quibron Plus (Bristol).
Tedral-25, Tab. (Parke-Davis).
T-E-P Compound, Tab. (Stanlabs).
Theofedral, Tab. (Redford).
Theofenal, Susp., Tab. (Rugby).

ephedrine hydrochloride nasal jelly.
See: Efedron Nasal (Hyrex).

•**ephedrine sulfate,** U.S.P. 23.
Use: Adrenergic (bronchodilator, nasal decongestant).
See: Ectasule Minus Jr. and Sr., Cap. (Fleming).
Slo-Fedrin, Cap. (Dooner).

ephedrine sulfate. (Various Mfr.) Inj. 50 mg/1mL Amp.
Use: Adrenergic (bronchodilator, nasal decongestant).

ephedrine sulfate w/combinations.
See: B.M.E., Elix. (Brothers).
Bronkaid, Tab. (Sanofi Winthrop Products).
Bronkolixir, Elix. (Sanofi Winthrop).
Bronkotabs (Sanofi Winthrop).
Ectasule, Cap. (Fleming).
Ectasule Minus, Cap. (Fleming).
Eponal, Prep. (Cenci).
Marax DF, Syr. (Roerig).
Marax, Tab., Syr. (Roerig).
Neogen, Supp. (Premo).
Pazo, Oint., Supp. (Bristol-Myers).
Rectacort, Supp. (Century).
Va-Tro-Nol, Nose Drops (Richardson-Vicks).
Wyanoids, Preps. (Wyeth-Ayerst).

ephedrine sulfate and phenobarbital capsules.
Use: Bronchodilator, sedative, hypnotic.

1-ephenamine penicillin g. Compenamine.

Ephenyllin. (CMC) Theophylline 130 mg, ephedrine HCl 24 mg, phenobarbital 8 mg/Tab. Bot. 100s, 500s, 1000s. *Rx.*
Use: Bronchodilator, decongestant, sedative, hypnotic.

Ephrine Nasal Spray. (Walgreen) Phenylephrine HCl 0.5%. Bot. 20 ml. *otc.*
Use: Decongestant.

Epi-C. (Lafayette Pharm.) Barium sulfate 150%. Susp. Bot. 450 ml.
Use: Diagnostic aid.

•**epicillin.** (EH-pih-SILL-in) USAN.
Use: Antibacterial.
See: Dexacillin.

epidermal growth factor (human). (Chiron)
Use: Accelerate corneal healing. [Orphan drug]

Epi-Derm Balm. (Pedinol) Methyl salicylate, menthol, propylene glycol, alcohol. Bot. gal. *otc.*
Use: Analgesic, topical.

EpiEZPen Autoinjector. (Center Laboratories) Epinephrine injection 1:2000. Delivers single dose of 0.3 mg. *Rx.*
Use: Emergency kit, anaphylaxis.

EpiEZPen Jr. Autoinjector. (Center Laboratories) Epinephrine injection 1:2000. Delivers single dose of 0.15 mg. *Rx.*
Use: Emergency kit, anaphylaxis.

Epifoam. (Schwarz Pharm) Hydrocortisone acetate 1%, pramoxine HCl 1% in base of propylene glycol, cetyl alcohol, PEG-100 stearate, glyceryl stearate, laureth-23, polyoxyl-40 stearate, methylparaben, propylparaben, trolamine, or hydrochloric acid to adjust pH, purified water, butane, propane inert propellant. Aerosol container 10 g. *Rx.*
Use: Corticosteroid, topical.

Epiform-HC. (Delta) Hydrocortisone 1%, iodohydroxyquin 3% in cream base. Tube 20 g. *Rx.*
Use: Corticosteroid, antifungal, topical.

Epifrin Sterile Ophthalmic Solution. (Allergan) Epinephrine HCl 0.5%, 1% or 2%. Bot. w/dropper 15 ml. *Rx.*
Use: Agent for glaucoma.

E-Pilo. (Ciba Vision) Pilocarpine HCl 1%, 2%, 3%, 4% or 6%, epinephrine bitartrate 1%. Soln. Bot. 10 ml w/dropper-tip plastic vial. *Rx.*
Use: Agent for glaucoma.

Epilyt. (Stiefel) Propylene glycol, glycerin, oleic acid, quaternium-26, lactic acid, BHT. Lotion. Bot. 118 ml. *otc.*
Use: Emollient.

•**epimestrol.** (EH-pih-MESS-trole) USAN.
Use: Anterior pituitary activator.

Epinal. (Alcon) Epinephrine borate 0.5%, 1%. Dropper Bot. 7.5 ml *Rx.*
Use: Agent for glaucoma.

epinephran.
See: Epinephrine, Preps. (Various Mfr.).

•**epinephrine,** (epp-ih-NEFF-rin) U.S.P. 23.
Use: Asthma, hayfever, acute allergic states, cardiac arrest, acute hypersensitivity reactions, adrenesgic (vasoconstrictor).
See: Asthma Meter, Aerosol (Rexall).
Asmolin, Vial (Lincoln).
Emergency Ana-Kit (Bayer).
W/Chlorobutanol, sodium bisulfite.
W/Lidocaine HCl.
See: Ardecaine 1%, 2%, Inj. (Burgin-Arden).

epinephrine. (Abbott) Epinephrine 0.01 mg/ml/Soln (Pediatric Inj). Box. 5 ml single-dose Abboject Syringe. *otc, Rx.*
Use: Asthma, hayfever, acute allergic states, cardiac arrest, acute hypersensitivity reactions, adrenergic (vasoconstrictor).

•**epinephrine bitartrate.** , U.S.P. 23.
Use: Adrenergic, ophthalmic.

epinephrine borate.
Use: Adrenergic, ophthalmic.
See: Epinal Ophth. Soln. (Alcon).

epinephrine hydrochloride. (Ciba Vi-

sion) 0.1%. Soln. 1 ml Dropperettes (12s). *Rx.*
Use: Adrenergic, ophthalmic. Emergency kit, anaphylaxis.
See: Adrenalin Cl, Soln. (Parke-Davis).
Ana-Guard Epinephrine, Inj. (Burgin-Arden).
EpiEZPen (Center Labs).
EpiEZPen Jr. (Center Labs).
EpiPen (Center Labs).
EpiPen Jr. (Center Labs).
Epifrin, Ophth. Soln. (Allergan).
Epinal, Ophth. Soln. (Alcon).
Sus-Phrine, Amp., Vial (Berlex).
Vaponefrin Solution & Nebulizer, Vial (Medeva).
W/Benzalkonium Cl, sodium Cl, sodium metabisulfite.
See: Glaucon, Soln. (Alcon).
W/Pilocarpine HCl.
See: Epicar, Soln. (Pilkington Barnes Hind).

epinephrine, racemic.
See: Asthmanefrin Solution (SK-Beecham).

epinephrine-related compounds.
See: Sympathomimetic Agents.

•**epinephryl borate,** (EPP-ih-NEFF-rill) U.S.P. 23.
Use: Adrenergic.

epinephryl borate ophthalmic solution.
Use: Adrenergic (ophthalmic).
See: Epinal (Alcon).
Eppy (Pilkington Barnes Hind).

Epipen Auto-Injector. (Center) Epinephrine injection 1:1000. Delivers dose of 0.3 mg. Pkg. 1s, 2s, 2 ml injectors. *Rx.*
Use: Emergency kit.

Epipen Jr. Auto-Injector. (Center) Epinephrine injection 1:2000. Delivers dose of 0.15 mg. Pkg. 1s, 2s, 2 ml injectors. *Rx.*
Use: Emergency kit.

epiphenethicillin.

•**epipropidine.** (EPP-ih-PRO-pih-deen) USAN.
Use: Antineoplastic.

epirenan.
See: Epinephrine (Various Mfr.).

•**epirizole.** (eh-PEER-IH-zole) USAN.
Use: Analgesic, anti-inflammatory.

•**epirubicin hydrochloride.** (EH-pih-ROO-bih-sin) USAN.
Use: Antineoplastic.
See: Pharmorubicin (Pharmacia & Upjohn).

•**epitetracycline hydrochloride,** U.S.P. 23.

Use: Antibiotic, antibacterial.

•**epithiazide.** (EH-pih-THIGH-azz-ide) USAN.
Use: Antihypertensive, diuretic.

Epitol. (Lemmon) Carbamazepine 200 mg/Tab. Bot. 500s, 1000s, UD 100s. *Rx.*
Use: Anticonvulsant.

Epivir. (Glaxo Wellcome) Lamivudine 150 mg/Tab. Bot. 60s. Lamivudine 10 mg/ml/Oral soln. Bot. 240 ml. *Rx.*
Use: Treatment of HIV infection.

EPO.
See: Epogen (Amgen).
Procrit (Ortho Biotech).

•**epoetin alfa.** (eh-POE-eh-tin) USAN.
Use: Recombinant human erythropoietin. [Orphan drug]
See: Epogen (Amgen).
Procrit (Ortho Biotech).

•**epoetin beta.** (eh-POE-eh-tin) USAN.
Use: Recombinant human erythropoietin, hematinic antianemic. [Orphan drug]

Epogen. (Amgen) Epoetin Alfa (Erythropoietin; EPO) 2,000 units, 3,000 units, 4,000 units, 10,000 units. Preservative free w/ 2.5 mg albumin (human) per ml. Vial 1 ml and 10,000 units in 2 ml multidose vials (1% benzyl alcohol). *Rx.*
Use: Recombinant human erythropoietin.

•**epoprostenol.** (EH-poe-PROSTE-eh-nole) USAN. Formerly Prostacyclin, PGI_2, Prostagland in I_2, Prostaglandin X, PGX.
Use: Inhibitor (platelet). [Orphan drug]

•**epoprostenol sodium.** (EH-poe-PROSTE-eh-nole) USAN.
Use: Inhibitor (platelet).
See: Flolan (Glaxo Wellcome).

•**epostane.** (EH-poe-stain) USAN.
Use: Interceptive.

epoxytropine tropate methylbromide.
See: Methscopolamine Bromide (Various Mfr.).

Eppy/N. (Pilkington Barnes Hind) Epinephryl borate ophthalmic soln. 0.5%, 1% or 2%. Bot. 7.5 ml. *Rx.*
Use: Agent for glaucoma.

•**epristeride.** USAN.
Use: Inhibitor (alpha reductase).

Epromate. (Major) Aspirin 325 mg, meprobamate 200 mg Tab. Bot. 100s, 500s. *c-iv.*
Use: Salicylate analgesic, antianxiety agent.

•**eprosartan.** USAN.
Use: Antihypertensive.

- **eprosartan mesylate.** (eh-pro-SAHR-tan) USAN.
  Use: Antihypertensive.
Epsal. (Press) Saturated soln. of epsom salts 80% in ointment form. Jar 0.5 oz, 2 oz. *otc.*
  Use: Drawing ointment.
Epsivite 100. (Standex) Vitamin E 100 IU/Cap. Bot. 100s. *otc.*
  Use: Vitamin E supplement.
Epsivite 200. (Standex) Vitamin E 200 IU/Cap. Bot. 100s. *otc.*
  Use: Vitamin E supplement.
Epsivite 400. (Standex) Vitamin E 400 IU/Cap. Bot. 100s. *otc.*
  Use: Vitamin E supplement.
Epsivite Forte. (Standex) Vitamin E 1000 IU/Cap. Bot. 100s. *otc.*
  Use: Vitamin E supplement.
epsom salt.
  See: Magnesium Sulfate.
E.p.t. Stick Test. (Parke-Davis) Reagent in-home kit for urine testing. Pregnancy test. Kit 1s. *otc.*
  Use: Diagnostic aid.
eptoin.
  See: Phenytoin Sodium (Various Mfr.).
Equagesic. (Wyeth-Ayerst) Meprobamate 200 mg, aspirin 325 mg/Tab. Bot. 100s, UD 100s. *c-iv.*
  Use: Antianxiety agent, salicylate analgesic.
Equal. (Nutrasweet) Aspartame. **Packet:** 0.035 oz. (1 g). Box 50s, 100s, 200s. **Tab.:** Bot. 100s. *otc.*
  Use: Artificial sweetener.
Equalactin. (Numark) Polycarbophil 500 mg (as calcium polycarbophil)/ Chew. tab. *otc.*
  Use: Antidiarrheal or laxative.
Equanil. (Wyeth-Ayerst) Meprobamate 200 mg or 400 mg/Tab. **200 mg:** Bot. 100s. **400 mg:** Bot. 100s, 500s, Redipak 25s. *c-iv.*
  Use: Antianxiety agent.
Equazine M. (Rugby) Aspirin 325 mg, meprobamate 200 mg, tartrazine tab. Bot. 100s, 500s. *c-iv.*
  Use: Salicylate analgesic, antianxiety agent.
Equilet. (Mission) Calcium carbonate 500 mg/Chew. tab. Strip packed in 100s. *otc.*
  Use: Antacid.
- **equilin,** U.S.P. 23.
  Use: Estrogen.
Equipertine Capsules. (Sanofi Winthrop) Oxypertine. *Rx.*
  Use: Antianxiety agent, tranquilizer.

Eradacil Capsules. (Sanofi Winthrop) Rosoxacin.
  Use: Antigonococcal agent.
Eramycin. (Wesley) Erythromycin 250 mg (as stearate)/FC tab. Bot. 100s, 500s. *Rx.*
  Use: Anti-infective, erythromycin.
- **erbulozole.** (ehr-BYOO-low-zole) USAN.
  Use: Radiosensitizer; antineoplastic (adjunct).
Ercaf. (Geneva Pharm.) Ergotamine tartrate 1 mg, caffeine 100 mg/Tab. Bot. 100s, 1000s. *Rx.*
  Use: Agent for migraine.
Ergamisol. (Janssen) Levamisole (base) 50 mg/Tab. Blister pack 36s. *Rx.*
  Use: Antineoplastic agent.
Ergo Caff. (Rugby) Ergotamine tartrate 1 mg, caffeine 100 mg/Tab. Bot. 100s. *Rx.*
  Use: Agent for migraine.
- **ergocalciferol,** U.S.P. 23.
  Use: Treatment of refractory rickets; familial hypophosphatemia; hypoparathyroidism, vitamin (antirachitic).
  See: Calciferol.
    Drisdol, Liq., Cap. (Sanofi Winthrop).
    Geltabs, Cap. (Pharmacia & Upjohn).
ergocornine. (Various Mfr.) Ergot alkaloid. *Rx.*
  Use: Peripheral vascular disorders.
ergocristine. (Various Mfr.) Ergot alkaloid. *Rx.*
  Use: Vascular disorders.
ergocryptine. (Various Mfr.) Ergot alkaloid. *Rx.*
  Use: Peripheral vascular disorders.
- **ergoloid mesylates,** (err-GO-loyd) U.S.P. 23.
  Use: Psychotherapeutic, cognition adjuvant.
  See: Hydergine Prods. (Sandoz).
ergoloid mesylates.
  Use: Psychotherapeutic, cognition adjuvant.
Ergomar. (Medeva) Ergotamine tartrate 2 mg/Sublingual Tab. Pkg. 20s. *Rx.*
  Use: Agent for migraine.
ergometrine maleate.
  See: Ergonovine (Various Mfr.).
Ergonal. (Vita Elixir) Ergot powder 259.2 mg, aloin 8.1 mg, apiol fluid green 290 mg, oil pennyroyal 28 mg/Cap. Bot. 24s. *Rx.*
  Use: Oxytocic.
ergonovine. (Various Mfr.) Ergobasine, erolklinine, ergometrine, ergostetrine, ergotocine. *Rx.*
  Use: Oxytocic.

See: Ergonovine Maleate.

● **ergonovine maleate, U.S.P. 23.**
Use: Oxytocic.
See: Methergine, Ing., Tab. (Sandoz).

ergosterol, activated or irradiated.
See: Ergocalciferol, U.S.P. 23.

ergostetrine.
See: Ergonovine (Various Mfr.).

Ergot Alkalside Dihydrogenated.
See: ergoloid mesylates.

● **ergotamine tartrate, U.S.P. 23.**
Use: Analgesic (specific in migraine).
See: Ergomar, Tab. (Medeva).
Ergostat, Tab. (Parke-Davis).
Gynergen, Amp., Tab. (Sandoz).
Medihaler-Ergotamine, Vial (3M).
W/Belladonna alkaloids, acetophenetidin, caffeine.
See: Wigraine, Tab., Supp. (Organon).
W/Belladonna alkaloids, pentobarbital.
See: Cafergot P-B, Supp., Tab. (Sandoz).
W/Belladonna alkaloids, phenobarbital.
See: Bellergal, Tab. (Sandoz).
W/Caffeine.
See: Cafergot, Tab., Supp. (Sandoz).
W/Caffeine, homatropine methylbromide.
See: Ergotatropin, Tab. (Cole).
W/Cyclizine HCl, caffeine.
See: Migral Tab. (Glaxo Wellcome).
W/1-Hyoscyamine sulfate, phenobarbital.
See: Ergkatal, Tab. (Gilbert).

● **ergotamine tartrate and caffeine suppositories.**
Use: Vascular headache; analgesic specific in migraine.
See: Cafergot, Supp. (Sandoz).

ergotamine tartrate and caffeine tablets.
Use: Vascular headache; Analgesic specific in migraine.
See: Cafergot, Tab. (Sandoz).

ergot, fluid extract. (Various Mfr.) Ergot 1 g/ml Bot. 4 oz, pt.

ergotidine.
See: Histamine (Various Mfr.).

ergotocine.
See: Ergonovine (Various Mfr.).

Ergotrate Maleate. (Bedford Labs) Ergonovine maleate 0.2 mg/ml. Inj. Vial 1 ml. *Rx.*
Use: Oxytocic.

ergot-related products.
See: Cafergot, Supp., Tab. (Sandoz).
Cafergot P-B, Tab., Supp. (Sandoz).
DHE-45, Amp. (Sandoz).
Ergonovine (Various Mfr.).
Ergotamine (Various Mfr.).
Ergotrate (Various Mfr.).

Gynergen, Amp., Tab. (Sandoz).
Hydergine, Sub. Tab. (Sandoz).
Hydro-Ergot, Tab. (Interstate).
Methergine, Amp., Tab. (Sandoz).
Trigot, Sublingual Tab. (Squibb).
Wigraine, Supp., Tab. (Organon).

eriodictin.
See: Vitamin P & Rutin.

eriodictyon. Flext., Aromatic Syrup.
Use: Pharmaceutic aid (flavor).
See: Vitamin P & Rutin.

E-R-O. (Scherer) Propylene glycol, glycerol. Bot. w/dropper tip 15 ml. *otc.*
Use: Otic preparation.

● **ersofermin.** (EER-so-FEER-min) USAN.
Use: Wound healing agent.
See: Trofak (Synergen).

Ertine. (Approved) Hexachlorophene, benzocaine, cod liver oil, allantoin, boric acid, lanolin. Tube 1.5 oz. *Rx.*
Use: Burn and first aid remedy.

erwinia asparaginase. *Rx.*
Use: Antineoplastic. [Orphan drug]

erwina L-asparaginase.
Use: Acute lymphocytic leukemia.
See: Erwinase (Porton).

Eryc. (Parke-Davis) Erythromycin enteric coated 250 mg/Tab. Bot. 40s, 100s, 500s, UD 100s. *Rx.*
Use: Anti-infective, erythromycin.

Erycette. (Ortho) Erythromycin 2%. Pkg. 60 pledgets. *Rx.*
Use: Antiacne.

Eryderm 2%. (Abbott) Erythromycin topical soln. 2%. Bot. 60 ml. *Rx.*
Use: Antiacne.

Erygel. (Allergan-Herbert) Erythromycin 2%. Gel Tube 30 g, 60 g, *Erygel 6* in 5 g (6s). *Rx.*
Use: Anti-infective, external.

Erymax. (Allergan-Herbert) Erythromycin 2% Soln. 59 ml, 118 ml. *Rx.*
Use: Antiacne.

Erypar. (Parke-Davis) Erythromycin stearate 250 mg or 500 mg/Filmseal. **250 mg:** Bot. 100s, 500s. **500 mg:** Bot. 100s. *Rx.*
Use: Anti-infective, erythromycin.

Eryped. (Abbott) Erythromycin ethylsuccinate granules for oral susp. representing erythromycin activity of 400 mg/5 ml. Bot. 60 ml, 100 ml, 200 ml, UD 5 ml, 100s. *Rx.*
Use: Anti-infective, erythromycin.

Ery-Tab. (Abbott) Erythromycin enteric coated 250 mg, 333 mg or 500 mg/Tab. **250 mg:** Bot. 30s, 40s, 100s, 500s, UD 100s. **333 mg:** Bot. 100s, 500s, UD 100s. **500 mg:** Bot. 100s, UD 100s. *Rx.*

Use: Anti-infective, erythromycin.

Erythra-Derm. (Paddock) Erythromycin 2%, alcohol 66%. Soln. Bot. 60 ml. *Rx.*
Use: Antiacne.

•**erythrityl tetranitrate, diluted,** (eh-RITH-rih-till TEH-trah-NYE-trate) U.S.P. 23.
Use: Coronary vasodilator.
See: Cardilate (Glaxo Wellcome).

erythrityl tetranitrate tablets. (eh-RITH-rih-till TEH-trah-NYE-trate) (Various Mfr.) Erythritol, erythrol tetranitrate, nitroerythrite, tetranitrin, tetranitrol.
Use: Coronary vasodilator.
See: Anginar, Tab. (Pasadena Research Labs.). Cardilate, Tab. (Glaxo Wellcome).
W/Phenobarbital.
See: Cardilate-P, Tab. (Glaxo Wellcome).

Erythrocin Lactobionate, I.V. (Abbott Hospital Prods) Erythromycin lactobionate. Pow. 500 mg/vial w/benzyl alcohol 90 mg; 1 g/vial w/benzyl alcohol 180 mg. Pkg. Vial 5s. *Rx.*
Use: Anti-infective, erythromycin.

Erythrocin Lactobionate Piggyback. (Abbott Hospital Prods) Erythromycin lactobionate for injection, 500 mg/dispensing vial. 5 mg/ml of erythromycin after reconstitution w/90 mg benzyl alcohol. Pow. Pkg. 5100 ml dispensing vials. *Rx.*
Use: Anti-infective, erythromycin.

•**erythromycin,** (eh-RITH-row-MY-sin) U.S.P. 23.
Use: Antibiotic, antibacterial.
See: AK-Mycin, Oint. (Akorn).
A/T/S, Gel (Hoechst Marion Roussel).
Del-Mycin, Soln. (Del Ray).
Emgel, Gel (Glaxo).
E-Mycin, Tab. (Pharmacia & Upjohn).
Erymax, Soln. (Allergan Herbert).
EryDerm, Soln. (Abbott).
Ery-sol, Soln. (Dermol).
Erythrocin, Prep. (Abbott).
Erythromycin, Gel (Glades).
Erythromycin Base, Filmtab (Abbott).
Ilotycin, Prep. (Dista).
PCE, Tab. (Abbott).
Robimycin, Tab. (Robins).
Romycin, Topical Soln. (Roberts).
RP-Mycin, Tab. (Solvay).
T-Stat, Pads (Westwood-Squibb).
Theramycin Z, Soln. (Medicis).

erythromycin. (Pharmacia & Upjohn) Tab. 100 mg. Bot. 100s; 250 mg. Bot. 25s, 100s. (Various Mfr.) 5 mg/g Oint. Tube 3.5 g, 3.75 g, UD 1 g.

Use: Antibiotic, antibacterial.

erythromycin. (Glades) Erythromycin 2%, alcohol 95% / Gel. Tube 30 g, 60 g. *Rx.*
Use: Antiacne.

•**erythromycin acistrate.** (eh-RITH-row-MY-sin ass-IH-strate) USAN.
Use: Antibiotic, antibacterial.

erythromycin and benzoyl peroxide topical gel. (eh-RITH-row-MY-sin and BEN-zoyl per-OX-ide)
Use: Antibiotic, keratolytic.

erythromycin base filmtab. (Abbott) Erythromycin base 250 mg or 500 mg/ Tab. **250 mg:** Bot. 100s, 500s, UD 100s. **500 mg:** Bot 100s. *Rx.*
Use: Anti-infective, erythromycin.

•**erythromycin estolate,** (eh-RITh-row-MY-sin ESS-toe-late) U.S.P. 23. Erythromycin 2-propionate dodecyl sulfate. Lauryl sulfate salt of the propionic acid ester of erythromycin. *Formerly Erythromycin Propionate Lauryl Sulfate.*
Use: Antibiotic, erythromycin; antibacterial.
See: Ilosone, Preps. (Dista).

•**erythromycin ethylsuccinate,** (eh-RITH-row-MY-sin ETH-il-SUX-i-nate) U.S.P. 23.
Use: Antibiotic, erythromycin; antibacterial.
See: E.E.S. Prods. (Abbott).
E-mycin E, Liq. (Pharmacia & Upjohn).
Pediamycin Prods. (Ross).
Pediazole, Liq. (Ross).
Wyamycin-E, Liq. (Wyeth-Ayerst).

erythromycin ethylsuccinate and sulfisoxazole acetyl for oral suspension. (eh-RITH-row-MY-sin Eth-ill-SUCK-sih-nate and sull-fih-SOX-ah-zole ASS-eh-till)
Use: Anti-infective.
See: Pediazole, Susp. (Ross).

•**erythromycin gluceptate, sterile,** (eh-RITH-row-MY-sin glue-SEP-tate) U.S.P. 23.
Use: Anti-infective, erythromycin; antibacterial.
See: Ilotycin Gluceptate, Amp. (Dista).

erythromycin glucoheptonate.
See: Erythromycin Gluceptate, U.S.P. 23. Ilotycin Glucoheptonate, Amp. (Dista).

•**erythromycin lactobionate for injection,** (eh-RITH-row-MY-sin lack-toe-BYE-oh-nate) U.S.P. 23.
Use: Anti-infective, erythromycin; antibacterial.

See: Erythrocin Lactobionate, Vial (Abbott).

erythromycin 2-propionate dodecyl sulfate. Erythromycin Estolate, U.S.P. 23.
Use: Anti-infective, erythromycin.

erythromycin pledgets. (eh-RITH-row-MY-sin)
Use: Anti-infective, erythromycin.

erythromycin pledgets. (Glades) Erythromycin 2%, alcohol 68.5%/Pledgets. Bot. 60s. *Rx.*
Use: Anti-infective, erythromycin.

•**erythromycin propionate.** USAN.
Use: Antibacterial.

erythromycin propionate lauryl sulfate.
Use: Anti-infective, erythromycin.
See: Erythromycin Estolate. Ilosone, Preps. (Dista).

•**erythromycin salnacedin.** (eh-RITH-row-MY-sin sal-NAH-seh-din) USAN.
Use: Antiacne.

•**erythromycin stearate,** (eh-RITH-row-MY-sin STEE-ah-rate) U.S.P. 23.
Use: Anti-infective, erythromycin; antibacterial.
See: Erypar Filmseal, Tab. (Parke-Davis).
Wyamycin-S, Tab. (Wyeth-Ayerst).

erythromycin sulfate.
Use: Anti-infective, erythromycin.

erythromycin topical. (Various Mfr.) 2% Gel. Tube 30 g, 60 g. 2% Soln. Bot. 60 ml. *Rx.*
Use: Antiacne.
See: Benzamycin (Dermik).
Emgel (Glaxo).
Erygel (Allergan Herbert).

erythropoietin (recombinant human). *Rx.*
Use: Antianemic. [Orphan drug]

erythrosine sodium, U.S.P. XXII.
Use: Diagnostic aid (dental disclosing agent).

Eryzole. (Alra) Erythromycin ethylsuccinate 200 mg, acetyl sulfisoxazole 600 mg/5 ml when reconstituted. Gran for Susp. 100 ml, 150 ml, 200 ml. *Rx.*
Use: Anti-infective.

esclabron. Guaithylline.
Use: Antiasthmatic.

Eserdine Forte Tabs. (Major) Methyclothiazide, reserpine 0.5 mg/Tab. Bot. 100s. *Rx.*
Use: Diuretic, antihypertensive.

Eserdine Tabs. (Major) Methyclothiazide, reserpine 0.25 mg/Tab. Bot. 100s, 250s. *Rx.*

Use: Diuretic, antihypertensive.

Eserine. Physostigmine as alkaloid, salicylate or sulfate salt. *Rx.*
Use: Agent for glaucoma.

Eserine Salicylate. (Alcon) Physostigmine 0.5%. Soln. 2 ml. *Rx.*
Use: Agent for glaucoma.

Eserine Sulfate Sterile Ophthalmic Ointment. (Ciba Vision) Physostigmine sulfate 0.25%. Tube 3.5 g. *Rx.*
Use: Agent for glaucoma.

Eserine Sulfate. (Ciba Vision) Physostigmine sulfate 0.25%. Oint. Tube 3.5 g. *Rx.*
Use: Agent for glaucoma.

Esgic Capsules. (Forest) Butalbital 50 mg, caffeine 40 mg, acetaminophen 325 mg/Cap. Bot. 100s. *Rx.*
Use: Sedative, hypnotic, analgesic.

Esgic Tablets. (Forest) Butalbital 50 mg, caffeine 40 mg, acetaminophen 325 mg/Tab. Bot. 100s. *Rx.*
Use: Sedative/hypnotic, analgesic.

Esgic-Plus. (Forest) Acetaminophen 500 mg, butalbital 50 mg, caffeine 40 mg/Tab. Bot. 100s, 500s. *Rx.*
Use: Analgesic, sedative, hypnotic.

Esidrix. (Novartis) Hydrochlorothiazide 25 mg, 50 mg/Tab. **25 mg:** Bot. 100s, 1000s, UD 100s. **50 mg:** Bot. 100s, 360s, 720s, 1000s, UD 100s. *Rx.*
Use: Diuretic, antihypertensive. W/ Apresoline.
See: Apresoline-Esidrix, Tab. (Novartis).

Esimil. (Novartis) Hydrochlorothiazide 25 mg, guanethidine monosulfate 10 mg/Tab. Bot. 100s. *Rx.*
Use: Diuretic, antihypertensive.

Eskalith. (SK-Beecham) Lithium carbonate. **Cap.:** 300 mg. Bot. 100s, 500s; **Tab.:** 300 mg. Bot. 100s. *Rx.*
Use: Antipsychotic.

Eskalith CR. (SK-Beecham) Lithium carbonate 450 mg/CR tab. Bot. 100s. *Rx.*
Use: Antipsychotic.

•**esmolol hydrochloride.** (ESS-moe-lahl) USAN.
Use: Short-acting beta-adrenergic blocker.
See: Brevibloc, Inj. (DuPont Merck).

E-Solve. (Syosset) Alcohol 75%, propylene glycol, diethanolamide, polysorbate 80, talc, titanium dioxide, iron oxides, povidone, water soluble cellulose gum. Lot. Bot. 50 ml. *otc.*
Use: Lotion base.

•**esorubicin hydrochloride.** (ESS-oh-

ROO-bih-sin) USAN.
Use: Antineoplastic.

Esoterica Dry Skin Treatment Lotion.
(SK-Beecham) Bot. 13 fl oz. *otc.*
Use: Emollient.

Esoterica Facial. (SK-Beecham) Hydroquinone 2%, padimate O 3.3%, oxybenzone 2.5%, sodium bisulfites, parabens, EDTA. Cream, Tube 85 g. *otc.*
Use: Topical drug.

Esoterica Medicated Fade Cream, (SK-Beecham) Hydroquinone 2%, padimate O 3.3%, oxybenzone 2.5%. Cream. Jar 90 g. *otc.*
Use: Skin bleaching agent.

Esoterica Medicated Fade Cream, Facial. (SK-Beecham) Hydroquinone 2%, padimate O 3.3%, oxybenzone 2.5% in cream base. Jar 90 g, scented or unscented. *otc.*
Use: Skin bleaching agent.

Esoterica Medicated Fade Cream, Regular. (SK-Beecham) Hydroquinone 2%. Cream. Jar 90 g. *otc.*
Use: Skin bleaching agent.

Esoterica Sensitive Skin Formula. (SK-Beecham) Hydroquinone 1.5% with mineral oil, sodium bisulfite, parabens, EDTA. Cream. Jar 85 g. *otc.*
Use: Skin bleaching agent.

Espotabs. (Combe) Yellow phenolphthalein 97.2 mg/Tab. Bot. 12s, 30s, 60s. *otc.*
Use: Laxative.

•**esproquin hydrochloride.** (ESS-prokwin) USAN.
Use: Adrenergic.

Essential-8. Liquid amino acid protein supplement.
Use: Protein supplement.
See: Vivonex Diets, Liq. (Procter & Gamble).

Estar. (Westwood Squibb) Tar equivalent to 5% coal tar, U.S.P. in a hydro-alcoholic gel w/alcohol 13.8%. Tube 3 oz. *otc.*
Use: Antipsoriatic, antipruritic.

•**estazolam.** (ess-TAZZ-OH-lam) USAN.
Use: Sedative, hypnotic.
See: ProSom (Abbott).

Ester-C Plus. (Solgar) Vitamin C 500 mg, citrus bioflavonoid complex 25 mg, acerola 10 mg, rutin 5 mg, rose hips 10 mg, calcium 62 mg/Cap. Bot. 50s. *otc.*
Use: Vitamin/mineral supplement.

Ester-C Plus, Extra Potency. (Solgar) Vitamin C 1000 mg, citrus bioflavonoid complex 200 mg, acerola 25 mg, rutin 25 mg, rose hips 25 mg, calcium 125

mg/Tab. Bot. 30s. *otc.*
Use: Vitamin/mineral supplement.

esterified estrogens.
See: estrogens, esterified.

•**esterifilcon a.** (ess-TER-ih-FILL-kahn A) USAN.
Use: Contact lens material (hydrophilic).

Estilben.
See: Diethylstilbestrol Dipropionate (Various Mfr.).

Estinyl. (Schering-Plough) Ethinyl estradiol. **0.02 mg, 0.05 mg/Tab., coated:** Bot. 100s, 250s; **0.5 mg/Tab.:** Bot. 100s. *Rx.*
Use: Estrogen.

estopen.
See: Benzylpenicillin 2-diethylaminoethyl ester HI.

Estrace. (Bristol-Myers) Estradiol micronized 0.5 mg, 1 mg or 2 mg/Tab. Bot. 100s. *Rx.*
Use: Estrogen.

Estrace Vaginal Cream. (Bristol-Myers) 17β Estradiol 0.1 mg/gm. Tube 42.5 g. *Rx.*
Use: Estrogen.

Estracon. (Freeport) Conjugated estrogens 1.25 mg/Tab. Bot. 1000s. *Rx.*
Use: Estrogen.

Estraderm Transdermal. (Novartis) Estradiol. **0.05:** Each 10 × 10 cm. system contains 4 mg of estradiol for nominal delivery of 0.05 mg estradiol/day. Patient calendar packs of 8 and 24 systems. Ctn 6s. **0.1:** Each 20 × 20 cm. system contains 8 mg estradiol for nominal delivery of 0.1 mg estradiol/day. Patient calendar packs of 8 and 24 systems. Ctn. 6s. *Rx.*
Use: Estrogen.

•**estradiol,** (ESS-truh-DIE-ole) U.S.P. 23. The form now known to be physiologically active is the "beta" form rather than the "alpha" form.
Use: Estrogen.
See: Aquagen, Vial, Aq. (Remsen).
Estrace, Tab., Vaginal Creme (Bristol-Myers).
Estraderm, Transdermal (Novartis).
Estring, Vaginal ring (Pharmacia & Upjohn).
Femogen, Susp., Tab. (Fellows-Testagar).
Progynon, Pellets (Schering-Plough).
W/Estriol, estrone. Hormonin No. 1 and 2, Tab. (Schwarz Pharma).
W/Estrone, estriol.
See: Sanestro, Tab. (Sandia).
W/Estrone, potassium estrone sulfate.
See: Tri-Estrin, Inj. (Keene).

W/Progesterone, testosterone, procaine HCl, procaine base.
See: Horm-Triad, Vial (Bell).
W/Testerone.
W/Testosterone and chlorobutanol in cottonseed oil.
See: Depo-Testadiol, Vial (Pharmacia & Upjohn).
Transdermal.
Estraderm, Patch (Novartis).
Climara, Patch (Berlex).
Vivelle, Patch (Novartis).
estradiol cyclopentylpropionate, Estradiol 17-beta(3-cyclopentyl)propionate.
Estradiol Cypionate, U.S.P. 23. W/ Testosterone cypionate.
See: Depo-Testadiol, Vial (Pharmacia & Upjohn).
•**estradiol cypionate,** (ESS-trah-DIE-ole SIP-ee-oh-nate) U.S.P. 23.
Use: Estrogen.
See: Estradiol cyclopentylpropionate.
Depo-Estradiol Cypionate, Inj. (Pharmacia & Upjohn).
Depogen, Inj. (Hyrex).
D-Est, Inj. (Burgin-Arden).
Estro-Cyp, Vial (Keene).
Estroject-L.A., Vial (Mayrand).
Hormogen Depot, Inj. (Roberts).
Span-F, Inj. (Scrip).
W/Testosterone cypionate.
See: D-Diol, Inj. (Burgin-Arden).
Dep-Tesestro, Inj. (Zeneca).
Duo-Cyp, Vial (Keene).
Duracrine, Inj. (Ascher).
Menoject, L.A., Vial (Mayrand).
T.E. Ionate P.A., Inj. (Solvay).
W/Testosterone cypionate, chlorobutanol.
See: Depo-Testadiol (Pharmacia & Upjohn).
Span F.M., Inj. (Scrip).
T.E. Ionate P.A., Inj. (Solvay).
estradiol cypionate. (Forest) Estradiol cypionate 5 mg/ml/Inj. Vial. 10 ml. *Rx.*
Use: Estrogen.
estradiol dipropionate.
Use: Estrogen.
•**estradiol enanthate.** (ESS-trah-DIE-ole eh-NAN-thate) USAN.
Use: Estrogen.
estradiol, ethinyl.
See: Ethinyl Estradiol.
estradiol monobenzonate.
See: Estradiol Benzoate.
estradiol phosphate.
See: Estradurin, Secule (Wyeth-Ayerst).
•**estradiol undecylate.** (ESS-trah-DIE-ole UHN-DEH-sill-ate) USAN. Estradiol 17-undecanoate.
Use: Estrogen.

See: Delestrec.
estradiol vaginal cream. (ESS-trah-DIE-ole)
Use: Estrogen.
•**estradiol valerate,** (ESS-trah-DIE-ole VAL-eh-rate) U.S.P. 23.
Use: Estrogen.
See: Ardefem 10, 20, Inj. (Burgin-Arden).
Deladiol, Inj. (Steris).
Delestrogen, Vial (Bristol-Myers).
Depogen, Inj. (Sig).
Dioval, Preps. (Keene).
Duragen, Inj. (Roberts Hauck).
Duratrad, Inj. (Ascher).
Estate, Inj. (Savage).
Estra-L, Inj. (Taylor Pharmaceuticals).
Gynogen L.A., Inj. (Forest).
Span-Est, Inj. (Scrip).
Valergen, Inj. (Hyrex).
W/Benzyl alcohol.
See: Estate, Vial (Savage).
Reposo E-40, Vial (Paddock).
W/Hydroxyprogesterone caproate.
See: Hy-Gestradol, Inj. (Taylor Pharmaceuticals).
Hylutin-Est, Inj. (Hyrex).
W/Testosterone cypionate.
See: Depo-Testadiol, Inj. (Pharmacia & Upjohn).
W/Testosterone enanthate.
See: Ardiol 90/4, 180/8, Inj. (Burgin-Arden).
Deladumone, Vial (Squibb Mark).
Delatestadiol, Vial (Dunhall).
Duoval-P.A., I.M. (Solvay).
Estra-Testrin, Inj. (Taylor Pharmaceuticals).
Span-Est-Test 4, Inj. (Scrip).
Teev, Inj. (Keene).
Tesogen L.A., Inj. (Sig).
Valertest, Inj. (Hyrex).
W/Testosterone enanthate, benzyl alcohol, sesame oil.
See: Repose-TE (Paddock).
estradiol valerate. (Various Mfr.) Inj. 10 mg/mL. 20 mg/mL. Vial 10 mL. 40 mg/mL. Vial 10 mL.
Use: Estrogen.
Estra-L. (Taylor Pharmaceuticals) Estradiol valerate in castor oil. **20 mg/ml:** Vial 10 ml. **40 mg/ml:** Vial 10 ml. *Rx.*
Use: Estrogen.
Estralutin.
See: Relutin (Solvay).
•**estramustine.** (ESS-truh-muss-TEEN) USAN.
Use: Antineoplastic.
•**estramustine phosphate sodium.** (Ess-truh-muss-TEEN) USAN.

Use: Antineoplastic.
See: Emcyt, Cap. (Pharmacia & Upjohn).

Estratab. (Solvay) **Tab.**: Esterified estrogens, principally sodium estrone sulfate 0.3 mg, 0.625 mg, 1.25 mg or 2.5 mg/Tab. Bot. 100s, 1000s. *Rx.*
Use: Estrogen.

Estratest. (Solvay) Esterified estrogens 1.25 mg, methyltestosterone 2.5 mg/Tab. Bot. 100s, 1000s. *Rx.*
Use: Estrogen, androgen combination.

Estratest H.S. (Solvay) Esterified estrogens 0.625 mg, methyltestosterone 1.25 mg/Tab. Bot. 100s. *Rx.*
Use: Estrogen, androgen combination.

•**estrazinol hydrobromide.** (ESS-trazz-ih-nahl) USAN.
Use: Estrogen.

estrin.
See: Estrone.

Estrinex. (Pharmacia & Upjohn)
See: Toremifene.

Estring. (Pharmacia & Upjohn). Estradiol 2 mg/Vaginal ring. Single packs. *Rx.*
Use: Treatment of postmenopausal atrophy of the vagina or lower urinary tract.

•**estriol,** U.S.P. 23.
Use: Estrogen.

Estrobene DP.
See: Diethylstilbestrol Dipropionate (Various Mfr.).

Estro-Cyp. (Keene) Estradiol cypionate 5 mg/ml in oil. Inj. Vial 10 ml. *Rx.*
Use: Estrogen.

Estrofem. (Taylor Pharmaceuticals) Estradiol cypionate 5 mg/ml in oil. Inj. Vial 10 ml.
Use: Estrogen.

•**estrofurate.** (ESS-troe-FYOOR-ate) USAN.
Use: Estrogen.

estrogen-androgen therapy.
See: Androgen-Estrogen Therapy.

estrogenic substances, conjugated. (Water-soluble) A mixture containing the sodium salts of the sulfate esters of the estrogenic substances, principally estrone and equilin that are of the type excreted by pregnant mares. *Rx.*
Cream.
See: Premarin Vaginal Cream (Wyeth-Ayerst).
Intravenous.
See: Estroject, Vial (Mayrand).
Premarin (Wyeth-Ayerst).
Tab.

See: Aquagen, Inj. (Remsen).
Ces (Zeneca).
Estroquin, Tab. (Sheryl).
Estrosan, Tab. (Recsei).
Evestrone, Tab. (Delta).
Genisis, Tab. (Organon).
Menotabs, Tab. (Fleming).
Orapin (Standex).
Prelestrin, Tab. (Taylor Pharmaceuticals).
Premarin, Tab. (Wyeth-Ayerst).
Tag-39 H, Tab. (Solvay).
W/Ethinyl estradiol.
See: Demulen, Tab. (Searle).
W/Meprobamate.
See: Milprem, Tab. (Wallace).
PMB 200, Tab. (Wyeth-Ayerst).
PMB 400, Tab. (Wyeth-Ayerst).
W/Methyltestosterone.
See: Estratest, Tab. (Solvay).
Estratest H.S., Tab (Solvay).
Premarin with Methyltestosterone, Tab. (Wyeth-Ayerst).

estrogenic substances in aqueous suspension. (Wyeth-Ayerst) Sterile estrone suspension 2 mg/ml. Vial 10 ml. *Rx.*
Use: Estrogen.

estrogenic substance aqueous. (Various) Estrogenic substance or estrogens (mainly estrone) 2 mg/ml/Inj. Vial 10 or 30 ml. *Rx.*
Use: Estrogen.

estrogenic substances mixed. May be a crystalline or an amorphous mixture of the naturally occurring estrogens obtained from the urine of pregnant mares.
Aqueous Susp.
See: Gravigen Inj. (Bluco).
Cap.
See: Urestrin, Cap. (Pharmacia & Upjohn).
W/Androgen therapy, vitamins, iron, d-desoxyephedrine HCl.
See: Mediatric, Preps. (Wyeth-Ayerst).
W/Methyltestosterone.
See: Premarin w/methyltestosterone, Tab. (Wyeth-Ayerst).
W/Testosterone.
See: Andrestraq, Vial (Schwarz Pharma).

•**estrogens, conjugated,** (ESS-truh-janz KAHN-juh-gay-tuhd) U.S.P. 23.
Use: Estrogen.
See: Conest, Tab. (Century).
Congens, Tab. (Blaine).
Estrocon, Tab. (Savage).
Ganeake, Tab. (Geneva Pharm.).
Menotab, Tab. (Fleming).

PMB, Tab. (Wyeth-Ayerst).
Premarin, Tab., I.V. (Wyeth-Ayerst).
Premarin Vaginal Cream (Wyeth-Ayerst).
Premarin with Methyltestosterone, Tab. (Wyeth-Ayerst).
Sodestrin and Sodestrin-H, Tab. (Solvay).
Tag-39, Tab. (Solvay).
Zeste, Tab. (Ascher).

estrogens equine.
See: Estrogen. PMB, Tab. (Wyeth-Ayerst).
Premarin, Tab., I.V. (Wyeth-Ayerst).
Premarin Vaginal Cream (Wyeth-Ayerst).
Premarin with Methyltestosterone, Tab. (Wyeth-Ayerst).

•**estrogens, esterified,** U.S.P. 23.
Use: Estrogen.
See: Amnestrogen, Tab. (Squibb).
Estratab (Solvay).
Evex, Tab. (Syntex).
Menest, Tab. (SK-Beecham).
Ms-Med, Tab. (Dunhall).

estrogens, esterified & androgens.
Use: Estrogen & androgen supplementation.
See: Estratest.

estrogens, natural.
Use: Estrogen.
See: Depogen, Vial (Hyrex).
Estradiol, Preps. (Various Mfr.).
Estrone, Preps. (Various Mfr.).
Estrogenic Substance (Various Mfr.).
PMB, Tab. (Wyeth-Ayerst).
Premarin, Tab., I.V. (Wyeth-Ayerst).
Premarin Vaginal Cream (Wyeth-Ayerst).
Premarin with Methyltestosterone, Tab. (Wyeth-Ayerst).

estrogens, synthetic.
See: Dienestrol, Preps. (Various Mfr.).
Diethylstilbestrol, Preps. (Various Mfr.).
Hexestrol, Preps. (Various Mfr.).
Meprane, Tab. (Reed & Carnrick).
TACE, Cap. (Hoechst Marion Roussel).
Vallestril, Tab. (Searle).

Estrogestin A. (Harvey) Estrogenic substance 1 mg, progesterone 10 mg/ml in peanut oil. Vial 10 ml. *Rx.*
Use: Estrogen, progestin combination.

Estrogestin C. (Harvey) Estrogenic substance 1 mg, progesterone 12.5 mg/ml in peanut oil. Vial 10 ml. *Rx.*
Use: Estrogen, progestin combination.

•**estrone,** U.S.P. 23. Femidyn, follicular hormone, folliculin, follicunodis, cris-

tallovar, glandubolin, hiestrone, ketohydroxy-estratriene, ketohydroxyestrin.
1 mg equals 10,000 IU.
Use: Estrogen.
See: Aquest, Inj. (Dunhall).
Bestrone Suspension, Inj. (Bluco).
Estrogenic Substances in Aqueous Susp. (Wyeth-Ayerst).
Estrone aqueous, Inj. (Various).
Estrone 5, Inj. (Keene).
Kestrone 5, Inj. (Hyrex).
Foygen, Vial (Foy).
Menagen, Cap. (Parke-Davis).
Menformon (A), Vial (Organon).
Par-Supp, Vag. Supp. (Parmed).
Propagon-S, Inj. (Spanner).
Theelin, Vial, Aqueous and Oil (Parke-Davis).
W/Hydrocortisone acetate.
See: Estro-V HC, Supp. (PolyMedica).
W/Estradiol, potassium estrone sulfate.
Tri-Orapin (Standex).
W/Estradiol, vitamin B_{12}.
See: Ovulin, Inj. (Sig).
W/Estriol, estradiol. Hormonin, Tab. (Schwarz Pharma).
W/Estrogens.
See: Estrogenic Mixtures, Preps. (Various Mfr.).
Estrogenic Substances, Preps. (Various Mfr.).
W/Lactose.
See: Estrovag, Supp. (Fellows-Testagar).
W/Potassium estrone sulfate.
See: Mer-Estrone, Inj. (Keene).
Sodestrin, Inj. (Solvay).
Spanestrin-P, Vial (Savage).
W/Progesterone.
See: Duovin-S, Inj. (Spanner).
W/Testosterone.
See: Andesterone, Vial (Lincoln).
Anestro, Inj. (Roberts).
Di-Hormone, Susp. (Paddock).
Di-Met Susp. (Organon).
Diorapin (Standex).
Dl-Steroid, Vial (Kremers-Urban).
Estratest, Tab. (Solvay).
W/Testosterone, progesterone.
See: Tripole-F, Inj. (Spanner).
W/Testosterone, sodium carboxymethylcellulose, sodium Cl.
See: Tostestro, Inj. (Jones Medical).
W/Testosterone, vitamins.
See: Android-G, Vial (ICN Pharm.).
Geratic Forte, Inj. (Keene Pharm.).
Geriamic, Tab. (Vortech).
Geritag, Inj., Cap. (Solvay).
W/Testosterone, vitamin and mineral formula, amino acids.
See: Geramine, Tab., Inj. (ICN Pharm.).

W/Testosterone propionate.

Estrone "5". (Keene) Estrone 5 mg/ml, sodium carboxymethylcellulose, povidone, benzyl alcohol, methyl and propyl parabens. Inj. Vial 10 ml. *Rx.*
Use: Estrogen.

estrone aqueous. (Various) Estrone aqueous 2 mg and 5 mg/ml/Inj. Vial 10 ml or 30 ml. *Rx.*
Use: Estrogen.

estrone sulfate, piperazine.
See: Ogen, Tab., Vaginal Cream (Abbott).

estrone sulfate, potassium.
See: Estrogen, Vial (Med. Chem.).
Kaytron, Inj. (Taylor Pharmaceuticals).

•**estropipate,** (ESS-troe-PIH-pate) U.S.P. 23. *Formerly Piperazine Estrone Sulfate.* Estrone hydrogen sulfate compound with piperazine (1:1). Piperazine estrone sulfate.
Use: Estrogen.
See: Ogen, Tab., Vaginal Cream (Abbott).
Ortho-Est (Ortho Pharma).

estropipate. (Various Mfr.) Estropipate 0.625 mg, 1.25 mg and 2.5 mg/Tab. Bot. 50s, 100s. *Rx.*
Use: Estrogen.

Estroquin Tablet. (Sheryl) Purified conjugated estrogens 1.25 mg/Tab. Bot. 100s. *Rx.*
Use: Estrogen.

Estrostep 21. (Parke-Davis) Norethindrone acetate 1 mg, ethinyl estradiol 20 mcg/Triangular tablet. Norethindrone acetate 1 mg, ethinyl estradiol 30 mcg/Square tablet. Norethindrone acetate 1 mg, ethinyl estradiol 35 mcg/Round tablet. Box. 21s. *Rx.*
Use: Oral contraceptive.

Estrostep Fe. (Parke-Davis) Norethindrone acetate 1 mg, ethinyl estradiol 20 mcg/Triangular tablet. Norethindrone acetate 1 mg, ethinyl estradiol 30 mcg/Square tablet. Norethindrone acetate 1 mg, ethinyl estradiol 35 mcg/Round tablet. Ferrous fumarate 75 mg. Box. 28s. *Rx.*
Use: Oral contraceptive.

•**etafedrine hydrochloride.** (EH-tah-FED-rin) USAN.
Use: Bronchodilator, adrenergic.
See: Mercodol w/Decapryn, Liq. (Merrell Dow).
Nethamine (Merrell Dow).

•**etafilcon a.** (EH-tah-FILL-kahn A) USAN.
Use: Contact lens material (hydrophilic.)
See: Acuvine (Vistacon).

Etalent. (Roger) Ethaverine HCl 100 mg/Cap. Bot. 50s, 500s. *Rx.*
Use: Peripheral vasodilator.

•**etanidazole.** (ETT-ah-NIDE-ah-zole) USAN.
Use: Antineoplastic (hypoxic cell radiosensitizer).
See: Radinyl (Roberts).

E-Tapp Elixir. (Edwards) Brompheniramine maleate 4 mg, phenylephrine HCl 5 mg, phenylpropanolamine HCl 5 mg/5 ml, alcohol 2.3%. Bot. gal. *otc.*
Use: Antihistamine, decongestant.

•**etarotene.** (ett-AHR-oh-teen) USAN.
Use: Keratolytic.

•**etazolate hydrochloride.** (eh-TAY-zoe-late) USAN.
Use: Antipsychotic.

Eterna 27 Cream. (Revlon) Pregnenolone acetate 0.5% in cream base. *otc.*
Use: Emollient.

•**eterobarb.** (ee-TEER-oh-barb) USAN.
Use: Anticonvulsant.

•**ethacrynate sodium for injection,** (ETH-ah-KRIN-ate) U.S.P. 23.
Use: Diuretic.
See: Edecrin Sodium I.V., Inj. (Merck).

•**ethacrynic acid,** (eth-uh-KRIN-ik) U.S.P. 23.
Use: Diuretic.
See: Edecrin, Tab. (Merck).

•**ethambutol hydrochloride,** (eth-AM-byoo-tahl) U.S.P. 23.
Use: Antibacterial, (tuberculostatic).
See: Myambutol HCl (Lederle).

Ethamicort.
See: Hydrocortamate.

•**ethamivan.** (eth-AM-ih-van) USAN.
Use: Stimulant (central and respiratory).

Ethamolin. (Schwarz Pharma) Ethanolamine oleate 5%. Inj. Amp. 2 ml. *Rx.*
Use: Sclerosing agent.

•**ethamsylate.** (ETH-AM-sill-ate) USAN.
Use: Hemostatic.

ethanol. (Various Mfr.) Alcohol, anhydrous. Alcohol, U.S.P. 23.

ethanolamine. Olamine.

•**ethanolamine oleate.** (ETH-ah-nahl-ah-MEEN OH-lee-ate) USAN.
Use: Sclerosing agent. [Orphan drug]
See: Ethamolin (Reed & Carnrick).

ethasulfate sodium. Sodium 2-Ethyl-1-hexanol sulfate.

ethaverine hydrochloride. The ethyl analog of papaverine HCl, 6,7-diethoxy-1-(3,4-diethoxybenzyl) isoquinoline HCl. Diquinol HCl, Preparin HCl, Perperine HCl. The tetraethyl homolog of papaverine is 2 to 4 times more active

and less than half as toxic as the parent drug. *Rx.*
Use: Antispasmodic.
See: Etalent, Cap. (Roger).
Ethaquin, Tab. (Ascher).
Neopavrin, Tab., Elix. (Savage).
Spasodil, Tab. (Rand).
•**ethchlorvynol,** (eth-klor-VIH-nahl) U.S.P. 23.
Use: Hypnotic, sedative.
See: Placidyl, Cap. (Abbott).
Serensil, Prods. (Novartis).
ethenol, homopolymer. Polyvinyl Alcohol, U.S.P. 23.
ethenzamide. o-Ethoxybenzamide.
•**ether,** U.S.P. 23. Ethyl ether.
Use: General anesthetic; inhalation.
•**ethinyl estradiol,** U.S.P. 23.
Use: Estrogen. Turner's syndrome [Orphan drug]
See: Estinyl, Tab. (Schering-Plough).
Feminone, Tab. (Pharmacia & Upjohn).
Lynoral, Tab. (Organon).
Menolyn, Tab. (Arcum).
Ovogyn, Tab. (Taylor Pharmaceuticals).
ethinyl estradiol w/combinations.
See: Ardiatric, Tab. (Burgin-Arden).
Brevicon, Tab. (Syntex).
Demulen, Tab. (Searle).
Desogen, Tab. (Organon).
GenCept, Tab. (Gencon).
Halodrin, Tab. (Pharmacia & Upjohn).
Jenest-28, Tab. (Organon).
Loestrin, Tab. (Parke-Davis).
Loestrin 1.5/30, Tab. (Parke-Davis).
Lo/Ovral, Tab. (Wyeth-Ayerst).
Modicon 21 and 28, Tab. (Ortho).
Nelulen, Tab. (Watson Labs).
Nordette, Tab. (Wyeth-Ayerst).
Norinyl, Prods. (Syntex).
Norlestrin, Tab. (Parke-Davis).
Norlestrin Fe, Tab. (Parke-Davis).
Ortho-Cept, Tab. (Ortho).
Ortho-Cyclen, Tab. (Ortho).
Ortho-Novum 1/35, 21 and 28 (Ortho).
Ortho Tri-Cyclen, Tab. (Ortho).
Os-Cal-Mone, Tab. (Hoechst Marion Roussel).
Ovcon-35, Tab. (Bristol-Myers).
Ovcon-50, Tab. (Bristol-Myers).
Ovlin, Vial (Zeneca).
Ovral, Tab. (Wyeth-Ayerst).
Triphasil, Tab. (Wyeth-Ayerst).
ethinyl estradiol and dimethisterone tablets.
Use: Estrogen, progestin combination.

ethinyl estrenol.
See: Lynestrenol (Organon).
•**ethiodized oil injection,** U.S.P. 23.
Use: Diagnostic aid (radiopaque medium).
See: Ethiodol, Inj. (Savage).
•**ethiodized oil I-131.** (eth-EYE-oh-dized OIL I 131) USAN. Radioactive iodine addition to ethyl ester of poppyseed oil. Ethiodal-131.
Use: Antineoplastic, radioactive agent.
Ethiodol. (Savage) Ethiodized oil. Fatty acid ethyl ester of poppy-seed oil, iodine 37%. Inj. Amp. 10 ml, Box 2s.
Use: Diagnostic aid.
Ethiofos. (eh-THIGH-oh-foss)
See: Amifostine.
•**ethionamide,** (eh-THIGH-ohn-ah-mid) U.S.P. 23.
Use: Antibacterial (tuberculostatic).
See: Trecator S.C., Tab. (Wyeth-Ayerst).
ethisterone.
See: Anhydrohydroxyprogesterone (Various Mfr.).
Ethmozine. (Roberts) Moricizine HCl 200 mg, 250 mg or 300 mg/Tab. Bot. 21s, 100s, UD 100s. *Rx.*
Use: Antiarrhythmic.
Ethocaine.
See: Procaine HCl (Various Mfr.).
ethocylorvynol. β-Chlorovinyl ethyl ethynyl carbinol. Ethchlorvynol, U.S.P. 23.
ethodryl.
See: Diethylcarbamazine Citrate.
ethoheptazine citrate.
ethohexadiol. Ethyl hexanediol, 2-ethyl-hexane-1,3-diol, Rutgers 612. Used in Comp. Dimethyl Phthalate.
Use: Insect repellent.
•**ethonam nitrate.** (ETH-oh-nam NYE-trate) USAN.
Use: Fungicide, antifungal.
•**ethosuximide,** (ETH-oh-SUX-ih-mide) U.S.P. 23.
Use: Anticonvulsant.
See: Zarontin, Cap., Syr. (Parke-Davis).
ethosuximide. (Copley) Ethosuximide 250 mg/5 ml/Syrup. Bot. 483 ml. *Rx.*
Use: Anticonvulsant.
•**ethotoin,** U.S.P. 23.
Use: Anticonvulsant.
See: Peganone (Abbott)
ethovan. Ethyl Vanillin.
•**ethoxazene hydrochloride.** (eth-OX-ah-zeen) USAN.
Use: Analgesic.
ethoxzolamide.

Use: Carbonic anhydrase inhibitor.

Ethrane. (Ohmeda) Enflurane. Volatile Liq. Bot. 125 ml, 250 ml. *Rx.*
Use: General anesthetic.

•**ethybenztropine.** (ETH-ih-BENZ-troe-peen) USAN. Methylbenztropine.
Use: Anticholinergic.

•**ethyl acetate,** N.F. 18.
Use: Flavor; Pharamaceutic aid, solvent.

ethyl aminobenzoate. Anesthesin, anesthrone, benzocaine, parathesin.
Use: Local anesthetic.
See: Benzocaine (Various Mfr.).

ethyl biscoumacetate.

ethyl bromide. (Various Mfr.) Bromoethane. *Rx.*
Use: General anesthetic.

ethyl carbamate.
See: Urethan (Various Mfr.).

•**ethylcellulose,** N.F. 18.
Use: Tablet binder, pharamaceutic aid.

ethylcellulose aqueous dispersion.
Use: Tablet binder, pharamaceutic aid.

ethyl chaulmoograte.
Use: Hansen's disease, sarcoidosis.

•**ethyl chloride,** U.S.P. 23. Chloroethane.
Use: Anesthetic, topical.
See: Gebauer-Spra-Pak. Stratford-Cook-Spray, 100 g.

ethyl chloride. (Various) Ethyl chloride 100 g chloroethane/Spray. Bot. 105 ml, 120 ml. *Rx.*
Use: Local anesthetic.

•**ethyl dibunate.** (ETH-ill DIE-byoo-nate) USAN.
Use: Cough suppressant, antitussive.

ethyl diiodobrassidate. Iodobrassid. Lipoiodine.

ethyldimethylammonium bromide.
See: Ambutonium Bromide.

ethylene. (Various Mfr.) Ethene. *Rx.*
Use: General anesthetic.

•**ethylenediamine,** U.S.P. 23.
Use: Component of aminophylline.

ethylenediamine solution. (67% w/v).
Use: Solvent (Aminophylline Inj.).

ethylenediaminetetraacetic acid.
See: Edathamil, EDTA (Various Mfr.).

ethylenediamine tetraacetic acid disodium salt.
See: Endrate Disodium, Amp. (Abbott).

•**ethylestrenol.** (ETH-ill-ESS-tree-nahl) USAN.
Use: Anabolic.

ethylhydrocupreine hydrochloride.
Use: Antiseptic.

ethylmorphine hydrochloride.

Use: Narcotic.

ethyl nitrite spirit. Ethyl nitrite. Sweet Spirit of Niter. Spirit of Nitrous Ether.

•**ethyl oleate,** N.F. 18.
Use: Pharmaceutic aid (vehicle).

ethyl oxide; ethyl ether,
Use: Solvent.

ethylpapaverine hydrochloride.
See: Ethaverine HCl (Various Mfr.).

•**ethylparaben,** N.F. 18. Ethyl p-Hydroxybenzoate.
Use: Pharmaceutic aid (antifungal preservative).

ethylstibamine. Astaril, neostibosan.
Use: Antimony therapy.

ethyl vanillate.

•**ethyl vanillin,** N.F. 18.
Use: Pharmaceutic aid (flavor).

•**ethynerone.** (eth-EYE-ner-ohn) USAN.
Use: Progestin.

•**ethynodiol diacetate,** (eh-THIN-oh-die-ole die-ASS-eh-tate) U.S.P. 23.
Use: As progesterone, progestin.
See: Ovulen, Tab. (Searle).
W/Ethinyl estradiol.
Demulen, Preps. (Searle).
Nelulen, Tab. (Watson Labs).
W/Mestranol.
See: Ovulen, Tab. (Searle).

ethynodiol diacetate and ethinyl estradiol tablets.
Use: Oral contraceptive.

ethynodiol diacetate and mestranol tablets.
Use: Oral contraceptive.

ethynylestradiol.
See: Ethinyl Estradiol, U.S.P. (Various Mfr.).
Mestranol (Various Mfr.).

ethynylestradiol 3-methyl ether.
See: Enovid, Tab. (Searle).

Ethyol. (Alza/US Bioscience) Pow. for Inj. Lyophilized: 500 mg (anhydrous basis) 500 mg mannitol in 10 ml single-use vials. *Rx.*
Use: Cyto-protective agent.

•**etibendazole.** (eh-tie-BEN-dah-ZOLE) USAN.
Use: Anthelmintic.

Eticylol. (Novartis) Ethinyl estradiol. *Rx.*
Use: Estrogen.

•**etidocaine.** (eh-TIE-doe-cane) USAN.
Use: Local anesthetic.
See: Duranest, Inj. (Astra).
Duranest-MPF, Inj. (Astra).

•**etidronate disodium,** (eh-TIH-DROE-nate) U.S.P. 23. The disodium salt of (1-Hydroxyethylidene) diphosphonic acid.

Use: Bone resorption inhibitor. Treatment of symptomatic Paget's disease of bone (osteitis deformans). Degenerative metabolic bone disease [Orphan drug]
See: Didronel, Tab. (Procter & Gamble).

•**etidronic acid.** USAN.
Use: Calcium regulator.

•**etifenin.** (EH-tih-FEN-in) USAN.
Use: Diagnostic aid.

•**etintidine hydrochloride.** (ett-IN-tih-DEEN) USAN.
Use: Antagonist to histamine H_2 receptors.

•**etocrylene.** (EH-toe-KRIH-leen) USAN.
Use: Ultraviolet screen.

•**etodolac.** (EE-toe-DOE-lak) USAN.
Use: Nonsteroidal anti-inflammatory, analgesic.
See: Lodine (Wyeth-Ayerst).

•**etofenamate.** (EH-toe-FEN-am-ate) USAN.
Use: Analgesic, anti-inflammatory.

•**etoformin hydrochloride.** (EH-toe-FORE-min) USAN.
Use: Antidiabetic

•**etomidate.** (eh-TAHM-ih-date) USAN.
Use: Sedative, hypnotic.
See: Amidate (Abbott).

etomide hydrochloride. (ETT-oh-mide) Bandol. Carbiphene HCl.

•**etonogestrel.** (ETT-oh-no-JESS-trell) USAN.
Use: Progestin.

•**etoperidone hydrochloride.** (EH-toe-PURR-ih-dohn) USAN.
Use: Antidepressant.
See: Vepesid, Inj., Cap. (Bristol).

Etopophoso. (Bristol-Myers Oncology) Etoposide phosphate 119.3 mg (100 mg etoposide), dextran 40 300mg/Pow. for Inj. Vials. Single dose. *Rx.*
Use: Antineoplastic.

•**etoposide,** (EH-toe-POE-side) U.S.P. 23.
Use: Antineoplastic.
See: Etopophos, Pow. for Inj. (Bristol-Myers Oncology). Vepesid, Inj., Cap. (Bristol).

etoposide. (EH-toe-POE-side) (Gensia) Etoposide 20 mg/ml, alcohol 30.5%, benzyl alcohol 30 mg, polysorbate 80 mg, PEG 300 650 mg, citric acid 2 mg/ml. Inj. Vials 5 ml, 25 ml. *Rx.*
Use: Antineoplastic.

•**etoposide phosphate.** (ee-toe-POE-side) USAN.
Use: Antineoplastic.

•**etoprine.** (ETT-oh-preen) USAN.
Use: Antineoplastic.

etoquinol sodium. Name used for Actinoquinol sodium.

etoval.
See: Butethal, N.F. (Various Mfr.).

•**etoxadrol hydrochloride.** (eh-TOX-ah-drole) USAN.
Use: Anesthetic.

•**etozolin.** (EAT-oh-zoe-lin) USAN.
Use: Diuretic.

Etrafon (2-10). (Schering-Plough) Perphenazine 2 mg, amitriptyline HCl 10 mg/Tab. Bot. 100s, 500s, UD 100s. *Rx.*
Use: Psychotherapeutic combination.

Etrafon (2-25). (Schering-Plough) Perphenazine 2 mg, amitriptyline HCl 25 mg/Tab. Bot. 100s, 500s, UD 100s. *Rx.*
Use: Psychotherapeutic combination.

Etrafon-A (4-10). (Schering-Plough) Perphenazine 4 mg, amitriptyline HCl 10 mg/Tab. Bot. 100s, UD 100s. *Rx.*
Use: Psychotherapeutic combination.

Etrafon Forte Tablets (4-25). (Schering-Plough) Perphenazine 4 mg, amitriptyline HCl 25 mg/Tab. Bot. 100s, 500s, UD 100s. *Rx.*
Use: Psychotherapeutic combination.

•**etretinate.** (eh-TRETT-ih-nate) USAN.
Use: Antipsoriatic.
See: Tegison, Cap. (Hoffman-LaRoche).

etrynit. Propatyl nitrate.
Use: Coronary agent.

•**etryptamine acetate.** (ee-TRIP-tah-meen) USAN.
Use: Central stimulant.
See: Monase (Pharmacia & Upjohn).

ETS-2%. (Paddock) Erythromycin topical 2%. Soln. Bot. 60 ml. *Rx.*
Use: Antiacne.

ettriol trinitrate.
See: Propatyl nitrate.

etybenzatropine. Ethybenztropine.

etynodiol acetate. Ethynodiol Diacetate.

eubasin.
See: Sulfapyridine (Various Mfr.).

eucaine hydrochloride. (Novartis) Menthol 8%, eucalyptus oil, SD 3A alcohol. Gel. Tube 60 g. *otc.*
Use: Rubs and liniments.

Eucalyptamint Maximum Strength. (Novartis) Menthol 16%, lanolin, eucalyptus oil. Oint. Tube 60 ml. *otc.*
Use: Rubs and liniments.

•**eucalyptol.** USAN. NF XVI.
Use: Pharmaceutic aid (flavor), antitussive, nasal decongestant.
See: Vicks Sinex, Nasal Spray (Richardson-Vicks).
Vicks Va-Tro-Nol, Nose Drops (Richardson-Vicks).

Vicks Prods. (Richardson-Vicks).

eucalyptus oil.
Use: Flavor, antitussive, nasal decongestant, expectorant, topical analgesic.
See: Vicks Prods. (Richardson-Vicks). Victors Regular, Cherry Loz. (Richardson-Vicks).

•**eucatropine hydrochloride,** U.S.P. 23. (Glogau) Crystal, Bot. g.
Use: Pharmaceutical necessity for ophthalmic dosage form; anticholinergic (ophthalmic).

eucatropine hydrochloride. (Glogau). Crystal, Bot. g.
Use: Pharmaceutical necessity for ophthalmic dosage form; anticholinergic (ophthalmic).

Eucerin. (Beiersdorf) Unscented moisturizing formula. **Creme:** Jar 120 g, lb. **Lot.:** Bot. 240 ml, 480 ml. *otc.*
Use: Emollient.

Eucerin Cleansing. (Beiersdorf) Sodium laureth sulfate, cocoamphocarboxyglycinate, cocamidopropyl betaine, cocamide MEA, PEG-7 glyceryl cocoate, PEG-5 lanolate, PEG-120 methyl glucose dioleate, lanolin alcohol, imidazolidinyl urea. Soap free. Lot. Bot. 240 ml. *otc.*
Use: Skin cleanser.

Eucerin Dry Skin Care Daily Facial. (Beiersdorf) Ethylhexyl p-methoxycinnamate, titanium dioxide, 2-phenylbenzimidazole-5-sulfonic acid, 2-ethylhexyl salicylate, mineral oil, cetearyl alcohol, castor oil, lanolin alcohol, EDTA. SPF 20. Lot. Bot. 120 ml. *otc.*
Use: Sunscreen.

Eucerin Plus. (Beiersdorf) Mineral oil, hydrogenated castor oil, 5% sodium lactate, 5% urea, glycerin, lanolin alcohol. Lot. Bot. 177 ml. *otc.*
Use: Emollient.

eucodal.
See: Oxycodone.

Eucoran.
See: Nikethamide (Various Mfr.).

eucupin dihydrochloride. Isoamylhydrocupreine dihydrochloride.

Eudal-SR. (UAD) Pseudoephedrine 120 mg, guaifenesin 400 mg/SR Tab. Bot. 100s. *Rx.*
Use: Decongestant, expectorant.

euflavine.
See: Acriflavine (Various Mfr.).

•**eugenol,** U.S.P. 23.
Use: Dental analgesic, oral anesthetic.
See: Benzodent, Oint. (Richardson-Vicks).

eukadol.
See: Dihydrohydroxycodeinone, Preps. (No Mfr. currently lists).

Eulcin. (Leeds) Methscopolamine bromide 2.5 mg, butabarbital sodium 10 mg, aluminum hydroxide gel, dried, 250 mg, magnesium trisilicate 250 mg/Tab. Bot. 100s. *Rx.*
Use: Anticholinergic, antispasmodic, sedative, hypnotic, antacid.

Eulexin. (Schering-Plough) Flutamide 125 mg/Cap. 100s, 500s, UD 100s. *Rx.*
Use: Antineoplastic.

Eumydrin Drops. (Sanofi Winthrop) Atropine methonitrate. *Rx.*
Use: Anticholinergic, antispasmodic.

euneryl.
See: Phenobarbital (Various Mfr.).

Euphorbia Compound. (Sherwood) Euphorbia pilulifera fluidextract 1.5 ml, iobelia tincture 2.2 ml, nitroglycerin spirit 0.29 ml, sodium iodide 1.04 g, sodium bromide 1.04 g, alcohol 24%/30 ml. Bot. pt, gal. *Rx.*
Use: Sedative, hypnotic, expectorant.

euphorbia pilulifera.
W/Cocillana, squill, antimony potassium tartrate, senega.
See: Cylana, Syr. (Jones Medical).
W/Phenyl salicylate and various oils.
See: Rayderm, Oint. (Velvet Pharmacal).

Eupractone. (Baxter) Dimethadione.

Euprax. Albution.

•**euprocin hydrochloride.** USAN.
Use: Anesthetic (topical).
See: Eucupin HCl.

euquinine. Quinine ethyl carbonate.
Use: Antimalarial, antipyretic.

Eurax Cream. (Westwood Squibb) Crotamiton 10% in vanishing-cream base of glyceryl monostearate, anhydrous lanolin, PEG 6-32, glycerin, polysorbate 80, water, benzyl alcohol, mineral oil, white wax, quaternium-15, fragrance. Tube 60 g. *Rx.*
Use: Scabicide, pediculicide.

Eurax Lotion. (Westwood Squibb) Crotamiton 10% in emollient-lotion base of glyceryl monostearate, anhydrous lanolin, PEG 6-32, glycerin, polysorbate 80, water, benzyl alcohol, light mineral oil, carboxymethylcellulose, simethicone, quaternium-15, fragrance. Bot. 60 g, 454 g. *Rx.*
Use: Scabicide, pediculicide.

Evac-Q-Kit. (Pharmacia & Upjohn) Each kit contains: **Evac-Q-Mag:** Magnesium citrate 300 ml, citric acid, potassium

citrate. **Evac-Q-Tabs:** 2 tab. phenol-phthalein 130 mg/Tab. **Evac-Q-Sert:** 2 supp. containing potassium bitartrate, sodium bicarbonate/supp. in polyethylene glycol base. Patient instruction sheet. *otc.*
Use: Bowel evacuant.

Evac-Q-Kwik. (Pharmacia & Upjohn) Each kit contains: **Evac-Q-Mag:** magnesium citrate 300 ml, citric acid, potassium citrate in cherry-flavored base. **Evac-Q-Tabs:** 2 tab. phenolphthalein 130 mg. **Evac-Q-Kwik Supp.:** bisacodyl 10 mg. *otc.*
Use: Bowel evacuant.

Evac Suppositories. (Burgin-Arden) Sodium bicarbonate, sodium biphosphate, dioctyl sodium sulfosuccinate 50 mg/Supp. *otc.*
Use: Laxative.

Evac Tablets. (Burgin-Arden) Guar gum 300 mg, danthron 50 mg, sodium 100 mg/Tab. *otc.*
Use: Laxative.

Evactol. (Delta) Docusate sodium 100 mg, sodium carboxymethyl cellulose 200 mg/Cap. Pkg. 10s, Bot. 10s, 30s, 100s. *otc.*
Use: Laxative.

Evac-U-Gen. (Walker Corp.) Yellow phenolphthalein 97.2 mg w/corn syrup, lactose, saccharin/Chew. Tab. Bot. 35s, 100s. *otc.*
Use: Laxative.

Evac-U-Lax. (Roberts) Yellow phenolphthalein 80 mg/Chew. tab. Bot. 100s. *otc.*
Use: Laxative.

Evalose. (Copley) Lactulose 10 g/15 ml, galactose < 1.6 g, lactose < 1.2 g, other sugars ≤ 1.2 g/Syrup. Bot. 240 ml, 960 ml. *Rx.*
Use: Laxative.

evans blue, U.S.P. XXII.
Use: Diagnostic aid (blood volume determination).

Evans Blue Dye. (New World Trading Corp.) Evans blue dye 5 ml/Inj.*Rx.*
Use: Diagnostic aid.

Everone. (Hyrex) Testosterone enanthate in oil 100 mg or 200 mg/ml. Vial 10 ml. *c-III.*
Use: Androgen.

Evicyl Tablets. (Sanofi Winthrop) Inositol hexanicotinate. *Rx.*
Use: Hypolipidemic, peripheral vasodilator.

Eviron. (Delta) Ferrous fumarate 160 mg, copper 1 mg, ascorbic acid 75 mg/Tab. *otc.*

Use: Vitamin/mineral supplement.

E-Vital Creme. (Taylor Pharmaceuticals) Vitamins E 100 IU, A 250 IU, D 100 IU, d-panthenol 0.2%, allantoin 0.1%/g. Jar 2 oz, lb. *otc.*
Use: Emollient.

Ewin Ninos Tablets. (Sanofi Winthrop) Aspirin. *otc.*
Use: Salicylate analgesic.

Exact. (Advanced Polymer Systems) Benzoyl peroxide 5%, cetyl and steryl alcohol, parabens. Cream Jar 18 g. *otc.*
Use: Antiacne.

Exact Liquid. (Advanced Polymer Systems) Salicylic acid 2%, propylene glycol, aloe vera gel, disodium EDTA, menthol, parabens, glycerin, diazolidinyl urea. Liq. Bot. 118 ml. *otc.*
Use: Antiacne.

●**exametazime.** (EX-ah-MET-ah-zeen) USAN.
Use: Diagnostic aid (regional cerebral perfusion imaging).

●**exaprolol hydrochloride.** (EX-ah-PRO-lahl) USAN.
Use: Anti-adrenergic (β-receptor).

Ex-Caloric Wafers. (Eastern Research) Carboxymethylcellulose 181 mg, methylcellulose 272 mg/Wafer. Bot. 100s, 500s, 5000s. *otc.*
Use: Nonprescription diet aid.

Excedrin Aspirin Free. (Bristol-Myers) Acetaminophen 500 mg, caffeine 65 mg/Cap. Bot. 24s, 50s, 100s. *otc.*
Use: Nonnarcotic analgesic combination.

Excedrin Extra Strength. (Bristol-Myers) Acetaminophen 250 mg, aspirin 250 mg, caffeine 65 mg. **Capl.:** Bot. 24s, 50s, 80s. **Tab.:** Bot. 12s, 30s, 60s, 100s, 165s, 225s. *otc.*
Use: Analgesic combination.

Excedrin P.M. Aspirin Free. (Bristol-Myers) Acetaminophen 500 mg, diphenhydramine citrate 25 mg. **Tab.:** Bot. 10s, 30s, 50s, 80s. **Capl.:** Bot. 30s, 50s. **Liquigels:** Bot. 20s, 40s. **Liq.:** Acetaminophen 167 mg or 1000 mg, diphenhydramine HCl 8.3 mg/5 ml or 50 mg/30 ml, alcohol 10%, sucrose. Bot. 180 ml. *otc.*
Use: Analgesic, sleep aid.

Excedrin Sinus. (Bristol-Myers) Pseudoephedrine HCl 30 mg, acetaminophen 500 mg/Tab. Capl. Bot. 24s. *otc.*
Use: Decongestant, analgesic.

Excita Extra. (Schmid) Nonoxynol 9 8% (Ribbed). Condom. Box 3s, 12s, 36s.. *otc.*

Use: Condom with spermicide.

exemestane. (Pharmacia & Upjohn) *Use:* Hormonal therapy of metastatic breast carcinoma. [Orphan drug]

Exgest LA Tablets. (Schwarz Pharma) Phenylpropanolamine HCl 75 mg, guaifenesin 400 mg. Bot. 100s or 500s. *Rx.* *Use:* Decongestant, expectorant.

Exidine-2 Scrub. (Baxter) Chlorhexidine gluconate 2%, isopropyl alcohol 4%. Soln. Bot. 120 ml. *otc.* *Use:* Antiseptic, germicide.

Exidine-4 Scrub. (Baxter) Chlorhexidine glucoante 4%, isopropyl alcohol 4%. Soln. Bot. 120 ml, 240 ml, 480 ml, 887 ml, 1 gal. *otc.* *Use:* Antiseptic, germicide.

Exidine Skin Cleanser. (Xttrium) Chlorhexidine gluconate 4%, isopropyl alcohol 4%. Bot. 120 ml, 240 ml, 16 oz, 32 oz, gal. *otc.* *Use:* Antiseptic, germicide.

Ex-Lax. (Sandoz) Yellow phenolphthalein 90 mg/chocolate Chew. Tab. or unflavored pill. Chocolate Tab. 6s, 18s, 48s, 72s. Unflavored pill 8s, 30s, 60s. *otc.* *Use:* Laxative.

Ex-Lax Chocolated. (Sandoz) Yellow phenolphthalein 90 mg/Chew. Tab. In 6s, 18s, 48s, 72s. *otc.* *Use:* Laxative.

Ex-Lax Extra Gentle. (Sandoz) Phenolphthalein 65 mg, docusate sodium 75 mg/Tab. Pkg. 24s, 48s. *otc.* *Use:* Laxative.

Ex-Lax Gentle Nature. (Sandoz) Calcium salts of sennosides A&B. Tab. 16s. *otc.* *Use:* Laxative.

Ex-Lax Maximum Relief. (Sandoz) Yellow phenolphthalein 135 mg. Tab. Pkg. 24s. *otc.* *Use:* Laxative.

Ex-Lax Unflavored. (Sandoz) Yellow phenolphthalein 90 mg/Tab. 8s, 30s, 60s. *otc.* *Use:* Laxative.

Exna. (Robins) Benzthiazide 50 mg/Tab. Bot. 100s. *Rx.* *Use:* Diuretic, antihypertensive.

Exocaine Plus. (Del Pharm.) Methyl salicylate 30%. Jar 4 oz, Tube 1.3 oz. *otc.* *Use:* Analgesic, topical.

exol. Di-isobutyl ethoxy ethyl dimethyl benzyl ammonium Cl.

exonic ot. Dioctyl Sodium Sulphosuccinate. *Use:* Laxative.

Exosurf Neonatal. (Glaxo Wellcome) Colfosceril palmitate; dipalmitoylphosphatidylcholine (DPPC). Lyophilized pow. Vial 10 ml. *Rx.* *Use:* Synthetic lung surfactant.

Expectorant DM Cough Syrup. (Weeks & Leo) Dextromethorphan HBr 15 mg, guaifenesin 100 mg/5 ml, alcohol 7.125%. Bot. 6 oz. *otc.* *Use:* Antitussive, expectorant.

Expendable Blood Collection Unit ACD. (Baxter) Citric acid 540 mg, sodium citrate 1.49 g, dextrose 1.65 g/67.5 ml. *Rx.* *Use:* Anticoagulant.

Exsel. (Allergan Herbert) Selenium sulfide 2.5% in shampoo/lotion base. Bot. 4 oz. *Rx.* *Use:* Antiseborrheic.

Exten Strone 10. (Schlicksup) Estradiol valerate 10 mg/ml. Vial 10 ml. *Rx.* *Use:* Estrogen.

Extendryl Chewable Tablets. (Fleming) Chlorpheniramine maleate 2 mg, phenylephrine HCl 10 mg, methscopolamine nitrate 1.25 mg/Chew. tab. Bot. 100s, 1000s. *Rx.* *Use:* Antihistamine, decongestant, anticholinergic, antispasmodic.

Extendryl Junior. (Fleming) Chlorpheniramine maleate 4 mg, phenylephrine HCl 10 mg, methscopolamine nitrate 1.25 mg/TD Cap. 100s, 1000s. *Rx.* *Use:* Antihistamine, decongestant, anticholinergic, antispasmodic.

Extendryl S.R. (Fleming) Chlorpheniramine maleate 8 mg, phenylephrine HCl 20 mg, methscopolamine nitrate 2.5 mg/TD Cap. Bot. 100s, 1000s. *Rx.* *Use:* Antihistamine, decongestant, anticholinergic, antispasmodic.

Extendryl Syrup. (Fleming) Chlorpheniramine maleate 2 mg, phenylephrine HCl 10 mg, methscopolamine nitrate 1.25 mg/5 ml. Bot. 473 ml, gal. *Rx.* *Use:* Antihistamine, decongestant, anticholinergic, antispasmodic.

Extenzyme Soflens Protein Cleaner. (Allergan) Papain, sodium Cl, sodium carbonate, sodium borate, edetate disodium. Vial w/Tab. 24s. Refill 36s. *otc.* *Use:* Soft contact lens care.

Extra Action Cough. (Rugby) Dextromethorphan HBr 15 mg, guaifenesin 100 mg w/alcohol 1.4%, corn syrup, saccharin. Syr. Bot. 118 ml. *otc.* *Use:* Antitussive, expectorant.

Extra Strength Adprin-B. (Pfeiffer) Aspirin with calcium carbonate 500 mg,

magnesium carbonate, magnesium oxide/Tab, buffered. *otc.*
Use: Analgesic.

Extra Strength Alka-Seltzer Effervescent. (Bayer) Sodium bicarbonate (heat-treated) 1985 mg, aspirin 500 mg, citric acid 1000 mg, sodium 588 mg/Tab. Bot. 12s and 24s. *otc.*
Use: Antacid.

Extra Strength Alkets Antacid. (Roberts Pharm) Calcium carbonate 750 mg/Tab. Chew. Bot. 96s. *otc.*
Use: Antacid.

Extra Strength Aspirin Capsules. (Walgreen) Aspirin 500 mg/Cap. Bot. 80s. *otc.*
Use: Salicylate analgesic.

Extra Strength Bayer Plus. (Bayer) Aspirin buffered with calcium carbonate, magnesium carbonate, magnesium oxide 500 mg / Capl. Bot. 30s, 60s. *otc.*
Use: Salicylate analgesic.

Extra Strength Bayer Enteric 500 Aspirin. (Bayer) Aspirin 500 mg. Tab. Enteric coated. Bot. 60s. *otc.*
Use: Salicylate analgesic.

Extra Strength Doan's PM. (Novartis) Magnesium salicylate 500 mg, diphenhydramine HCl 25 mg / Capl. Pkg. 20s. *otc.*
Use: Nonprescription sleep aid.

Extra Strength Exedrine Capsules and Tablets. (Bristol-Myers) Acetaminophen 250 mg, aspirin 250 mg, caffeine 65 mg. Cap. Bot. 24s, 50s, 80s. Tab. Bot. 30s, 60s, 100s, 165s, 225s, Pkg. 12s. *otc.*
Use: Analgesic combination.

Extra Strength 5 mg Biotin Forte. (Vitaline) Vitamins B_1 10 mg, B_2 10 mg, B_3 40 mg, B_5 10 mg, B_6 25 mg, B_{12} 10 mcg, C 100 mg, biotin 5 mg, FA 800 mcg/Tab. Bot. 60s, 1000s. *otc.*
Use: Vitamin/mineral supplement.

Extra Strength Gas-X. (Sandoz Consumer) Simethicone 125 mg/Tab. Pkg. 18s. *otc.*
Use: Antiflatulent.

Extra Strength Tylenol Headache Plus. (McNeil-CPC) Acetaminophen 500 mg, calcium carbonate 250 mg/Capl. Bot. 24s, 50s, 100s. *otc.*
Use: Nonnarcotic analgesic combination.

Extra Strength Tylenol PM. (McNeil-CPC) Diphenhydramine 25 mg, acetaminophen 500 mg / **Tab.:** 24s, 50s; **Capl.:** 24s, 50s; **Gelcap:** 20s, 40s. *otc.*
Use: Nonprescription sleep aid.

Extra Strength Vicks Cough Drops. (Richardson-Vicks) Menthol 8.4 mg (menthol flavor) or menthol 10 mg (cherry and honey lemon flavors), corn syrup, sucrose / Loz. Pkg. 9s, 30s. *otc.*
Use: Mouth and throat product.

Extreme Cold Formula. (Major) Pseudoephedrine HCl 30 mg, chlorpheniramine maleate 1 mg, dextromethorphan HBr 15 mg, acetaminophen 500 mg/Cap. Bot. 10s. *otc.*
Use: Decongestant, antihistamine, antitussive, analgesic.

Eye Drops. (Bausch & Lomb) Tetrahydrozoline HCl 0.05%. Drop. Bot. 15 ml. *otc.*
Use: Ophthalmic vasoconstrictor, mydriatic.

Eye Face and Body Wash Station. (Lavoptik) Sodium Cl 0.49 g, sodium biphosphate 0.4 g, sodium phosphate 0.45 g/100 ml, benzalkonium Cl 0.005%. Bot. 32 oz.
Use: Emergency wash.

Eye Irrigating Solution. (Rugby) Sodium Cl, sodium phosphate mono- and dibasic, benzalkonium Cl, EDTA. Soln. Bot. 118 ml. *otc.*
Use: Extraocular irrigating solution.

Eye Irrigating Wash. (Roberts Hauck) Boric acid, potassium Cl, sodium carbonate anhydrous, EDTA 0.01%, benzalkonium Cl. Soln. Bot. 120 ml. *otc.*
Use: Ophthalmic irrigation solution.

Eye-Lube-A. (Optopics) Glycerin 0.25%, EDTA, NaCl, benzalkonium chloride. Soln. Bot. 15 ml. *otc.*
Use: Ocular lubricant.

Eye Mo. (Sanofi Winthrop) Boric acid, benzalkonium Cl, phenylephrine HCl, zinc sulfate. *otc.*
Use: Astringent, ophthalmic.

Eye Scrub. (Ciba-Vision) PEG-200 glyceryl monotallawate, disodium laureth sulfosuccinate, cocoamidopropylamineoxide, PEG-78 glyceryl monococoate, benzyl alcohol, EDTA/Soln. Bot. 240 ml. *otc.*
Use: Ophthalmic cleansing solution.

Eye-Sed Ophthalmic Solution. (Scherer) Zinc sulfate 0.25%. Bot. 15 ml. *otc.*
Use: Astringent, ophthalmic.

Eyesine. (Akorn) Tetrahydrozoline HCl 0.05%. Drops. Bot. 15 ml. *otc.*
Use: Vasoconstrictor, mydriatic (ophthalmic).

Eye-Stream. (Alcon) Sodium Cl 0.64%, potassium Cl 0.075%, magnesium Cl

hexahydrate 0.03%, calcium Cl dihydrate 0.048%, sodium acetate trihydrate 0.39%, sodium citrate dihydrate 0.17%, benzalkonium Cl 0.013%. Bot. 30 ml, 118 ml. *otc.*
Use: Irrigating agent, ophthalmic.

Eye Wash. (Bausch & Lomb) Boric acid, potassium Cl, EDTA, sodium carbonate, benzalkonium Cl 0.01%. Soln. Bot. 118 ml. *otc.*
Use: Irrigating agent, ophthalmic.

Eye Wash. (Goldline) Boric acid, potassium Cl, EDTA, anhydrous sodium carbonate, benzalkonium Cl 0.1%. Soln. Bot. 118 ml. *otc.*
Use: Ophthalmic irrigation solution.

Eye Wash. (Lavoptik) Sodium Cl 0.49%, sodium biphosphate 0.4%, sodium phosphate 0.45%, benzalkonium Cl 0.005%. Soln. Bot. 180 ml with eye cup. *otc.*
Use: Ophthalmic irrigation solution.

EZ-Detect. (Biomerica) Occult blood screening test. Kit 3s.
Use: Diagnostic aid.

EZ Detect Strep-A Test. (Biomerica) Coated stick test for detection of group A streptococci taken directly from a throat swab.
Use: Diagnostic aid.

Eze Pain. (Halsey) Acetaminophen 2.5 gr, salicylamide, caffeine/Cap. Bot. 21s. *otc.*
Use: Analgesic combination.

Ezide. (Econo Med) Hydrochlorothiazide 50 mg/Tab. Bot. 100s, 1000s. *Rx.*
Use: Diuretic.

Ezol. (Stewart-Jackson) Butalbital 50 mg, caffeine 40 mg, acetaminophen 325 mg. Bot. 100s. *Rx.*
Use: Sedative, hypnotic, analgesic.

Ezol #3. (Stewart-Jackson) Acetaminophen 650 mg, codeine 30 mg. Bot. 100s. *c-III.*
Use: Narcotic analgesic combination.

F

Faces Only Moisturizing Sunblock by Coppertone. (Schering Plough) Ethylhexyl p-methoxycinnamate, oxybenzone. SPF 15. Lot. Bot. 55.5 ml. *otc.*
Use: Sunscreen.

Fact Home Pregnancy Test. (Advanced Care) Accurate test for pregnancy in 45 minutes, for use as early as 3 days after a missed period. 1 Test kit 1s.
Use: Diagnostic aid.

factor VII-A recombinant, DNA origin. *Rx.*
Use: Antihemophilic, von Willebrand's disease. [Orphan drug]

factor VIII.
See: Antihemophilic factor.

•**factor IX complex,** U.S.P. 23.
Use: Hemostatic.
See: Alpha Nine SD. (Alpha Therapeutics).
  Konyne 80. (Bayer)
  Mononine. (Centeon)
  Profilnine SD (Alpha Therapeutics).
  Proplex T. (Baxter).

factor IX, coagulation.
See: Coagulation factor ix.

factor XIII (placenta-derived). *Rx.*
Use: Congenital Factor XIII deficiency. [Orphan drug]
See: Fibrogammin.

Fact Plus. (Advanced Care Products) Reagent in-home kit for urine testing. Pregnancy test. Kit 1s, 2s.
Use: Diagnostic aid.

Factrel. (Wyeth-Ayerst) Gonadorelin HCl 100 mcg or 500 mcg/Vial w/Amp. of 2 ml sterile diluent. *Rx.*
Use: Diagnostic aid.

•**fadrozole hydrochloride.** (FAHD-rah-ZOLE) USAN.
Use: Antineoplastic.

Falgos Tablets. (Sanofi Winthrop) Acetylsalicylic acid. *otc.*
Use: Salicylate analgesic.

•**famciclovir.** (fam-SIGH-kloe-veer) USAN.
Use: Antiviral.
See: Famvir, Tab. (SK-Beecham).

Falmonox. (Sanofi Winthrop) Teclozan. Susp., Tab. *Rx.*
Use: Amebicide.

•**famotidine,** (fah-MOE-tih-den) U.S.P. 23.
Use: Antagonist (to histamine H_2 receptors).
See: Pepcid, Tab., Susp., Inj. (Merck).

•**famotine hydrochloride.** (FAM-oh-teen) USAN.

Use: Antiviral.

•**fampridine.** (FAHM-prih-DEEN) USAN.
Use: Symptomatic treatment of multiple sclerosis.

Famvir. (SmithKline Beecham) Famciclovir 125 mg, lactose/Tab. Bot 30s, UD 100s. Famciclovir 250 mg, lactose/Tab. Bot. 30s. Famciclovir 500 mg, lactose/Tab. Bot. 30s, UD 50s. *Rx.*
Use: Management of acute herpes zoster (shingles).

•**fananserin.** USAN.
Use: Antipsychotic, antischizophrenic (dual dopamine D_4 and serotonin 5-HT_2 receptor antagonist).

•**fanetizole mesylate.** (fan-EH-tih-zole) USAN.
Use: Immunoregulator.

Fansidar. (Roche) Sulfadoxine 500 mg, pyrimethamine 25 mg/Tab. Box 25s. *Rx.*
Use: Antimalarial.

•**fantridone hydrochloride.** (FAN-trih-dohn) USAN.
Use: Antidepressant.

Faramals. (Faraday) Vitamins A 10,000 IU, D 2000 IU, B_1 6 mg, B_2 4 mg, B_6 0.5 mg, folic acid 0.1 mg, C 100 mg, calcium pantothenate 5 mg, niacinamide 30 mg, E 5 IU, B_{12} 3 mcg/Tab. Bot. 100s, 250s, 500s, 1000s. *otc.*
Use: Vitamin/mineral supplement.

Faramals-M. (Faraday) Faramals plus calcium 103 mg, cobalt 0.1 mg, copper 1 mg, iodine 0.15 mg, iron 10 mg, magnesium 6 mg, molybdenum 0.2 mg, phosphorus 80 mg, potassium 5 mg, zinc 1.2 mg/Tab. Bot. 100s, 250s, 500s, 1000s. *otc.*
Use: Vitamin/mineral supplement.

Faramins. (Faraday) Vitamins B_1 20 mg, B_2 6 mg, C 40 mg, niacinamide 20 mg, calcium pantothenate 3 mg, B_6 0.5 mg, powdered whole dried liver 125 mg, dried debittered yeast 125 mg, choline dihydrogen citrate 20 mg, inositol 20 mg, dl-methionine 20 mg, folic acid 0.1 mg, B_{12} 10 mcg, ferrous gluconate 30 mg, dicalcium phosphate 250 mg, copper sulfate 5 mg, magnesium sulfate 10 mg, manganese sulfate 5 mg, cobalt sulfate 0.2 mg, potassium Cl 2 mg, potassium iodide 0.15 mg/Tab. Bot. 100s, 250s, 500s, 1000s. *otc.*
Use: Vitamin/mineral supplement.

Faratol. (Faraday) Vitamins A 12,500 IU, D 1000 IU, B_1 20 mg, B_2 6 mg, B_6 0.5 mg, B_{12} 15 mcg, folic acid 0.1 mg, niacinamide 10 mg, calcium pantothenate 3 mg, C 60 mg, E 5 IU, choline dihy-

drogen citrate 20 mg, inositol 20 mg, dl-methionine 20 mg, whole dried liver 100 mg, dried debittered yeast 100 mg, dicalcium phosphate 200 mg, ferrous gluconate 30 mg, potassium iodide 0.2 mg, magnesium sulfate 7.2 mg, copper sulfate 5 mg, manganese sulfate 3.4 mg, cobalt sulfate 0.2 mg, potassium Cl 1.3 mg, zinc sulfate 2 mg, molybdenum 0.2 mg in a base of alfalfa/Tab. Bot. 100s, 250s, 500s, 1000s. *otc.*
Use: Vitamin/mineral supplement.

Farbee with Vitamin C. (Major) Vitamins B_1 15 mg, B_2 10.2 mg, B_3 50 mg, B_5 10 mg, B_5 5 mg, C 300 mg/Capl. Bot. 100s, 130s, 1000. *otc.*
Use: Vitamin supplement.

Farbital Compound Capsules. (Major) Butalbital, caffeine, aspirin. Bot. 100s. *c-III.*
Use: Sedative, hypnotic, salicylate analgesic.

Farbital Compound with Codeine #3. (Major) Butalbital, caffeine, aspirin, codeine 30 mg. Bot. 1000s. *c-III.*
Use: Sedative, hypnotic, salicylate analgesic.

Farbital Tabs. (Major) Butalbital. Bot. 100s. *c-III.*
Use: Sedative, hypnotic.

farnoquinone.

Fastin. (SK-Beecham) Phentermine HCl 30 mg/Cap. Bot. 100s, 450s. Pack 150s. (5 × 30s). *c-IV.*
Use: Anorexiant.

fat emulsion, intravenous.
See: Liposyn 10% (Abbott).
Liposyn 20% (Abbott).
Travamulsion 10% (Baxter).
Travamulsion 20% (Baxter).
Intralipid 10% (Pharmacia & Upjohn).
Intralipid 20% (Pharmacia & Upjohn).
Soyacal 10% (Alpha Therapeutics).
Soyacal 20% (Alpha Therapeutics).
Liposyn II 10% (Abbott).
Liposyn II 20% (Abbott).

•**fat, hard, NF 18.**
Use: Pharmaceutic aid (suppository base).

Father John's Medicine Plus. (Oakhurst) Phenylephrine HCl 2.5 mg, chlorpheniramine maleate 1 mg, dextromethorphan HBr 7.5 mg, guaifenesin 30 mg, ammonium Cl 100 mg, sodium citrate/5 ml. Bot. 120 ml, 240 ml. *otc.*
Use: Decongestant, antihistamine, antitussive, expectorant.

Fattibase. (Paddock) Preblended fatty acid suppository base composed of

triglycerides of coconut oil and palm kernel oil. Jar 1 lb, 5 lb.
Use: Fatty acid suppository base.

fazadinium bromide.
Use: Neuromuscular blocking agent.

•**fazarabine.** (fah-ZAY-rah-BEAN) USAN.
Use: Antineoplastic.

F.C.A.H. Capsules. (Scherer) Chlorpheniramine maleate 4 mg, acetaminophen 162 mg, salicylamide 162 mg/Cap. Bot. 100s, 500s. *otc.*
Use: Antihistaminic, analgesic.

Feberin. (Arcum) Ferrous gluconate 3 gr, vitamins C 25 mg, B_1 2 mg, B_6 1 mg, B_2 1 mg, niacinamide 5 mg/Tab. Bot. 100s, 1000s. *otc.*
Use: Vitamin/mineral supplement.

febrile antigens. (Laboratory Diagnostics) Group O antigens (somatic) are dyed blue and group H antigens (flagellars) are dyed red for clear identification for detection of bacterial agglutinins, bacterial infections. Vial 5 ml.
Use: Diagnostic aid.

Febrinol. (Eon Labs) Acetaminophen 325 mg/Tab. Bot. 100s, 1000s. *otc.*
Use: Analgesic.

Fe-Brone. (Forest Pharm) Vitamins B_{12} 1 IU, folic acid 1 mg, ferrous sulfate exsiccated (powdered) 200 mg, ferrous sulfate exsiccated (timed) 200 mg, C acid 100 mg, B_6 0.5 mg, B_1 2 mg, B_2 1 mg, copper 0.9 mg, zinc 0.5 mg, manganese 0.3 mg/Cap. Bot. 30s, 100s, 1000s. *Rx.*
Use: Vitamin/mineral supplement.

Fedahist Gyrocaps. (Schwarz Pharma) Pseudoephedrine HCl 65 mg, chlorpheniramine maleate 10 mg/SR Cap. Bot. 100s. *Rx.*
Use: Decongestant, antihistamine.

Fedahist Timecaps. (Schwarz Pharma) Pseudoephedrine HCl 120 mg, chlorpheniramine maleate 8 mg/SR Cap. Bot. 100s. *Rx.*
Use: Decongestant, antihistamine.

Fedahist Tablets. (Schwarz Pharma) Pseudoephedrine HCl 60 mg, chlorpheniramine maleate 4 mg, sorbitol (alcohol and sugar free)/Tab. Bot. 100s. *Rx.*
Use: Decongestant, antihistamine.

Feen-a-Mint Dual Formula. (Schering Plough) Docusate sodium 100 mg, yellow phenolphthalein 65 mg/Tab. Box 15s, 30s, 60s. *otc.*
Use: Laxative.

Feen-a-Mint Gum. (Schering Plough) Yellow phenolphthalein 97.2 mg/Chew-

ing gum Tab. Box 5s, 16s, 40s. *otc.*
Use: Laxative.

Feen-a-Mint Mint. (Schering Plough) Yellow phenolphthalein 97.2 mg/Chewable mint tab. Box 20s. *otc.*
Use: Laxative.

Feen-a-Mint Pills. (Schering Plough) Docusate sodium 100 mg, yellow phenolphthalein 65 mg/Tab. Box 15s, 30s, 60s. *otc.*
Use: Laxative.

Feg-I. (Western Research) Ferrous gluconate 300 mg/Tab. Handicount 28s (36 bags of 28 tab.). *otc.*
Use: Iron supplement.

Feiba VH Immuno. (Immuno-U.S.) Freeze-dried anti-inhibitor coagulant complex. Heparin free. Vapor heated. Inj. Vial with diluent and needle. *Rx.*
Use: Antihemophilic.

•**felbamate.** (FELL-buh-MATE) USAN.
Use: Antiepileptic; treatment of Lennox-Gastaut Syndrome. [Orphan drug]
See: Felbatol (Wallace Labs).

Felbatol. (Wallace Labs) Felbamate, lactose 400 mg or 600 mg/tab., Felbamate, 600 mg/5 ml/susp. **Tab.:** Bot. 100s and UD 100s. **Susp.:** 240 ml and 960 ml. *Rx.*
Use: Antiepileptic. Due to 10 cases of aplastic anemia associated with felbamate use (including 2 deaths), the FDA and Carter-Wallace recommend that use of the drug be suspended unless the physician decides that withdrawal would pose an even greater risk to the patient. Patients should not discontinue the drug on their own. There has been no product recall at this time (5/95).

•**felbinac.** (FELL-bih-nak) USAN.
Use: Anti-inflammatory.

Feldene. (Pfizer Laboratories) Piroxicam 10 mg or 20 mg/Cap. **10 mg:** Bot 100s. **20 mg:** Bot. 100s, 500s, UD 100s. *Rx.*
Use: Nonsteroidal anti-inflammatory drug; analgesic.

Fellobolic Injection. (Forest Pharm) Methandriol dipropionate 50 mg/ml. Vial 10 ml. *Rx.*

•**felodipine.** (feh-LOW-dih-peen) USAN.
Use: Vasodilator.
See: Plendil, Tab. (Merck).

•**felypressin.** USAN.
Use: Vasoconstrictor.

Femagene. (Tennessee) Boric acid, sodium borate, lactic acid, menthol, methylbenzethonium Cl, parachlorometaxylenol, lactose, surface-active

agents. Pow. 6 oz. *otc.*
Use: Feminine hygiene.

Femazole Tabs. (Major) Metronidazole 250 mg or 500 mg/Tab. **250 mg:** Bot. 100s, 250s, 500s. **500 mg:** Bot. 50s, 100s. *Rx.*
Use: Anti-infective.

Femcal. (Freeda). Calcium carbonate 250 mg, vitamin D_3 100 IU, B_1 100 mg, Mg, Mn, Si, kosher, sugar free/Tab. Bot. 100s and 250s. *otc.*
Use: Mineral/electrolyte supplement.

Femcaps. (Buffington) Acetaminophen, caffeine, ephedrine sulfate, atropine sulfate/Tab. Sugar, lactose and salt free Dispens-a-Kit 500s, Aidpaks 100s. *Rx.*
Use: Analgesic, bronchodilator, anticholinergic, antispasmodic.

Femcet. (Whitby) Acetaminophen 325 mg, butalbital 50 mg, caffeine 40 mg/Cap. Bot. 100s. *Rx.*
Use: Analgesic, sedative, hypnotic.

femergin.
See: Ergotamine Tartrate (Various Mfr.)

Femicine. (Lake) Pulsatilla 28x, mercurius vivus 28x, sulphur 28x, polyethylene glycol. Supp. 10s, 15s w/applicator. *otc.*
Use: Vaginal preparation.

Femidyn.
See: Estrone (Various Mfr.)

Femilax. (G & W Labs) Docusate sodium 100 mg, phenolphthalein 65 mg/Tab. Bot. 30s, 60s, 90s. *otc.*
Use: Laxative.

Feminique Disposable Douche. (Schmid) Sodium benzoate, sorbic acid, lactic acid, octoxynol-9. Twin-pack Bot. 120 ml. *otc.*
Use: Douche.

Feminique Disposable Douche. (Schmid) Vinegar and water. Soln. Twin-packs. Bot. 180 ml. *otc.*
Use: Douche.

Feminone. (Pharmacia & Upjohn) Ethinyl estradiol 0.05 mg/Tab. Bot. 100s. *Rx.*
Use: Estrogen.

Femiron. (SK-Beecham) Iron 20 mg/Tab. Bot 40s, 120s. *otc.*
Use: Iron supplement.

Femiron Multi-Vitamins and Iron. (Menley & James) Iron 20 mg, vitamins A 5000 IU, D 400 IU, B_1 1.5 mg, riboflavin 1.7 mg, B_3 20 mg, C 60 mg, B_6 2 mg, B_{12} 6 mcg, B_5 10 mg, folic acid 0.4 mg, E 15 mg/Tab. Bot. 35s, 60s, 90s. *otc.*
Use: Vitamin/mineral supplement.

Femizol-M. (Lake Consumer Products) Miconazole nitrate 2%/Vaginal cream. Tube, with applicator. 45 g. *otc.*
Use: Vaginal antifungal.

Femotrone. (Bluco) Progesterone in oil 50 mg/ml. Vial 10 ml. *Rx.*
Use: Progestin.

FemPatch. (Parke-Davis) Estradiol 10.3 mg (0.025 mg/day)/Patch. Box. 4s. *Rx.*
Use: Estrogen replacement.

Femstat 3. (Procter-Syntex) 2% butoconazole nitrate, parabens, cetyl alcohol, mineral oil, steryl alcohol/Cream. Three 5 g prefilled applicators and 20 g with applicators. *otc.*
Use: Antifungal, vaginal.

•**fenalamide.** (fen-AL-am-IDE) USAN.
Use: Smooth muscle relaxant.

fenamisal. Phenyl aminosalicylate.

•**fenamole.** (FEN-ah-mole) USAN.
Use: Anti-inflammatory.

Fenaprin Tablets. (Sanofi Winthrop) Aspirin, chlormezanone. *Rx.*
Use: Salicylate analgesic, antianxiety agent.

Fenarol. (Sanofi Winthrop) Chlormezanone 100 mg or 200 mg/Tab. Bot. 100s.
Use: Antianxiety agent.

fenarsone.
See: Carbarsone (Various Mfr.)

•**fenbendazole.** (FEN-BEND-ah-zole) USAN.
Use: Anthelmintic.
See: Panacure (Hoechst-Roussel)

•**fenbufen.** (FEN-byoo-fen) USAN.
Use: Anti-inflammatory.
See: Cinopal (Lederle)

•**fencibutirol.** (fen-sih-BYOO-tih-role). USAN.
Use: Choleretic.

•**fenclofenac.** (FEN-kloe-fen-ACK) USAN.
Use: Anti-inflammatory.

•**fenclonine.** (fen-KLOE-neen) USAN. Under study by Pfizer.
Use: Serotonin inhibitor.

•**fenclorac.** (FEN-kloe-rack) USAN.
Use: Anti-inflammatory.

Fend. (Mine Safety Appliances).
A-2– Water soluble cream which forms a physical barrier to water insoluble irritants. Tube 3 oz, Jar lb.
E-2– This cream combines the functions of the water soluble Fend A-2 and water insoluble Fend I-2 creams. Tube 3 oz, Jar lb.
I-2– Water insoluble cream which forms a physical barrier to water soluble irritants. Tube 3 oz, Jar lb.

S-2– A silicone cream which forms a barrier against a combination of water soluble and water insoluble irritants. Tube 3 oz, Jar lb.
X– Industrial cold cream which rubs well into the skin and serves as a skin conditioner. Tube 3 oz, Jar lb.
Use: Skin protectant.

Fendol. (Buffington) Salicylamide, caffeine, acetaminophen, phenylephrine HCl/Tab. Sugar, lactose and salt free. Dispens-A-Kit 500s. Bot. 100s. *otc.*
Use: Analgesic combination.

•**fendosal.** (FEN-doe-sal) USAN.
Use: Anti-inflammatory.

Fenesin. (Dura) Guaifenesin 600 mg/SR Tab. Bot. 100s, 600s. *Rx.*
Use: Expectorant.

Fenesin DM. (Dura Pharm) Dextromethorphan HBr 30 mg, guaifenesin 600 mg/Tab. Bot. 100s. *Rx.*
Use: Antitussive, expectorant.

•**fenestrel.** (feh-NESS-trell) USAN. Under study.
Use: Estrogen.

•**fenethylline hydrochloride.** (FEN-ETH-ill-in) USAN.
Use: Stimulant (central).

•**fenfluramine hydrochloride.** (fen-FLURE-uh-meen) USAN.
Use: Anorexic.
See: Pondimin, Tab. (Robins).

•**fengabine.** (FEN-GAH-bean) USAN.
Use: Mood regulator.

•**fenimide.** (FEN-ih-mid) USAN.
Use: Tranquilizer, antipsychotic.

•**fenisorex.** (fen-EYE-so-rex) USAN.
Use: Anorexigenic, anorexic.

•**fenmetozole hydrochloride.** (FEN-MET-oh-zole) USAN.
Use: Antidepressant, antagonist (to narcotics).

•**fenmetramide.** (fen-MEH-trah-mide) USAN.
Use: Antidepressant.

fennel oil.
Use: Pharmaceutic aid (flavor).

•**fenobam.** (FEN-oh-bam) USAN.
Use: Sedative, hypnotic.

•**fenoctimine sulfate.** (fen-OCK-tih-MEEN) USAN.
Use: Gastric antisecretory.

fenofibrate.
Use: Antihyperlipidemic.
See: Lipidil, Cap. (Fournier).

•**fenoldopam mesylate.** (feh-NAHL-doe-pam) USAN.
Use: Antihypertensive, dopamine agonist.

See: Corlopam (SK-Beecham).

•**fenoprofen.** (FEN-oh-PRO-fen) USAN.
Use: Anti-inflammatory, analgesic.

•**fenoprofen calcium,** (FEN-oh-PRO-fen) U.S.P. 23.
Use: Anti-inflammatory, analgesic.
See: Nalfon, Cap., Tab. (Lilly).

•**fenoterol.** (FEN-oh-TER-ahl) USAN.
Use: Bronchodilator.

•**fenpipalone.** (FEN-PIP-ah-lone) USAN.
Use: Anti-inflammatory.

•**fenprinast hydrochloride.** (fen-PRIH-nast) USAN.
Use: Bronchodilator (antiallergic).

•**fenprostalene.** (FEN-PRAHST-ah-leen) USAN.
Use: Luteolysin.

•**fenquizone.** (FEN-kwih-zone) USAN.
Use: Diuretic.

•**fenretinide.** (fen-RET-ih-nide) USAN.
Use: Antineoplastic.

•**fenspiride hydrochloride.** (fen-SPIH-rid) USAN.
Use: Bronchodilator, anti-adrenergic (α-receptor).

fentanyl.
Use: Narcotic analgesic.
See: Duragesic, Transdermal (Janssen).

•**fentanyl citrate,** (FEN-tuh-nill) U.S.P. 23.
Use: Narcotic analgesic.
See: Sublimaze, Inj. (Janssen).
Oralet (Abbott).

fentanyl citrate. (Various Mfr.) 0.05 mg/ml. Inj. Amp. 2 ml, 5 ml, 10 ml, 20 ml. Vial. 30 ml, 50 ml.
Use: Narcotic analgesic.

Fentanyl Citrate and Droperidol. (Astra) Fentanyl 0.05 mg, droperidol 2.5 mg/ml. Inj. Amp and Vial 2 ml, 5 ml. *c-ii.*
Use: General anesthetic.
See: Innovar, Inj. (Janssen).

Fentanyl Oralet. (Abbott) Fentanyl 200 mcg, 300 mcg, 400 mg sucrose, liquid glucose/2 oz. 25s. *c-ii.*
Use: General anesthetic.

Fentanyl Transdermal System. (FEN-tuh-nill) *c-ii.*
See: Duragesic-25 (Janssen).
Duragesic-50 (Janssen).
Duragesic-75 (Janssen).
Duragesic-100 (Janssen).

•**fentiazac.** (fen-TIE-azz-ACK) USAN.
Use: Anti-inflammatory.

•**fenticlor.** (FEN-tih-Klor) USAN.
Use: Antiseptic (topical), fungicide.

•**fenticonazole nitrate.** (FEN-tih-KOE-nah-zole) USAN.
Use: Antifungal.

Fenton Elixir. (Sanofi Winthrop) Ferrous gluconate. *otc.*
Use: Iron supplement.

Fenylhist. (Roberts) Diphenhydramine HCl 25 mg or 50 mg/Cap. Bot. 1000s. *otc.*
Use: Antihistamine.

fenyramidol hydrochloride. Phenyramidol HCl.

•**fenyripol hydrochloride.** (FEH-nee-rih-pahl) USAN. α-(2-pyrimidinylaminomethyl) benzyl alcohol hydrochloride.
Use: Skeletal muscle relaxant.

Feocyte. (Dunhall) Iron 110 mg, vitamins C 100 mg, B_6 2 mg, B_{12} 50 mcg, copper sulfate, folic acid 0.8 mg, desiccated liver 15 mg/Prolonged Action Tab. Bot. 100s. *Rx.*
Use: Vitamin/mineral supplement.

Feocyte Injectable. (Dunhall) Peptonized iron 15 mg, vitamin B_{12} 200 mcg, liver injection N.F. beef 10 units, sodium citrate 10 mg, benzyl alcohol 2%/ml. Vial 10 ml. *Rx.*
Use: Vitamin/mineral supplement.

Feosol Capsules. (SK-Beecham) Dried ferrous sulfate 159 mg (50 mg iron)/SR Cap. Bot. 30s, 100s, 500s, UD 100s. *otc.*
Use: Iron supplement.

Feosol Elixir. (SK-Beecham) Ferrous sulfate (44 mg iron) 220 mg/5 ml, alcohol 5%. Bot. 16 oz. *otc.*
Use: Iron supplement.

Feosol Tablets. (SK-Beecham) Dried ferrous sulfate 200 mg (65 mg iron)/Tab. Bot. 100s, 1000s, UD 100s. *otc.*
Use: Iron supplement.

Feostat. (Forest) **Tab.:** Ferrous fumarate 100 mg (33 mg iron)/Chew. tab. Bot. 100s, 1000s. **Drops:** Ferrous fumarate 45 mg (15 mg iron)/0.6 ml. Bot. 60 ml. *otc.*
Use: Iron supplement.

Feostat Suspension. (Forest) Ferrous fumarate 100 mg (33 mg iron)/5 ml. Bot. 240 ml. *otc.*
Use: Iron supplement.

FE-Plus Protein. (Miller) Iron (as an iron-protein complex) 50 mg/Tab. Bot. 100s. *otc.*
Use: Iron supplement.

Ferancee. (J & J-Merck) Elemental iron 67 mg (as fumarate), vitamin C 150 mg Tab. Bot. 100s. *otc.*
Use: Vitamin/mineral supplement.

Ferancee-HP. (J & J-Merck) Elemental iron 110 mg (from 330 mg ferrous fumarate), ascorbic acid 350 mg, so-

dium ascorbate 281 mg/Tab. Bot. 60s. *otc.*
Use: Vitamin/mineral supplement.

Feratab. (Upsher-Smith) Ferrous sulfate 300 mg (60 mg iron)/Tab. Bot. 100s. *otc.*
Use: Iron supplement.

Ferate-C. (Pal-Pak) Ferrous fumarate 150 mg, ascorbic acid 200 mg, docusate sodium 25 mg/Tab. Bot. 100s, 1000s. *otc.*
Use: Vitamin/mineral supplement, stool softener.

Fer-Gen-Sol Drops. (Goldline) Ferrous sulfate 7 H_2O 75 mg/0.6 ml base. Drops. Bot. 50 ml. *otc.*
Use: Iron supplement.

Feridex I.V. (Berlex) Iron 11.2 mg, mannitol 61.3 mg/ml, dextran 5.6 to 9.1 mg/ml/Inj. Vial. 5 ml. *Rx.*
Use: Radiopaque agent.

Fer-in-Sol. (Bristol-Myers) **Drops:** Elemental iron 15 mg/0.6 ml, alcohol 0.02%. Bot. w/dropper 50 ml. **Syr.:** 18 mg/5 ml. Alcohol 5%. Bot. 16 fl oz.
Use: Iron supplement.

Fer-Iron. (Rugby) Ferrous sulfate 75 mg (iron 15 mg)/0.6 ml. Drops. Bot. 50 ml. *otc.*
Use: Iron supplement.

Ferocyl. (Hudson) Ferrous fumarate 150 mg (iron 50 mg), docusate sodium 100 mg/TR Cap. Bot. 100s. *otc.*
Use: Iron supplement, stool softener.

Fero-Folic 500. (Abbott) Ferrous sulfate controlled-release (equivalent to 105 mg iron), vitamin C 500 mg, folic acid 0.8 mg/Filmtab. Bot. 100s, 500s. *Rx.*
Use: Vitamin/mineral supplement.

Fero-Grad 500 Filmtab. (Abbott) Sodium ascorbate 500 mg, ferrous sulfate equivalent to 105 mg iron/CR Filmtab. Bot. 30s, 100s, 500s, UD 100s. *otc.*
Use: Iron supplement.

Fero-Gradumet Filmtab. (Abbott) Ferrous sulfate 525 mg controlled-release equivalent to 105 mg iron/Filmtab. Bot. 100s. *otc.*
Use: Iron supplement.

Ferolix. (Century) Ferrous sulfate 5 gr, alcohol 5%/10 ml Elix. Bot. 8 oz, pt, gal. *otc.*
Use: Iron supplement.

Ferosan Forte. (Sandia) Ferrous fumarate 300 mg, liver-stomach concentrate 150 mg, vitamin B_{12} w/intrinsic factor concentrate 7.5 mcg, intrinsic factor concentrate 150 mg, B_{12} 7.5 mcg, ascorbic acid 75 mg, folic acid 1 mg,

sorbitol 50 mg/Tab. Bot. 100s. *Rx.*
Use: Vitamin/mineral supplement.

Ferosan Syrup. (Sandia) Ferrous fumarate 91.2 mg, B_1 10 mg, B_6 3 mg, B_{12} 25 mcg/5 ml 16 oz, gal. *otc.*
Use: Vitamin/mineral supplement.

Ferospace. (Hudson) Ferrous sulfate 250 mg (iron 50 mg)/TR Cap. Bot. 100s. *otc.*
Use: Iron supplement.

Ferotrinsic. (Rugby) Iron 110 mg (from ferrous fumarate), vitamins B_{12} 15 mcg, C 75 mg, intrinsic factor (as concentrate or from stomach preparations) 240 mg, folic acid 0.5 mg/Cap. 100s, 500s, 1000s. *Rx.*
Use: Vitamin/mineral supplement.

Feroweet. (Barth's) Vitamins B_1 6 mg, B_2 12 mg, niacin 4 mg, iron 30 mg, B_{12} 10 mcg, B_6 95 mcg, pantothenic acid 50 mcg/3 Cap. Bot. 100s, 500s, 1000s. *otc.*
Use: Vitamin/mineral supplement.

Ferracomp. (Roberts) Liver 2 mcg, vitamins B_{12} 15 mcg, B_1 10 mg, B_2 5 mg, B_6 1 mg, calcium pantothenate 1 mg, niacinamide 10 mg, iron 31.3 mg/ml. Vial 30 ml. *otc.*
Use: Vitamin/mineral supplement.

Ferralet. (Mission) Ferrous gluconate 320 mg (37 mg iron)/Tab. Bot. 100s. *otc.*
Use: Iron supplement.

Ferralet Plus. (Mission) Ferrous gluconate equivalent to 46 mg iron, C 400 mg, folic acid 0.8 mg, vitamin B_{12} 25 mcg/Tab. Bot. 60s. *otc.*
Use: Vitamin/mineral supplement.

Ferralet S.R. (Mission) Ferrous gluconate 320 mg (iron 37 mg)/SR Tab. Bot. 30s. *otc.*
Use: Iron supplement.

Ferra-TD. (Goldline) Ferrous sulfate 250 mg (iron 50 mg)/TR Cap. Bot. 100s, 1000s. *otc.*
Use: Iron supplement.

Ferrets. (Pharmics) Ferrous fumarate 325 mg, iron 106 mg/Tab. Bot. 100s. *otc.*
Use: Iron supplement.

ferric ammonium citrate. Ammonium iron (Fe^{+++}) citrate.
Use: Iron supplement.

ferric ammonium sulfate. (Various Mfr.)
Use: Astringent.

ferric ammonium tartrate. (Various Mfr.)
Use: Iron supplement.

ferric cacodylate. (Various Mfr.)
Use: Leukemias & iron deficiency.

ferric chloride. (Various Mfr.)
Use: Astringent.

•**ferric chloride Fe 59.** USAN.
Use: Radioactive agent.

ferric citrochloride tincture. Iron (3+) chloride citrate.
Use: Hematinic.

•**ferric fructose.** (FER-ik FRUKE-tose) USAN. Fructose iron complex with potassium (2:1).
Use: Hematinic.

ferric glycerophosphate. Glycerol phosphate iron (3+) salt.
Use: Pharmaceutic necessity.

ferric hypophosphite. Iron (3+) phosphinate.
Use: Pharmaceutic necessity.

•**ferriclate calcium sodium.** (fer-ih-KLATE) USAN.
Use: Hematinic.

•**ferric oxide,** N.F. 18.
Use: Pharmaceutic aid (color).

ferric oxide, yellow.
Use: Pharmaceutic aid (color).

ferric "peptonate". (Various Mfr.)
See: Iron Peptonized.

ferric pyrophosphate, soluble. Iron (3+) citrate pyrophosphate.

ferric quinine citrate, "green". (Various Mfr.)
Use: Iron supplement.

ferric subsulfate solution. (Various Mfr.)
Use: Local use on the skin.

•**ferristene.** (FER-ih-steen) USAN.
Use: Diagnostic aid (paramagnetic).

Ferrizyme. (Abbott Diagnostics) Enzyme immunoassay for qualitative determination of ferritin in human serum or plasma. Test kit 100s.
Use: Diagnostic aid, paramagnetic.

ferrocholate.
See: Ferrocholinate.

ferrocholinate. Ferrocholate. Ferrocholine. A chelate prepared by reacting equimolar quantities of freshly precipitated ferric hydroxide with choline dihydrogen citrate.
Use: Iron supplement.
See: Chel-Iron, Preps. (Kinney).

ferrocholine.
See: Ferrocholinate.
Kelex, Tabseal. (Nutrition).

Ferro-Cyte. (Spanner) Iron peptonate 20 mg, liver injection (20 mg/ml) 0.25 ml, vitamins B_1 22 mg, B_2 0.5 mg, B_6 2.5 mg, B_{12} 30 mcg, niacinamide 25 mg, panthenol mg/ml. Inj. Multiple dose vial 10 ml. *Rx.*
Use: Vitamin/mineral supplement.

Ferro-Docusate TR. (Parmed) Ferrous fumarate 150 mg (iron 50 mg), docu-

sate sodium 100 mg/TR Cap. Bot. 100s. *otc.*
Use: Iron supplement, stool softener.

Ferro-Dok TR. (Major) Ferrous fumarate 150 mg (iron 50 mg), docusate sodium 100 mg/TR Cap. Bot. 100s. *otc.*
Use: Iron supplement, stool softener.

Ferro-DSS. (Geneva Pharm) Ferrous fumarate 150 mg (iron 50 mg), docusate sodium 100 mg/TR Cap. Bot. 100s. *otc.*
Use: Iron supplement, stool softener.

Ferrodyl Chewable Tablets. (Arcum) Ferrous fumarate 320 mg, vitamin C 200 mg/Tab. Bot. 100s, 1000s. *otc.*
Use: Vitamin/mineral supplement.

Ferromar. (Marnel) Ferrous fumarate 201.5 mg (iron 65 mg), vitamin C 200 mg/SR Capl. Bot. 100s. *otc.*
Use: Iron Supplement.

Ferroneed. (Hanlon) Ferrous gluconate 300 mg, ascorbic acid 60 mg/Cap. Bot. 100s. *otc.*
Use: Vitamin/mineral supplement.

Ferroneed T-Caps. (Hanlon) Ferrous fumarate 250 mg, thiamine HCl 5 mg, ascorbic acid 50 mg/TD Cap. Bot. 100s. *otc.*
Use: Vitamin/mineral supplement.

Ferronex. (Taylor) Iron from ferrous gluconate 2.9 mg, Vitamins B_{12} equivalent 1 mcg, B_2 0.75 mg, B_3 50 mg, B_5 1.25 mg, B_{12} 15 mcg, procaine 2%/ml. Inj. Vial 30 ml. *Rx.*
Use: Vitamin/mineral supplement.

Ferro-Sequels. (Lederle) Ferrous fumarate 150 mg (equivalent to 50 mg elemental iron), dioctyl sodium sulfosuccinate 100 mg/TD Cap. Bot. 30s, 100s, 1000s, UD 10×10s. *otc.*
Use: Iron supplement.

Ferrospan Capsules. (Imperial Lab.) Ferrous fumarate 200 mg, ascorbic acid 100 mg/Tab. Bot. 100s, 1000s. *otc.*
Use: Vitamin/mineral supplement.

Ferrosyn Injection. (Standex) Cyanocobalamin 30 mcg, liver 2 mcg, ferrous gluconate 100 mg, riboflavin 1.5 mg, panthenol 2.5 mg, niacinamide 100 mg, procaine 2%. Vial 30 ml. *Rx.*
Use: Vitamin/mineral supplement.

Ferrosyn S.C. (Standex) Iron 60 mg, vitamin B_{12} 5 mcg, magnesium 0.6 mg, copper 0.3 mg, manganese 0.1 mg, potassium 0.5 mg, zinc 0.15 mg/Tab. Bot. 100s, 1000s. *otc.*
Use: Vitamin/mineral supplement.

Ferrosyn See Tabs. (Standex) Iron 34 mg, ascorbic acid 60 mg/Tab. Bot. 100s, 1000s. *otc.*

Use: Vitamin/mineral supplement.

Ferrosyn Tab. (Standex) Iron 60 mg, vitamin B_{12} 5 mcg, magnesium 0.6 mg, copper 0.3 mg, manganese 0.1 mg, potassium 0.5 mg, zinc 0.15 mg/Tab. Bot. 100s. *otc.*
Use: Vitamin/mineral supplement.

ferrous bromide. (FER-uhs) (Various Mfr.)
Use: In chorea & tuberculous cervical adenitis.

ferrous carbonate mass. Vallet's mass. (Various Mfr.)
Use: Iron supplement.

ferrous carbonate, saccharated. (Various Mfr.)
Use: Iron supplement.

•**ferrous citrate Fe 59,** USAN.
Use: Radioactive agent.

•**ferrous fumarate,** U.S.P. 23.
Use: Hematinic.
See: Childron, Susp. (Fleming).
Eldofe, Tab. (Canright).
El-Ped-Ron, Liq. (Zeneca).
Farbegen, Cap. (Hickam).
Feco-T, Cap. (Blaine).
Ferretts, Tab. (Pharmics).
Fumasorb, Tab. (Hoechst Marion Roussel).
Fumerin, Tab. (Laser).
Ircon, Tab. (Key).
Laud-Iron, Tab., Susp. (Amfre-Grant).
Maniron, Meltab. (Jones Medical)).
W/Ascorbic Acid.
See: C-Ron, Preps. (Solvay).
Cytoferin, Tab. (Wyeth-Ayerst).
Eldofe-C, Tab. (Canright).
Ferancee, Tab. (J & J-Merck).
Ferancee-HP, Tab. (Stuart).
Ferrodyl Chewable Tab. (Arcum).
Ferromar, SR Cap. (Marnel).
Min-Hema Chewable, Tab. (Scrip).
W/Ascorbic acid and folic acid.
See: Fer-Regules, Cap. (Quality Generics).
Ferro-Docusate T.R., Cap. (Parmed)
Ferro Dok TR, Cap. (Major)
Ferro-DSS S.R., Cap. (Geneva Pharm)
Ferro-Sequels, Cap. (Lederle).
W/Norethindrone, mestranol.
See: Ortho Novum Fe-28, Fe-28, 1 mg Fe-28, Tab. (Ortho).
W/Vitamins and minerals.
See: Stuart Formula, Tab. (Stuart).
Stuart Prenatal, Tab. (Stuart).
Stuartnatal 1 + 1, Tab. (Stuart).
Theron, Tab. (Stuart).
Vitanate, Tab. (Century).

ferrous fumarate and docusate so-

dium extended-release tablets.
Use: Iron supplement.

•**ferrous gluconate,** U.S.P. 23.
Use: Hematinic.
See: Entron, Cap., Tab. (LaCrosse).
Fergon Prods. (Sanofi Winthrop Products).
W/Ascorbic acid, desiccated liver, vitamin B complex.
See: I.L.X. w/B_{12}, Tab. (Kenwood).
Stuart Hematinic, Liq. (Stuart).
W/Polyoxyethylene glucitan monolaurate.
See: Simron, Cap. (Hoechst Marion Roussel).

ferrous iodide. (Various Mfr.)
Use: In chronic tuberculosis.

ferrous iodide syrup. (Various Mfr.)
Use: In chronic tuberculosis.

ferrous lactate. (Various Mfr.)
Use: Iron supplement.

•**ferrous sulfate,** U.S.P. 23.
Use: Hematinic.
See: Feosol, Spansule, Tab., Elix. (SK-Beecham).
Fer-iron, Drops (Rugby).
Fero-Gradumet, Tab. (Abbott).
Ferolix, Elix. (Century).
Ferrous Sulfate Filmseals, Tab. (Parke-Davis).
Fesotyme SR, Cap. (Zeneca).
Irospan, Cap., Tab. (Fielding).
Mol-Iron, Prods. (Schering Plough).
W/Ascorbic acid.
See: Fero-Grad-500, Tab. (Abbott).
Mol-Iron W/Vitamin C, Tab., Chronosules (Schering Plough).
W/Ascorbic acid, folic acid.
See: Fero-Folic-500, Tab. (Abbott).
W/Cyanocobalamin, ascorbic acid, folic acid.
See: Intrin, Cap. (Merit).
W/Folic acid.
See: Folvron, Cap. (Lederle).
W/Maalox.
See: Fermalox, Tab. (Rhone-Poulenc Rorer Consumer).

•**ferrous sulfate, dried,** U.S.P. 23.
Use: Antianemic.
See: Fer-In-Sol (B-M Squibb Nutritionals).
Feosol (SmithKline-Beecham).
Ferrous Sulfate (Various).
Ferra-TD (Goldline).
Slow Fe (Novartis).

•**ferrous sulfate Fe 59.** USAN.
Use: Radioactive agent.

Ferrous Sulfate Filmseals. (Parke-Davis) Ferrous sulfate 5 gr/DR Tab. Bot. 1000s, UD 100s. *otc.*
Use: Iron supplement.

Fertility Tape. (Weston Labs.) Regular, extrasensitive, less-sensitive. W/Fertility Testor, cervical glucose test. Pkg. test 60s.
Use: Diagnostic aid.

Fertinex. (Serono) Urofollitropin 75 IU/Pow. for Inj., lyophilized. Ampules. 1, 20, 100 amps with diluent. Urofollitropin 150 IU/Pow. for Inj., lyophilized. Ampules. Single with diluent. *Rx.*
Use: Induction of ovulation.

•**ferumoxides.** (feh-roo-MOX-ides) USAN.
Use: Diagnostic aid (paramagnetic).
See: Ferides (Advanced Magnetics)

•**ferumoxsil.** (feh-roo-MOX-sill) USAN.
Use: Diagnostic aid (paramagnetic).
See: Gastromark (Advanced Magnetics).

Ferusal. (Eon Labs) Ferrous sulfate 325 mg/Tab. *otc.*
Use: Iron supplement.

Festalan. (Hoechst Marion Roussel) Lipase 6000 units, amylase 30,000 units, protease 20,000 units, atropine methylnitrate 1 mg/EC Tab. Bot. 100s, 1000s. *Rx.*
Use: Digestive enzyme.

Fetinic. (Roberts) Iron 3.6 mg, vitamins B_{12} equivalent 2 mcg, B_1 10 mg, B_2 0.5 mg, B_3 10 mg, B_5 1 mg, B_6 1 mg, B_{12} 15 mcg, chlorobutanol 0.5%, benzyl alcohol 2%/ml. Vial 30 ml. *Rx.*
Use: Vitamin/mineral supplement.

Fetinic-MW. (Roberts) Iron 66 mg (from ferrous fumarate), vitamins B_{12} 5 mcg, C 60 mg/SR Cap. Bot. 100s. *otc.*
Use: Vitamin/mineral supplement.

•**fetoxylate hydrochloride.** (fee-TOX-ih-LATE) USAN.
Use: Relaxant (smooth muscle).

Feverall, Children's. (Upsher-Smith) Acetaminophen 120 mg/Supp. Pkg. 6s. *otc.*
Use: Analgesic.

Feverall, Infants'. (Upsher-Smith) Acetaminophen 80 mg. Supp. Pkg. 6s. *otc.*
Use: Analgesic.

Feverall, Junior Strength. (Upsher-Smith) Acetaminophen 325 mg/Supp. Pkg. 6s. *otc.*
Use: Analgesic.

Feverall Sprinkle. (Upsher-Smith) Acetaminophen 80 mg or 160 mg/Cap. Bot. 20s. *otc.*
Use: Analgesic.

•**fexofenadine hydrochloride.** (fex-oh-FEN-ah-deen)USAN.
Use: Antihistamine.
See: Allegra, Tab. (Hoechst Marion Roussel).

•**fezolamine fumarate.** (feh-ZOLE-ah-MEEN) USAN.
Use: Antidepressant.

FGN-1. (Cell Pathways) *Rx.*
Use: Treatment of adenomatous polyposis coli. [Orphan drug]

•**fiacitabine.** (fih-AH-sit-ah-BEEN) USAN.
Use: Antiviral.

•**fialuridine.** (fie-al-YOUR-ih-deen) USAN.
Use: Antiviral.

fiau. (Oclassen) *Rx.*
Use: Treatment of hepatitis B. [Orphan drug]

Fiberall. (Novartis Consumer Health) Calcium carbophil 1250 mg (equiv. to 1000 mg polycarbophil). Chew. Tab. Lemon-flavor. Pkg. 18s. *otc.*
Use: Laxative.

Fiberall Natural Flavor. (Novartis Self-Mediation) **Pow.:** Psyllium hydrophilic mucilloid 3.4 g, wheat bran, sodium < 10 mg, potassium 60 mg, calories 6/5.9 g, saccharin. Can 150 g, 300 g, 450 g. **Wafer:** Psyllium hydrophilic mucilloid 3.4 g, wheat bran, oats, sucrose. Box 14s. *otc.*
Use: Laxative.

Fiberall Orange Flavor. (Novartis Consumer Health) Psyllium hydrophilic mucilloid 3.4 g, wheat bran, sodium < 10 mg, potassium 60 mg, calories 6/5.9 g Pow. Can 150 g, 300 g, 450 g. *otc.*
Use: Laxative.

Fibercon. (Lederle) Calcium polycarbophil 500 mg/Tab. Bot. 36s, 60s. *otc.*
Use: Laxative.

Fiber Guard. (Wyeth-Ayerst) All natural high fiber supplement 530 mg/Tab. Bot. 100s, 200s. *otc.*
Use: Fiber supplement.

Fiberlan. (Elan) Protein 50 g, fat 40 g, carbohydrates 160 g, Na 920 mg, K 1.56 g, fiber 14 g/per L. With vitamins A, C, B, B_2, B_3, D, E, B_5, B_6, B_{12}, K, Ca, Fe, folic acid, P, I, Mg, Zn, Cu, biotin, Mn, choline, Cl, Se, Cr, Mo. Liq. Bot. 237 ml. *otc.*
Use: Nutritional therapy.

Fiber-Lax. (Rugby) Calcium polycarbophil 625 mg (equiv. to 500 mg polycarbophil)/Tab. Bot. 60s. *otc.*
Use: Laxative.

Fibermed High-Fiber Snacks. (Purdue Frederick) One serving (15 snacks) contains 5 g dietary fiber. Box 8 oz. Packs of 24 × 1.3 oz. *otc.*
Use: Fiber supplement.

Fibermed High-Fiber Supplement. (Purdue Frederick) Each supplement

contains 5 g dietary fiber. Box 14s. Institutional pack, Box 144s of two supplements. *otc.*
Use: Fiber supplement.

Fibernorm. (G & W) Calcium polycarbophil 625 mg/Tab. Bot. 60s. *otc.*
Use: Laxative.

Fiber Rich. (Columbia) Phenylpropanolamine HCl 75 mg/Tab. Bot. 24s. *otc.*
Use: Nonprescription diet aid.

Fibrad. (Ross) Fiber 7 g, sodium 15 mg, potassium < 25 mg. Pow. Bot. 414 g. *otc.*
Use: Nongelling dietary fiber source for enteral use.

Fibre Trim Tablets. (Schering Plough) Grain and citrus fruit concentrated dietary fiber. Bot. 100s, 250s. *otc.*
Use: Nonprescription diet aid.

Fibre Trim w/Calcium Tablets. (Schering Plough) Grain and citrus fruit concentrated dietary fiber w/calcium. Bot. 90s, 225s. *otc.*
Use: Nonprescription diet aid.

fibrin hydrolysate.
See: Aminosol, Soln. (Abbott).

●**fibrinogen I 125.** (FIE-BRIN-oh-jen I 125) USAN.
Use: Diagnostic aid.

fibrinogen (human). Partially purified fibrinogen prepared by fractionation from normal human plasma. *Rx.*
Use: Coagulant (clotting factor). [Orphan drug]

fibrinolysin (human) with desoxyribonuclease. Plasmin. An enzyme prepared by activating a human blood plasma fraction with streptokinase. *Rx.*
Use: Topical enzyme preparation.
See: Elase, Oint., Pow. (Parke-Davis).

fibrinolysis inhibitor.
See: Amicar Syr., Tab., Vial (Lederle).

fibronectin.
Use: Treatment of nonhealing corneal ulcers or epithelial defects. [Orphan drug]

●**filaminast.** (fih-LAM-in-ast) USAN.
Use: Anti-asthmatic (selective phosphodiesterase IV inhibitor).

Filaxis. (Amlab) Vitamins A 25,000 IU, D 1250 IU, C 150 mg, E 5 IU, B_1 12 mg, B_2 5 mg, B_6 0.5 mg, B_{12} 5 mcg, calcium pantothenate 5 mg, niacinamide 100 mg, iron 15 mg, iodine 0.15 mg, magnesium 10 mg, potassium 5 mg, calcium 75 mg, phosphorous 60 mg/Tab. Bot. 30s, 100s. Available w/B_{12}. Bot. 30s, 60s, 100s. *otc.*
Use: Vitamin/mineral supplement.

●**filgrastim (G-CSF).** (fill-GRAH-stim) USAN.
Use: Biological response modifier, antineoplastic adjunct, antineutropenic, hematopietic stimulant. [Orphan drug]
See: Neupogen (Amgen).

●**filipin.** (FIH-lih-pin) USAN.
Use: Antifungal.

Finac. (C & M Pharmacal) Salicylic acid 2%, isopropyl alcohol 22.5%, propylene glycol, acetone in lotion base. Bot. 60 ml. *otc.*
Use: Antiacne.

●**finasteride.** (fih-NASS-teer-ide) USAN.
Use: Benign prostatic hypertrophy therapy, antineoplastic, antineutropenic, inhibitor (alpha-reductase).
See: Proscar, Tab. (Merck).

Fiogesic. (Sandoz) Phenylpropanolamine HCl 25 mg, pyrilamine maleate 12.5 mg, pheniramine maleate 12.5 mg, calcium carbaspirin 382 mg (equiv. to 300 mg ASA)/Tab. Bot. 100s. *otc.*
Use: Decongestant, antihistamine, analgesic.

Fiorgen Tabs PF. (Goldline) Butabarbital 50 mg, aspirin 325 mg, caffeine 40 mg/Tab. Bot. 100s, 1000s. *c-III.*
Use: Sedative, hypnotic, salicylate, analgesic.

Fioricet. (Sandoz) Acetaminophen 325 mg, butalbital 50 mg, caffeine 40 mg/Tab. Bot. 100s, 500s. SandoPak 100s. *Rx.*
Use: Analgesic, sedative, hypnotic.

Fioricet w/Codeine. (Sandoz) Codeine phosphate 30 mg, acetaminophen 325 mg, caffeine 40 mg, butalbital 50 mg/Cap. Bot. 100s, Control pak 25s. *c-III.*
Use: Narcotic analgesic combination.

Fiorinal. (Sandoz) Butalbital (Sandoptal) 50 mg, caffeine 40 mg, aspirin 325 mg/Tab. or Cap. **Tab.:** Bot. 100s, 1000s. Sandopak 100s. **Cap.:** Bot. 100s, 500s. Control Pak 25s. *c-III.*
Use: Sedative, hypnotic, salicylate analgesic.

Fiorinal with Codeine No. 3 Capsules. (Sandoz) Butalbital 50 mg, caffeine 40 mg, aspirin 325 mg, codeine phosphate 30 mg/Cap. Bot. 100s. Control Pak 25s. *c-III.*
Use: Sedative, hypnotic, analgesic combination.

Fiorpap. (Creighton) Butalbital 50 mg, acetaminophen 325 mg, caffeine 40 mg/Tab. Bot 100s, 500s. *Rx.*
Use: Analgesic.

fire ant venom, allergenic extract, im-

ported.
Use: Skin test, immunotherapy. [Orphan drug]

Firmdent. (Moyco) Formerly Moy. Karaya gum 94.6%, sodium borate 5.36% Pkg. 3 oz. *otc.*
Use: Denture adhesive.

First Aid Cream. (Johnson & Johnson) Cetyl alcohol, glyceryl stearate, isopropyl palmitate, stearyl alcohol, synthetic beeswax. Tube 0.8 oz, 1.5 oz, 2.5 oz. *otc.*
Use: Antiseptic, skin protectant.

First Aid Cream. (Walgreen) Benzocaine 3%, allantoin 0.2%, benzyl alcohol 4%, phenol 0.25%. Tube 1.5 oz. *otc.*
Use: Anesthetic, antiseptic.

First Choice. (Polymer Technology International) 50s.
Use: In vitro reagent test strips for blood glucose monitoring.

First Response Ovulation Predictor. (Tambrands) Monoclonal antibody-based enzyme immunoassay test for hLH in urine. Test kit 1s. *otc.*
Use: Diagnostic aid.

First Response Pregnancy Test. (Tambrands) Reagent in-home kit for urine testing. Test kit 1s.
Use: Diagnostic aid.

fish oil concentrate, natural. Natural fish oil concentrate containing EPA (Eicosapentaenoicacid) and DHA (Docosahexaenoic acid).
Use: Fish oil.
See: Comega, Cap. (Upsher-Smith).

Fitacol. (Standex) Atropine sulfate 0.2 mg, phenylpropanolamine 12.5 mg, chlorpheniramine maleate 0.5 mg, chlorobutanol 0.5 mg, water q.s./ml. Bot. pt. *Rx.*
Use: Anticholinergic, antispasmodic, decongestant, antihistamine.

Fitacol Stankaps. (Standex) Belladonna alkaloidal salts 0.16 mg (atropine sulfate 0.024 mg, scopolamine HBr 0.014 mg, hyoscyamine sulfate 0.122 mg), phenylpropanolamine HCl 50 mg, chlorpheniramine maleate 1 mg, pheniramine maleate 12.5 mg/Cap. Bot. 100s. *Rx.*
Use: Anticholinergic, antispasmodic, decongestant, antihistamine.

5-FC.
See: Flucytosine.

5-FU.
See: Fluorouracil.

523 Tablets. (Enzyme Process) Pancreatin 200 mg 4x/Tab. Tryspin, chymotrypsin, amylase, lipase enzymes from pancreatin, raw beef pancreas. Bot. 100s, 250s.
Use: Digestive enzyme.

Fixodent. (Procter & Gamble) Calcium sodium poly (vinyl methyl ether-maleate), carboxymethylcellulose sodium in a petrolatum base. Tube 0.75 oz, 1.5 oz, 2.5 oz. *otc.*
Use: Denture adhesive cream.

FK-506.
See: ProGra (Fujisawa).

FK-565.
Use: Immunomodulator.

Flagyl Capsules. (Searle) Metronidazole 375 mg/Cap. Bot. 50s, 100s, UD 100s. *Rx.*
Use: Anti-infective.

Flagyl Tablets. (Searle) Metronidazole 250 mg or 500 mg/Tab. **250 mg:** Bot. 50s, 100s, 250s, 1000s, 2500s, UD 100s; **500 mg:** Bot. 50s, 100s, 500s, UD 100s. *Rx.*
Use: Anti-infective.

Flagyl I.V. (Searle) Metronidazole HCl sterile lyophilized powder in single-dose vials equivalent to 500 mg metronidazole. Carton 10s. *Rx.*
Use: Anti-infective.

Flagyl I.V. RTU. (Searle) Metronidazole ready-to-use, premixed, 500 mg/100 ml Soln. Vial (glass), Box 6s; Container, (plastic), Box 24s. *Rx.*
Use: Anti-infective.

Flanders Buttocks Ointment. (Flanders) Zinc oxide, castor oil, balsam peru, boric acid in an emollient base. 60 g. *otc.*
Use: Minor skin irritations.

Flarex. (Alcon) Fluorometholone acetate 0.1%. Susp. Bot. 2.5 ml, 5 ml, 10 ml Drop-Tainers. *Rx.*
Use: Corticosteroid, ophthalmic.

Flatulence Tablets. (Pal-Pak) Nux vomica 16.2 mg, cascara sagrada extract 64.8 mg, ginger 48.6 mg, capsicum 16.2 mg/Tab. w/asafetida. *otc.*
Use: Laxative, antiflatulent.

Flatulex. (Dayton) **Tab.:** Simethicone 80 mg, activated charcoal 250 mg/Tab. Bot. 100s. **Drops:** Simethicone 40 mg/0.6 ml. Bot. 30 ml with calibrated dropper. *otc.*
Use: Antiflatulent.

Flatus. (Foy) Nux vomica extract 0.25 gr, cascara extract 1 gr, ginger ¾ gr, capsicum gr/Tab. w/asafetida qs. Bot. 1000s. *otc.*
Use: Antiflatulent, laxative.

Flav-A-D. (Kirkman Sales) Vitamins A

5000 IU, D 1000 IU, C 100 mg/Tab. Bot. 100s, 1000s. Also w/fluoride. Bot. 100s, 1000s. *otc, Rx.*
Use: Vitamin supplement.

flavine.
See: Acriflavine Hydrochloride (Various Mfr.)

Flavinoid-C. (Barth's) **Tab.:** Vitamin C 150 mg, hesperidin complex 10 mg, citrus bioflavonoid 50 mg, rutin 20 mg/ Tab. Bot. 100s, 500s, 1000s. **Liq.:** Vitamin C 100 mg, bioflavonoid complex 100 mg/5 ml. Bot. 4 oz. *otc.*
Use: Vitamin supplement.

•**flavodilol maleate.** (FLAY-voe-DILL-ole) USAN.
Use: Antihypertensive.

flavolutan.
See: Progesterone (Various Mfr.)

flavonoid compounds.
See: Bio-Flavonoid Compounds; Vitamin P.

Flavons-500. (Freeda) Citrus bioflavonoids complex 500 mg, hesperidin complex/Tab. Bot. 100s, 250s, 500s. *otc.*
Use: Vitamin supplement.

Flavorcee. (NBTY) Ascorbic acid 100 mg or 250 mg/Chew. Tab. **100 mg:** Bot. 100s; **250 mg:** Bot. 250s. *otc.*
Use: Vitamin C supplement.

flavored diluent. (Roxane) Flavored vehicle for the immediate administration of crushed tablet or capsule product. Bot. 500 ml, UD 15 ml × 100.
Use: Flavored vehicle.

•**flavoxate hydrochloride.** (flay-VOKES-ate) USAN.
Use: Urinary antispasmodic, smooth muscle relaxant.
See: Urispas, Tab. (SK-Beecham).

flavurol. Merbromin.
Use: Antiseptic.

•**flazalone.** (FLAY-zah-lone) USAN.
Use: Anti-inflammatory.

•**flecainide acetate,** (fleh-CANE-ide) U.S.P. 23.
Use: Cardiac depressant (antiarrhythmic).
See: Tambocor (3M Pharm)

Fleet Babylax. (Fleet) Glycerin 4 ml in disposable pre-lubricated rectal applicator. Liq. pkg. 6s. *otc.*
Use: Laxative.

Fleet Bagenema. (Fleet) Castile soap or Fleets bisacodyl prep. *otc.*
Use: Laxative.

Fleet Bisacodyl Prep Packets. (Fleet) Bisacodyl 10 mg/10 ml packet. 36 packets/box. *otc.*

Use: Laxative.

Fleet Enema. (Fleet) Sodium biphosphate 19 g, sodium phosphate 7 g/118 ml. Bot. w/rectal tube 4.5 oz. Pediatric size 67.5 ml, 135 ml. *otc.*
Use: Laxative.

Fleet Flavored Castor Oil Emulsion. (Fleet) 1 oz delivers 30 ml castor oil. Bot. 1.5 oz, 3 oz. *otc.*
Use: Laxative.

Fleet Glycerin Suppositories. (Fleet) Adult: Jar 12s, 24s, 50s. Child Size: Jar 12s. *otc.*
Use: Laxative.

Fleet Laxative. (Fleet) Bisacodyl. **EC Tab.:** 5 mg/Tab. Bot. 24s. **Supp.:** 10 mg. Box 4s. *otc.*
Use: Laxative.

Fleet Medicated Wipes. (Fleet) Hamamelis water 50%, alcohol 7%, glycerin 10%, benzalkonium Cl, methylparaben. Rectal pads. 100s. *otc.*
Use: Perianal hygiene product.

Fleet Mineral Oil Enema. (Fleet) Mineral oil 4.5 fl oz in an unbreakable vinyl squeeze bottle. *otc.*
Use: Laxative.

Fleet Pain Relief. (Fleet) Pramoxine HCl 1%, glycerin 12%. Pads. 100s. *otc.*
Use: Anorectal preparation.

Fleet Phospho-Soda. (Fleet) Sodium phosphate 18 g, sodium biphosphate 48 g/100 ml (96.4 mEq sodium/20 ml). Bot. 45 ml, 90 ml, 240 ml. *otc.*
Use: Laxative.

Fleet Prep Kits. (Fleet) A series of different laxative kits for use prior to barium enema, bowel surgery, proctoscopy, colonoscopy, etc. w/complete patient instruction form:

Prep Kit #1: Fleet Phospho-Soda 45 ml, Fleet Bisacodyl Tablets 45 mg, Fleet Bisacodyl Suppository 110 mg. *otc.*

Prep Kit #2: Fleet Phospho-Soda 45 ml, Fleet Bisacodyl Tablets 45 mg, 1 Fleet Bagenema set for large volume enema, including optional Castile Soap Packet. 20 ml. *otc.*

Prep Kit #3: Fleet Phospho-Soda 45 ml, Fleet Bisacodyl Tablets 45 mg, Fleet Bisacodyl Enema 130 ml. 10 mg. *otc.*

Prep Kit #4: Fleet Flavored Castor Oil Emulsion 45 ml, Fleet Bisacodyl Tablets 45 mg, Fleet Bisacodyl Suppository 110 mg. *otc.*

Prep Kit #5: Fleet Flavored Castor Oil Emulsion 45 ml, Fleet Bisacodyl Tablets 45 mg, 1 Fleet Bagenema set for large volume enema, including optional Castile Soap Packet. 20 ml. *otc.*

Prep Kit #6: Fleet Flavored Castor Oil Emulsion 45 ml, Fleet Bisacodyl Tablets 45 mg, Fleet Bisacodyl Enema 130 ml. 10 mg. *otc.*
Use: Laxative.

Fleet Relief Anesthetic Hemorrhoidal Ointment. (Fleet) Pramoxine HCl 1%. Six disposable pre-filled applicators. Tube 30 g. *otc.*
Use: Anorectal preparation.

•**fleroxacin.** (fler-OX-ah-SIN) USAN.
Use: Antibacterial.
See: Megalone (Hoffman-LaRouche).

•**flestolol sulfate.** (FLESS-toe-lahl) USAN.
Use: Anti-adrenergic (β-receptor).

•**fletazepam.** (FLET-AZE-eh-pam) USAN.
Use: Relaxant (skeletal muscle).

Fletcher's Castoria for Children. (Mentholatum) Senna 6.5%, alcohol 3.5%. Liq. Bot. 75 ml, 150 ml. *otc.*
Use: Laxative.

Flex-All 454. (Chattem) Menthol 7%, alcohol, allantoin, aloe vera gel, boric acid, carbomer 940, diazolidinyl urea, eucalyptus oil, glycerin, iodine, parabens, methyl salicylate, peppermint oil, polysorbate 60, potassium iodide, propylene glycol, thyme oil, triethanolamine. Gel Tube. 240 g. *otc.*
Use: Analgesic, topical.

Flex Anti-Dandruff Shampoo. (Revlon) Zinc pyrithione 1% in liquid shampoo. *otc.*
Use: Antiseborrheic.

Flex Anti-Dandruff Styling Mousse. (Revlon) Zinc pyrithione 0.1%. Aerosol foam. *otc.*
Use: Antiseborrheic.

Flexaphen. (Trimen) Chlorzoxazone 250 mg, acetaminophen 300 mg/Cap. Bot 100s. *Rx.*
Use: Skeletal muscle relaxant.

Flex-Care Especially for Sensitive Eyes. (Alcon) EDTA 0.1%, chlorhexidine gluconate 0.005%, sodium Cl, sodium borate, boric acid. Soln. Bot. 118 ml, 237 ml, 355 ml, 360 ml. *otc.*
Use: Contact lens care.

Flexeril. (Merck) Cyclobenzaprine HCl 10 mg/Tab. Bot. 100s, UD 100s. *Rx.*
Use: Muscle relaxant.

flexible hydroactive dressings/granules.
See: Intra Site (Smith & Nephew). Shur-Clens (SK-Beecham).

DuoDerm (ConvaTec)
Sorbsan (Dow B. Hickam).

Flexoject. (Mayrand) Orphenadrine citrate 30 mg/ml. Inj. Vial 10 ml, amps 2 ml. *Rx.*
Use: Muscle relaxant.

Flexon. (Keene) Orphenadrine citrate 30 mg/ml. Inj. Vial 10 ml. *Rx.*
Use: Muscle relaxant.

Flexsol. (Alcon Lenscare) Sterile, buffered, isotonic aqueous soln. of sodium Cl, sodium borate, boric acid, adsorbobase. Bot. 6 oz. *otc.*
Use: Soft contact lens care.

Flintstones Children's Tablets. (Bayer) Vitamin A 2500 IU, E 15 mg, C 60 mg, folic acid 0.3 mg, B_1 1.05 mg, B_2 1.2 mg, B_3 13.5 mg, B_6 1.05 mg, B_{12} 4.5 mcg, D 400 IU/Chew. Tab. Bot. 60s, 100s. *otc.*
Use: Vitamin supplement.

Flintstones Complete. (Bayer) Elemental iron 18 mg, vitamins A 5000 IU, D 400 IU, E 30 mg, B_1 1.5 mg, B_2 1.7 mg, B_3 20 mg, B_5 10 mg, B_6 2 mg, B_{12} 6 mcg, C 60 mg, folic acid 0.4 mg, biotin 40 mcg, Ca, Cu, I, Mg, P, zinc 15 mg/Chew. Tab. Bot. 60s, 120s. *otc.*
Use: Vitamin/mineral supplement.

Flintstones Plus Calcium. (Bayer) Vitamin A 2500 IU, D IU 400, E 15 IU, C 60 mg, folic acid 0.3 mg, B_1 1.05 mg, B_2 1.2 mg, B_3 13.5 mg, B_6 1.05 mg, B_{12} 4.5 mcg, Ca 200 mg/Tab. Chewable. Bot. 60s. *otc.*
Use: Vitamin/mineral supplement.

Flintstones Plus Extra C. (Bayer) Vitamins A 2500 IU, D 400 IU, E 15 mg, C 250 mg, folic acid 0.3 mg, B_1 1.05 mg, B_2 1.2 mg, niacin 13.5 mg, B_6 1.05 mg, B_{12} 4.5 mcg/Tab. Bot. 60s, 100s. *otc.*
Use: Vitamin supplement.

Flintstones Plus Iron. (Bayer) Vitamins A 2500 IU, E 15 mg, C 60 mg, folic acid 0.3 mg, B_1 1.05 mg, B_2 1.2 mg, niacin 13.5 mg, B_6 1.05 mg, B_{12} 4.5 mcg, D 400 IU, iron 15 mg/Chew. Tab. Bot. 60s, 100s. *otc.*
Use: Vitamin/mineral supplement.

Flo-Coat. (Lafayette Pharm) Barium sulfate 100%. Susp. Bot. 1850 ml.
Use: Radiopaque agent.

•**floctafenine.** (FLOCK-tah-FEN-een) USAN.
Use: Analgesic.

Flolan. (Glaxo Wellcome) Epoprostenol sodium 0.5 or 1.5 mg, mannitol, NaCl/Vial. Pow. for Inj. 17 ml. *Rx.*

Use: Antihypertensive.

Flonase. (Glaxo Wellcome) Fluticasone proprionate 50 mcg/actuation. Bot. 9 g (60 actuations), 16 g (120 actuations). *Rx.*
Use: Intranasal steroid.

Flor-D Chewable Tab. (Derm Pharm) Fluoride 1 mg, vitamins A 4000 IU, D 400 IU, C 75 mg, B_1 1.5 mg, B_2 1.8 mg, niacinamide 15 mg, B_6 1 mg, B_{12} 3 mcg, calcium pantothenate 10 mg/Tab. Bot. 100s. *Rx.*
Use: Vitamin/mineral supplement.

Flor-D Drops. (Derm Pharm) Fluoride 0.5 mg, vitamins A 3000 IU, D 400 IU, C 60 mg, B_1 1 mg, B_2 1.2 mg, niacinamide 8 mg/0.6 ml. Bot. 60 ml. *Rx.*
Use: Vitamin/mineral supplement.

•**flordipine.** (FLORE-dih-peen) USAN.
Use: Antihypertensive.

Florical. (Mericon) Sodium fluoride 8.3 mg, calcium carbonate 364 mg (equivalent to 145.6 mg calcium)/Cap. Bot. 100s, 500s. *otc.*
Use: Mineral supplement.

Florida Foam. (Hill) Benzalkonium Cl, aluminum subacetate, boric acid 2%. Bot. 8 oz. *otc.*
Use: Soap substitute, antiseborrheic, antifungal, antiacne.

Florida Sunburn Relief. (Pharmacel) Benzyl alcohol 3%, phenol 0.4%, camphor 0.2%, menthol 0.15%. Lot. Bot. 60 ml. *otc.*
Use: Sunburn relief.

Florinef Acetate Tablets. (Apothecon) Fludrocortisone acetate, 0.1 mg/Tab. Bot. 100s. *Rx.*
Use: Mineralocorticoid.

Florone Cream. (Dermik) Diflorasone diacetate 0.5 mg/g (0.05%) w/stearic acid, sorbitan mono-oleate, polysorbate 60, sorbic acid, citric acid, propylene glycol, purified water. Tube 15 g, 30 g, 60 g. *Rx.*
Use: Corticosteroid, topical.

Florone E. (Dermik) Diflorasone diacetate 0.5 mg. Tube 15 g, 30 g, 60 g. *Rx.*
Use: Corticosteroid, topical.

Florone Ointment. (Dermik) Diflorasone diacetate 0.5 mg/g (0.05%) w/polyoxypropylene 15-stearyl ether, stearic acid, lanolin alcohol and white petrolatum. Tube 15 g, 30 g, 60 g. *Rx.*
Use: Corticosteroid, topical.

Floropryl. (Merck) Isoflurophate 0.025% in sterile ophthalmic ointment in polyethylene-mineral oil gel. Tube 3.5 g. *Rx.*
Use: Agent for glaucoma.

Florvite Chewable Tablets. (Everett) Vitamins, fluoride 0.5 mg/Chew. tab. Bot 100s. *Rx.*
Use: Dental caries preventative.

Florvite Half Strength. (Everett) Elemental fluoride 0.5 mg, vitamins A 2500 IU, D 400 IU, E 15 mg, B_1 1.05 mg, B_2 1.2 mg, B_3 13.5 mg, B_6 1.05 mg, B_{12} 4.5 mcg, C 60 mg, folic acid 0.3 mg/Chew. Tab. Bot. 100s. *Rx.*
Use: Vitamin/mineral supplement, dental caries preventative.

Florvite + Iron Drops. (Everett) Elemental fluorine. **0.25 mg:** Vitamins A 1500 IU, D 400 IU, E 5 mg, B_1 0.5 mg, B_2 0.6 mg, B_3 8 mg, B_6 0.4 mg, C 35 mg, iron 10 mg/ml. **0.5 mg:** Vitamins A 1500 IU, D 400 IU, E 5 mg, B_1 0.5 mg, B_2 0.6 mg, B_3 8 mg, B_6 0.4 mg, C 35 mg, iron 10 mg/ml/Liq. Bot. 50 ml. *Rx.*
Use: Vitamin/mineral supplement, dental caries preventative.

Florvite + Iron Chewable. (Everett) Fluoride 1 mg, iron 12 mg, vitamins A 2500 IU, D 400 IU, E 15 mg, B_1 1.05 mg, B_2 1.2 mg, B_3 13.5 mg, B_6 1.05 mg, B_{12} 4.5 mcg, C 60 mg, folic acid 0.3 mg, Cu, Zn 10 mg, sucrose/Chew. tab. Bot. 100s. *Rx.*
Use: Vitamin/mineral supplement, dental caries preventative.

Florvite Pediatric Drops. (Everett) Elemental fluorine. **0.25 mg/ml:** vitamins A 1500 IU, D 400 IU, E 5 mg, B_1 0.5 mg, B_2 0.6 mg, B_3 8 mg, B_6 0.4 mg, B_{12} 2 mcg, C 35 mg/ml. **0.5 mg/ml:** vitamins A 1500 IU, D 400 IU, E 5 mg, B_1 0.5 mg, B_2 0.6 mg, B_3 8 mg, B_6 0.4 mg, B_{12} 2 mcg, C 35 mg, iron 10 mg/ml Bot. 50 ml. *Rx.*
Use: Vitamin/mineral supplement, dental caries preventative.

Florvite Tablets. (Everett) Fluoride 1 mg, vitamins A 2500 IU, D 400 IU, E 15 mg, B_1 1.05 mg, B_2 1.2 mg, B_3 13.5 mg, B_6 1.05 mg, B_{12} 4.5 mcg, C 60 mg, folic acid 0.3 mg/Chew. tab. Bot. 100s, 1000s. *Rx.*
Use: Vitamin/mineral supplement, dental caries preventative.

Florvite Drops. (Everett) Fluoride 0.25 mg or 0.5 mg, A 1500 IU, D 400 IU, E 5 IU, B_1 0.5 mg, B_2 0.6 mg, B_3 8 mg, B_6 0.4 mg, B_{12} 2 mcg, C 35 mg/Drop. Bot. 50 ml. *Rx.*
Use: Vitamin/mineral supplement, dental caries preventative.

•**flosequinan.** (flow-SEH-kwih-NAHN) USAN.
Use: Antihypertensive (vasodilator).

See: Manoplax (Knoll Pharm).

Flovent. (Glaxo Wellcome) Fluticasone propionate 44 mcg/Actuation/Aerosol spray. Canister. 7.9 g (60 actuations) and 13 g (120 actuations). Fluticasone propionate 110 mcg/actuation/Aerosol spray. Canister 13 g (120 actuations). Fluticasone propionate 220 mcg/actuation/Aerosol spray. Canister. 13 g (120 actuations). *Rx.*
Use: Management of seasonal and perennial allergic rhinitis.

●**floxacillin.** (FLOX-ah-SILL-in) USAN.
Use: Antibacterial.

Floxin. (Ortho) **Tab.:** Ofloxacin, 200 mg, 300 mg or 400 mg. Bot. 50s, 100s. **Inj.:** 200 mg flexible container; 400 mg Vial 10 ml, 20 ml; Bot. 100 ml; flexible container. *Rx.*
Use: Anti-infective, fluoroquinolone.

●**floxuridine,** (flox-YUR-ih-deen) U.S.P. 23.
Use: Antiviral, antineoplastic.
See: FUDR, Vial (Roche).

●**fluazacort.** (flew-AZE-ah-kort) USAN.
Use: Anti-inflammatory.

●**flubanilate hydrochloride.** (flew-BAN-ill-ate) USAN.
Use: Antidepressant; stimulant, CNS.

●**flubendazole.** (FLEW-BEN-dah-zole) USAN.
Use: Antiprotozoal.

flucarbril.
Use: Muscle relaxant, analgesic.

●**flucindole.** (flew-SIN-dole) USAN.
Use: Antipsychotic.

●**flucloronide.** (flew-KLOR-oh-nide) USAN.
Use: Glucocorticoid.

Flu, Cold & Cough Medicine. (Major) Pseudoephedrine HCl 60 mg, chlorpheniramine 4 mg, dextromethorphan HBr 20 mg, acetaminophen 500 mg. Pow. Pck. 6s. *otc.*
Use: Decongestant, antihistamine, antitussive, analgesic.

●**fluconazole.** (flew-KOE-nuh-sole) USAN.
Use: Antifungal.
See: Diflucan (Roerig).

●**flucrylate.** (FLEW-krih-late) USAN.
Use: Surgical aid (tissue adhesive).

●**flucytosine,** (flew-SITE-oh-seen) U.S.P. 23.
Use: Antifungal.
See: Ancobon, Cap. (Roche).

●**fludalanine.** (flew-DAL-AH-neen) USAN.
Use: Antibacterial.

Fludara. Fludarabine 50 mg. Pow. for recon. Vial. 6 ml. *Rx.*

Use: Antineoplastic.

●**fludarabine phosphate.** (flew-DAR-uh-BEAN) USAN.
Use: Antineoplastic. [Orphan drug]
See: Fludara, Pow. (Berlex).

●**fludazonium chloride.** (FLEW-dazz-OH-nee-uhm) USAN.
Use: Anti-infective, topical.

●**fludeoxyglucose F 18 injection,** (FLEW-dee-OX-ee-GLUE-kose F 18) U.S.P. 23.
Use: Diagnostic aid (brain disorders, thyroid disorders, liver disorders, cardiac disease and neoplastic disease), radioactive agent.

●**fludorex.** (FLEW-doe-rex) USAN.
Use: Anorexic, antiemetic.

●**fludrocortisone acetate,** (flew-droe-CORE-tih-sone) U.S.P. 23.
Use: Adrenocortical steroid (salt-regulating).
See: Florinef Acetate, Tab. (Apothecon).

●**flufenamic acid.** (FLEW-fen-AM-ik) USAN.
Use: Anti-inflammatory.

●**flufensal.** (flew-FEN-ih-sal) USAN.
Use: Analgesic.

Fluidex. (Columbia) Natural botanical ingredients. Tab. Bot. 36s, 72s.
Use: Diuretic.

Flu-Imune. (Lederle) Influenza virus vaccine. Vial 5 ml (10 doses). (Purified surface antigen). *Rx.*
Use: Vaccine, viral.

fluitran. Trichlormethiazide.

Flumadine. (Forest) **Tab.:** Rimantadine HCl 100 mg. Bot. 20s, 100s, 500s, 1000s. **Syr.:** Rimantadine HCl 50 mg/5ml. Bot. 60 ml, 240 ml, 480 ml. *Rx.*
Use: Antiviral.

●**flumazenil.** (flew-MAZ-ah-nil) USAN.
Use: Antagonist (to benzodiazepine).
See: Mazicon (Roche).
Romazicon, Inj. (Roche).

flumecinol.
Use: Hyperbilirubinemia in newborns. [Orphan drug]
See: Zixoryn.

●**flumequine.** (FLEW-meh-kwin) USAN.
Use: Antibacterial.

●**flumeridone.** (FLEW-MER-ih-dohn) USAN.
Use: Antiemetic.

●**flumethasone.** (FLEW-meth-ah-zone) USAN.
Use: Corticosteroid; glucocorticoid.
See: Locorten [21-pivalate] (Novartis).

●**flumethasone pivalate,** (FLEW-meth-ah-zone PIH-vah-late) U.S.P. 23.

Use: Glucocorticoid.
flumethiazide.
Use: Diuretic.
See: Rautrax, Tab. (Squibb).
•**flumetramide.** (flew-MEH-trah-mide)
USAN.
Use: Relaxant (skeletal muscle).
•**flumezapine.** (FLEW-MEZZ-ah-peen)
USAN.
Use: Antipsychotic, neuroleptic.
•**fluminorex.** (flew-MEE-no-rex) USAN.
Use: Anorexic.
•**flumizole.** (FLEW-mih-zole) USAN.
Use: Anti-inflammatory.
•**flumoxonide.** (flew-MOX-OH-nide)
USAN.
Use: Adrenocortical steroid.
flunarizine. *Rx.*
Use: Alternating hemiplegia. [Orphan
drug]
See: Sibelium.
•**flunarizine hydrochloride.** (flew-NAR-ih-
zeen) USAN.
Use: Vasodilator.
•**flunidazole.** (FLEW-nih-dah-ZOLE)
USAN.
Use: Antiprotozoal.
•**flunisolide,** (flew-NIH-sole-ide) U.S.P.
23.
Use: Glucocorticoid.
See: Nasalide (Syntex).
•**flunisolide acetate.** (flew-NIH-sole-ide)
USAN. Fluoxolonate.
Use: Anti-inflammatory.
•**flunitrazepam.** (flew-NYE-TRAY-zeh-
pam) USAN.
Use: Sedative, hynoptic.
•**flunixin.** (flew-NIX-in) USAN.
Use: Anti-inflammatory, analgesic.
•**flunixin meglumine,** U.S.P. 23.
Use: Anti-inflammatory, analgesic.
Fluocet. (NMC Labs) Fluocinolone aceto-
nide cream 0.025% or 0.01%. Tube 15
g, 60 g. *Rx.*
Use: Corticosteroid, topical.
fluocinolide. (flew-oh-SIN-oh-lide)
See: Fluocinonide.
•**fluocinolone acetonide,** (flew-oh-SIN-
oh-lone ah-SEE-toe-nide) U.S.P. 23.
Use: Glucocorticoid, corticosteroid (topical).
See: Fluonid, Cream, Oint., Soln. (Aller-
gan Herbert).
Synalar, Cream, Oint., Soln. (Syntex).
W/Neomycin sulfate.
See: Neo-Synalar (Syntex).
•**fluocinonide,** (FLEW-oh-SIN-oh-nide)
U.S.P. 23. *Formerly Fluocinolide.*

Use: Glucocorticoid, corticosteroid (topical).
See: Lidex, Cream, Oint., Soln. (Syntex).
Lidex-E, Cream (Syntex).
Metosyn.
Topsyn, Gel (Syntex).
fluocinonide. (Fougera) 0.05%. Tube 15
g, 60 g.
Use: Glucocorticoid, corticosteroid (topical).
fluocinonide topical solution. (Fougera) 0.05%. Soln. Bot. 60 ml.
Use: Corticosteroid, topical.
•**fluocortin butyl.** (FLEW-oh-CORE-tin
BYOO-tuhl) USAN.
Use: Anti-inflammatory.
•**fluocortolone.** (FLEW-oh CORE-toe-
lone) USAN.
Use: Corticosteroid, glucocorticoid.
See: Ultralanum [21-hexanoate]
•**fluocortolone caproate.** USAN.
Use: Glucocorticoid.
Fluogen. (Parke-Davis) Influenza virus
vaccine, trivalent–Immunizing antigen,
ether extracted. Vial 5 ml, UD syringe
0.5 ml. The 5 ml vial contains sufficient
product to deliver ten 0.5 ml doses.
Rx.
Use: Vaccine, viral.
Fluonex. (Zeneca) Fluocinonide 0.05%.
Cream. Tube. 15 g, 30 g. *Rx.*
Use: Corticosteroid, topical.
Fluonid. (Allergan Herbert) Fluocinolone
Acetonide. **Soln.:** 0.01%. Bot. 20 ml,
60 ml. *Rx.*
Use: Corticosteroid, topical.
Fluoracaine. (Akorn) Proparacaine HCl
0.5%, fluorescein sodium 0.25%. Drop-
per Bot. 5 ml. *Rx.*
Use: Local anesthetic, ophthalmic.
•**fluorescein,** U.S.P. 23.
Use: Diagnostic aid (corneal trauma in-
dicator).
See: Fluorescite (Alcon).
•**fluorescein sodium,** U.S.P. 23. *Formerly
Fluorescein, soluble.*
Use: Diagnostic aid (corneal trauma in-
dicator).
See: AK-Fluor, Amp., Vial (Akorn).
Fluor-I-Strip. (Wyeth-Ayerst).
Fluorets, Strips (Akorn).
Ful-Glo, Strips (Pilkington Barnes
Hind).
Funduscein, Amp. (Ciba Vision).
Plak-Lite Soln. (Internat. Pharm).
fluorescein sodium. (Various Mfr.) 2%
Ophth. Soln. Bot. 1 ml, 2 ml, 15 ml.
Use: Diagnostic aid (corneal trauma in-
dicator).

fluorescein sodium i.v.
See: Fluorescite, Amp. (Alcon).

Fluorescein Sodium 2% Solution. (Alcon) Drop-Tainer 15 ml, Steri-Unit 2 ml 12s.
Use: Diagnostic aid, ophthalmic.

Fluorescein Sodium 2%. (Ciba Vision) A sterile aqueous solution containing fluorescein sodium 2%. Dropperette 1 ml, Box 12s.
Use: Diagnostic aid, ophthalmic.

Fluorescein Sodium w/Proparacaine Hydrochloride. (Taylor) Proparacaine HCl 0.5%, fluorescein sodium 0.25%. Ophthalmic soln. Bot. 5 ml. *Rx.*
Use: Local anesthetic, diagnostic aid, ophthalmic.

Fluorescein Sodium/Sodium Hyaluronate.
See: Sodium Hyaluronate and Fluorescein Sodium Healon Yellow (Pharmacia & Upjohn).

Fluorescite. (Alcon) Fluorescein as sodium salt. Inj. Soln. **10%:** Amp. 5 ml with syringes; **25%:** Amp 2 ml. *Rx.*
Use: Diagnostic aid, ophthalmic.

Fluoresoft. (Various Mfr.) Fluorexon 0.35%. Soln. Pipette 0.5 ml, Box 12s. *otc.*
Use: Diagnostic aid, ophthalmic.

Fluorets. (Akorn) Fluorescein sodium 1 mg. Strip. Box 100s. *otc.*
Use: Diagnostic aid, ophthalmic.

fluorexon.
See: Fluoresoft (Holles).

fluoride. (Kirkman Sales) Fluoride 1 mg (sodium fluoride 2.21 mg). Tab. Bot. 1000s. *Rx.*
Use: Dental caries preventative.

Fluoride Lozenges. (Kirkman Sales) Fluoride 1 mg (sodium fluoride 2.21 mg). Loz. Bot. 1000s. *Rx.*
Use: Dental caries preventative.

fluoride sodium.
See: Dentafluor Chewable, Tab. (Western Pharm).
Karidium, Top. Soln., Tab. (Young Dental).
Karigel, Gel (Young Dental).

fluoride therapy.
See: Adeflor Preps. (Pharmacia & Upjohn).
Cari-Tab, Softab Tab. (Stuart).
Coral Prods. (Young Dental).
Fluorineed, Chew. Tab. (Hanlon).
Fluorinse, Liq. (Pacemaker).
Fluora, Loz. (Kirkman Sales).
Gal-Kam, Preps. (Scherer).
Luride Preps. (Colgate Oral).

Mulvidren-F, Softab Tab. (Stuart).
Point Two, Rinse (Colgate Oral).
Poly-Vi-Flor, Drops, Tab. (Bristol-Myers).
Soluvite-F, Drops (Pharmics).
Tri-Vi-Flor, Drops, Tab. (Bristol-Myers).

Fluorigard. (Colgate Oral) Fluoride 0.02% (from sodium fluoride 0.05%), alcohol 6%, tartrazine. Bot. 180 ml, 300 ml, 480 ml. *Rx.*
Use: Dental caries preventative.

Fluori-Methane Spray. (Gebauer) Dichlorodifluoromethane 15%, trichloromonofluoromethane 85%. Bot. 4 oz. *Rx.*
Use: "Painful motion" syndromes.

Fluorineed. (Hanlon) Fluoride 1 mg/ Chew. Tab. Bot. 100s, 1000s. *Rx.*
Use: Dental caries preventative.

Fluorinse. (Oral-B) Fluoride 0.09% from sodium fluoride 0.2%. Bot. 480 ml. *Rx.*
Use: Dental caries preventative.

Fluorinse. (Pacemaker) Fluoride mouthwash. Pack. Fluoride ion level 0.05% or 0.2%. UD Bot. 32 oz. Concentrate 1 oz, 4 oz, gal. *Rx.*
Use: Dental caries preventative.

Fluor-I-Strip. (Wyeth-Ayerst) Fluorescein sodium 9 mg/ophthalmic strip. Box. 300s. *Rx.*
Use: Diagnostic aid, ophthalmic.

Fluor-I-Strip-A.T. (Wyeth-Ayerst) Fluorescein sodium 1 mg/ophthalmic strip. Box 300s. *Rx.*
Use: Diagnostic aid, ophthalmic.

Fluoritab. (Fluoritab) Sodium fluoride 2.2 mg equivalent to 1 mg of fluorine (as fluoride ion) w/inert organic filler 75.8 mg/Tab. Bot. 100s; Liq. dropper bot. (fluorine 0.25 mg from 0.55 mg sodium fluoride/Drop) 19 ml. *Rx.*
Use: Dental caries preventative.

5-fluorocytosine.
See: Ancobon, Cap. (Roche).

•**fluorodopa F 18,** (FLEW-roe-DOE-pah) U.S.P. 23.
Use: Diagnostic aid (brain imaging), radioactive agent.

fluorogestone acetate.
Use: Progestin.

fluorohydrocortisone acetate. 9-α-Fluorohydrocortisone.
See: Fludrocortisone Acetate (Various Mfr.)

•**fluorometholone,** U.S.P. 23.
Use: Glucocorticoid.
See: Fluor-Op, Susp. (Ciba Vision).
FML, Liquifilm, Ophth. Susp., Oint. (Allergan).

Oxylone, Cream Ophth. Susp. (Pharmacia & Upjohn).
W/Neomycin sulfate.
See: Neo-Oxylone, Oint. (Pharmacia & Upjohn).
•**fluorometholone acetate.** (flure-oh-METH-oh-LONE) USAN.
Use: Glucocorticoid, anti-inflammatory.
Fluor-Op. (Ciba Vision) Fluorometholone 0.1%. Susp. Bot. 5 ml, 10 ml, 15 ml. Rx.
Use: Corticosteroid, ophthalmic.
fluorophene.
Use: Antiseptic.
Fluoroplex Topical. (Allergan Herbert) **Soln.:** Fluorouracil 1% in a propylene glycol base. Plastic bot. w/dropper 30 ml. **Cream:** Fluorouracil 1% in emulsion base w/benzyl alcohol 0.5%, emulsifying wax, mineral oil, isopropyl myristate, sodium hydroxide, purified water. Tube 30 g. Rx.
Use: Topical treatment of multiple actinic (solar) keratoses.
fluoroquinolones.
Use: Anti-infective.
See: Ciloxan (Alcon).
Cipro (Bayer).
Cipro I.V. (Bayer).
Floxin (Ortho).
Maxaquin (Searle).
Noroxin (Merck).
Penetrex (Rhone-Poulenc Rorer).
•**fluorosalan.** (FLEW-oh-row-SAH-lan) USAN.
Use: Antiseptic, disinfectant.
fluorothyl. Bis (2, 2, 2-trifluoroethyl) ether.
See: Flurothyl.
•**fluorouracil,** (FLURE-oh-YUR-uh-sill) U.S.P. 23.
Use: Antineoplastic. [Orphan drug]
See: Adrucil, Inj. (Pharmacia & Upjohn).
Efudex, Soln., Cream (Roche).
Fluoroplex, Soln., Cream (Allergan Herbert Labs.).
fluorouracil. (Roche) Amp. 10 ml, 500 mg. Box 10s.
Use: Antineoplastic. [Orphan drug.]
Fluothane. (Wyeth-Ayerst) Halothane. Bot. 125 ml, 250 ml. Rx.
Use: Inhalation anesthetic.
•**fluotracen hydrochloride.** (FLEW-oh-TRAY-sen) USAN.
Use: Antipsychotic, antidepressant.
•**fluoxetine.** (flew-OX-eh-teen) USAN.
Use: Antidepressant.
See: Prozac, Pulv., Liq. (Dista).
•**fluoxetine hydrochloride.** (flew-OX-eh-teen) USAN.

Use: Antidepressant.
See: Prozac (Dista).
Flu-Oxinate. (Taylor) Benoxinate HCl 0.4%, fluorescein sodium 0.25%. Ophthalmic Soln. Bot. 5 ml. Rx.
Use: Local anesthetic, diagnostic aid, ophthalmic.
•**fluoxymesterone, U.S.P. 23.**
Use: Androgen.
See: Android-F, Tab. (Zeneca).
Halotestin, Tab. (Pharmacia & Upjohn).
Ora-Testryl, Tab. (Squibb Mark).
W/Ethinyl estradiol.
See: Halodrin, Tab. (Pharmacia & Upjohn).
fluoxymestrone. (Various) 10 mg/Tab. Bot. 100s c-III.
Use: Androgen.
•**fluparoxan hydrochloride.** (flew-pah-ROX-an) USAN
Use: Antidepressant.
•**fluperamide.** (flew-purr-ah-mide) USAN.
Use: Antiperistaltic.
•**fluperolone acetate.** (FLEW-per-oh-lone) USAN.
Use: Corticosteroid, glucocorticoid.
•**fluphenazine decanoate,** (flew-FEN-uh-zeen) U.S.P. 23.
Use: Antipsychotic.
See: Prolixin Decanoate Soln. (Apothecon, Bristol-Myers).
•**fluphenazine enanthate,** U.S.P. 23.
Use: Tranquilizer, antipsychotic.
See: Prolixin Enanthate Prods. (Bristol-Myers).
•**fluphenazine hydrochloride,** (flew-FEN-uh-zeen) U.S.P. 23.
Use: Tranquilizer, antipsychotic.
See: Permitil, Preps. (Schering Plough).
Prolixin, Tab., Elix., Vial (Bristol-Myers).
•**flupirtine maleate.** (flew-PIHR-teen) USAN.
Use: Analgesic.
•**fluprednisolone.** (FLEW-pred-NIH-so-lone) USAN.
Use: Glucocorticoid.
•**fluprednisolone valerate.** (FLEW-pred-NIH-so-lone VAL-eh-rate) USAN.
Use: Glucocorticoid.
•**fluproquazone.** (FLEW-PRO-kwah-zone) USAN.
Use: Analgesic.
•**fluprostenol sodium.** (flew-PROSTE-een-ole) USAN.
Use: Prostaglandin.
See: Equimate (Bayer).
•**fluquazone.** (FLEW-kwah-zone) USAN.

Use: Anti-inflammatory.

•**fluradoline hydrochloride.** (FLURE-ade-OLE-een) USAN.
Use: Analgesic.

Flura-Drops. (Kirkman Sales) Fluoride. **Drops:** 0.25 mg (from 0.55 mg sodium fluoride). Bot. 30 ml. **Rinse:** 0.02% (from 0.05% sodium fluoride). Bot. 480 ml. *Rx.*
Use: Dental caries preventative.

Flura-Loz. (Kirkman Sales) Sodium fluoride 2.2 mg providing 1 mg fluoride/Loz. Bot. 100s, 1000s. *Rx.*
Use: Dental caries preventative.

•**flurandrenolide,** (FLURE-an-DREEN-oh-lide) U.S.P. 23.
Use: Corticosteroid, topical; glucocorticoid.
See: Cordran, Preps. (Dista).

flurandrenolone. (FLURE-an-DREE-nahl-ohn)
Use: Corticosteroid; glucocorticoid.

Flura-Tablets. (Kirkman Sales) Sodium fluoride 2.21 mg, equivalent to 1 mg fluoride ion/Tab. Bot. 100s, 1000s. *Rx.*
Use: Dental caries preventative.

Flurate. (Bausch & Lomb) Benoxinate HCl 0.4%, fluorescein sodium 0.25%, chlorobutanol 1%, povidone/Soln. Bot. 5 ml. *Rx.*
Use: Ophthalmic diagnostic agent.

•**flurazepam hydrochloride,** (flure-AZE-uh-pam) U.S.P. 23.
Use: Hypnotic, anticonvulsant, muscle relaxant, sedative, hypnotic.
See: Dalmane, Cap. (Roche).

•**flurbiprofen,** (FLURE-bih-PRO-fen) U.S.P. 23.
Use: Anti-inflamatory, analgesic.
See: Ansaid (Pharmacia & Upjohn).

flurbiprofen. (FLURE-bih-PRO-fen) (Various Mfr.) Flurbiprofen 50 mg or 100 mg. Tab. 100s, 500s. *Rx.*
Use: Nonsteroidal anti-inflamatory drug; analgesic.
See: Ansaid (Pharmacia & Upjohn).

•**flurbiprofen sodium,** (FLURE-bih-PRO-fen) U.S.P. 23.
Use: Nonsteroidal anti-inflamatory drug; analgesic; prostaglandin synthesis inhibitor.
See: Ocufen, Drops (Allergan).

flurbiprofen sodium ophthalmic. (FLURE-bih-PRO-fen) (Various) Flurbiprofen sodium 0.03%, polyvinyl alcohol 1.4%, thimerosal 0.005%, EDTA/Soln. Bot. 2.5 ml *Rx.*
Use: Nonsteroidal anti-inflammatory drug; analgesic.

Fluress. (Pilkington Barnes Hind) Fluorescein sodium 0.25%. Bot. 5 ml. *Rx.*
Use: Local anesthetic, diagnostic aid.

•**fluretofen.** (flure-EH-TOE-fen) USAN.
Use: Anti-inflammatory, antithrombotic.

flurfamide. (FLURE-fah-MIDE)
Use: Enzyme inhibitor.

•**flurocitabine.** (FLEW-row-SIGH-tah-bean) USAN.
Use: Antineoplastic.

Fluro-Ethyl. (Gebauer) Ethyl Cl 25%, dichlorotetrafluoroethane 75%/Spray. Can 270 g. *Rx.*
Use: Anesthetic, topical.

•**flurofamide.** USAN. *Formerly Flurfamide.*
Use: Enzyme inhibitor (urease).

•**flurogestone acetate.** (FLEW-row-JEST-ohn) USAN.
Use: Progestin.

Flurosyn. (Rugby) **Cream:** Fluocinolone acetonide 0.01% or 0.025%. Tube 15 g, 60 g, 425 g. **Oint:** Fluocinolone acetonide 0.025% in a white petrolatum base. Tube 15 g, 60 g. *Rx.*
Use: Corticosteroid, topical.

•**flurothyl.** (FLURE-oh-thill) USAN.
Use: Stimulant (central).

•**fluroxene.** (flure-OX-een) USAN. N.F. XIV. Fluoromar.
Use: General inhalation anesthetic.

Flu-Shield. (Wyeth Lederle) Influenza virus vaccine, trivalent - Immunizing antigen, ether extracted. Vial 5 ml, 0.5 ml. Tubex. *Rx.*
Use: Vaccine, viral.

•**fluspiperone.** (FLEW-spih-per-OHN) USAN.
Use: Antipsychotic.

•**fluspirilene.** (flew-SPIRE-ih-leen) USAN.
Use: Tranquilizer, antipsychotic.
See: Imap (McNeil).

•**flutamide,** U.S.P. 23.
Use: Antiandrogen.
See: Eulexin Cap. (Schering Plough).

Flutex. (Syosset) Triamcinolone acetonide. **Cream:** 0.025%, 0.1%, 0.5% Tube 15 g, 30 g, 60 g, 120 g, 240 g. **Oint.:** 0.025%, 0.1%, 0.5% Tube 30 g, 60 g, 120 g. *Rx.*
Use: Corticosteroid, topical.

•**fluticasone propionate.** (flew-TICK-ah-SONE) USAN.
Use: Anti-inflammatory.
See: Cutivate (Glaxo). Flonase, spray. (Allen & Hanburys).

Flutra. Trichlormethiazide.
Use: Diuretic.

•**flutroline.** (FLEW-troe-LEEN) USAN.
Use: Antipsychotic.

•**fluvastatin sodium.** (FLEW-vah-STAT-in) USAN.
Use: Antihyperlipidemic inhibitor (HMG-CoA reductase).
See: Lescol, Cap. (Sandoz).

Fluvirin. (Evans Medical) Influenza virus vaccine. Vial 5 ml, 0.5 ml pre-filled syringes. *Rx.*
Use: Agent for immunization.

•**fluvoxamine maleate.** (flew-VOX-ah-meen) USAN.
Use: Antidepressant; antiobsessional agent.
See: Luvox, Tab. (Solvay).

•**fluzinamide.** (flew-ZIN-ah-mide) USAN.
Use: Anticonvulsant.

Fluzone. (Pasteur-Merieux-Connaught) Influenza virus vaccine. Vial 5 ml (10 doses) (Whole-virus); Vial 5 ml, 25 ml, syringes 0.5 ml (Split-virus). *Rx.*
Use: Agent for immunization.

FML Forte. (Allergan) Fluorometholone 0.25%. Susp. Bot. 2 ml, 5 ml, 10 ml, 15 ml. *Rx.*
Use: Corticosteroid, ophthalmic.

FML Liquifilm. (Allergan) Fluorometholone 0.1%. Bot. 1 ml, 5 ml, 10 ml, 15 ml. *Rx.*
Use: Corticosteroid, ophthalmic.

FML-S. (Allergan) Fluorometholone 0.1%, sulfacetomide sodium 10%. Susp. Dropper Bot. 5 ml, 10 ml. *Rx.*
Use: Corticosteroid, ophthalmic.

FML S.O.P. (Allergan) Fluorometholone 0.1% Oint. Tube 3.5 g. *Rx.*
Use: Corticosteroid, ophthalmic.

Foamicon. (Invamed) Aluminum hydroxide 80 mg, magnesium trisilicate 20 mg, alginic acid, calcium stearate, compressible sugar, sodium bicarbonate, sucrose. Chew. Tab. Bot. 100s. *otc.*
Use: Antacid.

•**focofilcon a.** (FOE-koe-FILL-kahn A) USAN.
Use: Contact lens material (hydrophilic).

Foille. (Blistex) Benzocaine 2%, benzyl alcohol 4% in a bland vegetable oil base. Oint. Tube 30 g. *otc.*
Use: Local anesthetic, topical.

Foillecort. (Blistex) Hydrocortisone acetate 0.5%. Cream. Tube 3.5 g. *otc.*
Use: Corticosteroid, topical.

Foille Medicated First Aid. (Blistex) **Aerosol:** Benzocaine 5% with chloroxylenol 0.1% in a bland vegetable oil base with benzyl alcohol. Spray 92 g. **Oint.:** Benzocaine 5%, chloroxylenol 0.1% in a bland vegetable oil base. Tube 30 g. **Lot.:** Benzocaine 5%, chloroxylenol 0.1% in a bland vegetable oil base with benzyl alcohol 30 ml. **Oint:** Benzocaine 5%, chloroxylenol, benzyl alcohol, EDTA, corn oil. 3.5 g, 28 g. **Spray:** Benzocaine 5%, chloroxylenol, benzyl alcohol, corn oil. 92 ml. *otc.*
Use: Local anesthetic, topical.

Foille Plus. (Blistex) **Cream:** Benzocaine 5%, benzyl alcohol 4% in a nonstaining washable base. Tube 3.5 g. **Soln.:** Benzocaine 5%, benzyl alcohol, alcohol 77.8%. Aerosol spray 105 g. **Spray:** Benzocaine 5%, chloroxylenol, alcohol. 105 ml. *otc.*
Use: Local anesthetic, topical.

Folabee. (Vortech) Liver inj. B_{12} equivalent to 10 mcg, crystalline B_{12} 100 mcg, folic acid 0.4 mg. Inj. Vial 10 ml. *Rx.*
Use: Anemia.

folacin.
See: Folic acid.

folacine.
See: Folic acid. (Various Mfr.)

folate, sodium.
See: Folvite, Soln. (Lederle).

Folex PFS Injection. (Pharmacia & Upjohn) Methotrexate sodium 25 mg/ml. Preservative free. Inj. Vial. 2 ml, 4 ml, 8 ml. *Rx.*
Use: Antineoplastic.

•**folic acid,** U.S.P. 23.
Use: Anemia; vitamin (hematopoietic).
See: Folvite, Tab., Soln. (Lederle).

folic acid. (Various Mfr.) Tab. **0.4 mg:** Bot. 100s. **0.8 mg:** Bot. 100s. **1 mg:** Bot. 30s, 100s, 1000s, UD 100s. *Rx.*
Use: Treatment of folic acid deficiency.

folic acid. (Fujisawa) 5 mg/ml w/ benzyl alcohol 1.5%, EDTA. Inj. Vials 10 ml. *Rx.*
Use: Treatment of folic acid deficiency.

folic acid antagonists.
See: Methotrexate Inj., Tab. (Lederle).

folic acid salts.
See: Folvite, Tab., Soln. (Lederle).

folinic acid. Leucovorin Calcium, U.S.P. 23. (Various Mfr.)

Fol-Li-Bee. (Foy) Liver inj. equivalent to cyanocobalamin 10 mcg, folic acid 1 mg, cyanocobalamin 100 mcg/ml, phenol 0.5% pH adjusted w/sodium hydroxide and/or HCl. Vial 10 ml multidose, Monovials. *Rx.*
Use: Anemia.

follicle stimulating hormone, human. Menotropins, Pergonal.

follicormon.
See: Estradiol Benzoate. (Various Mfr.).

follicular hormones.
See: Estrone (Various Mfr.).

folliculin.
See: Estrone (Various Mfr.).

Foltrin. (Eon Labs) Liver and stomach concentrate 240 mg, B_{12} 15 mcg, iron 110 mg, C 75 mg, folic acid 0.5 mg/Cap. Bot. 100s, 1000s. Rx.
Use: Vitamin/mineral supplement.

•**fomepizole.** (foe-MEH-pih-ZOLE) USAN.
Use: Antidote (alcohol dehydrogenase inhibitor).

•**fomivirsen sodium.** USAN.
Use: Antiviral (CMV retinitis).

fonatol.
See: Diethylstilbestrol (Various Mfr.).

•**fonazine mesylate.** (FAH-nazz-een) USAN
Use: Serotonin inhibitor.

fontarsol.
See: Dichlorophenarsine Hydrochloride.

Foralicon Plus Elixir. (Forbes) Vitamins B_{12} 16.7 mcg, B_6 4 mg, iron 200 mg (equivalent to elemental iron 24 mg), niacinamide 40 mg, folic acid 0.8 mg, sorbitol soln. q.s./15 ml. Bot. 8 oz, 16 oz. Rx.
Use: Vitamin/mineral supplement.

Forane. (Ohmeda) Isoflurane. Gas. Volume 100 ml. Rx.
Use: General anesthetic.

•**forasartan.** (far-ah-SAHR-tan) USAN.
Use: Antihypertensive.

Fordustin. (Sween) Cornstarch based powder with deodorizing action. Bot. 3 oz, 8 oz. otc.
Use: Baby powder.

Formadon Solution. (Gordon) Formalin solution 3.7% to 4% (10% of U.S.P. strength) in an aqueous perfumed base. Bot. 1 oz, 4 oz, 0.5 gal, gal.
Use: Bromhidrosis, hyperhidrosis.

•**formaldehyde solution,** U.S.P. 23. A 37% aqueous solution.
Use: For poison ivy, fungus infections of the skin, hyperhidrosis and as an astringent, disinfectant.

formalin.
See: Formaldehyde Solution (Various Mfr.).

Formalyde-10. (Pedinol) Formaldehyde 10%, FDA-40 alcohol. Spray Bot. 60 ml. Rx.
Use: Bromhidrosis, hyperhidrosis.

Forma-Ray Solution. (Gordon) Formalin 7.4% to 8% (20% of USP strength) in aqueous, scented, tinted solution. Bot. 1.5 oz, 4 oz. otc.

Use: Drying agent following laser treatment for verrucae, excessive perspiration and odor.

formic acid.
W/Silicic acid.
See: Nyloxin, Inj. (Becton Dickinson).

•**formocortal.** (FORE-moe-CORE-tal) USAN.
Use: Glucocorticoid.

Formula 44 Cough Control Discs. (Procter & Gamble).
See: Vicks Formula 44 Cough Discs (Procter & Gamble).

Formula 44 Cough Mixture. (Procter & Gamble) Chlorpheniramine maleate 2 mg, dextromethorphan HBr 15 mg, alcohol 10%/5 ml. Liq. Bot. 120 ml, 240 ml. otc.
Use: Antihistamine, antitussive.

Formula 44D Decongestant Cough Mixture. (Procter & Gamble) Pseudoephedrine HCl 20 mg, dextromethorphan HBr 10 mg, guaifenesin 67 mg, alcohol 10%/5 ml. Liq. Bot. 120 ml, 240 ml. otc.
Use: Decongestant, antitussive, expectorant.

Formula 44M Cough and Cold. (Procter & Gamble) Pseudoephedrine HCl 15 mg, dextromethorphan HBr 7.5 mg, chlorpheniramine maleate 1 mg, acetaminophen 125 mg/5 ml, alcohol 20%, saccharin, sucrose. Liq. Bot. 120 ml, 240 ml. otc.
Use: Decongestant, antitussive, antihistamine, analgesic.

Formula No. 81. (Fellows) Liver (beef) for inj. 1 mcg, ferrous gluconate 100 mg, niacinamide 100 mg, B_2 1.5 mg, panthenol 2.5 mg, B_{12} 3 mcg, procaine HCl 25 mg/2 ml. Vial 30 ml. otc.
Use: Vitamin/mineral supplement.

Formula 405. (Doak) Sodium tallowate, sodium cocoate, Doak Additive A, PPF-20 methyl glucose ether, titanium dioxide, trochbrocarbanilide, pentasodium pentatate, EDTA. Bar 100 g. otc.
Use: Therapeutic skin cleanser.

Formula 1207. (Thurston) Iodine, liver fraction No. 2, caseinates/Tab. Bot. 100s, 250s. otc.
Use: Mineral supplement.

Formula B. (Major) Vitamins B_1 15 mg, B_2 15 mg, B_3 100 mg, B_5 18 mg, B_6 4 mg, B_{12} 5 mcg, C 500 mg, folic acid 0.5 mg/Tab. Bot 250 g. Rx.
Use: Vitamin supplement.

Formula B Plus. (Major) Iron 27 mg, A 5000 IU, E 30 IU, B_1 20 mg, B_2 20 mg,

B_3 100 mg, B_5 25 mg, B_6 25 mg, B_{12} 50 mcg, C 500 mg, folic acid 0.8 mg, biotin 0.15 mg, Cr, Cu, Mg, Mn, Zn/Tab. Bot 100s, 500s. *Rx.*
Use: Iron with vitamin supplement.

formyl tetrahydropteroylglutamic acid. Leucovorin Calcium, U.S.P. 23.

Formula VM-2000 Tablets. (Solgar) Iron 5 mg, A 12,500 IU, D 200 IU, E 100 IU, B_1 50 mg, B_2 50 mg, B_3 50 mg, B_5 50 mg, B_6 50 mg, B_{12} 50 mcg, C 150 mg, folic acid 0.2 mg, B, Ca, Cr, Cu, I, K, Mg, Mn, Mo, Se, Zn 7.5 mg, betaine, biotin 50 mcg, choline, bioflavonoids, amino acids, hesperidin, inositol, l-gluta-thione, PABA, rutin/Tab. Bot. 30s, 60s, 90s, 180s. *otc.*
Use: Vitamin/mineral supplement.

Forta Drink Powder. (Ross) Whey protein concentrate, sucrose, vitamins A, B_1, B_2, B_3, B_5, B_6, B_{12}, C, D, E, folic acid, biotin, Ca, Cu, Fe, I, Mg, Mn, P, Zn. Can. 482 g. *otc.*
Use: Nutritional supplement.

Forta-Flora. (Barth's) Whey-lactose 90%, pectin. **Pow.** Jar lb. **Wafer:** Bot. 100s.

Forta Instant Cereal. (Ross) Lactose-free oat or bran cereal provides 6.25 g dietary fiber/serving. Can 1 lb 1 oz. *otc.*
Use: Nutritional supplement.

Forta Instant Pudding. (Ross) Lactose-free in pudding base. Can 1 lb 12 oz. Vanilla, chocolate, butterscotch flavors. *otc.*
Use: Nutritional supplement.

Forta Pudding Mix. (Ross) Milk protein isolate, sucrose, hydrolyzed corn-starch, modified tapioca starch, partially hydrogenated soybean oil, vitamins A, B_1, B_2, B_3, B_5, B_6, B_{12}, C, D, E, folic acid, biotin, Ca, Fe, P, I, Mg, Zn, Cu, Mn, tartrazine. Can 794 g. *otc.*
Use: Nutritional supplement.

Forta Shake Powder. (Ross) Nonfat dry milk, sucrose, vitamins A, B_1, B_2, B_3, B_5, B_6, B_{12}, C, D, E, folic acid, biotin, Ca, Cu, Fe, I, Mg, Mn, P, Zn, tartrazine. Can lb, pkt. 1.4 oz. Can 1 lb 2.7 oz, pkt. 1.6 oz. *otc.*
Use: Nutritional supplement.

Forta Soup Mix. (Ross) Milk protein isolate, sodium and calcium caseinate, hydrolyzed cornstarch, modified tapioca starch, powdered shortening (partially hydrogenated coconut oil), vitamins A, B_1, B_2, B_3, B_5, B_6, B_{12}, C, D, E, folic acid, biotin, Ca, Cu, Fe, I, Mg, Mn, P, Zn. Chicken flavor. Can. 454 g. *otc.*
Use: Nutritional supplement.

Fortaz. (Glaxo Wellcome) Ceftazidime powder for parenteral administration 500 mg, 1 g, 2 g, or 6 g Vial. **Pow.: 500 mg:** Tray 25s. **1 g:** Tray 25s, Infusion Pack Tray 10s. **2 g:** Tray 10s, Infusion Pack Tray 10s. **6 g:** Pharmacy Bulk Pkg. Tray 6s. **Inj.:** 1 g, 2 g Vial 50 ml, premixed, frozen. *Rx.*
Use: Anti-infective, cephalosporin.

Forte L.I.V. (Foy) Cyanocobalamin 15 mcg liver injection equivalent to vitamin B_{12} activity 1 mcg, ferrous gluconate 50 mg, B_2 0.75 mg, panthenol 1.25 mg, niacinamide 50 mg, citric acid 8.2 mg, sodium citrate 118 mg/ml, procaine HCl 2%. Bot. 30 ml. *otc.*
Use: Vitamin/mineral supplement.

Fortel Midstream. (Biomerica) Reagent in-home urine test for pregnancy. 1 test stick per kit.
Use: Pregnancy test.

Fortel Ovulation. (Biomerica) Monoclonal antibody-based home test to predict ovulation. Kit 1s.
Use: Diagnostic aid.

Fortel Plus. (Biomerica) Reagent in-home urine pregnancy test. Kit contains urine collection cup, dropper, test device.
Use: Pregnancy test.

Fortral. (Sanofi Winthrop) Pentazocine as solution and tablets. *c-iv.*
Use: Narcotic agonist/antagonist analgesic.

Fortramin. (Thurston) Vitamins E 200 IU, A 6000 IU, D 600 IU, B_1 4.5 mg, B_2 4.5 mg, B_6 4.5 mg, B_{12} 5 mcg, C 2.75 mg, rutin 8 mg, hesperidin complex 10 mg, lemon bioflavonoids 15 mg, d-calcium pantothenate 50 mg, para-aminobenzoic acid 7.5 mg, biotin 10 mg, folic acid 24 mcg, niacinamide 20 mg, desiccated liver 25 mg, iron 3 mg, calcium 75 mg, phosphorous 34 mg, manganese 10 mg, copper 0.5 mg, zinc 0.5 mg, iodine 0.375 mg, potassium 500 mg, magnesium 5 mg/Tab. Bot. 100s, 250s. *otc.*
Use: Vitamin/mineral supplement.

40 Winks. (Roberts Med.) Diphenhydramine HCl 50 mg/Cap. Bot. 30s. *otc.*
Use: Sleep aid.

Fosamax. (Merck) Alendronate sodium 10 mg or 40 mg, lactose/Tab. Bot. 30s, 100s, UD 100s. *Rx.*
Use: Bone resorption inhibitor.

•**fosarilate.** (FOSS-ah-RILL-ate) USAN.
Use: Antiviral.

•**fosazepam.** (foss-AZZ-eh-pam) USAN.
Use: Hypnotic, sedative.

•**foscarnet sodium.** (foss-CAR-net) USAN.
Use: Antiviral.
See: Foscavir, Inj. (Astra).

Foscavir. (Astra) Foscarnet sodium 24 mg/ml. Inj. Bot. 250 ml, 500 ml. *Rx.*
Use: Anti-infective, antiviral.

•**fosfomycin.** (foss-foe-MY-sin) USAN.
Use: Anti-infective; antibacterial.
See: Monurol (Zambon).

•**fosfomycin tromethamine.** (foss-foe-MY-sin troe-METH-ah-meen) USAN.
Use: Antibacterial.
See: Monurol, Granules (Forest).

•**fosfonet sodium.** (FOSS-foe-net) USAN.
Use: Antiviral.

Fosfree. (Mission) Iron 14.5 mg, A 1500 IU, D 150 IU, B_1 5 mg, B_2 2 mg, B_3 10 mg, B_5 1 mg, B_6 3 mg, B_{12} 2 mcg, C 50 mg, Ca/Tab. Bot. 100s. *Rx.*
Use: Vitamin/mineral supplement.

fosinopril. (FAH-sen-oh-PRIL)
Use: Angiotensin-converting enzyme inhibitor, antihypertensive.
See: Monopril (Bristol-Myers).

•**fosinopril sodium.** USAN.
Use: Antihypertensive, enzyme inhibitor (angiotensin-converting).
See: Monopril, Tab. (B-M Squibb).

•**fosinoprilat.** USAN.
Use: Antihypertensive.

•**fosphenytoin sodium.** (FOSS-FEN-ih-toe-in) USAN.
Use: Anticonvulsant.
See: Cerebyx, Inj. (Parke-Davis).

•**fosquidone.** (FOSS-kwih-dohn) USAN.
Use: Antineoplastic.

•**fostedil.** (FOSS-teh-dill) USAN.
Use: Vasodilator (calcium channel blocker).

Fostex. (Bristol-Myers) Benzoyl peroxide 10%, EDTA, urea. Bar. 106 g. *otc.*
Use: Antiacne.

Fostex Acne Cleasing. (Westwood Squibb) Salicylic acid 2%, EDTA, stearyl alcohol. Cream. 118 g. *otc.*
Use: Antiacne.

Fostex Acne Medication Cleansing. (Westwood Squibb) Salicyclic acid 2%, EDTA. Bar. 106 g. *otc.*
Use: Antiacne.

Fostex 10% BPO. (Westwood Squibb) Benzoyl peroxide 10%, EDTA. Gel 42.5 g. *otc.*
Use: Antiacne.

Fostex 10% Wash. (Bristol-Myers) Benzoyl peroxide 10% with water base. Liq. Bot. 150 ml. *otc.*
Use: Antiacne.

•**fostriecin sodium.** (FOSS-try-eh-SIN) USAN.
Use: Antineoplastic.

Fostril. (Westwood Squibb) Sulfur, zinc oxide, parabens, EDTA. Lot. Tube 28 ml. *otc.*
Use: Antiacne.

Fototar Cream. (Zeneca) Coal tar 1.6% (from 2% coal tar extract) in emollient moisturizing cream base. Tube 90 g, 480 g. *otc.*
Use: Chronic skin disorders.

4-Way Cold Tablets. (Bristol-Myers) Aspirin 324 mg, phenylpropanolamine HCl 12.5 mg, chlorpheniramine maleate 2 mg/Tab. Bot. 36s, 60s, Card 15s. *otc.*
Use: Analgesic, decongestant, antihistamine.

4 Hair Softgel. (Marlyn) Iron 2.5 mg, A 1250 IU, E 10 IU, B_3 5mg, B_5 2.5 mg, B_6 1.5 mg, B_{12} 44 mcg, C 25 mg, folic acid 33.3 mg, biotin 250 mcg, I, Mg, Cu, Zn 7.5 mg, choline bitartrate, inositol, Mn, Methionine, PABA, B_1, L-cysteine, tyrosine, Si/Cap. Bot 60s. *otc.*
Use: Vitamin/mineral supplement.

4 Nails Softgel. (Marlyn) Ca 167 mg, iron 3 mg, A 833 IU, D 67, E 10 mg, B_1 3.3 mg, B_2 1.7 mg, B_3 8.3 mg, B_5 8.3 mg, B_6 8.3 mg, B_{12} 8.3 mg, C 10 mg, folic acid 33.3 mg, biotin 8.3 mcg, P, I, Mg, Cu, Zn 3.3 mg, Cr, Mn, methionine, inositol, choline bitartrate, Se, PABA, protein isolate, gelatin, lecithin, unsaturated fatty acid, predigested protein L-cysteine, B mucopolysaccharides, silicon amino acid chelate, S/Cap. Bot. 60s. *otc.*
Use: Vitamin/mineral supplement.

4-Way Fast Acting Nasal Spray. (Bristol-Myers) Phenylephrine HCl 0.5%, naphazoline HCl 0.05%, pyrilamine maleate 0.2%, buffered isotonic aqueous soln., thimerosal. Atomizer 15 ml, 30 ml. *otc.*
Use: Decongestant, antihistamine.

4-Way Long Acting Nasal Spray. (Bristol-Myers) Oxymetazoline HCl 0.05% in isotonic buffered soln. Spray Bot. 15 ml. *otc.*
Use: Decongestant.

Fowler's Solution. Potassium Arsenite Solution (Various Mfr.).

Foxalin. (Standex) Digitoxin 0.1 mg, sodium carboxymethylcellulose/Cap. Bot. 100s. *Rx.*
Use: Cardiac glycoside.

foxglove.
See: Digitalis (Various Mfr.).

Foygen Aqueous. (Foy) Estrogenic sub-

stance or estrogens 2 mg/ml with sodium carboxymethylcellulose, povidone, benzyl alcohol, methyl and propyl parabens. Inj. Vial 10 ml. *Rx.*
Use: Estrogen.

Foyplex Injection. (Foy) Sterile injectable soln. of nine water-soluble vitamins. Packaged as 2 separate solutions for extemporaneous combination. *Rx.*
Use: Parenteral nutritional supplement.

Fragmin. (Pharmacia & Upjohn) Dalteparin sodium 2500 anti-factor Xa IU/0.2 ml. Soln. Bot. 16 ml. 5000 anti-factor Xa IU/0.2 ml/Soln. Vials. Single dose. *Rx.*
Use: Anticoagulant.

Freamine III. (McGaw) Amino acid 8.5% or 10%. Bot. 500 ml, 1000 ml. *Rx.*
Use: Parenteral nutritional supplement.

Freamine III w/Electrolytes. (McGaw) Amino acid 3% with electrolytes. Bot. 1000 ml. *Rx.*
Use: Parenteral nutritional supplement.

Freamine 8.5% III w/Electrolytes. (McGraw) Sodium 60 mEq/L, potassium 60 mEq/L, magnesium 10 mEq/L, Cl 60 mEq/L, phosphate 40 mEq/L, acetate 125 mEq/L. Soln. Bot. 500 ml, 1000 ml. *Rx.*
Use: Parenteral nutritional supplement.

Freamine HBC. (American McGaw) High branched 6.9% amino acid formulation for hypercatabolic patients. Bot. 1000 ml. *Rx.*
Use: Parenteral nutritional supplement.

Free and Clear. (Pharmaceutical Specialties) Ammonium laureth sulfate, disodium cocamide MEA sulfosuccinate, cocamidopropyl hydroxysultaine, cocamide DEA, PEG-120 methyl glucose dioleate, EDTA, potassium sorbate, citric acid. Shampoo. Bot. 240 ml. *otc.*
Use: Therapeutic skin cleanser.

Freedavite. (Freeda) Iron 10 mg (from ferrous fumarate), vitamins A 5000 IU, D 400 IU, E 3 IU, B_1 5 mg, B_2 3 mg, B_3 25 mg, B_5 5 mg, B_6 2 mg, B_{12} 2 mcg, C 60 mg, choline, inositol, potassium iodide, Ca, Cu, K, Mg, Mn, Se, Zn 0.2 mg. Bot. 100s, 250s. *otc.*
Use: Vitamin/mineral supplement.

Freedox. (Pharmacia & Upjohn) Tirilazad.
Use: A 21 aminosteroid antioxidant.

Freezone. (Whitehall Robins) Salicylic acid 13.6%, alcohol 20.5%, ether 64.8% in flexible collodion base. Bot. 9.3 ml 13 oz. *otc.*
Use: Keratolytic.

•**frentizole.** (FREN-tih-zole) USAN.
Use: Immunoregulator.

FreshBurst Listerine. (Warner Lambert) Thymol 0.064%, eucalyptol 0.092%, methyl salicylate 0.06%, menthol 0.042%, alcohol 21.6%. Rinse. Bot. 250 ml. *otc.*
Use: Mouthwash.

Fresh n' Feminine. (Walgreen) Benzethonium Cl 0.2% Bot. 8 oz. *otc.*
Use: Vaginal preparation.

•**fructose,** U.S.P. 23. (Abbott) (Cutter) Soln. 10%. Bot. 1000 ml.
Use: Nutrient.
See: Frutabs, Tab. (Pfanstiehl).

fructose. (Cutter) Soln. 10%. Bot. 1000 ml.
Use: Nutrient.

fructose and sodium chloride injection.
Use: Fluid, nutrient and electrolyte replenisher.

Fruity Chews. (Goldline) Vitamins A 2500 IU, D 400 IU, E 15 mg, B_1 1.05 mg, B_2 1.2 mg, B_3 13.5 mg, B_6 1.05 mg, B_{12} 4.5 mcg, C (as sodium ascorbate and ascorbic acid) 60 mg, folic acid 0.3 mg/ Chew. Tab. Bot. 100s. *otc.*
Use: Vitamin/mineral supplement.

Fruity Chews with Iron. (Goldline) Elemental iron 12 mg, vitamins A 2500 IU, D 400 IU, E 15 mg, B_1 1.05 mg, B_2 1.2 mg, B_3 13.5 mg, B_6 1.05 mg, B_{12} 4.5 mcg, C (as sodium ascorbate and ascorbic acid) 60 mg, folic acid 0.3 mg, zinc 8 mg/Chew. Tab. Bot. 100s. *otc.*
Use: Vitamin/mineral supplement.

frusemide.
See: Lasix.

Frutabs. (Pfanstiehl) Fructose 2 g. Tab. Bot. 100s.
Use: Carbohydrate.

FTA-ABS. (Wampole-Zeus) Fluorescent treponemal antibody-absorbed test in vitro for confirming a positive reagin test for syphillis. Test 100s.
Use: Diagnostic aid.

AFT-ABS/DS. (Wampole-Zeus) Fluorescent treponemal antibody-absorbed test in vitro for confirming a positive reagin test for syphilis. Test 100s.
Use: Diagnostic aid.

•**fuchsin, basic,** U.S.P. 23. Basic Fuchsin is a mixture of rosaniline and pararosaniline HCl. Basic Magenta.
Use: Anti-infective (topical).

FUDR. (Roche) Floxuridine 500 mg sterile pow. for inj. Vial 5 ml. *Rx.*
Use: Antineoplastic.

Ful-Glo. (Pilkington Barnes Hind) Fluorescein sodium 0.6 mg/Strip. Box 300s. *otc.*

Use: Diagnostic aid, ophthalmic.

Fuller. (Birchwood) Pkg. 1 shield.
Use: Anorectal protective garment.

Fulvicin P/G. (Schering Plough) Griseo-fulvin ultramicrosize 125 mg, 165 mg, 250 mg or 330 mg/Tab. Bot. 100s. *Rx.*
Use: Antifungal.

Fulvicin-U/F. (Schering Plough) Griseo-fulvin microsize 250 mg or 500 mg/Tab. Bot. 60s, 250s. *Rx.*
Use: Antifungal.

•**fumaric acid,** N.F. 18.
Use: Acidifier.

Fumasorb. (Milance) Ferrous fumarate 200 mg (iron 66 mg)/Tab. Bot. 30s, 60s. *otc.*
Use: Iron supplement.

Fumatinic Capsules. (Laser) Iron 90 mg (from ferrous fumarate), vitamins C 100 mg, B_{12} 15 mcg, folic acid 1 mg/SR Cap. Bot. 100s. *Rx.*
Use: Vitamin/mineral supplement.

Fumerin. (Laser) Ferrous fumarate 195 mg equivalent to iron 64 mg/Tab. Bot. 100s, 1000s. *otc.*
Use: Iron supplement.

Fumeron. (Eon Labs) Ferrous fumarate 330 mg, vitamin B_1 5 mg/TR Cap. *otc.*
Use: Vitamin/mineral supplement.

•**fumoxicillin.** USAN.
Use: Antibacterial.

Funduscein. (Ciba Vision) Fluorescein sodium. Inj. **10%:** Amp. 5 ml. **25%:** Amp. 3 ml. *Rx.*
Use: Diagnostic aid, ophthalmic.

Fungacetin Ointment. (Blair) Triacetin (glyceryl triacetate) 25% in a water-miscible ointment base. Tube 30 g. *Rx.*
Use: Antifungal, topical.

Fungatin. (Major) Tolnaftate 1%. Cream Tube 15 g. *otc.*
Use: Antifungal, topical.

fungicides.
See: Aftate, Prods. (Schering Plough).
Amphotericin B (Fujisawa).
Ancobon (Roche).
Arcum, Preps. (Arcum).
Asterol.
Basic Fuchsin (Various Mfr.).
Desenex, Prods. (Novartis).
Dichlorophene.
Diflucan (Roerig).
Fungizone Intravenous (Squibb).
Fulvicin P/G (Schering Plough).
Fulvicin U/F (Schering Plough).
Grifulvin V (Ortho Derm).
Grisactin, Prods. (Wyeth-Ayerst).
Griseofulvin Ultramicrosize (Various Mfr.).

Gris-PEG (Allergan Herbert).
Miconazole Nitrate (Various Mfr.).
Monistat I.V. (Janssen).
Mycostatin (Apothecon).
Nifuroxime (Various Mfr.).
Nilstat (Lederle).
Nitrofurfuryl Methyl Ether (Various Mfr.).
Nizoral (Janssen).
Nystatin (Various Mfr.).
Phenylmercuric Preps. (Various Mfr.).
Sporanox, Cap. (Janssen).
Undecylenic Acid (Various Mfr.).

•**fungimycin.** (FUN-jih-MY-sin) USAN.
Use: Antifungal.

Funginail. (Kramer) Resorcinol 1%, sali-cyclic acid 2%, parachlorometaxylenol 2%, benzocaine 0.5%, acetic acid 2.5%, propylene glycol, hydroxypropyl methylcellulose, alcohol 0.5%. Bot. 30 ml. *otc.*
Use: Antifungal, topical.

Fungizone. (Bristol-Meyers Squibb) Amphotericin B 3%, thimerosal, titanium dioxide. **Lot.:** Plastic bot. 30 ml. **Cream, Oint:** Tube 20 g. **Oral Susp.:** 100 mg amphotericin B/ml, 0.55% alco-hol, parabens, sodium metabisulfite/Bot. 24 ml w/dropper. *Rx.*
Use: Antifungal, topical.

Fungizone Intravenous. (Squibb) Amphotericin B 50 mg, sodium desoxy-cholate 41 mg, sodium phosphate 25.2 mg/Vial (lyophilized). *Rx.*
Use: Antifungal.

Fungizone for Laboratory Use in Tissue Culture. (Squibb) Amphotericin B 50 mg, sodium desoxycholate 41 mg/Vial 20 ml.
Use: Laboratory.

Fungoid. (Pedinol) Clotrimazole 1%, polyethylene glycol 400/Soln. Bot. 30 ml. *otc.*
Use: Antifungal, topical.

Fungoid Af. (Pedinol) Undecylenic acid 25%/Soln. Bot. 30 ml. *otc.*
Use: Antifungal, topical.

Fungoid Creme. (Pedinol) Miconazole nitrate 2%, mineral oil. Tube 56.7 g. *Rx.*
Use: Antifungal, topical.

Fungoid HC Creme. (Pedinol) Micona-zole nitrate 2%, hydrocortisone 1%. In 56.7 g, 1 g dual packets. *Rx.*
Use: Antifungal, topical.

Fungoid Tincture. (Pedinol) Miconazole nitrate 2%, alcohol. Soln. Bot. with brush applicator 7.39 ml, 29.57 ml. *Rx.*
Use: Antifungal, topical.

Furacin Soluble Dressing. (Roberts) Nitrofurazone 0.2% in a water-soluble, non-drying, ointment-like base of polyethylene glycols. Jar 454 g, Tube 28 g, 56 g. *Rx.*
Use: Burn preparation.

Furacin Topical Cream. (Roberts) Furacin 0.2% in a water miscible, self-emulsifying cream w/glycerin, cetyl alcohol, mineral oil, ethoxylated fatty alcohol, methylparaben, propylparaben, water. Tube 28 g. *Rx.*
Use: Burn preparation.

Furacin Topical Solution. (Roberts) Nitrofurazone 0.2%. Bot. 480 ml. *Rx.*
Use: Burn preparation.

Furadantin Oral Suspension. (Procter & Gamble) Nitrofurantoin 5 mg/ml. Bot. 60 ml, 470 ml. *Rx.*
Use: Urinary anti-infective.

furalazine hydrochloride.
Use: Antimicrobial compound.

furaltadone.

Furanite Tabs. (Major) Nitrofurantoin 50 mg or 100 mg/Tab. Bot. 100s.
Use: Urinary anti-infective. *Rx.*

•**furaprofen.** (FYOOR-ah-PRO-fen) USAN. *Formerly Enprofen*
Use: Anti-inflammatory.

•**furazolidone,** U.S.P. 23.
Use: Anti-infective (topical), antiprotozoal (Trichomonas, topical).
See: Furoxone Tab., Susp. (Procter & Gamble).

•**furazolium chloride.** (FYOOR-ah-zoe-lee-uhm). USAN.
Use: Antibacterial.

•**furazolium tartrate.** (FYOOR-ah-ZOE-lee-uhm) USAN.
Use: Antibacterial.

furazosin hydrochloride. (FYOOR-ah-zoe-sin) Under study.
Use: Antihypertensive.

•**furegrelate sodium.** (fyoor-eh-GRELL-ate) USAN.
Use: Inhibitor (thromboxane synthetase).

furethidine.

•**furobufen.** (FER-oh-BYOO-fen) USAN.
Use: Anti-inflammatory.

•**furodazole.** USAN.
Use: Anthelmintic.

Furonatal FA. (Lexis) Vitamins A 8000 IU, D 400 IU, E 30 IU, C 60 mg, folic acid 1 mg, B_1 2 mg, B_2 2.8 mg, B_6 2.5 mg, B_{12} 8 mcg, niacinamide 20 mg, iron 65 mg, calcium 125 mg/Tab. Bot. 100s, 1000s. *Rx.*
Use: Vitamin/mineral supplement.

•**furosemide,** (fyu-ROH-se-mide) U.S.P. 23.
Use: Diuretic.
See: Fumide, Tab. (Everett).
Furomide, Vial (Hyrex).
Lasix, Tab., Inj., Soln. (Hoechst Marion Roussel).

furosemide. (Roxane) Furosemide. **10 mg/ml:** Soln. Dropper bot. 60 ml. **40 mg/5 ml:** Soln. Bot. 5 ml, 10 ml, 500 ml. *Rx.*
Use: Diuretic.

furosemide. (Various Mfr.) **Tab.: 20 mg or 80 mg:** Bot. 100s, 500s, 1000s, UD 100s; **40 mg:** Bot. 60s, 100s, 500s, 1000s, UD 100s. **Oral Soln.:** 10 mg/ml Bot. 60 ml, 120 ml. **Inj.:** 10 mg/ml Vial 10 ml; single dose vial 2 ml, 10 ml; partial fill single dose vial 4 ml. *Rx.*
Use: Diuretic.

Furoxone. (Procter & Gamble) Furazolidone. **Tab.:** 100 mg. Bot. 20s, 100s. **Liq.:** 50 mg/15 ml. Bot. 60 ml, 473 ml. *Rx.*
Use: Anti-infective.

•**fursalan.** (FYOOR-sal-an) USAN. Under study.
Use: Disinfectant.

•**fusidate sodium.** (FEW-sih-DATE) USAN.
Use: Antibacterial.
See: Fucidine (Squibb).

•**fusidic acid.** (few-SIH-dik) USAN.
Use: Antibacterial.

G

G-4.
See: Dichlorophene.
G-11. (Givaudan) Hexachlorophene Pow. for mfg.
See: Hexachlorophene, U.S.P. 23.
gabapentin. (GAB-uh-PEN-tin) USAN.
Use: Anticonvulsant; amyotrophic lateral sclerosis. [Orphan drug]
See: Neurontin, Cap. (Warner Lambert).
gabbromicina.
See: Aminosidine.
Gacid Tab. (Arcum) Magnesium trisilicate 500 mg, aluminum hydroxide 250 mg/Tab. Bot. 100s, 1000s. *otc.*
Use: Antacid.
•**gadobenate dimeglumine.** (gad-oh-BEN-ate die-meh-GLUE-meen) USAN.
Use: Diagnostic aid (paramagnetic), brain tumors, spine disorders.
•**gadodiamide.** (GAD-oh-DIE-ah-mide) USAN.
Use: Diagnostic aid (paramagnetic).
See: Omniscan, Vial (Sanofi Winthrop).
gadodiamide/caltiamide.
Use: Radiopaque agent.
See: Omniscan (Sanofi Winthrop).
•**gadopentetate dimeglumine,** (GAD-oh-PEN-teh-tate die-meh-GLUE-meen) U.S.P. 23.
Use: Radiopaque agent; diagnostic aid.
See: Magnevist (Berlex).
•**gadoteridol.** (GAD-oh-TER-ih-dahl) USAN.
Use: Diagnostic aid (paramagnetic).
See: ProHance, Inj. (Bracco DXS).
•**gadoversetamide.** (gad-oh-ver-SET-ah-mide) USAN.
Use: Diagnostic aid (paramagnetic, brain disorders, spine disorders).
•**galdansetron hydrochloride.** (gahl-DAN-seh-trahn) USAN.
Use: Antiemetic.
•**gallamine triethiodine,** U.S.P. 23.
Use: Neuromuscular blocking agent.
•**gallium citrate Ga-67 injection,** (GAL-ee-uhm SIH-trate) U.S.P. 23.
Use: Diagnostic aid (radiopaque medium); radioactive agent.
•**gallium nitrate.** (GAL-ee-uhm NYE-trate) USAN.
Use: Calcium regulator; treatment of cancer-related hypercalcemia. [Orphan drug]
See: Ganite, Inj. (Fujisawa).
gallochrome.
See: Merbromin (Various Mfr.).

gallotannic acid.
See: Tannic Acid, Preps. (Various Mfr.).
gallstone solubilizing agents.
See: Actigall, Cap. (Novartis).
Chenix, Tab. (Solvay).
Moctanin. (Ethitek).
Gamazole Tabs. (Major) Sulfamethoxazole 500 mg/Tab. Bot. 100s, 500s, 1000s. *Rx.*
Use: Anti-infective, sulfonamide.
•**gamfexine.** (gam-FEX-ine) USAN.
Use: Antidepressant.
Gammimune N 5%. (Bayer) Immune globulin IV (human) 5%. Inj. in maltose 10% 500 mg, 2.5 g, 5 g, 10 g. *Rx.*
Use: Immune serum.
Gamimune N 10%. (Bayer) Immune globulin IV (human) 10%. Inj. 5 g, 10 g, 20 g. Vial 50 ml, 100 ml, 200 ml. *Rx.*
Use: Immune serum.
Gammagard S/D. (Baxter) Immune globulin IV (human) 2.5 g, 5 g or 10 g/Bot. Freeze-dried, solvent/detergent treated w/ sterile water for injection. 500 mg. *Rx.*
Use: Immune serum.
gamma benzene hexachloride.
See: lindane.
gamma globulin.
See: Immune Globulin Intramuscular.
Immune Globulin Intravenous.
gamma-hydroxybutyrate.
Use: Narcolepsy. [Orphan drug]
gamma interferon, 1-b.
See: Actimmune (Genentech).
gammalinolenic acid.
Use: Juvenile rheumatoid arthritis. [Orphan drug]
Gammar-P IV. (Centeon) Immune globulin (human). Sucrose 5%, albumin 3% (1 g or 5 g). In 1 g single-dose vial with 20 ml sterile water for inj.; 2.5 g single-dose vial with 50 ml sterile water for inj.; 5 g single-dose vial with 100 ml sterile water for inj.; 5 g pharmacy bulk pack, 10 g. *Rx.*
Use: Immune serum.
Gamulin Rh. (Centeon) Rho (D) Immune globulin (Human). Vial, syringe 1 dose. *Rx.*
Use: Rh-negative mothers after delivery of an Rh-positive infant.
•**ganciclovir.** (gan-SIGH-kloe-VIHR) USAN.
Use: Antiviral.
See: Cytovene, Cap., Pow for Inj., (Roche).
ganciclovir intravitreal free implant.
Use: Cytomegalovirus retinitis. [Orphan drug]

•**ganciclovir sodium.** USAN.
Use: Antiviral.
See: Cytovene (Roche).

G and W products. (G & W) G and W markets the following products under the G & W brand name:
Aminophylline Rectal Supp., 250 mg, 500 mg.
Aspirin Rectal Supp., 125 mg, 300 mg, 600 mg.
Bisacodyl Supp., 10 mg.
Glycerin Supp., Adult and Infant Sizes.
Hemorrhoidal Rectal Ointment.
Hemorrhoidal Rectal Supp., Formula C-116 and Formula C-119.
Hemorrhoidal Rectal Supp. w/Hydrocortisone Acetate 10 mg or 25 mg/Supp.
Vaginal Sulfa Cream.

Ganeake. (Geneva Pharm) Conjugated Estrogens, 0.625 mg, 1.25 mg or 2.5 mg/Tab. Bot. 100s, 1000s. *Rx.*
Use: Estrogen.

ganglionic blocking agents.
See: Arfonad, Amp. (Roche).
Dibenzyline HCl, Cap. (SK-Beecham).
Hexamethonium Cl and Bromide (Various Mfr.).
Hydergine, Amp., Tab. (Sandoz).
Inversine, Tab. (Merck).
Priscoline HCl, Tab., Vial (Novartis).
Regitine, Amp., Tab. (Novartis).

gangliosides as sodium salts.
Use: Retinitis pigmentosa.
See: Cronassial (FIDIA Pharm).

•**ganirelix acetate.** (gah-nih-RELL-ix ASS-eh-tate) USAN.
Use: Gonad-stimulating principle.

Ganite. (Fujisawa). Gallium nitrate. 25 mg/ml. Vial. 20 ml. *Rx.*
Use: Treatment of cancer-related hypercalcemia.

Gantanol. (Roche) Sulfamethoxazole. **Tab.:** 0.5 g/Tab. Bot. 100s, 500s, Tel-E-Dose 100s. **Susp:** 0.5 g/5 ml (cherry flavor) Bot. 1 pt. *Rx.*
Use: Anti-infective, sulfonamide.

Gantanol DS. (Roche) Sulfamethoxazole 1 g/Tab. Bot. 100s. *Rx.*
Use: Anti-infective, sulfonamide.

Gantrisin Injectable. (Roche) Sulfisoxazole diolamine 4 mg/ml. *Rx.*
W/sodium metabisulfite 2 mg. Pkg. 10s.
Use: Anti-infective, sulfonamide.

Gantrisin, Lipo. (Roche) Acetyl Sulfisoxazole. *Rx.*
Use: Anti-infective, sulfonamide.
See: Lipo Gantrisin, Susp. (Roche).

Gantrisin Solution. (Roche) Sulfisoxazole diolamine 4%. Soln. Bot. 15 ml w/dropper. *Rx.*
Use: Anti-infective, sulfonamide (ophthalmic).

Garamycin. (Schering Plough) **Cream:** Gentamicin sulfate 1.7 mg (equivalent to gentamicin base 1 mg). Methylparaben 1 mg, butylparaben 4 mg as preservatives, stearic acid, propylene glycol monostearate, isopropyl myristate, propylene glycol, polysorbate 40, sorbitol soln., water/g. Tube 15 g. **Oint.:** Gentamicin sulfate 1.7 mg (equivalent to gentamicin base 1 mg), methylparaben 0.5 mg, propylparaben 0.1 mg in petrolatum base/g. Tube 15 g. *Rx.*
Use: Anti-infective, topical.

Garamycin Injectable. (Schering Plough) Gentamicin sulfate. Inj. equivalent to 40 mg gentamicin base, methylparaben 1.8 mg, propylparaben 0.2 mg, as preservatives, sodium bisulfite 3.2 mg, disodium edetate 0.1 mg/ml Vial 2 ml (80 mg), 20 ml (800 mg); Syringe 1.5 ml (60 mg), 2 ml (80 mg); **Pediatric Inj.:** 10 mg/ml w/methylparaben 1.3 mg, propylparaben 0.2 mg, sodium bisulfite 3.2 mg, edetate disodium 0.1 mg/ml. Vial 2 ml (20 mg). *Rx.*
Use: Anti-infective, aminoglycoside.

Garamycin Intrathecal Injection. (Schering Plough) Gentamicin sulfate equivalent to 2 mg/ml gentamicin base, 8.5 mg sodium Cl/ml. Amp. 2 ml. *Rx.*
Use: Anti-infective, aminoglycoside.

Garamycin I.V. Piggyback. (Schering Plough) Gentamicin sulfate equivalent to 1 mg gentamicin base, 8.9 mg sodium Cl, (no preservatives). Inj. Bot. 60 ml (60 mg), 80 ml (80 mg). *Rx.*
Use: Anti-infective, aminoglycoside.

Garamycin Ophthalmic Ointment-Sterile. (Schering Plough) Gentamicin sulfate 3 mg/g. Tube 3.5 g. *Rx.*
Use: Anti-infective, ophthalmic.

Garamycin Ophthalmic Solution, Sterile. (Schering Plough) Gentamicin sulfate 3 mg/ml. Dropper Bot. 5 ml. *Rx.*
Use: Anti-infective, ophthalmic.

Garamycin Pediatric Injection. (Schering Plough) Gentamicin sulfate equivalent to 10 mg per ml as sulfate. Vials 2 ml. *Rx.*
Use: Anti-infective, aminoglycoside.

gardenal.
See: Phenobarbital. (Various Mfr.).

gardinol type detergents. Aurinol, Cyclopon, Dreft, Drene, Duponol, Lissa-

pol, Maprofix, Modinal, Orvus, Sando-pan, Sadipan.
Use: Detergents.

gardol. Sodium Lauryl Sarcosinate.

Garfield. (Menley & James) Vitamin A 2500 IU, D 400 IU, E 15 IU, C 60 mg, folic acid 0.3 mg, Vitamin B_1 1.05 mg, B_2 1.2 mg, B_3 13.5 mg, B_6 1.05 mg, B_{12} 4.5 mcg, sucrose, lactose. Chew. Tab. Bot. 60s. *otc.*
Use: Vitamin supplement.

Garfield Complete w/ Minerals. (Menley & James) Vitamin A 5000 IU, D 400 IU, E 30 IU, C 60 mg, folic acid 0.4 mg, B_1 1.5 mg, B_2 1.7 mg, B_3 20 mg, B_6 2 mg, B_{12} 6 mcg, biotin 40 mcg, B_5 10 mg, iron 18 mg, Ca, Cu, P, I, Mg, zinc 15 mg, aspartame, phenylalanine, sorbital/Chew. Tab. Bot. 60s. *otc.*
Use: Vitamin/mineral supplement.

Garfield Plus Extra C. (Menley & James) Vitamin A 2500 IU, D 400 IU, E 15 IU, C 250 mg, folic acid 0.3 mg, B_1 1.05 mg, B_2 1.2 mg, B_3 13.5 mg, B_6 1.05 mg, B_{12} 4.5 mcg, sucrose, lactose/Chew. Tab. Bot. 60s. *otc.*
Use: Vitamin supplement.

Garfield Plus Iron. (Menley & James) Vitamin A 2500 IU, D 400 IU, E 15 IU, C 60 mg, folic acid 0.3 mg, B_1 1.05 mg, B_2 1.2 mg, B_3 13.5 mg, B_6 1.05 mg, B_{12} 4.5 mcg, iron 15 mcg, sucrose, lactose. Chew. Tab. Bot. 60s. *otc.*
Use: Vitamin/mineral supplement.

Garfields Tea. (Last) Senna leaf powder 68.3%. Bot. 2 oz. *otc.*
Use: Laxative.

Garitabs. (Halsey) Iron 50 mg, vitamins B_1 5 mg, B_2 5 mg, C 75 mg, niacinamide 30 mg, B_5 2 mg, B_6 0.5 mg, B_{12} 3 mcg Bot. 1000s. *otc.*
Use: Vitamin/mineral supplement.

Gari-Tonic Hematinic. (Halsey) Vitamins B_1 5 mg, niacinamide 100 mg, B_2 5 mg, pantothenic acid 4 mg, B_6 1 mg, B_{12} 6 mcg, choline bitartrate 100 mg, iron 100 mg/30 ml Bot. 16 oz. *otc.*
Use: Vitamin/mineral supplement.

garlic. Allium.
Use: Intestinal antispasmodic.
See: Allimin, Tab. (Mosso).

garlic capsules. (Miller) Garlic 166 mg/Cap. Bot. 100s. *otc.*
Use: Intestinal antispasmodic.

garlic concentrate.
W/Parsley Concentrate.
See: Allimin, Tab. (Mosso).

garlic oil.
See: Natural Garlic Oil, Cap. (Spirt).

garlic oil capsules. (Kirkman Sales) Bot. 100s. *otc.*

Gas-Ban. (Roberts Med) Calcium carbonate 300 mg, simethicone 40 mg/Tab. Bot. UD 8s, 1000s. *otc.*
Use: Antacid.

Gas-Ban-DS. (Roberts Med) Aluminum hydroxide 400 mg, magnesium hydroxide 400 mg, simethicone 40 mg/5 ml. Liq. Bot. 150 ml. *otc.*
Use: Antacid.

Gas Permeable Daily Cleaner. (Pilkington Barnes Hind) Potassium sorbate 0.13%, EDTA 2%, ethoxylated polyoxypropylene glycol, tris (hydroxymethyl) amino methane, hydroxymethylcellulose. Thimerosal free. Sol. Bot. 30 ml. *otc.*
Use: Gas permeable contact lens care.

Gas Permeable Lens Starter System. (Pilkington Barnes Hind) Daily cleanser, Bot. 3 ml, Wetting and soaking soln., Bot. 60 ml, Hydra-Mat II spin cleansing unit. Kit. *otc.*
Use: Gas permeable contact lens care.

Gas Permeable Wetting & Soaking Solution. (Pilkington Barnes Hind) Sterile aqueous, isotonic soln. of low viscosity, buffered to physiological pH. Bot. 60 ml, 120 ml. *otc.*
Use: Gas permeable contact lens care.

gastric acidifiers.
See: Acidulin, Pulv. (Lilly)
Glutamic Acid HCl (Various Mfr.).

Gastroccult. (SmithKline Diagnostics) Occult blood screening test. In 40s.
Use: Diagnostic aid.

Gastrocrom. (Medeva) Cromolyn sodium 100 mg/Cap. Bot. 100s. *Rx.*
Use: Mastocytosis.
See: Cromolyn Sodium.

Gastrografin. (Squibb) Diatrizoate methyl-glucamine 66%, sodium diatrizoate 10%. Soln. Bot. 120 ml.
Use: Radiopaque agent.

gastrointestinal tests.
See: Entero-test, Cap. (HDC)
Entero-Test, Ped. Cap. (HDC).
Gastro-Test (HDC).

Gastrosed. (Roberts/Hauck) Hyoscyamine sulfate. 0.125 mg/ml. Dropper Bot. 5 ml. Alcohol free. **Tab.:** 0.125 mg. Bot. 100s. *Rx.*
Use: Anticholinergic, antispasmodic.

Gastro-Test. (HDC Corp.) To determine stomach pH and to diagnose and locate gastric bleeding. Test 25s.
Use: Diagnostic aid.

Gas-X. (Sandoz Consumer) Simethicone

80 mg/Chew. Tab. Pkg. 12s, 30s. *otc.*
Use: Antiflatulent.

Gas-X, Extra Strength. (Sandoz Consumer) Simethicone 125 mg, sorbitol/ Chew. Tab. Box 18s. *otc.*
Use: Antiflatulent.

•**gauze, absorbent,** U.S.P. 23.
Use: Surgical aid.

•**gauze, petrolatum,** U.S.P. 23.
Use: Surgical aid.

Gaviscon. (SK-Beecham) Aluminum hydroxide 80 mg, magnesium trisilicate 20 mg, alginic acid, sodium bicarbonate, sucrose, calcium stearate. Chew. Tab. Bot. 30s, 100s. *otc.*
Use: Antacid.

Gaviscon-2 Double Strength Tablets. (SK-Beecham) Aluminum hydroxide 160 mg, magnesium trisilicate 40 mg, alginic acid, sodium bicarbonate, sucrose, Chew. Tab. Bot. 48s. *otc.*
Use: Antacid.

Gaviscon Extra Strength Relief Formula Liquid. (SK-Beecham) Aluminum hydroxide 254 mg, magnesium carbonate 237.5 mg, parabens, EDTA, saccharin, sorbitol, simethicone, sodium alginate/5 ml. Bot. 355 ml. *otc.*
Use: Antacid.

Gaviscon Extra Strength Relief Formula Tablets. (SK-Beecham) Aluminum hydroxide 160 mg, magnesium carbonate 105 mg, alginic acid, sodium bicarbonate, sucrose, calcium stearate. Chew. Tab. Bot. 30s, 100s. *otc.*
Use: Antacid.

Gaviscon Liquid. (SK-Beecham) Aluminum hydroxide 31.7 mg, magnesium carbonate 119.3 mg/5 ml Bot. 177 ml, 355 ml. *otc.*
Use: Antacid.

GBA.
See: Gamma hydroxybutyrate.

G.B.H. Lotion. (Century) Gamma benzene hexachloride 1%. Bot. 2 oz, pt, gal.
Use: Scabicide/pediculicide.

G.B.S. (Forest) Dehydrocholic acid 125 mg, phenobarbital 8 mg, homatropine methylbromide 2.5 mg/Tab. 100s, 1000s. *Rx.*
Use: Hydrocholeretic.

G-CSF.
See: Neupogen (Amgen).

Gebauer's 114. (Gebauer) Dichlorotetrafluoroethane 100%. Can 8 oz.
Use: Local anesthetic.

Gee-Gee. (Jones Medical) Guaifenesin 200 mg/Tab. Bot. 1000s. *otc.*
Use: Expectorant.

Geladine. (Barth's) Gelatin, protein, vitamin D/Cap. Bot. 100s, 500s. *otc.*

Gelamal. (Halsey) Magnesium-aluminum hydroxide gel. Bot. 12 oz. *otc.*
Use: Antacid.

•**gelatin,** N.F. 18.
Use: Pharmaceutic aid (encapsulating, suspending agent, tablet binder, tablet coating agent).

•**gelatin film, absorbable,** U.S.P. 23.
Use: Local hemostatic.
See: Gelfilm (Pharmacia & Upjohn).

gelatin film, sterile.
See: Neupogen (Amgen).

gelatin powder, sterile.
See: Gelfoam Powder (Pharmacia & Upjohn).

gelatin sponge.
See: Gelfilm (Pharmacia & Upjohn).

•**gelatin sponge, absorbable,** U.S.P. 23.
Use: Local hemostatic.
See: Gelfoam, Paks (Pharmacia & Upjohn).

gelatin, zinc.
See: Zinc gelatin. (Various Mfr.).

Gel-Clean. (Pilkington Barnes Hind) Gel formulated with nonionic surfactant. Tube 30 g. *otc.*
Use: Hard contact lens care.

Gelfilm. (Pharmacia & Upjohn) Sterile, absorbable gelatin film. Envelope 1s. 100 mm × 125 mm. Also available as Ophth. Sterile 25 × 50 mm. Box 6s. *Rx.*
Use: Hemostatic, topical.

Gelfoam. (Pharmacia & Upjohn) **Sterile Sponges:**
> **Size 12-3 mm.** 20 × 60 mm (12 sq. cm) × 3 mm. *Rx.*
> Box 4 sponges in individual envelopes. *Rx.*
> **Size 12-7 mm.** 20 × 60 mm (12 sq. cm.) × 7 mm.
> Box 12 sponges in individual envelopes, jar 4 sponges. *Rx.*
> **Size 50-10 mm.** 62.5 × 80 mm (50 sq. cm.) × 10 mm. Box 4 sponges in individual envelopes. *Rx.*
> **Size 100-10 mm.** 80 × 125 mm (100 sq. cm.) × 10 mm. *Rx.*
> Box 6 sponges in individual envelopes. *Rx.*
> **Size 200-10 mm.** 80 × 250 mm (200 sq. cm.) × 10 mm.
> Box 6 sponges in individual envelopes. *Rx.*
> **Compressed Size 100.** (intended primarily for application in the dry state). 80 × 125 mm. Boxes of 6

sponges in individual envelopes. *Rx.*
Packs: Packs size 2 cm. (Designed particularly for nasal packing). 2 × 40 cm. Single jar. (Packing cavities). *Rx.*
Size 6 cm. 6 × 40 cm. Box 6 sponges in individual envelopes. *Rx.*
Use: Hemostatic, topical.
Gelfoam Dental Pack. (Pharmacia & Upjohn) Size 4, 20 mm × 20 mm × 7 mm. Jar 15 sponges. *Rx.*
Use: Hemostatic, topical.
Gelfoam Powder. (Pharmacia & Upjohn) Sterile Jar 1 g. *Rx.*
Use: Hemostatic, topical.
Gelfoam Prostatectomy Cones. (Pharmacia & Upjohn) Prostatectomy cones (for use with Foley catheter). 13 cm, 18 cm in diameter. Box 6s. *Rx.*
Use: Hemostatic.
Gel Jet Gelatin Capsules. (Kirkman Sales) Bot. 100s, 250s.
Gel-Kam. (Scherer) Fluoride 0.1% (stannous fluoride 0.4%). Cinnamon flavor. Gel. Bot. w/applicator tip 69 g, 105 g, 129 g. *Rx.*
Use: Dental caries preventative.
Gelocast. (Beiersdorf) Unna's Boot medicated bandage: Semi-rigid cast impregnated with zinc oxide mixtures. Box 4 inches × 10 yd, 3 inches × 10 yd.
Use: Unna's cast dressing.
Gelpirin. Acetaminophen 125 mg, aspirin 240 mg, caffeine 32 mg. Tab. Bot. 100s, 1000s. *otc.*
Use: Analgesic combination.
Gelpirin CCF. (Alra) Acetaminophen 325 mg, guaifenesin 25 mg, chlorpheniramine maleate 1 mg, phenylpropanolamine HCl 12.5 mg/Tab. Bot. 50s. *otc.*
Use: Analgesic, expectorant, decongestant.
gelsemium. (Various Mfr.) Pkg. oz.
Use: For neuralgia.
W/APC.
See: APC Combinations.
gelsemium w/combinations.
See: Briacel, Tab. (Briar).
Bricor, Tab. (Briar).
Cystitol, Tab. (Briar).
Ricor, Tab. (Vortech).
Sodadide, Tab. (Scrip).
UB, Tab. (Scrip).
Urisan-P, Tab. (Sandia).
Uriseptic w/Gelsemium, Tab. (Rugby).
Urothyn Improved, Tab. (Solvay).
Urseptic, Tab. (Century).
U-Tract, Tab. (Jones Medical).
gelsolin, recombinant human. (Biogen) *Rx.*

Use: Treatment of cystic fibrosis. [Orphan drug]
Gel-Tin. (Young Dental) Fluoride 0.1% (from stannous flouride 0.4%) Gel Bot. 57 g, 623 g. *Rx.*
Use: Dental caries preventative.
•**gemcadiol.** (JEM-kah-DIE-ole) USAN.
Use: Antihyperlipoproteinemic.
•**gemcitabine.** (JEM-sit-ah-BEAN) USAN.
Use: Antineoplastic.
•**gemcitabine hydrochloride.** (JEM-sit-ah-BEAN) USAN.
Use: Antineoplastic.
See: Gemzar (Lilly).
Gemcor. (Upsher-Smith) Gemfibrozil 600 mg/Tab. Bot. 60s, 500s, 1000s. *Rx.*
Use: Treatment of hypercholesterolemia.
•**gemeprost.** (JEH-meh-PRAHST) USAN.
Use: Prostaglandin.
•**gemfibrozil,** (gem-FIE-broe-ZILL) U.S.P. 23. (Various Mfr.) 300 mg/Cap., Bot. 100s, 500s, 1000s. 600 mg/Tab., Bot. 60s, 100s, 500s, 1000s,
Use: Treatment of hypercholesterolemia; antihyperlipidemic.
See: Lopid, Cap. (Parke-Davis).
gemfibrozil, (Various Mfr.) 300 mg/Cap., Bot. 100s, 500s, 1000s. 600 mg/Tab., Bot. 60s, 100s, 500s, 1000s.
Use: Treatment of hypercholesterolemia; antihyperlipidemic.
Gemzar. (Lilly) Gemcitabine HCl 20 mg/ml/Pow for Inj. Vials 10 and 50 ml. *Rx.*
Use: Antineoplastic.
Genabid. (Goldline) Papaverine HCl 150 mg/TR Cap. Bot. 100s, 1000s. *Rx.*
Use: Peripheral vasodilator.
Genac Tablets. (Goldline) Triprolidine HCl 2.5 mg, pseudoephedrine HCl 60 mg/Tab. Bot. 24s, 100s. *otc.*
Use: Antihistamine, decongestant.
Genacol Tablets. (Goldline) Pseudoephedrine HCl 30 mg, chlorpheniramine maleate 2 mg, dextromethorphan HBr 10 mg, acetaminophen 325 mg/Tab. Bot. 50s. *otc.*
Use: Decongestant, antihistamine, antitussive, analgesic.
Genagesic Tabs. (Goldline) Propoxyphene HCl 165 mg, acetaminophen 650 mg/Tab. Bot. 100s, 500s. *c-iv.*
Use: Narcotic analgesic combination.
Genahist. (Goldline) Diphenhydramine HCl 25 mg/Cap or Tab. Bot. 24s. *otc.*
Use: Antihistamine.
Genahist Liquid. (Goldline) Diphenhydramine 12.5 mg/5 ml. Elix. 120 ml. *otc.*

Use: Antihistamine.

Genallerate Tablets. (Goldline) Chlorpheniramine maleate 4 mg, lactose/Tab. Bot. 24s. *otc.*
Use: Antihistamine.

Genamin Cold Syrup. (Goldline) Phenylpropanolamine HCl 6.25 mg, chlorpheniramine maleate 1 mg. Alcohol free. In 118 ml. *otc.*
Use: Decongestant, antihistamine.

Genamin Expectorant. (Goldline) Phenylpropanolamine 12.5 mg, guaifenesin 100 mg, alcohol 5%. In 120 ml. *otc.*
Use: Decongestant, expectorant.

Genapap Children's Chewable Tabs. (Goldline) Acetaminophen 80 mg/Tab. Bot. 30s. *otc.*
Use: Analgesic.

Genapap Children's Elixir. (Goldline) Acetaminophen 160 mg/5 ml. Cherry flavor. Bot. 120 ml. *otc.*
Use: Analgesic.

Genapap Extra Strength Caplets. (Goldline) Acetaminophen 500 mg/Cap. Bot. 50s, 100s. *otc.*
Use: Analgesic.

Genapap Infants' Drops. (Goldline) Acetaminophen 100 mg/ml, alcohol 7%. Soln. Dropper bot. 15 ml. *otc.*
Use: Analgesic.

Genapap Tablets. (Goldline) Acetaminophen 325 mg/Tab. Bot. 100s. *otc.*
Use: Analgesic.

Genapax. (Key) Gentian violet 5 mg/tampon. Box 12s.
Use: Antifungal, vaginal.

Genaphed Tablets. (Goldline) Pseudoephedrine HCl 30 mg/Tab. Bot. 24s, 100s. *otc.*
Use: Decongestant.

Genasal. (Goldline) Oxymetazoline 0.05%. Soln. 15 ml, 30 ml. *otc.*
Use: Decongestant.

Genasoft Capsules. (Goldline) Docusate sodium 100 mg/Cap. Bot. 60s. *otc.*
Use: Laxative, stool softener.

Genasoft Plus Capsules. (Goldline) Docusate sodium 100 mg, casanthranol 30 mg/Cap. Bot. 60s. *otc.*
Use: Laxative, stool softener.

Genaspor Antifungal Cream. (Goldline) Tolnaftate 1%. Bot. 15 g. *otc.*
Use: Antifungal, topical.

Genasyme Tablets. (Goldline) Simethicone 80 mg/Tab. Bot. 100s. *otc.*
Use: Antiflatulent.

Genatap Elixir. (Goldline) Brompheniramine maleate 2 mg, phenylpropanolamine HCl 12.5 mg/5 ml. Bot. 118 ml. *otc.*
Use: Antihistamine, decongestant.

Genaton. (Goldline) Aluminum hydroxide 80 mg, magnesium trisilicate 20 mg, alginic acid, sodium bicarbonate, sodium 18.4 mg, sucrose, sugar. Chew. Tab. Bot. 100s. *otc.*
Use: Antacid.

Genaton Extra Strength Tablets. (Goldline) Aluminum hydroxide 160 mg, magnesium carbonate 105 mg, alginic acid, sodium bicarbonate, sodium 29.9 mg, sucrose, calcium stearate. Chew. Tab. Bot. 100s. *otc.*
Use: Antacid.

Genaton Liquid. (Goldline) Aluminum hydroxide 31.7 mg, magnesium carbonate 137.3 mg, sodium alginate, sodium 13 mg, EDTA, saccharin, sorbitol/5 ml. Bot. 355 ml. *otc.*
Use: Antacid.

genatropine hydrochloride. (jen-AT-row-peen) Atropine-N-oxide HCl. Aminoxytropine Tropate HCl.
See: X-tro, Cap. (Xttrium).

Genatuss DM Syrup. (Goldline) Dextromethorphan HBr 10 mg, guaifenesin 100 mg. Bot. 120 ml. *otc.*
Use: Antitussive, expectorant.

Genatuss Syrup. (Goldline) Guaifenesin 100 mg/5 ml, alcohol 3.5%. Bot. 120 ml. *otc.*
Use: Expectorant.

Gen-Bee with C. (Goldline) Vitamins B_1 15 mg, B_2 10.2 mg, B_3 50 mg, B_5 10 mg, B_6 5 mg, C 300 mg/Cap. Bot. 130s, 1000s. *otc.*
Use: Vitamin supplement.

Gencalc 600 Tablets. (Goldline) Calcium 600 mg (from calcium carbonate 1.5 g)/Tab. Bot. 60s. *otc.*
Use: Calcium supplement.

Gencept. (Gencon) **0.5/35:** Norethindrone 0.5 mg, ethinyl estradiol, 35 mcg/Tab (with 7 inert tabs) Pkgs 21s and 28s; **1/35:** norethindrone 1 mg, ethinyl estradiol 35 mcg/Tab (with 7 inert tabs) Pkgs 21s and 28s; **10/11:** norethindrone 0.5 mg and 1 mg, ethinyl estradiol 35 mcg/Tab (with 7 inert tabs). Pkg 21s and 28s. *Rx.*
Use: Oral contraceptives.

Gencold Capsules. (Goldline) Phenylpropanolamine HCl 75 mg, chlorpheniramine maleate 8 mg/SR Tab. Pkg. 10s. *otc.*
Use: Decongestant, antihistamine.

Gendecon. (Goldline) Phenylephrine HCl 5 mg, chlorpheniramine maleate 2 mg, acetaminophen 325 mg/Tab. Bot. 50s. *otc.*
Use: Decongestant, antihistamine, analgesic.

Genebs Extra Strength Caplets. (Goldline) Acetaminophen 500 mg/Cap. Bot. 100s, 1000s. *otc.*
Use: Analgesic.

Genebs Extra Strength Tablets. (Goldline) Acetaminophen 500 mg/Tab. Bot. 100s, 1000s. *otc.*
Use: Analgesic.

Genebs Tablets. (Goldline) Acetaminophen 325 mg/Tab. Bot. 100s, 1000s. *otc.*
Use: Analgesic.

Generet-500. (Goldline) Iron 105 mg, Vitamins B_1 6 mg, B_2 6 mg, B_3 30 mg, B_5 10 mg, B_6 5 mg, B_{12} 25 mcg, C (as sodium ascorbate) 500 mg. TR Tab. Bot. 60s. *otc.*
Use: Vitamin/mineral supplement.

Generix-T. (Goldline) Iron 15 mg, vitamins A 10,000 IU, D 400 IU, E 5.5 mg, B_1 15 mg, B_2 10 mg, B_3 100 mg, B_5 10 mg, B_6 2 mg, B_{12} 7.5 mcg, C 150 mg, Cu, I, Mg, Mn, zinc 1.5 mg/Tab. Bot. 100s. *otc.*
Use: Vitamin/mineral supplement.

Genex Caps. (Goldline) Phenylpropanolamine HCl 18 mg, acetaminophen 325 mg/Cap. Bot. 100s, 1000s. *otc.*
Use: Decongestant, analgesic.

Geneye. (Goldline) Tetrahydrozoline HCl 0.05%. Drop. Bot. 15 ml. *otc.*
Use: Ophthalmic vasoconstrictor, mydriatic.

Geneye AC Allergy Formula. (Goldline) Tetrahydrozoline HCl 0.05%, zinc sulfate 0.25%, benzalkonium chloride 0.01%, EDTA/Drop. In 15 ml. *otc.*
Use: Ophthalmic decongestant, antihistamine.

Geneye Extra. (Goldline) Tetrahydrozoine HCl 0.05%, PEG 400, benzalkonium Cl, EDTA/Drop. 15 ml. *otc.*
Use: Ophthalmic vasoconstrictor.

genital herpes treatment.
See: Acyclovir.
Zovirax Cap., Oint. (Glaxo Wellcome).

Genite. (Goldline) Pseudoephedrine HCl 10 mg, doxylamine succinate 1.25 mg, dextromethorphan HBr 5 mg, acetaminophen 167 mg, alcohol 25%/5 ml. Bot. 177 ml. *otc.*
Use: Decongestant, antihistamine, antitussive, analgesic.

genitourinary irrigants.
See: Acetic acid for irrigation (Various Mfr.).
Glycine (Aminoacetic Acid) For Irrigation (Various Mfr.).
Neosporin G.U. Irrigant, Soln. (Burroughs-Wellcome).
Renacidin, Pow., Soln. (Guardian).
Resectisol, Soln. (McGaw).
Sorbitol (Various Mfr.).
Sorbitol-Mannitol (Abbott).
Sodium Chloride for Irrigation (Various Mfr.).
Sterile Water for Irrigation (Various Mfr.).
Suby's Solution G (Various Mfr.).

Gen-K Powder. (Goldline) Potassium Cl. Pow. 20 mEq/packet. Box 30s. *Rx.*
Use: Potassium supplement.

Gen-K Tabs. (Goldline) Effervescent potassium. Bot. 30s. *Rx.*
Use: Potassium supplement.

Genna Tablets. (Goldline) Senna concentrate 217 mg/Tab. Bot. 100s, 1000s. *otc.*
Use: Laxative.

Gennin Tablets. (Goldline) Buffered aspirin 5 gr. Bot. 100s. *otc.*
Use: Salicylate analgesic.

genophyllin.
See: Aminophylline (Various Mfr.).

Genoptic Liquifilm Sterile Ophthalmic Solution. (Allergan) Gentamicin sulfate 3 mg/ml. Bot. 1 ml, 5 ml. *Rx.*
Use: Anti-infective, ophthalmic.

Genoptic S.O.P. Sterile Ophthalmic Ointment. (Allergan) Gentamicin sulfate 3 mg/g. Oint. Tube 3.5 g. *Rx.*
Use: Anti-infective, ophthalmic.

Genora 0.5/35 Tablets. (Rugby) Norethindrone 0.5 mg, ethinyl estradiol 0.035 mg/Tab. Pkg. 21s; 28s (7 inert tab.) *Rx.*
Use: Oral contraceptive.

Genora 1/35-21 Tablets. (Rugby) Norethindrone 1 mg, ethinyl estradiol 0.035 mg/Tab. Pkg. 126s (6-pak). *Rx.*
Use: Oral contraceptive.

Genora 1/35-28 Tablets. (Rugby) Norethindrone 1 mg, ethinylestradiol 0.035 mg/Tab., 7 inert tab. Pkg. 168s (6-pak). *Rx.*
Use: Oral contraceptive.

Genora 1/50-21 Tablets. (Rugby) Norethindrone 1 mg, mestranol 0.05 mg/Tab. Pkg. 126s (6-pak). *Rx.*
Use: Oral contraceptive.

Genora 1/50-28 Tablets. (Rugby) Norethindrone 1 mg, mestranol 0.05 mg/

Tab., 7 inert tab. Pkg. 168s (6-pak). *Rx.*
Use: Oral contraceptive.

Genotropin. (Pharmacia & Upjohn)
Somatropin 1.5 mg/Cartridge. 5s.
Somatropin 5.8 mg/Cartridge 1s, 5s.
Pow. for Inj. *Rx.*
Use: Growth hormone.

Genprep Ointment. (Goldline) Live yeast
cell derivative supplying 2000 units skin
respiratory factor/oz of ointment w/
shark liver oil 3%, phenylmercuric nitrate 1:10,000. Tube 2 oz. *otc.*
Use: Anorectal preparation.

Genpril. (Goldline) Ibuprofen 200 mg.
Tab. 50s, 100s. *otc.*
Use: Nonsteroidal anti-inflammatory
drug, analgesic.

Genprin. (Goldline) Aspirin 325 mg. Tab.
100s. *otc.*
Use: Salicylate analgesic.

gensalate sodium. Sodium gentisate.
(Sodium salt of 2,5-dihydroxybenzoic
acid).
Use: Analgesic.

Gensan Tablets. (Goldline) Aspirin 400
mg, caffeine 32 mg/Tab. Bot. 100s. *otc.*
Use: Analgesic combination.

Gentacidin Ophthalmic Ointment.
(Ciba Vision) Gentamicin 3 mg/g. Oint.
Tube 3.5 g. *Rx.*
Use: Anti-infective, ophthalmic.

Gentacidin Ophthalmic Solution. (Ciba
Vision) Gentamicin sulfate 3 mg/ml.
Soln. Bot. 5 ml. *Rx.*
Use: Anti-infective, ophthalmic.

Gentafair. (Bausch & Lomb) **Oint.:**
Gentamicin 3 mg/g with liquid lanolin,
white petrolatum, mineral oil, parabens.
Tube 3.75 g, 15 g. **Soln.:** Gentamicin
3 mg/ml, polyoxyl 40 stearate, polyeth-
ylene glycol. Dropper bot. 5 ml, 15 ml.
Rx.
Use: Anti-infective, ophthalmic.

Gentak. (Akorn) **Oint.:** Gentamicin 3 mg/
g. Tube 3.5 g. **Soln.:** Gentamicin 3 mg/
ml. Bot. 5 ml, 15 ml. *Rx.*
Use: Anti-infective, ophthalmic.

**gentamicin impregnated PMMA beads
on surgical wire.** *Rx.*
Use: Chronic osteomyelitis. [Orphan
drug]

gentamicin liposome injection. *Rx.*
Use: Mycobacterium avium-intracellu-
lare infection. [Orphan drug]

•**gentamicin sulfate,** (JEN-tuh-MY-sin)
U.S.P. 23.
Use: Antibacterial.
See: Apogen, Inj. (SK-Beecham).
Garamycin, Preps. (Schering Plough).

Genoptic, Preps. (Allergan).
Gentaciden, Preps. (Ciba Vision).
Gentak, Preps. (Akorn).

gentamicin sulfate. (Schering Plough)
Produced by *Micromonospora pur-
purea.* (Various Mfr.) **Ophthalmic Oint.:**
3 mg/g Tube 3.5 g; **Ophthalmic Soln.:**
3 mg/ml Bot. 5 ml, 15 ml.
Use: Antibacterial.

**gentamicin and prednisolone acetate
ophthalmic suspension.**
Use: Anti-infective, anti-inflammatory.

gentisate sodium.

•**gentisic acid ethanolamide,** N.F. 18.
Use: Pharmaceutic aid; complexing
agent.

Gentlax. (Blair) Standardized senna con-
centrate 326 mg, malt extract, sucrose/
Gran. 180 g. *otc.*
Use: Laxative.

Gentlax S Tablets. (Blair) Standardized
senna concentrate 187 mg, docusate
sodium 50 mg. Tab. Bot. 30s, 60s. *otc.*
Use: Laxative.

**Gentle Nature Natural Vegetable Laxa-
tive.** (Sandoz Consumer) Sennosides
A and B as calcium salts. 20 mg/Tab.
Box 16s, 32s. *otc.*
Use: Laxative.

Gentle Shampoo. (Ulmer) Bot. 4 oz, gal.
otc.
Use: Mild, neutral shampoo.

Gentran 40. (Baxter) Dextran 40 10% w/
sodium Cl 0.9% or Dextran 40 10% w/
dextrose 5%. Inj. Plastic Bot. 500 ml.
Rx.
Use: Plasma expander.

Gentran 70. (Baxter) Dextran 70 6% w/
sodium Cl 0.9%. Inj. Plastic Bot. 500
ml. *Rx.*
Use: Plasma expander.

Gentran 75. (Baxter) Dextran 75 6% in
sodium Cl 0.9%. Inj. Bot. 500 ml. *Rx.*
Use: Plasma expander.

Gentrasul. (Bausch & Lomb) Gentamicin
3 mg. **Oint.:** 3.5 g. **Soln.:** Dropper bot.
5 ml. *Rx.*
Use: Anti-infective, ophthalmic.

Gentz Rectal Wipes. (Roxane) Pramoxine HCl 1%, alcloxa 0.2%, witch hazel 50%, propylene glycol 10%. Box
100s, 120s (individually wrapped disposable wipes). *otc.*
Use: Anorectal preparation.

Genuine Bayer Aspirin. (Bayer) Aspirin
325 mg/FC Tab. Bot. 12s, 24s, 50s,
200s, 300s. *otc.*
Use: Salicylate analgesic.

Gen-Xene. (Alra) Clorazepate dipotas-

sium 3.75 mg, 7.5 mg or 15 mg/Tab.
Bot. 30s, 100s, 500s, UD 100s. *c-iv.*
Use: Antianxiety agent, anticonvulsant.

Geocillin. (Roerig) Carbenicillin indanyl sodium 382 mg/Tab. Bot. 100s, UD 100s. *Rx.*
Use: Anti-infective, penicillin.

Geopen. (Roerig) Carbenicillin disodium. Inj. **Vial:** 1 g, 2 g, 5 g. Pkg. 10s. **Piggyback Vial:** 2 g, 5 g, 10 g. **Bulk Pharmacy Pack:** 30 g. *Rx.*
Use: Anti-infective, penicillin.

• **gepirone hydrochloride.** (jeh-PIE-rone) USAN.
Use: Tranquilizer.

Gera Plus. (Towne) Iron 50 mg, vitamins B_1 5 mg, B_2 5 mg, C 75 mg, niacinamide 30 mg, calcium pantothenate 2 mg, B_6 0.5 mg, B_{12} 3 mcg/Tab. Bot. 100s. *otc.*
Use: Vitamin/mineral supplement.

Geravim. (Major) Vitamins B_1 0.83 mg, B_2 0.42 mg, B_3 8.3 mg, B_5 1.67 mg, B_6 0.17 mg, B_{12} 0.17 mg, I, Fe 2.5 mg, Zn 0.3 mg, choline, Mn, alcohol 18%. Liq. Bot. pt., gal. *otc.*
Use: Vitamin/mineral supplement.

Geravite Elixir. (Roberts) Elix.: Vitamins B_1 0.3 mg, B_2 0.4 mg, B_3 33.3 mg, B_{12} 3.3 mcg, L-lysine, alcohol 15%, parabens, sorbitol, sucrose. Bot. 480 ml. *otc.*
Use: Vitamin/mineral supplement.

Gerber Baby Formula Low Iron. (Bristol-Myers) Protein (from non-fat milk) 14.7 g, carbohydrate (from lactose) 71.3 g, fat (from palm olein, soy, coconut and high oleic sunflower oils) 36 g, linoleic acid 5.9 g, vitamins A, D, E, K, C, B_1, B_2, B_3, B_5, B_6, B_{12}, folic acid, biotin, choline, inositol, Ca, P, Mg, Fe 3.4 mg, Zn, Mn, Cu, I, Na 220 mg, K 720 mg, Cl, taurine, calories per L 666.7. **Ready to use liq.:** Bot. 943 ml. **Concentrated liq.:** Bot. 433 ml. **Pow.:** Can 457 g and 914 g. *otc.*
Use: Nutritional therapy.

Gerber Baby Formula with Iron. (Bristol-Myers) Protein (from non-fat milk) 14.7 g, carbohydrate (from lactose) 71.3 g, fat (from palm olein, soy, coconut and high oleic sunflower oils) 36 g, with linoleic acid 5.9 g, vitamins A, D, E, K, C, B_1, B_2, B_6, B_{12}, B_3, folic acid, B_5, biotin, choline, inositol, Ca, P, Mg, Fe 12 mg, Zn, Mn, Cu, I, Na 220 mg, K 720 mg, Cl, taurine, calories per L 666.7./ concentrated Liq. Bot. 943 ml. *otc.*
Use: Nutritional therapy.

Geref. (Serono) Sermorelin acetate 50 mcg (lyophilized). Pow. for Inj. Amp. 2

ml w/sodium Cl. 0.9%.
Use: Diagnostic aid.

Geri-All-D. (Barth's) Vitamins A 10,000 IU, D 400 IU, B_1 7 mg, B_2 14 mg, C 200 mg, niacin 4.17 mg, B_{12} 25 mcg, E 50 IU, B_6 0.35 mg, pantothenic acid 0.63 mg, trace minerals and other factors. 2 Cap. Bot. 1 mo., 3 mo. and 6 mo. supply of Geri-All regular and Geri-All-D. *otc.*
Use: Vitamin/mineral supplement.

geriatric supplements w/multivitamins/ minerals.
See: Geravite, Elix. (Roberts).
  Gerimed, Tab. (Fielding).
  Geriplex FS, Caps. (Parke-Davis).
  Hep-Forte, Cap. (Marlyn).
  Megadose, Tab. (Arco).
  Mega VM-80, Tab. (NBTY).
  Optivite P.M.T., Tab. (Optimox).
  Strovite Plus, Tab. (Everett).
  Ultra-Freeda, Tab. (Freeda).
  Ultra-Freeda Iron Free, Tab. (Freeda).
  Vigortol, Liq. (Rugby).
  Viminate, Elix. (Various Mfr.).
  Viopan-T, Tab. (Trimen).
  Vita-Plus G Softgels (Scot-Tussin).

Geriatroplex. (Morton) Cyanocobalamin 30 mcg, liver inj. 0.1 ml vitamins B_{12} activity 2 mcg, ferrous gluconate 50 mg, B_2 1.5 mg, calcium pantothenate 2.5 mg, niacinamide 100 mg, citric acid 16.4 mg, sodium citrate 23.6 mg/2 ml. Vial 30 ml. *otc.*
Use: Vitamin/mineral supplement.

Geri-Derm. (Barth's) Vitamins A 400,000 IU, D 40,000 IU, E 200 IU, panthenol 800 mg/4 oz. Jar 4 oz. *otc.*
Use: Skin supplement.

Geridium Tablets. (Goldline) Phenazopyridine HCl 100 mg or 200 mg/Tab. Bot. 100s, 1000s. *Rx.*
Use: Urinary analgesic, anti-infective.

Gerifort Plus. (A.P.C.) Vitamins A 10,000 IU, B_1 5 mg, B_2 6 mg, B_6 2 mg, C 75 mg, D-2 1000 IU, niacinamide 60 mg, iron 10 mg, calcium 115 mg, phosphorous 83 mg, iodine 0.1 mg, calcium pantothenate 10 mg, d-alpha tocopheryl acid succinate 3 IU, cobalamin concentrate 3 mcg, choline bitartrate 70 mg, inositol 35 mg, biotin 15 mcg, Zn 0.2 mg, magnesium 2 mg, manganese 0.5 mg, potassium 0.15 mg/Amcap. Bot. 100s. *otc.*
Use: Vitamin/mineral supplement.

Gerilets. (Abbott) Vitamins A 5000 IU, D 400 IU, E 45 IU, C 90 mg (from sodium ascorbate), folic acid 0.4 mg, B_1 2.25 mg, B_2 2.6 mg, niacin 30 mg, B_6 3

mg, B_{12} 9 mcg, biotin 0.45 mg, pantothenic acid 15 mg, iron 27 mg (from ferrous sulfate)/Tab. Bot. 100s. *otc.*
Use: Vitamin/mineral supplement.

Gerimal. (Rugby) Ergoloid mesylates 0.5 mg or 1 mg/**Sublingual Tab.**: Bot. 100s, 500s, 1000s; 1 mg/**Oral Tab.**: Bot. 100s, 500s, 1000s. *Rx.*
Use: Psychotherapeutic agent.

Gerimed. (Fielding) Vitamins A 5000 IU, D 400 IU, E 30 mg, B_1 3 mg, B_2 3 mg, B_3 25 mg, B_6 2 mg, B_{12} 6 mcg, C 120 mg, calcium 370 mg, zinc 15 mg, Mg, P/ Tab. Bot. 60s. *otc.*
Use: Vitamin/mineral supplement.

Gerineed. (Hanlon) Vitamins A 5000 IU, B_1 20 mg, B_2 5 mg, niacinamide 20 mg, B_6 0.5 mg, calcium pantothenate 5 mg, B_{12} 5 mcg, rutin 25 mg, C 50 mg, E 10 IU, choline 50 mg, inositol 50 mg, calcium lactate 1.64 mg, iron sulfate 10 mg, copper 1 mg, iodine 0.5 mg, manganese 1 mg, magnesium sulfate 1 mg, potassium sulfate 5 mg, zinc sulfate 0.5 mg/Cap. Bot. 100s. *otc.*
Use: Vitamin/mineral supplement.

Geriot. (Goldline) Iron 50 mg (from ferrous sulfate), A 6000 IU, D 400 IU, E 30 IU, B_1 1.5 mg, B_2 1.7 mg, B_3 20 mg, B_5 10 mg, B_6 2 mg, B_{12} 6 mcg, C 60 mg, folic acid 0.4 mg, biotin 45 mcg, Ca, Cl, Cr, Cu, I, K, Mg, Mn, Mo, Ni, P, Se, Si, Sn, V, Zn, vitamin K/Tab. Bot. 100s. *otc.*
Use: Vitamin/mineral supplement.

Geri-Plus. (Approved) Vitamins A 12,500 IU, D 1200 IU, B_1 15 mg, B_2 10 mg, C 75 mg, niacinamide 30 mg, calcium pantothenate 2 mg, B_6 0.5 mg, E 5 IU, Brewer's yeast 10 mg, B_{12} 15 mcg, iron 11.58 mg, desiccated liver 15 mg, choline bitartrate 30 mg, inositol 30 mg, calcium 59 mg, phosphorous 45 mg, zinc 0.68 mg, francium dicalcium phosphate 200 mg, Mn, enzymatic factors, amino acids/Cap. Bot. 50s, 100s, 1000s. *otc.*
Use: Vitamin/mineral supplement.

Geri-Plus Elixir. (Approved) Vitamins B_1 25 mg, B_2 10 mg, B_6 1 mg, niacinamide 100 mg, calcium pantothenate 5 mg, B_{12} 20 mcg, iron ammonium citrate 100 mg, choline 200 mg, inositol 100 mg, magnesium Cl 2 mg, manganese citrate 2 mg, zinc acetate 2 mg, amino acids/fl oz. Bot. pt. *otc.*
Use: Vitamin/mineral supplement.

Geritol Complete Tablets. (SK-Beecham) Vitamins A 6000 IU, E 30 IU, C 60 mg, folic acid 400 mcg, B_1 1.5

mg, B_2 1.7 mg, B_3 20 mg, B_6 2 mg, B_{12} 6 mcg, D 400 IU, K, biotin 45 mcg, B_5 10 mg, iron 18 mg, Ca, Cl, Cr, Cu, I, K, Mg, Mn, Mo, Ni, P, Se, Si, Sn, V, Zn, vitamin K /Tab. Bot. 14s, 40s, 100s, 180s. *otc.*
Use: Vitamin/mineral supplement.

Geritol Extended Caplets. (SmithKline-Beecham) Capl.: Iron 10 mg, vitamins A 3333 IU, D 200 IU, E 15 IU, B_1 1.2 mg, B_2 1.4 mg, B_3 15 mg, B_6 2 mg, B_{12} 2 mg, C 60 mg, folic acid 0.2 mg, vitamin K, Ca, I, Mg, Se, Zn 15 mg. Bot. 40s, 100s. *otc.*
Use: Vitamin/mineral supplement.

Geritol Tonic Liquid. (SK-Beecham) Iron 18 mg, Vitamins B_1 2.5 mg, B_2 2.5 mg, B_3 50 mg, B_5 2 mg, B_6 0.5 mg, methionine 25 mg, choline bitartrate 50 mg/15 ml. Alcohol 12%. Bot. 120 ml, 360 ml. *otc.*
Use: Vitamin/mineral supplement.

Gerivite. (Goldline) Liq.: Vitamins B_1 0.8 mg, B_2 0.4 mg, B_3 8.3 mg, B_5 1.7 mg, B_6 0.2 mg, B_{12} 0.2 mcg, iron 0.3 mg, Zn 0.3 mg, choline, I Mg, Mn, alcohol 18%, methylparaben, sorbitol. Bot. 473 ml. *otc.*
Use: Vitamin/mineral supplement.

Gerivites. (Rugby) Iron (from ferrous sulfate) 50 mg, A 5000 IU, D 400 IU, E 30 IU, B_1 1.5 mg, B_2 1.7 mg, B_3 20 mg, B_5 10 mg, B_6 2 mg, B_{12} 300 mcg, C 60 mg, folic acid 400 mg, Ca, Cl, Cr, Cu, I, K, Mg, Mn, Mo, Ni, Se, Si, P, Zn 15 mg/Tab. 40s. *otc.*
Use: Vitamin/mineral supplement.

Gerix Elixir. (Abbott) Vitamins B_1 6 mg, B_2 6 mg, niacin 100 mg, iron 15 mg, B_6 1.6 mg, cyanocobalamin 6 mcg, alcohol 20%/30 ml. Bot. 480 ml. *otc.*
Use: Vitamin/mineral supplement.

germanin. (CDC) *Rx.*
Use: Anti-infective.
See: Suramin sodium (Naphuride sodium).

Germicin. (CMC) Benzalkonium Cl 50%. Bot. pt., gal. *otc.*
Use: Antiseptic, germicide.

Ger-O-Foam. (Geriatric) Methylsalicylate 30%, benzocaine 3%, volatile oils. Aerosol can 4 oz. *otc.*
Use: Analgesic, anesthetic.

Geroton Forte. (Kenwood/Bradley) Vitamin B_1 1.7 mg, B_2 1.9 mg, B_3 2.22 mg, B_5 1.11 mg, B_6 0.22 mg, B_{12} 0.67 mcg, Zn 1.7 mg, Mg, Mn, alcohol 13%. Liq. Bot. 473 ml. *otc.*
Use: Vitamin/mineral supplement.

Gerterol Depo. (Fellows) Medroxyprogesterone acetate 50 mg or 100 mg/ml. Vial 5 ml. *Rx.*
Use: Progestin.

Gesic. (Lexalabs) Aspirin 226.8 mg, caffeine 32.4 mg, codeine 32.4 mg/Tab. Bot. 100s. *c-III.*
Use: Narcotic analgesic combination.

•**gestaclone.** (JEST-ah-klone) USAN.
Use: Progestin.

•**gestodene.** (JEST-oh-deen) USAN.
Use: Progestin.

Gestoneed. (Hanlon) Calcium lactate 1069 mg, vitamins C 100 mg, nicotinic acid 18 mg, B_2 2.4 mg, B_1 1.8 mg, B_6 9 mg, D 500 IU, A 6000 IU/Cap. Bot. 100s. *otc.*
Use: Vitamin/mineral supplement.

•**gestonorone caproate.** (jess-TOE-noreohn CAP-row-ate) USAN. 17-Hydroxy-19-norpregn-4-ene-3,20-dione hexanoate.
Use: Progestin.

•**gestrinone.** (JESS-trih-nohn) USAN.
Use: Progestin.

Gets-It. (Oakhurst) Salicyclic acid, zinc Cl, collodion in ether ≈ 35%, alcohol ≈ 28%. Liq. Bot. 12 ml. *otc.*
Use: Keratolytic.

•**gevotroline hydrochloride.** (jeh-VOE-troe-LEEN) USAN.
Use: Antipsychotic.

Gevrabon. (Lederle) Vitamins B_1 0.83 mg, B_2 0.42 mg, B_3 8.3 mg, B_5 1.67 mg, B_6 0.17 mg, B_{12} 0.17 mcg, Fe 2.5 mg, choline, I, Mg, Mn, Zn 0.3 mg, alcohol 18%. Liq. Bot. 480 ml. *otc.*
Use: Vitamin/mineral supplement.

Gevral. (Lederle) Vitamins A 5000 IU, B_1 1.5 mg, B_2 1.7 mg, B_6 2 mg, B_{12} 6 mcg, folic acid 0.4 mg, C 60 mg, E 30 mg, B_3 20 mg, Ca, P, iron 18 mg, Mg, I, lactose, parabens, sucrose/Tab. Bot. 100s. *otc.*
Use: Vitamin/mineral supplement.

Gevral Protein. (Lederle) Calcium caseinate, sucrose, protein 15.6 g, carbohydrate 7.05 g, fat 0.52 g, sodium 50 mg, potassium 13 mg, calories 95.3/26 g. Pow. Can. 8 oz, 5 lb. *otc.*
Use: Nutritional supplement.

GG-Cen Capsules. (Schwarz Pharma) Guaifenesin 200 mg/Cap. Bot. 24s, 100s. *otc.*
Use: Expectorant.

GI stimulants.
See: Clopra, Tab. (Quantum).
Maxolon, Tab. (SK-Beecham).
Metoclopramide, Tab. (Various Mfr.).

Metoclopramide HCl, Inj. (Quad).
Octamide, Tab. (Pharmacia & Upjohn).
Reclomide, Tab. (Major).
Reglan, Inj., Syr., Tab. (Robins).

GL-2 Skin Adherent. (Gordon) Ready to use. Bot. pt, qt, gal. *otc.*

GL-7 Skin Adherent. (Gordon) Plastic material which may be used full strength or diluted with 3 to 10 parts 99% isopropyl alcohol, acetone or naphtha. Pkg. pt, qt, gal. *otc.*

Glandosane Mouth Moisturizer. (Kenwood) Sodium carboxymethylcellulose 0.51 g, sorbitol 1.52 g, sodium Cl 0.043 g, potassium Cl 0.061 g, calcium Cl 0.007 g, magnesium Cl 0.003 g, dipotassium hydrogen phosphate 0.017 g/50 ml. Soln. Bot. 50 ml. *otc.*
Use: Saliva substitute.

glandubolin.
See: Estrone (Various Mfr.).

glatiramer acetate.
Use: Treatment of relapsing-remitting multiple sclerosis.
See: Copaxone.

glauber's salt.
See: Sodium Sulfate (Various Mfr.).

Glaucon Solution. (Alcon) Epinephrine HCl 1% or 2%. Drop-Tainers. 10 ml. *Rx.*
Use: Agent for glaucoma.

GlaucTabs. (Akorn) Methazolamide 25 mg, 50 mg. Tab. Bot. 100s. *Rx.*
Use: Diuretics.

•**glaze, pharmaceutical,** N.F. 18.
Use: Pharmaceutic aid (tablet coating).

•**glemanserin.** (gleh-MAN-ser-in) USAN.
Use: Antianxiety.

•**gliamilide.** (glie-AM-ih-lide) USAN.
Use: Antidiabetic.

glibenclamide.
See: Glyburide.

•**glibornuride.** (glie-BORN-you-ride) USAN.
Use: Oral hypoglycemic agent; antidiabetic.

•**glicetanile sodium.** (glie-SET-AH-nile) USAN. **Formerly Glydanile Sodium.**
Use: Antidiabetic.

•**gliflumide.** (GLIH-flew-mide) USAN.
Use: Antidiabetic.

glim.
See: Gardinol Type Detergents (Various Mfr.).

•**glimepiride.** (GLIE-meh-pie-ride) USAN.
Use: Hypoglycemic.
See: Amaryl, Tab. (Hoescht Marion Roussel).

•**glipizide,** (GLIP-ih-zide) U.S.P. 23.
Use: Antidiabetic.
See: Glucotrol, Tab. (Pratt).

glipizide. (GLIP-ih-zide) (Various Mfr.) 5
or 10 mg/Tab. 100s, 500s, UD 100s.
Rx.
Use: Antidiabetic.

globulin, cytomegalovirus immune.
See: CytoGam, Vial (MedImmune).

globulin, gamma.
See: Immune Globulin Intramuscular.
Immune Globulin Intravenous.

globulin, hepatitis b immune.
See: BayHep B (Bayer).
H-BIG, Vial (Abbott).

•**globulin, immune,** U.S.P. 23. *Formerly
Globulin, Immune Human Serum.*
Use: IM, measles prophylactic and po-
lio; passive immunizing agent.
See: Gammagee, Vial (Merck).
Gammar-IM (Centeon).

globulin, immune, IV.
Use: Immunodeficiency; immune throm-
bocytopinea purpura; Kawasaki syn-
drome.
See: Gamimune-N (Bayer).
Gammagard S/D (Hyland).
Gammar-P IV (Centeon).
Iveegam (Immuno).
Polygam S/D (American Red Cross).
Sandoglobulin (Sandoz).
Venoglobulin-I (Alpha).
Venoglubulin-S (Alpha).

globulin, rabies immune.
Use: Passive immunization.
See: Bayrab (Bayer).
Imogam Rabies (Pasteur-Merieux-
Connaught).

•**globulin, rho(d) immune.**
Use: Prevention of Rh isoimmuniza-
tion; immune thrombocytopenic pur-
pura.
See: BayRhoD (Centeon).
Gamulin Rh (Bayer).
Mini-Gamulin Rh (Centeon).
MICRhoGAM (Ortho).
RhoGAM (Ortho).
WinRho SD (Univax Biologics).

•**globulin serum, anti-human,** U.S.P. 23.

globulin, tetanus immune.
Use: Passive immunization.
See: Baytet (Bayer).

globulin, vaccinia immune.
Use: Passive immunization.

globulin, varicella-zoster immune.
Use: Passive immunization.

•**gloximonam.** (GLOX-ih-MOE-nam)
USAN.
Use: Antibacterial.

glubionate calcium.
See: Neo-Calglucon, Syrup (Sandoz).

•**glucagon,** (GLUE-kuh-gahn) U.S.P. 23.
Use: Emergency treatment of hypogly-
cemia.

glucagon. (Lilly) 1 unit/ml w/diluent. 10
units w/10 ml diluent. Glucagon HCl 1
mg or 10 mg w/diluent; soln. contains
lactose, glycerin 1.6% w/phenol 0.2%
as a preservative. Vial.
Use: Hypoglycemic shock; antidiabetic.

Glucagon Emergency Kit. (Lilly) Glucagon 1 mg or 10 mg, lactose w/diluent.
Inj. 1 ml, 10 ml. *Rx.*

Glucamide. (Lemmon) Chlorpropamide
100 mg or 250 mg/Tab. Bot. 100s,
250s, 500s, 1000s, UD 100s. *Rx.*
Use: Antidiabetic.

Gluceana Liquid. (Ross) Calcium and
sodium caseinate, amino acids, hydrolyzed cornstarch, fructose, soy fiber,
safflower oil, soy oil, soy lecithin, vita-
mins A, B_1, B_2, B_3, B_5, B_6, B_{12}, C, D, E,
K, folic acid, Cl, Ca, P, Mg, I, Mn, Cu,
Zn, Fe, Se, Cr, Mo, biotin, choline. Can
8 oz. Ready-to-use. *otc.*
Use: Nutritional supplement.

•**gluceptate sodium.** (GLUE-sep-tate)
USAN.
Use: Pharmaceutic aid.

**d-glucitol(d-Sorbitol)/Homatropine
methylbromide.**
See: ProBilagol, Liq. (Purdue Frederick).

glucocerebrosidase-beta-glucosidase.
Use: Treatment of Gaucher's disease.
See: Ceredase, Inj. (Genzyme).

glucocerebrosidase (PEG).
See: PEG-glucocerebrosidase.

**glucocerebrosidase, recombinant ret-
roviral vector.** (Genetic Therapy) *Rx.*
Use: Treatment for Gaucher's disease.
[Orphan drug]

glucocorticoids.
See: Cortical Hormone Products.

Glucolet Automatic Lancing Device.
(Bayer) To obtain sample for blood glucose testing. Automatic spring loaded
lancing device.
Use: Diagnostic aid.

Glucolet Endcaps. (Bayer) To obtain
sample for blood glucose testing. Controls depth of lancet penetration. Regular or super puncture.
Use: Diagnostic aid.

Glucometer II Blood Glucose Meter.
(Bayer) Electronic meter for blood glu-
cose testing. *otc.*
Use: Diagnostic aid.

d-gluconic acid, calcium salt. Calcium Gluconate.

gluconic acid salts.
See: Calcium Gluconate.
Ferrous Gluconate.
Magnesium Gluconate.
Potassium Gluconate.

•**gluconolactone,** U.S.P. 23.
Use: Chelating agent.

Glucophage. (Bristol-Myers Squibb) Metformin HCl 500 mg or 850 mg/Tab. Bot. 100s. *Rx.*
Use: Antidiabetic.

•**glucosamine.** (glue-KOSE-ah-meen) USAN.
Use: Pharmaceutic aid.
W/Nystatin, oxytetracycline.
See: Terrastatin, Cap., Soln. (Pfizer).
W/Tetracycline HCl, nystatin.
See: Tetrastatin Cap., Susp. (Pfizer).
W/Tetracycline.
See: Tetracyn, Cap., Syr. (Roerig).
W/Oxytetracycline.
See: Terramycin, Prep (Pfizer).

glucose.
See: Glutose, Gel. (Paddock).
Insta-Glucose, Gel. (ICN).
Pal-A-Dex, Pow. (Baker).

Glucose-40 Ophthalmic Ointment. (Ciba Vision) Liquid glucose 40% in white petrolatum, anhydrous lanolin with parabens. Tube 3.5 g. *Rx.*
Use: Hyperosmolar preparation.

glucose elevating agents.
See: B-D Glucose, Chew. Tab. (Becton Dickinson).
Insta-Glucose, Gel. (ICN).
Glucagon, Pow. for Inj. (Lilly).
Glutose, Gel. (Paddock).
Insta-Glucose, Gel. (ICN).
Insulin Reaction, Gel. (Sherwood).
Proglycem, Cap., Oral. Susp. (Medical Market).

glucose enzymatic test strip.
Use: Diagnostic aid (in vitro, reducing sugars in urine).

glucose (hk) reagent strips. Reagent strip test for detection of glucose in serum or plasma. Bot. 50s.
Use: Diagnostic aid.

Glucose & Ketone Urine Test. (Major) Reagent test for glucose and ketones in urine. Bot. 100s.
Use: Diagnostic aid.

•**glucose, liquid,** N.F. 18.
Use: As a 5% to 50% solution as nutrient; for acute hepatitis and dehydration; to increase blood volume; pharmaceutic aid (tablet binder, tablet coating agent).

d-glucose, monohydrate. Dextrose.

glucose oxidase. W/peroxidase, potassium iodide.
See: Diastix, Vial, Tab. (Bayer).

glucose polymers.
See: Polycose, Pow., Liq. (Ross).

Glucose Reagent Strips. (Bayer) A quantitative strip test for glucose in serum or plasma. Seralyzer reagent strips. Bot. 50s.
Use: Diagnostic aid.

glucose test.
See: Combistix (Bayer).
First Choice, Strips (Polymer Technology Int.).
Glucose Reagent Strips (Bayer).

glucose tolerance test preparation.
See: Glucola (Bayer).

Glucostix Reagent Strips. (Bayer) Cellulose strip containing glucose oxidase and indicator system. Bot. 50s, 100s, UD 25s. *otc.*
Use: Diagnostic aid.

glucosulfone sodium, inj..
See: Sodium Glucosulfone Injection.

Gluco System Lancets. (Bayer) Disposable lancets for use in Miles Diagnostic Autolet or Glucolet.
Use: Diagnostic aid.

Glucotrol. (Roerig) Glipizide 5 mg or 10 mg, lactose/Tab. Bot. 100s, 500s, UD 100s. *Rx.*
Use: Antidiabetic.

Glucotrol-XL. (Pfizer) Glipizide 5 mg or 10 mg. ER Tab. Bot. 100s, 500s. *Rx.*
Use: Antidiabetic.

Glucovite. (Pal-Pak) Ferrous gluconate 260 mg, vitamins B_1 1 mg, B_2 0.5 mg, C 10 mg/Tab. Bot. 1000s, 5000s. *otc.*
Use: Vitamin/mineral supplement.

glucurolactone. Gamma lactone of glucofuranuronic acid.
See: Preltron-Oral, Tab. (Taylor).

glucuronate sodium.
See: Preltron, Inj. (Taylor).

Glu-K. (Western Research) Potassium gluconate 486 mg/Tab. Bot. 1000s. *otc.*
Use: Potassium supplement.

gluside.
See: Saccharin (Various Mfr.).

glutamate sodium.
W/Niacin, vitamins, minerals.
See: L-Glutavite, Cap. (Rydelle).

•**glutamic acid.** USAN.
Use: Dietary Supp.
See: Glutamic Acid Tablets (Various Mfr.).
Glutamic Acid Powder (J.R. Carlson).

Glutamic Acid Tablets. (Various Mfr.) 500 mg. In 100s, 500s. *otc.*
Use: Dietary supplement.

Glutamic Acid Powder. (J.R. Carlson) Bot. 100 g. *otc.*
Use: Dietary supplement.

glutamic acid hydrochloride. Acidogen, aciglumin, glutasin. *otc.*
Use: Gastric acidifier.

glutamic acid salts.
See: Calcium Glutamate (Various Mfr.).

glutamine.
Use: Treatment of short bowel syndrome. [Orphan drug]

•**glutaral concentrate,** U.S.P. 23.
Use: Disinfectant.
See: Cidex (Surgikos).

glutaraldehyde.
Use: Sterilizing, disinfecting agent.
See: Cidex (J&J Medical).
Cidex-7 (J&J Medical).
Cidex Plus (J&J Medical).

Glutarex-1. (Ross) Protein 15 g, fat 23.9 g, carbohydrates 46.3 g, linoleic acid 1800 mg, Fe 9 mg, Na 190 mg, K 675 mg, Ca, vitamins A, B_1, B_2, B_3, B_5, B_6, B_{12}, C, D, E, K, biotin, choline, folic acid, inositol, Cl, Cu, I, Mg, Mn, P, Se, Zn and 480 Cal per 100 g. Lysine and tryptophan free. Pow. Can 350 g. *otc.*
Use: Nutritional supplement.

Glutarex-2. (Ross) Protein 30 g, fat 15.5 g, carbohydrates 30 g, Fe 13 mg, Na 880 mg, K 1370 mg, Ca, vitamins A, B_1, B_2, B_3, B_5, B_6, B_{12}, C, D, E, K, biotin, choline, folic acid, inositol, Cl, Cu, I, Mg, Mn, P, Se, Zn and 410 Cal per 100 g. Lysine and tryptophan free. Pow. Can 325 g. *otc.*
Use: Nutritional supplement.

l-glutathione.
Use: Treatment of AIDS-associated cachexia. [Orphan drug]
See: Cachexon (Telluride Pharm).

•**glutethimide,** (glue-TETH-ih-mide) U.S.P. 23.
Use: Sedative, hypnotic.

Glutofac. (Kenwood/Bradley) Capl.: Vitamins A 500 IU, E 30 IU, B_1 15 mg, B_2 10 mg, B_3 50 mg, B_5 20 mg, B_6 50 mg, C 300 mg, Zn 5 mg, Ca, Cr, Cu, Fe, K, Mg, Mn, P, Se/Tab. Bot. 90s. *otc.*
Use: Vitamin/mineral supplement.

Glutol. (Paddock) Dextrose 100 g/180 ml. Bot. 180 ml.
Use: Diagnostic aid.

Glutose. (Paddock) Liquid glucose (40% dextrose). Concentrated glucose for insulin reactions. Gel. Bot. 60 g. *otc.*

Use: Glucose elevating agent.

Glyate. (Geneva Pharm) Guaifenesin 100 mg/5 ml, alcohol 3.5%. Syr. Bot. 118 ml, 480 ml. *otc.*
Use: Expectorant.

•**glyburide,** (glie-BYOO-ride) U.S.P. 23.
Use: Antidiabetic.
See: DiaBeta (Hoechst Marion Roussel).
Glynase, Tab. (Pharmacia & Upjohn).
Micronase, Tab. (Pharmacia & Upjohn).

glyburide. (Various Mfr.) **1.25 mg:** Tab. Bot. 50s, 100s. **2.5 & 5 mg:** Tab. Bot. 100s, 500s, 1000s, UD 100s.
Use: Antidiabetic.

glycarnine iron.
See: Ferronord, Tab. (Rydelle).

Glycate Chewables. (Forest) Glycine 150 mg, calcium carbonate 300 mg/Tab. Bot. 1000s. *otc.*
Use: Antacid.

•**glycerin,** (GLIH-suh-rin) U.S.P. 23.
Use: Pharmaceutic aid (humectant, solvent).
See: Corn Huskers Lot. (Warner Lambert).
Ophthalgan Ophthalmic, Soln. (Wyeth-Ayerst).
Osmoglyn (Alcon).
W/ Dimethicone.
See: Dermasil, Lot. (Chesebrough-Ponds).
W/Urea.
See: Kerid Ear Drops (Blair).

glycerin. (Various Mfr.) Various concentrations from 10% to > 95% for use as sterile allergen-extract diluents.

glycerin suppositories. (Various Mfr.) Glycerin, sodium stearate. *otc.*
Use: Rectal evacuant, cathartic.

glycerol.
See: Glycerin.

•**glycerol, iodinated.** USAN.
Use: Expectorant.

•**glyceryl behenate,** N.F. 18.
Use: Pharmaceutic aid (tablet/capsule lubricant).

glyceryl guaiacolate.
Use: Expectorant.
See: Guaifenesin, U.S.P. 23.

glyceryl guaiacolate carbamate. Methocarbamol.
See: Robaxin, Tab., Inj. (Robins).
Robaxin 750, Tab. (Robins).

glyceryl guaiacolether.
See: Guaifenesin.

•**glyceryl monostearate,** N.F. 18.
Use: Pharmaceutic aid (emulsifying agent).

Glyceryl-T. (Rugby) Theophylline 150 mg, guaifenesin 90 mg/Cap. Bot. 100s. *Rx.*
Use: Bronchodilator, expectorant.
Glyceryl-T Liquid. (Rugby) Theophylline 150 mg, guaifenesin 90 mg/15 ml. Liq. Bot. 480 ml. *Rx.*
Use: Bronchodilator, expectorant.
glyceryl triacetate.
See: Triacetin.
glyceryl triacetin. (Various Mfr.) Triacetin.
See: Enzactin, Aerosal, Pow., Cream (Wyeth-Ayerst).
Fungacetin, Oint, Liq. (Blair Labs.).
glyceryl trierucate.
Use: Adrenoleuko-dystrophy. [Orphan drug]
glyceryl trinitrate ointment.
See: Nitrol, Oint. (Kremers-Urban).
glyceryl trinitrate tablets.
See: Nitroglycerin (Various Mfr.)
Nitroglyn, Tab. (Key Corp.).
glyceryl trioleate.
Use: Adrenoleuko-dystrophy. [Orphan drug]
Glycets-Antacid Tablets. (Weeks & Leo) Calcium carbonate 350 mg, simethicone 25 mg/Chew. Tab. Bot. 100s. *otc.*
Use: Antacid, antiflatulent.
glycinato dihydroxyaluminum hydrate.
See: Dihydroxyaluminum Aminoacetate, U.S.P. 23.
•**glycine,** U.S.P. 23. U.S.P. XXI. *Formerly Aminoacetic Acid.*
Use: Myasthenia gravis treatment, irrigating solution.
W/Aluminum hydroxide-magnesium carbonate coprecipitated gel.
See: Glycogel, Tab., Susp. (Schwarz Pharma).
W/Calcium Carbonate.
See: Antacid No. 6, Tab. (Jones Medical).
Glycate Chewables, Tab. (O'Neal).
P.H. Tab. (Scrip).
Titralac, Liq., Tab. (3M).
W/Calcium carbonate, amylolytic, proteolytic cellulolytic enzymes.
See: Co-gel, Tab. (Arco).
W/Chlortrimeton, sodium salicylate.
See: Corilin, Liq. (Schering Plough).
W/Glutamic acid, alanine.
See: Prostall, Cap. (Metabolic Prods.).
W/Magnesium trisilicate, calcium carbonate.
See: P.H. Tab., Chewable, Mix (Scrip).
glycine, aluminum salt.
See: Dihydroxyaluminum Aminoacetate, U.S.P. 23.

glycine hydrochloride. (Various Mfr.)
Use: Gastric acidifier.
glycobiarsol, U.S.P. XXI. Bismuthyl-N-Glycolylarsanilate, Chemo Puro, Pow. for Mfr. (Hydrogen N-glycoloylarsanilato) oxobismuth.
Use: Amebiasis, Trichomonas vaginalis, Monilia albicans.
glycocoll. Glycine.
See: Aminoacetic Acid (Various Mfr.).
glycocyamine. Guanidoacetic acid.
Glycofed Tablets. (Pal-Pak) Pseudoephedrine 30 mg, guaifenesin 100 mg. Bot. 1000s. *otc.*
Use: Decongestant, expectorant.
•**glycol distearate.** (GLIE-kole dih-STEE-ah-rate) USAN.
Use: Pharmaceutic aid (thickening agent).
glycol monosalicylate.
W/Oil of mustard, camphor, menthol, methyl salicylate.
See: Musterole, Oint., Cream (Schering Plough).
glycophenylate bromide.
See: Mepenzolate Methylbromide.
•**glycopyrrolate,** (glie-koe-PIE-row-late) U.S.P. 23.
Use: Anticholinergic.
See: Robinul, Tab., Inj. (Robins).
Robinul Forte, Tab. (Robins).
Glycotuss. (Pal-Pak) Guaifenesin 100 mg/Tab. Bot. 100s, 1000s. *otc.*
Use: Expectorant.
Glycotuss-DM. (Pal-Pak) Guaifenesin 100 mg, dextromethorphan HBr 10 mg/Tab. Bot. 100s, 1000s. *otc.*
Use: Expectorant, antitussive.
glycyrrhiza. Pure extract, Fluidextract. Licorice root.
Use: Flavoring agent.
glycyrrhiza extract, pure.
Use: Flavoring agent.
glycyrrhiza fluidextract.
Use: Flavoring agent.
W/Camphorated opium tincture, tartar emetic, glycerin.
See: Brown Mixture. (Jones Medical).
W/Pepsin-papain complex, pancreas, malt diastase, charcoal, ox bile.
See: Pepsocoll, Tab. (Western Research Labs.).
glydanile sodium. (GLIE-dah-neel SO-dee-uhm)
Use: Antidiabetic.
•**glyhexamide.** (glie-HEX-ah-mid) USAN.
Use: Antidiabetic.
glylorin. (Cellergy Pharm)
See: Monolaurin.

•**glymidine sodium.** USAN.
Use: Oral hypoglycemic agent; antidiabetic.

glymol.
See: Petrolatum Liquid (Various Mfr.)

Glynase PresTab. (Pharmacia & Upjohn) Glyburide (micronized) **1.5 mg:** Tab. Bot. 100s, UD 100s. **3 mg:** Tab. Bot. 100s, 500s, 1000s, UD 100s. **6 mg:** Tab. Bot. 100s, 500s. *Rx.*
Use: Antidiabetic.

•**glyoctamide.** (glie-OCKT-am-id) USAN.
Use: Hypoglycemic agent; antidiabetic.

Gly-Oxide. (SKB Consumer Healthcare) Carbamide peroxide 10% in flavored anhydrous glycerol. Liq. Bot. 15 ml, 60 ml. *otc.*
Use: Mouth and throat product.

glyoxyldiureide.
See: Allantoin (Various Mfr.).

•**glyparamide.** (glie-PAR-am-ide) USAN.
Use: Oral hypoglycemic agent; antidiabetic.

Glypressin. (Ferring)
See: Terlipressin.

Glyset. (Bayer Corp.) Miglitol 25 mg, 50 mg, 100 mg/Tab. Bot. 100s, 1000s, UD 100. *Rx.*
Use: Treatment of diabetes.

Glytuss. (Mayrand) Guaifenesin 200 mg/Tab. Bot. 100s. *otc.*
Use: Expectorant.

GM-CSF. Granulocyte macrophage colony stimulating factor.
See: Leukine (Immunex).

G-Myticin Creme and Ointment. (Pedinol) Gentamicin sulfate equivalent to gentamicin base 1 mg. Tube 15 g. *Rx.*
Use: Anti-infective, topical.

gododiamide.
Use: Diagnostic aid.

Go-Evac. (Copley) Polyethylene glycol 3350 59 g, sodium sulfate 5.685 g, sodium bicarbonate 1.685 g, sodium chloride 1.465 g, potassium chloride 0.743 g/L. Pow. Jug 4 L. *Rx.*
Use: Bowel evacuants.

Golacol. (Arcum) Codeine sulfate 30 mg, papaverine HCl 30 mg, emetine HCl 2 mg, ephedrine HCl 15 mg, q.s./30 ml. Alcohol 6.25%. Syr. Bot. 4 oz, 16 oz, gal. Orange flavor. *c-III.*
Use: Antitussive, bronchodilator.

Gold Alka-Seltzer Effervescent. (Bayer) Sodium bicarbonate (heat treated) 958 mg, citric acid 832 mg, potassium bicarbonate 312 mg/Tab. 20s, 36s. *otc.*
Use: Antacid.

•**gold (Au¹⁹⁸). colloidal injection.** USAN. U.S.P. XX.
Use: Antineoplastic, diagnostic aid (liver imaging), radioactive agent.
See: Radio Gold (Au¹⁹⁸).

gold Au 198 injection.
Use: Antineoplastic; diagnostic for liver scanning.

gold compounds.
See: Gold Sodium Thiosulfate (Various Mfr.).
Ridaura, Cap. (SK-Beecham).
Solganal, Vial (Schering Plough).

Gold Seal Calcium 600. (Walgreen) Calcium 1200 mg/Tab. Bot. 60s. *otc.*
Use: Calcium supplement.

Gold Seal Calcium 600 with Vitamin D. (Walgreen) Calcium 1200 mg, vitamin D/Tab. Bot. 60s. *otc.*
Use: Calcium supplement.

Gold Seal Chewable Vitamin C. (Walgreen) Ascorbic acid 250 mg or 500 mg/Tab. Bot. 100s. *otc.*
Use: Vitamin C supplement.

Gold Seal Ferrous Gluconate. (Walgreen) Iron 37 mg/Tab. Bot. 100s. *otc.*
Use: Iron supplement.

Gold Seal Ferrous Sulfate Tablets. (Walgreen) Ferrous sulfate 325 mg/Tab. Bot. 100s, 1000s. *otc.*
Use: Iron supplement.

Gold Seal Time Release Ferrous Sulfate. (Walgreen) Iron 50 mg/Tab. Bot. 100s. *otc.*
Use: Iron supplement.

•**gold sodium thiomalate,** (gold thigh-oh-MAL-ate) U.S.P. 23.
Use: Antirheumatic.
See: Aurolate, Inj. (Taylor).
Myochrysine, Amp. (Merck).

gold sodium thiomalate. (King) 50 mg/ml. Inj. Vial 10 ml.
Use: Antirheumatic.

gold sodium thiosulfate. Sterile, Auricidine, Aurocidin, Aurolin, Auropin, Aurosan, Novacrysin, Solfocrisol and Thiochrysine.
Use: Antirheumatic.

gold thioglucose.
See: Aurothioglucose, U.S.P. 23.

Golden-West Compound. (Golden-West) Gentian root, licorice root, cascara sagrada, damiana leaves, senna leaves, psyllium seed, buchu leaves, crude pepsin. Box 1.5 oz. *otc.*
Use: Laxative.

Goldicide Concentrate. (Pedinol) Bot. (Conc.) oz. Ctn. 10s.
Use: Chemical disinfection of surgical

and podiatry instruments.

Golytely. (Braintree) Pow. for oral soln. after reconstitution containing PEG-3350 236 g, sodium sulfate 22.74 g, sodium bicarbonate 6.74 g, sodium Cl 5.86 g, potassium Cl 2.97 g when made up to 4 L. Disposable container 4800 ml. *Rx.*
Use: Bowel evacuant.

gonacrine.
See: Acriflavine (Various Mfr.).

•**gonadorelin acetate.** (go-NAD-oh-RELL-in) USAN. *Formerly Luteinizing Hormone-releasing Factor Diacetate Tetrahydrate.*
Use: Gonad-stimulating principle. [Orphan drug]
See: Cryptolin Prods. (Hoechst Marion Roussel).

•**gonadorelin hydrochloride.** (go-NAD-oh-RELL-in) USAN. *Formerly Luteinizing Hormone-releasing Factor Dihydrochloride.*
Use: Gonad-stimulating principle.

gonadotropic substance.
See: Gonadotropin Chorionic.

gonadotropins.
See: Pergonal, Pow. for Inj. (Serona).

•**gonadotropin, chorionic,** U.S.P. 23.
Use: Gonad-stimulating principle. In the female: Chronic cystic mastitis, functional sterility, dysmenorrhea, premenstrual tension, threatened abortion. In the male: Cryptorchidism, hypogenitalism, dwarfism, impotency, enuresis.
See: Android HCG, Inj. (Zeneca).
Antuitrin "S", Vial (Parke-Davis).
A.P.L., Secules (Wyeth-Ayerst).
Corgonject, Vial (Mayrand).
Follutein Pow. (Squibb).
Libigen, Vial (Savage).
Pregnyl, Amp. (Organon).
W/Vitamin B_1, glutamic acid, procaine HCl.
See: Glukor, Vial (Zeneca).

gonadotropin, pituitary ant. lobe. Extracted from anterior lobe of equine pituitaries (not pregnant mare urine) (rat unit = 1 Fevold-Hisaw unit).

gonadotropin releasing hormone analog.
See: Lupron, Inj. Susp. (TAP Pharm)
Zoladex, Implant (Zeneca)

gonadotropin releasing hormones.
See: Lutrepulse, Pow. for Inj. (Ortho).
Supprelin, Inj. (Ortho).
Synarel, Soln. (Syntex).

gonadotropin serum. Pregnant mare's serum.

Gonak. (Akorn) Hydroxypropyl methylcellulose 2.5%. Soln. Bot. 15 ml. *otc.*
Use: Ophthalmic preparation.

Gonic. (Roberts) Chorionic gonadotropin 10,000 units w/diluent/vial. Pow. for inj. Vial 10 ml. *Rx.*
Use: Chorionic gonadotropin.

gonioscopic hydroxypropyl methylcellulose.
See: Goniosol Lacrivial, Soln. (Smith, Miller & Patch).

Gonioscopic Solution. (Alcon) Hydroxyethyl cellulose. Drop-Tainer 15 ml. *Rx.*
Use: Ophthalmic preparation.

Goniosol. (Ciba Vision) Gonioscopic hydroxypropyl methylcellulose 2.5%. Bot. 15 ml. *otc.*
Use: Ophthalmic preparation.

Gonodecten Test Kit. (United States Packaging) Tube test for urethral discharge from males, for detection of *Neisseria gonorrhoeae.* Test kit 10s, 25s.
Use: Diagnostic aid.

gonorrhea tests.
See: Biocult-GC (Orion Diagnostica).
Gonodecten Test Kit (United States Packaging).
Gonozyme Diagnostic Kit (Abbott).
Isocult for Neisseria gonorrhoeae (SmithKline Diagnostics).
MicroTrak Neisseria gonorrhoeae Culture Test (Syva).

Gonozyme. (Abbott Diagnostics) Enzyme immunoassay for detection of *Neisseria gonorrhoeae* in urogenital swab specimens. Test kit 100s.
Use: Diagnostic aid.

Good Samaritan Ointment. (Good Samaritan) Tube 1.25 oz. *otc.*
Use: Counterirritant.

Goody's Headache Powders. (Goody) Aspirin 520 mg, acetaminophen 260 mg, caffeine 32.5 mg/dose. Pow. Pkg. 2s, 6s, 24s, 50s. *otc.*
Use: Analgesic.

Gordobalm. (Gordon) Chloroxylenol, methyl salicylate, menthol, camphor, thymol, eucalyptus oil, isopropyl alcohol 16%, fast-drying gum base. Bot. 4 oz, gal. *otc.*
Use: Analgesic, topical.

Gordochom. (Gordon) Undecylenic acid 25%, chloroxylenol 3%, penetrating oil base. Liq. Bot. 15 ml, 30 ml w/applicator. *otc.*
Use: Antifungal, topical.

Gordofilm. (Gordon) Salicylic acid 16.7%, lactic acid 16.7% in flexible col-

Iodian. Bot. 15 ml. *otc.*
Use: Keratolytic.

Gordogesic Cream. (Gordon) Methyl salicylate 10% in absorption base. Jar 2.5 oz, 1 lb. *otc.*
Use: Analgesic, topical.

Gordomatic Crystals. (Gordon) Sodium borate, sodium bicarbonate, sodium Cl, thymol, menthol, eucalyptus oil. Jar 8 oz, 7 lb. *otc.*
Use: Counterirritant.

Gordomatic Lotion. (Gordon) Menthol, camphor, propylene glycol, isopropyl alcohol. Bot. 1 oz, 4 oz, gal. *otc.*
Use: Counterirritant.

Gordomatic Powder. (Gordon) Menthol, thymol camphor, eucalyptus oil, salicylic acid, alum bentonite, talc. Shaker can 3.5 oz. Can 1 lb, 5 lb. *otc.*
Use: Counterirritant.

Gordon's Urea. (Gordon) Urea 40% in petrolatum base. Jar oz. *Rx.*
Use: Emollient.

Gordophene. (Gordon) Neutral coconut oil soap 15%, glycerin with Septi-Chlor (trichlorohydroxy diphenyl ether) broad spectrum antimicrobial and bacteriostatic agent. Bot. 4 oz, gal.
Use: Surgical soap.

Gordo-Vite A Creme. (Gordon) Vitamin A 100,000 IU/oz. in water soluble base. Jar 0.5 oz, 2.5 oz, 4 oz, lb, 5 lb. *otc.*
Use: Emollient.

Gordo-Vite A Lotion. (Gordon) Vitamin A 100,000 IU/oz. Plastic bot. 4 oz, gal. *otc.*
Use: Emollient.

Gordo-Vite E Creme. (Gordon) Vitamin E 1500 IU/oz in water soluble base. Jar 2.5 oz, lb. *otc.*
Use: Emollient.

Gormel Cream. (Gordon) Urea 20% in emollient base. Jar 0.5 oz, 2.5 oz, 4 oz, 1 lb, 5 lb. *otc.*
Use: Emollient.

•**goserelin.** (GO-suh-REH-lin) USAN.
Use: LHRH agonist.
See: Zoladex (Zeneca).

goserelin acetate. (GO-suh-REH-lin ASS-uh-TATE)
Use: Gonadotropin-releasing hormone analog.
See: Zoladex, Implant (Zeneca).

gossypol.
Use: Antineoplastic. [Orphan drug]

gotamine. (Vita Elixir) Ergotamine tartrate 1 mg, caffeine 100 mg/Tab. *Rx.*
Use: Agent for migraine.

gout, agents for.

See: Allopurinol, Tab. (Various Mfr.).
Anturane, Tab., Cap. (Novartis).
Benemid, Tab. (Merck).
ColBenemid, Tab. (Merck).
Colchicine, Inj. (Lilly).
Colchicine, Tab. (Various Mfr.).
Col-Probenecid, Tab. (Various Mfr.).
Proben-C, Tab. (Various Mfr.).
Probenecid, Tab. (Various Mfr.).
Probenecid w/Colchicine, Tab. (Various Mfr.).
Sulfinpyrazone, Tab., Cap. (Various Mfr.).
Zyloprim, Tab. (Glaxo Wellcome).

•**govafilcon a.** (GO-vaff-ILL-kahn A) USAN.
Use: Contact lens material (hydrophilic).

GP-500. (Marnel) Pseudoephedrine HCl 120 mg, guaifenesin 500 mg. Tab. Bot. 100s. *Rx.*
Use: Decongestant, expectorant.

•**gramicidin,** U.S.P. 23.
Use: Antibacterial.
W/Neomycin.
See: Spectrocin Oint. (Squibb).
W/Neomycin sulfate, polymyxin B sulfate, thimerosal.
See: Neo-Polycin Ophthalmic Soln. (Merrell Dow).
W/Neomycin sulfate, polymyxin B sulfate, benzocaine.
See: Tricidin, Oint. (Amlab).
W/Neomycin, triamcinolone, nystatin.
See: Mycolog Cream, Oint. (Squibb).
W/Polymyxin B sulfate, neomycin sulfate.
See: AK-Spore Ophth. Soln. (Akorn).
Neosporin, Ophthalmic Soln. (Glaxo Wellcome).
Neosporin-G Cream (Glaxo Wellcome).
Ocutricin Ophth. Soln. (Bausch & Lomb).
W/Polymyxin B sulfate, neomycin sulfate, hydrocortisone acetate.
See: Cortisporin, Cream (Glaxo Wellcome).

•**granisetron.** (gran-IH-SEH-trahn) USAN.
Use: Antiemetic.
See: Kytril, Vial (SK-Beecham).

•**granisetron hydrochloride.** (gran-IH-SEH-trahn) USAN.
Use: Antiemetic.
See: Kytril Injection (SmithKline Beecham).

Granulderm. (Copley) Trypsin 0.1 mg, balsam Peru 72.5 mg, castor oil 650 mg/0.82 ml. Aerosol Spray 113.4 g. *Rx.*
Use: Enzyme preparation, topical.

Granulex. (Hickam) Trypsin 0.1 mg, balsam Peru 72.5 mg, castor oil 650 mg w/

emulsifier/0.82 ml. Spray can 2 oz, 4 oz. *Rx.*
Use: Wound-healing agent.

granulocyte-colony stimulating factor.
See: Neupogen (Amgen).

granulocyte macrophage-colony stimulating factor.
See: Leukine (Immunex).

gratus strophanthin. Ouabain.

Gravineed. (Hanlon) Vitamins C 100 mg, E 10 IU, B_1 3 mg, B_2 2 mg, B_6 10 mg, B_{12} 5 mcg, A 4000 IU, D 400 IU, niacin 10 mg, folic acid 0.1 mg, iron fumarate 40 mg, calcium 67 mg/Cap. Bot. 100s. *otc.*
Use: Vitamin/mineral supplement.

Green mint. (Block) Urea, glycine, polysorbate 60, sorbitol, alcohol 12.2%, peppermint oil, menthol, chlorophyllin-copper complex. Bot. 7 oz, 12 oz. *otc.*
Use: Mouth and throat product.

green soap.
Use: Detergent.

Green Soap. (Paddock) Soybean oil, potassium salt, ethanol. Liq. Bot. 3780 ml. *otc.*
Use: Therapeutic skin cleanser.

•**grepafloxacin hydrochloride.** USAN.
Use: Antibacterial.

Grifulvin V. (Ortho Derm) Griseofulvin microsize. **Tab:** 250 mg. Bot. 100s; 500 mg. Bot. 100s, 500s. **Susp:** 125 mg/5 ml. Bot. 120 ml. *Rx.*
Use: Antifungal.

Grisactin Ultra. (Wyeth-Ayerst) Griseofulvin ultramicrosize 125 mg, 250 mg or 330 mg/Tab. Bot. 100s. *Rx.*
Use: Antifungal.

•**griseofulvin,** (griss-ee-oh-FULL-vin) U.S.P. 23.
Use: Antifungal.
See: Fulvicin P/G, Tab. (Schering Plough).
Fulvicin-U/F, Tab. (Schering Plough).
Grifulvin V, Tab., Susp. (Ortho).
Grisactin, Cap., Tab. (Wyeth-Ayerst).
Grisactin Ultra, Tab. (Wyeth-Ayerst).

griseofulvin. (Various Mfr.) 165 mg or 330 mg. Tab. Bot. 100s.
Use: Antifungal.

griseofulvin microcrystalline.
Use: Antifungal.
See: Fulvicin U/F, Tab. (Schering Plough).
Grifulvin V, Tab., Susp. (Ortho).
Grisactin, Cap., Tab. (Wyeth-Ayerst).

griseofulvin ultramicrosize. (Various Mfr.) Griseofulvin ultramicrosize 165 mg and 330 mg/Tab. Bot. 100s.

Use: Antifungal.
See: Fulvicin P/G, Tab. (Schering Plough).
Grisactin Ultra, Tab. (Wyeth-Ayerst)
Gris-PEG, Tab. (Allergan Herbert).

Gris-Peg Tablets. (Allergan Herbert) Griseofulvin ultramicrosize 125 mg or 250 mg/Tab. **125 mg:** Bot. 100s. **250 mg:** Bot. 100s, 500s. *Rx.*
Use: Antifungal.

growth hormone. Extract of human pituitaries containing predominantly growth hormone.
See: Crescormon.

growth hormone releasing factor. *Rx.*
Use: Long-term treatment of growth failure. [Orphan drug]

g-strophanthin. Ouabain.

guaiacol carbonate. (Various Mfr.) (Duotal).
Use: Expectorant.

guaiacol glyceryl ether.
See: Guaifenesin.

guaiacol potassium sulfonate.
See: Bronchial, Syr. (DePree).
W/Ammonium Cl, sodium citrate, benzyl alcohol, carbinoxamine maleate.
See: Clistin Expectorant, Syr. (McNeil).
W/Dextromethorphan HBr.
Bronchial DM, Syr. (DePree).
W/Pheniramine maleate, pyrilamine maleate, codeine phosphate.
See: Tritussin, Syr. (Towne). *Rx.*

guaianesin.
See: Guaifenesin.
Use: Expectorant.

•**guaiapate.** (GWIE-ah-pate) USAN.
Use: Antitussive.

Guaifed Capsules. (Muro) Guaifenesin 250 mg, pseudoephedrine HCl 120 mg/TR Cap. Bot. 100s, 500s. *Rx.*
Use: Expectorant, decongestant.

Guaifed PD Capsules. (Muro) Pseudoephedrine HCl 60 mg, guaifenesin 300 mg/TR Cap. Bot. 100s, 500s. *Rx.*
Use: Decogestant, expectorant.

Guaifed Syrup. (Muro) Pseudoephedrine HCl 30 mg, guaifenesin 200 mg. Bot. 118 ml, 473 ml. *Rx.*
Use: Decongestant, expectorant.

•**guaifenesin,** (GWHY-fen-ah-sin) U.S.P. 23. *Formerly Glyceryl Guaiacolate.*
Synonyms:
Glyceryl Guaiacolate.
Glyceryl Guaiacol Ether.
Guaianesin.
Guaifylline.
Guayanesin.
Use: Expectorant.

See: Anti-tuss, Liq. (Century).
Consin-GG, Syr. (Wisconsin).
Diabetic Tussin Ex, Liq. (Health Care Products).
Dilyn, Liq., Tab. (Zeneca).
2/G, Liq. (Merrell Dow).
G-100, Syr. (Bock).
GG-Cen, Syr. (Schwarz Pharma).
Glycotuss, Tab., Syr. (Pal-Pak).
Glytuss, Tab. (Mayrand).
G-Tussin, Syr. (Quality Generics).
Humibid L.A., Tab. (Adams).
Hytuss, Tab., Cap. (Hyrex).
Robitussin, Syr. (Robins).
Tursen, Tab. (Wren).
Wal-Tussin, Syr. (Walgreen).

W/Combinations:

See: Actified C Expectorant, Liq. (Glaxo Wellcome).
Actol Exp., Syr., Tab. (SK-Beecham).
Airet G.G., Cap., Elix. (Baylor Labs).
Ambenyl-D, Liq. (Hoechst Marion Roussel).
Anatuss DM, Syr., Tab. (Mayrand).
Anti-tuss D.M., Liq. (Century).
Antitussive Guaiacolate, Syr. (Med. Chem.).
Asbron G, Tab., Elix. (Sandoz).
Bur-Tuss Expectorant (Burlington).
Brexin, Cap., Liq. (Savage).
Bri-stan, Liq. (Briar).
Broncholate, Cap., Elix. (Bock).
Bronchovent, Tab. (Mills).
Bronkolate-G, Tab. (Parmed).
Bronkolixir, Elix. (Sanofi Winthrop).
Bronkotabs, Tab. (Sanofi Winthrop).
Bro-Tane, Expectorant (Scrip).
Cerylin, Liq. (Rugby).
Cheracol-D, Syr. (Pharmacia & Upjohn).
Chlor-Trimeton, Expectorant (Schering Plough).
Colrex, Expectorant (Solvay).
Conar-A, Susp., Tab. (SK-Beecham).
Conar Expectorant, Liq. (SK-Beecham).
Congestac, Tab. (SK-Beecham).
Consin-DM, Syr. (Wisconsin).
Coricidin Children's Cough Syr. (Schering Plough).
Cortane D.C., Exp. (Standex).
Dextro-Tuss GG, Liq. (Ulmer).
Dilaudid, Syr. (Knoll).
Dilor-G, Tab., Liq. (Savage).
Dilyn, Liq. (Zeneca).
Dimacol, Cap. (Robins).
Dimetane Expectorant, Liq. (Robins).
Dimetane Expectorant-DC, Liq. (Robins).
DM Plus, Liq. (West-Ward).
Donatussin, Syr. (Laser).

Duovent, Tab. (3M).
Emfaseem, Liq., Tab. (Saron).
Entex, Cap., Liq. (Procter & Gamble).
Formula 44D Decongestant Cough Mixture, Syr. (Procter & Gamble).
G-100/DM, Syr. (Bock).
G-Bron Elix. (Laser).
2G/DM, Liq. (Merrell Dow).
Glycotuss-DM, Tab. (Pal-Pak).
Guiatussin w/Codeine, Liq. (Rugby).
Guistrey Fortis, Tab. (Jones Medical).
Histussinol, Syr. (Bock).
Hycoff-A, Syr. (Saron).
Hycotuss Expectorant, Liq. (DuPont Merck).
Hylate, Tab., Syr. (Hyrex).
Isoclor Expectorant (DuPont Merck).
Lardet Expectorant, Tab. (Standex).
Mudrane GG, Tab., Elix. (ECR Pharm).
Neospect, Tab. (Lemmon).
Novahistine Cough Formula, Liq. (Merrell Dow).
Novahistine DMX, Liq. (Merrell Dow).
Novahistine, Expectorant (Merrell Dow).
Panaphyllin, Susp. (Panamerican).
Partuss-A, Tab. (Parmed).
Partuss AC (Parmed).
Phenatuss, Liq. (Dalin).
PMP, Expectorant, Syr. (Schlicksup).
Polaramine Expectorant (Schering Plough).
Poly-Histine Expectorant (Bock).
Polytuss-DM, Liq. (Rhode).
P.R. Syrup, Liq. (Fleming).
Queltuss, Syr., Tab. (Westerfield).
Quibron, Cap., Liq. (Bristol).
Quibron-300, Cap. (Bristol).
Quibron Plus, Cap., Elix. (Bristol).
Rentuss, Cap., Syr. (Wren).
Rhinex DM (Lemmon).
Robitussin AC, CF, DAC, DM, PE (Robins).
Robitussin-DM Cough Calmers, Loz. (Robins).
Robitussin Cold & Cough, Cap. (Robins).
Robitussin Severe Congestion, Cap. (Robins).
Rondec-DM, Syr. (Ross).
Rymed, Prods. (Edwards).
Santussin, Cap. (Sandia).
Scotcof, Liq. (Scott/Cord).
Silexin, Cough Syr. (Clapp).
Slo-Phyllin GG, Cap., Syr. (Dooner).
Sorbase Cough Syr. (Fort David).
Sorbase II Cough Syr. (Fort David).
Spen-Histine Expectorant (Rugby).
Sudafed Cough Syr. (Glaxo Wellcome).

Tolu-Sed, Liq. (Scherer).
Tolu-Sed DM, Liq. (Scherer).
Triaminic Expectorant (Sandoz Consumer).
Trihista-Phen, Liq. (Recsei).
Tri-Histin Expectorant (Recsei).
Tri-Mine, Expectorant (Rugby).
Trind-DM, Liq. (Bristol-Myers).
Trind, Liq. (Bristol-Myers).
Tussafed, Expectorant (Calvital).
Tussar-2, Syr. (Rhone-Poulenc Rorer).
Tussar SF, Liq. (Rhone-Poulenc Rorer).
Tussend, Liq. (Merrell Dow).
Verequad, Tab., Susp. (Knoll).
Vicks Cough Syr. (Procter & Gamble).
Vicks Formula 44D Decongestant Cough Mixture, Syr. (Procter & Gamble).
Wal-Tussin DM, Syr. (Walgreen).
guaifenesin and codeine phosphate syrup.
Use: Expectorant, antitussive.
guaifenesin/phenylpropanolamine hydrochloride.
See: Phenylpropanolamine hydrochloride & guaifenesin tablets.
guaifenesin & pseudoephedrine hydrochloride & codeine phosphate syrup. (Schein) Pseudoephedrine HCl 30 mg, codeine phosphate 10 mg, guaifenesin 100 mg, alcohol 1.4 %. Bot. 473 ml. *c-v.*
Use: Decongestant, antitussive, expectorant.
Guaifenex. (Ethex) Guaifenesin 100 mg, phenylpropanolamine HCl 20 mg, phenylephrine HCl 5 mg, parabens, sorbitol/5 ml. Liq. Bot. 118 ml, 473 ml. *Rx.*
Use: Expectorant, decongestant.
Guaifenex DM. (Ethex) Guaifenesin 600 mg, dextromethorphan HBr 30 mg/ER Tab. Bot. 100s, 500s, 1000s. *Rx.*
Use: Expectorant, antitussive.
Guaifenex LA. (Ethex) Guaifenesin 600 mg, lactose/ER Tab. Bot. 100s. *Rx.*
Use: Expectorant.
Guaifenex PPA 75. (Ethex) Guaifenesin 600 mg, phenylpropanolamine HCl 75 mg, lactose/ER Tab. Bot. 100s. *Rx.*
Use: Expectorant, decongestant.
Guaifenex PSE 120. (Ethex) Guaifenesin 600 mg, pseudoephedrine HCl 120 mg/ER Tab. Bot. 100s. *Rx.*
Use: Expectorant, decongestant.
Guaifenex PSE 60. (Ethex) Guaifenesin 600 mg, pseudoephedrine HCl 60 mg, lactose/ER Tab. Bot. 100s. *Rx.*
Use: Expectorant, decongestant.

Guaimax-D. (Schwarz Pharma) Pseudoephedrine HCl 120 mg, guaifenesin 600 mg. ER Tab. Bot. 100s. *Rx.*
Use: Decongestant, expectorant.
Guaipax Tablets. (Vitarine) Phenylpropanolamine HCl 75 mg, guaifenesin 400 mg/Tab. Bot. 100s, 500s, 1000s. *Rx.*
Use: Decongestant, expectorant.
Guaiphotol. (Foy) Iodine $\frac{1}{30}$ gr, calcium cresoate 4 gr/Tab. Bot. 1000s. *Rx.*
Use: Expectorant.
Guaitab Tablets. (Muro) Pseudoephedrine HCl 60 mg, guaifenesin 400 mg, lactose/Tab. Bot. 100s. *otc.*
Use: Decongestant, expectorant.
•**guaithylline.** (GWIE-thill-in) USAN.
Use: Bronchodilator, expectorant.
Guai-Vent/PSE. (Dura) Pseudoephedrine HCl 120 mg, guaifenesin 600 mg/SR Tab. 100s. *Rx.*
Use: Expectorant.
guamide.
See: Sulfaguanidine (Various Mfr.).
•**guanabenz.** (GWAHN-uh-benz) USAN.
Use: Antihypertensive.
See: Wytensin, Tab. (Wyeth-Ayerst).
•**guanabenz acetate,** (GWAHN-uh-benz) U.S.P. 23.
Use: Antihypertensive.
guanabenz acetate. (Various Mfr.) 4 mg or 8 mg/Tab. Bot. 30s, 100s, 500s.
Use: Antihypertensive.
•**guanacline sulfate.** (GWAHN-ah-kleen) USAN.
Use: Antihypertensive.
•**guanadrel sulfate,** (GWAHN-uh-drell) U.S.P. 23.
Use: Antihypertensive.
See: Hylorel, Tab. (Medeva).
•**guancydine.** (GWAHN-sigh-deen) USAN.
Use: Antihypertensive.
•**guanethidine monosulfate,** (gwahn-ETH-ih-deen MAH-no-SULL-fate) U.S.P. 23.
Use: Antihypertensive. Reflex sympathetic dystrophy and causalgia [Orphan drug]
W/Hydrochlorothiazide.
See: Esimil, Tab. (Novartis).
•**guanethidine sulfate.** (gwahn-ETH-ih-deen) USAN. U.S.P. XXI.
Use: Antihypertensive.
See: Ismelin, Tab. (Novartis).
W/Hydrochlorothiazide.
See: Esimil, Tab. (Novartis).
•**guanfacine hydrochloride,** (GWAHN-fay-seen) U.S.P. 23.

Use: Antihypertensive.
See: Tenex, Tab. (Robins).

guanidine hydrochloride. (Key) Guanidine HCl 125 mg/Tab. Bot. 100s. *Rx.*
Use: Cholinergic muscle stimulant.

guanisoquin. (GWAN-eye-so-KWIN)
Use: Antihypertensive.

•**guanisoquin sulfate.** (GWAHN-eye-so-kwin) USAN.
Use: Antihypertensive.

•**guanoclor sulfate.** (GWAHN-oh-klahr) USAN.
Use: Antihypertensive.

•**guanoctine hydrochloride.** (GWAHN-ock-teen) USAN.
Use: Antihypertensive.

•**guanoxabenz.** (gwahn-OX-ah-benz) USAN.
Use: Antihypertensive.

•**guanoxan sulfate.** (GWAHN-ox-an) USAN.
Use: Antihypertensive.

•**guanoxyfen sulfate.** (GWAHN-OX-ehfen) USAN.
Use: Antihypertensive, antidepressant.

Guardal. (Morton) Vitamins A 10,000 IU, B_1 20 mg, B_2 8 mg, C 50 mg, niacinamide 10 mg, calcium d-pantothenate 5 mg, iron 10 mg, dried whole liver 100 mg, yeast 100 mg, choline bitartrate 30 mg, B_6 0.5 mg, B_{12} 8 mcg, mixed tocopherols 5 mg, dicalcium phosphate anhydrous 150 mg, magnesium sulfate dried 7.2 mg, sodium 1 mg, potassium Cl 1.3 mg/Tab. Bot. 100s. *otc.*
Use: Vitamin/mineral supplement.

Guardex. (Archer-Taylor) Tube 4 oz, 1 lb, 4.5 lb. *otc.*
Use: Emollient.

•**guar gum,** N.F. 18.
Use: Pharmaceutic aid (tablet binder; tablet disintegrant).
W/Danthron, docusate sodium.
See: Guarsol, Tab. (Western Research).
W/Standardized senna concentrate.
See: Gentlax B, Granules, Tab. (Blair).

guayanesin.
Use: Expectorant.
See: Guaifenesin (Various Mfr.).

Guiacough CF Liquid. (Schein) Phenylpropanolamine HCl 12.5 mg, dextromethorphan HBr 10 mg, guaifenesin 100 mg. Bot. 118 ml. *otc.*
Use: Decongestant, antitussive, expectorant.

Guiacough PE Liquid. (Schein) Pseudoephedrine HCl 30 mg, guaifenesin 100 mg, alcohol 1.4%. Bot. 118 ml. *otc.*
Use: Decongestant, expectorant.

Guiamid Expectorant. (Vangard) Guaifenesin 100 mg/5 ml, alcohol 3.5%. Bot. pt, gal. *otc.*
Use: Expectorant.

Guiaphed Elixir. (Various Mfr.) Theophylline 45 mg, ephedrine sulfate 36 mg, guaifenesin 150 mg, phenobarbital 12 mg, alcohol 19%/15 ml Liq. Bot. 480 ml. *Rx.*
Use: Antiasthmatic combination.

Guiatuss A.C. Syrup. (Various Mfr.) Codeine phosphate 10 mg, guaifenesin 100 mg, alcohol 3.5%/5 ml. Syr. Bot. 120 ml, pt, gal. *c-v.*
Use: Antitussive, expectorant.

Guiatuss CF Syrup. (Barre National) Phenylpropanolamine HCl 12.5 mg, dextromethorphan HBr 10 mg, guaifenesin 100 mg/Syr. Bot. 120 ml. *otc.*
Use: Antitussive, expectorant.

Guiatuss DAC Liquid. (Various Mfr.) Pseudoephedrine HCl 30 mg, codeine phosphate 10 mg, guaifenesin 100 mg, alcohol. Liq. Bot. 120 ml, 480 ml. *c-v.*
Use: Decongestant, antitussive, expectorant.

Guiatuss D.M. Liquid. (Various Mfr.) Dextromethorphan HBr 10 mg, guaifenesin 100 mg. Bot. 120 ml, 240 ml, pt, gal. *otc.*
Use: Antitussive, expectorant.

Guiatuss Syrup. (Various Mfr.) Guaifenesin 100 mg/5 ml. Syr. Bot. 120 ml, 240 ml, pt, gal. *otc.*
Use: Expectorant.

Guiatuss PE. (Barre-National) Pseudoephedrine HCl 30 mg, guaifenesin 100 mg, alcohol 1.4%. Liq. Bot. In 120 ml. *otc.*
Use: Decongestant, expectorant.

Guiatussin w/Codeine Expectorant. (Rugby) Codeine phosphate 10 mg, guaifenesin 100 mg/5 ml, alcohol 3.5%. Syr. Bot. 120 ml, pt, gal. *c-v.*
Use: Antitussive, expectorant.

Guiatussin w/Dextromethorphan. (Rugby) Dextromethorphan HBr 15 mg, guaifenesin 100 mg, alcohol 1.4%. Liq. Bot. 480 ml. *otc.*
Use: Antitussive, expectorant.

Guaivent. (Ethex) Guaifenesin 250 mg, pseudoephedrine HCl 120 mg, 100s, 500s. *Rx.*
Use: Expectorant.

Guaivent PD. (Ethex) Guaifenesin 300 mg, pseudoephedrine HCl 60 mg, parabens, sucrose. 100s, 500s. *Rx.*
Use: Expectorant.

Guistrey Fortis. (Jones Medical) Guai-

fenesin 100 mg, phenylephrine HCl 10 mg, chlorpheniramine maleate 1 mg/Tab. Bot. 1000s. *otc.*
Use: Expectorant, decongestant, antihistamine.

Gulfasin Tabs. (Major) Sulfisoxazole 500 mg/Tab. Bot. 100s, 250s, 1000s.
Use: Anti-infective, sulfonamide.

guncotton, soluble. Pyroxylin.

•**gusperimus trihydrochloride.** USAN.
Use: Immunosuppressant.

Gustalac. (Geriatric) Calcium carbonate 300 mg, defatted skim milk pow. 200 mg/Tab. Bot. 100s, 250s, 1000s. *otc.*
Use: Antacid/calcium supplement.

Gustase. (Geriatric) Gerilase (standard amylolytic enzyme) 30 g, geriprotase (standard proteolytic enzyme) 6 mg, gericellulase (standard cellulolytic enzyme) 2 mg/Tab. Bot. 42s, 100s, 500s. *otc.*
Use: Digestive aid.

Gustase Plus. (Geriatric) Phenobarbital 8 mg, homatropine methylbromide 2.5 mg, gerilase 30 mg, geriprotase 6 mg, gericellulase 2 mg/Tab. Bot. 42s, 100s, 500s. *Rx.*
Use: Sedative, hypnotic, anticholinergic, antispasmodic, digestive aid.

•**gutta percha,** U.S.P. 23.
Use: Dental restoration agent.

G-vitamin.
See: Riboflavin (Various Mfr.).

G-Well Lotion. (Goldline) Lindane 1%. Bot. 2 oz, pt. *Rx.*
Use: Scabicide.

G-Well Shampoo. (Goldline) Lindane 1%. Bot. 2 oz, pt, gal. *Rx.*
Use: Pediculicide.

Gynecort 10, Extra Strength. (Combe) Hydrocortisone acetate 1%, parabens, zinc pyrithione. Cream. Tube 15 g. *otc.*
Use: Corticosteroid, topical.

Gyne-Lotrimin Combination Pack. (Schering Plough) **Vaginal Tab.:** Clotrimazole 100 mg. Pkg. 7s; **Topical Cream:** Clotrimazole 1%. Tube 7 g. *otc.*
Use: Antifungal, vaginal.

Gyne-Lotrimin Vaginal Cream 1%. (Schering Plough) Clotrimazole ≈ 5 g/applicatorful. Tube 45 g, 45 g twin-packs w/applicator. *otc.*
Use: Antifungal, vaginal.

Gyne-Lotrimin Vaginal Tablets. (Schering Plough) Clotrimazole 100 mg/Tab. Box 7 Tab. w/applicator, Box 6s. *otc.*
Use: Antifungal, vaginal.

Gyne-Moistrin. (Schering Plough) Propylene glycol, parabens. Gel. Tube 45 g, 75 g. *otc.*
Use: Vaginal preparation.

gynergon.
See: Estradiol (Various Mfr.)

Gyne-Sulf. (G & W) Sulfathiazole 3.42%, sulfacetamide 2.86%, sulfabenzamide 3.7%, urea 0.64%. Cream. Tube with applicator 82.5 g. *Rx.*
Use: Anti-infective, vaginal.

Gynogen L.A. 10. (Forest) Estradiol valerate in sesame oil 10 mg/ml. Vial 10 ml. *Rx.*
Use: Estrogen.

Gynogen L.A. 20. (Forest) Estradiol valerate in castor oil 20 mg/ml. Vial 10 ml. *Rx.*
Use: Estrogen.

Gynogen L.A. 40. (Forest) Estradiol valerate in castor oil 40 mg/ml. Inj. Vial 10 ml. *Rx.*
Use: Estrogen.

Gynol II Contraceptive. (Advanced Care) Nonoxynol-9 in 2% concentration. Starter 75 g tube w/applicator. Refill 75 g, 114 g/Tube. *otc.*
Use: Contraceptive.

Gynol II Extra Strength Contraceptive. (Advanced Care) Nonoxynol-9 3%. Jelly. 75 g, 114 g. *otc.*
Use: Contraceptive, spermicide.

Gyno-Petraryl. (Janssen) Econazole nitrate. *Rx.*
Use: Antifungal, vaginal.

Gynovite Plus. (Optimox) Vitamins A 833 IU, D 67 IU, E 67 mg (as d-alpha tocopheryl acid succinate), B_1 1.7 mg, B_2 1.7 mg, B_3 3.3 mg, B_5 1.7 mg, B_6 3.3 mg, B_{12} 21 mcg, C 30 mg, calcium 83 mg, iron 3 mg, folic acid 0.07 mg, boron, betaine, biotin, Cr, Cu, hesperidin, I, inositol, Mg, Mn, PABA, pancreatin, rutin, Se, Zinc 2.5 mg. Tab. Bot. 100s. *otc.*
Use: Vitamin/mineral supplement.

H

Habitrol. (Novartis) Nicotine transdermal system. Dose absorbed in 24 hours, 21 mg, 14 mg, 7; total nicotine content (respectively) 52.5 mg, 35 mg, 17.5. Patch. Box 30 systems. *Rx.*
Use: Smoking deterrent.

haemophilus b conjugate vaccine.
Use: Vaccine, bacterial.
See: HibTITER, Inj. (Wyeth Lederle).
OmniHIB, Pow. for Inj. (SmithKline Beecham)
Pedvax HIB, Pow. (Merck).
ProHIBIT, Inj. (Pasteur-Merieux-Connaught).
W/DTP vaccine.
See: ActHIB/DTP, Set of DTwP vial plus Hib Pow. for Inj. (Pasteur-Merieux-Connaught).
Tetramune, vial (Wyeth Lederle).

haemophilus influenzae type b and hepatitis vaccines, combined.
See: Comvax (Merck).

Hair Booster Vitamin. (NBTY) Vitamin B_3 35 mg, B_5 100 mg, B_{12} 6 mcg, folic acid 0.4 mg, zinc 15 mg, Cu, iron 18 mg, I, Mn, choline bitartrate, inositol, PABA, protein/Tab. Bot. 60s. *otc.*
Use: Vitamin/mineral supplement.

• **halazepam.** USAN. U.S.P. XXII.
Use: Sedative, hypnotic.

• **halazone,** U.S.P. 23.
Use: Disinfectant.

• **halcinonide,** (hal-SIN-oh-nide) U.S.P. 23. Corticosteroid halcinonide.
Use: Corticosteroid, anti-inflammatory (topical).
See: Halog Cream, Oint., Soln. (Westwood Squibb).

Halcion. (Pharmacia & Upjohn) Triazolam 0.125 mg or 0.25 mg/Tab. **0.125 mg:** Bot. 100s, Visipak 100s. (4 × 25s). **0.25 mg:** Bot. 100s, UD 100s, Visipak 100s. (4 × 25s). *c-iv.*
Use: Sedative, hypnotic.

Haldol. (McNeil Pharm) Haloperidol. **Tab.:** 0.5 mg, 1 mg, 2 mg, 5 mg or 10 mg/Tab. Bot. 100s, 1000s, UD blisterpacks 10 × 10s. 20 mg/Tab. Bot. 100s, UD blisterpacks 10 10s. **Conc. Soln.:** 2 mg/ml. Bot. 15 ml, 120 ml, 240 ml. **Inj.:** (w/methylparaben 1.8 mg, propylparaben 0.2 mg, lactic acid) amp. 5 mg/ml. Box 101 ml, multidose vial of 10 ml Prefilled Syringe 101 ml. *Rx.*
Use: Antipsychotic.

Haldol Concentrate. (McNeil-CPC) Haloperidol 2 mg/ml. Bot. 15, 120, 240 ml. *Rx.*

Use: Antipsychotic.

Haldol Decanoate. (McNeil Pharm) Haloperidol 70.5 mg/ml to provide Haldol 50 mg/ml. Inj. Amp. 1 ml. Box 3s, 10s. *Rx.*
Use: Antipsychotic.

Haldrone. (Lilly) Paramethasone acetate 1 mg or 2 mg/Tab. Bot. 100s. *Rx.*
Use: Corticosteroid.

Halenol, Children's. (Halsey) Acetaminophen 160 mg/5 ml. Elix. Bot. 120 ml, 240 ml, pt, gal. *otc.*
Use: Analgesic.

Halercol. (Mallard) Vitamins A 5000 IU, D 400 IU, E 1.36 mg, B_1 1.5 mg, B_2 2 mg, B_3 20 mg, B_5 1 mg, B_6 0.1 mg, B_{12} 1 mcg, C 37.5 mg/Cap. Bot. 100s. *otc.*
Use: Vitamin supplement.

Haley's M-O. (Bayer) Mineral oil 25%, milk of magnesia in emulsion base. Flavored or regular. Bot. 240 ml, 480 ml, 960 ml. *otc.*
Use: Laxative.

Halfan. (SmithKline Beecham) Halofantrine. *Rx.*
Use: Antimalarial.

Halfort-T. (Halsey) Vitamins C 300 mg, B_1 15 mg, B_2 10 mg, niacin 100 mg, B_6 5 mg, B_{12} 4 mcg, pantothenic acid 20 mg/Tab. Bot. 100s. *otc.*
Use: Vitamin supplement.

Halfprin 81. (Kramer) Aspirin 81 mg. EC Tab. Bot. 90s. *otc.*
Use: Salicylate analgesic.

Half Strength Entrition Entri-Pak. (Biosearch) Protein 17.5 g (Na and Ca caseinates), carbohydrate 68 g (maltodextrin), fat 17.5 g (corn oil, soy lecithin, mono- and diglycerides), sodium 350 mg, potassium 600 mg, m Osm/ 120 kg H_2O, calories 0.5/ml, vitamins A, B_1, B_2, B_3, B_5, B_6, B_{12}, C, D, E, K, P, Ca, Mg, I, Fe, Zn, Mn, Cu, Cl, biotin, choline, folic acid. Liq. Pouch 1 L. *otc.*
Use: Nutritional therapy.

Half Strength Florvite with Iron. (Everett) Flouride 0.5 mg, Vitamins A 2500 IU, D 400 IU, E 15 IU, B_1 1.05 mg, B_2 1.2 mg, B_3 13.5 mg, B_6 1.05 mg, B_{12} 4.5 mcg, C 60 mg, folic acid 0.3 mg, Cu, iron 12 mg, Zn 10 mg, sucrose/Tab. Bot. 100s. *Rx.*
Use: Vitamin/mineral supplement; dental caries preventative.

Half Strength Introlan. (Elan) Protein 22.5 g, fat 18 g, carbohydrates 70 g, Na 345 mg, K 585 mg/L. Vitamins A, C, B_1, B_2, B_3, D, E, B_6, B_{12}, B_5, K, Ca, Fe,

folic acid, P, I, Mg, Zn, Cu, biotin, Mn, choline, Cl, Se, Cr, Mo. Liq. In 1000 ml New Pak closed systems with and without color check. *otc.*
Use: Nutritional supplement.

Hali-Best. (Barth's) Vitamins A 10,000 IU, D 400 IU/Cap. Bot. 100s, 500s. *otc.*
Use: Vitamin supplement.

halibut liver oil.
Use: Vitamin supplement.

haliver oil.
See: Halibut Liver Oil (Various Mfr.).

Halls Mentho-Lyptus Decongestant Liquid. (Warner Lambert) Dextromethorphan HBr 15 mg, phenylpropanolamine HCl 37.5 mg, menthol 14 mg, eucalyptus oil 12.7 mg/10 ml, alcohol 22%. Bot. 90 ml. *otc.*
Use: Antitussive, decongestant.

Hall's Mentho-Lyptus Cough Lozenges. (Warner Lambert) Menthol and eucalyptus oil in varying amounts and flavors. Stick-Pack 9s. Bag 30s. *otc.*
Use: Mouth and throat product.

Halls-Plus Maximum Strength. (Warner Lambert) Menthol 10 mg, corn syrup, sugar. Cherry, honey-lemon and regular flavors. Tab. Pkg. 10s, 25s. *otc.*
Use: Mouth and throat product.

Hall's Sugar Free Mentho-Lyptus. (Warner Lambert) Menthol 5 mg or 6 mg, eucalyptus oil 2.8 mg/Tab. Pkg. 25s. *otc.*
Use: Mouth and throat product.

• **halobetasol propionate.** (hal-oh-BEH-tah-sahl PRO-pee-oh-nate) USAN.
Use: Corticosteroid, anti-inflammatory (topical).
See: Ultravate (Westwood Squibb).

• **halofantrine hydrochloride.** (HAY-low-FAN-trin) USAN.
Use: Antimalarial. [Orphan drug]
See: Halfan (SmithKline Beecham).

Halofed. (Halsey) **Tab.:** Pseudoephedrine HCl 30 mg or 60 mg. Bot. 100s, 1000s. **Syr.:** Pseudoephedrine HCl 30 mg/5 ml. Bot. 120 ml, 240 ml, pt, gal. *otc.*
Use: Decongestant.

• **halofenate.** (HAY-low-FEN-ate) USAN.
Use: Antihyperlipopoteinemic, uricosuric.
See: Livipas (Merck).

• **halofuginone hydrobromide.** (HAY-low-FOO-jin-ohn HIGH-droe-BROE-mide) USAN.
Use: Antiprotozoal.

Halog Cream. (Westwood Squibb) Hal-cinonide 0.025% or 0.1%, in specially formulated cream base consisting of glyceryl monostearate, cetyl alcohol, myristyl stearate, isopropyl palmitate, polysorbate 60, propylene glycol, purified water. **0.1%:** Tube 15 g, 30 g, 60 g, Jar 240 g. **0.025%:** Tube 15 g, 60 g. *Rx.*
Use: Corticosteroid, topical.

Halog E Cream. (Westwood Squibb) Halcinonide 0.1% in hydrophilic vanishing cream base consisting of propylene glycol dimethicone 350, castor oil, cetearyl alcohol, ceteareth-20, propylene glycol stearate, white petrolatum, water. Tube 15 g, 30 g, 60 g. *Rx.*
Use: Corticosteroid, topical.

Halog Ointment. (Westwood Squibb) Halcinonide 0.1%, in Plastibase (plasicized hydrocarbon gel), PEG 400, PEG 6000 disteareate, PEG 300, PEG 1540, butylated hydroxy toluene. Tube 15 g, 30 g, 60 g, Jar 240 g. *Rx.*
Use: Corticosteroid, topical.

Halog Solution. (Westwood Squibb) Halcinonide 0.1%, edetate disodium, PEG 300, purified water, butylated hydroxy toluene as preservative. Bot. 20 ml, 60 ml. *Rx.*
Use: Corticosteroid, topical.

• **halopemide.** (hay-LOW-PEH-mid) USAN.
Use: Antipsychotic.

• **haloperidol,** (HAY-low-PURR-ih-dahl) U.S.P. 23. Serenace Soln.
Use: Antipsychotic, tranquilizer; antidyskinetic (in Gilles de la Tourette's disease).
See: Haldol, Tab., Conc., Inj. (McNeil).

• **haloperidol decanoate.** (HAY-low-PURR-ih-dahl deh-KAN-oh-ate) USAN.
Use: Antipsychotic.

• **halopredone acetate.** (HAY-low-PREH-dohn) USAN.
Use: Anti-inflammatory (topical).

• **haloprogesterone.** (HAL-oh-pro-jeh-STEE-rone) USAN.
Use: Progestin.

• **haloprogin,** (hal-oh-PRO-jin) U.S.P. 23.
Use: Antimicrobic, topical; antibacterial.
See: Halotex, Cream, Soln. (Westwood Squibb).

Halotestin. (Pharmacia & Upjohn) Fluoxymesterone 2 mg, 5 mg or 10 mg. Tartrazine, lactose, sucrose. **2 mg:** Bot. 100s; **5 mg:** Bot. 100s; **10 mg:** Bot. 30s, 100s. *c-III.*
Use: Androgen.

W/Ethinyl estradiol.

See: Halodrin, Tab. (Pharmacia & Upjohn).

Halotex Cream. (Westwood Squibb) Haloprogin 1% in water dispersible base composed of PEG-400, PEG-4000, diethyl sebacate, polyvinylpyrrolidone. Tube 15 g, 30 g. *Rx.*
Use: Antifungal, topical.

Halotex Solution. (Westwood Squibb) Haloprogin 1% in a clear colorless vehicle of diethyl sebacate w/alcohol 75%. Bot. 10 ml, 30 ml. *Rx.*
Use: Antifungal, topical.

• **halothane,** U.S.P. 23. Fluothane.
Use: General anesthetic, inhalation.
See: Fluothane, Liq. (Wyeth-Ayerst). Halothane, 250 ml Liq. (Abbott).

Halotussin. (Halsey) Guaifenesin 100 mg/5 ml. Bot. 4 oz, 8 oz, pt, gal. *otc.*
Use: Expectorant.

Halotussin-DM. (Halsey) Dextromethorphan HBr 10 mg, guaifenesin 100 mg. In 120 ml, 240 ml, pt, gal. *otc.*
Use: Antitussive, expectorant.

Halotussin-DM Sugar-Free Liquid. (Halsey) Dextromethorphan HBr 10 mg, guaifenesin 100 mg. In 120 ml, 240 ml, 480 ml, gal. *otc.*
Use: Antitussive, expectorant.

• **halquinols.** (HAL-kwin-oles) USAN.
Use: Antimicrobial, anti-infective (topical).
See: Quinolor (Squibb).
Tarquinor (Squibb).

Haltran Tablets. (Roberts) Ibuprofen 200 mg/ Tab. Bot. 30s, 50s. Blister pkg. 12s. *otc.*
Use: Nonsteroidal anti-inflammatory, analgesic.

HAMA. Hydroxy-aluminum magnesium aminoacetate.

hamamelis water.
See: Succus Cineraria Maritima, Soln. (Walker Pharm).
Witch hazel (Various Mfr.).
Tucks (Parke-Davis).

• **hamycin.** (HAY-MY-sin) USAN.
Use: Antifungal.

Hang-Over-Cure. (Silvers) Calcium carbonate, glycine, thiamine HCl, pyridoxine HCl, aspirin. Cont. Tab. 6 g. *otc.*
Use: Antacid, analgesic combination.

Haniform. (Hanlon) Vitamins A 25,000 IU, D 1000 IU, B_1 10 mg, B_2 5 mg, C 150 mg, niacinamide 150 mg/Cap. Bot. 100s. *otc.*
Use: Vitamin supplement.

Haniplex. (Hanlon) Vitamins B_1 20 mg,

B_2 10 mg, B_6 1 mg, calcium pantothenate 10 mg, B_{12} 5 mcg, niacin 20 mg, liver concentrate 50 mg, C 150 mg/Cap. Bot. 100s. *otc.*
Use: Vitamin/mineral supplement.

Harbolin. (Arcum) Hydralazine HCl 25 mg, hydrochlorothiazide 15 mg, reserpine 0.1 mg/Tab. Bot. 100s, 1000s. *Rx.*
Use: Antihypertensive combination.

hard fat.
Use: Pharmaceutic necessity.

hartshorn. Ammonium Carbonate.

Haugase. (Madland) Trypsin, chymotrypsin. Bot. 50s, 250s.
Use: Enzyme preparation.

Havab. (Abbott Diagnostics) Radioimmunoassay or enzyme immunoassay for detection of antibody to hepatitis A virus. Test kit 100s.
Use: Diagnostic aid.

Havab EIA. (Abbott Diagnostics) Enzyme immunoassay for the detection of antibody to hepatitis A virus.
Use: Diagnostic aid.

Havab-M. (Abbott Diagnostics) Radioimmunoassay for the detection of specific Ig antibody to hepatitis A virus. Test kit 100s.
Use: Diagnostic aid.

Havab-M EIA. (Abbott Diagnostics) Enzyme immunoassay for the detection of Ig antibody to hepatitis A virus.
Use: Diagnostic aid.

Havrix. (SK-Beecham) Hepatitis A vaccine. **Adult:** 1440 ELISA units/ml. Vials 1 ml, Syr. 1 ml. **Pediatric:** 720 ELu/ 0.5 ml. Single-dose vial, prefilled syringe. *Rx.*
Use: Vaccine, inactivated.

Hawaiian Tropic Aloe Paba Sunscreen. (Tanning Research) Padimate 0, oxybenzone. Cream Bot. 120 g. *otc.*
Use: Sunscreen.

Hawaiian Tropic Baby Faces. (Tanning Research) SPF 20. Octyl methoxycinnamate, octocrylene, benzophenone-3, menthyl anthranilate, PABA free, waterproof. Gel Tube 120 g. *otc.*
Use: Sunscreen.

Hawaiian Tropic Baby Faces Sunblock. (Tanning Research) Octyl methoxycinnamate, benzophenone-3, octyl salicylate, titanium dioxide, octocrylene, PABA free, waterproof. **SPF 35:** Lot. Bot. 60 ml, 120 ml, 300 ml. **SPF 50:** Lot. Bot. 120 ml. *otc.*
Use: Sunscreen.

Hawaiian Tropic Cool Aloe with I.C.E. (Tanning Research) Lidocaine, men-

thol, aloe, SD alcohol 40, diazolidinyl urea, EDTA, vitamins A and E, tartrazine. Gel. Jar 360 g. *otc.*
Use: Emollient.

Hawaiian Tropic Dark Tanning. (Tanning Research) **Gel:** Phenylbenzimidazole sulfonic acid. SPF 2. Bot. 240 ml. **Oil:** 2-ethylhexyl methoxycinnamate, octyl dimethyl PABA, waterproof. Bot. 240 ml. *otc.*
Use: Sunscreen.

Hawaiian Tropic Dark Tanning with Sunscreen. (Tanning Research) **Oil:** Ethylhexyl p-methoxycinnamate, octyl dimethyl PABA. Waterproof. SPF 4. Bot. 240 ml. **Gel:** Phenylbenzimidazole, sulfonic acid. PABA free. SPF 4. Tube 240 g. *otc.*
Use: Sunscreen.

Hawaiian Tropic Just for Kids Sunblock. (Tanning Research) **SPF 30:** Homosalate, octyl methoxycinnamate, benzophenone-3, menthyl anthranilate, octyl salicylate. PABA free. Waterproof. Lot. Bot. 88.7 ml. **SPF 45:** Octyl methoxycinnamate, benzophenone-3, octyl salicylate, octocrylene, titanium dioxide. PABA free. Waterproof. Lot. Bot. 88.7 ml.
Use: Sunscreen.

Hawaiian Tropic Lip Balm Sunblock. (Tanning Research) Padimate 0, oxybenzone. Stick 4 g. *otc.*
Use: Sunscreen.

Hawaiian Tropic 8 Plus. (Tanning Research) Octyl methoxycinnamate, benzophenone-3, menthyl anthranilate. PABA free. Waterproof. SPF 8+. Gel 120 g. *otc.*
Use: Sunscreen.

Hawaiian Tropic 10 Plus. (Tanning Research) Octyl methoxycinnamate, benzophenone-3, menthyl anthranilate. PABA free. Waterproof. SPR 10+. Gel 120 g. *otc.*
Use: Sunscreen.

Hawaiian Tropic 15 Plus. (Tanning Research) Octyl methoxycinnamate, octocrylene, benzophenone-3, menthyl anthranilate, PABA free, waterproof. Gel Tube 120 g. *otc.*
Use: Sunscreen.

Hawaiian Tropic 15 Plus Sunblock. (Tanning Research) Menthyl anthranilate, octyl methoxycinnamate, benzophenone-3. PABA free. Waterproof. Lot. Bot. 7.5 ml, 15 ml, 60 ml, 120 ml, 240 ml, 300 ml. *otc.*
Use: Suncreen.

Hawaiian Tropic 15 Plus Sunblock Lip Balm. (Tanning Research) Padimate O, oxybenzone. SPF 15, waterproof. Stick 4.2 g. *otc.*
Use: Sunscreen.

Hawaiian Tropic 45 Plus Sunblock Lip Balm. (Tanning Research) Octyl methoxycinnamate, benzophenone-3, octyl salicylate, titanium dioxide, menthyl anthranilate. PABA free. Waterproof. SPF 45+. Lip balm 4.2 g. *otc.*
Use: Sunscreen.

Hawaiian Tropic Protective Tanning. (Tanning Research) Titanium dioxide. PABA free. Waterproof. SPF 6. Lot. Bot. 240 ml. *otc.*
Use: Sunscreen.

Hawaiian Tropic Protective Tanning Dry. (Tanning Research) SPF 6. **Oil:** 2-ethylhexyl p-methoxycinnamate, homosalate, menthyl anthranilate. Waterproof. Bot. 180 ml. **Gel:** Phenylbenzimidazole, sulfonic acid, benzophenone-4. Tube 180 g. *otc.*
Use: Sunscreen.

Hawaiian Tropic Self Tanning Sunblock. (Tanning Research) Octyl methoxycinnamate, benzophenone-3, aloe, cetyl alcohol, stearyl alcohol, cocoa butter, parabens, vitamin E. PABA free. SPF 15. Cream 93.75 ml. *otc.*
Use: Sunscreen.

Hawaiian Tropic Sport Sunblock. (Tanning Research) SPF 15, SPF 30. Methoxycinnamate, octocrylene, benzophenone-3, octyl salicylate, titanium dioxide. PABA free. Waterproof. Lot. Bot. 88.7 ml. *otc.*
Use: Sunscreen.

Hawaiian Tropic Sunblock. (Tanning Research) Titanium dioxide, octyl methoxycinnamate, benzophenone-3, octyl salicylate, octocrylene. PABA free. Waterproof. **SPF 30+:** Lot. Bot. 120 ml. **SPF 45+:** Lot. Bot. 120 ml, 300 ml. *otc.*
Use: Sunscreen.

Hawaiian Tropic Swim n Sun. (Tanning Research) Padimate O, oxybenzone. Lot. Bot. 120 ml. *otc.*
Use: Sunscreen.

Hayfebrol Liquid. (Scot-Tussin) Pseudoephedrine HCl 30 mg, chlorpheniramine 2 mg/Syr. Bot. 118 ml. *otc.*
Use: Decongestant, antihistamine.

Hazogel Body and Foot Rub. (Vortech) Witch hazel 70%, isopropanol 20% in a neutralized resin vehicle. Bot. 4 oz. *otc.*
Use: Astringent, antipruritic.

H-Big Hepatitis B Immune Globulin (Human). (North American Biologicals) Hepatitis B immune globulin (human). Vial 1 ml, 5 ml. Syr. 0.5 ml. *Rx.*
Use: Immune serum.

HC, 1%. (C & M Pharm) Hydrocortisone 1%, petrolatum base. Oint. Tube 15, 20, 30, 60, 120, 240 g, lb. *otc.*
Use: Corticosteroids, topical.

HC Derma-Pax. (Recsei) Hydrocortisone 0.5% in liquid base. Dropper Bot. 2 oz. *otc.*
Use: Corticosteroid, topical.

HCG.
See: Chorionic Gonadotropin.

HCG-Nostick. (Organon Teknika) Sol Particle Immunoassay (SPIA) for detection of hCG in urine. Stick 30s.
Use: Pregnancy test.

HD 85. (Lafayette) High density barium suspension 85% w/v. Bot. 4 x 2000 ml.
Use: Radiopaque agent.

HD 200 Plus. (Lafayette Pharm) Barium sulfate 98%. Pow. Bot. 312 g.
Use: Radiopaque agent.

Head & Shoulders Conditioner. (Procter & Gamble) Pyrithione zinc 0.3%. Bot. 4 oz, 11 oz. *otc.*
Use: Antiseborrheic.

Head & Shoulders Dry Scalp. (Procter & Gamble) Pyrithione zinc 1%, regular and conditioning formulas. Shampoo. Bot. 210 ml, 330 ml, 450 ml. *otc.*
Use: Antiseborrehic.

Head & Shoulders Intensive Treatment Dandruff Shampoo. (Procter & Gamble) Selenium sulfide 1%, regular and conditioning forumlas. Shampoo. Bot. 120 ml, 210 ml, 330 ml. *otc.*
Use: Antiseborrehic.

Head & Shoulders Shampoo. (Procter & Gamble) Pyrithione zinc 1%. **Cream:** Tube 51 g, 75 g, 120 g, 210 g. **Lot:** 120 ml, 210 ml, 330 ml, 450 ml. *otc.*
Use: Antiseborrheic.

Healon. (Pharmacia & Upjohn) Sodium hyaluronate 10 mg/ml Inj. Syringe 0.4 ml, 0.55 ml, 0.85 ml, 2 ml. *Rx.*
Use: Surgical aid, ophthalmic.

Healon GV. (Pharmacia & Upjohn) Sodium hyaluronate 14 mg/ml Inj. Syringe 0.55 ml, 0.85 ml. *Rx.*
Use: Surgical aid, ophthalmic.

Healon Yellow. (Pharmacia & Upjohn) Sodium hyaluronate 10 mg, fluorescein sodium 0.005 mg/ml Inj. Syringe 0.55 ml, 0.85 ml.
Use: Surgical and diagnostic aid, ophthalmic.

Healthbreak. (Lemar Labs) Silver acetate 6 mg. Chewing gum. Pack 24s. *otc.*
Use: Smoking deterrent.

Heartburn Antacid. (Walgreen) Aluminum hydroxide dried gel 80 mg, magnesium trisilicate 60 mg/ Tab. Bot. 100s. *otc.*
Use: Antacid.

heavy metal poisoning, antidote.
See: BAL., Amp. (Becton Dickinson). Calcium Disodium Versenate, Amp., Tab. (3M).

Heb Cream Base. (Pilkington Barnes Hind) Washable, hypoallergenic, odorless base. Jar lb.
Use: Extemporaneous prescription compounding.

Heet Liniment. (Whitehall Robins) Methyl salicylate 15%, camphor 3.6%, oloeoresin capsicum 0.025%, alcohol 70%. Bot. 2⅓ oz, 5 oz. *otc.*
Use: Analgesic, topical.

●**hefilcon a.** (heh-FILL-kahn A) USAN.
Use: Contact lens material (hydrophilic).

●**helfilcon b.** (heh-FILL-kahn B) USAN.
Use: Contact lens material (hydrophilic).

Helidac. (Procter & Gamble) Bismuth subsalicylate 264.4 mg/Tab. Metronidazole 250 mg/Tab. Tetracycline 500 mg/Cap. Box. 4s, 8s (bismuth subsalicylate only). *Rx.*
Use: Treatment of active duodenal ulcer due to *H. Pylori.*

Helistat. (Hoechst Marion Roussel) Absorbable collagen hemostatic sponge. 1"×2" and 3"×4" in 10s, 9"×10" in 5s. *Rx.*
Use: Collagen hemostat.

●**helium, U.S.P. 23.**
Use: Diluent for gases.

Helixate. (Centeon) Concentrated recombitant hemophilic factor. After reconstitution, also contains glycine 10 to 30 mg, imidazole ≤ 500 mcg/1000 IU, polysorbate 80 ≤ 600 mcg/1000 IU, Calcium Cl 2 to 5 mM, sodium 100 to 130 mEq/ L, chloride 100 to 130 mEq/L, albumin (human) 4 to 10 mg/ml. IU 250, 500, 1000. *Rx.*
Use: Antihemophilic.

Hemabate. (Pharmacia & Upjohn) Carboprost tromethamine equivalent to 250 mcg carboprost, tromethamine 83 mcg/ ml. Inj. Amp 1 ml. *Rx.*
Use: Abortifacient.

Hema-Chek Slides. (Bayer) Fecal occult blood test containing slide tests, devel-

oper and applicators. Pkg. 100s, 300s, 1000s.
Use: Diagnostic aid.

Hema-Combistix Reagent Strips. (Bayer) Four-way strip test for urinary pH, glucose, protein and occult blood. Strip. Bot. 100s.
Use: Diagnostic aid.

Hemaferrin Tablets. (Western Research) Ferrous fumarate 150 mg, desiccated liver 50 mg, docusate sodium 25 mg, betaine HCl 100 mg, folic acid 0.4 mg, vitamins C 50 mg, B_6 2 mg, manganese 2 mg, B_{12} 5 mcg, copper 1 mg, zinc 2 mg, molybdenum 0.4 mg/Tab. 28 Pack 1000s. *otc.*
Use: Vitamin/mineral supplement, stool softener.

Hemafolate. (Canright) Ferrous gluconate 293 mg, liver fraction II 250 mg, gastric substance 100 mg, vitamins C 50 mg, B_{12} 10 mcg/Tab. Bot. 100s, 1000s. *otc.*
Use: Vitamin/mineral supplement.

Hemalive Liquid. (Barth's) Vitamins B_1 3.15 mg, B_2 3.33 mg, niacin 22.5 mg, B_6 0.81 mg, B_{12} 6 mcg, biotin 3.6 mcg, iron 60 mg, choline, inositol, liver fraction No. 1, pantothenic acid/15 ml. Bot. 8 oz, 24 oz. *otc.*
Use: Vitamin/mineral supplement.

Hemalive Tablets. (Barth's) Vitamins B_{12} 25 mcg, iron 75 mg, B_1 2.5 mg, B_2 5 mg, niacin 1.4 mg, C 30 mg, liver 240 mg, B_6, pantothenic acid, aminobenzoic acid, choline, inositol, biotin, Mg, Mn, Cu/3 Tab. Bot. 100s, 500s, 1000s. *otc.*
Use: Vitamin/mineral supplement.

Hemaneed. (Hanlon) Hematinic B_{12}, intrinsic factor, Fe/Cap. Bot. 100s. *otc.*
Use: Vitamin/mineral supplement.

Hemaspan Tablets. (Bock) Iron 110 mg (from ferrous fumarate), ascorbic acid 200 mg, docusate sodium 20 mg/Tab. Bot. 100s, 1000s. *otc.*
Use: Vitamin/mineral supplement, stool softener.

Hemastix Reagent Strips. (Bayer) Cellulose strip, impregnated with a peroxide and orthotolidine for detection of hematuria and hemoglobinuria. Strip Bot. 50s.
Use: Diagnostic aid.

Hematest Reagent Tablets. (Bayer) Reagent Tab. for blood in the feces. Bot. 100s.
Use: Diagnostic aid.

Hematinic. (Canright) Ferrous gluconate 180 mg, desiccated liver 200 mg, vita-

mins B_{12} 1 mcg, C 25 mg, B_1 3.3 mg, copper gluconate 0.3 mg/Tab. Bot. 100s, 1000s. *otc.*
Use: Vitamin/mineral supplement.

hematinics.
See: Iron Products.
  Ferric Compounds.
  Ferrous Compounds.
  Liver Products.
  Vitamin B_{12}.
  Vitamin Products.

Hematrin. (Towne) Iron 50 mg, vitamins B_{12} 10 mcg, B_1 10 mg, B_2 10 mg, B_6 2 mg, C 150 mg, copper 2 mg, niacinamide 50 mg, calcium pantothenate 5 mg, desiccated liver 200 mg/Captab. Bot. 60s, 100s. *otc.*
Use: Vitamin/mineral supplement.

heme arginate. *Rx.*
Use: Acute porphyria; myelodysplastic syndromes. [Orphan drug]

Hemeselect. (SmithKline Diagnostics) Occult blood screening test. Box 40 test kits.
Use: Fecal testing.

Hemiacidrin. Citric acid, glucono-delta-lactone, magnesium carbonate.
Use: Genitourinary irrigant.
See: Renacidin, Pow. (Guardian).
  Renacidin, Soln. (Guardian).

Hemex. (Vogarell) Oint. Tube 1.25 oz. Supp. Box 12s.
Use: Anorectal preparation.

hemin. *Rx.*
Use: Acute intermittent porphyria. [Orphan drug]
See: Panhematin, Inj. (Abbott).

hemin and zinc mesoporphyrin. *Rx.*
Use: Acute porphyric syndromes. [Orphan drug]

hemisine.
See: Epinephrine (Various Mfr.).

Hemoccult Sensa. (SmithKline Diagnostics) Occult blood screening tests.
Use: Fecal testing.

Hemoccult Slides. (SmithKline Diagnostics) Occult blood detection (fecal). In 100s, 1000s and tape dispensers (test 100s).
Use: Diagnostic aid.

Hemoccult II. (SmithKline Diagnostics) Occult blood detection (fecal). In 102s, kit 100s.
Use: Diagnostic aid.

Hemocyte. (U.S. Pharm) Ferrous fumarate 324 mg (FE 106 mg)/Tab. Bot. 100s. *Rx.*
Use: Iron supplement.

Hemocyte-F. (U.S. Pharm) Iron 106 mg

(from ferrous fumarate), folic acid 1 mg/
Tab. 100s. *Rx.*
Use: Iron supplement.

Hemocyte Plus. (U.S. Pharm) Iron 106
mg (from ferrous fumarate), sodium
ascorbate 200 mg, vitamins B_1 10 mg,
B_2 6 mg, B_6 5 mg, B_{12} 15 mcg, folic
acid 1 mg, B_3 30 mg, B_5 10 mg, zinc
18.2 mg, Mg, Mn sulfate, Cu/Tabule.
Bot. 100s. *Rx.*
Use: Vitamin/mineral supplement.

Hemocyte Plus Elixir. (US Pharm) Polysaccharide iron complex 12 mg, vitamin B_3 13.3 mg, B_5 3.3 mg, B_6 1.3 mg,
B_{12} 4 mcg, folic acid 0.33 mg, zinc 5
mg, Mn 1.3 mg/15 ml. Bot. 473 ml. *Rx.*
Use: Vitamin/mineral supplement.

Hemofil M. (Baxter) Stable dried preparation of Antihemophilic Factor in concentrated form. Albumin (human) 12.5 mg/
ml when reconstituted. Bot. 10 ml, 20
ml, 30 ml with diluent. *Rx.*
Use: Antihemophilic.

Hemofil T. (Baxter) Antihemophilia Factor (Human), method four, dried, heat-
treated 225-375 IU/10 ml; 450-650 IU/
20 ml; 675-999 IU/30ml; 1000-1600
IU/30 ml. *Rx.*
Use: Treatment of Hemophilia A, for
prevention and control of hemorrhagic
episodes.

Hemoglobin Reagent Strips. (Bayer)
Seralyzer reagent strips. Bot. 50s.
Quantitive strip test for hemoglobin in
whole blood.
Use: Diagnostic aid.

Hemopad. (Astra) Fibrous absorbable
collagen hemostat. 2.5 cm×5 cm, 5
cm×8 cm, 8 cm×10 cm. *Rx.*
Use: Collogen hemostat.

hemorheologic agent. Pentoxifylline.
See: Trental, Tab. (Hoechst Marion
Roussel).

Hemorid for Women. (Thompson Medical) **Lotion:** Mineral oil, petrolatum, diazolidinyl urea, cetyl alcohol, glycerin,
parabens. Bot. 118 ml. **Cream:** white
petrolatum 30%, mineral oil 20%, pramoxine HCl 1%, phenylephrine HCl
0.25%, aloe vera gel, parabens, cetyl
and stearyl alcohols. In 28.3 g. **Supp:**
zinc oxide 11%, phenylephrine HCl
0.25%, hard fat 88.25%, aloe vera. In
12s. *otc.*
Use: Perianal hygiene product.

Hemorrhoidal HC. (Various Mfr.) Hydrocortisone acetate 25 mg/Supp. Bot.
12s, 24s, 50s, 100s, UD 12s. *Rx.*
Use: Anorectal preparation.

Hemorrhoidal Ointment. (Goldline) Live
yeast cell derivative supplying skin respiratory factor 2000 units/oz of ointment w/shark liver oil 3%, phenyl mercuric nitrate 1:10,000. *otc.*
Use: Anorectal preparation.

Hemorrhoidal Suppositories. (Goldline)
Bismuth subgallate 2.25%, bismuth resorcin compound 1.75%, benzyl benzoate 1.2%, balsam Peru 1.8%, zinc oxide 11%/Supp. Box 12s. *otc.*
Use: Anorectal preparation.

Hemorrhoidal Uniserts. (Upsher-Smith)
Bismuth subgallate 2.25%, bismuth resorcin compound 1.75%, benzyl benzoate 1.2%, balsam Peru 1.8%, zinc oxide
11%/Supp. Carton 12s, 50s. *otc.*
Use: Anorectal preparation.

hemostatics, local.
See: Absorbable Gelatin Sponge (Phar-
macia & Upjohn).
Gelfilm (Pharmacia & Upjohn).
Gelfoam, Preps. (Pharmacia & Up-
john).
Helistat (Hoechst Marion Roussel).
Hemotene (Astra).
Oxidized Cellulose.
Thrombin (Various Mfr.).

hemostatic topical. Thrombin.
See: Thrombinar, Pow. (Centeon).
Thrombostat, Pow. (Parke-Davis).

hemostatin.
See: Epinephrine (Various Mfr.).

Hemotene. (Astra) Absorbable collagen
hemostat. 1 g. Pkg. 5s. *Rx.*
Use: Hemostatic, topical.

Hemozyme Elixir. (Barrows) Vitamins
B_1 5 mg, B_2 5 mg, B_6 1 mg, panthenol 4 mg, niacinamide 100 mg, B_{12} 3
mcg, iron 100 mg, choline bitartrate 100
mg, dl-methionine 100 mg, yeast extract, alcohol 12%/fl oz. Bot. 12 oz. *otc.*
Use: Vitamin/mineral supplement.

Hem-Prep. (G & W) Phenylephrine HCl
0.25%, zinc oxide 11%. Supp. Bot.
12s. *otc.*
Use: Anorectal preparation.

Hem-Prep Ointment. (G & W) Phenylephrine HCl 0.025%, zinc oxide 11%,
white petrolatum. Oint. 42.5 g. *otc.*
Use: Anorectal preparation.

Hemril-HC Uniserts. (Upsher-Smith)
Hydrocortisone acetate 25 mg/Supp.
12s. *Rx.*
Use: Anorectal preparation.

Hemril Uniserts. (Upsher-Smith) Bismuth subgallate 2.25%, bismuth resorcin compound 1.75%, benzyl benzoate 1.2%, balsam Peru 1.8%, zinc ox-

ide 11%/Supp. 12s, 50s. *otc.*
Use: Anorectal preparation.

henbane.
See: Hyoscyamus (Various Mfr.).

Henydin-M. (Arcum) Thyroid desiccated pow. 0.5 gr, vitamins B₁ 1 mg, B₂ 0.5 mg, B₆ 0.5 mg, niacinamide 2.5 mg/Tab. Bot. 100s, 1000s. *Rx.*
Use: Vitamin supplement.

Henydin-R. (Arcum) Thyroid desiccated pow. 1 gr, vitamins B₁ 2 mg, B₂ 1 mg, B₆ 1 mg, niacinamide 5 mg/Tab. Bot. 100s, 1000s. *Rx.*
Use: Vitamin supplement.

heparin, 2-0-desulfated. (HEP-uh-rin) *Rx.*
Use: Treatment of cystic fibrosis. [Orphan drug]
See: Aeropin.

heparin antagonist.
See: Protamine Sulfate (Various Mfr.).

heparin calcium. *Rx.*
Use: Anticoagulant.
See: Calciparine, Inj. (DuPont Merck).

•**heparin calcium,** U.S.P. 23.
Use: Anticoagulant.

heparin lock flush solution. (Winthrop Pharm) **10 USP units/1 ml:** Cartridge 2 ml HEP-PAK containing 1 cartridge heparin lock flush Soln. (1 ml) and 2 cartridges sodium Cl Inj. HEP-PAK-2 containing 1 cartridge heparin lock flush soln. (1 ml) and 1 cartridge sodium Cl Inj. **10 USP units/2 ml:** Cartridge 2 ml. **100 USP units/1 ml:** Cartridge 2 ml HEP-PAK containing 1 cartridge heparin lock flush soln (1 ml) and 2 cartridges sodium Cl Inj. HEP-PAK-2 containing 1 cartridge of heparin lock flush soln (1 ml) and 1 cartridge sodium Cl Inj. **100 USP units/2 ml:** Cartridge 2 ml. *Rx.*
Use: Maintaining patency of indwelling IV catheter.

heparin lock flush solution. (Wyeth-Ayerst) Heparin sodium 10 units or 100 units/1 ml vial. Pkg. 50 Tubex 1 ml, 2 ml. *Rx.*
Use: Clearing intermittent infusion sets.

•**heparin sodium.** U.S.P. 23.
Use: I.M., I.V. or S.C., anticoagulant in prevention and treatment of thrombosis or embolism. Note: Protamine sulfate is antidote.
See: Hepathrom, Amp., Vial (Fellows-Testagar).
Heprinar, Inj. (Centeon).
Lipo-Hepin, Amp., Vial (3M).
Lipo-Hepin/BL, Amp., Vial (3M).
Liquaemin, Vial (Organon).

W/Vit. B₁₂, folic acid, niacinamide, choline Cl.
See: Heparin-B, Vial (Medical Chem.).

heparin sodium. (Pharmacia & Upjohn) 1000 units/ml. Vial 10 ml, 30 ml 5000 units/ml. Vial 1 ml, 10 ml 10,000 units/ml. Vial 1 ml, 4 ml (Winthrop Pharm) 5000 USP units/1 ml. Carpuject 1 ml fill in 2 ml cartridge.
Use: I.M., I.V. or S.C., anticoagulant in prevention and treatment of thrombosis or embolism. Note: Protamine sulfate is antidote.

heparin sodium and 0.45% sodium chloride. (Abbott) 12,500, 25,000 units in 250 ml Inj. *Rx.*
Use: Anticoagulant.

heparin sodium and 0.9% sodium chloride. (Baxter) Inj.: 1000 units in 500 ml Viaflex. 2000, 5000 units in 1000 ml Viaflex. *Rx.*
Use: Anticoagulant.

heparin sodium lock flush solution. *Rx.*
Use: Anticoagulant.
See: Heparin Lock Flush, Inj. (Various).
Hep-Lock, Inj. (Elkins-Sinn).
Hep-Lock U/P, Inj. (Elkins-Sinn).

Hepatamine. (McGaw) Amino acid 8%. Inj. Bot. 500 ml. *Rx.*
Use: Parenteral nutritional supplement.

Hepatic-Aid II Instant Drink Powder. (McGaw) Amino acids (high BCAA, low AAA), maltodextrin, sucrose, partially hydrogenated soybean oil, lecithin, mono and diglycerides. In 3 oz packet of 12s. *otc.*
Use: Nutritional supplement.

hepatitis A vaccine, inactivated. (hep-uh-TIGHT-iss) *Rx.*
Use: Agent for immunization.
See: Havrix, Inj. (SK-Beecham).
Voqta, Inj. (Merck).

hepatitis B and haemophilus type b vaccines, combined.
See: Comvax (Merck).

•**hepatitis B immune globulin,** (hep-uh-TIGHT-iss) U.S.P. 23.
Use: Passive immunizing agent.
See: BayHep B, Vial, Syr. (Bayer).
H-BIG, Vial, syr. (North American Biologicals).
Hep-B-Gammagee, Inj. (Merck).

hepatitis B immune globulin IV. (hep-uh-TIGHT-iss)
Use: Prophlaxis against hepatitis B virus reinfection in liver transplant patients. [Orphan drug]

hepatitis B vaccine, recombinant. (hep-uh-TIGHT-iss) *Rx.*

Use: Agent for immunization.
See: Engerix-B (SmithKline Beecham).
Recombivax-HB, Inj. (Merck).
•**hepatitis B virus vaccine inactivated,** (hep-uh-TIGHT-iss) U.S.P. 23.
Use: Active immunizing agent.
Hepfomin R Injection. (Keene) Liver inj. equivalent to cyanocobalamin 10 mcg, folic acid 0.4 mg, cyanocobalamin 100 mcg. Vial 10 ml. *Rx.*
Use: Parenteral nutritional supplement.
Hep-Forte. (Marlyn) Vitamins A 1200 IU, E 10 mg, B_1 1 mg, B_2 1 mg, B_3 10 mg, B_5 2 mg, B_6 0.5 mg, B_{12} 1 mcg, C 10 mg, folic acid 0.06 mg, zinc 0.5 mg, choline, inositol, biotin, dl-methionine, desiccated liver, liver concentrate, liver fraction number 2/Cap. Bot. 100s, 300s, 500s. *otc.*
Use: Vitamin/liver supplement.
Hep-Lock. (Elkins-Sinn) Sterile heparin sodium soln. in saline 10 units or 100 units/ml. Dosette 1 ml, 2 ml, multiple dose vial 10 ml, 30 ml. *Rx.*
Use: Maintenance of patency of heparin lock catheters.
Hep-Lock PF. (Elkins-Sinn) Preservative-free heparin flush soln. 10 units/ml or 100 units/ml. Vial 1 ml. *Rx.*
Use: Maintenance of patency of heparin lock catheters.
heprofax.
See: Mucoplex (Stuart).
Heptalac. (Copley) Lactulose 10 g/15 ml, galactose < 1.6 g, lactose < 1.2 g, other sugars ≤ 1.2 g/ Syrup. Bot. 473 ml, 1920 ml. *Rx.*
Use: Laxative.
Herbal Cellulex. (NBTY) Vitamin C 83 mg, K 33 mg, iron 9 mg/Tab. Bot. 90s. *otc.*
Use: Vitamin supplement.
Herbal Laxative. (NBTY) Senna concentrate 125 mg, cascara sagrada 20 mg, buckthorn bark PDR. Tab. Bot. 100s. *otc.*
Use: Laxative.
Hermal Bath Oil. (Hermal) Soybean oil-based bath oil. Bot. 8 oz, 32 oz. *otc.*
Use: Emollient.
Herpecin-L. (Campbell) Allantoin, octylp-(dimethylamino)-benzoate (Padimate O), titanium dioxide, pyridoxine HCl in a balanced, acidic lipid system. Lip balm. Tube 2.5 g. *otc.*
Use: Cold sore treatment.
herpes simplex virus gene. (Genetic Therapy) *Rx.*
Use: Treatment of brain tumors. [Orphan drug]

Herplex. (Allergan) Idoxuridine 0.1%. Soln. Bot. w/dropper 15 ml. *Rx.*
Use: Antiviral.
Herrick Lacrimal Plug. (Lacrimedics) Silicone plug 0.3 mm or 0.5 mm Pkg. 2 plugs. *Rx.*
Use: Punctal plug.
HES. Hetastarch.
Use: Plasma expander.
See: Hespan, Inj. (DuPont Merck).
Hespan Injection. (DuPont Merck) Hetastarch 6 g, sodium Cl 0.9%/100 ml. Bot. 500 ml. *Rx.*
Use: Plasma volume expander.
hesperidin.
Use: Capillary fragility and permeability, hemorrhage.
See: Vitamin P; also Rutin.
W/Combinations.
   See: A.C.N., Tab. (Person & Covey).
   Ceebec, Tab. (Person & Covey).
   Hesper Bitabs, Tab. (Hoechst Marion Roussel).
   Nialex, Tab. (Mallard).
   Norimex-Plus, Cap. (Vortech).
   Pregent, Tab. (Beutlich).
   Vita Cebus, Tab. (Cenci).
Hesperidin w/C. (Various Mfr.).
Use: Vitamin supplement.
See: Min-Hest, Cap. (Scrip).
hesperidin methyl chalcone.
Use: Vitamin P supplement.
•**hetacillin.** (HET-ah-SILL-in) USAN.
Use: Antibacterial.
•**hetacillin potassium,** U.S.P. 23.
Use: Antibacterial.
•**hetaflur.** (HEH-tah-flure) USAN.
Use: Dental caries prophylactic.
•**hetastarch.** (HET-uh-starch) USAN.
Use: Plasma volume extender.
See: Hespan, Inj. (DuPont Merck).
•**heteronium bromide.** (HET-er-oh-nee-uhm) USAN. Hetrum Cl.
Use: Anticholinergic.
Hexabamate #1. (Rugby) Tridihexethyl Cl 25 mg, meprobamate 200 mg/Tab. Bot. 100s, 500s. *Rx.*
Use: Anticholinergic combination.
Hexabamate #2. (Rugby) Tridihexethyl Cl 25 mg, meprobamate 400 mg/Tab. Bot. 100s, 500s. *Rx.*
Use: Anticholinergic combination.
Hexa-Betalin. (Lilly) Pyridoxine HCl. Inj. Vial 100 mg/ml. Ctn. 10s, vial 10 ml. *Rx.*
Use: Vitamin B_6 supplement.
Hexabrix Solution. (Mallinckrodt) Ioxaglate meglumine 39.3%, ioxaglate sodium 19.6% (32% iodine). Vial 20 ml,

30 ml, 50 ml, 100 ml fill in bot. 150 ml, 200 ml fill in bot. 250 ml, bot. 150 ml.
Use: Radiopaque agent.

hexachlorcyclohexane.
See: Benzene Hexachloride, Gamma.

•**hexachlorophene (I.N.N.),** U.S.P. 23.
Use: Antiseptic; anti-infective (topical), detergent.
See: Derl.
   Gamophen, Leaves, Bar (Arbrook).
   pHisoHex Prods. (Winthrop Pharm).
W/Soya protein complex.
See: Soy-Dome Cleanser, Liq. (Bayer).

hexachlorophene cleansing emulsion.
Use: Anti-infective, topical detergent.

hexachlorophene liquid soap, detergent liquid.
See: pHisoHex Liq. Prods. (Winthrop Pharm).
Use: Anti-infective, topical detergent.

hexacose. Mixture of C-6 alcohols derived from oxidation of tetracosane–$C_{24}H_{50}$.
See: Hexathricin, Aerospra (Lincoln).

hexadecadrol.
See: Dexamethasone.

hexadienol. Hexacose.

Hexadrol. (Organon) Dexamethasone.
Tab.: 4 mg. Bot. 100s, UD 100s, Strip 10 X 10s. **Elix.:** 0.5 mg/5 ml, alcohol 5%. Bot. 120 ml. *Rx.*
Use: Corticosteroid.

Hexadrol Phosphate. (Organon) Dexamethasone sodium phosphate 4 mg/ml, 10 mg/ml or 20 mg/ml, benzyl alcohol. **4 mg/ml:** Vial 1 ml, 5 ml, disposable syringe 1 ml. **10 mg/ml:** Vial 10 ml, disposable syringe 1 ml. **20 mg/ml:** Vial 5 ml, disposable syringe 5 ml. *Rx.*
Use: Corticosteroid.

•**hexafluorenium bromide.** (HEK-sah-flure-EE-nee-uhm) USAN. U.S.P. XXI.
Use: Skeletal muscle relaxant, synergist (succinycholine).

hexafluorodiethyl ether. Name used for Flurothyl.

hexahydroxycyclohexane.
See: Inositol, Preps. (Various Mfr.).

hexakose. Mixture of tetracosanes and oxidation products.
See: Hexathricin, Aerospra (Lincoln).
W/Benzethonium Cl, p-chloro-m-xylenol, ethyl p-aminobenzoate and tyrothricin.
See: Hexathricin, Aeropak (Lincoln).

Hexalen. (US Bioscience) Altretamine.
Rx.
Use: Antineoplastic.

hexamarium bromide.

hexamethonium.
W/Rauwiloid.
See: Rauwiloid w/hexamethonium, Tab. (3M).

hexamethonium chloride. (Various Mfr.) Hexamethylene (bistrimethylammonium) Cl.

hexamethylamine.
See: Hexastat. Hypotensive.

hexamethylenamine.
See: Methenamine (Various Mfr.).

hexamethylenetetramine.
See: Methenamine, U.S.P. 23. Hexamethylenetetramine Mandelate.

hexamethylmelamine. Altretamine.
Use: Antineoplastic.
See: Hexalen.

hexamethylpararosaniline chloride.
See: Bismuth Violet, Soln. (Table Rock).

hexamethylrosaniline chloride.
See: Gentian Violet.

hexamine.
See: Methenamine (Various Mfr.).

hexapradol hydrochloride. a-(1-Aminohexyl) benzhydrol HCl.
Use: CNS stimulant.

Hexate. (Davis & Sly) Atropine sulfate $\frac{1}{2000}$ gr, extract of hyoscyamus 0.25 gr, methylene blue gr, methanamine 0.5 gr, benzoic acid 0.5 gr, salol 0.5 gr./Tab. Bot. 1000s. *Rx.*
Use: Urinary anti-infective.

Hexavitamin Tablets. (Various Mfr.) Vitamins A 5000 IU, B₁ 2 mg, B₂ 3 mg, C 75 mg, D 400 IU, B₃ 20 mg/Tab. or Cap. Bot. 100s, 1000s, UD 100s. *otc.*
Use: Multivitamin.
See: Hepicebrin, Tab. (Lilly).

Hexavitamin Tablets. (Forest Pharm) Vitamin A 1.5 mg, D 10 mcg, C 75 mg, B₁ 2 mg, B₂ 3 mg, nicotinamide 20 mg/SC Tab. Bot. 1000s. *otc.*
Use: Vitamin supplement.

Hexavitamins SC. (Halsey)
Use: Vitamin supplement.

hexcarbacholine bromide.

•**hexedine.** (HEX-eh-deen) USAN.
Use: Anti-infective, antibacterial.

hexene-ol. Hexacose.

hexenol. Hexacose.

hexitol irrigants.
Use: Genitourinary irrigants.
See: Resectisol, Soln. (McGaw).
   Sorbitol, Soln. (McGaw).
   Sorbitol, Soln. (Baxter).
   Sorbitol-Mannitol, Soln. (Abbott).

hexobarbital, U.S.P. XXI.
See: Sombulex, Tab. (3M).

W/Dihydrohydroxycodeinone HCl, dihydrohydroxy-codeinone terephthalate, homatropine terephthalate, aspirin, phenacetin, caffeine.
See: Percobarb, Cap. (DuPont).

W/Dihydrohydroxycodeinone terephthalate, dihydrohydroxycodeinone HCl, homatropine terephthalate, aspirin, phenacetin, caffeine.
See: Percobarb-Demi, Cap. (DuPont).

•**hexobendine.** (HEX-oh-BEN-deen) USAN. Hexobendine HCl.
Use: Vasodilator.

hexoestrol.
See: Hexestrol (Various Mfr.).

Hexopal. (Winthrop Products) Inositol hexanicotinate. *Rx.*
Use: Hypolipidemic, peripheral vasodilator.

•**hexoprenaline sulfate.** USAN.
Use: Bronchodilator; tocolytic.

•**hexylene glycol,** N.F. 18.
Use: Pharmaceutic aid (humectant, solvent).

•**hexylresorcinol,** U.S.P. 23.
Use: Anthelmintic (intestinal roundworms and trematodes), minor throat irritations.
See: Listerine Antiseptic Throat Loz. (Warner Lambert).
Sucrets Sore Throat Loz. (SK-Beecham).

H.H.R. (Geneva Pharm) Hydralazine HCl 25 mg, hydrochlorothiazide 15 mg, reserpine 0.1 mg/Tab. Bot. 100s, 1000s. *Rx.*
Use: Antihypertensive.

Hibiclens. (J & J Merck) Chlorhexidine gluconate 4%, isopropyl alcohol 4%, in a non-alkaline base. Bot. 4 oz, 8 oz, 16 oz, 32 oz, gal. Packette 15 ml. *otc.*
Use: Antiseptic, germicide.

Hibiclens Sponge Brush. (J & J Merck) Chlorhexidine gluconate impregnated sponge brush. Unit-of-use 22 ml sponge brushes. *otc.*
Use: Antiseptic, germicide.

Hibistat. (J & J Merck) Chlorhexidine gluconate 0.5%. **Liq.:** Isopropyl alcohol 70%, emollients. Bot. 4 oz, 8 oz. **Towelettes:** Unit-of-use pocket-size towelette impregnated with 5 ml Hibistat. *otc.*
Use: Antiseptic, germicide.

Hibplex. (Standex) Vitamins B_1 100 mg, B_2 2 mg, B_3 100 mg, panthenol 2 mg/ml. Vial 30 ml. *otc.*
Use: Vitamin supplement.

HibTITER Vaccine. (Wyeth Lederle) Purified Haemophilus b saccharide 10 mcg, diphtheria CRM_{197} protein 25 mcg. Inj. 0.5 ml, 2.5 ml, 5 ml vials. *Rx.*
Use: Agent for immunization.

Hi B with C. (Towne) Vitamin C 300 mg, B_1 15 mg, B_2 10.2 mg, niacin 50 mg, B_6 5 mg, pantothenic acid 10 mg/Cap. Bot. 100s. *Rx.*
Use: Vitamin supplement.

Hi-Cor 1.0. (C & M Pharmacal) Hydrocortisone 1% in a nonionic, ester-free, salt-free, paraben-free washable base. Tube 30 g, Jar 60 g, lb. *Rx.*
Use: Corticosteroid, topical.

Hi-Cor 2.5. (C & M Pharmacal) Hydrocortisone 2.5% in a nonionic, ester-free, saltfree, parabenfree washable base. Tube 30 g. Jar 60 g. *Rx.*
Use: Corticosteroid, topical.

hiestrone.
See: Estrone (Various Mfr.).

High B12. (Barth's) Vitamin B_{12}, desiccated liver. Cap. Bot. 100s, 500s. *otc.*
Use: Vitamin supplement.

High Potency Cold Cap. (Weeks & Leo) Salicylamide 325 mg, chlorpheniramine maleate 4 mg, dextromethorphan HBr 15 mg, caffeine 16.2 mg/Tab. Bot. 18s. *otc.*
Use: Salicylate analgesic, antihistamine, antitussive.

High Potency N-Vites. (Nion) Vitamins B_1 15 mg, B_2 10 mg, B_3 100 mg, B_5 20 mg, B_{12} 10 mcg, C 500 mg/Tab. Bot. 100s. *otc.*
Use: Vitamin supplement.

High Potency Pain Relievers. (Weeks & Leo) Acetaminophen 300 mg, salicylamide 300 mg/Cap. Bot. 20s, 40s. *otc.*
Use: Analgesic.

High Potency Tar. (C & M) Coal tar topical solution 25%. Shampoo, gel. Bot. 240 ml. *otc.*
Use: Antiseborrheic.

High Potency Vitamins and Minerals. (Burgin-Arden) Vitamins A 25,000 IU, D 400 IU, B_1 10 mg, B_2 5 mg, C 150 mg, niacinamide 100 mg, calcium 103 mg, phosphorous 80 mg, iron 10 mg, B_6 1 mg, B_{12} 5 mcg, magnesium 5.5 mg, manganese 1 mg, potassium 5 mg, zinc 1.4 mg/Tab. Bot. 100s. *otc.*
Use: Vitamin/mineral supplement.

Hill-Shade Lotion. (Hill) Para-aminobenzoic acid, alcohol 65%. SPF 22. *otc.*
Use: Sunscreen.

Hi-Po-Vites Tablets. (Hudson) Iron 6 mg, vitamins A 10,000 IU, D 400 IU, E 13

mg, B$_1$ 25 mg, B$_2$ 25 mg, B$_3$ 50 mg, B$_5$ 12.5 mg, B$_6$ 15 mg, B$_{12}$ 50 mcg, C 150 mg, folic acid 0.4 mg, Ca, Cr, Cu, I, K, Mg, Mn, Mo, P, Se, Zn 5 mg, biotin 1 mg, bioflavonoids, bone meal, PABA, choline bitartrate, betaine, inositol, lecithin, desiccated liver, rutin/Tab. Bot. 100s. otc.
Use: Vitamin/mineral supplement.

• hioxifilcon a. USAN.
Use: Contact lens material (hydrophilic).

hippramine.
See: Methenamine hippurate.

hipputope. (Squibb) Radio-iodinated sodium iodohippurate (^{131}I) Inj. Bot. 1 m Ci, 2 m Ci.
Use: Diagnostic aid.

Hipotest. (Marlop Pharm) Ca 53.5 mg, iron 50 mg, vitamins A 10,000 IU, D 400 IU, E 2.5 mg, B$_1$ 25 mg, B$_2$ 25 mg, B$_3$ 50 mg, B$_5$ 13 mg, B$_6$ 15 mg, B$_{12}$ 50 mcg, C 150 mg, choline, betaine, PABA, rutin, bioflavonoids, biotin 1 mg, dessicated liver, bone meal, Cu, Mg, Mn, Zn 2.2 mg, I, P, lecithin/Tab. Bot. 100s. otc.
Use: Vitamin/mineral supplement.

Hiprex. (Hoechst Marion Roussel) Methenamine hippurate 1 g/Tab. Bot. 100s. Rx.
Use: Urinary anti-infective.

Hismanal. (Janssen) Astemizole 10 mg/Tab. 100s, UD 100s. Rx.
Use: Antihistamine.

Histacon. (Marsh Labs) Chlorpheniramine maleate 12 mg, ephedrine HCl 15 mg/SR Tab. Bot. 100s, 1000s. otc.
Use: Antihistamine, decongestant.

Histacon Syrup. (Marsh Labs) Chlorpheniramine maleate 3 mg, ephedrine HCl 4 mg/5 ml, alcohol 5%. Bot. pt.
Use: Antihistamine, decongestant.

Histagesic D.M. (Jones Medical) Phenylpropanolamine HCl 25 mg, chlorpheniramine maleate 4 mg, dextromethorphan HBr 10 mg, acetaminophen 324 mg/Tab. Bot. 100s, 1000s. otc.
Use: Decongestant, antihistamine, antitussive, analgesic.

Histagesic Modified. (Jones Medical) Acetaminophen 324 mg, phenylephrine HCl 10 mg, chlorpheniramine maleate 4 mg/Tab. otc.
Use: Analgesic, decongestant, antihistamine.

Histagesic Modified Tablets. (Jones Medical) Phenylephrine HCl 10 mg, chlorpheniramine maleate 4 mg, acetaminophen 324 mg/Tab. Bot. 1000s. otc.

Use: Decongestant, antihistamine, analgesic.

Histalet. (Solvay) Syr.: Pseudoephedrine HCl 45 mg, chlorpheniramine maleate 3 mg/5 ml. Bot. 473 ml. Rx.
Use: Decongestant, antihistamine.

Histalet Forte. (Major). Phenylpropanolamine HCl 50 mg, phenylephrine HCl 10 mg, chlorpheniramine maleate 4 mg, pyrilamine maleate 25 mg, lactose, sugar. Tab. Bot. 100s, 250s. Rx.
Use: Decongestant, antihistamine.

Histalet X. (Solvay) Syr.: Pseudoephedrine HCl 45 mg, guaifenesin 200 mg/5 ml, alcohol 15%. Bot. 480 ml.
Tab.: Pseudoephedrine HCl 120 mg, guaifenesin 400 mg/Tab. Bot. 100s. Rx.
Use: Decongestant, expectorant.

Histamic Capsules. (Lexis) Phenylpropanolamine HCl 50 mg, phenylephrine HCl 25 mg, phenyltoloxamine citrate 30 mg, chlorpheniramine maleate 12 mg/SR Cap. Bot. 100s, 1000s. otc.
Use: Decongestant, antihistamine.

Histamic Tablets. (Lexis) Phenylpropanolamine HCl 40 mg, phenylephrine HCl 10 mg, phenyltoloxamine citrate 15 mg, chlorpheniramine maleate 5 mg/Tab. Bot. 100s, 1000s. otc.
Use: Decongestant, antihistamine.

Histamine.
Use: Diagnostic aid.

• histamine dihydrochloride, U.S.P. 23.
W/Methyl nicotinate, oleoresincapicum, glycomonosalicylate.
Use: Analgesic, topical.
W/Menthol, thymol, methyl salicylate.
See: Imahist Unction (Gordon).

histamine H$_2$ antagonists.
See: Axid Pulvules, Cap. (Lilly).
Cimetidine HCl, Inj. (Endo).
Pepcid, Tab., Pow. (Merck).
Pepcid IV, Inj. (Merck).
Tagamet, Tab., Liq., Inj. (SK-Beecham).
Zantac, Tab. Syr. Inj. (Glaxo and Roche).

• histamine phosphate, U.S.P. 23.
Use: Stimulant (gastric secretory).

Histapco. (Apco) Chlorpheniramine maleate 4 mg, ipecac and opium pow. 0.25 gr, (contains opium 0.025 gr), camphor monobromated ⅛ gr, salicylamide 2 gr, phenacetin 1.5 gr, caffeine alkaloid gr, atropine sulfate gr/Tab. Rx.
Use: Antihistamine, analgesic, anticholinergic combination.

Histatab Plus. (Century) Chlorpheniramine maleate 2 mg, phenylephrine

HCl 5 mg/Tab. Bot. 100s. *otc.*
Use: Antihistamine, decongestant.

Histatime Forte. (Major) Phenyl-propanolamine HCl 50 mg, phenyleph-rine HCl 10 mg, chlorpheniramine ma-leate 4 mg, pyrilamine maleate 25 mg/ Cap. Bot. 100s. *Rx.*
Use: Decongestant, antihistamine.

Histatrol. (Center) 2.75 mg/ml histamine phosphate, equivalent ot 1 ml/ml hista-mine base, in 50% glycerin w/v, 5 ml vial; available in a Multitest dosage form or dropper bottle; 0.275 mg/ml hista-mine phosphate, equivalent to 0.1 mg/ ml histamine base, 5 ml vial.
Use: Skin test control.

Hista-Vadrin Syrup. (Scherer) Phenyl-propanolamine HCl 20 mg, chlorphenir-amine maleate 2 mg, phenylephrine HCl 2.5 mg, alcohol 2%/5 ml. Bot. pt. *Rx.*
Use: Decongestant, antihistamine.

Hista-Vadrin Tablets. (Scherer) Phenyl-propanolamine HCl 40 mg, chlorphenir-amine maleate 6 mg, phenylephrine HCl 5 mg/Tab. Bot. 100s. *Rx.*
Use: Decongestant, antihistamine.

Hista-Vadrin T.D. Capsules. (Scherer) Phenylpropanolamine HCl 50 mg, chlorpheniramine maleate 4 mg, bella-donna alkaloids 0.2 mg/Cap. Bot. 50s, 250s. *otc.*
Use: Decongestant, antihistamine com-bination.

Histerone Injection. (Roberts) Testoster-one aqueous susp. 50 mg or 100 mg/ ml. Vial 10 ml. *c-III.*
Use: Androgen.

•**histidine,** (HISS-tih-deen) U.S.P. 23.
Use: Amino acid.

histidine monohydrochloride.
Use: I.M., peptic and jejunal ulcers.

Histine-1. (Freeport) Diphenhydramine HCl 10 mg, alcohol 12% to 14%/4 ml. Bot. 4 oz. *otc.*
Use: Antihistamine with anticholinergic, antitussive, antiemetic and sedative effects.

Histine-2. (Freeport) Diphenhydramine HCl 12.5 mg/5 ml w/alcohol 5%. Bot. 4 oz. *otc.*
Use: Antihistamine with anticholinergic, antitussive, antiemetic and sedative effects.

Histine-4. (Freeport) Chlorpheniramine maleate 4 mg/Tab. Bot. 1000s. *otc.*
Use: Antihistamine.

Histine-8. (Freeport) Chlorpheniramine maleate 8 mg/TR Tab. Bot. 1000s. *otc.*

Use: Antihistamine.

Histine-12. (Freeport) Chlorpheniramine maleate 12 mg/TR Tab. Bot. 1000s. *otc.*
Use: Antihistamine.

Histine-25. (Freeport) Diphenhydramine HCl 25 mg/Cap. Bot. 1000s. *otc.*
Use: Antihistamine with anticholinergic, antitussive, antiemetic and sedative effects.

Histine-50. (Freeport) Diphenhydramine HCl 50 mg/Cap. Bot. 1000s. *otc.*
Use: Antihistamine with anticholinergic, antitussive, antiemetic and sedative effects.

Histine DM Syrup. (Ethex) Phenyl-propanolamine HCl 12.5 mg, brom-pheniramine maleate 2 mg, dextro-methorphan HBr 10 mg, parabens, saccharin. Bot. 120 ml or 480 ml. *Rx.*
Use: Decongestant, antihistamine, anti-tussive.

Histinex HC. (Ethex) Hydrocodone bitar-trate 2 mg, phenylephrine HCl 5 mg, chlorpheniramine maleate 2 mg/5 ml. Syrup. Alcohol and sugar free. Bot. 473 ml. *c-III.*
Use: Antitussive, decongestant, antihis-tamine.

Histinex PV. (Ethex) Hydrocodone bitar-trate 2.5 mg, pseudoephedrine HCl 30 mg, chlorpheniramine maleate 2 mg, parabens, saccharin, sorbitol/5ml. Syrup. Alcohol and sugar free. Bot. 120 ml, 480 ml. *c-III.*
Use: Antitussive, decongestant, antihis-tamine.

Histolyn-Cyl. (ALK Biologicals) Histo-plasmin sterile filtrate from yeast cells of *Histoplasma capsulatum.* Vial 1.3 ml. *Rx.*
Use: Skin test.

•**histoplasmin.** U.S.P. 23. (Parke-Davis) An aqueous solution containing stan-dardized sterile culture filtrate of *Histo-plasma capsulatum* grown on liquid synthetic medium.
Use: Diagnostic aid (dermal reactivity indicator).
See: Hisotlyn-CYL, Inj. (ALK Labs).

histoplasmin, diluted. (Parke-Davis) 1:100 w/v. Standardized sterile filtrate from cultures of *Histoplasma capsula-tum,* 0.5% phenol, polysorbate 80. 1 ml/Inj. *Rx.*
Use: In vivo diagnostic.

Histosal. (Ferndale) Pyrilamine maleate 12.5 mg, phenylpropanolamine HCl 20 mg, acetaminophen 324 mg, caffeine 30 mg/Tab. Bot. 100s. *otc.*

Use: Antihistamine, decongestant, analgesic.

•**histrelin.** (hiss-TRELL-in) USAN.
Use: LHRH agonist. Treatment of porphyria [Orphan drug]
See: Supprelin, Inj. (Ortho).

histrelin acetate. *Rx.*
Use: Central prococious puberty. [Orphan drug]

Histussin D. (Bock) Hydrocodone bitartrate 5 mg, pseudoephedrine HCl 60 mg/5 ml/Liq. Bot. 480 ml. *c-III.*
Use: Antitussive, decongestant.

Histussin-HC Syrup. (Bock) Phenylephrine HCl 5 mg, chlorpheniramine maleate 2 mg, hydrocodone bitartrate 2.5 mg. In 480 ml. *c-III.*
Use: Decongestant, antihistamine, narcotic analgesic.

Hitone. (Lafayette) Barium sulfate suspension 125% w/v. Bot. 2000 ml. Case 4s.
Use: Radiopaque agent.

Hi-Tor. (Barth's) Vitamins B_{12} 15 mcg, niacin 1.5 mg, B_1 6 mg, B_2 12 mg, B_6 54 mcg, pantothenic acid 150 mcg, choline 3.75 mg, inositol 5.25 mg/Tab. Bot. 100s, 500s, 1000s. *otc.*
Use: Vitamin supplement.

Hi-Tor 900. (Barth's) Vitamins B_1 13.5 mg, B_2 5.2 mg, niacin 15 mg, B_6 0.6 mg, pantothenic acid 1.2 mg, biotin, B_{12} 2.5 mcg, iron 0.9 mg, protein 7.5 g, inositol 50 mg, choline 40 mg, aminobenzoic acid 0.15 to 2.4 mg/15 g. Bot. 1 lb, 3 lb. *otc.*
Use: Vitamin/mineral supplement.

HIVAB HIV-1/HIV-2 (rDNA) EIA. (Abbott) Enzyme immunoassay for qualitative detection of antibodies to human immunodeficiency viruses Type 1 or Type 2 in human serum or plasma. Test kits 100s, 1000s, 5000s.
Use: Diagnostic aid.

Hi-Vegi-Lip Tablets. (Freeda) Pancreatin 2400 mg, lipase 12,000 units, protease 60,000 units, amylase 60,000 units/Tab. Bot. 100s, 250s. *otc.*
Use: Digestive aid.

Hivid. (Roche) Zalcitamine 0.375 mg or 0.75 mg/Tab. Bot. 100s. *Rx.*
Use: Antiviral (Phase II/III AIDS).

HIV-neutralizing antibodies. *Rx.*
Use: AIDS treatment. [Orphan drug]

Hiwolfia. (Jones Medical) Rauwolfia 25 mg, 50 mg or 100 mg/Tab. Bot. 100s, 1000s.
Use: Antihypertensive.

HMG-CoA Reductase Inhibitors. *Rx.*

Use: Antihyperlipidemic.
See: Lescol, Cap. (Sandoz).
Mevacor, Tab. (Merck).
Pravachol, Tab. (Bristol-Myers Squibb).
Zocor, Tab. (Merck).

HMM.
See: Hexamethylmelamine.

HMS Liquifilm. (Allergan) Medrysone 1%. Ophth. Susp. Bot. 5 ml, 10 ml. *Rx.*
Use: Anti-inflammatory, ophthalmic.

HN_2. Mechlorethamine HCl.
Use: Alkylating agent.
See: Mustargen, Pow. (Merck).

H_2 OEX. (Fellows) Benzthiazide 50 mg/Tab. Bot. 100s, 1000s. *Rx.*
Use: Diuretic.

Hold. (SK-Beecham) Dextromethorphan HBr 5 mg/Loz. Plastic tube 10 Loz. *otc.*
Use: Antitussive.

Hold DM. (Menley & James) Dextromethorphan HBr 5 mg, corn syrup, sucrose. Loz. Pkg. 10s. *otc.*
Use: Antitussive.

Hold Lozenges (Children's Formula). (SK-Beecham) Phenylpropanolamine HCl 6.25 mg, dextromethorphan HBr 3.75 mg/Loz. Roll 10s. *otc.*
Use: Decongestant, antitussive.

holocaine hydrochloride. (Various Mfr.) Phenacaine HCl.
Use: Local anesthetic.

homarylamine hydrochloride. N-Methyl-3,4-methylenedioxyphenethylamine HCl.

•**homatropine hydrobromide,** U.S.P. 23. (Various Mfr.) 5% Soln. Bot. 1 ml, 2 ml, 5 ml.
Use: Mydriatic, cycloplegic, anticholinergic (ophthalmic).
See: AK-Homatropine, Soln. (Akorn).
Homatropine HBr, Soln. (Ciba Vision).
Isopto Homatropine, Soln. (Alcon).
Murocoll, Liq. (Muro).

homatropine hydrobromide. (Various Mfr.) 5% Soln. Bot. 1 ml, 2 ml, 5 ml. *Rx.*
Use: Mydriatic, cycloplegic.

homatropine hydrochloride.
Use: Mydriatic, cyclopegic; anticholinergic, topical.

•**homatropine methylbromide,** U.S.P. 23.
Use: Anticholinergic.

homatropine methylbromide w/combinations.
Use: Anticholinergic.
See: Dranochol, Tab. (Marin).
Homapin, Tab. (Mission).

Hycodan, Tab., Pow., Syr. (DuPont).
Panitol H.M.B., Tab. (Wesley).
Spasmatol, Tab. (Pharmed).
Tapuline, Tab. (Wesley).

homatropine methylbromide and phenobarbital combinations.
Use: Anticholinergic.
See: Gustase-Plus, Tab. (Geriatric).

Hominex-1. (Ross) Protein 15 g, fat 23.9 g, carbohydrate 46.3 g, linoleic acid 1800 mg, Fe 9 mg, Na 190 mg, K 675 mg, Ca, vitamins A, B$_1$, B$_2$, B$_3$, B$_5$, B$_6$, B$_{12}$, C, D, E, K, biotin, choline, folic acid, inositol, Cl, Cu, I, Mg, Mn, P, Se, Zn and 480 Cal per 100 g. Methionine free. Pow. Can 350 g. *otc.*
Use: Nutritional supplement.

Hominex-2. (Ross) Protein 30 g, fat 15.5 g, carbohydrate 30 g, Fe 13 mg, Na 880 mg, K 1370 mg, Ca, vitamins A, B$_1$, B$_2$, B$_3$, B$_5$, B$_6$, B$_{12}$, C, D, E, K, biotin, choline, folic acid, inositol, Cl, Cu, I, Mg, Mn, P, Se, Zn and 410 Cal per 100 g. Methionine free. Pow. Can 325 g. *otc.*
Use: Nutritional supplement.

Homogene-S. (Spanner) Testosterone 25 mg, 50 mg or 100 mg/ml. Vial 10 ml. *c-III.*
Use: Androgen.

●**homosalate.** (hoe-moe-SAL-ate) USAN.
Formerly Homomenthyl Salicylate.
Use: Ultraviolet sunscreen.
W/Combinations.
See: Coppertone, Prods. (Schering Plough).

honey bee venom.
See: Albay (Bayer).
Pharmalgen (ALK Laboratories).
Venomil (Bayer).

●**hoquizil hydrochloride.** (HOE-kwih-zill) USAN.
Use: Bronchodilator.

hormofollin.
See: Estrone (Various Mfr.).

hornet venom.
See: Albay (Bayer).
Parmalgen (ALK Laboratories).
Venomil (Bayer).

Hospital Foam Cleaner. (Health & Medical Techniques) 0-phenylphenol 0.1%, 4-chloro-2-cyclopentyl-phenol 0.08%, lauric diethanolamide 0.2%, triethanolamine dodecylbenzenesulfonate 0.3%. Aerosol spray 19 oz.
Use: Germicidal, disinfectant.

Hospital Lotion. (Paddock) Diisobutylcresoxyethoxy-ethyl dimethyl benzyl ammonium Cl, menthol, lanolin, mineral and vegetable oils. Bot. 4 oz, 8 oz, gal. *otc.*

Use: Emollient.

12-Hour Antihistamine Nasal Decongestant. (URL) Pseudoephedrine sulfate 120 mg, dexbrompheniramine maleate 6 mg, sugar, sucrose. Tab. Pkg. 10s. *otc.*
Use: Decongestant, antihistamine.

12-Hour Cold. (Hudson) Phenylpropanolamine HCl 75 mg, chlorpheniramine maleate 4 mg/Cap. Pkg. 10s. *otc.*
Use: Decongestant, antihistamine.

HPA-23. (antimoniotungstate) An experimental compound developed at the Pasteur Institute in Paris to stop or slow the reproduction of the Acquired Immune Deficiency Syndrone (AIDS) virus, at least temporarily.

H.P. Acthar Gel. (Centeon) Repository corticotropin injection highly purified 40 U.S.P. units/1 ml. Vial 1 ml, 5 ml; 80 U.S.P. units/1 ml. Vial 1 ml, 5 ml. *Rx.*
Use: Corticosteroid.

H-R Lubricating Jelly. (Carter-Wallace) Hydroxypropyl methycellulose, parabens. Jelly 150 g. *otc.*
Use: Lubricating agent.

HRC-Tylaprin Elixir. (Cenci) Acetaminophen 120 mg, alcohol 7%/5 ml. Bot. 2 oz, 4 oz. *otc.*
Use: Analgesic.

H.S. Need. (Hanlon) Chloral hydrate 3¾ gr, 7.5 gr/Cap. Bot. 100s. *Rx.*
Use: Sedative.

HSV-1. (Wampole-Zeus) Herpes simplex virus type I test system. For the qualitative and semi-quantitative detection of HSV-1 antibody in human serum. Test 100s.
Use: Diagnostic aid.

HSV-2. (Wampole-Zeus) Herpes simplex virus type II antibody test. For the qualitative and semi-quantitative detection of HSV-2 antibody in human serum. Test 100s.
Use: Diagnostic aid.

H.T. Factorate. (Centeon) Antihemophilic factor (human) dried, heat treated for I.V. administration only. Single-dose vial w/diluent and needles. *Rx.*
Use: Classical hemophilia treatment.

H.T. Factorate Generation II. (Centeon) Antihemophilic factor (human) dried, heat treated for I.V. administration only. Single dose vial w/diluent and needles. *Rx.*
Use: Classical hemophilia treatment.

HTSH EIA. (Abbott Diagnostics) Enzyme immunoassay for the quantitative determination of human thyroid stimulating

hormone (HTSH) in human serum or plasma.
Use: Diagnostic aid.

HTSH RIAbead. (Abbott Diagnostics) Immunoradiometric assay for the quantitative measurement of human thyroid stimulating hormone (HTSH) in serum.
Use: Diagnostic aid.

Hulk Hogan Multi-Vitamins Plus Extra C. (S.G. Labs) Vitamins A 2500 IU, E 15 IU, D_3 400 IU, B_1 1.05 mg, B_2 1.2 mg, B_3 13.5 mg, B_6 1.05 mg, B_{12} 4.5 mcg, C 300 mg, folic acid 300 mcg, sucrose. Tab. chew. Bot. 60s. *otc.*
Use: Vitamin/mineral supplement.

Humalog. (Eli Lilly) Insulin lispro 100 units/ml. Inj. Vial, 10 ml. Cartridge 1.5 ml. *Rx.*
Use: Treatment of diabetes.

human antihemophilic factor.
See: Antihemophilic.

human growth hormone.
Use: With glutamine in the treatment of short bowel syndrome. [Orphan drug]

human growth hormone function test.
See: R-Gene 10, Inj. (Pharmacia & Upjohn).

human immunodeficiency virus immune globulin. *Rx.*
Use: AIDS treatment. [Orphan drug]

human insulin. Insulin Human, U.S.P. 23.
Use: Hypoglycemic.
See: Humulin Prods. (Lilly).

human serum albumin.
See: Albumotope (Squibb).

human t-lymphotropic virus type III antigens.
See: t-lymphotropic virus type III gp 160 antigens.

Humate-P. (Centeon). Pasteurized, purified lyophilized concentrate of antihemophilic factor (human). Inj. single dose vial. *Rx.*
Use: Antihemophilic.

Humatin Capsules. (Parke-Davis) Paromomycin sulfate 250 mg/Cap. Bot. 16s. *Rx.*
Use: Amebicide.

Humatrope. (Lilly) Somatropin (recombinant DNA origin). Inj. 5 mg/vial. *Rx.*
Use: Growth hormone.

Humegon. (Organon) Follicle-stimulating hormone activity 75 IU or 150 IU, lutienizing hormone activity 75 IU or 150 IU. Powd. for Inj. Vial 2 ml NaCl. *Rx.*
Use: Gonadotropin.

Humibid DM. (Adams) Dextromethorphan HBr 30 mg, guaifenesin 600 mg/Tab. Bot. 100s. *Rx.*

Use: Antitussive, expectorant.

Humibid L.A. (Adams Labs) Guaifenesin 600 mg/SR Tab. Bot. 100s. *Rx.*
Use: Expectorant.

Humibid Sprinkle. (Adams Labs) Dextromethorphan HBr 15 mg, guaifenesin 300 mg/SR Cap. Bot. 100s. *Rx.*
Use: Expectorant, antitussive.

Humist. (Scherer) Sodium Cl 0.65%, chlorobutanol 0.35%. Soln. Bot. 45 ml. *Rx.*
Use: Decongestant combination.

Humorsol. (Merck) Demecarium bromide 0.125% or 0.25% ophthalmic soln. 5 ml Ocumeter. *Rx.*
Use: Agent for glaucoma.

Humulin 50/50. (Lilly) Isophane insulin suspension (50%) and insulin injection (50%), 100 units/ml Inj. Vial 10 ml. *otc.*
Use: Antidiabetic.

Humulin 70/30. (Lilly) Isophane insulin suspension (70%) and insulin injection (30%), 100 units/ml/Inj. Bot. 10 ml. *otc.*
Use: Antidiabetic.

Humulin I. (Lilly) Lente human insulin (recombinant DNA origin) 100 units/ml. Inj. Bot. 10 ml. *otc.*
Use: Antidiabetic.

Humulin N. (Lilly) NPH human insulin (recombinant DNA origin) 100 units/ml. Vial 10 ml. *otc.*
Use: Antidiabetic.

Humulin R. (Lilly) Regular human insulin (recombinant DNA origin) 100 units/ml. Vial 10 ml. *otc.*
Use: Antidiabetic.

Humulin U. (Lilly) Ultralente human insulin (recombinant DNA origin) 100 units/ml. Inj. Bot. 10 ml. *otc.*
Use: Antidiabetic.

Hurricaine. (Beutlich) Benzocaine 20%. Liq.: 0.25 ml, 3.75 ml, 30 ml. Gel: 3.75 ml, 30 g. Spray: 60 ml. *otc.*
Use: Anesthetic, topical.

Hurricaine Topical Anesthetic Spray Kit. (Beutlich) Benzocaine 20%. Kit: Aerosol 60 g plus 200 disposable extension tubes. *otc.*
Use: Anesthetic, topical.

HVS 1 & 2. (Chemi-Tech) Benzalkonium Cl in a specially formulated base. Soln. Bot. 15 ml. *otc.*
Use: Cold sores, fever blisters, herpes virus.

Hyacide. (Niltig) Benzethonium Cl 0.1%, sodium nitrite 0.55%. Soln. Bot. oz. *otc.*
Use: Antiseptic.

Hyalex. (Miller) Magnesium salicylate 260 mg, magnesium p-aminobenzoate 163 mg, vitamins A 1500 IU, C 30 mg, D 100 IU, E 3 IU, B_{12} 2 mcg, pantothenic acid 5 mg, zinc 0.7 mg/Tab. Bot. 100s. *otc.*
Use: Vitamin/mineral supplement.

hyalidase.
See: Hyaluronidase (Various Mfr.).

•**hyaluronidase injection,** (high-uhl-yur-AHN-ih-dase) U.S.P. 23. Hyalidase, Hydase Enzymes which depolymerize hyaluronic acid. Hyalase, Rondase.
Use: Hypodermoclyses, promotion of diffusion, spreading agent.
See: Alidase, Vial (Searle).
  Wydase, Vial (Wyeth-Ayerst).

hyamagnate. Hydroxy-Aluminum-Magnesium-Aminoacetate, Sodium-free.

Hybec Forte. (Amlab) Vitamins B_1 100 mg, B_2 20 mg, B_6 2.5 mg, niacinamide 25 mg, C 200 mg, B_{12} 10 mcg, calcium pantothenate 5 mg, iron 10 mg, choline bitartrate 24 mg, inositol 10 mg, biotin 5 mcg, liver 50 mg, yeast 100 mg/Tab. Bot. 30s, 100s. *otc.*
Use: Vitamin/mineral supplement.

Hybolin Decanoate. (Hyrex) Nandrolone decanoate 50 mg or 100 mg/ml in oil. Vial 2 ml. *c-III.*
Use: Anabolic steroid.

Hybolin Improved. (Hyrex) Nandrolone phenpropionate 25 mg or 50 mg/ml in oil. Vial 2 ml. *c-III.*
Use: Anabolic steroid.

Hycamtin. (SmithKline Beecham) Topotecan HCl 4 mg (free base), mannitol 48 mg/Pow. for Inj. vial. single dose. *Rx.*
Use: Treatment of ovarian cancer.

•**hycanthone.** (HIGH-kan-thone) USAN.
Use: Antischistosomal.

Hyclorite. Sodium Hypochlorite soln., U.S.P. 23.

HycoClear Tuss. (Ethex) Hydrocodone bitartrate 5 mg, guaifenesin 100 mg/5 ml. Syrup. Alcohol, dye, sugar free. Bot. 118 ml, 473 ml. *c-III.*
Use: Antitussive, expectorant.

Hycodan. (DuPont Merck) Hydrocodone bitartrate 5 mg, homatropine methylbromide 1.5 mg/5 ml or Tab. **Syr.:** Bot. 473 ml. **Tab.:** Bot. 100s, 500s. *c-III.*
Use: Antitussive combination.

Hycomine Compound Tablets. (DuPont Merck) Hydrocodone bitartrate 5 mg, chlorpheniramine maleate 2 mg, phenylephrine HCl 10 mg, acetaminophen 250 mg, caffeine (anhydrous) 30 mg/Tab. Bot. 100s, 500s. *c-III.*

Use: Antitussive, antihistamine, decongestant, analgesic.

Hycomine Pediatric Syrup. (DuPont Merck) Hydrocodone bitartrate 2.5 mg, phenylpropanolamine HCl 12.5 mg/5 ml. Bot. 480 ml. *c-III.*
Use: Antitussive, decongestant.

Hycomine Syrup. (DuPont Merck) Hydrocodone bitartrate 5 mg, phenylpropanolamine HCl 25 mg/5 ml. Syr. Bot. pt, gal. *c-III.*
Use: Antitussive, decongestant.

Hycort Cream. (Everett) Hydrocortisone 1% in a cream base. Tube oz. *Rx.*
Use: Corticosteroid, topical.

Hycort Ointment. (Everett) Hydrocortisone 1% in ointment base. Tube oz. *Rx.*
Use: Corticosteroid, topical.

Hycortole. (Lemmon) Hydrocortisone. **Cream:** 0.5%: 5 g, 20 g; 1%: 5 g, 20 g, 4 oz; 2.5%: Tube 5 g, 20 g; **Oint.:** 1% or 2.5%. Tube 5 g, 20 g.
Use: Corticosteroid, topical.

Hycotuss Expectorant. (DuPont Merck) Hydrocodone bitartrate 5 mg, guaifenesin 100 mg, alcohol 10%(v/v)/5 ml. Bot. 480 ml. *c-III.*
Use: Antitussive, expectorant.

hydantoin derivatives.
Use: Anticonvulsant.
See: Dilantin, Preps. (Parke-Davis). Diphenylhydantoin Sodium, U.S.P. Ethotoin.
  Mesantoin, Tab. (Sandoz).
  Phenantoin.

hydase.
Use: Hypodermoclyses, promotion of diffusion.
See: Hyaluronidase (Various Mfr.).

Hydeltrasol Injection. (Merck) Prednisolone sodium phosphate 20 mg/ml w/ niacinamide 25 mg, sodium hydroxide to adjust pH, disodium edetate 0.5 mg, sodium bisulfite 1 mg, phenol 5 mg, water for injection q.s. 1 ml. Vial 2 ml, 5 ml. *Rx.*
Use: Corticosteroid.

Hydergine LC Liquid Capsules. (Sandoz) Ergoloid mesylates 1 mg/Cap. Bot. 100s, 500s. SandoPak 100s, 500s. *Rx.*
Use: Psychotherapeutic.

Hydergine Liquid. (Sandoz) Equal parts of dihydroergocornine, dihydroergocristine, dihydroergocryptine. (Ergoloid Mesylates). 1 mg/ml. Bot. 100 ml w/ dropper. *Rx.*
Use: Psychotherapeutic.

Hydergine, Oral. (Sandoz) Equal parts of dihydroergocornine, dihydroergocristine, dihydroergocryptine (Ergoloid Mesylates). 1 mg/Tab. Bot. 100s, 500s. SandoPak (UD) 100s, 500s. *Rx.*
Use: Psychotherapeutic.

Hydergine, Sublingual. (Sandoz) Equal parts of dihydroergocornine, dihydroergocristine, dihydroergocryptine (Ergoloid Mesylates). 0.5 mg or 1 mg/Tab. Bot. 100s, 1000s, SandoPak (UD) 100s. *Rx.*
Use: Psychotherapeutic.

Hydoril. (Cenci) Hydrochlorthiazide 25 mg or 50 mg/Tab. Bot. 100s, 1000s. *Rx.*
Use: Diuretic.

hydrabamine phenoxymethyl penicillin.
See: Penicillin V Hydrabamine.

hydracrylic acid beta lactone.
See: Propiolactone.

hydralazine. (Solopak) Hydralazine HCl 20 mg/ml Inj. Vial 1 ml. *Rx.*
Use: Antihypertensive.

•**hydralazine hydrochloride,** (high-DRAL-uh-zeen) U.S.P. 23.
Use: Antihypertensive.
See: Apresoline, Amp., Tab. (Novartis).
Dralzine, Tab. (Lemmon).
W/Hydrochlorothiazide.
See: Apresazide, Cap. (Novartis).
Apresoline-Esidrix, Tab. (Novartis).
Hydralazide, Tab. (Zenith).
Hydroserpine Plus, Tab. (Zenith).
W/Reserpine.
See: Dralserp, Tab. (Lemmon).
Serpasil-Apresoline, Tab. (Novartis).
W/Reserpine, hydrochlorothiazide (Esidrix).
See: Harbolin, Tab. (Arcum).
Ser-Ap-Es, Tab. (Novartis).
Unipres, Tab. (Solvay).

hydralazine hydrochloride. (Various Mfr.) **10 mg, 25 mg, 50 mg:** Tab. Bot. 100s, 1000s, UD 100s; **100 mg:** Tab. Bot. 100s, 1000s.
Use: Antihypertensive.

•**hydralazine polistirex.** (high-DRAL-ah-zeen pahl-ee-STIE-rex) USAN.
Use: Antihypertensive.

Hydra Mag Tablets. (Pal-Pak) Aluminum hydroxide gel, dried, 195 mg, magnesium trisilicate 195 mg, kaolin 162 mg/Tab. Bot. 1000s. *otc.*
Use: Antacid.

Hydramyn. (LuChem) Diphenhydramine HCl 12.5 mg/5 ml, alcohol 5%. Syr. Bot. pt. *otc.*
Use: Antihistamine.

Hydrap-ES. (Parmed) Hydrochlorothiazide 15 mg, reserpine 0.1 mg, hydralazine HCl 25 mg/Tab. Bot. 100s, 500s, 1000s. *Rx.*
Use: Antihypertensive.

Hydraserp. (Geneva Pharm) Hydrochlorothiazide 25 mg or 50 mg, reserpine 0.1 mg/Tab. Bot. 100s, 1000s. *Rx.*
Use: Antihypertensive combination.

hydrastine hydrochloride. (Penick) Pow. Bot. oz.
Use: Uterine hemostatic.

Hydrate. (Hyrex) Dimenhydrinate 50 mg/ml w/propylene glycol 50%, benzyl alcohol 5%. Amp. 1 ml. Box 25s, 100s; Vial 10 ml. *Rx.*
Use: Antiemetic, antivertigo, antihistamine.

Hydrazide Capsules. (Goldline) **25/25:** Hydrochlorothiazide 25 mg, hydralazine 25 mg/Cap. **50/50:** Hydrochlorothiazide 50 mg, hydralazine 50 mg/Cap. Bot. 100s. *Rx.*
Use: Antihypertensive.

Hydra-Zide Capsules. (Par Pharm) Hydralazine HCl 50 mg, hydrochlorothiazide 50 mg/Cap. Bot. 100s, 500s, 1000s. *Rx.*
Use: Antihypertensive.

hydrazone.
Use: Pulmonary tuberculosis.
See: Rimactane, Cap. (Novartis).

Hydrea. (Squibb Mark) Hydroxyurea. 500 mg/Cap. Bot. 100s. *Rx.*
Use: Antineoplastic.

hydriodic acid. (Various Mfr.).
Use: Expectorant.

hydriodic acid therapy.
See: Aminoacetic Acid HI.

Hydrisea Lotion. (Pedinol) Dead sea salts concentrate 8%, sodium, potassium, calcium magnesium Cl, propylene glycol stearate, polysorbate 40, silicone oil, coloring agent. Bot. 4 oz. *otc.*
Use: Hyperkeratotic, emollient.

Hydrisinol Creme and Lotion. (Pedinol) Sulfonated hydrogenated castor oil. **Cream:** Spout Cap Jar 4 oz, lb. **Lot.:** Bot. 8 oz. *otc.*
Use: Emollient.

Hydro-12. (Table Rock) Crystalline hydroxocobalamin 1000 mcg/ml Pkg. 10 ml. *Rx.*
Use: Vitamin B_{12} supplement.

Hydro-Ban Capsules. (Whiteworth Towne) Juniper oil 10 mg, uva ursi 50 mg, buchu extract 50 mg, parsley piert extract 50 mg, iron 6 mg/Cap. Bot. 42s. *otc.*

Use: Diuretic with iron.

Hydrocare Cleaning and Disinfecting. (Allergan) Tris(2-hydroxyethyl) tallow ammonium Cl, thimerosal 0.002%, bis(2-hydroxyethyl) tallow ammonium Cl, sodium bicarbonate, sodium phosphates, hydrochloric acid, propylene glycol, polysorbate 80, polyhema. Soln. Bot. 240 ml, 360 ml. *otc.*
Use: Soft contact lens disinfective.

Hydrocare Preserved Saline. (Allergan) Isotonic, buffered, NaCl, sodium hexametaphosphate, boric acid, sodium borate, EDTA 0.01%, thimerosal 0.001%. Soln. Bot. 240 ml, 360 ml. *otc.*
Use: Soft contact lens rinsing/storage solution.

Hydrocet. (Carnrick) Hydrocodone bitartrate 5 mg, acetaminophen 500 mg/ Cap. Bot. 100s. *c-III.*
Use: Narcotic analgesic combination.

hydrochlorate. Same as Hydrochloride.

•**hydrochloric acid, N.F 18.**
Use: Well diluted, achlorhydria; pharmaceutic aid (acidifying agent).

hydrochloric acid. (Various Mfr.) Muriatic Acid, Absolute 38%. Diluted 10%.

hydrochloric acid therapy.
Use: Well diluted, achlorhydria; pharmaceutic aid (acidifying agent).
Use: Gastric acidifier.
See: Betaine HCl (Various Mfr.).
Glutamic Acid HCl (Various Mfr.).
Glycine HCl (Various Mfr.).

Hydrochloroserpine. (Freeport) Hydralazine HCl 25 mg, hydrochlorthiazide 15 mg, reserpine 0.1 mg/Tab. Bot. 1000s.
Use: Antihypertensive combination.

•**hydrochlorothiazide,** (high-droe-klor-oh-THIGH-uh-zide) U.S.P. 23.
Use: Diuretic.
See: Chlorzide, Tab. (Foy).
Delco-Retic, Tab. (Delco).
Diu-Scrip, Cap. (Scrip).
Esidrix, Tab. (Novartis).
Hydromal, Tab. (Mallard).
HydroDiuril, Tab. (Merck).
Hydrozide-50, Tab. (Mayrand).
Oretic, Tab. (Abbott).
Thiuretic, Tab. (Parke-Davis).
Zide, Tab. (Solvay).
W/Deserpidine.
See: Oreticyl, Tab. (Abbott).
W/Enalapril.
See: Vaseretic, Tab. (Merck).
W/Guanethidine monosulfate.
See: Esimil, Tab. (Novartis).
W/Hydralazine HCl.
See: Apresazide, Cap. (Novartis).

Apresoline-Esidrix, Tab. (Novartis).
Hydralazide, Tab. (Zenith).
W/Labetalol.
See: Trandide, Tab. (Glaxo).
W/Lisinopril.
See: Prinzide, Tab. (Merck).
W/Methyldopa.
See: Aldoril, Tab. (Merck).
W/Propranolol.
See: Inderide, Tab. (Wyeth-Ayerst).
W/Reserpine.
See: Aquapres-R, Tab. (Castal).
Hydropres, Tab. (Merck).
Hydroserp, Tab. (Zenith).
Hydroserpine, Tab. (Geneva Pharm).
Hydrotensin-50, Tab. (Mayrand).
Hyperserp, Tab. (Zeneca).
Mallopress, Tab. (Mallard).
Serpasil-Esidrix, Tab. (Novartis).
W/Reserpine, Hydralazine HCl.
See: Harbolin, Tab. (Arcum).
Hydroserpine Plus, Tab. (Zenith).
Ser-Ap-Es, Tab. (Novartis).
Unipres, Tab. (Solvay).
W/Spironolactone.
See: Aldactazide, Tab. (Searle).
W/Timolol maleate.
See: Timolide, Tab. (Merck).
W/Triamterene.
See: Dyazide, Cap. (SK-Beecham).

hydrochlorothiazide/amiloride.
See: Amiloride hydrochloride and hydrochlorthiazide tablets.

hydrochlorothiazide/hydralazine. (Various Mfr.) Hydrochlorothiazide 25 mg, hydralazine HCl 25 mg/Cap, or hydrochlorothiazide 50 mg, hydralazine HCl 50 mg/Cap. Bot. 100s, 500s, 1000s. *Rx.*
Use: Antihypertensive.

hydrochlorothiazide/reserpine. (Various Mfr.) *Rx.*
See: Reserpine and hydrochlorothiazide.

hydrocholeretics.
See: Bile Salts (Various Mfr.).
Dehydrocholic Acid (Various Mfr.).
Desoxycholic Acid (Various Mfr.).
Ox Bile Extract (Various Mfr.).

hydrocholeretic combinations.
See: G.B.S., Tab. (Forest).

Hydrocil Instant. (Solvay) Blond psyllium coating containing psyllium 3.5 g/3.7 g dose. Tan granular, instant mix, sugar-free, low sodium, low potassium powder. UD packets. 3.7 g in 30s, 500s, Jar 250 g. *otc.*
Use: Laxative.

Hydro Cobex. (Taylor) Hydroxocobalamin 1000 mcg/Vial 30 ml. *Rx.*

Use: Vitamin B_{12} supplement.

hydrocodone w/acetaminophen. (HIGH-droe-KOE-dohn with ass-eet-ah-MEE-no-fen) (Pharmics) Hydrocodone bitartrate 7.5 mg, acetaminophen 500 mg. Tab. Bot. 100s, 500s. *c-III.*
Use: Narcotic analgesic combination.

• **hydrocodone bitartrate,** (HIGH-droe-KOE-dohn by-TAR-TRATE) U.S.P. 23. Dihydrocodeinone bitartrate.
Use: Antitussive.
W/Combinations.
See: Hydrocet, Cap. (Carnrick).
Hydrocodone/APAP, Tab. (Pharmics).
Medipain 5, Cap. (ECR Pharm).
Panacet 5/500, Tab. (ECR Pharm).
Panasal 5/500, Tab. (ECR Pharm).
Pandel, Cream (Savage).
Tyrodone, Liq. (Major).
Vicodin, Tab. (Knoll).

hydrocodone bitartrate and acetaminophen capsules. (Various) Hydrocodone bitartrate 5 mg, acetaminophen 500 mg/Cap. Bot. 100s, 500s. *c-III.*
Use: Narcotic/analgesic combination.

hydrocodone bitartate and acetaminophen caplets. (Various Mfr.) Hydrocodone bitartrate 7.5 mg, acetaminophen 650 mg. 100s, 500s. *c-III.*
Use: Narcotic/analgesic combination.

hydrocodone bitartrate and acetaminophen tablets. (Watson) Hydrocodone bitartrate 5 mg, acetaminophen 500 mg/Tab. Bot. 100s, 500s. (King Pharm) Hydrocodone bitartrate 7.5 mg, acetaminophen 650 mg/capl. Bot. 100s, 500s. *c-III.*
Use: Narcotic/analgesic combination.

hydrocodone bitartrate and phenylpropanolamine hydrochloride pediatric syrup. (Rosemont) Phenylpropanolamine HCl 12.5 mg, hydrocodone bitartrate 2.5 mg/Syr. Bot. 118 ml, pt, gal. *c-III.*
Use: Pediatric antitussive combination.

hydrocodone comp. syrup. (Various Mfr.) Hydrocodone bitartrate 5 mg, homatropine methylbromide 1.5 mg. Bot. 473 ml, gal. *c-III.*
Use: Antitussive.

Hydrocodone CP. (Morton Grove) Hydrocodone bitartrate 2.5 mg, phenylephrine 5 mg, chlorpheniramine maleate 2 mg/5 ml/Liq. bot. 473 ml. *c-III.*
Use: Antitussive.

Hydrocodone GF Syrup. (Morton Grove) Hydrocodone bitartrate 5 mg, guaifenesin 100 mg/5 ml/Syrup. Bot. 473 ml. *c-III.*
Use: Antitussive with expectorant.

Hydrocodone HD. (Morton Grove) Hydrocodone bitatrate 1.67 mg, phenylephrine HCl 5 mg, chlorpheniramine maleate 2 mg/5 ml/Liq. Bot. 473 ml. *c-III.*
Use: Antitussive with expectorant.

Hydrocodone PA Syrup. (Morton Grove) Hydrocodone bitartrate 5 mg, phenylpropanolamine HCl 25 mg/5 ml/Syrup. Bot. 473 ml. *c-III.*
Use: Decongestant, antitussive.

Hydrocodone PA Pediatric. (Morton Grove) Hydrocodone bitartrate 2.5 mg, phenylpropanolamine HCl 12.5 mg/5 ml/Syrup. Bot. 473 ml. *c-III.*
Use: Decongestant, antitussive.

• **hydrocodone polistirex.** (high-droe-KOE-dohn pahl-ee-STIE-rex) USAN.
Use: Antitussive.

hydrocodone resin complex.
Use: Antitussive.
W/Phenyltoloxamine resin complex.
See: Tussionex, Prods. (Medeva).

hydrocortamate hydrochloride. 17-Hydroxycorticoster-one-21-diethylaminoaceate HCl.
Use: Anti-inflammatory, topical.
See: Ulcortar, Oint. (Ulmer).

• **hydrocortisone,** (HIGH-droe-CORE-tih-sone) U.S.P. 23. Compound F. Cortisoln. (Pharmacia & Upjohn) Micronized non-sterile powder for prescription compounding.
Use: Anti-inflammatory (topical), glucocorticoid.
See: Acticort Lotion 100. (Cummins).
Aeroseb-HC, Aerosol (Allergan Herbert).
Alphaderm, Cream (Procter & Gamble).
Caldecort Spray (Novartis).
Cetacort, Lot. (Galderma).
Cort-Dome, Cream, Lot., Supp. (Bayer).
Cortef, Tab., Cream, Oint. (Pharmacia & Upjohn).
Cortenema, Enema (Solvay).
Cortril, Oint. (Pfizer).
Delacort, Lot. (Mericon).
Dermacort, Cream, Lot. (Solvay).
Dermol HC, Cream, Oint. (Dermol).
Dermolate, Prods. (Schering Plough).
Ecosone, Cream (Star).
Eldecort, Cream (Zeneca).
HC Derma-Pax, Liq. (Recsei).
HI-COR-1.0, Cream, (C & M Pharmacal).
HI-COR-2.5, Cream (C & M Pharmacal).
Hycort, Cream, Oint. (Everett).

Hycortole,Cream, Oint. (Premo).
Hydrocortone, Tab. (Merck).
Hytone, Cream, Oint., Lot. (Dermik).
KeriCort-10, Cream (Bristol-Myers Squibb).
Lexocort, Pow., Lot. (Lexington).
Lipo-Adrenal Cortex, Vial (Pharmacia & Upjohn).
Maso-Cort, Lot. (Mason).
Microcort, Lot. (Alto Pharm).
My Cort, Cream (Scrip).
Optef, Soln. (Pharmacia & Upjohn).
Proctocort, Oint. (Solvay).
Scalpicin, Liq. (Combe).
Signef, Supp. (Forest Pharm).
Synacort, Cream (Syntex).
T/Scalp, Liq. (Neutrogena).
Tarcortin, Cream (Reed & Carnrick).
Texacort 25, 50, Lot. (Rydelle).
Ulcort, Cream, Lot. (Ulmer).

hydrocortisone. (Pharmacia & Upjohn).
Micronized nonsterile powder for prescription compounding.
Use: Anti-inflammatory (topical), glucocorticoid.

hydrocortisone w/combinations.
See: Achromycin W/Hydrocortisone, Oint., Ophth. Oint. (Lederle).
Acrisan w/Hydrocortisone, Liq. (Recsei).
Bafil, Cream. (Scruggs).
Barseb HC, Scalp Lot. (Pilkington Barnes Hind).
Barseb Thera-spray, Aerosol (Pilkington Barnes Hind).
Bro-Parin, Otic Susp. (3M).
Calmurid HC, Cream (Pharmacia & Upjohn).
Carmol HC, Cream (Ingram).
Coidocort, Cream (Coast).
Cor-Tar-Quin, Cream, Lot. (Bayer).
Cortef, Preps. (Pharmacia & Upjohn).
Cortin, Cream (C & M Pharm).
Cortisporin, Prep. (Glaxo Wellcome).
Derma-Cover-HC, Liq., Oint. (Scrip).
Dermarex, Cream (Hyrex-Key).
Dicort, Cream, Supp. (Hickam).
Doak Oil Forte, Liq. (Doak).
Drotic No. 2, Drops (Ascher).
Fostril HC, Lot. (Westwood Squibb).
HC-Form, Jelly (Recsei).
HC-Jel, Jelly (Recsei).
Heb-Cort., Cream, Lot. (Pilkington Barnes Hind).
Heb-Cort MC, Lot. (Pilkington Barnes Hind).
Heb-Cort. V, Cream, Lot. (Pilkington Barnes Hind).
Hi-Cort N Cream (Blaine).
Hill-Cortac, Cream, Lot. (Hill).
Hysone, Oint. (Mallard).

Kleer, Spray (Scrip).
Loroxide-HC, Lot. (Dermik).
Maso-Form, Cream (Mason).
Mity-quin, Cream (Solvay).
Myci-Cort, Liq., Spray (Misemer).
My-Cort, Drops, Lot., Oint., Spray (Scrip).
Neocort, Oint. (H.V.P.).
Neo-Cort Dome, Cream, Lot., Drops (Bayer).
Neo Cort Top, Oint. (Standex).
Neo-Domeform-HC, Cream, Lot., Susp. (Bayer).
Nutracort, Cream, Gel, Lot. (Galderma).
1 + 1 Creme, 1 + 1-F Creme (Dunhall).
Ophthel, Liq. (Zeneca).
Ophthocort, Oint. (Parke Davis).
Orlex HC Otic (Baylor).
Oto, Drops (Solvay).
Otobiotic, Soln. (Schering Plough).
Otocalm-H Ear Drops (Parmed).
Otostan H.C. (Standex).
Pyocidin-Otic, Soln. (Berlex).
Racet Forte, Cream (Lemmon).
Racet LCD, Cream (Lemmon).
Rectal Medicone-HC (Medicone).
Sherform-HC, Creme (Sheryl).
Stera-Form, Creme (Mayrand).
Steramine Otic, Drops (Mayrand).
Syntar HC Cream, Oint. (Zeneca).
Tarcortin, Cream (Reed & Carnrick).
Tenda HC, Cream (Dermik).
Terra-Cortril, Preps. (Pfipharmics).
Theracort, Lot. (C & M Pharm).
Vanoxide-HC, Lot. (Dermik).
V-Cort, Cream (Scrip).
Vioform-Hydrocortisone, Preps. (Novartis).
Vio-Hydrocort, Oint., Cream (Quality Generics).
Vytone, Cream, (Dermik).

•**hydrocortisone acetate,** U.S.P. 23.
See: Anucort-HC, Supp. (G & W Labs).
Anuprep HC, Supp. (Great Southern).
Anusol-HC, Supp. (Parke-Davis).
Caldecort, Cream (Novartis).
Caldecort Light, Cream (Novartis).
Cortef Acetate, Ophth. Oint., Inj. (Pharmacia & Upjohn).
Cortifoam, Aerosol (Reed & Carnrick).
Cortiprel, Cream (Taylor).
Cortril Acetate, Aqueous Susp., Oint. (Pfipharmecs).
Ferncort, Lot. (Ferndale).
Fernisone Inj., Vial (Ferndale).
Gynecort, Oint. (Combe).
Hemril-HC Uniserts, Supp. (Upsher-Smith).

Hydro-Can (Paddock).
Hydrocort, Vial (Dunhall).
Hydrocortone Acetate, Inj. (Merck).
Hydrosone, Inj. (Sig).
Maximum Strength Corticaine, Cream (Whitby).
Maximum Strength Dermarest Dricort Creme (Del).
My-Cort, Lot. (Scrip).
Pramosone Cream, Lot. (Ferndale).
Span-Ster, Inj. (Scrip).
Tucks-HC (Parke-Davis).

hydrocortisone acetate. (Pharmacia & Upjohn) Micronized non-sterile powder for prescription compounding.
Use: Anti-inflammatory (topical), glucocorticoid.

hydrocortisone acetate w/combinations.
See: Anusol-HC, Cream, Supp. (Warner-Chilcott).
Biotic-Opth W/HC, Oint. (Scrip).
Biotres HC, Cream (Central).
Carmol HC, Cream (Ingram).
Chloromycetin-Hydrocortisone Ophth. Susp. (Parke-Davis).
Coly-Mycin-S Otic, Soln. (Warner-Chilcott).
Cor-Oticin, Liq. (Maurry).
Cortaid, Cream, Lot., Oint. (Pharmacia & Upjohn).
Cortef Acetate, Inj., Oint., Susp. (Pharmacia & Upjohn).
Corticaine Cream (Glaxo).
Derma Medicone-HC, Oint. (Medicone).
Dicort, Supp. (Hickam).
Doctient HC, Supp. (Suppositoria).
Epifoam, Aerosol (Reed & Carnrick).
Estro-V HC, Supp. (PolyMedica).
Eye-Cort, Soln. (Mallard).
Furacin-HC Otic (Eaton).
Furacin HC Urethral Inserts (Eaton).
Furacort Cream (Eaton).
Komed HC, Lot. (Pilkington Barnes Hind).
Lida-Mantle HC, Cream (Bayer).
Mantadil, Cream (Glaxo Wellcome).
Neo-Cortef, Preps. (Pharmacia & Upjohn).
Neo-Hytone Cream (Dermik).
Neopolycin-HC, Oint., Ophth. Oint. (Hoechst Marion Roussel).
Ophthocort, Oint. (Parke-Davis).
Proctofoam-HC, Aerosol (Reid and Carnrick).
Pyracort, Liq. (Lemmon).
Racet Forte, Cream (Lemmon).
Rectacort, Supp. (Century).
Rectal Medicone-HC, Supp. (Medicone).

Wyanoids HC, Supp. (Wyeth-Ayerst).

hydrocortisone and acetic acid otic solution.
Use: Anti-inflammatory, otic.

•**hydrocortisone buteprate,** (HIGH-droe-CORE-tih-sone BYOO-teh-prate) USAN.
Use: Anti-inflammatory; glucocorticoid.

•**hydrocortisone butyrate,** (HIGH-droe-CORE-tih-sone BYOO-tih-rate) U.S.P. 23.
Use: Glucocorticoid.
See: Locoid, Soln. (Ferndale).

hydrocortisone cypionate, U.S.P. XXII. Oral Susp., U.S.P. XXII. Hydrocortisone Cypionate.
Use: Glucocorticoid.

hydrocortisone diethylaminoacetate hcl.
See: Hydrocortamate.

hydrocortisone dypropionate.
See: Cortef, Fluid (Pharmacia & Upjohn).

•**hydrocortisone hemisuccinate,** U.S.P. 23.
Use: Adrenocortical steroid.

hydrocortisone I.V.
See: A-Hydro Cort, Vial (Abbott).
Solu-Cortef, Vial (Pharmacia & Upjohn).

hydrocortisone/iodochlorhydroxyquin. (Various Mfr.) **Cream:** Hydrocortisone 0.5% or 3%, iodochlorhydroxyquin 3%. 15 g, 30 g, 480 g. **Oint.:** Hydrocortisone 1%, iodochlorhydroxyquin 3%. 20 g, 30 g. *otc, Rx.*
Use: Corticosteroid, topical.

hydrocortisone/neomycin. (Various Mfr.) Hydrocortisone 1%, neomycin sulfate 0.5%. Oint. 20 g. *otc, Rx.*
Use: Corticosteroid, topical.

hydrocortisone phosphate.
See: Hydrocortone Phosphate, Inj. (Merck).

•**hydrocortisone sodium phosphate,** U.S.P. 23. Hydrocortisone Sodium Phosphate.
Use: Adrenocortical steroid (anti-inflammatory); glucocorticoid.

•**hydrocortisone sodium succinate,** U.S.P. 23. Hydrocortisone Sodium Succinate.
Use: Adrenocortical steroid (anti-inflammatory); glucocorticoid.
See: A-hydroCort, Vial (Abbott).
Solu-Cortef, Vial (Pharmacia & Upjohn).

•**hydrocortisone valerate,** (HIGH-droe-CORE-tih-sone VAL-eh-rate) U.S.P. 23.

Use: Corticosteroid, topical; glucocorticoid.
See: Westcort Cream, Oint. (Westwood Squibb).

Hydrocortone Acetate Saline Suspension. (Merck) Hydrocortisone acetate 25 mg or 50 mg/ml, sodium Cl 9 mg, polysorbate 80 4 mg, sodium carboxymethylcellulose 5 mg/ml, benzyl alcohol 9 mg q.s. water for injection to 1 ml. Vial 5 ml. *Rx.*
Use: Corticosteroid.

Hydrocortone Phosphate Injection. (Merck) Hydrocortisone sodium phosphate equivalent to hydrocortisone 50 mg/ml, creatinine 8 mg, sodium citrate 10 mg/ml, sodium hydroxide to adjust pH, sodium bisulfite 3.2 mg, methylparaben 1.5 mg, propylparaben 0.2 mg, water for injection q.s./ml. Vial 2 ml multiple dose, 10 ml multiple dose. Disposable syringe 2 ml single dose. *Rx.*
Use: Corticosteroid.

Hydrocortone Tablets. (Merck) Hydrocortisone 10 mg or 20 mg/Tab. Bot. 100s. *Rx.*
Use: Corticosteroid.

Hydrocream Base. (Paddock) Petrolatum, mineral oil, woolwax alcohol, imidazolidinyl urea, methyl propylparabens. Cream. Jar lb.
Use: Emollient.

Hydro-Crysti 12. (Roberts Hauck) Hydroxocobalamin, crystalline (vitamin B_{12}) 1000 mcg/ml Inj. Vial 30 ml. *Rx.*
Use: Vitamin B_{12} supplement.

HydroDIURIL. (Merck) Hydrochlorothiazide **25 mg/Tab.:** Bot. 100s, 1000s, UD 100s; **50 mg/Tab.:** Bot. 100s, 1000s, UD 100s; **100 mg/Tab.:** Bot. 100s. *Rx.*
Use: Diuretic.

Hydro-D Tablets. (Halsey) Hydrochlorothiazide. 25 mg or 50 mg/Tab. Bot. 1000s. *Rx.*
Use: Diuretic.

Hydro-Ergot. (Interstate) Hydrogenated ergot alkaloids 0.5 mg or 1 mg/Tab. Bot. 100s. *Rx.*
Use: Psychotherapeutic.

•**hydrofilcon a.** (HIGH-droe-FILL-kahn A) USAN.
Use: Contact lens material (hydrophilic).

•**hydroflumethiazide,** U.S.P. 23. Di-Ademil; Hydrenox; Naclex; Rontyl.
Use: Antihypertensive, diuretic.
See: Diucardin, Tab. (Wyeth-Ayerst).
Saluron, Tab. (Bristol).
W/Reserpine.
See: Salutensin, Tab. (Bristol).

Salutensin-Demi, Tab. (Bristol).
hydrogen dioxide.
See: Hydrogen Peroxide.
hydrogen iodide.
Use: Expectorant.
See: Hydriodic acid.

•**hydrogen peroxide concentrate,** U.S.P. 23.
Use: Anti-infective (topical) when diluted.

hydrogen peroxide solution 30%. Perhydrol, hydrogen pioxide. Bot. 0.25 lb, 0.5 lb, 1 lb.
Use: Dentistry, preparing the 3% solution.

hydrogen peroxide topical solution. (Various Mfr.) (3%). 4 oz, 8 oz, pt.
Use: Anti-infective, topical.

Hydrogesic. (Edwards) Hydrocodone bitartrate 5 mg, acetaminophen 500 mg/ Cap. Bot. 100s. *c-III.*
Use: Narcotic analgesic combination.

Hydroloid-G Sublingual. (Major) Ergoloid mesylates. **0.5 mg/Tab.:** Bot. 100s, 250s, 500s, UD 100s. **1 mg/Tab.:** Bot. 100s, 250s, 1000s, UD 100s. *Rx.*
Use: Psychotherapeutic.

Hydroloid-G Tabs. (Major) Ergoloid mesylates 1 mg/Tab. Bot. 100s, 250s, 1000s, UD 100s. *Rx.*
Use: Psychotherapeutic.

Hydromal. (Mallard) Hydrochlorothiazide 50 mg/Tab. Bot. 1000s. *Rx.*
Use: Diuretic.

Hydromet. (Barre-National) Hydrocodone bitartrate 5 mg, homatropine MBr 1.5 mg/Syr. Bot. 473 ml, gal. *c-III.*
Use: Antitussive.

hydromorphone. (HIGH-droe-MORE-phone) *c-II.*
Use: Narcotic analgesic.

•**hydromorphone hydrochloride,** (HIGH-droe-MORE-phone) U.S.P. 23. Dihydromorphinone HCl. *Formerly Dihydromorphinone Hydrochloride.*
Use: Analgesic (narcotic).
See: Dilaudid Prods. (Knoll).
W/sodium citrate, antimony potassium tartrate and chloroform. Inj.
See: Dilocol, Liq. (Table Rock).

hydromorphone sulfate.
Use: Narcotic analgesic.

Hydromox. (Lederle) Quinethazone 50 mg/Tab. Bot. 100s, 500s. *Rx.*
Use: Diuretic.

Hydromox-R. (Lederle) Quinethazone 50 mg, reserpine 0.125 mg/Tab. Bot. 100s, 500s. *Rx.*
Use: Antihypertensive combination.

Hydropane. (Halsey) Hydrocodone bitartrate 5 mg, homatropine methylbromide 1.5 mg. Pt, gal. *c-iii.*
Use: Antitussive combination.

Hydropel. (C & M Pharmacal) Silicone 30%, hydrophobic starch derivative 10%, petrolatum. Jar. 2 oz, lb. *otc.*
Use: Emollient.

Hydrophen Pediatric Syrup. (Rugby) Phenylpropanolamine HCl 12.5 mg, hydrocodone bitartrate 2.5 mg/5 ml. Bot. 480 ml. *c-iii.*
Use: Decongestant, antitussive.

Hydrophen Syrup. (Rugby) Phenylpropanolamine HCl 25 mg, hydrocodone bitartrate 5 mg/5 ml. Bot. pt, gal. *c-iii.*
Use: Decongestant, antitussive.

Hydrophed Tablets. (Rugby) Theophylline 130 mg, ephedrine sulfate 25 mg, hydroxyzine HCl 10 mg/Tab. Bot. 100s, 1000s. *Rx.*
Use: Antiasthmatic combination.

hydrophilic ointment. Stearyl alcohol, white petrolatum, propylene glycol, sodium lauryl sulfate, water. Jar lb. (Fougera).
Use: Ointment base.

hydrophilic ointment base. Oil in water emulsion bases. (Emerson) 1 lb.
Use: Ointment base.
See: Aquaphilic Ointment (Medco).
  Cetaphil, Cream, Lot. (Texas Pharmacal).
  Dermovan, Cream (Texas Pharmacal).
  Lanaphilic Ointment (Medco).
  Polysorb, Oint. (Savage).
  Unibase, Oint. (Parke-Davis).

Hydropine. (Rugby) Hydroflumethiazide 25 mg, reserpine 0.125 mg/Tab. Bot. 100s. *Rx.*
Use: Antihypertensive combination.

Hydropine H.P. Tablets. (Rugby) Hydroflumethiazide 50 mg, reserpine 0.125 mg/Tab. Bot. 100s, 500s, 1000s. *Rx.*
Use: Antihypertensive combination.

Hydropres-50. (Merck) Hydrochlorothiazide 50 mg, reserpine 0.125 mg/Tab. Bot. 100s, 1000s. *Rx.*
Use: Antihypertensive combination.

●**hydroquinone,** U.S.P. 23.
Use: Depigmentor.
See: Artra Skin Tone Cream (Schering Plough).
  Black and White Bleaching Cream (Schering Schering Plough).
  Derma-Blanch, Cream (Chattem).
  Eldopaque Cream, Oint. (Zeneca).
  Eldopaque Forte Cream, Oint. (Zeneca).

  Eldoquin, Cream, Lot. (Zeneca).
  Esoterica Medicated Cream Prods. (SK-Beecham).
  Melpaque HP, Cream (Stratus).
  Melquin HP, Cream (Stratus).
  Nuquin HP, Cream, Gel (Stratus).

hydroquinone. (Glades) Hydroquinone 3%, SD Alcohol 45%, propylene glycol, isopropyl alcohol 4%/Soln. 30 ml with applicator. Hydroquinone 4%, padimate 0.5%, dioxybenzone 3%, EDTA, sodium metabisulfite, hydroalcoholic base.
Use: Depigmentor.

hydroquinone monobenzyl ether.
See: Benoquin, Oint., Lot. (Zeneca).

Hydrosal. (Hydrosal Co.) Aluminum acetate 5%. **Susp.:** Bot. 16 oz, gal. **Oint.:** 54 g, 113.4 g, Jar 54 g, 454 g. *otc.*
Use: Astringent.

Hydroserp. (Zenith) Hydrochlorothiazide 25 mg or 50 mg, reserpine 0.125 mg or 0.1 mg/Tab. Bot. 100s, 1000s. *Rx.*
Use: Antihypertensive combination.

Hydroserp-50. (Freeport) Hydrochlorothiazide 50 mg, reserpine 0.125 mg/Tab. Bot. 1000s. *Rx.*
Use: Antihypertensive combination.

Hydroserpine #1. (Various Mfr.) Hydrochlorothiazide 25 mg, reserpine. Bot. 100s, 1000s. *Rx.*
Use: Antihypertensive combination.

Hydroserpine #2. (Various Mfr.) Hydrochlorothiazide 50 mg, reserpine. Bot. 100s, 250s, 400s, 1000s. *Rx.*
Use: Antihypertensive combination.

Hydrosine 25 Tablets. (Major) Hydrochlorothiazide 25 mg, reserpine 0.125 mg/Tab. Bot. 100s. Tartrazine. *Rx.*
Use: Antihypertensive combination.

Hydrosine 50 Tablets. (Major) Hydrochlorothiazide 50 mg, reserpine 0.125 mg/Tab. Bot. 100s. *Rx.*
Use: Antihypertensive combination.

Hydrosone. (Sig) Hydrocortisone acetate 25 mg or 50 mg, lactose/ml. Vial 5 ml. *Rx.*
Use: Corticosteroid.

HydroStat IR. (Richwood) Hydromorphone HCl 1 mg, 2 mg, 3 mg, or 4 mg, lactose/Tab. Bot. 100s. *c-ii.*
Use: Narcotic analgesic.

Hydrotensin-50. (Mayrand) Hydrochlorothiazide 50 mg, reserpine 0.125 mg/Tab. Bot. 100s, 1000s. *Rx.*
Use: Antihypertensive combination.

Hydro-Tex Cream. (Syosset) Hydrocortisone 0.5% or 1%. Greaseless base. Cream 30 g, 60 g, 120 g. *otc.*

Use: Corticosteroid, topical.

Hydro-T Tabs. (Major) Hydrochlorothiazide. **25 mg/Tab:** Bot. 100s, 1000s, UD 100s; **50 mg/Tab:** Bot. 100s, 1000s, UD 100s; **100 mg/Tab:** Bot. 100s, 250s, 1000s, UD 100s. *Rx.*
Use: Diuretic.

hydroxindasol hydrochloride.

hydroxocobalamin, (high-DROX-oh-koe-BAL-ah-meen) U.S.P. 23. Vitamin B_{12a} and B_{12b}. Hydrovit; Neo-Cytamen.
Use: Treatment of megaloblastic anemia, vitamin (hematopoietic).
See: AlphaRedisol, Inj. (Merck).
  Alpha-Ruvite, Vial (Savage).
  Cobavite L.A., Vial (Lemmon).
  Droxomin, Inj. (Solvay).
  Hydrobexan, Vial (Keene).
  Rubesol-L.A. 1000, Inj. (Central).
  Span-12, Inj. (Scrip).
  Sytobex-H, Vial (Parke-Davis).
  Twelve-Span, Vial (Foy).

hydroxocobalamin, crystalline. (Various Mfr.) 1000 mcg/ml Inj. 30 ml. *Rx.*
Use: Vitamin B_{12} supplement.
See: Hydroxocobalamin (Various).
  Alphamin (Vortech).
  AlphaRedisol (Merck).
  Codroxomin (Forest).
  Hybalamin (Mallard).
  Hydrobexan (Keene).
  Hydro Cobex (Taylor).
  Hydro-Crysti (Roberts).
  LA-12 (Hyrex).

hydroxocobalamin/sodium thiosulfate. *Rx.*
Use: Cyanide poisoning antidote. [Orphan drug]

•**hydroxyamphetamine hydrobromide,** U.S.P. 23.
Use: Pupil dilator; adrenergic (ophthalmic).
See: Paredrine (Pharmics).

2-hydroxybenzamide.
See: Salicylamide.

hydroxy bis(acetato)aluminum. Aluminum Subacetate Topical Soln.

hydroxybis (salicylato) aluminum diacetate.
See: Aluminum aspirin.

hydroxybutyrate, sodium/gamma.
See: sodium gamma-hydroxybutyrate acid.

hydroxycholecalciferol. (D_3).
Use: Hypocalcemia.
See: Calcifediol.

•**hydroxychloroquine sulfate,** (high-drox-ee-KLOR-oh-kwin) U.S.P. 23.
Use: Antimalarial, lupus erythematosus suppressant.

hydroxychloroquine sulfate. (Copley) 200 mg/Tab. Bot. 100s, 500s.
Use: Antimalarial, lupus erythematosus suppressant.

hydroxydione sodium.

•**hydroxyethyl cellulose,** N.F. 18.
Use: Pharmaceutic aid (suspending, viscosity-increasing agent).
See: Gonioscopic, Soln. (Alcon).

hydroxyethyl starch. (HES).
Use: Plasma volume expander.
See: Hespan, Inj. (DuPont Merck).

hydroxyisoindolin. Under study.
Use: Antihypertensive.

hydroxymagnesium aluminate.
Use: Antacid.
See: Magaldrate.

hydroxymycin. An antibiotic substance obtained from cultures of *Streptomyces paucisporogenes*.

•**hydroxyphenamate.** (high-DROX-ee-FEN-ah-mate) USAN.
Use: Tranquilizer (minor).

•**hydroxyprogesterone caproate,** U.S.P. 23.
Use: Progestin.
See: Delalutin, Vial (Squibb).
  Duralutin, Inj. (Roberts/Hauck).
  Gesterol L.A. 250, Inj. (Forest).
  Hy-Gestrone, Vial (Taylor).
  Hylutin, Inj. (Hyrex).
  Hyprogest 250, Inj. (Keene).
W/Estradiol valerate.
See: Hy-Gestradol, Inj. (Taylor).
  Hylutin-Est., Inj. (Hyrex).

hydroxyprogesterone caproate. (Various Mfr.) **125 mg/ml:** Inj. Vial 10 ml; **250 mg/ml:** Inj. Vial 5 ml.
Use: Progestin.

•**hydroxypropyl cellulose, low-substituted,** N.F. 18.
Use: Topical protectant, tablet coating agent.

•**hydroxypropyl methylcellulose,** U.S.P. 23. The propylene glycol ether of methylcellulose available in the 2208, 2906 and 2910 forms.
Use: Pharmaceutic aid (suspending, viscosity-increasing agent; tablet excipient).
See: Anestacon (Alcon).
  Econopred, Susp. (Alcon).
  Occucoat, Soln. (Storz).
W/benzalkonium Cl.
See: Gonak, Soln. (Akorn).
  Goniosol (Ciba Vision).
  Isopto Tears (Alcon).
  Ultra Tears, Soln. (Alcon).

•**hydroxypropyl methylcellulose phthal-**

ate, N.F. 18.
Use: Pharmaceutic aid (coating agent).
•**hydroxypropyl methylcellulose phthalate 200731,** N.F. 18.
Use: Pharmaceutic aid (coating agent).
•**hydroxypropyl methylcellulose phthalate 220824,** N.F. 18.
Use: Pharmaceutic aid (coating agent).
hydroxystearin sulfate. Sulfonate hydrogenated castor oil.
L-5 Hydroxytryptophan (L-5HTP). (Bolar) *Rx.*
Use: Postanoxic intention myoclonus.
[Orphan drug]
•**hydroxyurea,** (high-DROX-ee-you-REE-uh) U.S.P. 23. Hydroxycarbamide (I.N.N.).
Use: Antineoplastic. Sickle cell anemia
[Orphan drug]
See: Hydrea, Cap. (Squibb Mark).
•**hydroxyzine hydrochloride,** (high-DROX-ih-zeen) U.S.P. 23.
Use: Tranquilizer (minor), antihistamine.
See: Atarax, Syr., Tab. (Roerig).
Hyzine-50, Inj. (Hyrex).
Rezine, Tab. (Marnel).
Vistazine 25, Inj. (Keene).
Vistazine 50, Inj. (Keene).
Vistaril Isoject. (Roerig).
Vistaril, Cap., Susp. (Pfizer Laboratories).
W/Ephedrine sulf., theophylline.
See: Marax DF, Syr. (Roerig).
Marax Tab. (Roerig).
Theo-Drox, Tab. (Quality Generics).
W/Pentaerythritol tetranitrate.
See: Cartrax 10, 20, Tab. (Roerig).
hydroxyzine hydrochloride. (Abbott).
100 mg/2 ml Inj. Amp. 500 mg/10 ml
Abboject Syringe. Vial.
Use: Tranquilizer (minor), antihistamine.
•**hydroxyzine pamoate,** U.S.P. 23.
Use: Tranquilizer (minor), antihistamine.
See: Hy-Pam 25 Cap. (Lemmon).
Vistaril, Cap., Susp. (Pfizer).
Hydro-Z-50 Tablets. (Mayrand) Hydrochlorothiazide 50 mg/Tab. Bot. 100s, 1000s. *Rx.*
Use: Diuretic.
Hy-Flow Solution. (Ciba Vision) Polyvinyl alcohol with hydroxyethylcellulose, benzalkonium Cl, EDTA. Bot. 60 ml. *otc.*
Use: Hard contact lens care.
Hy-Gestrone. (Taylor) Hydroxyprogesterone caproate. **125 mg/ml.:** Vial 10 ml. **250 mg/ml.:** Vial 5 ml. *Rx.*
Use: Progestin.
Hygienic Cleansing. (Rugby) Witch hazel 50%, glycerin, benzalkonium Cl,

methylparaben. Pads. 100s. *otc.*
Use: Anorectal preparation.
Hygienic Powder.
See: Bo-Car-Al, Pow. (SK-Beecham).
Hygroton. (Rhone-Poulenc Rorer) Chlorthalidone 25 mg, 50 mg or 100 mg/Tab. Lactose (25, 50 mg). Bot. 100s. *Rx.*
Use: Diuretic.
Hylidone Tabs. (Major) Chlorthalidone. **25 mg or 50 mg/Tab:** Bot. 100s, 250s, 1000s, UD 100s. **100 mg/Tab:** Bot. 100s, 250s, 500s, 1000s. *Rx.*
Use: Diuretic.
Hyliver Plus. (Hyrex) Folic acid 0.4 mg, liver 10 mcg, vitamin B_{12} 100 mcg/ml. Vial 10 ml with phenol. *Rx.*
Use: Vitamin supplement.
Hylorel Tablets. (Medeva) Guanadrel sulfate 10 mg or 25 mg/Tab. Bot. 100s. *Rx.*
Use: Antihypertensive.
Hylutin Injectable. (Hyrex) Hydroxyprogesterone caproate in oil 250 mg/ml. Castor oil with benzyl benzoate and benzyl alcohol. Vial 5 ml. *Rx.*
Use: Progestin.
•**hymecromone.** (HIGH-meh-KROE-mone) USAN.
Use: Choleretic.
hymenoptera venom/venom protein. Purified venoms of honeybee, wasp, white faced hornet, yellow hornet, yellow jacket and mixed vespids (both hornets and yellow jackets). *Rx.*
Use: Allergenic extract.
See: Albay (Miles).
Phamalgen (ALK).
Venomil (Bayer).
HY-N.B.P. Ointment. (Jones Medical) Bacitracin zinc 400 units, neomycin sulfate 5 mg, polymixin B sulfate 10,000 units/g. Tube ⅛ oz. *Rx.*
Use: Anti-infective, topical.
hyoscine hydrobromide. Scopolamine HBr, U.S.P. 23.
Use: Intestinal antispasmodic.
hyoscine-hyoscyamine-atropine.
Use: Anticholinergic.
See: Atropine w/hyoscyamine w/hyoscine.
•**hyoscyamine,** U.S.P. 23. Levo form of atropine.
Use: Anticholinergic.
See: Bellafoline, Amp., Tab. (Sandoz).
Cysto-Spaz, Tab. (PolyMedica).
hyoscyamine-atropine-hyoscine.
Use: Anticholinergic.
See: Atropine w/hyoscyamine w/hyoscine.

- **hyoscyamine hydrobromide,** U.S.P. 23.
Daturine HBr.
Use: Anticholinergic.
W/Physostigine salicylate.
See: Pyatromine-H Inj. (Kremers-Urban).

hyoscyamine hydrochloride. (Various Mfr.).

hyoscyamine maleate.
See: Bellafoline, Amp., Tab. (Sandoz).

hyoscyamine salts.
Use: Anticholinergic.
W/Atropine salts.
See: Atropine W/Hyoscyamine.

- **hyoscyamine sulfate,** U.S.P. 23.
Use: Anticholinergic.
See: Anaspaz, Tab. (Ascher).
Cystospaz-M, Cap. (PolyMedica).
Donnamar, Tab. (Marnel).
ED-SPAZ, Tab. (Edwards).
Gastrosed, Drops, Tab. (Roberts).
Levsin/SL, Sublingual Tab. (Schwarz Pharma Kremers Urban).
W/Atropine sulfate, hyoscine HBr, phenobarbital.
See: DeTal, Elix., Tab. (DeLeon).
Donnatal, Prods. (Robins).
Hyonal C.T., Tab. (Paddock).
Maso-Donna, Elix., Tab. (Mason).
Peece, Tab. (Scrip).
Sedamine, Tab. (Dunhall).
Spasaid, Cap. (Century).
Spasquid, Elix. (Geneva Pharm).
W/Atropine sulfate, hyoscine HBr, phenobarbital, pepsin, pancreatin, bile salts.
See: Donnazyme, Tab. (Robins).
W/Atropine sulfate. Scopolamine HCl, phenobarbital.
See: Ultabs, Tab. (Burlington).
W/Belladonna Alkaloids.
See: Belladonna Prods.
W/Butabarbital.
See: Cystospaz-SR, Cap. (PolyMedica).
W/Methenamine, atropine sulfate, methylene blue, salol, benzoic acid, gelsemium.
See: Uriprel, Tab. (Taylor).
W/Phenobarbital, simethicone, atropine sulfate, scopolamine HBr.
See: Kinesed, Tab. (Stuart).

hyoscyamine sulfate. (Various Mfr.)
0.375 mg/ER Cap. 100s. *Rx.*
Use: Anticholinergic.

hyoscyamine sulfate. (Goldline) 0.125 mg/ml, alcohol 5%/Soln. Bot. with dropper. 15 ml. *Rx.*
Use: Anticholinergic.

hyoscyamus extract.
W/A.P.C.
See: Valacet Junior, Tab. (Pal-Pak).

W/A.P.C., gelsemium extract.
See: Valacet, Tab. (Pal-Pak).

hyoscyamus products and phenobarbital combinations.
Use: Anticholinergic, sedative.
See: Anaspaz PB, Tab. (Taylor).
Donnatal, Preps. (Robins).
Elixiral, Elix. (Vita Elixir).
Floramine, Tab. (Lemmon).
Kinesed, Tab. (Stuart).
Neoquess, Tab. (O'Neal).
Nevrotose, Cap. (Pal-Pak).

Hyosophen Elixir. (Rugby) Atropine sulfate 0.0194 mg, scopolamine HBr 0.0065 mg, hyoscyamine HBr or sulfate 0.1037 mg, phenobarbital 16.2 mg, alcohol 23%, sugar, sorbitol. 120 ml, pt, gal. *Rx.*
Use: GI anticholinergic.

Hyosophen Tablets. (Rugby). Atropine sulfate 0.0194 mg, scopolamine HBr 0.0065 mg, hyoscyamine HBr or SO_4 0.1037 mg, phenobarbital 16.2 mg. In 1000s. *Rx.*
Use: Anticholinergic combination.

Hypaque-76. (Winthrop Pharm) Diatrizoate meglumine 66%, diatrizoate sodium 10%, iodine 37%, EDTA. Vial 30 ml, 50 ml, 100 ml.
Use: Radiopaque agent.

Hypaque-Cysto. (Winthrop Pharm) Diatrizoate meglumine 30% soln., iodine 14.1%. 250 ml in 500 ml dilution bottle. Pediatric: 100 ml in 300 ml dilution bottle.
Use: Radiopaque agent.

Hypaque-M 75%. (Winthrop Pharm) Diatrizoate meglumine 50%, diatrizoate sodium 25%, iodine 38.5%, EDTA. Vial 20 ml, 50 ml.
Use: Radiopaque agent.

Hypaque-M 90%. (Winthrop Pharm) Diatrizoate meglumine 60%, diatrizoate sodium 30%, EDTA. Vial 50 ml.
Use: Radiopaque agent.

Hypaque Meglumine 30%. (Winthrop Pharm) Diatrizoate meglumine 30%, iodine 14.1%. Bot. 100 ml, 300 ml w/ and w/o I.V. infusion set.
Use: Radiopaque agent.

Hypaque Meglumine 60%. (Winthrop Pharm) Diatrizoate meglumine 60%, iodine 28%, EDTA. Vial 20 ml, 30 ml, 50 ml, 100 ml.
Use: Radiopaque agent.

Hypaque Oral. (Winthrop Pharm) **Pow.:** Diatrizoate sodium oral pow. containing iodine 600 mg/g. Can 250 g, Bot. 10 g. **Liq.:** Soln. 41.66%. Bot. 120 ml.
Use: Radiopaque agent.

Hypaque Sodium 20%. (Winthrop Pharm) Diatrizoate sodium 20%, iodine 12%, EDTA. Vial 100 ml.
Use: Radiopaque agent.

Hypaque Sodium 25%. (Winthrop Pharm) Diatrizoate sodium 25%, iodine 15%. Bot. 300 ml, w/ and w/out I.V. infusion set.
Use: Radiopaque agent.

Hypaque Sodium 50%. (Winthrop Pharm) Diatrizoate sodium 50%, iodine 30%. **Vial:** 20 ml, 30 ml, 50 ml. **Dilution Bottle:** 200 ml with EDTA.
Use: Radiopaque agent.

Hyperab.
See: Bayrab, Vial. (Bayer).

HyperHep.
See: BayHep B, Vial. (Bayer).

hypericin. (VIMRx Pharm/NIH) *Rx.*
Use: Antiviral, phase I AIDS.

hyperlipidemia, agents for.
See: Atromid-S (Wyeth-Ayerst).
Choloxin (Knoll Pharm).
Cholybar (Parke-Davis).
Clofibrate (Various).
Colestid (Pharmacia & Upjohn).
Lescol (Sandoz).
Lopid (Parke-Davis).
Lorelco (Hoechst Marion Roussel).
Mevacor (Merck).
Pravachol (Bristol-Myers Squibb).
Questran (Bristol-Myers).
Questran Light (Bristol-Myers).
Zocor (Merck).

Hyperlyte. (American McGaw) Sodium 25 mEq, potassium 40.5 mEq, calcium 5 mEq, magnesium 8 mEq, chloride 33.5 mEq, acetate 40.6 mEq, gluconate 5 mEq, 6050 mOsm/L. Inj. Vial 25 ml fill in 50 ml. *Rx.*
Use: Parenteral nutritional supplement.

Hyperlyte CR. (American McGaw) Sodium 25 mEq, potassium 20 mEq, calcium 5 mEq, magnesium 5 mEq, chloride 30 mEq, acetate 30 mEq, 5500 mOsm/L. Inj. Super-vial 150 ml, 250 ml fill. *Rx.*
Use: Parenteral nutritional supplement.

Hyperlyte R. (American McGaw) Sodium 25 mEq, potassium 20 mEq, calcium 5 mEq, magnesium 5 mEq, chloride 30 mEq, acetate 25 mEq, 4200 mOsm/L. Inj. Vial 25 ml fill in 50 ml. *Rx.*
Use: Parenteral nutritional supplement.

Hyperopto 5%. (Professional Pharmacal) Sodium Cl 5%. Oint. Tube 3.5 g. *otc.*
Use: Ophthalmic preparation.

Hyperopto Ointment. (Professional Pharmacal) Sodium HCl 50 mg, D.I. water 150 mg, anhydrous lanolin 150 mg, liquid petrolatum 50 mg, white petrolatum 599 mg, methylparaben 7 mg, propylparaben 3 mg/g. Tube 3.5 g. *otc.*
Use: Ophthalmic preparation.

hyperosmolar agents.
Use: Laxative.
See: Glycerin, USP (Various).
Sani-Supp, Supp. (G & W Labs).
Fleet Babylax, Liq. (Fleet).

Hyperstat I.V. Injection. (Schering Plough) Diazoxide 15 mg/ml. 20 ml. *Rx.*
Use: Antihypertensive.

hypertension diagnosis.
See: Regitine, Amp., Tab. (Novartis).

hypertensive emergency drugs.
See: Arfonad, Inj. (Roche).
Diazoxide Injection (Quad).
Hyperstat IV, Inj. (Schering Plough).
Nitropress, Inj. (Abbott).

Hyper-Tet.
See: Baytet, Vial. (Bayer).

Hy-Phen Tablets. (Ascher) Hydrocodone bitartrate 5 mg, acetaminophen 500 mg. Bot. 100s. *c-III.*
Use: Antitussive, analgesic.

Hyphylline. Dyphylline. *Rx.*
See: Neothylline, Elix., Amp., Tab. (Lemmon).

hypnogene.
See: Barbital (Various Mfr.).

Hypnomidate. (Janssen) Etomidate. *Rx.*
Use: General anesthetic.

hypnotics.
See: Sedatives.

"hypo".
See: Sodium Thiosulfate (Various Mfr.).

Hypo-Bee. (Towne) Vitamins B_1 50 mg, B_2 20 mg, B_6 5 mg, B_{12} 15 mcg, niacinamide 25 mg, calcium pantothenate 5 mg, C 300 mg, E 200 IU, iron 10 mg/Tab. Bot. 30s, 100s. *otc.*
Use: Vitamin/mineral supplement.

hypochlorite preps.
See: Antiformin.
Dakin's Soln.
Hyclorite.

Hypoclear. (Bausch & Lomb) Isotonic soln. with sodium Cl 0.9%. Aerosol soln. 240 ml, 300 ml. *otc.*
Use: Soft contact lens care.

hypoglycemic agents.
See: Chlorpropamide.
Diabeta, Tab. (Hoechst Marion Roussel).
Diabinese, Tab. (Pfizer).
Dymelor, Tab. (Lilly).
Glucotrol, Tab. (Roerig).

Glynase, Tab. (Pharmacia & Upjohn).
Micronase, Tab. (Pharmacia & Upjohn).
Orinase, Tab., Vial (Pharmacia & Upjohn).
Phenformin HCl.
Tolbutamide.
Tolinase, Tab. (Pharmacia & Upjohn).
α-hypophamine. Oxytocin.
•hypophosphorous acid, N.F. 18.
   Use: Pharmaceutic aid (antioxidant).
HypoTears Ophthalmic Liquid. (Ciba Vision) Polyvinyl alcohol 1%, PEG-400, dextrose 1%, benzalkonium Cl 0.01%, EDTA. Bot. 15 ml, 30 ml. otc.
   Use: Ophthalmic lubricant.
HypoTears Ophthalmic Ointment. (Ciba Vision) White petrolatum, light mineral oil. Tube 3.5 g. otc.
   Use: Ophthalmic lubricant.
Hypo-Tears PF. (Ciba Vision) Polyvinyl alcohol 1%, PEG 400, dextrose and EDTA. Soln. In 0.6 ml. otc.
   Use: Artificial tear solution.
hypotensive agents.
   See: Hypertension Therapy.
HypRh$_O$ D.
   See: BayRh$_O$ D, Vial. (Bayer).
HypRh$_O$ D Mini-Dose. (Bayer) RH$_O$ (D) Immune Globulin Micro-Dose. Each package contains a single dose syringe. Rx.
   Use: Immune serum.
Hyprogest 250. (Keene) Hydroxyprogesterone caproate 250 mg, castor oil with benzyl benzoate and benzyl alcohol/ ml. Inj. Vial 5 ml. Rx.
   Use: Progestin.
Hyrexin-50. (Hyrex) Diphenhydramine HCl 50 mg/ml. Vial 10 ml. Rx.
   Use: Antihistamine.
Hyscorbic Plus Tablets. (Bock) Vitamins E 45 IU, C 600 mg, folic acid 400 mcg, B$_1$ 20 mg, B$_2$ 10 mg, niacinamide 100 mg, B$_6$ 10 mg, B$_{12}$ 25 mcg, pantothenic acid 25 mg, copper 3 mg, zinc 23.9 mg/Tab. Bot. 60s. otc.
   Use: Vitamin/mineral supplement.
Hyserp. (Freeport) Reserpine alkaloid 0.25 mg/Tab. Bot. 1000s. Rx.
   Use: Antihypertensive.
Hyskon. (Pharmacia & Upjohn) Dextran 70 32% in 10% w/v dextrose. Bot. 100 ml, 250 ml. Rx.
   Use: Diagnostic aid. For distending the uterine cavity and in irrigating and visualizing its surfaces.
Hysone. (Roberts Med) Clioquinol 30 mg, hydrocortisone 10 mg/g. Cream. Tube. 20 g. otc.

   Use: Antifungal, corticosteroid, topical.
hysteroscopy fluid.
   Use: Diagnostic aid.
   See: Hyskon (Pharmacia & Upjohn).
Hytakerol. (Winthrop Pharm) Dihydrotachysterol. Cap.: 0.125 mg. Bot. 50s.
Soln.: 0.25 mg/ml in oil. Bot. 15 ml. Rx.
   Use: Treatment of tetany and hypoparathyroidism.
Hytinic. (Hyrex) Polysaccharide-iron complex 150 mg/Cap. Bot. 50s, 500s. otc.
   Use: Iron supplement.
Hytinic Injection. (Hyrex) Ferrous gluconate 3 mg, liver equivalent to vitamins B$_{12}$ 1 mcg, vitamins B$_2$ 0.75 mg, B$_3$ 50 mg, B$_5$ 1.25 mg, B$_{12}$ equivalent 15 mcg. Vial 30 ml. Rx.
   Use: Vitamin/mineral supplement.
Hytone Cream. (Dermik) Hydrocortisone in cream base. 1%: Tube 1 oz, Jar 4 oz. 2.5%: Tube 1 oz, 2 oz. Rx.
   Use: Corticosteroid, topical.
Hytone Lotion 1%. (Dermik) Hydrocortisone 1% (10 mg/ml). Bot. 120 ml. Rx.
   Use: Corticosteroid, topical.
Hytone Lotion 2.5%. (Dermik) Hydrocortisone 2 1/2% (25 mg/ml) in lotion base. Bot. 60 ml. Rx.
   Use: Corticosteroid, topical.
Hytone Ointment. (Dermik) Hydrocortisone in ointment base, mineral oil, white petrolatum. 1%: Tube 28.3 g, 113.4 g. 2.5%: Tube 28.3 g. Rx.
   Use: Corticosteroid, topical.
Hytone Spray. (Dermik) Hydrocortisone 1%. 45 ml. Rx.
   Use: Corticosteroid, topical.
Hytrin. (Abbott) Terazosin HCl. 1 mg, 2 mg or 5 mg. Bot. 100s, 500s, UD 100s. 10 mg: Tab. Bot. 100s, UD 100s. 1 mg, 2 mg, 5 mg, 10 mg: Cap. Bot. 100s, UD 100s. Rx.
   Use: Antihypertensive.
Hytuss Tablets. (Hyrex) Guaifenesin 100 mg/Tab. Bot. 100s, 1000s. otc.
   Use: Expectorant.
Hytuss-2X. (Hyrex) Guaifenesin 200 mg/ Cap. Bot. 100s, 1000s. otc.
   Use: Expectorant.
Hyzaar. (Merck) Losartan potassium 50 mg, hydrochlorothiazide 12.5 mg, potassium 4.24 mg, lactose/Tab. Bot. 30s, 90s, 100s, UD 100s. Rx.
   Use: Antihypertensive.
Hyzine-50. (Hyrex) Hydroxyzine HCl 50 mg as HCl/ml. Vial 10 ml. Rx.
   Use: Antianxiety agent.

I

•**ibafloxacin.** (ih-BAH-FLOX-ah-sin) USAN.
Use: Antibacterial.

ibenzmethyzin. Name used for Procarbazine Hydrochloride.

Iberet. (Abbott) Ferrous sulfate 105 mg, ascorbic acid 150 mg, vitamins B_{12} 25 mcg, B_1 6 mg, B_2 6 mg, niacinamide 30 mg, B_5 10 mg, B_6 5 mg/CR Filmtab. Bot. 60s. *Rx.*
Use: Vitamin/mineral supplement.

Iberet-500. (Abbott) Ascorbic acid 500 mg, ferrous sulfate 105 mg, vitamins B_1 6 mg, B_2 6 mg, B_3 30 mg, B_5 10 mg, B_6 5 mg, B_{12} 25 mcg/CR Filmtab. Bot. 60s, 100s, Abbo-Pac 100s. *Rx.*
Use: Vitamin/mineral supplement.

Iberet-500 Liquid. (Abbott) Ferrous sulfate 78.75 mg, vitamins B_1 4.5 mg, B_2 4.5 mg, B_3 22.5 mg, B_5 7.5 mg, B_6 3.75 mg, B_{12} 18.75 mcg, C 375 mg, sorbitol, parabens/5 ml. Bot. 240 ml. *Rx.*
Use: Vitamin/mineral supplement.

Iberet-Folic-500 Filmtab. (Abbott) Ferrous sulfate 105 mg, vitamin C 500 mg, B_3 30 mg, B_5 10 mg, B_1 6 mg, B_2 6 mg, B_5 5 mg, B_{12} 25 mcg, folic acid 0.8 mg/CR Filmtab. Bot. 60s. *Rx.*
Use: Vitamin/mineral supplement.

Iberet Liquid. (Abbott) Ferrous sulfate 78.75 mg, vitamins C 112.5 mg, B_{12} 18.75 mcg, B_1 4.5 mg, B_2 4.5 mg, B_3 22.5 mg, B_5 7.5 mg, B_6 3.75 mg/15 ml. Bot. 240 ml. *Rx.*
Use: Vitamin/mineral supplement.

•**ibopamine.** (EYE-BOE-pah-meen) USAN.
Use: Dopaminergic (peripheral).

IBU. (Knoll) Ibuprofen 400, 600 or 800 mg/Tab. 100s, 500s. *Rx.*
Use: Nonsteroidal anti-inflammatory drug; analgesic.

•**ibufenac.** (eye-BYOO-feh-nak) USAN. (p-Isobutylphenyl-acetic acid).
Use: Antirheumatic (anti-inflammatory, analgesic and antipyretic).
See: Dytransin.

Ibuprin. (Thompson Medical) Ibuprofen 200 mg. Bot. 50s, 100s. *otc.*
Use: Nonsteroidal anti-inflammatory, analgesic.

•**ibuprofen,** (eye-BYOO-pro-fen) U.S.P. 23.
Use: Anti-inflammatory, analgesic.
See: Advil, Tab. (Whitehall).
Arthritis Foundation, Tab. (McNeil-CPC).
Bayer Select Pain Relief Formula, Capl. (Bayer).
Children's Advil, Susp. (Wyeth-Ayerst).
Genpril, Tab. (Goldline).
Haltran, Tab. (Pharmacia & Upjohn).
IBU, Tab. (Knoll).
Ibuprin, Tab. (Thompson Med).
Ibuprohm, Tab. (Ohm Labs).
Junior Strength Advil, Tab. (Whitehall-Robins).
Junior Strength Motrin, Tab. (McNeil).
Menadol, Tab. (Rugby).
Midol IB, Tab. (Bayer).
Motrin, Tab., Drops, Chew. Tab., Susp. (Pharmacia & Upjohn).
Motrin IB, Tab. (Pharmacia & Upjohn).
Nuprin, Tab. (BM Squibb).
Rufen, Tab. (Knoll Pharm).
Saleto, Tab. (Roberts).

ibuprofen. (Various Mfr.) 200, 300, 400, 600, 800 mg/Tab. 12s, 15s, 21s, 30s, 40s, 50s, 60s, 100s, 360s, 500s, UD 100s. *otc. Rx.*
Use: Nonsteroidal anti-inflammatory, analgesic.

•**ibuprofen aluminum.** (eye-BYOO-pro-fen) USAN.
Use: Anti-inflammatory.

•**ibuprofen piconol.** (eye-BYOO-pro-fen PIK-oh-nahl) USAN.
Use: Topical anti-inflammatory.

ibuprofen suspension. (Various Mfr.) 100 mg/5 ml. UD 50s. *Rx.*
Use: Nonsteroidal anti-inflammatory drug, analgesic.

Ibuprohm. (Ohm Labs.) Ibuprofen 200 mg. **Tab.:** Bot. 24s, 50s, 100s, 165s, 250s, 500s, 1000s. 400 mg/Bot. 50s, 100s, 500s, 1000s. 200 mg **Cap.:** Bot. 24s, 50s, 100s, 250s. *otc, Rx.*
Use: Nonsteroidal anti-inflammatory drug, analgesic.

•**ibutilide fumarate.** USAN.
Use: Cardiac depressant (antiarrhythmic).
See: Corvert, Soln. (Pharmacia & Upjohn).

ICAPS Plus. (Ciba Vision) Vitamin A 6000 IU, C 200 mg, E 60 IU, B_2 20 mg, Zn 14.25 mg, Cu, Se, Mn/Tab. Sugar free. Bot. 60s, 120s. *otc.*
Use: Vitamin and mineral supplement.

ICAPS Time Release. (Ciba Vision) Vitamin A 7000 IU, C 200 mg, E 100 IU, B_2 20 mg, Zn 14.25 mg, Cu, Se/Tab. Sugar free. Bot. 60s, 120s. *otc.*
Use: Vitamin/mineral supplement.

•**icatibant acetate.** USAN.
Use: Bradykinin antagonist.

Ice Mint. (Westwood Squibb) Stearic acid, synthetic cocoa butter, lanolin oil, camphor, menthol, beeswax, mineral oil, sodium borate, aromatic oils, emulsifiers, water. Jar 4 oz. *otc.*
Use: Emollient, counterirritant.

I-Chlor 0.5%. (Americal) Chloramphenicol 5 mg/ml. Bot. 7.5 ml, 15 ml. *Rx.*
Use: Anti-infective, ophthalmic.

•**ichthammol,** U.S.P. 23. Ichthynate.
Use: Topical anti-infective.
W/Aluminum hydroxide, phenol, zinc oxide, camphor, eucalyptol.
See: Almophen, Oint. (Jones Medical).
W/Benzocaine, resin cerate, carbolic acid, thymol, camphor, juniper tar, hexachlorophene.
See: Boil-Ease Anesthetic Drawing Salve (Del Pharm).
W/Hydrocortisone acetate, benzocaine, oxyquinoline sulfate, ephedrine HCl.
See: Derma Medicone-HC (Medicone).
W/Naftalan, calamine, amber pet.
See: Naftalan, Oint. (Paddock).

ichthammol. (Lilly). 10%, 20% Oint.

ichthammol. (NMC) Ichthammol 10% or 20% in a lanolin-petrolatum base. Oint. Tube 28.4 g. *otc.*
Use: Topical antiseptic.

ichthynate.
See: Ichthammol.

•**icopezil maleate.** USAN.
Use: Alzheimer's disease treatment (cognition enhancer), cognition adjuvant, acetylcholinesterase inhibitor.

•**icotidine.** (eye-KOE-tih-DEEN) USAN.
Use: Antagonist (to histamine H_2 and H_1 receptors).

•**ictasol.** (IK-tah-sahl) USAN.
Use: Disinfectant.

Ictotest Reagent Tablets. (Bayer) Reagent Tab. For urinary bilirubin. Bot. 100s.
Use: Diagnostic aid.

Icy Hot Balm. (Richardson-Vicks) Methyl salicylate 29%, menthol 7.6%. Jar 3.5 oz, 7 oz. *otc.*
Use: Analgesic, topical.

Icy Hot Cream. (Richardson-Vicks) Methyl salicylate 30%, menthol 10%. Tube 0.25 oz, 1.25 oz, 3 oz. *otc.*
Use: Analgesic, topical.

Icy Hot, Extra Strength. (Richardson-Vicks) Methyl salicylate 30%, menthol 10%, ceresin, cyclomethicone, hydrogenated castor oil, PEG-150 distearate, propylene glycol, stearic acid, stearyl alcohol. Stick 52.5 g. *otc.*
Use: Rub, liniment.

Icy Hot Stick. (Richardson-Vicks) Methyl salicylate 15%, menthol 8%. Stick 1.75 oz. *otc.*
Use: Analgesic, topical.

I.D.A. Capsules. (Goldline) Isometheptene mucate 65 mg, dichloralphenazone 100 mg, acetaminophen 324 mg/Cap. Bot. 100s. *Rx.*
Use: Analgesic.

Idamycin. (Pharmacia & Upjohn) Idarubicin HCl. Lactose 50 mg/5 mg. Lactose 100 mg/10 mg. Lactose 200 mg/20 mg Pow. for Inj. *Rx.*
Use: Antibiotic.

Idamycin PFS. (Pharmacia & Upjohn) Idarubicin HCl 1 mg/ml Inj. Vial. 5, 10 and 20s. *Rx.*
Use: Antibiotic (anthracycline).

•**idarubicin hydrochloride,** (eye-DUH-RUE-bih-sin) U.S.P. 23.
Use: Antineoplastic. [Orphan drug]
See: Idamycin, Pow. for Inj. (Pharmacia & Upjohn).

•**idoxifene.** (ih-dox-ih-feen) USAN.
Use: Antineoplastic, hormone replacement therapy (estrogen receptor antagonist), osteoporosis treatment and prevention .

•**idoxuridine,** (EYE-dox-YOU-rih-deen) U.S.P. 23. Uridine; Dendroid; Kerecid; Ophthalmidine.
Use: Treatment of herpes simplex; antiviral (ophthalmic).
See: Herplex, Ophthalmic Soln. (Allergan).
Stoxil, Ophthalmic Soln., Oint. (SK-Beecham).

I-Drops. (Americal) Tetrahydrozoline HCl 0.5%. Ophthalmic soln. Bot. 0.5 oz
Use: Ophthalmic vasoconstrictor/mydriatic.

IDU. Idoxuridine. *Rx.*
Use: Antiviral drug, ophthalmic.
See: Herplex Liquifilm, Soln. (Allergan).
Stoxil, Soln. (SK-Beecham).
Stoxil, Oint. (SK-Beecham).

Ifen. (Everett) Ibuprofen 400 mg or 600 mg/Tab. Bot. 100s, 500s. *Rx.*
Use: Nonsteroidal anti-inflammatory, analgesic.

•**ifetroban.** USAN.
Use: Antithrombotic.

•**ifetroban sodium.** (ih-FEH-troe-ban) USAN.
Use: Antithrombotic.

Ifex. (Bristol-Myers) Ifosfamide 1 g or 3 g. Pow. for Inj. Vial single dose. *Rx.*
Use: Antineoplastic.

•**ifosfamide,** (eye-FOSS-fuh-MIDE) U.S.P. 23.

Use: Antineoplastic.

ifosfamide, sterile. (eye-FOSS-fah-MIDE)
Use: Antineoplastic.

I-Gent. (Americal) Gentamicin sulfate 3 mg/ml. Ophthalmic soln. Bot. 5 ml. *Rx.*
Use: Anti-infective, ophthalmic.

Igepal Co-430. (General Aniline & Film) Non-oxynol 4. *otc.*
Use: Spermicide.

Igepal Co-730. (General Aniline & Film) Non-oxynol 15. *otc.*
Use: Spermicide.

Igepal Co-880. (General Aniline & Film) Non-oxynol 30. *otc.*
Use: Spermicide.

igG monoclonal anti-CD4.
See: Chimeric m-t412 (human-m urine) igG monoclonal anti-cd4

IGIV. (Various Mfr.) Immune globulin IV. *Rx.*
Use: Immunomodulator (Phase II/III pediatric HIV), immune serum.
See: Gamimune N, Inj. (Bayer).
Gammagard S/D, Pow. (Baxter).
Gammar-P IV, Pow. (Centeon).
Iveegam, Pow. (Immuno).
Polygam S/D (American Red Cross).
Sandoglobulin, Pow. (Sandoz).
Venoglobulin-I, Pow. (Alpha Therapeutic).
Venoglobulin-S (Alpha).

I-Homatrine 5%. (Americal) Homatropine hydrobromide 5%. Ophthalmic soln. Bot. 5 ml. *Rx.*
Use: Cycloplegic mydriatic.

IL-2. (Various Mfr.) Interleukin-2. *Rx.*
Use: Cytokine agent.
See: Proleukin (Chiron).

•**ilepcimide.** USAN. *Formerly antiepilepsirine.*
Use: Anticonvulsant.

Iletin I. (Lilly) Regular and modified insulin products from beef and pork. *otc.*
Regular: 100 units/ml. Vial 10 ml
Lente: 100 units/ml. Vial 10 ml.
Semilente: 40 units or 100 units/ml. Vial 10 ml.
NPH: 100 units/ml. Vial 10 ml.
Use: Antidiabetic.

Iletin II. (Lilly) Special insulin products prepared from purified beef or purified pork. *otc.*
Lente: 100 units/ml. Vial 10 ml.
NPH: 100 units/ml. Vial 10 ml.
Use: Antidiabetic.

Iletin II Concentrated. (Lilly) Purified pork regular insulin 500 units/ml. Vial 20 ml. *Rx.*

Use: Antidiabetic.

•**ilmofosine.** (ill-MOE-fose-een) USAN.
Use: Antineoplastic.

•**ilonidap.** (ile-OHN-ih-dap) USAN.
Use: Anti-inflammatory.

Ilopan. (Pharmacia & Upjohn) Dexpanthenol 250 mg/ml. Amp. 2 ml, Disp. Syringe 2 ml. *Rx.*
Use: GI stimulant.

Ilopan-Choline. (Pharmacia & Upjohn) Ilopan 50 mg, choline bitartrate 25 mg/ Tab. Bot. 100s, 500s. *Rx.*
Use: GI stimulant.

•**iloperidone.** (ill-oh-PURR-ih-dohn) USAN.
Use: Antipsychotic.

iloprost infusion solution. (Berlex) Raynaud's phenomenon secondary to systemic sclerosis. [Orphan drug]

Ilosone. (Dista) Erythromycin estolate.
Cap.: (Erythromycin base) 250 mg/ Pulv. Bot. 24s, 100s, UD 100s, Blister pkg. 10 × 10s. **Liq.:** 125 mg or 250 mg/ 5 ml. Bot. 100 ml, 16 fl oz. **Tab.:** 500 mg. Bot. 50s. **Susp.:** 125 mg or 250 mg/ 5 ml. Bot. 10 ml. *Rx.*
Use: Anti-infective, erythromycin.

Ilosone Chewable. (Dista) Erythromycin estolate 125 mg or 250 mg/Tab. Bot. 50s. *Rx.*
Use: Anti-infective, erythromycin.

Ilotycin Gluceptate I.V. (Dista) Erythromycin gluceptate. Vial. I.V. 1 g, vial 30 ml. Box 1s. *Rx.*
Use: Anti-infective, erythromycin.

Ilotycin Ophthalmic Ointment. (Dista) Erythromycin 5 mg/g. Tube 3.5 g. *Rx.*
Use: Anti-infective, ophthalmic.

Ilozyme. (Pharmacia & Upjohn) Pancrelipase equivalent to lipase 11,000 units, protease 30,000 units, amylase 30,000 units/Tab. Bot. 250s. *Rx.*
Use: Digestive enzymes.

I-Lube. (Americal) Petrolatum ophthalmic ointment. Tube 0.125 oz.
Use: Ophthalmic lubricant.

I.L.X. B12 Elixir. (Kenwood/Bradley) Liver fraction 98 mg, iron 102 mg, vitamins B_1 5 mg, B_2 2 mg, B_3 10 mg, B_{12} 10 mcg/15 ml. Bot. 240 ml. *otc.*
Use: Vitamin/mineral supplement.

I.L.X. B12 Tablets and Caplets. (Kenwood/Bradley) Iron 37.5 mg, vitamins C 120 mg, B_{12} 12 mcg, desiccated liver 130 mg, B_1 2 mg, B_2 2 mg, B_3 20 mg/ Tab. Bot. 100s. *otc.*
Use: Vitamin/mineral supplement.

I.L.X. Elixir. (Kenwood/Bradley) Iron 70 mg, liver concentrate 98 mg, vitamins

B_1 5 mg, B_2 2 mg, B_3 10 mg/15 ml. Bot. 240 ml. *otc.*
Use: Vitamin/mineral supplement.

•**imafen hydrochloride.** USAN.
Use: Antidepressant.

Imagent GI. (Alliance) Perflubron Liq. In 200 ml.
Use: Radiopaque agent.

•**imazodan hydrochloride.** (ih-MAY-zoe-DAN) USAN.
Use: Cardiotonic.

•**imciromab pentetate.** (im-SIHR-ah-mab PEN-teh-tate) USAN.
Use: Monoclonal antibody (antimyosin). [Orphan drug]
See: Myoscint (Centocor).

Imdur. (Key) Isosorbide mononitrate 60 or 120 mg. ER Tab. Bot. 30s, 100s, UD 100s. *Rx.*
Use: Antianginal.

Imenol. (Sig) Guaiacol 0.1 g, eucalyptol 0.08 g, iodoform 0.02 g, camphor 0.05 g/ml. Vial 30 ml. *Rx.*
Use: Expectorant.

l-methorphinan levorphanol.
See: Levo-Dromoran, Amp., Tab., Vial (Roche).

Imferon. (Fisons) An iron-dextran complex containing iron 50 mg/ml. Amp. 2 ml. Box 10s. Vial (w/phenol 0.5%) 10 ml. Box 2s. *Rx.*
Use: Iron supplement.

imidazole carboxamide. *Rx.*
Use: Antineoplastic.
See: Dacarbazine, Inj. (Various Mfr.). DTIC-Dome, Inj. (Bayer).

•**imidecyl iodine.** (IH-mih-DEH-sill) USAN.
Use: Anti-infective, topical.

•**imidocarb hydrochloride.** (ih-MIH-doe-KARB) USAN.
Use: Antiprotozoal (Babesia).

•**imidoline hydrochloride.** (im-ID-oh-leen) USAN.
Use: Tranquilizer, antipsychotic.

•**imidurea,** N.F. 18.
Use: Antimicrobial.

•**imiglucerase.** (ih-mih-GLUE-ser-ACE) USAN.
Use: Enzyme replenisher, treatment for Gaucher's disease (glucocerebrosidase). [Orphan drug]
See: Cerezyme (Genzyme).

•**imiloxan hydrochloride.** (ih-mill-OX-ahn) USAN.
Use: Antidepressant.

imipemide. (ih-MIH-peh-MIDE)
Use: Anti-infective.
See: Imipenem, U.S.P 23.

•**imipenem,** (ih-mih-PEN-em) U.S.P. 23.
Formerly imipemide.
Use: Antibacterial.
W/Cilastatin for Injection.
See: Primaxin, Inj (Merck).

•**imipramine hydrochloride,** (im-IPP-ruh-meen) U.S.P. 23. Berkomine, IA-Pram, Impamin, Iprogen, Norpramine, & Tofranil HCl salts.
Use: Antidepressant.
See: Janimine, Tab. (Abbott).
Presamine, Tab. (Rhone-Poulenc Rorer).
Tofranil, Tab., Amp. (Geigy).
W.D.D., Tab. (Solvay).

imipramine pamoate. *Rx.*
Use: Antidepressant.
See: Tofranil-PM, Cap. (Geigy).

•**imiquimod.** (ih-mih-KWIH-mahd) USAN.
Use: Immunomodulator.
See: Aldara Cream (3M Pharmaceuticals).

Imitrex. (Glaxo Wellcome) Sumatriptan succinate. 12 mg/ml. Inj. Unit-of-use syringes: 0.5 ml in 1 ml; Single-dose vial: 6 mg; SELFdose system kit: 2 unit-of-use syringes, 1 SELFdose unit. *Rx.*
Use: Agent for migraine.

Imitrex Tablets. (Cerenex) Sumatriptan succinate 25 mg or 50 mg/Tab. Pkg. 9s. *Rx.*
Use: Agent for migraine.

Immun-Aid. (McGaw) A custard flavored liquid containing 18.5 g protein, 60 g carbohydrate, 11 g fat per liter. With appropriate vitamins and minerals. Pow. Packets 123 g. 24s. *otc.*
Use: Full enteral nutrition for immunocompromised patients.

immune globulin. (ih-MYOON GLAH-byoo-lin) Immune Serum Globulin Human. Gamma-globulin fraction of normal human plasma. Vial 10 ml. Tubex 1 ml, 2 ml w/thimerosal 1:10,000. *Rx.*
Use: Modification of active measles, prophylaxis of hepatitis; treatment of immune deficiencies; prevention of infection associated with bone marrow transplantation (BMT); decrease frequency of certain pediatric HIV-related infections and conjunctive therapy for Kawasaki syndrome (Iveegam only).
See: Gamimune N (Bayer).
Gammagard S/D (Baxter).
Gammar-P IV (Centeon).
Iveegam (Immuno).
Polygam S/D (American Red Cross).
Sandoglobulin (Sandoz).
Venoglobulin-I (Alpha Therapeutics).

Venoglobulin-S (Alpha Therapeutics).

immune globulin, cytomegalovirus.
See: CytoGam, Vial (MedImmune).

immune globulin, hepatitis B.
See: BayHep B, Vial, Syr. (Bayer).
H-BIG, Vial, Syr. (North American Biologicals).

immune globulin IM.
Use: Immune serum.
See: Gammar-IM (Centeon).

•**immune globulin intravenous pentetate.** (ih-MYOON GLAH-byoo-lin in-trah-VEE-nuhs PEN-teh-tate) USAN.
Use: Diagnostic aid.

immune globulin IV.
Use: Immune serum. [Orphan drug]
See: Gamimune N, Inj. (Bayer).
Gammagard, Pow. (Baxter).
Gammar-P IV, Pow. (Centeon).
Iveegam, Pow. (Immuno).
Polygam S/D (American Red Cross).
Sandoglobulin, Pow. (American Red Cross, Sandoz).
Venoglobulin-I, Pow. (Alpha Therapeutic).
Venoglobulin-S (Alpha).

immune globulin, rabies.
Use: Passive immunization.
See: Bayrab (Bayer).
Imogam Rabies (Pasteur-Merieux-Connaught).

immune globulin, Rh$_o$(D).
See: Gamulin Rh (Centeon).
BayRho D (Bayer).
MICRhoGAM (Ortho Diagnostics).
Mini-Gamulin Rh (Centeon).
RhoGAM (Ortho Diagnostics).
WinRho SD (Univax Biologics).

immune globulin, tetanus.
Use: Passive immunization.
See: Bay Tet (Bayer).

immune globulin, vaccinia.
Use: Passive immunization.

immune globulin, varicella-zoster.
Use: Passive immunization.

immune serums.
See: Cytomegalovirus Immune Globulin Intravenous (Human) (Massachusetts Public Health Biologic Laboratories).
Immune Serum Globulin (Human).

immune serum (animal).
See: Botulism Antitoxin, Vial (Connaught).
Diphtheria Antitoxin.

Immunex CRP. (Wampole) Two-minute latex agglutination slide test for the qualitative detection of C-Reactive protein in serum. Kit 100s.

Use: Diagnostic aid.

Immuno-C. (Biomune Systems)
See: Bovine Whey Protein Concentrate.

immunosuppressive drugs.
See: Atgam (Pharmacia & Upjohn).
Imuran (Glaxo Wellcome).
Orthoclone OKT3, Inj. (Ortho).
Prograf (Fujisawa).
Sandimmune, Cap., Oral Soln. or IV Soln. (Sandoz).

Immunorex. (Antigen Laboratories) Allergenic extracts, various. Vial. *Rx.*
Use: Agent for immunization.

Imodium A-D Liquid. (McNeil) Loperamide 1 mg/5 ml, alcohol 5.25%. *otc.*
Use: Antidiarrheal.

Imodium Capsules. (Janssen) Loperamide 2 mg/Cap. Bot. 100s, 500s, UD 100s. *Rx.*
Use: Antidiarrheal.

Imogam Rabies Immune Globulin. (Pasteur-Merieux-Connaught) Rabies immune globulin (human) 150 IU/ml. Vials 2 ml, 10 ml. *Rx.*
Use: Rabies prophylaxis agent.

Imovax Rabies I.D. (Connaught) Rabies vaccine 0.25 IU/0.1 ml for I.D. administration for pre-exposure treatment only. Wistar rabies virus strain PM-1503-3M grown in human diploid cell culture. Powd. Inj. in single dose syringe w/1 vial diluent. *Rx.*
Use: Rabies prophylaxis agent.

Imovax Rabies Vaccine. (Connaught) Merieux rabies vaccine, Wistar rabies virus strain PM-1503-3M grown in human diploid cell cultures. Rabies Vaccine ≥ 2.5 IU/ml. Powd. Inj. In single dose vial with disposable needle and syring containing diluent and disposable needle for administration. *Rx.*
Use: Rabies prophylaxis agent.

Impact. (Approved) Belladonna alkaloids 0.16 mg, phenylpropanolamine HCl 50 mg, chlorpheniramine maleate 1 mg, pheniramine maleate 12.5 mg/Cap. Pack 12s, 24s. Vial 15s, 30s, Bot. 1000s. *Rx.*
Use: Anticholinergic, antispasmodic, decongestant, antihistamine.

Impromen. (Janssen) Bromperidol decanoate. *Rx.*
Use: Antipsychotic.

Impromen Decanoate. (Janssen) Bromperidol decanoate. *Rx.*
Use: Antipsychotic.

•**impromidine hydrochloride.** (im-PRAH-mid-deen) USAN.

Use: Diagnostic aid (gastric secretion indicator).

Improved Congestant Tablets. (Rugby) Chlorpheniramine maleate 2 mg, acetaminophen 325 mg/Tab. Bot. 100s, 1000s. *otc.*
Use: Antihistamine, analgesic.

Imreg-1. (Imreg) *Rx.*
Use: Immunomodulator.

Imreg-2. (Imreg)
Use: Immunomodulator.

Imuran. (Glaxo Wellcome) **Tab.:** Azathioprine 50 mg/Tab. Bot. 100s, UD 100s. **Inj.:** Azathioprine 100 mg/20 ml. Vial. *Rx.*
Use: Immunosuppressant.

Imuthiol. (Connaught) Diethyldithiocarbamate. *Rx.*
Use: Immunomodulator.

Inapsine. (Janssen) Droperidol 2.5 mg/ml. Amp. 2 ml, 5 ml, 10 ml. Box 10s. Multi-dose Vial w/methylparaben 1.8 mg, propylparaben 0.2 mg, lactic acid/10 ml. Box 10s. *Rx.*
Use: General anesthetic.
W/Fentanyl citrate.
See: Innovar, Inj. (Janssen).

•**indacrinone.** (IN-dah-KRIH-nohn) USAN.
Use: Antihypertensive, diuretic.

indalone.
See: Butopyronoxyl (Various Mfr.).

indandione derivative. *Rx.*
Use: Anticoagulant.
See: Anisindione (Various Mfr.).

•**indapamide,** (IN-DAP-uh-mide) U.S.P. 23.
Use: Antihypertensive, diuretic.
See: Lozol, Tab. (Rhone-Poulenc Rorer).

indapamide. (IN-DAP-uh-mide) (Arcola) Indapamide 2.5 mg, lactose/Tab. Bot. 100s, 1000s. *Rx.*
Use: Antihypertensive, diuretic.

•**indecainide hydrochloride.** (in-deh-CANE-ide) USAN.
Use: Cardiac depressant (antiarrhythmic).
See: Decabid (Lilly).

•**indeloxazine hydrochloride.** (in-DELL-OX-ah-zeen) USAN.
Use: Antidepressant.

Inderal Injection. (Wyeth-Ayerst) Propranolol HCl 1 mg/ml. Amp. 1 ml. Box 10s. *Rx.*
Use: Beta-adrenergic blocking agent.

Inderal-LA. (Wyeth-Ayerst) Propranolol HCl 80 mg, 120 mg or 160 mg/SR Cap. Bot. 100s, 1000s, UD 100s. *Rx.*
Use: Beta-adrenergic blocking agent.

Inderal Tablets. (Wyeth-Ayerst) Propranolol HCl 10 mg, 20 mg, 40 mg, 60 mg or 80 mg/Tab. Bot. 100s, 1000s, UD 100s. *Rx.*
Use: Beta-adrenergic blocking agent.

Inderide. (Wyeth-Ayerst) Propranolol HCl 40 mg, hydrochlorothiazide 25 mg/Tab. Bot. 100s, 1000s, UD 100s. Propranolol HCl 80 mg, hydrochlorothiazide 25 mg/Tab. Bot. 100s. *Rx.*
Use: Antihypertensive combination.

Inderide LA Capsules. (Wyeth-Ayerst) Propranolol HCl/hydrochlorothiazide Long Acting Caps: 80 mg/50 mg, 120 mg/50 mg or 160 mg/50 mg. Bot. 100s. *Rx.*
Use: Antihypertensive combination.

indian gum.
See: Karaya Gum.

indigo carmine. (Becton Dickinson) Sodium indigotindisulfonate 8 mg/ml. Amp. 5 ml. Box 10s, 100s.
Use: Diagnostic aid.
See: Sodium indigotindisulfonate.

indigo carmine solution. (Becton Dickinson) Indigotindisulfonate sodium inj. (0.8% aqueous soln. sodium salt of indigotindisulfonic acid) 40 mg/5 ml. Amp. 5 ml, 10s.
Use: Diagnostic aid.

•**indigotindisulfonate sodium,** U.S.P. 23. Indigo Carmine.
Use: Diagnostic aid (cystoscopy).
See: Sodium Indigotindisulfonate.

indinavir. USAN.
Use: Antiviral (HIV-protease inhibitor).

•**indinavir sulfate.** (in-DIN-ah-veer) USAN.
Use: Antiviral.
See: Crixivan, Cap. (Merck).

•**indium chlorides In 113m.** (IN-dee-uhm) USAN. U.S.P. XX.
Use: Radioactive agent.

•**indium In 111 altumomab pentetate.** (IN-dee-uhm ahl-TOO-mah-mab PEN-teh-tate) USAN.
Use: Radiodiagnostic monoclonal antibody (anticarcinoembryonic antigen), radioactive agent. [Orphan drug]

•**indium In 111 chloride solution,** U.S.P. 23.
Use: Radioactive agent.

indium In 111 murine monoclonal antibody fab to myosin.
Use: Diagnostic aid in myocarditis. [Orphan drug]

•**indium In 111 oxyquinoline.** (In-dee-uhm OX-ee-KWIN-oh-lin) U.S.P. 23.
Use: Radioactive agent, diagnostic aid.

•**indium In 111 pentetate injection,** U.S.P. 23.
Use: Diagnostic aid (radionuclide cisternography), radioactive agent.

•**indium In 111 pentetreotide.** USAN.
Use: Diagnostic aid, radioactive agent.

•**indium In 111 satumomab pendetide.** (IN-dee-uhm sat-YOU-mah-mab PEN-deh-TIDE) USAN.
Use: Radiodiagnostic monoclonal antibody (ovarian and colorectal carcinoma), radioactive agent.

Indochron E-R. (Inwood) Indomethacin 75 mg. SR Cap. Bot. 60s, 100s. *Rx.*
Use: Nonsteroidal anti-inflammatory drug, analgesic.

Indocin. (Merck) Indomethacin. **Cap.:** 25 mg. Bot. 100s, 1000s, UD 100s. Unit-of-use 100s; 50 mg. Bot. 100s, UD 100s. **Supp.:** 50 mg. Pkg. 30s. **Oral Susp.:** 25 mg/5 ml, alcohol 1%, sorbitol 0.1%. Bot. 237 ml. *Rx.*
Use: Nonsteroidal anti-inflammatory, analgesic.

Indocin I.V. (Merck) Indomethacin sodium trihydrate equivalent to 1 mg indomethacin/Vial. Vial single dose. *Rx.*
Use: Agent for patent ductus arteriosus.

Indocin SR. (Merck) Indomethacin 75 mg/SR Cap. Unit-of-Use 30s, 60s.
Use: Nonsteroidal anti-inflammatory, analgesic.

•**indocyanine green,** U.S.P. 23. A tricarbocyanine dye.
Use: Diagnostic aid (cardiac output determination, hepatic function determination).
See: Cardio-Green, Inj. (Beckton-Dickinson).

Indogesic. (Century) Acetaminophen 32.5 mg, butalbital 50 mg/Tab. Bot. 100s, 1000s. *Rx.*
Use: Analgesic, sedative, hypnotic.

Indoklon. Hexafluorodiethyl ether. Flurothyl. Bis-(2,2,2-trifluoroethyl)ether. *Rx.*
Use: Shock inducing agent (convulsant).

•**indolapril hydrochloride.** (in-DAHL-ah-PRILL) USAN.
Use: Antihypertensive.

Indo-Lemmon. (Lemmon) Indomethacin 25 mg or 50 mg/Cap. Bot. 100s, 500s, 1000s. *Rx.*
Use: Nonsteroidal anti-inflammatory, analgesic.

•**indolidan.** (in-DOE-lih-DAN) USAN.
Use: Cardiotonic.

Indometh Caps. (Major) Indomethacin 25 mg or 50 mg/Tab. **25 mg:** Bot. 100s, 1000s. **50 mg:** Bot. 100s, 500s. *Rx.*
Use: Nonsteroidal anti-inflammatory, analgesic.

•**indomethacin,** (in-doe-METH-ah-sin) U.S.P. 23.
Use: Anti-inflammatory, analgesic.
See: Indochron E-R, Cap. (Inwood).
Indocin, Cap., S.R. Cap., I.V., Oral Susp., Supp. (Merck).
Indo-Lemmon, Cap. (Lemmon).

indomethacin. (Various Mfr.) **Cap.: 25 mg:** 60s, 100s, 500s, 1000s, UD 100s; **50 mg:** 23s, 72s, 100s, 250s, 500s, UD 100s; **SR Cap.:** 75 mg. Bot. 60s, 100s.
Use: Anti-inflammatory.

indomethacin. (Roxane) Indomethacin 25 mg/5ml. Oral susp. Bot. 500 ml. *Rx.*
Use: Nonsteroidal anti-inflammatory, analgesic.

•**indomethacin sodium,** (in-doe-METH-ah-sin) U.S.P. 23.
Use: Anti-inflammatory, analgesic.

indomethacin sodium trihydrate. *Rx.*
Use: Patent ductus arteriosus.
See: Indocin I.V., Pow. (Merck).

•**indoprofen.** (in-doe-PRO-fen) USAN.
Use: Analgesic, anti-inflammatory.

•**indoramin.** (in-DAHR-ah-min) USAN.
Use: Antihypertensive.

•**indoramin hydrochloride.** (in-DAHR-ah-min) USAN.
Use: Antihypertensive.

•**indorenate hydrochloride.** (in-DAHR-en-ATE) USAN.
Use: Antihypertensive.

•**indoxole.** (IN-dox-OLE) USAN.
Use: Antipyretic, anti-inflammatory.

•**indriline hydrochloride.** (IN-drih-leen) USAN.
Use: Stimulant (central).

I-Neocort. (American) Neomycin sulfate 5 mg, hydrocortisone acetate 15 mg/5 ml. Ophthalmic susp. Bot. 5 ml. *Rx.*
Use: Anti-infective, corticosteroid.

I-Neospor. (American) Polymixin B sulfate, gramicidin, neomycin sulfate ophthalmic soln. Bot. 10 ml. *Rx.*
Use: Anti-infective, ophthalmic.

Infalyte Oral Solution. (B-M Squibb) Electrolyte mixture with 30 g/L rice syrup solids containing 4.2 calories/fl. oz. In 1 liter. *otc.*
Use: Nutritional supplement.

Infanrix. (SK-Beecham) Diphtheria 25 Lf units, tetanus toxoid 10 Lf units, acellular pertussis vaccine (pertussis toxin

25 mcg, filamentous hemagglutinin 25 mcg, pertactin 8 mcg) and aluminum ≤ 0.625 mg/0.5 ml. With 2-phenoxyethanol 5 mg/ml. Vial 0.5 ml. *Rx.*
Use: Vaccine.

infant foods.
Use: Nutritional supplement.
See: Enfamil (Bristol-Myers).
    Enfamil Human Milk Fortifier (Bristol-Myers).
    Enfamil Premature 20 Formula (Bristol-Myers).
    RCF Liquid (Ross).
    Similac (Ross).
    Similac PM 60/40 Liquid (Ross).

infant foods, hypoallergenic.
Use: Nutritional supplement.
See: Alimentation (Ross).
    Isomil (Ross).
    Isomil SF (Ross).
    I-Soyalac (Mt. Vernon Foods).
    Nutramigen (Bristol-Myers).
    Pregestimil Powder (Bristol-Myers).
    ProSobee (Bristol-Myers).
    Soyalac (Mt. Vernon Foods).

Infant's Feverall. (Upsher-Smith) Acetaminophen 80 mg/Supp. 6s. *otc.*
Use: Analgesic.

Infant's No-Aspirin Drops. (Walgreen) Acetaminophen 80 mg/0.8 ml. Nonalcoholic. Bot. 15 ml. *otc.*
Use: Analgesic.

Infant's Silapap. (Silarx) Acetaminophen 80 mg/0.8 ml. Drops. Bot. 15 ml. Alcohol free. *otc.*
Use: Analgesic, antipyretic.

Infarub Cream. (Whitehall Robins) Methyl salicylate 35%, menthol 10% in vanishing cream base. Tube 1.25 oz, 3.5 oz. *otc.*
Use: Analgesic, topical.

Infatuss. (Scott/Cord) Dextromethorphan HBr 7.2 mg, chlorpheniramine maleate 1.1 mg, phenylpropanolamine HCl 4.8 mg, ammonium Cl 50 mg/5 ml. Bot. 4 oz, pt, gal. *otc.*
Use: Antitussive, antihistamine, decongestant, expectorant.

Infectrol Ointment. (Bausch & Lomb) Dexamethasone 0.1%, neomycin sulfate equivalent to 0.35% neomycin base and 10,000 units polymyxin B sulfate/ g. White petrolatum, lanolin, mineral oil, parabens. Oint. Tube 3.5, 3.75 g. *Rx.*
Use: Corticosteroid, anti-infective, topical.

Infectrol Suspension. (Bausch & Lomb) Dexamethasone 0.1%, neomycin sulfate equivalent to 0.35% neomycin base and 10,000 units polymyxin B sulfate/

ml. Hydroxypropyl methylcellulose, polysorbate 20, benzalkonium chloride. Drop. Bot. 5 ml. *Rx.*
Use: Corticosteroid, anti-infective, ophthalmic.

InFe D. (Schein) Iron 50/ml (as dextran), sodium chloride 0.9%. Inj. Amp 2 ml. Vial 10 ml. *Rx.*
Use: Parenteral iron supplement.

Inflamase Forte. (Ciba Vision) Prednisolone sodium phosphate 1%. Bot. 5 ml, 10 ml, 15 ml. *Rx.*
Use: Corticoisteroid, ophthalmic.

Inflamase Mild. (Ciba Vision) Prednisolone sodium phosphate 0.125%. Bot. 3 ml, 5 ml, 10 ml. *Rx.*
Use: Corticosteroid, ophthalmic.

•**influenza virus vaccine,** (in-flew-ENzuh) U.S.P. 23.
Use: Active immunizing agent.
See: Fluogen, Inj. (Parke-Davis).
    Flu-Shield, Inj. (Wyeth Lederle).
    Fluvirin, Inj. (Evans Medical).
    Fluzone, Inj. (Connaught).

influenza virus vaccine. Types A and B. A/Texas/36/91 (H1N1) 15 mcg, A/ Beijing/353/89 (H3N2) 15 mcg, B/ Panama/45/90 15 mcg/0.5 ml. Vial. 0.5 ml, 5 ml.
Use: Agent for immunization.
See: Fluogen, Inj. (Parke-Davis).
    Flu-Shield, Inj. (Wyeth Lederle).
    Fluvirin, Inj. (Adams).
    Fluzone, Inj. (Connaught).

Infrarub. (Whitehall Robins) Methyl salicylate 35%, menthol 10%. Cream. Jar 37.5, 90 g. *otc.*
Use: Analgesic, topical.

Infumorph 200. (Elkins-Sinn) Morphine sulfate 10 mg/ml/Inj. Ampuls 20 ml. Preservative free. *c-ii.*
Use: Narcotic analgesic.

Infumorph 500. (Elkins-Sinn) Morphine sulfate 25 mg/ml/Inj. Ampuls 20 ml. Preservative free. *c-ii.*
Use: Narcotic analgesic.

Ingadine Tabs. (Major) Guanethidine sulfate 10 mg or 25 mg/Tab. Bot. 100s, 1000s. *Rx.*
Use: Antihypertensive.

INH. (Ciba) Isoniazid 300 mg/Tab. *Rx.*
Use: Antituberculous agent.
See: Rimactane/INH, Dual Pack (Ciba).

Inhal-Aid. (Key)
Use: Drug delivery system for metered dose inhalers.

Inhibace. (Roche/Glaxo Wellcome) Cilazapril. *Rx.*
Use: Antihypertensive.

Innerclean Herbal Laxative. (Last) Senna leaf powder, psyllium seed, buckthorne, anise seed, fennel seed. Bot. 1 oz, 2 oz. *otc.*
Use: Laxative.

Innertabs. (Last) Senna leaf powder and psyllium seed tablets. Bot. 80s, 200s. *otc.*
Use: Laxative.

Innogel Plus. (Hogil Pharm) Pyrethrins 0.3%, piperonyl butoxide technical 3%. Gel. Kits contain 3 pre-dosed gel paks and a comb. *otc.*
Use: Pediculicide.

Innovar Injection. (Janssen) Fentanyl citrate 0.05 mg, droperidol 2.5 mg/ml. Amp. 2 ml, 5 ml. Box of 10s. *c-II.*
Use: Narcotic analgesic, general anesthetic.

Inocor Lactate. (Sanofi Winthrop) Amrinone lactate (base equivalent) 5 mg/ml, sodium metabisulfite 0.25 mg/Inj. Amp. 20 ml. Box 5s. *Rx.*
Use: Short-term management of congestive heart failure.

• **inocoterone acetate.** (ih-NO-koe-ter-ohn) USAN.
Use: Antiacne.

in-111 murine mab. (2B8-MX-DTPA).
Use: B-cell non-Hodgkin's lymphoma. [Orphan drug]

inophylline.
See: Aminophylline (Various Mfr.).

inosine pranobex. (Newport Pharmaceuticals) Isoprinosine. *Rx.*
Use: Antiviral. [Orphan drug]

Inosiplex. (Newport Pharmaceuticals) Isoprinosine. *Rx.*
Use: Antiviral.

inosit.
See: Inositol (Various Mfr.).

inositol. 1,2,3,5/4,6-Cyclohexanehexol. Commercial solvents (Bios 1,Hexahydroxycyclohexane, Inosit, Dambose).
Use: Lipotropic.
W/Choline bitartrate, vitamins, minerals.
W/Methionine, choline bitartrate, liver desiccated, vitamin B$_{12}$.
See: Limvic, Tab. (Briar).
W/Panthenol, choline Cl, vitamins, minerals, estrone, testosterone.
See: Geramine, Inj. (ICN Pharm).
W/Panthenol, choline Cl, vitamins, minerals, estrone, testosterone, polydigestase.
See: Geramine, Tab. (ICN Pharm).

• **inositol niacinate.** (in-OH-sih-tole NIE-ah-sin-ate) USAN. Myo-Inositol hexanicotinate. Meso-inositol hexanicotinate,

hexanicotinate. Meso-inositol hexanicotinate. Hexopal; Mesonex.
Use: Peripheral vasodilator.

inositol nicotinate.
See: Inositol Niacinate.

Inotropin. (Faulding) Dopamine 40 mg/ml, sodium metabisulfite 1%/Inj. In 5 ml. *Rx.*
Use: Vasopressor.

Inspirease. (Key). *Rx.*
Use: Drug delivery system for metered-dose inhalers.

Insta-Char. (Kerr) **Regular:** Aqueous suspension activated charcoal 50 g/8 oz. **Pediatric:** Aqueous suspension activated charcoal 15 g/4 oz. *otc.*
Use: Antidote.

Insta-Glucose. (ICN) Undiluted USP glucose. UD tube containing liquid glucose 31 g. *otc.*
Use: Glucose elevating agent.

Inst-E-Vite. (Barth's) Vitamin E 100 IU or 200 IU/Cap. **100 IU:** Bot 100s, 500s, 1000s. **200 IU:** Bot. 100s, 250s, 500s. *otc.*
Use: Vitamin E supplement.

Insulatard NPH Human. (Nordisk-USA) Human insulin isophane suspension 100 IU/ml. *otc.*
Use: Antidiabetic.

• **insulin,** (IN-suh-lin) U.S.P. 23.
Use: Antidiabetic.
See: Iletin Prods. (Lilly).
Insulin Prods. (Squibb).

insulin. (IN-suh-lin) (Nordisk) Insulatard NPH Mixtard Velosulin. *otc.*
Use: Antidiabetic.

• **insulin I-125.** USAN.
Use: Radioactive agent.

• **insulin I-131.** USAN.
Use: Radioactive agent.

• **insulin, dalanated.** USAN.
Use: Antidiabetic.

• **insulin human,** (IN-suh-lin) U.S.P. 23.
Use: Antidiabetic.
See: Humulin (Lilly).

• **insulin human zinc suspension,** U.S.P. 23.
Use: Antidiabetic.

• **insulin human zinc, extended, suspension,** U.S.P. 23.
Use: Antidiabetic.

• **insulin human, isophane, suspension,** U.S.P. 23.
Use: Antidiabetic.

• **insulin, isophane,suspension,** U.S.P. 23.
Use: Antidiabetic.
See: NPH (Novo Nordisk).

insulin-like growth factor-1. *Rx.*
Use: Amyotrophic lateral sclerosis. [Orphan drug]
•**insulin lispro.** (IN-suh-lin LICE-pro) USAN.
Use: Antidiabetic.
See: Humalog, Tab. (Bayer Corp.).
•**insulin, neutral.** (IN-suh-lin) USAN.
Use: Antidiabetic.
insulin novo rapitard. Biphasic Insulin.
insulin, protamine zinc suspension, (IN-suh-lin PRO-tah-meen zingk)
U.S.P. XXII. 40 or 100 units/ml. Vials 10 ml.
Use: Antidiabetic.
insulin, regular.
Use: Antidiabetic.
See: Regular Iletin I (Beef and Pork), Inj. (Lilly).
Regular Insulin (Pork), Inj. (Novo Nordisk).
Pork Regular Iletin II (Pork), Inj. (Lilly).
Regular Purified Pork Insulin, Inj. (Novo Nordisk).
Velosulin (Pork), Inj. (Novo Nordisk).
Humulin R, Inj. (Lilly).
Humulin BR, Inj. (Lilly).
Novolin R, Inj. (Novo Nordisk).
Velosulin, Inj. (Novo Nordisk).
Novolin R PenFill, Cartridges (Novo Nordisk).
insulin, regular concentrate.
Use: Antidiabetic.
See: Semilente Iletin I (Beef or Pork), Inj. (Lilly).
Semilente Insulin (Beef), Inj. (Novo Nordisk).
insulin suspension, isophane.
Use: Antidiabetic.
See: Humulin 50/50, Inj. (Lilly).
Humulin 70/30, Inj. (Lilly).
Mixtard, Inj. (Novo Nordisk).
Novolin 70/30, Inj. (Novo Nordisk).
Novolin 70/30 PenFill, Cartridge (Novo Nordisk).
insulin suspension, lente.
Use: Antidiabetic.
See: Lente Insulin, Cial (Novo Nordisk).
Lente L, Vial (Novo Nordisk).
Novolin L, Vial (Novo Nordisk).
Lente Iletin I (Beef and Pork), Inj. (Lilly).
Lente Insulin (Beef), Inj. (Novo Nordisk).
Lente Iletin II (Pork), Inj. (Lilly).
Lente Iletin II (Beef), Inj. (Lilly).
Lente Purified Pork Insulin, Inj. (Novo Nordisk).
Humulin L, Inj. (Lilly).
Novolin L, Inj. (Novo Nordisk).

insulin suspension, NPH.
Use: Antidiabetic.
See: NPH Iletin I (Beef and Pork), Inj. (Lilly).
NPH Insulin (Beef), Inj. (Novo Nordisk).
Beef NPH Iletin II, Inj. (Lilly).
NPH-N Purified (Pork), Inj. (Novo Nordisk).
Pork NPH Iletin II, Inj. (Lilly).
Insulatard NPH (Pork), Inj. (Novo Nordisk).
Humulin N, Inj. (Lilly).
Insulatard NPH, Inj. (Novo Nordisk).
Novolin N, Inj. (Novo Nordisk).
Novolin N PenFill, Cartridge (Novo Nordisk).
insulin suspension, PZI. *otc.*
Use: Antidiabetic.
See: Humulin U Ultralente, Inj. (Lilly).
insulin suspension semilente. *otc.*
Use: Antidiabetic.
See: Semilente Iletin I (Beef or Pork), Inj. (Lilly).
Semilente Insulin (Beef), Inj. (Novo Nordisk).
insulin suspension, ultralente. *otc.*
Use: Antidiabetic.
See: Ultralente Insulin (Beef), Inj. (Novo Nordisk).
Humulin U Ultralente, Inj. (Lilly).
•**insulin zinc suspension,** U.S.P. 23.
Use: Antidiabetic.
See: Humulin L, Bot. (Lilly).
Lente Insulin, Vial (Lilly).
Lente Insulin, Vial (Novo Nordisk).
Lente L, Vial (Novo Nordisk).
Novolin L, Vial (Novo Nordisk).
•**insulin zinc suspension, extended,** U.S.P. 23.
Use: Antidiabetic.
See: Humulin U Ultralente, Bot. (Lilly).
Ultralente U, Vial (Novo Nordisk).
•**insulin zinc, prompt, suspension,** U.S.P. 23.
Use: Antidiabetic.
Intal Inhaler. (Fisons) Cromolyn sodium inhalation aerosol 800 mcg/actuation. Canister 8.1 g, 14.2 g. *Rx.*
Use: Respiratory inhalant product.
Intal Nebulizer Solution. (Fisons) Cromolyn sodium 20 mg in 2 ml distilled water for use with a power operated nebulizer unit. Box 60s, 120s, Amp. 2 ml. *Rx.*
Use: Respiratory inhalant product.
Integrin Caps. (Sanofi Winthrop) Oxypertine. *Rx.*
Use: Anxiolytic, tranquilizer.

Intensol. (Roxane) A system of concentrated solutions of drugs w/calibrated dropper:
    Chlorpromazine HCl 30 mg or 100 mg/ml.
    Dexamethasone 1 mg/ml.
    Dihydrotachysterol 0.2 mg/ml.
    Hydrochlorothiazide 100 mg/ml.
    Prednisone 5 mg/ml.
    Thioridazine HCl 30 mg or 100 mg/ml.

interferon. (IN-ter-FEER-ahn) A family of naturally occurring, small protein molecules with molecular weights of approximately 15,000 to 21,000 daltons. They are formed by the interaction of animal cells with viruses capable of conferring on animal cells resistance to virus infection. Three major classes of interferons have been identified: alpha, beta, and gamma. Interferon was first derived from human white blood cells and originally used in Finland.
    Use: Antineoplastic, antiviral. Treatment of breast cancer lymphoma, multiple melanoma and malignant melanoma.
    See: Actimmune (Genentech).
    Alferon-N (Purdue-Frederick).
    Avonex (Biogen).
    Betaseron (Berlex).
    Intron-A, Inj. (Schering Plough).
    Roferon-A (Roche).

• **interferon alfa-2a.** (IN-ter-FEER-ahn AL-fuh-2a) USAN.
    Use: Antineoplastic, antiviral; biological response modifier. [Orphan drug]
    See: Roferon-A (Roche).

• **interferon alfa-2b.** (IN-ter-FEER-ahn AL-fuh-2b) USAN.
    Use: Antineoplastic, antiviral; biological response modifier. [Orphan drug]
    See: Intron-A (Schering Plough).

• **interferon alfa-n1.** USAN.
    Use: Antiviral, antineoplastic; biological response modifier. [Orphan drug]
    See: Wellferon (Glaxo Wellcome).

• **interferon alfa-n3.** (IN-ter-FEER-ahn AL-fuh n3) *Formerly Leukocyte Interferon.*
    Use: Antiviral, antineoplastic; biological response modifier.
    See: Alferon-N (Purdue-Frederick).

interferon beta. (IN-ter-FEER-ahn BAY-tuh) *Rx.*
    Use: Cytokine agent; treatment of multiple sclerosis.
    See: Betaseron (Berlex).

• **interferon beta-1a.** (in-ter-FEER-ohn BAY-tah-1a) USAN
    Use: Antineoplastic, biological response modifier, immunomodulator, antineo-blast. [Orphan drug]
    See: Avonex (Berlex).

• **interferon beta-1b.** USAN.
    Use: Immunomodulator.
    See: Betaseron (Berlex).

interferon beta (recombinant). *Rx.*
    Use: Immune therapy. [Orphan drug]
    See: r-IFN-beta, R-Frone.

• **interferon gamma-1b.** (IN-ter-FEER-ahn GAM-uh-1b). USAN.
    Use: Antineoplastic, antiviral, immunoregulator, biological response modifier. [Orphan drug]
    See: Actimmune (Genentech).

interleukin-1 receptor antagonist, human recombinant. *Rx.*
    Use: Juvenile rheumatoid arthritis, graft-v-host disease in transplant patients. [Orphan drug]

interleukin-2. *Rx.*
    Use: Cytokine agent. [Orphan drug]
    See: Proleukin (Chiron).

interleukin-2, recombinant liposome encapsulated. *Rx.*
    Use: Antineoplastic. [Orphan drug]

interleukin-2 PEG. (Cetus). *Rx.*
    Use: Cytokine agent.

interleukin-3, recombinant human. (Sandoz). *Rx.*
    Use: Cytokine agent. [Orphan drug]

Intralipid 10% I.V. Fat Emulsion. (Pharmacia & Upjohn) IV fat emulsion containing soybean oil 10%, egg yolk phospholipids 1.2%, glycerin 2.25% and water for injection. I.V. Flask 50 ml, 100 ml, 250 ml, 500 ml. *Rx.*
    Use: Parenteral nutritional supplement.

Intralipid 20% I.V. Fat Emulsion. (Pharmacia & Upjohn) IV fat emulsion containing soybean oil 20%, egg yolk phospholipids 1.2%, glycerin 2.25% and water for injection. I.V. Flask 50 ml, 100 ml, 250 ml, 500 ml. *Rx.*
    Use: Parenteral nutritional supplement.

intranasal steroids.
    See: Beconase AQ Nasal (Allen & Hanburys).
    Beconase Inhalation (Allen & Hanburys).
    Decadron Phosphate Turbinaire (Merck).
    Flonase (Allen & Hanburys).
    Nasalide (Syntex).
    Nasacort (Rhone-Poulenc Rorer).
    Vancenase Nasal Inhaler (Schering Plough).
    Rhinocort (Astra).
    Vancenase AQ Nasal (Schering Plough).

Intrasite. (Smith & Nephew) Graft T starch copolymer 2%, water 8%, propylene glycol 20%. Sterile amorphous interactive hydrogel dressing. 25 g. *Rx.*
Use: Wound dressing.

intrauterine progesterone system. *Rx.*
Use: Contraceptive.
See: Progestasert (Alza).

intraval sodium.
See: Pentothal Sodium, Preps. (Abbott).

•**intrazole.** USAN. 1-(p-Chlorobenzoyl)-3-(1H-tetrazol-5-ylmethyl) indole.
Use: Anti-inflammatory.

•**intriptyline hydrochloride.** (in-TRIP-tih-leen) USAN.
Use: Antidepressant.

Introlite. (Ross) Protein 22.2 g, carbohydrate 70.5 g, fat 18.4 g, sodium 930 mg, potassium 1570 mg/L with 200 mOsm/kg water, with appropriate vitamins and minerals, 0.53 Cal/ml. Liq. *otc.*
Use: Nutritional supplement.

Intron-A for Injection. (Schering Plough) **Pow. for Inj.:** 3 million/1 ml vial diluent/Multidose vial; 3 million IU/1 ml vial diluent with ⅝-inch, 25-gauge needle/Multidose vial, Pkg. 6s.; 5 million IU/1 ml vial diluent with ⅝ inch, 25-gauge needle/Multidose vial, Pkg. 6s.; 10 million IU/2 ml vial diluent/Multidose vial; 10 million IU/1 ml syringe diluent with ⅝-inch, 25-gauge needle/Multidose vial, Pkg. 6s.; 18 million IU/3.8 ml vial diluent/Multidose vial; 25 million IU/5 ml vial diluent/Multidose vial; 50 million IU/1 ml vial diluent/Multidose vial. **Soln:** 10 million IU/2 ml, 18 million IU/3 ml, 25 million IU/5 ml Multidose vial. *Rx.*
Use: Antineoplastic.

Intropaque Liquid. (Lafayette) Barium sulfate 60% w/v suspension. Bot. gal. Case 4 Bot.
Use: Radiopaque agent.

Intropin 200 mg. (DuPont Merck) Dopamine HCl 40 mg/ml, sodium bisulfite 1% as an antioxidant. Vial 5 ml. Box 20s; Amp. 5 ml. Box 20s; Prefilled additive Syr. 5 ml. Box 5s. *Rx.*
Use: Vasopressor used in shock.

Intropin 400 mg. (DuPont Merck) Dopamine HCl 80 mg/ml, sodium bisulfite 1% as an antioxidant. Vial 5 ml. Box 20s.; Prefilled additive Syringe 5 ml. Box 5s. *Rx.*
Use: Vasopressor used in shock.

Intropin 800 mg. (DuPont Merck) Dopamine HCl 160 mg/ml, sodium bisulfite 1% as an antioxidant. Vial 5 ml. Box 20s.; Prefilled additive syringe 5 ml. Box 5s. *Rx.*

Use: Vasopressor used in shock.

inulin. (DuPont Merck) Purified inulin 5 g/50 ml sodium Cl 0.9%, sodium hydroxide to adjust pH. Amp. 50 ml.
Use: Diagnostic aid.

•**inulin,** U.S.P. 23.
Use: Diagnostic aid (renal function determination).

Inversine. (Merck) Mecamylamine HCl 2.5 mg, lactose/Tab. Bot. 100s. *Rx.*
Use: Antihypertensive.

invert sugar. (Abbott) 10% soln. Bot. 1000 ml. *otc, Rx.*
Use: Parenteral nutritional supplement.
See: Travert, Soln. (Baxter).

invert sugar-electrolyte solutions. *Rx.*
Use: Parenteral nutritional supplement.
See: Ionosol G and 10% Invert Sugar (Abbott).
    Multiple Electrolyte 2 w/5% Invert Sugar (McGaw).
    5% Travert and Electrolyte No. 2 (Baxter).
    Ionosol B and 10% Invert Sugar (Abbott).
    10% Travert and Electrolyte No. 2 (Baxter).
    Multiple Electrolyte 2 w/10% Invert Sugar (McGaw).
    Ionosol D and 10% Invert Sugar (Abbott).

invert sugar injection.
Use: Replenisher (fluid and nutrient).

Invirase. (Roche) Saquinavir 200 mg, lactose/Cap. 270s. *Rx.*
Use: Antiviral.

•**iobenguane I 123 injection,** (EYE-oh-BEN-gwane) U.S.P. 23.
Use: Radioactive agent.

•**iobenguane sulfate I 123.** USAN.
Use: Diagnostic aid, radioactive adrenomedullary disorders and neuroendocrine tumors); radioactive agent.

•**iobenzamic acid.** (EYE-oh-ben-ZAM-ik) USAN. Osbil.
Use: Diagnostic aid (radiopaque medium; cholecystographic).

Iobid DM. (Iomed) Dextromethorphan HBr 30 mg, guaifenesin 600 mg/SR Tab. Bot. 100s, 500s. *Rx.*
Use: Antitussive, expectorant.

•**iocanlidic acid I 123.** USAN.
Use: Diagnostic aid for assessment of viable myocardium.

Iocare Balanced Salt Solution. (Ciba Vision) Sodium Cl 0.64%, potassium Cl 0.075%, magnesium Cl 0.03%, calcium Cl 0.048%, sodium acetate 0.39%, sodium citrate 0.17%, sodium hydrox-

ide or hydrochloric acid. Soln. Bot. 15 ml. *Rx.*
Use: Intraocular irrigation solution.

• **iocarmate meglumine.** (EYE-oh-CAR-mate meh-GLUE-meen) USAN.
Use: Diagnostic aid (radiopaque medium).

• **iocarmic acid.** (EYE-oh-CAR-mik) USAN. Dimer X is a sterile solution of the meglumine salt.
Use: Diagnostic aid (radiopaque medium).

• **iocetamic acid,** U.S.P. 23.
Use: Diagnostic aid (radiopaque medium).

Iocon Gel. (Galderma) Polyoxyethylene ethers, coal tar solution, Iopol (a cationic polymer), alcohol 1%, benzalkonium Cl in a non-ionic/amphoteric base. Tube 3.5 oz . *otc.*
Use: Antiseborrheic.

i-octadecanol.
See: Stearyl Alcohol, N.F. 18.

Iodal HD. (Iomed) Hydrocodone bitartrate 1.67 mg, phenylephrine HCl 2 mg, chlorpheniramine maleate 2 mg/5 ml. Liq. Bot. 473 ml. *c-III.*
Use: Antitussive, decongestant, antihistamine.

• **iodamide.** (EYE-oh-dah-mide) USAN.
Use: Diagnostic aid (radiopaque medium).

• **iodamide meglumine.** (EYE-oh-dah-MIDE meh-GLUE-meen) USAN.
Use: Diagnostic aid (radiopaque medium).
W/Combinations:
See: Renovue-65, Vial (Squibb).
Renovue-Dip, Vial (Squibb).

Iodex. (KM Lee) Iodine 4.7% in petrolatum ointment base. Jar 1 oz, 14 oz. *otc.*
Use: Antiseptic, germicide.

Iodex w/Methyl Salicylate. (KM Lee) Iodine 4.7%, methyl salicylate 4.8% in petrolatum ointment base. *otc.*
Use: Antiseptic, analgesic (topical).

iodinated I-125 albumin injection.
Use: Diagnostic aid (blood volume determination), radioactive agent.
See: albumin, iodinated I 125.

iodinated I-131 albumin aggregated injection.
Use: Radioactive agent.
See: albumin, aggregated iodinated I 131 serum.

iodinated I-131 albumin injection.
Use: Diagnostic aid (blood volume determination and intrathecal imaging), radioactive agent.

See: albumin, iodinated I-131.

iodinated glycerol and codeine phosphate liquid. (Various Mfr.) Codeine phosphate 10 mg, iodinated glycerol 30 mg/Liq. Bot. pt and gal. *c-v.*
Use: Narcotic antitussive, expectorant.

iodinated glycerol/theophylline.
See: Iophylline (Various Mfr.).

iodinated human serum albumin.
See: Albumotope (Squibb).

• **iodine,** (EYE-uh-dine) U.S.P. 23.
Use: Anti-infective, topical; source of iodine.
See: Kelp, Tab. (Quality Generics).

iodine cacodylate, colloidal. Cacodyne Iodine.

iodine 131: capsules diagnostic - capsules therapeutic - solution therapeutic oral.
See: Iodotope (Squibb).

iodine combination.
See: Calcidrine, Syr. (Abbott).

iodine I^{123} murine monoclonal antibody to alpha-fetoprotein. (Immunomedics)
Use: Diagnostic aid. [Orphan drug]

iodine I^{123} murine monoclonal antibody to hCG. (Immunomedics)
Use: Diagnostic aid. [Orphan drug]

iodine I^{131} 6b-iodomethyl-19-norcholesterol.
Use: Diagnostic aid. [Orphan drug]

iodine I^{131} metaiodobenzylguanidine sulfate.
Use: Diagnostic aid. [Orphan drug]

iodine I^{131} murine monoclonal antibody to alpha-fetoprotein. (Immunomedics) *Rx.*
Use: Antineoplastic. [Orphan drug]

iodine I^{131} murine monoclonal antibody to hCG. (Immunomedics) *Rx.*
Use: Antineoplastic. [Orphan drug]

iodine I^{131} murine monoclonal antibody IgG2a to B cell. (Immunomedics) *Rx.*
Use: Antineoplastic. [Orphan drug]

iodine-iodophor.
See: Betadine, Preps. (Purdue Frederick).
Isodine, Preps. (Blair).

iodine povidone.
See: Efodine, Oint. (Fougera).
Iodophor.
Mallsol, Liq. (Roberts).

iodine products, anti-infective.
See: Anayodin.
Betadine, Preps. (Purdue Frederick).
Chiniofon.
Diodoquin, Tab. (Searle).

Diiodo-Hydroxyquinoline (Various Mfr.).

Isodine, Preps. (Blair).

Prepodyne, Soln., Scrub (West).

Quinoxyl.

Surgidine, Liq. (Continental).

Vioform, Preps. (Ciba).

iodine products, diagnostic.
See: Chloriodized Oil (Various Mfr.).
Ethyl Iodophenylundecylate (Various Mfr.).
Iodized Oil.
Iodoalphionic Acid (Various Mfr.).
Iodobrassid.
Iodohippurate Sodium (Various Mfr.).
Iodopanoic Acid (Various Mfr.).
Iodophthalein Sodium (Various Mfr.).
Iodopyracet, Preps. (Various Mfr.).
Lipiodol Lafay, Amp., Vial (Savage).
Methiodal Sodium (Various Mfr.).
Pantopaque, Amp. (Lafayette).
Sodium Acetrizoate (Various Mfr.).
Sodium Iodomethamate (Various Mfr.).
Telepaque, Tab. (Sanofi Winthrop).

iodine products, nutritional.
See: Calcium Iodobehenate (Various Mfr.).
Entodon.
Hydriodic Acid (Various Mfr.).
Iodobrassid (Various Mfr.).
Potassium Iodide (Various Mfr.).

iodine ration, (Barth's) Iodine (from kelp) 0.15 mg, trace minerals/Tab. Bot. 90s, 180s, 360s. otc.
Use: Mineral supplement.

iodine ration. (Nion) Iodine (from kelp) 0.15 mg/3 Tab. Bot. 175s, 500s. otc.
Use: Mineral supplement.

iodide, sodium, I-123 capsules. (EYE-uh-dine SO-dee-uhm)
Use: Diagnostic aid (thyroid function determination).

iodide, sodium, I-123 tablets.
Use: Diagnostic aid (thyroid function determination).

iodide, sodium, I-125 capsules.
Use: Diagnostic aid (thyroid function determination), radioactive agent.

iodide, sodium, I-125 solution.
Use: Diagnostic aid (thyroid function determination), radioactive agent.

iodide, sodium, I-131 capsules.
Use: Antineoplastic, diagnostic aid (thyroid function determination), radioactive agent.

iodide, sodium, I-131 solution.
Use: Antineoplastic, diagnostic aid (thyroid function determination), radioactive agent.

iodine soluble.
See: Burnham Soluble Iodine, Soln. (Burnham).

iodine surface active complex.
See: Ioprep, Soln. (Arbrook).

iodine tincture, strong.
Use: Anti-infective, topical.

•**iodipamide,** U.S.P. 23. Adipiodone (I.N.N.).
Use: Pharmaceutic necessity for Iodipamide Meglumine Injection.

•**iodipamide meglumine injection,** U.S.P. 23.
Use: Diagnostic aid (radiopaque medium).

iodipamide methylglucamine. Also sodium salt inj.
W/Diatrizoate methylglucamine.
See: Sinografin, Vial (Squibb).

•**iodipamide sodium I 131.** USAN.
Use: Radioactive agent.

iodipamide sodium injection.
See: Cholografin Sodium, Soln. (Various Mfr.).

•**iodixanol.** (EYE-oh-DIX-an-ole) USAN
Use: Diagnostic aid (radiopaque medium).

iodized oil. A vegetable oil containing not less than 38% and not more than 42% of organically combined iodine.
Use: Diagnostic aid.
See: Lipiodol Lafay, Amp., Vial (Savage).

iodized poppy-seed oil.
See: Lipiodol Lafay, Amp., Vial (Savage).

iodoalphionic acid. Biliselectan dikol, pheniodol.

•**iodoantipyrine I 131.** USAN.
Use: Radioactive agent.

iodobehenate calcium. Calcium iododocosanoate.
Use: Antigoitrogenic.

iodobrassid. Ethyl Diiodobrassidate. Lipoiodine.

•**iodocetylic acid I 123.** (eye-OH-doe-SEE-till-ik) USAN.
Use: Diagnostic aid, radioactive agent.

•**iodocholesterol I-131.** (EYE-oh-DOE-koe-LESS-teh-role) USAN.
Use: Radioactive agent.

iodochlorhydroxyquin. Clioquinol, U.S.P. 23.

Iodo Cream. (Day-Baldwin) Clioquinol 3%. Tube 1 oz, Jar 1 lb. otc.
Use: Antifungal, topical.

Iodo H-C. (Day-Baldwin) Clioquinol 3%, hydrocortisone 1%. **Oint.:** Tube 20 g,

Jar 1 lb. **Cream:** Tube 20 g, Jar 1 lb.
Rx.
Use: Antifungal, corticosteroid.

•**iodohippurate sodium I 123 injection,** (EYE-oh-doe-HIP-you-rate) U.S.P. 23.
Use: Radioactive agent, diagnostic aid (renal function determination).

•**iodohippurate sodium I 125.** USAN.
Use: Radioactive agent.
See: Hipputope I 125 (Squibb).

•**iodohippurate, sodium I 131 injection,** U.S.P. 23.
Use: Diagnostic aid (renal function determination), radioactive agent.
See: Hipputope (Squibb).

iodo-hippuric acid.
See: Hipputope (Squibb).

iodol. 2,3,4,5-Tetraiodopyrrole.

Iodo Ointment. (Day-Baldwin) Clioquinol 3%. Tube oz, Jar lb. *Rx.*
Use: Antifungal, topical.

Iodo-Pak. (SoloPak) Iodine 100 mcg/ml. Inj. Vial 10 ml. *Rx.*
Use: Parenteral nutritional supplement.

iodopanoic acid.
Use: Diagnostic aid (radiopaque medium).

Iodopen. (Fujisawa) Sodium iodide 118 mcg/ml. Vial 3 ml, 10 ml. *Rx.*
Use: Parenteral nutritional supplement.

iodophene. Iodophthalein.

iodophene sodium.
See: Iodophthalein Sodium (Various Mfr.).

iodophor.
See: Betadine, Preps. (Purdue Frederick).
Isodine, Preps. (Blair).

iodophthalein sodium. Tetraiodophenolphthalein Sodium, Tetraiodophthalein Sodium, Tetiothalein Sodium (Antinosin, Cholepulvis, Cholumbrin, Foriod, Iodophene, Iodorayoral, Nosophene Sodium, Opacin, Photobiline, Piliophen, Radiotetrane).
Use: Radiopaque agent.

iodopropylidene glycerol.
See: Organidin, Elix., Tab., Soln. (Wampole).

•**iodopyracet I 125.** USAN.
Use: Radioactive agent.

•**iodopyracet I 131.** USAN.
Use: Radioactive agent.
See: Diodrast (R)-131.

iodopyracet inj. (Diatrast, Diodone, Iopyracil, Neo-Methiodal, NeoSkiodan).
Use: Radiopaque medium.

iodopyracet compound. Diodrast.

iodopyracet concentrated. Diodrast.

iodopyrine. Antipyrine iodide.
Use: Iodides, analgesic.

•**iodoquinol,** (EYE-oh-doe-KWIH-nole) U.S.P. 23. *Formerly Diiodohydroxyquin.*
Use: Antiamebic.
See: Floraquin (Searle).
Sebaquin, Shampoo (Summers Labs).
W/9-Aminoacridine HCl.
See: Vagitric, Cream (ICN Pharm).
Yodoxin, Tab., Pow. (Glenwood).
W/Hydrocortisone alcohol.
See: Vytone, Cream (Dermik).
W/Hydrocortisone, coal tar solution.
See: Cor-Tar-Quin, Cream, Lot. (Bayer).
W/Stilbestrol, sulfadiazine, tartaric acid, boric acid, etc.
See: Gynben, Vag. Insert, Cream (I. C. N).
Gynben Insufflate, Pow. (I. C. N).
W/Surfactants.
See: Lycinate, Supp. (Hoechst Marion Roussel).
W/Sulfanilamide, diethylstilbestrol.
See: Amide V/S, Vaginal Insert. (Scrip).
D.I.T.I. Creme (Dunhall).

Iodotope (Diagnostic). (Squibb) Sodium iodide I-131 for oral use. 7, 14, 28, 70, 106 units Ci/Vial of 5, 10, 15, 20 Cap.
Use: Diagnostic aid.

Iodotope (Therapeutic). (Bracco Diagnostics) Sodium iodide I-131. 1 to 50 mCi Cap./7, 14, 28, 70, 106 mCi, EDTA 1 mg/solution. *Rx.*
Use: Antithyroid.

•**iodoxamate meglumine.** (EYE-oh-DOX-ah-mate meh-GLUE-meen) USAN.
Use: Diagnostic aid (radiopaque medium).

•**iodoxamic acid.** (EYE-oh-dox-AM-ik) USAN.
Use: Diagnositc aid (radiopaque medium).

iodoxyl.
See: Sodium Iodomethamate (Various Mfr.).

Iofed. (Iomed) Brompheniramine maleate 12 mg, pseudoephedrine HCl 120 mg/ER Cap. Bot. 100s. *Rx.*
Use: Antihistamine, decongestant.

Iofed PD. (Iomed) Brompheniramine maleate 6 mg, pseudoephedrine HCl 60 mg/ER Cap. Bot. 100s. *Rx.*
Use: Antihistamine, decongestant.

•**iofetamine hydrochloride I 123.** (EYE-oh-FET-ah-meen) USAN.
Use: Diagnostic aid, radioactive agent.

•**ioglicic acid.** (eye-oh-GLIH-sick) USAN.

Use: Diagnostic aid (radiopaque medium).

●**ioglucol.** (EYE-oh-GLUE-kahl) USAN.
Use: Diagnostic aid (radiopaque medium).

●**ioglucomide.** (EYE-oh-GLUE-koe-mide) USAN.
Use: Diagnostic aid (radiopaque medium).

●**ioglycamic acid.** (EYE-oh-glie-KAM-ik) USAN. Biligram, Bilivistan.
Use: Diagnostic aid (radiopaque medium, cholecystographic).

●**iogulamide.** (EYE-oh-GULL-ah-mide) USAN.
Use: Diagnostic aid (radiopaque medium).

●**iohexol.** (EYE-oh-HEX-ole) U.S.P. 23.
Use: Diagnostic aid (radiopaque medium).

Iohist D. (Iomed) Phenylopropanolamine HCl 12.5 mg, phenyltoloxamine citrate 4 mg, pyrilamine maleate 4 mg, pheniramine maleate 4 mg, alcohol 4 %/5 ml. Pt. *Rx.*
Use: Decongestant, antihistamine.

Iohist DM. (Iomed) Dextromethorphan HBr 10 mg, phenylpropanolamine HCl 12.5 mg, brompheniramine maleate 2 mg/5ml. Syrup. Alcohol and sugar free. Bot. pt. *Rx.*
Use: Antitussive, decongestant, antihistamine.

Iohydro Cream. (Freeport) Hydrocortisone 1%, clioquinol 3%, pramoxine HCl 0.5%/0.5 oz. Tube 0.5 oz.
Use: Corticosteroid, antifungal, local anesthetic, topical.

●**iomeprol.** (EYE-oh-MEH-prole) USAN
Use: Diagnostic aid (radiopaque medium).

●**iomethin I 125.** (EYE-oh-METH-in) USAN.
Use: Diagnostic aid (neoplasm); radioactive agent.

●**iomethin I 131.** (EYE-o-METH-in) USAN.
Use: Diagnostic aid (neoplasm); radioactive agent.

Ionamin. (Pfizer) Phentermine. Resin base 15 mg and 30 mg lactose/Cap. Bot. 100s, 400s. *c-iv.*
Use: Anorexiant.

Ionax Astringent Cleanser. (Galderma) Isopropyl alcohol 48%, acetone, salicylic acid. Bot. 240 ml. *otc.*
Use: Antiacne.

Ionax Foam. (Galderma) Benzalkonium Cl, propylene glycol. Aerosol can 150 ml. *otc.*

Use: Antiacne.

Ionax Scrub. (Galderma) SD Alcohol 40, benzalkonium Cl. Tube 60 g, 120 g. *otc.*
Use: Antiacne.

ionaze.
See: Propazolamide.

I-131 radiolabeled b1 monoclonal antibody. (Coulter) *Rx.*
Use: Treatment for non-Hodgkin's B-cell lymphoma. [Orphan drug]

ion-exchange resins.
See: Polyamine Methylene Resin. Resins, Sodium Removing.

Ionil Plus Shampoo. (Galderma) Salicylic acid 2%, water, sodium laureth sulfate, lauramide dea, quaternium-22, talloweth-60 myristyl glycol, laureth-23, tea lauryl sulfate, glycol disterate, laureth-4, tea-abietoyl hydrolyzed collagen, DMDM hydantoin, tetrasodium EDTA, sodium hydroxide, fragrance, FD&C; blue No. 1. Bot. 4 oz, 8 oz. *otc.*
Use: Antiseborrheic.

Ionil Rinse. (Galderma) Conditioners with benzalkonium Cl in water base. Bot. 16 oz. *otc.*
Use: Hair rinse.

Ionil Shampoo. (Galderma) Salicylic acid, benzalkonium Cl, alcohol 12%, polyoxyethylene ethers. Plastic bot. w/ dispenser cap 4 oz, 8 oz, 16 oz, 32 oz. *otc.*
Use: Antiseborrheic.

Ionil T. (Galderma) A nonionic/cationic foaming shampoo w/coal tar, salicylic acid, benzalkonium Cl, alcohol 12%, polyoxyethylene ethers. Plastic bot. 4 oz, 8 oz, 16 oz, 32 oz. *otc.*
Use: Antiseborrheic.

Ionil T Plus Shampoo. (Galderma) Owentar II (equivalent to 2% coal tar), water, sodium laureth sulfate, lauramide dea, quaternium-22, laureth-23, talloweth-60 myristyl glycol, tea lauryl sulfate, glycol disterate, laureth-4, tea abietoyl hydrolyzed collagen, DMDM hydantoin, disodium EDTA, fragrance, FD&C; blue No.1, FD&C; yellow No. 70. Bot. 4 oz, 8 oz. *otc.*
Use: Antiseborrheic.

Ionosol D-CM. (Abbott Hospital Prods) Sodium Cl 516 mg, potassium Cl 89.4 mg, calcium Cl anhydrous 27.8 mg, magnesium Cl anhydrous 14.2 mg, sodium lactate 560 mg/100 ml. Bot. 1000 ml. *Rx.*
Use: Parenteral nutrient.

●**iopamidol,** (EYE-oh-PAM-ih-dahl) U.S.P. 23.

Use: Diagnostic aid (radiopaque medium).
See: Isovue-300, Inj. (Squibb).
Isovue-370, Inj. (Squibb).
Isovue-M 200, Inj. (Squibb).
Isovue-M 300, Inj. (Squibb).

• **iopanoic acid,** U.S.P. 23.
Use: Diagnostic aid (radiopaque medium).
See: Telepaque, Tab. (Sanofi Winthrop).

• **iopentol.** (EYE-oh-PEN-tole) USAN.
Use: Diagnostic aid (radiopaque medium).

Iophen. (Various Mfr.) 30 mg/Tab., 100s. 60 mg/5 ml/Elixer, 120 and 480 ml. 50 mg/ml/Soln., 30 ml. *Rx.*
Use: Expectorant.

• **iophendylate,** U.S.P. 23. Benzenedecanoic acid, iodo-t-methyl-, ethyl ester.
Use: Diagnostic aid (radiopaque medium).

iophendylate injection. Ethiodan, Myodil. Ethyl Iodophenylundecylate.
Use: Diagnostic aid (radiopaque medium).
See: Pantopaque, Amp. (LaFayette).

iophenoxic acid. (EYE-oh-pro-SEH-mik Acid) Tab.

Iophylline. (Various Mfr.) Theophylline 120 mg, iodinated glycerol 30 mg/15 ml. Elixir. Bot. 480 ml. *Rx.*
Use: Antiasthmatic combination.

Iopidine. (Alcon) Apraclonidine 0.5% or 1%, benzalkonium Cl 0.01%. Dispenser Bot. 0.25 ml (1%), Drop-Tainer 5 ml (0.5%). *Rx.*
Use: Agent for glaucoma.

iopodate sodium.
See: Ipodate Sodium.

Ioprep. (Johnson & Johnson) Nonylphenoxypolyethylenoxy (4) ethanol and nonylphenoxypolyethyleneoxy (15) ethanol iodine complex 5.5%, nonylphenoxypolyethyleneoxy (30) ethanol 10%. Solution provides 1% available iodine. Plastic bot. gal.
Use: Antiseptic.

• **ioprocemic acid.** (EYE-oh-pro-SEH-mik acid) USAN.
Use: Diagnostic aid; radiopaque medium.

• **iopromide.** (eye-oh-PRO-mide) USAN.
Use: Diagnostic aid (radiopaque medium).
See: Ultravist, Inj. (Berlex).

• **iopronic acid.** (eye-oh-PRO-nik Acid) USAN.
Use: Diagnostic aid (radiopaque medium, cholecystographic).

• **iopydol.** (eye-oh-PIE-dahl) USAN.
Use: Diagnostic aid (radiopaque medium, bronchographic).

• **iopydone.** (eye-oh-PIE-dohn) USAN.
Use: Diagnostic aid (radiopaque medium, bronchographic).

Iosal II. (Iomed) Pseudoephedrine HCl 60 mg, guaifenesin 600 mg/Tab. ER. 100s. *Rx.*
Use: Expectorant.

• **iosefamic acid.** (EYE-oh-seh-FAM-ik) USAN.
Use: Diagnostic aid; radiopaque medium.

• **ioseric acid.** (eye-oh-SEH-rik) USAN.
Use: Diagnostic aid (radiopaque medium).

Iosopan. (Goldline) Magaldrate 540 mg/5 ml. Liq. Bot. 355 ml. *otc.*
Use: Antacid.

Iosopan Plus. (Goldline) Magaldrate 540 mg, simethicone 40 mg/5 ml. Liq. Bot. 355 ml. *otc.*
Use: Antacid.

• **iosulamide meglumine.** (eye-oh-SULL-ah-mide meh-GLUE-meen) USAN.
Use: Diagnostic aid (radiopaque medium).

• **iosumetic acid.** (eye-oh-sue-MEH-tick) USAN.
Use: Diagnostic aid (radiopaque medium).

• **iotasul.** (EYE-oh-tah-sull) USAN.
Use: Diagnostic aid (radiopaque medium).

• **iotetric acid.** (eye-oh-TEH-trick) USAN.
Use: Diagnostic aid (radiopaque medium).

iothalamate meglumide and iothalmate sodium injection.
Use: Diagnostic aid (radiopaque medium).

• **iothalamate meglumine injection,** U.S.P. 23.
Use: Diagnostic aid (radiopaque medium).

• **iothalamate sodium injection,** (eye-oh-THAL-am-ate) U.S.P. 23.
Use: Diagnostic aid (radiopaque medium).

• **iothalamate sodium I 125,** (eye-oh-THAL-am-ate) U.S.P. 23.
Use: Radioactive agent.

• **iothalamate sodium I 131,** (eye-oh-THAL-am-ate) USAN.
Use: Radioactive agent.

• **iothalamic acid,** (eye-oh-THAL-am-ik) U.S.P. 23
Use: Diagnostic aid (radiopaque medium).

Iothiouracil sodium. Sodium salt of 5-iodo-2-thiouracil.

• **iotrolan.** (EYE-oh-TRAHL-an) USAN.
Formerly Iotrol.
Use: Diagnostic aid, (radiopaque medium).

• **iotroxic acid.** (EYE-oh-TRAHK-sick) USAN.
Use: Diagnostic aid (radiopaque medium).

Iotussin HC. (Iomed Labs) Hydrocodone bitartrate 2.5 mg, phenylephrine HCl 5 mg, chlorpheniramine maleate 2 mg/5ml. Alcohol and sugar free. Syr. Bot. 473 ml. *c-III.*
Use: Antitussive, decongestant, antihistamine.

• **iotyrosine I 131.** USAN.
Use: Radioactive agent.

• **ioversol.** (EYE-oh-ver-SAHL) USAN.
Use: Diagnostic aid (radiopaque medium).
See: Optiray 350, Inj. (Mallinckrodt Medical).

• **ioxaglate meglumine.** (eye-ox-AGG-late meh-GLUE-meen) USAN.
Use: Diagnostic aid (radiopaque medium).
See: Hexabrix, Inj. (Wallace).

ioxaglate meglumine/ioxaglate sodium.
Use: Radiopaque agent.
See: Hexabrix (Mallinckrodt).

• **ioxaglate sodium.** (eye-ox-AGG-late) USAN.
Use: Diagnostic aid (radiopaque medium).

• **ioxaglic acid,** (eye-ox-AGG-lick) U.S.P. 23.
Use: Diagnostic aid (radiopaque medium).

• **ioxilan.** (eye-OX-ee-lan) USAN
Use: Diagnostic aid.

• **ioxotrizoic acid.** (eye-OX-oh-TRY-zoe-ik) USAN.
Use: Diagnostic aid (radiopaque medium).

• **ipazilide fumarate.** (ih-PAZZ-ih-LIDE) USAN
Use: Cardiac depressant (antiarrhythmic).

• **ipecac,** (IPP-uh-kak) U.S.P. 23.
Use: Emetic.
W/Combinations.
See: Balmial Cough Syrup, Syr. (Clapp).
Creozets, Loz. (Creomulsion Co.).
Derfort, Cap. (Cole).
Ipsatol/DM, Cough Syr. (Key).

Ipsatol, Syr. (Key).
Mallergan, Liq. (Roberts)
Polyectin, Liq. (T.E. Williams).
Rubacac, Tab. (Scrip).
Spenlaxo, Tab. (Rugby).
Terpium, Tab. (Scrip).

ipecac. (Various Mfr.) 1.5% to 1.75% alcohol/Syrup. 15, 30 ml. *otc.*
Use: Antidote.

ipecac. (Various Mfr.) 2% alcohol/Syrup. 15, 30 ml. *Rx.*
Use: Antidote.

• **ipexidine mesylate.** (eye-PEX-ih-DEEN) USAN.
Use: Dental caries prophylactic.

I-Pilopine. (Akorn) Pilocarpine HCl 1%. Ophthalmic soln. Bot. 15 ml. *Rx.*
Use: Agent for glaucoma.

• **ipodate calcium,** U.S.P. 23.
Use: Diagnostic aid (radiopaque medium).
See: Oragrafin calcium, Granules (Squibb).

• **ipodate sodium,** U.S.P. 23.
Use: Diagnostic aid (radiopaque medium).
See: Bilivist, Cap. (Berlex).
Oragrafin sodium, Cap., Vial (Squibb).

Ipol. (Connaught) Suspension of 3 types of poliovirus (Types 1, 2 and 3) grown in monkey kidney cell cultures. Inj. Single-dose syringe 0.5 ml. *Rx.*
Use: Vaccine.

Ipran. (Major) Propranolol HCl 10 mg, 20 mg, 40 mg, 60 mg, 80 mg, 90 mg/Tab. **10 mg, 20 mg, 40 mg:** Bot. 100s, 250s, 1000s, UD 100s; **60 mg:** Bot. 100s, 500s; **80 mg:** Bot. 100s, 500s, 1000s, UD 100s; **90 mg:** Bot. 100s, 500s. *Rx.*
Use: Beta-adrenergic blocking agent.

• **ipratropium bromide.** (IH-pruh-TROE-pee-uhm) USAN.
Use: Bronchodilator.
See: Atrovent, Aerosol (Boehringer Ingelheim).

ipratropium bromide. (Dey) 0.02% (500 mcg/vial/Soln. for Inhalation. Vials. 25 and 60 unit dose (2.5 ml each). *Rx.*
Use: Anticholinergic.

ipratropium bromide/albuterol sulfate. (Boehringer Ingelheim)
Use: Secondary treatment of chronic obstructive pulmonary disease (COPD).
See: Combivent, Inhalation aerosol. (Boehringer Ingelheim).

I-Pred. (Akorn) Prednisolone sodium phosphate 0.5% or 1%. Ophthalmic soln. Bot. 5 ml. *Rx.*

Use: Corticosteroid, ophthalmic.

I-Prednicet. (Akorn) Prednisolone acetate 1%. Ophthalmic soln. Bot. 5 ml, 10 ml. *Rx.*
Use: Corticosteroid, ophthalmic.

• **iprindole.** (IH-prin-dole) USAN. Prondol hydrochloride.
Use: Antidepressant.

• **iprofenin.** (IH-pro-FEN-in) USAN.
Use: Diagnostic aid (hepatic funtion determination).

• **ipronidazole.** (ih-pro-NIH-dah-zole) USAN. Ipropran (Roche).
Use: Antiprotozoal (Histomonas).

• **iproplatin.** (IH-pro-PLAT-in) USAN.
Use: Antineoplastic.

iproveratril. Name used for verapamil.

• **iproxamine hydrochloride.** (IH-PROX-ah-meen) USAN.
Use: Vasodilator.

• **ipsapirone hydrochloride.** (ipp-sah-PIE-rone) USAN.
Use: Antianxiety.

Ipsatol Cough Formula Liquid for Children and Adults. (Kenwood) Guaifenesin 100 mg, dextromethorphan HBr 10 mg, phenylpropanolamine HCl 9 mg/5 ml. Bot. 118 ml. *otc.*
Use: Expectorant, antitussive, decongestant.

IPV.
Use: Poliomyelitis immunization.
See: IPOL (Connaught).
Polio Virus Vaccine, Inactivated.

• **irbesartan.** (ihr-beh-SAHR-tan) USAN.
Use: Antihypertensive (angiotensin II receptor antagonist).

Ircon. (Key) Ferrous fumarate 200 mg/Tab. Bot. 100s. *otc.*
Use: Iron supplement.

Ircon-FA. (Kenwood) Ferrous fumarate 82 mg, folic acid 0.8 mg/Tab. Bot. 100s. *otc.*
Use: Iron supplement.

Irgasan CF3. Cloflucarban.
Use: Antiseptic, topical.

• **iridium Ir 192.** USAN.
Use: Radioactive agent.
See: Iriditope (Squibb).

Irigate Eye Wash. (Optopics) Sodium Cl, sodium phosphate mono- and dibasic, benzalkonium Cl, EDTA. Soln. Bot. 118 ml. *otc.*
Use: Ophthalmic irrigation solution.

• **irinotecan hydrochloride.** (eye-rih-no-TEE-can) USAN.
Use: Antineoplastic (DNA topoisomerase I inhibitor).
See: Camptosar, Inj. (Pharmacia & Upjohn).

irisin. A polysaccharide found in several species of iris.

irocaine.
See: Procaine HCl (Various Mfr.).

Irodex. (Keene) Iron dextran complex 50 mg/ml. Vial 10 ml. *Rx.*
Use: Iron supplement.

Iromin-G. (Mission) Ferrous gluconate 260 mg (iron 30 mg), vitamins B_{12} (crystalline on resin) 2 mcg, C 100 mg, A acetate 4000 IU, D 400 IU, B_1 5 mg, B_2 2 mg, B_6 20.6 mg, B_3 10 mg, B_5 1 mg, folic acid 0.8 mg, Ca/Tab. Bot. 100s. *otc.*
Use: Vitamin/mineral supplement.

iron (2+) fumarate. Ferrous Fumarate, U.S.P. 23.

iron (2+) gluconate.
See: Ferrous Gluconate, U.S.P. 23.

iron bile salts.
See: Bilron, Pulvules (Lilly).

iron carbonate complex.
See: Polyferose.

iron choline citrate complex.
See: Chel-Iron, Tab. (Kinney).
Kelex, Tabseals (Nutrition Control).

• **iron dextran injection,** (iron DEX-tran) U.S.P. 23.
Use: Hematinic.
See: Ferrodex, Inj. (Keene Pharm).
Hydextran, Inj. (Hyrex).
Imferon, Amp., Vial (Merrell Dow).

Iron-Folic 500. (Major) Ferrous sulfate 105 mg, B_1 6 mg, B_2 6mg, B_3 30 mg, B_5 10 mg, B_{12} 25 mcg, C 500 mg, folic acid 0.8 mg/Tab. Bot. 100s, 500s. *otc.*
Use: Iron with vitamin supplement.

iron/liver combinations, injection.
See: Rogenic (Forest).
Hemocyte (US Pharm).
Hytinic (Hyrex).
Licoplex DS (Keene).
Hemocyte-V (US Pharm).
Liver-Iron B Complex w/Vitamin B_{12} (Akorn).

iron/liver combination, oral.
See: Arcotinic, Tab. (Arco).
Feocyte, Tab. (Dunhill).
Rogenic, Tab. (Forest).
I-L-X B_{12}, Tab. (Kenwood).
Livitamin, Cap. (SK-Beecham).
Liquid Geritonic (Geriatric Pharm).
I-L-X B_{12} Elixir (Kenwood).
I-L-X Elixir (Kenwood).
Arcotinic Liquid (Arco).
Livitamin Liquid (SK-Beecham).

iron oxide mixture with zinc oxide.
Calamine, U.S.P. 23.

iron peptonized.

See: Saferon, Tab. (ICN Pharm).

iron products, injection.
See: InFeD (Schein).

iron protein complex.

•**iron sorbitex injection,** (SORE-bih-tex)
U.S.P. 23. *Formerly iron sorbitol.*
Use: Hematinic.
See: Jectofer, Amp. (Astra).

iron sulfate. W/Maalox.
See: Fermalox, Tab. (Rhone-Poulenc
Rorer).

iron w/vitamin B$_{12}$ and ifc.
See: Pronemia Hematinic Capsules
(Lederle).
Contrin Capsules (Geneva Pharm).
Ferotrinsic Capsules (Rugby).
Livitrinsic-f Capsules (Goldline).
Trinsicon Capsules (Whitby).
Fergon Plus Caplets (Sanofi Win-
throp).
TriHEMIC 600 Tablets (Lederle).
Heptuna Plues Capsules (Roerig).
Livitamin w/Intrinsic Factor Capsules
(Savage).
Chromagen Capsules (Savage).

Ironco-B. (Pal-Pak) Ferrous sulfate 120.4
mg, manganese sulfate 21.6 mg, dical-
cium phosphate 129.6 mg, vitamins
B$_1$ 1 mg, B$_2$ 1 mg, niacin 6 mg, D 100
IU/Tab. Bot. 100s, 1000s. *otc.*
Use: Vitamin/mineral supplement.

Irospan. (Fielding) Ferrous sulfate 200
mg, vitamin C 150 mg/Cap. Bot. 60s.
Tab. Bot. 100s. *otc.*
Use: Vitamin/mineral supplement.

irradiated ergosterol.
See: Calciferol.

Irrigate Eye Wash. (Optopics) Sodium
Cl, mono- and dibasic sodium phosphate, benzalkonium Cl, EDTA. Bot. 118
ml. *otc.*
Use: Ophthalmic irrigation solution.

irrigating solutions, physiological.
Use: Sterile irrigating solutions.
See: 0.45% Sodium Chloride Irrigation
(Abbott).
0.9% Sodium Chloride Irrigation (Ab-
bott).
Tis-U-Sol (Baxter).
Lactated Ringer's Irrigation (Abbott).
Physiolyte (American McGaw).
PhysioSol (Abbott).

irrigating solutions, urinary.
Use: Sterile irrigating solutions.
See: Neosporin G.U. Irrigant (Glaxo
Wellcome).
Renacidin (Guardian).
Resectisol (McGaw).
Sorbitol-Mannitol (Abbott).

Acetic Acid (Various Mfr.).
Glycine (Aminoacetic acid) (Various
Mfr.).
Sodium Chloride (Various Mfr.).
Sterile Water (Various Mfr.).

•**irtemazole.** (ihr-TEH-mah-zole) USAN.
Use: Uricosuric.

isacen.
See: Oxyphenisatin, Preps. (Various
Mfr.).

•**isamoxole.** (eye-SAH-MOX-ole) USAN.
Use: Antiasthmatic.

iscador. (Hiscia).
Use: Antiviral agent-Phase I.

•**isepamicin.** (eye-SEP-ah-MY-sin) USAN.
Use: Antibacterial (aminoglycoside).

ISG. Immune globulin intramuscular. *Rx.*
Use: Immune serum.
See: Gammar-IM, Inj. (Centeon).

Ismelin. (Ciba) Guanethidine monosul-
fate 10 mg or 25 mg/Tab. Bot. 100s.
Rx.
Use: Antihypertensive.

ISMO. (Wyeth-Ayerst) Isosorbide mononi-
trate 20 mg/Tab. Bot. 100s, UD 100s.
Rx.
Use: Antianginal.

Ismotic. (Alcon Surgical) Isosorbide solution. W/sodium 4.6 mEq, potassium 0.9
mEq/220 ml, alcohol, saccharin, sorbitol. In 220 ml. *Rx.*
Use: Osmotic diuretic.

iso-alcoholic elixir.
Use: Vehicle.

**isoamylhydrocupreine dihydrochlor-
ide.**
See: Eucupin Dihydrochloride.

isoamyl nitrate.
See: Amyl Nitrite, U.S.P. 23.

isoamyne.
See: Amphetamine (Various Mfr.).

Iso-B. (Tyson) B$_1$ 25 mg, B$_2$ 25 mg, B$_3$
75 mg, B$_5$ 125 mg, B$_6$ 50 mg, B$_{12}$ 100
mcg, FA 0.2 mg, pyridoxal 5 phosphate
2.5 mg, PABA 50 mg, inositol 50 mg,
choline bitartrate 125 mg, biotin 100
mcg/Cap. Bot. 120s. *otc.*
Use: Vitamin/mineral supplement.

isobornyl thiocyanoacetate, technical.
Use: Pediculicide.
See: Barc, Liq. (Del Pharm).
W/Anhydrous soap.
W/Docusate sodium and related terpe-
nes.
See: Barc, Cream (Del Pharm).

isobucaine hydrochloride, U.S.P. XXI.
Use: Local anesthetic (dental).

**isobucaine hydrochloride & epineph-
rine injection,** U.S.P. XXI.

Use: Local anesthetic, dental.

• **isobutamben.** (EYE-so-BYOO-tam-ben) USAN. Isobutyl p-aminobenzoate. Isocaine. Cycloform.
Use: Topical anesthetic.

• **isobutane,** N.F. 18.
Use: Aerosol propellant.

isobutylallylbarbituric acid.
W/Aspirin, phenacetin, caffeine.
See: Buff-A-Comp, Tab., Cap. (Mayrand).
Fiorinal, Tab., Cap. (Sandoz).
Palgesic, Tab., Cap. (Pan Amer.).
Tenstan, Tab. (Standex).
W/Codeine phosphate.
See: Fiorinal w/codeine, Cap. (Sandoz).

isobutyl p-aminobenzoate.
See: Isobutamben, U.S.A.N.

isobutyramide. (Vertex) *Rx.*
Use: Treatment of sickle cell disease and beta-thalassemia. [Orphan drug]

isocaine. Isobutamben, USAN.

Isocaine Hydrochloride. (Novocal)
Mepivacaine HCl 3%: 1.8 ml (dental cartridge). 2%: w/levonordefrin 1:20,000, sodium bisulfite. 1.8 ml (dental cartridge). *Rx.*
Use: Local anesthetic, dental.
See: Isocaine HCl, Inj. (Novocol).

Isocal. (Bristol-Myers) Lactose-free isotonic liquid containing as a percentage of the calories protein 13% as caseinate and soy protein; fat 37% as soy oil and medium chain triglycerides; carbohydrate 50% as corn syrup solids w/vitamins and minerals for the tube fed patient. Bot. 8 fl oz, 12 fl oz, 32 fl oz. *otc.*
Use: Nutritional supplement.

Isocal HCN. (Bristol-Myers) High calorie, nitrogen nutritionally complete food. Protein 15%, fat 45%, carbohydrate 40%. Can 8 fl oz. *otc.*
Use: Nutritional supplement.

Isocal HN. (Bristol-Myers) ≈ 1 Kcal/ml with protein 44 g, fat 45 g, carbohydrates 124 g/L. In 237 ml. *otc.*
Use: Nutritional supplement.

• **isocarboxazid,** U.S.P. 23.
Use: Antidepressant.
See: Marplan (Hoffman-LaRoche).

Isocet. (Rugby) Acetaminophen 325 mg, caffeine 40 mg, butalbital 50 mg/Tab. Bot. 100s. *Rx.*
Use: Nonnarcotic analgesic combinations.

Isoclor Expectorant. (Fisons) Codeine phosphate 10 mg, pseudoephedrine HCl 30 mg, guaifenesin 100 mg/5 ml, alcohol 5%. Bot. pt. *c-v.*
Use: Antitussive, decongestant, expectorant.

isococaine. Pseudococaine.

Isocom. (Nutripharm) Isometheptene mucate 65 mg, dichloralphenazone 100 mg, acetaminophen 325 mg/Cap. Bot. 50s, 100s, 250s. *Rx.*
Use: Agent for migraine.

• **isoconazole.** (EYE-so-CONE-ah-zole) USAN.
Use: Antibacterial, antifungal.

Isocult Test for Bacteriuria. (SmithKline Diagnostics)
Use: Diagnostic aid.

Isocult Test for Candida. (SmithKline Diagnostics)
Use: Diagnostic aid.

Isocult Test for Neisseria Gonorrhoeae. (SmithKline Diagnostics)
Use: Diagnostic aid.

Isocult Test for N Gonorrhoeae and Candida. (SmithKline Diagnostics)
Use: Diagnostic aid.

Isocult Test for Pseudomonas Aeruginosa. (SmithKline Diagnostics)
Use: Diagnostic aid.

Isocult Test for Staphylococcus Aureus. (SmithKline Diagnostics)
Use: Diagnostic aid.

Isocult Test for Throat Streptococci. (SmithKline Diagnostics)
Use: Diagnostic aid.

Isocult Test for Trichomonas Vaginalis. (SmithKline Diagnostics)
Use: Diagnostic aid.

Isocult Test for T Vaginalis and Candida. (SmithKline Diagnostics)
Use: Diagnostic aid.

Iso D. (Dunhall) Isosorbide dinitrate. **Cap.:** 40 mg. Bot. 100s, 1000s. **Tab.:** 5 mg (sublingual). Bot. 100s. *Rx.*
Use: Antianginal agent.

isoephedrine hydrochloride. d-Isoephedrine HCl.
See: Pseudoephedrine HCl.
W/Chlorpheniramine maleate.
See: Isoclor, Tab., Expectorant Timesule, Liq. (Arnar-Stone).
W/Chlorprophenpyridamine maleate.
See: Isoclor, Tab. (Arnar-Stone).
W/Theophylline sodium glycinate, guaifenesin.
See: Iso-Tabs 60 Tab. (Solvay).

d-isoephedrine sulfate.
See: Pseudoephedrine Sulfate.

• **isoetharine.** (EYE-so-ETH-uh-reen) USAN.

Use: Bronchodilator.

•**isoetharine hydrochloride,** (EYE-so-ETH-uh-reen) U.S.P. 23.
Use: Bronchodilator.
See: Bronkosol, Soln. (Sanofi Winthrop).

isoetharine inhalation solution.
Use: Bronchodilator.

•**isoetharine mesylate,** (EYE-so-ETH-uh-reen) U.S.P. 23.
Use: Bronchodilator.
See: Bronkometer, Aerosol (Sanofi Winthrop).

•**isoflupredone acetate.** (eye-so-FLEW-PREH-dohn) USAN.
Use: Anti-inflammatory.

•**isoflurane,** (EYE-so-FLEW-rane) U.S.P. 23.
Use: Anesthetic (inhalation).

•**isoflurophate,** U.S.P. 23.
Use: Cholinergic (ophthalmic).
See: Floropryl, Oint. (Merck).

iso-iodeikon.
See: Phentetiothalein Sodium (No Mfr. currently lists).

Isoject. (Roerig) A purified, sterile, disposable injection system.
Permapen (benzathine pencillin G) aqueous soln. 1,200,000 units/2 ml. 10s.
Terramycin (oxytetracycline) intramuscular soln. 250 mg/2 ml. 10s.
Use: Injection system.

I-Sol Solution. (Dey Labs) Sodium Cl 0.64%, potassium Cl 0.075%, calcium Cl 0.048%, magnesium Cl 0.03%, sodium acetate 0.39%, sodium citrate 0.17%, sodium hydroxide or hydrochloric acid. Soln. Bot. 20 ml, 200 ml. *otc.*
Use: Ophthalmic irrigation solution.

Isolan. (Elan) Protein 40 g, fat 36 g, carbohydrates 144 g, Na 690 g, K 1.17 g/L, with appropriate vitamins and minerals. Lactose free. Liq. In 237 ml Tetra Pak containers and 1000 ml New Pak closed systems with and without Color Check. *otc.*
Use: Nutritional supplement.

Isolate Compound Elixir. (Various Mfr.) Theophylline 45 mg, ephedrine sulfate 12 mg, isoproterenol HCl 2.5 mg, potassium iodide 150 mg, phenobarbital 6 mg/15 ml, alcohol 19%. Elix. Bot. pt, gal. *Rx.*
Use: Antiasthmatic combination.

•**isoleucine,** (EYE-so-LOO-seen) U.S.P. 23. (Pfaltz & Bauer) Pow. 10 g.
Use: Amino acid.

Isollyl Improved. (Rugby) Aspirin 325 mg, caffeine 40 mg, butalbital 50 mg/Tab. or Cap. Bot. 100s, 1000s. *c-III.*
Use: Salicylate analgesic, sedative/hypnotic.

Isolyte G with Dextrose. (American McGaw) Sodium 65 mEq, potassium 17 mEq, chloride 150 mEq, NH₄ 70 mEq, dextrose 50 g, 170 Cal, 555 mOsm/L. Bot. 1000 ml. *Rx.*
Use: Parenteral nutritional supplement.

Isolyte H with 5% Dextrose. (American McGaw) Sodium 70 mEq, potassium 13 mEq, magnesium 3 mEq, chloride 40 mEq, acetate 16 mEq, dextrose 50 g, 170 Cal, 370 mOsm/L. Inj. Soln. 1000 ml. *Rx.*
Use: Parenteral nutritional supplement.

Isolyte M with 5% Dextrose. (American McGaw) Sodium 38 mEq, chloride 44 mEq, phosphate 15 mEq, acetate 20 mEq, dextrose 50 g, 175 Cal, 405 mOsm/L. Inj. Soln. 1000 ml. *Rx.*
Use: Parenteral nutritional supplement.

Isolyte P with 5% Dextrose. (American McGaw) Sodium 25 mEq, potassium 19 mEq, magnesium 3 mEq, chloride 23 mEq, phosphate 3 mEq, acetate 23 mEq, dextrose 50 g, 175 Cal, 350 mOsm/L. Inj. Soln. 250 ml, 500 ml, 1000 ml. *Rx.*
Use: Parenteral nutritional therapy.

Isolyte R with 5% Dextrose. (American McGaw) Sodium 41 mEq, potassium 16 mEq, calcium 5 mEq, magnesium 3 mEq, chloride 40 mEq, acetate 24 mEq, dextrose 50 g, 175 Cal, 380 mOsm/L. Inj. Soln. 1000 ml. *Rx.*
Use: Parenteral nutritional supplement.

Isolyte S Ph 7.4. (American McGaw) Sodium 140 mEq, potassium 5 mEq, magnesium 3 mEq, chloride 98 mEq, acetate 27 mEq, gluconate 23 mEq, 295 mOsm/L. Inj. Soln. 500 ml, 1000 ml. *Rx.*
Use: Parenteral nutritional supplement.

Isolyte S with 5% Dextrose. (American McGaw) Sodium 140 mEq, potassium 5 mEq, magnesium 3 mEq, chloride 98 mEq, acetate 27 mEq, gluconate 23 mEq, dextrose 50 g, 185 Cal, 550 mOsm/L. Inj. Soln. 1000 ml. *Rx.*
Use: Parenteral nutritional supplement.

•**isomazole hydrochloride.** (eye-SO-mah-ZOLE) USAN.
Use: Cardiotonic.

isomeprobamate.
See: Carisoprodol (Various Mfr.).

•**isomerol.** (EYE-so-MER-ole) USAN. *Formerly Parahydrecin.*
Use: Antiseptic.

isometheptane mucate, dichloral-phenazone and acetaminophen. (eye-so-meth-EPP-teen MYOO-kate, die-klor-uhl-FEN-uh-zone and ASS-et-ah-MEE-noe-fen)

isometheptene/dichloralphenazone/ acetaminophen. *Use:* Migraine combinations. *See:* Isometheptene/Dichloral-phenazone/Acetaminophen, Cap. (Various Mfr.). Isocam, Cap. (Nutripharm). Isopap, Cap. (Geneva Pharm). Midchlor, Cap. (Schein). Midrin, Cap. (Carnrick). Migratine, Cap. (Major).

•**isometheptene mucate,** U.S.P. 23. *See:* Midrin, Cap. (Carnick).

Isomil. (Ross) Soy protein isolate infant formula containing 20 calories/fl oz. **Pow.:** Can 14 oz. **Concentrated Liq.:** Can 13 fl oz. **Ready-to-feed:** Can 32 fl oz. **Nursing Bottles:** Hospital use. Bot. 8 fl oz. *otc.* *Use:* Nutritional supplement.

Isomil DF. (Ross) Protein 17.9 g, carbo-hydrates 67.3 g, fat 36.7 g, Fe 12 mg, Na 293 mg, K 720 mg, with appropriate vitamins and minerals. 676 cal/L. Lactose free. Liq. 960 ml prediluted, ready-to-use cans. *otc.* *Use:* Nutritional supplement.

Isomil SF. (Ross) Low osmolar sucrose-free soy protein isolate infant formula containing 20 calories/fl oz. **Concentrated Liq.:** Can 13 fl oz. **Ready-to-feed:** Can 32 fl oz. **Nursing Bottles:** Hospital use. Bot. 8 fl oz. *otc.* *Use:* Enteral nutritional supplement.

Isomune-CK. (Roche Diagnostics) Rapid immunochemical separation method of the heart specific CK-MB isoenzyme for quantitation when used with an appropriate CK substrate reagent. Test kit 100s, 250s. *Use:* Diagnostic aid.

Isomune-LD. (Roche Diagnostics) Rapid immunochemical separation method of the heart specific LD-1 isoenzyme for quantitation when used with an appropriate LD substrate reagent. Test kit 40s, 100s. *Use:* Diagnostic aid.

•**isomylamine hydrochloride.** (EYE-so-MILL-ah-meen) USAN. *Use:* Smooth muscle relaxant.

isomyn. *See:* Amphetamine (Various Mfr.).

Isonate Sublingual. (Major) Isosorbide 2.5 mg or 5 mg/Sublingual Tab. Bot.

100s, 1000s, UD 100s. *Rx.* *Use:* Antianginal.

Isonate Tablets. (Major) Isosorbide 5 mg, 10 mg, 20 mg or 30 mg/Tab. **5 mg or 10 mg:** Bot. 100s, 1000s, UD 100s. **20 mg or 30 mg:** Bot. 100s, 1000s. *Rx.* *Use:* Antianginal.

Isonate TD-Caps. (Major) Isosorbide 40 mg/TD Cap. Bot. 100s, 1000s. *Rx.* *Use:* Antianginal.

Isonate T.R. Tabs. (Major) Isosorbide 40 mg/TD Tab. Bot. 100s, 1000s. *Rx.* *Use:* Antianginal.

isoniazid. (eye-so-NYE-uh-zid) (Carolina Medical Products) Isoniazid 50 mg/5 ml. Syr. Bot. pt. *Rx.* *Use:* Antituberculous agent.

•**isoniazid,** (eye-so-NYE-uh-zid) U.S.P. 23. Isonicotinic acid hydrazide, isonico-tinyl hydrazide. Cotinazin; I.N.H.; My-basan; Neumandin; Nicetal; Nydrazid; Pycazide; Rimifon; Tubomel; Vazadrine. *Use:* Antibacterial (tuberculostatic). *See:* Dow-Isoniazid, Tab. (Merrell Dow). INH, Tab. (Ciba). Niconyl, Tab. (Parke-Davis). Nydrazid, Inj. (Squibb Mark). Nydrazid, Tab. (Squibb Marsam). Triniad, Tab. (Kasar). Uniad, Tab. (Kasar). W/Calcium paraminosalicylate. *See:* Calpas-INH, Tab. (American Chem. & Drug). W/Calcium p-aminosalicylate, vitamin B_6. *See:* Calpas Isoxine, Tab. (American Chem. & Drug). Calpas-INAH-6, Tab. (American Chem. & Drug). W/Pyridoxine HCl. (vitamin B_6). *See:* Niadox, Tab. (Pilkington Barnes Hind). Teebaconin w/B_6 (Consoln. Mid.). Triniad Plus 30, Tab. (Kasar). Uniad-Plus, Tab. (Kasar). W/Pyridoxine HCl, sodium aminosalicy-late. *See:* Pasna, Tri-Pack 300, Granules (Pilkington Barnes Hind). W/Rifampin. *See:* Rimactane/INH DuoPack (Ciba). W/Sodium aminosalicylate, pyridoxine. *See:* Pasna Tri-Pack, Granules (Pilk-ington Barnes Hind).

isoniazid. (Various Mfr.) 50 mg/Tab. Bot. 100s, 500, 1000s. *Use:* Antibacterial (tuberculostatic).

isonicotinic acid hydrazide. *See:* Isoniazid, U.S.P. 23. (Various Mfr.).

isonicotinyl hydrazide. *See:* Isoniazid, U.S.P. 23. (Various Mfr.).

isonipecaine hydrochloride.
See: Meperidine Hydrochloride, U.S.P. 23. (Various Mfr.).

Isopap. (Geneva Pharm) Isometheptene mucate 65 mg, dichloralphenazone 100 mg, APAP 325 mg/Cap. Bot. 100s. *Rx.*
Use: Migraine combination.

isopentaquine.
Use: Antimalarial.

isophane insulin suspension.
Use: Hypoglycemic agent.
See: Humulin, Vial (Lilly).
insulin, isophane.
Novolin, Vial (Novo Nordisk).
NPH Insulin, Vial (Novo Nordisk).
NPH Iletin, Vial (Lilly).

isophane insulin suspension and insulin injection.
Use: Antidiabetic agent.
See: Humulin 50/50 (Lilly).
Humulin 70/30 (Lilly).
Novolin 70/30 (Novo Nordisk).
Novolin 70/30 Penfill (Novo Nordisk).

isopregnenone.
See: Duphaston, Tab. (Philips Roxane).
Dydrogesterone.

isoprinosine. (Newport Pharmaceuticals)
Use: Antiviral, immunomodulator.
See: Inosine pranobex, inosiplex, methisoprinol.

•**isopropamide iodide,** U.S.P. 23. Tyrimide.
Use: Anticholinergic.
See: Darbid, Tab. (SK-Beecham).
W/Prochlorperazine maleate.
See: Iso-Perazine, Cap. (Lemmon).

isoprophenamine hydrochloride. Name used for Clorprenaline HCl.

isopropicillin potassium.
Use: Anti-infective.

•**isopropyl alcohol,** U.S.P. 23.
Use: Topical anti-infective; pharmaceutic aid (solvent).

isopropyl alcohol, azeotropic.

isopropyl alcohol spray. (Morton) Isopropyl alcohol w/propellant. Aerosol Can 6 oz. *otc.*
Use: Anti-infective.

isopropylarterenol hydrochloride.
Use: Asthma, vasoconstrictor and allergic states.

isopropylarterenol sulfate.
See: Isoproterenol Sulfate.

•**isopropyl myristate,** N.F. 18.
Use: Pharmaceutic aid (emollient).

iso-noradrenaline.
See: Isoproterenol.

isopropyl-noradrenaline hydrochloride.
See: Isoproterenol HCl, U.S.P. 23.

•**isopropyl palmitate,** N.F. 18.
Use: Pharmaceutic aid (oleaginous vehicle).

isopropyl phenazone. 4-Isopropyl antipyrine. Larodon.

isopropyl rubbing alcohol.
Use: Rubefacient, solvent.

isoproterenol. (eye-so-pro-TER-uh-nahl)
See: Norisidrine (Abbott).
W/Butabarbital, theophylline, ephedrine HCl.
See: Medihaler-Iso, Vial (3M).

•**isoproterenol hydrochloride,** U.S.P. 23.
Use: Bronchodilator, vasopressor used in shock.
See: Isuprel HCl, Prods. (Sanofi Winthrop).
Norisodrine, Aerotrol, Syr. (Abbott).
Proternol, Tab. (Key Pharm).
Vapo-Iso, Soln. (Fisons).
W/Aminophylline, ephedrine sulfate, phenobarbital.
See: Asminorel, Tab. (Solvay).
W/Clopane (clopentamine) HCl, propylene glycol, ascorbic acid.
See: Aerolone Compound, Soln. (Lilly).
W/Phenobarbital sodium, ephedrine sulfate, theophylline hydrous.
See: Iso-asminyl, Tab. (Cole).
W/Phenylephrine bitartrate.
See: Duo-Medihaler, Vial (3M).

isoproterenol hydrochloride and phenylephrine bitartrate inhalation aerosol.
Use: Bronchodilator.
See: Duo-Medihaler, Vial (3M).

isoproterenol inhalation solution.
Use: Bronchodilator.

•**isoproterenol sulfate,** U.S.P. 23.
Use: Bronchodilator.
See: Medihaler-Iso, Vial (3M).
W/Calcium iodide (anhydrous), alcohol.
See: Norisodrine, Syr. (Abbott).

Isoptin. (Knoll Pharm) Verapamil HCl 5 mg/2 ml. Inj. 2 ml and 4 ml amps, vials and disp. syringes. *Rx.*
Use: Calcium channel blocking agent.

Isoptin SR Tablets. (Knoll Pharm) Verapamil HCl **120 mg, 180 mg/SR Tab.:** Bot. 100s, 500s, UD 100s. **240 mg/ SR Tab.:** Bot. 100s, 500s, UD 100s. *Rx.*
Use: Calcium channel blocking agent.

Isoptin Tablets. (Knoll Pharm) Verapamil HCl 40 mg, 80 mg or 120 mg/Tab. Bot. 100s, 500s, 1000s, UD 100s. *Rx.*
Use: Calcium channel blocking agent.

Isopto Alkaline. (Alcon) Hydroxypropyl methylcellulose 1%, benzalkonium Cl 0.01%. Sterile ophthalmic soln. Dropper bot. 15 ml. *otc.*
Use: Artificial tear solution.

Isopto Atropine. (Alcon) Atropine sulfate 0.5% or 1%. **0.5%:** Drop-Tainer 5 ml. **1%:** Drop-Tainer 5 ml, 15 ml. *Rx.*
Use: Cycloplegic mydriatic.

Isopto Carbachol. (Alcon) Carbachol U.S.P. 0.75%, 1.5%, 2.25% or 3%, in a sterile buffered solution of methylcellulose 1%. **2.25%:** Drop-Tainer 15 ml. **0.75%, 1.5% or 3%:** Drop-Tainer 15 ml, 30 ml. *Rx.*
Use: Agent for glaucoma.

Isopto Carpine. (Alcon) Pilocarpine HCl 0.25%, 0.5%, 1%, 2%, 3%, 4%, 5%, 6%, 8% or 10%. Soln. Bot. 15 ml, 30 ml (except 0.25%, 5% and 10%). *Rx.*
Use: Agent for glaucoma.

Isopto Cetamide. (Alcon) Sodium sulfacetamide 15%. Soln. Drop-Tainer 5 ml, 15 ml. *Rx.*
Use: Anti-infective, ophthalmic.

Isopto Cetapred. (Alcon) Sulfacetamide sodium 10%, prednisolone 0.25%. Susp. Drop-Tainer 5 ml, 15 ml. *Rx.*
Use: Anti-infective, corticosteroid, ophthalmic.

Isopto Frin. (Alcon) Phenylephrine HCl 0.12% in a methylcellulose soln. Drop-Tainer 15 ml. *Rx.*
Use: Ophthalmic vasoconstrictor/mydriatic.

Isopto Homatropine. (Alcon) Homatropine HBr 2% or 5%. Soln. Drop-Tainer 5 ml, 15 ml. *Rx.*
Use: Cycloplegic mydriatic.

Isopto Hyoscine. (Alcon) Hyoscine HBr 0.25%. Soln. Drop-Tainer 5 ml, 15 ml. *Rx.*
Use: Cycloplegic mydriatic.

Isopto Plain. (Alcon) Hydroxypropyl methylcellulose 2910 0.5%, benzalkonium Cl 0.01%, sodium Cl, sodium phosphate, sodium citrate. Drop-Tainer 15 ml. *otc.*
Use: Artificial tear solution.

Isopto Tears. (Alcon) Hydroxypropyl methylcellulose 0.5%, benzalkonium Cl 0.01%, sodium Cl, sodium phosphate, sodium citrate. Bot. Drop-Tainer 15 ml, 30 ml. *otc.*
Use: Artificial tear solution.

Isordil Sublingual. (Wyeth-Ayerst) Isosorbide dinitrate 2.5 mg, 5 mg or 10 mg/Tab. **2.5 mg or 5 mg:** Bot. 100s, 500s, Redi-pak 100s. **10 mg:** Bot. 100s. *Rx.*

Use: Antianginal.

Isordil Tembids. (Wyeth-Ayerst) Isosorbide dinitrate 40 mg/Tab. or Cap. **SR Tab.:** Bot. 100s, 500s, 1000s. **SR Cap.:** Bot. 100s, 500s. *Rx.*
Use: Antianginal.

Isordil Titradose Tablets. (Wyeth-Ayerst) Isosorbide dinitrate 5 mg, 10 mg, 20 mg, 30 mg or 40 mg/Tab. **5 mg.:** Bot. 100s, 500s, 1000s, Redi-pak 100s. **10 mg:** Bot. 100s, 500s, 1000s, Redi-pak 100s. **20 mg:** Bot. 100s, 500s, Redi-pak 100s. **30 mg:** Bot. 100s, 500s. Redi-pak 100s. **40 mg:** Bot. 100s, Redi-pak 100s. *Rx.*
Use: Antianginal agent.

Isorgen-G. (Grafton) Isosorbide 5 mg or 10 mg/Tab. Bot. 1000s. *Rx.*
Use: Antianginal agent.

• **isosorbide concentrate.** (EYE-sos-ORE-bide) U.S.P. 23.
Use: Diuretic.

• **isosorbide dinitrate diluted,** (EYE-sos-ORE-bide die-NYE-trate) U.S.P. 23.
Use: Coronary vasodilator.
See: Dilatrate-SR, Cap. (Reed & Carnrick).
Iso-Bid, Cap. (Geriatric).
Iso-D, Tab., Cap. (Dunhall).
Isordil, Tab. (Wyeth-Ayerst).
Isordil Tembids Cap., Tab. (Wyeth-Ayerst).
Nitromed, Tab. (U.S. Ethicals).
Onset, Tab. (Bock).
Sorbitrate, Tab. (Stuart).
Sorquad, Tab. (Solvay).
W/Phenobarbital.
See: Sorbitrate w/Phenobarbital, Tab. (Stuart).

isosorbide dinitrate. (Various Mfr.) **Sublingual:** 2.5 mg, 5 mg, 10 mg. **2.5 mg:** Bot. 100s, 500s, 1000s, UD 100s. **5 mg:** Bot. 100s, 1000s, UD 100s. **10 mg:** Bot. 100s, 1000s. **Oral:** 5 mg, 10 mg, 20 mg, 30 mg/Tab. 40 mg/SR Tab. **5 mg:** Bot. 100s, 1000s, UD 100s. **10 mg:** Bot. 100s, 500s, 1000s, UD 100s. **20 mg:** Bot. 90s, 100s, 120s, 180s, 240s, 360s, 500s, 1000s, UD 100s. **30 mg:** Bot. 100s, 500s, 1000s, UD 100s. **40 mg:** Bot. 90s, 100s, 250s, 1000s, UD 100s. *Rx.*
Use: Coronary vasodilator.

• **isosorbide mononitrate.** (EYE-sos-ORE-bide MAH-no-NYE-trate) USAN.
Use: Coronary vasodilator.
See: Imdur, ER Tab. (Key).
ISMO, Tab. (Wyeth-Ayerst).
Monoket, Tab. (Schwarz Pharma Kremers Urban).

isosorbide oral solution.
Use: Diuretic.

Isosource. (Sandoz Nutrition) Protein (Ca and Na caseinate, soy protein isolate) 43.2 g, carbohydrate (maltodextrin) 1755 g, fat (MCT, canola oil, lecithin) 443.9 g, Na 760 mg, K 1182 mg, mOsm/kg H_2O 390, Cal/ml 1.2, vitamins A, B_1, B_2, B_3, B_5, B_6, B_{12}, C, D, E, K, FA, biotin, choline, Ca, Cl, Cu, Fe, I, Mg, Mn, P, Zn, Se, Cr, Mo. Liq. Bot. 250 ml, 1000 ml. *otc.*
Use: Nutritional therapy.

Isosource HN. (Sandoz Nutrition) Protein (Ca and Na caseinate, soy protein isolate) 56.1 g, carbohydrate (maltodextrin) 165 g, fat (MCT, canola oil, lecithin) 43.9 g, Na 760 mg, K 1772 mg, mOsm/kg H_2O 390, Cal/ml 1.2, vitamins A, B_1, B_2, B_3, B_5, B_6, B_{12}, C, D, E, K, FA, biotin, choline, Ca, P, I, Fe, Mg, Cu, Zn, Cl, Mn, Se, Cr, Mo. Liq. Bot. 250 ml, 1000 ml. *otc.*
Use: Nutritional therapy.

•**isostearyl alcohol.** (EYE-so-STEE-rill) USAN.
Use: Pharmaceutic aid (emollient, solvent).

•**isosulfan blue.** (EYE-so-SULL-fan) USAN.
Use: Diagnostic aid; lymphangiography.

Isotein HN. (Sandoz Nutrition) Vanilla Flavor. Maltodextrin, delactosed lactalbumin, partially hydrogenated soy oil with BHA, fructose, medium chain triglycerides, artificial flavor, sodium caseinate, mono and diglycerides, sodium Cl, vitamins, minerals. Pow. Packet 2.75 oz. *otc.*
Use: Nutritional supplement.

•**isotiquimide.** (eye-so-TIH-kwih-MIDE) USAN.
Use: Antiulcerative.

•**isotretinoin,** (EYE-so-TREH-tin-NO-in) U.S.P. 23.
Use: Keratolytic.
See: Accutane, Cap. (Roche).

isovorin. (Lederle)
See: L-Leucovorin.

Isovue-128. (Bracco DXS) Iopamidol 26% (12.8% iodine). Inj. Vial 50 ml.
Use: Radiopaque agent.

Isovue-200. (Bracco DXS) Iopamidol 41% (20% iodine). Inj. Vial 50. Bot. 100 ml, 200 ml.
Use: Radiopaque agent.

Isovue 300 Injection. (Squibb) Iopamidol 612 mg, tromethamine 1 mg, edetate calcium disodium 0.39 mg/ml. Vial 50 ml, Box 10s. Bot. 100 ml, Box 10s.
Use: Radiopaque agent.

Isovue 370 Injection. (Squibb) Iopamidol 755 mg, tromethamine 1 mg, edetate calcium disodium 0.48 mg/ml. Vial 50 ml, Box 10s; Bot. 100 ml, Box 10s; 150 ml, Box 10s; 200 ml, Box 10s.
Use: Radiopaque agent.

Isovue-m 200 Injection. (Squibb) Iopamidol 408 mg, tromethamine 1 mg, edetate calcium disodium 0.26 mg/ml. Vial 20 ml, Box 10s.
Use: Radiopaque agent.

Isovue-M 300 Injection. (Squibb) Iopamidol 612 mg, tromethamine 1 mg, edetate calcium disodium 0.39 mg/ml. Vial 20 ml, Box 10s.
Use: Radiopaque agent.

•**isoxepac.** (EYE-SOX-eh-pack) USAN.
Use: Anti-inflammatory.

•**isoxicam.** (eye-SOX-ih-kam) USAN.
Use: Anti-inflammatory.

•**isoxsuprine hydrochloride,** (eye-SOX-you-preen) U.S.P. 23.
Use: Vasodilator.
See: Vasodilan, Tab. (Bristol-Myers).

I-Soyalac. (Mt. Vernon Foods) P-soy protein isolate, l-methionine, CHO-sucrose, tapioca dextrin. F-soy oil, soy lecithin. Corn free. Protein 20.2 g, carbohydrate 63.4 g, fat 35.5 g, iron 12 mg, 640 Cal/serving (1 qt). Concentrate 390 ml, ready to use 1 qt. *otc.*
Use: Nutritional supplement.

•**isradipine.** (iss-RAHD-ih-peen) USAN.
Use: Calcium channel blocker.
See: DynaCirc (Sandoz).

I-Sulfacet. (American) Sulfacetamide sodium 10%, 15% or 30% ophthalmic soln. Bot. 2 ml, 5 ml, 15 ml. *Rx.*
Use: Anti-infective, ophthalmic.

I-Sulfalone Suspension. (American) Sulfacetamide sodium 100 mg, prednisolone acetate 5 mg. Ophthalmic susp. Bot. 5 ml, 15 ml. *Rx.*
Use: Anti-infective, ophthalmic.

Isuprel Inhalation Solution. (Sanofi Winthrop) Isoproterenol HCl inhalation soln. 1:200 or 1:100. Bot. 10 ml, 60 ml. *Rx.*
Use: Bronchodilator.

Isuprel Mistometer. (Sanofi Winthrop) Isoproterenol HCl. Complete nebulizing unit of aerosol soln. containing 10 ml or 15 ml of isoproterenol HCl w/inert propellants, alcohol 33%, ascorbic acid. Measured dose of approximately 131 mcg. Aerosol Unit. Bot. 15 ml, 22.5 ml.

Refill 15 ml, 22.5 ml. *Rx.*
Use: Bronchodilator.

Isuprel Sterile Injection. (Sanofi Winthrop) Isoproterenol HCl 0.2 mg/ml with sodium metabisulfite in 1:5000 solution in 1 and 5 ml amps.; 0.02 mg/ml with sodium metabisulfite in 1:50,000 solution in 10 ml with needle. *Rx.*
Use: Adjunct treatment of shock, cardiac standstill, bronchospasm during anesthesia.

isuprene.
See: Isoproterenol (Various Mfr.).

• **itasetron.** (eye-tah-SEH-trahn) USAN.
Use: Antianxiety agent; antidepressant; antiemetic, anxiolytic.

• **itazigrel.** (ih-TAY-zih-GRELL) USAN.
Use: Platelet aggregation inhibitor.

Itchaway. (Moyco) Zinc undecylenate 20%, undecylenic acid 2%. Pow. Can 1.5 oz. *otc.*
Use: Antifungal, topical.

Itch-X. (Ascher & Co.) Pramoxine HCl 1%. Gel: Benzyl alcohol, aloe vera gel, diazolidinyl urea, SD alcohol 40, parabens. 35.4 g. Spray: Benzyl alcohol, aloe vera gel, SD alcohol 40. In 60 ml. *otc.*
Use: Local anesthetic, topical.

itobarbital.
W/Acetaminophen.
See: Panitol, Tab. (Wesley).

• **itraconazole.** (ih-truh-KAHN-uh-zole) USAN.
Use: Antifungal.
See: Sporanox, Cap. (Janssen).

I-Trol. (Akorn) Neomycin sulfate-polymyxin B sulfate-dexamethasone 0.1%. Ophthalmic susp. Bot. 5 ml. *Rx.*
Use: Anti-infective, corticosteroid, ophthalmic.

I-Valex-1. (Ross) Protein 15 g, fat 23.9 g, carbohydrates 46.3 g, linoleic acid 1800 mg, Fe 9 mg, Na 190 mg, K 675 mg, with appropriate vitamins and minerals. 480 Cal per 100 g. Leucine free. Pow. Can 350 g. *otc.*
Use: Nutritional supplement.

I-Valex-2. (Ross) Protein 30 g, fat 15.5 g, carbohyrates 30 g, Fe 13 mg, Na 880 mg, K 1370 mg, with appropriate vitamins and minerals. 410 Cal per 100 g. Leucine free. Pow. Can 325 g. *otc.*
Use: Nutritional supplement.

Ivarest. (Blistex) Calamine 14%, benzocaine 5%. **Cream:** 60 g. **Lot.:** 120 ml. *otc.*
Use: Topical treatment of poison ivy, oak, sumac.

Iveegam. (Immune) Immune globulin 50 mg/ml IgG/Pow. for Inj. in 1000 mg with diluent, double-ended spike and filter needle; and 2500 and 5000 mg with diluent, double-ended spike and infusion set with filter. *Rx.*
Use: Immune serum.

• **ivermectin.** (eye-VER-MEK-tin) USAN.
Use: Antiparasitic.
See: Cardomec (Merck).
Equalan (Merck).
Ivomec (Merck).

Ivocort. (Roberts) Micronized hydrocortisone alcohol 0.5% or 1%. Bot. 4 oz. *otc.*
Use: Corticosteroid, topical.

Ivy-Chex. (Jones Medical) Polyvinyl pyrrolidone-vinyl acetate, benzalkonium Cl 1:1000 in alcohol acetone base. Aerosol can 4 oz. *otc.*
Use: Treatment or prevention of poison ivy, poison oak, poison sumac dermatitis.

Ivy Dry. (Ivy) Tannic acid 10%, isopropyl alcohol 12.5% Liq. 4 oz, Cream 1 oz, Super 6 oz. *otc.*
Use: Relief of itching.

Ivy-Rid. (Roberts) Polyvinyl pyrrolidone-vinyl acetate, benzalkonium Cl. Spray can 2.75 oz. *otc.*
Use: Relief of itching and discomfort of poison ivy, poison oak and poison sumac.

I-Wash. (Akorn) Phosphate buffered saline soln. Bot. 4 oz, 8 oz. *otc.*
Use: Eye wash.

I-White. (Akorn) Phenylephrine 0.12%, polyvinyl alcohol, hydroxyethyl cellulose. Soln. Bot. 15 ml. *otc.*
Use: Ophthalmic vasoconstrictor, mydriatic.

Izonid tablets. (Major) Isoniazid 300 mg/Tab. Bot. 100s. *Rx.*
Use: Antituberculous agent.

J

jalovis.
See: Hyaluronidase (Various Mfr.).

Janimine. (Abbott) Imipramine HCl 10 mg, 25 mg or 50 mg/Tab. Bot. 100s, 1000s. Rx.
Use: Antidepressant.

japan agar.
See: Agar (Various Mfr.).

japan gelatin.
See: Agar (Various Mfr.).

japan isinglass.
See: Agar (Various Mfr.).

japanese encephalitis vaccine.
Use: Vaccine.
See: JE-VAX.

JE-VAX. (Connaught) Japanese encephalitis virus vaccine 2-3 mcg nitrogen content per ml.. Pow. for Inj. single-dose vial with 1.3 ml diluent; 10-dose vial with 11 ml diluent. Rx.
Use: Vaccine, viral.

Jenamicin. (Roberts) Gentamicin sulfate 40 mg/ml. Vial 2 ml. Rx.
Use: Antibacterial, aminoglycoside.

Jenest-28. (Organon) 7 white tablets nor-ethindrone 0.5 mg, ethinyl estradiol 35 mcg; 14 peach tablets norethindrone 1 mg, ethinyl estradiol 35 mcg; 7 inert tablets. Cyclic dispenser of 28. Rx.
Use: Oral contraceptive.

Jeri-Bath. (Dermik) Concentrated moisturizing bath oil. Plastic Bot. 8 oz. otc.
Use: Bath dermatological.

Jets. (Freeda) Lysine 300 mg, vitamins C 25 mg, B_{12} 25 mcg, B_6 5 mg, B_1 10 mg/Chew. tab. Bot. 30s, 250s, 500s. otc.
Use: Vitamin supplement.

Jevity Liquid. (Ross) Calcium and sodium caseinates, soy fiber, hydrolyzed cornstarch, MCT (fractionated coconut oil) soy oil, corn oil, soy lecithin, vitamins A, B_1, B_2, B_3, B_5, B_6, B_{12}, C, D, E, K, folic acid, biotin, choline, Ca, P, Mg, Fe, Mn, Cu, Zn, I, Cl. In 240 ml. otc.
Use: Nutritional supplement.

Jiffy. (Block) Benzocaine, menthol, eugenol in glycerin-water base with SD alcohol 38-B 76%. Bot. 0.125 oz. otc.
Use: Local anesthetic, topical.

J-Liberty. (J Pharmacal) Chlordiazepoxide HCl 5 mg, 10 mg or 25 mg/Cap. c-iv.
Use: Antianxiety agent.

Johnson's Baby Cream. (Johnson & Johnson) Dimethicone 2%. Jar 4 oz, 6 oz, Tube 2 oz. otc.
Use: Skin protectant.

Johnson's Baby Sunblock Cream. (Johnson and Johnson) Octyl methoxycinnamate, octyl salicylate, oxybenzone, titandium dioxide, benzyl alcohol, cetyl alcohol. PABA free. SPF 15. Waterproof. Cream. Bot. 60 Gm. otc.
Use: Sunscreen.

Johnson's Baby Sunblock Extra Protection. (Johnson & Johnson) Octyl methoxycinnamate, octyl salicylate, titanium dioxide, oxybenzone, C12-15 alcohols benzoate, cetyl alcohol, EDTA, vitamin E. Lot. Bot. 120 ml. otc.
Use: Sunscreen.

Johnson's Baby Sunblock Lotion. (Johnson & Johnson) **SPF 30:** Benzo-phenone-3, octyl methoxycinnamate, octyl salicylate, titanium dioxide. PABA free. Waterproof. Bot. 120 ml. **SPF 15:** Octyl methoxycinnamate octyl salicylate, oxybenzone, titanium dioxide, benzyl alcohol, cetyl alcohol. PABA free. Waterproof. Bot. 60 Gm. otc.
Use: Sunscreen.

Johnson's Medicated Powder. (Johnson & Johnson) Bentonite, kaolin, talc, zinc oxide. Pow. Small, Medium, Large. otc.
Use: Diaper rash product.

•**josamycin.** (JOE-sah-MYsin) USAN.
Use: Antibacterial.

Junior Strength Advil. (Whitehall-Robins) Ibuprofen 100 mg, sucrose/Tab. Bot. 24s. otc.
Use: Nonsteroidal anti-inflammatory agent, analgesic.

Junior-Strength Feverall. (Upsher-Smith) Acetaminophen 120 mg or 325 mg/Supp. Pkg 6s. otc.
Use: Analgesic.

Junior Strength Motrin. (McNeil) Ibuprofen 100 mg, phenylalanine 6 mg, aspartame/Chew. Tab. Bot. 24s. otc.
Use: Nonsteroidal anti-inflammatory, analgesic.

Junior Strength Panadol. (Bayer) Acetaminophen 160 mg. Capl. 30s. otc.
Use: Analgesic.

•**juniper tar,** U.S.P. 23.
Use: Local antieczematic, pharmaceutic necessity.

Junyer-All. (Barth's) Vitamins A 6000 IU, D 400 IU, B_1 3 mg, B_2 6 mg, C 120 mg, niacin 1 mg, E 12 IU, B_{12} 10 mcg, calcium 217 mg, phosphorus 97.5 mg, red bone marrow 10 mg, organic iron 15 mg, iodine 0.1 mg, beef peptone 20 mg/2 Cap. Bot. 10 month, 3 month, 6 month supply. otc.
Use: Vitamin supplement.

Just Tears. (Blairex) Benzalkonium chloride, EDTA, NaCl, polyvinyl alcohol 1.4%. Soln. Bot. 15 ml. *otc.*
Use: Ocular lubricant.

juvocaine.
See: Procaine HCl (Various Mfr.)

K

K-1. Phytonadione.
Use: Vitamin K.
See: Mephyton, Tab. (Merck).
Aqua MEPHYTON, Inj. (Merck).
KonaKion, Inj. (For IM use only)
(Roche).

K-4. Menadiol sodium diphosphate.
Use: Vitamin K.
See: SynKayvite, Tab., Inj. (Roche).

K+8. (Alra) Potassium chloride 8 mEq.
ER Tab. Bot. 100s, 500s. *Rx.*
Use: Potassium replacement product.

K+10. (Alra) Potassium Cl 10 mEq/Tab.
Bot. 100s, 500s, 1000s. *Rx.*
Use: Potassium supplement.

K 34. Hexachlorophene.

K + Care. (Alra) Potassium chloride, saccharin. Soln. Pkt. 15, 20, 25 mEq, 30s, 100s. *Rx.*
Use: Potassium replacement product.

Kabikinase. (Pharmacia & Upjohn) Streptokinase 250,000 IU, 600,000 IU or 750,000 IU or 1,500,000 IU/vial. Pow. for inj. Vial 5 ml, 10 ml. *Rx.*
Use: Thrombolytic enzyme.

Kadian. (Zeneca) Morphine sulfate 20 mg, 50 mg and 100 mg/SR Cap. Bot. 60s, 100s, 500s (except 100 mg) and UD 100s. *c-II.*
Use: Narcotic agonist analgesic.

Kaergona.
See: Menadione (Various Mfr.).

Kala. (Freeda) Soy-based acidophilus 2 million units/Tab. Bot. 100s, 250s and 500s. *otc.*
Use: Nutritional supplement.

•**kalafungin.** (kal-ah-FUN-jin) USAN.
Use: Antifungal.

Kalory-Plus. (Tyler) Thyroid 3 gr, amphetamine sulfate 15 mg, atropine sulfate 1/180 gr, aloin 0.25 gr, phenobarbital 0.25 gr/TR cap. Bot. 100s, 1000s.
Use: Anorexiant.

Kaltostat. (SK Beecham) Calcium-sodium alginate fiber, 3"×4¾" sterile dressing. In 1s. *otc.*
Use: Hydroactive dressing.

Kaltostat Forte. (SK Beecham) Calcium-sodium alginate fiber, 4"×4" sterile dressing. In 1s. *otc.*
Use: Hydroactive dressing.

Kamfolene. (Wade) Camphor, menthol, methyl salicylate, oils turpentine and eucalyptus, carbolic acid 2%, calamine, zinc oxide in lanolin base. Jar 2 oz, lb. *otc.*
Use: Antiseptic.

•**kanamycin sulfate,** (kan-uh-MY-sin) U.S.P. 23. An antibiotic obtained from *Streptomycin kanamyceticus.*
Use: Antibacterial.
See: Kantrex, Cap., Vial (Bristol).
Klebcil, Inj. (SK Beecham).

Kank-A. (Blistex) Benzocaine 5%, cetylpyridinium chloride, castor oil, benzoin compound. Liq. Bot. 3.75 ml. *otc.*
Use: Local anesthetic, topical.

Kantrex. (Bristol) Kanamycin sulfate.
Cap.: 0.5 g. Bot. 20s, 100s. **Vial:** 0.5 g/2 ml or 1 g/3 ml. **Pediatric Inj.:** 75 mg/2 ml. **Disposable Syringe:** 500 mg/2 ml. *Rx.*
Use: Anti-infective, aminoglycoside.

Kaochlor 10% Liquid. (Pharmacia & Upjohn) Potassium and chloride 20 mEq/ 15 ml (potassium Cl 10%), alcohol 5%, saccharin, FD&C; Yellow No. 5. Bot. pt. *Rx.*
Use: Potassium supplement.

Kaochlor-Eff. (Pharmacia & Upjohn) Elemental potassium 20 mEq, chloride 20 mEq/Tab. Supplied by: Potassium Cl 0.6 g, potassium citrate 0.22 g, potassium bicarbonate 1 g, betaine HCl 1.84 g, saccharin 20 mg, artificial fruit flavor, tartrazine (color)/Tab. Sugar free. Carton 60s. *Rx.*
Use: Potassium supplement.

Kaochlor S-F 10% Liquid. (Pharmacia & Upjohn) Potassium 20 mEq, chloride 20 mEq/15 ml, saccharin, flavoring, alcohol 5%. Sugar free. Bot. 4 oz, pt. *Rx.*
Use: Potassium supplement.

Kaodene Non-Narcotic. (Pfeiffer) Kaolin 3.9 g, pectin 194.4 mg/30 ml, bismuth subsalicylate. Alcohol free. Liq. Bot. 120 ml. *otc.*
Use: Antidiarrheal.

Kaodene with Codeine. (Pfeiffer) Codeine phosphate 32.4 mg, kaolin 3.9 g, pectin 194.4 mg, sodium carboxymethylcellulose, bismuth subsalicylate/ 30 ml. Susp. Bot. 120 ml.
Use: Antidiarrheal.

•**kaolin,** (KAY-oh-lin) U.S.P. 23.
Use: Adsorbent.
W/Atropine sulfate, phenobarbital.
W/Belladonna, phenobarbital.
See: Bellkata, Tab. (Ferndale).
W/Bismuth compound.
See: Kaomine, Pow. (Lilly).
W/Bismuth subgallate.
See: Diastop, Liq. (ICN Pharm).
W/Bismuth subgallate, pectin, zinc phenolsulfonate, opium pow.
See: Diastay, Tab. (ICN Pharm).

W/Bismuth subsalicylate, salol, methyl salicylate, benzocaine, pectin.

W/Cornstarch, camphor, zinc oxide, eucalyptus oil.
See: Mexsana, Pow. (Schering Plough).

W/Furazolidone, pectin.
See: Furoxone, Liq. (Eaton).

W/Hyoscyamine sulfate, sodium benzoate, atropine sulfate, hyoscine HBR, pectin.
See: Donnagel, Susp. (Robins).

W/Neomycin sulfate, pectin.
See: Pecto-Kalin, Liq. (Harvey).

W/Pectin.
See: Kaopectate, Liq. (Pharmacia & Upjohn).
Kapectin, Liq. (Approved).
Pecto-Kalin, Susp. (Lemmon).
Pectokay Mixture (Jones Medical).

W/Pectin, belladonna alkaloids.

W/Pectin, bismuth subcarbonate.
See: B-K-P Mixture, Liq. (Sutliff & Case).

W/Pectin, bismuth subcarbonate, belladonna.
See: Kay-Pec, Liq. (Case).

W/Pectin, bismuth subcarbonate, opium pow.
See: KBP/O, Cap. (Cole).

W/Pectin, bismuth subsalicylate.

W/Pectin, bismuth subsalicylate, paregoric, zinc sulfocarbolate.

W/Pectin, hyoscyamine sulfate, atropine sulfate, hyoscine HBr.
See: Kapigam, Liq. (Solvay).
Palsorb Improved, Liq. (Roberts).

W/Pectin, pow. opium extract.
See: Pecto-Kalin, Susp. (Lemmon).

W/Pectin, opium pow., bismuth subgallate, zinc phenolsulfonate.
See: Cholactabs, Tab. (Philips Roxane).
B.P.P., Tab. (Lemmon).

W/Pectin, paregoric (equivalent).
See: Duosorb, Liq. (Solvay).
Kaoparin, Liq. (McKesson).
Kapectin, Liq. (Approved).
Ka-Pek w/Paregoric, Liq. (APC).
Parepectolin, Susp. (Rhone-Poulenc Rorer).

W/Pectin, zinc phenolsulfonate.
See: Pectocel, Susp. (Lilly).

W/Phenobarbital, atropine sulfate, aluminum hydroxide gel.
See: Kao-Lumin, Tab. (Philips Roxane).

W/Salol, zinc sulfocarbolate, aluminum hydroxide, bismuth subsalicylate, pectin.
See: Wescola Antidiarrheal-Stomach Upset (Western Research).

kaolin colloidal.
W/Bismuth subcarbonate.

See: Bisilad, Susp. (Central).

W/Magnesium trisilicate, aluminum hydroxide dried gel.
See: Kamadrox, Tab. (ICN Pharm).
Kathmagel, Tab. (Mason).

W/Pectin, aromatics.
See: Paocin, Susp. (SK Beecham).

W/Pectin, belladonna alkaloids.
See: Kamabel, Liq. (Towne).

kaolin w/pectin. (KAY-oh-lin with PECK-tin) (Various Mfr.) Kaolin 90 g, pectin 2 g/30 ml. Susp. Bot. 180, pt, UD 30 ml. *otc.*
Use: Antidiarrheal combinations.

Kaon Cl⁻10 controlled release tablets. (Pharmacia & Upjohn) Potassium Cl 750 mg/Tab. Bot. 100s, 500s, 1000s. Stat-Pak 100s. *Rx.*
Use: Potassium supplement.

Kaon Cl 20%. (Pharmacia & Upjohn) Potassium and chloride 40 mEq (to potassium Cl 3 g)/15 ml, saccharin, flavoring, alcohol 5%. Bot. pt. *Rx.*
Use: Potassium supplement.

Kaon Cl Controlled Release Tablets. (Pharmacia & Upjohn) Potassium Cl 500 mg/Tab., FD&C Yellow No. 5. Bot. 100s, 250s, 1000s. *Rx.*
Use: Potassium supplement.

Kaon Elixir. (Pharmacia & Upjohn) Elemental potassium 20 mEq (as potassium gluconate 4.68 g)/15 ml, aromatics, grape and lemon-lime flavors, alcohol 5%, saccharin. Unit pkg. pt, gal. *Rx.*
Use: Potassium supplement.

Kaon Tablets. (Pharmacia & Upjohn) Elemental potassium 5 mEq obtained from potassium gluconate 1.17 g/SC Tab. Bot. 100s, 500s. *Rx.*
Use: Potassium supplement.

Kaopectate. (Pharmacia & Upjohn) Kaolin 5.85 g, pectin 130 mg/oz. Bot. 8 oz, 12 oz, 16 oz, 1 gal, UD pkg. 3 oz. *otc.*
Use: Antidiarrheal.

Kaopectate Advanced Formula. (Pharmacia & Upjohn) Attapulgite 750 mg/15 ml, sucrose. Liq. Bot. 354 ml. *otc.*
Use: Antidiarrheal combination.

Kaopectate Children's. (Pharmacia & Upjohn) Attapulgite 600 mg/15 ml. Bot. 180 ml. *otc.*
Use: Antidiarrheal combination.

Kaopectate Maximum Strength. (Pharmacia & Upjohn) Attapulgite 750 mg, Capl. Pkg. 12s, 20s. *otc.*
Use: Antidiarrheal combination.

Kaopectate Tablet Formula. (Pharmacia & Upjohn) Attapulgite 750 mg/Tab.

Blister pak 12s, 20s. *otc.*
Use: Antidiarrheal.

Kaophen Tablets. (Pal-Pak) Phenobarbital 6.5 mg, belladonna extract 0.1 mg, kaolin 388.8 mg/Tab. Bot. 100s, 1000s.
Use: Antidiarrheal.

Kao-Spen. (Century) Kaolin 5.2 g, pectin 260 mg/30 ml. Susp. Bot. 120 ml, pt, gal. *otc.*
Use: Antidiarrheal.

Kao-Tin. (Major) Kaolin 5.85 g, pectin 130 mg/30 ml. Susp. Bot. 120 ml, 240 ml, pt, gal. *otc.*
Use: Antidiarrheal.

Kapectin. (Approved) Kaolin 90 gr, pectin 2 gr/oz. Bot. gal.
Use: Antidiarrheal.

Kapectolin. (Various Mfr.) Kaolin 90 g, pectin 2 g/30 ml. Susp. Bot. 360 ml. *otc.*
Use: Antidiarrheal.

Ka-Pek. (APC) Kaolin 90 gr, pectin 4.5 gr/fl oz. Bot. 6 oz, gal. *otc.*
Use: Antidiarrheal.

kapilin.
See: Menadione (Various Mfr.).

karaya gum. (Penick) Indian Gum. Sterculia gum,
See: Tri-Costivin (Prof. Lab.).
W/Frangula.
See: Saraka, Gran. (Schering Plough).
W/Psyllium seed, plantago ovata, brewers yeast.
See: Plantamucin Gran. (ICN Pharm).
W/Cortex rhamni frangulae.
See: Movicol (Norgine).
W/Refined psyllium mucilloid.
See: Hydrocil regular (Solvay).

karaya powder. (Sween) Bot. 3 oz.
Use: Ostomy care product.

Kareon.
See: Menadione (Various Mfr.).

Karidium. (Lorvic) **Tab.:** Sodium fluoride 2.21 mg, sodium Cl 94.49 mg, disintegrant 0.5 mg. Bot. 180s, 1000s. **Liq.:** Sodium fluoride 2.21 mg, sodium Cl 10 mg, purified water q.s./8 drops. Bot. 30 ml, 60 ml. *Rx.*
Use: Dental caries preventative.

Karigel. (Lorvic) Fluoride ion 0.5%, pH 5.6. Gel. Bot. 30 ml, 130 ml, 250 ml. *Rx.*
Use: Dental caries preventative.

Karigel-N. (Lorvic) Fluoride ion 0.5% in neutral pH gel. Bot. 24 ml, 125 ml. *Rx.*
Use: Dental caries preventative.

•**kasal.** (KAY-sal) USAN. Approximately $Na_8AP_2(OH)_2(PO_4)_4$ with about 30% of dibasic sodium phosphate; sodium aluminum phosphate, basic.
Use: Food additive.

Kasof. (J & J - Merck) Docusate potassium 240 mg/Cap. Bot. 30s, 60s. *otc.*
Use: Laxative.

kasugamycin. Under study.
Use: Anti-infective.

Kaviton.
See: Menadione, U.S.P. 23. (Various Mfr.).

Kay Ciel Elixir. (Forest) Potassium Cl 1.5 g/15 ml. (20 mEq/15 ml), alcohol 4%. Bot. 120 ml, 473 ml, gal. *Rx.*
Use: Potassium supplement.

Kay Ciel Powder. (Forest) Potassium chloride 1.5 g/Packette. (20 mEq/Packet), 4% alcohol. Box 30s, 100s, 500s. *Rx.*
Use: Potassium supplement.

Kayexalate. (Sanofi Winthrop) Sodium polystyrene sulfonate sodium content ≈100 mg/g. Jar lb. *Rx.*
Use: Potassium removing resin.

K-C. (Century) Kaolin 5.2 g, pectin 260 mg, bismuth subcarbonate 260 mg/30 ml. Susp. Bot. 120 ml, pt, gal. *otc.*
Use: Antidiarrheal.

K + Care Et. (Alra) Potassium bicarbonate 25 mEq/Effervescent tab. Bot. 30s, 100s, 1000s. *Rx.*
Use: Potassium supplement.

K-C Liquid. (Century) Kaolin 5.2 g, pectin 260 mg, bismuth subcarbonate 260 mg/oz. Bot. 4 oz, pt, gal. *otc.*
Use: Antidiarrheal.

K-C Suspension. (Century Pharm) Kaolin 5.2 g, pectin 260 mg, bismuth subcarbonate 260 mg/30 ml. Bot. 120 ml, pt, gal. *otc.*
Use: Antidiarrheal.

KC-20 Elixir. (Scruggs) Bot. pt, gal.

KCl-20. (Western Research) Potassium Cl 1.5 g (potassium 20 mEq, chloride 20 mEq)/Packet. Box 30s. *Rx.*
Use: Potassium supplement.

K-Dur 10 & 20. (Key) **10:** Potassium Cl 750 mg (10 mEq)/SR Tab. **20:** Potassium Cl 1500 mg (20 mEq)/SR Tab. Bot. 100s. *Rx.*
Use: Potassium supplement.

KE.
See: Cortisone Acetate (Various Mfr.).

Keelamin. (Mericon) Zinc 20 mg, manganese 5 mg, copper 3 mg/Tab. Bot. 100s. *otc.*
Use: Mineral supplement.

Keflex Capsules. (Dista) Cephalexin 250 mg, 500 mg/Capl. Bot. 20s, 100s, UD 100s. *Rx.*

Use: Anti-infective, cephalosporin.

Keflex Oral Suspension. (Dista) Cephalexin 125 mg and 250 mg/5 ml. Bot. 60 ml, 100 ml, 200 ml, UD 5 ml. *Rx.*
Use: Anti-infective, cephalosporin.

Keflex for Pediatric Drops. (Dista) Cephalexin 100 mg/ml. Dropper bot. 10 ml. *Rx.*
Use: Anti-infective, cephalosporin.

Keflex Pediatric Oral Suspension. (Dista) Cephalexin 100 mg/ml. Bot. 10 ml w/calibrated dropper. *Rx.*
Use: Anti-infective, cephalosporin.

Keftab. (Dista) Cephalexin HCl monohydrate 500 mg/Tab. Bot. 100s. *Rx.*
Use: Anti-infective, cephalosporin.

Kefurox. (Lilly) Cefuroxime sodium 750 mg or 1.5 g/Vial. ADD-vantage and Faspak **750 mg:** Vial 10 ml, 100 ml. **1.5 g:** Vial 20 ml, 100 ml. **7.5 g:** Vial. Pharmacy bulk pkg. *Rx.*
Use: Anti-infective, cephalosporin.

Kefzol. (Lilly) Cefazolin sodium. Powd. for Inj. **In Vials:** 250 mg, 500 mg, 1 g. **In 100 ml Bulk Vials:** 10 g, 20 g. *Rx.*
Use: Cephalosporin.

Kell E. (Canright) di-α Tocopheryl 100 IU, 200 IU or 400 IU. Bot. 100s. *otc.*
Use: Vitamin E supplement.

Kellogg's Tasteless Castor Oil. (SK Beecham) Castor oil 100%. Bot. 2 oz. *otc.*
Use: Laxative.

Kelp. (Arcum) Tab. Bot. 100s, 1000s.

Kelp Plus. (Barth's) Iodine from kelp plus 16 trace minerals/Tab. Bot. 100s, 500s, 1000s.

Kelp Tablets. (Faraday) Iodine from kelp 0.15 mg/Tab. Bot. 100s.

Kemadrin. (Glaxo Wellcome) Procyclidine HCl 5 mg/Tab. Bot. 100s. *Rx.*
Use: Antiparkinsonian.

kemithal. Thialbarbital. 5-Allyl-5-cyclohex-2-enyl-2-thiobarbituric acid.

Kenac Cream. (NMC Labs) Triamcinolone acetonide cream 0.025% or 0.1%. Tube 15 g, 60 g, 80 g, Jar 240 g. *Rx.*
Use: Corticosteroid, topical.

Kenac Ointment. (NMC Labs) Triamcinolone acetonide ointment 0.1%. Tube 15 g, 80 g. *Rx.*
Use: Corticosteroid, topical.

Kenaject-40. (Mayrand) Triamcinolone acetonide 40 mg/ml/Inj. Vial 5 ml. *Rx.*
Use: Corticosteroid.

Kenakion. (Harriett Lane Home of Johns Hopkins Hospital) Vitamin K-1 oxide. *Rx.*
Use: Vitamin K-induced kernicterus.

Kenalog. (Westwood Squibb) Triamcinolone acetonide. **0.1% Cream:** Tube 15 g, 60 g, 80 g, Jar 240 g, in aqueous lotion base w/propylene glycol, cetyl and stearyl alcohols, glyceryl monostearate, sorbitan monopalmitate, polyoxyethylene sorbitan monolaurate, methylparaben, propylparaben, polyethylene glycol monostearate, simethicone, sorbic acid. **0.5% Cream:** Tube 20 g. **0.1% Oint.:** (w/base of polyethylene, mineral oil) Tube 15 g, 60 g, 80 g; Jar 240 g, **0.5% Oint.:** Tube 20 g. **0.1% Lot.:** Bot. 15ml, 60 ml. **Spray:** 6.6 mg/100 g, alcohol 10.3%. Can 23 g, 63 g. *Rx.*
Use: Corticosteroid, topical.

Kenalog 0.025%. (Westwood Squibb) Triamcinolone acetonide. **Cream:** Tube 15 g, 80 g, Jar 240 g. **Lot.:** In aqueous lotion base w/propylene glycol, cetyl and stearyl alcohols, glyceryl monostearate, sorbitan monopalmitate, polyoxyethylene sorbitan monolaurate, methylparaben, propylparaben, polyethylene glycol monostearate, simethicone, sorbic acid, tinted in an isopropyl palmitate vehicle with alcohol (4.7%). Bot. 60 ml. **Oint.:** Plastibase (w/base of polyethylene and mineral oil gel). 15 g, 80 g, 240 g. *Rx.*
Use: Corticosteroid, topical.

Kenalog H. (Westwood Squibb) Triamcinolone acetonide cream USP 0.1%. Each g of cream provides 1 mg of triamcinolone acetonide in a specially formulated hydrophilic vanishing cream base containing propylene glycol, dimethicone 350, castor oil, cetearyl alcohol and ceteareth-20, propylene glycol stearate, white petrolatum, purified water. Tube 15 g, 60 g. *Rx.*
Use: Corticosteroid, topical.

Kenalog-10 Injection. (Squibb Mark) Sterile triamcinolone acetonide suspension 10 mg/ml, sodium Cl for isotonicity, benzyl alcohol 0.9% (w/v) as a preservative, sodium carboxymethylcellulose 0.75%, polysorbate 80 0.04%. Sodium hydroxide or HCl acid may be present to adjust pH to 5 to 7.5. Nitrogen packed at the time of manufacture. Vial 5 ml. *Rx.*
Use: Corticosteroid.

Kenalog-40 Injection. (Squibb Mark) Sterile triamcinolone acetonide suspension 40 mg/ml, sodium chloride for isotonicity, benzyl alcohol 0.9% (w/v) as a preservative, sodium carboxymethylcellulose 0.75%, polysorbate 80 0.04%.

Sodium hydroxide or HCl acid may be present to adjust pH to 5 to 7.5. Nitrogen packed at the time of manufacture. Vial 1 ml, 5 ml, 10 ml. *Rx.*
Use: Corticosteroid.

Kenalog in Orabase. (Apothecon) Triamcinolone acetonide 0.1% in Orabase. Triamcinolone acetonide 1 mg/g. Tube 5 g. *Rx.*
Use: Corticosteroid, topical.

Kendall's "Compound B".
See: Corticosterone (Various Mfr.).

Kendall's "Compound E".
See: Cortisone Acetate (Various Mfr.).

Kendall's "Compound F".
See: 17-Hydroxycorticosterone (Various Mfr.).

Kendall's "Desoxy Compound B".
See: Desoxycorticosterone Acetate (Various Mfr.).

Kenonel. (Marnel) Triamcinolone acetonide 0.1%. Cream. Tube 20 g. *Rx.*
Use: Corticosteroid, topical.

Kenwood Therapeutic Liquid. (Kenwood Bradley) Vitamins A 3333 IU, D 133 IU, E 1.5 IU, C 50 mg, B_1 2 mg, B_2 1 mg, B_3 20 mg, B_5 2 mg, B_6 0.33 mg, Ca, K, Mg, Mn, P/Liq. Bot. 240 ml. *otc.*
Use: Vitamin/mineral supplement.

Keralyt Gel. (Westwood Squibb) Salicylic acid 6% in a gel base of propylene glycol w/alcohol 19.4%, hydroxypropyl cellulose, water. Tube 1 oz. *otc.*
Use: Keratolytic.

keratolytics.
See: Condylox (Oclassen).

Keri Creme. (Westwood Squibb) Cream containing water, mineral oil, talc, sorbitol, ceresin, lanolin alcohol, magnesium stearate, glyceryl oleate/propylene glycol, isopropyl myristate, methylparaben, propylparaben, fragrance, quaternium-15. Tube 2.5 oz. *otc.*
Use: Emollient.

Keri Facial Soap. (Westwood Squibb) Sodium tallowate, sodium cocoate, water, mineral oil, octyl hydroxystearate, fragrance, glycerin, titanium dioxide, PEG-75, lanolin oil, docusate sodium, PEG-4 dilaurate, propylparaben, PEG-40 stearate, glyceryl monostearate, PEG-100 stearate, sodium Cl, BHT, EDTA. Bar 3.25 oz. *otc.*
Use: Therapeutic skin cleanser.

Keri Light Lotion. (Westwood Squibb) Water, stearyl alcohol, ceteareath-20, cetearyl octanoate, glycerin, stearyl heptanoate, stearyl alcohol, Carbomer 934, sodium hydroxide, squalane, methylparaben, propylparaben, fragrance. Bot. 6.5 oz, 13 oz. *otc.*
Use: Emollient.

Keri Lotion. (Westwood Squibb) Mineral oil, lanolin oil, water, propylene glycol, glyceryl stearate, PEG-100 stearate, PEG 40 stearate, PEG-4 dilaurate, laureth-4, parabens, docusate sodium, triethanolamine, quaternium 15, carbomer 934, fragrance. Bot. 6.5 oz, 13 oz, 20 oz. *otc.*
Use: Emollient.

Kerlone. (Searle) Betaxolol HCl 10 mg or 25 mg/Tab. Bot. 100s, UD 100s. *Rx.*
Use: Beta-adrenergic blocking agent.

Kerocaine.
See: Procaine HCl (Various Mfr.).

Kerodex. (Wyeth-Ayerst) *otc.*
No. 51: Water-miscible. Tube 4 oz, Jar lb.
No. 71: Water-repellent. Tube 4 oz, Jar lb.
Use: Emollient.

kerohydric. A de-waxed, oil-soluble fraction of lanolin.
Use: Emollient, cleanser.
See: Alpha-Keri, Soap, Spray (Westwood Squibb).
Keri, Cream, Lot. (Westwood Squibb).
W/Docusate sodium, sodium alkyl polyether sulfonate, sodium sulfoacetate, sulfur, salicylic acid, hexachlorophene.
See: Sebulex, Cream, Liq. (Westwood Squibb).

Kerr Insta-Char. (Kerr) **Regular:** Aqueous suspension activated charcoal 50 g/8 oz. **Pediatric:** Aqueous suspension activated charcoal 15 g/4 oz. *otc.*
Use: Antidote.

Kerr Triple Dye. (Kerr) Gentian violet, proflavine hemisulfate, brilliant green in water. Dispensing bot. 15 ml. Single Use Dispos-A-Swab 0.65 ml, Box 10s, Case 10 × 50 Box. *otc.*
Use: Antiseptic.

Kestrone 5. (Hyrex) Estrone 5 mg/ml, sodium carboxymethylcellulose, povidone, benzyl alcohol, parabens/Inj. Vial 10 ml. *Rx.*
Use: Estrogen.

Ketalar. (Parke-Davis) Ketamine HCl, sodium Cl, benzethonium Cl. **10 mg/ml:** Vial 20 ml, 25 ml and 50 ml. Pkg. 10s; **50 mg/ml:** Vial 10 ml. **100 mg/ml:** Vial 5 ml. Pkg. 10s. *Rx.*
Use: General anesthetic.

• **ketamine hydrochloride,** (KEET-uh-MEEN) U.S.P. 23.
Use: Anesthetic.

See: Ketaject, Vial (Bristol).
Ketalar, Inj. (Parke-Davis).
•**ketanserin.** (KEET-AN-ser-in) USAN.
Use: Serotonin antagonist.
•**ketazocine.** (key-TAY-zoe-seen) USAN.
Use: Analgesic.
•**ketazolam.** (keet-AZE-oh-lam) USAN.
Use: Tranquilizer (minor).
•**kethoxal.** (KEY-thox-al) USAN.
Use: Antiviral.
•**ketipramine fumarate.** (key-TIH-prah-MEEN) USAN.
Use: Antidepressant.
•**ketoconazole,** (KEY-toe-KOE-nuh-zole) U.S.P. 23.
Use: Antifungal.
See: Nizoral, Prods. (Janssen).
Ketodestrin.
See: Estrone (Various Mfr.).
Keto-Diastix Reagent Strips. (Bayer) Dip and read reagent strip test for glucose and ketones in urine. Two test areas: glucose levels from 30 mg to 5000 mg/dL; Ketone test (acetoacetic acid) negative 5 mg, 40 mg, 80 mg, 160 mg/dL. Strip Bot. 50s, 100s.
Use: Diagnostic aid.
ketohexazine. 4, 6-Diethyl-3(2H)-pyridazinono (Lederle).
Use: Hypnotic.
ketohydroxyestratriene.
See: Estrone.
ketohydroxyestrin.
See: Estrone (Various Mfr.).
ketone tests.
Use: Diagnostic aid.
See: Acetest Reagent, Tab. (Bayer).
Chemstrip K, Reagent paper (Boehringer Mannheim).
Ketostix Strips, Reagent Strips (Bayer).
Ketonex-1. (Ross) Protein 15 g, fat 23.9 g, carbohydrates 46.3 g, linoleic acid 1800 mg, Fe 9 mg, Na 190 mg, K 675 mg. With appropriate vitamins and minerals. 480 Cal/100 g. Isoleucine, leucine and valine free. Pow. Can 350 g. *otc.*
Use: Nutritional supplement.
Ketonex-2. (Ross) Protein 30 g, fat 15.5 g, carbohydrates 30 g, Fe 13 mg, Na 880 mg, K 1370 mg. With appropriate vitamins and minerals. 410 Cal/100 g. Isoleucine, leucine and valine free. Pow. Can 325 g. *otc.*
Use: Nutritional supplement.
•**ketoprofen,** (KEY-to-pro-fen) U.S.P. 23.
Use: Anti-inflammatory.
See: Orudis, Cap. (Wyeth-Ayerst).

Oruvail, Cap. (Wyeth-Ayerst).
Actron, Tab (Bayer).
ketoprofen. (Various Mfr.) 25 mg, 50 mg, 75 mg. Cap. Bot. 100s, 500s.
Use: Anti-inflammatory.
•**ketorfanol.** (key-TAR-fan-AHL) USAN.
Use: Analgesic.
•**ketorolac tromethamine,** (KEY-TOR-oh-lak tro-METH-uh-meen) U.S.P. 23.
Use: Analgesic.
See: Toradol (Syntex).
ketorolac tromethamine. (Ethex). 10 mg, lactose/Tab. Bot. 100s. *Rx.*
Use: Analgesic.
ketorolac tromethamine.
Use: Ophthalmic non-steroidal anti-inflammatory agent.
See: Acular (Allergan).
Ketostix Reagent Strips. (Bayer) Sodium nitroprusside, sodium phosphate, glycine. Stick test for ketones in urine (measures acetoacetic acid). Bot. 50s, 100s, UD 20s.
Use: Diagnostic aid.
•**ketotifen fumarate.** (KEY-toe-TIE-fen) USAN.
Use: Antiasthmatic.
Key-Plex. (Hyrex) Vitamins B_1 50 mg, B_2 5 mg, B_{12} 1000 mcg, pyridoxine HCl 5 mg, d-panthenol 6 mg, niacinamide 125 mg, ascorbic acid 50 mg/ml. Vial 10 ml. *Rx.*
Use: Parenteral nutritional supplement.
Key-Pred. (Hyrex) Prednisolone. **25 mg/ml:** Vial 10 ml, 30 ml; **50 mg/ml:** Vial 10 ml. *Rx.*
Use: Corticosteroid.
Key-Pred-SP. (Hyrex) Prednisolone sodium phosphate 20 mg/ml. Vial 10 ml. *Rx.*
Use: Corticosteroid.
K-G Elixir. (Geneva Pharm) Potassium (as potassium gluconate) 20 mEq/15 ml, alcohol 5%. Elix. Bot. pt. *Rx.*
Use: Potassium replacement.
kharophen.
See: Acetarsone (Various Mfr.).
khellin.
Use: Coronary vasodilator.
Kiddie Powder. (Gordon) Pure fine Italian talc. Can 3.5 oz. *otc.*
Use: Antifungal.
Kiddi-Vites, Improved. (Geneva Pharm) Vitamins A 5000 IU, D 500 IU, B_1 1 mg, B_2 1.5 mg, B_{12} 2 mcg, C 50 mg, B_6 1 mg, pantothenate 2 mg, niacinamide 10 mg/Tab. Bot. 100s, 1000s. *otc.*
Use: Vitamin supplement.

kidney function agents.
See: Biotel Kidney (Biotel).
Indigo Carmine Soln. (Various Mfr.).
Inulin, Amp. (Arnar-Stone).
Iodohippurate, Sodium.
Mannitol Soln., Amp. (Merck).
Methylene Blue (Various Mfr.).
Phenolsulfonphthalein (Various Mfr.).
Kie Syrup. (Laser) Potassium iodide 150 mg, ephedrine HCl 8 mg/5 ml. Syr. Bot. pt, gal. *Rx.*
Use: Expectorant, decongestant.
kinate. Hexahydrotetra hydroxybenzoate salt, quinic acid salt.
Kinevac. (Squibb) Sincalide 5 mcg/vial. For gallbladder, pancreatic secretion and cholecystography.
Use: Diagnostic aid.
Kin White. (Whiteworth Towne) Tri-amcinolone acetonide. **Cream:** 0.025% or 1%. Tube 15 g, 80 g. **Oint.:** 1%. Tube 15 g, 80 g. *Rx.*
Use: Corticosteroid, topical.
•**kitasamycin.** USAN. An antibiotic substance obtained from cultures of *Streptomyces kitasatoensis.* Under study.
Use: Antibacterial.
Klaron. (Dermik) Sodium sulfacetamide 10%, propylene glycol, polyethylene glycol 400, methylparaben, EDTA/Lot. Bot. 59 ml. *Rx.*
Use: Treatment of acne.
Klavikordal. (U.S. Ethicals) Nitroglycerin 2.6 mg/SR Tab. Bot. 100s, 1000s. *Rx.*
Use: Antianginal.
KLB6 Complete. (NBTY) Vitamins A 833.3 IU, E 5 mg (as IU), B_3 3.3 mg, C 10 mg, soya lecithin 200 mg, kelp 25 mg, cider vinegar 40 mg, wheat bran 83.3 mg, D 66.7 IU, FA 0.067 mg, B_1 0.25 mg, B_2 0.28 mg, B_6 8.3 mg, B_{12} 1 mcg, biotin 0.05 mg/Tab. Bot. 100s. *otc.*
Use: Vitamin supplement.
KLB6 Softgels. (NBTY) Vitamin B_6 mcg, soya lecithin 100 mg, kelp 25 mg, cider vinegar 80 mg/Capl. Bot. 100s. *otc.*
Use: Vitamin supplement.
K-Lease. (Pharmacia & Upjohn) Potassium chloride 10 mEq (750 mg). ER Cap. Bot. 100s, 500s, 1000s, 2500s, UD 100s. *Rx.*
Use: Potassium supplement.
Kleer Compound. (Scrip) Acetaminophen 300 mg, phenylpropanolamine HCl 35 mg, guaifenesin. Tab. Bot. 100s. *otc.*
Use: Analgesic, decongestant, expectorant.

Kleer Improved. (Scrip) Atropine sulfate 0.2 mg, chlorpheniramine maleate 5 mg/ml. *Rx.*
Use: Anticholinergic, antihistamine.
Klerist-D. (Nutripharm) **Cap. SR:** Pseudoephedrine HCl 120 mg, chlorpheniramine maleate 8 mg. Bot. 100s, 500s. **Tab.:** Pseudoephedrine HCl 60 mg, chlorpheniramine maleate 4 mg. Bot. 24s, 100s. *Rx.*
Use: Decongestant, antihistamine.
Kler-Ro Liquid. (Ulmer) Surgical cleanser and laboratory detergent. Bot. gal.
Use: Antiseptic.
Kler-Ro Powder. (Ulmer) Surgical cleanser and laboratory detergent. Can 2 lb, Bot. 6 lb.
Use: Antiseptic.
KL4-Surfactant.
Use: Treatment of acute respiratory distress syndrome. [Orphan drug]
Klonopin. (Roche) Clonazepam 0.5 mg, 1 mg or 2 mg/Tab. Rx Pak 100s. *c-iv.*
Use: Anticonvulsant.
K-Lor. (Abbott) Potassium Cl equivalent to potassium 20 mEq and Cl 20 mEq/ 2.6 g for oral soln. w/saccharin. Pkg. 30s, 100s. 15 mEq/2 g Pkg. 100s. *Rx.*
Use: Potassium supplement.
Klor-Con 8. (Upsher-Smith) Potassium Cl 8 mEq/ER Tab. Bot. 100s, 500s. *Rx.*
Use: Potassium supplement.
Klor-Con 10. (Upsher-Smith) Potassium Cl 10 mEq/ER Tab. Bot. 100s, 500s. *Rx.*
Use: Potassium supplement.
Klor-Con/25 Powder. (Upsher-Smith) Potassium Cl for oral soln 25 mEq/Pkt. Carton 30s, 100s, 250s. *Rx.*
Use: Potassium supplement.
Klor-Con/EF. (Upsher-Smith) Potassium bicarbonate 25 mEq/Tab. Carton 30s, 100s. *Rx.*
Use: Potassium supplement.
Klor-Con Powder. (Upsher-Smith) Potassium Cl for oral soln. 20 mEq/Packet w/ saccharin. Packet 1.5 g. Box 30s, 100s. *Rx.*
Use: Potassium supplement.
Klorvess Effervescent Granules. (Sandoz) Potassium 20 mEq, Cl 20 mEq supplied by potassium Cl 1.125 g, potassium bicarbonate 0.5 g, L-lysine monohydrochloride 0.913 g/Packet. w/ saccharin. Box 30s. *Rx.*
Use: Potassium supplement.
Klorvess Effervescent Tablets. (San-

doz) Potassium Cl 1.125 g, potassium bicarbonate 0.5 g, L-lysine HCl 0.913 g/Effervescent Tab. Sodium and sugar free. w/saccharin. Pkg. 60s, 1000s. *Rx.*
Use: Potassium supplement.

Klorvess Liquid. (Sandoz) Potassium Cl 1.5 g (20 mEq)/15 ml, alcohol 0.75%. Bot. pt. *Rx.*
Use: Potassium supplement.

Klotrix. (Bristol-Myers) Potassium Cl 10 mEq/SR Tab. Bot. 100s, 1000s, UD 100s. *Rx.*
Use: Potassium supplement.

K-Lyte. (Bristol) Potassium bicarbonate and citrate 25 mEq, saccharin. Lime and orange flavors. Effervescent Tab. Pkg. 30s, 100s, 250s. *Rx.*
Use: Potassium supplement.

K-Lyte/Cl. (Bristol) Potassium Cl 25 mEq, saccharin. Citrus and fruit punch flavor. Effervescent Tab. Pkg. 30s, 100s, 250s. Bulk powder 225 g/Can. *Rx.*
Use: Potassium supplement.

K-Lyte/Cl 50. (Bristol) Potassium Cl 50 mEq, saccharin. Citrus and fruit punch flavors. Pkg. 30s, 100s. *Rx.*
Use: Potassium supplement.

K-Lyte DS. (Bristol) Potassium bicarbonate and citrate 50 mEq, saccharin. Lime and orange flavor. Effervescent Tab. Pkg. 30s, 100s. *Rx.*
Use: Potassium supplement.

K-Norm. (Fisons) Potassium Cl 10 mEq/ CR Cap. Bot. 100s, 500s. *Rx.*
Use: Potassium supplement.

Koate HP. (Bayer) A stable dried concentrate of Anti-hemophilic Factor. When reconstituted, contains heparin ≤ 5 U/ ml, PEG ≤ 1500 ppm, glycine ≤ 0.05 M glycine, polysorbate 80 ≤ 25 ppm, calcium chloride ≤ 3 mM, aluminum ≤ 1 ppm, histidine ≤ 0.06 M, albumin (human) ≤ 10 mg/ml. Includes Sterile Water for Injection, double-ended transfer needle, filter needle and administration set. Pow. Bot. 250, 500, 1000 and 1500 IU Factor VIII activity (approximate). *Rx.*
Use: Antihemophilic.

Kodonyl Expectorant. (Halsey) Bromodiphenhydramine HCl 3.75 mg, diphenhydramine HCl 8.75 mg, ammonium Cl 80 mg, potassium guaiacolsulfonate 80 mg, menthol 0.5 mg/5 ml. Bot. 16 oz. *otc.*
Use: Antihistamine, expectorant.

Kof-Eze. (Roberts Med) Menthol 6 mg. Loz. Pkg. 4s, Bot. 500s. *otc.*
Use: Mouth and throat product.

Kogenate. (Bayer) Recombinant antihemophilic factor (Factor VIII). Pow. for inj. Bot. 250 IU, 500 IU, 1000 IU. *Rx.*
Use: Antihemophilic.

Kolephrin Caplets. (Pfeiffer) Pseudoephedrine HCl 30 mg, chlorpheniramine maleate 2 mg, acetaminophen 325 mg/Capl. Bot. 24s, 36s. *otc.*
Use: Decongestant, antihistamine, analgesic.

Kolephrin/DM Caplets. (Pfeiffer) Pseudoephedrine HCl 30 mg, chlorpheniramine maleate 2 mg, dextromethorphan HBr 10 mg, acetaminophen 325 mg/Capl. Bot. 30s. *otc.*
Use: Decongestant, antihistamine, antitussive, analgesic.

Kolephrin GG/DM Expectorant. (Pfeiffer) Dextromethorphan HBr 10 mg, guaifenesin 150 mg/5 ml. Alcohol free. Bot. 120 ml. *otc.*
Use: Antitussive, expectorant.

Kolephrin NN Liquid. (Pfeiffer) Phenylpropanolamine HCl 12.5 mg, pyrilamine maleate 10 mg, dextromethorphan HBr 7.5 mg/5 ml. Alcohol free. Bot. 120 ml. *otc.*
Use: Decongestant, antihistamine, antitussive.

•**kolfocon a.** (KAHL-FOE-kahn-A) USAN.
Use: Contact lens material (hydrophobic).

•**kolfocon b.** (KAHL-FOE-kahn B) USAN.
Use: Contact lens material (hydrophobic).

•**kolfocon c.** (KAHL-FOE-kahn C) USAN.
Use: Contact lens material (hydrophobic).

•**kolfocon d.** (KAHL-FOE-kahn D) USAN.
Use: Contact lens material (hydrophobic).

Kolyum Liquid. (Fisons) Potassium ion 20 mEq, chloride ion 3.4 mEq from potassium gluconate 3.9 g, potassium Cl 0.25 g/15 ml or 5 g/15 ml. w/saccharin, sorbitol. **Liq.:** Bot. pt, gal. *Rx.*
Use: Potassium supplement.

Konakion. (Roche) Phytonadione-synthetic vitamin K₁, polysorbate 80, phenol, propylene glycol, sodium acetate, glacial acetic acid. Amp. 2 mg/0.5 ml. Box 10s. *Rx.*
Use: Prevention and treatment of hypoprothrombinemia.

Kondon's Nasal Jelly. (Kondon) Tube 20 g w/ephedrine alkaloid. Tube 20 g. *otc.*
Use: Decongestant.

Kondremul. (Fisons) Mineral oil 55%,

Irish moss. Emulsion Bot. pt. *otc*.
Use: Laxative.
W/Phenolphthalein 2.2 gr/Tbsp. Bot. pt.
W/Cascara 0.66 g/15 ml. Bot. 14 oz.

Konsto. (Freeport) Docusate sodium 100 mg/Cap. Bot. 1000s. *otc.*
Use: Laxative.

Konsyl Powder. (Konsyl Pharm) Psyllium hydrophyllic mucilloid. Canister 300 g, 450 g, Packet 6 g, Ctn. 25s. *otc.*
Use: Laxative.

Konsyl-D Powder. (Konsyl Pharm) Psyllium hydrophilic mucilloid, dextrose. Canister 325 g, 500 g, Packet 6.5 g, Ctn. 25s. *otc.*
Use: Laxative.

Konsyl-Fiber. (Konsyl Pharm) Calcium polycarbophil 625 mg. Tab. Bot. 90s. *otc.*
Use: Laxative.

Konsyl-Orange. (Konsyl Pharm) Psyllium fiber 3.4 g/Tbsp., orange flavor. Pow. 12 g, 538 g. *otc.*
Use: Laxative.

Konyne 80. (Bayer) Dried plasma fraction of coagulation factors II, VII, IX and X. Heparin free. Heat treated. Vial. 10 ml and 20 ml. *Rx.*
Use: Antihemophilic.

Kophane Cough and Cold Formula Liquid. (Pfeiffer) Phenylpropanolamine HCl 12.5 mg, chlorpheniramine maleate 2 mg, dextromethorphan HBr 10 mg. Bot. 120 ml. *otc.*
Use: Decongestant, antihistamine, antitussive.

Koro-Flex. (Holland-Rantos) Improved contouring spring natural latex diaphrag 60 mm-95 mm.
Use: Contraceptive.

Koromex Coil Spring Diaphragm. (Holland-Rantos) Diaphragm made of pure latex rubber, cadmium plated coil spring. Koromex Jelly and Cream/kit. 50 mm-95 mm at graduations of 5 mm.
Use: Contraceptive.

Koromex Combination. (Holland-Rantos) Diaphrag 50 mm-95 mm, Koromex Jelly and Cream/Kit.
Use: Contraceptive.

Koromex Cream. (Schmid) Octoxynol 3%. Tube 115 g w/ applicator. *otc.*
Use: Spermicide contraceptive.

Koromex Crystal Clear Gel. (Schmid) Nonoxynol-9 2%. Tube 126 g with or without applicator. *otc.*
Use: Contraceptive.

Koromex Foam. (Schmid) Nonoxynol-9 12.5%. In 40 g. *otc.*

Use: Spermicide contraceptive.

Koromex Jelly. (Schmid) Nonoxynol-9 3%. Vaginal Jelly. 126 g. *otc.*
Use: Spermicide contraceptive.

Korum. (Geneva) Acetaminophen 5 gr/ Tab. Bot. 1000s. *otc.*
Use: Analgesic.

Kotabarb. (Wesley) Phenobarbital 1/4 gr/ Tab. Bot. 1000s. *Rx.*
Use: Sedative, hypnotic.

Kovitonic Liquid. (Freeda) Iron 42 mg, vitamins B_1 5 mg, B_6 10 mg, B_{12} 30 mcg, folic acid 0.1 mg, l-lysine 10 mg/ 15 ml. Liq. Bot. 120 ml, 240 ml. *otc.*
Use: Vitamin/mineral supplement.

K-Pek. (Rugby) Attapulgite 600 mg/15 ml. Susp. Bot. 237 ml, pt, gal. *otc.*
Use: Antidiarrheal.

K-Phos M.F. (Beach) Potassium acid phosphate 155 mg, sodium acid phosphate 350 mg/Tab. Bot. 100s, 500s. *Rx.*
Use: Urinary acidifier.

K-Phos Neutral. (Beach) Dibasic sodium phosphate 852 mg, potassium acid phosphate 155 mg, sodium acid phosphate 130 mg/Tab. Bot. 100s, 500s. *Rx.*
Use: Phosphorus supplement.

K-Phos No. 2. (Beach) Potassium acid phosphate 305 mg, sodium acid phosphate, anhydrous 700 mg/Tab. Bot. 100s, 500s. *Rx.*
Use: Urinary acidifier.

K-Phos Original. (Beach) Potassium acid phosphate 500 mg/Tab. Bot. 100s, 500s. *Rx.*
Use: Urinary acidifier, phosphorus supplement.

K.P.N. (Freeda) Vitamins C 333 mg, Fe 11 mg, A 2667 IU, D 133 IU, E 10 mg, B_1 2 mg, B_2 2 mg, B_3 10 mg, B_5 3.3 mg, B_6 0.83 mg, B_{12} 2 mcg, C 33 mg, FA 0.27 mg, I, Cu, Mn, K, Mg, Zn 6.7 mg, bioflavonoids/Tab. Bot. 100s, 250s, 500s. *otc.*
Use: Vitamin/mineral supplement.

K-P Suspension. (Century) Kaolin 5.2 g, pectin 260 mg/oz. Bot. gal. *otc.*
Use: Antidiarrheal.

Kronofed-A. (Ferndale) Pseudoephedrine HCl 120 mg, chlorpheniramine maleate 8 mg/Cap. Bot. 100s, 500s. *Rx.*
Use: Decongestant, antihistamine.

Kronofed-A-Jr. (Ferndale) Pseudoephedrine HCl 60 mg, chlorpheniramine maleate 4 mg/Cap. Bot. 100s, 500s. *Rx.*

Use: Decongestant, antihistamine.

Kronohist Kronocaps. (Ferndale) Chlorpheniramine maleate 4 mg, pyrilamine maleate 25 mg, phenylpropanolamine HCl 50 mg/Cap. Bot. 100s, 1000s. *otc.*
Use: Antihistamine, decongestant.

•**krypton clathrate Kr 85.** USAN.
Use: Radioactive agent.

•**krypton Kr 81m,** (KRIP-tahn Kr 81 m) U.S.P. 23.
Use: Radioactive agent.

K-Tab. (Abbott) Potassium Cl (10 mEq) 750 mg/ER Tab. Bot. 100s, 1000s, UD 100s. *Rx.*
Use: Potassium supplement.

K.T.V. Tablets. (Knight) Vitamin B_{12}, minerals. Bot. 50s. *otc.*
Use: Vitamin/mineral supplement.

Kudrox Double Strength Suspension. (Schwarz Pharma Kremers Urban) Aluminum hydroxide 500 mg, magnesium hydroxide 450 mg, simethicone 40 mg/5 ml. Bot. 355 ml. *otc.*
Use: Antacid.

Kutapressin. (Kremers-Urban) Liver derivative complex composed of peptides and amino acids. Inj. Vial 20 ml. *Rx.*
Use: Liver derivative complex.

Kutrase. (Kremers-Urban) Amylase 30 mg, protease 6 mg, lipase 25 mg, cellulase 2 mg, l-hyoscyamine sulfate 0.0625 mg, phenyltoloxamine citrate 15 mg/Cap. Bot. 100s, 500s. *Rx.*
Use: Digestive aid.

Ku-Zyme. (Kremers-Urban) Amylase 30 mg, protease 6 mg, lipase 75 mg, cellulase 2 mg/Cap. Bot. 100s, 500s. *Rx.*
Use: Digestive aid.

Ku-Zyme HP. (Kremers-Urban) Lipase 8000 units, protease 30,000 units, amylase 30,000 units/Cap. Bot. 100s. *Rx.*
Use: Digestive aid.

Kwelcof. (Ascher) Hydrocodone bitartrate 5 mg, guaifenesin 100 mg/5 ml.
Bot. pt, UD 5 ml. Pkg. 10s, 100s. Alcohol, dye, sugar, and corn free. *c-III.*
Use: Antitussive, expectorant.

Kwikderm Cream. (NMC Labs) Tolnaftate 1%. Cream. Tube 15 g. *otc.*
Use: Antifungal, topical.

Kwikderm Solution. (NMC Labs) Tolnaftate 1%. Soln. Bot. 10 ml.
Use: Antifungal, topical.

Kwildane Shampoo. (Major) Gamma benzene hexachloride 1%. Bot. 60 ml, pt, gal.
Use: Pediculicide.

K-Y. (Johnson & Johnson) Glycerin, methylparaben, hydroxyethylcellulose. Jelly Tube 2.7 g, 5 g, 12 g, 60 g, 120 g. *otc.*
Use: Vaginal and rectal lubricant.

Kyodex Reagent Strips. (Kyoto) A disposable plastic reagent strip for determination of glucose in whole blood. Vial 25s.
Use: Diagnostic aid.

Kyotest UG Reagent Strips. (Kyoto) Reagent strips for glucose and ketones in urine.
Use: Diagnostic aid.

Kyotest UGK Reagent Strip. (Kyoto) Disposable reagent strip for measurement of glucose and ketones in the urine. Vial 50s, 100s.
Use: Diagnostic aid.

Kyotest UK Reagent Strips. (Kyoto) Reagent strip for ketones in urine. Vial 50s.
Use: Diagnostic aid.

KY Plus. (Johnson & Johnson) Nonoxynol-9 2%, methylparaben. Non-greasy. 113 g. *otc.*
Use: Vaginal and rectal lubricant.

Kytril. (SK-Beecham) Granisetron HCl. **Inj.:** 1.12 mg/ml. Inj. Single-use vial 1 ml. **Tab:** 1.12 mg/Tab. Pkg. 20s, unit-of-use 2s. *Rx.*
Use: Antiemetic (cancer therapy).

L

LA-12. (Hyrex) Hydroxocobalamin 1000 mcg/ml. Vial 30 ml. *Rx.*
Use: Vitamin B$_{12}$ supplement.

•**labetalol hydrochloride,** (la-BET-ul-lahl) U.S.P. 23.
Use: Antihypertensive, anti-adrenergic, (α-receptor, β-receptor).
See: Trandate Inj., Tab. (Glaxo).
W/Hydrochlorothiazide.
See: Trandate HCT, Tab. (Glaxo).
Normodyne, Inj., Tab. (Schering Plough).

Labstix Reagent Strips. (Bayer) Urine screening test. Bot 100s.
Use: Diagnostic aid.

Lac-Hydrin Lotion. (Westwood-Squibb) Lactic acid 12% neutralized w/ammonium hydroxide, light mineral oil, cetyl alcohol, parabens. Tube 5 oz, 12 oz. *Rx.*
Use: Emollient.

•**lacidipine.** (lah-SIH-dih-PEEN) USAN.
Use: Antihypertensive.

Laclede Cleaner. (Laclede) Container. 2 lb.
Use: Detergent for instruments and trays.

Laclede Disclosing Swab. (Laclede) Swabs 6″. 100s, 500s, 1000s.
Use: Dental swab.

Laclede Topi-Fluor A.P.F. Topical Cream. (Laclede) Fluoride ion 1.23% (from sodium fluoride) in orthophosphoric acid 0.98%. Jar 50 ml, 500 ml, 1000 ml, 2000 ml. *Rx.*
Use: Dental caries preventative.

Lacotein. (Christina) Protein digest 5% w/preservatives. Vial 30 ml (w/iodochin), Vial 30 ml. *Rx.*
Use: Protein supplement.

Lacril. (Allergan) Hydroxypropyl methylcellulose 0.5%, gelatin A 0.01%, chlorobutanol 0.5%, polysorbate 80, dextrose, magnesium Cl, sodium borate, sodium chloride. Soln. Dropper bot. 15 ml. *otc.*
Use: Lubricant, ophthalmic.

Lacri-Lube NP. (Allergan) White petrolatum 55.5%, mineral oil 42.5%, petrolatum/lanolin alcohol 2%. Oint. 0.7 g. *otc.*
Use: Lubricant, ophthalmic.

Lacri-Lube S.O.P. (Allergan) White petrolatum 56.8%, mineral oil 41.5%, lanolin alcohols, chlorobutanol. Tube 3.5 g, 7 g. *otc.*
Use: Lubricant, ophthalmic.

Lacrisert. (Merck) Hydroxypropyl cellulose 5 mg/insert. Pkg. 60s w/applicators. *Rx.*
Use: Artificial tear insert, ophthalmic.

LactAid. (McNeil) **Liq.:** Beta-D-galactosidase derived from *Kluyveromyces lactis* yeast (1000 Neutral Lactase units/ 5 drop dosage) in carrier of glycerol 50%, water 30%, inert yeast dry matter 20%. Units of 4, 12, 30 and 75 onequart dosages at 5 drops/dose. **Tab.:** Beta-D-galactosidase from *Aspergillis oryzae* (3300 FCC lactase units/Tab.) In 12s, 100s. *otc.*
Use: Digestive aid.

lactalbumin hydrolysate.
See: Aminonat.

lactase enzyme.
Use: Digestive aid.
See: LactAid, Capl. Liq. (McNeil).
Lactogest, Cap. (Thompson).
Lactrase, Cap. (Schwarz Pharma).
Dairy Ease, Tabs. (Sanofi Winthrop).
SureLac, Tab. (Caraco).

lactated ringer's injection.
Use: Electrolyte and fluid replenisher, systemic alkalizer.

•**lactic acid,** U.S.P. 23.
Use: Pharmaceutic necessity for sodium lactate injection.
W/Sodium pyrrolidone carboxylate.
See: LactiCare (Stiefel).
Lactinol, Lot. Creme (Pedinol).

Lacticare Lotion. (Stiefel) Lactic acid 5%, sodium pyrrolidone carboxylate 2.5% in an emollient lotion base. Bot. 8 oz, 12 oz, w/pump dispenser. *otc.*
Use: Emollient.

Lacticare-HC Lotion. (Stiefel) Hydrocortisone lotion 1% or 2.5%. **1%:** Bot 4 oz. **2.5%:** Bot. 2 oz. *Rx.*
Use: Corticosteroid, topical.

Lactinex. (Becton Dickinson) *Lactobacillus acidophilus & Lactobacillus bulgaricus* mixed culture. Tab. 250 mg, Bot. 50s. Gran. 1 g pk. Box 12s. *otc.*
Use: Antidiarrheal, nutritional supplement.

Lactinol. (Pedinol) Lactic acid 10%. Lot. Bot. 237 ml. *Rx.*
Use: Emollient.

Lactinol-E Creme. (Pedinol) Lactic acid 10%, Vitamin E 3500 IU/30 g. Cream 56.7 g. *Rx.*
Use: Emollient.

lactobacillus acidophilus. Preparation made from acid-producing bacterium.
Use: Antidiarrheal, nutritional supplement.
See: Bacid (Novartis).

DoFUS (Miller).
MoreDophilus (Freeda).
Pro-Bionate (Natren).
Superdophilus (Natren).

lactobacillus acidophilus & bulgaricus mixed culture.
See: Lactinex, Tab., Gran. (Becton Dickinson).

lactobacillus acidophilus, viable culture.
See: DoFus, Tab. (Miller).
Lactinex Granules, Tab. (Becton Dickinson).

lactobin. *Rx.*
Use: AIDS-associated diarrhea. [Orphan drug]

Lactocal-F. (Laser) Vitamin A 4000 IU, D 400 IU, E 30 IU, C 100 mg, folic acid 1 mg, B_1 3 mg, B_2 3.4 mg, B_3 20 mg, B_6 5 mg, B_{12} 12 mcg, calcium 200 mg, I, iron 65 mg, Mg, Cu, zinc 15 mg/Tab. Bot. 100s, 1000s. *Rx.*
Use: Vitamin/mineral supplement.

lactoflavin.
See: Riboflavin, U.S.P. 23. (Various Mfr.).

Lactofree. (Bristol-Myers) Protein 14.7 g, carbohydrates 69.3 g, fat 36.7 g, linoleic acid 6 g, Fe 12 mg, Na 200 mg, K 733.3 mg, with appropriate vitamins and minerals. Lactose free. 666.7 cal/L. Pow. Can 400 g. *otc.*
Use: Enteral nutritional supplement.

lactose. Milk sugar.
Use: Pharmaceutic aid (tablet and capsule diluent).
See: Natur-Aid, pow. (Scott/Cord).

•**lactose anhydrous,** N.F. 18.
Use: Pharmaceutic aid (tablet and capsule diluent).

•**lactose monohydrate,** N.F. 18.
Use: Pharmaceutic aid (tablet and capsule diluent).

Lactrase. (Rhone-Poulenc Rorer) Standardized enzyme lactase (β-D-galactosidase) 125 mg dispersed in maltodextrins. Cap. Bot. 100s. *otc.*
Use: Nutritional supplement.

Lactrodectus Mactans Antivenin.
(Merck) Antivenin 6000 units per vial (with 1:10,000 thimersol), supplied with a 2.5 ml vial of Sterile Water for Injection and a 1 mg vial (with 1:10,000 thimersol) of normal horse serum (1:10 dilution) for sensitivity testing. *Rx.*
Use: Antivenin (Black Widow spider).
See: antivenin (Lactrodectus Mactans).

•**lactulose concentrate,** (LAK-tyoo-lohs) U.S.P. 23.

Use: Laxative, treatment of hepatic coma and chronic constipation.
See: Cephulac, Syr. (Hoechst Marion Roussel).
Chronulac, Liq. (Hoechst Marion Roussel).

ladakamycin.
Use: Refractory acute myelogenous leukemia (AML) agent.
See: Azacitidine.

Ladogal. (Sanofi Winthrop) Danazol. *Rx.*
Use: Androgen.

Ladogar. (Sanofi Winthrop) Danazol. *Rx.*
Use: Androgen.

Lady Esther. (Menley & James) Mineral oil. Cream. 120 g. *otc.*
Use: Emollient.

L.A.E. 20. (Seatrace) Estradiol valerate 20 mg/ml. Vial 10 ml. *Rx.*
Use: Estrogen.

L.A.E. 40. (Seatrace) Estradiol valerate 40 mg/ml. Vial 10 ml. *Rx.*
Use: Estrogen.

Lamictal. (Glaxo Wellcome) Lamotrigine 25 mg, 100 mg, 150 mg or 200 mg/ Tab. Bot. 25s (25 mg), 60s (150 mg, 200 mg), 100s (100 mg). *Rx.*
Use: Anticonvulsant.

•**lamifiban.** (la-mih-FIE-ban) USAN.
Use: Antithrombotic, platelet aggregation inhibitor, fibrinogen receptor antagonist.

Lamisil. (Sandoz) Terbinafine HCl. 1%. Cream/Tube 15 and 30 g. 250 mg/Tab. Bot. 30s and 100s.
Use: Antifungal.

•**lamivudine.** (la-MIH-view-deen) USAN.
Use: Antiviral; treatment of HIV infection.
See: Epivir, Tab., Oral Soln. (Glaxo Wellcome).

•**lamotrigine.** (lah-MOE-trih-JEEN) USAN.
Use: Anticonvulsant; Lennox-Gestaut syndrome. [Orphan drug]
See: Lamictal, Tab. (Glaxo Wellcome)

Lampit. (Bayer 2502) Nifurtimox.
Use: Anti-infective.

Lamprene. (Novartis) Clofazimine 50 mg/ Cap. Bot. 100s. *Rx.*
Use: Leprostatic.

Lanabiotic. (Combe) Polymyxin B sulfate 5000 units, neomycin (as sulfate) 3.5 mg, bacitracin 500 units, lidocaine 40 mg/g. Oint. 15 g, 30 g. *otc.*
Use: Anti-infective, local anesthetic, topical.

Lanacane. (Combe) Spray: Benzocaine 20%, benzethonium Cl, ethanol, aloe extract. 113 ml. Cream: Benzocaine

6%, benzethonium Cl, aloe, parabens, castor oil, glycerin, isopropyl alcohol. 28 g, 56 g. *otc.*
Use: Topical anesthetic.

Lanacort 10. (Combe) Hydrocortisone acetate 1% **Cream.** Tube 15, 30 g. **Oint.** Tube 15 g. *otc.*
Use: Corticosteroid, topical.

Lanacort Cream. (Combe) Hydrocortisone acetate 0.5%. Tube 0.5 oz, 1 oz. *otc.*
Use: Corticosteroid, topical.

Lanaphilic Ointment. (Medco Lab) Sorbitol, isopropyl palmitate, stearyl alcohol, white petrolatum, lanolin oil, sodium lauryl sulfate, propylene glycol, methylparaben, propylparaben. Jar 16 oz. Also available w/urea 10% or 20%. *otc.*
Use: Emollient.

Lanaphilic w/Urea 10%. (Medco Labs) Urea, stearyl alcohol, white petrolatum, isopropyl palmitate, propylene glycol, sorbitol, sodium lauryl sulfate, lactic acid, parabens. Oint. Jar lb. *otc.*
Use: Emollient.

Laniazid. (Lannett) Isoniazid 50 mg/5 ml, sorbitol. Syrup. 480 ml. *Rx.*
Use: Antituberculosis drug.

•**lanolin,** U.S.P. 23. *Formerly Anhydrous lanolin.*
Use: Pharmaceutic aid (ointment base, absorbant).
See: Kerohydric (Westwood Squibb).
W/Coconut oil, pine oil, castor oil, cholesterols, lecithin and parachlorometaxylenol.
See: Sebacide, Liq. (Paddock).
W/Diiosbutylcresoxyethoxyethyl, dimethyl benzyl ammonium Cl, menthol.
See: Hospital Lot. (Paddock).

•**lanolin alcohols,** N.F. 18.
Use: Pharmaceutic aid (emulsifying agent).

•**lanolin, modified,** U.S.P. 23.
Use: Pharmaceutic aid (ointment base, absorbant).

Lanoline. (Glaxo Wellcome) Perfumed emollient. Oint. Tube 1.75 oz. *otc.*
Use: Pharmaceutic aid, ointment base, absorbant, emollient.

Lano-Lo Bath Oil. (Whorton) 8 oz.

Lanolor. (Numark) Cream. Jar 8 oz, tube 2 oz. *otc.*
Use: Emollient.

•**lanoteplase.** USAN.
Use: Thrombolytic (plasminogen activator).

Lanoxicaps. (Glaxo Wellcome) Digoxin

0.05 mg, 0.1 mg, 0.2 mg. Soln. in cap. Bot. 100s. *Rx.*
Use: Cardiac glycoside.

Lanoxin. (Glaxo Wellcome) Digoxin. **Tab. 0.125 mg:** Bot. 100s, 1000s, Unit-of-use 30s, UD 100s. **0.25 mg:** Bot. 100s, 1000s, 5000s, UD 100s, Unit-of-use 30s. **Pediatric Elix.:** 0.05 mg/ml, alcohol 10%. Bot. 60 ml. **Inj.:** (w/propylene glycol 40%, alcohol 10%, sodium phosphate 0.3%, anhydrous citric acid 0.08%) Amp. 0.5 mg/2 ml. Amp. 10s, 50s. **Pediatric Inj.:** 0.1 mg/ml. Amp. 1 ml 10s. *Rx.*
Use: Cardiac glycoside.

•**lanreotide acetate.** (lan-REE-oh-tide) USAN.
Use: Antineoplastic.

•**lansoprazole.** (lan-SO-pruh-zole) USAN.
Use: Gastric acid pump inhibitor, antiulcerative, maintenance of healing of erosive esophagitis and gastric ulcers.
See: Prevacid, Cap. (TAP Pharm).

Lanturil. (Sanofi Winthrop) Oxypertine. *Rx.*
Use: Anxiolytic, tranquilizer.

lanum. (Various Mfr.) Lanolin. *otc.*
Use: Pharmaceutic aid.

•**lapyrium chloride.** (LAH-pihr-ee-uhm KLOR-ide) USAN.
Use: Pharmaceutic aid (surfactant).

Lardet. (Standex) Phenobarbital 8 mg, theophylline 130 mg, ephedrine HCl 24 mg/Tab. Bot. 100s. *Rx.*
Use: Antiasthmatic combination.

Lardet Expectorant. (Standex) Phenobarbital 8 mg, theophylline 130 mg, ephedrine HCl 24 mg, guaifenesin 100 mg/Tab. Bot. 100s. *Rx.*
Use: Antiasthmatic combination.

Largon. (Wyeth-Ayerst) Propiomazine HCl 20 mg/ml w/ sodium formaldehyde sulfoxylate, sodium acetate buffer. Amp. 1 ml, 2 ml. Pkg. 25s, Tubex syringe 1 ml. *Rx.*
Use: Sedative, hypnotic.

Lariam. (Roche) Mefloquine HCl 250 mg/ Tab. UD 25s. *Rx.*
Use: Antimalarial.

Larodopa Capsules. (Roche) Levodopa 100 mg, 250 mg or 500 mg/Cap. **100 mg:** Bot. 100s. **250 mg:** Bot. 100s, 500s. **500 mg:** Bot. 100s, 500s. *Rx.*
Use: Antiparkinsonian.

Larodopa Tablets. (Roche) Levodopa 100 mg, 250 mg or 500 mg. **100 mg:** Bot. 100s. **250 mg and 500 mg:** Bot. 100s, 500s. *Rx.*
Use: Antiparkinsonian.

Larotid. (SK-Beecham) Amoxicillin. **Cap.: 250 mg:** Bot. 100s, 500s, UD 100s, unit-of-use 18s. **500 mg:** Bot. 50s, 500s. **Oral Susp.:** 125 mg or 250 mg (as trihydrate)/5 ml. Bot. 80 ml, 100 ml, 150 ml. **Pediatric drops:** 50 mg (as trihydrate)/ml. Bot. 15 ml. *Rx.*
Use: Anti-infective, penicillin.

Larynex. (Dover) Benzocaine. Sugar, lactose and salt free. Loz. UD Box 500s. *otc.*
Use: Local anesthetic.

Lasix. (Hoechst Marion Roussel) Furosemide. **Tab.:** 20 mg or 40 mg/Tab. Bot. 100s, 500s, 1000s, UD 100s. **Inj.:** 10 mg/ml. 2 ml/Amp. Box 5s, 50s, 4 ml/Amp. Box 5s, 25s; 10 ml/Amp. Box 5s, 25s; Syringe 2 ml, 4 ml, 10 ml. Box 5s. Single Use Vial 2 ml, 4 ml, 10 ml. **Oral Soln.:** 10 mg/ml. Alcohol 11.5%. Dropper Bot 60 ml, Bot. 120 ml. *Rx.*
Use: Diuretic.

lassar's paste.
See: Zinc Oxide Paste, U.S.P. 23. (Various Mfr.).

•**latanoprost.** (lah-TAN-oh-prahst) USAN.
Use: Antiglaucoma agent.
See: Xalatan (Pharmacia & Upjohn).

Latest-CRP Kit. (Fisher) Measures C-reactive protein in serum. Kit 1s.
Use: Diagnostic aid.

•**laureth 4.** (LAH-reth 4) USAN.
Use: Pharmaceutic aid (surfacant).

•**laureth 9.** (LAH-reth 9) USAN. Mixture of polyoxyethylene lauryl ethers having a statistical average of 9 ethylene oxide groups per molecule.
Use: Surfactant, emulsifier, spermaticide.

•**laureth 10s.** (LAH-reth 10s) USAN.
Use: Spermaticide.

•**laurocapram.** (LAHR-oh-KAH-pram) USAN.
Use: Pharmaceutic aid (excipient).

lauromacrogol 400. Laureth 9.

•**lauryl isoquinolinium bromide.** (LAH-rill EYE-so-KWIN-oh-lih-nee-uhm) USAN.
Use: Anti-infective.

lauryl sulfoacetate.
See: Lowila, Cake, Liq., Oint. (Westwood Squibb).

Lavacol. (Parke-Davis Prods) Ethyl alcohol 70%. Bot. pt. *otc.*
Use: Anti-infective, topical.

Lavatar. (Doak) Coal tar distillate 25.5% in a bath oil base. Liq. Bot. 4 oz, pt. *otc.*
Use: Antipsoriatic, antipruritic.

lavender oil.
Use: Perfume.

•**lavoltidine succinate.** (lahv-OLE-tih-DEEN) USAN. *Formerly Loxotidine.*
Use: Anti-ulcerative; histamine H_2-receptor blocker.

Lavoptik Emergency Wash. (Lavoptik) Eye, face, body wash. 32 oz/Emergency station. *otc.*
Use: Emergency wash.

Lavoptik Eye Wash. (Lavoptik) Sodium Cl 0.49%, sodium biphosphate 0.4%, sodium phosphate 0.45%/100 ml w/ benzalkonium Cl 0.005%. Bot. 6 oz. *otc.*
Use: Irrigating agent, ophthalmic.

Lavoris. (Procter & Gamble) Zinc Cl, glycerin, poloxamer 407, saccharin, polysorbate 80, flavors, clove oil, alcohol, citric acid, water. Bot. 6 oz, 12 oz, 18 oz, 24 oz. *otc.*
Use: Mouthwash.

Laxative Caps. (Weeks & Leo) Docusate sodium 100 mg, casanthranol 30 mg/Cap. Bot. 30s, 60s. *otc.*
Use: Laxative.

laxatives.
See: Agar-Gel (Various Mfr.).
Aloe (Various Mfr.).
Aloin (Various Mfr.).
Bile Salts (Various Mfr.).
Bisacodyl, Tab., Supp. (Various Mfr.).
Bisacodyl Tannex (Pilkington Barnes Hind).
Carboxymethylcellulose Sodium (Various Mfr.).
Casanthranol, Cap., Tab. (Various Mfr.).
Cascara Sagrada (Various Mfr.).
Cascara Sagrada Fluidextract, Liq. (Parke-Davis).
Cascara Tab. (Various Mfr.).
Castor Oil (Various Mfr.).
Citrucel (SK-Beecham).
Correctol, Tab. (Schering Plough).
Docusate Sodium (Various Mfr.).
Ex-Lax, Tab., Pow. (Ex-Lax. Inc.).
Feen-a-Mint, Gum, Mints (Schering Plough).
Karaya Gum (Penick).
Liquid Petrolatum, Liq. (Various Mfr.).
Magnesia Maga (Various Mfr.).
Maltsupex (Wallace).
Methylcellulose (Various Mfr.).
Mucilloid of Psyllium Seed W/Dextrose (Searle).
Mylanta Natural Fiber Supplement (J & J-Merck).
Nature's Remedy (SK-Beecham).
Nujol, Liq. (Schering Plough).
Oxyphenisatin Acetate (Various Mfr.).

Petrolatum, Liq. (Various Mfr.).

Petrolatum, Liq., Emulsion (Various Mfr.).

Phenolphthalein (Various Mfr.).

Plantago ovata, Coating (Various Mfr.).

Poloxalkol, Cap., Soln. (Various Mfr.).

Prune Concentrate, Tab., Cap. (Various Mfr.).

Prune Preps. (Various Mfr.).

Psyllium Granules W/Dextrose (Med. Chem.).

Psyllium Husk Pow. (Pharmacia & Upjohn).

Psyllium Hydrocolloid, Pow. (Stuart).

Psyllium Hydrophilic Mucilloid (Various Mfr.).

Psyllium Seed, Gel, Gran. (Various Mfr.).

Regutol, Tab. (Schering Plough).

Restore (Inagra).

Sakara, Gran. (Schering Plough).

Senna, Alexandrian, Liq., Tab. (Various Mfr.).

Senna, Cassia angustifolia, Tab. (Brayten).

Senna Conc., Standardized, Gran., Tab., Pow., Supp. (Various Mfr.).

Senna Fruit Extract, Liq. (Various Mfr.).

Sennosides A & B, Tab. (Sandoz).

Sodium Biphosphate (Various Mfr.).

Sodium Phosphate (Various Mfr.).

Unifiber (Dow B. Hickam).

Laxinate 100. (Roberts) Dioctyl sodium sulfosuccinate 100 mg/Cap. Bot. 100s, 1000s. *otc.*
Use: Laxative.

Lax-Pills. (G & W) Yellow phenolphthalein 90 mg/Tab. Bot. 30s, 60s. *otc.*
Use: Laxative.

layor carang.
See: Agar (Various Mfr.).

•**lazabemide.** (lazz-AH-bem-ide) USAN.
Use: Antiparkinsonian.

Lazer Creme. (Pedinol) Vitamins E 3500 units, A 100,000 units/oz. Jar 2 oz. *otc.*
Use: Emollient.

Lazerformalyde Solution. (Pedinol) Formaldehyde 10%, polysorbate 20, hydroxyethyl cellulose. Bot. 3 oz. *Rx.*
Use: Antiperspirant drying agent for presurgical removal of warts or nonsurgical laser treatment of warts.

Lazersporin-C Solution. (Pedinol) Neomycin sulfate 3.5 mg, polymyxin B sulfate 10,000 units, hydrocortisone 1%. Bot. 10 ml. *Rx.*
Use: Anti-infective combination, topical.

l-bulgaricus. (Antidiarrheal).
See: Bacid (Medeva).
Lactinex B (Becton Dickinson).
More-Dophilus (Freeda).

LC-65 Daily Contact Lens Cleaner. (Allergan) Daily cleaning solution for all hard, soft (hydrophilic), rigid gas permeable contact lenses. Bot. 15 ml, 60 ml. *otc.*
Use: Contact lens care.

L-Caine E. (Century) Lidocaine HCl 1% or 2%, epinephrine 1:100,000/ml. Inj. 20 ml, 50 ml. *Rx.*
Use: Local anesthetic.

L-Caine Viscous. (Century) Lidocaine HCl 2% with sodium carboxymethylcellulose. Soln. Bot. 100 ml. *Rx.*
Use: Local anesthetic.

l-carnitine. Amino acid derivative 250 mg/Cap. Bot. 60s.
Use: Nutritional supplement.
See: Vitacarn.
Carnitor (Sigma-Tau).

L.C.D. (Almay) Alcohol extractions of crude coal tar. Cream, soln. Bot. 4 oz, pt. *otc.*
Use: Antipsoriatic, antipruritic (topical).
See: Coal Tar Topical Soln., U.S.P. 23.

LCR. *Rx.*
Use: Antineoplastic.
See: Vincristine sulfate.

LCx Neisseria gonorrhoeae Assay. (Abbott) Reagent kit for the detection of *Neisseria gonorrhoeae* in female endocervical, male urethral and urine swab specimens. Kit. 100s. *Rx.*
Use: Diagnostic aid.

l-cysteine.
See: Cysteine.

l-deprenyl.
See: Selegiline HCl.

LDH Reagent Strip. (Bayer) A quantitative strip test for LDH in serum or plasma. Seralyzer reagent strip. Bot. 25s. *Rx.*
Use: Diagnostic aid.

Leber Tabulae. (Paddock) Aloe 0.09 g, extract of rhei 0.03 g, myrrh 0.01 g, frangula 5 mg, galbanum 2 mg, olibanum 3 mg/Tab. Bot. 100s, 500s, 1000s.

Lec-E-Plex. (Barth's) Vitamin E 100 IU, 200 IU or 400 IU/Cap. w/lecithin. Bot. 100s, 500s, 1000s. *otc.*
Use: Vitamin E supplement.

•**lecimibide.** USAN.
Use: Antihyperlipidemic.

lecithin. (Various Mfr.) Lecithin. **Cap.:** 520 mg. Bot. 100s, 250s, 1000s; 650 mg. Bot. 90s, 100s, 250s, 500s. **Pow.:** 120 g, kg, lb. *otc.*

Use: Nutritional supplement.

●**lecithin,** N.F. 18.
Use: Pharmaceutic aid (emulsifying agent).
W/Choline base, cephalin, lipositol.
See: Alcolec Cap., Gran. (American Lecithin).
W/Coconut oil, pine oil, castor oil, lanolin, cholesterols, parachlorometaxylenol.
See: Sebacide, Liq. (Paddock).
W/Vitamins.
See: Acletin, Cap. (Associated Concentrates).
Lec-E-Plex, Cap. (Barth's).

lecithin. (Arcum) 1200 mg/Cap. Bot. 100s, 1000s; Gran. Bot. 8 oz; Pow. Bot. 4 oz.
Use: Pharmaceutic aid (emulsifying agent).
(Barth's) 8 gr/Cap. Bot. 100s, 500s, 1000s; Gran. Can 8 oz, 16 oz; Pow. Can 10 oz.
(Cavendish) Tab. (0.5 gr) Bot. 500s.
(Quality Generics) 1200 mg, Cap. 100s.
(De Pree) Cap. Bot. 100s.
(Pfanstiehl) 25 g, 100 g, 500 g/Pkg.

Legatrin PM. (Columbia) Acetaminophen 500 mg, diphenhydramine HCl 50 mg/ Capl. Bot. 30s, 50s. *otc.*
Use: Sleep aid.

lemon oil.
Use: Pharmaceutic aid (flavor).

lenetran. Mephenoxalone.
Use: Tranquilizer.

lenicet.
See: Aluminum Acetate, Basic (Various Mfr.).

●**leniquinsin.** (LEN-ih-KWIN-sin)
USAN. 6,7-Dimethoxy-4-(vera-trylideneamino) quinoline. Under study.
Use: Antihypertensive.

Lenium Medicated Shampoo. (Sanofi Winthrop) Selenium sulfide. *otc.*
Use: Antiseborrheic.

●**lenograstim.** (leh-no-GRAH-stim) USAN.
Use: Antineutropenic, hematopoietic stimulant, immunomodulator (granulocyte colony-stimulating factor).

●**lenperone.** (LEN-per-OHN) USAN.
Use: Antipsychotic.

Lens Clear. (Allergan) Sterile, isotonic solution surfactant cleaner w/sorbic acid 0.1%, edetate disodium 0.2%. Bot. 15 ml. *otc.*
Use: Soft contact lens care.

Lens Drops. (Ciba Vision) Sodium chloride, borate buffer, carbamide, po-

loxamer 407, EDTA 0.2%, sorbic acid 0.15%. Soln. Bot. 15 ml. *otc.*
Use: Rewetting solution.

Lensept Disinfecting Solution. (Ciba Vision) Micro-filtered hydrogen peroxide with sodium stannate 3%, sodium nitrate, phosphate buffers. Soln. Bot. 237, 355 ml. *otc.*
Use: Disinfecting solution.

Lensept Rinse and Neutralizer. (Ciba Vision) Sodium chloride, sodium borate decahydrate, boric acid, bovine catalase, sorbic acid, EDTA. Soln. Bot. 237 ml. System includes lens cup and holder. *otc.*
Use: Rinsing and neutralizing solution.

Lens Fresh. (Allergan) Sterile, buffered, isotonic aqueous soln. W/hydroxyethyl cellulose, sodium Cl, boric acid, sodium borate, sorbic acid 0.1%, edetate disodium 0.2%. Bot. 0.5 oz. *otc.*
Use: Contact lens care.

Lensine Extra Strength. (Ciba Vision) Cleaning agent with benzalkonium Cl 0.01%, EDTA 0.1%. Soln. Bot. 45 ml. *otc.*
Use: Hard contact lens care.

Lens Lubricant. (Bausch & Lomb) Povidone and polyoxyethylene with thimerosal 0.004%, EDTA 0.1% Soln. Bot. 15 ml. *otc.*
Use: Lens lubricant.

Lens Plus. (Allergan) Isotonic soln. w/ sodium Cl 0.9%. Aerosol 3 oz, 8 oz, 12 oz. Preservative free. *otc.*
Use: Soft contact lens care.

Lens Plus Daily Cleaner. (Allergan) Buffered solution with cocoamphocarboxyglycinate, sodium lauryl sulfate, hexylene glycol, sodium chloride, sodium phosphate. Preservative free. Soln. Bot. 15 ml or 30 ml. *otc.*
Use: Soft contact lens cleansing solution.

Lens Plus Oxysept Disinfecting Solution. (Allergan) Hydrogen peroxide with sodium stannate 3%, sodium nitrate and phosphate buffer. Soln. Bot. 240 ml. *otc.*
Use: Contact lens solution.

Lens Plus Oxysept 2 Neutralizing. (Allergan) Catalase with buffering agents used to neutralize the Lens Plus Oxysept 1 disinfecting solution in a chemical lens care system. For soft contact lens. Tabs. Box 12s. Bot. 36s. *otc.*
Use: Soft contact lens care.

Lens Plus Oxysept Rinse and Neutralizer. (Allergan) Isotonic with sodium chloride, mono- and dibasic sodium

phosphates, catalytic neutralizing agent, EDTA. Soln. Bot. 15 ml. *otc.*
Use: Soft contact lens care.

Lens Plus Preservative Free. (Allergan) Isotonic sodium chloride 9%. Soln. Bot. 90, 240, 360 ml. *otc.*
Use: Soft contact lens care.

Lens Plus Rewetting Drops. (Allergan) Sterile, non-preserved isotonic solution w/sodium Cl, boric acid. 0.35 ml (30s). *otc.*
Use: Soft contact lens care.

Lens Plus Rewetting Drops. (Allergan) Isotonic solution with sodium chloride and boric acid. Thimerosol and preservative free. Soln. Bot. 0.3 ml (30s). *otc.*
Use: Soft contact lens care.

Lens Plus Sterile Saline. (Allergan) Sodium Cl, boric acid, nitrogen. Soln. Bot. 90 ml, 240 ml, 360 ml. Aerosol. *otc.*
Use: Soft contact lens care.

Lensrins. (Allergan) Sterile preserved saline for heat disinfection, rinsing and storage of soft (hydrophilic) contact lenses; rinsing solution for chemical disinfection. Soln. Bot. 8 oz. *otc.*
Use: Soft contact lens care.

Lens-Wet. (Allergan) Isotonic, buffered soln. of polyvinyl alcohol, thimerosal 0.002%, EDTA 0.01%. Bot. 0.5 fl oz. *otc.*
Use: Contact lens care.

Lente Ilentin I. (Lilly) Insulin zinc suspension 100 units/ml. Beef and pork. Inj. Vial. 10 ml. *otc.*
Use: Antidiabetic.

Lente Iletin II. (Lilly) Insulin zinc suspension 100 units/ml. Purified pork. Inj. Bot. 10 ml. *otc.*
Use: Antidiabetic.

lente insulin. Susp. of zinc insulin crystals. *otc.*
See: Iletin Lente, Vial (Lilly).

lente insulin. (Novo Nordisk) Insulin zinc susp. 100 units/ml Beef. Inj. Vial 10 ml. *otc.*
Use: Antidiabetic.

lente I. (Novo Nordisk) Insulin zinc suspension 100 units/ml. Purified pork. Inj. Vial 10 ml. *otc.*
Use: Antidiabetic.

lentinan. (Lenti-Chemico Pharmaceuticals)
Use: Immunomodulator.

lepromin. (Louisiana State University) Lepromin, 30 to 40 million acid-fast bacilli per ml. Vial 5 ml, 10 ml, 20 ml, 50 ml.

leprostatics.

Use: Bactericidal.
See: Dapsone, Tab. (Jacobus).
Lamprene, Cap. (Novartis).

leptazol.
See: Pentylenetetrazol.

•**lergotrile.** (LER-go-trill) USAN.
Use: Enzyme inhibitor (prolactin).

•**lergotrile mesylate.** (LER-go-trill) USAN.
Use: Enzyme inhibitor (prolactin).

Lerton Ovules. (Vita Elixir) Caffeine 250 mg/Cap. *otc.*
Use: CNS Stimulants.

Lescol. (Sandoz) Fluvastatin sodium 20 mg or 40 mg. Cap. Bot. 30s, 100s. *Rx.*
Use: Antihyperlipidemic.

Lesterol. (Dram) Nicotinic acid 500 mg/Tab. Bot. 250s. *otc.*
Use: Antihyperlipidemic.

•**letimide hydrochloride.** (LET-ih-mide) USAN.
Use: Analgesic.

•**letrozole.** (let-ROW-zahl) USAN.
Use: Antineoplastic.

letusin. (Lilly).

•**leucine,** (LOO-SEEN) U.S.P. 23.
Use: Amino acid.

leucomax. (Various Mfr.). *Rx.*
Use: Cytokine agent.

l-leucovorin. *Rx.*
Use: Antineoplastic. [Orphan drug]
See: Isovorin.

•**leucovorin calcium,** (loo-koe-VORE-in) U.S.P. 23. (Various Mfr.) **Tab.:** 5 mg. Bot. 30s, 100s, UD 50s.
Use: Antagonist of amithopterin, antianemic (folate-deficiency), antidote to folic acid antagonists, antineoplastic. [Orphan drug]
See: Wellcovorin, Inj., Tab. (Glaxo Wellcome).

leucovorin calcium. (Various Mfr.) **Tab.:** 15 mg or 25 mg as calcium. Pkg. 12s, 24s, 25s, UD 50s. **Inj.:** 3 mg/ml as calcium w/ benzyl alcohol 0.9%. Amps 1 ml. **Pow. for Inj.:** 50 mg/vial, 100 mg/vial, 350 mg/vial. *Rx.*
Use: Folic acid antagonist overdosage.

Leukeran. (Glaxo Wellcome) Chlorambucil 2 mg/Tab. Bot. 50s. *Rx.*
Use: Antineoplastic.

Leukine. (Immunex) Sargramostin. 250 mcg or 500 mcg. Pow. for Inj. Lyophilized. Soln. Vials of 500 mcg/1 ml. *Rx.*
Use: Adjunct in bone marrow transplantation.

leukocyte protease inhibitor, recombinant secretory. *Rx.*
Use: Alpha-1 antitrypsin deficiency; cystic fibrosis. [Orphan drug]

leukocyte protease inhibitor, secretory. *Rx.*
Use: Bronchopulmonary dysplasia. [Orphan drug]

• **leukocyte typing serum,** U.S.P. 23.
Use: Diagnositc aid (blood, in vitro).

leupeptin.
Use: Adjunct to nerve repair. [Orphan drug]

• **leuprolide acetate.** (loo-PRO-lide) USAN.
Use: Antineoplastic, LHRH agonist, central precocious puberty [Orphan drug]
See: Lupron, Inj. (TAP Pharm).
Lupron Depot, Microspheres for Inj. (TAP Pharm).
Lurpon Depot-Ped, Microspheres for inj. (TAP Pharm).
Lupron Depot-3 Month, Microspheres for Inj. (TAP Pharm).

leurocristine.
See: Vincristine Sulfate (Lilly).

leurocristine sulfate (1:1) (salt). Vincristine Sulfate, U.S.P. 23.
Use: Antineoplastic.

Leustatin. (Ortho Biotech) Cladribine. Soln. 1 mg/ml. Vial. 20 ml single-use. *Rx.*
Use: Antineoplastic.

leutinizing hormone (recombinant) human.
Use: With recombinant human follicle stimulating hormone for chronic anovulation due to hypogonadotropic hypogonadism. [Orphan drug]

levamfetamine. (LEV-am-FET-ah-meen) F.D.A.
Use: Anorexic.

levamfetamine. (LEV-am-FET-ah-meen)
See: Levamphetamine succinate.

• **levamfetamine succinate.** (LEV-am-FET-ah-meen) USAN.
Use: Anorexic.

• **levamisole hydrochloride,** (lev-AM-ih-sole) U.S.P. 23.
Use: Biologic response modifier; antineoplastic.
See: Ergamisole (Janssen).

Levaquin. (McNeil Pharmaceutical) Levofloxacin 250 mg and 500 mg/Tab. Bot. 50s, 100s. Levofloxacin 500 mg/Inj. Vial. 20 ml. Levofloxacin 250 mg and 500/Inj. (premix). 50 ml flexible containers with 5% Dextrose solution (250 mg). 100 ml flexible containers with 5% Dextrose Solution. *Rx.*
Use: Fluoroquinolone.

levarterenol. *Rx.*
Use: Vasopressor (for shock).
See: Levophed, Inj. (Sanofi Winthrop).

levarterenol bitartrate.
See: Norepinephrine Bitartate, U.S.P. 23.

Levatol. (Schwarz Pharma) Penbutolol sulfate 20 mg. Tab. Bot. 100s. *Rx.*
Use: Beta-adrenergic blocking agent.

Levbid. (Schwarz Pharma) Hyoscyamine sulfate 0.375 mg/DR Tab. Bot. 100s. *Rx.*
Use: Anticholinergic.

• **levcromakalim.** (lev-KROE-mah-KAY-lim) USAN.
Use: Antihypertensive; antiasthmatic.

• **levcycloserine.** (LEV-sigh-kloe-SER-een) USAN.
Use: Enzyme inhibitor (Gaucher's disease).

• **levdobutamine lactobionate.** (LEV-dah-BYOOT-ah-meen LACK-toe-BYE-oh-nate) USAN.
Use: Cardiotonic.

Leviron. (Approved) Desiccated liver 7 gr, iron and ammonium citrate 3 gr, vitamins B_1 1 mg, B_2 0.5 mg, B_6 0.5 mg, calcium pantothenate 0.3 mg, niacinamide 2.5 mg, B_{12} 1 mcg/Cap. Bot. 100s, 1000s. *otc.*
Use: Vitamin/mineral supplement.

Levlen 21 Tablets. (Berlex) Levonorgestrel 0.15 mg, ethinyl estradiol 0.03 mg/Tab. Slidecase 21s, Box 3s. *Rx.*
Use: Oral contraceptive.

Levlen 28 Tablets. (Berlex) Levonorgestrel 0.15 mg, ethinyl estradiol 0.03 mg/Tab. (21 active, 7 inert). Slidecase 28s, Box 3s. *Rx.*
Use: Oral contraceptive.

levo-amphetamine. Alginate (l-isomer) alpha-2-phenylaminopropane succinate.
See: Levamphetamine.

levo-amphetamine succinate.
See: Pedestal, Cap., Tab. (Len-Tag).

• **levobetaxolol hydrochloride.** (LEE-voe-beh-TAX-oh-lahl) USAN.
Use: Antiadrenergic (β-receptor).

levobunolol hydrochloride, (LEE-voe-BYOO-no-lahl) U.S.P. 23.
Use: Antiadrenergic (β-receptor).

levobunolol hydrochloride. (LEE-voe-BYOO-no-lahl) (Various Mfr.) 0.25% or 0.5% Ophth. Soln. Bot. 5 ml, 10 ml, 15 ml. *Rx.*
Use: Beta-adrenergic blocking agent for glaucoma.
See: AKBeta, Ophth. Soln. (Akorn).
Betagan, Ophth. Soln. (Allergan).

•**levocabastine hydrochloride.** (LEE-voe-cab-ASS-teen) USAN.
Use: Antihistamine.
See: Livostin, Ophth. Susp. (Ciba Vision).

•**levocarnitine,** (LEE-voe-CAR-nih-teen) U.S.P. 23.
Use: Carnitine replenisher. [Orphan drug]
See: Carnitor, Liq., Tab. (Sigma-Tau).
L-Carnitine, Cap. (R & D Labs).
Vitacarn, Liq. (McGaw).

•**levodopa,** (LEE-voe-DOE-puh) U.S.P. 23.
Use: Antiparkinsonian.
See: Bio Dopa, Cap. (Bio-Deriv.).
Dopar, Cap. (Procter & Gamble).
Larodopa, Tab. or Cap. (Roche).
Levopa, Cap. (Zeneca).
Parda, Cap. (Parke-Davis).

levodopa and carbidopa. (LEE-voe-DOE-puh and CAR-bih-doe-puh)
Use: Antiparkinsonian.
See: Sinemet-10/100, Tab. (DuPont Merck).
Sinemet-25/100, Tab. (DuPont Merck).
Sinemet-25/250, Tab. (DuPont Merck).
Sinemet CR, SR Tab., (DuPont Merck).

Levo-Dromoran. (Roche) Levorphanol tartrate. **Amp.:** 2 mg/ml w/methyl and propyl parabens, sodium hydroxide to adjust pH. Amp. 1 ml, Box 10s. **Vial:** 2 mg/ml w/phenol 0.45%, sodium hydroxide to adjust pH. Vial 10 ml. **Tab.:** 2 mg. Bot. 100s. *c-II.*
Use: Narcotic analgesic.

levo-epinephrine bitartrate.
See: Lyophrin, Soln. (Alcon).

•**levofloxacin.** (lee-voe-FLOX-ah-sin) USAN.
Use: Antibacterial.
See: Levaquin, Tab. Inj. (McNeil).

•**levofuraltadone.** (LEE-voe-fer-AL-tah-dohn) USAN.
Use: Antibacterial, antiprotozoal.

•**levoleucovorin calcium.** (LEE-voe-loo-koe-VORE-in) USAN.
Use: Antidote to folic acid antagonist.
See: Isovorin (Immunex).

•**levomethadyl acetate.** (LEE-voe-METH-uh-dill) USAN.
Use: Narcotic analgesic.

•**levomethadyl acetate hydrochloride.** USAN.
Use: Narcotic analgesic, treatment of heroin addicts. [Orphan drug]

•**levonantradol hydrochloride.** (LEE-voe-NAN-trah-DAHL) USAN.
Use: Analgesic.

•**levonordefrin,** U.S.P. 23.
Use: Adrenergic (vasoconstrictor).

•**levonorgestrel,** (LEE-voe-nor-JESS-truhl) U.S.P. 23.
Use: Progestin.
See: Norplant (Wyeth-Ayerst).

levonorgestrel and ethinyl estradiol tablets.
Use: Oral contraceptive.
See: Nordette, Tab. (Wyeth-Ayerst).

Levophed. (Breon) Norepinephrine bitartrate 1 mg/ml Amp. 4 ml. *Rx.*
Use: Vasopressor used in shock.

Levophed Bitartrate. (Sanofi Winthrop) Norepinephrine bitartrate w/sodium Cl, sodium metabisulfite 1 mg or 2 mg/ml. Amp. 4 ml. Box 10s. *Rx.*
Use: Vasopressor used in shock.

Levoprome. (Lederle) Methotrimeprazine 20 mg/ml w/benzyl alcohol 0.9%, disodium edetate 0.065%, sodium metabisulfite 0.3%. Vial 10 ml. *Rx.*
Use: Analgesic.

•**levopropoxyphene napsylate.** (lee-voe-pro-POX-ee-feen NAP-sih-late) USAN. U.S.P. XXII.
Use: Antitussive.

•**levopropylcillin potassium.** USAN.
Use: Antibacterial.

Levora. (SCS) Ethinyl estradiol 0.03 mg, levonorgestrel 0.15 mg. Tab. Bot. 21s, 28s. *Rx.*
Use: Oral contraceptive.

levorenine.
See: Epinephrine, U.S.P. 23. (Various Mfr.).

levorotatory alkaloids of Belladolla.
Use: Anticholinergic; antispasmatic.
See: Bellafoline (Sandoz).

Levoroxine. (Bariatric) Sodium levothyroxine 0.05 mg, 0.1 mg, 0.2 mg or 0.3 mg/Tab. Bot. 100s, 500s. *Rx.*
Use: Thyroid hormone.

•**levorphanol tartrate,** U.S.P. 23.
Use: Narcotic analgesic.
See: Levo-Dromoran, Amp., Tab., Vial (Roche).

Levo-T. (Lederle) Levothyroxine sodium 0.025, 0.05, 0.075, 0.1, 0.125, 0.15, 0.2 or 0.3 mg. Tab. Bot. 100s (all strengths), 1000s (0.05, 0.1, 0.15 and 0.2 mg only). *Rx.*
Use: Thyroid hormone.

Levothroid. (Forest) Levothyroxine sodium. **Tab.:** 25 mcg, 50 mcg, 75 mcg, 88 mcg, 100 mcg, 112 mcg, 125 mcg,

137 mcg, 150 mcg, 175 mcg, 200 mcg or 300 mcg/Tab. Bot. 100s (all strengths), UD 100s (50 mcg, 100 mcg, 150 mcg, 200 mcg, 300 mcg only). **Inj.:** 200 mcg or 500 mcg. Vial 6 ml. *Rx.*
Use: Thyroid hormone.

levothyroxine sodium. (lee-voe-thigh-ROX-een) (Various Mfr.) Levothyroxine sodium 200 mcg, 500 mcg/Vial. Pow. for Inj. 6 ml, 10 ml. *Rx.*
Use: Thyroid hormone.

•**levothyroxine sodium,** (lee-voe-thigh-ROX-een) U.S.P. 23.
Use: Thyroid hormone.
See: Eltroxin, Tab. (Roberts).
  Levoid, Tab., Vial (Nutrition Control Products).
  Levo-T, Tab. (Lederle).
  Levothroid, Tab., Inj. (Forest).
  Levoxine, Inj. (Daniels).
  Levoxyl, Tab. (Daniels).
  Synthroid, Tab., Inj. (Boots).
W/Mannitol.
See: Levoxine, Inj. (Daniels).
  Synthroid, Inj. (Knoll Pharm).
W/Sodium liothyronine.
Use: Thyroid hormone.
See: Thyrolar, Tab. (Rhone-Poulenc Rorer).

levothyroxine sodium. (Various Mfr.) 0.1 mg, 0.15 mg, 0.2 mg, 0.3 mg/Tab. Bot. 100s, 1000s, UD 100s.
Use: Thyroid hormone.

•**levoxadrol hydrochloride.** (lev-OX-ah-drole) USAN.
Use: Local anesthetic; smooth muscle relaxant.

Levoxyl. (Daniels) Levothyroxine sodium 0.025 mg, 0.05 mg, 0.75 mg, 0.088 mg, 0.1 mg, 0.112 mg, 0.125 mg, 0.137 mg, 0.15 mg, 0.175 mg, 0.2 mg, 0.3 mg/Tab. Bot. 100s, 1000s, UD 100s. *Rx.*
Use: Thyroid hormone.

Levsin. (Schwarz Pharma) L-hyoscyamine sulfate. **Tab.:** 0.125 mg. Bot. 100s, 500s. **Soln.:** 0.125 mg/ml, alcohol 5%. Bot. 15 ml. **Elix.:** 0.125 mg/5 ml, alcohol 20%. Bot. pt. **Inj.:** 0.5 mg/ml. Vial 1 ml, 10 ml. *Rx.*
Use: Anticholinergic, antispasmodic.

Levsin-PB Drops. (Schwarz Pharma) Hyoscyamine sulfate 0.125 mg, phenobarbital 15 mg/ml, alcohol 5%. Liq. Bot. 15 ml. *Rx.*
Use: Anticholinergic, antispasmodic, sedative, hypnotic.

Levsin/SL. (Schwarz Pharma) Hyoscyamine sulfate 0.125 mg/Tab. Sublingual. Bot. 100s, 500s. *Rx.*
Use: Gastrointestinal anticholinergic, antispasmodic.

Levsinex Timecaps. (Schwarz Pharma) L-hyoscyamine sulfate 0.375 mg/TR Cap. Bot. 100s, 500s. *Rx.*
Use: Anticholinergic, antispasmodic.

levulose. Fructose.

levulose-dextrose.
See: Invert Sugar.

•**lexipafant.** (lex-IH-pah-fant) USAN.
Use: Platelet activating factor (PAP) antagonist.

•**lexithromycin.** (lex-ith-row-MY-sin) USAN.
Use: Antibacterial.

Lextron. (Lilly) Liver-stomach concentrate 50 mg, iron 30 mg, vitamins B_{12} (activity equivalent) 2 mcg, B_1 1 mg, B_2 0.25 mg w/other factors of vitamin B complex present in the liver-stomach concentrate/Pulv. Bot. 84s. *otc.*
Use: Vitamin/mineral supplement.

Lexxel. (Astra Merck) Enalapril maleate 5 mg, felodipine 5 mg/ER Tab. Bot. 30s, 100s, UD 100s. *Rx.*
Use: Antihypertensive combination.

l-glutathione.
See: Glutathione.

L'Homme. (Armenpharm) Vitamins A 4000 IU, D 400 IU, B_1 1 mg, B_2 1.2 mg, B_{12} 2 mcg, calcium pantothenate 5 mg, B_3 10 mg, C 30 mg, calcium 100 mg, phosphorus 76 mg, iron 10 mg, manganese 1 mg, magnesium 1 mg, zinc 1 mg. Bot. 100s. *otc.*
Use: Vitamin/mineral supplement.

•**liarozole fumarate.** (lie-AHR-oh-zole) USAN.
Use: Antipsoriatic.

•**liarozole hydrochloride.** (lie-AHR-oh-zole) USAN.
Use: Antineoplastic.

Li Ban Spray. (Pfizer) Synthetic pyrethroid 0.5%, related compounds 0.065%, aromatic petroleum hydrocarbons 0.664%. Bot. 5 oz, Box 6s. *otc.*
Use: Control of lice, fleas on bedding, furniture, etc. (Not to be used on humans or animals).

•**libenzapril.** (lie-BENZ-ah-prill) USAN.
Use: ACE inhibitor.

Librax. (Roche) Clidinium bromide (Quarzan) 2.5 mg, chlordiazepoxide HCl (Librium) 5 mg, parabens, lactose/Cap. Bot. 100s, 500s, Teledose 100s (10 strips of 10). *Rx.*
Use: Anticholinergic combination.

Libritabs. (Roche) Chlordiazepoxide 5 mg, 10 mg or 25 mg/Tab. **10 mg:** Bot. 100s, 500s; **25 mg:** Bot. 100s. *c-IV.*
Use: Antianxiety agent.

Librium. (Roche) Chlordiazepoxide HCl 5 mg, 10 mg or 25 mg/Cap. Bot. 100s, 500s, Tel-E-Dose (10 strips of 10; 4 cards of 25) in RNP (Reverse Numbered Package). *c-iv.*
Use: Antianxiety agent.

Librium Injectable. (Roche) Chlordiazepoxide HCl 100 mg/dry filled amp. plus special I.M. diluent, 2 ml for IM administration/compound w/benzyl alcohol 1.5%, polysorbate 80 4%, propylene glycol 20%, w/maleic acid and sodium hydroxide to adjust pH to approx. 3. Amp. 5 ml w/2 ml diluent, Box 10s. *c-iv.*
Use: Antianxiety agent.

Lice-Enz. (Copley) Pyrethrins 0.3%, piperonylbutoxide 3%. Shampoo. Bot. 60 g. *otc.*
Use: Miscellaneous pediculicide.

•**licryfilcon a.** USAN.
Use: Contact lens material (hydrophilic).

•**licryfilcon b.** USAN.
Use: Contact lens material (hydrophilic).

Lida-Mantle-HC Creme. (Bayer) Lidocaine 3%, hydrocortisone acetate 0.5% in cream base. Tube oz. *Rx.*
Use: Corticosteroid, local anesthetic, topical.

•**lidamidine hydrochloride.** (LIE-DAM-ih-deen) USAN.
Use: Antiperistaltic.

Lidex Cream. (Syntex) Fluocinonide 0.05%. Cream. In 15 g, 30 g, 60 g, 120 g. *Rx.*
Use: Corticosteroid, topical.

Lidex-E. (Syntex) Fluocinonide 0.05% in aqueous emollient base. Tube 15 g, 30 g, 60 g, 120 g. *Rx.*
Use: Corticosteroid, topical.

Lidex Gel. (Syntex) Fluocinonide 0.05% in gel base. Tube 15 g, 30 g, 60 g, 120 g. *Rx.*
Use: Corticosteroid, topical.

Lidex Ointment. (Syntex) Fluocinonide 0.05% in ointment base. Tube 15 g, 30 g, 60 g, 120 g. *Rx.*
Use: Corticosteroid, topical.

Lidex Topical Solution. (Syntex) Fluocinonide 0.05%. Soln. Bot. 20 ml, 60 ml. *Rx.*
Use: Corticosteroid, topical.

•**lidocaine,** (LIE-doe-cane) U.S.P. 23.
Use: Topical anesthetic.
See: Dermaflex, Gel (Schering Plough). Solarcaine Aloe Extra Burn Relief, Cream, Gel, Spray (Schering Plough).
Xylocaine, Oint. (Astra).
Zilactin-L, Liq. (Zila).

lidocaine and epinephrine injection.
Use: Local anesthetic.
See: L-Caine E, Vial (Century).
Norocaine 1%, 2% w/Epinephrine. (Vortech).
Xylocaine W/Epinephrine, Soln. (Astra).

•**lidocaine hydrochloride,** (LIE-doe-cane) U.S.P. 23.
Use: Cardiac depressant (antiarrhythmic), local anesthetic.
See: Anestacon, Jelly (PolyMedica).
Ardecaine 1%, 2%, Inj. (Burgin-Arden).
Dilocaine, Inj. (Hauck).
Dolicaine, I.M. (Solvay).
Duo-Track Kit, Inj. (Astra).
L-Caine, Inj., Liq. (Century).
Lidoject-1, Inj. (Mayrand).
Lidoject-2, Inj. (Mayrand).
Nervocaine, Inj. (Keene).
Norocaine, Inj. (Vortech).
Octocaine HCl, Inj. (Novocol).
Stanacaine (Standex).
Xylocaine HCl, Oint., Liq., Soln., Jelly (Astra).
Xylocaine 10% Oral, Spray (Astra).
Xylocaine Viscous, Soln. (Astra).
W/Benzalkonium Cl.
See: Medi-Quik, Aerosol (Reckitt & Coleman).
Medi-Quick Pump Spray (Reckitt & Coleman).
W/Benzalkonium Cl, phenol, menthol, eugenol, thyme oil, eucalyptus oil.
See: Unguentine Spray (Procter & Gamble).
W/Cetyltrimethylammonium bromide, hexachlorophene.
See: Aerosept, Aerosol (Dalin).
W/Hydrocortisone, clioquinol.
See: Bafil, Lot. (Scruggs).
Hil-20 Lot. (Solvay).
W/Dextrose.
W/Methylparaben, sodium Cl.
W/Methyl parasept.
See: L-Caine, Inj. (Century).
W/Methyl parasept, epinephrine.
See: L-Caine-E, Inj. (Century).
W/Orthohydroxyphenyl mercuric Cl, menthol, camphor, allantoin.
See: Kip First Aid preps. (Schmid).
W/Parachlorometaxylenol, phenol, zinc oxide.
See: Unguentine Plus, Cream (Procter & Gamble).
W/Polymyxin B sulfate.
See: Lidosporin, Otic soln. (Glaxo Wellcome).

lidocaine hydrochloride.
(Abbott) **0.2%, 0.4%, 0.8%:** w/5%

Dextrose. 250 ml single-dose container; **1%, 2%.** Abboject syringe 5 ml; Vial 1 g, 2 g. Premixed: 0.2%, 0.4% in 5% dextrose. Inj. containers (flexible or glass) 500 ml. **1%:** 2 ml, 5 ml single-dose amp. **1.5%:** 20 ml single-dose amp. **2%:** 10 ml/ 20 ml vial (for dilution to prepare I.V. drip soln.) **5%:** w/ 7.5% Dextrose amp. 2 ml.
(Maurry) 2%. Vial.
Use: Injection for infiltration block anesthesia and I.V. drip for cardiac arrhythmias.

Lidocaine HCl. (Abbott) Lidocaine HCl. 1%: 2 ml, 5 ml, 20 ml, 30 ml, 50 ml. 1.5%: 20 ml. w/Epinephrine 1:200,000. 5 ml. 2%: 5 ml, 20 ml, 30 ml, 50 ml. *Rx.*
Use: Local anesthetic.

lidocaine hydrochloride and dextrose injection.

lidocaine hydrochloride and epinephrine bitartrate injection.

lidocaine hydrochloride and epinephrine injection.

Lidocaine 2% Viscous. (Various Mfr.) Lidocaine HCl 2%. Soln. 100 ml, UD 20 ml. *Rx.*
Use: Local anesthetic.

•**lidofenin.** (LIE-doe-FEN-in) USAN.
Use: Diagnostic aid (hepatic function determination).

•**lidofilcon a.** (lih-DAH-FILL-kahn A) USAN.
Use: Contact lens material (hydrophilic).

•**lidofilcon b.** (lih-DAH-FILL-kahn B) USAN.
Use: Contact lens material (hydrophilic).

•**lidoflazine.** (LIE-dah-FLAY-zeen) USAN.
Use: Coronary vasodilator.

Lidoject-1. (Mayrand) Lidocaine HCl 1%. Vial 50 ml. *Rx.*
Use: Local anesthetic.

Lidoject-2. (Mayrand) Lidocaine HCl 2%. Vial 50 ml. *Rx.*
Use: Local anesthetic.

Lidopen Auto-Injector. (Survival Technology) Lidocaine HCl 10%. Auto-injection device. *Rx.*
Use: Antiarrhythmic.

Lidox Caps. (Major) Chlordiazepoxide HCl 10 mg, clidinium bromide 2.5 mg. Cap. Bot. 100s, 500s, 1000s, UD 100s. *Rx.*
Use: Anticholinergic combination.

Lidoxide. (Interstate) Chlordiazepoxide HCl 5 mg, clidinium bromide 2.5 mg/ Tab. Bot. 100s, 500s. *Rx.*

Use: Anticholinergic combination.

lid scrubs.
Use: Ophthalmic cleansing solutions.
See: I-Scrub, Soln. (Cooper Pharm).
Lid Wipes-SPF, Soln. (Akorn).
OcuClenz, Soln. (Storz/Lederle).
OCuSOFT, Soln. (Cynacon/OCu-SOFT).

Lid Wipes-SPF. (Akorn) PEG-200 glyceryl monotallowate, PEG-80 glyceryl monococoate, laureth-23, cocoamidopropylamine oxide, NaCl, glycerin, sodium phosphate, sodium hydroxide. Soln. Pads UD 30s. *otc.*
Use: Ophthalmic cleansing solution.

•**lifarizine.** (lih-FAR-ih-ZEEN) USAN.
Use: Cerebral anti-ischemic; platelet aggregation inhibitor.

Lifer-B. (Burgin-Arden) Cyanocobalamin 30 mcg, liver inj. 0.1 ml, ferrous gluconate 100 mg, riboflavin 1.5 mg, panthenol 2.5 mg, niacinamide 100 mg, citric acid 16.4 mg, sodium citrate 23.6 mg/ml. Vial 30 ml. *Rx.*
Use: Vitamin/mineral supplement.

Life Saver Kit. (Whiteworth Towne) Ipecac syrup two 1 oz bottles, activated charcoal pow. 1 oz, poison treatment instruction booklet. *otc.*
Use: Antidote kit, poisons.

Life Spanner. (Spanner) Vitamins A 12,500 IU, D 400 IU, E 5 IU, B$_1$ 10 mg, B$_2$ 5 mg, B$_6$ 2 mg, B$_{12}$ 5 mcg, niacinamide 50 mg, calcium pantothenate 10 mg, biotin 10 mcg, C 100 mg, hesperidin complex 10 mg, rutin 20 mg, choline bitartrate 40 mg, inositol 30 mg, betaine anhydrous 15 mg, l-lysine monohydrochloride 25 mg, iron 30 mg, copper 1 mg, manganese 1 mg, potassium 5 mg, calcium 105 mg, phosphorus 82 mg, magnesium 5.56 mg, zinc 1 mg/ Cap. Bot. 100s. *otc.*
Use: Vitamin/mineral supplement.

•**lifibrate.** (lih-FIE-brate) USAN.
Use: Antihyperlipoproteinemic.

•**lifibrol.** (lie-FIB-rahl) USAN.
Use: Hypercholesterolemic.

Lifol-B. (Burgin-Arden) Liver inj. 10 mcg, folic acid 1 mg, cyanocobalamin 100 mcg, phenol 0.5%/ml. Inj. Vial 10 ml. *Rx.*
Use: Nutritional supplement.

Lifolex. (Taylor) Liver 10 mcg, cyanocobalamin 100 mcg, folic acid 5 mg/ml. Inj. Vial 10 ml. *Rx.*
Use: Nutritional supplement.

Lilly Bulk Products. (Lilly) The following products are supplied by Eli Lilly under the U.S.P., N.F. or chemical name as a service to the health professions:

Ammoniated Mercury Oint.
Amyl Nitrite.
Analgesic Balm.
Apomorphine HCl.
Aromatic Elix.
Aromatic Ammonia.
Atropine Sulfate.
Bacitracin Oint.
Belladonna Tincture.
Benzoin.
Boric Acid.
Calcium Gluceptate.
Calcium Gluconate.
Calcium Gluconate with Vitamin D.
Calcium Hydroxide.
Calcium Lactate.
Carbarsone.
Cascara, Aromatic, fluidextract.
Cascara Sagrada fluidextract.
Citrated Caffeine.
Cocaine HCl.
Codeine Phosphate.
Codeine Sulfate.
Colchicine.
Compound Benzoin.
Dibasic Calcium Phosphate.
Diethylstilbestrol.
Ephedrine Sulfate.
Ferrous Gluconate.
Ferrous Sulfate.
Folic Acid.
Glucagon for Inj.
Green Soap Tincture.
Heparin Sodium.
Histamine Phosphate.
Ipecac.
Isoniazid.
Isopropyl Alcohol, 91%.
Liver, Vial for Inj.
Magnesium Sulfate.
Mercuric Oxide, Yellow.
Methadone HCl.
Methenamine for Timed Burning.
Methyltestosterone.
Milk of Bismuth.
Morphine Sulfate.
Myrrh.
Neomycin Sulfate.
Niacin.
Niacinamide.
Nitroglycerin.
Opium (Deodorized).
Ox Bile Extract.
Pancreatin.
Papaverine HCl.
Paregoric.
Penicillin G Potassium.
Phenobarbital.
Phenobarbital Sodium.

Potassium Cl.
Potassium Iodide.
Powder Papers (Glassine).
Progesterone.
Propylthiouracil.
Protamine Sulfate.
Pyridoxine HCl.
Quinidine Gluconate.
Quinidine Sulfate.
Quinine Sulfate.
Riboflavin.
Silver Nitrate.
Sodium Bicarbonate.
Sodium Chloride.
Sodium Salicylate.
Streptomycin Sulfate.
Sulfadiazine.
Sulfapyridine.
Sulfur.
Terpin Hydrate.
Terpin Hydrate and Codeine.
Testosterone Propionate.
Thiamine HCl.
Thyroid.
Tubocurarine HCl.
Tylosterone.
Whitfield's Oint.
Wild Cherry Syrup.
Zinc Oxide.
Zinc Oxide Paste.

limarsol.
See: Acetarsone. (City Chemical).

Limbitrol. (Roche) Chlordiazepoxide 5 mg, amitriptyline HCl 12.5 mg/Tab. Bot. 100s, 500s, Tel-E-Dose 100s, Prescription pak 50s. *c-iv.*
Use: Psychotherapeutic.

Limbitrol DS. (Roche) Chlordiazepoxide 10 mg, amitriptyline HCl 25 mg/Tab. Bot. 100s, 500s, Tel-E-Dose 100s, Prescription pak 50s. *c-iv.*
Use: Psychotherapeutic.

•**lime,** U.S.P. 23.
Use: Pharmaceutical necessity.

lime solution, sulfurated, U.S.P. XXI.
Use: Scabicide.

lime sulfur solution. Calcium polysulfide, calcium thiosulfate.
Use: Wet dressing.
See: Vlem-Dome, Liq. Concentrate (Bayer).

•**linarotene.** (lin-AHR-oh-teen) USAN.
Use: Antikeratolytic.

Lincocin. (Pharmacia & Upjohn) Lincomycin HCl 500 mg/Cap. Bot. 24s, 100s. **Pediatric:** 250 mg/Cap. Bot. 24s. *Rx.*
Use: Anti-infective.

Lincocin Sterile Solution. (Pharmacia & Upjohn) Lincomycin HCl equivalent

to 300 mg or 600 mg lincomycin base, benzyl alcohol 9.45 mg/ml. Vial 2 ml in 5s, 25s, 100s; 10 ml U-Ject. *Rx.*
Use: Anti-infective.

•**lincomycin.** (LIN-koe-MY-sin) USAN. Antibiotic produced by *Streptomyces lincolnensis.*
Use: Antibacterial; infections due to gram-positive organisms.

•**lincomycin hydrochloride,** U.S.P. 23.
Use: Antibacterial.
See: Lincocin, Cap., Soln., Syr. (Pharmacia & Upjohn).

•**lindane,** (LIN-dane) U.S.P. 23. Gamma-benzene-hexachloride, hexachlorocyclohexane.
Use: Pediculicide, scabicide.
See: Kwell, Cream, Lot., Shampoo (Schwarz Pharma).

lindane. (Fidelity Lab.) Pow. 50%, Pkg. 1 lb, 5 lb. (Imperial) Pow. 50%, Pkg. 1 lb, 4 lb; 12%, Pkg. 1 lb, 4 lb.
Use: Pediculicide, scabicide.

Lindora. (Westwood Squibb) Sodium laureth sulfate, water, cocamide DEA, sodium Cl, lactic acid, tetra sodium EDTA, benzophenone-4, FD&C Blue No. 1, fragrance. Bot. 8 oz. *otc.*
Use: Skin cleanser.

Linodil Capsules. (Sanofi Winthrop) Inositol hexanicotinate. *Rx.*
Use: Hyperlipidemic, peripheral vasodilator.

•**linogliride.** (lie-no-GLIE-ride) USAN.
Use: Antidiabetic.

•**linogliride fumarate.** (lih-no-GLIE-ride) USAN.
Use: Antidiabetic.

linolenic acid w/vitamin E.
See: Petropin, Cap. (Lannett).

linomide. (Pharmacia & Upjohn).
Use: Immunomodulator.

•**linopirdine.** (lih-no-PIHR-deen) USAN.
Use: Treatment of Alzheimer's disease (cognition enhancer).

Lioresal. (Novartis) Baclofen 10 mg or 20 mg/Tab. Bot. 100s, UD 100s. *Rx.*
Use: Muscle relaxant.

•**liothyronine I 125.** (lie-oh-THIGH-row-neen) USAN.
Use: Radioactive agent.

•**liothyronine I 131.** (lie-oh-THIGH-row-neen) USAN.
Use: Radioactive agent.

•**liothyronine sodium,** (lie-oh-THIGH-row-neen) U.S.P. 23.
Use: Thyroid hormone.
See: Cytomel, Tab. (SK-Beecham). Triostat, Inj. (SK-Beecham).

liothyronine sodium. (Various Mfr.) 10 mg/ml. Tab. Bot. 100s.
Use: Thyroid hormone.

liothyronine sodium injection. *Rx.*
Use: Myxedema coma/precoma. [Orphan drug]

•**liotrix tablets,** (LIE-oh-trix) U.S.P. 23. A combination of sodium levothyroxine and sodium 1-triiodothyronine in a ratio of 4 to 1 by weight.
Use: Thyroid hormone.
See: Euthroid, Tab. (Parke-Davis). Thyrolar, Tab. (Rhone-Poulenc Rorer).

lipase. W/Amylase, Protease.
Use: Digestive enzyme.
W/Amylase, bile salts, wilzyme, pepsin, pancreatin, calcium.
See: Enzyme, Tab. (Barth's).
W/Alpha-amylase W-100, proteinase W-300, cellase W-100, estrone, testosterone, vitamins, minerals.
See: Geramine, Tab. (Zeneca).
W/Alpha-Amylase, proteinase, cellase.
See: Kutrase (Schwarz Pharma). Ku-Zyme (Schwarz Pharma).
W/Amylolytic, proteolytic, cellulolytic enzymes.
See: Arco-Lase, Tab. (Arco).
W/Amylolytic, proteolytic, cellulolytic enzymes, phenobarbital, hyoscyamine sulfate, atropine sulfate.
See: Arco-Lase Plus, Tab. (Arco).
W/Pancreatin, protease, amylase.
See: Dizymes, Cap. (Recsei).
W/Pepsin, homatropine methylbromide, amylase, protease, bile salts.
See: Digesplen, Tab., Elix., Drops (Med. Prod.).
Use: Antihyperlipidemic.

lipids.
Use: Intravenous nutritional therapy.
See: Intralipid 10%, Soln. (Clintec). Intralipid 20%, Soln. (Clintec). Liposyn II 10%, Soln. (Abbott). Liposyn II 20%, Soln. (Abbott). Liposyn III 10%, Soln. (Abbott). Liposyn III 20%, Soln. (Abbott).

Lipisorb. (Bristol-Myers) Protein 35 g/L, fat 48 g/L, carbohydrates 115 g/L, Na 733.3 mg/L, K 1250 mg/L, H_2O 320 mOsm/kg. With appropriate vitamins and minerals. 1 calorie/ml. Vanilla flavored. Pow. Can 1 lb. *otc.*
Use: Nutritional supplement.

Lipitor. (Parke-Davis) Atorvastatin calcium 10 mg, 20 mg and 40 mg/Tab. Bot. 90s, 5000s (10 mg only) and UD 100s. *Rx.*
Use: Antihyperlipidemic.

Lipkote by Coppertone. (Schering

Plough) Padimate O, oxybenzone. SPF 15. Lip balm 4.2 g. *otc.*
Use: Sunscreen.

Lipkote SPF 15 Ultra Sunscreen Lipbalm. (Schering Plough) Tube 0.15 oz,. *otc.*
Use: Sunscreen.

Lip Medex. (Blistex) Petrolatum, camphor 1%, phenol 0.54%, cocoa butter, lanolin. Oint. 210 g. *otc.*
Use: Treatment of fever blisters and sore, dry cracked lips.

lipocholine. See: Choline dihydrogen citrate. (Various Mfr.).

Lipoflavonoid Caplets. (Numark) vitamins C 100 mg, B_1 0.33 mg, B_2 0.33 mg, B_3 3.33 mg, B_6 0.33 mg, B_{12} 1.66 mcg, B_5 1.66 mg, choline 111 mg, bioflavonoids 100 mg, inositol 111 mg. Bot. 100s, 500s. *otc.*
Use: Vitamin supplement.

Lipoflavonoid Capsules. (Numark) Choline 111 mg, inositol 111 mg, vitamins B_1 0.3 mg, B_2 0.3 mg, B_3 3.3 mg, B_5 1.7 mg, B_6 0.3 mg, B_{12} 1.7 mcg, C 100 mg, lemon bioflavonoid complex. Cap. Bot. 100s, 500s. *otc.*
Use: Vitamin supplement.

Lipogen Caplets. (Goldline) Choline 111 mg, inositol 111 mg, vitamins B_1 0.33 mg, B_2 0.33 mg, B_3 3.33 mg, B_5 1.7 mg, B_6 0.33 mg, B_{12} 1.7 mcg, C 20 mg, A 1667 IU, E 10 IU, Zn 30 mg, Cu, Se. Bot. 60s. *otc.*
Use: Vitamin/mineral supplement.

Lipogen Capsules. (Various Mfr.) Choline 111 mg, inositol, vitamins B_1 0.33 mg, B_2 0.33 mg, B_3 3.33 mg, B_5 1.7 mg, B_6 0.33 mg, B_{12} 1.7 mcg, C 100 mg/Cap. Bot. 60s. *otc.*
Use: Vitamin supplement.

lipolytic enzyme.
W/Proteolytic enzyme, amylolytic enzyme, cellulolytic enzyme, methyl polysiloxane, ox bile, betaine HCl.
See: Zymme, Cap. (Scrip).

Lipomul. (Pharmacia & Upjohn) Corn oil 10 g/15 ml w/d-Alpha tocopheryl acetate, butylated hydroxy-anisole, polysorbate 80, glyceride phosphates, sodium saccharin, sodium benzoate 0.05%, benzoic acid 0.05%, sorbic acid 0.07%. Bot. pt. *otc.*
Use: Nutritional supplement.

Lipo-Nicin/300 mg. (Zeneca) Niacin 300 mg, vitamin C 150 mg, B_1 25 mg, B_2 2 mg, B_6 10 mg/TR Cap. 100s. *Rx.*
Use: Peripheral vasodilator.

Lipo-Nicin/100 mg. (Zeneca) Nicotinic acid 100 mg, niacinamide 75 mg, vitamins C 150 mg, B_1 25 mg, B_2 2 mg, B_6 10 mg/Tab. Bot. 100s, 500s. *Rx.*
Use: Peripheral vasodilator combination.

Liponol Capsules. (Rugby) Choline, inositol 83 mg, methionine 110 mg, vitamins B_1 3 mg, B_2 3 mg, B_3 10 mg, B_5 2 mg, B_6 2 mg, B_{12} 2 mcg, desiccated liver 56 mg, liver concentrate 30 mg, sorbitol, lecithin/Cap. Bot. 60s. *otc.*
Use: Nutritional supplement.

liposomal doxorubicin.
See: doxorubicin hydrochloride.

Liposyn. (Abbott Hospital Prods) Intravenous fat emulsion containing safflower oil 10%, egg phosphatides 1.2%, glycerin 2.5% in water for inj. **10%:** Single-dose container 50 ml, 100 ml, 200 ml, 500 ml; Syringe Pump Unit 50 ml single-dose. **20%:** Single-dose container 200 ml, 500 ml Syringe Pump Unit 25 ml or 50 ml single-dose. *Rx.*
Use: Parenteral nutritional supplement.

Liposyn II. (Abbott Hospital Prods) Intravenous fat emulsion: **10%:** Safflower oil 5%, soybean oil 5%. Bot. 100 ml, 200 ml, 500 ml. **20%:** Safflower oil 10%, soybean oil 10% w/egg phosphatides 1.2%, glycerin 2.5%. 200 ml, 500 ml. Bot. Syringe pump unit 25 ml, 50 ml. *Rx.*
Use: Parenteral nutritional supplement.

Liposyn III. (Abbott) Oil, soybean, egg yolk phospholipids. **10%:** 100, 200, 500 ml. **20%:** 100, 500 ml. *Rx.*
Use: Parenteral nutritional supplement.

Lipo-Tears. (Spectra) Mineral oil, petrolatum. Preservative free. Drops. Bot. 1 ml (in 30s). *otc.*
Use: Ocular lubricant.

Lipotriad Caplets. (Numark) Zn 30 mg, vitamin A 5000 IU, C 60 mg, E 30 IU, Cu, Se, B_3 20 mg, B_1 1.5 mg, B_2 1.7 mg, B_6 2 mg, B_{12} 6 mcg, B_5 10 mg, choline bitartrate, inositol. Bot. 60s. *otc.*
Use: Vitamin/mineral supplement.

lipotropics with vitamins.
Use: Nutritional supplement.
See: Lipotriad, Liq. (Numark).
  Lipogen, Cap. (Various Mfr.).
  Lipotriad, Cap. (Numark).
  Lipoflavonoid, Cap. (Numark).
  Cholinoid, Cap. (Goldline).
  Akoline, C.B., Cap. (Akorn).
  Akoline, C.B., Cap. (Akorn).
  Liponol, Cap. (Rugby).
  Methatropic, Cap. (Goldline).
  Cholidase, Tab. (Freeda).

Lipoxide Caps. (Major) Chlordiazepoxide HCl 5 mg, 10 mg or 25 mg/Cap.

Bot. 100s, 500s, 1000s. *c-iv.*
Use: Antianxiety agent.

Liqua-Gel. (Paddock) Boric acid, glycerine, propylene glycol, methylparaben, propylparaben, Irish moss extract, methylcellulose. Bot. 4 oz, 16 oz. *otc.*

Liquibid. (ION) Guaifenesin 600 mg, dye free. SR Tab. Bot. 100s. *Rx.*
Use: Expectorant.

Liqui-Char. (Jones Medical) Acitvated charcoal. **Liq. Bot.:** 12.5 g/60 ml, 15 g/75 ml. **Squeeze container:** 25 g/120 ml, 50 g/240 ml, 30 g/120 ml. *otc.*
Use: Antidote.

Liqui-Doss. (Ferndale) Docusate sodium 60 mg, mineral oil. Bot. pt. *otc.*
Use: Laxative.

Liquid Barosperse. (Lafayette Pharm) Barium sulfate 60%. Susp. Bot. 355 ml.
Use: Radiopaque agents.

Liquid Geritonic. (Geriatric Pharm) Fe 105 mg, liver fraction 1 375 mg, B_1 3 mg, B_2 3 mg, B_3 30 mg, B_6 0.3 mg, B_{12} 9 mcg, inositol 60 mg, glycine 180 mg, yeast concentrate 375 mg, Ca, I, K, Mg, Mn, P, alcohol 20%. Liq. Bot. 240 ml, gal. *otc.*
Use: Iron and liver combination.

Liquid Lather. (Ulmer) Gentle wash for hands, body, face, hair. Bot. 8 oz, gal. *otc.*
Use: Cleanser.

liquid petrolatum emulsion.
See: Mineral Oil Emulsion, U.S.P. 23.

Liquid Pred Syrup. (Muro) Prednisone 5 mg/5 ml in syrup base. Alcohol 5%, saccharin, sorbitol. Bot. 120 ml, 240 ml. *Rx.*
Use: Corticosteroid.

Liquifilm Forte. (Allergan) Polyvinyl alcohol 3%, thimerosal 0.002%, EDTA, sodium Cl. Soln. Bot. 15 ml, 30 ml. *otc.*
Use: Artificial tears.

Liquifilm Tears. (Allergan) Polyvinyl alcohol 1.4%, chlorobutanol 0.5%, sodium Cl. Bot. 15 ml, 30 ml. *otc.*
Use: Artificial tears.

Liquifilm Wetting Solution. (Allergan) Polyvinyl alcohol, hydroxypropyl methylcellulose, edetate disodium, sodium Cl, potassium Cl, benzalkonium Cl 0.004%. Bot. 60 ml. *otc.*
Use: Hard contact lens care.

Liqui-Histine-D Elixir. (Liquipharm) Phenylpropanolamine HCl 12.5 mg, pyrilamine maleate 4 mg, phenyltoloxamine citrate 4 mg, pheniramine maleate 4 mg/5ml. Liq. Bot. 473 ml. *Rx.*

Use: Decongestant, antihistamine.

Liqui-Histine DM. (Liquipharm) Dextromethorphan HBr 10 mg, phenylpropanolamine HCl 12.5 mg, brompheniramine maleate 2 mg/5 ml. Alcohol free. Syr. Bot. 473 ml. *Rx.*
Use: Antitussive, decongestant, antihistamine.

Liquimat. (Galderma) Sulfur 5%, SD alcohol 40 22%, cetyl alcohol in drying makeup base. Plastic Bot. 45 ml. *otc.*
Use: Antiacne.

Liquipake. (Lafayette) Barium sulfate suspension 100% w/v for dilution. Bot. 1850 ml, Case 4s.
Use: Radiopaque agent.

Liquiprin. (Menley & James) Acetaminophen 80 mg/1.66 ml, saccharin. Soln. Bot. 35 ml w/dropper. *otc.*
Use: Analgesic.

liquor carbonis detergens.
See: Coal Tar Topical Soln., U.S.P. 23. (Various Mfr.)

•**lisadimate.** (liss-AD-ih-mate) USAN.
Use: Sunscreen.

•**lisinopril,** (lie-SIN-oh-pril) U.S.P. 23.
Use: Antihypertensive.
See: Prinivil, Tab. (Merck).
Zestril, Tab. (Zeneca).
W/Hydrochlorothiazide
See: Prinzide, Tab. (Merck).

•**lisofylline.** (lie-SO-fih-lin) USAN.
Use: Immunomodulator.

Listerine Antiseptic. (Warner-Wellcome) Thymol 0.06%, eucalyptol 0.09%, methyl salicylate 0.06%, menthol 0.04%. Alcohol 26.9% (regular flavor), 21.6% (cool mint flavor), sorbitol, saccharin. Bot. 90 ml, 180 ml, 360 ml, 540 ml, 720 ml, 960 ml, 1440 ml. *otc.*
Use: Mouthwash, antiseptic.

Listerine Antiseptic Throat Lozenges. (Warner-Wellcome) Hexylresorcinol 2.4 mg/Loz. Box 24s. *otc.*
Use: Throat preparation.

Listerine Maximum Strength Antiseptic Throat Lozenges. (Warner-Wellcome) Hexylresorcinol 4 mg/Loz. Box 24s. *otc.*
Use: Throat preparation.

Listermint Arctic. (Warner-Wellcome) Glycerin, poloxamer 335, PEG 600, sodium lauryl sulfate, sodium benzoate, benzoic acid, zinc chloride, saccharin. Liq. 946 ml. *otc.*
Use: Antiseptic mouthwash.

Lite Pred. (Horizon) Prednisolone sodium phosphate 0.125%. Soln. Bot. 5 ml. *Rx.*

Use: Corticosteroid, ophthalmic.

Lithane. (Bayer) Lithium carbonate 300 mg, tartrazine. Tab. Bot. 100s. *Rx.*
Use: Antipsychotic.

•**lithium carbonate,** (LITH-ee-uhm CARboe-nate) U.S.P. 23. Carbonic acid, dilithium salt.
Use: Antipsychotic, manic depressive state; antimanic; antidepressant.
See: Eskalith, Cap., Tab. (SK-Beecham).
Lithane, Tab. (Bayer).
Lithobid, Tab. (Novartis).
Lithotabs, Tab. (Solvay).

lithium carbonate capsules and tablets. (Roxane) Lithium carbonate. **Tab.:** 300 mg. Bot. 100s, 1000s, UD 100s. **Cap.:** 150 mg, 300 mg or 600 mg. Bot. 100s, 1000s, UD 100s. *Rx.*
Use: Antipsychotic, manic depressive state; antimanic; antidepressant.

•**lithium citrate,** (LITH-ee-uhm) U.S.P. 23.
Use: Antimanic.
See: Cibalith-Si, Liq. (Novartis).
Lithonate-S, Liq. (Solvay).

•**lithium hydroxide,** (LITH-ee-uhm high-DROX-ide) U.S.P. 23.
Use: Antipsychotic, manic depressive state; antimanic; antidepressant.

Lithonate. (Solvay) Lithium carbonate 300 mg/Cap. Bot. 100s, 1000s, Unit-of-use 90s, 100s, 120s, UD 100s. *Rx.*
Use: Antipsychotic.

Lithostat. (Mission) Acetohydroxamic acid 250 mg/Tab. Bot. 100s. *Rx.*
Use: Urinary anti-infective.

Lithotabs. (Solvay) Lithium carbonate 300 mg/Tab. Bot. 100s, 1000s, UD 100s. *Rx.*
Use: Antipsychotic.

Livec. (Enzyme Process) Vitamins A 5000 IU, B_1 1.5 mg, B_2 1.7 mg, niacin 20 mg, C 60 mg, B_6 2 mg, pantothenic acid 10 mg, E 30 IU, B_{12} 6 mcg, calcium 250 mg, iron 5 mg, D 400 IU, folacin 0.075 mg/3 Tab. Bot. 100s, 300s. *otc.*
Use: Vitamin/mineral supplement.

Liverbex. (Spanner) Liver 2 mcg, vitamins B_1, B_2, B_6, B_{12}, niacinamide, pantothenate/ml. Vial 30 ml. *otc.*
Use: Nutritional supplement.

Liver Combo No. 5. (Rugby) Liver vitamin B_{12} equivalent 10 mcg, crystalline B_{12} 100 mcg, folic acid 0.4 mg/ml. Inj. Vial 10 ml. *Rx.*
Use: Parenteral nutritional supplement.

liver, crude. (Various Mfr.) Vitamin B_{12} 2 mcg/ml. Inj. Vials 30 ml. *Rx.*

Use: Parenteral nutritional supplement.

liver derivative complex.
See: Kutapressin, Inj. (Schwarz Pharma).

liver desiccated. Desiccated liver substance.

liver extract. Dry liver extract w/Vitamin B_{12}, folic acid.

liver function agents.
See: Bromsulphalein, Amp. (Becton Dickinson).
Iodophthalein (Various Mfr.).
Sulfobromophthalein Sodium U.S.P. 23 (Gotham).

Livergran. (Rawl) Desiccated whole liver 9 g, vitamins B_1 18 mg, B_2 36 mg, niacinamide 90 mg, choline bitartrate 216 mg, B_6 3.6 mg, calcium pantothenate 3.6 mg, inositol 90 mg, biotin 6 mcg, vitamins B_{12} 5.4 mcg, methionine 198 mg, arginine 242 mg, cystine 72 mg, glutamic acid 675 mg, histidine 99 mg, isoleucine 333 mg, leucine 495 mg, lysine 297 mg, phenylalanine 189 mg, threonine 333 mg, tryptophan 45 mg, tyrosine 180 mg, valine 306 mg/3 Tsp. Bot. 15 oz. *otc.*
Use: Nutritional supplement.

liver injection. (Various Mfr.) Liver extract for parenteral use. *Rx.*
Use: Parenteral liver supplement.

liver injection. (Arcum; Lederle) Vitamin B_{12} 20 mcg/ml. Vial 10 ml. *Rx.*
Use: Nutritional supplement.

Liver Injection, Crude. (Lilly) 2 mcg/ml. Vial 30 ml; (Medwick) 2 mcg/ml. Vial 30 ml. *Rx.*
Use: Liver supplement.

Liver Iron Vitamins Inj. (Arcum) Liver inj. (10 mcg B_{12} activity/ml) 0.1 ml, crude liver inj. (2 mcg B_{12} activity/ml) 0.125 ml, green ferric ammonium citrate 20 mg, niacinamide 50 mg, vitamin B_6 0.3 mg, B_2 0.3 mg, procaine HCl 0.5%, phenol 0.5%/2 ml. Vial 30 ml. *Rx.*
Use: Nutritional supplement.

Liver, Refined. (Medwick) 20 mcg/ml. Vial 10 ml, 30 ml. *Rx.*
Use: Nutritional supplement.

liver vasoconstrictor.
See: Kutapressin, Vial, Amp. (Schwarz Pharma).

Livifol. (Dunhall) Vitamin B_{12} activity from liver inj. equivalent to cyanocobalamin 10 mcg, folic acid 1 mg, cyanocobalamin 100 mcg/ml. Vial 10 ml. *Rx.*
Use: Vitamin supplement.

Livitrinsic-F Capsules. (Goldline) Iron 110 mg, vitamins B_{12} 15 mcg, C 75

mg, intrinsic factor concentrate 240 mg, folic acid 0.5 mg/Cap. Bot. 100s, 1000s. *Rx.*
Use: Vitamin/mineral supplement.

Livostin. (Ciba Vision) Levocabastine HCl 0.05%. Susp. Dropper Bot. 2.5 ml, 5 ml, 10 ml. *otc.*
Use: Antiallergy, ophthalmic.

•**lixazinone sulfate.** (lix-AZE-ih-NOHN) USAN.
Use: Cardiotonic (phosphodiesterase inhibitor).

Lixoil. (Lixoil Labs.) Sulfonated fatty oils and one or more esters of higher fatty acids. Bot. 16 oz. *otc.*
Use: Dermatologic.

LKV-Drops. (Freeda) Vitamins A 5000 IU, D 400 IU, E 2 mg, B_1 1.5 mg, B_2 1.5 mg, B_3 10 mg, B_5 2 mg, B_6 2 mg, B_{12} 6 mcg, C 50 mg, biotin 50 mcg/0.6 ml. Bot. 60 ml. *otc.*
Use: Vitamin supplement.

LKV Infant Drops. (Freeda) Vitamins A 2500 IU, D 400 IU, E 5 IU, B_1 1 mg, B_2 1 mg, B_3 10 mg, B_5 3 mg, B_6 1 mg, B_{12} 4 mcg, C 50 mg, biotin 75 mcg/ 0.5 ml. Bot. 60 ml. *otc.*
Use: Vitamin supplement.

lld factor.
See: Vitamin B_{12}, Preps. (Various Mfr.).

l-leucovorin.
Use: Antineoplastic.
See: Isovorin.

lm-427. Ribabutin.
Use: CDC anti-infective agent.

LMD. (Abbott) Dextran 40 10%. 500 ml. With 0.9% sodium chloride or in 5% dextrose. *Rx.*
Use: Plasma volume expander.

LMWD-Dextran 40. (Pharmachem) Normal saline 0.9%, dextrose 10%. *Rx.*
Use: Plasma volume expander.

Lobac. (Seatrace) Salicylamide 200 mg, phenyltoloxamine 20 mg, acetaminophen 300 mg/Cap. Bot. 100s. *Rx.*
Use: Muscle relaxant, analgesic.

Lobak Tablets. (Sanofi Winthrop) Chlormezanone 250 mg, acetaminophen 300 mg/Tab. In 40s, 100s, 1000s. *Rx.*
Use: Antianxiety, analgesic.

Lobana Body. (Ulmer) Mineral oil, triethanolamine stearate, stearic acid, lanolin, cetyl alcohol, potassium stearate, propylene glycol parabens. Lot. Bot. 120, 240 ml, gal. *otc.*
Use: Emollient.

Lobana Body Shampoo. (Ulmer) Chloroxylenol. Bot. 240 ml, gal. *otc.*
Use: Hair & body cleanser.

Lobana Conditioning Shampoo. (Ulmer) Bot. 8 oz, gal. *otc.*
Use: Shampoo for hair and scalp.

Lobana Derm-Ade Cream. (Ulmer) Vitamin A, D, E cream. Jar 2 oz, 8 oz. *otc.*
Use: Minor skin irritations.

Lobana Liquid Lather. (Ulmer) Sodium laureth sulfate, sodium lauroyl sarcosinate, sodium myristyl sarcosonate, lauramide DEA, linoleamide DEA, octyl hydroxystearate, polyquaternium 7, tetrasodium EDTA, quaternium 15, sodium chloride, citric acid. Liq. Bot. 240 ml, gal. *otc.*
Use: Cleanser.

Lobana Peri-Gard. (Ulmer) Water-resistant ointment containing vitamin A & D. Jar 2 oz, 8 oz. *otc.*
Use: Skin protectant.

Lobana Perineal Cleanser. (Ulmer) Sprayer 4 oz, 8 oz. Bot. gal. *otc.*
Use: Urine and fecal cleanser.

lobelia fluidextract.
W/Hyoscyamus fluidextract, grindelia fluidextract, potassium iodide.
See: L.S. Mixture, Liq. (Paddock).

lobeline sulfate.
See: Lobidram, Tab. (Dram).
Nikoban, Loz., Gum. (Thompson).

•**lobenzarit sodium.** (low-BENZ-ah-RIT) USAN.
Use: Antirheumatic.

Lobidram. (Dram) Lobeline sulfate 2 mg/ Tab. Pkg. 15s, 30s. *otc.*
Use: Withdrawal symptoms of smoking.

•**lobucavir.** (lah-BYOO-kah-vihr) USAN.
Use: Antiviral.

Locoid. (Ferndale) **Cream:** Hydrocortisone butyrate 0.1%. Tube 15 g, 45 g. **Oint.:** Hydrocortisone butyrate 0.1%. Tube 15 g, 45 g. **Soln.:** Hydrocortisone butyrate 0.1%, isopropyl alcohol 50%, glycerin, povidone. Bot. 20 ml, 60 ml. *Rx.*
Use: Corticosteroid, topical.

•**lodelaben.** (low-DELL-ah-ben) USAN.
Formerly Declaben.
Use: Antiarthritic; emphysema therapy adjunct.

Lodine. (Wyeth-Ayerst) Etodolac 200, 300 or 400 mg, lactose/Cap. Bot. 100s, UD 100s. *Rx.*
Use: Nonsteroidal anti-inflammatory, analgesic.

Lodine XL. (Wyeth-Ayerst) Etodolac 400 mg and 600 mg, lactose/ER Tab. Bot. 100s and UD 100s. *Rx.*
Use: Nonsteroidal anti-inflammatory, analgesic.

Lodosyn. (Merck) Carbidopa 25 mg/Tab. Bot. 100s. *Rx.*
Use: Antiparkinsonian.

•**Iodoxamide ethyl.** (low-DOX-ah-mide ETH-uhl) USAN.
Use: Antiasthmatic, antiallergic; bronchodilator.

•**Iodoxamide tromethamine.** (low-DOX-ah-mide troe-METH-ah-meen) USAN.
Use: Antiasthmatic, antiallergic; bronchodilator; vernal keratoconjunctivitis [Orphan drug]
See: Alomide, Soln. (Alcon).

Lodrane LD. (ECR Pharm) Brompheniramine maleate 6 mg, pseudoephedrine HCl 60 mg/SR Cap. Bot. 100s. *Rx.*
Use: Antihistamine, decongestant.

Loestrin 21 1/20. (Parke-Davis) Norethindrone acetate 1 mg, ethinyl estradiol 20 mcg Tab. Petipac compact 21 Tab. Ctn. 5 compacts or Ctn. 5 refills. *Rx.*
Use: Oral contraceptive.

Loestrin 21 1.5/30. (Parke-Davis) Norethindrone acetate 1.5 mg, ethinyl estradiol 30 mcg/Tab. Petipac compact. Ctn. 5 compacts or Ctn. 5 refills. *Rx.*
Use: Oral contraceptive.

Loestrin Fe 1/20. (Parke-Davis) **White Tab.:** Norethindrone acetate 1 mg, ethinyl estradiol 20 mcg/Tab.; **Brown Tab.:** Ferrous fumarate 75 mg (7 tabs.) Carton 5 petipac compacts 28 Tab., carton of 5 refills 28 Tab. *Rx.*
Use: Oral contraceptive.

Loestrin Fe 1.5/30. (Parke-Davis) **Green Tab.:** Norethindrone acetate 1.5 mg, ethinyl estradiol 30 mcg. **Brown Tab.:** Ferrous fumarate 75 mg (7 tabs.). Carton 5 petipac compacts 28 Tab., carton of 5 refills 28 Tab. *Rx.*
Use: Oral contraceptive.

•**Iofemizole hydrochloride.** (low-FEM-ih-ZOLE) USAN.
Use: Anti-inflammatory; analgesic; antipyretic.

Lofenalac. (Bristol-Myers) Corn syrup solids 49.2%, casein hydrolysate 18.7% (enzymic digest of casein containing amino acids and small peptides), corn oil 18%, modified tapioca starch 9.57%, protein equivalent 15%, fat 18%, carbohydrate 60%, minerals (ash) 3.6%, phenylalanine 75 mg/100 g pow., Vitamins A 1600 IU, D 400 IU, E 10 IU, C 52 mg, folic acid 100 mcg, B_1 0.5 mg, B_2 0.6 mg, niacin 8 mg, B_6 0.4 mg, B_{12} 2 mcg, biotin 0.05 mg, pantothenic acid 3 mg, Vitamin K-1 100 mcg, choline 85 mg, inositol 30 mg, calcium 600 mg, phosphorus 450 mg, iodine 45 mcg, iron 12 mg, magnesium 70 mg, copper 0.6 mg, zinc 4 mg, manganese 1 mg, chloride 450 mg, potassium 650 mg, sodium 300 mg/qt. at normal dilution of 20 k cal/fl oz, Can 2 1/2 lb. *otc.*
Use: Nutritional supplement.

•**Iofentanil oxalate.** (low-FEN-tah-NILL OX-ah-late) USAN.
Use: Narcotic analgesic.

•**Iofepramine hydrochloride.** (low-FEH-prah-MEEN) USAN.
Use: Antidepressant.

•**Iofexidine hydrochloride.** (low-FEX-ih-DEEN) USAN.
Use: Antihypertensive.

Logen Liquid. (Goldline) Diphenoxylate HCl w/atropine sulfate. Bot. 2 oz. *c-v.*
Use: Antidiarrheal.

Logen Tablets. (Goldline) Diphenoxylate HCl, atropine sulfate. Bot. 100s, 500s, 1000s. *c-v.*
Use: Antidiarrheal.

Lomanate. (Various Mfr.) Diphenoxylate HCl 2.5 mg, atropine sulfate 0.025 mg/ 5 ml. Bot. 60 ml. *c-v.*
Use: Antidiarrheal.

•**Iomefloxacin.** (low-MEH-FLOX-ah-sin) USAN.
Use: Antibacterial.

•**Iomefloxacin hydrochloride.** (low-MEH-FLOX-ah-sin) USAN.
Use: Antibacterial.
See: Maxaquin, Tab. (Searle).

•**Iomefloxacin mesylate.** (low-MEH-FLOX-ah-sin) USAN.
Use: Antibacterial.

•**Iometraline hydrochloride.** (low-MET-rah-LEEN) USAN.
Use: Antipsychotic, antiparkinsonian.

•**Iometrexol sodium.** (LOW-meh-TREX-ole) USAN.
Use: Antineoplastic.

•**Iomofungin.** (low-moe-FUN-jin) USAN.
Use: Antifungal.

Lomotil. (Searle) Diphenoxylate HCl 2.5 mg, atropine sulfate 0.025 mg/Tab. or 5 ml. **Tab.:** Bot. 100s, 500s, 1000s, 2500s, UD 100s. **Liq.:** Bot. w/dropper 2 oz. *c-v.*
Use: Antidiarrheal.

•**Iomustine.** (LOW-muss-teen) USAN. CCNU; NSC-79037.
Use: Antineoplastic.
See: CeeNu, Cap. (Bristol).

Lonalac. (Bristol-Myers) Protein as casein 21%, fat as coconut oil 49%, carbohydrate as lactose 30%, vitamins A 1440 IU, B_1 0.6 mg, B_2 2.6 mg, nia-

cin 1.2 mg, calcium 1.69 g, phosphorus 1.5 g, chloride 750 mg, potassium 1.88 g, sodium 38 mg, magnesium 135 mg/qt. Pow. Can 16 oz. *otc.*
Use: Nutritional supplement.

•**lonapalene.** (low-NAP-ah-LEEN) USAN.
Use: Antipsoriatic.

Long Acting Nasal Spray. (Weeks & Leo) Oxymetazoline HCl 0.05%. Soln. Bot. 0.75 oz. *otc.*
Use: Decongestant.

Long Acting Neo-Synephrine II Nose Drops and Nasal Spray. (Sanofi Winthrop Products) Xylometazoline HCl 0.1% (adult strength) or 0.05% (child strength). Bot. 1 oz, Spray 0.5 oz (adult strength). *otc.*
Use: Decongestant.

Long Acting Neo-Synephrine II Vapor Spray. (Sanofi Winthrop Products) Xylometazoline HCl 0.1%. Mentholated. Spray Bot. 0.5 fl oz. *otc.*
Use: Decongestant.

Loniten. (Pharmacia & Upjohn) Minoxidil 2.5 mg or 10 mg/Tab. **2.5 mg:** Unit-of-use Bot. 100s. **10 mg:** Bot. 500s, Unit-of-use Bot. 100s. *Rx.*
Use: Antihypertensive.

Lonox. (Geneva Pharm) Diphenoxylate HCl 2.5 mg, atropine sulfate 0.025 mg/Tab. Bot. 100s, 500s, 1000s, UD 100s. *c-v.*
Use: Antidiarrheal.

Lo/Ovral. (Wyeth-Ayerst) Norgestrel 0.3 mg, ethinyl estradiol 0.03 mg/Tab. Pilpak dispenser 6s, Tab. 21s. *Rx.*
Use: Oral contraceptive.

Lo/Ovral-28. (Wyeth-Ayerst) Tab. 21s, each containing norgestrel 0.03 mg, ethinyl estradiol 0.03 mg, 7 pink inert. Tab. Pilpak dispenser 6s, Tab 28s. *Rx.*
Use: Oral contraceptive.

•**loperamide hydrochloride,** (low-PURR-ah-mide) U.S.P. 23.
Use: Antiperistaltic.
See: Imodium, Cap. (Ortho).

Lopid. (Parke-Davis) Gemfibrozil. 600 mg/Tab. Bot. 60s. *Rx.*
Use: Antihyperlipidemic agent.

Lopressor. (Novartis) Metoprolol tartrate. **Tab.:** 50 mg or 100 mg. Bot. 100s, 1000s, UD 100s, Gy-Pak 60s, 100s. **Amp.:** 5 mg/5 ml. *Rx.*
Use: Beta-adrenergic blocking agent.

Lopressor HCT. (Novartis) Metoprolol tartrate, hydrochlorothiazide. **Tab.:** 50/25 mg, 100/25 mg or 100/50 mg. Bot. 100s. *Rx.*
Use: Antihypertensive combination.

Loprox. (Hoechst Marion Roussel) Ciclopirox olamine 1% in cream base. Tube 15 g, 30 g, 90 g. *Rx.*
Use: Antifungal, topical.

Lopurin. (Knoll Pharm) Allopurinol 100 mg or 300 mg/Tab. Bot. 100s, 1000s, UD 100s. *Rx.*
Use: Agent for gout.

Lorabid. (Lilly) Loracarbef.

•**loracarbef.** (LOW-ra-CAR-beff) U.S.P. 23.
Use: Antibacterial.
See: Lorabid, Cap., Pow. (Lilly).

•**lorajmine hydrochloride.** (lahr-AZH-meen) USAN.
Use: Cardiac depressant (antiarrhythmic).

•**loratadine.** (lore-AT-uh-DEEN) USAN.
Use: Antihistamine.
See: Claritin, Tab. (Schering Plough).

•**lorazepam,** (lore-AZE-uh-pam) U.S.P. 23.
Use: Minor tranquilizer.
See: Alzapam, Tab. (Ultra).
Ativan, Tab., Inj. (Wyeth-Ayerst).

lorazepam. (lore-AZE-uh-pam) (Purepac) Lorazepam. **0.5 mg:** Tab. Bot. 100s, 500s. **1 mg, 2 mg:** Tab. Bot. 100s, 500s, 1000s. *c-IV.*
Use: Antianxiety, sedative, hypnotic.

lorazepam. (lore-AZE-uh-pam) (Various Mfr.) Lorazepam, benzyl alcohol 2%. Inj. 2 mg/ml, 4 mg/ml. Vial 1 ml, 10 ml. *c-IV.*
Use: Antianxiety, sedative, hypnotic.

Lorazepam Intensol. (Roxane) Lorazepam 2 mg/ml. Concentrated oral soln. Alcohol and dye free. Dropper Bot. 30 ml. *c-IV.*
Use: Antianxiety, sedative, hypnotic.

•**lorbamate.** (lore-BAM-ate) USAN.
Use: Muscle relaxant.

•**lorcainide hydrochloride.** (lahr-CANE-ide) USAN.
Use: Cardiac depressant; antiarrhythmic.

Lorcet. (UAD) Hydrocodone bitartrate 5 mg, acetaminophen 500 mg/Tab. Bot. 100s. *c-III.*
Use: Narcotic analgesic combination.

Lorcet HD. (UAD) Hydrocodone bitartrate 5 mg, acetaminophen 500 mg/Cap. Bot. 500s. *c-III.*
Use: Narcotic analgesic combination.

Lorcet Plus. (UAD) Hydrocodone bitartrate 7.5 mg, acetaminophen 650 mg/Tab. Bot. 100s., 500s, UD 100s. *c-III.*
Use: Narcotic analgesic combination.

Lorcet 10/650. (UAD) Hydrocodone bitartrate 10 mg, acetaminophen 650 mg/

Tab. Bot. 20s, 100s, UD 100s. *c-III.*
Use: Narcotic analgesic combination.

●**lorcinadol.** (LORE-sin-ah-dole) USAN.
Use: Analgesic.

●**loreclezole.** (lahr-EH-kleh-zole) USAN.
Use: Antiepileptic.

Lorelco. (Hoechst Marion Roussel) Probucol 250 mg/Tab. Bot. 120s. *Rx.*
Use: Antihyperlipidemic.

●**lormetazepam.** (LORE-met-AZE-eh-pam) USAN.
Use: Sedative, hypnotic.

●**lornoxicam.** (lore-NOX-ih-kam) USAN.
Use: Anti-inflammatory; analgesic.

Loroxide. (Dermik) Benzoyl peroxide 5.5%, cetyl alcohol, parabens, EDTA, 1% silica, 64% calcium phosphate. Lot. Bot. 25 g. *otc.*
Use: Antiacne.

Lorprn. (Whitby) Aspirin 325 mg, caffeine 40 mg, butalbital 50 mg/Cap. Bot. 100s. *c-III.*
Use: Narcotic analgesic combination.

Lortab 2.5/500. (Whitby) Hydrocodone 2.5 mg, acetaminophen 500 mg/Tab. Bot. 100s, 500s. *c-III.*
Use: Narcotic analgesic combination.

Lortab 5/500. (Whitby) Hydrocodone 5 mg, acetaminophen 500 mg/Tab. Bot. 100s, 500s, UD 100s. *c-III.*
Use: Narcotic analgesic combination.

Lortab 7/500. (Whitby) Hydrocodone 7.5 mg, acetaminophen 500 mg/Tab. Bot. 100s, 500s, UD 100s. *c-III.*
Use: Narcotic analgesic combination.

Lortab 10/500. (UCB Pharma) Hydrocodone bitartrate 10 mg, acetaminophen 500 mg/Tab. Bot. 100s, 500s. *c-III.*
Use: Narcotic analgesic combination.

Lortab ASA. (Whitby) Hydrocodone bitartrate 5 mg, aspirin 500 mg/Tab. Bot. 100s. *c-III.*
Use: Narcotic analgesic combination.

Lortab Elixir. (UCB Pharma) Hydrocodone 2.5 mg, acetaminophen 167 mg/5 ml w/alcohol 7%, parabens, saccharin, sorbitol, sucrose. Bot. 473 ml. *c-III.*
Use: Narcotic analgesic combination.

●**lortalamine.** (lahr-TAHL-ah-MEEN) USAN.
Use: Antidepressant.

●**lorzafone.** (LAHR-zah-FONE) USAN.
Use: Minor tranquilizer.

●**losartan potassium.** (low-SAHR-tan) USAN.
Use: Antihypertensive; treatment of CHF (angiotensin II receptor blocker).
See: Cozaar, Tab. (Merck).

Losec.
See: Prilosec.

Losopan Liquid. (Goldline) Magaldrate 540 mg/5 ml. Bot. 12 oz. *otc.*
Use: Antacid.

Losopan Plus Liquid. (Goldline) Magaldrate 540 mg, simethicone 20 mg/5 ml. Bot. 12 oz. *otc.*
Use: Antacid, antiflatulent.

Losotron Plus Liquid. (Various Mfr.) Magaldrate 540 mg, simethicone 20 mg/5 ml. Bot. 360 ml. *otc.*
Use: Antacid, antiflatulent.

●**losoxantrone hydrochloride.** (low-SOX-an-trone) USAN.
Use: Antineoplastic.

●**losulazine hydrochloride.** (low-SULL-ah-zeen) USAN.
Use: Antihypertensive.

Lotawin Capsules. (Sanofi Winthrop) Oxypertine. *Rx.*
Use: Anxiolytic, tranquilizer.

●**loteprednol etabonate.** (low-TEH-PRED-nole ett-AB-ohn-ate) USAN.
Use: Topical anti-inflammatory.

Lotensin. (Novartis) Benazepril HCl 5 mg, 10 mg, 20 mg, or 40 mg, lactose/Tab. Bot. 100s, UD 100s. *Rx.*
Use: Antihypertensive.

lotio alba. White lotion. *otc.*
Use: Antiacne, antiseborrheic.
W/Sulfur, calamine, alcohol.
See: Sulfa-Lo, Lot. (Whorton).

lotio alsulfa. (Doak) Colloidal sulfur 5%. Bot. 4 oz. *otc.*
Use: Antiacne, antiseborrheic.

Lotion-Jel. (C.S. Dent) Benzocaine in gel base. Tube 0.2 oz. *otc.*
Use: Local anesthetic, topical.

Lotrel. (Novartis) Amlodipine 2.5 mg or 5 mg, benazepril HCl 10 mg/Cap. or amlodipine 5 mg, benazepril HCl 20 mg/Cap. Bot. 100s. *Rx.*
Use: Antihypertensive combination.

Lotrimin. (Schering Plough) Clotrimazole 1%. **Cream:** Tube 15 g, 30 g, 45 g, 90 g. **Lot.:** Bot. 30 ml. **Soln.:** 1%. Bot. 10 ml, 30 ml. *Rx.*
Use: Antifungal, topical.

Lotrimin AF. (Schering Plough).

Lotrisone. (Schering Plough) Clotrimazole 1%, betamethasone dipropionate 0.05%/g. Tube 15 g, 45 g. *Rx.*
Use: Antifungal, topical.

Lo-Trop. (Vangard) Diphenoxylate HCl 2.5 mg, atropine sulfate 0.025 mg/Tab. Bot. 100s, 1000s. *c-v.*
Use: Antidiarrheal.

•**lovastatin.** (LOW-vuh-STAT-in) U.S.P. 23. *Formerly Mevinolin.*
Use: Antihypercholesteremic; antihyperlipidemic; HMG-CoA reductase inhibitor.
See: Mevacor, Tab. (Merck).

Love Longer. (Schmid) Benzocaine 7.5% in water-soluble lubricant base. Tube 0.5 oz. *otc.*
Use: Local anesthetic, topical.

Lovenox. (Rhone-Poulenc Rorer) Enoxaparin sodium. 30 mg/0.3 ml. Inj. Pk. 10 prefilled syringes w/26 guage x ½-inch needle. *Rx.*
Use: Anticoagulant.

•**loviride.** USAN.
Use: Antiviral for chronic oral treatment of HIV-seropositive patients (nonnucleoside reverse transcriptase inhibitor).

Lowila Cake. (Westwood-Squibb) Sodium lauryl sulfoacetate, dextrin, boric acid, urea, sorbitol, mineral oil, PEG 14 M, lactic acid, cellulose gum, docusate sodium, water, fragrance. Cake 112.5 g. *otc.*
Use: Skin cleanser.

Low-Quel. (Halsey) Diphenoxylate HCl 2.5 mg, atropine sulfate 0.025 mg/Tab. Bot. 100s. *c-v.*
Use: Antidiarrheal.

Lowsium. (Rugby) Magaldrate 540 mg/5 ml. Susp. Bot. 360 ml. *otc.*
Use: Antacid.

Lowsium Plus. (Rugby) **Tab.:** Magaldrate 480 mg, simethicone 20 mg. Bot. 60s. **Susp.:** Magaldrate 540 mg, simethicone 40 mg/5 ml. Bot. 360 ml. *otc.*
Use: Antacid, antiflatulent.

•**loxapine.** (LOX-ah-peen) USAN.
Use: Minor tranquilizer.

loxapine hydrochloride. *Rx.*
Use: Tranquilizer.
See: Daxolin Concentrate, Liq. (Bayer).
Loxitane-C Oral Concentrate (Lederle).
Loxitane, Inj. (Lederle).

•**loxapine succinate,** (LOX-ah-peen) U.S.P. 23. (Various Mfr.) 5 mg, 10 mg, 25 mg or 50 mg. Cap. Bot. 100s.
Use: Minor tranquilizer.
See: Loxitane, Cap. (Lederle).

loxapine succinate. (Various Mfr.) 5 mg, 10 mg, 25 mg, 50 mg. Cap. Bot. 100s.
Use: Minor tranquilizer.

Loxitane-C. (Lederle) Loxapine HCl oral concentrate 25 mg/ml. Bot. 120 ml w/ dropper. *Rx.*
Use: Antipsychotic.

Loxitane Capsules. (Lederle) Loxapine succinate. **5 mg/Cap.:** Bot. 100s, UD 10 × 10s. **10 mg, 25 mg or 50 mg/ Cap.:** Bot. 100s, 1000s, UD 10 10s. *Rx.*
Use: Antipsychotic.

Loxitane IM. (Lederle) Loxapine HCl (base equivalent) 50 mg/ml. Amp 1 ml. Box 10s. *Rx.*
Use: Antipsychotic.

•**loxoribine.** (LOX-ore-ih-BEAN) USAN.
Use: Immunostimulant; vaccine adjuvant.

L₂-oxothiazolidine₄-carboxylic acid.
Use: Treatment of adult respiratory distress syndrome.
See: Procysteine.

Lozol. (Rhone-Poulenc Rorer) Indapamide 2.5 mg/Tab. Bot. 100s, 1000s, 2500s, Strip dispenser 100s. *Rx.*
Use: Diuretic, antihypertensive.

l-pam.
See: Alkeran (Glaxo Wellcome).

l-sarcolysin.
See: Alkeran, Tab. (Glaxo Wellcome).

l-threonine.
Use: Antispasmodic.

l-triiodothyronine sod.
See: Cytomel, Tab. (SK-Beecham).
Liothyronine Sod.

Lubafax. (Glaxo Wellcome) Surgical lubricant, sterile; water soluble, nonstaining. Foil wrapper 2.7 g, 5 g. Box 144s.
Use: Surgical lubricant.

Lubath. (Warner-Lambert Prods) Mineral oil, PPG-15, stearyl ether, oleth-2, nonoxynol-5, fragrance, FD&C; Green No. 6. Bot. 4 oz, 8 oz, 16 oz. *otc.*
Use: Emollient.

Lubinol. (Purepac) Light, heavy and extra heavy mineral oil. Bot. pt, qt, gal. (Extra heavy Bot.) 8 oz, pt, qt, gal. *otc.*
Use: Emollient.

Lubraseptic Jelly. (Guardian) Water-soluble amyl phenyl phenol complex 0.12%, phenylmercuric nitrate, 0.007%. Bellows-type tube 10 g, 24s.
Use: Urethral instillation, urologic and proctologic exams.

Lubrasol Bath Oil. (Pharmaceutical Specialties) Mineral oil, lanolin oil, PEG-200 dilaurate, oxybenzone. Bot. 240 ml, 480 ml, gal. *otc.*
Use: Emollient.

Lubricating Gel. (Lake) Chlorhexidine gluconate, methylparaben, glycerin. Gel. Tub. 113.4 g, 3 g individual packets. *otc.*
Use: Vaginal preparation.

Lubricating Jelly. (Taro) Glycerin, propylene glycol. Jelly. 60 g, 125 g. *otc.*
Use: Vaginal preparation.

Lubriderm Cream. (Warner-Lambert Prods.)

Lubriderm Lotion. (Warner-Lambert Prods) Water, mineral oil, petrolatum, sorbitol, lanolin, lanolin alcohol, stearic acid, TEA, cetyl alcohol, fragrance (if scented), butylparaben, methylparaben, propylparaben, sodium Cl. Bot. (scented), 4 oz, 8 oz, 16 oz; (unscented) 8 oz, 16 oz. *otc.*
Use: Emollient.

Lubriderm Lubath Oil. (Warner-Lambert) Mineral oil, PPG-15 stearyl ether, oleth-2, nonoxynol-5. Lanolin free. Bot. 240 ml, pt. *otc.*
Use: Emollient.

Lubrin. (Kenwood/Bradley) Glycerin, caprylic/capric triglyceride. Pkg. 5s, 12s, 40s. *otc.*
Use: Vaginal lubricant.

LubriTears. (Bausch & Lomb) White petrolatum, mineral oil, lanolin, chlorobutanol 0.5%. Oint. Tube 3.5 g. *otc.*
Use: Ocular lubricant.

LubriTears Solution. (Bausch & Lomb) Hydroxypropyl methylcellulose 2906 0.3%, dextran 70 0.1%, EDTA, KCl, NaCl, benzalkonium chloride 0.01%. Bot. 15 ml. *otc.*
Use: Artificial tears.

• **lucanthone hydrochloride.** (LOO-kanthone) USAN.
Use: Antischistosomal.

Ludens Cough Drops. (Luden's).

Ludiomil. (Novartis) Maprotiline 25 mg, 50 mg or 75 mg/Tab. Bot. 100s, Accu-Pak 100s. *Rx.*
Use: Antidepressant.

• **lufironil.** (loo-FIHR-ah-nill) USAN.
Use: Collagen inhibitor.

Lufyllin. (Wallace) Dyphylline. Inj. **Amp.:** (500 mg/2 ml) Box 25s. **Elix.:** 100 mg/15 ml; alcohol 20%. Bot. pt, gal. **Tab.:** 200 mg. Bot. 100s, 1000s, UD 100s. *Rx.*
Use: Bronchodilator.

Lufyllin-400. (Wallace) Dyphylline 400 mg/Tab. Bot. 100s, 1000s. *Rx.*
Use: Bronchodilator.

Lufyllin-EPG. (Wallace) Ephedrine HCl 16 mg, dyphylline 100 mg, phenobarbital 16 mg, guaifenesin 200 mg/Tab. or 10 ml. Tab. Bot. 100s. *Rx.*
Use: Antiasthmatic combination.

Lufyllin-EPG Elixir. (Wallace) Dyphylline 150 mg, ephedrine HCl 24 mg, guaifenesin 300 mg, phenobarbital 24 mg, alcohol 5.5%/15 ml. Elix. Bot. 480 ml. *Rx.*
Use: Antiasthmatic combination.

Lufyllin-GG. (Wallace) **Tab.:** Dyphylline 200 mg, guaifenesin 200 mg/Tab. Bot. 100s, 3000s, UD 100s. **Elix.:** Dyphylline 100 mg, guaifenesin 100 mg, alcohol 17%/15 ml. Elix. Bot. pt, gal. *Rx.*
Use: Bronchodilator, expectorant.

Lugol's Solution. Strong iodine soln, U.S.P. 23. (Lyne). Iodine 5 g, potassium iodide 10 g, in purified water to make 100 ml. Bot. 15 ml. (Wisconsin) Bot. pt. *otc, Rx.*
Use: Antithyroid, antiseptic, topical.

Luminal Injection. (Sanofi Winthrop) Phenobarbital 130 mg/ml. Amp 1 ml. Box 100s.
Use: Sedative, hypnotic.

Lumopaque Capsules. (Sanofi Winthrop) Tyropanoate sodium.
Use: Radiopaque agent.

lung surfactants.
Use: Surfactant replacement therapy in neonatal respiratory distress syndrome.
See: Exosurf (Glaxo Wellcome). Survanta (Ross).

Lupron Depot. (TAP Pharm) Leuprolide acetate 11.25 mg. Lyophilized microspheres for injection. Single-use kit. Leuprolide acetate 3.75 or 7.5 mg. Preservative free. Microspheres for inj. Single-dose vials. *Rx.*
Use: Hormone.

Lupron Depot-Ped. (TAP Pharm) Leuprolide acetate 7.5, 11.25 or 15 mg. Preservative free. Microspheres for inj. *Rx.*
Use: Hormone.

Lupron Depot-3 Month. (TAP Pharm) Leuprolide acetate 11.25 mg/Lyophilized microspheres for injection. Single-use kit. Leuprolide acetate 22.5 mg. Preservative free. Microspheres for inj. *Rx.*
Use: Hormone.

Lupron Injection. (TAP) Leuprolide acetate 1 mg/0.2 ml. Vial 2.8 ml. *Rx.*
Use: Antineoplastic.

Luramide Tabs. (Major) Furosemide 20 mg, 40 mg or 80 mg/Tab. Bot. 100s, 1000s. *Rx.*
Use: Diuretic.

Luride Drops. (Colgate Oral) Sodium fluoride equivalent to 0.5 mg of fluoride/Drop. Plastic dropper bot. 50 ml. *Rx.*
Use: Dental caries preventative.

Luride Gel. (Colgate) Fluoride (from sodium fluoride and hydrogen fluoride) 1.2%. 7 g. *Rx.*
Use: Dental caries preventative.

Luride Lozi-Tabs. (Colgate Oral) Sodium fluoride 0.25 mg/Tab. Sugar free. Bot. 120s. *Rx.*
Use: Dental caries preventative.

Luride-F Lozi Tablets. (Colgate Oral) Sodium fluoride in Lozi base tab. available as fluoride. **0.25 mg:** Bot. 120s; **0.5 mg:** Bot. 120s, 1200s; **1 mg:** Bot. 120s, 1000s, 5000s. *Rx.*
Use: Dental caries preventative.

Luride Prophylaxis Paste. (Colgate Oral) Acidulated phosphate sodium fluoride containing 0.4% fluoride ion w/ silicon dioxide abrasive. UD 3 g, Jar 50 g. *otc.*
Use: Teeth cleaner.

Luride-SF Lozi Tablets. (Colgate Oral) Sodium fluoride 1 mg fluoride/Tab. Bot. 120s. *Rx.*
Use: Dental caries preventative.

Luride Topical Gel. (Colgate Oral) Fluoride 1.2%. Tube 7 g. *Rx.*
Use: Dental caries preventative.

Luride Topical Solution. (Colgate Oral) Acidulated phosphate sodium fluoride w/pH 3.2. Bot. 250 ml. *otc.*
Use: Dental caries preventative.

Lurline PMS. (Fielding) Acetaminophen 500 mg, pamabrom 25 mg, pyridoxine 50 mg/Tab. Bot. 24s, 50s. *otc.*
Use: Analgesic combination.

•**lurosetron mesylate.** (loo-ROW-set-rahn MEH-sih-late) USAN.
Use: Antiemetic.

Lurotin Caps. (BASF Wyandotte) Beta-carotene 25 mg/Cap. Bot. 100s. *otc.*
Use: Nutritional supplement.

•**lurtotecan dihyrochloride.** USAN.
Use: Antineoplastic (DNA topoisomerase I inhibitor).

luteogan.
See: Progesterone (Various Mfr.).

luteosan.
See: Progesterone (Various Mfr.).

lutocylol. (Novartis) Ethisterone.

Lutolin-F. (Spanner) Progesterone 25 mg or 50 mg/ml. Vial 10 ml.
Use: Progestin.

Lutolin-S. (Spanner) Progesterone 25 mg/ml. Vial 10 ml. *Rx.*
Use: Progestin.

•**lutrelin acetate.** (loo-TRELL-in ASS-eh-tate) USAN.
Use: LHRH agonist.

lutren.
See: Progesterone (Various Mfr.).

Lutrepulse. (Ortho) Gonadorelin acetate 0.8 mg or 3.2 mg/vial. Pow. for reconstitution (lyophilized). Vial 10 ml. *Rx.*
Use: Gonadotropin-releasing hormone.

lututrin.
See: Lutrexin, Tab. (Becton Dickinson).

Luvox. (Solvay) Fluvoxamine maleate 50 mg or 100 mg/Tab. Bot. 100s, 1000s, UD 100s. *Rx.*
Use: Antidepressant.

•**lyapolate sodium.** USAN. Sodium ethenesulfonate polymer. Peson (Hoechst Marion Roussel).
Use: Anticoagulant.

•**lycetamine.** (lie-SEET-ah-meen) USAN.
Use: Antimicrobial (topical).

lycine hydrochloride.
See: Betaine HCl (Various Mfr.).

Lydia E. Pinkham Herbal Compound. (Numark) Vitamin C, iron. Bot. 8 fl oz, 16 fl oz.

Lydia E. Pinkham Tablets. (Numark) Vitamin C, iron, calcium. 72s, 150s. *otc.*

•**lydimycin.** (lie-dih-MY-sin) USAN.
Use: Antifungal.

Lymphazurin. (Hirsch) Isosulfan blue 10 mg, sodium monohydrogen phosphate 6.6 mg, potassium dihydrogen phosphate 2.7 mg/ml. Vial 5 ml.
Use: Radiopaque agent.

lymphocyte immune globulin.
Use: Management of rejection in renal transplant.
See: Atgam, Inj. (Pharmacia & Upjohn).

•**lynestrenol.** (lin-ESS-tree-nahl) USAN.
Use: Progestin.

lynoestrenol. Lynestrenol.

Lyphocin P. (Fujisawa) Vancomycin HCl 500 mg. Vial 10 ml. *Rx.*
Use: Anti-infective.

lypholized vitamin B complex and vitamin C with B$_{12}$. (McGuff) B$_1$ 50 mg, B$_2$ 5 mg, B$_3$ 125 mg, B$_5$ 6 mg, B$_6$ 5 mg, B$_{12}$ 1000 mcg, C 50 mg/ml/Inj. Vial 10 ml. *Rx.*
Use: Parenteral vitamin supplement.

Lypholyte. (Fujisawa) Multiple electrolye concentrate. Vial 20 ml, 40 ml, Maxivial 100 ml, 200 ml. *Rx.*
Use: Parenteral electrolyte replacement.

Lypholyte II. (Fujisawa) Na$^+$ 35 mEq/L, K$^+$ 20 mEq/L, Ca^{++} 4.5 mEq/L, Mg^{++} 5 mEq/L, Cl 35 mEq/L, acetate 29.5 mEq/L. Single dose flip-top vial 20 ml, 40 ml; flip-top vial 100 ml, 200 ml. *Rx.*
Use: Parenteral nutritional supplement.

•**lypressin nasal solution,** (LIE-PRESS-in) U.S.P. 23. 8-Lysine vasopressin. Syntopressin.
Use: Antidiuretic; vasoconstrictor.
See: Diapid Nasal Spray (Sandoz).

lysidin. Methyl glyoxalidin.

•**lysine.** (LIE-SEEN) USAN.
Use: Nutrient, rapid weight gain; amino acid.

l-lysine.
Use: Dietary supplement; amino acid.
See: Enisyl (Person & Covey).
L-Lysine (Various Mfr.).

L-Lysine. (Various Mfr.) 312 mg, 500 mg/ Tab. Bot. 100s. 1000 mg/Tab. Bot. 60s. 500 mg/Cap. Bot. 100s and 250s. *otc.*
Use: Dietary supplement; amino acid.

•**lysine acetate,** (LIE-SEEN) U.S.P. 23. $C_6H_14N_2O_2\text{-}C_2H_4O_2$

Use: Amino acid.

•**lysine hydrochloride,** U.S.P. 23.
Use: Amino acid.
See: Enisyl, Tab. (Person & Covey).

lysivane.
See: Parsidol, Tab. (Warner-Chilcott).

Lysodren. (Bristol-Myers Oncology) Mitotane 500 mg/Tab. Bot. 100s. *Rx.*
Use: Antineoplastic.

•**lysostaphin.** (LIE-so-STAFF-in) USAN. Antibiotic derived from *Staphylococcus staphylolyticus.*
Use: Antibiotic; antibacterial enzyme.

Lyteers. (Pilkington Barnes Hind).

Lytren. (Bristol-Myers) Water, dextrose, sodium citrate, citric acid, sodium Cl, potassium citrate. Ready-To-Use Bot. 8 fl. oz. *otc.*
Use: Fluid/electrolyte replacement.

M

Maagel. (Approved) Aluminum and magnesium hydroxide. Bot. 12 oz, gal. *otc.*
Use: Antacid.

Maalox Antacid. (Rhone-Poulenc Rorer) Calcium carbonate 1000 mg, sodium ≤ 0.4 mEq. Capl. Bot. 50s. *otc.*
Use: Antacid.

Maalox Anti-Diarrheal Caplets. (Rhone-Poulenc Rorer) Loperamide HCl 2 mg/ Tab. Pkg. 12s. *otc.*
Use: Anti-diarrheal.

Maalox Anti-Gas. (Rhone-Poulenc Rorer) Simethicone 80 mg, sucrose/ Chew. Tab. Bot. 12s. *otc.*
Use: Antiflatulent

Maalox Daily Fiber Therapy. (Rhone-Poulenc Rorer) Psyllium hydrophilic mucilloid fiber 3.4 g/dose, sucrose and 35 cal/12 g in regular; aspartame, 21 mg/tsp phenylalanine and 9 cal/5.8 g in sugar free. Pow. Can 283 g (sugar free), 369 g, 3 single-dose (12 g) packets. *otc.*
Use: Laxative.

Maalox Extra Strength Plus Suspension. (Rhone-Poulenc Rorer) Magnesium hydroxide 450 mg, aluminum hydroxide 500 mg, simethicone 40 mg/ 5 ml. Susp. Bot. 148, 355, 769 ml. *otc.*
Use: Antacid, antiflatulent.

Maalox Extra Strength Plus Tablets. (Rhone-Poulenc Rorer) Magnesium hydroxide 350 mg, aluminum hydroxide 350 mg, simethicone 30 mg. Chew. Tab. Bot. 38s, 75s. *otc.*
Use: Antacid, antiflatulent.

Maalox Extra Strength Suspension. (Rhone-Poulenc Rorer) Aluminum hydroxide 500 mg, magnesium hydroxide 450 mg, simethicone 40 mg, parabens, saccharin, sorbitol/5 ml. Susp. Bot. 148 ml, 355 ml, 769 ml. *otc.*
Use: Antacid, antiflatulent.

Maalox Extra Strength Tablets. (Rhone-Poulenc Rorer) Magnesium hydroxide 350 mg, dried aluminum hydroxide gel 350 mg/Tab. Bot. 38s, 75s. *otc.*
Use: Antacid.

Maalox Heartburn Relief Liquid. (Rhone-Poulenc Rorer) Aluminum hydroxide, magnesium carbonate 140 mg, magnesium carbonate 175 mg, tartrazine, saccharin, magnesium alginate, parabens, sorbitol/5 ml. Bot. 296 ml. *otc.*
Use: Antacid.

Maalox HRF. (Rhone-Poulenc Rorer) Aluminum hydroxide/magnesium carbonate codried gel 280 mg, magnesium carbonate 350 mg/10 ml, saccharin, tartrazine. Liq. Bot. 355 ml. *otc.*
Use: Antacid.

Maalox Plus Tablets. (Rhone-Poulenc Rorer) Magnesium hydroxide 200 mg, dried aluminum hydroxide gel 200 mg, simethicone 25 mg/Tab. Bot. 50s, 100s, 144s. *otc.*
Use: Antacid, antiflatulent.

Maalox Suspension. (Rhone-Poulenc Rorer) Magnesium hydroxide 200 mg, aluminum hydroxide 225 mg/5 ml, Susp. Bot. 148 ml, 355 ml, 769 ml. *otc.*
Use: Antacid.

Maalox Tablets. (Rhone-Poulenc Rorer) Magnesium hydroxide 200 mg, dried aluminum hydroxide gel 200 mg/Tab. Bot. 100s. *otc.*
Use: Antacid.

Maalox Therapeutic Concentrate Suspension. (Rhone-Poulenc Rorer) Magnesium hydroxide 300 mg, aluminum hydroxide 600 mg/5 ml, Susp. Bot. 355 ml. *otc.*
Use: Antacid.

Maalox Therapeutic Concentrate Tablets. (Rhone-Poulenc Rorer) Magnesium hydroxide 300 mg, aluminum hydroxide 600 mg. Tab. Bot. 48s. *otc.*
Use: Antacid.

MacPac. (Procter & Gamble) Nitrofurantoin macrocrystals 50 mg or 100 mg/ Cap. UD 28s. *Rx.*
Use: Urinary anti-infective.

macroaggregated albumin.
See: Albumotope-LS. (Squibb).

Macrobid. (Procter & Gamble) Nitrofurantoin 100 mg (as 25 mg nitrofurantoin macrocrystals and 75 mg nitrofurantoin monohydrate). Cap. Bot. 100s. *Rx.*
Use: Urinary anti-infective.

Macrodantin. (Procter & Gamble) Nitrofurantoin macrocrystals **25 mg/Cap.:** Bot. 100s. **50 mg or 100 mg/Cap.:** Bot. 100s, 500s, 1000s, UD 100s. *Rx.*
Use: Urinary anti-infective.

Macrodex. (Pharmacia & Upjohn) Dextran 6% w/v in normal saline, 6% w/v in dextrose 5% in water. Bot. 500 ml. *Rx.*
Use: Plasma volume expander.

macrogol stearate 2000. Polyoxyl 40 Stearate.

Macrotec. (Squibb) Technetium Tc99m Medronate kit. Vial Kit 10s.
Use: Radiopaque agent.

Macrotin. W/Phenobarbital, hyoscyamus extract, caulophyllin, helonin, pulsatilla extract.
See: Tranquilans, Tab. (Noyes).

•**maduramicin.** (mad-UHR-ah-MY-sin) USAN.
Use: Anticoccidal.

•**mafenide.** (MAY-feh-NIDE) USAN.
Use: Antibacterial.

•**mafenide acetate,** (MAY-feh-NIDE) U.S.P. 23.
Use: Anti-infective (topical).
See: Sulfamylon Cream (Dow B. Hickam).

mafenide acetate solution. *Rx.*
Use: Prevent graft loss on burn wounds. [Orphan drug]

•**mafilcon a.** (MAY-fill-kahn A) USAN.
Use: Contact lens material (hydrophilic).

Mafylon Cream. (Sanofi Winthrop) Mafenide acetate. *Rx.*
Use: Burn preparation.

•**magaldrate,** (MAG-al-drate) U.S.P. 23. (Wyeth-Ayerst) Monalium Hydrate. Aluminum Magnesium Hydroxide.
Use: Antacid.
See: Iosopan (Goldline).
Monalium Hydrate.
Riopan, Tab., Susp. (Wyeth-Ayerst).

magaldrate and simethicone.
Use: Antacid, antiflatulant.
See: Lowsium. (Rugby).
Lowsium Plus. (Rugby).
Riopan Plus. (Wyeth-Ayerst).

magaldrate plus suspension. (Various Mfr.) Magaldrate 540 mg, simethicone 40 mg/5 ml. Susp. Bot. 360 ml. *otc.*
Use: Antacid, antiflatulant.

Magalox Plus. (Invamed) Dried aluminum hydroxide 200 mg, magnesium hydroxide 200 mg, simethicone 25 mg, sugar/Tab. Chewable. Bot. 100s. *otc.*
Use: Antacid.

Magan. (Pharmacia & Upjohn) Magnesium salicylate (anhydrous) 545 mg/Tab. Bot. 100s, 500s. *Rx.*
Use: Salicylate analgesic.

Mag-Cal Tablets. (Fibertone) Calcium 416.7 mg (as carbonate), calcium 166.7 mg (as elemental), vitamin D 66.7 IU, magnesium 83.3 mg, copper 0.167 mg, manganese 0.83 mg, potassium 1.67 mg, zinc 0.167 mg/Tab. Bot. 90s, 180s. *otc.*
Use: Vitamin/mineral supplement.

Mag-Cal Mega. (Freeda) Mg 800 mg, Ca 400 mg, kosher, sugar free/Tab. Bot. 100s and 250s. *otc.*
Use: Vitamin/mineral supplement.

Magdrox. (Vita Elixir) Magnesium hydroxide, aluminum hydroxide. *otc.*
Use: Antacid.

Magmalin Lozenge. (Pal-Pak) Magnesium hydroxide 0.2 g, aluminum hydroxide gel, dried 0.2 g/Loz. Bot. 1000s. *otc.*
Use: Antacid.

Magnacal Liquid. (Biosearch) Protein-calcium, sodium caseinate, carbohydrate-maltodextrin, sucrose, fat (partially hydrogenated), soy oil, lecithin, mono- and diglycerides. 1.5 Cal/ml, 590 mOsm/kg H_2O. Protein 70 g, CHO 250 g, fat 80 g, sodium 1000 mg, potassium 1250 mg/L. Can 120 ml, 240 ml. *otc.*
Use: Nutritional supplement.

Magnalox Liquid. (Schein) Aluminum hydroxide 225 mg, magnesium hydroxide 200 mg/5 ml. Liq. Bot. 360 ml. *otc.*
Use: Antacid.

Magnalum. (Global Pharms) Magnesium hydroxide 3.75 gr, aluminum hydroxide 2 gr/Tab. Bot. 1000s. *otc.*
Use: Antacid.

Magnaprin Arthritis Strength Tablets. (Rugby) Aspirin 325 mg, dried aluminum hydroxide gel 150 mg, magnesium hydroxide 150 mg/Tab. Bot. 100s, 500s. *otc.*
Use: Analgesic.

Magnaprin Tablets. (Rugby) Aspirin 325 mg, dried aluminum hydroxide gel 75 mg, magnesium hydroxide 75 mg/Tab. Bot. 100s, 500s. *otc.*
Use: Analgesic.

magnesia tablets.
Use: Antacid.

magnesia & alumina oral suspension. (Philips Roxane) Oral Susp. 6 fl oz. 25s.
Use: Antacid.
See: Maalox, Liq. (Rhone-Poulenc Rorer).

magnesia & alumina tablets.
Use: Antacid.
See: Maalox, Tab. (Rhone-Poulenc Rorer).

magnesia magma. Milk of Magnesia, U.S.P. 23.
Use: Antacid, cathartic, laxative.
See: Magnesium Hydroxide, Preps.

magnesium acetylsalicylate. Apyron, Magnespirin, Magisal, Novacetyl.
Use: Salicylate analgesic.

magnesium aluminate hydrated.
Use: Antacid.
See: Riopan, Susp., Tab. (Wyeth-Ayerst).

magnesium aluminum hydroxide.
Use: Antacid.
See: Maalox, Susp. (Rhone-Poulenc Rorer).
Malogel, Gel (Quality Generics).
Medalox, Gel (Med. Chem.).
W/APC.
See: Buffadyne, Tab. (Lemmon).
W/Calcium carbonate.
See: Camalox, Susp. (Rhone-Poulenc Rorer).
W/Simethicone.
See: Maalox Plus, Susp. (Rhone-Poulenc Rorer).

•**magnesium aluminum silicate,** NF 18.
Use: Pharmaceutic aid, suspending agent.

•**magnesium carbonate,** U.S.P. 23.
Use: Antacid.

magnesium carbonate. (Baker, d.T.) Pow. 4 oz, 1 lb, 5 lb.
Use: Antacid.

magnesium carbonate and sodium bicarbonate for oral suspension.
Use: Antacid.

magnesium carbonate w/combinations.
Use: Antacid.
See: Algicon, Tab. (Rhone-Poulenc Rorer).
Alkets, Tab. (Pharmacia & Upjohn).
Antacid No. 2, Tab. (Jones Medical).
Bismatesia, Can (Noyes).
Bufferin, Tab. (Bristol-Myers).
Di-Gel, Tab., Liq. (Schering Plough).
Magnagel, Liq., Tab. (Roberts).
Marblen, Susp., Tab. (Fleming).

•**magnesium chloride,** U.S.P. 23. Magnesium Cl hexahydrate.
Use: Electrolyte replenisher, pharmaceutical necessity for hemodialysis and peritoneal dialysis.
W/Potassium Cl, calcium Cl, red phenol.
See: Electrolytic replenisher, Vial (Invenex).

•**magnesium citrate oral solution,** (mag-NEE-zee-uhm) U.S.P. 23.
Use: Cathartic; laxative.

•**magnesium gluconate,** U.S.P. 23.
Use: Magnesium supplement, replenisher.
See: Almora, Tab. (Forest Pharm).

•**magnesium gluconate.** USAN. (Western Research) Magnesium gluconate 500 mg/Tab. Bot. 1000s. *otc.*
Use: Magnesium supplement.

magnesium glycinate.
W/Gastric mucin, aluminum hydroxide gel.
See: Mucogel, Tab. (Inwood).

•**magnesium hydroxide,** U.S.P. 23.
Use: Antacid, cathartic, laxative.
See: Magnesia Magma (Various Mfr.).
Milk of Magnesia (Various Mfr.).
Phillips' Milk of Magnesia (Bayer).
Phillips' Chewable, Tab. (Bayer).

magnesium hydroxide w/combinations.
See: Aludrox, Susp., Tab., Vial (Wyeth-Ayerst).
Ascriptin, Tab. (Rhone-Poulenc Rorer).
Ascriptin A/D, Tab. (Rhone-Poulenc Rorer).
Ascriptin Extra Strength, Tab. (Rhone-Poulenc Rorer).
Ascriptin w/Codeine, Tab. (Rhone-Poulenc Rorer).
Banacid, Tab. (Buffington).
Camalox, Susp., Tab. (Rhone-Poulenc Rorer).
Delcid, Susp. (Hoechst Marion Roussel).
Fermalox, Tab. (Rhone-Poulenc Rorer).
Kolantyl, Gel, Wafer (Hoechst Marion Roussel).
Laxsil Liquid, Liq. (Reed & Carnrick).
Maalox, Susp., Tab. (Rhone-Poulenc Rorer).
Maalox Plus, Susp., Tab. (Rhone-Poulenc Rorer).
Mylanta, Mylanta II, Liq., Tab. (Stuart).
Simeco, Liq. (Wyeth-Ayerst).
WinGel, Liq., Tab. (Sanofi Winthrop Products).

•**magnesium oxide,** (mag-NEE-zee-uhm OX-ide) U.S.P. 23.
Use: Pharmaceutic aid (sorbent).

magnesium oxide. (Manne) 420 mg/ Tab. Bot. 250s, 1000s. (Stanlabs) 10 gr/ Tab. Bot. 100s, 1000s.
Use: Pharm aid (sorbant).
See: Mag-Ox, Tab. (Blaine).
Mag-Ox 400, Tab. (Blaine).
Niko-Mag, Cap. (Scruggs).
Par-Mag, Cap. (Parmed).
Uro-Mag, Cap. (Blaine).
W/Calcium, Vitamin D.
See: Elekap, Cap. (Western Research).
W/Glutamic acid magnesium complex, N-acetyl-P-aminophenol, ascorbic acid, dl-methionine, lemon bioflavonoid complex, dl-α-tocopheryl acetate, glycine, soybean flour.
See: Ulcimins, Tab. (Miller).
W/Magnesium carbonate, calcium carbonate.
See: Alkets, Tab. (Pharmacia & Upjohn).

W/Ox bile (desiccated), hog bile (desiccated.).
See: Hyper-Cholate, Tab. (Roberts).
W/Phenobarbital, atropine sulfate.
See: Magnox, Tab. (Jones Medical).
•**magnesium phosphate,** U.S.P. 23.
Use: Antacid.
•**magnesium salicylate,** U.S.P. 23.
Use: Analgesic, antipyretic, antirheumatic.
See: Analate, Tab. (Winston).
Efficin, Tab. (Pharmacia & Upjohn).
Magan, Tab. (Pharmacia & Upjohn).
W/Phenyltoloxamine citrate.
See: Mobigesic, Tab. (Ascher).
•**magnesium silicate,** N.F. 18.
Use: Pharmaceutic aid (tablet excipient).
•**magnesium stearate,** N.F. 18.
Use: Pharmaceutic aid (tablet and capsule lubricant).
•**magnesium sulfate,** (mag-NEE-zee-uhm SULL-fate) U.S.P. 23.
Use: Anticonvulsant, electrolyte replenisher, laxative.
magnesium sulfate. (Abbott)–50% Amp. 2 ml Box 25s, 100s. Abboject Syringe (20 G X 2.5) 5 ml, 10 ml; 12.5% in Pintop Vial, 8 ml, 20 ml. (Atlas)–10% Amp. 10 ml Box 100s; 1 g/2 ml. Box 100s. (Baxter)–10%. Vial 10 ml, 20 ml. (CMC)–1 g/2 ml, 10% Amp. 10 ml, 20 ml; 25% Amp. 10 ml 50%. Vial 30 ml. (Quality Generics)–50% Amp. 2 ml, 100s. (Lilly)–10% Amp 20 ml Box 6s, 25s; 50% 1 g Amp. 2 ml, Box 12s, 100s. (Parke-Davis)–50% Amp. 2 ml, 10s. (Trent)–50% Amp. 2 ml, 10 ml. (Various Mfr.) Inj. 12.5% Vial 8 ml; 50% Amps 2 ml, 10 ml; Vial 10 ml, 20 ml, 50 ml; Disp. Syringe 5 ml, 10 ml; 2 ml fill in 5 ml vials.
•**magnesium trisilicate,** U.S.P. 23. Magnesium silicate hydrate.
Use: Antacid.
See: Trisomin, Tab. (Lilly).
magnesium trisilicate w/combinations.
See: Alsorb Gel C.T., Gel (Standex).
Arcodex Tablets, Tab. (Arcum).
Banacid, Tab. (Buffington).
Gacid, Tab. (Arcum).
Gaviscon, Tab. (Hoechst Marion Roussel).
Maracid 2, Tab. (Marin).
Magnevist. (Berlex) Gadopentetate dimeglumine 469.01 mg, meglumine 0.39 mg, diethylenetriamine pentaacetic acid 0.15 mg. Inj. Vial 20 ml.
Use: Radiopaque agent.

Magonate. (Fleming) Magnesium gluconate 500 mg/Tab. Bot. 100s, 1000s. otc.
Use: Magnesium supplement.
Mag-Ox 400. (Blaine) Magnesium oxide 400 mg/Tab. Bot. 100s, 1000s. otc.
Use: Antacid, magnesium supplement.
Magsal. (U.S. Pharm) Magnesium salicylate 600 mg, phenyltoloxamine citrate 25 mg/Tab. Bot. 100s. Rx.
Use: Analgesic combination.
Mag-Tab Sr. (Niche) Magnesium (as lactate) 84 mg/SR Capl. Bot. 60s, 100s. otc.
Use: Magnesium supplement.
Maigret-50. (Ferndale) Phenylpropanolamine HCl 50 mg/Tab. Bot. 100s.
Use: Decongestant.
Maintenance Vitamin Formula w/Minerals. (Towne) Vitamins A palmitate 10,000 IU, D 400 IU, B_1 5 mg, B_2 2.5 mg, C 75 mg, niacinamide 40 mg, B_6 1 mg, calcium pantothenate 4 mg, B_{12} 2 mcg, E 2 IU, choline bitartrate 31.4 mg, inositol 15 mg, calcium 75 mg, phosphorus 58 mg, iron 30 mg, magnesium 3 mg, manganese 0.5 mg, potassium 2 mg, zinc 0.5 mg/Cap. Bot. 100s. otc.
Use: Vitamin/mineral supplement.
majeptil. Thioproperazine. Psychopharmacologic agent; pending release.
Major-Gesic. (Major) Phenyltoloxamine citrate 30 mg, acetaminophen 325 mg/Tab. Bot. 100s. otc.
Use: Antihistamine, analgesic.
malagride.
See: Acetarsone.
Malaraquin. (Sanofi Winthrop) Chloroquine phosphate. Rx.
Use: Antimalarial.
Malatal Tablets. (Roberts) Atropine sulfate 0.0194 mg, scopolamine HBr 0.0065 mg, hyoscyamine HBr, SO_4 0.1037 mg, phenobarbital 16.2 mg/Tab. Bot. 1000s. Rx.
Use: Anticholinergic, antispasmodic, sedative, hypnotic.
•**malathion,** U.S.P. 23.
Use: Pediculicide.
•**malethamer.** (mal-ETH-ah-mer) USAN. Maleic anhydride ethylene polymer.
Use: Antidiarrheal, antiperistaltic.
•**malic acid,** N.F. 18.
Use: Pharmaceutic aid (acidifying agent).
malic acid with pectin.
See: Mallo-Pectin, Liq. (Roberts).
Mallamint. (Roberts) Calcium carbonate

420 mg/Tab. Bot. 100s. *otc.*
Use: Antacid.

Mallazine Drops. (Roberts Hauck) Tetrahydrozoline 0.05%. Soln. 15 ml. *otc.*
Use: Vasoconstrictor, mydriatic, ophthalmic.

Mallergan-VC w/Codeine Syrup. (Roberts) Phenylephrine HCl 5 mg, promethazine HCl 6.25 mg, codeine phosphate 10 mg/5 ml, alcohol 7%. Syr. Bot. 120 ml. *c-v.*
Use: Decongestant, antihistamine, antitussive.

Mallisol. (Roberts) Povidone-iodine. *otc.*
Use: Germicidal, antiseptic surgical scrub.

Malogen Injection Aqueous. (Forest Pharm) Testosterone. **25 mg/ml:** 10 ml, 30 ml; **50 mg/ml:** 10 ml; **100 mg/ml:** 10 ml. *c-III.*
Use: Androgen.

Malogen 100 L.A. in Oil inj. (Forest Pharm) Testosterone enanthate 100 mg/ml. 10 ml. *c-III.*
Use: Androgen.

Malogen 200 L.A. in Oil inj. (Forest Pharm) Testosterone enanthate 200 mg/ml. 10 ml. *c-III.*
Use: Androgen.

Malogen Cyp. (Forest Pharm) Testosterone cypionate in oil 100 mg or 200 mg/ml. Vial 10 ml. *c-III.*
Use: Androgen.

malonal.
See: Barbital (Various Mfr.).

•**malotilate.** (mal-OH-tih-LATE) USAN.
Use: Liver disorder treatment.

•**maltitol solution,** NF 18.
Use: Sweetener.

Malotrone Aqueous Injection. (Bluco) Testosterone, USP 25 mg or 50 mg/ml in aqueous susp. Vial 10 ml. *c-III.*
Use: Androgen.

•**maltodextrin,** N.F. 18.
Use: Pharmaceutic aid (coating agent, diluent, tablet binder, tablet and capsule, viscosity-increasing agent).

Maltsupex. (Wallace) Laxative derived from natural barley malt extract for relief of constipation in children and adults. **Liq.:** Bot. 8 oz, pt. **Pow.:** Jar 8 oz, lb. **Tab.:** Malt soup extract 750 mg/Tab. Bot. 100s. *otc.*
W/Psyllium seed husks.
Use: Laxative.
See: Syllamalt, Pow. (Wallace).

Mammol Ointment. (Abbott) Bismuth subnitrate 40%, castor oil 30%, anhydrous lanolin 22%, ceresin wax 7%,

balsam Peru 1%. Tube ⅞ oz. Ctn. 12s. *otc.*
Use: Skin protectant, emollient.

mandameth. (Major) Methenamine mandelate 0.5 g/EC Tab. Bot. 1000s. *Rx.*
Use: Urinary anti-infective.

mandelic acid.
Use: Urinary anti-infective.

mandelic acid salts.
See: Calcium mandelate (Various Mfr.).

mandelyltropeine.
See: Homatropine Salts (Various Mfr.).

Mandol. (Lilly) Cefamandole nafate. Vial: **1 g/10 ml:** Traypak 25s; **1 g/100 ml** or **2 g/20 ml:** Traypak 10s; **2 g/100 ml:** Traypak 10s. *Rx.*
Use: Anti-infective, cephalosporin.

Manganese.
Use: Dietary supplement.
See: Chelated manganese (Freeda).

•**manganese chloride,** U.S.P. 23.
Use: Manganese deficiency treatment, trace mineral supplement.

•**manganese gluconate.** U.S.P. 23.
Use: Manganese deficiency, trace mineral supplement.

manganese glycerophosphate. Glycerol phosphate manganese salt.
Use: Pharmaceutical necessity.

manganese hypophosphite. Manganese (2+) phosphinate.
Use: Pharmaceutical necessity.

•**manganese sulfate,** U.S.P. 23.
Use: Supplement (trace mineral).
W/Thyroid, ferrous sulfate, ferrous gluconate, sodium ferric pyrophosphate, extract of nux vomica.
See: Hemocrine, Tab. (Roberts).

Manga-Pak. (SoloPak) Manganese 0.1 mg/ml. Inj. Vial 10 ml, 30 ml. *Rx.*
Use: Parenteral nutritional supplement.

Maniron. (Jones Medical) Ferrous fumarate 3 mg/Tab. Bot. 100s, 1000s, 5000s. *otc.*
Use: Iron supplement.

Mann Astringent Mouth Wash Concentrate. (Mann) Bot. 4 oz, qt, 0.5 gal, gal. Also mint flavored. Bot. 4 oz, qt, 0.5 gal, gal. *otc.*
Use: Mouthwash.

Mann Body Deodorant. (Mann) Bot. 4 oz, 8 oz, pt, qt. *otc.*

Mann Breath Deodorant. (Mann) Bot. 1 oz, 4 oz, 8 oz, pt, qt, 0.5 gal. *otc.*

Mann Emollient. (Mann) Jar. 100 g. *otc.*
Use: Emollient.

Mann Eugenol U.S.P. Extra. (Mann) 0.06 lb, 0.13 lb, 0.25 lb, 0.5 lb, 1 lb. *otc.*
Use: With zinc oxide as protective pack.

Mann Germicidal Solution. (Mann)
Regular: Bot. gal, 4 gal. **Conc.:** 12.8%.
Bot. pt, qt, 0.5 gal, gal. *otc.*
Use: Germicide.

Mann Hand Lotion. (Mann) Twin pack,
gal. *otc.*
Use: Emollient.

Mann Hemostatic. (Mann) Bot. 1 oz, 4
oz, 8 oz, pt, qt. *otc.*
Use: Hemostatic.

Mann Liquid Soap. (Mann) Concentrated cococastile. Bot. qt, 0.5 gal, gal.
otc.
Use: Emollient.

Mann Lubricant and Cleanser. (Mann)
Bot. pt, qt. *otc.*
Use: Emollient.

Mann Superfatted Bar Soap. (Mann)
Rich in lanolin. Cake. 12s. *otc.*
Use: Emollient.

Mann Talbot's Iodine. (Mann) Glycerin
base. Bot. 1 oz, 4 oz, 8 oz, pt, qt. *otc.*
Use: Antiseptic.

Mann Topical Anesthetic. (Mann) Bot.
1 oz, 4 oz, 8 oz, pt. W/stain to indi-
cate area treated. Bot. 1 oz, 4 oz, 8 oz.
otc.
Use: Local anesthetic, topical.

manna sugar.
See: Mannitol (Various Mfr.).

Mannan. (Rugby) Purified glucomannan
500 mg/Cap. Bot. 90s. *otc.*
Use: Nutritional supplement.

Mannest. (Manne) Conjugated estrogens
0.625 mg, 1.25 mg or 2.5 mg/Tab. Bot.
100s, 200s. *Rx.*
Use: Estrogen.

mannite.
See: Mannitol, U.S.P. 23.

•**mannitol,** U.S.P. 23. Manna Sugar, D-
Mannitol, Mannite.
Use: Diagnostic aid (renal function de-
termination), diuretic.
See: Osmitrol (Baxter).
W/Sorbitol.
See: Cystosol, Liq. (Baxter).
Cytal, Liq. (Bayer).

mannitol injection. (Abbott) 15% or
20%. Abbo-Vac Single dose container
500 ml.
Use: Diagnostic aid (renal function determination), diuretic.
See: Mannitol Solution, Amp. (Merck).

mannitol hexanitrate.
Use: Coronary vasodilator.
See: Vascunitol, Tab. (Apco).
W/Reserpine, rutin, ascorbic acid.
See: Ruhexatal W/Reserpine, Tab.
(Lemmon).

**mannitol hexanitrate & phenobarbital
tab.** (Jones Medical; Quality Generics) Mannitol hexanitrate 0.5 g, phenobarbital 0.25 g/Tab. Bot. 1000s. *c-iv.*
Use: Vasodilator.

**mannitol hexanitrate with phenobarbi-
tal combinations.**
See: Manotensin,Tab. (Dunhall).
Ruhexatal, Tab. (Lemmon).
Vascused, Tab. (Apco).
Vermantin, Tab. (Trout).

mannitol in sodium chloride injection.
Use: Diuretic.

Manotensin. (Dunhall) Mannitol hexani-
trate 32 mg, phenobarbital 16 mg/Tab.
Bot. 100s, 1000s. *c-iv.*
Use: Vasodilator combination.

Mantadil. (Glaxo Wellcome) Chlorocycli-
zine HCl 2%, hydrocortisone acetate
0.5%, liquid and white petrolatum, wax,
methylparaben 0.25%. Cream Tube
15 g. *Rx.*
Use: Antipruritic, anti-inflammatory, anesthetic.

Mantoux Test.
See: Tuberculin, U.S.P. 23. Test.

manvene.
Use: Antineoplastic.

MAOI.
See: Monoamine Oxidase Inhibitors.

Maolate Tablets. (Pharmacia & Upjohn)
Chlorphenesin carbamate 400 mg/Tab.
Bot. 50s, 500s. *Rx.*
Use: Muscle relaxant, mild tranquilizer.

Maox 420. (Manne Co.) Magnesium oxide 420 mg/Tab. Bot. 250s, 1000s. *otc.*
Use: Antacid.

Mapap Cold Formula. (Major) Aceta-
minophen 325 mg, pseudoephedrine
HCl 30 mg, dextromethorphan HBr 15
mg, chlorpheniramine maleate 2 mg.
Tab. Pkg. 24s. *otc.*
Use: Antitussive combination.

Mapap Extra Strength. (Major) Acetaminophen 500 mg/Tab. Bot. 30s, 60s,
100s, 200s, 1000s and UD 100s. *otc.*
Use: Analgesic.

Mapap Infant Drops. (Major) Acetamino-
phen 100 mg/ml, alcohol free/Drops.
Bot. 15 and 30 ml. *otc.*
Use: Analgesic.

Mapap Regular Strength. (Major) Acetaminophen 325 mg/Scored Tab. Bot.
100s, 1000s and UD 100s. *otc.*
Use: Analgesic.

maphenide.
See: Sulfbenzamine HCl.

Maprofix.
See: Gardinol Type Detergents (Various Mfr.).

●**maprotiline.** (map-ROW-tih-leen) USAN.
Use: Antidepressant.
See: Ludiomil, Tab. (Novartis).

●**maprotiline hydrochloride,** (map-ROW-tih-leen) U.S.P. 23.
Use: Antidepressant.

Maracid 2. (Marin) Magnesium trisilicate 150 mg, aluminum hydroxide dried gel 90 mg, aminoacetic acid 75 mg/Tab. Bot. *otc.*
Use: Antacid, adsorbant.

Maranox. (C.S. Dent) Acetaminophen 325 mg/Tab. Bot. 8s. *otc.*
Use: Analgesic.

Marax-DF Syrup. (Roerig) Hydroxyzine HCl 7.5 mg, ephedrine sulfate 18.75 mg, theophylline 97.5 mg/15 ml. Color free, dye free. Bot. pt, gal. *Rx.*
Use: Antiasthmatic combination.

Marax Tab. (Roerig) Hydroxyzine HCl 10 mg, ephedrine sulfate 25 mg, theophylline 130 mg/Tab. Bot. 100s, 500s. *Rx.*
Use: Antiasthmatic combination.

Marbaxin 750. (Vortech) Methocarbamol 750 mg/Tab. Bot. 500s. *Rx.*
Use: Skeletal muscle relaxant.

Marblen Liquid. (Fleming) Magnesium carbonate 400 mg, calcium carbonate 520 mg/5 ml. Bot. 473 ml. *otc.*
Use: Antacid.

Marblen Tablets. (Fleming) Calcium carbonate 520 mg, magnesium carbonate 400 mg. Tab. Bot. 100s, 1000s. *otc.*
Use: Antacid.

Marcaine. (Sanofi Winthrop) Bupivacaine in sterile isotonic soln. containing sodium Cl pH adjusted 4.0 to 6.5 w/sodium hydroxide or hydrochloric acid. Multiple-dose vial also contains methylparaben 1 mg/ml as preservative. **0.25%:** Amp. 50 ml. Box 5s. Vial: Single dose 10 ml, 30 ml. Box 10s; multiple dose 50 ml. Box 1s. **0.5%:** Amp. 30 ml. Box 1s. Vial: Single dose 10 ml, 30 ml. Box 10s; multiple dose 50 ml. Box 1s. **0.75%:** Amp. 30 ml. Box 5s. Vial (single dose) 10 ml, 30 ml. Box 10s. *Rx.*
Use: Local anesthetic.

Marcaine with Epinephrine. (1:200,000). (Sanofi Winthrop) **Bupivacaine 0.25%:** with epinephrine 1:200,000 in sterile isotonic soln. containing sodium Cl. Each 1 ml contains bupivacaine HCl 2.5 mg, epinephrine bitartrate 0.0091 mg, sodium metabisulfite 0.5 mg, monothioglycerol 0.001 ml, ascorbic acid 2 mg and edetate calcium disodium 0.1 mg. In Multiple Dose Vial, each 1 ml also contains methylparaben 1 mg as antiseptic preservative. pH adjusted to between 3.4 and 4.5 with sodium hydroxide or hydrochloric acid. Amp. 50 ml, 5s, Single Vial 10 ml, 30 ml. 10s, Multiple Dose Vial 50 ml 1s. **Bupivacaine 0.5%:** with epinephrine 1:200,000 in sterile isotonic soln. containing sodium Cl. Each 1 ml contains bupivacaine HCl 5 mg and epinephrine bitartrate 0.0091 mg, with sodium metabisulfite 0.5 mg, monothioglycerol 0.001 ml and ascorbic acid 2 mg, edetate calcium disodium 0.1 mg. In Multiple Dose Vial, each 1 ml also contains methylparaben 1 mg antiseptic preservative. pH adjusted to between 3.4 and 4.5 with sodium hydroxide or hydrochloric acid. Amp. 3 ml 10s, 30 ml 5s. Single Dose Vial 10 ml, 30 ml 10s. Multiple Dose Vial 50 ml 1s. **Bupivacaine 0.75%:** with epinephrine 1:200,000 in sterile isotonic soln. containing sodium Cl. Each 1 ml contains bupivacaine HCl 7.5 mg, epinephrine bitartrate 0.0091 mg with sodium metabisulfite 0.5 mg, monothioglycerol 0.001 ml, ascorbic acid 2 mg as antioxidants, edetate calcium disodium 0.1 mg. pH adjusted to between 3.4 and 4.5 with sodium hydroxide or hydrochloric acid. Amp 30 ml in 5s. *Rx.*
Use: Local anesthetic.

Marcaine Spinal. (Sanofi Winthrop) Bupivacaine HCl 15 mg/2 ml (0.75%) and dextrose 165 mg/2 ml (8.25%). Amp. 2 ml. *Rx.*
Use: Local anesthetic.

Marcillin. (Marnel) **Cap.:** Ampicillin trihydrate 500 mg. Bot. 100s; **Pow. for Susp.:** Ampicillin trihydrate 250 mg/100 ml. *Rx.*
Use: Anti-infective, penicillin.

Marcof Expectorant. (Marnel) Hydrocodone bitartrate 5 mg, potassium guaiacolsulfonate 300 mg/5 ml. Liq. Bot. 480 ml. *c-III.*
Use: Narcotic antitussive, expectorant.

Mardon. (Armenpharm) Propoxyphene HCl. **Cap.:** 32 mg Bot. 100s, 1000s. **65 mg:** Bot. 100s, 500s, 1000s. [c-iv] c-iv.
Use: Narcotic analgesic.

Mardon Compound. (Armenpharm) Propoxyphene compound 65 mg, aspirin 3.5 gr, phenacetin 2.5 gr, caffeine 0.5 gr/Cap. Bot. 100s, 500s, 1000s. *c-iv.*
Use: Narcotic analgesic combination.

Marezine Tablets. (Himmel) Cyclizine HCl 50 mg/Tab. Bot. 100s. Box 12s. *otc.*

Use: Anticholinergic.
W/Ergotamine tartrate, caffeine.
See: Migral, Tab. (Glaxo Wellcome).
marfanil.
See: Sulfbenzamine HCl (Various Mfr.).
Margesic. (Marnel) Butalbital 50 mg, acetaminophen 325 mg, caffeine 40 mg/Cap. Bot. 100s. *Rx.*
Use: Analgesic, sedative, hypnotic.
Margesic H. (Marnel) Hydrocodone bitartrate 5 mg, acetaminophen 500 mg/ Cap. Bot. 100s. *c-III.*
Use: Narcotic analgesic combination.
Margesic No. 3. (Marnel) Codeine phosphate 30 mg, acetaminophen 300 mg/ Tab. Bot. 100s. *c-III.*
Use: Narcotic analgesic combination.
Marhist. (Marlop) Chlorpheniramine maleate 20 mg, phenylephrine HCl 2.5 mg, methscopolamine nitrate in special base/Cap. Bot. 30s, 100s. Expectorant Bot. 4 oz, pt, gal. *Rx.*
Use: Antihistamine, decongestant, anticholinergic.
•**marimastat.** USAN.
Use: Antineoplastic (matrix matalloproteinase inhibitor).
Marine Lipid Concentrate. (Vitaline) Omega-3 1200 mg, EPA 360 mg, DHA 240 mg, E 5 IU/Cap., sodium free. Bot. 90s. *otc.*
Use: Fish oil.
Marinol Capsules. (Roxane) Dronabinol 2.5 mg, 5 mg or 10 mg/Cap. Bot. 25s. *c-II.*
Use: Antiemetic.
Marlin Salt System. (Marlin) Sodium Cl 250 mg/Tab. Bot. 200s with bot. 27.7 ml. *otc.*
Use: Soft contact lens care.
Marlyn Formula 50. (Marlyn) Vitamin B₆ w/18 amino acids/Cap. Bot. 100s, 250s, 1000s. *otc.*
Use: Nutritional supplement.
Marmine. (Vortech) Dimenhydrinate 50 mg/ml. Inj. Vial 1 ml, 10 ml. *Rx.*
Use: Antiemetic/antivertigo agent.
Marnal. (Vortech) Aspirin 325 mg, caffeine 40 mg, butalbital 50 mg/Tab. Bot. 100s. *c-III.*
Use: Analgesic, sedative, hypnotic.
Marnatal-F. (Marnal) Calcium 250 mg, iron 60 mg, vitamins A 4000 IU, D 400 IU, E 30 mg, B₁ 3 mg, B₂ 3.4 mg, B₃ 20 mg, B₆ 5 mg, B₁₂ 12 mcg, C 100 mg, folic acid 1 mg, Mg, Zn 25 mg, Cu, I/ Tab. Bot. 30s, 100s. *Rx.*
Use: Vitamin/mineral supplement; dental caries preventative.

Marpres. (Marnel) Hydrochlorothiazide 15 mg, reserpine 0.1 mg, hydralazine HCl 25 mg/Tab. Bot. 100s, 1000s. *Rx.*
Use: Antihypertensive.
Marthritic. (Marnel) Salsalate 750 mg. Tab. Bot. 100s. *Rx.*
Use: Salicylate analgesic.
•**masoprocol.** (mass-OH-prah-KOLE) USAN.
Use: Antineoplastic.
See: Actinex, cream. (Schwarz Pharma).
Masse Breast Cream. (Advanced Care) Water, glyceryl monostearate, glycerin, cetyl alcohol, lanolin, peanut oil, Span-60, stearic acid, Tween-60, sodium benzoate, propylparaben, methylparaben, potassium hydroxide. Tube 2 oz. *otc.*
Use: Emollient.
Massengill Baking Soda Freshness. (SK-Beecham) Sanitized water, sodium bicarbonate. Soln. Bot. 180 ml. *otc.*
Use: Vaginal preparation.
Massengill Feminine Cleansing Wash. (SK-Beecham) Sodium laureth sulfate, magnesium laureth sulfate, sodium oleth sulfate, magnesium oleth sulfate, PEG-120 methyl glucose dioleate, parabens. Liq. Bot. 240 ml. *otc.*
Use: Vaginal preparation.
Massengill Feminine Deodorant Spray. (SK-Beecham) Aerosol Bot. 3 oz. *otc.*
Use: Vaginal preparation.
Massengill Disposable Douche. (SK-Beecham) Water, S.D. alcohol 40, lactic acid, sodium lactate, octoxymol-9, cetylpyridium Cl, propylene glycol, diazolidinyl urea, EDTA, parabens, fragrance, color. Bot. 180 ml. *otc.*
Use: Vaginal preparation.
Massengill Extra Cleansing w/Puraclean. (SK-Beecham) Vinegar, water, cetylpyridinium chloride, diazolidinyl urea, EDTA. Soln. Bot. 180 ml. *otc.*
Use: Vaginal preparation.
Massengill Liquid. (SK-Beecham) Lactic acid, S.D. alcohol 40, octoxynol-9, water, sodium bicarbonate. Bot. 120 ml. *otc.*
Use: Vaginal preparation.
Massengill Medicated. (SK-Beecham) Povidone-iodine 0.3% when added to sanitized fluid. Bot. 6 oz. *otc.*
Use: Vaginal preparation.
Massengill Medicated Disposable Douche w/Cepticin. (SK-Beecham) Povidone-iodine 10%. Liq. Vial 5 ml w/ 180 ml bot. of sanitized water. *otc.*

Use: Vaginal preparation.

Massengill Medicated Douche w/Cepticin. (SK-Beecham) Povidone-iodine 12%. Liq. concentrate. Bot. 120 ml, 240 ml. *otc.*
Use: Vaginal preparation.

Massengill Powder. (SK-Beecham) Ammonium alum, PEG-8, methyl salicylate, eucalyptus oil, menthol, thymol, phenol. Jar 120 g, 240 g, 480 g, 660 g. UD Packette 10s, 12s. *otc.*
Use: Vaginal preparation.

Massengill Soft Cloth. (SK-Beecham) Hydrocortisone 0.5%, diazolidinyl urea, DMDM hydantoin, isopropyl myristate, methylparaben, polysorbate 60, propylene glycol, propylparaben, sorbitan stearate, steareth-2, steareth-21. Towelettes 10s. *otc.*
Use: Vaginal preparation.

Massengill Unscented. (SK-Beecham) Water, SD alcohol 40, lactic acid, sodium lactate, octoxynol-9, cetylpyridium chloride, propylene glycol, diazolidinyl urea, parabens, EDTA. Soln. Bot. 180 ml.
Use: Vaginal preparation.

Massengill Vinegar-Water Disposable Douche. (SK-Beecham) Water and vinegar solution. Bot. 180 ml. *otc.*
Use: Vaginal preparation.

Massengill Vinegar & Water Extra Cleansing with Puraclean. (SK-Beecham) Vinegar, water, cetylpyridinium chloride, diazolidinyl urea, EDTA. Soln. Bot. 180 ml. *otc.*
Use: Vaginal preparation.

Massengill Vinegar & Water Extra Mild. (SK-Beecham) Vinegar, water, preservative free. Soln. Bot. 180 ml. *otc.*
Use: Vaginal preparation.

Master Formula. (Barth's) Vitamins A 10,000 IU, D 400 IU, C 180 mg, B_1 7 mg, B_2 14 mg, niacin 4.6 mg, B_6 292 mcg, pantothenic acid 210 mcg, B_{12} 25 mcg, biotin 2.9 mcg, E 50 IU, calcium 800 mg, phosphorus 387 mg, iron 10 mg, iodine 0.1 mg, choline 7.78 mg, inositol 11.6 mg, aminobenzoic acid 35 mcg, rutin 30 mg, citrus bioflavonoid complex 30 mg/4 Tab. Bot. 120s, 600s, 1200s.
Use: Vitamin/mineral supplement.

Mastisol. (Ferndale) Nonirritating medical adhesive. Bot. 4 oz.
Use: Skin dressing adhesive.

matrix metalloproteinase inhibitor.
Use: Corneal ulcers. [Orphan drug]

Matulane. (Roche) Procarbazine HCl 50 mg/Cap. Bot. 100s. *Rx.*
Use: Antineoplastic.

Mavik. (Knoll) Trandolapril 1 mg, 2 mg and 4 mg, lactose/Tab. Bot. 100s, UD 100s. *Rx.*
Use: Antihypertensive.

Maxair. (3M) Pirbuterol acetate aerosol 0.2 mg pirbuterol/actuation. Metered dose inhaler 25.6 g (300 inhalations). *Rx.*
Use: Sympathomimetic bronchodilator.

Maxaquin. (Searle) Lomefloxacin HCl 400 mg/Tab. Bot. 20s, UD 100s. *Rx.*
Use: Anti-infective, fluoroquinolone.

Max EPA Capsules. (Various Mfr.) Omega-3 polyunsaturated fatty acids 1000 mg/Cap. containing EPA 180 mg, DHA 60 mg/Cap. Bot. 50s, 60s, 100s. *otc.*
Use: Fish oil, nutritional supplement.

Maxidex. (Alcon) Dexamethasone 0.1%. Soln. Drop-Tainers 5 ml, 15 ml. *Rx.*
Use: Corticosteroid, ophthalmic.

Maxidex Ointment. (Alcon) Dexamethasone phosphate 0.05%. Tube 3.5 g. *Rx.*
Use: Corticosteroid, ophthalmic.

Maxiflor Cream & Ointment. (Allergan Herbert) Diflorasone diacetate 0.05%. Tubes 15 g, 30 g, 60 g. *Rx.*
Use: Corticosteroid, topical.

Maxilube Personal Lubricant. (Mission) Water, silicone oil, glycerin, carbomer 934, triethanolamine, sodium lauryl sulfate, parabens. Jelly 90 g. *otc.*
Use: Vaginal preparation.

Maximum Bayer Aspirin Tablets and Capsules. (Bayer) Aspirin (Acetylsalicylic Acid; ASA) 500 mg. **Tab.:** 10s, 30s, 60s, 100s. **Capl.:** 60s. *otc.*
Use: Salicylate analgesic.

Maximum Blue Label. (Vitaline) Vitamins A 2500 IU, D 16.7 IU, E 66.7 mg, B_1 16.7 mg, B_2 8.3 mg, B_3 31.7 mg, B_5 66.7 mg, B_6 16.7 mg, B_{12} 16.7 mcg, C 200 mg, folic acid 0.13 mg, zinc 5 mg, Ca, Cr, Cu, I, K, Mg, Mn, Mo, Se, Si, V, biotin 50 mcg, SOD, l-lysine/Tab. Bot. 180s. *otc.*
Use: Vitamin/mineral supplement.

Maximum Green Label. (Vitaline) Vitamins A 2500 IU, D 16.7 IU, E 66.7 mg, B_1 16.7 mg, B_2 8.3 mg, B_3 31.7 mg, B_5 66.7 mg, B_6 16.7 mg, B_{12} 16.7 mcg, C 200 mg, folic acid 0.13 mg, zinc 5 mg, Ca, Cr, I, K, Mg, Mn, Mo, Se, Si, V, biotin 50 mcg, SOD, l-lysine/Tab. Bot. 180s. *otc.*
Use: Vitamin/mineral supplement.

Maximum Pain Relief Pamprin. (Chat-

tem) Acetaminophen 250 mg, magnesium salicylate 250 mg, pamabrom 25 mg/Capl. Bot. 16s, 32s. *otc.*
Use: Nonnarcotic analgesic combination.

Maximum Red Label. (Vitaline) Iron 3.3 mg, vitamins A 2500 IU, D 67 IU, E 66.7 mg, B_1 16.7 mg, B_2 8.3 mg, B_3 31.7 mg, B_5 66.7 mg, B_6 16.7 mg, B_{12} 16.7 mcg, C 200 mg, folic acid 0.13 mg, Zn 5 mg, Ca, Cr, Su, I, K, Mg, Mo, Se, Si, V, biotin 50 mcg, choline, inositol, bioflavonoids, l-lysine, PABA/Tab. Bot. 180s. *otc.*
Use: Vitamin/mineral supplement.

Maximum Strength Allergy Drops. (Bausch & Lomb) Naphazoline HCl 0.03%. Soln. Bot. 15 ml. *otc.*
Use: Vasoconstrictor/mydriatic, ophthalmic.

Maximum Strength Anbesol Mouth and Throat. (Whitehall Robins) **Gel:** Benzocaine 20%, alcohol 60%, saccharin. Tube 7 g. **Liq.:** Benzocaine 20%, alcohol 50%, saccharin. Bot. 9 ml. *otc.*
Use: Topical anesthetic.

Maximum Strength Aqua-Ban. (Thompson) Pamabrom 50 mg, lactose/Tab. Bot. 30s. *otc.*
Use: Diuretic.

Maximum Strength Arthriten. (Alva-Amco) Acetaminophen 250 mg, magnesium salicylate 250 mg, caffeine anhydrous 32.5 mg, magnesium carbonate, magnesium oxide, calcium carbonate. Sugar free/Tab. Bot. 40s. *otc.*
Use: Analgesic.

Maximum Strength Benadryl. (Parke-Davis) **Cream:** Diphenhydramine HCl 2%, parabens in a greaseless base. Jar 15 g. **Spray, non-aerosol:** Diphenhydramine HCl 2%, alcohol 85%. Bot. 60 ml. *otc.*
Use: Antihistamine, topical.

Maximum Strength Benadryl Itch Relief. (Warner Lambert) Diphenhydramine HCl. **Cream:** 2%, zinc acetate 1%, parabens, aloe vera. 14.2 g. **Stick:** 2%, zinc acetate 1%. Alcohol 73.5%, aloe vera. 14 ml. *otc.*
Use: Antihistamine.

Maximum Strength Clearasil Clearstick.
See: Clearasil.

Maximum Strength Clearasil Clearstick for Sensitive Skin.
See: Clearasil.

Maximum Strength Comtrex.
See: Comtrex.

Maximum Strength Cortaid. (Pharmacia & Upjohn) Hydrocortisone 1% in parabens, mineral oil, white petrolatum. Oint. Tube 15 g, 30 g. *otc.*
Use: Corticosteroid, topical.

Maximum Strength Cortaid Faststick. (Pharmacia & Upjohn) Hydrocortisone 1%, alcohol 55%, methylparaben. Stick, roll-on. 14 g. *otc.*
Use: Corticosteroid, topical.

Maximum Strength Corticaine. (Whitby) Hydrocortisone acetate 1%, glycerin, menthol, EDTA, parabens. Cream. Tube 30 g. *otc.*
Use: Corticosteroid, topical.

Maximum Strength Dermarest Dricort Creme. (Del) Hydrocortisone (as acetate) 1%, white petrolatum. Cream. Tube 14 g. *otc.*
Use: Corticosteroid, topical.

Maximum Strength Desenex Antifungal. (Novartis) Miconazole nitrate 2%, EDTA. Cream. Tube 14 g. *otc.*
Use: Antifungal, topical.

Maximum Strength Dexatrim. (Thompson) Phenylpropanolamine HCl 75 mg. ER Tab. Pkg. 20s. *otc.*
Use: Nonprescription diet aid.

Maximum Strength Dexatrim with Vitamin C. (Thompson) Phenylpropanolamine HCl, vitamin C 180 mg/Cap. Bot. 20s. *otc.*
Use: Nonprescription diet aid.

Maximum Strength Diet Aid Plus Vitamin C. (Columbia) Phenylpropanolamine HCl 75 mg, vitamin C 180 mg/Cap. Bot. 20s. *otc.*
Use: Nonprescription diet aid.

Maximum Strength Dristan. (Whitehall Robins) Pseudoephedrine HCl 30 mg, acetaminophen 500 mg/Cap. Bot. 24s, 48s, 100s. *otc.*
Use: Decongestant, analgesic.

Maximum Strength Dristan Cold. (Whitehall Robins) Pseudoephedrine HCl 30 mg, brompheniramine maleate 2 mg, acetaminophen 500 mg/Capl. Pkg. 16s, bot. 36s. *otc.*
Use: Decongestant, antihistamine, analgesic.

Maximum Strength Dynafed. (BDI) Acetaminophen 500 mg, pseudoephedrine 30 mg/Tab. Bot. 36s. *otc.*
Use: Analgesic, decongestant.

Maximum Strength Flexall 454. (Chattem) Menthol 16%, aloe vera gel, eucalyptus oil, methylsalicylate, SD alcohol 38-B, thyme oil. Gel. Tube 90 g. *otc.*

Use: Rub/liniment.

Maximum Strength Grapefruit Diet Plan w/Diadex. (Columbia) Phenyl-propanolamine HCl 37.5 mg, grapefruit extract, sugar/Cap. Bot. 20s. *otc.*
Use: Nonprescription diet aid.

Maximum Strength Halls-Plus. (Warner-Lambert) Menthol 10 mg, corn syrup, sucrose. Loz. Pkg. 10s, 20s. *otc.*
Use: Anesthetic.

Maximum Strength Kericort-10. (Bristol-Myers Squibb) Hydrocortisone 1%, parabens, cetyl alcohol, stearyl alcohol. Cream. Tube 56.7 g. *otc.*
Use: Corticosteroid, topical.

Maximum Strength Meted. (GenDerm) Sulfur 5%, salicylic acid 3%. Shampoo. Bot. 118 ml. *otc.*
Use: Antiseborrheic combination.

Maximum Strength Midol Multi-Symptom. (Bayer) Acetaminophen 325 mg, pyrilamine maleate 12.5 mg/Tab. Bot. 30s. *otc.*
Use: Nonnarcotic analgesic combination.

Maximum Strength Midol PMS. (Bayer) Acetaminophen 500 mg, pamabrom 25 mg, pyrilamine maleate 15 mg/Capl. Pkg. 8s, 16s. Bot. 32s. Gelcaps. Pkg. 12s, 24s.
Use: Analgesic combination.

Maximum Strength Nasal Decongestant. (Taro Pharm) Oxymetazoline HCl 0.05%, 0.002% phenylmercuric acetate, benzalkonium chloride. Spray. Bot. 15 ml, 30 ml. *otc.*
Use: Decongestant.

Maximum Strength Neosporin. (Glaxo Wellcome) Polymyxin B sulfate 10,000 units, neomycin 3.5 mg, bacitracin 500 units/g, white petrolatum. Oint. Tube 15 g. *otc.*
Use: Anti-infective, topical.

Maximum Strength No-Aspirin Sinus Medication. (Walgreen) Acetaminophen 500 mg, pseudoephedrine HCl 30 mg/Tab. Bot. 50s. *otc.*
Use: Analgesic, decongestant.

Maximum Strength Nytol. (Block) Diphenhydramine HCl 50 mg/Tab., lactose. Pkg. 8s, 16s. *otc.*
Use: Nonprescription sleep aid.

Maximum Strength Orajel Gel. (Del Pharm) Benzocaine 20%, saccharin. Tube. 9.45 g. *otc.*
Use: Local anesthetic, oral.

Maximum Strength Orajel Liquid. (Del Pharm) Benzocaine 20%, ethyl alcohol 44.2%, phenol, tartrazine, saccharin. Liq. Bot. 13.3 ml. *otc.*
Use: Local anesthetic, oral.

Maximum Strength Ornex. (Menley & James) Pseudoephedrine HCl 30 mg, acetaminophen 500 mg/Cap. Bot. 24s, 48s. *otc.*
Use: Decongestant, analgesic.

Maximum Strength Sine-Aid. (McNeil-CPC) Pseudoephedrine HCl 30 mg, acetaminophen 500 mg/Cap., Tab. or Gelcap. **Cap. & Tab.:** Bot. 50s. **Gelcaps:** Bot. 40s. *otc.*
Use: Decongestant, analgesic.

Maximum Strength Sinutab Nighttime. (Parke-Davis Consumer) Pseudo-ephedrine HCl 10 mg, diphenhydramine HCl 8.33 mg, acetaminophen 167 mg/ 5 ml. Alcohol free. In 120 ml. *otc.*
Use: Decongestant, antihistamine, analgesic.

Maximum Strength Sinutab without Drowsiness. (Warner Lambert) Pseudoephedrine HCl 30 mg, acetaminophen 500 mg/Tab. or Capl. Bot. 24s, 48s (tab. only). *otc.*
Use: Decongestant, analgesic.

Maximum Strength Sleepinal. (Thompson) **Cap.:** Diphenhydramine HCl 50 mg, lactose. Pkg. 16s. **Soft gel:** diphenhydramine HCl 50 mg, sorbitol. Pkg. 16s. *otc.*
Use: Nonprescription sleep aid.

Maximum Strength Sudafed Severe Cold Formula. (Glaxo Wellcome) Dextromethorphan HBr 15 mg, pseudoephedrine HCl 30 mg, acetaminophen 500 mg/Tab. 10s. *otc.*
Use: Antitussive, decongestant, analgesic.

Maximum Strength Sudafed Sinus. (Warner Lambert) Pseudoephedrine HCl 30 mg, acetaminophen 500 mg/ Tab. or Capl. Bot. 24s, 48s. *otc.*
Use: Decongestant, analgesic.

Maximum Strength Thera-Flu Non-Drowsy.
See: Thera-Flu.

Maximum Strength Tylenol Allergy Sinus. (McNeil-CPC) Pseudoephedrine HCl 30 mg, chlorpheniramine maleate 2 mg, acetaminophen 500 mg/Tab. Bot. 24s, 60s. *otc.*
Use: Decongestant, antihistamine, analgesic.

Maximum Strength Tylenol Cough Liquid. (McNeil-CPC) Dextromethorphan HBr 7.5 mg, acetaminophen 250 mg, alcohol 10%. Bot. 120 ml. *otc.*
Use: Antitussive, analgesic.

Maximum Strength Tylenol Cough w/ Decongestant Liquid. (McNeil-CPC) Pseudoephedrine HCl 15 mg, dextromethorphan HBr 7.5 mg, acetaminophen 250 mg, alcohol 10%. Bot. 120 ml. *otc.*
Use: Decongestant, antitussive, analgesic.

Maximum Strength Tylenol Flu Gelcaps. (McNeil-CPC) Acetaminophen 500 mg, pseudoephedrine HCl 30 mg, dextromethorphan HBR 15 mg. Tab. Pkg. 10s. *otc.*
Use: Antitussive, decongestant, analgesic.

Maximum Strength Tylenol Flu Night-Time Gelcaps. (McNeil-CPC) Pseudoephedrine HCl 30 mg, chlorpheniramine maleate 2 mg, acetaminophen 500 mg/Cap. Pkg. 12s, 20s. *otc.*
Use: Decongestant, antihistamine, analgesic.

Maximum Strength Tylenol Flu Night-Time Powder. (McNeil-CPC) Pseudoephedrine HCl 60 mg, diphenhydramine HCl 50 mg, acetaminophen 1000 mg. Powd. Pkt. 6s. *otc.*
Use: Decongestant, antihistamine, analgesic.

Maximum Strength Tylenol Select Allergy Sinus. (McNeil-CPC) Pseudoephedrine HCl 30 mg, diphenhydramine HCl 25 mg, acetaminophen 500 mg. Cap. Bot. 24s. *otc.*
Use: Antihistamine, decongestant, analgesic.

Maximum Strength Tylenol Sinus. (McNeil-CPC) Pseudoephedrine HCl 30 mg, acetaminophen 500 mg/Tab., Capl. or Gelcap. **Tab. and Capl.:** Bot. 24s, 50s. **Gelcap:** Bot. 24s, 60s. *otc.*
Use: Decongestant, analgesic.

Maximum Strength Unisom Sleepgels. (Pfizer) Diphendhydramine HCl 50 mg, sorbitol. Cap. Pkg. 8s. *otc.*
Use: Nonprescription sleep aid.

Maximum Strength Wart Remover. (Stiefel) Salicylic acid 17%, alcohol 29%, castor oil, flexible collodion. Liq. 13.3 ml. *otc.*
Use: Keratolytic.

Maxipime. (BM Squibb) Cefepime HCl 500 mg/15 ml, 1 g/15 ml or 2 g/20 ml. Pow. for Inj. Vial, piggyback bottle. *Rx.*
Use: Cephalosporin.

maxiton.
See: Amphetamine (Various Mfr.).

Maxitrol Ointment. (Alcon) Dexamethasone 0.1%, neomycin 0.35%, polymyxin B sulfate 10,000 units/g. Tube 3.5 g. *Rx.*

Use: Anti-infective, ophthalmic.

Maxitrol Ophthalmic Suspension. (Alcon) Dexamethasone 0.1%, neomycin (as sulfate) 0.35%, polymyxin B sulfate 10,000 units/ml. Bot. 5 ml dropper tainer. *Rx.*
Use: Anti-infective, ophthalmic.

Maxivate. (Westwood Squibb) Betamethasone dipropionate 0.05%. Cream, Oint. Tube 15 g, 45 g. *Rx.*
Use: Corticosteroid, topical.

Maxi-Vite. (Goldline) Vitamins A 10,000 IU, D 400 IU, E 15 mg, B_1 10 mg, B_2 10 mg, B_3 100 mg, B_5 20 mg, B_6 5 mg, B_{12} 5 mcg, C 200 mg, Ca 53.5 mg, iron 1.5 mg, folic acid 0.4 mg, biotin 1 mcg, I, P, Cu, Mg, Mn, Zn 1.5 mg, PABA, rutin, glutamic acid, inositol, choline bitartrate, bioflavonoids, L-lysine, betaine, lecithin/Tab. Bot. 60s. *otc.*
Use: Vitamin/mineral supplement.

Maxolon Tablets. (SK-Beecham) Metoclopramide HCl 10 mg/Tab. Bot. 100s. *Rx.*
Use: Antiemetic, GI stimulant.

Maxovite. (Tyson) Vitamins A 2083 IU, D 16.7 IU, E 16.7 mg, B_1 5 mg, B_2 4.2 mg, B_3 4.2 mg, B_5 4.2 mg, B_6 54.2 mg, B_{12} 10.8 mcg, C 250 mg, folic acid 0.33 mg, Zn 5 mg, Ca, Cr, Cu, Fe, I, K, Mg, Mn, Se, biotin 11.7 mcg/Tab. Bot. 120s, 240s. *otc.*
Use: Vitamin/mineral supplement.

Maxzide. (Lederle) Hydrochlorothiazide 50 mg, triamterene 75 mg/Tab. Bot. 100s, 500s, UD 10 × 10s. *Rx.*
Use: Diuretic, antihypertensive.

Maxzide-25 mg. (Lederle) Triamterene 37.5 mg, hydrochlorothiazide 25 mg/Tab. Bot. 100s, UD 100s. *Rx.*
Use: Diuretic combination.

Mayotic. (Mayrand) Hydrocortisone 1%, neomycin sulfate 5 mg, polymyxin B sulfate 10,000 units/ml, thimerosal 0.01%. Susp. Bot. 10 ml w/dropper. *Rx.*
Use: Otic preparation.

•**maytansine.** (MAY-tan-SEEN) USAN.
Use: Antineoplastic.

May-Vita Elixir. (Mayrand) B_3 4.4 mg, B_5 1.1 mg, B_6 0.44 mg, B_{12} 1.33 mcg, FA 0.1 mg, Fe 4 mg, Mn, Zn 1.7 mg, alcohol 13%/Liq. Bot. 473 ml. *Rx.*
Use: Vitamin/mineral supplement.

Mazanor. (Wyeth-Ayerst) Mazindol 1 mg/Tab. Bot. 30s. *c-iv.*
Use: Anorexiant.

•**mazapertine succinate.** (mazz-ah-PURR-teen) USAN.
Use: Antipsychotic.

Mazicon. (Roche) Flumazenil 0.1 mg/ml. Inj. Vial 5 ml, 10 ml. *Rx.*
Use: Antidote.

•**mazindol,** (MAZE-in-dole) U.S.P. 23.
Use: Anorexic, appetite suppressant, Duchenne muscular dystrophy [Orphan drug]
See: Mazanor, Tab. (Wyeth-Ayerst). Sanorex, Tab. (Sandoz).

M-Caps. (Mill-Mark) Methionine 200 mg/ Cap. Bot. 50s, 1000s. *Rx.*
Use: Diaper rash product.

MCT Oil. (Bristol-Myers) Triglycerides of medium chain fatty acids. Lipid fraction of coconut oil; fatty acid shorter than C-8 < 6%, C_8(octanoic) 67%, C_{10}(decanoic) 23%, longer than C_{10} 4%. Bot. qt. *otc.*
Use: Enteral nutritional supplement.

MD-Gastroview. (Mallinckrodt) Diatrizoate meglumine 66%, diatrizoate sodium 10%. Soln. 120 ml, 240 ml.
Use: Radiopaque agent.

MD-60. (Mallinckrodt) Diatrizoate meglumine 52%, diatrizoate sodium 8% (29.2% iodine). Inj. Vial 30 ml, 50 ml.
Use: Radiopaque agent.

MD-76. (Mallinckrodt) Diatrizoate meglumine 66%, diatrizoate sodium 10% (37% iodine). Inj. Vial 50 ml, 100 ml, 150 ml, 200 ml.
Use: Radiopaque agent.

MDP-Squibb. (Squibb) Technetium Tc 99 medronate. Reaction vial pkg. 10s.
Use: Radiopaque agent.

meadinin. Mixture of Amoidin & Amidin alk. of Ammi Majus Linn.

measles prophylactic serum.
See: Immune Globulin (Intramuscular).

measles, mumps and rubella virus vaccine live, (MEE-zuhls, mumps and ru-BELL-uh vaccine)
Use: Immunizing agent (active).
See: M-M-R II, Inj. (Merck).

measles and rubella virus vaccine live.
See: M-R-Vax II, Inj. (Merck).

•**measles virus vaccine, live,** U.S.P. 23. Modified live-virus measles vaccine.
Use: Active immunizing agent.
See: Attenuvax, Inj. (Merck).
W/Mumps virus vaccine, rubella virus vaccine.
See: M-M-R II (Merck).
W/Rubella virus vaccine.
See: M-M-R II (Merck).

measles virus vaccine, live attenuated. Moraten line derived from Enders' attenuated Edmonston strain grown in cell cultures of chick embryos.

See: Attenuvax, Inj. (Merck).
W/Mumps virus vaccine, rubella virus vaccine.
See: M-M-R., Vial (Merck).
W/Rubella virus vaccine.
See: M-R-Vax, Inj. (Merck).

Mebaral. (Sanofi Winthrop) Mephobarbital. Tab. **0.5 gr, 0.75 gr or 1.5 gr:** Bot. 250s. *c-ɪv.*
Use: Sedative, anticonvulsant.

•**mebendazole,** (meh-BEND-uh-zole) U.S.P. 23.
Use: Anthelmintic.
See: Vermox, Tab. (Janssen).

mebendazole. (Copley) 100 mg/Chew. Tab. Pkg. 12s, 36s.
Use: Anthelmintic.

•**mebeverine hydrochloride.** (MEH-BEH-ver-een) USAN.
Use: Spasmolytic agent, smooth muscle relaxant.

•**mebrofenin,** (MEH-broe-FEN-in) U.S.P. 23.
Use: Diagnostic aid (hepatobiliary function determination).

•**mebutamate.** (MEH-byoo-TAM-at) USAN.
Use: Antihypertensive.

•**mecamylamine hydrochloride,** U.S.P. 23.
Use: Antihypertensive.
See: Inversine, Tab. (Merck).

•**mecetronium ethylsulfate.** (MEH-seh-TROE-nee-uhm ETH-ill-SULL-fate) USAN.
Use: Antiseptic.

•**mechlorethamine hydrochloride,** U.S.P. 23.
Use: Antineoplastic.
See: Mustargen, Vial (Merck).

mecholin hydrochloride.
See: Methacholine Cl, U.S.P. 23.

Mecholyl Ointment. (Gordon) Methacholine Cl 0.25%, methyl salicylate 10% in ointment base. Jar 4 oz, 1 lb, 5 lb. *otc.*
Use: Analgesic, topical.

Meclan. (Ortho Derm) Meclocycline sulfosalicylate 1%. Cream Tube 20 g, 45 g. *Rx.*
Use: Antiacne.

meclastine. Clemastine.

•**meclizine,** (MEK-lih-zeen) U.S.P. 23.
Use: Antinauseant, antiemetic.
See: Antivert, Chew. Tab. (Roerig). Antrizine (Major). Bonine, Tab. (Roerig). Dizmiss (JMI Canton) Dramamine II, Tab. (Pharmacia & Upjohn).

Meclizine HCl (Various Mfr.).
Meni-D (Seatrace).
Ru-Vert-M (Reid-Rowell).
Vergon, Cap. (Marnel).
Meclizine HCl. (Various) **Tab.: 12.5 mg:**
Bot. 30s, 60s, 100s, 500s, 1000s & UD
100s. **25 mg:** In 12s, 20s, 30s, 60s,
100s, 500s, 1000s & UD 32s & 100s. **50
mg:** 100s. **Chew Tab.: 25 mg:** Bot.
20s, 30s, 60s, 100s, 1000s & UD 100s.
otc, Rx.
Use: Antinauseant.
•**meclocycline.** (meh-kloe-SIGH-kleen)
USAN.
Use: Antibacterial.
•**meclocycline sulfosalicylate,** (meh-
kloe-SIGH-kleen SULL-foe-sah-LIH-sih-
late) U.S.P. 23.
Use: Antibacterial.
See: Meclan, Cream (Ortho).
•**meclofenamate sodium,** (mek-loe-FEN-
uh-mate) U.S.P. 23.
Use: Anti-inflammatory.
meclofenamate sodium. (Mylan) Meclofenamate sodium 50 mg or 100 mg/
Cap. Bot. 100s, 500s.
Use: Anti-inflammatory.
•**meclofenamic acid.** (MEH-kloe-fen-AM-
ik Acid) USAN.
Use: Anti-inflammatory.
•**mecloqualone.** (MEH-kloe-KWAH-lone)
USAN.
Use: Sedative, hypnotic.
•**meclorisone dibutyrate.** (MEH-KLAHR-
ih-sone die-BYOO-tih-rate) USAN.
Use: Anti-inflammatory (topical.)
•**mecobalamin.** (MEH-koe-BAHL-ah-min)
USAN.
Use: Vitamin (hematopoietic).
mecodrin.
See: Amphetamine (Various Mfr.).
•**mecrylate.** (MEH-krih-late) USAN.
Use: Surgical aid (tissue adhesive).
mecysteine. Methyl Cysteine.
Meda Cap. (Circle) Acetaminophen 500
mg/Cap. Bot. 25s, 60s, 100s. *otc.*
Use: Analgesic.
Medacote. (Dal-Med) Pyrilamine maleate 1%, dimethyl polysiloxane, zinc oxide, menthol, camphor in a greaseless
base. Lot. Bot. 120 ml. *otc.*
Use: Antihistamine, topical.
Medadyne. (Dal-Med) **Liq.:** Methylbenzethonium chloride, benzocaine,
tannic acid, camphor, chlorothymol,
menthol, benzyl alcohol, alcohol 61%.
Bot. 15 ml, 30 ml. **Throat Spray:** Lidocaine, cetyl dimethyl ammonium chloride, ethyl alcohol. Bot. 30 ml. *otc.*

Use: Mouth and throat product.
Meda-Hist Expectorant. (Medwick) Bot.
4 oz, pt, gal.
Use: Decongestant, antitussive.
Medalox Gel. (Med. Chem.) Magnesium
aluminum hydroxide gel. Bot. 12 oz, pt,
gal. *otc.*
Use: Antacid.
Medamint. (Dal-Med) Benzocaine 10 mg/
Loz. Pkg. 12s, 24s. *otc.*
Use: Mouth and throat product.
Meda Cap. (Circle) Acetaminophen 500
mg/Cap. Bot. 100s. *otc.*
Use: Analgesic.
Meda Tab. (Circle) Acetaminophen 325
mg/Tab. Bot. 100s. *otc.*
Use: Analgesic.
Medatussin Pediatric. (Dal-Med)
Dextromethorphan HBr 5 mg, guai-
fenesin 50 mg, potassium citrate, citric
acid, sorbitol, saccharin. Syr. Bot. 120
ml. *otc.*
Use: Antitussive, expectorant.
Medatussin Plus Cough. (Dal-Med)
Phenylpropanolamine HCl 25 mg,
chlorpheniramine maleate 2 mg, phenyltoloxamine citrate 25 mg, dextromethorphan HBr 20 mg, guaifenesin
100 mg. Bot. pt. gal. *otc.*
Use: Decongestant, antihistamine, antitussive, expectorant.
•**medazepam hydrochloride.** (med-AZE-
eh-pam) USAN. Under study.
Use: Tranquilizer (minor).
Medent. (Stewart-Jackson) Pseudoephedrine HCl 120 mg, guaifenesin 500
mg/Tab. Bot. 100s.
Use: Decongestant, expectorant.
Medicaine Cream. (Walgreen) Benzocaine 3%, resorcinol 2%. Tube 1.25
oz. *otc.*
Use: Antipruritic.
Medicated Acne Cleanser. (C & M) Sulfur 4%, resorcinol 2%, SD alcohol 40
11.65%, methylparaben. Lot. Bot. 120
ml. *otc.*
Use: Antiacne.
Medicated Healer. (Walgreen) Strong
ammonia soln. 10%, camphor 2.6%.
Bot. 6 oz. *otc.*
Use: Emollient.
Medicated Powder. (Johnson &
Johnson) Zinc oxide, talc, fragrance,
menthol. Plastic container 3 oz, 6 oz, 11
oz. *otc.*
Use: Antipruritic.
Medicone Derma. (Medicone) Benzo-
caine 2%, zinc oxide 13.73%, 8-hy-
droxyquinoline sulfate 1.05%, ichtham-

mol 1%, menthol 0.48%, petrolatum-lanolin base 79.87%. Oint. Tube 42.5 g. *otc.*
Use: Local anesthetic, topical.

Medicone Dressing. (Medicone) Cod liver oil 125 mg, zinc oxide 125 mg, 8-hydroxyquinoline-sulfate 0.5 mg, benzocaine 5 mg, menthol 1.8 mg/g w/ petrolatum, lanolin, talcum, paraffin, perfume. Tube 1 oz, 3 oz, Jar lb. *otc.*
Use: Local anesthetic, topical.

Medicone Ointment. (EE Dickinson) Benzocaine 20%. Oint. 30 g. *otc.*
Use: Anorectal preparation.

Medicone Rectal. (Medicone) Benzocaine 130 mg, hydroxyquinoline sulfate 16 mg, zinc oxide 195 mg, menthol 9 mg, balsam Peru 65 mg. In a vegetable and petroleum oil base. Supp. 12s, 24s. *otc.*
Use: Anorectal preparation.

Medicone-HC Rectal. (Medicone) Hydrocortisone acetate 10 mg, benzocaine 2 gr, oxyquinoline sulfate 0.25 gr, zinc oxide 3 gr, menthol 1/2 gr, balsam Peru 1 gr, in a cocoa butter base/Supp. Box 12s. *Rx.*
Use: Anorectal preparation.

Medicone Suppositories. (EE Dickinson) Phenylephrine HCl 0.25%, hard fat 88.7%, parabens. Pkg. 12s, 24s. *otc.*
Use: Anorectal preparation.

Medigesic Plus. (U.S. Pharm Corp.) Acetaminophen 325 mg, caffeine 40 mg, butalbital 50 mg/Cap. Bot. 100s. *Rx.*
Use: Analgesic, sedative, hypnotic.

Medihaler-Duo.
See: Duo-Medihaler. (3M)

Medihaler-Iso. (3M) Isoproterenol sulfate 2 mg/ml. Soln. Oral adapter w/ 15 ml. Oral adapter w/22.5 ml vial. Refill vial 15 ml and 22.5 ml. *Rx.*
Use: Antiasthmatic.

Medi-Ject UD Vials. (Century) Tamperproof rubber stoppered vial containing 1 ml sterile soln. Single dose use.
See: Ulti-ject disposable syringe prods.
Atropine sulfate 0.4 mg/ml.
Atropine sulfate 1.2 mg/ml.
Scopolamine HBr 400 mcg/ml.

Medilax. (Mission) Phenolphthalein 120 mg, aspartame, phenylalanine 1.5 mg/ Chew. Tab. Bot. 24s. *otc.*
Use: Laxative.

Medipain 5. (Medi-Plex) Hydrocodone bitartrate 5 mg, acetaminophen 500 mg. Cap. Bot. 100s. *c-III.*
Use: Narcotic analgesic combination.

Medipak. (Armenpharm) First-aid kit.

Medi-Phite. (Med Chem.) Vitamins B_1 and B_{12}. Syr. Bot. 4 oz, pt, gal. *otc.*
Use: Vitamin supplement.

Mediplast. (Beiersdorf) Salicylic acid plaster 40%. Box 25s. *otc.*
Use: Keratolytic.

Mediplex Tabules. (U.S. Pharm) Vitamins E 60 IU, B_1 25 mg, B_2 10 mg, B_3 100 mg, B_5 25 mg, B_6 10 mg, B_{12} 25 mcg, C 300 mg, Zn 4 mg, Cu, Mg, Mn/ Tab. Bot. 100s. *otc.*
Use: Vitamin/mineral supplement.

Mediquell. (Parke-Davis Prods) Dextromethorphan HBr 15 mg/Chewy square. Pkg. 12s, 24s. *otc.*
Use: Antitussive.

Medi-Quik Aerosol. (Mentholatum) Lidocaine 2.5%, benzalkonium Cl 0.1%, ethanol 38%. Aerosol 3 oz. *otc.*
Use: Antiseptic, local anesthetic, topical.

Medi-Quick Antibiotic Ointment. (Mentholatum) Bacitracin neomycin, polymyxin in ointment base. Tube 0.5 oz. *otc.*
Use: Anti-infective, topical.

Meditussin-X Liquid. (Roberts) Codeine phosphate 50 mg, ammonium Cl 520 mg, potassium guaiacolsulfonate 520 mg, pyrilamine maleate 50 mg, phenylpropanolamine HCl 50 mg, dl-desoxyephedrine HCl 2 mg, tartar emetic 5 mg, phenyltoloxamine dihydrogen citrate 30 mg/30 ml. Bot. pt, gal. *c-v.*
Use: Antitussive, expectorant, antihistamine.

•**medorinone.** (MEH-doe-RIH-nohn) USAN.
Use: Cardiotonic.

Medotar. (Medco Lab) Coal tar 1%, polysorbate 80 0.5%, octoxynol 5, zinc oxide, starch, white petrolatum. Jar lb. *otc.*
Use: Antipsoriatic, antipruritic.

Medotopes. (Squibb) Radiopharmaceuticals.
See: A-C-D Solution Modified (Squibb).
Acid Citrate Dextrose Anticoagulant Solution Modified (Squibb).
Aggregated Albumin (Squibb).
Albumotope (Squibb).
Angiotensin Immutope Kit (Squibb).
Cobalt-Labeled Vitamin B_{12} (Squibb).
Cobalt Standards for Vitamin B_{12} (Squibb).
Cobatope (Squibb).
Digoxin (^{125}I) Immutope Kit (Squibb).
Gastrin (^{125}I) Immutope Kit (Squibb).
Gold-198 (Squibb).

Hipputope (Squibb).

Human Serum Albumin (Squibb).

Iodine 131: Capsules Diagnostic-Capsules Therapeutic-Solution Therapeutic Oral (Squibb).

Iodinated Human Serum Albumin (Squibb).

Iodo-hippuric Acid (Squibb).

Macroaggregated Albumin (Squibb).

Macrotec (Squibb).

Minitec (Squibb).

Phosphorus-32: Solution Oral, Therapeutic-Sodium Phosphate Solution U.S.P. for oral or IV use therapeutic or diagnostic (Squibb).

Red Cell Tagging Solution (Squibb).

Renotec (Squibb).

Rose Bengal (Squibb).

Rubratope-57: Diagnostic Capsules-Diagnostic Kit (Squibb).

Rubratope-60: Diagnostic Capsules-Diagnostic Kit (Squibb).

Selenomethionine (Squibb).

Sethotope (Squibb).

Technetium 99m (Squibb).

Technetium 99m-Iron-Ascorbate (DTPA) (Squibb).

Technetium 99m Sulfur Colloid Kit (Squibb).

Tesuloid (Squibb).

Thyrostat-FTI (Squibb).

Thyrostat-3 (Squibb).

Thyrostat-4 FTI (Squibb).

Medralone 40. (Keene) Methylprednisolone acetate 40 mg/ml. Vial 5 ml. *Rx.*
Use: Corticosteroid.

Medralone 80. (Keene) Methylprednisolone acetate 80 mg/ml. Vial 5 ml. *Rx.*
Use: Corticosteroid.

•**medrogestone.** (MEH-droe-JEST-ohn) USAN. *Formerly Metrogestone.*
Use: Progestin.
See: Colprone (Wyeth-Ayerst).

Medrol. (Pharmacia & Upjohn) Methylprednisolone. **Tab.:** 2 mg. Bot. 100s; 4 mg Bot. 30s, 100s, 500s, UD 100s; 8 mg Bot. 25s; 16 mg Bot. 50s; 24 mg Bot. 25s; 32 mg Bot. 25s. **Dosepak:** 4 mg Pkg. 21s. **Alternate Daypak:** 16 mg Pkg. 14s. *Rx.*
Use: Corticosteroid.

•**medronate disodium.** (MEH-droe-nate die-SO-dee-uhm) USAN. *Formerly Disodium Methylene Diphosphonate; MDP.*
Use: Pharmaceutic aid.

•**medronic acid.** (meh-DRAH-nik Acid) USAN.
Use: Pharmaceutic aid.

Medrosphol Hg-197.

See: Merprane.

•**medroxalol.** (meh-DROX-ah-LAHL) USAN.
Use: Antihypertensive.

•**medroxalol hydrochloride.** (meh-DROX-ah-LAHL) USAN.
Use: Antihypertensive.

medroxyprogesterone acetate. (meh-DROX-ee-pro-JESS-tuh-rone) (Lederle) Medroxyprogesterone acetate 10 mg/Tab. Bot. 50s, 250s. *Rx.*
Use: Progestin.

•**medroxyprogesterone acetate,** (meh-DROX-ee-pro-JESS-tuh-rone) U.S.P. 23.
Use: Progestin.
See: Amen, Tab. (Carnrick).
  Curretab, Tab. (Solvay).
  Cycrin, Tab. (ESI Pharma).
  depCorlutin (Forest).
  Depo-Provera, Vial (Pharmacia & Upjohn).
  P-Medrate-P.A., Inj. (Solvay).
  Provera, Tab. (Pharmacia & Upjohn).

medroxyprogesterone acetate. (meh-DROX-ee-pro-JESS-tuh-rone) (CMC) 50 mg, 100 mg/ml. Vial 5 ml.
Use: Progestin.

medroxyprogesterone acetate. (Various Mfr.) Medroxyprogesterone acetate 10 mg/Tab. Bot. 50s, 100s and 250s. *Rx.*
Use: Progestin.

MED-Rx. (Iomed) Pseudoephedrine HCl 60 mg, guaifenesin 600 mg/CR Tab. Box 28s. Guaifenesin 600 mg/CR Tab. Box 28s. *Rx.*
Use: Decongestant, expectorant.

MED-Rx DM. (Iomed) Pseudoephedrine 60 mg, guaifenesin 600 mg/CR Tab. Bot. 28s. Dextromethorphan hydrobromide 30 mg, guaifenesin 600 mg/CR Tab. Bot. 28s. *Rx.*
Use: Antitussive, expectorant.

•**medrysone.** (MEH-drih-sone) USAN. U.S.P. XXII.
Use: Glucocorticoid.
See: HMS Liquifilm, Ophth. Soln. (Allergan).

•**mefenamic acid.** (MEH-fen-AM-ik) USAN. U.S.P. 23.
Use: Anti-inflammatory, analgesic.
See: Ponstel, Kapseal (Parke-Davis).

•**mefenidil.** (meh-FEN-ih-dill) USAN.
Use: Cerebral vasodilator.

•**mefenidil fumarate.** (meh-FEN-ih-dill) USAN.
Use: Cerebral vasodilator.

•**mefenorex hydrochloride.** (meh-FEN-

oh-rex) USAN. Under study.
Use: Anorexic.

• **mefexamide.** (meh-FEX-am-IDE) USAN.
Use: Stimulant (central).

• **mefloquine.** (MEH-flow-kwin) USAN.
Use: Antimalarial.

• **mefloquine hydrochloride.** (MEH-flow-kwin) USAN.
Use: Antimalarial. [Orphan drug]
See: Lariam (Roche).

Mefoxin. (Merck) Sterile cefoxitin sodium 1 g, 2 g or 10 g/Vial. **1 g, 2 g:** Vial, ADD-Vantage Vial, Infusion bottle. **10 g:** Bulk bot. *Rx.*
Use: Anti-infective, cephalosporin.

Mefoxin in 5% Dextrose. (Merck) Cefoxitin sodium 1 g or 2 g in Dextrose in Water 5%. Inj. Containers 50 ml. *Rx.*
Use: Anti-infective, cephalosporin.

• **mefruside.** (MEFF-ruh-side) USAN. (FBA)
Use: Diuretic.

Mega-B. (Arco) Vitamins B_1 100 mg, B_2 100 mg, B_3 100 mg, B_5 100 mg, B_6 100 mg, B_{12} 100 mcg, folic acid 100 mcg, d-biotin 100 mcg, PABA 100 mg/Tab. Bot. 100s. *otc.*
Use: Vitamin supplement.

Megace. (Bristol-Myers) Megestrol acetate 20 mg or 40 mg/Tab. **20 mg/Tab.:** Bot. 100s; **40 mg/Tab.:** Bot. 100s, 250s, 500s. Megestrol acetate 40 mg/ml, alcohol ≤ 0.06%, sucrose. Susp. Bot. 236.6 ml. *Rx.*
Use: Antineoplastic, progestin.

• **megalomicin potassium phosphate.** (meh-GAL-OH-my-sin) USAN.
Use: Antibacterial.

Megaton. (Hyrex) Vitamins B_3 4.4 mg, B_5 1.1 mg, B_6 0.44 mg, B_{12} 1.33 mcg, FA 0.1 mg, Fe 4 mg, Mn, Zn 1.7 mg, alcohol 13%/Liq. Bot. 473 ml. *Rx.*
Use: Vitamin/mineral supplement.

Mega VM-80. (NTBY) Vitamins A 10,000 IU, D 1000 IU, E 100 mg, B_1 80 mg, B_2 80 mg, B_3 80 mg, B_5 80 mg, B_6 80 mg, B_{12} 80 mcg, C 250 mg, iron 1.2 mg, folic acid 0.4 mg, calcium 4.5 mg, zinc 3.58 mg, choline, inositol, biotin 80 mcg, PABA, bioflavonoids, betaine, hesperidin, Cu, I, K, Mg, Mn. Tab. Bot. 60s, 100s. *otc.*
Use: Vitamins/mineral supplement.

• **megestrol acetate,** (meh-JESS-trole) U.S.P. 23.
Use: Antineoplastic; palliative treatment of advanced carcinoma of the breast or endometrium. AIDS-related weight loss. [Orphan drug]

See: Megace (Bristol-Myers).
Pallace, Tab. (Bristol).

• **meglumine,** U.S.P. 23.
Use: Diagnostic (radiopaque medium).

meglumine, diatrizoate inj.
Use: Diagnostic aid; radiopaque medium.
See: Cardiografin, Vial (Squibb).
Cystografin, Vial (Squibb).
Gastrografin, Soln. (Squibb).
Hypaque-76, Inj. (Sanofi Winthrop).
Hypaque-M 75%, Inj. (Sanofi Winthrop).
Hypaque-M 90%, Inj. (Sanofi Winthrop).
Hypaque Meglumine, Vial (Sanofi Winthrop).
Reno-M-30, -60, Vial (Squibb).
Reno-M-Dip, Vial (Squibb).
W/Meglumine iodipamide.
See: Sinografin, Soln. (Squibb).
W/Sodium diatrizoate.
See: Gastrografin, Soln. (Squibb).
Renografin-60, Inj. (Squibb).
Renografin-76, Inj. (Squibb).
Renovist II, Inj. (Squibb).

meglumine, iodipamide inj.
Use: Diagnostic aid; radiopaque medium.
See: Cholografin, Vial (Squibb).
W/Meglumine diatrizoate.
See: Sinografin, Soln. (Squibb).

meglumine, iothalamate inj. U.S.P. 23.
Use: Diagnostic aid; radiopaque medium.

• **meglutol.** (MEH-glue-tahl) USAN.
Use: Antihyperlipoproteinemic.

mejeptil.
See: Thioperazine (SK-Beecham).

• **melafocon a.** (MEH-lah-FOE-kahn A) USAN.
Use: Contact lens material (hydrophobic).

Melanex. (Neutrogena) Hydroquinone 3% in solution containing alcohol 47.3%. Bot. 1 oz w/Appliderm applicator and pinpoint rod applicator. *Rx.*
Use: Skin bleaching agent.

melanoma vaccine.
Use: Stage III-IV melanoma. [Orphan drug]

melanoma cell vaccine.
Use: Invasive melanoma. [Orphan drug]

melarsoprol. (Mel B)
Use: Anti-infective.
See: Arsobol.

melatonin. *otc, Rx.*
Use: Treatment of circadian rhythm sleep disorders in blind patients. [Orphan drug]

Mel B.
See: Melarsoprol.
• **melengestrol acetate.** USAN.
Use: Antineoplastic, progestin.
Melfiat-105 Unicelles. (Solvay) Phendimetrazine tartrate 105 mg/SR Cap.
Bot. 100s. c-iv.
Use: Anorexiant.
Melhoral Child Tablet. (Sanofi Winthrop)
Acetylsalicylic acid. otc.
Use: Salicylate analgesic.
melitoxin.
See: Dicumarol (Various Mfr.).
• **melitracen hydrochloride.** (meh-lih-TRAY-sen) USAN.
Use: Antidepressant.
• **melizame.** (MEH-lih-zame) USAN.
Use: Sweetener.
Mellaril Concentrate. (Sandoz) Thioridazine HCl 30 mg/ml, alcohol 3%. Soln.
Bot. 4 oz. Concentrate 100 mg/ml. Pk. 4
oz. Rx.
Use: Antipsychotic.
Mellaril S. (Sandoz) Thioridazine 25 mg/
5 ml or 100 mg/5 ml. Susp. Bot. pt. Rx.
Use: Antipsychotic.
Mellaril Tablets. (Sandoz) Thioridazine
HCl 10 mg, 15 mg, 25 mg, 50 mg, 100
mg, 150 mg or 200 mg/Tab. Bot. 100s,
1000s. SandoPak pkg. 100s (except
150 mg). Rx.
Use: Antipsychotic.
mellose. Methylcellulose.
Melonex. Metahexamide.
Use: Oral antidiabetic.
Melpaque HP. (Stratus) Hydroquinone
4% in a sunblocking base of talc,
EDTA, sodium metabisulfite. Cream.
Tinted. Tube 14.2 g, 28.4 g. Rx.
Use: Skin bleaching agent.
• **melphalan,** (MELL-fuh-lan) U.S.P. 23.
Tab., U.S.P. 23.
Use: Antineoplastic. [Orphan drug]
See: Alkeran, Tab. (Glaxo Wellcome).
Alkeran, Pow. for Inj. (Glaxo Wellcome).
Melquin HP. (Stratus) Hydroquinone 4%,
mineral oil, propylparaben, sodium
metabisulfite. Vanishing base. Cream.
Tube 14.2 g, 28.4 g. Rx.
Use: Skin bleaching agent.
• **memotine hydrochloride.** (MEH-moe-teen) USAN.
Use: Antiviral.
• **menabitan hydrochloride.** (meh-NAB-ih-tan) USAN.
Use: Analgesic.
• **menadiol sodium diphosphate,** U.S.P.
23.

Use: Vitamin (prothrombogenic).
• **menadione,** U.S.P. 23.
Use: Orally & IM, Vitamin K therapy, vitamin (prothrombogenic).
W/Ascorbic acid.
See: Rependo, Cap. (Scruggs).
W/Ascorbic acid, hesperidin.
See: Hescor-K, Tab. (Madland).
W/Bioflavonoid citrus compound, ascorbic acid.
See: C.V.P. W/Vitamin K, Syr., Tab.
(Rhone-Poulenc Rorer).
menadione diphosphate sodium.
See: menadiol sodium diphosphate.
Menadol. (Rugby) Ibuprofen 200 mg/
Tab. Bot. 50s, 100s. otc.
Use: Nonsteroidal anti-inflammatory
drug, analgesic.
menaphthene or menaphthone.
See: Menadione (Various Mfr.).
menaquinone.
See: Menadione (Various Mfr.).
Menest. (SK-Beecham) Esterified estrogens, conjugated estrogens (equine)
0.3 mg, 0.625 mg or 1.25 mg/Tab.:
Bot. 100s. **2.5 mg/Tab.:** Bot. 50s. Rx.
Use: Estrogen combination.
Meni-D. (Seatrace) Meclizine 25 mg/Cap.
Bot. 100s. Rx.
Use: Antiemetic/antivertigo.
meningococcal polysaccharide vaccine group A, C, Y, W-135. (Pasteur-Merieux-Connaught) Serogroup A, C, Y
and W-135 capsular polysaccharides
50 mcg/0.5 ml. Pow. for Inj.
Use: Vaccine.
See: Menomune A/C/Y/W-135 (Pasteur-Merieux-Connaught).
• **meningococcal polysaccharide vaccine group A,** U.S.P. 23.
Use: Active immunizing agent.
• **meningococcal polysaccharide vaccine group C,** U.S.P. 23.
Use: Active immunizing agent.
• **menoctone.** USAN. Under study.
Use: Antimalarial.
• **menogaril.** (MEN-oh-gar-ILL) USAN.
Use: Antineoplastic.
Menoject L.A. (Mayrand) Testosterone
cypionate, estradiol cypionate. Vial 10
ml. Rx.
Use: Androgen, estrogen combination.
Menolyn. (Arcum) Ethinyl estradiol 0.05
mg/Tab. Bot. 100s, 1000s. Rx.
Use: Estrogen.
Menomune A/C/Y/W-135. (Pasteur-Merieux-Connaught) Serogroup A, C, Y
and W-135 capsular polysaccharides
50 mcg/0.5 ml. Pow. for Inj.

Use: Vaccine.

Menoplex Tablets. (Fiske) Acetaminophen 325 mg, phenyltoloxamine citrate 30 mg/ Tab. Bot. 20s. *otc.*
Use: Analgesic.

•**menotropins,** (MEN-oh-trope-inz) U.S.P. 23. *Formerly Human Follicle Stimulating Hormone.*
Use: Gonadotropin, gonad-stimulating principle.
See: Humegon, Inj. (Organon).
Pergonal, Inj. (Serono).

Menrium. (Roche) **Menrium 5-2:** Chlordiazepoxide 5 mg, water-soluble esterified estrogens 0.2 mg/Tab. **Menrium 5-4:** Chlordiazepoxide 5 mg, water-soluble esterified estrogens 0.4 mg/Tab. **Menrium 10-4:** Chlordiazepoxide 10 mg, water-soluble esterified estrogens 0.4 mg, lactose, sucrose/Tab. Bot. 100s. *Rx.*
Use: Estrogen.

Mentax. (Schering/Penederm) Butenafine HCl 1%, benzyl and cetyl alcohol/ Cream. Tube. 2 g, 15 g, 30 g. *Rx.*
Use: Antifungal.

Mentene. (Hoechst Marion Roussel) Velnacrine.
Use: Cholinesterase inhibitor for Alzheimer's disease.

•**menthol,** U.S.P. 23.
Use: Topical antipruritic, local analgesic, nasal decongestant, antitussive.
See: Benzedrex Inhaler (SK-Beecham).
Blue Gel Muscular Pain Reliever (Rugby).
Robitussin Liquid Center Cough Drops, Loz. (Robins).
Vicks Cough Silencers, Loz. (Procter & Gamble).
Vicks Formula 44 Cough Control Discs, Loz. (Procter & Gamble).
Vicks Inhaler (Procter & Gamble).
Vicks Blue Mint, Lemon, Regular and Wild Cherry Medicated Cough Drops ().
Vicks Medi-Trating Throat Loz. (Procter & Gamble).
Vicks Oracin Regular and Cherry, Loz. (Procter & Gamble).
Vicks Sinex, Nasal Spray (Procter & Gamble).
Vicks Vaporub, Oint. (Procter & Gamble).
Vicks Vaposteam, Liq. (Procter & Gamble).
Vicks Va-Tro-Nol, Nose Drops (Procter & Gamble).
Victors Regular and Cherry, Loz. (Procter & Gamble).

W/Combinations.
See: Eucalyptamint, Gel (Novartis).
Eucalyptamint Maximum Strength, Oint. (Novartis).
Halls Mentho-Lyptus, Prods. (Warner-Lambert).
Listerine Antiseptic, Liq. (Warner-Lambert).

Mentholatum. (Mentholatum) Menthol 1.35%, camphor 9%, titanium dioxide and fragrance in ointment base of petrolatum. Tube 0.4 oz, 1 oz. Jar 1 oz, 3 oz. *otc.*
Use: Analgesic, topical.

Mentholatum Deep Heating Lotion. (Mentholatum) Menthol 6%, methyl salicylate 20%, lanolin derivative in lotion base. Bot. 2 oz, 4 oz. *otc.*
Use: Analgesic, topical.

Mentholatum Deep Heating Rub. (Mentholatum) Menthol 5.8%, methyl salicylate 12.7%, eucalyptus oil, turpentine oil, anhydrous lanolin, vehicle and fragrance. Tube 1.25 oz, 3.33 oz, 5 oz. *otc.*
Use: Analgesic, topical.

Mentholin. (Apco) Methyl salicylate 30%, chloroform 20%, hard soap 3%, camphor gum 2.2%, menthol 0.8%, alcohol 35%. Bot. 2 oz. *otc.*
Use: Analgesic, topical.

menthyl valerate. Validol.
Use: Sedative.

•**meobentine sulfate.** USAN.
Use: Cardiac depressant (antiarrhythmic).

mepacrine hydrochloride.
Use: Anthelmintic, antimalarial.
See: Quinacrine HCl, U.S.P. 23.

meparfynol.

•**mepartricin.** (meh-PAR-trih-sin) USAN.
Use: Antifungal, antiprotozoal.

mepavlon.
See: Meprobamate, U.S.P. 23.

mepazine acetate & hydrochloride.

•**mepenzolate bromide,** U.S.P. 23.
Use: Anticholinergic.
See: Cantil, Tab., Liq. (Hoechst Marion Roussel).

W/Phenobarbital.
See: Cantil w/phenobarbital (Hoechst Marion Roussel).

mepenzolate methyl bromide. Mepenzolate bromide.
Use: Anticholinergic.

Mepergan. (Wyeth-Ayerst) Promethazine HCl 25 mg, meperidine HCl 25 mg/ ml. Inj. Vial 10 ml, Tubex 2 ml. Box 10s. *c-ii.*

Use: Narcotic analgesic combination.

Mepergan Fortis. (Wyeth-Ayerst)
Meperidine HCl 50 mg, promethazine
HCl 25 mg/Cap. Bot. 100s. *c-ii.*
Use: Narcotic analgesic combination.

•**meperidine hydrochloride,** (meh-
PEHR-ih-deen) U.S.P. 23.

meperidine hydrochloride. (meh-
PEHR-ih-deen) (Parke-Davis) 50 mg/
ml, 75 mg/ml or 100 mg/ml as 1 ml fill in
2 ml Steri-dose syringe.
Use: Narcotic analgesic.
See: Demerol HCl, Prods. (Sanofi Win-
throp).
W/Acetaminophen.
See: Demerol APAP, Tab. (Sanofi Win-
throp).
W/Promethazine HCl.
See: Mepergan, Preps. (Wyeth-Ayerst).

**meperidine hydrochloride and atro-
pine sulfate.**
Use: General anesthetic.
See: Atropine and Demerol, Inj. (Sanofi
Winthrop.).

mephenesin.
Use: Skeletal muscle relaxant.
See: Myanesin.
W/Acetaminophen, Vitamin C, butabarbi-
tal.
See: T-Caps, Cap. (Burlington).
W/Pentobarbital.
See: Nebralin, Tab. (Sandoz).
W/Salicylamide, butabarbital sodium.
See: Metrogesic, Tab. (Lexis).

mephenesin carbamate.
See: Methoxydone.

mephenoxalone.

•**mephentermine sulfate,** (meh-FEN-ter-
meen) U.S.P. 23.
Use: Vasoconstrictor and nasal decongestant. Also IV or IM; adrenergic (vasoconstrictor).
See: Wyamine Sulfate Inj. (Wyeth-
Ayerst).

•**mephenytoin,** (meh-FEN-ee-TOE-in)
U.S.P. 23.
Use: Anticonvulsant.
See: Mesantoin, Tab. (Sandoz).

•**mephobarbital,** U.S.P. 23.
Use: Anticonvulsant, sedative, hypnotic.
See: Mebaral, Tab. (Sanofi Winthrop).
W/Acetaminophen.
See: Koly-Tabs (Scrip).
W/Homatropine methylbromide, atropine
methylnitrate and hyoscine HBr.

mephone.
See: Mephentermine.

Mephyton. (Merck) Phytonadione (vitamin K$_1$) 5 mg/Tab. Bot. 100s. *Rx.*

Use: Anticoagulant.

Mepiben. (Schen Labs.) Methylpiperidyl
benzhydryl ether.
Use: Antihistamine.

mepiperphenidol bromide.
Use: Anticholinergic.

•**mepivacaine hydrochloride,** U.S.P. 23.
Use: Local anesthetic.
See: Carbocaine, Inj. (Sanofi Winthrop).
Carbocaine Dental, Inj. (Cook-Waite).
Carbocaine with Neo-Cobefrin, Inj.
(Cook-Waite).
Isocaine HCl, Inj. (Novocol).
Polocaine, Inj. (Astra).
Polocaine MPF, Inj. (Astra).

mepivacaine hydrochloride. (Goldline)
Mepivacaine HCl 1%, methylparaben.
Inj. Vial 50 ml. *Rx.*
Use: Local anesthetic.

**mepivacaine hydrochloride and levo-
nordefrin inj.**
Use: Local anesthetic.
See: Carbocaine, Cartridge, Vial (Cook-
Waite).

•**meprednisone,** (meh-PRED-nih-sone)
U.S.P. 23. Betaspred.
Use: Glucocorticoid.

•**meprobamate,** (meh-pro-BAM-ate)
U.S.P. 23. Oral susp., Tab.
Use: Minor tranquilizer, sedative, hyp-
notic.
See: Arcoban Tab. (Arcum).
Bamate, Tab. (Century).
Equanil Tab., Cap., (Wyeth-Ayerst).
Meprospan, Cap. (Wallace).
Miltown, Tab. (Wallace).
Tranmep, Tab. (Solvay).
W/Acetylsalicylic acid.
See: Equagesic, Tab. (Wyeth-Ayerst).
W/Benactyzine HCl.
See: Deprol, Tab. (Wallace).
W/Estrogens conjugated.
See: Milprem, Tab. (Wallace).
W/Pentaerythritol tetranitrate.
See: Miltrate, Tab. (Wallace).
W/Premarin.
See: PMB 200, Tab. (Wyeth-Ayerst).
W/Tridihexethyl Cl.
See: Milpath, Tab. (Wallace).
Pathibamate–200, 400, Tab. (Led-
erle).

meprobamate/aspirin. (Various Mfr.) Aspirin 325 mg, meprobamate 200 mg/
Tab. Bot. 100s, 500s. *Rx.*
Use: Nonnarcotic analgesic combination.

meprobamate/benactyzine.
Use: Miscellaneous psychotherapeutic
agent.
See: Deprol (Wallace).

meprobamate, n-isopropyl.
See: Carisoprodol.

Meprogesic Q. (Various Mfr.) Aspirin 325 mg, meprobamate 200 mg/Tab. Bot. 100s, 500s. Rx.
Use: Nonnarcotic analgesic combination.

Meprolone Tabs. (Major) Methylprednisolone 4 mg/Tab. Bot. 25s, 100s. Rx.
Use: Corticosteroid.

Mepron Suspension. (Glaxo Wellcome) Atovaquone 750 mg/5 ml. Bot. 210 ml. Rx.
Use: Anti-infective.

meprylcaine hydrochloride, U.S.P. XXII.
Use: Local anesthetic, dental.

•**meptazinol hydrochloride.** (mep-TAZE-ih-nahl) USAN.
Use: Analgesic.

mepyrapone.
See: Metopirone, Tab., Amp. (Novartis).

•**mequidox.** (MEH-kwih-dox) USAN. Under study.
Use: Antibacterial.

mequinolate. (meh-KWIN-ole-ate) Name used for Proquinolate.

meragidone sodium.

•**meralein sodium.** USAN.
Use: Anti-infective (topical).
See: Sodium Meralein.

merbaphen.

merbromin. otc.
Use: Antiseptic, topical.

•**mercaptopurine,** U.S.P. 23.
Use: Antineoplastic.
See: Purinethol, Tab. (Glaxo Wellcome).

mercarbolid. o-Hydroxy-phenylmercuric Cl.

mercazole.
See: Methimazole, U.S.P. 23.

mercocresols.
See: Mercresin, Tr. (Pharmacia & Upjohn).

•**mercufenol chloride.** (MER-cue-FEEN-ole) USAN.
Use: Anti-infective (topical).

mercupurin.
See: Mercurophylline Inj. (Various Mfr.).

mercuranine.
See: Merbromin.

mercurial, antisyphilitics. Mercuric Oleate Mercuric Salicylate.

mercuric oleate. Oleate of mercury.
Use: Parasitic and fungal skin diseases.

mercuric oxide ophthalmic ointment, yellow.
Use: Local anti-infective, ophthalmic.

mercuric salicylate. Mercury subsalicylate.
Use: Parasitic and fungal skin diseases.

mercuric succinimide. BisSuccinimidato-mercury.

mercuric sulfide, red. W/Colloidal sulfur, urea.
See: Teenac Cream, Oint. (Baxter).

mercurin.

mercurocal.
See: Merbromin Soln. (Premo).

Mercurochrome. (Various Mfr.) Merbromin 2%. Soln. Bot. 15 ml, 30 ml. otc.
Use: Antiseptic, topical.

mercurome.
See: Merbromin Soln.

•**mercury, ammoniated,** U.S.P. 23.
Use: Anti-infective (topical).

mercury bichloride.
See: Diamond, Tab. (Lilly).

mercury compounds.
See: Antiseptics, Mercurials.

mercury-197-203.
See: Chlormerodrin (Squibb).

mercury oleate. Mercury (2+) oleate. Pharmaceutic aid.

Merdex. (Faraday) Docusate sodium 100 mg/Tab. Vial 60 ml. otc, Rx.
Use: Laxative.

•**merisoprol Hg 197.** (mer-EYE-so-prole) USAN.
Use: Renal function determination, radioactive agent.

•**merisoprol acetate Hg 197.** (mer-EYE-so-prole) USAN.
Use: Radioactive agent.

•**merisoprol acetate Hg 203.** (mer-EYE-so-prole) USAN.
Use: Radioactive agent.

Meritene Powder. (Sandoz Nutrition) Vanilla flavor: Specially processed nonfat dry milk, corn syrup solids, sucrose, fructose, calcium caseinate, sodium Cl, natural and artificial flavors, lecithin, vitamins and minerals. Can 1 lb, 4.5 lb, 25 lb. Packet 1.14 oz. Vanilla, chocolate, eggnog, milk chocolate, plain flavors. otc.
Use: Nutritional supplement.

merodicein. Sodium meralein. W/Saligenin.
See: Thantis, Loz. (Becton Dickinson).

•**meropenem.** (meh-row-PEN-em) USAN.
Use: Antibacterial.
See: Merrem IV. (Zeneca).

merprane. 1-(Hydroxymercuri-197 Hg)-2-propanol.

Use: Diagnostic aid.

Merrem. (Zeneca) Meropenem 500 mg/ Pow. for injection. Vial 20 ml, 100 ml, 15 ml ADD-Vantage. Meropenem 1 g/ Pow. for injection. Vial 30 ml, 100 ml, 15 ml ADD-Vantage. *Rx.*
Use: Antibacterial.

mersol. (Century) Thimerosal tincture, N.F. ¹⁄₁₀₀₀. 1 oz, 4 oz, pt, gal. *otc.*
Use: Antiseptic.

Merthiolate. (Lilly) Thimerosal.
   Soln: 1:1000: 4 fl. oz, 16 fl oz, gal.
   Tincture: 1:1000: alcohol 50%, 0.75 oz, 4 fl oz, 16 fl oz, gal. *otc.*
Use: Antiseptic.

Meruvax II. (Merck) Lyophilized, live attenuated rubella virus of the Wistar Institute RA 27/3 strain. Each dose contains approximately 25 mcg of neomycin. Single dose Vial w/diluent. Pkg. 1s, 10s. *Rx.*
Use: Agent for immunization.
W/Attenuvax.
   See: M-R-Vax II, Vial (Merck).
W/Attenuvax, Mumpsvax.
   See: M-M-R II, Vial (Merck).
W/Mumpsvax.
   See: Biavax II, Vial (Merck).

Mervan. (Continental Pharma, Belgium) Alclofenac.
Use: Anti-inflammatory.

•**mesalamine.** (me-SAL-uh-MEEN) USAN.
Use: Anti-inflammatory.
   See: Asacol, DR Tab. (Procter & Gamble).
      Pentasa, CR Cap. (Hoechst Marion Roussel).
      Rowasa, Enema, Supp. (Solvay).

mesantoin. (Sandoz) 100 mg/Tab. Bot. 100s. *Rx.*
Use: Anticonvulsant.

Mescolor. (Horizon) Chlorpheniramine maleate 8 mg, pseudoephedrine HCl 120 mg, methscopolamine nitrate 2.5 mg, dye free/Tab. Bot. 100s. *Rx.*
Use: Antihistamine, decongestant, anticholinergic.

mescomine.
   See: Methscopolamine bromide (Various Mfr.)

•**meseclazone.** (meh-SAK-lah-zone) USAN.
Use: Anti-inflammatory.

•**mesifilcon a.** (MEH-sih-FILL-kahn A) USAN.
Use: Contact lens material, hydrophilic.

•**mesna.** (MESS-nah) USAN.
Use: Hemorrhagic cystitis prophylactic;

detoxifying agent. [Orphan drug]
   See: Mesnex, Inj. (B-M Squibb Oncology).

Mesnex. (B-M Squibb Oncology) Mesna 100 mg/ml, 0.25 mg/ml EDTA, benzyl alcohol 10.4 mg (10 ml)/Inj. Vial 2 ml, 10 ml. *Rx.*
Use: Antidote.

•**mesoridazine.** (MESS-oh-RID-ah-zeen) USAN.
Use: Tranquilizer, antipsychotic.

•**mesoridazine besylate,** (MESS-oh-RID-ah-zeen) U.S.P. 23.
Use: Antipsychotic.
   See: Serentil, Amp., Liq., Tab. (Boehringer-Ingelheim).

•**mesterolone.** (MESS-TER-oh-lone) USAN.
Use: Androgen.

mestibol. Monomestrol.

Mestinon. (Zeneca) Pyridostigmine bromide 60 mg/Tab. Bot. 100s, 500s. Timespan 180 mg/Tab. Bot. 100s, 500s. *Rx.*
Use: Cholinergic muscle stimulant.

Mestinon Injectable. (Zeneca) Pyridostigmine bromide 5 mg/ml, w/methyl and propyl parabens 0.2%, sodium citrate 0.02%, pH adjusted to approximately 5 w/citric acid, sodium hydroxide. Amp. 2 ml. Box 10s. *Rx.*
Use: Cholinergic muscle stimulant.

Mestinon Syrup. (Zeneca) Pyridostigmine bromide 60 mg/5 ml, alcohol 5%. Bot. pt. *Rx.*
Use: Cholinergic muscle stimulant.

Mestinon Timespan. (Zeneca) Pyridostigmine bromide 180 mg/Timespan Tab. Bot. 100s. *Rx.*
Use: Cholinergic muscle stimulant.

•**mestranol,** (MESS-trah-nole) U.S.P. 23.
Use: Oral contraceptive, estrogen.
W/Ethynodiol Diacetate.
   See: Ovulen, Tab. (Searle).
      Ovulen-21, Tab. (Searle).
      Ovulen-28, Tab. (Searle).
W/Norethindrone.
   See: Norinyl, Tab. (Syntex).
      Norinyl-1 Fe 28 (Syntex).
      Ortho-Novum, Tab. (Ortho).
W/Norethindrone, ferrous fumarate.
   See: Ortho Novum Fe-28, Fe-28, 1 mg Fe-28, Tab. (Ortho).
W/Norethynodrel.
   See: Enovid, Tab. (Searle).
      Enovid-E, Tab. (Searle).
      Enovid-E 21, Tab. (Searle).

•**mesuprine hydrochloride.** (MEH-suh-PREEN) USAN.

Use: Vasodilator, smooth muscle relaxant.

Metabolin. (Thurston) Vitamins A 833 IU, D 66 IU, B_1 833 mcg, B_2 500 mcg, B_6 0.083 mcg, calcium pantothenate 833 mcg, niacinamide 5 mg, folic acid 0.066 mcg, niacinamide 5 mg, p-aminobenzoic acid 0.416 mcg, inositol 833 mcg, B_{12} 500 mcg, C 5 mg, calcium 33.1 mg, phosphorus 14.6 mg, iron 2.5 mg, iodine 0.15 mg/Tab. Bot. 100s, 500s, 1000s. *otc.*
Use: Vitamin/mineral supplement.

• **metabromsalan.** (MET-ah-BROME-sah-lan) USAN.
Use: Germicide, disinfectant.

metabutethamine hydrochloride.
Use: Local anesthetic.

metabutoxycaine hydrochloride.
Use: Local anesthetic.

metacaraphen hydrochloride. Netrin.

metacordralone.
See: Prednisolone. (Various Mfr.).

metacortalone.
See: Meticortelone, Susp. (Schering Plough).

metacortandracin.
See: Prednisone, Tab. (Various Mfr.).

metacortin.
See: Meticorten, Tab. (Schering Plough).

• **metacresol,** U.S.P. 23.
Use: Antiseptic (topical), antifungal.

meta-delphene. Diethyltoluamide U.S.P. 23.

metaglycodol.
Use: Central nervous system depressant.

Metahydrin. (Hoechst Marion Roussel) Trichlormethiazide 2 mg or 4 mg/Tab. Bot. 100s. *Rx.*
Use: Diuretic.

• **metalol hydrochloride.** (MEH-ta-lahl) USAN. Under study.
Use: Anti-adrenergic β-receptor.

Metalone T.B.A. (Foy) Prednisolone tertiary butylacetate 20 mg, sodium citrate 1 mg, polysorbate 80 1 mg, d-sorbitol 450 mg/ml, benzyl alcohol 0.9%, water for inj. Vial 10 ml. *Rx.*
Use: Corticosteroid.

Metamucil. (Procter & Gamble) Psyllium hydrophilic mucilloid, sodium 1 mg, potassium 31 mg/Dose. **Regular Flavor:** w/ dextrose. Jar 7 oz, 14 oz, 21 oz. Packette 5.4 g. Box 100s. **Orange and Strawberry Flavors:** w/flavoring, sucrose and coloring. Jar 7 oz, 14 oz, 21 oz. *otc.*

Use: Laxative.

Metamucil Instant Mix. (Procter & Gamble) Psyllium hydrophilic mucilloid with citric acid, sucrose, potassium bicarbonate, sodium bicarbonate. Powder when combined with water forms an effervescent, flavored liquid. **Lemon Lime Flavor:** w/calcium carbonate. Cartons of 16, 30 or 100 packets of 3.4 g. **Orange Flavor:** w/flavoring and coloring. Ctn. 16 or 30 packets of 3.4 g. *otc.*
Use: Laxative.

Metamucil, Sugar Free. (Procter & Gamble) Psyllium hydrophilic mucilloid in sugar-free formula. **Regular Flavor:** Jar 3.7 oz, 7.4 oz, 11.1 oz. Packet 3.4 g. Box 100s. **Orange Flavor:** Jar 3.7 oz, 7.4 oz, 11.1 oz. *otc.*
Use: Laxative.

Metandren. (Novartis) Methyltestosterone. **Linguet:** 5 mg or 10 mg Bot. 100s. **Tab.:** 10 mg or 25 mg Bot. 100s. *Rx.*
Use: Androgen.

metaphenylbarbituric acid.
See: Mephobarbital.

metaphyllin.
See: Aminophylline (Various Mfr.).

Metaprel Syrup. (Sandoz) Metaproterenol sulfate 10 mg/5 ml. Bot. pt. *Rx.*
Use: Bronchodilator.

• **metaproterenol polistirex.** (MEH-tuh-pro-TEHR-uh-nahl pahl-ee-STIE-rex) USAN.
Use: Bronchodilator.

• **metaproterenol sulfate,** (MEH-tuh-pro-TEHR-uh-nahl) U.S.P. 23.
Use: Bronchodilator.
See: Alupent Inhalation (Novartis). Metaprel, Tab., Inhalation, Syr. (Sandoz). Prometa, Syr. (Muro).

• **metaraminol bitartrate,** (met-uh-RAM-in-ole by-TAR-trate) U.S.P. 23.
Use: Adrenergic.
See: Aramine, Amp., Vial (Merck).

Metasep. (MiLance) Parachlorometaxylenol 2%, isopropyl alcohol 9%. Shampoo 120 ml. *otc.*
Use: Antiseborrheic.

Metastron. (Medi-Physics/Amersham) Strontium-89 Cl 10.9 to 22.6 mg/ml. Preservative free. Inj. Vial 10 ml.
Use: Radiopharmaceutical.

Metatensin #2 & #4. (Hoechst Marion Roussel) Trichlormethiazide 2 mg or 4 mg, each containing reserpine 0.1 mg/Tab. Bot. 100s. *Rx.*

Use: Antihypertensive.

• **metaxalone.** (mex-TAX-ah-lone) USAN.
Use: Skeletal muscle relaxant.
See: Skelaxin (Carnrick).

metcaraphen hydrochloride.

Meted, Maximum Strength. (Gen-Derm)
Sulfur 5%, salicylic acid 3%. Shampoo.
Bot. 118 ml. *otc.*
Use: Antiseborrheic combination.

• **meteneprost.** (meh-TEN-eh-PRAHST)
USAN.
Use: Oxytocic, prostaglandin.

• **metesind glucuronate.** (MEH-teh-sind
glue-CURE-oh-nate) USAN.
Use: Antineoplastic (specific thymic-
lylate synthase inhibitor).

metethoheptazine.
Use: Analgesic.

• **metformin.** (MET-fore-min) USAN.
Use: Oral hypoglycemic; antidiabetic.
See: Glucophage, Tab. (Bristol-Myers
Squibb).

• **metformin hydrochloride.** (MET-fore-
min) USAN.
Use: Antidiabetic.

methacholine bromide. Mecholin bromide.
Use: Cholinergic.

• **methacholine chloride,** U.S.P. 23.
Use: Cholinergic.
See: Mecholyl Cl, Amp. (Mallinckrodt
Baker).
Provocholine, Amp. (Roche).

methacholine chloride.
Use: Diagnostic aid.
See: Provocholine, pow. for reconstitu-
tion. (Roche).

• **methacrylic acid copolymer,** N.F. 18.
Use: Pharmaceutic aid (tablet coating
agent).

• **methacycline.** (meth-ah-SIGH-kleen)
USAN.
Use: Antibacterial.
See: Rondomycin, Cap., Syr. (Wallace).

methadone hydrochloride diskets.
(METH-uh-dohn) (Lilly) Methadone HCl
40 mg/Dispersible Tab. Bot. 100s. *c-ii.*
Use: Narcotic agonist analgesic.

methadone hydrochloride intensol.
(METH-uh-dohn) (Lilly) Methadone HCl
10 mg/ml. Oral concentrate. Bot. 30
mg. *c-ii.*
Use: Narcotic agonist analgesic.

• **methadone hydrochloride,** (METH-uh-
dohn) U.S.P. 23.
Use: Narcotic analgesic, narcotic absti-
nence syndrome suppressant.
See: Dolophine HCl, Preps. (Lilly).

• **methadyl acetate.** USAN.
Use: Narcotic analgesic.

• **methafilcon b.** (METH-ah-FILL-kahn B)
USAN.
Use: Contact lens material (hydrophilic).

Methagual. (Gordon) Guaiacol 2%,
methyl salicylate 8% in petrolatum. Oint.
2 oz, lb. *otc.*
Use: Analgesic, topical.

methalamic acid. Name used for Iothalamic acid, U.S.P. 23.

methalgen. (Alra) Camphor, menthol,
mustard oil, methyl salicylate in non-
greasy cream base. Bot. 2 oz, Jar 4 oz,
lb. *otc.*
Use: Analgesic, topical.

methallatal.

• **methalthiazide.** (METH-al-THIGH-ah-
zide) USAN.
Use: Antihypertensive, diuretic.

methaminodiazepoxide. Chlordiazepoxide HCl, U.S.P. 23.
See: Librium, Cap., Amp. (Roche).

methamoctol.
Use: Adrenergic.

• **methamphetamine hydrochloride,**
(meth-am-FET-uh-meen) U.S.P. 23
Use: CNS stimulant.
See: Desoxyn, Gradumets, Tab. (Ab-
bott).
Methampex, Tab. (Lemmon).
Methamphetamine HCl, Tab. (Various
Mfr.).
W/Pamabrom, pyrilamine maleate, hom-
atropine methylbromide, hyoscyamine
sulfate, scopolamine HBr.
See: Aridol, Tab. (MPL).
W/Pentobarbital sodium, vitamins, miner-
als.
See: Fetamin, Tab. (Mission).

methamphetamine-dl hydrochloride.
See: dl-Methamphetamine HCl.

methampyrone.
See: Dipyrone.

methandriol. Methylandrostenediol.
(Various Mfr.)
See: Anabol, Inj. (Keene Pharm).

methandriol dipropionate.
See: Andriol Inj. (Solvay).
Arbolic, Inj. (Burgin-Arden).
Crestabolic, Vial (Nutrition).
Probolik (Hickam).

methandrostenolone.
See: Dianabol, Tab. (Novartis).

methantheline bromide, U.S.P. XXII.
Sterile, Tab., U.S.P. XXII.
Use: Parasympatholytic, anticholiner-
gic.
See: Banthine, Vial, Tab. (Roberts).

W/Phenobarbital.
See: Banthine w/Phenobarbital, Tab. (Roberts).

Methaphor. (Borden) Protein hydrolysate (l-leucine, l-isoleucine, l-methionine, l-phenylalanine, l-tyrosine); methionine, camphor, benzethonium Cl, in Dermabase vehicle/Oint. Tube 1.5 oz. *otc.*
Use: Dermatologic, amino acid preparation.

•**methaqualone.** (METH-ah-kwan-lone) USAN.
Use: Sedative, hypnotic.

Methatropic Capsules. (Goldline) Choline 115 mg, inositol 83 mg, methionine 110 mg, vitamins B_1 3 mg, B_2 3 mg, B_3 10 mg, B_5 2 mg, B_6 2 mg, B_{12} 2 mcg, desiccated liver 86 mg/Cap. Bot. 100s. *otc.*
Use: Vitamin supplement.

•**methazolamide,** U.S.P. 23.
Use: Carbonic anhydrase inhibitor.
See: Neptazane.
Neptazane, Tab. (Lederle).

methazolamide. (Various Mfr.) 25 mg or 50 mg/Tab. Bot. 100s. *Rx.*
Use: Carbonic anhydrase inhibitor.

Methblue 65. (Manne Co.) Methylene blue 65 mg/Tab. Bot. 100s, 1000s. *Rx.*
Use: Antiethemoglobinemic, antidote to cyanide poisoning.

Meth-Choline Capsules. (Schein) Choline 115 mg, inositol 83 mg, methionine 110 mg, vitamins B_1 3 mg, B_2 3 mg, B_3 10 mg, B_5 2 mg, B_6 2 mg, B_{12} 2 mcg, desiccated liver 56 mg, liver concentrate 30 mg/Cap. Bot. 100s, 250s, 1000s. *otc.*
Use: Vitamin supplement.

Meth-Dia-Mer Sulfa Tablets. Trisulfapyrimidines Tab., U.S.P. 23.
Use: Triple sulfonamide therapy.
See: Chemozine, Tab. (Tennessee Pharm).
Neotrizine, Tab. (Lilly).
Terfonyl, Susp., (Squibb).
Triple Sulfa, Tab. (Various Mfr.).

Meth-Dia-Mer Sulfonamides.
Use: Triple sulfonamide therapy.
W/Sulfacetamide.
See: Sulfa-Plex Vaginal Cream (Solvay).
W/Sulfacetamide, hexestrol.
See: Vagi-Plex, Cream (Solvay).

Meth-Dia-Mer Sulfonamides Suspension, Trisulfapyrimidines Oral Suspension, U.S.P. 23.
Use: Triple sulfonamide therapy.
See: Chemozine, Susp. (Tennessee Pharm).

Neotrizine, Susp. (Lilly).
Terfonyl, Susp. (Squibb).
Triple Sulfa, Susp. (CMC).

•**methdilazine,** U.S.P. 23.
Use: Antipuritic.
See: Tacaryl Chew. Tab. (Westwood Squibb).

•**methdilazine hydrochloride,** U.S.P. 23.
Use: Antipruritic.
See: Tacaryl, Tab. (Westwood Squibb).

•**methenamine,** (meh-THEN-uh-meen) U.S.P. 23. *Formerly Hexamethylenamine.* (Hexamethyleneamine, Cystamin, Cystogen, Hexamine, Hexamethylenetetramine.).
Use: Antibacterial (urinary).

methenamine w/combinations. (meh-THEN-uh-meen)
Use: Urinary anti-infective.
See: Cystamine, Tab. (Tennessee Pharm).
Cystex, Tab. (Numark).
Cystitol, Tab. (Briar).
Cysto, Tab. (Freeport).
Hexalol, Tab. (Schwartz Pharma).
Prosed/DS, Tab. (Star).
Urimar-T, Tab. (Marnel).
Urisan-P, Tab. (Sandia).
Urised, Tab. (PolyMedica).
Urogesic Blue, Tab. (Edwards).
Uro Phosphate, Tab. (ECR Pharm).
UTA, Tab. (Bentex).
U-Tract, Tab. (Jones Medical).
U-Tran, Tab. (Scruggs).

methenamine and monobasic sodium phosphate tablets, U.S.P. 23.
Use: Anti-infective, urinary.

methenamine anhydromethylene citrate. Formanol, Uropurgol, Urotropin.

•**methenamine hippurate,** (meh-THEN-uh-meen HIP-you-rate) U.S.P. 23. Tab., U.S.P. 23. A 1:1 complex of methenamine and hippuric acid.
Use: Antibacterial (urinary).
See: Hiprex, Tab. (Hoechst Marion Roussel).
Urex, Tab. (3M).

•**methenamine mandelate,** U.S.P. 23.
Use: Antibacterial (urinary).
See: Mandelamine, Tab. (Parke-Davis).

methenamine mandelate. (Various Mfr.) **Tab.:** 0.5 g or 1 g/Tab. 100s, 1000s. **Susp.:** 0.5 g/5 ml. Susp. BOt. 480 ml. *Rx.*
Use: Antibacterial (urinary).

methenamine mandelate w/combinations.
Use: Anti-infective, urinary.
See: Mandex, Tab. (Pal-Pak).
Thiacide, Tab. (Beach).

Urisedamine, Tab. (PolyMedica).

•**methenolone acetate.** (meth-EEN-oh-lone) USAN.
Use: Anabolic.

•**methenolone enanthate.** (meth-EEN-oh-lone eh-NAN-thate) USAN.
Use: Anabolic.

Metheponex. (Rawl) Choline 0.54 g, dl-methionine 1.80 g, inositol 0.27 g, whole desiccated liver 8.10 g, vitamins B_1 18 mg, B_2 36 mg, niacinamide 90 mg, B_6 3.6 mg, calcium pantothenate 3.6 mg, biotin 10.8 mcg, B_{12} 5.4 mcg and amino acid/daily therapeutic dose. Cap. Bot. 100s, 500s. *Rx.*
Use: Antidiabetic, nutritional supplement.

metheptazine.
Use: Analgesic.

Methergine. (Sandoz) Methylergonovine maleate. **Amp.:** 0.2 mg/ml, tartaric acid 0.25 mg/ml, sodium Cl 3 mg/ml. **Tab.:** 0.2 mg. Bot. 100s, 1000s, SandoPak pkgs. 100s. *Rx.*
Use: Oxytocic.

methestrol.
See: Promethestrol (Various Mfr.).

methetharimide bemegride. (METH-eh-toe-in) USAN.
Use: Anticonvulsant.

•**methetoin.** (METH-eh-toe-in) USAN.
Use: Anticonvulsant.

Methibon Capsules. (Barrows) Choline dihydrogen citrate 278 mg, dl-methionine 111 mg, inositol 83.3 mg, vitamin B_{12} 2 mcg, liver concentrate, desiccated liver 86.6 mg/Cap. Bot. 100s. *Rx.*
Use: Antidiabetic, nutritional supplement.

•**methicillin sodium, sterile,** (meth-ih-SILL-in) U.S.P. 23.
Use: Antibacterial.
See: Celbenin, Vial (SK-Beecham).
Staphcillin, Vial (Bristol).

•**methimazole,** (meth-IMM-uh-zole) U.S.P. 23.
Use: Thyroid inhibitor.
See: Tapazole, Tab. (Lilly).
Thiamazole (I.N.N.).

methiodal sodium, U.S.P. XXI. Sodium monoiodomethanesulfonate. Abrodil, Radiographol, Diagnorenol.
Use: Radiopaque medium.

Methiokaps. (Pal-Pak) dl-methionine 200 mg/Cap. Bot. 1000s. *Rx.*
Use: Diaper rash product.

methiomeprazine hydrochloride. (SK-Beecham)
Use: Antiemetic.

•**methionine C 11 injection,** U.S.P. 23.
Use: Radioactive agent.

•**methionine,** (meh-THIGH-oh-NEEN) U.S.P. 23.
Note: Also see Racemethionine, U.S.P. 23.
Use: Amino acid.

methionyl human stem cell factor (recombinant).
Use: Combination w/filgrastim to decrease the number of phereses required to collect blood progenitor cells following myelosuppressive/myeloblative therapy. [Orphan drug]

methionyl neurotrophic (brain-derived, recombinant) factor.
Use: Amyotrophic lateral sclerosis. [Orphan drug]

Methioplex. (Lincoln) Methionine 25 mg, vitamins B_1 50 mg, niacinamide 100 mg, B_2 2 mg, choline 50 mg, B_6 2 mg, panthenol 2 mg, benzyl alcohol 1%, distilled water q.s./ml. Vial 30 ml. *Rx.*
Use: Nutritional supplement.

•**methisazone.** (METH-eye-SAH-zone) USAN.
Use: Antiviral.

methitural sodium.
Use: Hypnotic; sedative.

•**methixene hydrochloride,** (meh-THIX-een) USAN.
Use: Smooth muscle relaxant.

•**methocarbamol,** (meth-oh-CAR-buh-mahl) U.S.P. 23.
Use: Skeletal muscle relaxant.
See: Delaxin, Tab. (Ferndale).
Robaxin, Tab., Inj. (Robins).
W/Aspirin.
See: Robaxisal, Tab. (Robins).

methocarbamol. (Various Mfr.) **Tab.:** 500 mg or 750 mg. Bot. 100s, 500s; **Inj.:** 100 mg/ml Vial 10 ml.
Use: Skeletal muscle relaxant.

Methocarbamol/ASA. (Various Mfr.) Methocarbamol 400 mg, aspirin 325 mg/Tab. Bot. 15s, 30s, 40s, 100s, 500s, 1000. *Rx.*
Use: Skeletal muscle relaxant combination.

methocel. Methylcellulose.

•**methohexital,** U.S.P. 23.
Use: Pharmaceutic necessity for Methohexital Sodium for Injection.

•**methohexital sodium for injection,** U.S.P. 23.
Use: General anesthetic; anesthetic (intravenous).
See: Brevital, Amp., Pow. (Lilly).

•**methopholine.** (METH-oh-foe-leen) USAN.

Use: Analgesic.
See: Versidyne.
Methopto 0.25%. (Professional Pharmacal) Methylcellulose pow. 2.5 mg (0.25% soln.), boric acid 12 mg, potassium Cl 7.3 mg, benzalkonium Cl 0.04 mg, glycerin 12 mg/ml w/sodium carbonate to adjust pH and purified water. Bot. 15 ml, 30 ml. *otc.*
Use: Artificial tear solution.
Methopto Forte 0.5%. (Professional Pharmacal) Methylcellulose pow. 5 mg (0.5% soln.), boric acid 12 mg, potassium Cl 7.3 mg, benzalkonium Cl 0.4 mg, glycerin 12 mg/ml w/sodium carbonate to adjust pH and purified water. Bot. 15 ml. *otc.*
Use: Artificial tear solution.
Methopto Forte 1%. (Professional Pharmacal) Methylcellulose pow. 10 mg (1% soln.), boric acid 12 mg, potassium Cl 7.3 mg, benzalkonium Cl 0.04 mg, glycerin 12 mg/ml w/sodium carbonate to adjust pH and purified water. Bot. 15 ml. *otc.*
Use: Artificial tear solution.
methopyraphone.
See: Metopirone, Tab., Amp. (Novartis).
methorate.
See: Dextromethorphan HBr.
Methorbate S.C. (Standex) Methenamine 40.8 mg, atropine sulfate 0.03 mg, hyoscyamine sulfate 0.03 mg, salol 18.1 mg, benzoic acid 4.5 mg, methylene blue 5.4 mg/Tab. Bot. 100s. *Rx.*
Use: Urinary anti-infective.
d-methorphan hydrobromide.
See: Dextromethorphan HBr (Various Mfr.).
methorphinan. Racemorphan HBr. Dromoran.
•**methotrexate,** (meth-oh-TREK-sate) U.S.P. 23. *Formerly Amethopterin.*
Use: Leukemia in children, antineoplastic, antipsoriatic, juvenile rheumatoid arthritis [Orphan drug]
See: Rheumatrex, Tab. (Lederle).
methotrexate. (Various Mfr.) Tab. 2.5 mg. Bot. 36s, 100s, UD 20s.
Use: Antineoplastic.
methotrexate. (Immunex) Inj.: 25 mg/ml as sodium, benzyl alcohol 0.9%, sodium Cl 0.26% and water for inj. Vials 2 ml or 10 ml. **Pow. for Inj.:** 20 mg or 1 g/vial as sodium. Single-use vials. *Rx.*
Use: Antipsoriatic.
methotrexate sodium for injection. (Lederle) 2.5 mg/ml Vial 2 ml; 25 mg/ml.

Vial 2 ml w/preservatives; 20 mg, 50 mg, 100 mg Vial cryodesiccated, preservative free; 50 mg, 100 mg, 200 mg Vial; 25 mg/ml solution preservative free.
Use: Leukemia therapy, psoriasis, osteogenic sarcoma [Orphan drug]
See: Folex, Inj. (Pharmacia & Upjohn) Folex PFS. Inj. (Pharmacia & Upjohn) Methotrexate, Inj., Pow. (Lederle).
Mexate, Inj. (Bristol).
methotrexate USP with laurocapram. *Rx.*
Use: Topical treatment of *Mycosis fungoides.* [Orphan drug]
•**methotrimeprazine,** (METH-oh-trih-MEP-rah-zeen) U.S.P. 23.
Use: Tranquilizer, analgesic.
See: Levoprome, Amp., Vial (Immunex).
methoxamine hydrochloride, U.S.P. XXII.
Use: Vasopressor used in shock.
See: Vasoxyl (Glaxo Wellcome).
•**methoxsalen,** U.S.P. 23.
Use: Pigmenting agent.
See: Meloxine, (Pharmacia & Upjohn) Oxsoralen, Cap., Lot. (Baxter). Oxsoralen-Ultra, Cap. (Baxter).
8-methoxsalen. *Rx.*
Use: Treatment of diffuse systemic sclerosis, rejection of cardiac allografts. [Orphan drug]
See: Uvadex.
methoxsalen topical solution.
Use: Pigmenting agent, topical.
methoxydone.
See: Mephenoxalone (Various Mfr.).
•**methoxyflurane,** (meth-OCK-sih-FLEW-rane) U.S.P. 23.
Use: Anesthetic (inhalation).
See: Penthrane, Liq. (Abbott).
methoxyphenamine hydrochloride, U.S.P. XXI.
Use: Adrenergic (bronchodilator).
W/Chlorpheniramine maleate, acetophenetidin, acetylsalicylic acid, caffeine.
See: Pyrroxate, Cap., Tab. (Pharmacia & Upjohn).
W/Dextromethorphan HCl, orthoxine, sodium citrate.
See: Orthoxicol, Syr. (Pharmacia & Upjohn).
W/Dextromethorphan HBr, phenylephrine HCl, chlorpheniramine maleate.
See: Statuss, Syr., Cap. (Baxter).
W/Medrol.
See: Medrol, Tab. (Pharmacia & Upjohn).

methoxypromazine maleate.
Use: CNS depressant.
methoxypsoralen, oral.
Use: Psoralen.
See: Oxsoralen (Baxter).
Oxsoralen-Ultra (Baxter).
8-MOP (Baxter).
methscopolamine bromide, U.S.P. XXII.
Tab., U.S.P. XXII.
Use: Anticholinergic.
See: Pamine, Tab., Vial (Pharmacia &
Upjohn).
Scoline, Tab. (Westerfield).
W/Amobarbital.
See: Scoline-Amobarbital, Tab. (West-
erfield).
W/Butabarbital sodium, dried aluminum
hydroxide gel and magnesium trisili-
cate.
See: Eulcin, Tab. (Leeds Pharmacal).
W/Phenobarbital.
See: Pamine PB, Preps. (Pharmacia &
Upjohn).
Synt-PB, Tab. (Scrip).
W/Phenylpropanolamine HCl, chlor-
pheniramine maleate.
See: Bobid, Cap. (Boyd).
Symptrol, Cap. (Saron).
methscopolamine nitrate. Scopolamine
Methyl Nitrate, Preps. (Various Mfr.)
Mescomine.
See: Cenahist, Cap. (Century).
Dallergy, Cap., Tab., Syr. (Laser).
Extendryl, Cap., Tab., Syr. (Fleming).
Histaspan-D, Cap. (Rhone-Poulenc
Rorer).
Sanhist T.D. 12, Tab. (Sandia).
Scotnord, Tab. (Scott/Cord).
Sinovan, Timed Cap. (Drug Ind.).
•**methsuximide,** U.S.P. 23.
Use: Anticonvulsant.
See: Celontin Kapseal (Parke-Davis).
Methyclodine. (Rugby) Methyclothiazide
5 mg, deserpidine 0.25 mg/Tab. Bot.
100s. *Rx.*
Use: Antihypertensive, diuretic.
•**methyclothiazide,** (METH-ee-kloe-
THIGH-ah-zide) U.S.P. 23.
Use: Diuretic, antihypertensive.
See: Enduron, Tab. (Abbott) Methyclo-
dine, Tab. (Rugby).
W/Deserpidine.
See: Enduronyl, Tab. (Abbott).
Enduronyl Forte, Tab. (Abbott).
W/Pargyline HCl.
See: Eutron, Tab. (Abbott).
methylacetylcholine.
See: Methacholine.
•**methyl alcohol,** N.F. 18.
Use: Pharmaceutic acid (solvent).

**methylamphetamine hydrochloride &
sulfate.**
See: Desoxyephedrine HCl (Various
Mfr.).
methylandrostenediol.
See: Hybolin, Vial (Hyrex).
Methandriol.
W/Adrenal cortex extract, Vitamin B₁₂.
See: Geri-Ace, Inj. (Baxter).
W/Carboxymethylcellulose sodium, thi-
merosal.
See: Cenabolic, Vial (Century).
W/Pentylenetetrazol, nicotinic acid, l-ly-
sine, dl-methionine, ethinyl estradiol,
thiamine, pyridoxine, riboflavin, vitamins
B₁₂, A, D, ascorbic acid.
See: Ardiatric, Tab. (Burgin-Arden).
•**methylatropine nitrate.** (METH-ill-AT-
row-peen) USAN.
Use: Anticholinergic.
•**methylbenzethonium chloride,** U.S.P.
23.
Use: Bactericide, local anti-infective
(topical).
See: Ammorid, Oint. (Kinney).
Benephen, Prods. (Halsted).
Cuticura Acne Cream (Purex).
Cuticura Medicated First Aid Cream
(Purex).
Diaparene Prods. (Bayer).
Fordustin, Pow. (Sween).
Surgi-Kleen, Liq. (Sween).
W/Cod liver oil.
See: Benephen, Prods. (Halsted).
Sween Cream (Sween).
W/Magnesium stearate.
See: Mennen Baby Pow. (Mennen).
W/Phenol, acetanilid, zinc oxide, cala-
mine and eucalyptol.
See: Taloin, Oint. (Warren-Teed).
W/Phenylmercuric acetate, methylpara-
ben.
See: Lorophyn, Supp. (Eaton).
Norforms, Aerosal, Supp. (Procter &
Gamble).
W/Zinc oxide, calamine, eucalyptol.
See: Taloin, Tube (Warren-Teed).
methylbenztropine.
See: Ethybenztropine (Sandoz).
methylbromtropin mandelate.
See: Homatropine Methylbromide,
U.S.P. 23.
•**methylcellulose,** U.S.P. 23. Cellulose
methylether. Mellose.
Use: Pharmaceutic aid (suspending
agent).
See: Cellothyl, Tab. (International Drug).
Cologel, Soln. (Lilly).
Isopto-Plain, Liq. (Alcon).
Melozets, Wafer (SK-Beecham).

W/Boric acid, glycerine, propylene glycol, methylparaben, propylparaben, irish moss extract.
See: Canfield Lubricating Jelly (Paddock).
W/Carboxymethylcellulose.
See: Ex-Caloric, Wafer (Eastern Research).
W/Dicyclomine HCl, magnesium trisilicate, aluminum hydroxide-magnesium carbonate, dried.
See: Triactin Tab. (Procter & Gamble).
W/Dicyclomine HCl, aluminum hydroxide and magnesium hydroxide.
See: Triactin Liq. (Procter & Gamble).
W/Phenylephrine HCl.
See: Vernacel (Professional Pharmacal).
W/Phenylephrine HCl, benzalkonium Cl.
See: Efricel % (Professional Pharmacal).
W/Polysorbate 80, boric acid.
See: Lacril Artificial Tears (Allergan).
methyl cysteine hydrochloride. Cysteine methyl ester hydrochloride.
Use: Mucolytic agent.
•**methyldopa,** (meth-ill-DOE-puh) U.S.P. 23. Formerly Alpha-Methyldopa.
Use: Antihypertensive.
See: Aldomet, Tab. (Merck).
methyldopa and chlorothiazide tablets.
Use: Antihypertensive.
See: Aldoclor, Tab. (Merck).
methyldopa and hydrochlorothiazide tablets.
Use: Antihypertensive.
See: Aldoril, Tab. (Merck).
methyldopa/hydrochlorothiazide. (Various Mfr.) Methyldopa 250 mg, hydrochlorothiazide 15 mg or 25 mg/Tab. Bot. 100s, 500s, 1000s, UD 100s. Rx.
Use: Antihypertensive combination.
methyldopa/hydrochlorothiazide. (Various Mfr.) Methyldopa 500 mg, hydrochlorothiazide 30 mg or 50 mg/Tab. Bot. 100s, 250s, 500s. Rx.
Use: Antihypertensive combination.
•**methyldopate hydrochloride,** (meth-ill-DOE-pate) U.S.P. 23.
Use: Antihypertensive.
See: Aldomet Ester HCl, Inj. (Merck).
methyldopate hydrochloride. (Fujisawa) Methyldopate HCl 250 mg/5 ml. Inj. Vial. 6 ml. Rx.
Use: Antihypertensive.
•**methylene blue,** U.S.P. 23. Methylthionine Cl.
Use: Antimethemoglobinemic, antidote to cyanide poisoning.

See: Methblue 65, Tab. (Manne Co.).
Urolene Blue, Tab. (Star).
Wright's Stain, Liq. (Becton Dickinson).
methylene blue. (Various) 10 mg/ml. Inj. Vial 1 ml, 10 ml. Rx.
Use: GU antiseptic, cyanide antidote.
methylene blue w/combinations.
See: Hexalol, Tab. (Schwartz Pharma).
Urised, Tab. (PolyMedica).
U-Tract, Tab. (Jones Medical).
•**methylene chloride,** N.F. 18.
Use: Pharmaceutic aid (solvent).
•**methylergonovine maleate,** U.S.P. 23.
Use: Oxytocic.
See: Methergine, Amp., Tab. (Sandoz).
methylethylamino-phenylpropanol hydrochloride.
See: Nethamine HCl. (Various Mfr.).
methylglucamine diatrizoate, inj., A water-soluble radiopaque iodine cpd. N-methylglucamine salt of Diatrizoate.
See: Diatrizoate (Various Mfr.).
Diatrizoate Meglumine Inj., U.S.P. 23.
methulglucamine iodipamide, inj.
See: Meglumine Iodipamide, Inj., U.S.P. 23. (Various Mfr.).
W/Diatrizoate methylglucamine.
See: Sinografin, Vial (Squibb).
methylglyoxal-bis-guanylhydrazone. Methyl GAG.
•**methyl isobutyl ketone,** N.F. 18.
Use: Pharmaceutic aid (alcohol denaturant).
methyliso-octenylamine.
See: Isometheptene HCl (Various Mfr.).
methylmercadone. Name used for Nifuratel.
•**methyl nicotinate.** USAN.
W/Histamine dihydrochloride, oleoresin capsicum, glycomonosalicylate.
See: Akes-N-Pain Rub, Oint. (Moore).
W/methyl salicylate, menthol.
See: Musterole Deep Strength Oint. (Schering Plough).
W/Methyl salicylate, menthol, camphor, dipropylene glycol salicylate, cassia oil, oleoresins capsicum, ginger.
See: Arthaderm, Lot. (Paddock).
Scrip-Gesic, Oint. (Scrip).
Methylone. (Paddock) Methylprednisolone acetate 40 mg/ml. Vial 5 ml. Rx.
Use: Corticosteroid.
•**methyl palmoxirate.** (METH-ill pal-MOX-ihr-ate) USAN.
Use: Antidiabetic.
•**methylparaben,** (meth-ill-PAR-ah-ben) N.F. 18.
Use: Pharmaceutic aid (antifungal agent).

•**methylparaben sodium,** (meth-ill-PAR-ah-ben) N.F. 18.
Use: Pharmaceutic aid antimicrobial preservative.

methylparafynol.

methylphenethylamine.
See: Amphetamine HCl (Various Mfr.).

•**methylphenidate hydrochloride,** (meth-ill-FEN-ih-date) U.S.P. 23.
Use: CNS stimulant.
See: Ritalin HCl, Tab., Vial (Novartis).

methylphenidate hydrochloride. (Various Mfr.) **Tab.:** 5 mg, 10 mg or 20 mg. Bot. 100s, 1000s; **SR Tab.:** 20 mg. Bot. 100s.
Use: CNS stimulant.

methylphenidylacetate hydrochloride.
See: Methylphenidate HCl (Various Mfr.).

methylphenobarbital.
See: Mephobarbital.

d-methylphenylamine sulfate.
See: Dextroamphetamine Sulfate, U.S.P. 23. (Various Mfr.).

methyl phenylethylhydantoin.
See: Mesantoin, Tab. (Sandoz).

methylphenylsuccinimide.
See: Milontin, Kapseal, Susp. (Parke-Davis).

methylphytyl naphthoquinone.
Use: Vitamin K supplement.
See: Phytonadione (Various Mfr.)

methyl polysiloxane.
See: Mylicon, Tab., Drops (Stuart).
Phasil, Tab. (Reed & Carnrick).
Silain, Tab. (Robins).
Simethicone (Various Mfr.)

methylpred-40. (Seatrace) Methylprednisolone acetate 40 mg/ml. Vial 5 ml, 10 ml. *Rx.*
Use: Corticosteroid.

•**methylprednisolone,** (METH-ill-pred-NIH-suh-lone) U.S.P. 23.
Use: Glucocorticoid.
See: A-Methapred, Inj. (Abbott).
Dura-Meth, Inj. (Foy).
Medralone 40, Inj. (Keene).
Medralone 80, Inj. (Keene).
Medrol, Tab. (Pharmacia & Upjohn).
W/Neomycin sulfate.
See: Neo-Medrol, Oint. (Pharmacia & Upjohn).
W/Sodium succinate.
See: Solu-Medrol, Vial (Pharmacia & Upjohn).

•**methylprednisolone acetate,** (METH-ill-pred-NIH-suh-lone) U.S.P. 23.
Use: Glucocorticoid.
See: Adlone, Inj. (UAD).

Depo-Medrol, Inj., Rectal (Pharmacia & Upjohn).
Depo-Pred., Vial (Hyrex).
Mepred-40, Susp. (Savage).
Mepred-80, Susp. (Savage).
Neo-Medrol, Preps. (Pharmacia & Upjohn).
Rep-Pred, Vial (Schwartz Pharma).

•**methylprednisolone hemisuccinate,** (METH-ill-pred-NIH-suh-lone) U.S.P. 23.
Use: Adrenocortical steroid.

•**methylprednisolone sodium phosphate.** (METH-ill-pred-NIH-suh-lone) USAN.
Use: Glucocorticoid.

•**methylprednisolone sodium succinate,** (METH-ill-pred-NIH-suh-lone) U.S.P. 23.
Use: Adrenocorticoid steroid, glucocorticoid.
See: Solu-Medrol, Mix-O-Vial (Pharmacia & Upjohn).

•**methylprednisolone suleptanate.** (METH-ill-pred-NIH-suh-lone sull-EPP-tah-NATE) USAN.
Use: Adrenocortical steroid, anti-inflammatory.

methylpromazine.

4-methylpyrazole. *Rx.*
Use: Methanol or ethylene glycol poisoning. [Orphan drug]

methylpyrimal.
See: Sulfamerazine (Various Mfr.).

methylrosaniline chloride.
Use: Anthelmintic, anti-infective.
See: Gentian Violet, U.S.P. 23. (Various Mfr.).

•**methyl salicylate,** N.F. 18.
Use: Pharmaceutic aid (flavor).

methyl salicylate w/combinations.
Use: Rubefacient rub (topical).
See: Analbalm, Liq. (Schwartz Pharma).
Analgesic Balm (Various Mfr.).
Banalg, Liniment (Forest).
Chloral-Methylol, Oint. (Ulmer).
Cydonol, Lot. (Gordon).
Emul-o-balm, Liq. (Medeva).
Gordobalm, Oint. (Gordon).
Listerine Antiseptic, Liq. (Warner-Lambert).
Musterole, Oint. (Schering Plough).
Pain Bust-R II, Cream (Continental).
Sloan's Liniment, Liq. (Warner-Lambert).

methyl sulfanil amidoisoxazole. Sulfamethoxazole.
See: Gantanol, Tab., Susp. (Roche Lab.).

●**methyltestosterone,** U.S.P. 23.
Use: Androgen.
See: Android-10 or 25, Tab. (Zeneca).
Arcosterone, Tab. (Arcum).
Metandren, Linguet, Tab. (Novartis).
Neo-Hombreol-M, Tab. (Organon).
Oreton-M, Tab., Buccal Tab. (Schering Plough).
Ostone, Tab. (Solvay).
Testred, Cap. (Zeneca).
Virilon, Cap. (Star).

Methyltestosterone. (Various Mfr.) 10 mg, 25 mg/Tab. Bot. 100s, 1000s. 10 mg/Tab., Buccal. Bot. 100s. *c-III.*
Use: Androgen.

methyltestosterone w/combinations.
Use: Androgen.
See: Android-5, 10 or 25, Tab. (Baxter).
Mediatric, Cap., Liq., Tab. (Wyeth-Ayerst).
Premarin w/Methyltestosterone, Tab. (Wyeth-Ayerst).
Virilon, Cap. (Star).

methylthionine chloride. Name used for Methylene Blue.

methylthionine hydrochloride. Name used for Methylene Blue.

methylthiouracil, U.S.P. XXI.
Use: Thyroid inhibition.

methyl violet.
See: Gentian Violet, Crystal Violet, Methylrosanaline Cl.

methyndamine. Name used for Tetrydamine.

●**methynodiol diacetate.** (meh-THIN-oh-die-ole die-ASS-eh-tate) USAN.
Use: Progestin.

●**methysergide.** (METH-ih-SIR-jide) USAN.
Use: Agent for migraine; vasoconstrictor.

●**methysergide maleate,** (METH-ih-SIR-jide) U.S.P. 23.
Use: Agent for migraine; vasoconstrictor.
See: Sansert, Tab. (Sandoz).

●**metiamide.** (meh-TIE-aim-id) USAN.
Histamine H₂ antagonist.
Use: Treatment for peptic ulcer; antagonist to histamine H₂ receptors.

●**metiapine.** (meh-TIE-ah-PEEN) USAN.
Use: Antipsychotic.

meticlopindol. Name used for Clopidol.

Meticorten. (Schering Plough) Prednisone 1 mg/Tab. Bot. 100s. *Rx.*
Use: Corticosteroid.

Metimyd Ophthalmic Oint. Sterile.
(Schering Plough) Prednisolone acetate 0.5% (5 mg), sulfacetamide sodium 10%. Tube 3.5 g. *Rx.*
Use: Corticosteroid, sulfonamide (topical).

Metimyd Ophthalmic Susp. Sterile.
(Schering Plough) Prednisolone acetate 0.5%, sulfacetamide sodium 10%. Bot. dropper 5 ml. *Rx.*
Use: Corticosteroid, sulfonamide, topical.

●**metioprim.** (meh-TIE-oh-PRIM) USAN.
Use: Antibacterial.

●**metipranolol.** (meh-tih-PRAN-oh-lahl) USAN.
Use: Antihypertensive (β-blocker, ophthalmic).
See: OptiPranolol (Bausch & Lomb).

metipranolol hydrochloride.
Use: Antihypertensive (β-blocker, ophthalmic).

metizoline. (meh-TIH-zoe-leen) F.D.A.
Use: Decongestant.

●**metizoline hydrochloride.** USAN.
Use: Adrenergic vasoconstrictor.

●**metkephamid acetate.** (MET-KEFF-am-id) USAN.
Use: Analgesic.

metoclopramide.

●**metoclopramide hydrochloride,** (MET-oh-kloe-PRA-mide) U.S.P. 23.
Use: Antiemetic, GI stimulant.
See: Reclomide, Tab. (Ultra).
Reglan, Amp. (Robins).

Metoclopramide Intensol. (Roxane)
Metoclopramide HCl 10 mg/ml, EDTA, sorbitol/Concentrated soln. Dropper Bot. 10 ml, 30 ml.
Use: Antiemetic, GI stimulant.

●**metocurine iodide,** (MEH-toe-CURE-een) U.S.P. 23. *Formerly Dimethyl Tubocurarine Iodide.*
Use: Neuromuscular blocking agent.
See: Metubine Iodide, Vial (Lilly).

metofurone. (MET-oh-fyoor-OHN) Name used for Nifurmerone.

●**metogest.** (MET-oh-JEST) USAN.
Use: Hormone.

●**metolazone,** (meh-TOLE-uh-ZONE) U.S.P. 23.
Use: Diuretic, antihypertensive.
See: Mykrox, Tab. (Medeva).
Zaroxolyn, Tab. (Medeva).

●**metopimazine.** (meh-toe-PIH-mazz-EEN) USAN.
Use: Antiemetic.

●**metoprine.** (MET-oh-preen) USAN.
Use: Antineoplastic.

●**metoprolol.** (meh-TOE-pro-lahl) USAN.
Use: Anti-adrenergic β-receptor.

•**metoprolol fumarate,** (meh-TOE-pro-lahl) U.S.P. 23.
Use: Antihypertensive.

•**metoprolol succinate.** (meh-TOE-pro-lahl) USAN.
Use: Antihypertensive; antianginal; treatment of myocardial infarction.
See: Toprol XL, Extended release Tab. (Astra).

•**metoprolol tartrate,** (meh-TOE-pro-lahl TAR-trate) U.S.P. 23.
Use: Antiadrenergic (β-receptor).
See: Lopressor, Tab. (Novartis).

metoprolol tartrate. (Various Mfr.) **Tab.**: 50 mg or 100 mg, lactose. Bot. 100s, 500s, 1000s, UD 100s. **Inj.**: 1 mg/ml. Amp. 5 ml.
Use: Antiadrenergic (β-receptor).

metoprolol tartrate and hydrochlorothiazide.
Use: Antihypertensive combination.
See: Lopressor HCT 100/50, Tab. (Novartis).
Lopressor HCT 100/25, Tab. (Novartis).
Lopressor HCT 50/25, Tab. (Novartis).

metoquine.
Use: Antimalarial.
See: Quinacrine HCl, U.S.P.

•**metoquizine.** (MET-oh-kwih-zeen) USAN.
Use: Antiulcer agent, anticholinergic.

Metreton Ophthalmic Solution. (Schering Plough) Prednisolone sodium phosphate 5.5 mg/ml. Bot. 5 ml. *Rx.*
Use: Corticosteroid, ophthalmic.

Metric 21. (Fielding) Metronidazole 250 mg/Tab. Bot. 100s. *Rx.*
Use: Anti-infective.

•**metrizamide.** (meh-TRIH-zam-ide) USAN.
Use: Myelography, diagnostic aid (radiopaque medium).
See: Amipaque, Inj. (Sanofi Winthrop).

•**metrizoate sodium.** USAN.
Use: Diagnostic aid (radiopaque medium).

Metrodin. (Serono) Urofollitropin 0.83 mg containing 75 IU follicle stimulating hormone (FSH) activity with sodium Cl 2 ml/Inj. Amp. 1, 10, 100. Urofollitropin 1.66 mg containing 150 IU FSH activity with sodium Cl 2 ml/Inj. Amp. 1. *Rx.*
Use: Ovulation stimulant.

Metrogel. (Galderma) Metronidazole 0.75%. Gel Tube 28.4 g. *Rx.*
Use: Antiacne.

Metrogel-Vaginal. (3M Pharm.) Metronidazole 0.75%, carbomer 934P, EDTA, parabens and propylene glycol. Gel/Tube (with applicator) 70 g. *Rx.*
Use: Anti-infective, vaginal.

Metrogesic. (Lexis) Salicylamide 325 mg, acetaminophen 162 mg, phenacetin 65 mg/Tab. Bot. 100s.
Use: Analgesic.

metrogestone. (MEH-troe-JEST-ohn)
Use: Progestin.

Metro I.V. (McGaw) Metronidazole 500 mg/100 ml. Inj. Vial 100 ml. Plastic containers 100 ml. *Rx.*
Use: Antibacterial.

•**metronidazole,** (meh-troe-NID-uh-zole) U.S.P. 23.
Use: Antiprotozoal (trichomonas); antitrichomonal. [Orphan drug]
See: Flagyl, Tab. (Searle).
Flagyl I.V., Vial (Searle).
Flagyl I.V. RTU, Vial (Searle).
MetroGel-Vaginal, Gel (3M Pharm.)
Metronid, Tab. (Ascher).
Metryl, Tab., Vial (Lemmon).

•**metronidazole hydrochloride.** (meh-troe-NIH-dah-zole) USAN.
Use: Antibacterial.
See: Flagyl I.V. (Searle).

•**metronidazole phosphate.** (meh-troe-NIH-dah-zole FOSS-fate) USAN.
Use: Anti-infective, antiprotozoal.

Metronidazole Redi-Infusion. (Elkins-Sinn) Metronidazole 500 mg/100 ml Vial. *Rx.*
Use: Amebicide.

Metrozole. (Lexis) Metronidazole 250 mg or 500 mg/Tab. **250 mg:** Bot. 100s, 250s; **500 mg:** Bot. 100s. *Rx.*
Use: Anti-infective, amebicide.

Metryl. (Lemmon) Metronidazole 250 mg/Tab. Bot. 100s, 250s, 500s, UD 100s. *Rx.*
Use: Anti-infective, amebicide.

Metryl 500. (Lemmon) Metronidazole 500 mg/Tab. Bot. 100s, 500s. *Rx.*
Use: Anti-infective, amebicide.

Metubine Iodide. (Lilly) Metocurine iodide 2 mg/ml. Vial 20 ml. *Rx.*
Use: Skeletal muscle relaxant.

•**meturedepa.** (meh-TOO-ree-DEH-pah) USAN.
Use: Antineoplastic.

Metussin. (Faraday) Dextromethorphan. Bot. 4 oz. *otc.*
Use: Antitussive.

Metussin Jr. (Faraday) Dextromethorphan. Bot. 4 oz. *otc.*
Use: Antitussive.

•**metyrapone,** (meh-TEER-ah-pone) U.S.P. 23.

Use: Diagnostic aid (pituitary function determination).
Adrenocortical enzyme inhibitor.
See: Metopirone, Amp. (Novartis).

• **metyrapone tartrate.** (meh-TEER-ah-pone) USAN.
Use: Diagnostic aid (pituitary function determination).

metyrapone tartrate injection.
Use: Diagnostic aid.

• **metyrosine,** U.S.P. 23.
Use: Antihypertensive.
See: Demser (Merck).

Mevacor. (Merck) Lovastatin Tab. **10 mg:** Bot. 60s; **20 mg:** Bot. 30s, 60s, 90s, 100s, 180s, 10,000s, UD 100s; **40 mg:** Bot. 60s, 90s, 10,000s. *Rx.*
Use: Antihyperlipidemic.

mevinolin.
See: Lovastatin.

Mexate-AQ. (Bristol-Myers/Bristol Oncology) Preservative-free liquid. Methotrexate 50 mg, 100 mg or 250 mg/Vial. *Rx.*
Use: Antineoplastic.

• **mexiletine hydrochloride,** (MEX-ih-leh-teen) U.S.P. 23.
Use: Cardiac depressant (antiarrhythmic).
See: Mexitil, Cap. (Boehringer Ingelheim).

mexiletine hydrochloride. (Various Mfr.) 150 mg, 200 mg or 250 mg/Cap. Bot. 100s, UD 100s (except 250 mg). *Rx.*
Use: Cardiac depressant (antiarrhythmic).

Mexitil. (Boehringer Ingelheim) Mexiletine HCl 150 mg, 200 mg or 250 mg/Cap. Bot. 100s, UD 100s. *Rx.*
Use: Antiarrhythmic.

• **mexrenoate potassium.** (mex-REN-oh-ate poe-TASS-ee-uhm) USAN.
Use: Aldosterone antagonist.

Mexsana Medicated Powder. (Schering Plough) Corn starch, kaolin, triclosan, zinc oxide. Can 3 oz, 6.25 oz, 11 oz. *otc.*
Use: Diaper rash product.

Meyenberg Goat Milk. (Jackson-Mitchell) Evaporated and powdered cans of goat milk. Foil pack 4 oz. (makes one quart). *otc.*
Use: Cows' milk allergies.

Mezlin. (Bayer) Mezlocillin sodium. Vial 1 g, 2 g, 3 g, 4 g. Infusion Bot. 2 g, 3 g, 4 g. *Rx.*
Use: Anti-infective, penicillin.

• **mezlocillin.** (MEZZ-low-SILL-in) USAN.
Use: Antibacterial.

• **mezlocillin sodium, sterile,** (MEZZ-low-SILL-in) U.S.P. 23.
Use: Antibacterial.
See: Mezlin, Inj. (Bayer).

MG Cold Sore Formula. (Outdoor Recreations) Menthol 1%, lidocaine, propylene glycol in alcohol base. Soln. Bot. 7.5 ml. *otc.*
Use: Cold sores, fever blisters.

MG-Oroate. (Miller) Magnesium (as magnesium orotate) 33 mg/Tab. Bot. 100s. *otc.*
Use: Magnesium supplement.

MG 217 Medicated Conditioner. (Triton) Coal tar solution 2%. Bot. 120 ml. *otc.*
Use: Antiseborrheic.

MG 217 Medicated Formula. (Triton) Coal tar solution 5%, colloidal sulfur 1.5%, salicylic acid 2% in a special base of cleansers, wetting agents and lanolin. Shampoo 120 ml, 240 ml. *otc.*
Use: Antiseborrheic, antipruritic.

MG 400. (Triton) Colloidal sulfur in Guy-Base II 5%, salicylic acid 3%. Shampoo. Bot. 240 ml, pt. *otc.*
Use: Antiseborrheic.

MG-Plus Protein. (Miller) Magnesium-protein complex made w/specially isolated soy protein 133 mg/Tab. Bot. 100s. *otc.*
Use: Magnesium supplement.

Miacalcin. (Sandoz) Calcitonin-salmon 200 IU, acetic acid 2.25 mg, phenol 5 mg, sodium acetate trihydrate 2 mg, sodium chloride 7.5 mg/ml. Inj. Vial 2 ml. *Rx.*
Use: Hormone.

Miacalcin Nasal Spray. (Sandoz) Calcitonin-salmon/activation (0.9 ml/dose) 200 IU, sodium chloride 8.5 mg/Spray. Bot. 2 ml. *Rx.*
Use: Antihypercalcemic.

Mi-Acid Gelcaps. (Major) Calcium carbonate 311 mg, magnesium carbonate 232 mg, parabens, EDTA. Bot. 50s. *otc.*
Use: Antacid.

Mi-Acid Liquid. (Major) Aluminum hydroxide 200 mg, magnesium hydroxide 200 mg, simethicone 20 mg/5 ml. Bot. 355 ml, 780 ml. *otc.*
Use: Antacid, antiflatulent.

Mi-Acid II Liquid. (Major) Aluminum hydroxide 400 mg, magnesium hydroxide 400 mg, simethicone 40 mg/5 ml. Bot. 355 ml. *otc.*
Use: Antacid, antiflatulent.

miadone.
See: Methadone HCl. (Various Mfr.).

●**mianserin hydrochloride.** (my-AN-ser-in) USAN. Under study.
Use: Serotonin inhibitor, antihistamine.

miaquin.
See: Camoquin, Tab. (Parke-Davis).

●**mibefradil dihydrochloride.** (mih-beh-FRAH-dill-die-HIGH-droe-KLOR-ide) USAN.
Use: Vasodilator.

●**mibolerone.** USAN.
Use: Anabolic, androgen.

Micanolol. (Bioglan Pharma) Anthralin 1%/Cream. Tube 50 g. *Rx.*
Use: Treatment of psoriasis.

micasorb. W/Red Veterinary Petrolatum.
See: RV Plus, Oint. (Baxter).

Micatin. (Advanced Care) Miconazole nitrate 2%. **Cream:** Tube 0.5 oz, 1 oz. **Spray powder:** Aerosol 3 oz. **Spray Liquid Aerosol:** Bot. 3.5 oz. *otc.*
Use: Antifungal, topical.

Mi-Cebrin. (Dista) Vitamins B_1 10 mg, B_2 5 mg, B_6 1.7 mg, pantothenic acid 10 mg, niacinamide 30 mg, B_{12} (activity equiv.) 3 mcg, C 100 mg, E 5.5 IU, A 10,000 IU, D 400 IU, iron 15 mg, copper 1 mg, iodine 0.15 mg, manganese 1 mg, magnesium 5 mg, zinc 1.5 mg/Tab. Pkg. 60s, 100s, 1000s, Blister pkg. 10 × 10s. *otc.*
Use: Vitamin/mineral supplement.

Mi-Cebrin T. (Dista) Vitamins B_1 15 mg, B_2 10 mg, B_6 2 mg, pantothenic acid 10 mg, niacinamide 100 mg, B_{12} 7.5 mcg, C 150 mg, E 5.5 IU, A 10,000 IU, D 400 IU, iron 15 mg, copper 1 mg, iodine 0.15 mg, manganese 1 mg, magnesium 5 mg, zinc 1.5 mg/Tab. Bot. 30s, 100s, 1000s, Blister pkg. 10 × 10s. *otc.*
Use: Vitamin/mineral supplement.

micofur. Anti 5-Nitro-2-Furaldoxime, Nifuroxime.
Use: Antifungal, anti-infective, topical.
See: Tricofuron, Vaginal Pow., Supp. (Eaton).

●**miconazole,** (my-KAHN-uh-zole) U.S.P. 23.
Use: Antifungal.
See: Monistat IV, Inj. (Janssen).

●**miconazole nitrate,** (my-CONE-ah-zole NYE-trate) U.S.P. 23.
Use: Antifungal.
See: Breezee Mist Antifungal, Pow. (Pedinol).
Fungoid Tincture, Soln. (Pedinol).
Maximum Strength Desenex Antifungal, Cream (Novartis).
Monistat, Cream, supp. (Ortho).

Monistat-3, Vaginal supp. (Ortho).
Monistat-7, Vaginal cream, supp. (Advanced Care).
Monistat-Derm, Prods. (Ortho).
Nibustat Prods. (Ortho).
Zeasorb-AF, Pow. (Stiefel).

miconazole nitrate. (Copley) Miconazole nitrate 2%. Cream. Tube 45 g (100 mg/dose for 7 doses). *otc.*
Use: Antifungal, vaginal.

miconazole nitrate. (Taro) Miconazole nitrate 2%, benzoic acid, mineral oil, apricot kernel oil. Cream. Tube 15 g, 30 g. *otc.*
Use: Antifungal, topical.

micoren. (Novartis) A respiratory stimulant; pending release.

Micrainin. (Wallace) Meprobamate 200 mg, aspirin 325 mg/Tab. Bot. 100s, UD 100s. *c-iv.*
Use: Analgesic combination.

MicRhoGAM. (Ortho Diagnostic) Rh_0 (D) immune globulin (Human) micro dose. Single-dose prefilled syringe. *Rx.*
Use: Agent for immunization.

Micrin Plus. (Johnson & Johnson) Water, S.D. alcohol 38-B, glycerin, poloxamer 407, flavor, sodium saccharin, glutamic acid buffer, cetylpyridinium Cl, FD & C Yellow #5, Blue #1. Bot. 12 oz, 24 oz. *otc.*
Use: Mouth preparation.

microbubble contrast agent. *Rx.*
Use: Aid in ID of intracranial tumors. [Orphan drug]

Microcult-GC Test. (Bayer) Miniaturized culture test for the detection of *Neisseria Gonorrhoeae.* Test Kit 25s.
Use: Diagnostic aid.

microfibrillar collagen hemostat.
Use: Hemostatic, topical.
See: Avitene (Alcon).
Hemopad (Astra).
Hemotene (Astra).

Micro-Guard. (Sween) Antimicrobial skin cream. Tube 0.5 oz, Jar 2 oz. *otc.*

Micro-K Extencaps. (Robins) Potassium Cl (8 mEq) 600 mg/Cap. Bot. 100s, 500s, Dis-Co pack 100s. *Rx.*
Use: Potassium supplement.

Micro-K 10 Extencaps. (Robins) Potassium Cl 750 mg (10 mEq)/Cap. Bot. 100s, 500s, Dis-co UD 100s. *Rx.*
Use: Potassium supplement.

Micro-K LS. (Robins) Potassium Cl 20 mEq (1500 mg). Extended release Susp. Packet 30s, 100s. *Rx.*
Use: Potassium supplement.

Microlipid. (Biosearch) Fat emulsion 50%, safflower oil, polyglycerol esters of fatty acids, soy lecithin, xanthan gum, ascorbic acid. Cal 4500, fat 500 g/L, 80 mOsm/Kg. H_2O. 120 ml. *Rx.*
Use: Nutritional supplement.

Micronase Tablets. (Pharmacia & Upjohn) Glyburide 1.25, 2.5 or 5 mg/Tab. **1.25 mg:** Bot. 100s. **2.5 mg:** Bot. 30s, 60s, 100s, UD 100s. **5 mg:** Bot. 30s, 60s, 90s, 100s, 500s, 1000s, UD 100s. *Rx.*
Use: Antidiabetic.

Micronefrin. (Bird) Racemic methylaminoethanol catechol HCl 2.25 g, sodium Cl, sodium bisulfite, potassium metabisulfite 0.99 g, chlorobutanol 0.5 g, benzoic acid 0.5 g, propylene glycol 8 mg/100 ml. Bot 15 ml, 30 ml. *Rx.*
Use: Antiasthmatic.

Micronized Glyburide. (Copley) 1.5 mg/Tab. Bot. 100s, UD 100s. 3 mg/Tab. Bot. 100s, 500s, 1000s, UD 100s. *Rx.*
Use: Treatment of diabetes.

Microsol. (Star) Sulfamethizole 0.5 g or 1 g/Tab. Bot. 100s, 1000s. *Rx.*
Use: Urinary anti-infective.

Microsol-A. (Star) Phenazopyridine 50 mg, sulfamethizole 0.5 g/Tab. Bot. 100s, 1000s. *Rx.*
Use: Urinary anti-infective.

Microstix Candida. (Bayer) Test for *Candida* species in vaginal specimens. Box 25s.
Use: Diagnostic aid.

Microstix-3 Reagent Strips. (Bayer) For recognition of nitrite in urine and for semi-quantitation of bacterial growth. Bot. 25s w/25 incubation pouches.
Use: Diagnostic aid.

Microtrak Chlamydia Trachomatis Direct Specimen Test. (Syva) To detect and identify chlamydia trachomatis. Slide test 60s.
Use: Diagnostic aid.

Microtrak HSV 1/HSV 2 Culture Confirmation/Typing Test. (Syva) For identification and typing of herpes simplex in tissue culture. Test kit 1s.
Use: Diagnostic aid.

Microtrak Neisseria Gonorrhea Culture Test. (Syva) For endocervical, urethral, rectal and pharyngeal cultures. Test kit 85s.
Use: Diganostic aid.

micrurus fulvius antivenin. (Wyeth-Ayerst) Inj. Combination package: One vial antivenin, one vial diluent (Bacteriostatic Water for Injection 10 ml.).

Use: Antivenin.

•**midaflur.** (MY-dah-flure) USAN.
Use: Sedative, hypnotic.

Midahist Expectorant. (Vangard) Codeine phosphate 10 mg, phenylpropanolamine HCl 18.75 mg, guaifenesin 100 mg/5 ml, alcohol 7.5%. Bot. pt, gal. *c-v.*
Use: Antitussive, decongestant, expectorant.

midamaline hydrochloride.
Use: Local anesthetic.

Midamor. (Merck) Amiloride 5 mg/Tab. Bot. 100s. *Rx.*
Use: Diuretic, antihypertensive.

Midaneed. (Hanlon) Vitamins A 5000 IU, D 500 IU, B_1 5 mg, B_2 3 mg, B_6 0.5 mcg, B_{12} 5 mcg, C 100 mg, niacinamide 10 mg, calcium pantothenate 5 mg/Cap. Bot. 100s. *otc.*
Use: Vitamin/mineral supplement.

Midatane DC Expectorant. (Vangard) Brompheniramine maleate 2 mg, guaifenesin 100 mg, phenylephrine HCl 5 mg, phenylpropanolamine HCl 5 mg, codeine phosphate 10 mg/5 ml, alcohol 3.5%. Bot. pt, gal. *c-v.*
Use: Antihistamine, expectorant, decongestant, antitussive.

Midatapp TR Tablets. (Vangard) Brompheniramine maleate 12 mg, phenylephrine HCl 15 mg, phenylpropanolamine HCl 15 mg/Tab. Bot. 100s, 500s, 1000s. *Rx.*
Use: Antihistamine, decongestant.

•**midazolam hydrochloride.** (meh-DAZE-oh-lam) USAN.
Use: Anesthetic (injectable).
See: Versed, Inj. (Roche).

•**midazolam maleate.** (meh-DAZE-oh-lam) USAN.
Use: Anesthetic, intravenous.

Midchlor. (Schein) Isometheptene mucate 65 mg, dichloralphenazone 100 mg, acetaminophen 325 mg/Cap. Bot. 100s. *Rx.*
Use: Agent for migraine.

•**midodrine hydrochloride.** (MIH-doe-DREEN) USAN.
Use: Antihypotensive, vasoconstrictor.
See: ProAmatine, Tab. (Roberts).

Midol for Cramps Caplets. (Bayer) Aspirin 500 mg, caffeine 32.4 mg, cinnamedrine HCl 14.9 mg/Tab. In 8s, 16s, 32s. *otc.*
Use: Analgesic combination.

Midol IB. (Bayer) Ibuprofen 200 mg. Tab. Bot. 50s. *otc.*
Use: Nonsteroidal anti-inflammatory drug, analgesic.

Midol Maximum Strength. (Bayer) Cinnamedrine HCl 14.9 mg, aspirin 500 mg, caffeine 32.4 mg/Tab. Bot. 12s, 30s, 60s. *otc.*
Use: Analgesic combination.

Midol Multi-Symptom, Maximum Strength. (Bayer) Acetaminophen 500 mg, pyrilamine maleate 15 mg. Capl. Bot. 32s. *otc.*
Use: Analgesic combination.

Midol Multi-Symptom, Regular Strength. (Bayer) Acetaminophen 325 mg, pyrilamine maleate 12.5 mg. Capl. Bot. 32s. *otc.*
Use: Analgesic combination.

Midol Multi-Symptom Menstrual, Maximum Strength. (Bayer) Acetaminophen 500 mg, caffeine 60 mg, pyrilamine maleate 15 mg. Capl. Pkg. 8s, 16s, 32s. Gelcaps. Pkg. 12s, 24s. *otc.*
Use: Analgesic combination.

Midol Original Formula. (Bayer) Cinnamedrine HCl 14.9 mg, aspirin 454 mg, caffeine 32.4 mg/Tab. Bot. 30s, 60s. Strip pack 12s. *otc.*
Use: Analgesic combination.

Midol PM. (Bayer) Acetaminophen 500 mg, diphenhydramine 25 mg. Capl. Pkg. 16s. *otc.*
Use: Analgesic combination.

Midol Teen. (Bayer) Acetaminophen 400 mg, pamabrom 25 mg/Cap. Pkg. 16s, 32s. *otc.*
Use: Analgesic combination.

Midrin. (Carnrick) Isometheptene mucate 65 mg, acetaminophen 325 mg, dichloralphenazone 100 mg/Cap. Bot. 50s, 100s. *Rx.*
Use: Agent for migraine.

•**mifobate.** (mih-FOE-bate) USAN.
Use: Antiatherosclerotic.

•**miglitol.** (mih-GLIH-tole) USAN.
Use: Antidiabetic.
See: Glycet, Tab. (Bayer Corp.).

migraine agents.
See: Sansert, Tab. (Sandoz).
Ergostat, Tab. (Parke-Davis).
Medihaler Ergotamine, Aerosol (3M).
D.H.E. 45, Inj. (Sandoz).
Imitrex (Glaxo).

migraine combinations.
See: Isometheptene/Dichloralphenazone/Acetaminophen. (Various Mfr.).
Isocom, Cap. (Nutripharm).
Isopap, Cap. (Geneva Pharm).
Midchlor, Cap. (Schein).
Midrin, Cap. (Carnrick).
Migratine, Cap. (Major).

Migratine. (Major) Isometheptene mucate 65 mg, dichloralphenazone 100 mg, acetaminophen 325 mg/Cap. Bot. 100s, 250s. *Rx.*
Use: Agent for migraine.

MIH.
Use: Antineoplastic.
See: Matulane (Roche).

•**milacemide hydrochloride.** (mill-ASS-eh-mide HIGH-droe-KLOR-ide) USAN.
Use: Anticonvulsant, antidepressant.

•**milameline hydrochloride.** USAN.
Use: Antidementia (partial muscarinic agonist).

mild silver protein.
See: Silver Protein, Mild.

•**milenperone.** (mih-LEN-per-OHN) USAN.
Use: Antipsychotic.

Miles Nervine. (Bayer) Diphenhydramine HCl 25 mg/Tab. Pkg. 12s, Bot. 30s. *otc.*
Use: Nonprescription sleep aid.

•**milipertine.** (MIH-lih-PURR-teen) USAN.
Use: Antipsychotic.

Milkinol. (Schwarz Pharma Kremers-Urban) Mineral oil in an emulsifying base. Bot. 240 ml. *otc.*
Use: Laxative.

milk of bismuth. (Various Mfr.) Bismuth hydroxide, bismuth subcarb.
Use: Orally, intestinal disturbances.

•**milk of magnesia,** (milk of mag-NEE-zhuh) U.S.P. 23. Formerly Magnesia Magma.
Use: Antacid, laxative.
See: Magnesium hydroxide (Various Mfr.).

milk of magnesia. (Various Mfr.). Magnesia (Magnesium hydroxide) 325 mg, 390 mg. **Tab.:** 250s, 1000s; **Liq.:** 120 ml, 360 ml, 720 ml, pt, qt, gal, UD 10 ml, 15 ml, 20 ml, 30 ml, 100 ml, 180 ml, 400 ml. **Susp.:** Pt, qt, gal, UD 15 and 30 ml.
Use: Antacid, laxative.

Milk of Magnesia-Concentrated. (Roxane) Magnesium hydroxide. Liq. Bot. 100 ml, 180 ml, 400 ml, UD 10 ml, 15 ml, 20 ml, 30 ml.
Use: Antacid.

Millazine. (Major) Thioridazine. **10 mg or 15 mg/Tab.:** Bot. 100s; **25 mg/Tab.:** Bot. 100s, 1000s; **100 mg, 150 mg or 200 mg/Tab.:** Bot. 100s, 500s. *Rx.*
Use: Antipsychotic agent.

•**milodistim.** USAN.
Use: Colony stimulating factor for cells of granulocyte and megakarocyte lineage hematopoietic stimulant (antineutropenic).

Milontin. (Parke-Davis) Phensuximide 0.5 g/Kapseal. Bot. 100s. *Rx.*
Use: Anticonvulsant.

Milophene. (Milex) Clomiphene citrate 50 mg/Tab. 30s. *Rx.*
Use: Ovulation stimulant.

Milpar. (Sanofi Winthrop) Magnesium hydroxide, mineral oil. *otc.*
Use: Antacid, laxative.

•**milrinone.** (MILL-rih-nohn) USAN.
Use: Cardiotonic, congestive heart failure.
See: Primacor (Sanofi Winthrop).

Milroy Artificial Tears. (Milton Roy) Bot. 22 ml. *otc.*
Use: Artificial tear solution.

Miltown. (Wallace) Meprobamate. **200 mg/Tab.** Bot. 100s. **400 mg/Tab.** Bot. 100s, 500s, 1000s. **600 mg/Tab.** Bot. 100s. *c-iv.*
Use: Antianxiety agent.
See: Meprospan (Wallace).

Miltown 600. (Wallace) Meprobamate 600 mg/Tab. Bot. 100s. *c-iv.*
Use: Antianxiety agent.

•**mimbane hydrochloride.** (MIM-bane) USAN. 1-Methyl-yohimbane HCl.
Use: Analgesic.

•**minaprine.** (MIN-ah-preen) USAN.
Use: Psychotropic.

•**minaprine hydrochloride.** (MIN-ah-preen) USAN.
Use: Antidepressant.

•**minaxolone.** (min-AX-oh-lone) USAN.
Use: Anesthetic.

mincard.
Use: Diuretic.

Mineral Ice, Therapeutic. (Bristol-Myers Products) Menthol 2%, ammonium hydroxide, carbomer 934, cupric sulfate, isopropyl alcohol, magnesium sulfate, thymol. Gel. Tube 105 g, 240 g, 480 g. *otc.*
Use: Liniment.

mineral-corticoids.
See: Desoxycorticosterone salts (Various Mfr.).

•**mineral oil,** U.S.P. 23.
Use: Laxative, pharmaceutic aid (solvent, oleaginous vehicle).
See: Petrolatum, Liq (Various Mfr.).

mineral oil emulsion.
Use: Cathartic.

mineral oil enema.
Use: Cathartic.

•**mineral oil, light,** N.F. 18.
Use: Pharmaceutic aid (tablet and capsule lubricant, vehicle).

Minibex. (Faraday) Vitamins B$_1$ 6 mg, B$_2$ 3 mg, B$_6$ 0.5 mg, C 50 mg, niacinamide 10 mg, calcium pantothenate 3 mg, B$_{12}$ 2 mcg, folic acid 0.1 mg/Cap. Bot. 100s, 250s, 1000s. *otc.*
Use: Vitamin/mineral supplement.

Minidyne 10%. (Pedinol) Povidone-iodine 10%, citric acid, sodium phosphate dibasic. Soln. Bot. 15 ml. *otc.*
Use: Antiseptic, germicide.

Mini-Gamulin Rh. (Centeon) Rh$_o$ (D) Immune Globulin (Human). Single-dose vial. *Rx.*
Use: Agent for immunization.

Minipress. (Pfizer Laboratories) Prazosin HCl 1 mg, 2 mg or 5 mg/Cap. **1 mg, 2 mg:** Bot. 250s, 1000s, UD 100s; **5 mg:** Bot. 250s, 500s, UD 100s. *Rx.*
Use: Antihypertensive.

Minitec. (Squibb) Sodium pertechnetate Tc 99 m generator.
Use: Radiopaque agent.

Minitec Generator (Complete with Components). (Squibb) Medotopes Kit.
Use: Diagnostic aid.

Mini Thin Asthma Relief. (BDI Pharm) Ephedrine HCl 25 mg, guaifenesin 100 mg or 200 mg/Tab. Bot. 60s (25/100 mg), 100s (25/200 mg). *otc.*
Use: Antiasthmatic.

Mini Thin Pseudo. (BDI Pharm) Pseudoephedrine HCl 60 mg/Tab. Bot. 60s. *otc.*
Use: Decongestant.

Minitran Transdermal Delivery System. (3M Pharm.) Nitroglycerin 9 mg, 18 mg, 36 mg or 54 mg. Patch 33s. *Rx.*
Use: Antianginal.

Minit-Rub. (Bristol-Myers) Methyl salicylate 15%, methol 3.5%, camphor 2.3% in anhydrous base. Tube 1.5 oz, 3 oz. *otc.*
Use: Analgesic, topical.

Minizide. (Pfizer) Prazosin HCl and polythiazide. **Minizide 1:** Prazosin 1 mg, polythiazide 0.5 mg/Cap. **Minizide 2:** Prazosin 2 mg, polythiazide 0.5 mg/Cap. **Minizide 5:** Prazosin 5 mg, polythiazide 0.5 mg/Cap. Bot. 100s. *Rx.*
Use: Antihypertensive.

Minocin. (Lederle) Minocycline HCl **Cap., pellet-filled 50 mg:** Bot. 100s, UD 10 × 10s; **100 mg:** Bot. 50s, 100s, UD 10 × 10s. **I.V.:** 100 mg/Vial. **Oral Susp.:** 50 mg/5 ml, propylparaben 0.1%, butylparaben 0.06%, alcohol 5% v/v. Bot. 2 oz. *Rx.*
Use: Anti-infective, tetracycline.

•**minocromil.** (MIH-no-KROE-mill) USAN.
Use: Antiallergic (prophylactic).

•**minocycline.** (mihn-oh-SIGH-kleen) USAN.
Use: Antibacterial.
See: Minocyn (Lederle).

•**minocycline hydrochloride,** (mihn-oh-SIGH-kleen) U.S.P. 23.
Use: Antibacterial. [Orphan drug]
See: Dynacin, Cap. (Medicis Dermatologics).
Minocin, Cap., Syr., Vial (Lederle).

minocycline hydrochloride. (Warner Chilcott) Cap. **50 mg:** Bot. 100s; **100 mg:** Bot. 50s.
Use: Antibacterial.

minoxidil. (min-OX-ih-dill) (Schein) Minoxidil 2.5 mg/Tab. Bot. 100s, 500s, 1000s. *Rx.*
Use: Antihypertensive.

minoxidil. (min-OX-ih-dill) (Rugby) Minoxidil 10 mg/Tab. Bot. 500s. *Rx.*
Use: Antihypertensive.

•**minoxidil,** (min-OX-ih-dill) U.S.P. 23.
Use: Antihypertensive, peripheral vasodilator, hair growth stimulant (topical).
See: Loniten, Tab. (Pharmacia & Upjohn).

Minoxidil for Men. (Lemmon) Minoxidil 2%, alcohol 60%/Soln (topical).
Pouches. 60 ml single and twin. *otc.*
Use: Male pattern baldness.

minoxidil, topical.
Use: Male pattern baldness.
See: Rogaine, Soln. (Pharmacia & Upjohn).

Mintezol. (Merck) Thiabendazole. **Susp.:** 500 mg/5 ml. Bot. 120 ml. **Chew. Tab.:** 500 mg. Pkg. 36s. *Rx.*
Use: Anthelmintic.

Minto-Chlor Syrup. (Pal-Pak) Codeine sulfate 10 mg, potassium citrate 219 mg, alcohol 2%. Gal. *c-v.*
Use: Antitussive, expectorant.

Mintox. (Major) Aluminum hydroxide 200 mg, magnesium hydroxide 200 mg. Tab. Bot. 100s. *otc.*
Use: Antacid.

Mintox Plus Extra Strength Liquid. (Major) Aluminum hydroxide 500 mg, magnesium hydroxide 450 mg, simethicone 40 mg/5 ml. Bot. 355 ml. *otc.*
Use: Antacid, antiflatulent.

Mintox Plus Tablets. (Major) Aluminum hydroxide 200 mg, magnesium hydroxide 200 mg, simethicone 25 mg. Chew. Tab. 100s. *otc.*
Use: Antacid, antiflatulent.

Mintox Suspension. (Major) Aluminum hydroxide 225 mg, magnesium hydroxide 200 mg, parabens, saccharin, sorbitol/5 ml. Susp. Bot. 355 ml, 780 ml. *otc.*
Use: Antacid, antiflatulent.

Mint Sensodyne. (Block) Potassium nitrate 5%, saccharin, sorbitol. Toothpaste. Tube 28.3 g. *otc.*
Use: Toothpaste for sensitive teeth.

Minute-Gel. (Oral-B) Acidulated phosphate fluoride 1.23% Gel. Bot. 16 oz. *Rx.*
Use: Dental caries preventative.

Miochol-E. (Ciba Vision) Acetylcholine Cl 1:100, mannitol 2.8% when reconstituted. Soln. In 2 ml univials. *Rx.*
Use: Agent for glaucoma.

•**mioflazine hydrochloride.** (MY-ah-FLAY-zeen) USAN.
Use: Vasodilator (coronary).

Miostat Intraocular Solution. (Alcon Surgical) Carbochol 0.01%. Vial 1.5 ml. Pkg. 12s. *Rx.*
Use: Agent for glaucoma.

miotics, cholinesterase inhibitors.
Use: Agents for glaucoma.
See: Humorsal, Soln. (Merck).
Eserine Sulfate, Oint. (Various Mfr.).
Isopto Eserine, Soln. (Alcon).
Eserine Salicylate, Soln. (Alcon).
Phospholine Iodide, Pow. (Wyeth-Ayerst).
Floropryl, Oint. (Merck).

•**mipafilcon a.** (mih-paff-ILL-kahn A) USAN.
Use: Contact lens material (hydrophilic).

Miradon. (Schering Plough) Anisindione 50 mg/Tab. Bot. 100s. *Rx.*
Use: Anticoagulant.

MiraFlow Extra Strength. (Ciba Vision) Isopropyl alcohol 15.7%, poloxamer 407, amphoteric 10. Thimerosal free. Soln. Bot. 12 ml. *otc.*
Use: Contact lens care.

Miral. (Armenpharm) Dexamethasone 0.75 mg/Tab. Bot. 100s, 1000s. *Rx.*
Use: Corticosteroid.

MiraSept. (Alcon) **Disinfecting Solution:** Hydrogen peroxide 3%, sodium stannate, sodium nitrate. Bot. 120 ml. **Rinse and neutralizer:** Boric acid, sodium borate, sodium Cl, sodium pyruvate, EDTA. Bot. 120 ml (2s). *otc.*
Use: Soft contact lens care.

•**mirfentanil hydrochloride.** (MIHR-FEN-tan-ill) USAN.
Use: Analgesic.

•**mirincamycin hydrochloride.** (mihr-IN-kah-MY-sin) USAN.
Use: Antibacterial, antimalarial.

•**mirisetron maleate.** (my-RIH-seh-trahn) USAN.

Use: Antianxiety.

• **mirtazapine.** (mihr-TAZZ-ah-PEEN) USAN.
Use: Antidepressant.
See: Remeron, Tab. (Organon).

• **misonidazole.** (MY-so-NIH-dah-zole) USAN.
Use: Antiprotozoal (trichomonas).

• **misoprostol.** (MY-so-PRAHST-ole) USAN.
Use: Antiulcerative.
See: Cytotec, Tab. (Searle).

Mission Prenatal. (Mission) Ferrous gluconate 260 mg (iron 30 mg), vitamins C 100 mg, B_1 5 mg, B_6 3 mg, B_2 2 mg, B_3 10 mg, B_5 1 mg, B_{12} 2 mcg, A 4000 IU, D 400 IU, Ca, zinc 15 mg/Tab. Bot. 100s. *otc.*
Use: Vitamin/mineral supplement.

Mission Prenatal F.A. (Mission) Ferrous gluconate 260 mg (iron 30 mg), vitamins C 100 mg, B_1 5 mg, B_6 10 mg, B_2 2 mg, B_3 10 mg, B_{12} 2 mcg, folic acid 0.8 mg, A acetate 4000 IU, D 400 IU, Ca, B_5 1 mg/Tab. Bot. 100s. *otc.*
Use: Vitamin/mineral supplement.

Mission Prenatal H.P. (Mission) Ferrous gluconate 260 mg (iron 30 mg), vitamins C 100 mg, B_1 5 mg, B_6 25 mg, B_2 2 mg, B_3 10 mg, B_5 1 mg, B_{12} 2 mcg, folic acid 0.8 mg, A 4000 IU, D 400 IU, Ca/Tab. Bot. 100s. *otc.*
Use: Vitamin/mineral supplement.

Mission Prenatal-RX. (Mission) Vitamins A 8000 IU, D 400 IU, C 240 mg, B_1 4 mg, B_2 2 mg, B_3 20 mg, B_5 10 mg, B_6 20 mg, B_{12} 8 mcg, folic acid 1 mg, iron 60 mg, calcium 175 mg, I, zinc 15 mg, Cu/Tab. Bot. 100s. *Rx.*
Use: Vitamin/mineral supplement.

Mission Surgical Supplement. (Mission) Vitamins C 500 mg, B_1 2.5 mg, B_2 2.6 mg, B_3 30 mg, B_5 16.3 mg, B_6 3.6 mg, B_{12} 9 mcg, A 5000 IU, D 400 IU, E 45 IU, iron 27 mg, zinc 22.5 mg/Tab. Bot. 100s. *otc.*
Use: Vitamin/mineral supplement.

Mithracin. (Bayer) Plicamycin 2500 mcg/Vial. Unit vial 10s. *Rx.*
Use: Antineoplastic, antihypercalcemic.

mithramycin. (MITH-rah-MY-sin)
Use: Antineoplastic.
See: Plicamycin.

• **mitindomide.** (my-TIN-doe-MIDE) USAN.
Use: Antineoplastic.

• **mitocarcin.** (MY-toe-CAR-sin) USAN. Antibiotic derived from *Streptomyces* species.

Use: Antineoplastic.

• **mitocromin.** (MY-toe-KROE-min) USAN. Produced by *Streptomyces virdochromogenes.*
Use: Antineoplastic.

• **mitogillin.** (MY-toe-GIH-lin) USAN. An antibiotic obtained from a "unique strain" of *Aspergillus restrictus.*
Use: Antitumorigenic antibiotic; antineoplastic.

mitoguazone. (CTRC Research) *Rx.*
Use: Treatment of diffuse non-Hodgkin's lymphoma. [Orphan drug]

mitolactol.
Use: Adjuvant therapy in the treatment of primary brain tumors. [Orphan drug]

• **mitomalcin.** (MY-toe-MAL-sin) USAN. Produced by *Streptomyces malayensis.* Under study.
Use: Antineoplastic.

• **mitomycin,** (MY-toe-MY-sin) U.S.P. 23. In literature as Mitomycin C. Antibiotic isolated from *Streptomyces caespitosis.*
Use: Anti-infective; antineoplastic.
See: Mutamycin, Inj. (Bristol).

• **mitosper.** (MY-toe-sper) USAN. Substance derived from *Aspergillus* of the glaucus group.
Use: Antineoplastic.

• **mitotane,** (MY-toe-TANE) U.S.P. 23. *Formerly o,p'-DDD.*
Use: Antineoplastic.
See: Lysodren, Tab. (Bristol-Myers Oncology).

• **mitoxantrone hydrochloride,** (MY-toe-ZAN-trone) U.S.P. 23.
Use: Antineoplastic. [Orphan drug]
See: Novantrone (Lederle).

Mitran. (Roberts) Chlordiazepoxide HCl 10 mg/Cap. Bot. 100s. *c-iv.*
Use: Antianxiety agent.

Mitrolan. (Robins) Calcium polycarbophil equivalent to polycarbophil 500 mg/Tab. Blister Pak 36s, 100s. *otc.*
Use: Laxative.

• **mivacurium chloride.** (mih-vah-CURE-ee-uhm) USAN.
Use: Blocking agent (neuromuscular).

Mixed Respiratory Vaccine. Each ml contains *Staphylococcus aureus* 1,200 million organisms, *Streptococcus* (both *viridans* and non-hemolytic) 200 million organisms, *Streptococcus (Diplococcus) pneumoniae* 150 million organisms, *Moraxella (Branhamella, Neisseria) catarrhalis* 150 million organisms, *Klebsiella pneumoniae* 150 million organisms, and *Haemophilus influenzae*

types a and b 150 million organisms. Vial. 20 ml.
Use: Bacterial vaccine.
See: MRV, Inj. (Bayer).

mixed vespid Hymenoptera venom. *Rx.*
Use: Agent for immunization.
See: Albay (Bayer).
Pharmalgen (ALK Laboratories).
Venomil (Bayer).

•**mixidine.** (MIX-ih-deen) USAN.
Use: Vasodilator (coronary).

mixture 612. Dimethyl Phthalate Solution, Compound.

M-M-R II. (Merck) Lyophilized preparation of live attenuated measles virus vaccine (Attenuvax), live attenuated mumps virus vaccine (Mumpsvax), live attenuated rubella virus vaccine (Meruvax II). See details under Attenuvax, Mumpsvax and Meruvax II. Single dose vial w/diluent. Pkg. 1s, 10s. *Rx.*
Use: Agent for immunization.

Moban. (DuPont Merck) Molindone HCl.
Liq.: 20 mg/ml concentrate. Bot. 4 oz/ w dropper. **Tab.:** 5 mg, 10 mg, 25 mg, 50 mg or 100 mg/Tab. Bot. 100s. *Rx.*
Use: Antipsychotic.

mobenol.
See: Tolbutamide, U.S.P. 23.

Mobidin. (Ascher) Magnesium salicylate, anhydrous 600 mg/Tab. Bot. 100s, 500s. *Rx.*
Use: Antiarthritic.

Mobigesic. (Ascher) Magnesium salicylate 325 mg, phenyltoloxamine citrate 30 mg/ Tab. Bot. 50s, 100s, Pkg. 18s. *otc.*
Use: Analgesic combination.

Mobisyl Creme. (Ascher) Trolamine salicylate in vanishing creme base. Tubes 100 g. *otc.*
Use: Analgesic, topical.

moccasin bite.
See: Antivenin (Crotalidae).

•**moclobemide.** (moe-KLOE-beh-mide) USAN.
Use: Antidepressant.

moctanin. (Ethitek) Glyceryl-l-mono-octanoate (80-85%), glyceryl-l-mono-decanoate (10-15%), glyceryl-l-2-di-octanoate (10-15%), free glyceryl (2.5% maximum). Bot. 120 ml. *Rx.*
Use: Gallstone-solubilizing agent.

•**modafinil.** (moe-DAFF-ih-nill) USAN.
Use: Analeptic treatment of narcolepsy and hypersomnia. [Orphan drug]

•**modaline sulfate.** (MODE-al-een) USAN
Use: Antidepressant.

Modane. (Pharmacia & Upjohn)

Phenolphthalein 130 mg/Tab. Pkg. 10s, 30s. Bot. 100s. *otc.*
Use: Laxative.

Modane Bulk. (Pharmacia & Upjohn) Powdered mixture of equal parts of psyllium and dextrose. Container 14 oz. *otc.*
Use: Laxative.

Modane Mild. (Pharmacia & Upjohn) Phenolphthalein 60 mg/Tab. Bot. 10s, 30s, 100s. *otc.*
Use: Laxative.

Modane Plus. (Pharmacia & Upjohn) Phenolphthalein 60 mg, docusate sodium 100 mg/Tab. Bot. 100s, Box 10s, 30s. *otc.*
Use: Laxative.

Modane Soft. (Pharmacia & Upjohn) Docusate sodium 100 mg/Cap. UD Pkg. 30s. *otc.*
Use: Laxative.

Modane Versabran. (Pharmacia & Upjohn) Psyllium hydrophilic mucilloid in wheat bran base. Dose 3.4 g, Bot. 10 oz. *otc.*
Use: Laxative.

•**modecainide.** (moe-deh-CANE-ide) USAN.
Use: Cardiac depressant (antiarrhythmic).

Modicon 21. (Ortho) Norethindrone 0.5 mg, ethinyl estradiol 35 mcg/Tab. Dialpak 21s. *Rx.*
Use: Oral contraceptive.

Modicon 28. (Ortho) Norethindrone 0.5 mg, ethinyl estradiol 35 mcg/Tab., 7 inert Tab. Dialpak 28s. *Rx.*
Use: Oral contraceptive.

modified burow's solution.
See: Burow's solution.

modinal.
See: Gardinol Type Detergents (Various Mfr.).

Modical. (Bristol-Myers) Maltodextrin. Pow. Can 13 oz. *otc.*
Use: Nutritional supplement.

Moduretic. (Merck) Hydrochlorothiazide 50 mg, amiloride 5 mg/Tab. Bot. 100s, UD 100s. *Rx.*
Use: Diuretic, antihypertensive.

moenomycin. Phosphorus-containing glycolipide antibiotic. Active against gram-positive organisms. Under study.

•**moexipril hydrochloride.** (moe-EX-ah-prill) USAN.
Use: Antihypertensive, ACE inhibitor.
See: Univasc, Tab. (Schwarz Pharma).

•**mofegiline hydrochloride.** (moe-FEH-jih-leen) USAN.

Use: Treatment of Parkinson's disease.

Moist Again. (Lake) Aloe vera, EDTA, methylparaben, glycerin. Gel. Tube 70.8 g. *otc.*
Use: Vaginal preparation.

Moi-Stir. (Kingswood) Dibasic sodium phosphate, magnesium, calcium, sodium Cl, potassium Cl, sorbitol, sodium carboxymethylcellulose, parabens. Soln. 120 ml with pump spray. *otc.*
Use: Saliva substitute.

Moi-Stir Swabsticks. (Kingswood) Dibasic sodium phosphate, magnesium, calcium, sodium Cl, potassium Cl, sorbitol, sodium carboxymethylcellulose, parabens. Soln. Pkt. 3s. *otc.*
Use: Saliva substitute.

Moisture Drops. (Bausch & Lomb) Hydroxypropyl methylcellulose 0.5%, povidone 0.1%, glycerin 0.2%, benzalkonium Cl 0.01%, EDTA, sodium Cl, boric acid, potassium Cl, sodium borate. Soln. Bot. 0.5 oz, 1 oz. *otc.*
Use: Artificial tear solution.

Moisturel Lotion. (Westwood Squibb) Petrolatum, glycerin, dimethicone steareth-2, cetyl alcohol, benzyl alcohol, laureth-23, carbomer-934, magnesium aluminum silicate, quaternium-15. Lot. Bot. 240 ml. *otc.*
Use: Emollient.

molar phosphate.
W/Fluoride ion.
See: Coral Prods. (Young Dental).
  Karigel, Gel. (Young Dental).

molecusol-carbamazepine.
See: PR-320.

•**molgramostim.** (mahl-GRAH-moe-STIM) USAN.
Use: Hematopoietic stimulant, antineutropenic.

•**molinazone.** (moe-LEEN-ah-zone) USAN.
Use: Analgesic.

•**molindone hydrochloride,** (moe-LIN-dohn) U.S.P. 23.
Use: Antipsychotic.
See: Lidone, Cap. (Abbott).
  Lidone Concentrate, Liq. (Abbott).
  Moban, Tab. (DuPont Merck).

Mol-Iron Tablets. (Schering Plough) Ferrous sulfate 195 mg, (equivalent 39 mg elemental iron)/Tab. Bot. 100s. *otc.*
Use: Iron supplement.
W/Vitamin C (Schering Plough) Ferrous sulfate 195 mg, ascorbic acid 75 mg/Tab. Bot. 100s.

Mollifene Ear Drops. (Pfeiffer) Glycerin, camphor, cajaput oil, eucalyptus oil, thyme oil. Soln. Bot. 24 ml. *otc.*
Use: Otic preparation.

•**molsidomine.** (mole-SIH-doe-meen) USAN.
Use: Antianginal, vasodilator (coronary).

molybdenum solution. (American Quinine) Molybdenum 25 mcg/ml (as 46 mcg/ml ammonium molybdate tetrahydrate). Inj. Vial 10 ml. *Rx.*
Use: Parenteral nutritional supplement.

Molycu. (Burns) Meprobamate 400 mg, copper 60 mg/ml. *Rx.*
Use: Antidote.

Moly-Pak. (SoloPak) Molybdenum 25 mcg. Inj. Vial 10 ml. *Rx.*
Use: Parenteral nutritional supplement.

Molypen. (Fujisawa) Ammonium molybdate tetrahydrate 46 mcg/ml. Vial 10 ml. *Rx.*
Use: Parenteral nutritional supplement.

Momentum. (Whitehall Robins) Aspirin 500 mg, phenyltoloxamine citrate 15 mg/Capl. Bot. 24s, 48s. *otc.*
Use: Analgesic.

Momentum Muscular Backache Formula. (Whitehall) Magnesium salicylate tetrahydrate 580 mg (equivalent to 467 mg magnesium salicylate anhydrous)/Cap. Box. 48s. *otc.*
Use: Nonnarcotic analgesic compound.

•**mometasone furoate.** (moe-MET-uh-SONE FYU-roh-ate) U.S.P. 23.
Use: Topical steroid.
See: Elocon Cream, Oint., Lot. (Schering Plough).

monacetyl pyrogallol. Eugallol. Pyrogallol Monoacetate.
Use: Keratolytic.

Monafed. (Monarch Pharmaceuticals) Guaifenesin 600 mg, lactose/SR Tab. Bot. 100s. *Rx.*
Use: Expectorant.

Monafed DM. (Monarch Pharmaceuticals) Guaifenesin 600 mg, dextromethorphan HBr 30 mg/ER Tab. Bot. 100s. *Rx.*
Use: Antitussive, expectorant.

monalium hydrate. Hydrated magnesium aluminate. Magalorate.
See: Riopan, Tab., Susp. (Wyeth-Ayerst).

•**monatepil maleate.** (moe-NAT-eh-pill) USAN.
Use: Antianginal; antihypertensive.

•**monensin,** (mah-NEN-sin) U.S.P. 23.
Use: Antiprotozoal, antibacterial, antifungal.

•**monensin sodium,** (mah-NEN-sin) U.S.P. 23.

Use: Antibacterial, antifungal, antiprotozoal.

Monistat Dual-Pak. (Ortho) Miconazole nitrate suppositories and cream. **200 mg/Supp.:** Pkg. 3s w/applicator; **Cream 2%.:** Tube 15 g, 30 g, 90 g. *Rx.*
Use: Antifungal, vaginal.

Monistat 3 Vaginal Suppositories. (Ortho) Miconazole nitrate 200 mg/Supp. Pkg. 3s w/applicator. *Rx.*
Use: Antifungal, vaginal.

Monistat IV. (Janssen) Miconazole 10 mg/ml, PEG 40, castor oil, lactate, methylparaben, propylparaben, water. Amp. 20 ml. *Rx.*
Use: Antifungal.

Monistat 7 Vaginal Cream. (Advanced Care) Miconazole nitrate 2% in water-miscible cream. Tube 45 g w/dose applicator. *otc.*
Use: Antifungal, vaginal.

Monistat 7 Vaginal Suppositories. (Advanced Care) Miconazole nitrate 100 mg/Supp. Pkg. 7s w/applicator. *otc.*
Use: Antifungal, vaginal.

Monistat 7 Combination Pack. (Advanced Care) **Vaginal Supp.:** Miconazole nitrate 100 mg. In 7s with applicator; **Topical Cream:** Miconazole nitrate 2%. Tube 9 g. *otc.*
Use: Antifungal, vaginal.

Monistat-Derm Cream. (Ortho) Miconazole nitrate 2%, pegoxol 7 stearate, peglicol 5 oleate, mineral oil, benzoic acid, butylated hydroxyanisole. Tube 15 g, 30 g, 90 g. *otc.*
Use: Antifungal, topical.

Monistat-Derm Lotion. (Ortho Derm) Miconazole nitrate 2%, pegoxol 7 stearate, peglicol 5 oleate, mineral oil, benzoic acid, butylated hydroxyanisole. Squeeze bot. 30 ml, 60 ml. *Rx.*
Use: Antifungal, topical.

monoamine oxidase inhibitors.
Use: Antidepressant.
See: Parnate, Tab. (SK-Beecham). Marplan, Tab. (Roche). Nardil, Tab. (Parke-Davis).

•**mono and di-acetylated monoglycerides,** N.F. 18. A mixture of glycerin esterfied mono- and di-esters of edible fatty acids followed by direct acetylation.
Use: Pharmaceutic aid (plasticizer).

•**mono and di-glycerides,** N.F. 18. A mixture of mono- and di-esters of fatty acids from edible oils.
Use: Fatty acids, pharmaceutic aid (emulsifying agent).

•**monobenzone,** U.S.P. 23.
Use: Depigmentor.
See: Benoquin, Oint., Lot. (Zeneca).

monobenzyl ether of hydroquinone.
See: Benoquin, Oint., Lot. (Zeneca).

monobromisovalerylurea.
See: Bromisovalum. (Various Mfr.).

Monocaps Tablets. (Freeda) Iron 14 mg, vitamins A 10,000 IU, D 400 IU, E 15 IU, B_1 15 mg, B_2 15 mg, B_3 41 mg, B_5 15 mg, B_6 15 mcg, B_{12} 15 mcg, C 125 mg, folic acid 0.1 mg, biotin 15 mg, PABA, L-lysine, Ca, Cu, I, K, Mg, Mn, Se, Zn 12 mg, lecithin/Tab. Bot. 100s, 250s, 500s. *otc.*
Use: Vitamin/mineral supplement.

Mono-Chlor. (Gordon) Monochloroacetic acid 80%. Bot. 15 ml.
Use: Cauterizing agent.

monochloroacetic acid.
Use: Cauterizing agent.
See: Monocete, Soln. (Pedinol). Mono-Chlor, Soln. (Gordon).

monchlorophenol-para.
See: Camphorated para-chlorophenol, Liq. (Novocol).

Monocid. (SK-Beecham) Cefonicid sodium 500 mg, 1 g or 10 g/Vial and piggyback vial. Pharmacy Bulk Vial. *Rx.*
Use: Anti-infective, cephalosporin.

Monoclate. (Centeon) Monoclonal antibody derived stable lyophilized concentrate of Factor VIII: R heat-treated. With albumin (human) 1% to 2%, mannitol 0.8%, histadine 1.2 mM. Inj. Vial 1 ml single dose with diluent. *Rx.*
Use: Antihemophilic.

Monoclate-P. (Centeon). Stable concentrate of Factor VIII: C. ≈ 300 to 450 mmol sodium ions and ≈ 2 to 5 mmol calcium (as chloride) per L. With albumin (human) 1% to 2%, mannitol 0.8%, histadine 1.2 mmol, ≤ 50 ng/100 AHF activity units mouse protein. Pow. for Inj. *Rx.*
Use: Antihemophilic.

monoclonal antibodies (murine) anti-idiotype melanoma associated antigen. *Rx.*
Use: Invasive cutaneous melanoma. [Orphan drug]

monoclonal antibodies (murine or human) B-cell lymphoma. (Idec)
Use: B-cell lymphoma. [Orphan Drug]

monoclonal antibodies PM-81. *Rx.*
Use: Adjunctive treatment for leukemia. [Orphan drug]

monoclonal antibodies PM-81 and AML-AML-2-23. *Rx.*

Use: Leukemic bone marrow transplantation. [Orphan drug]

monoclonal antibody 17-LA. *Rx.*
Use: Pancreatic cancer. [Orphan drug]

monoclonal antibody to CD4, 5a8. (Biogen) *Rx.*
Use: Post-exposure prophylaxis for HIV. [Orphan drug]

monoclonal antibody (human) against hepatitis B virus. *Rx.*
Use: Prophylaxis in hepatitis B reinfection in liver transplants. [Orphan drug]

monoclonal antibody for lupus nephritis. (Medclone) *Rx.*
Use: Immunization agent. [Orphan drug]

•**monoctanoin.** (MAHN-ahk-tuh-NO-in) USAN.
Use: Anticholelithic (dissolution of gallstones). [Orphan drug]
See: Moctanin, Inf. (Ethiteck).

monocycline hydrochloride.
See: Minocin I.V., Syr., Cap. (Lederle).

Mono-Diff Test. (Wampole).
Use: Mononucleosis test.

Monodox. (Oclassen) Doxycycline monohydrate equivalent to **50 mg** doxycycline. Cap. Bot. 100s or **100 mg** doxycycline. Cap. Bot. 50s, 250s. *Rx.*
Use: Anti-infective, tetracycline.

•**monoethanolamine,** N.F. 18.
Use: Pharmaceutic aid (surfactant).

Mono-Gesic Tablets. (Schwartz Pharma) Salsalate (salicylsalicylic acid) 750 mg/ Tab. Bot. 100s, 500s. *Rx.*
Use: Salicylate analgesic.

monoiodomethanesulfonate sodium.
See: Methiodal Sodium, U.S.P. 23.

Monojel. (Sherwood) Glucose 40% in UD 25 g. *otc.*
Use: Glucose-elevating agent.

Monoket. (Schwarz Pharma Kremers-Urban) Isosorbide mononitrate 10 mg or 20 mg. Tab. Bot. 60s, 100s, 180s, UD 100s. *Rx.*
Use: Antianginal.

Mono-Latex. (Wampole) Two minute latex agglutination slide test for the qualitative or semiquantitative detection of infectious mononucleosis heterophile antibodies in serum or plasma. Test kit 20s, 50s, 1000s.
Use: Diagnostic aid.

monolaurin.
Use: Treatment of congenital primary ichthyosis. [Orphan drug]
See: Glylorin.

monomercaptoundecahydrocloso-DO decaborate sodium.
Use: Treatment of glioblastoma multi-

forme. [Orphan drug]

Mononine. (Centeon) Factor IX 100 IU/ ml with nondetectable levels of Factors II, VII and X with histidine ≈ 10 mM, mannitol ≈ 3%, mouse protein ≤ 50 ng/100 IU Factor IX activity units. Pow. for inj. (lyophilized). Single-dose vials with diluent. *Rx.*
Use: Antihemophilic.

mononucleosis tests.
Use: Diagnostic aid.
See: Mono-Diff Test (Wampole).
Mono-Latex (Wampole).
Mono-Lisa (Orion Diagnostics).
Mono-Plus (Wampole).
Monospot (Ortho Diagnostics).
Monosticon (Organon Teknica).
Monosticon Dri-Dot (Organon Teknika).
Mono-Sure Test (Wampole).
Mono-Test (Wampole).
Mono-Test (FTB) (Wampole).

Monopar. Stilbazium Iodide.
Use: Anthelmintic.

monophen.
Use: Orally, cholecystography.

Mono-Plus. (Wampole) To diagnose infectious mononucleosis from serum, plasma or fingertip blood. Test kits of 24s.
Use: Diagnostic aid.

Monopril. (Bristol-Myers) Fosinopril sodium. 10 mg or 20 mg/Tab., lactose. In 100s, UD 100s. *Rx.*
Use: Antihypertensive; congestive heart failure.

•**monosodium glutamate,** N.F. 18.
Use: Pharmaceutic aid (flavor, perfume).

monosodium phosphate.
See: Sodium Biphosphate, U.S.P. 23.

Monospot. (Ortho Diagnostics) Diagnosis of infectious mononucleosis. Test kit 20s.
Use: Diagnostic aid.

monostearin. (Various Mfr.) Glyceryl monostearate.

Monosticon Dri Dot. (Organon Technica) Diagnosis of infectious mononucleosis. Test kit 40s, 100s.
Use: Diagnostic aid.

Mono-Sure Test. (Wampole) One-minute hemagglutination slide test for the differential qualitative detection and quantitative determination of infectious mononucleosis heterophile antibodies in serum or plasma. Kit 20s.
Use: Diagnostic aid.

Monosyl. (Arcum) Secobarbital sodium

1 gr, butabarbital 0.5 gr/Tab. Bot. 100s, 1000s. *c-II*.
Use: Sedative, hypnotic.

Monotard Human Insulin. (Squibb/ Novo) Human insulin zinc 100 units/ml. Susp. Vial 10 ml. *otc*.
Use: Antidiabetic.

●**monothioglycerol,** N.F. 18.
Use: Pharmaceutic aid (preservative).

Mono-Vacc Test O.T. (Pasteur-Merieux-Connaught) 5 tuberculin units by the mantoux method. Multiple puncture disposable device. Box 25s (tamper-proof).
Use: Tuberculin test.

monoxychlorosene. A stabilized, buffered, organic hypochlorous acid derivative.
See: Oxychlorosene (Guardian Chem.).

Monsel Solution. (Wade) Bot. 2 oz, 4 oz.
Use: Styptic solution.

●**montelukast sodium.** USAN.
Use: Antiasthmatic (leukotriene antagonist).

Monurol. (Forest) Fosfomycin tromethamine 3 g/Granules. Single-dose packet. *Rx*.
Use: Urinary anti-infective.

8-MOP. (Zeneca) Methoxsalen 10 mg/ Cap. Pkg. 8s. *Rx*.
Use: Psoralens.

●**morantel tartrate.** (moe-RAN-tell) USAN.
Use: Anthelmintic.

moranyl.
See: Suramin Sodium.

Morco. (Archer-Taylor) Cod liver oil ointment, zinc oxide, benzethonium Cl, benzocaine 1%. 1.5 oz, lb. *otc*.
Use: Antiseptic, antipruritic, topical.

More-Dophilus. (Freeda) Acidophilus-carrot derivative 4 billion units/g Pow. Bot. 120 g. *otc*.
Use: Antidiarrheal, nutritional supplement.

●**moricizine.** (MAHR-IH-sizz-een) USAN.
Use: Cardiac depressant (antiarrhythmic).
See: Ethmozine (DuPont Merck).

●**morniflumate.** (MAR-nih-FLEW-mate) USAN.
Use: Anti-inflammatory.

Moroline. (Schering Plough) Petrolatum. Jar 1.75 oz, 3.75 oz, 15 oz. *otc*.
Use: Skin protectant, lubricant.

Morpen Tabs. (Major) Ibuprofen 400 mg or 600 mg/Tab. Bot. 500s. *Rx*.
Use: Nonsteroidal anti-inflammatory, analgesic.

morphine acetate.
W/Terpin hydrate, ammonium hypophosphite, potassium guaiacol-sulfonate.
See: Broncho-Tussin Soln. (First Texas).

morphine and atropine sulfates tablets.
Use: Analgesic, parasympatholytic.

morphine hydrochloride. (Various Mfr.) Pow. Bot. 1 oz, 5 oz. *c-II*.
Use: Analgesic.

●**morphine sulfate,** (MORE-feen) U.S.P. 23.
Use: Narcotic analgesic, sedative. [Orphan drug]
See: Infumorph 200 & 500, Inj. (Elkins-Sinn).
   MS Contin, CR Tab. (Purdue Frederick).
   OMS Concentrate, Soln. (Upsher-Smith).
   Oramorph SR Tab. (Roxane).
   Roxanol, Supp. (Roxane).
   Roxanol Rescudose, Soln. (Roxane).
W/Tartar emetic, bloodroot, ipecac, squill, wild cherry.
See: Pectoral, Preps. (Noyes).

morphine sulfate. (Various Mfr.) Flake or Pow. Bot. ⅛ oz, 1 oz, 5 oz, H.T. gr, gr, 0.25 gr, 0.5 gr, 1 gr.
Use: Narcotic analgesic.

morphine sulfate. (IMS) **25 mg/ml:** Inj. 4, 10, 20, 40 ml *Select-A-Jet syringe systems.* **50 mg/ml:** Inj. 10, 20, 40 ml *Select-A-Jet syringe systems. c-II*.
Use: Narcotic analgesic.

●**morrhuate sodium injection,** U.S.P. 23.
Use: Sclerosing agent.

Morton Salt Substitute. (Morton Salt) Potassium Cl, fumaric acid, tricalcium phosphate, monocalcium phosphate. Sodium: < 0.5 mg/5 g (0.02 mEq/5 g), potassium 2800 mg/5 g (72 mEq/5 g) 88.6 g. *otc*.
Use: Salt substitute.

Morton Seasoned Salt Substitute. (Morton Salt) Potassium chloride, spices, sugar, fumaric acid, triacalcium phosphate, monocalcium phosphate. Sodium < 1 mg/5 g (< 0.04 mEq/5 g), potasium 2165 mg/5 g (56 mEq/5 g). Bot. 85.1 g. *otc*.
Use: Salt substitute.

Mosco. (Medtech) 17.6% Salicylic acid. Jar 10 ml. *otc*.
Use: Keratolytic.

Motilium. (Janssen) Domperidone maleate. *Rx*.
Use: Antiemetic.

Motion Aid Tablets. (Vangard) Dimenhydrinate 50 mg/Tab. Bot. 100s, 1000s, UD 10×10s. *otc, Rx.*
Use: Antiemetic, antivertigo.
Motion Cure. (Wisconsin Pharm) Meclizine 25 mg/Chew. Tab. 12s. *otc, Rx.*
Use: Antiemetic, antivertigo.
motion sickness agents.
See: Antinauseants.
Bucladin, Softab Tab. (Stuart).
Dramamine, Preps. (Searle).
Emetrol, Liq. (Rhone-Poulenc Rorer).
Marezine, Tab., Amp. (Glaxo Wellcome).
Scopolamine HBr (Various Mfr.).
Motofen. (Carnrick) Difenoxin HCl 1 mg, atropine sulfate 0.025 mg/Tab. Bot. 100s. *c-iv.*
Use: Antidiarrheal.
•**motretinide.** (MOE-TREH-tih-nide) USAN.
Use: Keratolytic.
Motrin. (McNeil) Ibuprofen. **Capl.:** 100 mg: Bot. 100s; **Tab:** 50 mg or 100 mg: Bot. 100s; **300 mg:** Bot. 500s, Unit-0f-Use 60s; **400 mg:** Bot. 500s, Unit-of-Use 100s, UD 100s; **600 mg:** Bot. 500s, Unit-of-Use 100s, UD 100s, **800 mg:** Bot. 500s, Unit-of-Use 100s, UD 100s. **Chew. Tab.: 50 mg:** 100s. **100 mg:** 100s. **Susp.:** 100 mg/5 ml, sucrose. 120, 480 ml. *Rx.*
Use: Nonsteroidal anti-inflammatory, analgesic.
Motrin, Children's. (McNeil-CPC) Ibuprofen 100 mg/5 ml, sucrose. Susp. Bot. 120 ml, 480 ml. *otc, Rx.*
Use: Nonsteroidal anti-inflammatory, analgesic.
Motrin IB. (Pharmacia & Upjohn) Ibuprofen 200 mg. **Tab.** or **Capl.** Bot. 24s, 50s, 100s, 165s. **Gelcaps:** parabens. Bot. 24s, 50s. *otc.*
Use: Nonsteroidal anti-inflammatory, analgesic.
Motrin IB Sinus. (Pharmacia & Upjohn) Pseudoephedrine HCl 30 mg, ibuprofen 200 mg. Capl. Pkg. 20s, Bot. 40s. *otc.*
Use: Decongestant, nonsteroidal anti-inflammatory.
Mouthkote. (Unimed) Xylitol, sorbitol, Mucoprotective Factor (MPF), Yerba Santa, saccharin. Alcohol free. Soln. Bot. 60, 240 ml and UD 5 ml. *otc.*
Use: Saliva substitute.
Mouthkote F/R. (Parnell) Sodium fluoride 0.04%, benzyl alcohol, sorbitol, menthol, EDTA. Rinse. Bot. 237 ml.
Use: Fluoride, topical. *otc.*

MouthKote O/R Rinse. (Unimed) Benzyl alcohol, menthol, sorbitol. Rinse. Sugar free. Bot. 240 ml. *otc.*
Use: Antiseptic.
MouthKote O/R Solution. (Unimed) Diphenhydramine HCl 1.25%, cetylpyridinium Cl, EDTA, saccharin. Soln. Bot. 40 ml. *otc.*
Use: Antiseptic.
MouthKote P/R. (Parnell) **Oint.:** Diphenhydramine HCl 25%. Tube 15 g. **Soln.:** Diphenhydramine HCl 1.25%, cetylpyridinium Cl, EDTA, saccharin. Bot. 40 ml. *otc.*
Use: Mouth and throat product.
•**moxalactam disodium for injection,** U.S.P. 23.
Use: Anti-infective.
See: Moxam, Inj. (Lilly).
Moxam. (Lilly) Moxalactam disodium. Vial 1 g/10 ml Traypak 10s; Vial 2 g/20 ml Traypak 10s; Vial 10 g/100 ml Traypak 6s. *Rx.*
Use: Anti-infective, cephalosporin.
•**moxazocine.** (MOX-AZE-oh-seen) USAN.
Use: Analgesic, antitussive.
•**moxnidazole.** (MOX-NIH-dazz-ole) USAN.
Use: Antiprotozoal (trichomonas).
Moxy Compound. (Major) Theophylline 130 mg, ephedrine 25 mg, hydroxyzine HCl 10 mg/Tab. Bot. 100s. *Rx.*
Use: Antiasthmatic compound.
Moyco Fluoride Rinse. (Moyco) Fluoride 2%. Flavor. Bot. 128 oz. with pump. *otc, Rx.*
Use: Dental caries preventative.
6-MP.
Use: Antimetabolite.
See: Purinethol, Tab. (Burroughs Wellcome).
M-Prednisol-40. (Taylor) Methylprednisolone acetate 40 mg/ml. Inj. Susp. Vial 5 ml. *Rx.*
Use: Corticosteroid.
M-Prednisol-80. (Taylor) Methylprednisolone acetate 80 mg/ml. Inj. Susp. Vial 5 ml. *Rx.*
Use: Corticosteroid.
MRV. (Bayer) 2000 million organisms/ml from *Staphylococcus aureus* (1200 million), *Streptococcus,* viradens and non-hemolytic (200 million), *Streptococcus pneumoniae* (150 million), *Branhamella catarrhalis* (150 million), *Klebsiella pneumoniae* (150 million), *Haemophilus influenzae* (150 million). Inj. Vial 20 ml. *Rx.*

Use: Agent for immunization.

M-R-VAX II. (Merck) Live attenuated measles virus vaccine (Attenuvax) and live attenuated rubella virus vaccine (Meruvax II). See details under Attenuvax and Meruvax II. Single dose vial w/diluent. Pkg. 1s, 10s. *Rx.*
Use: Agent for immunization.

MS Contin. (Purdue Frederick) Morphine. **CR Tab.: 15 mg or 100 mg:** Bot. 100s, UD 100s. **30 mg:** Bot. 50s, 100s, 250s, Card 25s. **60 mg or 200 mg:** Bot. 100s, UD 25s. *c-II.*
Use: Narcotic analgesic.

MSIR Tablets. (Purdue Frederick) Morphine 15 mg and 30 mg/IR Tab. Bot. 50s. Morphine sulfate 15 mg and 30 mg, lactose, sucrose/Cap. Bot. 50s. *c-II.*
Use: Narcotic analgesic.

MSL-109. (Sandoz) Monoclonal antibody.
Use: Antiviral. [Orphan Drug]

MS/L. (Richwood) Morphine sulfate 10 mg/5 ml. Soln. Bot. 500 ml. *c-II.*
Use: Narcotic agonist analgesic.

MS/L-Concentrate. (Richwood) Morphine sulfate 100 mg/5 ml. Soln. Bot. 120 ml w/calibrated dropper. *c-II.*
Use: Narcotic agonist analgesic.

MS/S. (Richwood) Morphine sulfate 5 mg, 10 mg, 20 mg or 30 mg/Supp. 12s. *c-II.*
Use: Narcotic agonist analgesic.

MSTA. (Pasteur-Merieux-Connaught) Mumps skin test antigen. Inj. Vial 1 ml.
Use: Diagnostic aid.

MTC. Mitomycin.
Use: Anti-infective.
See: Mutamycin, Pow. (Bristol-Myers Oncology).

M.T.E.-4. (Fujisawa) Zinc 1 mg, copper 0.4 mg, chromium 4 mcg, manganese 0.1 mg/ml. Vial 3 ml, 10 ml, MD Vial 30 ml. *Rx.*
Use: Mineral supplement.

M.T.E.-4 Concentrated. (Fujisawa) Zinc 5 mg, copper 1 mg, chromium 10 mcg, manganese 0.5 mg/ml. Vial 1 ml, MD Vial 10 ml. *Rx.*
Use: Mineral supplement.

M.T.E.-5. (Fujisawa) Zinc 1 mg, copper 0.4 mg, chromium 4 mcg, manganese 0.1 mg, selenium 20 mcg/ml. Vial 10 ml. *Rx.*
Use: Mineral supplement.

M.T.E.-5 Concentrated. (Fujisawa) Zinc 5 mg, copper 1 mg, chromium 10 mcg, manganese 0.5 mg, selenium 60 mcg/ml. Vial 1 ml, MD vial 10 ml. *Rx.*
Use: Mineral supplement.

M.T.E.-6. (Fujisawa) Zinc 1 mg, copper 0.4 mg, chromium 4 mcg, manganese 0.1 mg, selenium 20 mcg, iodide 25 mcg/ml. Vial 10 ml. *Rx.*
Use: Mineral supplement.

M.T.E.-6 Concentrate. (Fujisawa) Zinc 5 mg, copper 1 mg, chromium 10 mcg, manganese 0.5 mg, selenium 60 mcg, iodide 75 mcg/ml. Vial 1 ml. MD vial 10 ml. *Rx.*
Use: Mineral supplement.

M.T.E.-7. (Fujisawa) Zinc 1 mg copper 0.4 mg, manganese 0.1 mg, chromium 4 mcg, selenium 20 mcg, iodide 25 mcg, molybdenum 25 mcg/ml. Vial 10 ml. *Rx.*
Use: Mineral supplement.

MTP-PE. (Novartis) Muramyl-tripeptide. *Rx.*
Use: Immunomodulator.

MTX. *Rx.*
Use: Antineoplastic, antipsoriatic.
See: Methotrexate.

MUC 9 + 4 Pediatric. (Fujisawa) Vitamin A 2300 IU, D 400 IU, E 7 mg, B_1 1.2 mg, B_2 1.4 mg, B_3 17 mg, B_5 5 mg, B_6 1 mg, B_{12} 1 mcg, C 80 mg, biotin 20 mcg, folic acid 0.14 mg, K 200 mcg/5 ml, mannitol 375 mg. Pow. Vial. 10 ml. *Rx.*
Use: Parenteral nutritional supplement.

mucilloid of psyllium seed.
W/Dextrose.
See: Metamucil, Liq. (Searle).

mucin.
See: Gastric Mucin (Wilson).

mucin, vegetable.
W/Yeast or alkalized.
See: Plantamucin, Granules (Baxter).

Muco-Fen-DM. (Wakefield Pharm) Guaifenesin 600 mg, dextromethorphan HBr 30 mg/Tab. Bot. 1000s. *Rx.*
Use: Antitussive, expectorant.

Muco-Fen-LA. (Wakefield) Guaifenesin 600 mg, dye free/TR Tab. Bot. 100s. *Rx.*
Use: Expectorant.

mucolytics.
Use: Respiratory inhalant products.
See: Mucomyst, Soln. (Bristol-Myers).

Mucomyst. (Bristol) A sterile 20% solution of acetylcysteine for nebulization or direct instillation into the lung as a mucolytic agent. Approved as antidote for acetaminophen overdose. Vial. **4 ml:** Ctn. 12s; **10 ml:** Ctn. 3s with dropper; **30 ml:** Ctn. 3s. *Rx.*
Use: Respiratory inhalant.

Mucomyst-10. (Bristol) A sterile 10% solution of acetylcysteine for nebulization

or direct instillation into the lung as a mucolytic agent. Approved as antidote for acetaminophen overdose. Vial. **4 ml:** Ctn. 12s; **10 ml:** Ctn. 3s with dropper; **30 ml:** Ctn. 3s. *Rx.*
Use: Respiratory inhalant.

Mucosil 10 & 20 Solution. (Dey) Acetylcysteine sodium salt 10% or 20%. Soln. Vial 4 ml Box 12s. *Rx.*
Use: Respiratory inhalant.

Mudd. (Chattem) Natural hydrated magnesium aluminum silicate. Topical preparation. *otc.*
Use: Cleansing agent.

Mudrane. (ECR Pharm) Aminophylline (anhydrous) 130 mg, phenobarbital 8 mg, ephedrine HCl 16 mg, potassium iodide 195 mg/Tab. Bot. 100s. *Rx.*
Use: Antiasthmatic combination.

Mudrane-2. (ECR Pharm) Potassium iodide 195 mg, aminophylline (anhydrous) 130 mg/Tab. Bot. 100s. *Rx.*
Use: Antiasthmatic combination.

Mudrane GG. (ECR Pharm) Aminophylline (anhydrous) 130 mg, ephedrine HCl 16 mg, guaifenesin 100 mg, phenobarbital 8 mg/Tab. Bot. 100s. *Rx.*
Use: Antiasthmatic combination.

Mudrane GG-2. (ECR Pharm) Guaifenesin 100 mg, theophylline 111 mg/Tab. Bot. 100s. *Rx.*
Use: Antiasthmatic combination.

Mudrane GG Elixir. (ECR Pharm) Theophylline 20 mg, ephedrine HCl 4 mg, guaifenesin 26 mg, phenobarbital 2.5 mg/5 ml, alcohol 20%. Bot. pt, 0.5 gal. *Rx.*
Use: Antiasthmatic combination.

Multa-Gen 12 + E. (Jones Medical) Vitamin A 5000 IU, D 400 IU, B_1 2 mg, B_2 2 mg, B_6 0.5 mg, B_{12} 3 mcg, C 37.5 mg, E 15 IU, folic acid 0.2 mg, nicotinamide 20 mg/Cap. Bot. 60s, 500s, 1000s. *otc.*
Use: Vitamin supplement.

Multe-Pak-4. (SoloPak) Zinc 1 mg, copper 0.4 mg, manganese 0.1 mg, chromium 4 mg/ml. Vial 3 ml, 10 ml, 30 ml. *Rx.*
Use: Mineral supplement.

Multe-Pak-5. (SoloPak) Zinc 1 mg, copper 0.4 mg, manganese 0.1 mg, chromium 4 mg, selenium 20 mcg/ml. Vial 3 ml, 10 ml. *Rx.*
Use: Mineral supplement.

Multi-B-Plex. (Forest) Vitamins B_1 100 mg, B_2 1 mg, nicotinamide 100 mg, pantothenic acid 10 mg, B_6 10 mg/ml. Vial 10 ml, 30 ml. *Rx.*
Use: Vitamin supplement.

Multi-B-Plex Capsules. (Forest) Vitamins B_1 50 mg, B_2 5 mg, niacinamide 50 mg, calcium pantothenate 5.4 mg, B_6 0.2 mg, C 150 mg, B_{12} 1 mcg/Cap. Bot. 100s, 1000s. *otc.*
Use: Vitamin/mineral supplement.

Multi-Day. (NTBY) Vitamins A 5000 IU, D 400 IU, E 30 mg, B_1 1.5 mg, B_2 1.7 mg, B_3 20 mg, B_5 10 mg, B_6 2 mg, B_{12} 6 mcg, C 60 mg, FA 0.4 ml/Tab. Bot. 100s. *otc.*
Use: Vitamin supplement.

Multi-Day Plus Iron. (NTBY) Fe 18 mg, A 5000 IU, D 400 IU, E 15 mg, B_1 1.5 mg, B_2 1.7 mg, B_3 20 mg, B_6 2 mg, B_{12} 6 mcg, C 60 mg, FA 0.4 mg. Tab. Bot. 100s. *otc.*
Use: Vitamin supplement.

Multi-Day Plus Minerals. (NTBY). Fe 18 mg, A 6500 IU, D 400 IU, E 30 mg, B_1 1.5 mg, B_2 1.7 mg, B_3 20 mg, B_5 10 mg, B_6 2 mg, B_{12} 6 mcg, C 60 mg, FA 0.4 mg, Ca, Cl, Cr, Cu, I, K, Mg, Mn, Mo, P, Se, Zn 15 mg, biotin 30 mcg. Tab. Bot. 100s. *otc.*
Use: Vitamin supplement.

Multi-Day w/Calcium and Extra Iron Tablets. (NTBY) Fe 27 mg, A 5000 IU, D 400 IU, E 30 mg, B_1 1.5 mg, B_2 1.7 mg, B_3 20 mg, B_5 10 mg, B_6 2 mg, B_{12} 6 mcg, C 60 mg, FA 0.4 mg, Ca, Zn 15 mg, tartrazine/Tab. Bot. 100s. *otc.*
Use: Vitamin/mineral supplement.

Multi-Germ Oil. (Viobin) Corn, sunflower and wheat germ oils. Bot. 4 oz, 8 oz, pt, qt. *otc.*
Use: Nutritional supplement.

Multi-Jets. (Kirkman Sales) Vitamins A 10,000 IU, D_2 400 IU, B_1 20 mg, B_2 8 mg, C 120 mg, niacinamide 10 mg, calcium pantothenate 5 mg, B_6 0.5 mg, E 50 IU, desiccated liver 100 mg, dried debittered yeast 100 mg, choline bitartrate 62 mg, inositol 30 mg, dl-methionine 30 mg, B_{12} 7 mcg, iron 2.6 mg, calcium (dical phosphate) 58 mg, phosphorus (dical phosphate) 45 mg, iodine (potassium iodide) 0.114 mg, magnesium sulfate 1 mg, copper sulfate 1.99 mg, manganese sulfate 1.11 mg, potassium Cl iodide 79 mg/Tab. Bot. 100s. *otc.*
Use: Vitamin/mineral supplement.

Multilex Tablets. (Rugby) Iron 15 mg, vitamins A 10,000 IU, D 400 IU, E 5.5 mg, B_1 10 mg, B_2 5 mg, B_3 30 mg, B_5 10 mg, B_6 1.7 mg, B_{12} 3 mcg, C 100 mg, zinc 1.5 mg, Cu, I, Mg, Mn/Tab. Bot. 100s. *otc.*

Use: Vitamin/mineral supplement.

Multilex T/M Tablets. (Rugby) Iron 15 mg, vitamins A 10,000 IU, D 400 IU, E 5.5 mg, B_1 15 mg, B_2 10 mg, B_3 100 mg, B_5 10 mg, B_6 2 mg, B_{12} 7.5 mcg, C 150 mg, Cu, I, Mg, Mn, Zn 1.5 mg, sugar/Tab. Bot. 100s. *otc.*
Use: Vitamin/mineral supplement.

Multilyte. (Fujisawa) Vitamins A 5000 IU, D 400 IU, E 15 mg, B_1 3 mg, B_2 3.4 mg, B_3 36 mg, B_5 14 mg, B_6 4.4 mg, B_{12} 6 mcg, C 120 mg, FA 0.4 mg, Zn 10.5 mg, biotin 100 mcg, Ca, K, Mg, Mn, phenylalanine. Tab. Pkg. 12s. *otc.*
Use: Vitamin/mineral supplement.

Multilyte-20. (Fujisawa) Sodium 25 mEq/L, potassium 20 mEq/L, calcium 5 mEq/L, magnesium 5 mEq/L, chloride 30 mEq/L, acetate 25 mEq/L, gluconate 5 mEq/L. Vial 25 ml fill in 50 ml. *Rx.*
Use: Fluid/electrolyte replacement.

Multilyte-40. (Fujisawa) Sodium 25 mEq/L, potassium 40.5 mEq/L, calcium 5 mEq/L, magnesium 8 mEq/L, chloride 33.5 mEq/L, acetate 40.6 mEq/L, gluconate 5 mEq/L. Vial 25 ml fill in 50 ml. *Rx.*
Use: Fluid/electrolyte replacement.

Multi-Mineral Tablets. (NTBY) Ca 166.7 mg, P 75.7 mg, I 25 mcg, Fe 3 mg, Mg 66.7 mg, Cu 0.33 mg, Zn 2.5 mg, K 12.5 mg, Mn 8.3 mg/Tab. Bot. 100s. *otc.*
Use: Vitamin/mineral supplement.

Multipals. (Faraday) Vitamins A 5000 IU, D 400 IU, C 50 mg, B_1 3 mg, B_6 0.5 mg, B_2 3 mg, calcium pantothenate 5 mg, niacinamide 20 mg, B_{12} 2 mcg/Tab. Bot. 100s, 250s, 1000s. *otc.*
Use: Vitamin/mineral supplement.

Multipals-M. (Faraday) Vitamins A 6000 IU, D 400 IU, B_1 3 mg, B_2 3 mg, B_6 0.5 mg, B_{12} 5 mcg, C 60 mg, E 2 IU, niacinamide 20 mg, calcium pantothenate 5 mg, iron 10 mg, iodine 0.15 mg, copper 1 mg, magnesium 6 mg, manganese 1 mg, potassium 5 mg/Tab. Bot. 100s, 250s, 1000s. *otc.*
Use: Vitamin/mineral supplement.

Multiple Trace Element. (American Regent) Zinc sulfate 1 mg, copper sulfate 0.4 mg, manganese sulfate 0.1 mg, chromium Cl 4 mg/ml. Inj. Soln. Vial 10 ml. *Rx.*
Use: Mineral supplement.

Multiple Trace Element Concentrated. (American Regent) Zinc sulfate 5 mg, copper sulfate 1 mg, manganese sulfate 0.5 mg, chromium Cl 10 mcg/ml. Inj. Soln. Vial 10 ml. *Rx.*
Use: Mineral supplement.

Multiple Trace Element Neonatal. (American Regent) Zn 1.5 mg, Cu 0.1 mg, Mn 25 mcg, Cr 0.85 mcg/ml. Vial 2 ml single dose. *Rx.*
Use: Mineral supplement.

Multiple Trace Element Pediatric. (American Regent) Zinc sulfate 0.5 mg, copper sulfate 0.1 mg, manganese sulfate 0.03 mg, chromium Cl 1 mcg/ml. Inj. Soln. Vial 10 ml. *Rx.*
Use: Mineral supplement.

Multiple Vitamin Mineral Formula. (Kirkman Sales) Vitamins A 5000 IU, D_2 400 IU, C 50 mg, B_1 2.5 mg, B_2 2.5 mg, B_6 0.5 mg, B_{12} 1 mcg, niacinamide 15 mg, calcium pantothenate 5 mg, E 0.1 IU, calcium 100 mg, iron 7.5 mg, magnesium 2.5 mg, potassium 2.5 mg, zinc 0.15 mg, manganese 0.5 mg, iodine 0.07 mg/Tab. Bot. 100s. *otc.*
Use: Vitamin/mineral supplement.

Multiple Vitamins Chewable. (Kirkman Sales) Vitamins A 5000 IU, D 400 IU, C 50 mg, B_1 3 mg, B_2 2.5 mg, B_6 1 mg, B_{12} 1 mcg, niacinamide 20 mg/Tab. Bot. 100s. *otc.*
Use: Vitamin supplement.

Multiple Vitamins w/Iron. (Kirkman Sales) Vitamins A 5000 IU, D 400 IU, C 50 mg, B_1 3 mg, B_2 2.5 mg, B_6 1 mg, B_{12} 1 mcg, niacinamide 20 mg, iron 10 mg/Tab. Bot. 100s. *otc.*
Use: Vitamin/mineral supplement.

Multi 75. (Fibertone) Vitamins A 25,000 IU, D 500 IU, E 150 IU, B_1 75 mg, B_2 75 mg, B_3 75 mg, B_5 75 mg, B_6 75 mg, B_{12} 75 mcg, C 250 mg, FA 0.4 mg, Ca 50 mg, Fe 10 mg, Biotin, I, Mg, Zn 15 mg, Cu, PABA, K, Mn, Cr, Se, Mo, B, Si, choline bitartrate, inosol, rutin, lemon bioflavonoid complex, hesperidin, betaine, HCl/TR Tab. Bot. 60s, 90s. *otc.*
Use: Vitamin/mineral supplement.

Multistix 2 Reagent Strips. (Bayer) Urinalysis reagent strip test for nitrite and leukocytes. Bot. 100s.
Use: Diagnostic aid.

Multistix 7. (Bayer) Urinalysis reagent strip test for glucose ketone, blood, pH, protein, nitrite and leukocytes. Box 100s.
Use: Diagnostic aid.

Multistix 8. (Bayer) Urinalysis reagent strip test for detecting glucose, ketone, blood, pH, protein, nitrite, bilirubin and leukocytes. Box. 100s.
Use: Diagnostic aid.

Multistix 8 SG Reagent Strips. (Bayer) Urinalysis reagent strip test for glucose, ketone, specific gravity, blood, pH, pro-

tein nitrite, leukocytes. Box 100s.
Use: Diagnostic aid.

Multistix 9 Reagent Strips. (Bayer) Urinalysis reagent strip test for glucose, bilirubin, ketone, blood, pH, protein, urobilinogen, nitrite, leukocytes. Box 100s.
Use: Diagnostic aid.

Multistix 9 SG Reagent Strips. (Bayer) Urinalysis reagent strip test for glucose, bilirubin, ketone, specific gravity, blood, pH, protein, nitrite and leukocytes. Box 100s.
Use: Diagnostic aid.

Multistix 10 SG Reagent Strips. (Bayer) Reagent strip test for glucose, bilirubin, ketone, specific gravity, blood, pH, protein, urobilinogen, nitrite and leukocytes in urine. Box 100s.
Use: Diagnostic aid.

Multistix-N. (Bayer) Glucose, protein, pH, blood, ketones, bilirubin, urobilinogen, nitrate, leukocytes. Kit. 100s.
Use: In vitro diagnostic aid.

Multistix-N S.G. Reagent Strips. (Bayer) Urinalysis reagent strip test for pH, protein, glucose, ketones, bilirubin, blood nitrite, urobilinogen and specific gravity. Bot. 100s.
Use: Diagnostic aid.

Multistix Reagent Strips. (Bayer) Urinalysis reagent strip test for pH, protein, glucose, ketone, bilirubin and blood. Box 100s.
Use: Diagnostic aid.

Multistix S. G. Reagent Strips. (Bayer) Urinalysis reagent strip test for pH, glucose, protein, ketones, bilirubin, blood and urobilinogen. Box. 100s.
Use: Diagnostic aid.

Multi-Symptom Tylenol Cold. (McNeil-CPC) Pseudoephedrine HCl 30 mg, chorpheniramine maleate 2 mg, dextromethorphan HBr 15 mg, acetaminophen 325 mg/Capl. or Tab. Bot. 24s, 50s. *otc.*
Use: Decongestant, antihistamine, antitussive, analgesic.

Multi-Symptom Tylenol Cough. (McNeil) Dextromethorphan HBr 10 mg, acetaminophen 216.7 mg, alcohol 5%/5 ml. Liq. Bot. 120 ml. *otc.*
Use: Antitussive, analgesic.

Multi-Symptom Tylenol Cough with Decongestant. (McNeil) Dextromethorphan HBr 10 mg, acetaminophen 200 mg, pseudoephedrine HCl 20 mg, alcohol 5%, saccharin, sorbitol/5 ml. Liq. Bot. 120 ml. *otc.*
Use: Antitussive, analgesic, decongestant.

Multitest CMI. (Pasteur-Merieux-Connaught) One disposable applicator preloaded with seven glycerinated liquid antigens and glycerin negative control. 10 units/box.
Use: Diagnostic aid.

Multi-Thera Tablets. (NTBY) Vitamins A 5500 IU, D 400 IU, E 30 mg, B_1 3 mg, B_2 3.4 mg, B_3 30 mg, B_5 10 mg, B_6 3 mg, B_{12} 9 mcg, C 120 mg, folic acid 0.4 mg, biotin 15 mcg/Tab. Bot. 100s. *otc.*
Use: Vitamin supplement.

Multi-Thera-M. (NTBY) Iron 27 mg, vitamins A 5500 IU, D 400 IU, E 30 mg, B_1 3 mg, B_2 3.4 mg, B_3 30 mg, B_5 10 mg, B_6 3 mg, B_{12} 9 mcg, C 120 mg, folic acid 0.4 mg, biotin 15 mcg, zinc 15 mg, Ca, Cl, Cr, Cu, I, K, Mg, Mn, Mo, Se/Tab. Bot. 130s. *otc.*
Use: Vitamin/mineral supplement.

Multitrace-5 Concentrate. (American Regent) Zinc sulfate 5 mg, copper sulfate 1 mg, manganese sulfate 0.5 mg, chromium Cl 10 mcg, selenium 60 mcg, benzyl alcohol 0.9%. Inj. Soln. Vial 1 ml and 10 ml. *Rx.*
Use: Mineral supplement.

Multi-Vit Drops. (Barre) Vitamins A 500 IU, D 400 IU, E 5 mg, B_1 0.5 mg, B_2 0.6 mg, B_3 8 mg, B_6 0.4 mg, B_{12} 2 mcg, C 35 mg/ml. Bot. 50 ml. *otc.*
Use: Vitamin supplement.

Multi-Vit Drops w/Iron. (Barre-National) Iron 10 mg, vitamins A 1500 IU, D 400 IU, E 5 IU, B_1 0.5 mg, B_2 0.6 mg, B_3 8 mg, B_6 0.4 mg, C 35 mg/ml. Methylparaben. Bot. 50 ml. *otc.*
Use: Vitamin/mineral supplement.

Multi-Vita. (Rosemont) Vitamins A 1500 IU/ml, D 400 IU, E 5 mg, B_1 0.5 mg, B_2 0.6 mg, B_3 8 mg, B_6 0.4 mg, B_{12} 2 mcg, C 35 mg, alcohol free. Drop. Bot. 50 ml. *otc.*
Use: Vitamin supplement.

Multi-Vita Drops. (Rosemont) Vitamins A 1500 IU, D 400 IU, E 5 mg, B_1 0.5 mg, B_2 0.6 mg, B_3 8 mg, B_6 0.4 mg, B_{12} 2 mcg, C 35 mg/ml. Alcohol free. Bot. 50 ml. *otc.*
Use: Vitamin/mineral supplement.

Multi-Vita Drops w/Fluoride. (Rosemont) Fluoride 0.5 mg, vitamins A 1500 IU, D 400 IU, E 5 mg, B_1 0.5 mg, B_2 0.6 mg, B_3 8 mg, B_6 0.4 mg, B_{12} 2 mcg, C 35 mg/ml. Alcohol free. Bot. 50 ml. *Rx.*
Use: Vitamin supplement; dental caries preventative.

Multi-Vita Drops w/Iron. (Rosemont) Iron 10 mg, vitamins A 1500 IU, D 400

IU, E 5 mg, B$_1$ 0.5 mg, B$_2$ 0.6 mg, B$_3$ 8 mg, B$_6$ 0.4 mg, C 35 mg/ml. Alcohol free. Bot. 50 ml. *otc.*
Use: Vitamin/mineral supplement.

Multivitamin with Fluoride Drops. (Major) Fluoride 0.5 mg, vitamins A 1500 IU, D 400 IU, E 5 IU, B$_1$ 0.5 mg, B$_2$ 0.6 mg, B$_3$ 8 mg, B$_6$ 0.4 mg, B$_{12}$ 2 mcg, C 35 mg, F 0.25 mg/Drop. Bot. 50 ml. *Rx.*
Use: Vitamin supplement; dental caries preventative.

multi vitamin concentrate injection. (Fujisawa) Vitamins A 10,000 IU, D 1000 IU, E 5 IU, B$_1$ 50 mg, B$_2$ 10 mg, B$_3$ 100 mg, B$_5$ 25 mg, B$_6$ 15 mg, C 500 mg/Inj. Vial 5 ml. *Rx.*
Use: Vitamin supplement.

multi-vitamin infusion (neonatal formula). *Rx.*
Use: Nutritional supplement for low birth weight infants. [Orphan drug]

Multi-Vitamin Mineral w/Beta Carotene. (Mission) Iron 27 mg, A 5000 IU, D 400 IU, E 30 IU, B$_1$ 2.25 mg, B$_2$ 2.6 mg, B$_3$ 20 mg, B$_5$ 10 mg, B$_6$ 3 mg, B$_{12}$ 9 mcg, C 90 mg, folic acid 0.4 mg, biotin, 0.45 mg, Ca, Cl, Cr, Cu, I, K, Mg, Mn, Mo, P, Se, Zn 15 mg, Vitamin K/Tab. Bot. 130s. *otc.*
Use: Iron with vitamin supplement.

Multi-Vitamins Capsules. (Forest) Vitamins A 5000 IU, D 400 IU, B$_1$ 1.5 mg, B$_2$ 2 mg, B$_6$ 0.1 mg, C 37.5 mg, calcium pantothenate 1 mg, niacinamide 20 mg/Cap. Bot. 100s, 1000s, 5000s. *otc.*
Use: Vitamin/mineral supplement.

Multivitamins Capsules. (Solvay) Vitamins A 5000 IU, D 400 IU, B$_1$ 2.5 mg, B$_2$ 2.5 mg, C 50 mg, B$_3$ 20 mg, B$_5$ 5 mg, B$_6$ 0.5 mg, B$_{12}$ 2 mcg, E 10 IU/Cap. Bot. 100s, UD 100s. *otc.*
Use: Vitamin/mineral supplement.

Multivitamin with Fluoride Drops. (Major) Fluoride 0.5 mg, vitamins A 1500 IU, D 400 IU, E 4.1 IU, B$_1$ 0.5 mg, B$_2$ 0.6 mg, B$_3$ 8 mg, B$_6$ 0.4 mg, B$_{12}$ 2 mg, C 35 mg/Drop. Bot. 50 ml. *Rx.*
Use: Vitamin supplement; dental caries preventative.

multizine.
See: Trisulfapyrimidines Tab., U.S.P. 23.

Multorex. (Approved) Vitamins A 6000 IU, D 1250 IU, C 50 mg, E 5 IU, B$_1$ 3 mg, B$_2$ 3 mg, B$_6$ 0.5 mg, niacinamide 20 mg, calcium pantothenate 5 mg, B$_{12}$ 5 mcg, calcium 59 mg, phosphorus 45 mg/Cap. Bot. 100s, 250s, 1000s. *otc.*
Use: Vitamin/mineral supplement.

Mulvidren-F Softabs. (Wyeth-Ayerst) Fluoride 1 mg, vitamins A 4000 IU, D 400 IU, B$_1$ 1.6 mg, B$_2$ 2 mg, B$_3$ 10 mg, B$_5$ 2.8 mg, B$_6$ 1 mg, B$_{12}$ 3 mcg, C 75 mg, Saccharin/Tab. Bot. 100s. *Rx.*
Use: Vitamin/mineral supplement, dental caries preventative.

•**mumps skin test antigen,** U.S.P. 23.
Use: Diagnostic aid (dermal reactivity indicator).
See: MSTA, Inj. (Pasteur-Merieux-Connaught).

Mumpsvax. (Merck) Live mumps virus vaccine, Jeryl Lynn strain. Single-dose vial w/diluent Pkg. 1s, 10s. *Rx.*
Use: Agent for immunization.
W/Attenuvax, Meruvax II.
See: M-M-R II, Inj. (Merck).
W/Meruvax II.
See: Biavax II (Merck).

•**mumps virus vaccine live,** U.S.P. 23.
Use: Active immunizing agent.
See: Mumpsvax, Inj. (Merck).

mumps virus vaccine, live attenuated. Jeryl Lynn (B Level) strain.
W/Measles virus vaccine, rubella virus vaccine.
See: M-M-R, Inj. (Merck).

•**mupirocin,** (myoo-PIHR-oh-sin) U.S.P. 23.
Use: Antibacterial (topical and nasal).
See: Bactroban, Oint. (SK-Beecham).

•**mupirocin calcium.** (myoo-PIHR-oh-sin KAL-see-uhm) USAN.
Use: Antibacterial (topical).

•**muplestim.** USAN.
Use: Hematopoietic stimulant; antineutropenic.

muriatic acid.
See: Hydrochloric Acid, N.F. 18.

Muri-Lube. (Fujisawa) Mineral Oil "Light." Vial 2 ml, 10 ml. *Rx.*
Use: Lubricant for surgery.

Murine Ear Drops. (Ross) Carbamide peroxide 6.5% in anhydrous glycerin. Bot. 0.5 oz. *otc.*
Use: Otic preparation.

Murine Ear Wax Removal System. (Ross) Carbamide peroxide 6.5% in anhydrous glycerin w/ear washing syringe. Bot. 0.5 oz. and ear washer 1 oz. *otc.*
Use: Otic preparation.

Murine Eye Drops. (Ross) Polyvinyl alcohol 0.5%, povidone 0.6%, benzalkonium chloride, dextrose, EDTA, NaCl, sodium bicarbonate, sodium phosphate. Soln. Bot. 15 ml, 30 ml. *otc.*
Use: Artificial tear solution.

Murine Plus Eye Drops. (Ross) Tetra-hydrozoline HCl 0.05%. Drop. Bot. 15 ml, 30 ml. *otc.*
Use: Vasoconstrictor, ophthalmic.

Murine Regular Formula. (Ross) Sodium chloride, potassium chloride, sodium phosphate, glycerin, benzalkonium chloride 0.01%, EDTA 0.05%/Drop. Bot. 15, 30 ml. *otc.*
Use: Artificial tear solution.

Muro 128 Ointment. (Bausch & Lomb) Sodium Cl 5% in sterile ointment base. Tube 3.5 g. *otc.*
Use: Hyperosmolar agent.

Muro 128 Solution. (Bausch & Lomb) Sodium Cl 2% or 5%. Soln. Bot. 15 ml, 30 ml (5% only). *otc.*
Use: Hyperosmolar agent.

Murocel Solution. (Bausch & Lomb) Methylcellulose 1%, propylene glycol, sodium Cl, methylparaben 0.046%, propylparaben 0.02%, boric acid, sodium borate. Soln. Bot. 15 ml. *otc.*
Use: Artificial tear solution.

Murocoll-2. (Bausch & Lomb) Phenylephrine HCl 10%, scopolamine HBR 0.3% Bot. 5 ml. *Rx.*
Use: Mydriatic, cycloplegic, ophthalmic.

•**muromonab-cd3.** (MYOO-row-MOE-nab cd3) USAN.
Use: Monoclonal antibody (immunosuppressant).
See: Orthoclone OKT3, Inj. (Ortho).

Muroptic-5. (Optopics) Sodium Cl, hypertonic 5%. Soln. Bot. 15 ml. *otc.*
Use: Hyperosmolar agent.

Muro's Opcon A Solution. (Bausch & Lomb) Naphazoline HCl 0.025%, pheniramine maleate 0.3%. Bot. 15 ml. *otc.*
Use: Decongestant, antihistamine (ophthalmic).

Muro's Opcon Solution. (Bausch & Lomb) Naphazoline HCl 0.1%. Bot. 15 ml. *otc.*
Use: Decongestant, ophthalmic.

Muro Tears Solution. (Bausch & Lomb) Hydroxypropyl methylcellulose, dextran 40. Soln. Bot. 15 ml. *otc.*
Use: Artificial tear solution.

muscle adenylic acid. (Various Mfr.) Active form of adenosine 5-monophosphate.
See: Adenosine 5-monophosphate, Preps. (Various Mfr.).

muscle relaxants.
See: Arduan (Organon).
Curare (Various Mfr.).
Flexeril, Tab. (Merck).
Flaxedil Triethiodide, Vial (Davis & Geck).

Lioresal, Tab. (Novartis).
Mephenesin (Various Mfr.).
Meprobamate (Various Mfr.).
Metubine Iodine, Vial (Lilly).
Neostig, Tab. (Freeport).
Norflex, Tab., Inj. (3M).
Nuromax (Glaxo Wellcome).
Parafon Forte, Tab. (McNeil).
P-A-V, Cap. (T.E. Williams).
Rela, Tab. (Schering Plough).
Robaxin, Tab., Inj. (Robins).
Soma, Tab., Cap. (Wallace).
Succinylcholine Cl (Various Mfr.).
d-Tubocurarine Cl (Various Mfr.).

mustaral oil.
See: Allyl Isothiocyanate.

Mustargen. (Merck) Mechlorethamine HCl 10 mg/Vial, sodium Cl q.s. 100 mg/Vial. Treatment set vial 4s. *Rx.*
Use: Antineoplastic.

Musterole. (Schering Plough) **Regular:** Camphor 4%, menthol 2%. Jar 0.9 oz. **Extra Strength:** Camphor 5%, menthol 3%. Jar 0.9 oz., Tube 1 oz, 2.25 oz. *otc.*
Use: Analgesic, topical.

Musterole Deep Strength. (Schering Plough) Methyl salicylate 30%, menthol 3%, methyl nicotinate 0.5%. Jar 1.25 oz, Tube 3 oz. *otc.*
Use: Analgesic, topical.

Musterole Extra Strength. (Schering Plough) Camphor 5%, menthol 3%, methyl salicylate, lanolin, oil of mustard, petrolatum. 27, 30, 67.5 g. *otc.*
Use: Rub/liniment.

mustin.
See: Mechlorethamine HCl, Sterile.

mutalin. (Spanner) Protein and iodine. Vial 30 ml.

Mutamycin. (Bristol-Myers/Bristol Oncology) Mitomycin 5 mg, 20 mg or 40 mg/Vial. *Rx.*
Use: Antineoplastic.

•**muzolimine.** (MYOO-ZOLE-ih-meen) USAN.
Use: Diuretic, antihypertensive.

M.V.I.-12. (Astra) Vitamins A 3300 IU, D 200 IU, E 10 IU, B_1 3 mg, B_2 3.6 mg, B_3 40 mg, B_5 15 mg, B_6 4 mg, B_{12} 5 mcg, C 100 mg, biotin 60 mcg, FA 0.4 mg. Inj. Vials. 5 ml single dose or 50 ml multiple dose; Unit vial: 10 ml two-chambered vials *Rx.*
Use: Parenteral nutritional supplement.

M.V.I. Pediatric. (Astra) Vitamin A 2300 IU, D 400 IU, E 7 IU, B_1 1.2 mg, B_2 1.4 mg, B_3 17 mg, B_5 5 mg, B_6 1 mg, B_{12} 1 mcg, C 80 mg, biotin 20 mcg, FA 0.14

mg, vitamin K 200 mcg, mannitol 375 mg/Inj. Vial. *Rx.*
Use: Parenteral nutritional supplement.

M.V.M. (Tyson and Associates) Iron 3.6 mg, vitamins A 400 IU, E 60 IU, B$_1$ 20 mg, B$_2$ 10 mg, B$_3$ 10 mg, B$_5$ 100 mg, B$_6$ 31 mg, B$_{12}$ 160 mcg, C 50 mg, folic acid 0.08 mg, Ca, Cr, Cu, I, K, Mg, Mo, Zn 6 mg, biotin 160 mcg, PABA, Mn, Se, tryptophan/Cap. Bot 150s. *otc.*
Use: Vitamin/mineral supplement.

Myadec. (Parke-Davis) Iron 18 mg, A 5000 IU, D 400 IU, E 30 IU, B$_1$ 1.7 mg, B$_2$ 2 mg, B$_3$ 20 mg, B$_5$ 10 mg, B$_6$ 3 mg, B$_{12}$ 6 mcg, C 60 mg, folic acid 0.4 mg, biotin 30 mcg, vitamin K, Ca, P, I, Mg, Cu, zinc 15 mg, Mn, K, Cl, Cr, Mo, Se, Ni, Si, V, B, Sn/Tab. Bot. 130s. *otc.*
Use: Vitamin/mineral supplement.

myagen. Bolasterone.
Use: Anabolic agent.

Myambutol. (Lederle) Ethambutol HCl. Tab. **100 mg:** Bot. 100s. **400 mg:** Bot. 100s, 1000s, UD 10 × 10s. *Rx.*
Use: Antituberculous agent.

myanesin.
See: Mephenesin (Various Mfr.).

Myapap Drops. (Rosemont) Acetaminophen 80 mg/0.8 ml. Bot. 15 ml w/dropper. *otc.*
Use: Analgesic.

Myapap Elixir. (Rosemont) Acetaminophen 160 mg/5 ml. Bot. 4 oz, pt, gal. *otc.*
Use: Analgesic.

Myapap with Codeine Elixir. (Rosemont) Acetaminophen 120 mg, codeine phosphate 12 mg/5 ml. Bot. 4 oz, pt, gal. *c-v.*
Use: Analgesic, antitussive.

Mybanil. (Rosemont) Codeine phosphate 10 mg, bromodiphenhydramine HCl 12.5 mg/5 ml, alcohol 5%. Bot. 4 oz, pt, gal. *c-v.*
Use: Antitussive, antihistamine.

Mycadec DM Drops. (Rosemont) Pseudoephedrine 25 mg, carbinoxamine maleate 2 mg, dextromethorphan HBr 4 mg. Bot. 30 ml. *Rx.*
Use: Decongestant, antihistamine, antitussive.

Mycadec DM Syrup. (Rosemont) Carbinoxamine maleate 4 mg, pseudoephedrine HCl 60 mg, dextromethorphan HBr 15 mg/5 ml, alcohol 0.6%. Bot. 4 oz, pt, gal. *Rx.*
Use: Antihistamine, decongestant, antitussive.

Mycadec Drops. (Rosemont) Pseudoephedrine HCl 25 mg, dextromethorphan HBr 4 mg, carbinoxamine maleate 2 mg/ml. Bot. 30 ml. *Rx.*
Use: Decongestant, antitussive, antihistamine.

Mycartal. (Sanofi Winthrop) Pentaerythritol tetranitrate. *Rx.*
Use: Coronary vasodilator.

Mycelex. (Bayer) Clotrimazole. **Topical Cream:** 1%. Tube 15 g, 30 g, 90 g (2 × 45 g). **Topical Soln.:** 1%. Bot. 10 ml, 30 ml. *otc, Rx.*
Use: Antifungal, topical.

Mycelex-7. (Bayer) **Vaginal Tab.:** Clotrimazole 100 mg. Pkg. 7s with applicator; **Vaginal Cream:** Clotrimazole 1%. Tube 45 g (7 day therapy) with applicator. *otc.*
Use: Antifungal, vaginal.

Mycelex-7 Combination Pack. (Bayer) Clotrimazole. **Cream:** 1%. Tube 7 g; **Supp.:** 100 mg. Pkg. 7s w/applicator. *otc.*
Use: Antifungal, vaginal.

Mycelex-G. (Bayer) Clotrimazole. **Vaginal Tab.:** 100 mg. Pkg. 7s w/applicator. **Cream:** 1%. Tube 45 g, 90 g. *Rx.*
Use: Antifungal, vaginal.

Mycelex-G 500. (Bayer) Clotrimazole 500 mg/Vaginal Tab. w/applicator. *Rx.*
Use: Antifungal, vaginal.

Mycelex OTC. (Bayer) Clotrimazole 1%, benzyl alcohol 1%. Cream. Tube 15 g. *otc.*
Use: Anti-infective, topical.

Mycelex Troches. (Bayer) Clotrimazole 10 mg/Troche 70s, 140s. *Rx.*
Use: Antifungal, oral.

Mycelex Twin Pack. (Bayer) Clotrimazole 500 mg/Vaginal Tab. w/applicator. Topical cream 1%. Tube 7 g. *Rx.*
Use: Antifungal, vaginal.

Mychel-S. (Rachelle) Sterile chloramphenicol sodium succinate. Vial 1 g/15 ml. Box 5s. *Rx.*
Use: Anti-infective.

Mycifradin. (Pharmacia & Upjohn) Neomycin sulfate 125 mg/5 ml (equivalent to 87.5 mg neomycin). Oral soln. Bot. pt. *Rx.*
Use: Anti-infective.

Myciguent. (Pharmacia & Upjohn) Neomycin sulfate. **Cream:** 5 mg/g. Tube 0.5 oz. **Oint.:** 5 mg/g. Tube 0.5 oz, 1 oz, 4 oz. *otc.*
Use: Anti-infective, topical.

Mycinette. (Pfeiffer) Benzocaine 15 mg, sorbitol, saccharin, menthol. Loz. 12s. *otc.*

Use: Local anesthetic, antiseptic, expectorant.

Mycinette Sore Throat. (Pfeiffer) Phenol 1.4%, alum 0.3%, alcohol free, sugar free. Spray 180 ml. *otc.*
Use: Mouth/throat product.

Myci-Spray. (Misemer) Phenylephrine HCl 0.25%, pyrilamine maleate 0.15%/ml. Bot. 20 ml. *otc.*
Use: Decongestant, antihistamine.

Mycitracin. (Pharmacia & Upjohn) Bacitracin 500 units, neomycin sulfate 5 mg, polymyxin B sulfate 5000 units/g. Oint.: Tube 0.5 oz. Box 36s; 1 oz; UD ⅟₃₂ oz Box 144s. *otc.*
Use: Anti-infective, topical.

Mycitracin Plus. (Pharmacia & Upjohn) Polymyxin B sulfate 5000 units/g, neomycin 3.5 mg/g, bacitracin 500 units/g, lidocaine 40 mg, white petrolatum. Tube Oint. 15 g. *otc.*
Use: Anti-infective, topical.

Mycitracin Triple Antibiotic Maximum Strength. (Pharmacia & Upjohn) Polymyxin B sulfate 5000 units/g, neomycin 3.5 mg/g, bacitracin 500 units/g, parabens, mineral oil, white petrolatum. Oint. Tube 30 g, UD 0.94 g. *otc.*
Use: Anti-infective, topical.

Mycobutin. (Pharmacia & Upjohn) Rifabutin. 150 mg/Cap. Bot. 100s. *Rx.*
Use: Antituberculous.

Mycocide NS. (Woodward) Benzalkonium Cl, propylene glycol, methylparaben. Soln. Bot. 30 ml. *Rx.*
Use: Antiseptic, germicide.

Mycodone Syrup. (Rosemont) Hydrocodone bitartrate 5 mg, homatropine MBr 1.5 mg/5 ml. Bot. 4 oz, pt, gal. *c-III.*
Use: Antitussive.

Mycogen II Cream. (Goldline) Nystatin 100,000 units, triamcinolone acetonide 1 mg/g. Cream Tube 15 g, 30 g, 60 g, 120 g, lb. *Rx.*
Use: Antifungal, corticosteroid, topical.

Mycolog II Cream and Ointment. (Squibb) Triamcinolone acetonide 1 mg, nystatin 100,000 units/g. Ointment base w/Plastibase (polyethylene, mineral oil). Tube 15 g, 30 g, 60 g, Jar 120 g. *Rx.*
Use: Antifungal, corticosteroid, topical.

Mycogen II Ointment. (Goldline) Nystatin 100,000 units, triamcinolone acetonide 1 mg/g. Oint. Tube 15 g, 30 g, 60 g. *Rx.*
Use: Antifungal, corticosteroid, topical.

Mycomist. (Gordon) Chlorophyll, formalin, benzalkonium Cl. Bot. 4 oz, plastic Bot. 1 oz. *otc.*

Use: Antifungal for clothing.

•**mycophenolate mofetil.** (my-koe-FEN-oh-LATE MOE-feh-till) USAN.
Use: Immunomodulator.
See: CellCept, Cap. (Roche).

•**mycophenolic acid.** (MY-koe-fen-AHL-ik Acid) USAN.
Use: Antineoplastic.

Mycoplasma Pneumonia IFA IgM Test. (Wampole-Zeus) Indirect fluorescent assay for IgM antibodies to *Mycoplasma pneumoniae.* Box test 100s.
Use: Diagnostic aid.

Mycoplasma Pneumonia IFA Test. (Wampole-Zeus) Indirect fluorescent assay for antibodies to *Mycoplasma pneumoniae.* Box test 100s.
Use: Diagnostic aid.

Mycostatin. (Apothecon) Nystatin. **Tab.:** 500,000 units. Bot. 100s. **Cream:** 100,000 units/g in aqueous base. Tube 15 g, 30 g. **Oint.:** 100,000 units/g in Plastibase (polyethylene and mineral oil). Tube 15 g, 30 g. **Susp.:** 100,000 units/ml. In vehicle containing sucrose 50%, saccharin < 1% alcohol. Bot. 60 ml, 473 ml. **Troche:** 200,000 units. 30s. **Vaginal Tab:** 100,000 units, lactose 0.95 g, ethyl cellulose, stearic acid, starch. Pkg. 15s, 30s. **Pow.:** (topical) 100,000 units/g in talc. Shaker bot. 15 g. *Rx.*
Use: Antifungal.

Mycostatin Pastilles. (Bristol-Myers Oncology) Nystatin, 200,000 units/Troche. 30s. *Rx.*
Use: Antifungal, oral.

Myco Triacet. (Various Mfr.) Triamcinolone acetonide 0.1%, neomycin sulfate 0.25%, gramicidin 0.25 mg, nystatin 100,000 units/g. **Cream:** 15 g, 30 g, 60 g, 480 g. **Oint.:** 15 g, 30 g, 60 g. *Rx.*
Use: Corticosteroid, antifungal, topical.

Myco Triacet II Cream & Ointment. (Lemmon) Nystatin 100,000 units, triamcinolone acetonide 1 mg/g. **Cream:** White petrolatum and mineral oil. Tube 15 g, 30 g, 60 g. **Oint.:** Tube 15 g, 30 g, 60 g. *Rx.*
Use: Antifungal, corticosteroid, topical.

Mycotussin Expectorant. (Rosemont) Pseudoephedrine HCl 60 mg, hydrocodone bitartrate 5 mg, guaifenesin 200 mg/5 ml, alcohol 12.5%. Bot. 4 oz, pt, gal. *c-III.*
Use: Decongestant, antitussive, expectorant.

Mycotussin Liquid. (Rosemont) Pseudoephedrine HCl 60 mg, hydro-

codone bitartrate 5 mg/5 ml, alcohol 5%. Bot. 4 oz, pt, gal. *c-III*.
Use: Decongestant, antitussive.

Mydacol. (Rosemont) Vitamins B$_1$ 5 mg, B$_2$ 2.5 mg, niacinamide 50 mg, B$_6$ 1 mg, B$_{12}$ 1 mcg, pantothenic acid 10 mg, iodine 100 mcg, iron 15 mg, magnesium 2 mg, zinc 2 mg, choline 100 mg, manganese 2 mg/30 ml. Bot. pt, gal. *otc*.
Use: Vitamin/mineral supplement.

Mydfrin Ophthalmic 2.5%. (Alcon) Phenylephrine HCl 2.5%. Drop-Tainers. 3 ml, 5 ml. *Rx*.
Use: Mydriatic.

Mydriacyl. (Alcon) Tropicamide 0.5% or 1%. Soln. 3 ml (1% only), 15 ml Drop-Tainer. *Rx*.
Use: Cycloplegic mydriatic.

mydriatics.
  Parasympatholytic Types
  Atropine Salts (Various Mfr.).
  Homatropine Hydrobromide (Various Mfr.).
  Scopolamine Salts (Various Mfr.).
  Sympathomimetic Types
  Amphetamine Sulfate 3% (Various Mfr.).
  Clopane HCl, Liq. (Lilly).
  Ephedrine Sulfate (Various Mfr.).
  Epinephrine HCl (Various Mfr.).
  Neo-Synephrine HCl, Preps. (Sanofi Winthrop).
  Phenylephrine HCl. (Various Mfr.).

myelin. *Rx*.
Use: Multiple sclerosis. [Orphan drug]

Myelo-Kit. (Sanofi Winthrop) Omnipaque 180 or 240 in various sizes and one sterile myelogram tray.
Use: Radiopaque agent.

Myfedrine. (Rosemont) Pseudoephedrine 30 mg/5 ml. Liq. Bot. 473 ml. *otc*.
Use: Decongestant.

Myfedrine Plus Syrup. (Rosemont) Pseudoephedrine HCl 30 mg, chlorpheniramine maleate 2 mg/5 ml. Bot. 4 oz, pt, gal. *otc*.
Use: Decongestant, antihistamine.

Myfed Syrup. (Rosemont) Triprolidine HCl 1.25 mg, pseudoephedrine HCl 30 mg/5 ml. Bot. 4 oz, pt, gal. *otc*.
Use: Antihistamine, decongestant.

Mygel Liquid. (Geneva Pharm) Aluminum hydroxide 200 mg, magnesium hydroxide 200 mg, simethicone 20 mg, sodium 1.38 mg/5 ml. Liq. Bot. 360 ml. *otc*.
Use: Antacid, antiflatulent.

Mygel Suspension. (Geneva Pharm) Aluminum hydroxide 200 mg, magnesium hydroxide 200 mg, simethicone 20 mg/5 ml. Bot. 360 ml. *otc*.
Use: Antacid, antiflatulent.

Mygel II Suspension. (Geneva Pharm) Aluminum hydroxide 400 mg, magnesium hydroxide 400 mg, simethicone 40 mg/5 ml. Bot. 360 ml. *otc*.
Use: Antacid, antiflatulent.

Myhistine DH. (Rosemont) Codeine phosphate 10 mg, chlorpheniramine maleate 2 mg, pseudoephedrine HCl 30 mg/5 ml. Liq. Bot. 4 oz, pt, gal. *c-v*.
Use: Antitussive, antihistamine, decongestant.

Myhistine Elixir. (Rosemont) Chlorpheniramine maleate 2 mg, phenylephrine HCl 5 mg/5 ml, alcohol 5%. Liq. Bot. 4 oz, pt, gal. *otc*.
Use: Antihistamine, decongestant.

Myhistine Expectorant. (Rosemont) Codeine phosphate 10 mg, guaifenesin 100 mg, pseudoephedrine HCl 30 mg/5 ml, alcohol 7.5%. Liq. Bot. 4 oz, pt, gal. *c-v*.
Use: Antitussive, expectorant, decongestant.

Myhydromine Pediatric. (Rosemont) Phenylpropanolamine HCl 12.5 mg, hydrocodone bitartrate 2.5 mg/5 ml. Bot. pt, gal. *c-III*.
Use: Decongestant, antitussive.

Myhydromine Syrup. (Rosemont) Phenylpropanolamine HCl 25 mg, hydrocodone bitartrate 5 mg/5 ml. Bot. 4 oz, pt, gal. *c-III*.
Use: Decongestive, antitussive.
Use: Antihistamine.

Myidone Tabs. (Major) Primidone 250 mg/Tab. Bot. 100s, 1000s. *Rx*.
Use: Anticonvulsant.

Myidyl Syrup. (Rosemont) Triprolidine HCl 1.25 mg/5 ml, alcohol 4%. Bot. 120 ml, pt, gal. *Rx*.
Use: Antihistamine.

Mykacet Cream. (NMC Labs) Nystatin 100,000 units, triamcinolone acetonide 0.1%/g. Tube 15 g, 30 g, 60 g. *Rx*.
Use: Antifungal, corticosteroid, topical.

My-K Elixir. (Rosemont) Potassium 20 mEq/15 ml, alcohol 5%, saccharin. Bot. pt, gal. *Rx*.
Use: Potassium supplement.

My-K Formula 77D. (Rosemont) Phenylpropanolamine HCl 12.5 mg, dextromethorphan HBr 10 mg, guaifenesin 100 mg/5 ml, alcohol 10%. Liq. Bot. 180 ml. *otc*.

Use: Decongestant, antitussive, expectorant.

My-K Formula 77 Liquid. (Rosemont) Doxylamine succinate 3.75 mg, dextromethorphan HBr 7.5 mg/5 ml, alcohol 10%. Liq. Bot. 180 ml. *otc.*
Use: Antihistamine, antitussive.

Mykinac Cream. (NMC Labs) Nystatin 100,000 units/g in cream base. Tube 15 g, 30 g. *otc.*
Use: Antifungal, topical.

My-K Nasal Spray. (Rosemont) Oxymetazoline HCl 0.05%. Bot. 0.5 oz. *otc.*
Use: Decongestant.

Mykrox. (Medeva) Metolazone 0.5 mg/ Tab. Bot. 100s. *Rx.*
Use: Diuretic.

Mylagen Gelcaps. (Goldline) Calcium carbonate 311 mg, magnesium carbonate 232 mg. Pkg. 24s. *otc.*
Use: Antacid.

Mylagen Liquid. (Goldline) Magnesium hydroxide 200 mg, aluminum hydroxide 200 mg, simethicone 20 mg/5 ml. Bot. 355 ml. *otc.*
Use: Antacid, antiflatulent.

Mylagen II Liquid. (Goldline) Aluminum hydroxide 400 mg, magnesium hydroxide 400 mg, simethicone 40 mg/5 ml. Bot. 355 ml. *otc.*
Use: Antacid, antiflatulent.

Mylanta. (J & J-Merck) Calcium carbonate 600 mg. Loz. 18s, 50s. *otc.*
Use: Antacid.

Mylanta Double Strength. (J & J-Merck) **Chew. Tab.:** Magnesium hydroxide 400 mg, aluminum hydroxide dried gel 400 mg, simethicone 40 mg, Bot. 24s, 60s. **Liq.:** Magnesium hydroxide 400 mg, aluminum hydroxide dried gel 400 mg, simethicone 40 mg, sorbitol/5 ml. Bot. 150 ml, 360 ml. **Susp.:** Magnesium hydroxide 400 mg, aluminum hydroxide dried gel 400 mg, simethicone 40 mg, sodium 0.05 mEq/5 ml. Bot. 150 ml, 360 ml, 720 ml, UD 30, 150 ml. *otc.*
Use: Antacid.

Mylanta Gas. (J & J-Merck) Simethicone **40 mg:** Chew. Tab. Bot. 100s, UD 100s; **80 mg:** Chew. Tab. Pkg. 12s, Bot. 48s, 100s, UD 100s. *otc.*
Use: Antiflatulent.

Mylanta Gas, Maximum Strength. (J & J-Merck) Simethicone 125 mg/Chew. Tab. Pkg. 12s, Bot. 60s. *otc.*
Use: Antiflatulent.

Mylanta Gelcaps. (J & J-Merck) Calcium carbonate 311 mg, magnesium carbonate 232 mg. Bot. 24s, 50s. *otc.*

Use: Antacid.

Mylanta Liquid. (J & J-Merck) Magnesium hydroxide 200 mg, aluminum hydroxide 200 mg, simethicone 20 mg, sodium 0.68 mg/5 ml. Bot. 150 ml, 360 ml, 720 ml, UD 30 ml. *otc.*
Use: Antacid, antiflatulent.

Mylanta Natural Fiber Supplement. (J & J-Merck) Psyllium hydrophilic mucilloid fiber 3.4 g/dose, sucrose, orange flavor. Pow. Can 390 g. *otc.*
Use: Laxative.

Mylanta Soothing Antacids. (J & J-Merck) Calcium carbonate 600 mg, corn syrup, sucrose. Loz. Pkg. 18s. Bot. 50s. *otc.*
Use: Antacid.

Mylanta Tablets. (J & J-Merck) Magnesium hydroxide 200 mg, aluminum hydroxide 200 mg, simethicone 20 mg, sodium 0.77 mg, sorbitol/Chew. Tab. Bot. 12s, 40s, 48s, 100s, 180s. *otc.*
Use: Antacid, antiflatulent.

Mylanta-II Liquid. (J & J-Merck) Magnesium hydroxide 400 mg, aluminum hydroxide 400 mg, simethicone 40 mg, sodium 1.14 mg, sorbitol/5 ml. Bot. 0.5 oz, 12 oz, UD 30 ml, 100s. *otc.*
Use: Antacid, antiflatulent.

Mylanta-II Tablets. (J & J-Merck) Magnesium hydroxide 400 mg, aluminum hydroxide 400 mg, simethicone 40 mg, sodium 1.3 mg/Chew. Tab. Box 24s, 60s. *otc.*
Use: Antacid, antiflatulent.

Mylase 100. Alpha-amylase.
See: Diastase.
W/Prolase, cellulase, calcium carbonate, magnesium glycinate.
See: Zylase Tab. (Eon Labs).

Myleran. (Glaxo Wellcome) Busulfan 2 mg/Tab. Bot. 25s. *Rx.*
Use: Alkylating agent.

Mylicon. (Zeneca) Simethicone 40 mg. **Chew. Tab.:** Bot. 100s, 500s, UD 100s. **Drops:** 40 mg/0.6 ml. Bot. 30 ml. *otc.*
Use: Antiflatulent.

Mylicon-80. (Zeneca) Simethicone 80 mg/Chew. Tab. Bot. 100s, Box 12s, 48s, UD 100s. *otc.*
Use: Antiflatulent.

Mylicon-125. (Zeneca) Simethicone 125 mg/Chew. Tab. In 12s, 50s. *otc.*
Use: Antiflatulent.

Mylocaine 2% Viscous Solution. (Rosemont) Lidocaine HCl 2%. Bot. 100 ml. *Rx.*
Use: Local anesthetic.

Mylocaine 4% Solution. (Rosemont) Lidocaine HCl 4%. Bot. 50 ml, 100 ml. *Rx.*
Use: Local anesthetic.

Mymethasone Elixir. (Rosemont) Dexamethasone 0.5 mg/5 ml, alcohol 5%. Bot. 100 ml, 240 ml. *Rx.*
Use: Corticosteroid.

Myminic Expectorant. (Morton Grove) Phenylpropanolamine HCl 12.5 mg, guaifenesin 100 mg/5 ml, alcohol 5%. Bot. 4 oz, pt, gal. *otc.*
Use: Decongestant, expectorant.

Myminic Pediatric. (Rosemont) Phenylpropanolamine HCl 12.5 mg, guaifenesin 100 mg/5 ml, alcohol 5%. Liq. Bot. 4 oz, pt, gal. *otc.*
Use: Decongestant, expectorant.

Myminic Syrup. (Rosemont) Phenylpropanolamine HCl 12.5 mg, chlorpheniramine maleate 2 mg/5 ml. Alcohol free. Bot. 4 oz, pt, gal. *otc.*
Use: Decongestant, antihistamine.

Myminicol Liquid. (Morton Grove) Phenylpropanolamine HCl 12.5 mg, chlorpheniramine maleate 2 mg, dextromethorphan HBr 10 mg/5 ml. Liq. Bot. 4 oz, pt, gal. *otc.*
Use: Decongestant, antihistamine, antitussive.

Mynatal. (ME Pharm) Ca 300 mg, iron 65 mg, vitamins A 5000 IU, D 400 IU, E 30 mg, B_1 3 mg, B_2 3.4 mg, B_3 20 mg, B_5 10 mg, B_6 10 mg, B_{12} 12 mcg, C 120 mg, folic acid 1 mg, biotin 30 mcg, Cr, Cu, I, Mg, Mn, Mo, Zn 25 mg/Cap. Bot. 100s, 500s. *Rx.*
Use: Vitamin/mineral supplement.

Mynatal FC. (ME Pharm) Calcium 250 mg, iron 60 mg, vitamin A 5000 IU, D 400 IU, E 30 IU, B_1 3 mg, B_2 3.4 mg, B_3 20 mg, B_5 10 mg, B_6 10 mg, B_{12} 12 mcg, C 100 mg, folic acid 1 mg, biotin 30 mcg, calcium 25 mg, I, Mg, Cr, Cu, Mo, Mn. Capl. Bot. 100s. *Rx.*
Use: Vitamin/mineral supplement.

Mynatal PN Captabs. (ME Pharm) Ca 125 mg, iron 60 mg, vitamins A 4000 IU, D 400 IU, B_1 3 mg, B_2 3 mg, B_3 10 mg, B_6 2 mg, B_{12} 3 mcg, C 50 mg, folic acid 1 mg, Zn 18 mg/Tab. Bot. 100s. *Rx.*
Use: Vitamin/mineral supplement.

Mynatal PN Forte. (ME Pharm) Iron 60 mg, vitamin A 5000 IU, D 400 IU, E 30 IU, C 80 mg, B_1 3 mg, B_2 3.4 mg, B_3 20 mg, B_6 4 mg, B_{12} 12 mcg, folic acid 1 mg, calcium 250 mg, zinc 25 mg, I, Mg, Cu. Capl. Bot. 100s. *Rx.*
Use: Vitamin/mineral supplement.

Mynatal Rx. (ME Pharm) Calcium 200 mg, iron 60 mg, vitamin A 4000 IU, D 400 IU, E 15 mg, B_1 1.5 mg, B_2 1.6 mg, B_3 17 mg, B_5 7 mg, B_6 4 mg, B_{12} 2.5 mcg, C 80 mg, folic acid 1 mg, biotin 0.03 mg, zinc 25 mg, Mg, Cu. Capl. Bot. 100s. *Rx.*
Use: Vitamin/mineral supplement.

Mynate 90 Plus. (ME Pharm) Calcium 250 mg, iron 90 mg, vitamin A 4000 IU, D 400 IU, E 30 IU, B_1 3 mg, B_2 3.4 mg, B_3 20 mg, B_6 20 mg, B_{12} 12 mcg, C 120 mg, folic acid 1 mg, zinc 25 mg, DSS, I, Cu. Capl. Bot. 100s. *Rx.*
Use: Vitamin/mineral supplement.

Myo-B. (Sig) Adenosine-5-monophosphoric acid, vitamin B_{12}. Vial 10 ml. *Rx.*

Myocide NS. (Woodward) Benzalkonium chloride, propylene glycol, methylparaben/Soln. 30 ml. *otc.*
Use: Antiseptic.

myodil.
See: Iophendylate Inj., U.S.P. 23.

Myoflex Creme. (Rhone-Poulenc Rorer) Trolamine salicylate 10% in a vanishing cream base. Tube 2 oz, 4 oz, Jar 8 oz, lb, Pump dispenser 3 oz. *otc.*
Use: Analgesic, topical.

Myolin. (Roberts Hauck) Orphenadrine citrate 30 mg/ml. Inj. Vial 10 ml. *Rx.*
Use: Skeletal muscle relaxant.

Myorgal. (Mysuran.) Ambenonium Cl.
Use: Cholinergic.

Myotalis. (Vita Elixir) Digitalis 1.5 gr/EC Tab. *Rx.*
Use: Digitalis therapy.

Myoscint. (Centocor) Imciromab pentetate 0.5 mg for conjugation with indium-111. Kit.
Use: Radioimmunoscintigraphy.

Myotonachol. (Glenwood) Bethanechol Cl 10 mg or 25 mg/Tab. Bot. 100s. *Rx.*
Use: Urinary tract product.

Myotoxin. (Vita Elixir) **#1:** Digitoxin 0.1 mg/Tab. **#2:** Digitoxin 0.2 mg/Tab. *Rx.*
Use: Cardiac glycoside.

Myphentol Elixir. (Rosemont) Phenobarbital 16.2 mg, hyoscyamine SO_4 or HBr 0.1037 mg, atropine sulfate 0.0194 mg, scopolamine HBr 0.0065 mg/5 ml, alcohol 23%. Bot. 4 oz, pt, gal. *Rx.*
Use: Anticholinergic, antispasmodic, sedative, hypnotic.

Myphetane DC Cough Syrup. (Morton Grove) Codeine phosphate 10 mg, brompheniramine maleate 2 mg, phenylpropanolamine HCl 12.5 mg/5 ml, alcohol 1.2%. Bot. 4 oz, gal. *c-v.*

Use: Antitussive, antihistamine, decongestant.

Myphetane DX Cough Syrup. (Various Mfr.) Brompheniramine maleate 2 mg, pseudoephedrine HCl 30 mg, dextromethorphan HBr 10 mg/5 ml, alcohol 0.95%. Bot. 4 oz, pt, gal. *Rx.*
Use: Antihistamine, decongestant, antitussive.

Myphetane Elixir. (Rosemont) Brompheniramine maleate 2 mg/5 ml, alcohol 3%. *otc.*
Use: Antihistamine.

Myphetapp Elixer. (Rosemont) Brompheniramine maleate 2 mg, phenylpropanolamine HCl 12.5 mg/5 ml, alcohol 2.3%. Bot. 4 oz, pt. *otc.*
Use: Antihistamine, decongestant.

Myproic Acid Syrup. (Rosemont) Valproic acid 250 mg (as sodium valproate)/5 ml. Bot. pt. *Rx.*
Use: Anticonvulsant.

Myriatin Drops. (Sanofi Winthrop) Atropine methonitrate BP. *Rx.*
Use: Antispasmodic.

myristica oil.
Use: Flavor.

•**myristyl alcohol,** N.F. 18.
Use: Pharmaceutic aid (stiffening agent).

myristyl-picolinium chloride.
See: Wet Tone, Soln. (3M).

Myrj 45. (Zeneca) Mixture of free polyoxyethylene glycol and its mono- and di-stearates. Polyoxyl 8 stearate.
Use: Surface-active agent.

Myrj 52 and M2s. (Zeneca) Polyoxyethylene 40 stearate. Mixture of free polyoxyethylene glycol and its mono-and distearates.
Use: Surface-active agent.

Myrj 53. (Zeneca) Polyoxyl 50 stearate.
Use: Surface-active agent.

Mysoline. (Wyeth-Ayerst) Primidone, lactose, saccharin. **Tab.:** 50 mg Bot. 100s, 500s; 250 mg. Bot. 100s, 1000s, UD 100s. **Susp.:** 250 mg/5 ml. Bot. 240 ml. *Rx.*
Use: Anticonvulsant.

Mysuran. Ambenonium Cl.
Use: Cholinergic muscle stimulant.
See: Mytelase Cl, Cap. (Winthrop-Breon).

Mytelase. (Sanofi Winthrop) Ambenonium Cl 10 mg/Cap. Bot. 100s. *Rx.*
Use: Cholinergic muscle stimulant.

Myticin G Creme and Ointment.
See: g-myticin creme and ointment.

Mytomycin-C. (IOP) *Rx.*
Use: Treatment of refractory glaucoma as an adjunct to AB externo glaucoma surgery. [Orphan drug]

Mytrex. (Savage) Triamcinolone acetonide 0.1%, nystatin 100,000 units/g. Cream, Oint. 15 g, 30 g, 60 g, 120 g. *Rx.*
Use: Corticosteroid, antifungal, topical.

Mytussin AC Cough. (Morton Grove) Guaifenesin 100 mg, codeine phosphate 10 mg/5 ml, alcohol 3.5%. Bot. 4 oz, pt, gal. *c-v.*
Use: Expectorant, antitussive.

Mytussin DM Expectorant. (Morton Grove) Guaifenesin 100 mg, dextromethorphan HBr 10 mg/5 ml, alcohol 1.6%. Bot. 4 oz, pt, gal. *otc.*
Use: Expectorant, antitussive.

Mytussin DAC Syrup. (Rosemont) Guaifenesin 100 mg, pseudoephedrine HCl 30 mg, codeine phosphate 10 mg/5 ml. Bot. 4 oz, pt, gal. *c-v.*
Use: Expectorant, decongestant, antitussive.

Mytussin Syrup. (Rosemont) Guaifenesin 100 mg/5 ml, alcohol 3.5%. Bot. 4 oz, pt, gal. *otc.*
Use: Expectorant.

Myverol. (Eastman Kodak) Glyceryl monostearate.

My-Vitalife. (ME Pharm) Ca 130 mg, iron 27 mg, vitamins A 6500 IU, D 400 IU, E 30 mg, B_1 1.5 mg, B_2 1.7 mg, B_3 20 mg, B_5 10 mg, B_6 2 mg, B_{12} 6 mcg, C 60 mg, folic acid 0.4 mg, Cr, Cu, K, I, Mg, Mn, Mo, P, Se, Zn, 15 mg, vitamin K, biotin 30 mcg/Cap. Bot. 60s. *otc.*
Use: Vitamin/mineral supplement.

N

Na-Ana-Tal. (Churchill) Phenobarbital 0.25 g, phenacetin 2 g, aspirin 3 g, nicotinic acid 50 mg/Tab. Bot. 100s, Liq. Bot. 16 oz. *c-iv.*
Use: Sedative, hypnotic, analgesic.

● **nabazenil.** (nab-AZE-eh-nill) USAN.
Use: Anticonvulsant.

● **nabilone.** (NAB-ih-lone) USAN.
Use: Tranquilizer (minor).

● **nabitan hydrochloride.** (NAB-ih-tan) USAN. *Formerly Nabutan Hydrochloride.*
Use: Analgesic.

● **naboctate hydrochloride.** (NAB-ock-tate) USAN.
Use: Antiglaucoma agent, antinauseant.

● **nabumetone.** (nab-YOU-meh-TONE) USAN.
Use: Anti-inflammatory.
See: Relafen (S-K Beecham).

n-acetylcysteine.
See: Acetylcysteine.

n-acetyl-p-aminophenol. Acetaminophen, U.S.P. 23.

n¹-acetylsulfanilamide.
See: Acetylsulfanilamide.

● **nadide.** (NAD-ide) USAN. *Formerly Diphosphopyridine Nucleotide, Nicotinamide Adenine Dinucleotide.*
Use: Antagonist to alcohol and narcotics.

Nadinola (Deluxe) for Oily Skin. (Strickland) Hydroquinone 2%. Bot. 1.25 oz, 2.25 oz. *Rx.*
Use: Skin bleaching agent.

Nadinola for Dry Skin. (Strickland) Hydroquinone 2%. Bot. 1.25 oz, 2.25 oz. *Rx.*
Use: Skin bleaching agent.

Nadinola (Ultra) for Normal Skin. (Strickland) Hydroquinone 2%. Bot. 1.25 oz, 3.75 oz, Tube 1.85 oz. *Rx.*
Use: Skin bleaching agent.

● **nadolol,** (nay-DOE-lahl) U.S.P. 23.
Use: Antihypertensive, antianginal, beta-adrenergic blocker.
See: Corgard, Tab. (Bristol Labs).

nadolol. (nay-DOE-lahl) (Various Mfr.) Tab.: **20 mg:** 100s, UD 100s. **40 mg, 80 mg:** 100s, 1000s, UD 100s. **120 mg:** 100s, 1000s. **160 mg:** 100s. *Rx.*
Use: Beta-adrenergic blocker.

nadolol and bendroflumethiazide.
Use: Antihypertensive and antianginal beta blocker.
See: Corzide (Bristol-Myers).

naepaine hydrochloride.
Use: Local anesthetic.

● **nafamostat mesylate.** (naff-AM-oh-stat) USAN.
Use: Anticoagulant; antifibrinolytic.

● **nafarelin acetate.** (NAFF-uh-RELL-in) USAN.
Use: LHRH agonist; agonist, central precocious puberty [Orphan drug].
See: Synarel (Syntex).

Nafazair. (Bausch & Lomb) Naphazoline HCl 0.1%. Soln. Bot. 15 ml. *Rx.*
Use: Ophthalmic vasoconstrictor, mydriatic.

Nafazair A. (Bausch & Lomb) Naphazoline HCl 0.025%, pheniramine maleate 0.3%, benzalkonium chloride 0.01%, EDTA, boric acid, sodium borate. Bot. 15 ml. *Rx.*
Use: Ophthalmic decongestant combination.

Nafcil. (Bristol) Nafcillin sodium pow. for inj. Sodium 2.9 mEq/g. Vial 500 mg, 1 g, 2 g; Bulk vial 10 g; Piggyback vial 1 g, 2 g. *Rx.*
Use: Anti-infective, penicillin.

● **nafcillin, sodium,** (naff-SILL-in) U.S.P. 23.
Use: Antibacterial.
See: Nafcil, Inj. (Bristol).
Unipen, Vial, Cap., Pow., Tab. (Wyeth-Ayerst).

Na-Feen. (Pacemaker) Fluoride 1 mg/ Dose. Tab. Bot. 100s, 500s, 1000s; Liq. 2 oz. *Rx.*
Use: Dental caries preventative.

● **nafenopin.** (naff-EN-oh-pin) USAN.
Use: Antihyperlipoproteinemic.

● **nafimidone hydrochloride.** (naff-IH-mih-DOHN) USAN.
Use: Anticonvulsant.

● **naflocort.** (NAFF-lah-cort) USAN.
Use: Adrenocortical steroid (topical).

● **nafomine malate.** (NAFF-oh-meen) USAN.
Use: Muscle relaxant.

● **nafoxidine hydrochloride.** (naff-OX-ih-deen) USAN.
Use: Antiestrogen.

● **nafronyl oxalate.** (NAFF-row-NILL OX-ah-late) USAN.
Use: Vasodilator.

naftalan.
W/Ichthyol, calamine, amber petrolatum.
See: Nagtalan, Oint. (Paddock).

● **naftifine hydrochloride.** (NAFF-tih-FEEN) USAN.
Use: Antifungal.
See: Naftin, Cream (Allergan Herbert).

Naftin. (Allergan Herbert) Naftifine HCl 1%. Cream. 2 g, 15 g, 30 g. *Rx.*
Use: Antifungal, topical.

naganol.
See: Suramin Sodium. Naphuride Sodium.

Nailicure. (Purepac) Denatonium benzoate in a clear nail polish base. Bot. 0.33 oz. *otc.*
Use: Nail biting deterrent.

Nail Plus. (Faraday) Gelatin Cap. Bot. 100s, 200s.

•**nalbuphine hydrochloride.** (NAL-byoo-FEEN) USAN.
Use: Analgesic; antagonist to narcotics.
See: Nubain, Vial (DuPont Merck).

Naldecon-CX Adult Liquid. (Apothecon) Phenylpropanolamine 12.5 mg, guaifenesin 200 mg, codeine phosphate 10 mg/10 ml. Alcohol free. Bot. 4 oz, pt. *c-v.*
Use: Decongestant, expectorant, antitussive.

Naldecon-DX Adult Liquid. (Apothecon) Phenylpropanolamine HCl 12.5 mg, guaifenesin 200 mg, dextromethorphan HBr 10 mg/10 ml, saccharin, sorbitol. Alcohol free. Bot. 4 oz, pt. *otc.*
Use: Decongestant, expectorant, antitussive.

Naldecon-DX Children's Syrup. (Apothecon) Phenylpropanolamine HCl 6.25 mg, dextromethorphan HBr 5 mg, guaifenesin 100 mg/5 ml. Bot. 4 oz, 16 oz. *otc.*
Use: Decongestant, antitussive, expectorant.

Naldecon-DX Pediatric Drops. (Apothecon) Phenylpropanolamine HCl 6.25 mg, guaifenesin 50 mg, dextromethorphan HBr 5 mg/ml, alcohol free, saccharin, sorbitol. Bot. 30 ml. *otc.*
Use: Decongestant, expectorant, antitussive.

Naldecon-EX Children's Syrup. (Apothecon) Phenylpropanolamine HCl 6.25 mg, guaifenesin 100 mg/5 ml, saccharin, sorbitol. Bot. 118 ml, 480 ml. *otc.*
Use: Decongestant, expectorant.

Naldecon-EX Pediatric Drops. (Apothecon) Phenylpropanolamine HCl 6.25 mg, guaifenesin 50 mg/ml. Bot. 30 ml. w/dropper. *otc.*
Use: Decongestant, expectorant.

Naldecon Pediatric Drops. (Apothecon) Chlorpheniramine maleate 0.5 mg, phenyltoloxamine citrate 2 mg, phenylpropanolamine HCl 5 mg, phenylephrine HCl 1.25 mg/ml, sorbitol. Bot. 30 ml. *Rx.*
Use: Antihistamine, decongestant.

Naldecon Pediatric Syrup. (Apothecon) Chlorpheniramine maleate 0.5 mg, phenyltoloxamine citrate 2 mg, phenylpropanolamine HCl 5 mg, phenylephrine HCl 1.25 mg/5 ml, sorbitol. Bot. 473 ml. *Rx.*
Use: Antihistamine, decongestant.

Naldecon Senior DX. (Apothecon) Dextromethorphan HBr 10 mg, guaifenesin 200 mg/5 ml, saccharin, sorbitol, alcohol free. Liq. Bot. 118 ml. *otc.*
Use: Antitussive, expectorant.

Naldecon Senior EX. (Apothecon) Guaifenesin 200 mg/5 ml, saccharin, sorbitol. Liq. Bot. 118 ml. *otc.*
Use: Expectorant.

Naldecon Syrup. (Apothecon) Chlorpheniramine maleate 2.5 mg, phenyltoloxamine citrate 7.5 mg, phenylpropanolamine HCl 20 mg, phenylephrine HCl 5 mg/5 ml. Bot. 473 ml. *Rx.*
Use: Antihistamine, decongestant.

Naldecon Tablets. (Apothecon) Phenylephrine HCl 10 mg, phenylpropanolamine HCl 40 mg, phenyltoloxamine citrate 15 mg, chlorpheniramine maleate 5 mg/SR Tab. Bot. 100s, 500s. *Rx.*
Use: Decongestant, antihistamine.

Naldegesic Tablets. (Bristol) Pseudoephedrine HCl 15 mg, acetaminophen 325 mg/Tab. Bot. 100s. *otc.*
Use: Decongestant, analgesic.

Naldelate DX Adult Liquid. (Barre-National) Phenylpropanolamine HCl 12.5 mg, dextromethorphan HBr 10 mg, guaifenesin 200 mg. Bot. 120 ml or 480 ml. *otc.*
Use: Decongestant, antitussive, expectorant.

Naldelate Pediatric Syrup. (Various Mfr.) Phenylpropanolamine HCl 5 mg, phenylephrine HCl 1.25 mg, chlorpheniramine maleate 0.5 mg, phenyltoloxamine citrate 2 mg/5 ml. Bot. 120 ml, 473 ml, gal. *Rx.*
Use: Decongestant, antihistamine.

Naldelate Syrup. (Various Mfr.) Phenylpropanolamine HCl 20 mg, phenylephrine HCl 5 mg, chlorpheniramine maleate 2.5 mg, phenyltoloxamine citrate 7.5 mg/5 ml. Syr. Bot. 473 ml, gal. *Rx.*
Use: Decongestant, antihistamine.

Nalfon. (Dista) Fenoprofen calcium. **Cap.:** 200 mg. Rx Pak 100s. **300 mg.** Rx Pak 100s, Bot. 500s. *Rx.*
Use: Nonsteroidal anti-inflammatory, analgesic.

Nalgest. (Major) Phenylpropanolamine HCl 40 mg, phenylephrine HCl 10 mg, chlorpheniramine maleate 5 mg, phenyltoloxamine citrate 15 mg/Tab. Bot. 100s, 500s, 1000s. *Rx.*
Use: Decongestant, antihistamine.

Nalgest Pediatric Drops. (Major) Phenylpropanolamine HCl 5 mg, phenylephrine HCl 1.25 mg, chlorpheniramine maleate 0.5 mg, phenyltoloxamine citrate 2 mg, sorbitol/Drop. Bot. 30 ml. *Rx.*
Use: Decongestant, antihistamine.

Nalgest Pediatric Syrup. (Major) Phenylpropanolamine HCl 5 mg, phenylephrine HCl 1.25 mg, chlorpheniramine maleate 0.5 mg, phenyltoloxamine citrate 2 mg/5 ml. Syr. Bot. 473 ml, gal. *Rx.*
Use: Decongestant, antihistamine.

Nalgest Syrup. (Major) Phenylpropanolamine HCl 20 mg, phenylephrine HCl 5 mg, chlorpheniramine maleate 2.5 mg, phenyltoloxamine citrate 7.5 mg/5 ml. Syr. Bot. 473 ml. *Rx.*
Use: Decongestant, antihistamine.

• **nalidixate sodium.** (nal-ih-DIK-sate) USAN. Under study.
Use: Antibacterial.

• **nalidixic acid,** (nal-ih-DIK-sik) U.S.P. 23.
Use: Antibacterial.
See: NegGram, Capl., Susp. (Sanofi Winthrop).

Nallpen. (S-K Beecham) Nafcillin sodium monohydrate 500 mg, 1 g or 2 g/ Vial. Inj. Piggyback 1 g, 2 g, Bulk 10 g. *Rx.*
Use: Anti-infective, penicillin.

• **nalmefene.** (NAL-meh-FFEN) USAN.
Formerly Naletrene.
Use: Antagonist to narcotics.
See: Revex, Inj. (Ohmeda).

nalmetrene. (NAL-meh-treen)
Use: Antagonist to narcotics.

• **nalmexone hydrochloride.** (NAL-mex-ohn) USAN.
Use: Analgesic; antagonist to narcotics.

• **nalorphine hydrochloride,** U.S.P. 23.
See: Nalline (Merck).

• **naloxone hydrochloride,** (NAL-ox-ohn) U.S.P. 23.
Use: Narcotic antagonist.
See: Narcan, Amp. (DuPont Merck).

naloxone hydrochloride. (Various Mfr.) **0.02 mg/ml:** Amps 2 ml. **0.4 mg/ml:** Amps 1 ml, syringes 1 ml, vials 1 ml, 2 ml, 10 ml. *Rx.*
Use: Narcotic antagonist.

Nalspan. (Rosemont) Phenylpropanolamine HCl 20 mg, phenylephrine HCl 5 mg, chlorpheniramine maleate 2.5 mg, phenyltoloxamine citrate 7.5 mg/ml, alcohol free. Syr. Bot. pt. *otc.*
Use: Decongestant, antihistamine.

• **naltrexone.** (nal-TREX-ohn) USAN.
Use: Antagonist to narcotics. [Orphan drug]
See: ReVia, Tab. (DuPont Merck).

namazene. Phenothiazine.

namol xenyrate. (NAY-mahl ZEH-neh-rate)
See: Namoxyrate.

• **namoxyrate.** (nam-OX-ee-rate) USAN.
Use: Analgesic.
See: Namol Xenyrate (Warner-Chilcott).

namuron.
See: Cyclobarbital Calcium (Various Mfr.).

• **nandrolone cyclotate.** (NAN-drole-ohn SIH-kloe-tate) USAN.
Use: Anabolic.

• **nandrolone decanoate,** (NAN-drole-ohn deh-KAN-oh-ate) U.S.P. 23.
Use: Androgen.
See: Anabolin LA-100, Vial (Alto).
Androlone-D, Inj. (Keene).
Androlone-D 50, Inj. (Keene).
Deca-Durabolin, Amp., Vial (Organon).
Hybolin Decanoate, Inj. (Hyrex).

• **nandrolone phenpropionate,** (NAN-droe-lone fen-PRO-pee-oh-nate) U.S.P. 23.
Use: Androgen.
See: Anabolin IM, Vial (Alto).
Androlone, Inj. (Keene).
Androlone 50, Inj. (Keene).
Durabolin Inj. (Organon).
Hybolin Improved, Vial (Hyrex).
Nandrolin, Inj. (Solvay).

• **nantradol hydrochloride.** (NAN-trah-DAHL) USAN.
Use: Analgesic.

Naotin. (Drug Products) Sodium nicotinate. Amp. (equivalent to 10 mg nicotinic acid/ml) 10 ml, Box 25s, 100s. *Rx.*
Use: Vitamin B_3 supplement.

Napa. (Medco Research/Parke-Davis) Acecainide hydrochloride.
Use: Cardiac depressant (anti-arrhythmic).

• **napactadine hydrochloride.** (nap-ACK-tah-deen) USAN.
Use: Antidepressant.

• **napamezole hydrochloride.** (nap-am-EH-zole) USAN.
Use: Antidepressant.

Napamide Caps. (Major) Disopyramide phosphate 100 mg or 150 mg/Cap. Bot. 100s, 500s, UD 100s. *Rx.*
Use: Antiarrhythmic.

•**naphazoline hydrochloride,** U.S.P. 23.
Use: Adrenergic (vasoconstrictor).
See: AK-Con, Soln., (Akorn).
Albalon, Soln., (Allergan America).
Allerest Eye Drops, Soln. (Novartis).
Comfort Eye Drops, Soln., (Pilkington Barnes Hind).
Clear Eyes, Drops (Abbott).
Degest 2, Soln., (Pilkington Barnes Hind).
Estivin II, Soln. (Alcon).
Maximum Strength Allergy Drops (Bausch & Lomb).
Muro's Opcon, Soln. (Bausch & Lomb).
Nafazair, Soln. (Bausch & Lomb).
Naphcon, Drops (Alcon).
Privine HCl, Soln., Spray (Novartis).
VasoClear, Soln., (Ciba Vision).
Vasocon Regular, Liq. (Ciba Vision).
W/Antazoline phosphate, boric acid, phenylmercuric acetate, sodium Cl, sodium carbonate anhydrous.
See: Antazoline-V, Soln. (Rugby).
Vasocon-A Ophthalmic, Soln. (Ciba Vision).
W/Antazoline phosphate, polyvinyl alcohol.
See: Albalon-A Liquifilm, Ophth. (Allergan).
W/Methapyrilene HCl, cetylpyridinum Cl, thimerosal.
See: Vapocyn II Nasal Spray (Solvay).
W/Pheniramine maleate.
See: AK-Con-A, Soln., (Akorn).
Nafazair A, Soln., (Bausch & Lomb).
Naphazole-A, Soln., (Major).
Naphazoline Plus, Soln. (Parmed).
Naphcon A, Liq. (Alcon).
Naphoptic-A, Soln. (Optopics).
W/PEG 300, benzalkonium Cl.
See: Allergy Drops (Bausch & Lomb).
W/Phenylephrine HCl, pyrilamine maleate, phenylpropanolamine HCl.
See: 4-Way Nasal Spray (Bristol-Myers).
W/Polyvinyl alcohol.
See: Albalon, Ophth. Soln. (Allergan).
Albalon Liquifilm, Ophth. Soln. (Allergan).

naphazoline hydrochloride. (Various Mfr.) 0.1% Soln. Bot. 15 ml. *Rx.*
Use: Adrenergic (vasoconstrictor).

naphazoline hydrochloride & antazoline phosphate. (Various Mfr.) Naphazoline HCl 0.05%, antazoline phosphate 0.5%. Soln. 5 ml, 15 ml. *otc.*
Use: Ophthalmic decongestant, antihistamine.

naphazoline hydrochloride & pheniramine maleate. (Various Mfr.) Naphazoline HCl 0.025%, pheniramine maleate 0.3%. soln. bot. 15 ml. *otc.*
Use: Ophthalmic decongestant, antihistamine.

naphazoline plus. (Parmed) Naphazoline HCl 0.025%, pheniramine maleate 0.3%. Bot. 15 ml. *otc.*
Use: Ophthalmic decongestant combination.

Naphcon. (Alcon) Naphazoline HCl 0.012%. Bot. 15 ml. *otc.*
Use: Ophthalmic vasoconstrictor, mydriatic.

Naphcon A. (Alcon) Naphazoline HCl 0.025%, pheniramine maleate 0.3%. Bot. 15 ml. *otc.*
Use: Ophthalmic decongestant combination.

Naphcon Forte. (Alcon) Naphazoline HCl 0.1%/ml. Drop-Tainer Bot. 15 ml. *Rx.*
Use: Ophthalmic vasoconstrictor, mydriatic.

Napholine. (Horizon) Naphazoline HCl 0.1%. Soln. Bot. 15 ml. *Rx.*
Use: Ophthalmic vasoconstrictor, mydriatic.

Naphoptic-A. (Optopics) Naphazoline HCl 0.025%, pheniramine maleate 0.3%. Bot. 15 ml. *Rx.*
Use: Ophthalmic decongestant combination.

Naphthyl-B Salicylate. Betol, Naphthosalol, Salinaphthol.
Use: G.I. & G.U., antiseptic.

naphuride sodium. Suramin Sodium.

•**napitane mesylate.** (NAP-ih-tane) USAN.
Use: Antidepressant.

Naprelan. (Wyeth-Ayerst) Naproxen 375 or 500 mg/ER Tab. 100s (375 mg), 75s (500 mg). *Rx.*
Use: Analgesic.

•**napitane mesylate.** (NAP-ih-tane) USAN.
Use: Antidepressant.

Naprosyn. (Syntex) Naproxen. **Oral susp.:** 125 mg/5 ml, sorbitol. Bot. 480 ml. **250 mg/Tab.:** Bot. 100s, 500s, UD 100s; **375 mg/Tab.:** Bot. 100s, 500s, UD 100s; **500 mg/Tab.:** Bot. 100s, 500s, UD 100s. *Rx.*
Use: Nonsteroidal anti-inflammatory, analgesic.

•**naproxen,** (nah-PROX-ehn) U.S.P. 23.

Use: Anti-inflammatory, analgesic, antipyretic.
See: Naprosyn, Susp., Tab. (Syntex).

naproxen. (Various Mfr.) 250, 375, 500 mg/Tab. 100s, 500s, 1000s, UD 100s. *Rx.*
Use: Nonsteroidal anti-inflammatory, analgesic, antipyretic.

naproxen. (Roxane) 125 mg/5ml, methylparaben, sorbitol, sucrose, pineapple-orange flavor. Oral Susp. 500 ml, UD 15 ml and 20 ml.
Use: Nonsteroidal anti-inflammatory agent; analgesic.

•**naproxen sodium,** (nah-PROX-ehn) U.S.P. 23.
Use: Anti-inflammatory, analgesic, antipyretic.
See: Aleve, Tab. (Procter & Gamble).
Anaprox, Tab. (Syntex).
Anaprox DS, Tab. (Syntex).
Naprosyn, Tab., Susp. (Syntex).

naproxen sodium. (Various Mfr.) 200 mg, 250 mg, 500 mg/Tab. 100s, 500s, 1000s, UD 100s. *Rx.*
Use: Nonsteroidal anti-inflammatory, analgesic.

•**naproxol.** (nay-PROX-ole) USAN.
Use: Anti-inflammatory; analgesic; antipyretic.

Naqua. (Schering Plough) Trichlormethiazide 2 mg or 4 mg/Tab. Bot. 100s, 1000s. *Rx.*
Use: Diuretic.
W/Reserpine.
See: Naquival, Tab. (Schering Plough).

•**napsagatran.** USAN.
Use: Antithrombotic.

•**naranol hydrochloride.** (NARE-ah-nahl) USAN.
Use: Antipsychotic.

•**naratriptan hydrochloride.** (NAHR-ah-trip-tan) USAN.
Use: Antimigraine.

Narcan. (DuPont Merck) Naloxone HCl. **0.02 mg/ml:** Amp. 2 ml. **0.4 mg/ml:** Amp. 1 ml, Box 10s. Prefilled syringe 1 ml, Tray 10s; 1 ml, 2 ml, 10 ml multiple dose vials. **1 mg/ml:** Amp. 2 ml, Box 10s; Multiple dose vial 10 ml. *Rx.*
Use: Narcotic antagonist.

Nardil. (Parke-Davis) Phenelzine sulfate 15 mg/Tab. Bot. 100s. *Rx.*
Use: Antidepressant.

Naropin. (Astra USA) Ropivacaine HCL 2, 5, 7.5, and 10 mg/ml concentrations/Inj. Single-dose amps, vials and infusion bottles. *Rx.*
Use: Local anesthetic.

Nasabid. (Abana) Pseudoephedrine HCl 90 mg, guaifenesin 250 mg, sucrose. Cap. Bot. 100s. *Rx.*
Use: Decongestant, expectorant.

Nasacort. (Rhone-Poulenc Rorer) Each actuation: Triamcinolone acetonide 55 mcg. Cannister 10 mg. *Rx.*
Use: Intranasal steroid.

Nasacort AQ. (Rhone-Poulenc Rorer) Triamcinolone acetonide 55 mcg per actuation, benzalkonium chloride, EDTA/spray. Bot. 16.5 g. *Rx.*
Use: Intranasal steroid.

Nasadent. (Scherer) Sodium metaphosphate, glycerin, distilled water, dicalcium phosphate dihydrate, sodium carboxymethylcellulose, oil of spearmint, sodium benzoate, saccharin. *otc.*
Use: Ingestible dentifrice.

Nasahist B Injectable. (Keene) Brompheniramine maleate 10 ml/Vial. For IM, IV and SC administration. *Rx.*
Use: Antihistamine.

Nasahist Capsules. (Keene) Phenylpropanolamine HCl 40 mg, phenylephrine HCl 10 mg, chlorpheniramine maleate 12 mg/Cap. Bot. 100s. *Rx.*
Use: Decongestant, antihistamine.

NaSal Saline Nasal. (Sanofi Winthrop) Sodium Cl 0.65%. Drops, Spray. Bot. 15 ml. *otc.*
Use: Nasal moisturizer.

Nasalcrom Nasal Solution. (McNeil) Cromolyn sodium 40 mg/ml, benzalkonium Cl 0.01%, EDTA 0.01%. Metered dose spray. Delivers 5.2 mg/spray. Complete pkg. 13 ml. Refill 13 ml. *otc.*
Use: Nasal antiallergic.

Nasalide. (Syntex) Flunisolide 0.025% soln. Pump. Bot. 25 ml. *Rx.*
Use: Intranasal steroid.

Nasal Saline. (Sanofi Winthrop Products) Nasal spray and drops. Sodium Cl 0.65% buffered w/phosphates, preservatives. Bot. 15 ml. Spray Bot. 15 ml. *otc.*
Use: Nasal moisturizer.

Nasarel. (Roche) Flunisolide 0.025%/Spray Soln. 25 ml. *Rx.*
Use: Anti-inflammatory.

Nasatab LA. (ECR Pharmaceuticals) Guaifenesin 500 mg, pseudoephedrine HCl 120 mg/LA Tab. Dye free. Bot. 100s. *Rx.*
Use: Expectorant, decongestant.

Nasophen. (Premo) Phenylephrine HCl 0.25% or 1%. Bot. pt. *otc.*
Use: Decongestant.

Natabec. (Parke-Davis) Vitamins A 4000

IU, D 400 IU, B$_1$ 3 mg, B$_2$ 2 mg, B$_6$ 3 mg, C 50 mg, B$_{12}$ 5 mcg, B$_3$ 10 mg, elemental calcium 240 mg, elemental iron 30 mg/Kapseal. Bot. 100s. *otc.*
Use: Vitamin/mineral supplement.

Natabec-F.A. (Parke-Davis) Vitamins A 4000 IU, D 400 IU, B$_1$ 3 mg, B$_2$ 2 mg, B$_6$ 3 mg, C 50 mg, B$_{12}$ 5 mcg, B$_3$ 10 mg, elemental calcium 240 mg, elemental iron 30 mg, folic acid 0.1 mg/Kapseal, magnesium, bisulfites. Bot. 100s. *otc.*
Use: Vitamin/mineral supplement.

Natabec with Fluoride. (Parke-Davis) Vitamins A 4000 IU, D 400 IU, B$_1$ 3 mg, B$_2$ 2 mg, B$_6$ 3 mg, C 50 mg, B$_{12}$ 5 mcg, B$_3$ 10 mg, elemental calcium 240 mg, elemental iron 30 mg, elemental fluoride 1 mg/Kapseal. Bot. 100s. *Rx.*
Use: Vitamin supplement, dental caries preventative.

Natacyn. (Alcon) Natamycin 5%. Bot. 15 ml. *Rx.*
Use: Antifungal agent, ophthalmic.

Natalins. (B-M Squibb) Ca 200 mg, iron 30 mg, vitamins A 4000 IU, D 400 IU, E 15 IU, B$_1$ 1.5 mg, B$_2$ 1.6 mg, B$_3$ 17 mg, B$_6$ 2.6 mg, B$_{12}$ 2.5 mcg, C 70 mg, folic acid 0.5 mg, Mg, Cu, Zn 15 mg/ Tab. Bot. 100s. *otc.*
Use: Vitamin/mineral supplement.

Natalins RX. (B-M Squibb) Ca 200 mg, iron 60 mg, vitamins A 4000 IU, D 400 IU, E 15 mg, B$_1$ 1.5 mg, B$_2$ 1.6 mg, B$_3$ 17 mg, B$_5$ 7 mg, B$_6$ 4 mg, B$_{12}$ 2.5 mcg, C 80 mg, folic acid 1 mg, Cu, Mg, Zn 25 mg, biotin 30 mcg/Tab. Bot. 100s, 1000s. *Rx.*
Use: Vitamin/mineral supplement.

•**natamycin,** (NAT-uh-MY-sin) U.S.P. 23. An antibiotic produced by *Streptomyces natalensis.* Pimafucin.
Use: Antibacterial (ophthalmic).
See: Natacyn, Susp. (Alcon).

Natarex Prenatal. (Major) Ca 200 mg, iron 60 mg, vitamins A 4000 IU, D 400 IU, E 15 mg, B$_1$ 1.5 mg, B$_2$ 1.6 mg, B$_3$ 17 mg, B$_5$ 7 mg, B$_6$ 4 mg, B$_{12}$ 2.5 mcg, C 80 mg, folic acid 1 mg, Cu, Mg, Zn 25 mg, biotin 30 mcg/Tab. Bot 100s. *Rx.*
Use: Vitamin/mineral supplement.

Nata-San. (Sandia) Vitamins A 4000 IU, D 400 IU, B$_1$ 5 mg, B$_2$ 4 mg, B$_6$ 10 mg, nicotinic acid 10 mg, C 100 mg, B$_{12}$ activity 5 mcg, ferrous fumarate 200 mg (elemental iron 65 mg), calcium carbonate 500 mg (calcium 196 mg), copper (sulfate) 0.5 mg, magnesium (sulfate) 0.1 mg, manganese (sulfate) 0.1 mg, potassium (sulfate) 0.1 mg, zinc

(sulfate) 0.5 mg/Tab. Bot. 100s, 1000s. *otc.*
Use: Vitamin/mineral supplement.

Nata-San F.A. (Sandia) Vitamins A 4000 IU, D 400 IU, B$_1$ 5 mg, B$_2$ 4 mg, B$_6$ 10 mg, nicotinic acid 10 mg, C 100 mg, B$_{12}$ activity 5 mcg, folic acid 1 mg, iron 65 mg, calcium 200 mg, copper (sulfate) 0.5 mg, magnesium (sulfate) 0.1 mg, manganese (sulfate) 0.1 mg, potassium (sulfate) 0.1 mg, zinc (sulfate) 0.5 mg/Tab. Bot. 100s, 1000s. *Rx.*
Use: Vitamin/mineral supplement.

Natodine. (Faraday) Iodine in organic form as found in kelp 1 mg/Tab. Bot. 100s, 250s. *otc.*

Natrapel. (Tender) Citronella 10% in 15% Aloe Vera base. *otc.*
Use: Insect repellent.

Natrico. (Drug Products) Potassium nitrate 2 g, sodium nitrite 1 g, nitroglycerin 0.25 g, crataegus oxycantha 0.25 gr/Pulvoid. Bot. 100s, 1000s. *Rx.*
Use: Antihypertensive.

Naturacil. (Bristol-Myers) Psyllium seed husks 3.4 g, carbohydrate 9.6 g, sodium 11 mg, 54 cal./2 pieces. Carton 24s, 40s. *otc.*
Use: Laxative.

Natur-Aid. (Scott/Cord) Lactose, pectin and Carob-lemon juice. Pow. 90%. Bot. 8 oz. *otc.*
Use: Increase in normal intestinal flora.

Natural Diuretic Water Tablet. (Amlab) Buchu leaves 1 g, uva ursi 1 g, trilicum 1 g, parsley 1 g, juniper berries 1 g, asparagus 1 g, alfalfa powder 1 gr/ Tab. Bot. 100s. *otc.*
Use: Diuretic.

natural lung surfactant.
See: Survanta (Ross Laboratories).

natural vegetable powder. (Various Mfr.) Psyllium hydrophilic mucilloid 3.4 g, dextrose, sodium < 10 mg, 14 Cal/ Dose. Pow. 210 g, 420 g, 630 g. *otc.*
Use: Laxative.

natural vitamin a in oil.
See: Oleovitamin A, U.S.P.

Naturalyte. (UBI) Sodium 45 mEq, potassium 20 mEq, chloride 35 mEq, citrate 48 mEq, dextrose 25 g/L. Soln. Bot. 240 ml, 1 L. *otc.*
Use: Minerals/electrolytes, oral.

Nature's Aid Laxative Tabs. (Walgreen) Docusate sodium 100 mg, yellow phenolphthalein 65 mg/Tab. Bot. 60s. *otc.*
Use: Laxative.

Nature's Remedy Tablets. (SK-Beecham) Aloe 100 mg, cascara

sagrada 150 mg/FC Tab. Foil backed blister pkg. Box 12s, 30s, 60s. *otc.*
Use: Laxative.

Nature's Tears. (Rugby) Hydroxypropyl methylcellulose 2906 0.4%, KCl, NaCl, sodium phosphate, benzalkonium Cl 0.01%, EDTA. Soln. Bot. 15 ml. *otc.*
Use: Artificial tears.

Naturetin. (Bristol-Myers) Bendroflumethiazide. **5 mg/Tab.:** Bot. 100s, 1000s. **10 mg/Tab.:** Bot. 100s. *Rx.*
Use: Diuretic.

Natur-Lax Tablets. (Faraday) Rhubarb root, cape aloes, cascara sagrada extract, mandrake root, parsley, carrot. Protein coated tab. Bot. 100s. *otc.*
Use: Laxative.

Naus-A-Tories. (Table Rock) Pyrilamine maleate 25 mg, secobarbital 30 mg/ Supp. Box 12s. *c-ii.*
Use: Antiemetic.

Nausetrol. (Various Mfr.) Fructose, dextrose, orthophosphoric acid with controlled hydrogen ion concentration. Soln. Bot. 120 ml, pt, gal. *otc.*
Use: Antiemetic, antivertigo.

Navane. (Roerig) Thiothixene. **Cap.:** 1 mg, 2 mg, 5 mg, 10 mg or 20 mg. Bot. 100s, 1000s, UD 100s. **Liq.:** 5 mg/ml. Bot. 1 oz, 4 oz. **IM Soln.:** 2 mg/ml. Vial 2 ml. Pkg. 10s. *Rx.*
Use: Antipsychotic.

Navane Concentrate. (Roerig) Thiothixene HCl 5 mg/ml, alcohol 7%. Soln. Bot. 30 ml, 120 ml with dropper. *Rx.*
Use: Antipsychotic.

Navane Intramuscular for Injection. (Roerig) Thiothixene HCl 5 mg/ml. Lyophilized for reconstitution with 2.2 ml sterile water. Vial 2 ml. Pkg. vial 10s. *Rx.*
Use: Antipsychotic.

Navelbine. (Glaxo Wellcome) Vinorelbine tartrate 10 mg/ml. Inj. Vial 1 ml, 5 ml. *Rx.*
Use: Antineoplastic.

Navidrix. Cyclopenthiazide. 3-Cyclopentylmethyl derivative of hydrochlorothiazide. *Rx.*
Use: Diuretic.

•**naxagolide hydrochloride.** (nax-AH-go-LIDE) USAN.
Use: Antiparkisonian; dopamine agonist.

Nazafair. (Various Mfr.) Naphazoline HCl 0.1%. Soln. Bot. 15 ml. *Rx.*
Use: Ophthalmic vasoconstrictor, mydriatic.

N D Clear. (Seatrace) Chlorpheniramine maleate 8 mg, pseudoephedrine HCl 120 mg/T.D. Cap. Bot. 100s, 1000s. *Rx.*
Use: Antihistamine, decongestant.

n-diethyl meta-toluamide.
W/Red Veterinary Petrolatum.
See: RV Pellent, Oint. (ICN Pharm).

n-diethylvanillamide.
See: Ethamivan, Inj. (Various Mfr.).

ND-Gesic. (Hyrex) Acetaminophen 300 mg, pyrilamine maleate 12.5 mg, chlorpheniramine maleate 2 mg, phenylephrine HCl 5 mg/Tab. Bot. 100s, 1000s. *otc.*
Use: Analgesic, antihistamine, decongestant.

NDNA. (Wampole-Zeus) Anti-native DNA test by IFA. Confirmatory test for active SLE. Test 48s.
Use: Diagnostic aid.

ND-Stat. (Hyrex) Brompheniramine maleate 10 mg/ml. Vial 10 ml. *Rx.*
Use: Antihistamine.

•**nebacumab.** USAN. *Formerly Septomonab.*
Use: Monoclonal antibody (antiendotoxin).

Nebcin. (Lilly) Tobramycin sulfate. **Inj.:** 80 mg/2 ml. Vial 2 ml. **Pow. (after reconstitution):** 30 mg/ml or 40 mg/ml. Vial 1.2 g. **Pediatric Inj.:** 20 mg/2 ml. Vial 2 ml. **Hyporets:** 60 mg/1.5 ml or 80 mg/2 ml. *Rx.*
Use: Anti-infective, aminoglycoside.

•**nebivolol.** (neh-BIV-oh-lole) USAN.
Use: Antihypertensive (beta blocker).

•**nebramycin.** (neh-brah-MY-sin) USAN. A complex of antibiotic substances produced by *Streptomyces tenebrarius.*
Use: Antibacterial.

Nebupent. (Fujisawa) Pentamidine isethionate 300 mg. Aerosol single dose vial. *Rx.*
Use: Anti-infective.

Nebu-Prel. (Mahon) Isoproterenol sulfate 0.4%, phenylephrine HCl 2%, propylene glycol 10%. Liq. Vial 10 ml. *Rx.*
Use: Bronchodilator.

Nechlorin. (Interstate) Chlorpheniramine 5 mg, phenylpropanolamine 40 mg, phenylephrine 20 mg, phenyltoloxamine 15 mg/Tab. Bot. 100s.
Use: Antihistamine, decongestant.

•**nedocromil.** (NEH-doe-KROE-mill) USAN.
Use: Antiallergic (prophylactic).

•**nedocromil calcium.** (NEH-doe-KROE-mill) USAN.
Use: Antiallergic (prophylactic).
See: Tilade.

•**nedocromil sodium.** (NEH-doe-KROE-mill) USAN.
Use: Antiallergic (prophylactic).
See: Tilade, Aerosol (Fisons).

N.E.E.. (Lexis) Ethinyl estradiol 35 mcg, norethindrone 1 mg/Tab. 6 pcks. 21s, 28s. *Rx.*
Use: Oral contraceptive.

•**nefazodone hydrochloride.** (neff-AZE-oh-dohn) USAN.
Use: Antidepressant.
See: Serzone (Princeton).

•**neflumozide hydrochloride.** (neh-FLEW-moe-ZIDE) USAN.
Use: Antipsychotic.

•**nefocon a.** (NEE-FOE-kahn A) USAN.
Use: Contact lens material (hydrophilic).

•**nefopam hydrochloride.** (NEFF-oh-pam) USAN.
Use: Muscle relaxant; analgesic.

Negacide. (Sanofi Winthrop) Nalidixic acid. *Rx.*
Use: Urinary anti-infective.

NegGram. (Sanofi Winthrop) Nalidixic acid. **1 g/Capl.:** UD 100s; **250 mg/Capl.:** Bot. 56s. **500 mg/Capl.:** Bot. 56s, 500s. **250 mg/5 ml/Susp:** Bot. 480 ml. *Rx.*
Use: Urinary anti-infective.

•**nelezaprine maleate.** (neh-LEH-zah-PREEN) USAN.
Use: Muscle relaxant.

•**nelfinavir mesylate.** (nell-FIN-ah-veer) USAN.
Use: Antiviral.
See: Viracept, Tab., Pow. (Agouron).

Nelova 0.5/35. (Warner-Chilcott) Ethinyl estradiol 35 mcg, norethindrone 0.5 mg/Tab. 6 Pcks. 21 day and 28 day w/ 7 inert tabs. *Rx.*
Use: Oral contraceptive.

Nelova 1/35E. (Warner-Chilcott) Norethindrone 1 mg, ethinyl estradiol 35 mcg/Tab. 21 day and 28 day (with 7 inert tabs.). *Rx.*
Use: Oral contraceptive.

Nelova 1/50M. (Warner-Chilcott) Norethindrone 1 mg, mestranol 50 mcg/Tab. 21 day and 28 day (with 7 inert tabs). *Rx.*
Use: Oral contraceptive.

Nelova 10/11. (Warner-Chilcott) **Phase 1-** Norethindrone 0.5 mg, ethinyl estradiol 35 mcg/Tab.; **Phase 2-** Norethindrone 1 mg, ethinyl estradiol 35 mcg/Tab., 11 tabs. 21 day and 28 day (with 7 inert tabs). *Rx.*
Use: Oral contraceptive.

Nelulen. (Watson Labs) **1/35 E Tab.:** Ethynodiol diacetate 1 mg, ethinyl estradiol 35 mcg. Pcks 21s, 28s. **1/50 E Tab.:** Ethynodiol diacetate 1 mg, ethinyl estradiol 50 mcg. Pcks. 21s, 28s. *Rx.*
Use: Oral contraceptive.

nemazine. Under study.
Use: Anti-inflammatory.

•**nemazoline hydrochloride.** (neh-MAZZ-oh-leen) USAN.
Use: Nasal decongestant.

Nembutal Elixir. (Abbott) Pentobarbital 18.2 mg/5 ml, alcohol 18%. Bot. pt, gal. *c-II.*
Use: Sedative, hypnotic.

Nembutal Sodium. (Abbott) Pentobarbital sodium. **Inj.:** 50 mg/ml. Amp 2 ml; Vial 20 ml, 50 ml. Box 5s. **Cap.:** 50 mg: Bot. 100s; 100 mg: Bot. 100s, 500s. Display pack 100s. **Supp.:** 30 mg, 60 mg, 120 mg or 200 mg. Box 12s. *c-II.*
Use: Sedative, hypnotic.

neoarsphenamine.

Neo-Benz-All. (Xttrium) Benzalkonium Cl 20.1%. Packet 25 ml 15s. To make gal of 1:750 soln. Also Aqueous Neo-Benz-All 1:750 soln. Packet 20 ml, 50s. *otc.*
Use: Antiseptic, germicidal.

Neo Beserol. (Sanofi Winthrop) Aspirin, methocarbamol. *Rx.*
Use: Salicylate analgesic, skeletal muscle relaxant.

Neocalamine. (Various Mfr.) Red ferric oxide 30 g, yellow ferric oxide 40 g, zinc oxide 930 g. *otc.*
Use: Astringent, antiseptic.

Neo-Calglucon. (Sandoz) Glubionate calcium 1.8 g/5 ml. Syr. Bot. pt. *Rx.*
Use: Calcium supplement.

Neocate One +. (SHS) Protein 2.5 g (amino acids 3 g), carbohydrates 14.6 g (maltodextrin, sucrose), fat (fractionated) 3.5 g, coconut, canola, and high oleic sunflower oils, vitamins A, D, E, K, B_1, B_2, B_3, B_5, B_6, B_{12}, folic acid, biotin, C, choline, inositol, Ca, P, Mg, Fe, Zn, Mn, Cu, I, Mo, Cr, Se, Cl, Na 20 mg (0.9 mEq), K 93 mg (2.4 mEq), 835 mOsm/kg per 100 ml, 100 cal/ml. Liq. Bot. 237 ml. *otc.*
Use: Enteral nutritional therapy for children 1 to 10 years of age.

Neo-Cholex. (Lafayette) Fat emulsion containing 40%/w/v pure vegetable oil. Bot. 60 ml.
Use: Produce maximum cholecystokinetic activity in roentgen study.

Neocidin. (Major) Polymyxin B sulfate 10,000 units, neomycin sulfate 1.75 mg, gramicidin 0.025 mg/ml. Soln. Bot. 10 ml. *Rx.*
Use: Anti-infective, ophthalmic.

neo-cobefrin.
Use: Vasoconstrictor.

Neo-Cortef Cream. (Pharmacia & Upjohn) Hydrocortisone acetate 10 mg (1%), neomycin sulfate 5 mg (0.5%), methylparaben 1 mg, butylparaben 4 mg, polysorbate 80, propylene glycol, cetyl palmitate, glyceryl monostearate, emulsifier/g. When necessary, pH adjusted with sulfuric acid. Tube 20 g. *Rx.*
Use: Corticosteroid, anti-infective, topical.

Neo-Cortef Ointment. (Pharmacia & Upjohn) **0.5%:** Hydrocortisone acetate 5 mg, neomycin sulfate 5 mg, methylparaben 0.2 mg, butylparaben 1.8 mg in a bland base of white petrolatum, microcrystalline wax, mineral oil, cholesterol/g. Tube 20 g. **1%:** Hydrocortisone acetate 10 mg, neomycin sulfate 5 mg/g. Oint. Tube 5 g, 20 g. *Rx.*
Use: Corticosteroid, anti-infective, topical.

Neo-Cultol. (Fisons) Refined mineral oil jelly. Chocolate flavored. Bot. 6 oz. *otc.*
Use: Laxative.

Neocurb. (Pasadena Research) Phendimetrazine tartrate 35 mg/Tab. Bot. 100s, 1000s. *c-III.*
Use: Anorexient.

Neocylate. (Central) Potassium salicylate 280 mg, aminobenzoic acid 250 mg/Tab. Bot. 100s, 1000s. *otc.*
Use: Salicylate analgesic.

Neocyten. (Central) Orphenadrine citrate 30 mg/ml. Vial 10 ml. *Rx.*
Use: Skeletal muscle relaxant.

NeoDecadron Ophthalmic Solution. (Merck) Dexamethasone sodium phosphate equivalent to 0.1% dexamethasone phosphate, neomycin sulfate equivalent to 0.35% mg neomycin base. Ocumeter ophthalmic dispenser 5 ml. *Rx.*
Use: Corticosteroid, anti-infective, ophthalmic.

NeoDecadron Ophthalmic Ointment. (Merck) Dexamethasone sodium phosphate equivalent to 0.05% dexamethasone phosphate, neomycin sulfate equivalent to 0.35% neomycin base. Tube 3.5 g. *Rx.*
Use: Corticosteroid, anti-infective, ophthalmic.

NeoDecadron Topical Cream. (Merck) Dexamethasone sodium phosphate equivalent to 1 mg dexamethasone phosphate, neomycin sulfate equivalent to 3.5 mg neomycin base/g, stearyl alcohol, cetyl alcohol, mineral oil, polyoxyl 40 stearate, sorbitol soln, methyl polysilicone emulsion, creatinine, disodium edetate, sodium citrate, sodium hydroxide to adjust pH, purified water, methylparaben 0.15%, sodium bisulfite 0.25%, sorbic acid 0.1%. Tube 15 g, 30 g.
Use: Corticosteroid, anti-infective, topical.

Neo-Dexair. (Bausch & Lomb) Dexamethasone sodium phosphate 0.1%, neomycin sulfate 0.35%, polysorbate 80, EDTA, benzalkonium Cl 0.02%, sodium bisulfite 0.1%. Soln. Bot. 5 ml. *Rx.*
Use: Corticosteroid, anti-infective, ophthalmic.

Neo-Dexameth. (Major) Dexamethasone sodium phosphate 0.1%, neomycin sulfate 0.35%. Soln. Bot. 5 ml. *Rx.*
Use: Corticosteroid, anti-infective, ophthalmic.

Neo-Diaral. (Roberts) loperamide 2 mg/Cap. Bot. UD 8s, 250s. *otc.*
Use: Antidiarrheals.

neodrenal.
See: Isoproterenol.

Neo-Durabolic. (Roberts) Nandrolone decanoate injection. **50 mg/ml** or **100 mg/ml:** Vial 2 ml. **200 mg/ml:** Vial 1 ml. *c-III.*
Use: Anabolic steroid.

Neo-Fradin. (Pharma-Tek) Neomycin sulfate 125 mg/5 ml. Parabens. Soln. Bot. 480 ml. *Rx.*
Use: Amebicide.

Neogesic Tablets. (Pal-Pak) Aspirin 194.4 mg, acetaminophen 129.6 mg, caffeine 32.4 mg/Tab. Bot. 1000s. *otc.*
Use: Analgesic combination.

Neoloid. (Kenwood) Castor oil 36.4% (emulsified), sodium benzoate 0.1%, potassium sorbate 0.2%. Sugar free. Bot. 118 ml. *otc.*
Use: Laxative.

Neo-Mist Nasal Spray. (A.P.C.) Phenylephrine HCl 0.5%, cetalkonium Cl 0.02%. Spray Bot. 20 ml. *otc.*
Use: Decongestant, antiseptic.

Neo-Mist Pediatric 0.25% Nasal Spray. (A.P.C.) Phenylephrine HCl 0.25%, cetalkonium Cl 0.02%. Squeeze Bot. 20 ml. *otc.*
Use: Decongestant, antiseptic.

Neomixin. (Roberts) Bacitracin zinc 400 units, neomycin sulfate 3.5 mg, polymyxin B sulfate 5000 units in petrolatum base/g. Tube 15 g. *otc.*
Use: Anti-infective, topical.

neomycin base.
Use: Anti-infective.
W/Combinations.
See: Maxitrol, Oint., Susp. (Alcon).
Neo-Cort-Dome, Cream, Lot. (Bayer).
Neotal, Oint. (Roberts).

•**neomycin palmitate.** (NEE-oh-MY-sin PAL-mih-tate) USAN.
Use: Antibacterial.
See: Biozyme, Oint. (Centeon).

neomycin and polymyxin B sulfates, bacitracin, and hydrocortisone acetate ointment.
Use: Anti-infective, antifungal, anti-inflammatory, topical.

neomycin and polymyxin B sulfates, bacitracin, and hydrocortisone acetate ophthalmic ointment.
Use: Anti-infective, antifungal, anti-inflammatory, topical.

neomycin and polymyxin B sulfates and bacitracin ointment.
Use: Anti-infective, topical.

neomycin and polymyxin B sulfates and bacitracin ophthalmic ointment.
Use: Anti-infective, topical.

neomycin and polymyxin B sulfates, bacitracin zinc, and hydrocortisone acetate ophthalmic ointment.
Use: Anti-infective, corticosteroid, topical.

neomycin and polymyxin B sulfates, bacitracin zinc, and hydrocortisone ointment.
Use: Anti-infective, corticosteroid, topical.

neomycin and polymyxin B sulfates, bacitracin zinc, and hydrocortisone ophthalmic ointment.
Use: Anti-infective, corticosteroid, topical.

neomycin and polymyxin B sulfates, bacitracin zinc, and lidocaine ointment.
Use: Anti-infective, topical.
See: Lanabiotic, Oint. (Combe).

neomycin and polymyxin B sulfates and bacitracin zinc ointment.
Use: Anti-infective, topical.

neomycin and polymyxin B sulfates and bacitracin zinc ophthalmic ointment.
Use: Anti-infective, ophthalmic.

neomycin and polymyxin B sulfates and bacitracin zinc topical aerosol, U.S.P. XXI.
Use: Anti-infective, topical.

neomycin and polymyxin B sulfates and bacitracin zinc topical powder, U.S.P. XXI.
Use: Anti-infective, topical.

neomycin and polymyxin B sulfates cream.
Use: Anti-infective, topical.

neomycin and polymyxin B sulfates and dexamethasone ophthalmic ointment. (Various Mfr.) Dexamethasone 0.1%, neomycin sulfate 0.35%, polymyxin B sulfate 10,000 units. Tube 3.5 g.
Use: Anti-infective, corticosteroid, ophthalmic.

neomycin and polymyxin B sulfates and dexamethasone ophthalmic suspension. (Various Mfr.) Dexamethasone 0.1%, neomycin sulfate 0.35%, polymyxin B sulfate 10,000 units. Bot. 5 ml, 10 ml.
Use: Anti-infective, corticosteroid, ophthalmic.

neomycin and polymyxin B sulfates and gramicidin cream.
Use: Anti-infective, topical.

neomycin and polymyxin B sulfates, gramicidin, and hydrocortisone acetate cream.
Use: Anti-infective, corticosteroid, topical.

neomycin and polymyxin B sulfates and gramicidin ophthalmic solution.
Use: Anti-infective, ophthalmic.

neomycin and polymyxin B sulfates and hydrocortisone acetate cream.
Use: Anti-infective, corticosteroid, topical.

neomycin and polymyxin B sulfates and hydrocortisone acetate ophthalmic suspension.
Use: Anti-infective, corticosteroid, ophthalmic.

neomycin and polymyxin B sulfates and hydrocortisone ophthalmic suspension. (Various Mfr.) Hydrocortisone 1%, neomycin sulfate 0.35%, polymyxin B sulfate 10,000 units. Bot. 7.5 ml, 10 ml.
Use: Anti-infective, corticosteroid, ophthalmic.

neomycin and polymyxin B sulfates and hydrocortisone otic solution.
Use: Anti-infective, corticosteroid, otic.

neomycin and polymyxin B sulfates and hydrocortisone otic suspension.

(Steris) Polymyxin B sulfate equiv. to 10,000 polymyxin B units, neomycin sulfate equiv. to 3.5 mg neomycin base/ml. Hydrocortisone 1%, thimerosal 0.01%, cetyl alcohol, propylene glycol, polysorbate 80. Susp. Bot. 10 ml.
Use: Anti-infective, corticosteroid, otic.

neomycin and polymyxin B sulfates ophthalmic ointment.
Use: Anti-infective, ophthalmic.

neomycin and polymyxin B sulfates and prednisolone acetate ophthalmic suspension.
Use: Anti-infective, corticosteroid, ophthalmic.

neomycin and polymyxin B sulfates solution for irrigation.
Use: Irrigating solution, topical anti-infective.
See: Neosporin G.U. Irrigant (Glaxo Wellcome).

neomycin and polymyxin B sulfates ophthalmic solution.
Use: Anti-infective, ophthalmic.

• **neomycin sulfate.** (NEE-oh-MY-sin) U.S.P. 23.
Use: Antibacterial.
See: Mycifradin Sulfate, Tab., Soln. (Pharmacia & Upjohn).
Myciguent, Oint., Ophth. Oint., Cream (Pharmacia & Upjohn).
Neo-fradin, Soln. (Pharma-Tek).
Neo-Tabs (Pharma-Tek).
W/Combinations.
See: AK-Spore, Preps. (Akorn).
Bacitracin Neomycin, Oint. (Various Mfr.).
Baximin, Oint. (Quality Generics).
Biotres HC, Oint. (Central).
B.N.P., Ophthalmic Oint. (Solvay).
B.P.N., Oint. (Procter & Gamble).
Bro-Parin, Otic Susp. (3M).
Coracin, Oint. (Roberts).
Cordran-N, Oint., Lot. (Dista).
Cor-Oticin, Liq. (Maurry).
Cortisporin, Preps. (Glaxo Wellcome).
Epimycin A, Oint. (Delta).
Hi-Cort N, Cream (Blaine).
Hysoquen Oint. (Solvay).
Maxitrol, Ophth., Oint., Susp. (Alcon).
Mity-Mycin, Oint. (Solvay).
Mycifradin Sulfate Sterile, Vial (Pharmacia & Upjohn).
Mycitracin, Oint., Ophth. Oint. (Pharmacia & Upjohn).
My-Cort, Oint., Cream, Soln. (Scrip).
Neo-Cort Dome, Otic Soln. (Bayer).
Neo-Cortef, Preps. (Pharmacia & Upjohn).
Neo-Decadron, Ophth., Topical (Merck).
Neo-Delta-Cortef, Preps. (Pharmacia & Upjohn).
Neo-Hydeltrasol, Oint., Soln. (Merck).
Neo-Hytone, Cream (Dermik).
Neo-Medrol, Preps. (Pharmacia & Upjohn).
Neo-Nysta-Cort, Oint. (Bayer).
Neo-Oxylone, Oint. (Pharmacia & Upjohn).
Neosone, Ophth. Oint. (Pharmacia & Upjohn).
Neosporin, Preps. (Glaxo Wellcome).
Neotal, Ophth. Oint. (Roberts).
Neo-Thrycex, Oint. (Del Pharm).
Ocutricin, Preps. (Bausch & Lomb).
Otobione, Soln. (Schering Plough).
Otoreid-HC, Liq. (Solvay).
Spectrocin, Oint. (Squibb Mark).
Statrol Sterile, Ophthalmic Oint. (Alcon).
Tigo, Oint. (Burlington).
Tri-Bow, Oint. (Jones Medical).
Tricidin, Oint. (Amlab).
Trimixin, Oint. (Hance).

neomycin sulfate. (Pharmacia & Upjohn) Pow. micronized for compounding. Bot. 100 g.
Use: Antibacterial.

neomycin sulfate and bacitracin ointment.
Use: Anti-infective, topical.

neomycin sulfate and bacitracin zinc ointment.
Use: Anti-infective, topical.

neomycin sulfate and dexamethasone sodium phosphate cream.
Use: Anti-infective, corticosteroid, topical.

neomycin sulfate and dexamethasone sodium phosphate ophthalmic ointment.
Use: Anti-infective, corticosteroid, ophthalmic.

neomycin sulfate and dexamethasone sodium phosphate ophthalmic solution. (Various Mfr.) Dexamethasone sodium phosphate 0.1%, neomycin sulfate 0.35%. Bot. 5 ml.
Use: Anti-infective, corticosteroid, ophthalmic.

neomycin sulfate and fluocinolone acetonide cream.
Use: Anti-infective, corticosteroid, topical.

neomycin sulfate and fluoromethozone ointment.
Use: Anti-infective, corticosteroid, topical.

neomycin sulfate and flurandrenolide.
Use: Anti-infective, corticosteroid, topical

See: Cordran Prods. (Dista).

neomycin sulfate and gramicidin ointment.
Use: Anti-infective, topical.

neomycin sulfate and hydrocortisone.
Use: Anti-infective, corticosteroid, topical.

neomycin sulfate and hydrocortisone acetate.
Use: Anti-infective, corticosteroid.

neomycin sulfate and methylprednisolone acetate cream.
Use: Anti-infective, corticosteroid, topical.

neomycin sulfate, polymyxin B sulfate and gramicidin solution. (Various Mfr.)
Polymyxin B sulfate 10,000 units/g, neomycin sulfate 1.75 mg/g, gramicidin 0.025 mg/ml. Bot. 2 ml, 10 ml. *Rx.*
Use: Anti-infective, ophthalmic.

neomycin sulfate and prednisolone acetate ointment.
Use: Anti-infective, corticosteroid, topical.

neomycin sulfate and prednisolone acetate ophthalmic ointment.
Use: Anti-infective, corticosteroid, topical.

neomycin sulfate and prednisolone acetate ophthalmic suspension.
Use: Anti-infective, corticosteroid, topical.

neomycin sulfate and prednisolone sodium phosphate ophthalmic ointment.
Use: Anti-infective, corticosteroid, topical.

neomycin sulfate, sulfacetamide sodium, and prednisolone acetate ophthalmic ointment.
Use: Anti-infective, corticosteroid, topical.

neomycin sulfate and triamcinolone acetonide cream.
Use: Anti-infective, corticosteroid, topical.

neomycin sulfate and triamcinolone acetonide ophthalmic ointment.
Use: Anti-infective, corticosteroid, ophthalmic.

•**neomycin undecylenate.** (NEE-oh-MY-sin UHN-de-sih-LEN-ate) USAN.
Use: Antibacterial, antifungal.
See: Neodecyllin (Penick).

neomycorsone.
See: Neosone, Oint. (Pharmacia & Upjohn).

Neopap. (PolyMedica) Acetaminophen 125 mg/Supp. In 12s. *otc.*

Use: Analgesic.

Neopham 6.4%. (Pharmacia & Upjohn) Essential and non-essential amino acids 6.4%. Inj. 250 ml, 500 ml. *Rx.*
Use: Parenteral nutritional supplement.

Neo Picatyl. (Sanofi Winthrop) Glycobiarsoln. *Rx.*
Use: Amebicide.

neoquinophan.
See: Neocinchophen (Various Mfr.).

Neo Quipenyl. (Sanofi Winthrop) Primaquine phosphate. *Rx.*
Use: Antimalarial.

Neoral Capsules. (Sandoz) Cyclosporine 25 mg or 100 mg/Cap. 9.5% dehydrated alcohol. Bot. UD 30s. *Rx.*
Use: Immunosuppresive.

Neoral Oral Solution. (Sandoz) Cyclosporine 100 mg/ml. Bot. 50 ml. *Rx.*
Use: Immunosuppressant.

Neosar. (Pharmacia & Upjohn) Cyclophosphamide. For inj. **100 mg:** Cyclophosphamide 100 mg, sodium Cl 45 mg/Vial. Pkg. 12s. **200 mg:** Cyclophosphamide 200 mg, sodium Cl 90 mg/Vial. Pkg. 12s. **500 mg:** Cyclophosphamide 500 mg, sodium Cl 225 mg/Vial. Pkg 12s. *Rx.*
Use: Antineoplastic agent.

neo-skiodan.
Iodopyracet, Diodrast.

Neosporin Cream. (Glaxo Wellcome) Polymyxin B sulfate, neomycin sulfate. Tube 0.5 oz, foil packet 1/32 oz. Ctn. 144s. *otc.*
Use: Anti-infective, topical.

Neosporin G.U. Irrigant. (Glaxo Wellcome) Neomycin sulfate 40 mg, polymyxin B sulfate 200,000 units/ml. Amp. 1 ml. Box 10s, 50s, Multiple dose vial 20 ml. *Rx.*
Use: Genitourinary irrigant.

Neosporin Ointment. (Glaxo Wellcome) Polymyxin B sulfate 5000 units, bacitracin zinc 400 units, neomycin sulfate 5 mg/g. Tube 0.5 oz, 1 oz. Foil packet 1/32 oz. Box 144s. *otc.*
Use: Anti-infective, topical.

Neosporin, Maximum Strength. (Glaxo Wellcome) Polymyxin B sulfate 10,000 units, neomycin 3.5 mg, bacitracin 500 units/g, white petrolatum. Oint. Tube 15 g. *otc.*
Use: Topical anti-infective.

Neosporin Ophthalmic Ointment, Sterile. (Glaxo Wellcome) Polymyxin B sulfate 10,000 units, bacitracin zinc 400 units, neomycin sulfate 3.5 mg/g. Tube 3.5 g. *Rx.*

Use: Anti-infective, ophthalmic.

Neosporin Ophthalmic Solution, Sterile. (Glaxo Wellcome) Polymyxin B sulfate 10,000 units, neomycin sulfate 1.75 mg, gramicidin 0.025 mg/ml. Bot. 10 ml. Drop-dose. *Rx.*
Use: Anti-infective, ophthalmic.

Neosporin Plus. (Glaxo Wellcome) **Cream:** 10,000 polymyxin B sulfate, neomycin 3.5 mg and lidocaine 40 mg/g, methylparaben 0.25%, mineral oil, white petrolatum. Tube 15 g. **Oint.:** Polymyxin B sulfate 10,000 units, bacitracin zinc 500 units, neomycin 3.5 mg and lidocaine 40 mg per g. In a white petrolatum base. Tube 15 g. *otc.*
Use: Topical anti-infective.

neostibosan. Ethylstibamine.

neostigine and atropine sulfate.
Use: Cholinergic muscle stimulant.
See: Neostigine Min-I-Mix (IMS).

neostigmine. (nee-oh-STIGG-meen)
Use: Cholinergic.
See: Neostigmine Bromide (Lannett).
Neostigmine Methylsulfate (Various Mfr.).
Prostigmin (Roche).

•**neostigmine bromide,** U.S.P. 23.
Use: Cholinergic.
See: Prostigmin Bromide, Tab. (Hoffman-LaRoche).

neostigmine bromide. (Lannett) 15 mg/Tab. 100s and 1000s.
Use: Cholinergic.

•**neostigmine methylsulfate,** U.S.P. 23.
Use: Cholinergic.
See: Prostigmin methylsulfate, Vial (Hoffman-LaRoche).

neostigmine methylsulfate. (Various Mfr.) 1:1000 Inj. In 10 ml vials. 1:2000 Inj. In 1ml amps. and 10 ml vials. 1:4000 Inj. In 1 ml amps.
Use: Cholinergic.

Neostigmine Min-I-Mix. (IMS) Atropine sulfate 1.2 mg, neostigmine methylsulfate 2.5 mg. Inj. Vial.
Use: Cholinergic muscle stimulant.
Use: Ophthalmic vasoconstrictor/mydriatic.

Neostrate AHA for Age Spots and Skin Lightening. (NeoStrata) Hydroquinone 2%, glycolic acid, propylene glycol, sodium bisulfite, sodium sulfite, EDTA/Gel. 48 g. *otc.*
Use: Skin bleaching agent.

neo-strepsan.
See: Sulfathiazole (Various Mfr.).

Neo-Synephrine. (Sanofi Winthrop.) Phenylephrine HCl 2.5% or 10%. Soln.

Bot. 5 ml (10%), 15 ml (2.5%). *Rx.*
Use: Ophthalmic vasoconstrictor/mydriatic.

Neo-Synephrine Hydrochloride. (Sanofi Winthrop) Phenylephrine HCl.
Spray: 0.25% children and adult, 0.5% adult. **Regular:** Squeeze bot. 0.5 oz. **0.5% mentholated:** Squeeze bot. 0.5 oz. **Drops:** 0.125% infant; 0.25% children and adult; 0.5% adult; 1% adult extra strength. Bot. 1 oz; 0.25% and 1% also bot. 16 oz. **Jelly:** 0.5%. Tube 18.75 g. *otc.*
Use: Decongestant.

Neo-Synephrine Hydrochloride. (Sanofi Winthrop) Phenylephrine HCl.
Amp.: 1%, Carpuject sterile cartridge-needle unit 10 mg/ml. (1 ml fill in 2 ml cartridge) w/22 gauge, 1.25 inch needle. Dispensing Bin 50s; Vial 1 ml Box 25s. *Rx.*
Use: Vasopressor used in shock.

Neo-Synephrine Viscous Ophthalmic. (Sanofi Winthrop) Phenylephrine HCl 10%. Soln. Bot. 5 ml. *Rx.*
Use: Ophthalmic vasoconstrictor, mydriatic.

Neo-Tabs. (Pharma-Tek) Neomycin sulfate 500 mg (equivalent to 350 mg neomycin base)/Tab. Bot. 100s. *Rx.*
Use: Amebicide.

Neotal. (Roberts) Zinc bacitracin 400 units, polymyxin B sulfate 5000 units, neomycin sulfate 5 mg, petrolatum and mineral oil base/g. Tube 3.5 g. *Rx.*
Use: Anti-infective, ophthalmic.

Neo-Thrycex Oint. (Del Pharm) Bacitracin, neomycin sulfate, polymyxin B sulfate. Tube 0.5 oz. *Rx.*
Use: Anti-infective, topical.

Neothylline. (Lemmon) Dyphylline. **200 mg/Tab.:** Bot. 100s, 1000s. **400 mg/Tab.:** Bot. 100s, 500s. *Rx.*
Use: Bronchodilator.

Neothylline-GG. (Lemmon) Dyphylline 200 mg, guaifenesin 200 mg/Tab. Bot. 100s, 1000s. *Rx.*
Use: Bronchodilator, expectorant.

Neotrace-4. (Fujisawa) Zinc 1.5 mg, copper 0.1 mg, chromium 0.85 mcg, manganese 25 mcg/ml. Vial 2 ml. *Rx.*
Use: Mineral supplement.

Neotricin HC. (Bausch & Lomb) Hydrocortisone acetate 1%, neomycin sulfate 0.35%, bacitracin zinc 400 units, polymyxin B sulfate 10,000 units. Oint. Tube 3.5 g. *Rx.*
Use: Anti-infective, corticosteroid, ophthalmic.

Neotricin Ophthalmic Ointment.
(Bausch & Lomb) Polymyxin B sulfate
10,000 units, neomycin sulfate 3.5 mg,
bacitracin 400 units/g. In 3.5 g. *Rx.*
Use: Anti-infective, ophthalmic.

Neotricin Ophthalmic Solution.
(Bausch and Lomb) Polymyxin B sulfate 10,000 units, neomycin sulfate 1.75
mg, gramicidin 0.025 mg/ml. Dropper
bot. 10 ml. *Rx.*
Use: Anti-infective, ophthalmic.

Neo-Trobex Injection. (Forest) Vitamins
B_1 150 mg, B_6 10 mg, riboflavin 5-phos-
phate sodium 2 mg, niacinamide 150
mg, panthenol 10 mg, choline Cl 20 mg,
inositol 20 mg/ml. Vial 30 ml. *Rx.*
Use: Vitamin supplement.

Neotrol. (Horizon) Phenylephrine HCl
0.25%, pyrilamine maleate 0.2%, cetalkonium Cl 0.05%, tyrothricin 0.03%,
phenylmercuric acetate 1:50,000. Soln.
Squeeze Bot. 20 ml. *otc.*
Use: Decongestant, antihistamine.

**Neo-Vadrin Stress Formula Vitamins
Plus Zinc.** (Scherer) Vitamins E 45
IU, C 600 mg, folic acid 400 mcg, B_1 20
mg, B_2 10 mg, B_{12} 25 mcg, biotin 45
mcg, pantothenic acid 25 mg, copper 3
mg, zinc 23.9 mg/Tab. Bot. 60s. *otc.*
Use: Vitamin/mineral supplement.

Neo-Vadrin Time Release Vit. C. (Scherer) Vitamin C 500 mg/Cap. Bot. 50s,
100s. *otc.*
Use: Vitamin C supplement.

Neo-Vadrin Vitamin B_6 TR. (Scherer) Vitamin B_6 100 mg/Cap. Bot. 100s. *otc.*
Use: Vitamin B_6 supplement.

Neoval. (Halsey) Vitamins A 10,000 IU,
D 400 IU, B_1 10 mg, B_2 5 mg, B_6 2 mg,
B_{12} 3 mcg, C 100 mg, E 5 mg, pantothenic acid 10 mg, niacinamide 30 mg,
iron 15 mg, copper 1 mg, magnesium 5
mg, manganese 1 mg, zinc 1.5 mg, iodine 0.15 mg/Tab. Bot. 100s. *otc.*
Use: Vitamin/mineral supplement.

Neoval T. (Halsey) Vitamins A 10,000 IU,
D 400 IU, B_1 15 mg, B_2 10 mg, B_6 2
mg, C 150 mg, B_{12} 7.5 mcg, E 5 mg,
pantothenic acid 10 mg, E 5 mg, niacinamide 100 mg, iron 15 mg, magnesium 5 mg, manganese 1 mg, zinc 1.5
mg, copper 1 mg/Tab. Bot. 1000s. *otc.*
Use: Vitamin/mineral supplement.

Nephplex Rx. (Nephro-Tech) Iron 66 mg
(from ferrous fumarate), B_1 1.5 mg, B_2
1.7 mg, B_3 20 mg, B_5 10 mg, B_6 10
mg, B_{12} 6 mcg, C 60 mg, folic acid 1
mg, d-biotin 300 mcg/Tab. Bot. 100s.
Rx.
Use: Iron with vitamin supplement.

Nephramine. (McGaw) Amino acid concentration 5.4%, nitrogen 0.65 g/100
ml. **Essential amino acids:** Isoleucine
560 mg, leucine 880 mg, lysine 640
mg, methionine 880 mg, phenylalanine
880 mg, threonine 400 mg, tryptophan
200 mg, valine 640 mg, histidine 250
mg/100 ml. **Nonessential amino acids:** Cysteine <20 mg/100 ml, sodium 5
mEq, acetate 44 mEq, chloride 3 mEq/
L, sodium bisulfite. Inj. 250 ml. *Rx.*
Use: Parenteral nutritional supplement.

nephridine.
See: Epinephrine (Various Mfr.).

Nephro-Calci. (R & D) Calcium carbonate 1.5 g/Chew. Tab. (600 mg calcium). Bot. 100s, 200s, 500s, 1000s.
otc.
Use: Calcium supplement.

Nephrocaps Capsules. (Fleming) Vitamins B_1 1.5 mg, B_2 1.7 mg, B_3 20 mg,
B_5 5 mg, B_6 10 mg, B_{12} 6 mcg, C 100
mg, folic acid 1 mg, biotin 150 mcg/Cap.
Bot. 100s. *Rx.*
Use: Vitamin supplement.

Nephro-Fer. (R & D Labs) Ferrous fumarate 350 mg iron (iron 115 mg)/Tab. Bot.
100s. *otc.*
Use: Iron supplement.

Nephro-Fer RX. (R & D Labs) Iron 106.9
mg, folic acid 1 mg. Tab. Bot. 120s. *Rx.*
Use: Vitamin/mineral supplement.

Nephron FA. (Nephro-Tech) Fe 200 mg,
C 40 mg, B_1 1.5 mg, B_2 1.7 mg, B_3 20
mg, B_5 10 mg, B_6 10 mg, B_{12} 5 mcg,
biotin 300 mcg, FA 1 mg, docusate sodium 75 mg/Tab. Bot. 100s. *otc.*
Use: Iron with vitamins.

Nephron Inhalant and Vaporizer.
(Nephron) Racemic epinephrine HCl
2.25%. Bot. 0.25 oz, 0.5 oz, 1 oz. *otc.*
Use: Bronchodilator.

Nephro-Vite Rx. (R & D) Vitamins B_1 1.5
mg, B_2 1.7 mg, B_3 20 mg, B_5 10 mg,
B_6 10 mg, B_{12} 6 mcg, C 60 mg, folic acid
1 mg, d-biotin 300 mcg/Tab. Bot. 100s.
Rx.
Use: Vitamin/mineral supplement.

Nephro-Vite Rx + Fe. (R & D) Iron 100
mg, Vitamins B_1 1.5 mg, B_2 1.7 mg, B_3
20 mg, B_5 10 mg, B_6 10 mg, B_{12} 6
mcg, C 60 mg, folic acid 1 mg, d-biotin
300 mcg, lactose/Tab. Bot. 120s. *Rx.*
Use: Vitamin/mineral supplement.

**Nephro-Vite Vitamin B Complex and C
Supplement.** (R & D) Vitamins B_1 1.5
mg, B_2 1.7 mg, B_3 20 mg, B_5 10 mg,
B_6 10 mg, B_{12} 6 mcg, C 60 mg, folic acid
800 mcg, biotin 300 mcg/Tab. Bot.
100s. *otc.*

Use: Vitamin/mineral supplement.

Nephrox. (Fleming) Aluminum hydroxide 320 mg, mineral oil 10%/5 ml. Bot. pt. *otc.*
Use: Antacid.

Nepro. (Ross) Protein 6.6 g (as Ca, Mg and Na caseinates), fat 22.7 g (as 90% high-oleic safflower oil, 10% soy oil), carbohydrate 51.1 g (as sucrose, hydrolyzed corn starch), vitamins A, D, E, K, C, B_1, B_3, B_5, B_6, B_{12}, biotin, FA, Na, K, Cl, Ca, P, Mg, I, Mn, Cu, Zn, Fe 4.5 mg, Se/240 ml. Bot. 59.4 calories. Liq. Bot. 240 ml. *otc.*
Use: Enteral nutritional therapy for dialyzed patients with chronic or acute renal failure.

Neptazane. (Lederle) Methazolamide 25 mg or 50 mg/Tab. Bot. 100s. *Rx.*
Use: Carbonic anhydrase inhibitor.

neraval.
Use: General anesthetic.

•**nerelimomab.** USAN.
Use: Monoclonal antibody.

Nervine Nighttime Sleep-Aid. (Bayer) Diphenhydramine HCl 25 mg/Tab. Bot. 12s, 30s, 50s. *otc.*
Use: Nonprescription sleep aid.

Nervocaine. (Keene) Lidocaine HCl 1%/ Inj. Vial 50 ml. *Rx.*
Use: Local anesthetic.

Nesacaine. (Astra) Chloroprocaine HCl 1% or 2%, methylparaben, EDTA. Inj. Vial 30 ml. *Rx.*
Use: Local anesthetic.

Nesacaine-CE. (Astra) **Conc. 2%:** Chloroprocaine HCl 20 mg/ml in a sterile soln. containing sodium bisulfite, sodium Cl, HCl. Vial 30 ml. **Conc. 3%:** Chloroprocaine HCl 30 mg/ml in a sterile soln. containing sodium bisulfite, sodium Cl, HCl. Vial 30 ml. *Rx.*
Use: Local anesthetic.

Nesacaine-MPF. (Astra) Chloroprocaine HCl 2% or 3%. EDTA or preservative-free. Inj. Vial 30 ml. *Rx.*
Use: Local anesthetic.

Nesa Nine Cap. (Standex) Vitamins A 5000 IU, D 400 IU, C 37.5 mg, B_1 1.5 mg, B_2 2 mg, niacinamide 20 mg, B_6 0.1 mg, calcium pantothenate 1 mg, E 2 IU/Cap. Bot. 100s. *otc.*
Use: Vitamin/mineral supplement.

nesdonal sodium.
See: Thiopental Sodium U.S.P. 23. Pentothal Sodium, Prods. (Abbott).

Nestabs. (Fielding) Vitamins A 5000 IU, D 400 IU, E 30 mg, C 120 mg, B_1 3 mg, B_2 3 mg, B_3 20 mg, B_6 3 mg, B_{12} 8

mcg, calcium 200 mg, iron 36 mg, folic acid 0.8 mg, zinc 15 mg, l/Tab. Bot. 100s. *otc.*
Use: Vitamin/mineral supplement.

Nestabs FA Tablets. (Fielding) Vitamins A 5000 IU, D 400 IU, E 30 mg, C 120 mg, B_1 3 mg, B_2 3 mg, B_3 20 mg, B_6 3 mg, B_{12} 8 mcg, Ca 200 mg, iron 36 mg, folic acid 1 mg, zinc 15 mg, l/Tab. Bot. 100s. *Rx.*
Use: Vitamin/mineral supplement.

Nestrex. (Fielding) Pyridoxine 25 mg/ Tab., dextrose. Bot. 100s. *otc.*
Use: Vitamin B_6 supplement.

Nethamine.
W/Codeine phosphate, phenylephrine HCl, sodium citrate, doxylamine succinate.
See: Mercodol with Decapryn. Syr. (Hoechst Marion Roussel).

•**netilmicin sulfate,** (neh-TILL-MY-sin SULL-fate) U.S.P. 23.
Use: Antibacterial.
See: Netromycin (Schering Plough).

•**netrafilcon a.** (NET-rah-FILL-kahn A) USAN.
Use: Contact lens material (hydrophilic).

netrin. Under Study.
Use: Anticholinergic.
See: Metcaraphen HCl.

Netromycin. (Schering Plough) Netilmicin 100 mg/ml. Inj. Vial 1.5 ml Box 10s, 25s. Multi-dose vial 15 ml Box 5s. Disposable Syringe 1.5 ml Box 10s. *Rx.*
Use: Anti-infective, aminoglycoside.

neulactil.
See: Pericyazine.

Neupogen. (Amgen). Filgrastim (G-CSF) 300 mcg/ml. Vial 1 ml, 1.6 ml. *Rx.*
Use: Colony stimulating factor.

Neurodep-Caps. (Medical Products) Vitamins B_1 125 mg, B_6 125 mg, B_{12} 1000 mcg/Cap. Bot. 50s. *otc.*
Use: Vitamin supplement.

Neurodep Injection. (Medical Products) Vitamins B_1 50 mg, B_2 5 mg, B_3 125 mg, B_5 6 mg, B_6 5 mg, B_{12} 1000 mcg, C 50 mg/ml. Inj. Vial 10 ml. *Rx.*
Use: Parenteral vitamin supplement.

Neurontin. (Parke-Davis) Gabapentin 100 mg, 300 mg, 400 mg; lactose. Cap. Bot. 100s, UD 50s. *Rx.*
Use: Anticonvulsant.

neurosin.
See: Calcium glycerophosphate (Various Mfr.).

neutropin-1.
Use: Motor neuron disease/amyothro-

phic lateral sclerosis. [Orphan drug]

Neut (sodium bicarbonate 4% additive solution). (Abbott) Sodium bicarbonate 4%. Vial (2.4 mEq each of sodium and bicarbonate), disodium edetate anhydrous 0.05% as stabilizer. Pintop Vial 5 ml, 10 ml. Box 25s, 100s. *Rx.*
Use: Parenteral nutritional supplement.

neutral acriflavin.
See: Acriflavin (Various Mfr.).

Neutralin. (Dover) Calcium carbonate, magnesium oxide/Tab. Sugar, lactose and salt free. UD Box 500s. *otc.*
Use: Antacid.

neutral protamine hagedorn-insulin.
See: Insulin, N.P.H. Iletin (Lilly).

•**neutramycin.** (NEW-trah-MY-sin) USAN. A neutral macrolide antibiotic produced by a variant strain of *Streptomyces rimosus.*
Use: Antibacterial.

Neutrexin. (US Bioscience) Trimetrexate glucuronate 25 mg. Pow. for Inj. (lyophilized). Vial 5 ml w/wo 50 mg leucovorin. *Rx.*
Use: Anti-infective.

neutroflavin.
See: Acriflavine (Various Mfr.).

Neutrogena Acne Mask. (Neutrogena) Benzoyl peroxide 5% in sebum absorbing facial mask vehicle, SD alcohol 40, glycerin, titanium dioxide. Tube 60 g. *otc.*
Use: Antiacne.

Neutrogena Antiseptic Cleanser for Acne-Prone Skin. (Neutrogena) Benzethonium Cl, butylene glycol, methylparaben, menthol, peppermint oil, eucalyptus oil, cornmint oil, rosemary oil, witch hazel extract, camphor. Liq. Bot. 135 ml. *otc.*
Use: Antiacne.

Neutrogena Baby Cleansing Formula Soap. (Neutrogena) Triethanolamine, glycerin, stearic acid, tallow, coconut oil, castor oil, sodium hydroxide, oleic acid, laneth-10 acetate, cocamide DEA, nonoxynol 14, PEG-4 octoate. Bar 105 g. *otc.*
Use: Skin cleanser.

Neutrogena Body Lotion. (Neutrogena) Glyceryl stearate, isopropyl myristate, PEG-100 stearate, butylene glycol, imidazolidinyl urea, carbomer-934, parabens, sodium lauryl sulfate, triethanolamine, cetyl alcohol. Lot. Bot. 240 ml. *otc.*
Use: Emollient.

Neutrogena Body Oil. (Neutrogena) Iso-propyl myristate, sesame oil, PEG-40 sorbitan peroleate, parabens. Bot. 240 ml. *otc.*
Use: Emollient.

Neutrogena Chemical-Free Sunblocker. (Neutrogena) Titanium dioxide, parabens, diazolidinyl urea, shea butter. SPF 17. Lot. Bot. 120 ml. *otc.*
Use: Sunscreen.

Neutrogena Cleansing for Acne-Prone Skin. (Neutrogena) TEA-stearate, triethanolamine, glycerin, sodium tallowate, sodium cocoate, TEA-oleate, sodium ricinoleate, acetylated lanolin alcohol, cocamide DEA, TEA lauryl sulfate, tocopherol. Bar 105 g. *otc.*
Use: Skin cleanser.

Neutrogena Drying. (Neutrogena) Witch hazel, isopropyl alcohol, EDTA, parabens, tartrazine. Gel. Tube 22.5 g. *otc.*
Use: Antiacne.

Neutrogena Dry Skin Soap. (Neutrogena) Triethanolamine, stearic acid, tallow, glycerin, coconut oil, castor oil, sodium hydroxide, oleic acid, laneth-10 acetate, cocamide DEA, nonoxynol 14, PEG-14 octoate, BHT, O-tolyl biguanide. Bar 105 g, 165 g. Scented or unscented. *otc.*
Use: Skin cleanser.

Neutrogena Glow Sunless Tanning. (Neutrogena) Octyl methoxycinnamate, cetyl alcohol, diazolidinyl urea, parabens, EDTA. SPF 8. Lot. Bot. 120 ml. *otc.*
Use: Sunscreen.

Neutrogena Intensified Day Moisture. (Neutrogena) Octyl methoxycinnamate, 2-phenylbenzimidazole sulfonic acid, titanium dioxide, cetyl alcohol, diazolidinyl urea, parabens, EDTA. SPF 15. Cream 67.5 g. *otc.*
Use: Moisturizer, sunscreen.

Neutrogena Lip Moisturizer. (Neutrogena) Octyl methoxycinnamate, benzophenone-3, corn oil, castor oil, mineral oil, lanolin oil, petrolatum, lanolin, stearyl alcohol. SPF 15. Lip balm 4.5 g. *otc.*
Use: Lip moisturizer, sunscreen.

Neutrogena Moisture SPF 5. (Neutrogena) Octyl methoxycinnamate, petrolatum, cetyl alcohol, parabens, diazolidinyl urea, EDTA, cetyl alcohol. Lot. Bot 60 ml, 120 ml. *otc.*
Use: Moisturizer, sunscreen.

Neutrogena Moisture SPF 15. (Neutrogena) Octyl methoxycinnamate, benzophenone-3, glycerine, PEG 100 stearate, dimethicone, PEG-6000 mono-

stearate, triethanolamine, parabens, imidazolidinyl urea, carbomer 954, PABA free. Lot. Bot. 120 ml. *otc.*
Use: Sunscreen.

Neutrogena Non-Drying Cleansing. (Neutrogena) Glycerin, caprylic/capric triglyceride, PEG-20 almond glycerides, cetyl recinoleate, isohexadecane, TEA-cocoyl glutamate, PEG-20 methyl glucose sesquistearate, stearyl alcohol, cetyl alcohol, EDTA, dipotassium glycyrrhizate, stearyl glycyrrhetinate, bisabolol, parabens, acrylates/C 10-30 alkyl acrylate crosspolymer, triethanolamine, diazolidinyl urea. Lot. Bot. 165 ml. *otc.*
Use: Skin cleanser.

Neutrogena Norwegian Formula Emulsion. (Neutrogena) Glycerin base 2%. Pump dispenser 5.25 oz. *otc.*
Use: Emollient.

Neutrogena Norwegian Formula Hand Cream. (Neutrogena) Glycerin base 41%. Tube 2 oz. *otc.*
Use: Emollient.

Neutrogena No-Stick Sunscreen. (Neutrogena) SPF 30. Homosalate 15%, octyl methoxycinnamate 7.5%, benzophenone-3 6%, octyl salicylate 5%, EDTA, parabens, diazolidinyl urea/ Cream. Waterproof 118 g. *otc.*
Use: Sunscreen.

Neutrogena Oil-Free Acne Wash. (Neutrogena) Salicylic acid 2%, EDTA, propylene glycol, tartrazine, aloe extract. Liq. Bot. 180 ml. *otc.*
Use: Antiacne.

Neutrogena Oily Skin Formula Soap. (Neutrogena) Triethanolamine, glycerin, fatty acids. Bar 3.5 oz. *otc.*
Use: Skin cleanser.

Neutrogena Original Formula Soap. (Neutrogena) Triethanolamine, glycerin, fatty acids. Bar 3.5 oz, 5.5 oz. *otc.*
Use: Skin cleanser.

Neutrogena Soap. (Neutrogena) TEA-stearate, triethanolamine, glycerin, sodium tallowate, sodium cocoate, sodium ricinoleate, TEA-oleate, cocamide DEA, tocopherol. Bar 105 g, 165 g. *otc.*
Use: Skin cleanser.

Neutrogena Sunblock. (Neutrogena) **SPF 8:** Octyl methoxycinnamate, menthyl anthranilate, titanium dioxide, mineral oil. Cream 67.5 g. **SPF 15:** Octyl methoxycinnamate, octyl salicylate, menthyl anthranilate, mineral oil, titanium dioxide, propylparaben. Cream 67.5 g. **SPF 25:** Octyl methoxycinna-

mate, benzophenone-3, octyl salicylate, castor oil, cetearyl alcohol, propylparaben, shea butter. Stick 12.6 g. **SPF30:** Octocrylene, octyl methoxycinnamate, menthyl anthranilate, zinc oxide, mineral oil, vitamin E. Cream 67.5 g. *otc.*
Use: Sunscreen.

Neutrogena Sunscreen. (Neutrogena) Ethylhexyl p-methoxycinnamate 7%, oxybenzone 4%, titanium dioxide 2%. Tube 3 oz. *otc.*
Use: Sunscreen.

Neutrogena T/Gel. (Neutrogena) Coal tar extract 2%. Shampoo. Bot. 132 ml. *otc.*
Use: Antiseborrheic.

Neutrogena T/Sal. (Neutrogena) Salicylic acid 2%, solubilized coal tar extract 2%. Shampoo. Bot. 135 ml. *otc.*
Use: Antiseborrheic shampoo.

•**nevirapine.** (neh-VIE-rah-peen) USAN.
Use: Antiviral.
See: Viramune, Tab. (Roxane).

New-Decongest Pediatric Syrup. (Goldline) Phenylpropanolamine HCl 5 mg, phenylephrine HCl 1.25 mg, chlorpheniramine maleate 0.5 mg, phenyltoloxamine citrate 2 mg/5 ml. Syr. Bot. pt, gal. *Rx.*
Use: Decongestant, antihistamine.

New Decongestant. (Goldline) Phenylpropanolamine HCl 40 mg, phenylephrine HCl 10 mg, chlorpheniramine maleate 5 mg/ SR Tab. Bot. 100s, 1000s. *otc, Rx.*
Use: Decongestant, antihistamine.

•**nexeridine hydrochloride.** (NEX-eh-RIH-deen) USAN.
Use: Analgesic.

ng-29.
Use: Diagnostic aid. [Orphan drug]

N.G.T. (Geneva Pharm) Triamcinolone acetonide 0.1%, nystatin 100,000 units/g. Cream. Tube 15 g. *Rx.*
Use: Topical corticosteroid, antifungal.

Nia-Bid. (Roberts) Niacin 400 mg/TR Cap. Bot. 100s. *otc.*
Use: Vitamin B_3 supplement.

Niacal. (Jones Medical) Calcium lactate 324 mg, niacin 25 mg/Tab. Peppermint flavor. Bot. 100s, 1000s. *otc.*
Use: Vasodilator, vitamin supplement.

niacamide.
See: Nikethamide (Various Mfr.).

•**niacin,** (NYE-uh-sin) U.S.P. 23.
Use: Antihyperlipidemic; vitamin (enzyme co-factor).
See: Efacin, Tab. (Person & Covey).

Niac, Cap. (Cole).
Nicobid, Cap. (Rhone-Poulenc Rorer).
Nicolar, Tab. (Rhone-Poulenc Rorer).
Nico-400 (Hoechst Marion Roussel).
Ni Cord XL, Cap. (Scott/Cord).
Nicotinex, Elix. (Fleming).
Span Niacin 300, Tab. (Scrip).
niacin w/combinations.
See: Lipo-Nicin, Tab., Cap. (ICN Pharm).
Vasostim, Cap. (Dunhall).
•**niacinamide, U.S.P. 23.**
Use: Vitamin (enzyme co-factor).
W/Pentylenetetrazol, thiamine HCl, cyanocobalamin, alcohol.
See: Cenalene, Tab., Elix. (Central).
W/Potassium iodide.
See: Iodo-Niacin, Tab. (Cole).
W/Riboflavin.
See: Riboflavin and Niacinamide, Amp. (Lilly).
Niacor. (Upsher-Smith) Niacin 500 mg/Tab. Bot. 100s. *Rx.*
Use: Vitamin B$_3$ supplement.
Nialexo-C. (Roberts) Niacin 50 mg, vitamin C 30 mg/Tab. Bot. 100s. *otc.*
Use: Vitamin supplement.
Niarb Super. (Miller) Magnesium 100 mg, vitamin C 200 mg, niacinamide 200 mg (as ascorbate)/Tab. Bot. 100s. *otc.*
Use: Vitamin/mineral supplement.
Niazide. (Major) Trichlormethiazide 4 mg/Tab. Bot. 100s, 1000s. *Rx.*
Use: Diuretic.
niazo. Neotropin.
Use: Urinary antiseptic.
•**nibroxane.** (nye-BROX-ane) USAN.
Use: Antimicrobial (topical).
nicamindon.
See: Nicotinamide (Various Mfr.).
•**nicardipine hydrochloride.** (NYE-CAR-dih-peen) USAN.
Use: Vasodilator.
See: Cardene (Syntex).
nicardipine hydrochloride. (Mylan) 20 mg and 30 mg/Cap. 90s and 500s. *Rx.*
Use: Vasodilator.
N'ice. (SK-Beecham) Menthol 5 mg/Loz. in sugarless sorbitol base, saccharin. Pkg. 16s. *otc.*
Use: Local anesthetic.
N'ice 'n Clear. (SK-Beecham) Menthol 5 mg, sorbitol. Loz. Pkg. 16s. *otc.*
Use: Local anesthetic.
N'ice Throat Spray. (SK-Beecham) Menthol 0.12%, glycerin 25%, alcohol 23%, glucose, saccharin, sorbitol. Spray. 180 ml. *otc.*
Use: Mouth/throat product.

N'ice w/Vitamin C Drops. (SK-Beecham Consumer) Ascorbic acid 60 mg, menthol, sorbitol, tartrazine/Loz. Pks. 16s. *otc.*
Use: Vitamin supplement, local anesthetic.
•**nicergoline.** (nice-ERR-go-leen) USAN.
Use: Vasodilator.
Nichols Syphon Powder. (Last) Sodium bicarbonate, sodium Cl, sodium borate. Pouch 12.2 g (add to 32 oz. water to yield isotonic soln.).
•**niclosamide.** (nye-CLOSE-ah-mide) USAN.
Use: Antihelmintic.
Nico-400. (Jones Medical) Niacin 400 mg/Cap. Bot. 100s. *otc.*
Use: Vitamin B$_3$ supplement.
Nicobid. (Rhone-Poulenc Rorer) Nicotinic acid 125 mg, 250 mg or 500 mg/Tempule TR Cap. Bot. 100s, 500s. *otc.*
Use: Vitamin B$_3$ supplement.
nicobion.
See: Nicotinamide (Various Mfr.).
Nicoderm. (Hoechst Marion Roussel) Total nicotine content 36 mg or 114 mg/patch. 14 systems/box. *Rx.*
Use: Smoking deterrent.
nicoduozide. A mixture of nicothazone and isoniazid.
Nicolar. (Rhone-Poulenc Rorer) Niacin 500 mg/Tab. Bot. 100s. *Rx.*
Use: Vitamin B$_3$ supplement.
•**nicorandil.** (NIH-CAR-an-dill) USAN.
Use: Coronary vasodilator.
Ni Cord XL Caps. (Scott/Cord) Nicotinic acid 400 mg/Cap. Bot. 100s, 500s. *otc.*
Use: Vitamin B$_3$ supplement.
Nicorette. (SK-Beecham) Nicotine polacrilex 2 mg/Chew. piece. Box 96s. *Rx.*
Use: Smoking deterrent.
Nicorette DS. (SK-Beecham) Nicotine polacrilex 4 mg/Chew. gum. Box 96s. *Rx.*
Use: Smoking deterrent.
nicotamide.
See: Nicotinamide (Various Mfr.).
nicothazone. Nicotinaldehyde thiosemi-carbazone.
nicotilamide.
See: Nicotinamide (Various Mfr.).
nicotinamide. Niacinamide, U.S.P. 23. Vitamin B$_3$, Aminicotin, Dipegyl, Nicamindon, Nicotamide, Nicotilamide, Nicotinic Acid Amide.
nicotinamide adenine dinucleotide. Name used for Nadide.
nicotine transdermal systems.

Use: Smoking deterrent.
See: Habitrol (Basel Pharm)
  Nicoderm (Hoechst Marion Roussel).
  Nicotrol (Parke-Davis).
  Prostep (Lederle).
•**nicotine polacrilex.** (NIK-oh-TEEN PAHL-ah-KRILL-ex) U.S.P. 23.
Use: Smoking deterrent.
See: Nicorette (Hoechst Marion Roussel).
nicotine resin complex.
See: nicotine polacrilex.
Nicotinex Elixir. (Fleming) Niacin 50 mg/ 5 ml, alcohol 14%. Bot. pt, gal.
Use: Vitamin B$_3$ supplement.
nicotinic acid. Niacin, U.S.P. 23.
nicotinic acid w/combinations.
See: Niacin w/Combinations (Various Mfr.).
nicotinic acid amide. Niacinamide, U.S.P. 23.
See: Niacinamide (Various Mfr.).
•**nicotinyl alcohol.** (NIK-oh-TIN-ill AL-koe-hahl) USAN.
Use: Vasodilator (peripheral).
nicotinyl tartrate. 3-Pyridinemethanol tartrate.
See: Roniacol Timespan, Tab. (Roche).
Nicotrol. (McNeil CPC) Total nicotine content 8.3 mg, 16.6 mg or 24.9 mg/ patch. 14 systems/box. Nicotine 15 mg/ Patch. Kit. 7 patches. *Rx.*
Use: Smoking deterrent.
Nicotrol NS. (McNeil CPC) Nicotine 0.5 mg per actuation, methlyparaben, propylparaben, EDTA/Spray, pump. Bot. 10 ml. (200 sprays). *Rx.*
Use: Smoking deterrent.
nidroxyzone.
nieraline.
See: Epinephrine (Various Mfr.).
•**nifedipine,** (nye-FED-ih-peen) U.S.P. 23.
Use: Coronary vasodilator, interstitial cystitis. [Orphan drug]
See: Adalat, Cap. (Bayer).
  Adalat CC, ER Tab. (Bayer).
  Procardia, Cap. (Pfizer).
nifedipine. (Various Mfr.) Nifedipine 10 mg or 20 mg/Tab. In 100s, 300s and UD 100s. *Rx.*
Use: Calcium channel blocking agent.
Niferex. (Central) **Elix.:** Iron 100 mg/5 ml polysaccharide-iron complex, alcohol 10%. Sugar and dye free. Bot. 8 oz.
Tab.: Iron 50 mg. Bot. 100s. *otc.*
Use: Iron supplement.
Niferex-150. (Central) Polysaccharide iron complex equivalent to iron 150 mg/ Cap. Bot. 100s, 1000s. *otc.*

Use: Iron supplement.
Niferex-150 Forte Capsules. (Central) Elemental iron as polysaccharide-iron complex 150 mg, folic acid 1 mg, vitamin B$_{12}$ 25 mcg/Cap. Bot. 100s, 1000s. *Rx.*
Use: Vitamin/mineral supplement.
Niferex-PN. (Central) Iron 60 mg, folic acid 1 mg, vitamins C 50 mg, B$_{12}$ 3 mcg, A 4000 IU, D 400 IU, B$_1$ 3 mg, B$_2$ 3 mg, B$_6$ 2 mg, B$_3$ 10 mg, Zn 18 mg, Ca, sorbitol/Tab. Bot. 30s, 100s, 1000s. *Rx.*
Use: Vitamin/mineral supplement.
Niferex-PN Forte Tablets. (Central) Calcium 250 mg, iron 60 mg, vitamins A 5000 IU, D 400 IU, E 30 mg, B$_1$ 3 mg, B$_2$ 3.4 mg, B$_3$ 20 mg, B$_6$ 4 mg, B$_{12}$ 12 mcg, C 80 mg, folic acid 1 mg, Cu, I, Mg, zinc 25 mg/Tab. Bot. 100s. *Rx.*
Use: Vitamin/mineral supplement.
Niferex w/Vitamin C. (Central) Iron 50 mg, vitamin C 269 mg (as ascorbic acid 100 mg, as sodium ascorbate 169 mg)/Tab. Bot. 50s. *otc.*
Use: Vitamin/mineral supplement.
•**nifluridide.** (nye-FLURE-ih-DIDE) USAN.
Use: Ectoparasiticide.
•**nifungin.** (nih-FUN-jin) USAN. Substance derived from *Aspergillus giganteus.*
•**nifuradene.** (NYE-fyoor-ad-EEN) USAN.
Use: Antibacterial.
•**nifuraldezone.** (NYE-fer-AL-dee-zone) USAN. (Eaton).
Use: Antibacterial.
•**nifuratel.** (NYE-fyoor-at-ell) USAN.
Use: Antibacterial, antifungal, antiprotozoal (trichomonas).
•**nifuratrone.** (nye-FYOOR-ah-trone) USAN.
Use: Antibacterial.
•**nifurdazil.** (NYE-fyoor-dazz-ill) USAN.
Use: Antibacterial.
nifurethazone.
Use: Anti-infective.
•**nifurimide.** (nye-FYOOR-ih-MIDE) USAN.
Use: Antibacterial.
•**nifurmerone.** (NYE-fyoor-MER-ohn) USAN.
Use: Antifungal.
nifuroxime.
Use: Antifungal, anti-infective, topical, antiprotozoal.
See: Micofur.
W/Furazolidone.
See: Tricofuron, Pow., Supp. (Eaton).
•**nifurpirinol.** (nye-fer-PIHR-ih-nole) USAN.

Use: Antibacterial.

•**nifurquinazol.** (NYE-fyoor-KWIN-azz-ole) USAN.
Use: Antibacterial.

•**nifurthiazole.** (NYE-fyoor-THIGH-ah-zole) USAN.
Use: Antibacterial.

nifurtimox.
Use: CDC anti-infective agent.
See: Lampit (Bayer 2502).

Night-Time Effervescent Cold Tablets.
(Goldline) Phenylpropanolamine HCl 15 mg, diphenhydramine citrate 38.33 mg, aspirin 325 mg/Tab. Pkg. 20s. *otc.*
Use: Decongestant, antihistamine, analgesics.

Nighttime Pamprin. (Chattem) Diphenhydramine HCl 50 mg, acetaminophen 650 mg. Pow. Pkg. 4s. *otc.*
Use: Nonprescription sleep aid.

Night-Time Thera-Flu. (Sandoz) Pseudoephedrine HCl 60 mg, chlorpheniramine maleate 4 mg, dextromethorphan HBr 30 mg, acetaminophen 1000 mg. Powd. 6s. *otc.*
Use: Decongestant, antihistamine, antitussive, analgesic.

nigrin. Streptonigrin.
Use: Antineoplastic.

Niko-Mag. (Scruggs) Magnesium oxide 500 mg/Cap. Bot. 100s, 1000s. *otc.*
Use: Antacid.

Nikotime TD Caps. (Major) Niacin 125 mg or 250 mg/TD Cap. Bot. 100s, 1000s. *otc.*
Use: Vitamin B_3 supplement.

Nilandron. (Hoechst Marion Roussel) Nilutamide 50 mg/Tab. Bot. 90s. *Rx.*
Use: Treatment of prostate cancer.

Nilspasm. (Parmed) Phenobarbital 50 mg, hyoscyamine sulfate 0.31 mg, atropine sulfate 0.06 mg, scopolamine hydrobromide 0.0195 mg/Tab. Bot. 100s, 1000s. *Rx.*
Use: Sedative, hypnotic, anticholinergic, antispasmodic.

Nilstat Ointment & Cream. (Lederle) Nystatin 100,000 units/g. **Cream base** w/ Emulsifying wax, isopropyl myristate, glycerin, lactic acid, sodium hydroxide, sorbic acid 0.2%. Tube 15 g, Jar 240 g. **Oint. base:** w/light mineral oil, Plastibase 50 W. Tube 15 g. *Rx.*
Use: Antifungal, topical.

Nilstat Oral. (Lederle) Nystatin 500,000 units/FC Tab. Bot. 100s, UD 10 × 10s. *Rx.*
Use: Antifungal.

Nilstat Oral Suspension. (Lederle) Nystatin 100,000 units/ml, methylparaben 0.12%, propylparaben 0.03%, cherry flavor. Bot. 60 ml w/dropper, 16 fl oz. *Rx.*
Use: Antifungal.

Nilstat Powder. (Lederle) Nystatin pow. 150 million, 1 billion or 2 billion units/ Bot. *Rx.*
Use: Antifungal.

Nil Tuss. (Minnesota Pharm) Dextromethorphan HBr 10 mg, chlorpheniramine maleate 1.25 mg, phenylephrine HCl 5 mg, ammonium Cl 83 mg/5 ml. Syr. Bot. pt. *otc.*
Use: Antitussive, antihistamine, decongestant, expectorant.

•**nilutamide.** USAN.
Use: Antineoplastic.
See: Nilandron, Tab. (Hoechst Marion Roussel).

Nil Vaginal Cream. (Century) Sulfanilamide 15%, 9-aminoacridine HCl 0.2%, allantoin 1.5%. Bot. 4 oz. w/applicator. *otc.*
Use: Anti-infective, vaginal.

•**nilvadipine.** (NILL-vah-DIH-peen) USAN.
Use: Antagonist (calcium channel).

•**nimazone.** (nih-mah-ZONE) USAN.
Use: Anti-inflammatory.

Nimbex. (Glaxo Wellcome) Cisatracurium besylate 2 mg/ml, Vial 5 ml, 10 ml; 10 mg/ml, Vial 20 ml. Inj. *Rx.*
Use: Nondepolarizing neuromuscular blocker; muscle relaxant; adjunct to anesthesia.

Nimbus. (Bioamerica) Monoclonal antibody-based enzyme immunoassay. Screens for urinary chorionic gonadotropin. Pkg. 10s, 25s, 50s.
Use: Diagnostic aid.

•**nimodipine.** (NYE-MOE-dih-peen) USAN.
Use: Vasodilator.
See: Nimotop, Cap. (Bayer).

Nimotop. (Bayer) Nimodipine 30 mg Liq. Cap. Bot. UD 100s. *Rx.*
Use: For neurological deficits due to spasm following subarachnoid hemorrhage.

Nion B Plus C. (Nion) Vitamins B_1 15 mg, B_2 10.2 mg, B_3 50 mg, B_5 10 mg, C 300 mg/Capl. Bot 100s. *otc.*
Use: Vitamin supplement.

Niong. (U.S. Ethicals) Nitroglycerin 2.6 mg or 6.5 mg/CR Tab. Bot. 100s. *Rx.*
Use: Antianginal.

Nipent. (Parke-Davis) Pentostatin 10 mg/ Pow. Vial. Single dose. *Rx.*
Use: Antineoplastic.

Niratron. (Progress) Chlorpheniramine maleate 4 mg/Tsp. Bot. pt.
Use: Antihistamine.
•**niridazole.** (nye-RIH-dah-ZOLE) USAN.
Use: Antischistosomal.
•**nisbuterol mesylate.** (NISS-BYOO-teh-role) USAN.
Use: Bronchodilator.
•**nisobamate.** (NYE-so-BAM-ate) USAN.
Use: Minor tranquilizer, sedative, hypnotic.
•**nisoldipine.** (nye-SOLE-idh-peen) USAN.
Use: Vasodilator (coronary).
See: Sular, ER Tab. (Zeneca).
•**nisoxetine.** (NISS-OX-eh-teen) USAN.
Use: Antidepressant.
•**nisterime acetate.** (nye-STEER-eem) USAN.
Use: Androgen.
•**nitarsone.** (NITE-AHR-sone) USAN.
Use: Antiprotozoal (histomonas).
Nite Time Cold Formula. (Barre-National) Pseudoephedrine HCl 10 mg, doxylamine succinate 1.25 mg, dextromethorphan HBr 5 mg, acetaminophen 167 mg, alcohol 25%. Liq. Bot. 180 ml, 300 ml. *otc.*
Use: Decongestant, antihistamine, antitussive, analgesic.
•**nitrafudam hydrochloride.** (NIGH-trah-FEW-dam) USAN.
Use: Antidepressant.
•**nitralamine hydrochloride.** (nye-TRAL-ah-meen) USAN.
Use: Antifungal.
•**nitramisole hydrochloride.** (nye-TRAM-ih-sole) USAN.
Use: Anthelmintic.
•**nitrazepam.** (nye-TRAY-zeh-pam) USAN.
Use: Anticonvulsant, sedative, hypnotic.
Nitrazine Paper. (Squibb) Determines pH of a solution, in pH 4.5-7.5 range. 15 ft. roll with dispenser and color chart.
Use: Diagnostic aid.
•**nitrendipine.** (NIGH-TREN-dih-peen) USAN.
Use: Antihypertensive.
•**nitric acid,** N.F. 18.
Use: Pharmaceutic aid (acidifying agent).
nitric acid silver. Silver Nitrate, U.S.P. 23.
nitric oxide. (Ohmeda Pharmaceuticals) *Rx.*
Use: Treatment of primary pulmonary hypertension in the newborn. [Orphan drug]

Nitro-Bid IV. (Hoechst Marion Roussel) Nitroglycerin 5 mg/ml. Inj. Vial 1 ml box 10s; 5 ml Box 10s; 10 ml Box 5s. *Rx.*
Use: Antianginal.
Nitro-Bid Ointment. (Hoechst Marion Roussel) Nitroglycerin (glyceryl trinitrate) 2%, in lanolin and petrolatum base. Tube 20 g, 60 g, UD 1 g (100s). *Rx.*
Use: Antianginal.
Nitro-Bid Plateau Caps. (Hoechst Marion Roussel) Nitroglycerin 2.5 mg, 6.5 mg or 9 mg/SR Cap. Bot. 60s, 100s. *Rx.*
Use: Antianginal.
Nitrocap. (Freeport) Nitroglycerin 2.5 mg/TR Cap. Bot. 100s. *Rx.*
Use: Antianginal.
•**nitrocycline.** (NYE-troe-SIGH-kleen) USAN.
Use: Antibacterial.
•**nitrodan.** (NYE-troe-dan) USAN.
Use: Anthelmintic.
Nitrodisc. (Roberts) Nitroglycerin. Transcutaneous nitroglycerin discs releasing 16 mg, 24 mg or 32 mg/Patch. Carton 30s, 100s. *Rx.*
Use: Antianginal.
Nitro-Dur. (Key Pharm) Nitroglycerin. Transdermal system releasing 20 mg, 40 mg, 60 mg, 80 mg, 120 mg or 160 mg/Patch. Carton 30s, 100s, UD 30s, 100s. *Rx.*
Use: Antianginal.
Nitrofan Caps. (Major) Nitrofurantoin 50 mg or 100 mg/Cap. Bot. 100s, 500s. *Rx.*
Use: Urinary anti-infective.
•**nitrofurantoin,** (nye-troe-FYOOR-an-toyn) U.S.P. 23.
Use: Urinary antibacterial.
See: Furadantin, Soln. (Procter and Gamble Pharm).
nitrofurantoin macrocrystals. (Various Mfr.) 50 mg or 100 mg/Cap. Bot. 100s, 500s, 1000s. *Rx.*
Use: Urinary anti-infective.
See: Macrobid, Cap. (Procter and Gamble Pharm)
Macrodantin, Cap. (Procter and Gamble Pharm).
•**nitrofurazone,** U.S.P. 23.
Use: Topical anti-infective.
See: Furacin, Preps. (Roberts).
Nitrozone, Oint. (Century).
W/Allantoin, stearic acid.
See: Eldezol, Oint. (ICN Pharm).
nitrofurazone. (Various Mfr.) **Top. Soln:** 0.2%. Bot. Pt., gal. **Oint.:** 0.2%. Tube 480 g.

Use: Topical anti-infective.

nitrogard. (Parke-Davis) Transmucosal controlled-released nitroglycerin 1 mg, 2 mg or 3 mg/Tab. Bot. 100s. *Rx.*
Use: Antianginal.

•**nitrogen,** N.F. 18.
Use: Pharmaceutic aid (air displacement).

nitrogen monoxide. Laughing Gas, Nitrous Oxide.
Use: Inhalation anesthetic, analgesic.

nitrogen mustard.
See: Mustargen, Vial (Merck).

nitrogen mustard derivatives.
See: Leukemia Agents.
Leukeran, Tab. (Burroughs-Wellcome).
Mustargen HCl, Vial (Merck).
Triethylene Melamine, Tab. (Lederle).

nitroglycerin. (nye-troe-GLIH-suh-rin) (Various Mfr.) 5 mg/ml. Inj. Vial 5 ml, 10 ml. *Rx.*
Use: Antianginal.

•**nitroglycerin, diluted,** U.S.P. 23. *Formerly Glyceryl Trinitrate.*
Use: Vasodilator (coronary).

nitroglycerin in 5% dextrose. (Various Mfr.) **25 mg, 100 mg:** Inj. Soln. 250 ml. **50 mg:** Inj. Soln. 250, 500 ml. **200 mg:** Inj. Soln. 500 ml. *Rx.*
Use: Antianginal.

nitroglycerin injection. (Abbott) 25 mg/ml. Vial 5 ml, 10 ml.
Use: Vasodilator, treatment of angina.
See: Tridil, Inj. (DuPont Merck).

nitroglycerin, intravenous.
Use: Vasodilator.
See: Nitro-Bid IV (Hoechst Marion Roussel).

nitroglycerin ointment. (Various Mfr.) 2% in lanolin-petrolatum base. Tube 30 g, 60 g. *Rx.*
Use: Vasodilator.

nitroglycerin tablets. (Various Mfr.) Glyceryl Trinitrate, Glonoin, Nitroglycerol, Trinitrin, Trinitroglycerol Tab.
Use: Vasodilator.
See: Niglycon, Tab. (Consoln. Midland).
Niong, Tab. (U.S. Ethicals).
Nitrobid, Cap. (Hoechst Marion Roussel).
Nitrocels, Cap. (Winston).
Nitrodyl, Cap. (Bock).
Nitrogard (Parke-Davis).
Nitroglyn, Tab. (Key Pharm.)
Nitrol Oint. (Kremers-Urban).
Nitro-Lyn, Cap. (Lynwood).
Nitrong, Tab. (Wharton).
Nitrospan, Cap. (Rhone-Poulenc Rorer).

Nitro, TD Cap. (Fleming).
Nitro-Time, Cap. (Time-Cap Labs).
Trates, Cap. (Solvay).
Vasoglyn, Unicelles (Solvay).
W/Butabarbital.
See: Nitrodyl-B, Cap. (Bock).

nitroglycerin transdermal. (Various Mfr.) 16 mg - 62.5 mg, 32 mg - 125 mg or 75 mg - 187.5 mg (some systems have different release rates). Box 30s.
Use: Vasodilator.
See: Deponit 5 and 10 (Wyeth-Ayerst).
Nitrodisc (Searle).
NTS (Bolar).
Transderm-Nitro (Novartis).

nitroglycerol.
See: Nitroglycerin (Various Mfr.).

Nitroglyn. (Key) Nitroglycerin 2.5 mg, 6.5 mg or 9 mg/SR Cap. Bot. 100s. *Rx.*
Use: Antianginal.

Nitrolan. (Elan) Protein 60 g, fat 40 g, carbohydrates 160 g, sodium 690 mg, potassium 1.17 g/L, lactose free. With appropriate vitamins and minerals. Liq. In 237 ml Tetra Pak containers and 1000 ml New Pak closed systems with and without Color Check. *otc.*
Use: Nutritional supplement.

Nitrolin. (Schein) Nitroglycerin 2.5 mg or 9 mg/SR Cap. **2.5 mg:** Bot. 100s. **9 mg:** Bot. 60s. *Rx.*
Use: Antianginal.

Nitrolingual Spray. (Rhone-Poulenc Rorer) Nitroglycerin lingual aerosol 0.4 mg/metered dose. Canister 13.8 g containing 200 metered doses. *Rx.*
Use: Antianginal.

Nitrol IV. (Rhone-Poulenc Rorer) Nitroglycerin 0.8 mg/ml. Amp. 1 ml Box 25s; 10 ml Box 10s; 30 ml Box 5s. *Rx.*
Use: Antianginal.

Nitrol IV Concentrate. (Rhone-Poulenc Rorer) Nitroglycerin for infusion 50 mg/10 ml. Amp. Box 10s. *Rx.*
Use: Antianginal.

Nitrol Ointment. (Pharmacia & Upjohn) Nitroglycerin 2% in lanolin and petrolatum base. Tube 30 g, 60 g, Pack 6s. *Rx.*
Use: Antianginal.

Nitrol Ointment. (Savage) Nitroglycerin 2% in a lanolin-petrolatum base. Tube 60 g, UD 3 g (50s). *Rx.*
Use: Antianginal agent.

Nitro-Lyn. (Lynwood) Nitroglycerin 2.5 mg/Cap. Bot. 100s. *Rx.*
Use: Antianginal.

nitromannite.
See: Mannitol Hexanitrate (Various Mfr.).

nitromannitol.
See: Mannitol Hexanitrate (Various Mfr.).

Nitromed. (U.S. Ethicals) Nitroglycerin 2.6 mg or 6.5 mg/CR Tab. Bot. 100s. *Rx.*
Use: Antianginal.

•**nitromersol,** U.S.P. 23.
Use: Anti-infective (topical).

•**nitromide.** USAN.
Use: Antibacterial.

nitromifene citrate. (nye-TROE-mih-feen) USAN.
Use: Antiestrogen.

Nitronet. (U.S. Ethicals) Nitroglycerin 2.6 mg or 6.5 mg/CR Tab. Bot. 100s. *Rx.*
Use: Antianginal.

Nitrong Ointment. (Wharton) Nitroglycerin 2%. Oint. Tube 30 g, 60 g with dose applicator. *Rx.*
Use: Antianginal.

Nitrong Tablets. (Wharton) Nitroglycerin 2.6 mg, 6.5 mg or 9 mg/CR Tab. Bot. 30s, 60s (9 mg), 100s. *Rx.*
Use: Antianginal.

Nitropress. (Abbott) Sodium nitroprusside 50 mg/2 ml. Vial. *Rx.*
Use: Antihypertensive.

nitroprusside sodium. (nye-troe-PRUSS-ide SO-dee-uhm)
Use: Antihypertensive.
See: Nitropress, Pow. for Inj. (Abbott). Sodium Nitroprusside, Pow. for Inj. (Various Mfr.).

nitrosoureas.
Use: Alkylating agent (antineoplastic).
See: CeeNu (Bristol Myers Oncology). BiCNU (Bristol Myers Oncology). Zanosar (Pharmacia & Upjohn). Thiotepa (Lederle).

Nitrostat. (Parke-Davis) Nitroglycerin 0.3 mg, 0.4 mg or 0.6 mg/Tab. Bot. 25s, 100s, UD 100s. *Rx.*
Use: Antianginal.

Nitrostat IV. (Parke-Davis) Nitroglycerin for infusion. **0.8 mg/ml:** Amp. 10 ml. **5 mg/ml:** Amp. 10 ml, Vial 10 ml. **10 mg/ml:** Vial 10 ml. *Rx.*
Use: Antianginal.

Nitro-Time. (Time-Cap Labs) Nitroglycerin 2.5 mg, 6.5 mg or 9 mg, lactose, sucrose/ER Cap. Bot. 60s, 90s, 100s. *Rx.*
Use: Antianginal.

nitrous acid, sodium salt. Sodium Nitrite, U.S.P. 23.

•**nitrous oxide,** U.S.P. 23. Laughing Gas. Nitrogen Monoxide.
Use: Anesthesia (inhalation).

•**nivazol.** (NIH-vah-ZOLE) USAN.
Use: Glucocorticoid.

Nivea Moisturizing. (Beiersdorf) **Cream:** Mineral oil, petrolatum, lanolin alcohol, glycerin, microcrystalline wax, paraffin, magnesium sulfate, decyloleate, octyl dodecanol, aluminum stearate, citric acid, magnesium stearate. In 120 g, 180 g, 300 g, 480 g. **Lot.:** Mineral oil, lanolin, isopropyl myristate, cetearyl alcohol, glyceryl stearate, acrylamide/sodium acrylate copolymer, simethicone, methychloroisothiazolinone, methylisothiazolinone. In 180 ml, 300 ml, 450 ml. *otc.*
Use: Emollient.

Nivea Moisturizing Creme Soap. (Beiersdorf) Sodium tallowate, sodium cocoate, glycerin, petrolatum, titanium dioxide, NaCl, octyldodecanol, macadamia nut oil, aloe, sodium thiosulfate, lanolin alcohol, pentasodium pentetate, EDTA, BHT, beeswax. Bar 90 g, 150 g. *otc.*
Use: Skin cleanser.

Nivea Oil. (Beiersdorf) Emulsion of neutral aliphatic hydrocarbons. **Liq.:** Bot. 2 oz, 4 fl oz, pt, qt. **Cream:** Tube 1 oz, 2⅓ oz, Jar 4 oz, 6 oz, 1 lb, 5 lb. tin. **Soap:** Bath or toilet size. *otc.*
Use: Emollient.
See: Basic, soap (Beiersdorf).

Nivea Sun. (Beiersdorf) Octyl methoxycinnamate, octyl salicylate, benzophenone-3, 2-phenylbenzimidazole-5-sulfonic acid. Lot. Bot. 120 ml. *otc.*
Use: Sunscreen.

•**nivimedone sodium.** (nih-VIH-meh-dohn) USAN.
Use: Antiallergic.

Nix Creme Rinse. (Glaxo Wellcome) Permethrin 1%. Bot. 2 oz. *otc.*
Use: Pediculicide.

•**nizatidine.** (nye-ZAT-ih-deen) U.S.P. 23.
Use: Antiulcerative.
See: Axid, Cap. (Lilly).

Nizoral Cream. (Janssen) Ketoconazole 2% cream. Tube 15 g, 30 g. *Rx.*
Use: Antifungal, topical.

Nizoral Suspension. (Janssen) Ketoconazole 20 mg/ml. Saccharin. Bot. 4 oz. *Rx.*
Use: Antifungal.

Nizoral Tablets. (Janssen) Ketoconazole 200 mg/Tab. Bot. 100s. Box of 10 strips of 10 tablets. *Rx.*
Use: Antifungal.

n-methylhydrazine.
Use: Antineoplastic.

See: Procarbazine.

n-methylisatin beta-thiosemicarbazone. Under study.
Use: Smallpox protection.

N-Multistix. (Bayer) Glucose, protein, pH, blood, ketones, bilirubin, urobilinogen, nitrate, leukocytes. Kit 100s.
Use: In vitro diagnostic aid.

N-Multistix S. G. Reagent Strips. (Bayer) Urinalysis reagent strip test for pH, protein, glucose, ketones, bilirubin, blood, nitrite, urobilinogen and specific gravity. Bot. 100s.
Use: Diagnostic aid.

n, n-diethylvanillamide.
See: Ethamivan, Inj. (Various Mfr.).

No-Aspirin. (Walgreen) Acetaminophen 325 mg/Tab. Bot. 100s. *otc.*
Use: Analgesic.

No-Aspirin Extra Strength. (Walgreen) Acetaminophen 500 mg/Tab. or Cap. **Tab.:** Bot. 60s, 100s. **Cap.:** Bot. 50s, 100s. *otc.*
Use: Analgesic.

•**noberastine.** (no-BER-ast-een) USAN.
Use: Antihistamine.

•**nocodazole.** (no-KOE-DAH-zole) USAN.
Use: Antineoplastic.

NoDoz. (Bristol-Myers) Caffeine 100 mg, aspartame, phenylalanine 15 mg, spearmint flavor. Chew. Tab. Pkg. 12s, 30s.
Use: Analeptic.

No-Drowsiness Allerest. (Novartis) Pseudoephedrine HCl 30 mg, acetaminophen 500 mg/Tab. Bot. 20s. *otc.*
Use: Decongestant, analgesic.

No Drowsiness Sinarest. (Fisons) Pseudoephedrine HCl 30 mg, acetaminophen 500 mg/Tab. Bot. 24s. *otc.*
Use: Decongestant, analgesic.

nofetumomab merpentan.
See: Verluna (NeoRx, DuPont Merck).

•**nogalamycin.** (no-GAL-ah-MY-sin) USAN.
Use: Antineoplastic.

No-Hist Capsules. (Dunhall) Phenylephrine HCl 5 mg, phenylpropanolamine HCl 40 mg, pseudoephedrine HCl 40 mg/Cap. Bot. 100s. *Rx.*
Use: Decongestant.

No-Hist-S Syrup. (Dunhall) Phenylephrine HCl 5 mg, phenylpropanolamine HCl 40 mg, pseudoephedrine HCl 40 mg/5 ml. Bot. pt. *Rx.*
Use: Decongestant.

Nokane. (Wren) Salicylamide 4 g, N-acetyl-p-aminophenol 4 g, caffeine 0.5 gr/Tab. Bot. 40s. *otc.*

Use: Analgesic combination.

Nolahist. (Carnrick) Phenindamine tartrate 25 mg/Tab. Bot. 100s. *otc.*
Use: Antihistamine.

Nolamine. (Carnrick) Chlorpheniramine maleate 4 mg, phenindamine tartrate 24 mg, phenylpropanolamine HCl 50 mg/Tab. Bot. 100s, 250s. *Rx.*
Use: Antihistamine, decongestant.

Nolex LA. (Carnrick). Phenylpropanolamine 75 mg, guaifenesin 400 mg/SR Tab. Bot. 100s. *Rx.*
Use: Decongestant, expectorant.

•**nolinium bromide.** (no-LIN-ee-uhm) USAN.
Use: Antiulcerative, antisecretory.

Nolvadex. (Zeneca) Tamoxifen citrate 10 mg: 60s, 250s. 20 mg: 30s. *Rx.*
Use: Antineoplastic.

Nometic. Diphenidol.
Use: Antiemetic.

•**nomifensine maleate.** (NO-mih-FEN-seen) USAN.
Use: Antidepressant.

Nonamin. (Western Research) Calcium 100 mg, chloride 90 mg, magnesium 50 mg, zinc 3.75 mg, iron 4.5 mg, copper 0.5 mg, iodine 37.5 mcg, potassium 49 mg, phosphorus 100 mg/Tab. Bot. 1000s. *otc.*
Use: Mineral supplement.

Non-Drowsy Contac Sinus. (SK Beecham) Pseudoephedrine HCl 30 mg, acetaminophen 500 mg. Cap. Bot. 24s. *otc.*
Use: Decongestant, analgesic.

None. (Forest) Heparin sodium 1000 units/ml. No preservatives. Amps 5 ml. Box 25s. *Rx.*
Use: Anticoagulant.

nonoxynol. (nahn-OCK-sih-nahl) (Ortho) *otc.*
Use: Spermicide.
See: Emko, Preps. (Schering Plough).

•**nonoxynol 4.** (NAHN-ox-sih-nahl 4) USAN.
Use: Pharmaceutic aid (surfactant).

•**nonoxynol 9,** (NAHN-ox-sih-nahl 9) U.S.P. 23.
Use: Spermaticide, pharmaceutic aid (wetting and solubilizing agent).
See: Because, Foam (Schering Plough).
Conceptrol, Cream, Gel (Ortho).
Delfen, Foam (Ortho).
Emko Prods. (Schering Plough).
Encare, Insert (Eaton-Merz).
Gynol II, Jelly (Ortho).
Intercept, Inserts (Ortho).

Ortho-Creme, Cream (Ortho).
Ortho-Gynol, Jelly (Ortho).
●**nonoxynol 10,** (nahn-OCK-sih-nahl 10)
N.F. 18.
Use: Pharmaceutic aid (surfactant).
●**nonoxynol 15.** (NAHN-ox-sih-nahl 15)
USAN.
Use: Pharmaceutic aid (surfactant).
●**nonoxynol 30.** (NAHN-ox-sih-nahl 30)
USAN. Under study.
Use: Pharmaceutic aid (surfactant).
nonspecific protein therapy.
See: Protein, Nonspecific Therapy.
**nonsteroidal anti-inflammatory agents,
ophthalmic.**
See: Ocufen (Allergan).
Profenal (Alcon).
Voltaren (Ciba Vision Ophthalmics).
nonylphenoxypolyethoxy ethanol.
Nonoxynol.
Use: Spermicide.
See: Delfen Vaginal Foam (Ortho).
No Pain-HC. (Young Again Products)
Capsaicin 0.075%. Roll-on. 60 ml. *otc.*
Use: External analgesic.
●**noracymethadol hydrochloride.** (nahr-
ASS-ih-METH-ah-dole) USAN.
Use: Analgesic.
●**norbolethone.** (nahr-BOLE-eth-ohn)
USAN.
Use: Anabolic.
Norcet Tablets. (Holloway) Hydrocodone
bitartrate 5 mg, acetaminophen 500 mg/
Tab. Bot. 100s. *c-III.*
Use: Narcotic analgesic combination.
Norcuron. (Organon) Vecuronium bro-
mide 10 mg/5 ml. **With diluent:** Vial
5 ml lyophilized powder and 5 ml am-
pul of sterile water for injection. Box
10s. **Without diluent:** Vial 5 ml lyophilized powder. Box 10s. **Prefilled syringe:** Vial 10 ml lyophilized powder
and 10 ml syringe w/bacteriostatic water for injection. Box 10s. *Rx.*
Use: Skeletal muscle relaxant, adjunct
to anesthesia.
norcycline.
Use: Anti-infective.
Nordette. (Wyeth-Ayerst) Levonorgestrel
0.15 mg, ethinyl estradiol 0.03 mg/Tab.
6 Pilpak dispensers, 21 day and 28
day w/ 7 inert tabs. *Rx.*
Use: Oral contraceptive.
Norditropin. (Novo Nordisk) Somatropin
4 mg (≈ to 12 IU) or 8 mg (≈ to 24 IU),
glycine 8.8 mg, mannitol 44 mg. Powd.
for Inj. Vials with 2 ml water for injection.
Benzyl alcohol 1.5%. *Rx.*
Use: Growth hormone.

Norel Plus Capsules. (U.S. Pharmaceutical Corp.) Chlorpheniramine maleate
4 mg, phenyltoloxamine dihydrogen citrate 25 mg, phenylpropanolamine HCl
25 mg, acetaminophen 325 mg/Cap.
Bot. 100s. *Rx.*
Use: Antihistamine, decongestant, analgesic.
●**norepinephrine bitartrate,** (NOR-eh-pih-
NEFF-reen) U.S.P. 23.
Use: Adrenergic (vasoconstrictor).
See: Levophed Bitartrate, Soln., Amp.
(Sanofi Winthrop).
Norethin 1/50 M. (Roberts) Norethin-
drone 1 mg, mestranol 50 mcg/Tab. 21
day and 28 day (with 7 inert tabs.). *Rx.*
Use: Oral contraceptive.
Norethin 1/35 E. (Roberts) Norethin-
drone 1 mg, ethinyl estradiol 35 mg/Tab.
21 day and 28 day (with 7 inert tabs.).
Rx.
Use: Oral contraceptive.
●**norethindrone,** U.S.P. 23.
Use: Progestin.
See: Micronor, Tab. (Ortho).
Norlutin, Tab. (Parke-Davis).
Nor-QD, Tab. (Syntex).
W/Ethinyl estradiol.
See: Brevicon 21 and 28, Tab. (Syn-
tex).
GenCept, Tab. (Gencon).
Jenest-28, Tab. (Organon).
Modicon 21 and 28, Tab. (Ortho).
Ortho-Novum 21 and 28, Prods. (Or-
tho).
Ovcon-35, Tab. (Bristol-Myers).
Ovcon-50, Tab. (Bristol-Myers).
W/Mestranol.
See: Norinyl, Prods. (Syntex).
Ortho-Novum, Prods. (Ortho).
W/Mestranol, ferrous fumarate.
See: Norinyl-I Fe 28, Prods. (Syntex).
●**norethindrone acetate,** U.S.P. 23.
Use: Progestin.
See: Aygestin, Tab. (Wyeth-Ayerst).
Norlutate, Tab. (Parke-Davis).
**norethindrone acetate and ethinyl
estradiol tablets.**
Use: Oral contraceptive.
See: Brevicon, Tab. (Syntex).
Gestest, Tab. (Squibb).
Loestrin, Prods. (Parke-Davis).
Norinyl, Prods. (Syntex).
Norlestrin, Prods. (Parke-Davis).
**norethindrone and ethinyl estradiol
tablets.**
Use: Oral contraceptive.
norethindrone and mestranol tablets.
Use: Oral contraceptive.

•**norethynodrel,** (nahr-eh-THIGH-no-drell) U.S.P. 23.
Use: Progestin.
See: Enovid, Prods. (Searle).

Norflex. (3M Pharm) Orphenadrine citrate 100 mg/SR Tab. Bot. 100s, 500s. *Rx.*
Use: Skeletal muscle relaxant.

Norflex Injectable. (3M Pharm) Orphenadrine citrate 30 mg, sodium bisulfite 2 mg, sodium Cl 5.8 mg, water for injection qs 2 ml. Amp. 2 ml 6s, 50s. *Rx.*
Use: Skeletal muscle relaxant.

•**norfloxacin,** (nor-FLOX-uh-SIN) U.S.P. 23.
Use: Antibacterial.
See: Chibroxin, Ophth. Soln. (Merck).
Noroxin, Tab. (Merck).

•**norflurane.** (nahr-FLEW-rane) USAN. Under study.
Use: Inhalation anesthetic.

Norforms. (Fleet) **Powd.:** Cornstarch, zinc oxide. 120 g. **Supp.:** PEG-18, PEG-32, PEG-20 stearate, methylparaben. 6s, 12s, 24s w/applicator. *otc.*
Use: Vaginal preparation.

Norgesic Forte Tablets. (3M) Orphenadrine citrate 50 mg, aspirin 770 mg, caffeine 60 mg, lactose/Tab. Bot. 100s, 500s, UD 100s. *Rx.*
Use: Skeletal muscle relaxant, salicylate analgesic.

Norgesic Tablets. (3M) Orphenadrine citrate 25 mg, aspirin 385 mg, caffeine 30 mg, lactose/Tab. Bot. 100s, 500s, UD 100s. *Rx.*
Use: Skeletal muscle relaxant, salicylate analgesic.

•**norgestimate.** (nore-JEST-ih-mate) USAN. *Formerly Dexnorgestrel Acetine.*
Use: Progestin.
W/ Ethinyl estradiol.
See: Ortho-Cyclen, Tab. (Ortho).
Ortho Tri-Cyclen, Tab. (Ortho).

•**norgestomet.** (nore-JESS-toe-met) USAN.
Use: Progestin.

•**norgestrel,** (nahr-JESS-trell) U.S.P. 23.
Use: Oral contraceptive, progestin.
See: Ovrette, Tab. (Wyeth-Ayerst).

norgestrel and ethinyl estradiol tablets.
Use: Oral contraceptive.
See: Lo/Ovral, Tab. (Wyeth-Ayerst).
Ovral-Prep. (Wyeth-Ayerst).

Norinyl 1 + 35. (Syntex) Norethindrone 1 mg, ethinyl estradiol 0.035 mg/Tab. Wallette 21 and 28 day (7 inert tabs). *Rx.*

Use: Oral contraceptive.

Norinyl 1 + 50. (Syntex) Norethindrone 1 mg, mestranol 0.05 mg/Tab. Wallette 21 and 28 day (7 inert tabs). *Rx.*
Use: Oral contraceptive.

Norinyl 2 mg. (Syntex) Norethindrone 2 mg, mestranol 0.1 mg/Tab. Memorette Disp. of 20s. Refill folders of 20s. *Rx.*
Use: Oral contraceptive.

Norisodrine Aerotrol. (Abbott) Norisodrine HCl (isoproterenol HCl) 0.25% (2.8 mg/ml) in inert chlorofluorohydrocarbon propellants, alcohol 33%, ascorbic acid 0.1% as preservative. Aerotrol 15 ml. Box 12s. *Rx.*
Use: Bronchodilator.

Norisodrine with Calcium Iodide Syrup. (Abbott) Isoproterenol sulfate 3 mg, calcium iodide, anhydrous 150 mg/5 ml, alcohol 6%. Bot. pt. *Rx.*
Use: Bronchodilator.

Norlestrin-21 1/50 Tablets. (Parke-Davis) Norethindrone acetate 1 mg, ethinyl estradiol 50 mcg/Tab. (yellow). Compact 21s. Pkg. 5 compacts. Pkg. 5 refills; Ctn. 10×5 refills. *Rx.*
Use: Oral contraceptive.

Norlestrin-28 1/50 Tablet. (Parke-Davis) Norethindrone acetate 1 mg, ethinyl estradiol 50 mcg/Tab. (yellow). Compact 21 yellow, 7 white (inert) tablets. Pkg. 5 compacts. Pkg. 5 refills; Ctn. 10×5 refills. *Rx.*
Use: Oral contraceptive.

Norlestrin-21 2.5/50 Tablets. (Parke-Davis) Norethindrone acetate 2.5 mg, ethinyl estradiol 50 mcg/Tab. (pink). Compact 21s. Pkg. 5 compacts. Pkg. 5 refills; Ctn. 10×5 refills. *Rx.*
Use: Oral contraceptive.

Norlestrin Fe 1/50 Tablets. (Parke-Davis) Norethindrone acetate 1 mg, ethinyl estradiol 50 mcg/Tab. (yellow). Compact 21 yellow tab., 7 brown 75 mg ferrous fumarate tab. Pkg. 5 compacts. Pkg. 5 refills; Ctn. 10×5 refills. *Rx.*
Use: Oral contraceptive.

Norlestrin Fe 2.5/50 Tablets. (Parke-Davis) Norethindrone acetate 2.5 mg, ethinyl estradiol 50 mcg/Tab. (pink). Compact 21 pink tab., 7 brown 75 mg ferrous fumarate tab. Pkg. 5 compacts. Pkg. 5 refills; Ctn. 10×5 refills. *Rx.*
Use: Oral contraceptive.

Normaderm Cream & Lotion. (Doak) Buffered lactic acid in vanishing bases. **Cream:** Jar 3¾ oz, 16 oz. **Lot.:** Bot. 4 oz, 16 oz, 128 oz. *otc.*
Use: Emollient, acid restorer for skin.

normal human serum albumin. Albumin Human, U.S.P. 23.

normal human serum albumin. (Immuno-US). 5%/Inj.: 50, 250, 500 ml. 25%/Inj.: 20, 50, 100 ml. *Rx.*
Use: Shock treatment.

normal saline.
See: 0.2% Sodium chloride (Solopak).
0.45% sodium chloride (1/2 normal saline) (Various Mfr.).
0.9% Sodium chloride (Normal saline) (Various Mfr.).
3% Sodium chloride (Various Mfr.).
5% Sodium chloride (Various Mfr.).

Normaline Kit. (Apothecary Products) Salt tablets for normal saline 250 mg/Tab. Preservative free. 200s with Bot. 27.7 ml. *otc.*
Use: Ophthalmic preparation.

Normodyne. (Schering Plough) Labetalol HCl. **Inj.:** 5 mg/ml. Amp. 20 ml, 40 ml, 60 ml. **Tab.:** 100 mg, 200 mg or 300 mg. Bot. 100s, 500s, UD 100s. Calendar pak 56s. *Rx.*
Use: Antihypertensive.

Normol. (Alcon Lenscare) Sterile, isotonic solution of thimerosal 0.004%, chlorhexidine gluconate 0.005%, edetate disodium 0.1%. Bot. 8 oz. *otc.*
Use: Soft contact lens care.

Normosol-M in D5-W. (Abbott Hospital Prods) Dextrose 5 g, sodium Cl 234 mg, potassium acetate 128 mg, magnesium acetate 21 mg, sodium bisulfite 30 mg/100 ml. Bot. 500 ml, 1000 ml in Abbo-Vac (glass) or Life Care (flexible) containers. *Rx.*
Use: Parenteral nutritional supplement.

Normosol-R; Normosol-R pH 7.4; 500 ml., 1000 ml. Normosol-R D5-W. (Abbott Hospital Prods) Sodium Cl 526 mg, sodium acetate 222 mg, sodium gluconate 502 mg, potassium Cl 37 mg, magnesium Cl 14 mg, pH of Normosol-R and Normosol R in D5-W adjusted with HCl/100 ml. Bot. 1000 ml, 500 ml. in Life Care (flexible) containers. *Rx.*
Use: Parenteral nutritional supplement.

Normotensin. (Marcen) IM soln. for inj. Mucopolysaccharide 20 mg, sodium nucleate 25 mg, epinephrine-neutralizing factor 25 units, sodium citrate 10 mg, inositol 5 mg, phenol 0.5%/ml. Multi-dose vial 10 ml, 30 ml.
Use: Antihypertensive.

Norolon. (Sanofi Winthrop) Chloroquine phosphate. *Rx.*
Use: Antimalarial.

Noroxin. (Roberts) Norfloxacin 400 mg/Tab. Bot. 100s, UD 20s, UD 100s. *Rx.*

Use: Urinary anti-infective.

Norpace. (Searle) Disopyramide phosphate 100 mg or 150 mg/Cap. Bot. 100s, 500s, 1000s, UD 100s. *Rx.*
Use: Antiarrhythmic.

Norpace CR. (Searle) Disopyramide phosphate 100 mg or 150 mg/CR Cap. Bot. 100s, 500s, UD 100s. *Rx.*
Use: Antiarrhythmic.

Norphyl. (Vita Elixir) Aminophylline 100 mg/Tab. *Rx.*
Use: Bronchodilator.

Norplant. (Wyeth-Ayerst) Levonorgestrel 36 mg. Implant kit 6s. *Rx.*
Use: Progestin contraceptive system.

Norpramin. (Hoechst Marion Roussel) Desipramine HCl 10 mg, 25 mg, 50 mg, 75 mg, 100 mg or 150 mg/Tab. **10 mg:** Bot. 100s; **25 mg:** Bot. 100s, 1000s, UD 100s; **50 mg:** Bot. 100s, 1000s, UD 100s; **75 mg:** Bot. 100s; **100 mg:** Bot. 100s. **150 mg:** Bot. 50s. *Rx.*
Use: Antidepressant.

nortesterionate.

Nortriptyline. (nor-TRIP-tih-leen) (Schein) 10 mg, 25 mg, 50 mg or 75 mg. Cap. Bot. 100s; **25 mg:** Bot. 500s also. *Rx.*
Use: Antidepressant.

nortriptyline. (Various Mfr.) 10, 25, 50 and 75 mg/Cap. 100s, 500s. *Rx.*
Use: Antidepressant.

•**nortriptyline hydrochloride,** (nor-TRIP-tih-leen) U.S.P. 23.
Use: Antidepressant.
See: Aventyl HCl, Liq., Pulvule (Lilly). Pamelor, Cap., Liq. (Sandoz).

Norval. Docusate sodium.
Use: Laxative.

Norvasc. (Pfizer) Amlodipine **2.5 mg:** Bot. 100s; **5 mg:** Bot. 100s, UD 100s; **10 mg:** Bot. 100s, UD 100s. *Rx.*
Use: Calcium channel blocker.

Norvir. (Abbott) Ritonavir 100 mg. Soln.: 80 mg/ml ritonavir, saccharin. *Rx.*
Use: Antiviral.

Norwich Extra Strength. (Procter & Gamble) Aspirin 500 mg/Tab. Bot. 150s. *otc.*
Use: Salicylate, analgesic.

Norzine. (Purdue Frederick) **Tab.:** Thiethylperazine maleate 10 mg. Bot. 100s. **Supp.** Thiethylperazine maleate 10 mg. Pkg 12s. **Inj.:** Thiethylperazine maleate 5 mg/ml. 2 ml. *Rx.*
Use: Antiemetic, antivertigo.

Nosalt. (SK-Beecham) Potassium Cl, potassium bitartrate, adipic acid, mineral oil, fumaric acid. Sodium < 10 mg/5 g

(0.43 mEq/5 g), potassium 2502 mg/5 g (64 mEq/5 g). Pkg. 330 g. *otc.*

Nosalt Seasoned. (SK-Beecham) Potassium Cl, dextrose, onion and garlic, spices, lactose, cream of tartar, paprika, silica, disodium inosinate, disodium guanylate, turmeric. Sodium < 5 mg/5 g (0.2 mEq/5 g), potassium 1328 mg/5 g (34 mEq/5 g). Pkg. 240 g. *otc.*
Use: Salt substitute.

•**noscapine,** U.S.P. 23.
Use: Antitussive.

noscapine hydrochloride. l-Narcotine hydrochloride.
Use: Antitussive.
See: Conar Prods. (S-K Beecham).
W/Chlorpheniramine maleate, phenylephrine HCl, N-acetyl-p-aminophenol, salicylamide, vitamin C.
See: Noscaps, Cap. (Table Rock).
W/Phenylephrine HCl.
See: Conar Liq. (S-K Beecham).
W/Phenylephrine HCl, guaifensin.
See: Conar, Expectorant (S-K Beecham).

Noscaps. (Table Rock) Noscapine 7.5 mg, chlorpheniramine maleate 1 mg, phenylephrine HCl 5 mg, N-acetyl-p-aminophenol 150 mg, salicylamide 150 mg, vitamin C 20 mg/Cap. Bot. 100s, 500s. *otc.*
Use: Antihistamine, decongestant, analgesic, vitamin C.

Noskote. (Schering Plough) Oxybenzone 3%, homosalate 8%. SPF 8. Cream 13.2 g, 30 g. *otc.*
Use: Sunscreen.

Noskote Sunblock. (Schering Plough) Padimate O 8%, oxybenzone 3%, benzyl alcohol. SPF 15. Cream. Tube 30 g. *otc.*
Use: Sunscreen.

Nostril. (Boehringer Ingelheim) Phenylephrine HCl 0.25% or 0.5%, benzalkonium Cl 0.004% in buffered aqueous soln. Bot. 15 ml, pump spray. *otc.*
Use: Decongestant.

Nostrilla. (Boehringer Ingelheim) Oxymetazoline HCl 0.05%, benzalkonium Cl 0.02%. Bot. 15 ml, pump spray. *otc.*
Use: Decongestant.

Novacet. (Genderm) Sodium sulfacetamide 100 mg, sulfur 50 mg, benzyl alcohol, cetyl alcohol, sodium thiosulfate, EDTA. Lot. Bot. 30 ml. *Rx.*
Use: Antiacne.

Nova-Dec. (Rugby) Iron 18 mg, vitamins A 5000 IU, D 400 IU, E 30 IU, B_1 1.7 mg, B_2 2 mg, B_3 20 mg, B_5 10 mg, B_6 3 mg, B_{12} 6 mcg, C 60 mg, folic acid 0.4 mg, Ca, Cr, Cu, I, Mg, Mo, Mn, P, Se, K, Zn 15 mg, vitamin K, Cl, Ni, Sn, V, B, biotin 30 mcg/Tab. Bot. 130s. *otc.*
Use: Vitamin/mineral supplement.

Novadyne Expectorant. (Various Mfr.) Pseudoephedrine 30 mg, codeine phosphate 10 mg, guaifenesin 100 mg, alcohol 7.5%. Bot. 120 ml, pt, gal. *c-iii.*
Use: Decongestant, antitussive, expectorant.

Novagest Expectorant w/Codeine. (Major) Pseudoephedrine HCl 30 mg, codeine phosphate 10 mg, guaifenesin 100 mg/5 ml, alcohol 8.2%. Liq. Bot. 118 ml. *c-v.*
Use: Decongestant, antitussive, expectorant.

Novahistine DH. (SK-Beecham) Pseudoephedrine HCl 30 mg, codeine phosphate 10 mg, chlorpheniramine maleate 2 mg/5 ml, alcohol 5%, saccharin, sorbitol. Bot. 4 oz, pt. *c-v.*
Use: Decongestant, antitussive, antihistamine.

Novahistine DMX. (SK-Beecham) Pseudoephedrine HCl 30 mg, dextromethorphan HBr 10 mg, guaifenesin 100 mg/10 ml, alcohol 10%, saccharin, sorbitol, sugar. Bot. 4 oz. *otc.*
Use: Decongestant, antitussive, expectorant.

Novahistine Elixir. (SK-Beecham) Phenylephrine HCl 5 mg, chlorpheniramine maleate 2 mg/5 ml, alcohol 5%, sorbitol. Bot. 118 ml. *otc.*
Use: Decongestant, antihistamine.

Novahistine Expectorant. (SK-Beecham) Pseudoephedrine HCl 30 mg, codeine phosphate 10 mg, guaifenesin 100 mg/5 ml, alcohol 7.5%, saccharin, sorbitol. Bot. 4 oz, pt. *c-v.*
Use: Decongestant, antitussive, expectorant.

novamidon.
See: Aminopyrine (Various Mfr.).

Novamine. (Clintec Nutrition) Amino acid concentration 11.4%, for infusion. Nitrogen 1.8 g/100 ml. Essential amino acids (mg/100 ml): Isoleucine 570, leucine 790, lysine 900, methionine 570, phenylalanine 790, threonine 570, tryptophan 190, valine 730. Nonessential amino acids (mg/100 ml): Alanine 1650, arginine 1120, histidine 680, proline 680, serine 450, tyrosine 30, glycine 790, glutamic acid 570, aspartic acid 330, acetate 114 mEq/L, sodium metabisulfite 30 mg/100 ml. In 250 ml, 500 ml, 1 L. *Rx.*

Use: Parenteral nutritional supplement.

Novamine 15%. (Clintec Nutrition) Amino acids 15%: Lysine 1.18 g, leucine 1.04 g, phenylalanine 1.04 g, valine 960 mg, isoleucine 749 mg, methionine 749 mg, threonine 749 mg, tryptophan 250 mg, alanine 2.17 g, arginine 1.47 g, glycine 1.04 g, histidine 894 mg, proline 894 mg, glutamic acid 749 mg, serine 592 mg, aspartic acid 434 mg, tyrosine 39 mg, nitrogen 2.37 g/100 ml. Inj. 500 ml, 1000 ml. *Rx.*
Use: Parenteral nutritional supplement.

Novamine Without Electrolytes. (Clintec Nutrition) Amino acid concentration 8.5%, for infusion. Nitrogen 1.35 g/100 ml. Essential amino acids (mg/100 ml): Isoleucine 420, leucine 590, lysine 673, methionine 420, phenylalanine 590, threonine 420, tryptophan 140, valine 550. Nonessential amino acids (mg/100 ml): Alanine 1240, arginine 840, histidine 500, proline 500, serine 340, tyrosine 20, glycine 590, glutamic acid 420, aspartic acid 250, acetate 88 mEq/L, sodium bisulfite 30 mg/100 ml. In 500 ml, 1 L. *Rx.*
Use: Parenteral nutritional supplement.

Novantrone. (Immunex) Mitoxantrone HCl 2 mg base/ml. Inj. Vial 10 ml, 12.5 ml, 15 ml. *Rx.*
Use: Antineoplastic.

novatophan.
See: Neocinchophen (Various Mfr.).

novatropine.
See: Homatropine Methylbromide (Various Mfr.).

novobiocin calcium, U.S.P. XXII.
Use: Anti-infective.
See: Cathomycin Calcium.

novobiocin monosodium salt.
Use: Anti-infective.
See: Sodium Novobiocin.

•**novobiocin sodium,** U.S.P. 23.
Use: Antibacterial.
See: Albamycin, Cap. (Pharmacia & Upjohn).
Cathomycin Sodium.

Novocain. (Sanofi Winthrop) Procaine HCl. **1%:** 2 ml, 6 ml, 30 ml. **2%:** 30 ml. **10%:** 2 ml/Inj. *Rx.*
Use: Local anesthetic.

Novocain for Spinal Anesthesia. (Sanofi Winthrop) Procaine HCl 10% soln. Amp. 2 ml. Box 25s. *Rx.*
Use: Spinal anesthesia.

Novolin 70/30. (Novo Nordisk) Isophane susp. 70% (human), regular insulin 30% (human, semi-synthetic) 100 units/ml. Inj. Vial 10 ml. *otc.*
Use: Antidiabetic.

Novolin 70/30 Penfill. (Novo Nordisk) Isophane insulin suspension and insulin injection 100 U per ml human insulin. Cartridge 1.5 ml. *otc.*
Use: Antidiabetic.

Novolin L. (Novo Nordisk) Human insulin (semi-synthetic) 100 units/ml. An insulin-zinc suspension (Lente). Inj. Vial 10 ml. *otc.*
Use: Antidiabetic.

Novolin N. (Novo Nordisk) Human insulin NPH (semisynthetic) 100 units/ml. Isophane insulin suspension (insulin w/ protamine and zinc). Inj. Vial 10 ml. *otc.*
Use: Antidiabetic.

Novolin N Penfill. (Novo Nordisk) Isophane insulin suspension (NPH) 100 U per ml human insulin. Cartridge. 1.5 ml. *otc.*
Use: Antidiabetic.

Novolin R. (Novo Nordisk) Human insulin, regular (semisynthetic) 100 units/ml. Inj. Vial 10 ml. *otc.*
Use: Antidiabetic.

Novolin R Penfill. (Novo Nordisk) Semisynthetic human regular insulin 100 units/ml. Inj. 1.5 ml cartridges. *otc.*
Use: Antidiabetic.

Noxzema Antiseptic Cleanser Sensitive Skin Formula. (Noxell) Benzalkonium Cl 0.13%. Bot. 4 oz, 8 oz. *otc.*
Use: Skin cleanser.

Noxzema Antiseptic Skin Cleanser. (Noxell) SD-40 alcohol 63%. Bot. 4 oz, 8 oz. *otc.*
Use: Skin cleanser.

Noxzema Antiseptic Skin Cleanser Extra Strength Formula. (Noxell) SD-40 alcohol 36%, isopropyl alcohol 34%. Bot. 4 oz, 8 oz. *otc.*
Use: Skin cleanser.

Noxzema Clear-Ups. (Noxell) Salicylic acid 0.5% on pads. Jar 50s. *otc.*
Use: Antiacne.

Noxzema Clear Ups Acne Medicine Maximum Strength Lotion. (Noxell) Benzoyl peroxide 10%. Bot. 1 oz. Vanishing formula. *otc.*
Use: Antiacne.

Noxzema Clear Ups Maximum Strength. (Noxell) Salicylic acid 2% on pads. Jar 50s. *otc.*
Use: Antiacne.

Noxzema Medicated Skin Cream. (Noxell) Menthol, camphor, clove oil, eucalyptus oil, phenol. Jar 2.5 oz, 4 oz, 6 oz, 10 oz. Tube 4.5 oz. Bot. 6 oz., 14 oz.

Pump Bottle 10.5 oz. *otc.*
Use: Counterirritant.

Noxzema On-The-Spot. (Noxell) Benzoyl peroxide 10% in vanishing and tinted lotion. Bot. 0.25 oz. *otc.*
Use: Antiacne.

NP-27 Aerosol. (Thompson Medical) Tolnaftate 1%, alcohol 14.9%. Spray Can 100 ml. *otc.*
Use: Antifungal, topical.

NP-27 Cream. (Thompson Medical) Tolnaftate 1% in cream base. Tube 45 g. *otc.*
Use: Antifungal, topical.

NP-27 Liquid. (Thompson Medical) Tolnaftate 1%. Plastic bot. 2 oz. *otc.*
Use: Antifungal, topical.

NPH Iletin I. (Lilly) Insulin from beef and pork. 100 units/ml. Inj. Vial 10 ml. *otc.*
Use: Antidiabetic.

NPH Insulin. (Novo Nordisk) Isophane insulin suspension (NPH) 100 units per ml beef. Vial. 10 ml. *otc.*
Use: Antidiabetic.

NPH-N. (Novo Nordisk) Purified pork insulin 100 units/ml in isophane insulin suspension (insulin w/protamine and zinc). Inj. Vial 10 ml. *otc.*
Use: Antidiabetic.

NTBC.
Use: Tyrosinemia type 1. [Orphan drug]

n-trifluoroacetyladriamycin-14-valerate. (Anthra Pharm) *Rx.*
Use: Antineoplastic.

NTS Transdermal System. (Bolar) Nitroglycerin transdermal system 5 mg/24 hours or 15 mg/24 hours. Box 30s. *Rx.*
Use: Antianginal.

NTZ Long-Acting. (Sanofi Winthrop.) Oxymetazoline HCl 0.05%, benzalkonium Cl and phenylmercuric acetate 0.002% as preservatives. Drops. Bot. 1 oz. Spray Bot. 1 oz. *otc.*
Use: Decongestant.

Nubain. (DuPont Merck) Nalbuphine HCl, sodium metabisulfite 0.1%. **10 mg/ml:** Amp 1 ml. Vial 10 ml. Box 1s. **20 mg/ml:** Amp 1 ml. Syringe 1 ml calibrated. Vial 10 ml. *Rx.*
Use: Narcotic analgesic.

Nu-Bolic. (Seatrace) Nandrolone phenpropionate 25 mg/ml. Vial 5 ml. *c-iii.*
Use: Anabolic steroid.

nucite.
See: Inositol (Various Mfr.).

Nucofed. (Roberts) Codeine phosphate 20 mg, pseudoephedrine HCl 60 mg/5 ml or Cap. Syrup is alcohol-free. **Liq.:** Bot. pt. **Cap.:** Bot. 60s. *c-iii.*

Use: Antitussive, decongestant.

Nucofed Expectorant. (Roberts/Hauck) Codeine phosphate 20 mg, pseudoephedrine HCl 60 mg, guaifenesin 200 mg/5 ml, alcohol 12.5%, saccharin. Bot. 480 ml. *c-iii.*
Use: Antitussive, decongestant, expectorant.

Nucofed Pediatric Expectorant. (Roberts) Codeine phosphate 10 mg, pseudoephedrine HCl 30 mg, guaifenesin 100 mg/5 ml, alcohol 6%. Bot. pt. *c-v.*
Use: Antitussive, decongestant, expectorant.

Nucotuss Expectorant. (Barre-National) Pseudoephedrine HCl 60 mg, codeine phosphate 20 mg, guaifenesin 200 mg/5 ml, alcohol 12.5%, wintergreen flavor. Liq. Bot. 480 ml. *c-iii.*
Use: Decongestant, antitussive, expectorant.

Nucotuss Pediatric Expectorant. (Barre-National) Pseudoephedrine HCl 30 mg, codeine phosphate 10 mg, guaifenesin 100 mg/5 ml, strawberry flavor. Liq. Bot. 480 ml. *c-v.*
Use: Decongestant, antitussive, expectorant.

•**nufenoxole.** (NEW-fen-OX-ole) USAN.
Use: Antiperistaltic.

Nu-Iron. (Mayrand) Polysaccharide-iron complex. **Cap.:** Elemental iron 150 mg. Bot. 100s. **Elix.:** Elemental iron 100 mg/5 ml. Bot. 8 oz. *otc.*
Use: Iron supplement.

Nu-Iron 150. (Mayrand) Polysaccharide-Iron complex 100 mg/5 ml, alcohol 10%. Elix. 237 ml. *otc.*
Use: Iron supplement.

Nu-Iron Plus Elixir. (Mayrand) Polysaccharide iron complex 300 mg, folic acid 3 mg, vitamin B_{12} 75 mcg/15 ml. Bot. 237 ml. *Rx.*
Use: Vitamin/mineral supplement.

Nu-Iron-V. (Mayrand) Polysaccharide iron 60 mg, folic acid 1 mg, vitamins A 4000 IU, C 50 mg, D 400 IU, B_1 3 mg, B_2 3 mg, B_3 10 mg, B_6 2 mg, B_{12} 3 mcg, Ca/Tab. Bot. 100s. *Rx.*
Use: Vitamin/mineral supplement.

Nul-Tach. (Davis & Sly) Potassium 16 mg, magnesium 13 mg, ascorbic acid 250 mg/Tab. Bot. 100s. *Rx.*
Use: Paroxysmal tachycardia.

Nulytely. (Braintree) PEG 3350 420 g, sodium bicarbonate 5.72 g, sodium chloride 11.2 g, potassium chloride 1.48 g. Pow. Jugs. 4 L. *Rx.*
Use: Laxative.

Numorphan. (DuPont Merck) Oxymorphone HCl. **1 mg/ml.:** Amp. 1 ml. Box 10s. **1.5 mg/ml.:** Amp. 1 ml, Box 10s. Vial 10 ml, Box 1s. **Rectal Supp.:** 5 mg. Box 6s. *c-II.*
Use: Narcotic analgesic.

Numotizine Cataplasm. (Hobart) Guaiacol 0.26 g, beechwood creosote 1.302 g, methyl salicylate 0.26 g/100 g. Jar 4 oz. *otc.*
Use: Analgesic, topical.

Numotizine Cough Syrup. (Hobart) Guaifenesin 5 g, ammonium Cl 5 g, sodium citrate 20 g, menthol 0.04 g/fl oz. Bot. 3 oz, pt, gal. *otc.*
Use: Expectorant.

Numzident. (Purepac) Benzocaine 10%, PEG-400 NF 47.86%, PEG-3350 NF 10%, saccharin. Gel. 15 g. *otc.*
Use: Local anesthetic, dental.

Num-Zit. (Purepac) Benzocaine, menthol, glycerin, methylparaben, alcohol 12%. Liq. Bot. 22.5 ml. *otc.*
Use: Local anesthetic, dental.

Num-Zit Gel. (Purepac) Benzocaine, menthol. Tube 10 g. *otc.*
Use: Local anesthetic, dental.

Numzit Teething Gel. (Goody's) Benzocaine 7.5%, peppermint oil 0.018%, clove leaf oil 0.09%, PEG-400 66.2%, PEG-3350 26.1%, saccharin 0.036%. Tube. 14.1 g. *otc.*
Use: Local anesthetic, oral.

Numzit Teething Lotion. (Goody's) Benzocaine 0.2%, alcohol 12.1%, saccharin 0.02%, glycerin 2%, kelgin MU 0.5%, methylparaben. Lot. Bot. 15 ml. *otc.*
Use: Local anesthetic, oral.

nunol.
See: Phenobarbital (Various Mfr.).

Nupercainal. (Novartis) **Oint.:** Dibucaine 1%, acetone, sodium bisulfite, lanolin, mineral oil, white petrolatum. 30 g, 60 g. **Cream:** Dibucaine 0.5%, acetone, sodium bisulfite, glycerin. 42.5 g. **Supp.:** Cocoa butter, zinc oxide, sodium bisulfite. 12s, 24s. *otc.*
Use: Local anesthetic, topical (Oint., Cream); Anorectal preparation (Supp.).

Nuprin Caplets. (Bristol-Myers) Ibuprofen 200 mg/Capl. Bot. 24s, 50s, 100s. *otc.*
Use: Nonsteroidal anti-inflammatory, analgesic.

Nuprin Tablets. (Bristol-Myers) Ibuprofen 200 mg/Tab. Blister Pak 8s. Bot. 24s, 50s, 100s. *otc.*

Use: Nonsteroidal anti-inflammatory, analgesic.

Nuquin HP. (Stratus) **Cream:** 4% hydroquinone, 30 mg dioxybenzone, 20 mg oxybenzone per g. Vanishing base. Stearyl alcohol, EDTA, sodium metabisulfite. Tube 14.2 g, 28.4 g, 56.7 g. **Gel:** 4% hydroquinone, 30 mg dioxybenzone per g. Alcohol, sodium metabisulfite, EDTA. Tube 14.2 g, 28.4 g. *Rx.*
Use: Skin bleaching agent.

Nuromax. (Glaxo Wellcome) Doxacurium chloride 1 mg/ml. Inj. Vial 5 ml. *Rx.*
Use: Neuromuscular blocking agent.

Nu-Salt. (Cumberland Pkg.) Potassium Cl, potassium bitartrate, calcium silicate, natural flavor derived from yeast. Sodium 0.85 mg/5 g (< 0.04 mEq/5 g), potassium 2640 mg/5 g (68 mEq/5 g). Pkg. 90 g. *otc.*
Use: Salt substitute.

Nu-Tears. (Optopics) Polyvinyl alcohol 1.4%, EDTA, NaCl, benzalkonium chloride, potassium chloride. Soln. Bot. 15 ml. *otc.*
Use: Artificial tears.

Nu-Tears II. (Optopics) Polyvinyl alcohol 1%, PEG-400 1%, EDTA, benzalkonium chloride. Soln. Bot. 15 ml. *otc.*
Use: Artificial tears.

Nu-Thera. (Kirkman Sales) Vitamins A 10,000 IU, D 400 IU, B_1 10 mg, B_2 5 mg, niacinamide 100 mg, B_6 1 mg, B_{12} 5 mcg, C 150 mg, calcium 103 mg, phosphorus 80 mg, iron 10 mg, magnesium 5.5 mg, manganese 1 mg, potassium 5 mg, zinc 1.4 mg/Cap. Bot. 100s. *otc.*
Use: Vitamin/mineral supplement.

nutmeg oil.
Use: Pharmaceutic aid (flavor).

Nutracort. (Galderma) Hydrocortisone 1%. **Cream:** Jar 4 oz. Tube 30 g, 60 g. *Rx.*
Use: Corticosteroid, topical.

Nutraderm. (Galderma) Oil-in-water emulsion. **Lot.:** Plastic bot. 8 oz, 16 oz. **Cream:** Tube 1.5 oz, 3 oz, Jar lb. *otc.*
Use: Emollient.

Nutraderm Bath Oil. (Galderma) Mineral oil, PEG-4 dilaurate, lanolin oil, butylparaben, benzophenone-3, fragrance, D & C Green No. 6. Bot. 8 oz. *otc.*
Use: Emollient.

Nutraloric. (Nutraloric) A chocolate, vanilla or strawberry flavored liquid containing, when mixed with whole milk to make 1 L, 91.7 g protein, 175 g car-

bohydrates, 125 g fat, 875 mg sodium, 3166.7 mg potassium, 2.2 calories/ml. Pow. Can 480 g. *otc.*
Use: Nutritional supplement.

Nutrament Drink Box. (Drackett) Protein 10 g, fat 7 g, carbohydrate 35 g, vitamins, minerals/240 calories/8 oz. Drink Box. *otc.*
Use: Nutritional supplement.

Nutrament Liquid. (Drackett) Protein 16 g, fat 10 g, carbohydrates 52 g, vitamins, minerals/360 calories/12 oz. Can. *otc.*
Use: Nutritional supplement.

Nutramigen. (Bristol-Myers) Hypoallergenic formula that supplies 640 calories/qt. Protein 18 g, fat 25 g, carbohydrates 86 g, vitamins A 2000 IU, D 400 IU, E 20 IU, C 52 mg, folic acid 100 mcg, B_1 0.5 mg, B_2 0.6 mg, niacin 8 mg, B_6 0.4 mg, B_{12} 2 mcg, biotin 50 mcg, pantothenic acid 3 mg, K-1 100 mcg, choline 85 mg, inositol 30 mg, calcium 600 mg, phosphorus 400 mg, iodine 45 mcg, iron 12 mg, magnesium 70 mg, copper 0.6 mg, zinc 5 mg, manganese 200 mg, chloride 550 mg, potassium 700 mg, sodium 300 mg/qt of formula (4.9 oz pow.). Can 16 oz, 390 ml concentrate and 1 qt ready-to-use. *otc.*
Use: Nutritional supplement.

Nutramin. (Thurston) Vitamins A 666 IU, D 66 IU, B_1 666 mcg, B_2 333 mcg, niacinamide 2 mg, folic acid 0.0444 mcg, calcium 16.6 mg, phosphorus 8.33 mg, iron 1.33 mg, iodine 0.15 mg/Tab. Bot. 200s, 500s, 1000s. *otc.*
Use: Vitamin/mineral supplement.

Nutramin Granular. (Thurston) Vitamins A 333 IU, D 333 IU, B_1 3.3 mg, B_2 1.6 mg, niacinamide 10 mg, folic acid 0.133 mg, calcium 250 mg, phosphorus 115 mg, iron 6.6 mg, iodine 0.15 mg/5 g. Bot. 10 oz, 32 oz. *otc.*
Use: Vitamin/mineral supplement.

Nutraplus. (Galderma) Urea 10% in emollient cream base or lotion base with preservatives. **Cream:** Tube 3 oz, Jar lb. **Lot.:** Bot. 8 oz, 16 oz. *otc.*
Use: Emollient.

Nutra-Soothe. (Pertussin) Colloidal oatmeal and light mineral oil. Emollient bath preparation. Pow. Pkts. 9s. *otc.*
Use: Bath dermatologic.

Nutravims. (Approved) Vitamins A 6000 IU, D 1250 IU, C 50 mg, E 5 IU, B_{12} 5 mcg, B_1 3 mg, B_2 3 mg, B_6 0.5 mg, niacinamide 20 mg, calcium pantothenate 5 mg, zinc 1.5 mg, manganese 1 mg, iodine 0.15 mg, potassium 5 mg, mag-

nesium 4 mg, iron 15 mg, calcium 59 mg, phosphorus 45 mg/Cap. Bot. 100s, 250s, 1000s. *otc.*
Use: Vitamin/mineral supplement.

Nutren 1.0 Liquid. (Clintec Nutrition) Potassium and sodium caseinate, maltodextrin, sucrose, MCT, corn oil, lecithin, vitamins A, B_1, B_2, B_3, B_5, B_6, B_{12}, C, D, E, K, folic acid, biotin, choline, Ca, Cl, Cu, Fe, I, Mg, Mn, P, Zn. 250 ml. *otc.*
Use: Nutritional supplement.

Nutren 1.5 Liquid. (Clintec Nutrition) Casein, maltodextrin, corn syrup, sucrose, MCT, corn oil, vitamins A, B_1, B_2, B_3, B_5, B_6, B_{12}, C, D, E, K, folic acid, biotin, choline, Ca, Cl, Cu, Fe, I, Mg, Mn, P, Zn. 250 ml. *otc.*
Use: Nutritional supplement.

Nutren 2.0 Liquid. (Clintec Nutrition) Casein, maltodextrin, corn syrup, sucrose, MCT, corn oil, vitamins A, B_1, B_2, B_3, B_5, B_6, B_{12}, C, D, E, K, folic acid, biotin, choline, Ca, Cl, Cu, Fe, I, Mg, Mn, P, Zn. 250 ml. *otc.*
Use: Nutritional supplement.

Nutrex. (Holloway) Calcium 162 mg, iron 27 mg, vitamins A 5000 IU, D 400 IU, E 30 mg, B_1 2.25 mg, B_2 2.6 mg, B_3 20 mg, B_5 10 mg, B_6 3 mg, B_{12} 9 mcg, C 90 mg, folic acid 0.4 mg, Cu, I, K, Mg, Mn, P, zinc 22.5 mg, biotin 45 mcg/Tab. Bot. 100s. *otc.*
Use: Vitamin/mineral supplement.

Nutricon Tablets. (Pasadena) Calcium 200 mg, iron 20 mg, vitamins A 2500 IU, D 200 IU, E 15 mg, B_1 1.5 mg, B_2 1.5 mg, B_3 10 mg, B_5 5 mg, B_6 2 mg, B_{12} 5 mcg, C 50 mg, folic acid 0.4 mg, Cu, I, Mg, zinc 3.75 mg, biotin 150 mcg/Tab. Bot. 120s. *otc.*
Use: Vitamin/mineral supplement.

Nutri-E. (Nutri Lab.) Vitamin E. **Cream:** 200 IU/g. Jar 1 oz, 2 oz. **Oil:** 1 oz. **Oint.:** 200 IU/g. Tube 1 oz, 1.5 oz. **Cap.:** 200 IU. Bot. 80s; 400 IU. Bot. 60s, 100s; 800 IU. Bot. 55s. *otc.*
Use: Vitamin E supplement.

Nutrilan. (Elan) A vanilla, chocolate or strawberry flavored liquid containing 38 g protein, 37 g fat, 143 g carbohydrates, 632.5 mg Na, 1.073 g K/L. With appropriate vitamins and minerals. In 237 ml Tetra Pak containers. *otc.*
Use: Nutritional supplement.

Nutrilipid. (McGaw) Soybean oil intravenous fat emulsion. **10%:** Calories 1.1/ml. In 250 ml, 500 ml. **20%:** Calories 2/ml. In 250 ml, 500 ml. *Rx.*
Use: Parenteral nutritional supplement.

Nutrilyte. (American Regent) Acetate 2.03 mEq, potassium 2.03 mEq, chloride 1.68 mEq, sodium 1.25 mEq, magnesium 0.4 mEq, calcium 0.25 mEq, gluconate 0.25 mEq per ml, ≈ 6212 mOsml/L. Concentrated soln. Bot. 20 ml, 100 ml. *Rx.*
Use: Parenteral nutritional supplement.

Nutrilyte II. (American Regent) Acetate 1.475 mEq, potassium 1 mEq, chloride 1.75 mEq, sodium 1.75 mEq, magnesium 0.25 mEq, calcium 0.225 mEq per ml, ≈ 6212 mOsml/L. Concentrated soln. Bot. 20 ml, 100 ml. *Rx.*
Use: Parenteral nutritional supplement.

Nutri-Plex Tablets. (Faraday) Vitamins B_1 5 mg, B_2 5 mg, B_6 5 mg, pantothenic acid 25 mg, B_{12} 12.5 mcg, niacinamide 50 mg, iron gluconate 30 mg, choline bitartrate 50 mg, inositol 50 mg, PABA 15 mg, C 150 mg/2 Tab. Bot. 100s, 250s. *otc.*
Use: Vitamin/mineral supplement.

Nutrisource Modular System. (Sandoz Nutrition) Individual Nutrisource modules available: protein, amino acids, amino acids-high branched chain, carbohydrate, lipid-medium chain triglycerides, lipid-long branched chain triglycerides, vitamins, minerals. Cans of liquid. Packets of powder. *otc.*
Use: Nutritional supplement.

Nutri-Val. (Marcen) Vitamins A 5000 IU, D 500 IU, B_1 10 mg, B_2 5 mg, B_{12} activity 5 mcg, B_6 5 mcg, C 50 mg, hesperidin 5 mg, niacinamide 15 mg, folic acid 0.2 mg, calcium pantothenate 50 mg, choline bitartrate 50 mg, betaine HCl 25 mg, lipo-K 0.4 mg, duodenum substance 50 mg, pancreas substance 50 mg, inositol 25 mg, Cy-yeast hydrolysates 50 mg, rutin 5 mg, 1-lysine HCl 5 mg, E 5 IU, Ossonate (glucuronic complex) 8 mg, glutamic acid 30 mg, lecithin 5 mg, iron 20 mg, iodine 0.15 mg, calcium 50 mg, phosphorus 40 mg, boron 0.1 mg, copper 1 mg, manganese 1 mg, magnesium 1 mg, potassium 5 mg, zinc 0.5 mg, biotin 0.02 mg/ Cap. Bot. 100s, 500s, 1000s. *otc.*
Use: Vitamin/mineral supplement.

Nutri-Vite Natural Multiple Vitamin and Minerals. (Faraday) Vitamins A 15,000 IU, D 400 IU, B_1 1.5 mg, B_2 3 mg, B_{12} 15 mcg, niacin 500 mcg, B_6 20 mcg, choline 1.75 mg, folic acid 13 mcg, pantothenic acid 50 mcg, p-aminobenzoic acid 12 mcg, inositol 1.72 mg, C 60 mg, citrus bioflavonoids 15 mg, E 50 IU, iron gluconate 15 mg, calcium 192 mg, phosphorus 85 mg, iodine 0.15 mg, red bone marrow 30 mg/3 Tab. Protein coated Tab. Bot. 100s, 250s. *otc.*
Use: Vitamin/mineral supplement.

Nutrizyme. (Enzyme Process) Vitamins A 5000 IU, D 400 IU, C 60 mg, B_1 1.5 mg, B_2 1.7 mg, niacinamide 20 mg, B_6 2 mg, pantothenate 10 mg, B_{12} 6 mcg, E 30 IU, iron 10 mg, copper 1 mg, zinc 1 mg, Folacin 0.025 mg/Tab. Bot. 90s, 250s. *otc.*
Use: Vitamin/mineral supplement.

Nutropin. (Genentech) Somatropin 5 mg (≈ 13 IU)/vial, 10 mg (≈ 26 IU)/vial. Pow. for inj. (lyophilized). Vials with 10 ml diluent. *Rx.*
Use: Growth hormone.

Nutropin AQ. (Genentech) Somatropin 10 mg/Inj. Vial 2 ml. *Rx.*
Use: Growth hormone.

Nutrox Capsules. (Tyson) Vitamins A 10,000 IU, E 150 IU, B_1 25 mg, B_2 25 mg, B_3 50 mg, B_5 22 mg, C 80 mg, L-cysteine, taurine, glutathione, zinc oxide 15 mg, Se/Cap. Bot. 90s. *otc.*
Use: Vitamin/mineral supplement.

Nuzine Ointment. (Hobart) Guaiacol 1.66 g, oxyquinoline sulfate 0.42 g, zinc oxide 2.5 g, glycerine 1.66 g, lanum (anhydrous) 43.76 g, petrolatum 50 g/ 100 g. Tube 1 oz. *otc.*
Use: Anorectal preparation.

Nycoff. (Dover) Dextromethorphan HBr/ Tab. UD Box 500s. Sugar, lactose and salt free. *otc.*
Use: Antitussive.

Nyco-White. (Whiteworth Towne) Nystatin, neomycin, gramcidin, triamcinolone. Cream. Tube 15 g, 30 g, 60 g. *Rx.*
Use: Anti-infective, topical.

Nyco-Worth. (Whiteworth Towne) Nystatin. Cream Tube 15 g. *Rx.*
Use: Antifungal, topical.

Nydrazid Injection. (Apothecon) Isoniazid 100 mg/ml, chlorobutanol 0.25%, sodium hydroxide or hydrochloric acid to adjust pH. Vial 10 ml. *Rx.*
Use: Antituberculous agent.

●**nylestriol.** (NYE-less-TRY-ole) USAN.
Use: Estrogen.

NyQuil Cough/Cold, Children's. (Procter & Gamble) Pseudoephedrine HCl 10 mg, chlorpheniramine maleate 0.67 mg, dextromethorphan HBr 5 mg/5 ml, sucrose, alcohol free, cherry flavor. Liq. 120 ml. *otc.*
Use: Decongestant, antihistamine, antitussive.

NyQuil Hot Therapy. (Procter & Gamble) Pseudoephedrine HCl 60 mg, doxylamine succinate 12.5 mg, dextromethorphan HBr 30 mg, acetaminophen 1000 mg. Powd. 6s. *otc.*
Use: Decongestant, antihistamine, antitussive, analgesic.

NyQuil Liquicaps. (Procter & Gamble) Pseudoephedrine HCl 30 mg, diphenhydramine HCl 25 mg, dextromethorphan HBr 15 mg, acetaminophen 250 mg/Cap. Bot. 20s. *otc.*
Use: Decongestant, antihistamine, analgesic, antitussive.

NyQuil Nighttime Cold/Flu Medicine. (Procter & Gamble) Pseudoephedrine HCl 10 mg, doxylamine succinate 2.1 mg, dextromethorphan HBr 5 mg, acetaminophen 167 mg/5 ml, alcohol 10%, sucrose, saccharin (cherry flavor), tartrazine (regular flavor). Liq. Bot. 295 ml. *otc.*
Use: Decongestant, antihistamine, antitussive, analgesic.

NyQuil Night Time Cold Medicine Liquid. (Procter & Gamble) Dextromethorphan HBr 30 mg, pseudoephedrine HCl 60 mg, doxylamine succinate 7.5 mg, acetaminophen 1000 mg/oz, alcohol 25%. Regular and cherry flavors. Regular flavor contains FDC Yellow #5 tartrazine. Bot. 6 oz, 10 oz, 14 oz. *otc.*
Use: Antitussive, decongestant, antihistamine, analgesic.

NyQuil Nighttime Head Cold Allergy Formula, Children's. (Procter & Gamble) Pseudoephedrine HCl, chlorpheniramine maleate per 5 ml, 0.67 mg, alcohol free, sorbitol, sucrose, grape flavor. Liq. Bot. 120 ml. *otc.*
Use: Decongestant, antihistamine.

Nyral. (Pal-Pak) Cetylpyridinium Cl 0.5 mg, benzocaine 5 mg/Loz. w/parabens. Pkg. 100s, 1000s. *otc.*
Use: Antiseptic.

• **nystatin,** (nye-STAT-in) U.S.P. 23. An antifungal antibiotic derived from cultures of *Streptomyces noursei.*
Use: Antifungal.
See: Mycostatin Preps. (Apothecon).
Nilstat, Tab., Cream, Oint., Pow. (Lederle).
Nilstat, Oral Drops (Lederle).
Nilstat, Vaginal Tab. (Lederle).
Nystatin, Bulk Pow. (Paddock).
Nystex, Cream, Oint., Susp. (Savage).

O-V Statin, Tab. (Squibb Mark).
W/Clioquinol.
See: Nystaform, Oint. (Bayer).
W/Demethylchlortetracycline.
See: Declostatin, Tab., Cap. (Lederle).
W/Gramicidin, neomycin, triamcinolone.
See: Mycolog, Cream, Oint. (Squibb).
W/Tetracycline phosphate buffered.
See: Achrostatin-V, Cap. (Lederle).
W/Tetracycline phosphate complex.
See: Tetrex-F, Cap. (Bristol).

nystatin. (Various Mfr.) 100,000 units/ml.
Oral Susp. Bot. 5 ml, 60 ml, 480 ml.
Vaginal Tab. Pkg. 15s or 30s.
Use: Antifungal.

nystatin and triamcinolone acetonide cream.
Use: Antifungal, corticosteroid, topical.

nystatin and triamcinolone acetonide ointment.
Use: Antifungal, corticosteroid, topical.

nystatin, neomycin sulfate, gramicidin and triamcinolone acetonide.
Use: Antifungal, antibacterial, corticosteroid, topical.
See: Mycolog, Prods. (Squibb).

Nystex Cream & Ointment. (Savage) Nystatin 100,000 units/g. Tube 15 g, 30 g. *Rx.*
Use: Antifungal, topical.

Nystex Oral Suspension. (Savage) Nystatin 100,000 units/ml in suspension. Bot. 60 ml. *Rx.*
Use: Antifungal, topical.

Nytcold Medicine. (Rugby) Pseudoephedrine HCl 10 mg, doxylamine succinate 1.25 mg, dextromethorphan HBr 5 mg, acetaminophen 167 mg, alcohol 25%, glucose, saccharin, sucrose, cherry flavor. Liq. Bot. 177 ml. *otc.*
Use: Decongestant, antihistamine, antitussive, analgesic.

Nytime Cold Medicine. (Rugby) Acetaminophen 1000 mg, doxylamine succinate 7.5 mg, pseudoephedrine HCl 60 mg, dextromethorphan HBr 30 mg/30 ml, alcohol 25%. Bot. 6 oz, 10 oz. *otc.*
Use: Analgesic, antihistamine, decongestant, antitussive.

Nytol. (Block) Diphenhydramine HCl 25 mg/Tab. Bot. 16s, 32s, 72s. *otc.*
Use: Nonprescription sleep aid.

Nytol, Maximum Strength. (Block) Diphenhydramine HCl 50 mg, lactose. Tab. Bot. 8s. *otc.*
Use: Nonprescription sleep aid.

O

O.A.D. (Sween) Ostomy deodorant. Bot. 1.25 oz, 4 oz, 8 oz. *otc.*
Use: Ostomy appliance deodorant.

Oasis. (Zitar) Artificial saliva. Bot. 6 oz. *otc.*
Use: To relieve xerostomia.

•**oatmeal, colloidal,** U.S.P. 23.
Use: Antipruritic (topical).

oatmeal, gum fraction.
See: Aveeno, Preps. (Rydelle).

Obe-Nix. (Holloway) Phentermine HCl 30 mg/Cap. (equivalent to 24 mg base) Bot. 100s. *c-iv.*
Use: Anorexiant.

Obepar. (Tyler) Vitamins A 3000 IU, D 300 IU, B$_1$ 3 mg, B$_2$ 2 mg, nicotinamide 10 mg, B$_6$ 3 mg, calcium pantothenate 2 mg, B$_{12}$ 3 mcg, C 37.5 mg, calcium 150 mg, iron 5 mg, magnesium 1 mg, manganese 0.1 mg, potassium 1 mg, zinc 0.15 mg/Cap. Bot. 100s. *otc.*
Use: Vitamin/mineral supplement.

Obephen. (Roberts) Phentermine HCl 30 mg (equivalent to 24 mg base) Cap. Bot. 1000s. *c-iv.*
Use: Anorexiant.

Obe-Tite. (Scott/Cord) Phendimetrazine tartrate 35 mg/Tab. Bot. 100s, 500s. *c-iii.*
Use: Anorexiant.

Obezine. (Western Research) Phendimetrazine tartrate 35 mg/Tab. Handicount 28 (36 bags of 28s). *c-iii.*
Use: Anorexiant.

•**obidoxime chloride.** (OH-bih-DOX-eem) USAN.
Use: Cholinesterase reactivator.

Obrical. (Canright) Calcium lactate 500 mg, vitamins D 400 IU, ferrous sulfate exsiccated 35 mg, B$_1$ 1 mg, B$_2$ 1 mg, C 10 mg/Tab. Bot. 100s, 1000s. *otc.*
Use: Vitamin/mineral supplement.

Obrical-F. (Canright) Ferrous sulfate 50 mg, calcium lactate 500 mg, vitamins D 400 IU, B$_1$ 1 mg, B$_2$ 1 mg, C 10 mg, folic acid 0.67 mg/Tab. Bot. 100s, 1000s. *otc.*
Use: Vitamin/mineral supplement.

Obrite. (Milton Roy) Contact lens and eye glass cleaner. Plastic spray Bot. 30 ml, 55 ml. *otc.*
Use: Contact lens and eye glass care.

OB-Tinic. (Roberts) Iron 65 mg, vitamins A 6000 IU, D 400 IU, E 30 IU, B$_1$ 1.1 mg, B$_2$ 1.8 mg, B$_3$ 15 mg, B$_6$ 2.5 mg, B$_{12}$ 5 mcg, C 60 mg, folic acid 1 mg, Ca/Tab. Bot. 100s. *Rx.*

Use: Vitamin/mineral supplement.

OBY-CAP. (Richwood) Phentermine HCl 30 mg/Cap. Bot. 100s, 500s. *c-iv.*
Use: Anorexiant.

Oby-Trim. (Rexar) Phentermine HCl 30 mg/Cap. Bot. 1000s. *c-iv.*
Use: Anorexiant.

O-Cal F.A. (Pharmics) **Tab.**: Ca 200 mg, iron 66 mg, vitamins A 5000 IU, D 400 IU, E 30 mg, B$_1$ 3 mg, B$_2$ 3 mg, B$_3$ 20 mg, B$_6$ 4 mg, B$_{12}$ 12 mcg, C 90 mg, folic acid 1 mg, fluoride 1.1 mg, Mg, I, Cu, Zn 15 mg. Bot. 100s. *Rx.*
Use: Vitamin/mineral supplement.

•**ocaperidone.** (oke-ah-PURR-ih-dohn) USAN.
Use: Antipsychotic.

Occlusal-HP. (Genderm) Salicylic acid 17%. Bot. 10 ml. *otc.*
Use: Keratolytic.

Occucoat. (Storz) Hydroxypropyl methylcellulose 2%. Soln. Syringe 1 ml with cannula. *Rx.*
Use: Ophthalmic preparation.

Ocean. (Fleming) Sodium Cl 0.65%, benzyl alcohol. Bot. 45 ml, pt. *otc.*
Use: Nasal membrane moisturizer.

Ocean Plus. (Fleming) Caffeine 2.5%, benzyl alcohol. Bot. 15 ml. *otc.*

•**ocfentanil hydrochloride.** (ock-FEN-tah-NILL) USAN.
Use: Analgesic (narcotic).

•**ocinaplon.** (oh-SIN-ah-plahn) USAN.
Use: Antianxiety.

OCL Solution. (Abbott Hospital Prods) Oral colonic lavage soln. Sodium Cl 146 mg, sodium bicarbonate 168 mg, sodium sulfate decahydrate 1.29 g, potassium Cl 75 mg, PEG-3350 6 g, polysorbate-80 30 ml/100 ml. 1.35 L 3-pack units. *Rx.*
Use: Laxative.

•**ocrylate.** (AH-krih-late) USAN.
Use: Surgical aid (tissue adhesive).

•**octabenzone.** (OCK-tah-BEN-zone) USAN.
Use: Ultraviolet screen.

octadecanoic acid.
See: Stearic Acid, N.F. 18.

octadecanoic acid, sodium salt.
See: Sodium Stearate, N.F. 18.

octadecanoic acid, zinc salt.
See: Zinc Stearate, N.F. 18.

octadecanol-l.
See: Stearyl Alcohol, N.F. 18.

Octamide. (Pharmacia & Upjohn) Metoclopramide 10 mg/Tab. Bot. 100s, 500s. *Rx.*
Use: GI stimulant, antiemetic.

Octamide PFS. (Pharmacia & Upjohn) Metoclopramide HCl 5 mg/ml, preservative free. Vial. Single dose; 2, 10, 30 ml. *Rx.*
Use: GI stimulant, antiemetic.

●**octanoic acid.** (OCK-tah-NO-ik) USAN.
Use: Antifungal.

octapeptide sequence.
Use: Antiviral.
See: Flumadine (Roche).

Octarex. (Approved) Vitamins A 5000 IU, D 1000 IU, B_1 1.5 mg, B_2 2 mg, B_6 0.1 mg, calcium pantothenate 1 mg, niacinamide 20 mg, C 37.5 mg, E 1 IU, B_{12} 1 mcg/Cap. Bot. 100s, 1000s. *otc.*
Use: Vitamin/mineral supplement.

Octavims. (Approved) Vitamins A 6000 IU, D 1250 IU, C 50 mg, E 5 IU, B_1 3 mg, B_2 3 mg, B_6 0.5 mg, niacinamide 20 mg, calcium pantothenate 5 mg, B_{12} 5 mcg, calcium 59 mg, phosphorus 45 mg/Cap. Bot. 100s, 250s, 1000s. *otc.*
Use: Vitamin/mineral supplement.

●**octazamide.** (OCK-TAY-zah-mide) USAN.
Use: Analgesic.

●**octenidine hydrochloride.** (OCK-TEN-ih-deen) USAN.
Use: Anti-infective (topical).

●**octenidine saccharin.** (OCK-TEN-ih-deen SACK-ah-rin) USAN.
Use: Dental plaque inhibitor.

●**octicizer.** (OCK-tih-SIGH-zer) USAN. Santicizer 141
Use: Pharmaceutic aid (plasticizer).

Octocaine HCl. (Novocol) Lidocaine HCl 2%, epinephrine 1:50,000 or 1:100,000. Inj. Dent. Cartridge 1.8 ml. *Rx.*
Use: Local anesthetic.

●**octocrylene.** (OCK-toe-KRIH-leen) USAN.
Use: Ultraviolet screen.

●**octodrine.** (OCK-toe-DREEN) USAN. Under study.
Use: Adrenergic (vasoconstrictor), local anesthetic.

octofollin.
See: Benzestrol, U.S.P. 23.

●**octoxynol 9,** (ock-TOXE-ih-nahl 9) N.F. 18.
Use: Pharmaceutic aid (surfactant).

OctreoScan. (Mallinckrodt) Oxidronate sodium 2 mg, stannous chloride (anhydrous) 0.16 mg, gentisic acid 0.56 mg, sodium chloride 30 mg/vial. Powd. lyophilized. In kits containing 5 ml or 30 ml vials and additive-free sodium pertechnate Tc-99m (for reconstitution). *Rx.*

Use: Diagnostic aid, radiopaque agent.

●**octreotide.** (ock-TREE-oh-tide) USAN.
Use: Antisecretory (gastric).

●**octreotide acetate.** (ock-TREE-oh-tide) USAN.
Use: Antidiarrheal, gastrointestinal tumor; antihypotensive, carcinoid crisis; growth hormone suppressant, acromegaly, antisecretory (gastric).

●**octriptyline phosphate.** (ock-TRIP-tih-leen FOSS-fate) USAN.
Use: Antidepressant.

●**octrizole.** (OCK-TRY-zole) USAN.
Use: Ultraviolet screen.

n-octyl bicyalohephene dicarbosimide.
See: Bansum, Bot. (Summers).

●**octyldodecanol,** N.F. 18.
Use: Pharmaceutic aid (oleaginous vehicle).

octylphenoxy polyethoxyethanol. A mono-ether of a polyethylene glycol. Igepal CA 630 (Antara).
W/Phenylmercuric acetate, methylparaben, sodium borate.
See: Lorophyn jelly, Supp. (Eaton).
W/Lactic acid, sodium lactate.
See: Jeneen premeasured liquid douche (Procter & Gamble).

OcuClear. (Schering-Plough) Oxymetazoline HCl 0.025%. Bot. 30 ml. *otc.*
Use: Vasoconstrictor, mydriatic (ophthalmic).

OcuClenz. (Storz) Disodium oleamido PEG-2 sulfosuccinate, cocoamphodiacetate, poloxamer 185, poloxamer 188, parabens, citric acid, EDTA. Soln. Bot. 120 ml and combo pack (120 ml and 50 pads). *otc.*
Use: Ophthalmic cleansing solution.

OcuCoat. (Storz) Hydroxypropyl methylcellulose 2%. Soln. Syringe 1 ml. *Rx.*
Use: Ophthalmic lubricant.

OcuCoat PF. (Storz Ophthalmics) Dextran 70 0.1%, hydroxypropyl methylcellulose, NaCl, KCl, dextrose, sodium phosphate. Preservative free. Drops. In 0.5 ml single-dose containers. *otc.*
Use: Ophthalmic lubricant.

Ocufen. (Allergan) Flurbiprofen sodium 0.03%. Bot. 2.5 ml, 5 ml, 10 ml w/dropper. *Rx.*
Use: Nonsteroidal anti-inflammatory, ophthalmic.

●**ocufilcon A.** (OCK-you-FILL-kahn A) USAN.
Use: Contact lens material (hydrophilic).

●**ocufilcon B.** (OCK-you-FILL-kahn B) USAN.
Use: Contact lens material (hydrophilic).

•**ocufilcon C.** (OCK-you-FILL-kahn C) USAN.
Use: Contact lens material (hydrophilic).

•**ocufilcon D.** (OCK-you-FILL-kahn D) USAN.
Use: Contact lens material (hydrophilic).

•**ocufilcon E.** (OCK-you-FILL-kahn E) USAN.
Use: Contact lens material (hydrophilic).

Ocuflox. (Allergan) Ofloxacin 3 mg/ml. Soln. Bot. 1 ml, 5 ml. *Rx.*
Use: Anti-infective, ophthalmic.

ocular lubricants.
Use: Ophthalmic.
See: Akwa Tears (Akorn).
Artificial Tears (Rugby).
Dey-Lube (Dey).
Dry Eyes (Bausch & Lomb).
Duolube (Bausch & Lomb).
Duratears Naturale (Alcon).
Hypotears (Novartis Vision).
Lacri-Lube NP (Allergan).
Lacri-Lube S.O.P. (Allergan).
Lipo-Tears (Spectra).
LubriTears (Bausch & Lomb).
OcuCoat PF (Storz Ophthalmics).
Puralube (Fougera).
Refresh PM (Allergan).
Tears Renewed (Akorn).
Vit-A-Drops (Vision Pharm).

Ocu-Lube. (Bausch & Lomb) Petrolatum sterile, preservative and lanolin free. Tube 3.5 g. *otc.*
Use: Ophthalmic lubricant.

Ocumeter.
See: Decadron Phosphate, Preps. (Merck).
Humorsol, Ophth. Soln. (Merck).
Neo-Decadron, Preps. (Merck).

Ocupress. (Otsuka America) Carteolol HCl 1%. Soln. Bot. 5 ml, 10 ml. *Rx.*
Use: Beta-adrenergic blocking agent, glaucoma agent.

Ocusert. (Alza) Pilocarpine ocular therapeutic system. *Rx.*
Pilo-20: Releases 20 mcg pilocarpine/hour for one week. Pkg. 8s.
Pilo-40: Releases 40 mcg pilocarpine/hour for one week. Pkg. 8s.
Use: Agent for glaucoma.

OCuSOFT. (OCuSOFT) PEG-80 sorbitan laurate, sodium trideceth sulfate, PEG-150 distearate, cocoamido propyl hydroxysultaine, lauroamphocarboxyglycinate, sodium laureth-13 carboxylate, PEG-15 tallow polyamine, quaternium-15. Soln. Pads UD 30s, Bot. 30 ml, 120 ml, 240 ml, Compliance kit (120 ml and 100 pads). *otc.*
Use: Ophthalmic cleansing solution.

OCuSoft VMS. Tab.: Vitamins A 5000 IU, E 30 IU, C 60 mg, Cu, Se, Zn 40 mg. Bot. 60s. *otc.*
Use: Vitamin/mineral supplements.

Ocusulf-10. (Optopics) Sodium sulfacetamide 10%. Soln. Bot. 2 ml, 5 ml, 15 ml. *Rx.*
Use: Anti-infective, ophthalmic.

Ocutricin. (Bausch & Lomb) **Oint.:** Polymyxin B sulfate 10,000 units, bacitracin zinc 400 units, neomycin sulfate 3.5 mg. Tube 3.5 g. *Rx.*
Use: Antibiotic, ophthalmic.

Ocuvite. (Lederle) Formerly distributed by Storz. Vitamins A 5000 IU, E 30 IU, C 60 mg, Zn 40 mg, Cu, Se 40 mcg, lactose/Tab. Bot. 60s. *otc.*
Use: Vitamin/mineral supplement.

Ocuvite Extra. (Storz) Vitamin A 6000 IU, C 200 mg, E 50 IU, Zn 40 mg, B_3 40 mg, B_2 3 mg, Cu, Se, Mn, l-glutathione. 50s. Tab. Bot. *otc.*
Use: Vitamin supplement.

Odara. (Lorvic) Alcohol 48%, carbolic acid less than 2%, zinc Cl, potassium iodide, glycerin, methyl salicylate, oil eucalyptus, tincture myrrh. Concentrated Liq. Bot. 8 oz. *otc.*
Use: Mouthwash, gargle.

oestergon.
See: Estradiol (Various Mfr.).

Oesto-Mins. (Tyson) Ascorbic acid 500 mg, Ca 250 mg, Mg 250 mg, K 45 mg, vitamin D 100 IU/4.5 g. Powd. 200 g. *otc.*
Use: Vitamin Supplement.

oestradiol.
See: Estradiol (Various Mfr.).

oestrasid.
See: Dienestrol (Various Mfr.).

oestrin.
See: Estrone (Various Mfr.).

oestroform.
See: Estrone (Various Mfr.).

oestromenin.
See: Diethylstilbestrol (Various Mfr.).

oestromon.
See: Diethylstilbestrol (Various Mfr.).

Off-Ezy Corn & Callous Remover. (Del Pharm) Salicylic acid 17% in a collodion-like vehicle of 65% ether and 21% alcohol. Kit. 13.5 ml with callous smoother and 3 corn cushions. *otc.*
Use: Keratolytic.

Off-Ezy Corn Remover. (Del Pharm.) Salicylic acid 13.57% in flexible collodion base, ether 65%, alcohol 21%. Bot. 0.45 oz. *otc.*
Use: Keratolytic.

Off-Ezy Wart Remover. (Del Pharm.) Salicylic acid 17% in flexible collodion base, ether 65%, alcohol 21%. Bot. 13.5 ml. *otc.*
Use: Keratolytic.

●**ofloxacin,** (oh-FLOX-uh-SIN) U.S.P. 23.
Use: Anti-infective. [Orphan drug], antibacterial.
See: Floxin (Ortho).
Ocuflox, Ophth. Soln. (Allergan).

●**ofornine.** (ah-FAR-neen) USAN.
Use: Antihypertensive.

Ogen. (Abbott) Estropipate. **Tab. 0.625:** Estropipate 0.75 mg/Tab. Bot. 100s. **Tab. 1.25:** Estropipate 1.5 mg/Tab. Bot. 100s. **Tab. 2.5:** Estropipate 3 mg/Tab. Bot. 100s. *Rx.*
Use: Estrogen.

Ogen Vaginal Cream. (Abbott) Estropipate 1.5 mg/g. Tube 1.5 oz w/applicator. *Rx.*
Use: Estrogen, vaginal.

Oilatum Soap. (Stiefel) Polyunsaturated vegetable oil 7.5%. Bar 120 g, 240 g. *otc.*
Use: Skin cleanser.

oil of camphor w/combinations.
See: Sloan's Liniment, Liq. (Warner-Lambert).

oil of cloves w/alcohol.
See: Buckley "Z.O.", Liq. (Crosby).

Oil of Olay Daily UV Protectant. (Procter & Gamble) SPF 15. **Cream:**Titanium dioxide, ethylhexyl p-methoxycinnamate, 2-phenylbenzimidazole- 5-sulfonic acid, glycerin, triethanolamine, imidazolidinyl urea, parabens, carbomer, PEG-10, EDTA, castor oil, tartrazine. Scented and unscented. 51 g. **Lot.:** Ethylhexyl p-methoxycinnamate, 2-phenylbenzimidazole-5sulfonic acid, titanium dioxide, cetyl alcohol, imidazolidinyl urea, parabens, EDTA, castor oil, tartrazine. Bot. 105 g, 157.7 g. *otc.*
Use: Sunscreen.

Oil of Olay Foaming Face Wash. (Procter & Gamble) Potassium cocoyl hydrolyzed collagen, glycerin, EDTA. Liq. Bot. 90 ml, 210 ml. *otc.*
Use: Antiacne.

oil of pine w/combinations.
See: Sloan's Liniment, Liq. (Warner-Lambert).

ointment base, washable.
See: Absorbent Base (Upsher-Smith).
Cetaphil, Cream, Lot. (Galderma).
Velvachol, Cream (Galderma).

●**ointment, bland lubricating ophthalmic,** U.S.P 23.

Use: Lubricant (ophthalmic).

●**ointment, hydrophilic,** U.S.P. 23.
Use: Pharmaceutic aid (oil-in-water emulsion ointment base).

●**ointment, rose water,** U.S.P 23.
Use: Pharmaceutic aid (emollient, ointment base).

●**ointment, white,** U.S.P. 23.
Use: Pharmaceutical aid (oleaginous ointment base).

●**ointment, yellow,** U.S.P. 23.
Use: Pharmaceutic aid (ointment base).

●**olaflur.** (OH-lah-flure) USAN.
Use: Dental caries prophylactic.

olamine.
See: Ethanolamine.

●**olanzapine.** (oh-LAN-zah-PEEN) USAN.
Use: Antipsychotic.
See: Zyprexa, Tab. (Eli Lilly & Co.).

old tuberculin.
See: MonoVacc Test (OT), Box (Connaught).
Tuberculin, Old, Tine Test, Jar (Wyeth Lederle).

oleandomycin phosphate. Phosphate of an antibacterial substance produced by *Streptomyces antibioticus.*
Use: Anti-infective.

oleandomycin salt of penicillin.
See: Pen-M (Pfizer) Under study.

oleandomycin, triacetyl. Troleandomycin, U.S.P. XX.

●**oleic acid,** N.F. 18.
Use: Pharmaceutic aid (emulsion adjunct).

●**oleic acid I 125.** USAN.
Use: Radioactive agent.

●**oleic acid I 131.** USAN.
Use: Radioactive agent.

oleovitamin A, Vitamin A, U.S.P. 23.

●**oleovitamin A & D,** U.S.P. 23.
Use: Vitamin A & D supplement.
See: Super-D, Perles, Liq. (Pharmacia & Upjohn).

oleovitamin D, synthetic.
Use: Vitamin D supplement.
See: Viosterol in Oil.

●**oleyl alcohol,** N.F. 18.
Use: Pharmaceutic aid (emulsifying agent, emollient).
See: Patanol, Soln. (Alcon).

●**olive oil,** N.F. 18.
Use: Emollient, pharmaceutic aid (setting retardant for dental cements).

●**olopatadine hydrochloride.** (oh-low-pat-AD-een) USAN.
Use: Antiallergic (allergic rhinitis, urticaria, allergic conjunctivitis, asthma).

See: Patanol, Soln. (Alcon).

• **olsalazine sodium.** (OLE-SAL-uh-zeen) USAN.
Use: Maintenance of remission of ulcertiave colitis in patients intolerant of sulfasalazine; anti-inflammatory (gastrointestinal).
See: Dipentum (Pharmacia & Upjohn).

• **olvanil.** (OLE-van-ill) USAN.
Use: Analgesic.

OM 401. *Rx.*
Use: Sickle cell disease. [Orphan drug]

omega-3 (n-3) polyunsaturated fatty acids. From cold water fish oils.
Use: Dietary supplement to reduce risk of coronary artery disease.
See: Cardi-Omega 3, Cap. (Thompson Medical).
Marine 500, 1000, Cap. (Murdock).
Max EPA, Cap. (Various Mfr.).
Promega, Cap. (Parke-Davis).
Proto-Chol, Cap. (Squibb).
Sea-Omega 50, Cap. (Rugby).

Omega Oil. (Block) Methyl nicotinate, methyl salicylate, capsicum oleoresin, histamine dihydrochloride, isopropyl alcohol 44%. Bot. 2.5 oz, 4.85 oz. *otc.*
Use: Analgesic, topical.

• **omeprazole,** (oh-MEH-pray-ZAHL) U.S.P. 23. (Astra Merck)
Use: Depressant (gastric acid secretory).
Agent for gastroesophageal reflux disease.
See: Prilosec, (Merck).

• **omeprazole sodium.** (oh-MEH-pray-ZOLE) USAN.
Use: Antisecretory (gastric).

Omnicol. (Delta) Dextromethorphan HBr 15 mg, chlorpheniramine maleate 4 mg, phenylephrine HCl 5 mg, phenindamine tartrate 4 mg, salicylamide 227 mg, acetaminophen 100 mg, caffeine alkaloid 10 mg, ascorbic acid 25 mg/Tab. Bot. 100s. Bot. pt. *otc.*
Use: Antitussive, antihistamine, decongestant, analgesic.

Omnihemin. (Delta) Iron 110 mg, vitamins C 150 mg, B_{12} 7.5 mcg, folic acid 1 mg, zinc 1 mg, copper 1 mg, manganese 1 mg, magnesium 1 mg/Tab. or 5 ml. **Cap.:** Bot. 100s; **Soln.:** Bot. pt. *Rx.*
Use: Vitamin/mineral supplement.

OmniHIB. (SK-Beecham) Purified capsular polysaccharide 10 mcg, tetanus toxoid 24 mcg/0.5 ml, sucrose 8.5%. Pow. for Inj. (lyophilized). Vial w/0.6 ml syringe of diluent. *Rx.*
Use: Agent for immunization.

OMNIhist L.A. (WE Pharm) Phenylephrine 20 mg, chlorpheniramine maleate 8 mg, methscopolamine nitrate 2.5 mg/Tab. Bot. 100s. *Rx.*
Use: Decongestant, antihistamine, anticholinergic.

Omninatal. (Delta) Iron 60 mg, copper 2 mg, zinc 15 mg, vitamins A 8000 IU, D 400 IU, C 90 mg, calcium 200 mg, folic acid 1.5 mg, B_1 2.5 mg, B_2 3 mg, niacinamide 20 mg, pyridoxine HCl 10 mg, pantothenic acid 15 mg, B_{12} 8 mcg/Tab. Bot. 100s. *Rx.*
Use: Vitamin/mineral supplement.

Omnipaque. (Sanofi Winthrop) Iohexol (46.4% iodine). Nonionic contrast medium. **180 mg/ml:** Vial 10 ml, 20 ml. **240 mg/ml:** Vial 10 ml, 100 ml. Bot. 200 ml. **300 mg/ml:** Vial 10 ml, 30 ml, 50 ml, 100 ml, 200 ml. **350 mg/ml:** Vial 50 ml, 100 ml. Bot. 200 ml.
Use: Radiopaque agent.

Omnipen. (Wyeth-Ayerst) Ampicillin, anhydrous 250 mg or 500 mg/Cap. Bot. 100s, 500s. *Rx.*
Use: Anti-infective, penicillin.

Omnipen. (Wyeth-Ayerst) Ampicillin trihydrate 125 mg or 250 mg/5 ml when reconstituted. Pow. for oral susp. **125 mg/5 ml:** Bot. 100 ml, 150 ml, 200 ml. **250 mg/5 ml:** Bot. 100 ml, 150 ml, 200 ml, UD 5 ml × 20. *Rx.*
Use: Anti-infective, penicillin.

Omnipen-N. (Wyeth-Ayerst) Ampicillin sodium pow. for inj. 125 mg, 250 mg, 500 mg, 1 g or 2 g/Vial. Pkg. 10s. Piggyback units 500 mg, 1 g, 2 g, Bulk 10 g/Vial. Pkg. 1s. *Rx.*
Use: Anti-infective, penicillin.

Omniscan. (Sanofi Winthrop) Gadodiamide 287 mg, caldiamide sodium 12 mg/ml. Inj. Vial 10 ml, 15 ml fill in 20 ml vials.
Use: Radiopaque agent.

Omnitabs. (Halsey) Vitamins A 5000 IU, D 400 IU, C 50 mg, B_1 3 mg, B_2 2.5 mg, niacin 20 mg, B_6 1 mg, B_{12} 1 mcg, pantothenic acid 0.9 mg/Tab. Bot. 100s. *otc.*
Use: Vitamin supplement.

Omnitabs with Iron. (Halsey) Vitamins A 5000 IU, D 400 IU, B_1 3 mg, B_2 2.5 mg, B_6 1 mg, B_{12} 1 mcg, C 50 mg, niacinamide 20 mg, calcium pantothenate 1 mg, iron 15 mg/Tab. Bot. 100s. *otc.*
Use: Vitamin/mineral supplement.

• **omoconazole nitrate.** USAN.
Use: Antifungal.

OMS Concentrate. (Upsher-Smith) Morphine sulfate 20 mg/ml. Soln. 30, 120 ml. *c-II.*

Use: Narcotic analgesic.

Oncaspar. (Enzon) Pegaspargase 750 IU/ml in a phosphate buffered saline solution. Inj. In single-use vials. *Rx.*
Use: Antineoplastic agent.

Oncet. (Wakefield) Hydrocodone bitartrate 5 mg, acetaminophen 500 mg/ Cap. Bot. 100s. *c-III.*
Use: Antitussive, analgesic.

oncorad ov103. *Rx.*
Use: Ovarian cancer. [Orphan drug]

Oncoscint CR/OV. (Cytogen)
See: Satumomab Pendetide.

Oncovin Solution. (Lilly) Vincristine sulfate for inj. 1 mg/ml, 2 mg/2 ml or 5 mg/ 5 ml. Ctn. 10s. Hyporets 1 mg/Pkg 3s; 2 mg/Pkg 3s. *Rx.*
Use: Antineoplastic.

•**ondansetron hydrochloride.** (ahn-DAN-SEH-trahn) USAN.
Use: Antianxiety, antiemetic, antischizophrenic.
See: Zofran (Cerenex).

Ondrox. (Unimed) **Tab.:** Ca 25 mg, iron 3 mg, vitamins A 2000 IU, D 100 IU, E 17 mg, B_1 0.25 mg, B_2 0.28 mg, B_3 3.33 mg, B_5 1.67 mg, B_6 0.33 mg, B_{12} 1 mcg, C 41.7 mg, folic acid 0.67, biotin 0.5 mcg, I, Mg, Cu, P, vitamin K, Cr, Mn, Mo, Se, V, B, Si, Zn 2.5 mg, inositol, bioflavonoids, N-acetylcysteine, L-glutathione, L-methionine, L-glutamine, taurine. Bot. 60s, 180s. *otc.*
Use: Vitamin/mineral supplements.

One-a-Day Essential. (Bayer) Vitamins A 5000 IU, E 30 IU, C 60 mg, folic acid 0.4 mg, B_1 1.5 mg, B_2 1.7 mg, B_3 20 mg, B_6 2 mg, B_{12} 6 mcg, B_5 10 mg, D 400 IU/Tab. Sodium free. Bot. 75s, 130s. *otc.*
Use: Vitamin supplement.

One-A-Day Extras Antioxidant. (Bayer) Vitamin E 200 IU, C 250 mg, A 5000 IU, Zn 7.5 mg, Cu, Se, Mn, tartrazine/ Softgel cap. Bot. 50s. *otc.*
Use: Vitamin Supplement.

One-A-Day Extras Vitamin C. (Bayer) Vitamin C 500 mg/Tab. Bot. 100s. *otc.*
Use: Vitamin supplement.

One-A-Day Extras Vitamin E. (Bayer) Vitamin E 400 IU/Softgel Cap. Bot. 60s. *otc.*
Use: Vitamin supplement.

One-A-Day Maximum Formula. (Bayer) Iron 18 mg, vitamins A 5000 IU, D 400 IU, E 30 IU, B_1 1.5 mg, B_2 1.7 mg, B_3 20 mg, B_5 10 mg, B_6 2 mg, B_{12} 6 mcg, C 60 mg, folic acid 0.4 mg, Ca, Cl, Cr, Cu, I, K, Mg, Mn, Mo, P, Se, Zn 15 mg, biotin 30 mcg/Tab. Bot. 60s, 100s. *otc.*

Use: Vitamin/mineral supplement.

One-A-Day Men's Vitamins. (Bayer) Vitamin A 5000 IU, C 200 mg, B_1 2.25 mg, B_2 2.55 mg, B_3 20 mg, D 400 IU, E 45 IU, B_6 3 mg, folic acid 0.4 mg, B_{12} 9 mcg, B_5 10 mg/Tab. Bot. 60s, 100s. *otc.*
Use: Vitamin/mineral supplement.

One-A-Day 55 Plus. (Bayer) Vitamin A 6000 IU, C 120 mg, B_1 4.5 mg, B_2 3.4 mg, B_3 20 mg, D 400 IU, E 60 IU, B_6 6 mg, folic acid 0.4 mg, biotin 30 mcg, B_5 20 mg, K 25 mcg, Ca 220 mg, I, Mg, Cu, Zn 15 mg, Cr, Se, Mo, Mn, K, Cl/ Tab. Bot. 50s, 80s. *otc.*
Use: Vitamin/mineral supplement.

One-A-Day Women's Formula. (Bayer) **Tab.:** Ca 450 mg, iron 27 mg, vitamins A 5000 IU, D 400 IU, E 30 mg, B_1 1.5 mg, B_2 1.7 mg, B_3 20 mg, B_5 10 mg, B_6 2 mg, B_{12} 6 mcg, C 60 mg, folic acid 0.4 mg, Zn 15 mg, tartrazine. Bot. 60s, 100s. *Rx.*
Use: Vitamin/mineral supplement.

One Step Midstream Pregnancy Test. (Biocare International Inc.) Stick for urine test. 1s. *otc.*
Use: Pregnancy test.

One-Tablet-Daily. (Various Mfr.) Vitamins A 5000 IU, D 400 IU, E 30 mg, B_1 1.5 mg, B_2 1.7 mg, B_3 20 mg, B_5 10 mg, B_6 2 mg, B_{12} 6 mcg, C 60 mg, folic acid 0.4 mg. Tab. Bot. 30s, 100s, 250s, 365s, 1000s. *otc.*
Use: Multivitamin.

One Tablet Daily. (Various Mfr.) Vitamins A 5000 IU, D 400 IU, E 30 mg, B_1 1.5 mg, B_2 1.7 mg, B_3 20 mg, B_5 10 mg, B_6 2 mg, B_{12} 6 mcg, C 60 mg, folic acid 0.4 mg/Tab. Bot. 365s, 1000s. *otc.*
Use: Vitamin supplement.

One Tablet Daily Plus Iron. (Various Mfr.) Iron 18 mg, vitamins A 5000 IU, D 400 IU, E 15 mg, B_1 1.5 mg, B_2 1.7 mg, B_3 20 mg, B_6 2 mg, B_{12} 6 mcg, C 60 mg, folic acid 0.4 mg/Tab. Bot. 100s, 250s, 365s. *otc.*
Use: Vitamin/mineral supplement.

One Tablet Daily with Iron. (Goldline) Iron 18 mg, A 5000 IU, D 400 IU, E 30 mg, B_1 1.5 mg, B_2 1.7 mg, B_3 20 mg, B_5 10 mg, B_6 2 mg, B_{12} 6 mcg, C 60 mg, folic acid 0.4 mg. Bot. 100s. *otc.*
Use: Vitamin/mineral supplement.

One-Tablet-Daily with Minerals. (Goldline) Iron 18 mg, vitamins A 5000 IU, D 400 IU, E 30 IU, B_1 1.5 mg, B_2 1.7 mg, B_3 20 mg, B_5 10 mg, B_6 2 mg, B_{12} 6 mcg, C 60 mg, folic acid 0.4 mg, Ca, Cl, Cr, Cu, I, K, Mg, Mn, Mo, P, Se, Zn 15 mg, biotin 30 mcg/Tab. Bot. 100s, 1000s. *otc.*

Use: vitamin/mineral supplement.

1000-BC, IM or IV. (Solvay) Vitamins B$_1$ 25 mg, B$_2$ 2.5 mg, B$_6$ 5 mg, panthenol 5 mg, B$_{12}$ 500 mcg, niacinamide 75 mg, C 100 mg/ml. Vial 10 ml. *Rx.*
Use: Vitamin supplement.

1+1-F Creme. (Dunhall) Hydrocortisone 1%, pramoxine HCl 1%, iodochlorhydroxyquin 3%. Tube 30 g. *Rx.*
Use: Corticosteroid, local anesthetic, antifungal, topical.

1-2-3 Ointment No. 20. (Durel) Burow's solution, lanolin, zinc oxide (Lassar's paste). Jar oz, 1 lb, 6 lb. *otc.*
Use: Anti-inflammatory agent, topical.

1-2-3 Ointment No. 21. (Durel) Burow's solution 1 part, lanolin 2, zinc oxide (Lassar's paste) 1.5, cold cream 1.5. Jar oz, 1 lb, 6 lb. *otc.*
Use: Anti-inflammatory agent, topical.

OncoScint CR/OV. (Cytogen) Satumomab pendetide labeled with indium-111, obtained separately. Kit with 1 mg/ 2 ml satumomab vial, vial of sodium acetate buffer, and filter.

Onoton Tablets. (Sanofi Winthrop) Pancreatin, hemicellulose, ox bile extracts. *otc.*
Use: Digestive aid.

•**ontazolast.** (ahn-TAH-zoe-last) USAN.
Use: Antiasthmatic (leukotriene antagonist).

ontosein.
See: Orgotein (Diagnostic Data).

Ony-Clear Nail. (Pedinol) Miconazole nitrate 2%, benzyl alcohol. Spray. 42.5 g. *Rx.*
Use: Antiacne, topical.

Opcon. (Bausch & Lomb) Naphazoline HCl 0.1%. Bot. 15 ml. *otc.*
Use: Vasoconstrictor, mydriatic, ophthalmic.

Opcon-A. (Bausch & Lomb)**Soln.:** 0.027% nephazoline HCl, 0.315% pheniramine maleate, 0.5% hydroxypropyl methylcellulose, 0.01% benzalkonium chloride, 0.1% EDTA, NaCl, boric acid, sodium buffers. 15 ml. *otc.*
Use: Vasoconstrictor, mydriatic, antihistamine (ophthalmic).

o,p'-ddd.
Use: Miscellaneous antineoplastic.
See: Lysodren (Bristol-Myers Oncology).

Operand. (Redi-Products) **Aerosal:** Iodine 0.5%. 90 ml. **Skin cleanser:** Iodine 1%. 90 ml. **Oint.:** Iodine 1%. 30 g, lb, packette 1.2 g and 2.7 g. **Perineal wash conc.:** Iodine 1%. 240 ml. **Prep soln.:** Iodine 1%. 60 ml, 120 ml, 240 ml, pt, qt. **Soln:** Prep pad 100s, swab stick 25s. **Surgical scrub:** Povidone-iodine 7.5%. 60 ml, 120 ml, 240 ml, pt, qt, gal, packette 22.5 ml. **Whirlpool conc.:** Iodine 1%. gal. *otc.*
Use: Antiseptic, germicide.

Operand Douche. (Redi-Products) Povidone-iodine. Soln. 60 ml, 240 ml, UD 15 ml. *otc.*
Use: Vaginal preparation.

o-phenylphenol. W/Amyl complex, phenylmercuric nitrate.
See: Lubraseptic Jelly (Guardian).

Ophthacet. (Vortech) Sodium sulfacetamide 10%. Soln. 15 ml. *Rx.*
Use: Anti-infective, ophthalmic.

Ophthaine Hydrochloride. (Apothecon) Proparacaine HCl 0.5%. Soln. Bot. w/ dropper 15 ml. *Rx.*
Use: Local anesthetic, ophthalmic.

Ophthalgan. (Wyeth-Ayerst) Glycerin ophthalmic soln. w/chlorobutanol 0.55% as preservative. Bot. 7.5 ml. *Rx.*
Use: Hyperosmolar preparation.

Ophtha P/S. (Misemer) Prednisolone acetate 0.5%, sodium sulfacetamide 10%, hydroxyethylcellulose, EDTA, polysorbate 80, sodium thiosulfate, benzalkonium chloride 0.025%. Susp. Bot. 5 ml. *Rx.*
Use: Corticosteroid, anti-infective, ophthalmic.

Ophtha P/S Ophthalmic Suspension. (Misemer) Sodium sulfacetamide 10%, prednisolone acetate 0.5%. Bot. 5 ml w/dropper. *Rx.*
Use: Corticosteroid, anti-infective, ophthalmic.

Ophthetic. (Allergan) Proparacaine HCl 0.5%. Bot. 15 ml. *Rx.*
Use: Local anesthetic, ophthalmic.

•**opipramol hydrochloride.** (oh-PIH-prah-mole) USAN.
Use: Antipsychotic, antidepressant, tranquilizer.

•**opium,** U.S.P. 23.
Use: Pharmaceutic necessity for powdered opium.

opium alkaloids, total, as the hydrochloride salt.
See: Pantopon, Amp. (Roche).

opium and belladonna. (Wyeth-Ayerst) Powdered opium 60 mg, extract of belladonna 15 mg/Supp. Box 20s. *c-II.*
Use: Narcotic analgesic, anticholinergic/antispasmodic.

•**opium powdered,** U.S.P. 23.
Use: Pharmaceutical necessity for Paregoric.

W/Albumin tannate, colloidal kaolin, pectin.
See: Ekrised, Tab. (Roberts).
W/Atropine sulfate, alcohol.
See: Stopit Liq. (Scrip).
W/Belladonna extract.
See: B & O, Supp. (PolyMedica).
W/Bismuth subgallate, kaolin, pectin, zinc phenolsulfonate.
See: Diastay, Tab. (ICN Pharm.).
W/Kaolin, pectin, bismuth subcarbonate.
See: KBP/O, Cap. (Cole).
W/Kaolin, pectin, hyoscyamine sulfate, atropine sulfate, hyoscine HBr.
See: Donnagel-PG, Susp. (Robins).
opium tincture.
W/Homatropine MBr, Pectin.
See: Dia-Quel, Liq. (I.P.C.).
W/Pectin.
See: Opecto, Elix. (Jones Medical).
Parelixir, Liq. (Purdue Frederick).
opium tincture, camphorated.
Use: Antidiarrheal.
See: Paregoric, U.S.P. 23.
W/Glycyrrhiza fluid extract, tartar emetic, glycerin.
See: Brown Mixture.
•**oprelvekin.** USAN.
Use: Hematopoietic stimulant.
Opti-Bon Eye Drops. (Barrows) Phenylephrine HCl, berberine sulfate, boric acid, sodium Cl, sodium bisulfite, glycerine, camphor water, peppermint water, thimerosal 0.004%. Bot. 1 oz. *otc.*
Use: Ophthalmic preparation.
Opticaps. (Approved) Vitamins A 32,500 IU, D 3250 IU, B_1 15 mg, B_2 5 mg, B_6 0.5 mg, C 150 mg, E 5 IU, calcium pantothenate 3 mg, niacinamide 150 mg, B_{12} 20 mg, iron 11.26 mg, choline bitartrate 30 mg, inositol 30 mg, pepsin 32.5 mg, diastase 32.5 mg, calcium 30 mg, phosphorus 25 mg, magnesium 0.7 mg, Fr. dicalcium phosphate 110 mg, manganese 1.3 mg, potassium 0.68 mg, zinc 0.45 mg, hesperidin compound 25 mg, biotin 20 mcg, Brewer's yeast 50 mg, wheat germ oil 20 mg, hydrolized yeast 81.25 mg, protein digest. 47.04 mg, amino acids 34.21 mg/Cap. Bot. 30s, 60s, 90s, 1000s. *otc.*
Use: Vitamin/mineral supplement.
Opticare PMS. (Standard Drug) Iron 2.5 mg, vitamins 2083 IU, D 17 IU, E 14 IU, B_1 4.2 mg, B_2 4.2 mg, B_3 4.2 mg, B_5 4.2 mg, B_6 50 mg, B_{12} 10.4 mcg, C 250 mg, folic acid 0.03 mg, Cr, Cu, I, K, Mg, Mn, Se, Zn 4.2 mg, biotin 10.4 mcg, choline bitartrate, bioflavonoids,

inositol, PABA, rutin, Ca, amylase activity, protease activity, lipase activity, betaine, tartrazine. Bot. 150s. *otc.*
Use: Vitamin/mineral supplement.
Opti-Clean. (Alcon) Tween 21, polymeric cleaners, hydroxyethylcellulose, thimerosal 0.004%, EDTA 0.1%. Bot 12 ml, 20 ml. *otc.*
Use: Contact lens care.
Opti-Clean II. (Alcon) Polymeric cleaning agent, Tween 21, EDTA 0.1%, polyquaternium-1 0.001%. Thimerosal free. Bot. 12 ml, 20 ml. *otc.*
Use: Contact lens care.
Opti-Clean II Especially For Sensitive Eyes. (Alcon) EDTA 0.1%, polyquaternium-1 0.001%, polymeric cleaners, Tween 21. Thimerosal free. Bot. 12 ml, 20 ml. *otc.*
Use: Contact lens care.
Opticyl. (Optopics) Tropicamide 0.5%, 1%. Soln. Bot. 2 ml, 15 ml. *Rx.*
Use: Mydriatic/cycloplegic, ophthalmic.
Opti-Free Enzymatic Cleanar. (Alcon) Highly purified pork pancrentin. Tab. Pkg. 6s, 12s, 18s. *otc.*
Use: Soft contact lens care.
Opti-Free Non-Hydrogen Peroxide-Containing System. (Alcon) Citrate buffer, NaCl, EDTA 0.05%, polyquaternium-1 0.001%. Soln. 118 ml, 237 ml, 355 ml. *otc.*
Use: Ophthalmic preparation.
Opti-Free Rewetting Solution. (Alcon) Citrate buffer, sodium Cl, EDTA 0.05%, polyquaternium-1 0.001%. Soln. Bot. 10 ml, 20 ml. *otc.*
Use: Soft contact lens care.
Opti-Free Surfactant Cleaning Solution. (Alcon) EDTA 0.01%, polyquaternium-1 0.001%, microclens polymeric cleaners, Tween 21. Thimerosal free. Soln. Bot. 12 ml, 20 ml. *otc.*
Use: Soft contact lens care.
Optigene. (Pfeiffer) Sodium Cl, sodium phosphate mono- and dibasic, benzalkonium Cl, EDTA. Soln. Bot. 118 ml. *otc.*
Use: Ophthalmic irrigation solution.
Optigene 3. (Pfeiffer) Tetrahydrozoline HCl 0.05%. Soln. Bot. 15 ml. *otc.*
Use: Vasoconstrictor, mydriatic (ophthalmic).
Optilets-500. (Abbott) Vitamins B_1 15 mg, B_2 10 mg, B_3 100 mg, B_5 20 mg, B_6 5 mg, C 500 mg, A 10,000 IU, D 400 IU, E 30 IU, B_{12} 12 mcg/Filmtab. Bot. 120s. *otc.*
Use: Vitamin/mineral supplement.
Optilets-M-500. (Abbott) Vitamins C 500

mg, B_3 100 mg, B_5 20 mg, B_1 15 mg, A 5000 IU, B_2 10 mg, B_6 5 mg, D 400 IU, B_{12} 12 mcg, E 30 IU, iron 20 mg, Mg, zinc 1.5 mg, Cu, Mn, I/Filmtab. Bot. 120s. *otc.*
Use: Vitamin/mineral supplement.

Optimine. (Schering-Plough) Azatadine maleate 1 mg/Tab. Bot. 100s. *Rx.*
Use: Antihistamine.

Optimoist. (Colgate Oral) Xylitol, calcium phosphate monobasic, citric acid, sodium hydroxide, sodium benzoate, acesulfame potassium, hydroxyethyl cellulose, sodium monofluoro phosphate, 2 ppm fluoride. Soln. Bot. 60 ml and 330 ml. Spray. *otc.*
Use: Saliva substitute.

Optimax Prenatal. (Optimax) **Tab.**: Ca 100 mg, iron 5 mg, vitamins A 833 IU, D 67 IU, E 2 mg, B_1 0.5 mg, B_2 0.6 mg, B_3 6.7 mg, B_5 3.3 mg, B_6 0.73 mg, B_{12} 0.87 mcg, C 30 mg, folic acid 0.13 mg, Cr, Cu, I, K, Mg, Mn, Se, Zn 3.17 mg. Bot. 360s. *otc.*
Use: Vitamin/mineral supplement.

Optimyd. (Schering-Plough) Prednisolone phosphate 0.5%, sodium sulfacetamide 10%, sodium thiosulfate. Soln-Sterile. Drop bot. 5 ml. *Rx.*
Use: Anti-infective, corticosteroid, ophthalmic.

Opti-One. (Alcon) EDTA 0.05%, polyquaternium-1 0.001%, sodium chloride, sodium citrate. Buffered, isotonic. Soln. 120 ml. *otc.*
Use: Soft contact lens care.

Opti-One Multi-Purpose. (Alcon) **Soln.**: 0.05% EDTA, 0.001% polyquaternium-1, NaCl. Buffered, isotonic. 118, 237, 355, 473 ml. *otc.*
Use: Soft contact lens care.

Opti-One Rewetting. (Alcon) EDTA 0.05%, polyquaternium-1 0.001%, sodium chloride, citrate buffer, isotonic. Drops. Bot. 10 ml. *otc.*
Use: Soft contact lens care.

OptiPranolol. (Bausch & Lomb) Metipranolol HCl 0.3%. Bot. 5 ml, 10 ml. *Rx.*
Use: Agent for glaucoma.

Optiray. (Mallinckrodt) Ioversol.
Use: Radiopaque agent.

Optiray 350. (Mallinckrodt Medical) Ioversol 74%, iodine 35%, tromethamine 3.6 mg, EDTA 0.2 mg/ml. Inj. 30 and 50 ml glass vials, 75 ml fill in 150 ml glass bottles, 100 ml fill in 150 ml glass bottles, 150 ml glass bottles, 200 ml fill in 250 ml glass bottles, 30 and 50 ml handheld plastic syringes, 50 ml fill in 125 ml power injector plastic syringes,

100 ml fill in 125 ml power injector plastic syringes and 125 ml power injector plastic syringes.
Use: Radiopaque agent.

Opti-Soft. (Alcon) Isotonic soln of sodium Cl, borate buffer, EDTA 0.1%, polyquaternium-1 0.001%. Thimerosal free. Soln. Bot. 237 ml, 355 ml. *otc.*
Use: Soft contact lens care.

Opti-Soft Especially for Sensitive Eyes. (Alcon) Buffered, isotonic. EDTA 0.1%, polyquaternium-1 0.001%, NaCl, borate buffer. For lenses w/ ≤ 45% water content. Soln. Bot. 118 ml, 237 ml, 355 ml. *otc.*
Use: Soft contact lens care.

Opti-Tears. (Alcon) Isotonic solution with dextran, sodium Cl, potassium Cl, hydroxypropyl methylcellulose, EDTA 0.1%, polyquaternium-1 0.001%. Thimerosal and sorbic acid free. Soln. Bot. 15 ml. *otc.*
Use: Contact lens care.

Optivite for Women. (Optimox) Vitamins A 2083 IU, D 16.7 IU, E 14 mg, B_1 4.2 mg, B_2 4.2 mg, B_3 4.2 mg, B_5 4.2 mg, B_6 50 mg, B_{12} 10.4 mcg, C 250 mg, iron 2.5 mg, folic acid 0.03 mg, zinc 4.2 mg, choline 52 mg, inositol 10 mg, Cr, Cu, I, K, Mg, Mn, Se, citrus bioflavonoids, PABA, rutin, pancreatin, biotin/Tab. Bot. 180s. *otc.*
Use: Vitamin/mineral supplement.

Optivite P.M.T. (Optimox) Vitamins A 2083 IU, D, E 16.7 mg, B_1 4.2 mg, B_2 4.2 mg, B_3 4.2 mg, B_5 4.2 mg, B_6 50 mg, B_{12} 10.4 mcg, C 250 mg, iron 2.5 mg, FA 0.03 mg, Zn 4.2 mg, choline, Ca, Cr, Cu, I, K, Mg, Mn, Se, bioflavonoids, betaine, PABA, rutin, pancreatin, biotin, inositol/Tab. Bot. 180s. *otc.*
Use: Vitamin/mineral supplement.

Opti-Zyme Enzymatic Cleaner Especially For Sensitive Eyes. (Alcon) Pork pancreatin tablets. Pak 8s, 24s, 36s, 56s. *otc.*
Use: Contact lens care.

ORA5. (McHenry) Copper sulfate, iodine, potassium iodide, alcohol 1.5%. Liq. Bot. 3.75 ml, 30 ml. *otc.*
Use: Mouth preparation.

Orabase. (Colgate Oral) Gelatin, pectin, sodium carboxymethylcellulose in hydrocarbon gel w/polyethylene and mineral oil. 0.75 g Packet Box 100s. Tube 5 g, 15 g. *otc.*
Use: Mouth preparation.

Orabase-B. (Colgate Oral) Benzocaine 20%, mineral oil. Paste. 5 g, 15 g. *otc.*
Use: Mouth and throat product.

Orabase Baby. (Colgate Oral) Benzo-
caine 7.5%, alcohol free, fruit flavor.
Gel. 7.2 g. *otc.*
Use: Local anesthetic, dental.

Orabase Gel. (Colgate-Palmolive)
Benzocaine 15%, ethyl alcohol, tannic
acid, salicylic acid, saccharin. Gel. 7
g. *otc.*
Use: Local anesthetic, dental.

Orabase HCA. (Colgate Oral) Hydrocortisone acetate 0.5%, polyethylene 5%,
mineral oil. Tube 5 g. *Rx.*
Use: Corticosteroid, dental.

Orabase Lip. (Colgate Oral) Benzocaine
5%, allantoin 1.5%, menthol 0.5%, petrolatum, lanolin, parabens, camphor,
phenol. Cream. 10 g. *otc.*
Use: Local anesthetic, dental.

Orabase-O. (Colgate Oral) Benzocaine
20% in a polyethylene, mineral oil
base. Gel. In 15 g. *otc.*
Use: Local anesthetic, dental.

Orabase Plain. (Colgate Oral) Gelatin,
pectin & sodium carboxymethyl cellulose in polyethylene and mineral gel.
Paste. 5, 15 g. *otc.*
Use: Mouth and throat product.

Orabase with Benzocaine. (Colgate
Oral) Benzocaine 20% in gel base.
Packet 0.75 g, Box 100s. Tube 5 g, 15
g. *otc.*
Use: Local anesthetic, dental.

Oracap Capsules. (Vangard) Phenylpropanolamine HCl 75 mg, chlorpheniramine maleate 12 mg/Cap. Bot. 100s,
1000s. *Rx.*
Use: Decongestant, antihistamine.

Oracit. (Carolina Medical Prod.) Sodium
citrate 490 mg, citric acid 640 mg/5 ml,
(sodium 1 mEq/ml equivalent to 1 mEq
bicarbonate), alcohol 0.25%. Soln. Bot.
pt, UD 15, 30 ml. *Rx.*
Use: Systemic alkalinizer.

Oraderm Lip Balm. (Schattner) Sodium
phenolate, sodium tetraborate, phenol,
base containing an anionic emulsifier.
⅛ oz. *otc.*
Use: Local anesthetic, antiseptic, dental.

Orafix Medicated. (SK-Beecham) Allantoin 0.2%, benzocaine 2%. Tube 0.75
oz. *otc.*
Use: Local anesthetic, denture adhesive.

Orafix Original. (SK-Beecham) Tube 1.5
oz, 2.5 oz, 4 oz. *otc.*
Use: Denture adhesive.

Orafix Special. (SK-Beecham) Tube 1.4
oz, 2.4 oz. *otc.*

Use: Denture adhesive.

Oragrafin Calcium Granules. (Squibb)
Ipodate calcium (61.7% iodine) 3 g/8
g Pkg. 25 × 1 dose pkg.
Use: Radiopaque agent.

Oragrafin Sodium Capsules. (Squibb)
Ipodate sodium (61.4% iodine) 0.5 g/
Cap. Bot. 100s, 144s. Unimatic pkg.
100s. Card 6s. Box 25s.
Use: Radiopaque agent.

Orahesive Powder. (Colgate Oral) Gelatin, pectin, sodium carboxymethylcellulose. Bot. 25 g. *otc.*
Use: Denture adhesive.

Orajel. (Del Pharm.) Benzocaine 10% in
a special base. Tube 0.2 oz, 0.5 oz. *otc.*
Use: Local anesthetic, dental.

Orajel Brace-Aid Gel. (Del Pharm)
Benzocaine 20%, saccharin. Tube. 14.1
g. *otc.*
Use: Mouth preparation, dental.

Orajel Brace-Aid Oral Hygienic Rinse.
(Del Pharm.) Carbamide peroxide 10%
in anhydrous glycerin. Tube oz. *otc.*
Use: Mouth preparation, dental.

Orajel D. (Del Pharm) Benzocaine 10%,
saccharin. Tube 9.45 g. *otc.*
Use: Local anesthetic, dental.

Orajel Mouth-Aid. (Del) Benzocaine
20%.
Liq.: Cetylpyridinium 0.1%, ethyl alcohol 70%, tartrazine, saccharin, 13.5
ml.
Gel: Benzalkonium Cl 0.02%, zinc Cl
0.1%, EDTA, saccharin. 5.6 g, 10
g. *otc.*
Use: Topical anesthetic.

Orajel Perioseptic. (Del Pharm.) Carbamide peroxide 15% in anhydrous glycerin, saccharin, methylparaben, EDTA.
Liq. Bot. 13.3 ml. *otc.*
Use: Mouth preparation.

Oral-B Muppets Fluoride Toothpaste.
(Oral-B) Fluoride 0.22%. Pump 4.3 oz.
otc.
Use: Dental caries preventative.

oralcid.
See: Acetarsone.

oral contraceptives.
See: Demulen, Tab. (Searle).
Desogen, Tab. (Organon).
Enovid-E, Tab. (Searle).
GenCept, Tab. (Gencon).
Jenest-28, Tab. (Organon).
Loestrin, Prods. (Parke-Davis).
Lo/Ovral, Prods. (Wyeth-Ayerst).
Miconor, Tab. (Ortho).
Modicon, Prods. (Ortho).
Nelulen, Tab. (Watson Labs).

Norethin 1/35 E Tab. (Roberts).
Norethin 1/50 M Tab. (Roberts).
Nordette, Tab. (Wyeth-Ayerst).
Norinyl, Prods. (Syntex).
Norlestrin, Prods. (Parke-Davis).
Norquen, Tab. (Syntex).
Ortho Cept, Tab. (Ortho).
Ortho-Cyclen, Tab. (Ortho).
Ortho Tri-Cyclen, Tab. (Ortho).
Ortho-Novum, Prods. (Ortho).
Ovcon-35, Tab. (Bristol-Myers).
Ovcon-50, Tab. (Bristol-Myers).
Ovral, Tab. (Wyeth-Ayerst).
Ovrette, Tab. (Wyeth-Ayerst).
Ovulen, Tab. (Searle).
Triphasil, Tab. (Wyeth-Ayerst).

Oral Drops/Canker Sore Relief. (Weeks & Leo) Carbamide peroxide 10% in anhydrous glycerin base. Bot. 30 ml. *otc.*
Use: Mouth preparation.

Oralone Dental. (Thames) Triamcinolone acetonide 0.1%. Paste 5 g. *Rx.*
Use: Corticosteroid, dental.

oral rehydration salts.
Use: Electrolyte combination.

Oramide. (Major) Tolbutamide 0.5 g/Tab. Bot. 100s, 1000s. *Rx.*
Use: Antidiabetic.

Oraminic II. (Vortech) Brompheniramine maleate 10 mg per ml/Inj. Vial. 10 ml multidose. *Rx.*
Use: Antihistamine.

Oramorph SR. (Roxane)
SR Tab.: Morphine sulfate.
30 mg: Lactose. 50s, 100s, 250s, UD 100s.
60 mg: Lactose. 100s, UD 25s.
100 mg: Lactose. 100s, UD 25s. *c-ii.*
Use: Narcotic analgesic.

orange flower oil, N.F. XVII.
Use: Flavor, perfume, vehicle.

orange flower water, N.F. XVI.
Use: Flavor, perfume.

orange oil, N.F. XVI.
Use: Flavor.

orange peel tincture, sweet, N.F. XVI.
Use: Flavor.

orange spirit, compound, N.F. XVI.
Use: Flavor.

orange syrup, N.F. XVI.
Use: Flavored vehicle.

Orap. (McNeil Pharm) Pimozide 2 mg/Tab. Bot. 100s. *Rx.*
Use: Antipsychotic.

Oraphen-PD. (Great Southern) Acetaminophen 120 mg per 5 ml, alcohol 5%, cherry flavor. Elix. 120 ml. *otc.*
Use: Analgesic.

orarsan.

See: Acetarsone.

Orasept. (Pharmakon Labs) Tannic acid 12.16%, methylbenzethonium HCl 1.53%, ethyl alcohol 53.31%, camphor, menthol, benzyl alcohol, spearmint oil, cassia oil. Liq. Bot. 15 ml. *otc.*
Use: Mouth and throat preparation.

Orasept, Throat. (Pharmakon) Benzocaine 0.996%, methylbenzethonium Cl 1.037%, sorbitol 70%, menthol, peppermint, saccharin. Throat spray. 45 ml. *otc.*
Use: Mouth and throat preparation.

Orasol. (Goldline) Benzocaine 6.3%, phenol 0.5%, alcohol 70%, povidone-iodine. Liq. Bot. 14.79 ml. *otc.*
Use: Local anesthetic, oral.

Orasone. (Solvay) Prednisone **1 mg, 5 mg, 10 mg or 20 mg/Tab.:** Bot. 100s, 1000s, UD 100s. **50 mg/Tab.:** Bot. 100s, UD 100s. *Rx.*
Use: Corticosteroid.

OraSure HIV-1. (Epitope) Collection kit: Cotton fiber on a stick with collection vial. Device for oral specimen collection. For professional use only.
Use: Diagnostic aid.

Oratuss TR. (Vangard) Caramiphen edisylate 20 mg, chlorpheniramine maleate 8 mg, phenylpropanolamine HCl 50 mg, isopropamide iodide 2.5 mg/TR Cap. Bot. 100s, 500s. *Rx.*
Use: Antitussive, antihistamine, decongestant, anticholinergic, antispasmodic.

Orazinc. (Mericon) Zinc sulfate 220 mg/Cap. Bot. 100s, 1000s. *otc.*
Use: Mineral supplement.

orbenin. Sodium cloxacillin.
Use: Anti-infective.
See: Cloxapen (SK-Beecham).

Orbiferrous. (Orbit) Ferrous fumarate 300 mg, vitamins B_{12} 12 mcg, C 50 mg, B_1 3 mg, defatted desiccated liver 50 mg/Tab. Bot. 60s, 500s. *otc.*
Use: Vitamin/mineral supplement.

Orbit. (Spanner) Vitamins A 6250 IU, D 400 IU, B_1 3 mg, B_2 3 mg, B_6 2 mg, B_{12} 5 mcg, C 75 mg, niacinamide 20 mg, calcium pantothenate 10 mg, E 15 IU, biotin 15 mcg, iron 20 mg/Tab. Bot. 100s. *otc.*
Use: Vitamin/mineral supplement.

•**orbofiban acetate.** (ore-boe-FIE-ban) USAN.
Use: Fibrinogen receptor antagonist; platelet aggregation inhibitor.

•**orconazole nitrate.** (ahr-KOE-nah-zole NYE-trate) USAN.

Use: Antifungal.

Ordrine. (Eon Labs) Chlorpheniramine maleate 12 mg, phenylpropanolamine HCl 75 mg/SR Cap. Bot. 100s, 1000s. *Rx.*
Use: Antihistamine, decongestant.

Ordrine AT Extended Release. (Eon Labs) Phenylpropanolamine HCl 75 mg, caramiphen edisylate 40 mg/Cap. Bot. 50s, 100s, 500s. *Rx.*
Use: Cough preparation.

Oretic. (Abbott) Hydrochlorothiazide 25 mg or 50 mg/Tab. Bot. 100s, 1000s, UD 100s. *Rx.*
Use: Diuretic.

Oreton Methyl. (Schering-Plough) Methyltestosterone. **Buccal Tab.:** 10 mg, Bot. 100s. **Tab.:** 10 mg or 25 mg. Bot. 100s. *c-III.*
Use: Androgen.

Orexin. (Roberts) Vitamins B$_1$ 8.1 mg, B$_6$ 4.1 mg, B$_{12}$ 25 mcg/Chew-Tab. Bot. 100s. *otc.*
Use: Vitamin supplement.

Organidin. (Wallace) **Tab.:** 30 mg. Rose, scored. In 100s. **Elix.:** 60 mg/5 ml. 21.75% alcohol, glucose, saccharin. In pt and gal. **Sol.:** 50 mg/ml. In 30 ml w/ dropper.
Use: Expectorant.

Organidin NR. (Wallace) **Tab:** guaifenesin 200 mg/Tab. Bot. 100s. **Liq:** guaifenesin 100 mg/5 ml. Liq. Bot. pt, gal. *Rx.*
Use: Expectorant.

Orgaran. (Organon) Danaparoid sodium 750 anti-Xa units/0.6 ml, sodium sulfite/ Inj. Box. Single-dose ampules and prefilled syringes. 10s. *Rx.*
Use: Anticoagulant.

Orglagen Tablets. (Goldline) Orphenadrine citrate 100 mg/Tab. Bot. 100s, 1000s. *Rx.*
Use: Skeletal muscle relaxant.

•**orgotein.** (ORE-go-teen) USAN. A group of soluble metalloproteins isolated from liver, red blood cells, and other mammalian tissues.
Use: Anti-inflammatory, antirheumatic.

orgotein. (Diagnostic Data) Pure water soluble protein with a compact conformation maintained by 4 g atoms of chelated divalent metals, produced from bovine liver as a Cu-Zn mixed chelate having superoxide dismutase activity. Ontosein, Palosein.

orgotein for injection.
Use: Familial amyotropic lateral sclerosis. [Orphan drug]

Original Alka-Seltzer Effervescent. (Bayer) **Tab.:** 1700 mg sodium bicarbonate, 325 mg aspirin, 1000 mg citric acid, 9 mg phenylalanine, 506 mg sodium, aspartame. 24s. *otc.*
Use: Antacid.

Original Eclipse Sunscreen. (Triangle Labs) Padimate O, glyceryl PABA, SPF 10. Lot. Bot. 120 ml. *otc.*
Use: Sunscreen.

Original Sensodyne. (Block) Strontium chloride hexahydrate 10%, saccharin, sorbitol. Toothpaste. Tube 59.5 g. *otc.*
Use: Mouth and throat preparation.

Orimune. (Wyeth Lederle) Poliovirus vaccine. Live, Oral, Trivalent. Sabin strains Types 1, 2, and 3. Dose of 0.5 ml Dispette disposable pipette 1 dose. 10s and 50s. *Rx.*
Use: Agent for immunization.

Orinase. (Pharmacia & Upjohn) Tolbutamide 500 mg/Tab. Bot. 200s, 500s, 1000s, Unit-of-Use. 100s. *Rx.*
Use: Antidiabetic.

Orinase Diagnostic. (Pharmacia & Upjohn) Tolbutamide sodium 1 g/Vial. Pow. for inj. Vial with 20 ml amp diluent.
Use: Diagnostic aid.

Orisul. (Novartis) Sulfaphenazole. A sulfonamide under study.

ORLAAM. (Bio Development) Levomethadyl acetate HCl 10 mg, methylparaben 1.8 mg and propylparaben 0.2 mg/ ml. Soln. Bot. 474 ml. *c-II.*
Use: Narcotic agonist analgesic.

•**orlistat.** (ORE-lih-stat) USAN.
Use: Inhibitor (pancreatic lipase).

•**ormaplatin.** (ORE-mah-PLAT-in) USAN.
Use: Antineoplastic.

Ormazine. (Roberts) Chlorpromazine HCl 25 mg/ml. Vial 10 ml. *Rx.*
Use: Antipsychotic.

•**ormetoprim.** (ore-MEH-toe-PRIM) USAN.
Use: Antibacterial.

Ornade. (SK-Beecham) Phenylpropanolamine HCl 75 mg, chlorpheniramine maleate 12 mg/Spansule. Bot. 50s, 500s. *Rx.*
Use: Decongestant, antihistamine.

Ornex. (SK-Beecham) Acetaminophen 325 mg, phenylpropanolamine HCl 12.5 mg/Capl. Blister Pak 24s, 48s. Bot. 100s. Dispensary pak 792s. *otc.*
Use: Analgesic, decongestant.

Ornex, Maximum Strength. (Menley & James) Pseudoephedrine HCl, acetaminophen 500 mg. Cap. Bot. 24s, 30s, 48s. *otc.*

Use: Decongestant, analgesic.

Ornex, No Drowsiness. (Menley & James) **Cap.:** 30 mg pseudoephedrine HCl, 325 mg acetaminophen. In 24s and 48s. *otc.*
Use: Decongestant, analgesic.

•**ornidazole.** (ahr-NIH-DAH-zole) USAN.
Use: Anti-infective.

Ornidyl. (Hoechst Marion Roussel) Eflornithine HCl 200 mg/ml. Inj. Vial. 100 ml. *Rx.*
Use: Antiprotozoal.

•**orpanoxin.** (AHR-pan-OX-in) USAN.
Use: Anti-inflammatory.

Orpeneed VK. (Hanlon) Penicillin, buffered 400,000 units/Tab. Bot. 100s. *Rx.*
Use: Anti-infective, penicillin.

•**orphenadrine citrate,** (ore-FEN-uh-dreen) U.S.P. 23.
Use: Skeletal muscle relaxant, antihistamine.
See: Banflex (Forest Pharm.).
Flexoject (Mayrand).
Flexon, Inj. (Keene).
Myolin (Roberts Hauck).
Norflex, Tab., Amp. (3M Pharm).
Orphanate, Inj. (Hyrex).
W/Aspirin, phenacetin, caffeine.
See: Norgesic, Tab. (3M).
Norgesic Forte, Tab. (3M).

orphenadrine citrate. (Various Mfr.) **Inj.:** 30 mg/ml. Amps 2 ml, vial 10 ml. **Tab.:** 100 mg. Bot. 30s, 100s, 500s, 1000s.
Use: Skeletal muscle relaxant, antihistamine.

orphenadrine hydrochloride.
See: Disipal, Tab. (3M).
W/Comb.
See: Estomul, Liq., Tab. (3M).

Orphengesic. (Various Mfr.) Orphenadrine citrate 25 mg, aspirin 385 mg, caffeine 30 mg/Tab. Bot. 100s, 500s, UD 100s. *Rx.*
Use: Skeletal muscle relaxant, salicylate analgesic.

Orphengesic Forte. (Various Mfr.) Orphenadrine citrate 50 mg, aspirin 770 mg, caffeine 60 mg/Tab. Bot. 100s, 500s. *Rx.*
Use: Skeletal muscle relaxant, salicylate analgesic.

Ortac-DM Liquid. (ION) Dextromethorphan 10 mg, phenylephrine HCl 5 mg, guaifenesin 100 mg/5 ml. Bot. 4 oz. *otc.*
Use: Antitussive, decongestant, expectorant.

ortal sodium. Sodium 5-ethyl-5-hexylbarbiturate. Hexethal sodium.

ortedrine.

See: Amphetamine (Various Mfr.).

orthesin.
See: Benzocaine.

Ortho All-Flex Diaphragm. (Ortho) Diaphragm kit (all flex arcing spring) in plastic compact, sizes 55, 60, 65, 70, 75, 80, 85, 90, 95 mm. *Rx.*
Use: Contraceptive.

orthocaine.
See: Orthoform.

Ortho-Cept. (Ortho) Desogestrel 0.15 mg, ethinyl estradiol 0.03 mg. Tab. Pkg. 28s w/ 7 inert tab. and 21s. *Rx.*
Use: Oral contraceptive.

Orthoclone OKT3. (Ortho) Muromonab-CD3 5 mg per 5 ml. Inj. 5 ml amps. *Rx.*
Use: Immunosuppressive drug.

Ortho-Cyclen. (Ortho) Norgestimate 250 mcg, ethinyl estradiol 35 mcg. Tab. Pkg. 21s, 28s. *Rx.*
Use: Oral contraceptive.

Ortho Diaphragm. (Ortho) Diaphragm kit, coil spring sizes 50, 55, 60, 65, 70, 75, 80, 85, 90, 95, 100, 105 mm. *Rx.*
Use: Contraceptive.

Ortho Diaphragm-White. (Ortho) Diaphragm kit, flat spring sizes 55, 60, 65, 70, 75, 80, 85, 90, 95 mm. *Rx.*
Use: Contraceptive.

Ortho Dienestrol Cream. (Ortho) Dienestrol 0.01%. Tube 78 g with or without applicator. *Rx.*
Use: Estrogen.

Ortho-Est. (Ortho) **Tab.:** 0.625 or 1.25 mg estropipate, lactose. 100s. *Rx.*
Use: Estrogen.

Orthoflavin. (Enzyme Process) Vitamins C 150 mg, E 25 mg/Tab. Bot. 100s, 250s. *otc.*
Use: Vitamin supplement.

Orthoform. Menthyl 3-amino-4-hydroxybenzoate.
Use: Local anesthetic.
W/Tyrothricin. (Columbus) Tyrothricin 0.5 mg, tetracaine HCl 0.5%, epinephrine 1/1000 Soln. 2%/g. Oint., Tube oz.
Use: Anti-infective, ophthalmic.

Ortho-Gynol Contraceptive. (Advanced Care) Oxtoxynol 9. Gel. Tube. 75 g w/ applicator and 75 g, 114 g refills. *otc.*
Use: Contraceptive.

ortho-hydroxybenzoic acid. Salicylic Acid, U.S.P. 23.

orthohydroxyphenylmercuric chloride.
Use: Antiseptic.
W/Benzocaine, ephedrine HCl.
See: Myrimgacaine, Liq. (Pharmacia & Upjohn).
W/Benzocaine, parachlorometaxylenol,

benzalkonium Cl, phenol.
See: Unguentine Aerosol (Procter & Gamble).
W/Benzoic acid, salicylic acid.
See: NP-27 Liq. (Procter & Gamble).
W/Benzoic acid, salicylic acid, sec.-amyl-tricresols.
See: Salicresin, Liq.(Pharmacia & Upjohn).
W/Zinc acetate, salicylic acid, phenol.
See: Zemacol, Medicated Skin Lotion (Procter & Gamble).

Ortho-Novum 1/35-21. (Ortho) Norethindrone 1 mg, ethinyl estradiol 0.035 mg/Tab. Dialpak 21s. *Rx.*
Use: Oral contraceptive.

Ortho-Novum 1/35-28. (Ortho) Norethindrone 1 mg, ethinyl estradiol 0.035 mg/Tab. w/ 7 inert Tab. Dialpak 28s. *Rx.*
Use: Oral contraceptive.

Ortho-Novum 1/50-21. (Ortho) Norethindrone 1 mg, mestranol 50 mcg/Tab. Dialpak 21s. *Rx.*
Use: Oral contraceptive.

Ortho-Novum 1/50-28. (Ortho) Norethindrone 1 mg, mestranol 50 mcg/Tab. w/ 7 inert Tab. Dialpak 28s. *Rx.*
Use: Oral contraceptive.

Ortho-Novum 7/7/7-21 Tablets. (Ortho) Norethindrone 0.5 mg, ethinyl estradiol 0.035 mg/Tab.; norethindrone 0.75 mg, ethinyl estradiol 0.035 mg/Tab.; norethindrone 1 mg, ethinyl estradiol 0.035 mg/Tab. Dialpak 21s. *Rx.*
Use: Oral contraceptive.

Ortho-Novum 7/7/7-28 Tablets. (Ortho) Same as Ortho-Novum 7/7/7/-21 w/ 7 inert tab. Dialpak 28s. *Rx.*
Use: Oral contraceptive.

Ortho-Novum 10/11-21 Tablets. (Ortho) Norethindrone 0.5 mg, ethinyl estradiol 0.035 mg/Tab; norethindrone 1 mg, ethinyl estradiol 0.035 mg/Tab. Dialpak 21s. *Rx.*
Use: Oral contraceptive.

Ortho-Novum 10/11-28 Tablets. (Ortho) Norethindrone 0.5 mg, ethinyl estradiol 0.035 mg/Tab; norethindrone 1 mg, ethinyl estradiol 0.035 mg/Tab; w/inert tab. Dialpak 28s. *Rx.*
Use: Oral contraceptive.

Ortho Personal Lubricant. (Advanced Care) Greaseless, water soluble and non-staining aqueous hydrocolloid gel. Acid buffered to vaginal pH. Tube 2 oz, 4 oz. *otc.*
Use: Lubricant.

Ortho Tri-Cyclen. (Ortho) 7 white tablets containing norgestimate 0.18 mg, ethinyl estradiol 35 mcg; 7 light blue tablets containing norgestimate 0.215 mg, ethinyl estradiol 35 mcg; 7 blue tablets containing norgestimate 0.25 mg, ethinyl estradiol 35 mcg. Tab. Pkg. 21s, 28s. *Rx.*
Use: Oral contraceptive.

Orthoxicol Cough Syrup. (Roberts) Phenylpropanolamine HCl 8.3 mg, chlorpheniramine maleate 1.3 mg, dextromethorphan HBr 6.7 mg, alcohol 8%, sorbitol, parabens. Bot. 60 ml, 120 ml, 480 ml. *otc.*
Use: Decongestant, antihistamine, antitussive.

orthoxine. Methoxyphenamine.

orticalm.
Use: Hypotensive, tranquilizer.
See: Serpasil, Prod. (Squibb).

Orudis. (Wyeth-Ayerst) Ketoprofen 25 mg, 50 mg or 75 mg/Cap. Bot. **25 mg or 50 mg:** 100s; **75 mg:** 100s, 500s, UD 100s. *Rx.*
Use: Nonsteroidal anti-inflammatory, analgesic.

Orudis KT. (Whitehall-Robins) **Tab.:** 12.5 mg ketoprofen, tartrazine, sugar. In 50s. *otc.*
Use: Analgesic, NSAID.

Oruvail. (Wyeth-Ayerst) **SR Tab.:** Ketoprofen 100 mg, 150 mg or 200 mg/SR Tab. Bot. 100s, Redipak 100s. **SR Cap.:** 100 mg, 150 mg. 100s, Redipak 100s. *Rx.*
Use: Nonsteroidal anti-inflammatory, analgesic.

orvus.
See: Gardinol Type Detergents (Various Mfr.).

osarsal.
See: Acetarsone.

Os-Cal 250. (Hoechst Marion Roussel) Oyster shell powder as calcium 250 mg, vitamin D 125 IU and trace minerals (Cu, Fe, Mg, Mn, Zn, silica)/Tab. Bot. 100s, 240s, 500s, 1000s. *otc.*
Use: Vitamin/mineral supplement.

Os-Cal 500. (SK-Beecham) Calcium 500 mg/Tab. Bot. 60s, 120s. *otc.*
Use: Calcium supplement.

Os-Cal 250 + D. (SK-Beecham) Calcium carbonate 625 mg, vitamin D 125 units/Tab. Bot. 100s. *otc.*
Use: Vitamin/mineral supplement.

Os-Cal 500 + D. (SK-Beecham) Calcium carbonate 1250 mg, vitamin D 125 units/Tab. Bot. 60s. *otc.*
Use: Vitamin/mineral supplement.

Os-Cal 500 Chewable Tablets. (Hoechst Marion Roussel) Calcium 500 mg/Tab. Bot. 60s. *otc.*

Use: Calcium supplement.

Os-Cal-Fortified. (SmithKline Beecham) Calcium 250 mg, iron 5 mg, Mg, Mn, zinc 0.5 mg, vitamin A 1668 IU, D 125 IU, B₁ 1.7 mg, B₂ 1.7 mg, B₃ 15 mg, B₆ 2 mg, C 50 mg, E 0.8 IU, parabens/Tab. Bot. 100s. *otc.*
Use: Vitamin/mineral supplement.

Os-Cal Fortified Multivitamin & Minerals. (SmithKline Beecham) **Tab.**: 1668 IU vitamin A, 125 IU D, 0.8 IU E, 1.7 mg B₁, 1.7 mg B₂, 15 mg B₃, 2 mg B₆, 50 mg C, 5 mg Fe, 250 mg Ca, 0.5 mg Zn, Mn, Mg, EDTA, parabens. In 100s. *otc.*
Use: Vitamin/mineral supplement.

Os-Cal Plus. (SK-Beecham) Calcium 250 mg, vitamins D 125 IU, A 1666 IU, C 33 mg, B₂ 0.66 mg, B₁ 0.5 mg, B₆ 0.5 mg, niacinamide 3.33 mg, zinc 0.75 mg, manganese 0.75 mg, iron 16.6 mg/Tab. Bot. 100s. *otc.*
Use: Vitamin/mineral supplement.

Osmitrol. (Baxter) Mannitol in water. **5%:** 1000 ml; **10%:** 500 ml, 1000 ml; **15%:** 150 ml, 500 ml; **20%:** 250 ml, 500 ml. Mannitol in 0.3% sodium **5%:** 1000 ml. Mannitol in 0.45% sodium **20%:** 500 ml. *Rx.*
Use: Osmotic diuretic.
See: Mannitol.

Osmoglyn. (Alcon Surgical) Glycerin 50% in flavored aqueous vehicle. Plastic bot. 6 oz. *Rx.*
Use: Osmotic diuretic.

Osmolite. (Ross) Isotonic liquid food containing 1.06 calories/ml. Two quarts (2000 calories) provides 100% US RDA vitamins and minerals for adults and children. Osmolality: 300 mOsm/kg water. Ready-to-Use: Bot. Can 8 fl oz, 32 fl oz. *otc.*
Use: Nutritional supplement.

Osmolite HN. (Ross) High nitrogen isotonic liquid food containing 1.06 calories/ml; 1400 calories provides 100% US RDA vitamins and minerals for adults and children. Osmolality: 300 mOsm/kg water. Ready-to-Use: Bot. 8 fl oz. Can 8 fl oz, 32 fl oz. *otc.*
Use: Nutritional supplement.

Osmotic Diuretics.
See: Mannitol (Various Mfr.).
Osmitrol (Baxter).
Ureaphil (Abbott).
Glyrol (Ciba Vision).
Osmoglyn (Alcon).
Ismotic (Alcon).

ospolot.
Use: Anticonvulsant drug; pending release.

Ossonate Capsule. (Marcen) Cartilage mucopolysaccharide extract, chondroitin sulfate 50 mg/Cap. Bot. 100s, 500s, 1000s.

Ossonate-Plus, Caps. (Marcen) Ossonate-mucopolysaccharide extract 50 mg, acetaminophen 300 mg, salicylamide 200 mg/Cap. Bot. 100s, 500s, 1000s. *otc.*
Use: Antiarthritic.

Ossonate-Plus, Inj. (Marcen) Ossonate cartilage mucopolysaccharide extract 12.5 mg, casein hydrolysates 80 mg, sulfur 20 mg, sodium citrate 5 mg, benzyl alcohol 0.5%, phenol 0.5%/ml. Multidose 10 ml vial. *Rx.*
Use: Skeletal muscle relaxant, pain reliever.

Ossonate-75. (Marcen) Chondroitin sulfate 37.5 mg, benzyl alcohol 0.5%, phenol 0.5%, sodium citrate 5 mg/ml. Vial 10 ml. *Rx.*
Use: Infantile and atopic eczemas, drug allergies, dermatoses associated with intestinal toxemias.

Osteocalcin. (Arcola) Calcitonin-salmon 200 IU, phenol 5 mg/ml. Inj. Vial 2 ml. *Rx.*
Use: Hormone for regulation of calcium and bone metabolism.

Osteo-D. (Lemmon)
See: Secalciferol.

Osteolate Injection. (Fellows) Sodium thiosalicylate 50 mg, benzyl alcohol 2%/ml. Vial 30 ml. *Rx.*
Use: Salicylate analgesic.

Osteo-Mins. (Tyson) Powd.: 500 mg vitamin C, 250 mg Ca, 250 mg Mg, 45 mg K, 100 IU D/4.5 g. Sugar free. 200 g. *otc.*
Use: Vitamin supplement.

Osteon/D. (Pasadena Research) Calcium 600 mg, phosphorus 400 mg, magnesium 240 mg, vitamin D 400 IU/6 Tab. Bot. 180s. *Rx.*
Use: Vitamin/mineral supplement.

Osti-Derm Lotion. (Pedinol) Aluminum sulfate, phenol, zinc oxide, camphor, glycerin, sorbitol, magnesium carbonate, bentonite 670, cabosil, acetic acid lelcoloid HVF, Tween 20, calcium carbonate. Lot. Bot. 42.5 g. *otc.*
Use: Antipruritic, astringent, topical.

Ostiderm Roll-On. (Pedinol) Aluminum chlorohydrate, aluminum sulfate, glycerin, phenol, camphor, alcohol, sorbitol, calcium carbonate, bentonite, hydroxypropylcellulose, polysorbate-20, EDTA, diazolidinyl urea, sodium benzoate, potassium sorbate. Bot. 88.7 ml. *otc.*

Use: Antipruritic, astringent, topical.

Osto-K. (Parthenon) Potassium 1 mEq (39 mg from gluconate, Cl and citrate), vitamin C 25 mg, sodium 0.52 mg/Tab. Bot. 60s. *otc.*
Use: Vitamin/mineral supplement.

osvarsan.
See: Acetarsone.

Otic-Care. (Parmed) Hydrocortisone 1%, neomycin sulfate 5 mg, polymyxin B sulfate 10,000 units/ml, glycerin, hydrochloric acid, propylene glycol, potassium metabisulfite. Soln. *Rx.*
Use: Otic preparation.

Otic Domeboro. (Bayer) Acetic acid 2%, aluminum acetate solution. Plastic dropper bot 2 oz. *Rx.*
Use: Otic preparation.

Otic-HC. (Roberts) Chloroxylenol 1 mg, pramoxine HCl 10 mg, hydrocortisone alcohol 10 mg, benzalkonium Cl 0.2 mg/ml. Bot. 12 ml. *Rx.*
Use: Otic preparation.

Otic-Neo-Cort Dome.
See: Neo-Cort Dome Otic Soln. (Bayer).

Otic-Plain. (Roberts) Chloroxylenol 1 mg, pramoxine HCl 10 mg, benzalkonium Cl 0.2 mg/ml. Bot. 12 ml. *Rx.*
Use: Otic preparation.

Otic Solution No. 1. (Foy) Hydrocortisone alcohol 10 mg, pramoxine HCl 10 mg, benzalkonium Cl 0.2 mg, acetic acid glacial 20 mg/ml w/propylene glycol q.s. *Rx.*
Use: Otic preparation.

Oti-Med. (Hyrex) **Drops:** 1 mg chloroxyphenol, 10 mg pramoxine HCl, 10 mg hydrocortisone, propylene glycol. 10 ml. *Rx.*
Use: Otic preparation.

Otobiotic Otic Solution. (Schering-Plough) Polymyxin B, hydrocortisone in propylene glycol and glycerin vehicle w/edetate disodium, sodium bisulfite, anhydrous sodium sulfite, purified water. Bot. w/dropper 15 ml. *Rx.*
Use: Otic preparation.

Otocain. (Holloway) Benzocaine 20%, benzethonium Cl 0.1%, glycerin 1%, polyethylene glycol. Soln. Bot. 15 ml. *Rx.*
Use: Otic preparation.

Otocalm-H Ear Drops. (Parmed) Pramoxine HCl 10 mg, hydrocortisone alcohol 10%, p-Chloro-m-Xylenol 1 mg, benzalkonium Cl 0.2 mg, acetic acid glacial 20 mg, propylene glycol/ml. Bot. 10 ml. *Rx.*
Use: Otic preparation.

Otocort Sterile Solution. (Lemmon) Neomycin sulfate equivalent to 3.5 mg neomycin base, polymyxin B sulfate 10,000 units, hydrocortisone 10 mg/ml, propylene glycol, glycerin, potassium metabisulfite, HCl, purified water. Bot. 10 ml. *Rx.*
Use: Otic preparation.

Otocort Sterile Suspension. (Lemmon) Neomycin sulfate equivalent to 3.5 mg neomycin base, polymyxin B sulfate 10,000 units, hydrocortisone 10 mg/ml, cetyl alcohol, propylene glycol, polysorbate 80, thimerosal, water for injection. Bot. 10 ml. *Rx.*
Use: Otic preparation.

Otogesic HC Solution. (Lexis) Polymyxin B sulfate 10,000 IU, neomycin sulfate 3.5 mg, hydrocortisone 10 mg/ml, potassium metabisulfite 0.1%. Bot. 10 ml. *Rx.*
Use: Otic preparation.

Otogesic HC Suspension. (Lexis) Polymyxin B sulfate 10,000 units, neomycin sulfate 3.5 mg, hydrocortisone 10 mg/ml, benzalkonium Cl 0.01%. Bot. 10 ml. *Rx.*
Use: Otic preparation.

Otomycin-HPN. (Misemer) Polymyxin B sulfate 10,000 units, neomycin sulfate 3.5 mg, hydrocortisone 10 mg/ml. Bot. w/dropper 10 ml. *Rx.*
Use: Otic preparation.

Otrivin. (Geigy) Xylometazoline HCl. **Nasal Drops:** 0.1% w/sodium Cl, phenylmercuric acetate 1:50,000. Dropper bot. 20 ml. **Nasal Spray:** 0.1% w/potassium phosphate monobasic, potassium Cl, sodium phosphate dibasic, sodium Cl, benzalkonium Cl 1:5000. Plastic squeeze spray 15 ml. **Ped. Nasal Soln. Drops:** 0.05%. Bot. 20 ml. *otc.*
Use: Decongestant.

ouabain octahydrate. Ouabain, U.S.P. 23.

Outgro. (Whitehall Robins) Chlorobutanol 5%, tannic acid 25%, isopropyl alcohol 83%. Bot. 13 oz. *otc.*
Use: Ingrown toenail preparation.

ovarian extract. Aqueous extract of whole ovaries of cattle.
Use: Estrogen.

ovarian substance. (Various Mfr.) Whole ovarian substance from cattle, sheep or swine. *Rx.*
Use: Estrogen.

Ovastat. (Medac)
See: Treosulfan.

Ovcon-35. (Bristol-Myers) Norethindrone

0.4 mg, ethinyl estradiol 0.035 mg/Tab. Ctn. 6×21s. *Rx.*
Use: Oral contraceptive.

Ovcon-35, 28 Day. (Bristol-Myers) Norethindrone 0.4 mg, ethinyl estradiol 0.035 mg, w/7 inert tab/Carton 6×28s. *Rx.*
Use: Oral contraceptive.

Ovcon-50. (Bristol-Myers) Norethindrone 1 mg, ethinyl estradiol 0.05 mg/Tab. Ctn. 6×21s. *Rx.*
Use: Oral contraceptive.

Ovcon-50, 28 Day. (Bristol-Myers) Norethindrone 1 mg, ethinyl estradiol 0.05 mg, w/7 inert tab/Carton. 6×28s. *Rx.*
Use: Oral contraceptive.

Ovide. (GenDerm) Malathion 0.5%. Lot. Bot. 59 ml. *Rx.*
Use: Scabicide, pediculicide.

ovifollin.
See: Estrone (Various Mfr.).

Ovlin. (Sig) **Tab.:** Ethinyl estradiol 0.02 mg, conjugated estrogens 0.2 mg/Tab. Bot. 100s, 1000s. **Inj.:** Estrone 2 mg, estradiol 0.05 mg, vitamin B_{12} 1000 mcg/ml. Vial 30 ml. *Rx.*
Use: Estrogen.

Ovocylin Dipropionate. (Novartis) Estradiol dipropionate. *Rx.*
Use: Estrogen.

Ovral. (Wyeth-Ayerst) Norgestrel 0.5 mg, ethinyl estradiol 0.05 mg/Tab. 6 Pilpak dispensers, 21 Tab. Tripak 63s. *Rx.*
Use: Oral contraceptive.

Ovral-28. (Wyeth-Ayerst) Norgestrel 0.5 mg, ethinyl estradiol 0.05 mg/Tab. w/7 inert Tab. Pilpak dispenser 6s containing 21 Tab, 7 inert Tab. *Rx.*
Use: Oral contraceptive.

Ovrette. (Wyeth-Ayerst) Norgestrel 0.075 mg/Tab. 6 Pilpak dispenser, Tab. 28s. *Rx.*
Use: Oral contraceptive.

Ovugen. (BioGenex) In vitro diagnostic test for measurement of LH urine to determine ovulation. Kits. 6s, 10s.
Use: Ovulation test.

Ovukit Self-Test. (Monoclonal Antibodies) Monoclonal antibody-based enzyme immunoassay test for hLH in urine. Kit 6, 9 day.
Use: Ovulation test.

ovulation stimulants.
See: Clomid (Merrell Dow).
Serophene (Serono).
Metrodin (Serono).

ovulation tests.
See: Answer Ovulation (Carter).
Clearplan Easy (Whitehall Robins).

OvuQUICK Self-Test (Monoclonal Antibodies).
Color Ovulation Test (Biomerica).
Conceive Ovulation Predictor (Quidel).
First Response Ovulation Predictor Test Kit (Carter Products).
Fortel Home Ovulation Test (Biomerica).
OvuGen (BioGenex).
OvuKIT Self-Test (Monoclonal Antibodies).

Ovulen-21. (Searle) Ethynodiol diacetate 1 mg, mestranol 0.1 mg/Tab. Compack Disp. 21s, 6×21, 24 ×21. Refill 21s, 12×21. *Rx.*
Use: Oral contraceptive.

Ovulen-28. (Searle) Ethynodiol diacetate 1 mg, mestranol 0.1 mg/Tab. w/7 inert Tab. Compack 28s: 21 active tab., 7 placebo tab. Compack dispenser 28s. Box 6×28. Refill 28s, Box 12×28. *Rx.*
Use: Oral contraceptive.

Ovustick Self-Test. (Monoclonal Antibodies) Home test for ovulation. Test kit 10s.
Use: Diagnostic aid.

Oxabid. (Jamieson-McKames) Magnesium oxide 140 mg or magnesium oxide heavy 400 mg/Cap. Bot. 100s. *otc.*
Use: Antacid.

•**oxacillin, sodium,** (ox-uh-SILL-in) U.S.P. 23.
Use: Antibacterial.
See: Bactocill, Cap., Vial (SK-Beecham).
Prostaphilin, Preps. (Bristol).
Sodium oxacillin.

oxadimedine hydrochloride.
Use: Antiarrhythmic.

oxafuradene. Name used for Nifuradene. (OX-ah-FYOOR-ah-deen)
Use: Platelet aggregation agent.

•**oxagrelate.** (OX-ah-greh-LATE) USAN.
Use: Platelet aggregation inhibitor.

oxaliplatin. (Axion) *Rx.*
Use: Treatment of ovarian cancer. [Orphan drug]

•**oxamarin hydrochloride.** (OX-ah-mah-rin) USAN.
Use: Hemostatic.

•**oxamisole hydrochloride.** (ox-AM-ih-sole) USAN.
Use: Immunoregulator.

•**oxamniquine,** (ox-AM-nih-kwin) U.S.P. 23.
Use: Antischistosomal, treatment of schistosomiasis.
See: Vansil, Cap. (Pfizer Laboratories).

oxanamide.
Use: Tranquilizer.

Oxandrin. (Bio-Technology) **Tab.:** 2.5 mg oxandrolone, lactose. In 100s. *c-III.*
Use: Anabolic steroid.

•**oxandrolone,** (ox-AN-droe-lone) U.S.P. 23.
Use: Androgen, anabolic. [Orphan drug]
See: Anavar, Tab. (Searle).

•**oxantel pamoate.** (OX-an-tell-PAM-oh-ate) USAN.
Use: Anthelmintic.

•**oxaprotiline hydrochloride.** (OX-ah-PRO-tih-leen) USAN.
Use: Antidepressant.

•**oxaprozin.** (OX-ah-pro-zin) USAN.
Use: Anti-inflammatory.
See: Daypro.

•**oxarbazole.** (ox-AHR-bah-zole) USAN.
Use: Antiasthmatic.

•**oxatomide.** (ox-AT-ah-mid) USAN.
Use: Antiallergic, antiasthmatic.

•**oxazepam,** (ox-AZE-uh-pam) U.S.P. 23.
Use: Sedative; tranquilizer (minor).
See: Serax, Cap., Tab. (Wyeth-Ayerst).

oxazolindinediones.
See: Paradione (Abbott).
Tridione (Abbott).

ox bile extract. Purified oxgall.
See: Bile Extract, Ox.

•**oxendolone.** (OX-en-doe-LONE) USAN.
Use: Antiandrogen (benign prostatic hypertrophy).

•**oxethazaine.** (OX-ETH-ah-zane) USAN.
Use: Topical anesthetic.

•**oxetorone fumarate.** (ox-EH-toe-rone) USAN.
Use: Agent for migraine.

•**oxfendazole.** (ox-FEN-DAH-zole) USAN.
Use: Anthelmintic.
See: Synanthic (Syntex).

•**oxfenicine.** (OX-FEN-ih-seen) USAN.
Use: Vasodilator.

ox gall.
See: Bile Extract, Ox.

•**oxibendazole.** (ox-ee-BEND-ah-zole) USAN.
Use: Anthelmintic.

•**oxiconazole nitrate.** (ox-ee-KAHN-ah-zole) USAN.
Use: Antifungal.
See: Oxistat Cream (Glaxo Dermatology).
Oxistat Lotion (Glaxo).

oxidized bile acids.
See: Bile Acids, Oxidized.

oxidized cellulose. Absorbable cellulose. Cellulosic acid.

Use: Local hemostatic.
See: Oxycel, **Pad, Pledg., Strip.** (Becton-Dickinson).
Surgicel, **Stip, Nu-knid.** (Johnson & Johnson).

•**oxidopamine.** (OX-ih-DOE-pah-meen) USAN.
Use: Adrenergic (ophthalmic).

•**oxidronic acid.** (OX-ih-DRAHN-ik) USAN.
Use: Regulator (calcium).

Oxi-Freeda. (Freeda) Vitamin A 5000 IU, E 150 mg, B_3 40 mg, C 100 mg, B_1 20 mg, B_2 20 mg, B_5 20 mg, B_6 20 mg, B_{12} 10 mcg, Zn 15 mg, Se, glutathione, L-cysteine. Tab. Bot. 100s, 250s. *otc.*
Use: Vitamin/mineral supplement.

•**oxifungin hydrochloride.** (OX-ih-FUN-jin) USAN.
Use: Antifungal.

•**oxilorphan.** (ox-ih-LORE-fan) USAN.
Use: Antagonist to narcotics.

•**oximonam.** (OX-ih-MOE-nam) USAN.
Use: Anti-infective, antibacterial.

•**oximonam sodium.** (OX-ih-MOE-nam) USAN.
Use: Anti-infective, antibacterial.

oxine.
See: Oxyquinoline sulfate (Various Mfr.).

•**oxiperomide.** (ox-ih-PURR-oh-mide) USAN.
Use: Antipsychotic.

Oxipor VHC Psoriasis Lotion. (Whitehall Robins) **Lot.:** Coal tar soln. 25%, alcohol 79%. 56 ml. *otc.*
Use: Antipsoriatic.

•**oxiramide.** (ox-EER-am-ide) USAN.
Use: Cardiac depressant (antiarrhythmic).

Oxistat. (Glaxo Derm.) Oxiconazole nitrate 1%. **Cream:** Tube 15 g, 30 g; **Lotion:** Bot. 30 ml. *Rx.*
Use: Antifungal, topical.

•**oxisuran.** (OX-ih-SUH-ran) USAN.
Use: Antineoplastic.

•**oxmetidine hydrochloride.** (ox-MEH-tih-DEEN) USAN.
Use: Antagonist to histamine H_2 receptors.

•**oxmetidine mesylate.** (ox-MEH-tih-DEEN) USAN.
Use: Antagonist to histimine H_2 receptors.

•**oxogestone phenpropionate.** (ox-oh-JESS-tone fen-PRO-pih-oh-nate) USAN.
Use: Progestin.

Oxolamine. (Arcum) Crystalline hydroxycobalamin 1000 mcg/ml. Vial 10 ml. *Rx.*

Use: Vitamin B$_{12}$ supplement.

•**oxolinic acid.** (ox-oh-LIH-nik Acid) USAN.
Use: Antibacterial.

oxophenarsine hydrochloride.
l-2-oxothiazolidine$_4$-carboxylic acid. *Rx.*
Use: Treatment of adult respiratory distress syndrome. [Orphan drug]
See: Procysteine.

Oxothiazolidine Carboxylate. (Clintec Nutritional/Ben Venise Labs) Phase I restoration of glutathione depletion in HIV, ARC, AIDS; prevention of inflammation-induced HIV replication. *Rx.*
Use: Immunomodulator.

oxpheneridine. 1-(β-phenyl-βhydroxyethyl)-4-carbethoxy-4- phenylpiperidine.

•**oxprenolol hydrochloride,** (ox-PREHno-lole) U.S.P. 23. Under study.
Use: Beta-adrenergic receptor blocking agent, vasodilator (coronary).

Oxsoralen Lotion. (ICN Pharm) Methoxsalen 1% in an inert lotion vehicle of alcohol 71%, propylene glycol, acetone, water. Bot. oz. *Rx.*
Use: Psoralen, topical.

Oxsoralen Ultra. (ICN Pharm) **Soft Cap.:** 10 mg methoxsalen. 50s, 100s. *Rx.*
Use: Psoralen, topical.

•**oxtriphylline,** U.S.P. 23. Oral Soln, ER Tab., U.S.P. 23. Choline theophyllinate.
Use: Bronchodilator.
See: Choledyl, Tab., Elix. (Parke-Davis).
W/Guaifenesin.
See: Brondecon, Tab., Elix. (Parke-Davis).

oxtriphylline and guaifenesin elixir. (Barre-National) Oxtriphylline 300 mg, guaifenesin 150 mg, alcohol 20%/15 ml. Elix. Bot. pt, gal. *Rx.*
Use: Bronchodilator, expectorant.

Oxy-5 Acne-Pimple Medication. (SK-Beecham) Benzoyl peroxide 5% in lotion base. Bot. fl oz. *otc.*
Use: Antiacne.

Oxy 5 Tinted. (SK-Beecham) Benzoyl peroxide 5%, titanium dioxide, sodium PCA, cetyl alcohol, silica, iron oxides, propylene glycol, citric acid, sodium laurel sulfate, stearyl alcohol, parabens. Lot. Bot. 30 ml. *otc.*
Use: Antiacne.

Oxy 10 Maximun Strength Advanced Formula. (SK-Beecham) Benzoyl peroxide 10%, EDTA. Gel. 30 g. *otc.*
Use: Antiacne.

Oxy 10 Wash. (SK-Beecham) Benzoyl peroxide 10%, parabens, diazolidinyl

urea. Liq. Bot. 120 ml. *otc.*
Use: Antiacne.

•**oxybenzone,** U.S.P. 23. Cyasorb UV 9 (Lederle).
Use: Ultraviolet screen.
W/Dioxybenzone, benzophenone.
See: Solbar, Lot. (Person & Covey).

oxybenzone with combinations.
See: Coppertone, Prods. (Schering-Plough).
Noskote, Cream (Schering-Plough).
Shade, Prods. (Schering-Plough).
Sunger, Prods. (Schering-Plough).
Super Shade, Lot. (Schering-Plough).

•**oxybutynin chloride,** (OX-ee-BYOO-tih-nin) U.S.P. 23.
Use: Anticholinergic.
See: Ditropan Syr., Tab. (Hoechst Marion Roussel).
Oxybutynin Cl (Bristol-Myers).

Oxycel. (Becton-Dickinson) Cellulosic acid in absorbable hemostatic agent prepared from cellulose. Resembles ordinary surgical gauze or cotton. Pledget 2 × 1 × 1 in. 10s. Pad 3 × 3 in. 8 ply. 10s. Strip 5 × 0.5 in. 4 ply. 18 × 2 in. 4 ply. 10s. 36 × 0.5 in. 4 ply. *Rx.*
Use: Hemostatic, topical.

Oxycet. (Halsey) Oxycodone HCl 5 mg, acetaminophen 325 mg/Tab. Bot. 100s, 500s, Hospital pack 250s. *c-II.*
Use: Narcotic analgesic combination.

Oxy-Chinol. (Ferndale) Potassium oxyquinoline sulfate 1 gr/Tab. Bot. 100s, 1000s. *otc.*
Use: Deodorizer, bacteriostatic.

•**oxychlorosene.** (OCK-sih-KLOR-ah-seen) USAN. Monoxychlorosene. Hydrocarbon derivative containing fourteen carbons and hypochlorous acid. The hydrocarbon chain also has a phenyl substituent which in turn holds a sulfonic acid group.
Use: Anti-infective (topical).
See: Clorpactin, Prod. (Scrip).

•**oxychlorosene sodium.** (OCK-sih-KLOR-ah-seen) USAN. Sodium salt of the complex derived from hypochlorous acid and tetradecylbenzene sulfonic acid. Action of active chlorine.
Use: Anti-infective (topical).

Oxy Clean Lathering Facial. (SK-Beecham) Sodium tetraborate decahydrate dissolving particles in a base of surfactant cleaning agents. Soap free. Scrub 79.5 g. *otc.*
Use: Anti-acne.

Oxy Clean Medicated Cleanser and Pads. (SK-Beecham) **Cleanser and reg. strength pads:** Salicylic acid

0.5%, SD alcohol 40 B 40%, citric acid, menthol, sodium lauryl sulfate. **Max. strength pads:** Salicylic acid 2%, SD alcohol 40 B 50%, citric acid, menthol, sodium lauryl sulfate. Cleanser 120 ml Pad. 50s. *otc.*
Use: Anti-acne.

Oxy Clean Medicated Pads for Sensitive Skin. (SK-Beecham) Salicylic acid 0.5%, SD alcohol 40B 16%. Jar 50s. *otc.*
Use: Anti-acne.

Oxy Clean Scrub. (SK-Beecham) Sodium tetraborate decahydrate dissolving particles in a base of surfactant cleaning agents, soap free. Lot. Bot. 79.5 g. *otc.*
Use: Anti-acne.

Oxy Clean Soap. (SK-Beecham) Salicylic acid 3.5%, sodium borate. Bar 97.5 g. *otc.*
Use: Anti-acne.

•**oxycodone.** (OX-ee-KOE-dohn) USAN.
Use: Narcotic analgesic.

oxycodone and aspirin. (Various Mfr.) Oxycodone HCl 4.5 mg, oxycodone terephthalate 0.38 mg, aspirin 325 mg/ Tab. Bot. 100s, 500s, 1000s, UD 25s. *c-II.*
Use: Narcotic analgesic combination.

oxycodone and acetaminophen capsules. (OX-ee-KOE-dohn and ass-cet-ah-MEE-noe-fen) (Various Mfr.) Oxycodone HCl 5 mg, acetaminophen 500 mg/Cap. Bot. 100s, 500s, 1000s, UD 25s. *c-II.*
Use: Narcotic analgesic combination.

oxycodone and acetaminophen tablets. (OX-ee-KOE-dohn and ass-cet-ah-MEE-noe-fen) (Various Mfr.) Oxycodone HCl 5 mg, acetaminophen 325 mg/Tab. Bot. 100s, 500s, 1000s, UD 25s. *c-II.*
Use: Narcotic analgesic combination.

•**oxycodone hydrochloride,** (OX-ee-KOE-dohn) U.S.P. 23.
Use: Narcotic analgesic.
See: Dihydrohydroxycodeinone HCl.
W/Acetaminophen, oxycodone terephthalate.
See: Percocet-5, Tab. (DuPont Merck).
Tylox, Cap. (McNeil).

•**oxycodone terephthalate,** (OX-ee-KOE-dohn teh-REFF-thah-late) U.S.P. 23.
Use: Analgesic (narcotic).

OxyContin. (Perdue Pharma) **CR-Tab.:** 10, 20, 40 mg oxycodone HCl. Lactose. 100s. *c-II.*
Use: Narcotic analgesic.

Oxy Cover. (SK-Beecham) Benzoyl peroxide 10%. Cream. 30 g. *otc.*
Use: Antiacne.

oxyethylated tertiary octylphenol-formaldehyde polymer.
See: Triton WR-1339 (Rohm & Haas).

oxyethylene oxypropylene polymer.
See: Poloxalkol.
W/Danthron, B₁, carboxymethyl cellulose.
See: Evactol, Cap. (Delta).

•**oxyfilcon A.** (OX-ee-FILL-kahn A) USAN.
Use: Contact lens material (hydrophilic).

•**oxygen,** U.S.P. 23.
Use: Gas, medicinal.

•**oxygen 93 percent,** U.S.P. 23.
Use: Gas, medicinal.

OxyIR. (Purdue Pharma.) Oxycodone HCl 5 mg/IR Tab. Bot. 100s. *c-II.*
Use: Narcotic analgesic.

Oxy Medicated Cleanser and Regular Strength Pads. (SK-Beecham) Salicylic acid 0.5%, SD alcohol 28%, citric acid, menthol, propylene glycol. Cleanser. Bot. 120 ml. Pads 50s, 90s. *otc.*
Use: Anti-acne.

Oxy Medicated Cleanser and Maximum Strength Pads. (SK-Beecham) Salicylic acid 2%, SD alcohol 44%, citric acid, menthol, propylene glycol. Cleanser. Bot. 120 ml. Pads 50s, 90s. *otc.*
Use: Anti-acne.

Oxy Medicated Cleanser and Sensitive Skin Pads. (SK-Beecham) Salicylic acid 0.5%, alcohol 22%, disodium lauryl sulfosuccinate, menthol, trisodium EDTA. Cleanser. Bot. 120 ml. Pads 50s, 90s. *otc.*
Use: Anti-acne.

Oxy Medicated Soap. (SK Beecham) Triclosan 1%, bentonite, cocoamphodipropionate, iron oxides, glycerin, magnesium silicate, sodium borohydride, sodium cocoate, sodium tallowate, talc, EDTA, titanium dioxide. Bar. 97.5 g. *otc.*
Use: Anti-acne.

oxymetazoline hydrochloride.
Use: Vasoconstrictors, mydriatics (ophthalmic).
See: Ocuclear (Schering-Plough).
Visine (Pfizer).

•**oxymetazoline hydrochloride,** (OX-ee-MET-azz-oh-leen) U.S.P. 23.
Use: Decongestant, adrenergic (vasoconstrictor).
See: Afrin, Nasal Spray, Soln. (Schering-Plough).
Duration Nasal Spray (Schering-Plough).

Duration Nose Drops (Schering-Plough).

Duration Nose Drops for Children (Schering-Plough).

St. Joseph Nasal Spray for Children (Schering-Plough).

St. Joseph Nose Drops for Children (Schering-Plough).

•**oxymetholone,** (OCK-sih-METH-oh-lone) U.S.P. 23.
Use: Androgen.
See: Anadrol, Tab. (Syntex).

•**oxymorphone hydrochloride,** U.S.P. 23.
Use: Analgesic (narcotic). [Orphan drug]
See: Numorphan Amp., Vial, Supp. (Du-Pont Merck).

Oxy Night Watch. (SK-Beecham) Salicylic acid 1%, cetyl alcohol, silica, propylene glycol, stearyl alcohol, sodium laureth sulfate, parabens, EDTA. Lot. Bot. 60 ml. *otc.*
Use: Antiacne.

Oxy Night Watch Maximum Strength. (SK-Beecham) Salicylic acid 2%, cetyl alcohol, EDTA, parabens, stearyl alcohol. Lot. Bot. 60 ml. *otc.*
Use: Antiacne.

Oxy Night Watch Sensitive Skin. (SK-Beecham) Salicylic acid 1%, cetyl alcohol, EDTA, stearyl alcohol, parabens. Lot. Bot. 60 ml. *otc.*
Use: Antiacne.

•**oxypertine.** (OX-ee-PURR-teen) USAN. Integrin hydrochloride.
Use: Psychotropic, antidepressant.

•**oxyphenbutazone,** U.S.P. 23.
Use: Antiarthritic, anti-inflammatory, analgesic, antipyretic, antirheumatic.
See: Oxalid, Tab. (Rhone-Poulenc Rorer).

oxyphencyclimine hydrochloride, U.S.P. XXII.
Use: Antispasmodic.
See: Daricon, Tab. (SK-Beecham).
W/Hydroxyzine HCl.
See: Enarax, Tab. (SK-Beecham).
W/Phenobarbital.
See: Daricon-PB, Tab. (SK-Beecham).

•**oxyphenisatin acetate.** (OX-ee-fen-EYE-sah-tin) USAN.
Use: Laxative.
See: Endophenolphthalein (Roche).
Isacen (No Mfr. currently lists).
Prulet, Tab. (Mission).
Prulet Liquitab. (Mission).

•**oxyphenudrine.**

•**oxypurinol.** (OX-ee-PYOO-ree-nahl) USAN.

Use: Xanthine oxidase inhibitor.

•**oxyquinoline.** (OX-ih-KWIN-oh-lin) USAN.
Use: Disinfectant.

oxyquinoline benzoate. (Merck) Pkg. lb. 8-Hydroxyquinoline benzoate.
W/Alkyl aryl sulfonate, disodium edetate, aminacrine HCl, copper sulfate, sodium sulfate.
See: Triva, Vaginal Jelly, Pow. (Boyle).
W/Benzoic acid, salicylic acid, sodium tetradecyl sulfate.
See: NP-27 Cream (Procter & Gamble).

•**oxyquinoline sulfate,** (OX-ih-KWIN-oh-lin) N.F. 18.
Use: Disinfectant, pharmaceutic aid (complexing agent).
See: Chinosol, Tab., Pow., Vial (Vernon).

oxyquinoline sulfate w/combinations.
See: Oxyzal Wet Dressing, Soln. (Gordon).
Rectal Medicone, Oint. (Medicone).
Rectal Medicone-HC, Oint. (Medicone).
Rectal Medicone Unguent, Oint. (Medicone).
Trapens, Tab. (Mills).
Triticoll, Tab. (Western Research).
Triva, Douche Pow. (Boyle).

Oxy ResiDON'T. (SK-Beecham) Triclosan 0.6%, diazolidinyl urea. Liq. Bot. 240 ml. *otc.*
Use: Antiseptic, germicide.

Oxy ResiDON'T Medicated Face Wash. (SK-Beecham) Cocamidopropyl betaine, sodium laureth sulfate, sodium cocoyl isethionate, triclosan, diazolidinyl urea. Liq. Bot. 240 ml. *otc.*
Use: Antiacne.

Oxy-Scrub. (SK-Beecham) Abradant cleanser containing dissolving abradant particles of sodium tetraborate decahydrate. Tube 2.65 oz. *otc.*
Use: Antiacne.

Oxysept. (Allergan) **Disinfecting Soln.:** Hydrogen peroxide 3%, sodium stannate, sodium nitrate, phosphate buffer. Bot. 240 ml or 360 ml. **Neutralizer Tab.:** Catalase, buffering agents. In 12s (w/Oxy-Tab cup) or 36s. *otc.*
Use: Soft contact lens care.

Oxysept 1. (Allergan) Microfiltered hydrogen peroxide 3% w/sodium stannate and sodium nitrate, preservative free, buffered. Soln. Bot. 355 ml. *otc.*
Use: Contact lens product.

Oxysept 2. (Allergan) Catalytic neutralizing agent, EDTA, sodium Cl, mono- and dibasic sodium phosphates. Buffered,

preservative free. Soln. In 15 ml single-use containers (25s). *otc.*
Use: Contact lens product.

•**oxytetracycline**, U.S.P. 23.
Use: Anti-infective, antibacterial.
See: Terramycin, Prods. (Pfizer Laboratories).

oxytetracycline and hydrocortisone acetate ophthalmic suspension.
Use: Anti-infective, anti-inflammatory.

oxytetracycline and nystatin capsules.
Use: Anti-infective, antifungal.

oxytetracycline and nystatin for oral suspension.
Use: Anti-infective, antifungal.

oxytetracycline and phenazopyridine hydrochlorides and sulfamethizole capsules.
Use: Anti-infective, urinary analgesic, antispasmodic.

•**oxytetracycline calcium**, U.S.P. 23.
Use: Anti-infective, antibacterial.

•**oxytetracycline hydrochloride**, U.S.P. 23. An antibiotic from *Streptomyces rimosus.*
Use: Anti-infective, antirickettsial, antibacterial.
See: Dalimycin, Cap. (Dalin).
Oxlopar, Cap. (Parke-Davis).
Oxy-Kesso-Tetra, Cap. (McKesson).
Terramycin HCl, Preps. (Pfizer Laboratories, Pfipharmecs).
Uri-tet, Cap. (American Urologicals).
Urobiotic (Roerig).

oxytetracycline hydrochloride and hydrocortisone ointment.
Use: Anti-infective, anti-inflammatory.

oxytetracycline hydrochloride and polymyxin B sulfate.
Use: Anti-infective.

oxytetracycline hydrochloride and polymyxin B sulfate ophthalmic ointment.
Use: Anti-infective.

oxytetracycline hydrochloride and polymyxin B sulfate topical powder.
Use: Anti-infective.

oxytetracycline hydrochloride and polymyxin B sulfate vaginal tablets.
Use: Anti-infective.

oxytetracycline-polymyxin B. Mix of oxytetracycline HCl and polymyxin B sulfate.
Use: Anti-infective.
See: Terramycin HCl w/Polymyxin B. Sulfate, Oint., Tab., Pow. (Pfizer Laboratories, Pfipharmecs).

oxytocics.

See: Ergotrate Maleate, **Inj.** (Bedford Labs).
Methergine, **Inj.** (Sandoz).

•**oxytocin**, (ox-ih-TOE-sin) U.S.P. 23.
Use: Oxytocic.
See: Pitocin, Amp. (Parke-Davis).
Syntocinon, Amp. (Sandoz).

oxytocin nasal solution. (ox-ih-TOE-sin)
Use: Oxytocic.

oxytocin, synthetic. (ox-ih-TOE-sin)
See: Pitocin, Amp. (Parke-Davis).
Syntocinon, Amp. (Sandoz).
Syntocinon Nasal Spray (Sandoz).

Oxy Wash. (SK-Beecham) Benzoyl peroxide 10%. Liq. Bot. 120 ml. *otc.*
Use: Antiacne.

Oxyzal Wet Dressing. (Gordon) Benzalkonium Cl 1:2000, oxyquinoline sulfate, distilled water. Dropper bot. 1 oz, 4 oz. *otc.*
Use: Minor skin irritations.

Oysco. (Rugby) Elemental calcium 500 mg/Tab. Bot. 60s. *otc.*
Use: Calcium supplement.

Oysco D. (Rugby) Ca 250 mg, D 125 IU. Tab. Bot. 100s, 250s, 1000s. *otc.*
Use: Vitamin/mineral supplement.

Oyst-Cal 500. (Goldline) Calcium carbonate 1.25 g (calcium 500 mg)/Tab. Bot. 60s, 120s. *otc.*
Use: Calcium supplement.

Oyst-Cal-D. (Goldline) Calcium 250 mg, vitamin D 125 IU/Tab. Bot. 100s, 1000s. *otc.*
Use: Vitamin/mineral supplement.

Oyster Calcium. (NBTY) Ca 275 mg, D 200 IU, A 800 IU. Tab. Bot. 100s. *otc.*
Use: Vitamin/mineral supplement.

Oyster Shell Calcium-500. (Vangard) Calcium carbonate 1.25 g, (calcium 500 mg). Tab. Bot. 100s, UD 100s, 640s. *otc.*
Use: Calcium supplement.

oyster shells.
See: Os-Cal, Tab. (Hoechst Marion Roussel).
W/Vitamin D-2.
See: Ostrakal, Tab. (ICN Pharm.).

Oystercal 500. (NBTY) Calcium carbonate 1.25 g (calcium 500 mg)/Tab. Bot. 100s. *otc.*
Use: Calcium supplement.

Oystercal-D. (NBTY) Calcium 250 mg, vitamin D 125 IU/Tab. Bot. 100s, 250s. *otc.*
Use: Vitamin/mineral supplement.

•**ozolinone.** (oh-ZOE-lih-NOHN) USAN.
Use: Diuretic.

P

P₁E₁; P₂E₁; P₃E₁; P₄E₁; P₆E₁. (Alcon) Pilocarpine HCl 1%, 2%, 3%, 4% or 6% respectively, with epinephrine bitartrate 1%. Plastic dropper vial 15 ml. *Rx.*
Use: Agent for glaucoma.

P and S Liquid. (Baker/Cummins) Bot. 4 oz, 8 oz. *otc.*
Use: Antiseborrheic.

P and S Plus. (Baker/Cummins) Coal tar solution 8% (crude coal tar 1.6%, ethyl alcohol 6.4%), salicylic acid 2%. Gel 105 g. *otc.*
Use: Tar-containing preparation, topical.

P and S Shampoo. (Baker/Cummins) Salicylic acid 2%, lactic acid 0.5% Bot. 4 oz. *otc.*
Use: Antiseborrheic.

Pabalate. (Robins) Sodium salicylate 300 mg, sodium aminobenzoate 300 mg/ EC Tab. Bot. 100s, 500s. *otc.*
Use: Antirheumatic.

Pabalate-SF. (Robins) Potassium salicylate 300 mg, potassium aminobenzoate 300 mg/Tab. Bot. 100s, 500s. *otc.*
Use: Antirheumatic.

PABA-Salicylate. (Various Mfr.) Sodium salicylate, p-aminobenzoate, vitamin C/ Tab. Bot. 100s, 500s. *otc.*
Use: Salicylate analgesic, vitamin combination.

PABA sodium. (Various Mfr.). Sodium p-aminobenzoate. *otc.*
Use: Vitamin supplement.

Pabasone. (Pinex) Sodium salicylate 5 gr, para-aminobenzoic acid 5 gr, ascorbic acid 20 mg/Tab. Bot. 100s. *otc.*
Use: Salicylate analgesic, vitamin supplement.

P-A-C. Preparations of phenacetin, aspirin, caffeine.
See: A.P.C. Preparations, Empirin Preparations.

p-acetylaminobenzaldehyde thiosemicarbazone. (Amithiozone, Antib, Berculon A, Benzothiozon, Conteben, Myuizone, Neustab, Tebethion, Thiomicid, Thioparamizone, Thiacetazone)
Use: Antituberculous.

P-A-C Revised Formula Analgesic. (Pharmacia & Upjohn) Aspirin 400 mg, caffeine 32 mg/Tab. Bot. 100s, 1000s. *otc.*
Use: Salicylate analgesic.

Pacemaker Prophylaxis Pastes with Fluoride. (Pacemaker) Silicone dioxide and diatomaceous earth, sodium fluoride 4.4%. Light abrasive, cinnamon/ cherry. Medium abrasive, orange. Heavy abrasive, mint. Paste Bot. 8 oz.
Use: Dental caries preventative.

Packer's Pine Tar Liquid Shampoo. (Rydelle) Pine tar. Bot. 6 fl oz. *otc.*
Use: Antiseborrheic.

Packer's Pine Tar Soap. (Rydelle) Bar 3.3 oz. *otc.*
Use: Tar-containing preparation, topical.

Paclin VK. (Armenpharm) Penicillin phenoxymethyl 125 mg or 250 mg/Tab. Bot. 100s, 1000s. *Rx.*
Use: Anti-infective, penicillin.

•**paclitaxel.** (pak-lih-TAX-uhl) USAN.
Use: Antineoplastic.
See: Taxol.

•**padimate a.** (PAD-ih-mate A) USAN.
Use: Ultraviolet screen.

•**padimate O,** (PAD-ih-mate O) U.S.P. 23.
Use: Ultraviolet screen.
See: Coppertone Prods. (Schering-Plough).
Eclipse Prods. (Sandoz).
Escalol 506 (Van Dyk).
Noskote Prods. (Schering-Plough).
Pabafilm (Galderma).
Shade Prods. (Schering-Plough).
Sunger Prods. (Schering-Plough).
Super Shade, Prods. (Schering-Plough).
Tropical Blend Sunscreen Lot. (Schering-Plough).

•**pagoclone.** (PAG-oh-klone) USAN.
Use: Antianxiety.

PAH.
See: Sodium Aminohippurate Inj. (Various Mfr.).

Pain-a-Lay. (Glessner) Antiseptic, anesthetic soln. Bot. 4 oz w/sprayer, Bot. 4 oz, 8 oz, 1 pt.
Use: Mouth and throat product.

Pain and Fever Capsules. (Lederle) Acetaminophen 500 mg/Cap. Bot. 50s, 100s. *otc.*
Use: Analgesic.

Pain and Fever Liquid. (Lederle) Acetaminophen 160 mg/5 ml (children's strength). Unit-of-use 4 oz, Bot. 16 oz. *otc.*
Use: Analgesic.

Pain and Fever Tablets. (Lederle) Acetaminophen 325 mg or 500 mg/Tab. **325 mg:** Bot. 100s, 1000s; **500 mg:** Bot. 50s, 100s. *otc.*
Use: Analgesic.

Pain Bust-R II. (Continental) Methyl sa-

licylate 17%, menthol 12%. Cream. Jar 90 g. *otc.*
Use: Rub and liniment.

Pain Doctor. (Fougera) Capsaicin 0.025%, methyl salicylate 25%, menthol 10%, parabens, propylene glycol. Cream. In 60g. *otc.*
Use: Topical anesthetic.

Pain Gel Plus. (Mentholatum Co.) Menthol 4%, aloe, vitamin E. Gel. Tube 57 g. *otc.*
Use: Rub or liniment.

Pain Relief, Aspirin Free. (Hudson) Acetaminophen 325 mg/Tab. Bot. 100s, 200s. *otc.*
Use: Analgesic.

Pain Relief Ointment. (Walgreen) Methyl salicylate 15%, menthol 10%. Tube 1.5 oz, 3 oz. *otc.*
Use: Analgesic, topical.

Pain Reliever. (Rugby) Acetaminophen 250 mg, aspirin 250 mg, caffeine 65 mg/Tab. Bot. 100s, 1000s. *otc.*
Use: Analgesic combination.

Pain Relievers-Tension Headache Relievers. (Weeks & Leo) Acetaminophen 325 mg, phenyltoloxamine citrate 30 mg/Tab. Bot. 40s, 100s. *otc.*
Use: Analgesic combination.

Palbar No. 2. (Roberts) Atropine sulfate 0.012 mg, scopolamine HBr 0.005 mg, hyoscyamine HBr 0.018 mg, phenobarbital 32.4 mg/Tab. Bot. 100s. *Rx.*
Use: Anticholinergic, antispasmodic, sedative, hypnotic.

•**paldimycin.** USAN.
Use: Antibacterial.

palestrol.
See: Diethylstilbestrol (Various Mfr.).

•**palinavir.** USAN.
Use: Antiviral.

palinum.
Use: Sedative, hypnotic.
See: Cyclobarbital Calcium (Various Mfr.).

palmidrol. N-(2-Hydroxyethyl) palmitamide.

Palmitate-A 5000. Vitamin A 5000 IU. Tab. Bot. 100s. *otc.*
Use: Vitamin supplement.

•**palmoxirate sodium.** (pal-MOX-ihr-ate) USAN.
Use: Antidiabetic.

•**palonosetron hydrochloride.** USAN.
Use: Antiemetic, antinauseant.

Pals. (Palisades) Chlorophyllin copper complex 100 mg. Tab. Bot. 30s, 100s, 1000s, UD 30s. *otc.*
Use: Systemic deodorizer.

PAM.
See: Melphalan.

•**pamabrom.** USAN.
W/Acetaminophen.
See: Pamprin, Tab. (Chattem Labs.).
W/Acetaminophen, pyrilamine maleate.
See: Cardui, Tab. (Chattem Labs.).
Sunril, Cap. (Schering-Plough).
W/Pyrilamine maleate, homatropine methylbromide, hyoscyamine sulfate, scopolamine HBr, methamphetamine HCl.
See: Aridol, Tabs. (MPL).

•**pamaqueside.** (pam-ah-KWEH-side) USAN.
Use: Antiatherosclerotic, hypocholesterolemic.

•**pamatolol sulfate.** (PAM-ah-TOE-lole) USAN.
Use: Anti-adrenergic (β-receptor).

Pamelor. (Sandoz) Nortriptyline HCl. Cap or Liq. **Cap.:** 10 mg, 25 mg, 50 mg or 75 mg base. **10 mg:** Bot. 100s, SandoPak 100s; **25 mg:** Bot. 100s, 500s, SandoPak 100s; **50 mg:** Bot. 100s, SandoPak 100s. **75 mg:** Bot. 100s. **Liq.:** Nortriptyline HCl equivalent to 10 mg base/5 ml. Bot. pt. *Rx.*
Use: Antidepressant.

•**pamidronate disodium.** (pam-IH-DROE-nate) USAN.
Use: Bone resorption inhibitor.
See: Aredia, Inj. (Novartis).

Pamine. (Kenwood/Bradley) Methscopolamine bromide 2.5 mg/Tab. Bot. 100s, 500s. *Rx.*
Use: Anticholinergic, antispasmodic.

p-aminobenzene-sulfonylacetylimide.
See: Sulfacetamide.

p-aminobenzoic acid, salts.
See: p-Aminobenzoate potassium and p-Aminobenzoate sodium.

p-aminosalicylic acid salts.
See: Aminosalicylic Acid Salts.

Pamprin. (Chattem) Acetaminophen 400 mg, pamabrom 25 mg, pyrilamine maleate 15 mg/Tab. Bot. 24s, 48s. *otc.*
Use: Analgesic combination.

Pamprin Extra Strength Multi-Symptom Relief Formula Tablets. (Chattem) Acetaminophen 400 mg, pamabrom 25 mg, pyrilamine maleate 15 mg/Tab. Bot. 12s, 24s, 48s. *otc.*
Use: Analgesic combination.

Pamprin Maximum Cramp Relief Formula Caplets. (Chattem) Acetaminophen 500 mg, pamabrom 25 mg, pyrilamine maleate 15 mg/Tab. Bot. 8s, 16s, 32s. *otc.*

Use: Analgesic combination.

Pamprin Multi-Symptom Caplets and Tablets. (Chattem) Acetaminophen 500 mg, pamabrom 25 mg, pyrilamine maleate 15 mg. Capl. Bot. 24s, 48s, Tab. Bot. 12s, 24s, 48s. *otc.*
Use: Analgesic combination.

Panacet 5/500. (ECR Pharm) Hydrocodone bitartrate 5 mg, acetaminophen 500 mg. Tab. Bot. 100s. *c-III.*
Use: Narcotic analgesic combination.

•**panadiplon.** (pan-ad-IH-pione) USAN.
Use: Antianxiety.

Panadol. (Bayer) Acetaminophen 500 mg/Tab. or Cap. **Tab:** Bot. 2s, 30s, 60s, 100s; **Cap:** Bot. 10s, 24s, 48s. *otc.*
Use: Analgesic.

Panadol Children's. (Bayer) Acetaminophen. **Tab.:** 80 mg. Bot. 30s. **Liq.:** 80 mg/0.8 ml. Bot. 2 oz, 4 oz. **Drops:** 80 mg/0.5 oz. Bot. 0.5 oz. *otc.*
Use: Analgesic.

Panadol, Infants' Drops. (Bayer) Acetaminophen 100 mg/ml. Bot. 15 ml with 0.8 ml dropper. *otc.*
Use: Analgesic.

Panadol Jr. (Bayer) Acetaminophen 160 mg/Caplet. Box. 30s. *otc.*
Use: Analgesic.

Panadyl. (Misemer) Pyrilamine maleate 25 mg, phenylpropanolamine HCl 50 mg, pheniramine maleate 25 mg/Tab. Bot. 100s, 1000s. *Rx.*
Use: Antihistamine, decongestant.

Panadyl Forte. (Misemer) Phenylpropanolamine HCl 50 mg, phenylephrine HCl 25 mg, chlorpheniramine maleate 8 mg/Tab. Bot. 100s. *Rx.*
Use: Antihistamine, decongestant.

Panafil. (Rystan) Papain pow. 10%, urea 10%, chlorophyllin copper complex 0.5%, hydrophilic base. Oint. Tube oz, Jar lb. *Rx.*
Use: Topical enzyme preparation.

Panafil White Ointment. (Rystan) Papain 10,000 units enzyme activity, hydrophilic base/g, urea 10%. Tube oz. *Rx.*
Use: Topical enzyme preparation.

Panalgesic Cream. (ECR Pharm) Methyl salicylate 35%, menthol 4%. Jar 4 oz. *otc.*
Use: Analgesic, topical.

Panalgesic Liquid. (ECR Pharm) Methyl salicylate 55.01%, menthol 1.25%, camphor 3.1%, in alcohol 22%, emollients, color. Bot. 4 oz, pt, 0.5 gal. *otc.*
Use: Analgesic, topical.

Panasal 5/500. (E.C. Robins) Hydrocodone bitartrate 5 mg, aspirin 500 mg. Tab. Bot. 100s. *c-III.*
Use: Narcotic analgesic combination.

Panasol. (Seatrace) Prednisone 5 mg/Tab. Bot. 100s. *Rx.*
Use: Corticosteroid.

Panasol-S. (Seatrace) Prednisone 1 mg/Tab. Bot. 100s, 1000s. *Rx.*
Use: Corticosteroid.

Panc-500. (Freeda) Hesperidin 100 mg, citrus bioflavonoids 100 mg, rutin 50 mg, vitamin C 500 mg/Tab. Bot. 100s, 250s, 500s. *otc.*
Use: Vitamin supplement.

•**pancopride.** (PAN-koe-pride) USAN.
Use: Antiemetic, antianxiety, peristaltic stimulant.

Pancrease. (Ortho McNeil) Enteric coated pancrelipase capsules. **Regular:** Lipase 4500 units, amylase 20,000 units, protease 25,000 units/Cap. Sugar. Dye free. Bot. 100s, 250s; **MT4:** Lipase 4500 units, amylase 12,000 units, protease 12,000 units/Cap. Bot. 100s; **MT10:** Lipase 10,000 units, amylase 30,000 units, protease 30,000 units/Cap. Bot. 100s; **MT16:** Lipase 16,000 units, amylase 48,000 units, protease 48,000 units/Cap. Bot. 100s; **MT20:** lipase 20,000 units, amylase 56,000 units, protease 44,000 units/Cap. Bot. 100s. **MT 25:** Lipase 25,000 units, amylase 70,000 units, protease 55,000 units. Cap. Bot. 100s; **MT 32:** Lipase 32,000 units, amylase 90,000 units, protease 70,000 units. Cap. Bot. 100s. *Rx.*
Use: Digestive enzyme.

pancreatic enzyme.
W/Pepsin, ox bile.
See: Nu' Leven, Nu' Leven Plus, Tab. (Lemmon).

pancreatic substance. Substance from fresh pancreas of hog or ox, containing the enzymes amylopsin, trypsin, steapsin.
W/Bile extract, dl-methionine, choline bitartrate.
See: Licoplex, Tab. (Mills).
W/Bile salts, lipase.
See: Cotazym-B, Tab. (Organon).
W/Bile, whole (desiccated), oxidized bile acids, homatropine methylbromide.
See: Pancobile, Tab. (Solvay).
W/Lipase.
See: Cotazym, Cap., Packet (Organon).

•**pancreatin,** U.S.P. 23. Pancreatic enzymes obtained from hog or cattle pancreatic tissue.

Use: Enzyme (digestant adjunct).
See: Depancol, Tab. (Warner-Chilcott).
Elzyme, Tab. (ICN Pharm).
Panteric, Tab. (Parke-Davis).

pancreatin w/combinations.
See: Entozyme, Tab. (Robins).
Nu'Leven, Tab. (Lemmon).
Ro-Bile, Tab. (Solvay).
Sto-Zyme, Tab. (Jalco).
Zypan, Tab. (Standard Process).

•**pancrelipase,** (pan-KREE-lih-pace) U.S.P. 23. *Formerly Lipancreatin.*
Preparation of hog pancreas with high content of steapsin and adequate amounts of pancreatic enzymes.
Use: Enzyme (digestant adjunct).
See: Accelerase, Cap. (Organon).
Cotazym, Cap., Packet (Organon).
Viokase, Pow., Tab. (Robins).
W/Mixed conjugated bile salts, cellulase.
See: Accelerase, Cap. (Organon).
Cotazym-B, Tab. (Organon).

Pancretide. (Baxter) Pancreatic polypeptide in normal saline.
Use: Fibrinolytic conditions.

pancuronium. (PAN-cue-ROW-nee-uhm)
See: Pancuronium Bromide (Organon).

•**pancuronium bromide.** (PAN-cue-ROW-nee-uhm) USAN.
Use: Neuromuscular blocking relaxant.
See: Pavulon, Inj. (Organon).

pancuronium bromide. (Various Mfr.) **1 mg/ml:** Vials 10 ml; **2 mg/ml:** Vials, amps, syringes 2 ml or 5 ml.
Use: Neuromuscular blocking relaxant.

Panex. (Roberts) Acetaminophen 325 mg/Tab. Bot. 1000s. *otc.*
Use: Analgesic.

Panex 500. (Roberts) Acetaminophen 500 mg/Tab. Bot. 1000s. *otc.*
Use: Analgesic.

Panhematin. (Abbott) Hemin 301 mg/2 ml when reconstituted, 300 mg sorbitol. Inj. Vial 2 ml. *Rx.*
Use: Agent for acute intermittent porphyria.

Panitol. (Wesley) Allylisobutyl barbituric acid 15 mg, acetaminophen 300 mg/Tab. Bot. 100s, 1000s. *Rx.*
Use: Sedative/hypnotic, analgesic.

Panmycin. (Pharmacia & Upjohn) Tetracycline HCl 250 mg/Cap. Bot. 100s, 1000s. *Rx.*
Use: Anti-infective, tetracycline.
See: Panmycin, Cap. (Pharmacia & Upjohn).

Panoxyl 5, 10 Acne Gel. (Stiefel) Benzoyl peroxide 5% or 10%, alcohol 20% in a hydroalcoholic gel base. Tube 56.7 g, 113.4 g. *Rx.*
Use: Antiacne.

Panoxyl AQ 2.5, 5, 10 Acne Gel. (Stiefel) Benzoyl peroxide 2.5%, 5% or 10%, methylparaben, EDTA in an aqueous gel base. Tube 56.7 g, 113.4 g. *Rx.*
Use: Antiacne.

Panoxyl Bar. (Stiefel) Benzoyl peroxide 5% cetostearyl alcohol, EDTA, glycerin, castor oil, mineral oil in a rich-lathering, mild surfactant cleansing base. Bar 113 g. *otc.*
Use: Antiacne.

Panoxyl-10 Bar. (Stiefel) Benzoyl peroxide 10% cetostearyl alcohol, castor oil, mineral oil, soap free in rich-lathering, mild surfactant cleansing base. Bar 113 g. *otc.*
Use: Antiacne.

panparnit hydrochloride. Caramiphen HCl.
Use: Antiparkinsonian.

Panscol. (Baker/Cummins) Salicylic acid 3%, lactic acid 2%, phenol (less than 1%). **Oint.:** Jar 3 oz. **Lot.:** Bot. 4 oz. *otc.*
Use: Emollient.

•**panthenol,** (PAN-theh-nahl) U.S.P. 23.
Alcohol corresponding to pantothenic acid. Pantothenol. Pantothenylol.
Use: Treatment of paralytic ileus and postoperative distention; vitamin.
See: Ilopan, Amp., Vial (Warren-Teed).
Panadon, Cream (Gordon Labs.).
Panthoderm Cream (Rhone-Poulenc Rorer).

panthenol w/combinations.
See: Lifer-B, Liq. (Burgin-Arden).
Nutricol, Cap., Inj. (Nutrition Control).

Panthoderm Cream. (Rhone-Poulenc Rorer) Dexpanthenol 2% in water-miscible cream. Tube 1 oz, Jar 2 oz, lb. *otc.*
Use: Emollient.

pantocaine.
See: Tetracaine HCl. (Various Mfr.).

Pantocrin-F. (Spanner) Plurigland, ovarian, anterior and posterior pituitary, adrenal, thyroid extracts. Vial 30 ml. *Rx.*
Use: Hormone.

Pantopaque. (Alcon Surgical) Iophendylate, ethyl iodophenylundecanoate. Amp. 3 ml 3s; 6 ml 6s; 1 ml 2s.
Use: Radiopaque agent.

•**pantoprazole.** (pahn-TOE-prazz-ole) USAN.
Use: Antiulcer.

pantothenic acid. As calcium or sodium salt.

Use: Vitamin B$_5$ supplement.
See: Vitamin preparations.

pantothenic acid salts.
See: Calcium Pantothenate.
Sodium Pantothenate.

pantothenol.
See: Panthenol, Preps. (Various Mfr.).

pantothenyl alcohol.
See: Panthenol, Preps. (Various Mfr.).

pantothenylol.
See: Panthenol, Preps. (Various Mfr.).

Panvitex Geriatric Capsules. (Forest Pharm) Safflower oil 340 mg, vitamins A 10,000 IU, D 400 IU, B$_1$ 5 mg, B$_6$ 1 mg, B$_2$ 2.5 mg, B$_{12}$ activity 2 mcg, C 75 mg, niacinamide 40 mg, calcium pantothenate 4 mg, E 2 IU, inositol 15 mg, choline bitartrate 31.4 mg, calcium 75 mg, phosphorus 58 mg, iron 30 mg, manganese 0.5 mg, potassium 2 mg, zinc 0.5 mg, magnesium 3 mg/Cap. Bot. 100s, 1000s. *otc.*
Use: Vitamin/mineral supplement.

Panvitex Plus Minerals Capsules. (Forest Pharm) Vitamins A 5000 IU, D 400 IU, B$_1$ 3 mg, B$_2$ 2.5 mg, niacinamide 20 mg, B$_6$ 1.5 mg, calcium pantothenate 5 mg, B$_{12}$ 2.5 mcg, C 50 mg, E 3 IU, calcium 215 mg, phosphorus 166 mg, iron 13.4 mg, magnesium 7.5 mg, manganese 1.5 mg, potassium 5 mg, zinc 1.4 mg/Cap. Bot. 100s, 1000s. *otc.*
Use: Vitamin/mineral supplement.

Panvitex Prenatal Capsules. (Forest Pharm) Ferrous fumarate 150 mg, cobalamin concentration 2 mcg, vitamins A 6000 IU, D 400 IU, B$_1$ 1.5 mg, B$_2$ 2.5 mg, niacinamide 15 mg, B$_6$ 3 mg, C 100 mg, calcium 250 mg, calcium pantothenate 5 mg, folic acid 0.2 mg/Cap. Bot. 100s, 1000s. *otc.*
Use: Vitamin/mineral supplement.

Panvitex T-M. (Forest Pharm) Vitamins A 10,000 IU, D 400 IU, B$_1$ 10 mg, B$_6$ 1 mg, B$_2$ 5 mg, B$_{12}$ 5 mcg, C 150 mg, niacinamide 100 mg, calcium 103 mg, phosphorus 80 mg, iron 10 mg, manganese 1 mg, potassium 5 mg, zinc 1.4 mg, magnesium 5.56 mg/Cap. Bot. 100s, 1000s. *otc.*
Use: Vitamin/mineral supplement.

PAP. (Abbott Diagnostics) Enzyme immunoassay for measurement of prostatic acid phosphatase. Test kit 100s.
Use: Diagnostic aid.

Papadeine #3. (Vangard) Codeine phosphate 30 mg, acetaminophen 300 mg/Tab. Bot. 100s, 1000s. *c-III.*
Use: Narcotic analgesic combination.

●**papain,** U.S.P. 23. A proteolytic substance derived from *Carlica papaya.*
Use: Proteolytic enzyme.
See: Papase, Tab. (Parke-Davis).
Softlens Enzymatic Contact Lens Cleaner (Allergan).

papain w/combinations.
See: Bilate, Tab. (Schwarz Pharma).
Cerophen, Tab. (Wendt-Bristol).
Digenzyme, Tab. (Burgin-Arden).
Panafil, Oint. (Rystan).

Pap-a-Lix. (Freeport) n-Acetyl-aminophenol 120 mg, alcohol 10%/5 ml. Bot. 4 oz, gal. *otc.*
Use: Analgesic.

●**papaverine hydrochloride,** (pap-PAV-uhr-een) U.S.P. 23.
Use: Smooth muscle relaxant.
See: BP-Papaverine, Cap. (Burlington).
Cerespan, Cap. (Rhone-Poulenc Rorer).
Cirbed, Cap. (Boyd).
Delapav, Time Cap. (Dunhall).
Myobid, Cap. (Laser).
P-200, Cap. (Knoll Pharm).
Pavabid, Cap. (Hoechst Marion Roussel).
Pavacap, Unicells (Solvay).
Pavacaps, Cap. (Freeport).
Pavacen Cenules, Cap. (Schwarz Pharma).
Pavaclor, Cap. (Pasadena Research).
Pavadel, Cap. (Canright).
Pavadyl, Cap. (Bock).
Pavakey 300, Cap. (Key).
Pavakey S.A., Cap. (Key).
Pava-lyn, Cap. (Lynwood).
Pava Par, Cap. (Parmed).
Pavasule, Cap. (Jalco).
Pavatest T.D., Cap. (Fellows-Testagar).
Pavatym, Cap. (Everett).
Pavatran T.D. Cap. (Mayrand).
Vasocap, Cap. (Keene).
Vazosan, Tab. (Sandia).

W/Codeine sulfate.
See: Copavin, Pulvule, Tab. (Lilly).

W/Codeine sulfate, aloin, sodium salicylate.
See: Copavin Compound, Elix. (Lilly).

W/Codeine sulfate, emetine HCl, ephedrine HCl.
See: Golacol, Syr. (Arcum).

W/Phenobarbital.
See: Pavadel-PB, Cap. (Canright).

Paplex Ultra. (Medicis) Salicylic acid 26% in flexible collodion. Bot. 15 ml. *otc.*
Use: Keratolytic.

para-aminobenzoic acid. (Various Mfr.).

Tab.: 100 mg or 500 mg. Bot. 100s, 250s (100 mg only); **Pow.:** 120 g. *otc.*
Use: Sunscreen, agent for scleroderma.
See: Potaba, Tab., Cap., Powd., envules. (Glenwood).

para-aminosalicylate sodium.
See: Aminosalicylate Sodium.

para-aminosalicylic acid. Aminosalicylic Acid, U.S.P. 23. *Rx.*
Use: Tuberculosis infections.

Parabaxin. (Parmed) Methocarbamol 500 mg or 750 mg/Tab. Bot. 100s. *Rx.*
Use: Skeletal muscle relaxant.

parabrom.
See: Pyrabrom.

parabromidylamine.
See: Brompheniramine, Dimetane, Preps. (Robins).

paracain.
See: Procaine Hydrochloride (Various Mfr.).

paracarbinoxamine maleate. Carbinoxamine.

Paracet Forte Tabs. (Major) Chlorzoxazone, acetaminophen. Bot. 100s, 1000s. *Rx.*
Use: Skeletal muscle relaxant.

paracetaldehyde.
See: Paraldehyde, U.S.P. 23.

parachloramine hydrochloride. Meclizine HCl, U.S.P. 23.
See: Bonine, Tab. (Pfizer).

parachlorometaxylenol.
Use: Phenolic antiseptic.
See: D-Seb, Liq. (Rydelle).
Nu-Flow, Liq. (Rydelle).
W/9-aminoacridine HCl, methyl-dodecylbenzyl-trimethyl ammonium Cl, pramoxine HCl, hydrocortisone, acetic acid.
See: Drotic No. 2, Drops (Ascher).
W/Benzocaine.
See: TPO 20 (DePree).
W/Coconut oil, pine oil, castor oil, lanolin, cholesterols, lecithin.
See: Sebacide, Liq. (Paddock).
W/Hydrocortisone, pramoxine HCl, benzalkonium Cl, acetic acid.
See: Oto Drops (Solvay).
W/Lidocaine, phenol, zinc oxide.
See: Unguentine Plus, Cream (Procter & Gamble).
W/Pramoxine HCl, hydrocortisone, benzalkonium Cl, acetic acid.
See: My Cort Otic #2, Drops (Scrip).
Steramine Otic, Drops (Mayrand).
W/Resorcinol, sulfur.
See: Rezamid, Lot. (Dermik).

•**parachlorophenol,** U.S.P. 23.
Use: Topical antibacterial.

•**parachlorophenol, camphorated,** U.S.P. 23.
Use: Anti-infective, topical (dental).

paracodin.
See: Dihydrocodeine.

Paraeusal Liquid. (Paraeusal) Liq. Bot. 2 oz, 6 oz, 12 oz.
Use: Minor skin irritations.

Paraeusal Solid. (Paraeusal) Oint. Jar 1 oz, 2 oz, 16 oz.
Use: Minor skin irritations.

•**paraffin,** N.F. 18.
Use: Pharmaceutic aid (stiffening agent).

•**paraffin, synthetic,** N.F. 18.
Use: Pharmaceutic aid (stiffening agent).

Paraflex. (McNeil Pharm) Chlorzoxazone 250 mg/Tab. Bot. 100s. *Rx.*
Use: Skeletal muscle relaxant.

Parafon Forte DSC. (McNeil Pharm) Chlorzoxazone 500 mg/Capl. Bot. 100s, 500s, UD 100s. *Rx.*
Use: Skeletal muscle relaxant.

paraform. Paraformaldehyde. (No Mfr. listed).

paraformaldehyde.
Use: Essentially the same as formaldehyde.
See: Formaldehyde (Various Mfr.).
Trioxymethylene (an incorrect term for paraformaldehyde).

paraglycylarsanilic acid. N-Carbamylmethyl-p-aminobenzenearsonic acid, the free acid of tryparsamide.

Parahist HD Liquid. (Pharmics) Phenylephrine HCl 5 mg, chlorpheniramine maleate 2 mg, hydrocodone bitartrate 1.67 mg, alcohol free. Bot. 473 ml. *c-III.*
Use: Decongestant, antihistamine, antitussive.

Para-Jel. (Approved) Benzocaine 5%, cetyl dimethyl benzyl ammonium Cl. Tube 0.25 oz. *otc.*
Use: Local anesthetic, topical.

•**paraldehyde,** U.S.P. 23.
Use: Sedative, hypnotic.
See: Paral, Cap., Liq., Amp. (Forest).

Paral Oral. (Forest) Paraldehyde 30 ml. Bot. 12s, 25s. *c-IV.*
Use: Sedative, hypnotic.

paramephrin.
See: Epinephrine (Various Mfr.).

paramethadione, U.S.P. XXII.
Use: Anticonvulsant.
See: Paradione, Cap., Soln. (Abbott).

•**paramethasone acetate,** (PAR-ah-meth-ah-zone) U.S.P. 23.

Use: Glucocorticoid.
See: Haldrone, Tab. (Lilly).

para-monochlorophenol.
See: Camphorated para-chlorophenol, Liq. (Novocol).

•**paranyline hydrochloride.** (PAR-ah-NYE-leen) USAN.
Use: Anti-inflammatory.

•**parapenzolate bromide.** (pa-rah-PEN-zoe-late BROE-mide) USAN.
Use: Anticholinergic.

Paraplatin. (Bristol-Myers Oncology) Carboplatin 50 mg, 150 mg or 450 mg. Inj. Vial. *Rx.*
Use: Antineoplastic.

pararosaniline embonate. Pararosaniline pamoate.

•**pararosaniline pamoate.** (par-ah-row-ZAN-ih-lin PAM-oh-ate) USAN.
Use: Antischistosomal.

parasympatholytic agents. Cholinergic blocking agents.
See: Anticholinergic Agents.
Antispasmodics.
Mydriatics.
Parkinsonism.

parasympathomimetic agents.
See: Cholinergic Agents.

Parathar. (Rhone-Poulenc Rorer) Teriparatide acetate hPTH activity 200 units with gelatin 20 mg pow. for inj. Vial 10 ml w/10 ml vial diluent.
Use: Diagnostic aid.

Paratrol Liquid. (Walgreen) Pyrethrins 0.2%, piperonyl butoxide technical 2%, deodorized kerosene 0.8%. Bot. 2 oz. *otc.*
Use: Pediculicide.

Parazone. (Interstate) Chlorzoxazone 250 mg, acetaminophen 300 mg/Tab. Bot. 100s, 1000s. *Rx.*
Use: Skeletal muscle relaxant, analgesic.

•**parbendazole.** (par-BEN-dah-ZOLE) USAN. Under study.
Use: Anthelmintic.

parbutoxate.

Parcillin. (Parmed) Crystalline potassium penicillin G 240 mg, 400,000 units/Tab. Bot. 100s, 1000s. Pow. for syr. 400,000 units/Tsp. 80 ml. *Rx.*
Use: Anti-infective, penicillin.

•**parconazole hydrochloride.** (par-KOE-nah-zole) USAN.
Use: Antifungal.

Par Decon. (Par) Phenylpropanolamine HCl 40 mg, phenylephrine HCl 10 mg, chlorpheniramine maleate 5 mg, phenyltoloxamine citrate 15 mg/Tab. Bot.

100s, 500s, 1000s. *Rx.*
Use: Antihistamine, decongestant.

Paredrine. (Pharmics) Hydroxyamphetamine HBr 1%. Bot. 15 ml. *Rx.*
Use: Pupil dilation.

•**paregoric,** U.S.P. 23.
Use: Antiperistaltic.

paregoric. (Various Mfr.) Morphine equivalent 2 mg/5 ml, 45% alcohol. Liq. Bot. 60 ml, pt, gal, UD 5 ml (40s, 50s, 100s). *c-III.*
Use: Antiperistaltic.

Paremyd. (Allergan) Hydroxyamphetamine HBr 1%, tropicamide 0.25%. Soln. Bot. 5 ml, 15 ml. *Rx.*
Use: Mydriatic, cycloplegic.

parenabol. Boldenone undecylenate.

Parepectolin. (Rhone-Poulenc Rorer) Attapulgite 600 mg/15 ml. Liq. Bot. 240 ml. *otc.*
Use: Antidiarrheal.

•**pareptide sulfate.** (PAR-epp-tide) USAN.
Use: Antiparkinsonian.

Par Estro. (Parmed) Conjugated estrogens 1.25 mg/Tab. Bot. 100s. *Rx.*
Use: Estrogen.

parethoxycaine hydrochloride.
W/Zirconium oxide, calamine.
See: Zotox, Spray, Cream (Del Pharm).

Par-F. (Pharmics) Iron 60 mg, calcium 250 mg, vitamins C 120 mg, A 5000 IU, D 400 IU, B_1 3 mg, B_2 3.4 mg, B_{12} 12 mcg, B_6 12 mg, B_9 20 mg, Cu, I, Mg, Zn 15 mg, E 30 IU, folic acid 1 mg/Tab. Bot. 100s. *Rx.*
Use: Vitamin/mineral supplement.

Par Glycerol. (Par) Iodinated glycerol 60 mg/5 ml. Alcohol 21.75%, peppermint oil, corn syrup, saccharin. Caramel-mint flavor. Elixir. Bot. Pt. *Rx.*
Use: Expectorant.

•**pargyline hydrochloride.** USAN. U.S.P. XXII
Use: Antihypertensive.

Parhist SR. (Parmed) Phenylpropanolamine HCl 75 mg, chlorpheniramine maleate 12 mg/Cap. Bot. 100s, 1000s. *Rx.*
Use: Decongestant, antihistamine.

Parkelp. (Phillip R. Park) Pacific sea kelp.
Tab.: Bot. 100s, 200s, 500s, 800s.
Gran.: Bot. 2 oz, 7 oz, 1 lb, 3 lb. *otc.*
Use: Iodine supplement.

parkinsonism, agents for. Parasympatholytic agents.
See: Akineton, Tab., Inj. (Knoll).
Artane, Elix., Tab., Sequels (Lederle).
Benztropine Mesylate, Tab. (Various Mfr.).

Caramiphen HCl.
Cogentin, Tab., Amp. (Merck).
Dopar, Cap. (Procter & Gamble).
Eldepryl, Tab. (Somerset).
Kemadrin, Tab. (Glaxo Wellcome).
Larodopa, Tab. (Roche).
Lodosyn, Tab. (Merck).
Parlodel, Tab., Cap. (Sandoz).
Permax, Tab. (Lilly).
Sinemet, Tab. (DuPont Pharma).
Symmetrel, Cap., Syr. (DuPont
Merck).
Trihexyphenidyl HCl (Various Mfr.).
Trihexy-2 (Geneva Pharm).

Parlodel. (Sandoz) Bromocriptine mesylate. Lactose. **Tab.:** 2.5 mg. Bot. 30s, 100s. **Cap.:** 5 mg. Bot. 30s, 100s. Rx.
Use: Antiparkinsonian.

Parmeth. (Parmed) Promethazine HCl 50 mg/Cap. Bot. 100s, 1000s. Rx.
Use: Antihistamine, antiemetic, antivertigo.

parminyl. W/Salicylamide, phenacetin, caffeine, acetaminophen.
See: Dolopar, Tab. (O'Neal).

Par-Natal-FA. (Parmed) Vitamins A 4000 IU, D 400 IU, thiamine HCl 2 mg, riboflavin 2 mg, pyridoxine HCl 0.8 mg, ascorbic acid 50 mg, niacinamide 10 mg, iodine 0.15 mg, folic acid 0.1 mg, cobalamin concentrate 2 mcg, iron 50 mg, calcium 240 mg/Cap. Bot. 100s, 1000s. otc.
Use: Vitamin/mineral supplement.

Par-Natal Plus 1 Improved. (Parmed) Elemental calcium 200 mg, elemental iron 65 mg, vitamins A 4000 IU, D 400 IU, E 11 mg, B_1 1.5 mg, B_2 3 mg, B_3 20 mg, B_6 10 mg, B_{12} 12 mcg, C 120 mg, folic acid 1 mg, zinc 25 mg, Cu/Tab. Bot. 500s. Rx.
Use: Vitamin/mineral supplement.

Parnate. (SK-Beecham) Tranylcypromine sulfate 10 mg/Tab. Bot. 100s. Rx.
Use: Antidepressant.

parodyne.
See: Antipyrine (Various Mfr.).

paroleine.
See: Petrolatum Liquid (Various Mfr.).

•**paromomycin sulfate,** (par-oh-moe-MY-sin) U.S.P. 23. An antibiotic substance obtained from cultures of certain *Streptomyces* species, one of which is *Streptomyces rimosus*.
Use: Antiamebic.

parothyl. (Interstate) Meprobamate 400 mg, tridihexethyl Cl 25 mg/Tab. Bot. 100s. c-iv.
Use: Antianxiety, anticholinergic, antispasmodic.

•**paroxetine.** (puh-ROX-eh-teen) USAN.
Use: Antidepressant.

paroxetine hydrochloride.
Use: Antidepressant.
See: Paxil, Tab. (SK-Beecham).

paroxyl.
See: Acetarsone (Various Mfr.).

parpanit.
See: Caramiphen HCl (Various Mfr.).

Parsidol. (Parke-Davis) Ethopropazine HCl 10 mg or 50 mg/Tab. Bot. 100s. Rx.
Use: Antiparkinsonian.

parsley concentrate. Rx.
W/Garlic concentrate.
See: Allimin, Tab. (Mosso).

Par-Supp. (Parmed) Estrone 0.2 mg, lactose 50 mg/Vaginal Supp. Pkg. 12s.
Use: Estrogen, vaginal.

Partapp TD. (Parmed) Phenylpropanolamine HCl 15 mg, phenylephrine HCl 15 mg, brompheniramine maleate 12 mg/TD Tab. Bot. 1000s.

Parten. (Parmed) Acetaminophen 10 gr/Tab. Bot. 100s, 1000s. otc.
Use: Analgesic.

•**partricin.** (PAR-trih-sin) USAN. Antibiotic produced by *Streptomyces aureofaciens.*
Use: Antifungal, antiprotozoal.

Partuss. (Parmed) Dextromethorphan hydrobromide 60 mg, potassium guaiacolsulfonate 8 gr, chlorpheniramine maleate 6 mg, ammonium Cl 8 gr, tartar emetic ¹⁄₁₂ gr, chloroform 2 min/30 ml. Bot. 4 oz, pt, gal. Rx.
Use: Antitussive, expectorant, antihistamine.

Partuss A.C. (Parmed) Guaifenesin 100 mg, pheniramine maleate 7.5 mg, codeine phosphate 10 mg, alcohol 3.5%/5 ml. Bot 4 oz. c-v.
Use: Expectorant, antihistamine, antitussive.

Partuss LA. (Parmed) Phenylpropanolamine HCl 75 mg, guaifenesin 400 mg/LA Tab. Bot. 100s, 500s. Rx.
Use: Decongestant, expectorant.

Parvlex. (Freeda) Iron 100 mg, vitamins B_1 20 mg, B_2 20 mg, B_3 20 mg, B_5 1 mg, B_6 10 mg, B_{12} 50 mcg, C 50 mg, folic acid 0.1 mg, Cu, Mn/Tab. Bot. 100s, 250s. otc.
Use: Vitamin/mineral supplement.

Pas-C. (Hellwig) Pascorbic. p-aminosalicylic acid 0.5 g with vitamin C/Tab. Bot. 1000s. Rx.
Use: Antituberculous agent.

Paser. (Jacobus) Aminosalicylic acid 4 g/

packet. Gran. Pkt. 30s. *Rx.*
Use: Adjunctive tuberculosis agent.
passiflora. Dried flowering and fruiting tops of Passiflora incarnata.
W/Phenobarbital, extract hyoscyamus.
See: Somlyn w/Pb, Cap. (Scrip).
W/Phenobarbital, jamaica dogwood.
See: Sominol, Phenobarbital, Tab. (O'Neal).
W/Phenobarbital, valerian, hyoscyamus.
See: Aluro, Tab. (Foy).
Patanol. (Alcon) Olopatadine HCl 0.1%/ Soln. Drop-Tainer. 5 ml. *Rx.*
Use: Ophthalmic antihistamine.
Path. (Parker) Buffered neutral formalin soln. 10%. Bot. 1 gal, 5 gal. Jar 4 oz.
Use: Tissue specimen fixative.
Pathilon. (Lederle) Tridihexethyl chloride 25 mg/Tab. Bot. 100s. *Rx.*
Use: Anticholinergic, antispasmodic.
Pathocil. (Wyeth-Ayerst) Sodium dicloxacillin monohydrate. **250 mg/Cap.:** Bot. 100s. **500 mg/Cap.:** Bot. 50s. **Pow. for oral susp.:** 62.5 mg/5 ml. Bot. to make 100 ml. *Rx.*
Use: Anti-infective, penicillin.
•**paulomycin.** (PAW-low-MY-sin) USAN.
Use: Antibacterial.
Pavabid Plateau. (Hoechst Marion Roussel) Papaverine HCl 150 mg/TR Cap. Bot. 100s, 250s, 1000s, UD 100s. *Rx.*
Use: Peripheral vasodilator.
Pavacaps. (Freeport) Papaverine HCl 150 mg/TR Cap. Bot. 1000s. *Rx.*
Use: Peripheral vasodilator.
Pavacen Cenules. (Schwarz Pharma) Papaverine HCl 150 mg/TR Cap. Bot. 100s. *Rx.*
Use: Peripheral vasodilator.
Pavadel. (Canright) Papaverine HCl 150 mg/Cap. Bot. 100s, 1000s. *Rx.*
Use: Peripheral vasodilator.
Pavadel PB. (Canright) Papaverine HCl 150 mg, phenobarbital 45 mg/Cap. Bot. 100s. *Rx.*
Use: Peripheral vasodilator.
Pavadyl Capsules. (Bock) Papaverine HCl 150 mg/Cap. Bot. 100s. *Rx.*
Use: Peripheral vasodilator.
Pavagen. (Rugby) Papaverine 150 mg/ TR Cap. Bot. 500s, 1000s, UD 100s. *Rx.*
Use: Peripheral vasodilator.
Pava-Lyn. (Lynwood) Papaverine HCl 150 mg/Cap. Bot. 100s. *Rx.*
Use: Peripheral vasodilator.
Pavatine Tabs. (Major) Papaverine 300 mg/Tab. Bot. 100s. *Rx.*
Use: Peripheral vasodilator.

Pavatine T.D. Caps. (Major) Papaverine 150 mg/TD Cap. Bot. 100s, 1000s. *Rx.*
Use: Peripheral vasodilator.
Pavulon. (Organon) Pancuronium bromide. **1 mg/ml:** Vial 10 ml, Box 25s. **2 mg/ml:** Amp. 2 ml, 5 ml, Box 25s. *Rx.*
Use: Muscle relaxant, adjunct to anesthesia.
Paxarel. (Circle) Acetylcarbromal 250 mg/Tab. Bot. 100s. *Rx.*
Use: Sedative, hypnotic.
Paxil. (SK-Beecham) Paroxetine 20 mg or 30 mg. Tab. **20 mg:** Bot. 30s, 100s, UD 100s; **30 mg:** Bot. 30s. *Rx.*
Use: Antidepressant.
•**pazinaclone.** USAN.
Use: Antianxiety.
Pazo Hemorrhoid Ointment. (Bristol-Myers) Zinc oxide 5%, ephedrine sulfate 0.2%, camphor 2% in lanolin-petrolatum base. Tube 28 g. *otc.*
Use: Anorectal preparation.
Pazo Hemorrhoid Suppositories. (Bristol-Myers) Ephedrine sulfate 3.8 mg, zinc oxide 96.5 mg, vegetable oil/Supp. Box 12s, 24s. *otc.*
Use: Anorectal preparation.
•**pazoxide.** (pay-ZOX-ide) USAN.
Use: Antihypertensive.
PB 100. (Schlicksup) Phenobarbital 1.5 gr/Tab. Bot. 1000s. *c-iv.*
Use: Sedative, hypnotic.
PBZ. (Novartis) Tripelennamine HCl. **Tab.:** 25 mg Bot. 100s. 50 mg Bot. 100s, 1000s. **Elix.:** Tripelennamine citrate (equivalent to HCl 25 mg)/5 ml. Bot. 473 ml. *Rx.*
Use: Antihistamine.
PBZ-SR. (Novartis) Tripelennamine HCl 100 mg/SR Tab. Bot. 100s. *Rx.*
Use: Antihistamine.
PCE Dispertab Tablets. (Abbott) Erythromycin particles 333 mg/Tab. Bot. 60s, 500s. *Rx.*
Use: Anti-infective, erythromycin.
p-chlorometaxylenol.
W/Benzocaine, benzyl alcohol, propylene glycol.
See: 20-Caine Burn Relief (Alto).
W/Hydrocortisone, pramoxine HCl.
See: Orlex HC, Otic (Baylor).
p-chlorophenol.
See: Parachlorophenol.
PCMX.
See: Parachlorometaxylenol.
PDP Liquid Protein. (Wesley Pharm) Protein 15 g (from protein hydrolysates), cal 60/30 ml. Bot. pt, qt, gal. *otc.*
Use: Protein supplement.

Peacock's Bromides. (Natcon) **Liq.:** Potassium bromide 6 gr, sodium bromide 6 gr, ammonium bromide 3 gr/5 ml. Bot. 8 oz. **Tab.:** Potassium bromide 3 gr, sodium bromide 3 gr, ammonium bromide 1.5 gr. Bot. 100s. *Rx.*
Use: Sedative, hypnotic.

•**peanut oil,** N.F. 18.
Use: Pharmaceutic aid (solvent).

Pectamol. (British Drug House) Diethylaminoethoxyethyl-a,a-diethylphenylacetate citrate. Bot. 4 fl oz, 16 fl oz, 80 fl oz, 160 fl oz.
Use: Antitussive.

•**pectin,** U.S.P. 23.
Use: Protectant, pharmaceutic aid (suspending agent).

pectin w/combinations.
See: Donnagel Susp. (Robins).
Donnagel-PG, Susp. (Robins).
Furoxone, Liq., Tab. (Eaton).
Infantol Pink, Liq. (Scherer).
Kaopectate, Liq. (Pharmacia & Upjohn).
Kapigam, Liq. (Solvay).
KBP/O, Cap. (Cole).
Parepectolin, Susp. (Rhone-Poulenc Rorer Consumer).
Pectokay, Liq. (Jones Medical).

Pedameth. (Forest) Racemethionine.
Cap.: 200 mg. Bot. 50s, 500s. **Liq.:** 75 mg/5 ml. Bot. pt. *Rx.*
Use: Diaper rash product.

Pedenex. (Approved) Caprylic acid, zinc undecylenate, sodium propionate. Tube 1.5 oz. Foot pow. spray 5 oz. *otc.*
Use: Antifungal, topical.

Pedia Care Allergy Formula. (McNeil-CPC) Chlorpheniramine maleate 1 mg/5 ml, sorbitol, sucrose. Alcohol free. Grape flavor. Syr. Bot. 120 ml. *otc.*
Use: Antihistamine.

Pedia Care Cold Allergy Chewable Tablets. (McNeil-CPC) Pseudoephedrine HCl 15 mg, chlorpheniramine maleate 1 mg, aspartame, phenylalanine 8 mg/Tab. Pkg. 18s. *otc.*
Use: Decongestant, antihistamine.

Pedia Care Cough-Cold. (McNeil-CPC) **Chew. Tab.:** Pseudoephedrine HCl 15 mg, chlorpheniramine maleate 1 mg, dextromethorphan HBr 5 mg, aspartame (phenylalanine 6 mg), dextrose, sucrose. Fruit flavor. Pkg. 16s. **Liq.:** Pseudoephedrine HCl 15 mg, chlorpheniramine maleate 1 mg, dextromethorphan HBr 5 mg/5 ml, sorbitol, sucrose. Alcohol free. Cherry flavor. Syr. Bot. 120 ml. *otc.*
Use: Decongestant, antihistamine, antitussive.

Pedia Care Infants' Decongestant. (McNeil-CPC) Pseudoephedrine HCl 7.5 mg/0.8 ml. Cherry flavor. Syr. Bot. 15 ml. *otc.*
Use: Decongestant.

Pedia Care NightRest Liquid. (McNeil-CPC) Pseudoephedrine HCl 15 mg, chlorpheniramine maleate 1 mg, dextromethorphan HBr 7.5 mg/5 ml, sorbitol, sucrose. Alcohol free. Cherry flavor. Syr. Bot. 120 ml. *otc.*
Use: Decongestant, antihistamine, antitussive.

Pediacof Syrup. (Sanofi Winthrop) Codeine phosphate 5 mg, phenylephrine HCl 2.5 mg, chlorpheniramine maleate 0.75 mg, potassium iodide 75 mg/5 ml, sodium benzoate 0.2%, alcohol 5%. Syr. Bot. 16 fl oz. *c-v.*
Use: Antitussive, decongestant, antihistamine, expectorant.

Pediacon DX Children's. (Goldline) Phenylpropanolamine HCl 6.25 mg, guaifenesin 100 mg, dextromethorphan HBr 5 mg, alcohol 5%/5 ml. Syrup. Bot. 118 ml. *otc.*
Use: Decongestant, expectorant, antitussive.

Pediacon DX Pediatric. (Goldline) Phenylpropanolamine HCl 6.25 mg, guaifenesin 50 mg, dextromethorphan HBr 5 mg/ml. 5% alcohol. Sugar free. Drops. Bot. 30 ml. *otc.*
Use: Decongestant, expectorant, antitussive.

Pediacon EX. (Goldline) Phenylpropanolamine 6.25 mg, guaifenesin 50 mg/ml. Sugar free. Drops. Bot. 30 ml. *otc.*
Use: Decongestant, expectorant.

Pediaflor Fluoride Drops. (Ross) Fluoride 0.5 mg/ml as sodium fluoride 1.1 mg/ml. Bot. 50 ml. *Rx.*
Use: Dental caries preventative.

Pedialyte. (Ross) Sodium 45 mEq, potassium 20 mEq, chloride 35 mEq, citrate 30 mEq, dextrose 25 g/L. 100 calories/L. **Plastic Bot.:** 8 fl oz. (unflavored), 32 fl oz. (unflavored, fruit). **Nursing Bot.:** Hospital use. Bot. 8 fl oz. *otc.*
Use: Minerals/electrolytes, oral.

Pedialyte Freezer Pops. (Ross) Na 45 mEq/L, K 20 mEq/L, Cl 35 mEq/L, citrate 30 mEq/L, dextrose 25 g/L, phenylalanine, aspartame/Liq. Box. 16s. *otc.*
Use: Minerals/electrolytes, oral.

Pediamycin Drops. (Ross) Erythromycin ethylsuccinate for oral suspension 100 mg/2.5 ml. Bot. 50 ml (Dropper enclosed). *Rx.*

Use: Anti-infective, erythromycin.

Pediapred Oral Liquid. (Medeva) Prednisolone sodium phosphate 6.7 mg/5 ml. Bot. 4 oz. *Rx.*
Use: Corticosteroid.

Pediasure. (Ross) Protein 30 g (Na caseinate, whey protein concentrate), carbohydrate 109.8 g (hydrolyzed corn-starch, sucrose), fat 49.8 g (hi-oleic safflower oil, soy oil, MCT [fractionated coconut oil], mono- and diglycerides, soy lecithin), sodium 380 mg, potassium 1308 mg/L, vitamins A, B_1, B_2, B_3, B_5, B_6, B_{12}, C, D, E, K, inositol, Cl, Ca, P, Mg, I, Mn, Cu, Zn, Fe, biotin, choline, folic acid. < 310 mosm/kg H_2O, 1 cal/ml. Gluten free. Vanilla flavor. Ready-to-use can 240 ml. *otc.*
Use: Nutritional supplement.

Pediatric Cough Syrup. (Weeks & Leo) Ammonium Cl 300 mg, sodium citrate 600 mg/oz. Bot. 4 oz. *otc.*
Use: Expectorant.

Pediatric Electrolyte. (Goldline) Dextrose 25 g, K 20 mEq, Cl 35 mEq, Na 45 mEq, citrate 48 mEq, calories 100/ L. Soln. Bot. 1 L. *otc.*
Use: Enteral nutritional supplement.

Pediatric Maintenance Solution. (Abbott) I.V. solution w/dose calculated according to age, weight, clinical condition. Bot. 250 ml. *Rx.*
Use: Fluids, electrolyte and nutrient replenisher.

Pediatric Multiple Trace Element. (American Regent) Zinc (as sulfate) 0.5 mg, copper (as sulfate) 0.1 mg, manganese (as sulfate) 0.03 mg, chromium (as chloride) 1 mcg/ml. Soln. Vial 10 ml. *Rx.*
Use: Parenteral nutritional supplement.

Pediatric Triban. (Great Southern) Trimethobenzamide HCl 100 mg, benzocaine 2%/Supp. Pkg. 10s. *Rx.*
Use: Antiemetic, antivertigo.

Pediazole Suspension. (Ross) Erythromycin ethylsuccinate 200 mg, sulfisoxazole acetyl 600 mg/5 ml. Bot. Granules reconstituted to 100 ml, 150 ml, 200 ml. *Rx.*
Use: Anti-infective, erythromycin.

Pedi-Bath Salts. (Pedinol) Colloidal sulfur, potassium iodide, balsam peru, sodium hyposulfate, sodium bicarbonate, pine needle oil. Bot. 170 g. *otc.*
Use: Bath dermatological, emollient.

Pedi-Boot Mist Kit. (Pedinol) Cetyl pyridinium Cl, triacetin, chloroxylenol. Bot. 2 oz. *otc.*
Use: Fungicide, sanitizer, deodorizer for shoes.

Pedi-Boro Soak Paks. (Pedinol) Astringent wet dressing w/aluminum sulfate, calcium acetate, coloring agent. Box 12s, 100s. *otc.*
Use: Minor skin irritations.

Pedi-Cort V Creme. (Pedinol) Clioquinol 3%, hydrocortisone 1%. Tube 20 g. *Rx.*
Use: Antifungal, corticosteroid, topical.

Pedicran with Iron. (Scherer) Vitamin B_{12} (crystallized) 25 mcg, ferric pyrophosphate, soluble (elemental iron 30 mg) 250 mg, thiamine mononitrate 10 mg, nicotinamide 10 mg, alcohol 1%/5 ml. Bot. 4 oz, pt. *otc.*
Use: Vitamin/mineral supplement.

pediculicides/scabicides.
See: A-200, Shampoo (SK-Beecham).
A-200 Pyrinate, Gel (SK-Beecham).
Barc, Liq. (Del Pharm).
Blue, Gel (Various Mfr.).
Elimite, Cream (Allergan Herbert).
Eurax, Preps. (Westwood Squibb).
G-well, Preps. (Goldline).
Kwell, Preps. (Reed & Carnrick).
Licetrol 400, Liq. (Republic).
Lindane, Preps. (Various Mfr.).
Nix, Liq. (Glaxo Wellcome).
Ovide, Lot. (GenDerm).
Pronto Concentrate, Shampoo (Del Pharm).
Pyrinyl, Liq. (Various Mfr.).
R & C, Shampoo (Reed & Carnrick).
RID, Liq. (Pfizer).
Scabene, preps. (Stiefel).
Step 2, Liq. (GenDerm).
Tisit, Preps. (Pfeiffer).
Tisit Blue, Gel (Pfeiffer).
Triple X Kit, Liq. (Carter Products).

Pedi-Dri. (Pedinol) Nystatin 100,000 u/g, corn starch, aluminum chlorhydroxide, menthol. Bot. 56.7 g. *Rx.*
Use: Antiperspirant, deodorant, fungicidal foot powder.

Pediotic. (Glaxo Wellcome) Hydrocortisone 1%, neomycin 3.5 mg (as sulfate), polymyxin B sulfate 10,000 units/ ml. Susp. Bot 7.5 ml with dropper. *Rx.*
Use: Otic preparation.

Pedi-Pro Foot Powder. (Pedinol) Aluminum chlorhydroxide, menthol, zinc undecylenate, chloroxylenol. Bot. 2 oz. *otc.*
Use: Fungicide, antiperspirant, deodorant.

Pedituss Cough. (Major) Phenylephrine HCl 2.5 mg, chlorpheniramine maleate 0.75 mg, codeine phosphate 5 mg, potassium iodide 75 mg/5 ml, alcohol 5%, saccharin, sorbitol, sucrose. Syr. Bot. pt., gal. *c-v.*

Use: Decongestant, antihistamine, antitussive, expectorant.

Pedi-Vit A Creme. (Pedinol) Vitamin A 100,000 units/oz. Jar 2 oz, 16 oz, 5 lb. *otc.*
Use: Emollient.

Pedolatum. (King) Salicylic acid, sodium salicylate. Oint. Pkg. 0.5 oz. *otc.*
Use: Analgesic, topical.

Pedric Senior. (Pal-Pak) Acetaminophen 320 mg. *otc.*
Use: Analgesic.

PedTE-PAK-4. (SoloPak) Zinc 1 mg, copper 0.1 mg, manganese 0.025 mg, chromium 1 mcg. Vial 3 ml. *Rx.*
Use: Parenteral nutritional supplement.

Pedtrace-4. (Fujisawa) Zinc 0.5 mg, copper 0.1 mg, chromium 0.85 mcg, manganese 0.25 mg/ml. Vial 3 ml, 10 ml. *Rx.*
Use: Parenteral nutritional supplement.

PedvaxHIB. (Merck) Purified capsular polysaccharide of *Haemophilus influenzae* type b, *Neisseria meningitidis* OMPC 250 mcg/dose when reconstituted, sodium chloride 0.9%, lactose 2 mg, thimerosal 1:20,000. Pow. for Inj. or Soln. Single-dose vial with vial of aluminum hydroxide diluent or single-dose vial. *Rx.*
Use: Agent for immunization.

•**pefloxacin.** (PEH-FLOX-ah-sin) USAN.
Use: Antibacterial.

•**pefloxacin mesylate.** (PEH-FLOX-ah-sin) USAN.
Use: Antibacterial.

•**pegademase bovine.** (peg-AD-ah-MASE BOE-vine) USAN.
Use: Replacement therapy (adenosine deaminase deficiency); modified enzyme for use in ADA deficiency. [Orphan drug]
See: Adagen (Enzon).

Peganone. (Abbott) Ethotoin 250 mg/Tab. or 500 mg/Cap. Bot. 100s. *Rx.*
Use: Anticonvulsant.

•**pegaspargase.** (peh-ASS-par-jase) USAN.
Use: Antineoplastic. [Orphan drug]
See: Oncaspar, Inj. (Enzon).

•**peglicol 5 oleate.** (PEG-lih-kahl 5 OH-lee-ate) USAN.
Use: Pharmaceutic aid (emulsifying agent).

PEG-glucocerebrosidase. (Enzon) *Rx.*
Use: Treatment of Gaucher's disease. [Orphan drug]

PEG-interleukin-2. (Cetus) *Rx.*
Use: Treatment of immunodeficiency in T-cell defects. [Orphan drug]

PEG-l-asparaginase. (Enzon) *Rx.*
Use: Antineoplastic.

P.E.G. Ointment. (Medco Lab) Polyethylene glycol. Jar 16 oz. *otc.*
Use: Water soluble ointment base.

•**pegorgotein.** (peg-AHR-gah-teen) USAN.
Use: Free oxygen radical scavenger.

•**pegoterate.** (PEG-oh-TEER-ate) USAN.
Use: Pharmaceutic aid (suspending agent).

•**pegoxol 7 stearate.** (peg-OX-ole 7 STEE-ah-rate) USAN.
Use: Pharmaceutic aid (emulsifying agent).

Pelamine. (Major) Tripelennamine HCl 50 mg/Tab. Bot. 100s, 1000s. *Rx.*
Use: Antihistamine.

•**pelanserin hydrochloride.** (peh-LAN-ser-in) USAN.
Use: Antihypertensive; vasodilator (serotonin S_2 and α_1 adrenergic receptor blocker).

•**peldesine.** (PELL-deh-seen) USAN.
Use: Antineoplastic, antipsoratic.

pelentan. Ethyl Biscoumacetate. (No Mfr. currently lists).

•**peliomycin.** (PEE-lee-oh-MY-sin) USAN. An antibiotic derived from *Streptomycin luteogriseus.*
Use: Antineoplastic.

•**pelretin.** (PELL-REH-tin) USAN.
Use: Antikeratinizer.

•**pelrinone hydrochloride.** (PELL-rih-nohn) USAN.
Use: Cardiotonic.

•**pemedolac.** (peh-MEH-doe-LACK) USAN.
Use: Analgesic.

•**pemerid nitrate.** (PEM-eh-rid) USAN.
Use: Antitussive.

•**pemirolast potassium.** (peh-mihr-OH-last) USAN.
Use: Antiallergic; inhibitor (mediator release).

•**pemoline.** (PEM-oh-leen) USAN.
Use: Stimulant (central); childhood attention-deficit syndrome (hyperkinetic syndrome).
See: Cylert Prods. (Abbott).

Penagen-VK. (Grafton) Penicillin V. **Tab.:** 250 mg. Bot. 100s. **Pow.:** 250 mg/100 ml. *Rx.*
Use: Anti-infective, penicillin.

•**penamecillin.** (PEN-ah-meh-SILL-in) USAN.
Use: Antibacterial.

•**penbutolol sulfate,** (pen-BYOO-toe-lole)
U.S.P. 23.
Use: Beta-adrenergic blocking agent.
See: Levatol (Reed and Carnrick).

•**penciclovir.** (pen-SIGH-kloe-VEER)
USAN.
Use: Antiviral.
See: Denavir, Cream. (SmithKline
Beecham).

Penecare. (Reed & Carnrick) **Cream:**
Isostearic acid, lactic acid, stearic acid,
PPG-12/SMDI copolymer, steareth-21,
steareth-2, mineral oil, magnesium aluminum silicate, imidurea. Tube. 120 g.
Lot.: Isostearic acid, lactic acid, stearic
acid, steareth-21, PPG-12/SMDI copolymer, steareth-2, magnesium aluminum silicate, imidurea. Bot. 240 ml.
otc.
Use: Emollient.

Penecort Cream. (Allergan Herbert)
Hydrocortisone 1% or 2.5%, benzyl alcohol, petrolatum, stearyl alcohol, propylene glycol, isopropyl myristate, polyoxyl 40 stearate, carbomer 934, sodium lauryl sulfate, edetate disodium
w/sodium hydroxide to adjust pH, purified water. **1%:** Tube 30 g, 60 g. **2.5%:**
Tube 30 g. *Rx.*
Use: Corticosteroid, topical.

Penetrex. (Rhone-Poulenc Rorer) Enoxa-
cin 200 mg or 400 mg/Tab. Bot. 50s.
Rx.
Use: Anti-infective, fluoroquinolone.

•**penfluridol.** (pen-FLEW-rih-dahl) USAN.
Use: Antipsychotic.

penfonylin.
See: Pentid, Prods. (Squibb).

•**penicillamine,** (PEN-ih-SILL-ah-meen)
U.S.P. 23.
Use: Chelating agent; metal complex-
ing agent, cystinuria, rheumatoid ar-
thritis.
See: Cuprimine, Cap. (Merck).
Depen, Tab. (Wallace).

penicillin. (pen-ih-SILL-in) Unless clari-
fied, it means an antibiotic substance
or substances produced by growth of
the molds *Penicillium notatum* or *P.
chrysogenum. Rx.*
Use: Anti-infective.

penicillin aluminum. *Rx.*
Use: Anti-infective, penicillin.

penicillin calcium. U.S.P. XIII. *Rx.*
Use: Anti-infective, penicillin.

penicillin, dimethoxy-phenyl. Methi-
cillin Sodium.
Use: Anti-infective, penicillin.
See: Staphcillin, Vial (Bristol-Myers).

•**penicillin g benzathine,** U.S.P. 23.
Benzathine penicillin G.
Use: Antibacterial.
See: Bicillin, Tab. (Wyeth-Ayerst).
Bicillin Long-Acting (Wyeth-Ayerst).
Permapen, Aqueous Susp. (Pfizer
Laboratories).

**penicillin G benzathine & procaine
combined.** (pen-ih-SILL-in G BENZ-
ah-theen and PRO-cane)
Use: Anti-infective, penicillin.
See: Bicillin C-R, Inj. (Wyeth-Ayerst).
Bicillin C-R 900/300, Inj. (Wyeth-
Ayerst).

•**penicillin G potassium,** (pen-ih-SILL-in)
U.S.P. 23. (Potassium Penicillin, Benzyl
Penicillin Pot.).
Use: Antibacterial.
See: Pfizerpen, Syr. (Pfizer Laborato-
ries).
Pfizerpen, Inj. (Roerig).

**penicillin G potassium w/combina-
tions.**
See: Pentid, Prods. (Squibb).

•**penicillin G procaine sterile,** (pen-ih-
SILL-in G PRO-cane) U.S.P. 23.
Use: Antibacterial.

penicillin G procaine combinations.
See: Bicillin C-R, Tubex (Wyeth-
Ayerst).
Bicillin C-R 900/300 Inj. (Wyeth-
Ayerst).
Duracillin F.A., Amp. (Lilly).
Duracillin Fortified, Vial (Lilly).

**penicillin G procaine and dihydro-
streptomycin sulfate intramammary
infusion,**
Use: Anti-infective.

**penicillin G procaine, dihydrostrepto-
mycin sulfate, chlorpheniramine maleate and dexamethasone suspension, sterile.** (pen-ih-SILL-in G PRO-
cane, die-HIGH-droe-STREP-toe-MY-
sin klor-fen-EAR-ah-meen MAL-ee-ate
and DEX-ah-METH-ah-sone)
Use: Anti-infective, antihistamine, anti-
inflammatory.

**penicillin G procaine, dihydrostrepto-
mycin sulfate, and prednisolone
suspension, sterile.**
Use: Anti-infective, anti-inflammatory.

**penicillin G procaine and dihydro-
streptomycin sulfate suspension,
sterile.**
Use: Anti-infective.

**penicillin G procaine, neomycin and
polymyxin B sulfates, and hydrocortisone acetate topical suspension.**
Use: Anti-infective, anti-inflammatory.

penicillin G procaine and novobiocin sodium intramammary infusion.
Use: Anti-infective.

penicillin G procaine w/aluminum stearate suspension, sterile.
Use: Anti-infective.

penicillin G, procaine, sterile. Sterile Susp., Intramammary infusion, U.S.P. 23. Procaine Penicillin.
Use: Anti-infective.
W/Parenteral, aqueous susp., (Procaine Penicillin, for Aqueous Inj.,) Procaine Penicillin and buffered Penicillin for aqueous, Inj.
See: Crysticillin A.S., Vial (Squibb).
Diurnal-Panicillin (Pharmacia & Upjohn).
Duracillin A.S., Preps. (Lilly).
Pfizerpen-A.S. (Roerig).
Tu-Cillin, Inj. (Solvay).
Wycillin, Susp. (Wyeth-Ayerst).
W/Parenteral, in oil w/aluminum monostearate. Penicillin Procaine in Oil Inj.

•**penicillin G sodium for injection,** U.S.P. 23.
Use: Antibacterial.

penicillin hydrabamine phenoxymethyl.
Use: Anti-infective.

penicillin O chloroprocaine.
Use: Anti-infective, penicillin.

penicillin O, sodium. Allylmercaptomethyl penicillin.
Use: Anti-infective.

penicillin, phenoxyethyl.
Use: Anti-infective, penicillin.
See: Phenethicillin, Penicillin potassium 152.

penicillin phenoxymethyl benzathine.
Use: Anti-infective, penicillin.
See: Penicillin V Benzathine.

penicillin phenoxymethyl hydrabamine.
Use: Anti-infective, penicillin.
See: Penicillin V Hydrabamine.

penicillin S benzathine and penicillin G procaine suspension, sterile.
Use: Anti-infective.

•**penicillin V,** U.S.P. 23. *Formerly Penicillin Phenoxymethyl.* A biosynthetic penicillin formed by fermentation, with suitable precursors of *Penicillin notatum.*
Use: Antibacterial.
See: Biotic Pow. (Scrip).
Compocillin-V, Water, Susp. (Ross).
Ledercillin VK (Lederle).
Penagen-VK, Tab., Pow. (Gafton).
Robicillin-VK (Robins).

Uticillin VK (Pharmacia & Upjohn).
V-Cillin, Preps. (Lilly).
V-Pen, Tab. (Century).

•**penicillin V benzathine,** (pen-ih-SILL-in V BEN-zah-theen) U.S.P. 23. *Formerly Penicillin Benzathine Phenoxymethyl.*
Use: Antibacterial.
See: Pen-Vee, Prods. (Wyeth-Ayerst).

•**penicillin V hydrabamine.** (pen-ih-SILL-in V HIGH-drah-BAM-een) USAN. U.S.P. XX. *Formerly Penicillin Hydrabamine Phenoxymethyl.*
Use: Antibacterial.
See: Compocillin-V Hydrabamine, Oral Susp. (Ross).

•**penicillin V potassium,** (pen-ih-SILL-in V) U.S.P. 23. *Formerly Penicillin Potassium Phenoxymethyl.*
Use: Antibacterial.
See: Beepen VK, Tab., Syr. (SK-Beecham).
Betapen VK., Soln., Tab. (Bristol-Myers).
Biotic-V-Powder (Scrip).
Bopen, V-K, Tab. (Boyd).
Dowpen VK, Tab. (Hoechst Marion Roussel).
Ledercillin VK, Oral Soln., Tab. (Lederle).
LV, Tab (ICN Pharm).
Pen-Vee-K, Soln., Tab. (Wyeth-Ayerst).
Pfizerpen VK, Pow., Tab. (Pfizer Laboratories).
Phenethicillin Potassium.
Repen-VK, Tab., Oral Susp. (Solvay).
Robicillin VK, Tab., Soln. (Robins).
Ro-Cillin VK, Soln., Tab. (Solvay).
Saropen-VK (Saron).
SK-Penicillin VK, Soln., Tab. (SK-Beecham).
Suspen, Liq. (Circle).
Uticillin VK, Tab., Soln. (Pharmacia & Upjohn).
V-Cillin K, Tab., Oral Soln. (Lilly).
Veetids, Soln., Tab. (Squibb Mark).

penidural.
Use: Anti-infective.

Pen-Kera Creme with Keratin Binding Factor. (Ascher) Bot. 8 oz. *otc.*
Use: Emollient.

Penntuss. (Medeva) Codeine (as polistirex) 10 mg, chlorpheniramine maleate 4 mg/5 ml. Bot. pt. *c-v.*
Use: Antitussive, antihistamine.

•**pentabamate.** (PEN-tah-BAM-ate) USAN.
Use: Tranquilizer (minor).

Pentacarinat. (Centeon) Pentamidine isethionate 300 mg. Inj. Single-dose vial. *Rx.*

Use: Anti-infective.
pentacosactride.
Use: Corticotrophic peptide.
See: Norleusactide (I.N.N.).
●**pentaerythritol tetranitrate diluted,** U.S.P. 23.
Use: Vasodilator.
See: Arcotrate Nos. 1 and 2, Tab. (Arcum).
Dilac-80, Cap. (Ascher).
Duotrate-45, Cap. (Hoechst Marion Roussel).
Kortrate, Cap. (Amid).
Maso-Trol, Tab. (Mason).
Metranil, Cap. (Meyer).
Nitrin, Tab. (Pal-Pak).
Penta-E, Tab. (Recsei).
Pentafin, Granucap, Tab. (Solvay).
Pentetra, Tab. (Paddock).
Peritrate, Tab. (Parke-Davis).
Petro-20 mg, Tab. (Foy).
Reithritol, Tab. (Jones Medical).
Tentrate, Tab. (Tennessee Pharm).
Tetracap-30, Cap. (Freeport).
Tetracap-80, Cap. (Freeport).
Tetratab, Tab. (Freeport).
Tetratab No. 1, Tab. (Freeport).
Tranite, Cap., Tab. (Westerfield).
Vasolate, Cap. (Parmed).
Vasolate-80, Cap. (Parmed).
pentaerythritol tetranitrate, diluted, U.S.P. 23.
Use: Vasodilator.
pentaerythritol tetranitrate w/combinations.
See: Arcotrate No. 3, Tab. (Arcum).
Bitrate, Tab. (Arco).
Dimycor, Tab. (Standard Drug).
Pentetra w/Phenobarbital, Tab. (Paddock).
Peritrate w/Nitroglycerin, Tab. (Parke-Davis).
Respet, Tab. (Westerfield).
●**pentafilcon a.** (PEN-tah-FILL-kahn A) USAN.
Use: Contact lens material (hydrophilic).
●**pentagastrin.** (PEN-tah-ASS-trin) USAN.
Use: Diagnostic aid (gastric secretion indicator).
See: Peptavlon, Amp. (Wyeth-Ayerst).
●**pentalyte.** USAN.
Use: Electrolyte combination.
Pentam 300. (Fujisawa) Pentamidine isethionate 300 mg/Vial. *Rx.*
Use: Anti-infective.
pentamethylenetetrazol.
See: Pentylenetetrazol, U.S.P.
pentamidine isethionate. (pen-TAM-ih-deen ice-uh-THIGH-uh-nate) (Abbott) 300 mg. Inj., lyophilized. Single-dose fliptop vials. *Rx.*

Use: Anti-infective. [Orphan drug]
See: Pentam 300, Inj. (Fujisawa).
pentamidine isethionate (inhalation). *Rx.*
Use: Anti-infective. [Orphan drug]
●**pentamorphone.** (PEN-tah-MORE-fone) USAN.
Use: Analgesic (narcotic).
pentamoxane hydrochloride.
Use: Tranquilizer.
●**pentamustine.** (PEN-tah-MUSS-teen) USAN.
Use: Antineoplastic.
pentaphonate. Dodecyltriphenylphosphonium pentachlorophenolate.
Use: Anti-infective.
●**pentapiperium methylsulfate.** (PEN-tah-PIP-ehr-ee-uhm METH-ill-SULL-fate) USAN.
Use: Anticholinergic.
pentapyrrolidinium bitartrate.
See: Pentolinium Tartrate.
pentaquine phosphate.
Pentasa. (Hoechst Marion Roussel) Mesalamine 250 mg. CR Cap. Bot. 240s, UD 80s. *Rx.*
Use: Ulcerative colitis, proctosigmoiditis or proctitis.
pentasodium colistinmethanesulfonate. Sterile Colistimethate Sodium, U.S.P. 23.
●**pentastarch.** (PEN-tah-starch) USAN.
Use: Leukopheresis adjunct (red cell sedimenting agent). [Orphan drug]
Penta-Stress. (Penta) Vitamins A 10,000 IU, D 500 IU, B_1 10 mg, B_2 10 mg, B_6 1 mg, calcium pantothenate 5 mg, niacinamide 50 mg, C 100 mg, E 2 IU, B_{12} 3.3 mcg/Cap. Bot. 90s, 1000s, Jar 250s. *otc.*
Use: Vitamin/mineral supplement.
Penta-Viron. (Penta) Calcium carbonate 500 mg, ferrous fumarate 100 mg, vitamins C 50 mg, D 167 IU, A 3.333 IU, B_1 3.3 mg, B_2 3.3 mg, B_6 2 mg, calcium pantothenate 1.6 mg, niacinamide 16.7 mg, E 2 IU/Cap. Bot. 100s, 1000s, Jar 250s. *otc.*
Use: Vitamin/mineral supplement.
Pentazine. (Century) Promethazine expectorant. Bot. 4 oz, 16 oz, gal. *Rx.*
Use: Antihistamine.
Pentazine Inj. (Century) Promethazine 50 mg/ml. Inj. Vial 10 ml. *Rx.*
Use: Antihistamine.
Pentazine w/Codeine. (Century) Promethazine expectorant. Bot. 4 oz, 16 oz, gal.
Use: Antihistamine.

Pentazine VC w/Codeine Liquid. (Century) Promethazine HCl 6.25 mg, codeine phosphate 10 mg. Liq. Bot. 118 ml, pt, gal. *c-v.*
Use: Antihistamine, antitussive.

•**pentazocine,** (pen-TAZ-oh-seen) U.S.P. 23.
Use: Analgesic.

•**pentazocine hydrochloride,** (pen-TAZ-oh-seen) U.S.P. 23.
Use: Analgesic.
W/ Acetaminophen.
See: Talacen, Cap. (Sanofi Winthrop).

pentazocine hydrochloride and aspirin tablets.
Use: Analgesic.
See: Talwin Compound, Tab. (Sanofi Winthrop).

•**pentazocine lactate injection,** (pen-TAZ-oh-seen LACK-tate) U.S.P. 23.
Use: Analgesic.
See: Talwin Injection, Inj. (Sanofi Winthrop).

pentazocine and naloxone hydrochloride tablets. (Royce) Pentazocine 50 mg, naloxone HCl 0.5 mg/Tab. Box. 100s, 500s, 1000s. *Rx.*
Use: Analgesic.
See: Talwin NX, Tab. (Sanofi Winthrop).

•**pentetate calcium trisodium.** (PEN-teh-tate KAL-see-uhm try-SO-dee-uhm) USAN.
Use: Chelating agent (plutonium).

•**pentetate calcium trisodium Yb 169.** (PEN-teh-tate KAL-see-uhm TRY-SO-dee-uhm Yb 169) USAN.
Use: Radioactive agent.

•**pentetate indium disodium In 111.** (PEN-teh-tate IN-dee-uhm) USAN.
Use: Diagnostic aid, radioactive agent.

•**pentetic acid,** (PEN-teh-tick) U.S.P. 23.
Use: Diagnostic aid.

Pentetra-Paracote. (Paddock) Pentaerythritol tetranitrate 30 mg or 80 mg/Cap. Bot. 100s, 500s, 1000s. *Rx.*
Use: Antianginal.

penthienate bromide.

Penthrane. (Abbott Hospital Prods) Methoxyflurane. Bot. 15 ml, 125 ml. *Rx.*
Use: General anesthetic.

•**pentiapine maleate.** (pen-TIE-ah-PEEN) USAN.
Use: Antipsychotic.

•**pentigetide.** (pent-EYE-jeh-TIDE) USAN.
Use: Antiallergic.

Pentina. (Freeport) Rauwolfia serpentina, 100 mg/Tab. Bot. 1000s. *Rx.*
Use: Antihypertensive.

•**pentisomicin.** (pent-IH-so-MY-sin) USAN.
Use: Anti-infective.

•**pentizidone sodium.** (pen-TIH-ZIH-dohn) USAN.
Use: Antibacterial.

•**pentobarbital,** (pen-toe-BAR-bih-tahl) U.S.P. 23.
Use: Sedative, hypnotic.
See: Nembutal, Elix., Gradumets (Abbott) Penta, Tab. (Dunhall).

pentobarbital combinations.
Use: Sedative/hypnotic.
See: Cafergot-PB, Supp., Tab. (Sandoz).
Nembutal, Preps. (Abbott).

•**pentobarbital, sodium,** (pen-toe-BAR-bih-tahl) U.S.P. 23.
Use: Hypnotic, sedative.
See: Maso-Pent, Tab. (Mason).
Nembutal Sodium, Preps. (Abbott).
Night-Caps, Cap. (Jones Medical).
W/Adiphenine HCl, phamasorb, aluminum hydroxide.
See: Spasmasorb, Tab. (Roberts).
W/Atropine sulfate, hyoscine HBr, hyoscyamine sulfate.
See: Eldonal, Elix., Tab., Cap. (Canright).
W/Ephedrine.
See: Ephedrine and Nembutal-25, Cap. (Abbott).
W/Ergotamine tartrate, caffeine alkaloid, bellafoline.
See: Cafergot-P.B., Tab. (Sandoz).
W/Homatropine methylbromide, dehydrocholic acid, ox bile extract.
See: Homachol, Tab. (Lemmon).
W/Pyrilamine maleate.
See: A-N-R, Rectorette (Roberts).
W/Seco-, buta-, phenobarbital.
W/Vitamin compounds, d-methamphetamine HCl.
See: Fetamin, Tab. (Mission).

pentobarbital sodium. (Various Mfr.) 100 mg/Cap. Bot. 100s.
Use: Hypnotic, sedative.

pentobarbital sodium. (Wyeth-Ayerst) 50mg/ml. Inj. Tubex 2 ml. *c-II.*
Use: Hypnotic, sedative.

pentobarbital, soluble.
See: Pentobarbital Sodium, U.S.P.

Pentol Tabs. (Major) Pentaerythritol tetranitrate. **10 mg/Tab.:** Bot. 1000s; **20 mg/Tab.:** Bot. 100s, 1000s; **80 mg/SA Tab.:** Bot. 250s, 1000s. *Rx.*
Use: Antianginal.

Pentolair. (Bausch & Lomb) Cyclopentolate HCl 1%. Soln. Squeeze Bot. 2 ml, 15 ml. *Rx.*

Use: Cycloplegic mydriatic.

pentolinium tartrate. Pentamethylene-1:5-bis (1'-methylpyrrolidinium bitartrate).
Use: Antihypertensive.

•**pentomone.** (PEN-toe-MONE) USAN.
Use: Prostate growth inhibitor.

•**pentopril.** (PEN-toe-prill) USAN.
Use: Enzyme inhibitor (angiotensin-converting).

•**pentosan polysulfate sodium.** (PEN-toe-san) USAN.
Use: Anti-inflammatory (interstitial cystitis).

pentosan sodium polysulfate.
Use: Treatment of interstitial cystitis. [Orphan drug]
See: Elmiron, Cap. (Ivax).

•**pentostatin.** (PEN-toe-STAT-in) USAN.
Use: Potentiator; leukemia. [Orphan drug]

Pentothal. (Abbott) **Pow. for Inj.:** Thiopental sodium 20 mg/ml. In 1, 2.5, 5 g kits, 400 mg syringes; 25 mg/ml. In 1, 2.5, 5 g, 500 mg kits, 250, 400, 500 mg syringes. **Rectal Susp.:** Thiopental sodium 400 mg/g. In 2 g syringe. *Rx.*
Use: Anesthetic.

•**pentoxifylline.** (pen-TOX-IH-fill-in) USAN.
Use: Vasodilator; oral hemorrheologic agent for peripheral vascular disease.
See: Trental (Hoechst Marion Roussel).

Pentrax Gold. (GenDerm) Solubilized coal tar extract 4%. Shampoo. Bot. 168 ml. *otc.*
Use: Antiseborrheic.

Pentrax Shampoo. (Rydelle) Tar extract 8.75%, detergents, conditioning agents. Bot. 4 oz, 8 oz. *otc.*
Use: Antiseborrheic.

•**pentrinitrol.** (pen-TRY-nye-TROLE) USAN.
Use: Vasodilator (coronary).

Pent-T-80. (Mericon) Pentaerythritol tetranitrate 80 mg/T.D. Cap. Bot. 100s, 1000s. *Rx.*
Use: Antianginal.

Pen-V. (Goldline) Penicillin 250 mg or 500 mg/Tab. Bot. 100s, 1000s. *Rx.*
Use: Anti-infective, penicillin.

Pen-Vee K. (Wyeth-Ayerst) Potassium phenoxymethyl penicillin. 250 mg or 500 mg/Tab. Bot. 100s, 500s, Redipak 100s. *Rx.*
Use: Anti-infective, penicillin.

Pen-Vee K for Oral Solution. (Wyeth-Ayerst) Penicillin V potassium. **125 mg/5 ml:** Bot. 100 ml, 200 ml. **250 mg/5 ml:** Bot. 100 ml, 150 ml, 200 ml. *Rx.*
Use: Anti-infective, penicillin.

Pepcid. (Merck) Famotidine. **Tab.:** 20 mg or 40 mg. Bot. 30s, 90s, 100s, UD 100s. **Oral Susp.:** 40 mg/5 ml. Bot. 400 mg. **I.V. Inj. Premixed:** 20 mg/50 ml in 0.9% NaCl. 50 ml *Galaxy* container. *Rx.*
Use: Histamine H_2 antagonist.

Pepcid AC Acid Controller. (J & J-Merck) Famotidine 10 mg/Tab. Pkg. 12s. *otc.*
Use: Histamine H_2 antagonist.

•**peplomycin sulfate.** (PEP-low-MY-sin) USAN.
Use: Antineoplastic.

•**peppermint,** N.F. 18.
Use: Pharmaceutic aid (flavor, perfume), antitussive, expectorant, nasal decongestant.
See: Vicks Prods. (Richardson-Vicks).

•**peppermint oil,** N.F. 18.
Use: Pharmaceutic aid (flavor).

•**peppermint spirit,** U.S.P. 23.
Use: Digestive aid, (flavor, perfume).

•**peppermint water,** N.F. 18.
Use: Pharmaceutic aid (vehicle, flavored).

Pepsamar Comp. Tablets. (Sanofi Winthrop) Aluminum hydroxide, magnesium hydroxide. *otc.*
Use: Antacid.

Pepsamar Esp Liquid. (Sanofi Winthrop) Aluminum hydroxide, glycerin. *otc.*
Use: Antacid.

Pepsamar Esp Tablets. (Sanofi Winthrop) Aluminum hydroxide, magnesium hydroxide, mannitol powder. *otc.*
Use: Antacid.

Pepsamar HM Tablets. (Sanofi Winthrop) Aluminum hydroxide, starch. *otc.*
Use: Antacid.

Pepsamar Liquid. (Sanofi Winthrop) Aluminum hydroxide. *otc.*
Use: Antacid.

Pepsamar Suspension. (Sanofi Winthrop) Aluminum hydroxide, magnesium hydroxide, sorbitol. *otc.*
Use: Antacid.

Pepsamar Tablets. (Sanofi Winthrop) Aluminum hydroxide. *otc.*
Use: Antacid.

Pepsicone Gel. (Sanofi Winthrop) Aluminum hydroxide, magnesium hydroxide, simethicone. *otc.*
Use: Antacid, antiflatulent.

Pepsicone Tablet. (Sanofi Winthrop) Aluminum hydroxide, magnesium hydrox-

ide, simethicone. *otc.*
Use: Antacid, antiflatulent.
pepsin.
Use: Digestive aid.
pepsin w/combinations.
See: Biloric, Cap. (Arcum).
Donnazyme, Tab. (Robins).
Entozyme, Tab. (Robins).
Enzobile, Tab. (Roberts).
Gourmase-PB, Cap. (Solvay).
Kanulase, Tab. (Sandoz).
Leber Taurine, Liq. (Paddock).
Nu'Leven, Tab. (Lemmon).
Ro-Bile, Tab. (Solvay).
Zypan, Tab. (Standard Process).
pepsin lactated, elixir.
See: Peptalac, Liq. (Jones Medical).
•**pepstatin.** USAN.
Use: Enzyme inhibitor (pepsin).
Peptamen Liquid. (Clintec Nutrition) En-
zymatically hydrolyzed whey proteins,
maltodextrin, starch, MCT, sunflower oil,
lecithin, vitamins A, B$_1$, B$_2$, B$_3$, B$_5$, B$_6$,
B$_{12}$, C, D, E, K, folic acid, biotin, cho-
line, Ca, Cl, Cu, Fe, I, Mg, Mn, P, Zn.
Can 500 ml. *otc.*
Use: Nutritional supplement.
Peptavlon. (Wyeth-Ayerst) Pentagastrin
0.25 mg, sodium Cl/ml. For evaluation
of gastric acid secretion. Amp. 2 ml,
Ctn. 10s.
Use: Diagnostic aid.
Peptenzyme. (Reed & Carnrick) Alcohol
16%. Pleasantly aromatic. Bot. pt.
Use: Pharmaceutic aid.
Pepto-Bismol Caplets. (Procter &
Gamble) Bismuth subsalicylate 262 mg,
< 2 mg sodium/Capl. Sugar free. Bot.
24s, 40s. *otc.*
Use: Antidiarrheal.
Pepto-Bismol Liquid. (Procter &
Gamble) Bismuth subsalicylate 262
mg/15 ml. Bot. 4 oz, 8 oz, 12 oz, 16 oz.
otc.
Use: Antidiarrheal.
**Pepto-Bismol Maximum Strength Liq-
uid.** (Procter & Gamble) 524 mg/15 ml.
Bot. 120 ml, 240 ml, 360 ml. *otc.*
Use: Antidiarrheal.
Pepto-Bismol Tablets. (Procter &
Gamble) Bismuth subsalicylate 262.5
mg/Chew. Tab. Pkg. 24s, 42s. *otc.*
Use: Antidiarrheal.
Perandren Phenylacetate. (Novartis)
Testosterone phenylacetate. *c-iii.*
Use: Androgen.
percaine.
Use: Local anesthetic.
See: Dibucaine HCl, U.S.P.

Perchloracap. (Mallinckrodt) Potassium
perchlorate 200 mg/Cap. Bot. 100s.
Use: Radiographic adjunct.
perchlorethylene.
See: Tetrachlorethylene, U.S.P. 23.
perchlorperazine.
See: Compazine, Preps. (SK-
Beecham).
Percocet. (DuPont) Oxycodone HCl 5
mg, acetaminophen 325 mg/Tab. Bot.
100s, 500s, UD 100s. *c-ii.*
Use: Narcotic analgesic combination.
Percodan. (DuPont) Oxycodone HCl 4.5
mg, oxycodone terephthalate 0.38 mg,
aspirin 325 mg/Tab. Bot. 100s, 500s,
1000s, UD 250s. *c-ii.*
Use: Narcotic analgesic combination.
W/Hexobarbital.
See: Percobarb, Cap. (DuPont).
Percodan-Demi. (DuPont) Oxycodone
HCl 2.25 mg, oxycodone terephthal-
ate 0.19 mg, aspirin 325 mg/Tab. Bot.
100s. *c-ii.*
Use: Narcotic analgesic combination.
Percogesic. (Richardson-Vicks) Aceta-
minophen 325 mg, phenyltoloxamine
citrate 30 mg/Tab. Bot. 24s, 50s, 90s.
otc.
Use: Analgesic, antihistamine.
Percomorph Liver Oil. (May be blended
with 50% other fish liver oils; each g
contains vitamins A 60,000 IU & D 8500
IU).
See: Oleum Percomorphum.
Percy Medicine. (Merrick Medicine) Bismuth subnitrate 959 mg, calcium
hydroxide 21.9 mg/10 ml, alcohol 5%.
otc.
Use: Antidiarrheal.
Perdiem. (Rhone-Poulenc Rorer) Blend
of psyllium 82%, senna 18% as active
ingredients in granular form. Sodium
content (0.08 mEq) 1.8 mg/rounded tsp.
(6 g). Canister 100 g, 250 g, UD 6 g.
otc.
Use: Laxative.
Perdiem Fiber. (Rhone-Poulenc Rorer)
Psyllium 100% as active ingredient in
granular form. Sodium content (0.08
mEq) 1.8 mg/rounded tsp. (6 g). Canister 100 g, 250 g, UD 6 g. *otc.*
Use: Laxative.
Pere-Diosate. (Towne) Docusate sodium
100 mg, casanthranol 30 mg/Cap. Bot.
100s. *otc.*
Use: Laxative.
Perestan. (Interstate) Docusate sodium
100 mg, casanthranol 30 mg/Cap. Bot.
100s, 1000s. *otc.*

Use: Laxative.

•**perfilcon a.** (per-FILL-kahn A) USAN.
Use: Contact lens material (hydrophilic).
See: Permalens (Ciba Vision).

•**perflenapent.** USAN.
Use: Diagnostic aid (ultrasound contrast agent).

•**perflisopent.** USAN.
Use: Diagnostic aid (ultrasound contrast agent).

•**perflubron,** (per-FLEW-brahn) U.S.P. 23.
Use: Contrast agent; blood substitute.
See: Imagent GI, Liq. (Alliance).

•**perfosfamide.** (per-FOSS-fam-ide) USAN.
Use: Antineoplastic. [Orphan drug]

pergalen.
See: Sodium Apolate.

•**pergolide mesylate.** (PURR-go-lide) USAN.
Use: Dopamine agonist.

Pergonal (menotropins). (Serono) Follicle stimulating hormone (FSH) and luteinizing hormone (LH) 75 IU or 150 IU. Inj. Amp 2 ml. *Rx.*
Use: Gonadotropin.

Pergrava. (Arcum) Vitamins A 2000 IU, D 300 IU, B_1 2 mg, B_2 2 mg, nicotinamide 10 mg, B_6 2 mg, B_{12} 5 mcg, C 60 mg, calcium 40 mg/Cap. Bot. 100s, 1000s. *otc.*
Use: Vitamin/mineral supplement.

Pergrava No. 2. (Arcum) Vitamins A 2000 IU, D 300 IU, B_1 2 mg, B_2 2 mg, nicotinamide 10 mg, B_6 2 mg, $\bar{C}$ 60 mg, calcium lactate monohydrate 200 mg, ferrous gluconate 31 mg, folic acid 0.1 mg/Cap. Bot. 100s, 1000s. *otc.*
Use: Vitamin/mineral supplement.

perhexiline. (per-HEX-ih-leen)
Use: Treatment of angina pectoris.

•**perhexiline maleate.** (per-HEX-ih-leen) USAN.
Use: Vasodilator (coronary).

perhydrol.
See: Hydrogen Peroxide 30% (Various Mfr.).

Peri Sofcap. (Alton) Docusate sodium with peristim. Bot. 100s, 1000s. *otc.*
Use: Laxative.

Periactin. (Merck) Cyproheptadine HCl 4 mg/Tab. Bot. 100s. *Rx.*
Use: Antihistamine.

Periactin Syrup. (Merck) Cyproheptadine HCl 2 mg/5 ml, alcohol 5%, sorbic acid 0.1%. Bot. 473 ml. *Rx.*
Use: Antihistamine.

Peri-Care. (Sween) Vitamins A and D in petroleum ointment base. Tube 0.5 oz,

1.75 oz. Jar 2 oz, 5 oz, 8 oz. *otc.*
Use: Emollient.

Peri-Colace. (Bristol-Myers) **Cap.:** Docusate sodium 100 mg, casanthranol 30 mg/Cap. Bot. 30s, 60s, 250s, 1000s, UD 100s. **Syr.:** Docusate sodium 60 mg, casanthranol 30 mg/15 ml, ethyl alcohol 10%. Bot. 8 oz, pt. *otc.*
Use: Laxative.

Peridex. (Procter & Gamble) Chlorhexidine gluconate 0.12%, alcohol 11.6%, glycerin, PEG-40 sorbitan diisostearate, flavor, sodium saccharin, FD&C blue No. 1, water. Bot. 480 ml. *Rx.*
Use: Mouth preparation.

Peridin-C. (Beutlich) Hesperidin methyl chalcone 50 mg, hesperidin complex 150 mg, ascorbic acid 200 mg/Tab. Bot. 100s, 500s. *otc.*
Use: Vitamin supplement.

Peri-Dos. (Goldline) Docusate sodium 100 mg, casanthranol 30 mg/Cap. Bot. 30s, 60s, 100s, 1000s. *otc.*
Use: Laxative.

Peries. (Xttrium) Medicated pads w/witch hazel, glycerin. Jar pad 40s. *otc.*
Use: Hygienic wipe and local compress.

Perimed. (Olin) Hydrogen peroxide 1.5%, povidone-iodine 6%, saccharin. Pouch 20 ml. *otc.*
Use: Mouth and gum preparation.

•**perindopril.** (per-IN-doe-prill) USAN.
Use: ACE inhibitor.

•**perindopril erbumine.** (per-IN-doe-prill ehr-BYOO-meen) USAN.
Use: Antihypertensive.
See: Aceon, Tab. (Ortho).

Perio-Eze-20. (Moyco) Oral paste.
Use: Analgesic for pain of gums and mucosa.

PerioGard. (Colgate Oral) Chlorhexidine gluconate 0.12%, alcohol 11.6%, glycerin, PEG-40, sorbitol diisostearate, saccharin. Rinse. 473 ml w/ 15 ml dose cup. *Rx.*
Use: Anesthetic, oral.

peristomal covering.
See: Stomahesive, wafer (Squibb).

Peritinic. (Lederle) Elemental iron 100 mg, docusate sodium 100 mg, vitamins B_1 7.5 mg, B_2 7.5 mg, B_6 7.5 mg, B_{12} 50 mcg, C 200 mg, niacinamide 30 mg, folic acid 0.05 mg, pantothenic acid 15 mg/Tab. Bot. 60s. *otc.*
Use: Vitamin/mineral supplement, laxative.

Peritrate. (Parke-Davis) Pentaerythritol tetranitrate. **10 mg/Tab.:** Bot. 100s, 1000s. **20 mg/Tab.:** Bot. 100s, 1000s,

UD 100s. **40 mg/Tab.**: Bot. 100s. *Rx.*
Use: Antianginal.

Peritrate S.A. (Parke-Davis) Pentaerythritol tetranitrate 80 mg (20 mg in immediate release layer, 60 mg in sustained release base)/Tab. Bot. 100s, 1000s, UD 100s. *Rx.*
Use: Antianginal.

Peri-Wash. (Sween) Bot. 4 oz, 8 oz, 1 gal, 5 gal, 30 gal, 55 gal.
Use: Anorectal preparation.

Peri-Wash II. (Sween) Bot. 4 oz, 8 oz, 1 gal, 5 gal, 30 gal, 55 gal.
Use: Anorectal preparation.

•**perlapine.** USAN.
Use: Sedative, hypnotic.

perlatan.
See: Estrone (Various Mfr.).

permanganic acid, potassium salt. Potassium permanganate, U.S.P. 23.

Permapen. (Roerig) Benzathine penicillin G 1,200,000 units/ml. Disp. syringe 2 ml. *Rx.*
Use: Anti-infective, penicillin.

Permax. (Athena Neurosciences) Pergolide mesylate. **0.05 mg, 0.25 mg/Tab.:** Bot. 30s. **1 mg/Tab.:** Bot. 100s. *Rx.*
Use: Antiparkinsonian.

•**permethrin.** (per-METH-rin) USAN. Synthetic pyrethrin.
Use: Pediculicide for treatment of head lice, ectoparasiticide.
See: Nix, Cream (Glaxo Wellcome).

Permitil. (Schering-Plough) Fluphenazine HCl. **2.5 mg or 5 mg/Tab:** Bot. 100s. **10 mg/Tab.:** Bot. 1000s. *Rx.*
Use: Antipsychotic.

Permitil Oral Concentrate. (Schering-Plough) Fluphenazine HCl 5 mg/ml. Bot. 120 ml w/calibrated dropper. Hospital use. *Rx.*
Use: Antipsychotic.

Pernox Lathering Abradant Scrub. (Westwood Squibb) Sulfur, salicylic acid. Lot. Bot. 141 g. *otc.*
Use: Antiacne.

Pernox Lotion. (Westwood Squibb) Microfine granules of polyethylene 20%, sulfur 2%, salicylic acid 2% in a combination of soapless cleansers and wetting agents. Bot. 6 oz. *otc.*
Use: Antiacne.

Pernox Medicated Lathering Scrub Cleanser. (Westwood Squibb) Polyethylene granules 26%, sulfur 2%, salicylic acid 1.5% w/soapless surface-active cleansers and wetting agents. Regular or lemon. Tube 2 oz, 4 oz. *otc.*
Use: Antiacne.

Pernox Scrub for Oily Skin. (Westwood Squibb) Sulfur, salicylic acid, EDTA. Cleanser. 56 g, 113 g. *otc.*
Use: Antiacne.

Pernox Shampoo. (Westwood Squibb) Sodium laureth sulfate, water, lauramide DEA, quaternium 22, PEG-75 lanolin/hydrolyzed animal protein, fragrance, sodium Cl, lactic acid, sorbic acid, disodium EDTA, FD&C yellow No. 6 and blue No. 1. Bot. 8 oz. *otc.*
Use: Cleanser and conditioner for oily hair.

peroxidase. W/Glucose oxidase, potassium, iodide.
See: Diastix Reagent Strips (Bayer).

peroxide, dibenzoyl. Benzoyl Peroxide, Hydrous.

peroxides.
See: Hydrogen Peroxide (Various Mfr.).
Urea Peroxide.
Zinc Peroxide.

Peroxin A5. (Dermol) Benzoyl peroxide 5%. Gel. Tube 45 g. *Rx.*
Use: Antiacne.

Peroxin A10. (Dermol) Benzoyl peroxide 10%. Gel. Tube 45 g. *Rx.*
Use: Antiacne.

Peroxyl Dental Rinse. (Colgate Oral) Hydrogen peroxide 1.5% in mint flavored base, alcohol 6%. Bot. 240 ml, pint. *otc.*
Use: Mouth preparation.

Peroxyl Gel. (Colgate Oral) Hydrogen peroxide 1.5% in a mint flavored base. Tube. 15 g. *otc.*
Use: Mouth preparation.

•**perphenazine,** (per-FEN-uh-ZEEN) U.S.P. 23.
Use: Antiemetic, antipsychotic, tranquilizer.
See: Trilafon, Prods. (Schering-Plough).

perphenazine/amitriptyline tablets. (per-FEN-uh-zeen am-ee-TRIP-tih-leen) (Various, eg, Bolar, Geneva, Goldline, Lemmon, Par, Rugby, Schein, Zenith). Perphenazine (mg): 2, 2; Amitriptyline (mg): 10, 25. Bot. 21s, 100s, 500s, 1000s; Bot. 100s, 500s, 1000s.
Use: Miscellaneous psychotherapeutic.
See: Etrafon, Prods. (Schering-Plough).
Triavil, Tab. (Merck).

Persa-Gel. (Ortho Derm) Benzoyl peroxide 5% or 10%, acetone base. Tube 45 g, 90 g. *Rx.*
Use: Antiacne.

Persa-Gel W 5%, 10%. (Ortho Derm) Benzoyl peroxide 5% or 10% in wa-

ter base. Tube 45 g, 90 g. *Rx.*
Use: Antiacne.

Persangue. (Arcum) Ferrous gluconate 192 mg, vitamins C 150 mg, B$_1$ 3 mg, B$_2$ 3 mg, B$_{12}$ 50 mcg/Cap. Bot. 100s, 500s. *otc.*
Use: Vitamin/mineral supplement.

Persantine. (Boehringer Ingelheim) Dipyridamole 25 mg, 50 mg or 75 mg/Tab. **25 mg or 50 mg:** Bot. 100s, 1000s, UD 100s. **75 mg:** Bot. 100s, 500s, UD 100s. *Rx.*
Use: Antiplatelet.

Persantine IV. (DuPont-Merck) Dipyridamole. Inj. For evaluation of coronary artery disease.
Use: Diagnostic aid.

persic oil, N.F. XVII.
Use: Vehicle.

pertechnetic acid, sodium salt. Sodium Pertechnetate Tc 99 m Solution.

Pertofrane. (Rhone-Poulenc Rorer) Desipramine HCl 25 mg or 50 mg/Cap. Bot. 100s, 1000s. *Rx.*
Use: Antidepressant.

Pertscan-99m. (Abbott Diagnostics) Radiodiagnostic. Inj. Tc-99m.
Use: Diagnostic aid.

Pertussin All-Night PM. (Pertussin Labs) Acetaminophen 167 mg, doxylamine succinate 1.25 mg, pseudoephedrine HCl 10 mg, dextromethorphan HBr 5 mg/5 ml, alcohol 25%. Liq. Bot. 240 ml. *otc.*
Use: Analgesic, antihistamine, decongestant, antitussive.

Pertussin CS. (Pertussin) Dextromethorphan HBr 3.5 mg, guaifenesin 25 mg/5 ml, 8.5% alcohol. Bot. 90 ml. *otc.*
Use: Antitussive, expectorant.

Pertussin ES. (Pertussin) Dextromethorphan HBr 15 mg/5 ml, alcohol 9.5%, sugar, sorbitol. Liq. Bot. 120 ml. *otc.*
Use: Antitussive.

Pertussin Syrup. (Pertussin) Dextromethorphan HBr 15 mg/5 ml, alcohol 9.5%. Bot. 3 oz, 6 oz. *otc.*
Use: Antitussive.

•**pertussis immune globulin,** U.S.P. 23.
Formerly Pertussis Immune Human Globulin.
Use: Immunizing agent (passive).

•**pertussis vaccine,** U.S.P. 23.
Use: Immunizing agent (active).
W/diphtheria and tetanus toxoids.
See: Acel-Imune, Vial (Wyeth Lederle).
Tri-Immunol, Vial (Wyeth Lederle).
Tripedia, Vial (Pasteur-Merieux-Connaught).

pertussis vaccine. (Michigan Department of public Health). Vial 5 mL.
Use: Immunizing agent (active).

•**pertussis vaccine adsorbed,** U.S.P. 23.
Use: Immunizing agent (active).

pertussis vaccine and diphtheria and tetanus toxoids, combined.
Use: Active immunizing agent.
See: Acel-Imune, Vial (Wyeth Lederle).
Tri-Immunol, Vial (Wyeth Lederle).
Tripedia, Vial (Pasteur-Merieux-Connaught).

peruvian balsam.
Use: Local protectant, rubefacient.
W/Benzocaine, zinc oxide, bismuth subgallate, boric acid.
See: Anocaine, Supp. (Roberts).
W/Benzocaine, zinc oxide, 8-hydroxyquinoline benzoate, menthol. Unit-of-Use 90s. **50 mg:** Bot. 100s, 1000s, UD 100s. **75 mg:** Bot. 100s.
See: Hemorrhoidal Oint. (Towne).
W/Ephedrine sulfate, belladonna extract, zinc oxide, boric acid, bismuth oxyiodide, subcarbonate.
See: Wyanoids, Preps. (Wyeth-Ayerst).
W/Lidocaine, bismuth subgallate, zinc oxide, aluminum subacetate.
See: Xylocaine, Supp. (Astra).
W/Oxyquinoline sulfate, pramoxine HCl, zinc oxide.
See: Zyanoid, Oint. (ICN Pharm).

peson. Sodium Lyapolate. Polyethenesulfonate sodium.
Use: Anticoagulant.

Peterson's Ointment. (Peterson) Carbolic acid, camphor, tannic acid, zinc oxide. Tube w/pipe 1 oz. Jar 16 oz. Can 1.4 oz, 3 oz. *otc.*
Use: Anorectal preparation.

Pethadol Tablets. (Halsey) Meperidine HCl 50 mg or 100 mg/Tab. Bot. 100s, 1000s. *c-ii.*
Use: Narcotic analgesic.

pethidine hydrochloride.
See: Meperidine HCl, U.S.P. 23.

PETN.
See: Pentaerythritol tetranitrate.

petrichloral. Pentaerythritol chloral.
Use: Sedative.

Petro-20. (Foy) Pentaerythritol tetranitrate 20 mg/Tab. Bot. 100s, 1000s. *Rx.*
Use: Antianginal.

•**petrolatum,** U.S.P. 23.
Use: Pharmaceutic aid (ointment base).
See: Lipkote, Stick (Schering-Plough).

petrolatum gauze.
Use: Surgical aid.

•**petrolatum, hydrophilic,** U.S.P. 23.

Use: Pharmaceutic aid (absorbent, ointment base) topical protectant.
See: Lipkote (Schering-Plough).

petrolatum, liquid. Mineral Oil, U.S.P. 23. Light Mineral Oil, U.S.P. 23. Adepsine Oil, Glymol, Liquid Paraffin, Parolein, White Mineral Oil, Heavy Liquid Petrolatum.
Use: Laxative.
See: Clyserol Oil Retention Enema (Fuller Labs).
Fleet Mineral Oil Enema (Fleet).
Mineral Oil (Various Mfr.).
Nujol, Liq. (Schering-Plough).
Saxol (Various Mfr.).

petrolatum, liquid, emulsion.
Use: Lubricant, laxative.
See: Milkinol, Liq. (Kremers-Urban).
W/Agar-Gel.
See: Agoral Plain, Liq. (Parke-Davis).
Petrogalar, Preps. (Wyeth-Ayerst).
W/Cascara.
See: Petrogalar w/Cascara, Emulsion (Wyeth-Ayerst).
W/Docusate sodium.
See: Milkinol, Liq. (Kremers-Urban).
W/Irish moss, casanthranol.
See: Neo-Kondremul (Medeva).
W/Milk of magnesia.
See: Haley's M. O., Liq. (Sanofi Winthrop Products).
W/Phenolphthalein.
See: Agoral, Emulsion (Parke-Davis).
Petrogalar w/Phenolphthalein, Emulsion (Wyeth-Ayerst).
Phenolphthalein in liquid Petrolatum Emulsion.

petrolatum, red veterinarian. (Zeneca) Also known as RVP.
See: Rubrapet, Oint. (Medco).
W/Micasorb.
See: RV Plus, Oint. (ICN Pharm).
W/N-diethyl metatoluamide.
See: RV Pellent, Oint. (Zeneca).
W/Zinc oxide, 2-ethoxyethyl p-methoxycinnamate.
See: RV Paque, Oint. (ICN Pharm).

•**petrolatum, white,** U.S.P. 23.
Use: Pharmaceutic aid (oleaginous ointment base) topical protectant.
See: Moroline, Oint. (Schering-Plough).

Petro-Phylic Soap. (Doak) Hydrophilic Petrolatum. Cake 4 oz.
Use: Emollient, anti-infective, external.

PF4RIA. (Abbott Diagnostics) Platelet factor 4 radioimmunoassay for the quantitative measurement of total PF4 levels in plasma.
Use: Diagnostic aid.

Pfeiffer's Allergy. (Pfeiffer) Chlorphenir-

amine maleate 4 mg/Tab. Bot. 24s. *otc.*
Use: Antihistamine.

Pfeiffer's Cold Sore. (Pfeiffer) Gum benzoin 7%, camphor, menthol, thymol, eucalyptol, alcohol 85%. Lot. Bot. 15 ml. *otc.*
Use: Cold sores, fever blisters, cracked lips.

Pfizerpen-AS. (Roerig) Procaine penicillin G 3,000,000 units in aqueous susp./ Vial. Carton 5s. Multi-Vial Pack, Carton 100s. *Rx.*
Use: Anti-infective, penicillin.

Pfizerpen for Injection. (Roerig) Potassium penicillin G, buffered. **Multi-Vial Pack:** 1,000,000 units or 5,000,000 units/Vial. Carton 10s, 100s; **Individual Vial:** 20,000,000 units/Vial 1s, 10s. *Rx.*
Use: Anti-infective, penicillin.

Pfizerpen VK Tablets. (Pfizer Laboratories) Penicillin V potassium 250 mg or 500 mg/Tab. **250 mg:** Bot. 1000s. **500 mg:** Bot. 100s. *Rx.*
Use: Anti-infective, penicillin.

PGA.
See: Folic Acid, U.S.P. 23.

PgE.
Use: Prostaglandin.
See: Alprostadil.

pHacid. (Baker/Cummins) Bot. 8 oz.
Use: Shampoo.

Phadiatop RIA Test. (Pharmacia & Upjohn) Determination of IgE antibodies specific to inhalant allergens in human serum. Kit 60s.
Use: Diagnostic aid.

Phanacol Cough. (Pharmakon) Phenylpropanolamine HCl 25 mg, dextromethorphan HBr 10 mg, guaifenesin 100 mg, acetaminophen 325 mg/5 ml. Syrup. Bot. 118 ml, 236 ml. *otc.*
Use: Antitussive, expectorant, decongestant.

Phanadex Cough Syrup. (Pharmakon) Phenylpropanolamine HCl 25 mg, pyrilamine maleate 40 mg, dextromethorphan HBr 15 mg, guaifenesin 100 mg/ 5 ml, sugar, potassium citrate, citric acid. Syr. Bot. 118 ml, 236 ml. *otc.*
Use: Decongestant, antihistamine, antitussive, expectorant.

Phanatuss Cough Syrup. (Pharmakon Labs) Dextromethorphan HBr 10 mg, guaifenesin 85 mg, potassium citrate 75 mg, citric acid 35 mg/5 ml, sorbitol, menthol. Syr. Bot. 118 ml. *otc.*
Use: Antitussive, expectorant.

pH Antiseptic Skin Cleanser. (Walgreen) Alcohol 63%. Bot. 16 oz. *otc.*

Use: Astringent, cleanser.

Pharazine. (Halsey) Bot. 4 oz, 16 oz, gal.
Use: A series of cough and cold products.

Pharmadine. (Sherwood Pharm) Povidone-iodine. **Oint.:** Pkt. 1 g, 1.5 g, 2 g, 30 g, 1 lb. **Perineal wash:** 240 ml. **Skin cleanser:** 240 ml. **Soln.:** 15 ml, 120 ml, 240 ml, pt, qt. **Soln., swabs:** 100s. **Soln., swabsticks:** 1 or 3/packet in 250s. **Spray:** 120 g. **Surgical scrub:** 30 ml, pt, qt, gal, foil-pack 15 ml. **Surgical scrub sponge/brush:** 25s. **Swabsticks, lemon glycerin:** 100s. **Whirlpool soln.:** gal. *otc.*
Use: Antiseptic.

Pharmaflur. (Pharmics) Sodium fluoride 2.21 mg. Tab. Bot. 1000s. *Rx.*
Use: Dental caries preventative.

Pharmalgen Hymenoptera Venoms. (ALK Laboratories) Freeze-dried venom or venom protein. Vials of 120 mcg or 1100 mcg for each of honey bee, white-faced hornet, yellow hornet, yellow jacket, or wasp. Vials of 360 mcg or 3300 mcg for mixed vespids (white-faced hornet, yellow hornet, yellow jacket). Diagnostic kit: 5 × 1 ml vial. Treatment kit: 6 × 1 ml vial or 1 × 1.1 mg multiple dose vial. Starter Kit: 6 × 1 ml, pre-diluted 0.01 mcg to 100 mcg/ ml.
Use: Hymenoptera venom.

Pharmalgen Standardized Allergenic Extracts. (ALK Laboratories) 100,000 allergenic units/Vial. Box 5 × 1 ml.
Use: Diagnostic aid, treatment kit.

Phazyme. (Reed & Carnrick) Simethicone 60 mg/Tab. Bot. 50s, 100s, 1000s. *otc.*
Use: Antiflatulent.

Phazyme-95. (Reed & Carnrick) Simethicone 95 mg/Tab. Bot. 100s. *otc.*
Use: Antiflatulent.

Phazyme 125. (Reed & Carnrick) Simethicone 125 ml. Cap. Bot. 50s. *otc.*
Use: Antiflatulent.

Phazyme Drops. (Reed & Carnrick) Simethicone 40 mg/0.6 ml, saccharin. Bot. 30 ml w/dropper. *otc.*
Use: Antiflatulent.

•**phemfilcon a.** (FEM-fill-kahn A) USAN.
Use: Contact lens material (hydrophilic).

phenacaine hydrochloride, U.S.P. XXI.
Use: Local anesthetic (ophthalmic).

W/Atropine, phenol, nut gall, zinc oxide.
See: Tanicaine, Oint., Supp. (Pharmacia & Upjohn).

W/Cod liver oil.
See: Morusan Oint. (SK-Beecham).

W/Ephedrine. (Pharmacia & Upjohn) Phenacaine HCl 1%, epinephrine 1:25,000. Ophth. oint. Tube 1 dr.

W/Mercarbolide. (Pharmacia & Upjohn) Holocaine HCl 2%, mercarbolide 1:3000. Ophth. oint., Tube w/applicator tip, 1 dr.

Phenacal. (NeuroGenesis/Matrix) D,L-phenylalanine 500 mg, L-glutamine 15 mg, L-tyrosine 25 mg, L-carnitine 10 mg, L-arginine pyroglutamate 10 mg, L-ornithine/L-aspartate 10 mg, chromium 0.033 mg, selenium 0.012 mg, vitamin B_1 0.33 mg, B_2 5 mg, B_3 3.3 mg, B_5 0.33 mg, B_6 0.33 mg, B_{12} 1 mcg, E 5 IU, biotin 0.05 mg, folic acid 0.066 mg, iron 1 mg, zinc 2.5 mg, calcium 35 mg, iodine 0.25 mg, copper 0.33 mg, magnesium 25 mg/Cap. Bot. 42s, 180s. *otc.*
Use: Nutritional supplement.

phenacetin. Acetophenetidin. Ethoxyacetanilide.
Use: Antipyretic, analgesic.
Note: This drug has been withdrawn from the market due to liver and kidney toxicity. This drug is no longer official in the U.S.P.

phenacetylcarbamide.
See: Phenurone, Tab. (Abbott).

phenacetylurea.
See: Phenurone, Tab. (Abbott).

phenacridane. (9(p-Hexloxphenyl)-10-methyl-acridinium Cl).
See: Micridium (Johnson & Johnson).

phenacyl homatrophinium hydrochloride. Not available.

Phenadex Children's Cough/Cold. (Barre-National) Phenylpropanolamine HCl 6.25 mg, dextromethorphan HBr 5 mg, guiafenesin 100 mg/5 ml, alcohol 5%. Syrup. Bot. 118 ml. *otc.*
Use: Decongestant, antitussive, expectorant.

Phenadex Pediatric Cough/Cold. (Barre-National) Phenylpropanolamine HCl 6.25 mg, dextromethorphan HBr 5 mg, guiafenesin 50 mg/5 ml. Sugar free. Drops. Bot. 30 ml. *otc.*
Use: Decongestant, antitussive, expectorant.

Phenadex Senior. (Barre-National) Dextromethorphan HBr 10 mg, guiafenesin 200 mg/5 ml. Liq. Bot. 118 ml. *otc.*
Use: Antitussive, expectorant.

Phenahist Injectable. (T.E. Williams) Atropine sulfate 0.2 mg, phenylpropanolamine HCl 12.5 mg, chlorphenir-

amine maleate 5 mg/ml. Vial 10 ml. *Rx.*
Use: Anticholinergic, antispasmodic, decongestant, antihistamine.

Phenahist-TR Tablets. (T.E. Williams) Phenylephrine HCl 25 mg, phenylpropanolamine HCl 50 mg, chlorpheniramine maleate 8 mg, hyoscyamine sulfate 0.19 mg, atropine 0.04 mg, scopolamine HBr 0.01 mg. Tab. Bot. 100s. *Rx.*
Use: Decongestant, antihistamine, anticholinergic/antispasmodic.

phenamazoline hydrochloride. 2-(Anilinomethyl)-2-imidazoline HCl.
Use: Vasoconstrictor.

Phenameth DM. (Major) Promethazine HCl 6.25 mg, dextromethorphan HBr 15 mg/5 ml, alcohol. Syr. Bot. 120 ml. *Rx.*
Use: Antihistamine, antitussive.

Phenameth Tablets. (Major) Promethazine 25 mg. Tab. Bot. 1000s. *Rx.*
Use: Antihistamine, antiemetic.

Phenameth VC w/Codeine. (Major) Phenylephrine HCl 5 mg, promethazine HCl 6.25 mg, codeine phosphate 10 mg/5 ml, alcohol 7%. Syr. Bot. pt, gal. *c-v.*
Use: Decongestant, antihistamine, antitussive.

Phenameth w/Codeine. (Major) Promethazine HCl 6.25 mg, codeine phosphate 10 mg/5 ml, alcohol 7%. Syr. Bot. 4 oz, pt, gal. *c-v.*
Use: Antihistamine, antitussive.

phenantoin. Mephenytoin. N-Methyl-5,5-phenylethylhydantoin.
See: Mesantoin, Tab. (Sandoz).

Phenapap Sinus Headache & Congestion. (Rugby) Pseudoephedrine HCl 30 mg, chlorpheniramine 2 mg, acetaminophen 325 mg. Tab. Bot. 30s, 100s, 1000s. *otc.*
Use: Decongestant, antihistamine, analgesic.

Phenaphen w/Codeine No. 3. (Robins) Codeine phosphate 30 mg, acetaminophen 325 mg/Tab. *c-iii.*
Use: Narcotic analgesic combination.

phenaphthazine. Sodium dinitro phenylazonaphthol disulfonate.
See: Nitrazine Paper, Roll (Squibb).

phenarsone sulfoxylate. (5-Arsono-2-hydroxyanilino)methanesulfinic acid disodium salt.
Use: Antiamebic.

Phenaspirin Compound. (Davis & Sly) Phenobarbital 0.25 gr, aspirin 3.5 gr. Cap. Bot. 1000s. *Rx.*

Use: Sedative, hypnotic, salicylate analgesic.

Phenate. (Roberts Medical) Phenylpropanolamine HCl 40 mg, chlorpheniramine maleate 4 mg, acetaminophen 325 mg. CR Tab. Bot. 100s, 1000s. *Rx.*
Use: Decongestant, antihistamine, analgesic.

Phenazine. (Keene) Promethazine HCl 50 mg. Vial 10 ml. *Rx.*
Use: Antihistamine, antiemetic.

phenazocine hydrobromide.
Use: Analgesic.

phenazone.
See: Antipyrine (Various Mfr.).

•**phenazopyridine hydrochloride,** (fen-AZZ-oh-PIH-rih-deen) U.S.P. 23.
Use: Analgesic (urinary tract).
See: Azogesic, Tab. (Century).
Azo-Pyridon, Tab. (Solvay).
Azo-Standard, Tab. (PolyMedica).
Azo-Sulfizin (Solvay).
Phen-Azo, Tab. (Vanguard).
Pyridium, Tab. (Parke-Davis).
Uri-Pak (Westerfield).

phenazopyridine hydrochloride w/ combinations.
See: Azo Gantanol, Tab. (Roche).
Azo Gantrisin, Tab. (Roche).
Azosulfisoxazole (Various Mfr.).
Pyridium Plus, Tab. (Parke-Davis).
Thiosulfil-A, Tab. (Wyeth-Ayerst).
Thiosulfil-A Forte, Tab. (Wyeth-Ayerst).
Triurisul, Tab. (Sheryl).
Uridium, Tab. (Ferndale; Pharmex).
Urisan-P, Tab. (Sandia).
Uritral, Cap. (Schwarz Pharma).
Urobiotic, Cap. (Pfizer).
Urogesic, Tab. (Edwards).
Urotrol, Tab. (Mills).

•**phenbutazone sodium glycerate.** (fen-BYOO-tah-zone GLIH-seh-rate) USAN.
Use: Anti-inflammatory.

•**phencarbamide.** (FEN-car-BAM-id) USAN.
Use: Anticholinergic, spasmolytic.
See: Escorpal (Farben-Fabriken).

Phenchlor-Eight. (Freeport) Chlorpheniramine maleate 8 mg. TR Cap. Bot. 1000s. *Rx.*
Use: Antihistamine.

Phenchlor S.H.A. (Rugby) Phenylpropanolamine HCl 50 mg, phenylephrine HCl 25 mg, chlorpheniramine maleate 8 mg, hyoscyamine sulfate 0.19 mg, atropine sulfate 0.04 mg, scopolamine HBr 0.01mg/SR. Tab. Bot. 100s, 500s. *Rx.*
Use: Decongestant, antihistamine, anticholinergic.

Phenchlor-Twelve. (Freeport) Chlorpheniramine maleate 12 mg. TR Cap. Bot. 1000s. *Rx.*
Use: Antihistamine.

• **phencyclidine hydrochloride.** (fen-SIGH-klih-deen) USAN.
Use: Anesthetic.

• **phendimetrazine tartrate,** U.S.P. 23.
Use: Appetite suppressant (systemic).
See: Adipost, Cap. (Ascher).
   Adphen, Tab. (Ferndale).
   Anorex, Cap., Tab. (Dunhall).
   Bacarate, Tab. (Solvay).
   Bontril PDM, Tab. (Carnrick).
   Bontril Slow Release, Cap. (Carnrick).
   Delcozine, Tab. (Delco).
   Di-Ap-Trol, Tab. (Foy).
   Elphemet, Tab. (Canright).
   Limit, Tab. (Bock).
   Melfiat, Tab. (Solvay).
   Melfiat 105, Cap. (Solvay).
   Obepar, Tab. (Parmed).
   Obe-Tite, Tab. (Scott/Cord).
   Phen-70, Tab. (Parmed).
   Phenzine, Tab. (Roberts).
   Prelu-2, Cap. (Boehringer Ingelheim).
   Reducto, Tab. (Arcum).
   Rexigen Forte, SR Cap. (ION).
   Slim-Tabs, Tab. (Wesley).
   Statobex, Prods. (Lemmon).
   Stodex, Tab., Cap. (Jalco).
   Trimtabs, Tab. (Mayrand).

Phendry. (LuChem) Diphenhydramine HCl 12.5 mg/5 ml, alcohol 14%. Elix. Bot. pt, gal. *otc.*
Use: Antihistamine.

Phendry Children's Allergy Medicine. (LuChem) Diphenhydramine HCl 12.5 mg/5 ml, alcohol 14%. Elix. Bot. 120 ml. *otc.*
Use: Antihistamine.

phenelzine dihydrogen sulfate.
See: Nardil, Tab. (Parke-Davis).

• **phenelzine sulfate,** (FEN-uhl-zeen) U.S.P. 23. Phenethylhydrazine sulfate. Monoamine oxidase inhibitor, beta-phenylethyl-hydrazinedihydrogen sulfate.
Use: Antidepressant.
See: Nardil, Tab. (Parke-Davis).

Phenerbel-S. (Rugby) Phenobarbital 40 mg, ergotamine tartrate 0.6 mg, l-alkaloids of belladonna 0.2 mg. Tab. Bot. 100s. *Rx.*
Use: Sedative, hypnotic, anticholinergic.

Phenergan-D. (Wyeth-Ayerst) Promethazine HCl 6.25 mg, pseudoephedrine HCl 60 mg. Tab. Bot. 100s. *Rx.*

Use: Antihistamine, decongestant.

Phenergan Fortis. (Wyeth-Ayerst) Promethazine HCl 25 mg/5 ml, alcohol 1.5%. Bot. pt. *Rx.*
Use: Antihistamine.

Phenergan Injection. (Wyeth-Ayerst) Promethazine HCl 25 mg or 50 mg/ml. Inj. Amp. 1 mg Pkg. 5s, 25s, Tubex 10s. *Rx.*
Use: Antihistamine.

Phenergan Plain. (Wyeth-Ayerst) Promethazine HCl 6.25 mg/5 ml, alcohol 7%, saccharin. Syr. Bot. 120 ml, 180 ml, 240 ml, pt, gal. *Rx.*
Use: Antihistamine.

Phenergan Suppositories. (Wyeth-Ayerst) Promethazine HCl 12.5 mg, 25 mg or 50 mg. Supp. Box. 12s, Redipak. *Rx.*
Use: Antihistamine.

Phenergan Syrup Plain. (Wyeth-Ayerst) Promethazine HCl 6.25 mg/5 ml. Bot. 4 oz, 6 oz, 8 oz, pt, gal. *Rx.*
Use: Antihistamine.

Phenergan Tablets. (Wyeth-Ayerst) Promethazine HCl 12.5 mg, 25 mg or 50 mg. Tab. Bot. 100s. Redipak 100s. *Rx.*
Use: Antihistamine.

Phenergan VC. (Wyeth-Ayerst) Promethazine HCl 6.25 mg, phenylephrine HCl 5 mg/5 ml. Syr. Bot. 118 ml, 473 ml. *Rx.*
Use: Antihistamine, decongestant.

Phenergan VC with Codeine. (Wyeth-Ayerst) Promethazine HCl 6.25 mg, codeine phosphate 10 mg, phenylephrine HCl 5 mg/5 ml, alcohol 7%. Bot. 4 oz, 6 oz, 8 oz, pt, gal. *c-v.*
Use: Antihistamine, antitussive, decongestant.

Phenergan with Codeine. (Wyeth-Ayerst) Promethazine HCl 6.25 mg, codeine phosphate 10 mg/5 ml. Bot. 4 oz, 6 oz, 8 oz, pt, gal. *c-v.*
Use: Antihistamine, antitussive.

Phenergan with Dextromethorphan. (Wyeth-Ayerst) Promethazine HCl 6.25 mg, dextromethorphan HBr 15 mg/5 ml, alcohol 7%. Bot. 4 oz, 6 oz, pt, gal. *Rx.*
Use: Antihistamine, antitussive.

pheneridine.
Use: Analgesic.

i-phenethylbiguanide monohydrochloride. Phenformin HCl.

Phenex-1. (Ross) Protein 15 g, fat 23.9 g, carbohydrates 46.3 g, linoleic acid 1800 mg, Fe 9 mg, Na 190 mg, K 675 mg, Cal 480/100 g. With appropriate

vitamins and minerals. Phenylalanine free. Pow. Can 350 g. *otc.*
Use: Nutritional supplement.

Phenex-2. (Ross) Protein 30 g, fat 15.5 g, carbohydrates 30 g, Fe 13 mg, Na 880 mg, K 1370 mg, Cal 410/100 g. With appropriate vitamins and minerals. Phenylalanine free. Pow. Can 325 g. *otc.*
Use: Nutritional supplement.

phenformin hydrochloride. *Rx.*
Use: Hypoglycemic.
Note: Withdrawn from market in 1978. Available under IND exemption.

Phenhist DH w/Codeine. (Rugby) Pseudoephedrine HCl 30 mg, chlorpheniramine maleate 2 mg, codeine phosphate 10 mg/5 ml, alcohol 5%. Liq. Bot. 120 ml, 480 ml. *c-v.*
Use: Decongestant, antihistamine, antitussive.

Phenhist Expectorant. (Rugby) Pseudoephedrine HCl 30 mg, codeine phosphate 10 mg, guaifenesin 100 mg/5 ml, alcohol 7.5%. Liq. Bot. 118 ml, pt, gal. *c-v.*
Use: Decongestant, antihistamine, antitussive.

pheniform.
See: Phenformin HCl.

•**phenindamine tartrate.** USAN.
Use: Antihistamine.
See: Nolahist, Tab. (Carnrick).
   Thephorin, Tab. (Roche).
W/Chlorpheniramine maleate, phenylpropanolamine HCl.
See: Nolamine, Tab. (Carnrick).
W/Phenylephrine HCl, aspirin, caffeine, aluminum hydroxide, magnesium carbonate.
See: Dristan, Tab. (Whitehall Robins).
W/Phenylephrine HCl, caramiphen ethanedisulfonate.
See: Dondril, Tab. (Whitehall Robins).
W/Phenylephrine HCl, chlorpheniramine maleate, drytane.
See: Comhist, Tab., Elix. (Baylor).
W/Phenylephrine HCl, chlorpheniramine maleate, belladonna alkaloids.
See: Comhist L.A., Cap. (Baylor Labs).
W/Phenylephrine HCl, pyrilamine maleate, chlorpheniramine maleate, dextromethorphan HBr.
See: Histalet, Histalet-DM, Histalet-Forte, Syr. (Solvay).

pheniodol.
See: Iodoalphionic Acid (Various Mfr.).

pheniprazine hydrochloride. (α-Methylphenethyl)-hydrazine monohydrochloride.

Use: Antihypertensive.

•**pheniramine maleate.** USAN.
Use: Antihistamine.
See: Inhiston, Tab. (Schering-Plough).
W/Combinations.
   Allerstat, Cap. (Lemmon).
   Chexit, Tab. (Sandoz Consumer).
   Citra Forte, Cap., Syr. (Boyle).
   Partuss AC (Parmed).
   Poly-Histine Cap., Elix., Lipospan (Bock).
   T.A.C., Cap. (Towne).
   Thor, Cap. (Towne).
   Tritussin, Syr. (Towne).

•**phenmetrazine hydrochloride,** U.S.P. 23.
Use: Anorexic.

•**phenobarbital,** (fee-no-BAR-bih-tahl) U.S.P. 23.
Use: Anticonvulsant, hypnotic, sedative.
See: Henomint, Elix. (Jones Medical).
   Hypnette, Supp., Tab. (Fleming).
   Orprine, Liq. (Medeva).
   Pheno-Square, Tab. (Roberts).
   Sedadrops, Liq. (Hoechst Marion Roussel).
   Solfoton, Tab., Cap. (ECR Pharm).

phenobarbital. (Various Mfr.) **Tab.: 15 mg, 30 mg:** Bot. 100s, 1000s, 5000s, UD 100s; **60 mg:** Bot. 100s, 1000s, UD 100s; **100 mg:** 100s, 1000s. **Elixir:** 20 mg/5 ml. Bot. Pt, gal, UD 5 ml, UD 7.5 ml.
Use: Anticonvulsant, hypnotic, sedative.

phenobarbital. (Pharmaceutical Associates) 15 mg/5 ml. Elixir. Bot. Pt, UD 5 ml, 10 ml, 20 ml. *c-iv.*
Use: Sedative, hypnotic, anticonvulsant.

phenobarbital w/aminophylline.
See: Aminophylline (Various Mfr.).

phenobarbital w/atropine sulfate.
See: Atropine Sulfate (Various Mfr.).
   P.A., Tab. (Scrip).

phenobarbital w/belladonna.
See: Belladonna Products and Phenobarbital Combinations.

phenobarbital with central nervous system stimulants.
See: Arcotrate No. 3, Tab. (Arcum).
   Bronkolixir, Elix. (Sanofi Winthrop).
   Bronkotab, Tab. (Sanofi Winthrop).
   Quadrinal, Susp., Tab. (Knoll).
   Sedamine, Tab. (Dunhall).
   Spabelin, Elix., Tab. (Arcum).

phenobarbital combinations.
See: Aminophylline w/Phenobarbital, Combinations.

Aspirin-Barbiturate, Combinations.

Atropine-Hyoscine-Hyoscyamine Combinations.

Atropine Sulfate w/Phenobarbital.

Belladonna Extract Combinations.

Belladonna Products and Phenobarbital Combinations.

Homatropine Methylbromide and Phenobarbital Combinations.

Hyoscyamus Products and Phenobarbital Combinations.

Mannitol Hexanitrate w/Phenobarbital Combinations.

Mephenesin and Barbiturates Combinations.

Phenobarbital w/Central Nervous System Stimulants.

Secobarbital Combinations.

Sodium Nitrite Combinations.

Theobromine w/Phenobarbital Combinations.

Theophylline w/Phenobarbital Combinations.

Veratrum Viride w/Phenobarbital Combinations.

phenobarbital w/homatropine methylbromide.
See: Homatropine Methylbromide and Phenobarbital Combinations.

phenobarbital w/hyoscyamus.
See: Hyoscyamus Products and Phenobarbital Combinations.

phenobarbital w/mannitol hexanitrate.
Use: Anticonvulsant, sedative, hypnotic.
See: Mannitol Hexanitrate w/Phenobarbital Combinations.

•**phenobarbital sodium,** U.S.P. 23.
Use: Anticonvulsant, sedative, hypnotic.
See: Luminal Sodium, Inj. (Sanofi Winthrop).

phenobarbital sodium. (Wyeth-Ayerst) Inj. **30 mg/ml, 60 mg/ml:** Tubex 1 ml; **65 mg/ml:** Vial 1 ml; **130 mg/ml:** Tubex 1 ml, vial 1 ml. *c-iv.*
Use: Anticonvulsant, sedative, hypnotic.

phenobarbital sodium in propylene glycol. Vitarine. Amp. 0.13 g: 1 ml, Box 25s, 100s. *c-iv.*
Use: Anticonvulsant, hypnotic, sedative.

phenobarbital and theobromine combinations.
See: Theobromine w/Phenobarbital Combinations.

phenobarbital w/theophylline.
See: Theophylline w/Phenobarbital Combinations.

phenobarbital w/veratrum viride.
See: Veratrum Viride w/Phenobarbital Combinations.

Pheno-Bella. (Ferndale) Belladonna extract 10.8 mg, phenobarbital 16.2 mg/ Tab. Bot. 100s, 1000s. *Rx.*
Use: Anticholinergic/antispasmodic, sedative/hypnotic.

Phenoject-50. (Mayrand) Promethazine HCl 50 mg/ml. Inj. Vial 10 ml. *Rx.*
Use: Antihistamine, antiemetic.

•**phenol,** U.S.P. 23.
Use: Pharmaceutic aid (preservative), topical antipruritic.
W/Aluminum hydroxide, zinc oxide, camphor, eucalyptol, ichthammol, thyme oil.
See: Almophen, Oint. (Jones Medical).
W/Benzocaine, triclosan.
See: Solarcaine Pump Spray (Schering-Plough).
W/Dextromethorphan.
See: Chloraseptic DM Lozenges (Eaton).
W/Resorcinol.
See: Black & White Ointment (Schering-Plough).
W/Resorcinol, boric acid, basic fuchsin, acetone.
See: Castellani's Paint, Liq. (Various Mfr.).

•**phenolate sodium.** (FEEN-oh-late) USAN.
Use: Disinfectant.

Phenolax. (Pharmacia & Upjohn) Phenolphthalein 64.8 mg/Wafer. Bot. 100s. *otc.*
Use: Laxative.

•**phenol, liquefied,** U.S.P. 23.
Use: Topical antipruritic.

•**phenolphthalein,** (fee-nahl-THAY-leen) U.S.P. 23.
Use: Laxative.
See: Alophen, Pill (Parke-Davis).
Espotabs, Tab. (Combe).
Evac-U-Lax, Wafer (Roberts).
Evasof, Tab. (Lemmon).
Ex-Lax, Prods. (Sandoz Consumer).
Feen-A-Mint, Tab., Gum (Schering-Plough).
Phenolax, Wafer (Pharmacia & Upjohn).
Veracolate, Tab. (Numark).

phenolphthalein. (Various Mfr.) Pkg. 1 oz, 0.25 lb, 1 lb.
Use: Laxative.

phenolphthalein w/combinations.
See: Correctol, Tab. (Schering-Plough).
Evac-Q-Kit, Tab., Supp. (Warren-Teed).
Dual Formula Feen-A-Mint Pills (Schering-Plough).
Feen-A-Mint, Gum, Mint, Pill (Schering-Plough).

4-Way Cold Tab. (Bristol-Myers).

phenolphthalein in liquid petrolatum emulsion. (Various Mfr.).
See: Petrolatum, Liq.

phenolphthalein. (Various Mfr.). Pkg. 1 oz, 0.25 lb., 1 lb.
Use: Laxative.

•**phenolphthalein yellow,** U.S.P. 23.
Use: Laxative.

phenolsulfonates.
See: Sulfocarbolates.

phenolsulfonic acid. Sulfocarbolic acid.
Note: Used in Sulphodine, Tab. (Strasenburgh).

phenoltetrabromophthalein. Disulfonate Disodium.
See: Sulfobromophthalein Sodium, U.S.P. 23.

phenolzine sulfate.

Pheno Nux Tablets. (Pal-Pak) Phenobarbital 16.2 mg, nux vomica extract 8.1 mg, calcium carbonate 194.4 mg/Tab. Bot. 1000s. *c-iv.*
Use: Sedative, hypnotic, antacid.

Phenoptic. (Optopics) Phenylephrine HCl 2.5%. Soln. Bot. 2 ml, 5 ml, 15 ml. *Rx.*
Use: Ophthalmic vasoconstrictor, mydriatic.

phenothiazine. Thiodiphenylamine.

Phenoturic. (Truett) Phenobarbital 40 mg/5 ml. Elix. Bot. pt, gal. *c-iv.*
Use: Sedative, hypnotic.

•**phenoxybenzamine hydrochloride,** (fen-ox-ee-BEN-zuh-meen) U.S.P. 23.
Use: Antihypertensive.
See: Dibenzyline, Cap. (SK-Beecham).

phenoxymethyl penicillin.
See: Penicillin V.

phenoxymethyl penicillin potassium.
See: Penicillin V Potassium.

phenoxynate. Mixture of phenylphenols 17-18%, octyl and related alkylphenols 2-3%.
See: Surtenol, Liq. (Guardian Chem).

•**phenprocoumon.** (fen-PRO-koo-mahn) USAN.
Use: Anticoagulant.
See: Liquamar, Tab. (Organon).

Phen-70. (Parmed) Phendimetrazine tartrate 70 mg/Tab. Bot. 100s, 1000s. *c-iii.*
Use: Anorexiant.

•**phensuximide,** U.S.P. 23.
Use: Anticonvulsant.
See: Milontin, Preps. (Parke-Davis).

Phental. (Armenpharm) Belladonna alkaloids, phenobarbital 0.25 gr/Tab. Bot. 1000s. *c-iv.*

Use: Anticholinergic, antispasmodic, sedative, hypnotic.

Phentamine. (Major) Phentermine HCl 30 mg/Cap. (equivalent to 24 mg base). Bot. 100s. *c-iv.*
Use: Anorexiant.

•**phentermine.** (FEN-ter-meen) USAN.
Use: Anorexic.
See: Adipex, Tab. (Lemmon).
    Adipex-8 C.T., Cap. (Lemmon).
    Adipex-P, Cap. (Lemmon).
    Fastin, Cap. (SK-Beecham).
    Parmine, Cap. (Parmed).
    Tora, Tab. (Solvay).
    Unifast Unicelles, Cap. (Solvay).
    Wilpowr, Cap. (Foy).

phentermine as resin complex.
See: Ionamin, Cap. (Medeva).

•**phentermine hydrochloride,** U.S.P. 23. Benzeneethanamine, α,α-dimethyl-, HCl.
Use: Appetite suppressant (systemic).
See: Zantryl, Cap. (ION).

phentetiothalein sodium. Iso-Iodeikon.
Use: Radiopaque agent.

phentolamine hydrochloride. (fen-TOLE-uh-meen)
Use: Antihypertensive.
See: Regitine HCl, Tab. (Novartis).

•**phentolamine mesylate,** U.S.P. 23. *Formerly Phentolamine Methanesulfonate.*
Use: Antiadrenergic.
See: Regitine Inj. (Novartis).

phentolamine methanesulfonate. Phentolamine mesylate, U.S.P. 23.

Phentolox w/APAP. (Global Pharms) Phenyltoloxamine citrate 30 mg, acetaminophen 325 mg/Tab. Bot. 1000s. *Rx.*
Use: Antihistamine, analgesic.

Phentox Compound. (Rosemont) Phenylpropanolamine HCl 20 mg, phenylephrine HCl 5 mg, chlorpheniramine maleate 2.5 mg, phenyltoloxamine citrate 7.5 mg/5 ml. Bot. pt, gal. *Rx.*
Use: Decongestant, antihistamine.

phentydrone.
Use: Systemic fungicide.

n-phenylacetamide.
See: Acetanilid (Various Mfr.).

phenylacetylurea.
See: Phenurone, Tab. (Abbott).

phenylalanine ammonia-lyase.
Use: Hyperphenylalaninemia. [Orphan drug]

•**phenyl aminosalicylate.** (FEN-ill ah-MEE-no-sah-LIH-sih-late) USAN. Phenyl 4 aminosalicylate. Fenamisal (I.N.N.) Phenypastebamin.

Use: Antibacterial (tuberculostatic).

•**phenylalanine,** (fen-ill-AL-ah-NEEN) U.S.P. 23.
Use: Amino acid.
See: Phenylketonuria therapy.

phenylalanine mustard.
See: Melphalan, U.S.P. 23. analgesic.

phenylazo-diamino-pyridine.
See: Phenazopyridine (Various Mfr.).

phenylazo-diamino-pyridine hcl or hbr.
See: Phenazopyridine HCl or HBr (Various Mfr.).

phenylazo-diaminopyridine hydrochloride.
See: Rodine, Tab. (Paddock).

phenylazo sulfisoxazole. (A.P.C.) Sulfisoxazole 0.5 g, phenylazopyridine 50 mg/Tab. Bot. 1000s. *Rx.*
Use: Anti-infective, sulfonamide.

phenylazo tablets. (A.P.C.) Phenylazodiamino-pyridine HCl 1.5 gr/Tab. Bot. 1000s. *Rx.*
Use: Urinary analgesic.

•**phenylbutazone,** U.S.P. 23.
Use: Antirheumatic.

phenylbutyrate sodium. *Rx.*
Use: Treatment of blood disorders. [Orphan drug]

phenylcarbinol.
See: Benzyl Alcohol, N.F. 18.

phenylcinchoninic acid. Name used for cinchophen.

•**phenylephrine hydrochloride,** (fen-ill-EFF-rin) U.S.P. 23.
Use: Sympathomimetic agent, vasoconstrictor, mydriatic, adrenergic (ophthalmic).
See: AK-Dilate (Akorn).
AK-Nefrin (Akorn).
Alcon-Efrin, Soln. (PolyMedica).
Allerest Nasal Spray (Novartis).
Coricidin Decongestant Nasal Mist (Schering-Plough).
Ephrine, Spray (Walgreen).
Isopto Frin (Alcon).
Mydfrin 2.5% (Alcon).
Neo-Synephrine HCl, Preps. (Sanofi Winthrop Products).
Phenoptic (Optopics).
Prefrin Liquifilm Ophth. Soln. (Allergan).
Pyracort-D, Spray (Lemmon).
Relief (Allergan).
Sinarest, Nasal Spray (Novartis).
Super-Anahist Nasal Spray (Warner-Lambert).
W/Combinations.
See: Acotus, Liq. (Whorton).
Anodynos Forte, Tab. (Buffington).
Bur-Tuss Expectorant (Burlington).
Cenahist, Cap. (Century).
Cenaid, Tab. (Century).
Chlor-Trimeton Expectorant (Schering-Plough).
Chlor-Trimeton Expectorant w/Codeine (Schering-Plough).
Conar, Susp., Expectorant (SK-Beecham).
Conar-A, Tab., Susp. (SK-Beecham).
Congespirin, Tab. (Bristol-Myers).
Coricidin Demilets (Schering-Plough).
Dallergy, Syr., Cap., Tab., Inj. (Laser).
Demazin, Syr. (Schering-Plough).
Dimetane Decongestant, Tab., Elix. (Robins).
Dimetane Expectorant, Liq. (Robins).
Dimetane Expectorant-DC, Liq. (Robins).
Dimetapp, Elix., Extentabs (Robins).
Doktors, Drops, Spray (Scherer).
Eldatapp, Tab., Liq. (ICN Pharm).
Entex, Prods. (Procter & Gamble).
Eye-Gene, Soln. (Pearson).
4 Way Tab., Spray (Bristol-Myers).
Furacin Nasal Soln. (Eaton).
Histabid, Cap. (Meyer).
Histapp Prods. (Upsher-Smith).
Histaspan-D, Cap. (Rhone-Poulenc Rorer).
Histaspan-Plus, Cap. (Rhone-Poulenc Rorer).
Mydfrin Ophthalmic, Liq. (Alcon).
Nasahist, Cap. (Keene).
Pediacof, Syr. (Sanofi Winthrop).
Phenoptic, Soln. (Muro).
Phenylzin Drops, Ophth. Soln. (Ciba Vision).
Prefrin-A Ophth. Soln. (Allergan).
Prefrin-Z Ophth. Soln. (Allergan).
Pyraphed, Soln. (Lemmon).
Pyristan, Cap., Elix. (Arcum).
Queledrine, Syr. (Abbott).
Rhinall, Liq. (Scherer).
Rhinex DM, Tab. (Lemmon).
Rymed, Prods. (Edwards).
Sinex, Nasal Spray (Richardson-Vicks).
Singlet, Tab. (Hoechst Marion Roussel).
Spectab, Tab. (Solvay).
Spec-T Sore Throat-Decongestant Loz. (Squibb).
Sucrets Cold Decongestant Loz. (SK-Beecham).
Tearefrin, Liq. (Ciba Vision).
Trind, Liq. (Bristol-Myers).
Trind-DM, Liq. (Bristol-Myers).
Tri-Ophtho, Soln. (Maurry).
Turbilixir, Liq. (Burlington).

Turbispan Leisurecaps, Cap. (Burlington).

Tussar-DM, Liq. (Rhone-Poulenc Rorer).

Tympagesic, Liq. (Pharmacia & Upjohn).

Vacon, Liq. (Scherer).

Vasocidin, Ophth. Soln. (Ciba Vision).

Vasosulf, Ophth. Soln. (Novartis).

phenylephrine hydrochloride. (Various Mfr.) **Ophth. Soln. 2.5%:** Bot. 15 ml; **10%:** Bot. 2 ml, 5 ml. **Inj. 1%:** Vial 5 ml. *Rx.*
Use: Sympathomimetic agent, vasoconstrictor, mydriatic, adrenergic (ophthalmic).

Phenylephrine tannate, chlorpheniramine tannate and pyrilamine tartrate. (Goldline) Phenylephrine tannate 25 mg, chlorpheniramine tannate 8 mg, pyrilamine tannate 25 mg/Tab. Bot. 100s, 500s. *Rx.*
Use: Decongestant, antihistamine.

•**phenylethyl alcohol,** U.S.P. 23. Betaphenylethanol. Benzylcarbinol. Phenethyl Alcohol.
Use: Pharmaceutic aid (antimicrobial).

phenyl-ethyl-hydrazine, beta. Phenelzine dihydrogen sulfate.
See: Nardil, Tab. (Parke-Davis).

phenylethylmalonylurea.
See: Phenobarbital (Various Mfr.).

Phenylfenesin L.A. (Goldline) Phenylpropanolamine HCl 75 mg, guaifenesin 400 mg/ER Tab. Bot. 100s. *Rx.*
Use: Decongestant, expectorant.

Phenylgesic Tabs. (Goldline) Phenyltoloxamine citrate 30 mg, acetaminophen 325 mg/Bot. 100s, 1000s. *otc.*
Use: Antihistamine, analgesic.

phenylic acid.
See: Phenol, U.S.P. 23.

•**phenylmercuric acetate,** N.F. 18.
Use: Pharmaceutic aid (antimicrobial), preservative (bacteriostatic).

W/9-Aminoacridine HCl, tyrothricin, urea, lactose.
See: Trinalis, Vaginal Supp. (Poly-Medica).

W/Benzocaine, chlorothymol, resorcin.
See: Lanacane Creme (Combe).

W/Boric acid, polyoxyethylenenonylphenol or oxyquinoline benzoate.
See: Koromex, Preps. (Holland-Rantos).

W/Methylbenzethonium Cl.
See: Norforms, Aerosol, Supp. (Procter & Gamble).

phenylmercuric acetate. (Various Mfr.) Bot. 1 lb, 5 lb, 10 lb.

Use: Pharmaceutic aid (antimicrobial), preservative (Bacteriostatic).

phenylmercuric borate. (F. W. Berk) Pkg. Custom packed.

W/Benzyl alcohol, benzocaine, butyl p-aminobenzoate.
See: Dermathyn, Oint. (Davis & Sly).

phenylmercuric chloride. Chlorophenylmercury.

•**phenylmercuric nitrate,** N.F. 18.
Use: Pharmaceutic aid (antimicrobial); preservative (bacteriostatic).
See: Preparation H, Oint., Supp. (Whitehall Robins).

W/Amyl, phenylphenol complex.
See: Lubraseptic Jelly (Guardian).

W/Undecylenic acid.
See: Bridex, Oint. (Briar).

phenylmercuric nitrate. (A.P.L.) **Oint. 1:1500,** 1 oz, 4 oz, lb. (Chicago Pharm.) Loz. w/benzocaine. Bot. 100s, 1000s. **Ophth. Oint., 1:3000,** Tube ⅛ oz. **Soln. 1:20,000,** Bot. pt, gal. **Vaginal supp.,** 1:5000, Box 12s.
Use: Pharmaceutic aid (antimicrobial), preservative (bacteriostatic).

phenylmercuric picrate.
Use: Germicide.

phenylphenol-o.

W/Amyl complex, phenylmercuric nitrate.
See: Lubraseptic Jelly. (Guardian).

•**phenylpropanolamine bitartrate,** U.S.P. 23.

•**phenylpropanolamine hydrochloride,** (fen-ill-pro-pan-OLE-uh-meen) U.S.P. 23.
Use: Adrenergic (vasoconstrictor).
See: Maximum Strength Dexatrim, ER Tab. (Thompson).
Obestat, Cap. (Lemmon).
Obestat 150, Cap. (Lemmon).
Propadrine HCl, Preps. (Merck).
Propagest, Tab. (Carnrick).
Spray-U-Thin (Caprice Greystoke).

phenylpropanolamine hydrochloride w/combinations.
See: Allerest, Prods. (Novartis).
Allerstat, Cap. (Lemmon).
A.R.M., Tab. (SK-Beecham).
Bayer, Prods. (Bayer).
BQ Cold, Tab. (Bristol-Myers).
Breacol Cough Medication, Liq. (Bayer).
Bur-Tuss Expectorant (Burlington).
Chexit, Tab. (Sandoz Consumer).
Comtrex, Cap., Liq., Tab. (Bristol-Myers).
Congespirin, Liq., Tab. (Bristol-Myers).
Contac, Prods. (SK-Beecham).

Cophene No. 2, Cap. (Dunhall).
Coricidin Cough Formula (Schering-Plough).
Coricidin "D" Decongestant, Tab. (Schering-Plough).
Coricidin Sinus Headache, Tab. (Schering-Plough).
Coryban-D, Cap. (Pfizer).
Dex-A-Diet, Prods. (Columbia).
Dezest, Cap. (Geneva Pharm).
Dimetane Expectorant, Liq. (Robins).
Dimetapp, Elix., Extentabs (Robins).
Entex, Cap., Liq. (Procter & Gamble).
Entex LA, Tab. (Procter & Gamble).
Halls Mentho-Lyptus Cough Formula, Liq. (Warner-Lambert).
Histabid, Cap. (Glaxo).
Histalet Forte T. D., Tab. (Solvay).
Hista-Vadrin, Syr., Tab., Cap. (Scherer).
Kleer Compound, Tab. (Scrip).
Meditussin-X, Liq. (Roberts).
Naldecon, Drop, Syr., Tab. (Bristol-Myers).
Nasahist, Cap., Inj. (Keene).
Nolamine, Tab. (Carnrick).
Ornade, Cap. (SK-Beecham).
Ornex, Cap. (SK-Beecham).
Panadyl, Tab., Cap. (Misemer).
Partuss-A, Tab. (Parmed).
Partuss T.D., Tab. (Parmed).
Pyristan, Cap., Elix. (Arcum).
Rhinex DM, Liq. (Lemmon).
Rymed, Prods. (Edwards).
Sanhist TD, Tab., Vial (Sandia).
Santussin, Cap., Susp. (Sandia).
Sinarest, Tab. (Pharmcraft).
Sine-Off, Tab. (SK-Beecham).
Sinulin, Tab. (Carnrick).
Spec-T Sore Throat-Decongestant, Loz. (Squibb).
St. Joseph Cold Tablets for Children (Schering-Plough).
Sto-Caps, Cap. (Jalco).
Sucrets Cold Decongestant Loz. (SK-Beecham).
Triaminic, Preps. (Sandoz Consumer).
Triaminicin, Chew. Tab. (Sandoz Consumer).
Triaminicol, Syr. (Sandoz Consumer).
Turbilixir, Liq. (Burlington).
Turbispan Leisurecaps, Cap. (Burlington).
Tusquelin, Syr. (Circle).
Tussagesic, Susp., Tab. (Sandoz Consumer).
U.R.I., Cap., Liq. (ICN).
phenylpropanolamine hydrochloride & chlorpheniramine maleate capsules.
(Various Mfr.) Chlorpheniramine ma-

leate 12 mg, pseudoephedrine HCl 75 mg/Cap. Bot. 50s, 100s, 1000s. *otc, Rx.*
Use: Antihistamine, decongestant.
phenylpropanolamine hydrochloride & guaifenesin tablets. (fen-ill-pro-pan-OLE-uh-meen HIGH-droe-KLOR-ide & GWH-fen-ah-sin) (Various Mfr.) Phenylpropanolamine HCl 75 mg, guaifenesin 400 mg. Tab. Bot. 100s, 500s. *c-III.*
Use: Decongestant, expectorant.
phenylpropanolamine hydrochloride & hydrocodone syrup. (Rosemont) Phenylpropanolamine HCl 25 mg, hydrocodone bitartrate 5 mg. Bot. 480 ml.
Use: Decongestant, antitussive.
•**phenylpropanolamine polistirex.** (fen-ill-pro-pan-OLE-ah-meen pahl-ee-STIE-rex) USAN.
Use: Adrenergic (vasoconstrictor).
phenylpropylmethylamine hydrochloride. Vonedrine HCl.
phenyl salicylate. Salol.
W/Atropine sulfate, hyoscyamine, methenamine, methylene blue, gelsemium, benzoic acid.
See: Renalgin, Tab. (Meyer).
U-Tract, Tab. (Jones Medical).
W/Euphorbia extract and various oils.
See: Rayderm Oint. (Velvet Pharmacal).
W/Methenamine, methylene blue, benzoic acid, hyoscyamine alkaloid, atropine sulfate.
See: Urised, Tab. (PolyMedica).
UTA, Tab. (ICN).
W/Methenamine, sodium biphosphate, methylene blue, hyoscyamine, alkaloid.
See: Urostat Forte, Tab. (ICN Pharm).
phenyl-tert-butylamine.
See: Phentermine.
phenylthilone.
Use: Anticonvulsant.
phenyltoloxamine citrate.
Use: Antihistamine.
See: Volaxin Modified, Tab. (ICN Pharm).
phenyltoloxamine citrate w/combinations.
See: Dengesic, Tab. (Scott-Alison).
Dilone, Tab. (Richardson-Vicks).
Meditussin-X, Liq. (Roberts).
Myocalm, Tab. (Parmed).
Naldecon, Preps. (Bristol-Myers).
Poly-histine Prods. (Bock).
S.A.C. Sinus, Tab. (Towne).
Scotgesic, Elix., Cap. (Scott/Cord).
phenyltoloxamine resin w/combinations.

See: Tussionex, Cap., Liq., Tab. (Medeva).

Phenylzin. (Ciba Vision) Zinc sulfate 0.25%, phenylephrine HCl 0.12%. Bot. 15 ml. *Rx.*
Use: Ophthalmic decongestant.

•**phenyramidol hydrochloride.** (FEN-ih-RAM-ih-dole) USAN.
Use: Analgesic; relaxant (skeletal muscle).

phenythilone.

•**phenytoin,** (FEN-ih-toe-in) U.S.P. 23.
Formerly Diphenylhydantoin.
Use: Anticonvulsant.
See: Dilantin Prods. (Parke-Davis).
Di-phenyl, TR Cap. (Drug. Ind.).
Ekko, Cap. (Fleming).
Toin, Unicelles (Solvay).

•**phenytoin sodium,** U.S.P. 23. *Formerly Diphenylhydantoin Sodium.* Alepsin, Dihydan soluble, Diphentoin, Silantin Sodium, Epanutin, Eptoin, Phenytoin soluble, Solantoin, Solantyl, Denyl Sodium, Soluble Phenytoin.
Use: Anticonvulsant, cardiac depressant (antiarrhythmic).
See: Dilantin Sodium, Preps. (Parke-Davis).
Ekko Jr. and Sr., Cap. (Fleming).

phenytoin sodium with phenobarbital.
Use: Anticonvulsant.
See: Dilantin with Phenobarbital Kapseals, Cap. (Parke-Davis).

pheochromocytoma, agents for.
See: Demser, Cap. (Merck).
Dibenzyline, Cap. (SK-Beecham).
Regitine, Inj. (Novartis) Pharm).

Pherazine DM. (Halsey) Promethazine 6.25 mg, dextromethorphan HBr 15 mg, alcohol 7%/5 ml. Bot. 4 oz, 6 oz, pt, gal. *Rx.*
Use: Antihistamine, antitussive.

Pherazine VC with Codeine Syrup. (Halsey) Phenylephrine HCl 5 mg, promethazine HCl 6.25 mg, codeine phosphate 10 mg, alcohol 7%/5 ml. Bot. pt, gal. *c-v.*
Use: Decongestant, antihistamine, antitussive.

Pherazine VC Syrup. (Halsey) Phenylephrine HCl 5 mg, promethazine HCl 6.25 mg, alcohol 7%/5 ml. Bot. pt, gal. *Rx.*
Use: Decongestant, antihistamine.

Pherazine w/Codeine. (Halsey) Promethazine HCl 6.25 mg, codeine phosphate 10 mg/5 ml, alcohol 7%, sorbitol, sucrose. Syr. Bot. 120 ml, pt, gal. *c-v.*

Use: Antihistamine, antitussive.

phetharbital.

phethenylate. Also sodium salt.

Phicon. (T.E. Williams) Pramoxine HCl 0.5%, vitamin A 7500 IU, E 2000 IU/ 30 g. Cream. Tube 60 g. *otc.*
Use: Local anesthetic, topical.

Phicon F. (T.E. Williams) Undecylenic acid 8%, pramoxine HCl 0.05%. Cream. 60 g. *otc.*
Use: Antifungal, local anesthetic, topical.

Phillips' Chewable. (Bayer) Magnesium hydroxide 311 mg. Tab. 100s, 200s.
Use: Laxative, antacid.

Phillip's Laxative Gelcaps. (Bayer) Phenolphthalein 90 mg, docusate sodium 83 mg, sorbitol. Bot. 30s. *otc.*
Use: Laxative.

Phillips' Laxcaps. (Bayer) Docusate sodium 83 mg, phenolphthalein 90 mg/ Cap. Bot. 8s, 24s, 48s. *otc.*
Use: Laxative.

Phillips' Milk of Magnesia. (Bayer) Magnesium hydroxide. Reg. and Mint. Bot. 4 oz, 12 oz, 26 oz; Tab. Bot. 30s, 100s, 200s. *otc.*
Use: Laxative, antacid.

Phillips' Milk of Magnesia Concentrated. (Bayer) Magnesium hydroxide 800 mg/5 ml, sorbitol, sugar. Liq. Bot. 240 ml. *otc.*
Use: Antacid.

Phish Omega. (Pharmics) Natural salmon oil concentrate containing EPA 120 mg, DHA 100 mg/Cap. Bot. 60s. *otc.*
Use: Fish oil.

Phish Omega Plus. (Pharmics) Natural fish oil concentrate containing EPA 300 mg, DHA 200 mg/Cap. Bot. 60s. *otc.*
Use: Fish oil.

PHisoDerm. (Chattem) Sodium octoxynol-2 ethane sulfonate, white petrolatum, water, mineral oil (with lanolin alcohol and oleyl alcohol), sodium benzoate, octoxynol-3, tetrasodium EDTA, methylcellulose, cocamide MEA, imidazolidinyl urea. **Regular:** 150 ml, 270 ml, 480 ml, gal. **Oily skin:** 150 ml, 480. *otc.*
Use: Skin cleanser, conditioner.

PHisoDerm for Baby. (Chattem) Sodium octoxynol-2 ethane sulfonate, petrolatum, octoxynol-3, mineral oil (with lanolin alcohol and oleyl alcohol), cocamide MEA, imidazolidinyl urea, sodium benzoate, tetrasodium EDTA, methylcellulose, hydrochloric acid. Liq.

Bot. 150 ml, 270 ml. *otc.*
Use: Skin cleanser, conditioner.

PHisoDerm Gentle Cleansing Bar.
(Chattem) Sodium tallowate, sodium cocoate, petrolatum, glycerin, lanolin, sodium Cl, BHT, trisodium EDTA, titanium dioxide. Bar 99 g. *otc.*
Use: Skin cleanser.

PHisoHex. (Sanofi Winthrop) Entsufon sodium, hexachlorophene 3%, petrolatum, lanolin cholesterols, methylcellulose, polyethylene glycol, polyethylene glycol monostearate, lauryl myristyl diethanolamine, sodium benzoate, water, pH adjusted with hydrochloric acid. Emulsion, Bot. 5 oz, pt, gal. Wall dispensers pt. Unit packets 0.25 oz. Box 50s, Pedal operated dispenser 30 oz. *otc.*
Use: Antiseptic, germicide skin cleanser.

PHisoMed. (Sanofi Winthrop) Hexachlorophene. *otc.*
Use: Antiseptic, germicide.

PHisoPuff. (Sanofi Winthrop) Nonmedicated cleansing sponge. Box sponge 1s. *otc.*
Use: Skin cleanser.

Phoschol. (American Lecithin) Phosphatidycholine (highly purified lecithin). **Softgel:** 565 mg or 900 mg. Bot. 100s, 300s. **Liq. Conc.:** 3000 mg/5 ml. Bot. 240 ml, 480 ml. *otc.*
Use: Oral nutritional supplement.

phoscolic acid.
Use: Adjuvant.

Phos-Flur Oral Rinse Supplement.
(Colgate Oral) Acidulated phosphate sodium fluoride 0.05%, fluoride 1 ml/5 ml. Bot. 250 ml, 500 ml, gal. *Rx.*
Use: Dental caries preventative.

Phoslo. (Braintree) Calcium acetate 667 mg (calcium 169 mg)/Tab. Bot. 200s. *Rx.*
Use: Minerals and electrolytes, oral.

phosphate.
See: Potassium Phosphate, Inj. (Abbott).
Sodium Phosphate, Inj. (Abbott).

phosphentaside. Adenosine-5-monophosphate. Adenylic acid.
W/Vitamin B$_{12}$, niacin.
See: Denylex Gel, Vial (Westerfield).
W/Vitamin B$_{12}$, niacin, B$_1$.
See: Adenolin, Vial (Lincoln).

phosphocol p32. (Mallinckrodt) Chromic phosphate P32: 15 mCi with a concentration of up to 5 mCi/ml and specific activity of up to 5 mCi/mg at time of

standardization. Susp. Vial 10 ml.
Use: Radiopharmaceutical.

phosphocysteamine. *Rx.*
Use: Cystinosis. [Orphan drug]

Phospholine Iodide. (Wyeth-Ayerst) Echothiophate Iodide for Ophthalmic Solution. 0.03%, 0.06%, 0.125% and 0.25% potencies/5 ml of sterile eye drops. Package: 1.5 mg for 0.03%; 3 mg for 0.06%; 6.25 mg for 0.125%; 12.5 mg for 0.25% w/5 ml diluent. *Rx.*
Use: Agent for glaucoma.

phospholipids, soy.
See: Granulestin Concentrate, Gran. (Associated Concentrates).

phosphonoformic acid.
See: Foscarnet sodium.

phosphorated carbohydrate solution.
See: Emetrol, Liq. (Bock).
Naus-A-Way, Soln. (Roberts).
Nausetrol, Soln. (Various Mfr.).

•**phosphoric acid,** N.F. 18.
Use: Pharmaceutic aid (solvent).

phosphoric acid, diluted.
Use: Pharmaceutic aid (solvent).

phosphorus.
Use: Phosphorus replacement.
See: Uro-KP-Neutral, Tab. (Star).
K-Phos Neutral, Tab. (Beach).
Neutra-Phos, Cap., Pow. (Baker Norton).
Neutra-Phos-K, Cap., Pow. (Baker Norton).

Phospho-Soda. (Fleet) Sodium biphosphate 48 g, sodium phosphate 18 g/100 ml. Bot. 1.5 oz, 3 oz, 8 oz. Flavored, unflavored. *otc.*
Use: Laxative.

Phosphotec. (Squibb) Technetium Tc 99m pyrophosphate kit. 10 vials/kit.
Use: Radiodiagnostic.

Photofrin. (QLT Photo) Porfimer sodium 75 mg. Freeze-dried cake or powder. *Rx.*
Use: Antineoplastic.

Photoplex Sunscreen. (Allergan Herbert) Butyl methoxydibenzoylmethane 3%, padimate O 7%. Lot. 120 ml. *otc.*
Use: Sunscreen.

Phrenilin Forte Capsules. (Schwarz Pharma) Acetaminophen 650 mg, butalbital 50 mg/Cap. Bot. 100s. *Rx.*
Use: Analgesic, sedative, hypnotic.

Phrenilin Tablets. (Schwarz Pharma) Butalbital 50 mg, acetaminophen 325 mg/Tab. Bot. 100s. *Rx.*
Use: Sedative/hypnotic, analgesic.

Phrenilin with Codeine #3. (Schwarz Pharma) Acetaminophen 325 mg, bu-

talbital 50 mg, codeine phosphate 30 mg/Cap. Bot. 100s. *c-III.*
Use: Narcotic analgesic combination, sedative, hypnotic.

Phresh 3.5 Finnish Cleansing Liquid. (3M Products) Water, cocamidopropyl betaine, lactic acid, polyoxyethylene distearate, polyoxyethylene monostearate, hydroxyethyl cellulose, sodium phosphate, methylparaben. Bot. 6 oz. *otc.*
Use: Soapless cleansing agent.

pH-Stabil Cream. (Hermal) Skin protection cream. Bot. 8 oz. Tube 2 oz. *otc.*
Use: Skin protectant.

Phthalamaquin. (Penick) Quinetolate.
Use: Antiasthmatic.

phthalazine, i-hydrazino-, monohydrochloride. Hydralazine Hydrochloride, U.S.P. 23.

phylcardin.
See: Aminophylline (Various Mfr.).

phyllindon.
See: Aminophylline (Various Mfr.).

Phyllocontin. (Purdue Frederick) Aminophylline 225 mg/CR Tab. Bot. 100s. *Rx.*
Use: Bronchodilator.

phylloquinone. 2-Methyl-3-phytyl-1,4-naphthoquinine, vitamin K.
See: Phytonadione, U.S.P., Inj., Tab. (Various Mfr.).
Vitamin K-1 (Various Mfr.).

Phylorinol Liquid. (Schaffer) Phenol 0.6%, boric acid, strong iodine solution, sorbitol 70% solution, sodium copper chlorophyll. 240 ml. *otc.*
Use: Mouth and throat product.

Phylorinol Mouthwash. (Shaffer) Phenol 0.6%, methyl salicylate, sorbitol. Mouthwash. 240 ml. *otc.*
Use: Mouth and throat product.

physiological irrigating solution.
See: TIS-U-SOL, Soln. (Baxter).
Physiosol, Soln. (Abbott).
Physiolyte, Soln. (American McGaw).

Physiolyte. (American McGaw) Sodium Cl 530 mg, sodium acetate 370 mg, sodium gluconate 500 mg, potassium Cl 37 mg, magnesium Cl 30 mg/100 ml. Soln. Bot. 500 ml, 2 L, 4 L. *Rx.*
Use: Irrigating solution.

Physiosol Irrigation. (Abbott Hospital Prods) Bot. 250 ml, 500 ml, 1000 ml glass or Aqualite (semi-rigid) containers. *Rx.*
Use: Irrigating solution.

•**physostigmine,** U.S.P. 23. An alkaloid.
Use: Cholinergic (ophthalmic).

•**physostigmine salicylate,** U.S.P. 23.

Physostigmine monosalicylate. Eserine salicylate.
Use: Cholinergic (ophthalmic); parasympathomimetic agent, Friedreich's and other inherited ataxias [Orphan drug]
See: Antilirium, Amp. (Forest).
Isopto-Eserine, Ophthalmic, Soln. (Alcon).

W/l-Hyoscyamine HBr.
See: Phyatromine-H, Amp., Vial (Kremers-Urban).

W/Pilocarpine, methylcellulose.
See: Isopto P-ES, Soln. (Alcon).

physostigmine salicylate. (Forest) Pow., Tube 1 gr, 5 gr, 15 gr.
Use: Cholinergic (ophthalmic).

•**physostigmine sulfate,** U.S.P. 23.
Use: Cholinergic (ophthalmic).

•**phytate persodium.** (FIE-tate per-SO-dee-uhm) USAN.
Use: Pharmaceutic aid.

•**phytate sodium.** (FIE-tate) USAN. Sodium salt of inositol hexaphosphoric acid.
Use: Chelating agent (calcium).

phytic acid. Inositol hexophosphoric acid.

phytonadiol sodium diphosphate.

•**phytonadione,** (fye-toe-nuh-DIE-ohn) U.S.P. 23.
Use: Vitamin (prothrombogenic).
See: Aquamephyton, Inj. (Merck).
Konakion, Amp. (Roche).
Mephyton, Tab. (Merck).

phytonadione. (IMS) 2 mg/ml (Vitamin K_1). Inj. 0.5 ml, Min-I-ject prefilled syringes. *Rx.*
Use: Vitamin (prothrombogenic).

•**picenadol hydrochloride.** (pih-SEN-AID-ole) USAN.
Use: Analgesic.

•**piclamilast.** (pih-KLAM-ill-ast) USAN.
Use: Antiasthmatic (type IV phosphodiesterase inhibitor).

•**picotrin diolamine.** (PIH-koe-trin die-OH-lah-meen) USAN.
Use: Keratolytic.

picric acid, trinitrophenol.
See: Butesyn Picrate, Oint. (Abbott).
Silver Salts (Various Prods.).

picrotoxin. Cocculin.
Use: Respiratory stimulant.

•**picumeterol fumarate.** (PIKE-you-MEH-teh-role) USAN.
Use: Bronchodilator.

P.I.D.
See: Phenindione (Various Mfr.).

• **pifarnine.** (pih-FAR-neen) USAN.
Use: Antiulcerative (gastric).

Pilagan. (Allergan) Pilocarpine nitrate 1%, 2% or 4%. Soln. Bot. 15 ml. *Rx.*
Use: Agent for glaucoma.

Pilocar. (Ciba Vision) Pilocarpine HCl 0.5%, 1%, 2%, 3%, 4% or 6%. Bot. 15 ml; Twinpack 2 × 15 ml 0.5%, 1%, 2%, 3%, 4% or 6%; 1 ml Dropperettes 1%, 2% or 4%. *Rx.*
Use: Agent for glaucoma.

• **pilocarpine,** (pie-low-CAR-peen) U.S.P. 23.
Use: Antiglaucoma, ophthalmic cholinergic, miotic.
See: Ocusert Pilo-20 and Pilo-40 (Novartis).

• **pilocarpine hydrochloride,** U.S.P. 23.
Use: Cholinergic (ophthalmic), topically as a miotic, xerostomia and keratoconjunctivitis sicca [Orphan drug]
See: Almocarpine (Wyeth-Ayerst).
Isopto-Carpine, Soln. (Alcon).
Mi-Pilo, Soln. (Pilkington Barnes Hind).
Pilocar, Soln. (Ciba Vision).
Pilomiotin, Soln. (Ciba Vision).
Piloptic, Soln. (Muro).
Salagen, Tab. (MGI Pharma).
W/Epinephrine HCl.
See: E-Carpine, Inj. (Alcon).
Epicar, Ophthalmic Soln. (Pilkington Barnes Hind).
W/Epinephrine bitartrate, mannitol, benzalkonium Cl.
See: E-Pilo, Soln. (Ciba Vision).
W/Physostigmine salicylate, methylcellulose.
See: Isopto P-ES, Soln. (Alcon).

pilocarpine hydrochloride. (Various Mfr.) Pilocarpine HCl. **0.5%:** 15 ml, 30 ml; **1%:** 2 ml, 15 ml, 30 ml, UD 1 ml; **2% and 4%:** 2 ml, 15 ml, 30 ml; **6%:** 15 ml; **8%:** 2 ml. *Rx.*
Use: Cholinergic (ophthalmic), topically as a miotic, xerostomia and keratoconjunctivitis sicca [Orphan drug]

• **pilocarpine nitrate,** U.S.P. 23.
Use: Cholinergic (ophthalmic).
See: P.V. Carpine (Allergan).
W/Phenylephrine HCl.
Use: Parasympathomimetic agent.
See: Pilofrin Liquifilm, Ophthalmic (Allergan).

Pilopine. (International Pharm) Pilocarpine HCl 1%, 2% or 4%. Soln. Bot. 15 ml. *Rx.*
Use: Agent for glaucoma.

Pilopine HS Gel. (Alcon) Pilocarpine HCl 4%. Tube 3.5 g. *Rx.*

Use: Agent for glaucoma.

Piloptic. (Optopics) Pilocarpine HCl 0.5%, 1%, 2%, 3%, 4% or 6%. Soln. Bot. 15 ml. *Rx.*
Use: Agent for glaucoma.

Pilostat. (Bausch & Lomb) Pilocarpine HCl 0.5%, 1%, 2%, 3%, 4% or 6%. Soln. Bot. 15 ml, twin pack 2 x 15 ml. *Rx.*
Use: Agent for glaucoma.

Pima Syrup. (Fleming) Potassium iodide 5 gr/5 ml. Bot. pt, gal. *Rx.*
Use: Expectorant.

• **pimagedine hydrochloride.** (pih-MAH-jeh-deen) USAN.
Use: Inhibitor (advanced glycosylation end-product formation inhibitors).

• **pimetine hydrochloride.** (PIM-eh-teen) USAN.
Use: Antihyperlipoproteinemic.

piminodine esylate.
Use: Analgesic.

piminodine ethanesulfonate.
Use: Narcotic analgesic.

• **pimobendan.** (pie-MOE-ben-dan) USAN.
Use: Cardiotonic.

• **pimozide,** (pih-moe-ZIDE) U.S.P. 23.
Use: Antipsychotic.
See: Orap, Tab. (McNeil Pharm).

• **pinacidil.** (pie-NASS-ih-DILL) USAN.
Use: Antihypertensive.

• **pinadoline.** (pih-nah-DOE-leen) USAN.
Use: Analgesic.

• **pindolol,** (PIN-doe-lahl) U.S.P. 23.
Use: Beta-adrenergic blocking agent, vasodilator.
See: Visken (Sandoz).

pine needle oil, N.F. XVI.
Use: Perfume; flavor.

pine tar, U.S.P. XXI.
Use: Local antieczematic; rubefacient.

Pinex Concentrate Cough Syrup. (Last) Dextromethorphan HBr 7.5 mg/5 ml (after diluting 3 oz. concentrate to make 16 oz. solution). Bot. 3 oz. *otc.*
Use: Antitussive.

Pinex Cough Syrup. (Last) Dextromethorphan HBr 7.5 mg/5 ml. Bot. 3 oz, 6 oz. *otc.*
Use: Antitussive.

Pinex Regular. (Pinex) Potassium guaiacolsulfonate, oil of pine and eucalyptus, extract of grindelia, alcohol 3%/ 30 ml. Syr. Bot. 3 oz, 8 oz. Also cherry flavored 3 oz. Super and concentrated 3 oz. *otc.*
Use: Expectorant.

Pink Bismuth. (Goldline) 130 mg/15 ml. Liq. Bot. 240 ml. *otc.*

Use: Antidiarrheal.

●**pinoxepin hydrochloride.** (pih-NOX-eh-PIN) USAN.
Use: Antipsychotic.

Pin-Rid. (Apothecary) **Soft gelcap:** Pyrantel pamoate 180 mg (equivalent to 62.5 mg pyrantel base). Pkg. 24s; **Liq.:** Pyrantel pamoate 144 mg/ml (equivalent to 50 mg/ml pyrantel base), saccharin, sucrose. Bot. 30 ml. *otc.*
Use: Anthelmintic.

Pin-X. (Effcon) Pyrantel base (as pamoate) 50 mg/ml, sorbitol. Liq. Bot. 30 ml. *otc.*
Use: Anthelmintic.

●**pioglitazone hydrochloride.** (PIE-oh-GLIH-tah-zone) USAN.
Use: Antidiabetic.

●**pipamperone.** (pih-PAM-peer-OHN) USAN. *Formerly Floropipamide.*
Use: Antipsychotic.

●**pipazethate.** (pip-AZZ-eh-thate) USAN.
Use: Cough suppressant; antitussive.

pipazethate hydrochloride.
Use: Antitussive.

●**pipecuronium bromide.** (pih-peh-cure-OH-nee-uhm) USAN.
Use: Neuromuscular blocking agent.

●**piperacetazine.** (pih-PURR-ah-SET-ah-zeen) USAN.
Use: Antipsychotic.

●**piperacillin,** U.S.P. 23.

●**piperacillin sodium,** (PIH-per-uh-SILL-in) U.S.P. 23.
Use: Antibacterial.
W/ Tazobactam
See: Zosyn, Inj. (Lederle).

●**piperamide maleate.** (PIH-per-ah-mid) USAN.
Use: Anthelmintic.

●**piperazine,** (pie-PEAR-ah-zeen) U.S.P. 23.
Use: Anthelmintic.

●**piperazine citrate,** (pie-PEAR-ah-zeen) U.S.P. 23. Piperazine Citrate Telra Hydrous Tripiperazine Dicitrate.
Use: Anthelmintic.
See: Bryrel, Syr. (Sanofi Winthrop).
Ta-Verm, Syr., Tab. (Table Rock).
Vermago, Syr. (Westerfield).

●**piperazine edetate calcium.** (pie-PEAR-ah-zeen EH-deh-tate) USAN.
Use: Anthelmintic.

piperazine estrone sulfate. (pie-PEAR-ah-zeen)
See: Estropipate.

piperazine hexahydrate. Tivazine.

piperazine phosphate.
Use: Anthelmintic.

piperazine tartrate.
See: Razine Tartrate, Tab. (Paddock).

piperidine phosphate.
Use: Psychiatric drug.

piperidinoethyl benzilate hydrochloride. No products listed.

piperidolate hydrochloride.
Use: Anticholinergic.

piperoxan hydrochloride. Fourneau 933. Benzodioxane. Diagnosis of hypertension.
Use: Diagnostic aid.

piperphenidol hydrochloride.

pipethanate hydrochloride.
Use: Tranquilizer.

●**pipobroman.** (PIP-oh-BROE-man) USAN.
Use: Antineoplastic.
See: Vercyte, Tab. (Abbott).

●**piposulfan.** (PIP-oh-SULL-fan) USAN.
Use: Antineoplastic.

●**pipotiazine palmitate.** (PIP-oh-TIE-ah-zeen PAL-mih-tate) USAN.
Use: Antipsychotic.
See: Piportil (Ives).

●**pipoxolan hydrochloride.** USAN. Rowapraxin.
Use: Muscle relaxant.

Pipracil. (Lederle) Piperacillin sodium 2 g, 3 g, 4 g or 40 g/Vial; 2 g, 3 g or 4 g/Infusion Bottle. Sterile. *Rx.*
Use: Anti-infective, penicillin.

●**piprozolin.** (PIP-row-ZOE-lin) USAN.
Use: Choleretic.

●**piquindone hydrochloride.** (PIH-kwin-dohn) USAN.
Use: Antipsychotic.

●**piquizil hydrochloride.** (PIH-kwih-zill) USAN.
Use: Bronchodilator.

●**piracetam.** (PIHR-ASS-eh-tam) USAN.
Use: Cognition adjuvant, cerebral stimulant, myoclonus [Orphan drug]

●**pirandamine hydrochloride.** (pih-RAN-dah-meen) USAN.
Use: Antidepressant.

●**pirazmonam sodium.** (pihr-AZZ-moe-nam SO-dee-uhm) USAN.
Use: Antimicrobial.

●**pirazolac.** (PIHR-AZE-oh-lack) USAN.
Use: Antirheumatic.

●**pirbenicillin sodium.** (pihr-ben-IH-SILL-in) USAN.
Use: Antibacterial.

●**pirbuterol acetate.** (pihr-BYOO-tuh-role) USAN.
Use: Bronchodilator.
See: Maxair, Aerosol (3M Pharm).

•**pirbuterol hydrochloride.** USAN.
Use: Bronchodilator.

•**pirenperone.** (PIHR-en-PURR-ohn)
USAN.
Use: Tranquilizer.

•**pirenzepine hydrochloride.** (PIHR-en-
zeh-PEEN) USAN.
Use: Antiulcerative.

•**piretanide.** (pihr-ETT-ah-nide) USAN.
Use: Diuretic.
See: Arlix, Prods. (Hoechst Marion
Roussel).

•**pirfenidone.** (PEER-FEN-ih-dohn)
USAN.
Use: Anti-inflammatory, antipyretic, an-
algesic.

piridazol.
See: Sulfapyridine, Tab. (Various Mfr.).

•**piridicillin sodium.** (pihr-RIH-dih-SILL-
in) USAN.
Use: Antibacterial.

piridocaine hydrochloride.

•**piridronate sodium.** (pihr-IH-DROE-
nate) USAN.
Use: Regulator (calcium).

•**piriprost.** (PIHR-ih-prahst) USAN.
Use: Antiasthmatic.

•**piriprost potassium.** (PIHR-ih-prahst)
USAN.
Use: Antiasthmatic.

piriton.
See: Chlorpheniramine (Various Mfr.).

•**piritrexim isethionate.** (pih-rih-TREX-im
eye-seh-THIGH-oh-nate) USAN.
Use: Antiproliferative. [Orphan drug]

•**pirlimycin hydrochloride.** (PIHR-lih-MY-
sin) USAN.
Use: Antibacterial.

•**pirmagrel.** (PIHR-mah-GRELL) USAN.
Use: Inhibitor (thromboxane synthetase).

•**pirmenol hydrochloride.** (PIHR-MEH-
nahl) USAN.
Use: Cardiac depressant (antiarrhythmic).

•**pirnabine.** (PIHR-NAH-bean) USAN.
Use: Antiglaucoma.

•**piroctone.** (pihr-OCK-TONE) USAN.
Use: Antiseborrheic.

•**piroctone olamine.** (pihr-OCK-TONE
OH-lah-meen) USAN.
Use: Antiseborrheic.

•**pirodavir.** (pih-ROW-dav-ihr) USAN.
Use: Antiviral.

•**pirogliride tartrate.** (PIHR-oh-GLIE-ride)
USAN.
Use: Antidiabetic.

•**pirolate.** (PIHR-oh-late) USAN.

Use: Antiasthmatic.

•**pirolazamide.** (PIHR-ole-aze-ah-mide)
USAN.
Use: Cardiac depressant (antiarrhyth-
mic).

•**piroxantrone hydrochloride.** (PIH-row-
ZAN-trone) USAN.
Use: Antineoplastic.

•**piroxicam,** (pihr-OX-ih-kam) U.S.P. 23.
Use: Anti-inflammatory.
See: Feldene, Cap. (Pfizer).

piroxicam. (Various Mfr.) 10 mg, 20 mg.
Cap. Bot. 100s, 500s, 1000s.
Use: Anti-inflammatory.

•**piroxicam betadex.** USAN.
Use: Analgesic, anti-inflammatory, antirheumatic.

•**piroxicam cinnamate.** (pihr-OX-ih-kam
SIN-ah-mate) USAN.
Use: Anti-inflammatory.

•**piroxicam olamine.** (pihr-OX-ih-kam
OH-lah-meen) USAN.
Use: Anti-inflammatory, analgesic.

•**piroximone.** (PIHR-ox-ih-MONE) USAN.
Use: Cardiotonic.

•**pirprofen.** (pihr-PRO-fen) USAN.
Use: Anti-inflammatory.

•**pirquinozol.** (PIHR-KWIN-oh-zole)
USAN.
Use: Antiallergic.

•**pirsidomine.** (pihr-SIH-doe-meen)
USAN.
Use: Vasodilator.

Piso's. (Pinex) Ipecac, ammonium Cl,
menthol in syrup base. Bot. 3 oz, 5
oz. *otc.*
Use: Expectorant.

pitayine.
See: Quinidine, Preps. (Various Mfr.).

Pitocin. (Parke-Davis) Oxytocin w/chloro-
butanol 0.5%, acetic acid to adjust pH.
Amp. 5 units/0.5 ml; 10 units/1 ml. Box
10s, Steri-dose syringe; 10 units/1 ml
10s. *Rx.*
Use: Oxytocic.

Pitressin Synthetic. (Parke-Davis) Vasopressin w/chlorobutanol 0.5%, pH adjusted with acetic acid. Amp. 0.5 ml, 1
ml (20 pressor units). Box 10s. *Rx.*
Use: Posterior pituitary hormones.

Pitts Carminative. (Del Pharm) Bot. 2
oz.
Use: Antiflatulent.

pituitary, anterior. The anterior lobe of
the pituitary gland supplies protein hormones classified under following head-
ings.
See: Corticotropin, Preps. (Various
Mfr.).

Gonadotropin, Preps. (Various Mfr.).
Growth Hormone.
Thyrotropic Principle.
pituitary function test.
See: Metopirone, Tab. (Novartis).
pituitary, posterior, hormones.
(a) Vasopressin. Pressor principle, β-hypophamine, postlobin-V.
See: Pitressin, Amp. (Parke-Davis).
(b) Oxytocin. Oxytocic principle. α-hypophamine, postiobin-O.
See: Oxytocin, Inj. (Various Mfr.).
Pitocin, Amp. (Parke-Davis).
Syntocinon, Amp. (Sandoz).
•**pituitary, posterior, injection,** U.S.P. 23.
Use: Hormone (antidiuretic).
See: Pituitrin, Obstetrical, Amp. (Parke-Davis).
Pituitrin, Surgical, Amp. (Parke-Davis).
•**pivampicillin hydrochloride.** (pihv-AM-pih-SILL-in) USAN.
Use: Antibacterial.
•**pivampicillin pamoate.** (pihv-AM-pih SILL-in PAM-oh-ate) USAN.
Use: Antibacterial.
•**pivampicillin probenate.** (pihv-AM-pih-SILL-in PRO-ben-ate) USAN.
Use: Antibacterial.
•**pivopril.** (PIH-voe-PRILL) USAN.
Use: Antihypertensive.
pix carbonis.
See: Coal Tar, Preps. (Various Mfr.).
pix juniperi.
Use: Sunscreen, moisturizer.
See: Juniper Tar, Comp. (Various Mfr.).
•**pizotyline.** (pih-ZOE-tih-leen) USAN.
Use: Anabolic, antidepressant, serotonin inhibitor (migraine).
placebo capsules. (Cowley) No. 3 orange red; No. 4 yellow. Bot. 1000s.
Use: Placebo.
placebo tablets. (Cowley) 1 gr white; 2 gr white; 3 gr white, red or yellow, pink, orange; 4 gr white; 5 gr white. Bot. 1000s.
Use: Placebo.
Placidyl. (Abbott) Ethchlorvynol. **200 mg/Cap.:** Bot. 100s. **500 mg/Cap.:** Bot. 100s, 500s, UD 100s. **750 mg/Cap.:** Bot. 100s. *c-IV.*
Use: Sedative, hypnotic.
•**plague vaccine,** U.S.P. 23.
Use: Active immunizing agent.
plague vaccine. (Greer Laboratories) 2000 million killed *Pasteurella pestis*/ml. Vial 20 ml.
Use: Active immunizing agent.

planocaine.
See: Procaine HCl, Preps. (Various Mfr.).
planochrome.
See: Merbromin, Soln. (Various Mfr.).
plantago, ovata coating.
See: Effersyllium, Prods. (Stuart).
Konsyl, Pow. (Burton, Parsons).
L.A. Formula, Pow. (Burton, Parsons).
Metamucil, Pow. (Searle).
W/Psyllium seed, gum karaya, Brewer's yeast.
See: Plantamucin, Gran. (ICN Pharm).
W/Vitamin B$_1$.
See: Siblin, Gran. (Parke-Davis).
•**plantago seed,** U.S.P. 23.
Use: Laxative.
plant protease concentrate.
See: Ananase, Tab. (Rhone-Poulenc Rorer).
Plaquenil Sulfate. (Sanofi-Winthrop) Hydroxychloroquine sulfate 200 mg/Tab. (equivalent to base 155 mg). Bot. 100s. *Rx.*
Use: Antimalarial, antirheumatic.
Plaquenil Tablet. (Sanofi Winthrop.) Hydroxychloroquine sulfate. *Rx.*
Use: Antimalarial, antirheumatic.
Plasbumin-5. (Bayer) Normal serum albumin (Human) 5% U.S.P. fractionated from normal serum plasma, heat treated against hepatitis virus. Albumin 12.5 g/250 ml. Vial 50 ml. Bot. with IV set 250 ml, 500 ml. *Rx.*
Use: Plasma protein fraction.
Plasbumin-25. (Bayer) Normal serum albumin (Human) 25% U.S.P. fractionated from normal serum plasma, heat treated against hepatitis virus. Albumin 12.5 g/50 ml. Vial 20 ml. Bot. with IV set 50 ml, 100 ml. *Rx.*
Use: Plasma protein fraction.
plasma.
See: Normal Human Plasma (Various Mfr.).
plasma expanders or substitutes.
See: Dextran 6% and LMD 10% (Abbott).
Macrodex, Soln. (Pharmacia & Upjohn).
Plasma-Lyte A Injection. (Baxter) Sodium 140 mEq, potassium 5 mEq, magnesium 3 mEq, chloride 98 mEq, acetate 27 mEq, gluconate 23 mEq/L w/pH adjusted to 7.4. Plastic bot. 500 ml, 1000 ml. *Rx.*
Use: Parenteral nutritional supplement.
Plasma-Lyte 148 Injection. (Baxter) Sodium 140 mEq, potassium 5 mEq, mag-

nesium 3 mEq, chloride 98 mEq, acetate 27 mEq, gluconate 23 mEq/L. Plastic bot. 500 ml, 1000 ml. *Rx.*
Use: Parenteral nutritional supplement.

Plasma-Lyte M and 5% Dextrose Injection. (Baxter) Sodium 40 mEq, potassium 16 mEq, calcium 5 mEq, magnesium 3 mEq, chloride 40 mEq, acetate 12 mEq, lactate 12 mEq/L. Plastic bot. 500 ml, 1000 ml. *Rx.*
Use: Parenteral nutritional supplement.

Plasma-Lyte R and 5% Dextrose Injection. (Baxter) Sodium 140 mEq, potassium 10 mEq, calcium 5 mEq, magnesium 3 mEq, chloride 103 mEq, acetate 47 mEq, lactate 8 mEq/L. Bot. 500 ml, 1000 ml. *Rx.*
Use: Parenteral nutritional supplement.

Plasma-Lyte 56 and 5% Dextrose. (Baxter) Sodium 40 mEq, potassium 13 mEq, magnesium 3 mEq, chloride 40 mEq, acetate 16 mEq/L. Plastic bot. 500 ml, 1000 ml. *Rx.*
Use: Parenteral nutritional supplement.

Plasma-Lyte 148 and 5% Dextrose. (Baxter) Dextrose 50 g, calories 190, sodium 140 mEq, potassium 5 mEq, magnesium 3 mEq, chloride 98 mEq, acetate 27 mEq, 547 mOsm, gluconate 23 mEq/L. Soln. Bot. 500 ml, 1000 ml. *Rx.*
Use: Parenteral nutritional supplement.

Plasma-Lyte 56 in Water. (Baxter) Sodium 40 mEq, potassium 13 mEq, magnesium 3 mEq, chloride 40 mEq, acetate 16 mEq/L. Plastic bot. 500 ml, 1000 ml. *Rx.*
Use: Parenteral nutritional supplement.

Plasma-Lyte R Injection. (Baxter) Sodium 140 mEq, potassium 10 mEq, calcium 5 mEq, magnesium 3 mEq, chloride 103 mEq, acetate 47 mEq, lactate 8 mEq/L. Bot. 1000 ml. *Rx.*
Use: Parenteral nutritional supplement.

Plasmanate. (Bayer) Plasma protein fraction (Human) 5%. U.S.P. Vial 50 ml. Bot. 250 ml, 500 ml with set. *Rx.*
Use: Plasma protein fraction.

Plasma-Plex. (Centeon) Plasma protein fraction 5%. Inj. Vial 250 ml, 500 ml. *Rx.*
Use: Plasma protein fraction.

•**plasma protein fraction,** U.S.P. 23. *Formerly Plasma Protein Fraction, Human.*
Use: Blood-volume supporter.
See: Plasmanate, Soln. (Bayer).
Plasma-Plex, Soln. (Centeon).
Plasmatein, Soln. (Abbott).
Protenate, Soln. (Baxter).

plasma protein fraction. (Baxter) For the plasma protein preparation obtained from human plasma using the Cohn fractionation technique Bot. 250 ml.
Use: Blood volume supporter.

Plasmatein. (Alpha Therapeutic) Plasma protein fraction 5%. Inj. Vial w/injection set 250 ml, 500 ml. *Rx.*
Use: Plasma protein fraction.

plasmochin naphthoate. Pamaquine naphthoate.
Use: Antimalarial.

•**platelet concentrate,** U.S.P. 23.
Use: Platelet replenisher.

Platelet Factor 4. (Abbott Diagnostics) Radioimmunoassay for quantitative measurement of total PF4 levels in plasma. Test kit 100s.
Use: Diagnostic aid.

Platinol. (Bristol-Myers/Bristol Oncology) Cisplatin 10 mg or 50 mg/Vial. *Rx.*
Use: Antineoplastic agent.

Platinol-AQ. (Bristol-Myers Oncology) Cisplatin (CDDP) 1 mg/ml. Inj. Vial. 50 ml, 100 ml. *Rx.*
Use: Antineoplastic.

Plegisol. (Abbott Hospital Prods) Calcium Cl dihydrate 17.6 mg, magnesium Cl hexahydrate 325.3 mg, potassium Cl 119.3 mg, sodium Cl 643 mg/100 ml. Approximately 260 mOsm/L. Single Dose Container 1000 ml without sodium bicarbonate. *Rx.*
Use: Cardioplegic solution.

Plendil. (Astra-Merck) Felodipine 2.5 mg, 5 mg or 10 mg/ER Tab. Bot. 30s, 100s, UD 100s. *Rx.*
Use: Calcium channel blocker.

Plewin Tablets. (Sanofi Winthrop) Glycobiarsol, chloroquine phosphate. *Rx.*
Use: Amebicide.

Plexolan Cream. (Last) Zinc oxide, lanolin. Tube 1.25 oz, 3 oz. Jar 16 oz. *otc.*
Use: Skin protectant.

Plexon. (Sig) Testosterone 10 mg, estrone 1 mg, liver 2 mcg, pyridoxine HCl 10 mg, panthenol 10 mg, inositol 20 mg, choline Cl 20 mg, vitamin B_2 2 mg, B_{12} 100 mcg, procaine HCl 1%, niacinamide 100 mg/ml. Vial 10 ml.
Use: Hormone, vitamin/mineral supplement.

Pliagel. (Alcon) Sodium Cl, potassium Cl, poloxamer 407, sorbic acid 0.25%, EDTA 0.5%. Soln. Bot. 25 ml. *otc.*
Use: Soft contact lens care.

•**plicamycin,** (PLY-kae-MY-sin) U.S.P. 23. Antibiotic derived from *Streptomyces*

agrillaceus & *S. tanashiensis. Formerly Mithramycin.*
Use: Antineoplastic.
See: Mithracin, Pow. (Bayer).

•**plomestane.** (PLOE-mess-TANE) USAN.
Use: Antineoplastic (aromatase inhibitor).

Plova. (Washington Ethical) Psyllium mucilloid. Pow. (flavored) 12 oz., (plain) 10 0.5 oz. *otc.*
Use: Laxative.

Pluravit Drops. (Sanofi Winthrop) Multivitamin.
Use: Vitamin supplement.

PMB 200. (Wyeth-Ayerst) Premarin (Conjugated Estrogens, U.S.P.) 0.45 mg, meprobamate 200 mg, lactose, sucrose/Tab. Bot. 60s. *Rx.*
Use: Estrogen, antianxiety.

PMB 400. (Wyeth-Ayerst) Premarin (Conjugated Estrogens, U.S.P.) 0.45 mg, meprobamate 400 mg, lactose, sucrose/Tab. Bot. 60s. *Rx.*
Use: Estrogen, antianxiety.

P.M.P. Compound. (Mericon) Chlorpheniramine maleate 4 mg, phenylephrine HCl 15 mg, salicylamide 300 mg, scopolamine methylnitrate 0.8 mg/Tab. Bot. 100s, 1000s. *Rx.*
Use: Antihistamine, decongestant, analgesic.

PMP Expectorant. (Mericon) Codeine phosphate 10 mg, phenylephrine HCl 10 mg, guaifenesin 40 mg, chlorpheniramine maleate 2 mg/5 ml. Bot. gal. *c-v.*
Use: Antitussive, decongestant, expectorant, antihistamine.

pneumococcal vaccine, polyvalent. (new-moe-KAH-kuhl) Purified capsular polysaccharides from 23 pneumococcal types. 25 mcg each of 23 polysaccharides per 0.5 ml.
Use: Agent for immunization.
See: Pneumovax 23, Inj. (Merck).
Pnu-Imune 23, Inj. (Wyeth Lederle).

Pneumomist. (ECR Pharm) Guaifenesin 600 mg. SR Tab. Bot. 100s. *Rx.*
Use: Expectorant.

Pneumotussin HC. (ECR Pharm) Hydrocodone bitartrate 5 mg, guaifenesin 100 mg/5 ml Syrup. Bot. 120 ml, 480 ml. *c-iii.*
Use: Antitussive, expectorant.

Pneumovax 23. (Merck) Pneumococcal vaccine polyvalent 0.5 ml/dose. Vial 5 dose, 1 dose X 5s. *Rx.*
Use: Agent for immunization.

PNS Unna Boot. (Pedinol) Non-sterile gauze bandage 10 yds X 3″. Box 12s.
Use: Ambulatory procedure in treatment of leg ulcers and varicosities.

Pnu-Imune 23. (Wyeth Lederle) Pneumococcal vaccine 0.5 ml dose. 5-dose vials. Lederject disposable syringe 5 X 1 dose. *Rx.*
Use: Agent for immunization.

•**pobilukast edamine.** USAN.
Use: Antiasthmatic (leukotriene antagonist).

pochlorin. Prophyrinic and chlorophyllic compound.
Use: Antihypercholesteremic agent.

Pod-Ben-25. (C & M Pharmacal) Podophyllin 25% in benzoin tincture. Bot. 1 oz. *Rx.*
Use: Keratolytic.

Podoben. (American) Podophyllum resin extract 25%. Bot. 5 ml. *Rx.*
Use: Keratolytic.

Podocon-25. (Paddock) Podophyllum resin 25% in benzoin tincture. Soln. 15 ml. *Rx.*
Use: Keratolytic.

•**podofilox.** (pah-dah-FILL-ox) USAN.
Use: Antimitotic.
See: Condylox (Oclassen).

Podofin. (Syosset Labs) Podophyllum resin 25% in benzoin tincture. Liq. Bot. 7.5 ml. *Rx.*
Use: Keratolytic.

podophyllin.
See: Podophyllum resin.

•**podophyllum,** U.S.P. 23.
Use: Pharmaceutic necessity.
W/Oxgall, cascara sagrada, dandelion root, tincture nux vomica.
See: Oxachol, Liq. (Philips Roxane).

•**podophyllum resin,** U.S.P. 23.
Use: Caustic.
See: Podoben, Liq. (Maurry).
W/Salicylic acid.
See: Ver-Var, Soln. (Galderma).

podophyllum resin. (Various Mfr.) Podophyllin. Pkg. 1 oz, 0.25 lb, 1 lb.
Use: Caustic

Point-Two Mouthrinse. (Colgate Oral) Sodium fluoride 0.2% in a flavored neutral liquid. Bot. 120 ml. *Rx.*
Use: Dental caries preventative.

Poison Antidote Kit. (JMI Canton) Charcoal suspension. Bot. 60 ml, 4s. Ipecac syrup, Bot. 30 ml, 1/Kit. *otc.*
Use: Antidote.

•**poison ivy extract, alum precipitated.** USAN.
Use: Ivy poisoning counteractant.

•**poison oak extract.** USAN.
Use: Antiallergic.

Poison Oak-n-Ivy Armor. (Tec Labs)
Trioctyl citrate, mineral oil, monostearyl
citrate, beeswax, 4-chloro-3,5-xylenol.
Lot. Bot. 59.1 ml. *otc.*
Use: Topical poison ivy treatment.

•**polacrilin.** USAN. Methacrylic acid with
divinylbenzene. A synthetic ion-exchange resin, supplied in the hydrogen
or free acid form. Amberlite IRP-64.
Use: Pharmaceutic aid.

•**polacrilin potassium,** N.F. 18. A synthetic ion-exchange resin, prepared
through the polymerization of methacrylic acid and divinylbenzene, further
neutralized with potassium hydroxide to
form the potassium salt of methacrylic
acid and divinylbenzene. Supplied as
a pharmaceutical-grade ion-exchange
resin in a particle size of 100- to 500-
mesh.
Use: Pharmaceutic aid (tablet disintegrant).
See: Amberlite IRP-88 (Rohm and
Haas).

Poladex Tabs. (Major) Dexchlorpheniramine maleate. **4 mg/Tab.:** Bot. 100s,
250s, 1000s; **6 mg/Tab.:** Bot. 100s,
1000s. *Rx.*
Use: Antihistamine.

polamethene resin caprylate. The phys-
iochemical complex of the acid-binding
ion exchange resin, polyamine-methylene resin and caprylic acid.

Polaramine. (Schering-Plough) Dexchlor-
pheniramine maleate (d-isomer of
Chlor-Trimeton). **Repetab:** 4 mg/Tab.
Bot. 100s; 6 mg/Tab. Bot. 100s, 1000s.
Syr.: 2 mg/5 ml. Bot. 16 oz. *Rx.*
Use: Antihistamine.

Polaramine Expectorant. (Schering-
Plough) Dexchlorpheniramine maleate
2 mg, pseudoephedrine sulfate 20 mg,
guaifenesin 100 mg/5 ml, alcohol 7.2%.
Bot. 16 oz. *Rx.*
Use: Antihistamine, decongestant, expectorant.

Poldeman AD Suspension. (Sanofi Winthrop) Kaolin. *otc.*
Use: Antidiarrheal.

Poldeman Suspension. (Sanofi Winthrop) Kaolin. *otc.*
Use: Antidiarrheal.

Poldemicina Suspension. (Sanofi Winthrop) Kaolin. *otc.*
Use: Antidiarrheal.

•**poldine methylsulfate.** (POLE-deen
METH-ill-SULL-fate) USAN. U.S.P. XX.
Use: Anticholinergic.

•**policapram.** (PAH-lee-CAP-ram) USAN.
Use: Pharmaceutic aid (tablet binder).

Polident Dentu-Grip. (Block) Carboxymethylcellulose gum, ethylene oxide
polymer. Pkg. 0.675 oz, 1.75 oz, 3.55
oz. *otc.*
Use: Denture adhesive.

•**polifeprosan 20.** (pahl-ee-FEH-pro-
SAHN 20) USAN.
Use: Pharmaceutic aid (biodegradable
polymer for controlled drug delivery).

•**poligeenan.** (PAHL-ih-JEE-nan) USAN.
Polysaccharide produced by limited hydrolysis of carragheen from red algae.
Use: Pharmaceutic aid (dispersing
agent).

•**poliglecaprone 25.** (poe-lih-GLEH-kah-
prone 25) USAN.
Use: Surgical aid (surgical suture material, absorbable).

•**poliglecaprone 90.** (poe-lih-GLEH-kah-
prone 90) USAN.
Use: Surgical aid (surgical suture coating, absorbable).

•**poliglusam.** (pahl-ee-GLUE-sam) USAN.
Use: Antihemorrhagic; wound healing;
hemostatic.

•**polignate sodium.** (poe-LIG-nate)
USAN.
Use: Enzyme inhibitor (pepsin).

Poli-Grip. (Block) Karaya gum, magnesium oxide in petrolatum mineral oil
base, peppermint and spearmint flavor.
Tube 0.75 oz, 1.5 oz, 2.5 oz. *otc.*
Use: Denture adhesive.

poliomyelitis vaccine, inactivated.
(Pasteur-Merieux-Connaught) (Purified,
Salk Type IPV) Amp. 5 x 1 ml. Vial 10
dose. *Rx.*
Use: Agent for immunization.
See: IPOL.
Poliovirus vaccine, inactivated.

poliomyelitis vaccine inactivated.
See: Poliovirus vaccine, inactivated.

•**poliovirus vaccine, inactivated,** (POE-
lee-oh-VYE-russ) U.S.P. 23. *Formerly*
Poliomyelitis Vaccine.
Use: Agent for immunization (active).
See: IPOL.

poliovirus vaccine, inactivated. (Pasteur-Merieux-Connaught) Amp. 1 ml.
Box 5s. Vial 10 dose. Subcutaneous administration.
Use: Agent for immunization (active).

•**poliovirus vaccine live oral,** U.S.P. 23.
Poliovirus vaccine, live, oral, type I, II
or III. Poliovirus vaccine, live, oral, trivalent.

Use: Agent for immunization (active).
See: Orimune Trivalent I, II & III, Vial (Wyeth Lederle).

poliovirus vaccine, live, oral, trivalent. Immunization against polio strains 1, 2 & 3. *Rx.*
Use: Agent for immunization.
See: Orimune (Wyeth Lederle).

•**polipropene 25.** (pahl-ee-PRO-peen 25) USAN.
Use: Pharmaceutic aid (tablet excipient).

•**polixetonium chloride.** (pahl-ix-eh-TOE-nee-uhm) USAN.
Use: Pharmaceutic aid (preservative).

Polocaine. (Astra) Mepivacaine. **1%, 2%:** Inj. Vial 50 ml. **3%:** Inj. Dental cartridge 1.8 ml. **2% w/levonordefrin 1:20,000:** Sodium bisulfite. Inj. Dental cartridge 1.8 ml.*Rx.*
Use: Local anesthetic.

Polocaine MPF. (Astra) Mepivacaine HCl. **1%, 1.5%:** Inj. Vial 30 ml. **2%:** Inj. Vial 20 ml. *Rx.*
Use: Local anesthetic.

Poloris Poultices. (Block) Benzocaine 7.5 mg, capsicum 4.6 mg in poultice base. Pkg. 5 unit, 12 unit. *Rx.*
Use: Local anesthetic.

•**poloxalene.** (PAHL-OX-ah-leen) USAN. Liquid nonionic surfactant polymer of polyoxypropylene polyoxyethylene type.
Use: Pharmaceutic aid (surfactant).

poloxalkol. Polyoxyethylene polyoxypropylene polymer.
See: Magcyl, Cap. (ICN Pharm).
W/Casanthrol.
See: Casakol, Cap. (Pharmacia & Upjohn).
W/Phenylephrine HCl, dextrose soln.
See: Isohalent, Soln. (ICN Pharm).

•**poloxamer,** N.F. 18.
Use: Pharmaceutic aid (ointment and suppository base, surfactant, tablet binder and coating agent, emulsifying agent).

poloxamer 182 d. (pahl-OX-ah-mer 182D)
Use: Pharmaceutic aid (surfactant).

poloxamer 182 lf. (pahl-OX-ah-mer 182LF)
Use: Food additive; pharmaceutic aid.

poloxamer 188. (pahl-OX-ah-mer 188)
Use: Cathartic; sickle cell crisis, severe burns [Orphan drug]

poloxamer 188 lf. (pahl-OX-ah-mer 188LF)
Use: Pharmaceutic aid (surfactant).

poloxamer 331. (pahl-OX-ah-mer 331)

Use: Food additive (surfactant); AIDS-related toxoplasmosis [Orphan drug]

poloxamer-iodine.
See: Prepodyne, Soln. (West).

polyamine-methylene resin.
See: Exorbin (Various Mfr.).

polyamine resin.
See: Polyamine-Methylene Resin (Various Mfr.).

polyanethol sulfonate, sodium.
See: Grobax, Vial (Roche Diagnostics).

polyanhydroglucose. Polyanhydroglucuronic acid.
See: Dextran, Inj., Soln. (Various Mfr.).

Polybase. (Paddock) Preblended polyethylene glycol suppository base for incorporation of medications where a water soluble base is indicated. Jar 1 lb, 5 lb.
Use: Suppository base.

polybenzarsol. Benzocal.

Poly-Bon Drops. (Barrows) Vitamins A 3000 IU, D 400 IU, C 60 mg, B_1 1 mg, B_2 1.2 mg, niacinamide 8 mg/0.6 ml. Bot. 50 ml. *otc.*
Use: Vitamin supplement.

•**polybutester.** (PAHL-ee-byoot-ESS-ter) USAN.
Use: Surgical aid (surgical suture material).

•**polybutilate.** (PAHL-ee-BYOO-tih-late) USAN.
Use: Surgical aid (surgical suture coating).

•**polycarbophil,** U.S.P. 23. A synthetic, loosely crosslinked, hydrophilic resin of the polycarboxylic type. Sorboquel.
Use: Laxative.

Polycillin. (Bristol-Myers) Ampicillin trihydrate. **250 mg/Cap.:** Bot. 100s, 500s, 1000s, UD 100s. **500 mg/Cap.:** Bot. 100s, 500s, UD 100s. **Pediatric Drops:** 100 mg/ml. Dropper bot. 20 ml. *Rx.*
Use: Anti-infective, penicillin.

Polycillin-N. (Bristol-Myers) Sodium ampicillin 125 mg, 250 mg, 500 mg, 1 g or 2 g/Vial. Pkg. 1s, 10s. Piggyback vial 500 mg, 1 g, 2 g. Bulk vial 10 g. *Rx.*
Use: Anti-infective, penicillin.

Polycillin Oral Suspension. (Bristol-Myers) Ampicillin trihydrate. **125 mg/5 ml:** Bot. 80 ml, 100 ml, 150 ml, 200 ml, UD 5 ml. **250 mg/5 ml:** Bot. 80 ml, 100 ml, 150 ml, 200 ml, UD 5 ml. **500 mg/ 5 ml:** Bot. 100 ml, UD 5 ml. *Rx.*
Use: Anti-infective, penicillin.

Polycillin-PRB Oral Suspension. (Bristol-Myers) Ampicillin trihydrate 3.5 g, probenecid 1 g/Bot. Bot 9s. *Rx.*

Use: Anti-infective, penicillin.

Polycitra-K. (Baker Norton) Potassium citrate monohydrate 1100 mg, citric acid monohydrate 334 mg, potassium ion 10 mEq/5 ml. Bot. 4 oz, pt. *Rx.*
Use: Systemic alkalinizer.

Polycitra-K Crystals. (Baker Norton) Potassium citrate monohydrate 3300 mg, citric acid 1002 mg, potassium ion 30 mEq, equivalent to 30 mEq bicarbonate/ UD pkg. Sugar free. Box 100s. *Rx.*
Use: Systemic alkalinizer.

Polycitra-LC. (Baker Norton) Potassium citrate monohydrate 550 mg, sodium citrate dihydrate 500 mg, citric acid monohydrate 334 mg, potassium ion 5 mEq, sodium ion 5 mEq/5 ml. Bot. 4 oz, pt. *Rx.*
Use: Systemic alkalinizer.

Polycitra Syrup. (Baker Norton) Potassium citrate monohydrate 550 mg, sodium citrate dihydrate 500 mg, citric acid monohydrate 334 mg, potassium ion 5 mEq, sodium ion 5 mEq/5 ml. Bot. 4 oz, pt. *Rx.*
Use: Systemic alkalinizer.

Polycose. (Ross) **Pow.:** Glucose polymers derived from controlled hydrolysis of corn starch. Calories 380, carbohydrate 94 g, water 6 g, sodium 110 mg, potassium 10 mg, chloride 223 mg, calcium 30 mg, phosphorus 5 mg/100 g. Can 12.3 oz. Case 6s. **Liq.:** Calories 200, carbohydrate 50 g, water 70 g, sodium 70 mg, potassium 6 mg, chloride 140 mg, calcium 20 mg, phosphorus 3 mg/100 ml. Bot. 4 oz. Case 48s. *otc.*
Use: Nutritional supplement.

polycycline intravenous.
See: Bristacycline, Cap., Vial (Bristol-Myers).

•**polydextrose.** (PAH-lee-DEX-trose) USAN.
Use: Food additive.

polydimethylsiloxane (silicone oil).
Use: Ophthalmic.
See: AdatoSil 5000, Inj. (Escalon Ophthalmics).

Polydine Ointment. (Century) Povidone-iodine in ointment base. Jar 1 oz, 4 oz, lb. *otc.*
Use: Anti-infective, topical.

Polydine Scrub. (Century) Povidone-iodine in scrub solution. Bot. 1 oz, 4 oz, 8 oz, pt, gal. *otc.*
Use: Antiseptic.

Polydine Solution. (Century) Povidone-iodine solution. Bot. 1 oz, 4 oz, 8 oz, pt, gal. *otc.*

Use: Antiseptic.

•**polydioxanone.** (PAHL-ee-die-OX-ah-nohn) USAN.
Use: Surgical aid (surgical suture material, absorbable).

Poly ENA Test System for RNP and SM. (Wampole-Zeus) Qualitative identification of auto antibodies to extractable nuclear antigens in human serum by gel precipitation technique. Aid in the diagnosis of SLE, MCTD, PSS, SS. Box test 48s.
Use: Diagnostic aid.

Poly ENA Test System for RNP, SM, SSA and SSB. (Wampole-Zeus) Qualitative identification of auto antibodies to extractable nuclear antigens in human serum by gel precipitation techniques. Aid in the diagnosis of SLE, MCTD, PSS, SS. Box test 96s.
Use: Diagnostic aid.

Poly ENA Test System for SSA and SSB. (Wampole-Zeus) Qualitative identification of auto antibodies to extractable nuclear antigens in human serum by gel precipitation techniques. Aid in the diagnosis of SLE, MCTD, PSS, SS. Box test 48s.
Use: Diagnostic aid.

polyestradiol phosphate.
See: Estradurin, Amp. (Wyeth-Ayerst).

•**polyethadene.** (PAHL-ee-ETH-ah-DEEN) USAN.
Use: Antacid.

polyethylene excipient, N.F. XVII.
Use: Pharmaceutic aid (stiffening agent).

•**polyethylene glycol,** (poli-eth-uh-leen gli-cawl) N.F. 18.
Use: Pharmaceutic aid (ointment and suppository base, tablet excipient, solvent, tablet and capsule lubricant).
See: P.E.G., Oint. (Medco).

polyethylene glycol 3350 and electrolytes for oral solution. (poli-eth-uh-leen gli-cawl)
Use: Rehydration.

•**polyethylene glycol monomethyl ether,** N.F. 18.
Use: Pharmaceutic aid (excipient).

•**polyethylene oxide,** N.F. 18.
Use: Pharmaceutic aid (suspending and viscosity agent, tablet binder).

•**polyferose.** (PAHL-ee-feh-rohs) USAN. An iron carbohydrate chelate containing approximately 45% of iron in which the metallic (Fe) ion is sequestered within a polymerized carbohydrate derived from sucrose.

Use: Hematinic.

Poly-F Fluoride Drops. (Major) Fluoride 0.5 mg, vitamins A 1500 IU, D 400 IU, E 5 mg, B$_1$ 0.5 mg, B$_2$ 0.6 mg, B$_3$ 8 mg, B$_6$ 0.4 mg, B$_{12}$ 2 mcg, C 35 mg/ml. Drops. Bot. 50 ml. *Rx.*
Use: Vitamin/mineral supplement.

Polygam S/D. (American Red Cross) Protein 50 mg (90% gamma globulin). Inj. Single-use vials 2.5 g, 5 g, 10 g. *Rx.*
Use: Immune globulin.

• **polyglactin 370.** (PAHL-ee-GLAHK-tin 370) USAN. Lactic acid polyester with glycolic acid.
Use: Surgical aid (surgical suture coating, absorbable).

• **polyglactin 910.** (PAHL-ee-GLAHK-tin 910). USAN.
Use: Surgical aid (surgical suture coating, absorbable).

• **polyglycolic acid.** (PAHL-ee-glie-KAHL-ik) USAN.
Use: Surgical aid (surgical suture material).
See: Dexon Sterile Suture (David & Geck).

• **polyglyconate.** (PAHL-ee-GLIE-koe-nate) USAN.
Use: Surgical aid (surgical suture material, absorbable).

Poly-Histine CS. (Bock) Brompheniramine maleate 2 mg, phenylpropanolamine HCl 12.5 mg, codeine phosphate 10 mg/5 ml, alcohol 0.95%. Bot. pt. *c-v.*
Use: Antihistamine, decongestant, antitussive.

Poly-Histine-D Capsules. (Bock) Phenylpropanolamine HCl 50 mg, phenyltoloxamine citrate 16 mg, pyrilamine maleate 16 mg, pheniramine maleate 16 mg/Cap. Bot. 100s. *Rx.*
Use: Decongestant, antihistamine.

Poly-Histine-D Elixir. (Bock) Phenylpropanolamine HCl 12.5 mg, phenyltoloxamine citrate 4 mg, pyrilamine maleate 4 mg, pheniramine 4 mg/5 ml. Bot. 473 ml. *Rx.*
Use: Antihistamine, decongestant.

Poly-Histine DM. (Bock) Dextromethorphan HBr 10 mg, phenylpropanolamine HCl 12.5 mg, brompheniramine maleate 2 mg/5 ml. Bot. pt. *Rx.*
Use: Antitussive, decongestant, antihistamine.

Poly-Histine-D Ped Caps. (Bock) Phenylpropanolamine HCl 25 mg, phenyltoloxamine citrate 8 mg, pheni-

ramine maleate 8 mg, pyrilamine maleate 8 mg/Cap. Bot. 100s. *Rx.*
Use: Decongestant, antihistamine.

Poly-Histine Elixir. (Bock) Phenyltoloxamine citrate 4 mg, pyrilamine maleate 4 mg, pheniramine maleate 4 mg/5 ml, alcohol 4%. Elix. Bot. pt. *Rx.*
Use: Antihistamine.

poly I; poly C12U. *Rx.*
Use: AIDS, antineoplastic. [Orphan drug]

• **polymacon.** (PAHL-ee-MAY-kahn) USAN.
Use: Contact lens material (hydrophilic).

polymeric oxygen. *Rx.*
Use: Sickle cell anemia. [Orphan drug]

• **polymetaphosphate P 32.** USAN.
Use: Radioactive agent.

polymethine blue dye.

polymonine.

Polymox. (Bristol-Myers) Amoxicillin trihydrate. **Cap.:** 250 mg. Bot. 100s, 500s, UD 100s; 500 mg. Bot. 50s, 100s, 500s, UD 100s. **Oral Susp.:** 125 mg or 250 mg/5 ml. Bot. 80 ml, 100 ml, 150 ml. Dosatrol 125 mg or 250 mg/Bot. 5 ml. **Ped. Drops:** 50 mg/ml. Bot. 15 ml. *Rx.*
Use: Anti-infective, penicillin.

polymyxin B. (Various Mfr.) (No pharmaceutical form available) Antimicrobial substances produced by *Bacillus polymyxa.*
W/Bacitracin zinc, neomycin sulfate, benzalkonium Cl.
See: Biotres, Oint. (Schwarz Pharma).

• **polymyxin B sulfate,** U.S.P. 23.
Use: Antibacterial.
See: Aerosporin, Pow., Soln. (Glaxo Wellcome).

polymyxin B sulfate and bacitracin zinc topical aerosol.
Use: Anti-infective, topical.

polymyxin B sulfate and bacitracin zinc topical powder.
Use: Anti-infective, topical.

polymyxin B sulfate and hydrocortisone otic solution.
Use: Anti-infective, anti-inflammatory, otic.

polymyxin B sulfate sterile. (Roerig) Polymyxin B sulfate 500,000 units Ophth Soln. Vial 20 ml for reconstitution. *Rx.*
Use: Anti-infective.

polymyxin B sulfate w/combinations.
See: AK-Poly-Bac Oint. (Akorn).
AK-Spore, Preps. (Akorn).
Aquaphor, Oint. (Beiersdorf).

Cortisporin, Preps. (Glaxo Wellcome).
Epimycin A, Oint. (Delta).
Maxitrol, Oint., Ophthalmic Oint. (Pharmacia & Upjohn).
Mycitracin, Oint., Ophthalmic Oint. (Pharmacia & Upjohn).
Neomixin, Oint. (Roberts).
Neosporin, Preps. (Glaxo Wellcome).
Neosporin G.U. Irrigant, Amp. (Glaxo Wellcome).
Neotal, Oint. (Roberts).
Neo-Thrycex, Oint. (Del Pharm).
Ocutricin, Preps. (Bausch & Lomb).
Otobiotic, Soln. (Schering-Plough).
Otoreid-HC, Liq. (Solvay).
Polysporin, Oint., Ophthalmic Oint. (Glaxo Wellcome).
Polytrim Ophth. Soln. (Allergan).
Pyocidin-Otic, Soln. (Berlex).
Statrol, Liq. (Alcon).
Statrol Sterile Ophthalmic Oint. (Alcon).
Terramycin, Preps. w/Polymyxin (Pfizer).
Tigo, Oint. (Burlington).
Tribotic, Oint. (Burgin-Arden).
Tribiotic Plus, Oint. (Thompson).
Trimixin, Oint. (Hance).

polymyxin-neomycin-bacitracin ointment. (Various Mfr.). *otc.*
Use: Anti-infective, topical.

polynoxylin. Poly[methylenedi(hydroxymethyl)urea]. Anaflex.

polyoxyethylene 8 stearate. Myrj 45. (Zeneca), Polyoxyl 8 Stearate.

polyoxyethylene (20) sorbitan monoleate.
See: Polysorbate 80, U.S.P. 23. (Various Mfr.).

polyoxyethylene 20 sorbitan trioleate. Tween 85. (Zeneca), Polysorbate 85.

polyoxyethylene 20 sorbitan tristearate. Tween 65. (Zeneca), Polysorbate 65.

polyoxyethylene 40 monostearate. Polyoxyl 40 Stearate.
See: Myrj 52 & Myrj 52S (Zeneca).

polyoxyethylene 50 stearate.
See: Polyoxyl 50 stearate.

polyoxyethyleneonylphenol.
W/Alkyldimethylbenzylammonium Cl, methylrosaniline Cl, polyethylene glycol tert-dodecylthioether.
See: Hyva, Vaginal Tab. (Holland-Rantos).

polyoxyethylene lauryl ether.
W/Benzoyl peroxide, ethyl alcohol.
See: Benzagel, Gel (Dermik).
Desquam-X, Preps. (Westwood Squibb).

W/Hydrocortisone, sulfur.
See: Fostril HC, Lot. (Westwood Squibb).
W/Sulfur.
See: Fostril, Lot. (Westwood Squibb).
Proseca, Oint. (Westwood Squibb).

polyoxyethylene nonyl phenol.
W/Sodium edetate, docusate sodium, 9-aminoacridine HCl.
See: Vagisec Plus, Supp. (Schmid).

polyoxyethylene sorbitan monolaurate. Polysorbate 20, N.F. 18.
W/Ferrous gluconate.
See: Simron, Cap. (Hoechst Marion Roussel).
W/Ferrous gluconate, vitamins.
See: Simron Plus, Cap. (Hoechst Marion Roussel).

•**polyoxyl 8 stearate.** (PAHL-ee-OX-ill 8 STEE-ah-rate) USAN. Polyoxyethylene 8 stearate.
Use: Pharmaceutic aid (surfactant).
See: Myrj 45 (Atlas).

•**polyoxyl 10 oleyl ether,** (PAHL-ee-OX-ill 10 EETH-ehr) N.F. 18.
Use: Pharmaceutic aid (surfactant).

•**polyoxyl 20 cetostearyl ether,** (PAHL-ee-OX-ill 20 SEE-toe-STEE-rill EETH-ehr) N.F. 18.
Use: Pharmaceutic aid (surfactant).

•**polyoxyl 35 castor oil,** (PAHL-ee-OX-ill) N.F. 18.
Use: Pharmaceutic aid (surfactant, emulsifying agent).

•**polyoxyl 40 hydrogenated castor oil,** (PAHL-ee-OX-ill 40 high-DRAH-jen-ATE-ehd) N.F. 18.
Use: Pharmaceutic aid (surfactant, emulsifying agent).

•**polyoxyl 40 stearate,** (PAHL-ee-OX-ill 40 STEE-ah-rate) N.F. 18. Macrogic Stearate 2,000 (I.N.N.) Polyoxyethylene 40 monostearate.
Use: Pharmaceutic aid (surfactant).
Use: Hydrophilic oint., surfactant; surface-active agent.
See: Myrj 52 (Atlas).
Myrj 52S (Atlas).
W/Polyethylene glycol, chlorobutanol.
See: Blink-N-Clean (Allergan).

•**polyoxyl 50 stearate,** (PAHL-ee-OX-ill 50 STEE-ah-rate) N.F. 18.
Use: Pharmaceutic aid (surfactant, emulsifying agent).

•**polyoxypropylene 15 stearyl ether.** USAN. *Formerly PPG-15 Stearyl Ether.*
Use: Pharmaceutic aid (solvent).

Poly-Pred Suspension. (Allergan) Prednisolone acetate 0.5%, neomycin sul-

fate equivalent to 0.35% neomycin base, polymyxin B sulfate 10,000 units/ml. Dropper bot. 5 ml, 10 ml. *Rx.*
Use: Corticosteroid, anti-infective, ophthalmic.

polypropylene glycol. An addition polymer of propylene oxide and water.
Use: Pharmaceutic aid (suspending agent).

polysaccharide-iron complex.
Use: Iron-containing products, oral.
See: Hytinic (Hyrox).
　Niferex (Schwarz Pharma).
　Niferex-150 (Schwarz Pharma).
　Nu-Iron (Mayrand).
　Nu-Iron 150 (Mayrand).

polysaccharide iron complex. (URL) iron 50 mg/Cap. Bot. 100s. *otc.*
Use: Iron supplement.

polysonic lotion. (Parker) Multi-purpose ultrasound lotion with high coupling efficiency. Bot. 8.5 oz, gal.
Use: For diagnostic and therapeutic medical ultrasound.

•**polysorbate 20,** (PAHL-ee-SORE-bate 20) N.F. 18.
Use: Pharmaceutic aid (surfactant).

•**polysorbate 40,** (PAHL-ee-SORE-bate 40) N.F. 18.
Use: Pharmaceutic aid (surfactant).

•**polysorbate 60,** (PAHL-ee-SORE-bate 60) N.F. 18.
Use: Pharmaceutic aid (surfactant).

•**polysorbate 65.** (PAHL-ee-SORE-bate 65) USAN.
Use: Pharmaceutic aid (surfactant).

•**polysorbate 80,** (PAHL-ee-SORE-bate 80) N.F. 18.
Use: Pharmaceutic aid (surfactant).

•**polysorbate 85.** (PAHL-ee-SORE-bate 85) USAN.
Use: Pharmaceutic aid (surfactant).

Polysorb Hydrate. (Fougera) Sorbitan sesquinoleate in a wax and petrolatum base. Cream. Tube 56.7 g, lb. *otc.*
Use: Emollients.

Polysporin Ointment. (Glaxo Wellcome) Polymyxin B sulfate 10,000 units, bacitracin zinc 500 units/g in special white petrolatum base. Tube 3.75 g. *otc.*
Use: Anti-infective, topical.

Polysporin Ophthalmic Ointment. (Glaxo Wellcome) Polymyxin B sulfate, 10,000 units, bacitracin zinc 500 units. Tube 3.5 g. *Rx.*
Use: Antibiotic, ophthalmic.

Polysporin Powder. (Glaxo Wellcome) Polymyxin B 10,000 units, zinc bacitracin 500 units, lactose base/g. Shaker vial 10 g. *Rx.*

Use: Anti-infective, topical.

polysulfides. Polythionate.

Polytabs-F Chewable Vitamin. (Major) Fluoride 1 mg, vitamins A 2500 IU, D 400 IU, E 15 mg, B_1 1.05 mg, B_2 1.2 mg, B_3 13.5 mg, B_6 1.05 mg, B_{12} 4.5 mcg, C 60 mg, folic acid 0.3 mg/Tab. Bot. 100s, 1000s. *Rx.*
Use: Vitamin/mineral supplement.

Polytar Bath. (Stiefel) A 25% polytar blend of four different vegetable and mineral tars in an emulsion base. Bot. 8 fl oz. *otc.*
Use: Tar-containing bath dermatological.

Polytar Shampoo. (Stiefel) A neutral soap containing 1% Polytar in a surfactant shampoo. Buffered. Plastic Bot. 6 fl oz, 12 fl oz, gal. *otc.*
Use: Antiseborrheic.

Polytar Soap. (Stiefel) A neutral soap containing 1% Polytar. Cake 4 oz. *otc.*
Use: Tar-containing preparation.

•**polytef.** (PAHL-ee-teff) USAN.
Use: Prosthetic aid.

•**polythiazide,** (PAHL-ee-THIGH-azz-ide) U.S.P. 23.
Use: Diuretic; antihypertensive.
See: Renese Tab. (Pfizer Laboratories).
W/Prazosin.
See: Minizide, Cap. (Pfizer Laboratories).
W/Reserpine.
See: Renese-R, Tab. (Pfizer Laboratories).

Polytinic. (Pharmics) Elemental iron 100 mg, vitamin C 300 mg, folic acid 1 mg/tab. Bot. 100s. *Rx.*
Use: Vitamin/mineral supplement.

Polytrim. (Allergan) Polymyxin B sulfate 10,000 units/g or ml, trimethoprim 1 mg/ml. Drop. Bot. 10 ml. *Rx.*
Use: Anti-infective, ophthalmic.

Polytuss-DM. (Rhode) Dextromethorphan HBr 15 mg, chlorpheniramine maleate 1 mg, guaifenesin 25 mg/5 ml. Bot. 4 oz, 8 oz. *otc.*
Use: Antitussive, antihistamine, expectorant.

•**polyurethane foam.** (PAHL-ih-you-ree-thane foam) USAN.
Use: Prosthetic aid (internal bone splint).

polyvidone.
See: Polyvinylpyrrolidone.

Poly-Vi-Flor 0.25 mg. (BM-Squibb) **Drops:** Vitamins A 1500 IU, D 400 IU, E 5 IU, C 35 mg, B_1 0.5 mg, B_2 0.6

mg, B_6 0.4 mg, B_3 8 mg, B_{12} 2 mcg, fluoride 0.25 mg/ml. Dropper bot. 50 ml. **Tab.:** Vitamins A 2500 IU, D 400 IU, E 15 IU, B_1 1.05 mg, B_2 1.2 mg, B_3 13.5 mg, B_6 1.05 mg, B_{12} 4.5 mcg, C 60 mg, folic acid, 0.3 mg, fluoride 0.25 mg, lactose, sucrose. Chewable. Bot. 100s. *Rx.*
Use: Vitamin/mineral supplement, dental caries preventative.

Poly-Vi-Flor 0.5 mg Chewable Tabs. (BM-Squibb) Vitamins A 2500 IU, D 400 IU, E 15 IU, C 60 mg, B_1 1.05 mg, B_2 1.2 mg, B_3 13.5 mg, B_6 1.05 mg, B_{12} 4.5 mcg, fluoride 0.5 mg, folic acid 0.3 mg/ Chew. tab. Bot. 100s. **With Iron:** Above formula plus iron 12 mg, copper, zinc 10 mg/Tab. Bot. 100s. *Rx.*
Use: Vitamin/mineral supplement, dental caries preventative.

Poly-Vi-Flor 1 mg Chewable Tablets. (BM-Squibb) Vitamins A 2500 IU, D 400 IU, E 15 IU, C 60 mg, B_1 1.05 mg, B_2 1.2 mg, B_3 13.5 mg, B_6 1.05 mg, B_{12} 4.5 mcg, fluoride 1 mg, folic acid 0.3 mg, sucrose/Chew. tab. Bot. 100s, 1000s. **With Iron:** Above formula plus iron 12 mg, copper 1 mg, zinc 10 mg/ Tab. *Rx.*
Use: Vitamin/mineral supplement, dental caries preventative.

Poly-Vi-Flor 0.5 mg Drops. (BM-Squibb) Vitamins A 1500 IU, D 400 IU, E 5 IU, C 35 mg, B_1 0.5 mg, B_2 0.6 mg, B_6 0.4 mg, niacin 8 mg, B_{12} 2 mcg, fluoride 0.5 mg/ml. Dropper bot. 30 ml, 50 ml. *Rx.*
Use: Vitamin/mineral supplement, dental caries preventative.

Poly-Vi-Flor 0.25 mg w/Iron. (BM-Squibb) **Drops:** Vitamins A 1500 IU, D 400 IU, E 5 IU, C 35 mg, B_1 0.5 mg, B_2 0.6 mg, B_6 0.4 mg, niacin 8 mg, fluoride 0.25 mg, iron 10 mg/ml. Bot. 50 ml. **Tab.:** Vitamins A 2500 IU, D 400 IU, E 15 IU, B_1 1.05 IU, B_2 1.2 mg, B_3 13.5 mg, B_6 1.05 mg, B_{12} 4.5 mcg, C 60 mg, folic acid 0.3 mg, fluoride 0.25 mg, Cu, iron 12 mg, zinc 10 mg, lactose, sucrose. Chewable. Bot. 100s. *Rx.*
Use: Vitamin/mineral supplement, dental caries preventative.

Poly-Vi-Flor 0.5 mg w/Iron. (Bristol-Myers) **Drops:** Vitamins A 1500 IU, D 400 IU, E 5 IU, C 35 mg, B_1 0.5 mg, B_2 0.6 mg, B_3 8 mg, B_6 0.4 mg, fluoride 0.5 mg, iron 10 mg/ml. Dropper bot. 50 ml. **Tab.:** Vitamins A 2500 IU, D 400 IU, E 15 IU, B_1 1.05 mg, B_2 1.2 mg, B_3 13.5 mg, B_6 1.05 mg, B_{12} 4.5 mcg, C 60

mg, folic acid 0.3 mg, fluoride 0.5 mg, iron 12 mg, Cu, zinc 10 mg, lactose, sucrose. Chewable. Bot. 100s. *Rx.*
Use: Vitamin/mineral supplement, dental caries preventative.

Poly-Vi-Flor 0.5 Tabs. (BM-Squibb) Fluoride 0.5 mg, vitamins A 2500 IU, D 400 IU, E 15 mg, B_1 1.05 mg, B_2 1.2 mg, B_3 13.5 mg, B_6 1.05 mg, B_{12} 4.5 mcg, C 60 mg, folic acid 0.3 mg, Cu, iron 12 mg, zinc 10 mg, sucrose. Tab. Bot. 100s. *Rx.*
Use: Vitamin/mineral supplement, dental caries preventative.

•**polyvinyl acetate phthalate,** N.F. 18.
Use: Pharmaceutic aid (coating agent).

•**polyvinyl alcohol,** U.S.P. 23. Ethanol, homopolymer.
Use: Pharmaceutic aid (viscosity-increasing agent).
See: Liquifilm Forte (Allergan).
Liquifilm Tears (Allergan).
W/Hydroxypropyl methylcellulose.
See: Liquifilm Wetting Soln. (Allergan).

polyvinylpyrrolidone, polyvidone, povidone.
W/Acetrizoate Sodium
See: Salpix, Vial (Ortho).

polyvinylpyrrolidone vinylacetate copolymers.
See: Ivy-Rid, Spray (Roberts).
W/Benzalkonium.
See: Ivy-Chex, Aerosol (Jones Medical).

Poly-Vi-Sol Drops. (BM-Squibb) Vitamins A 1500 IU, D 400 IU, C 35 mg, B_1 0.5 mg, B_2 0.6 mg, E 5 IU, B_6 0.4 mg, B_3 8 mg, B_{12} 2 mcg/ml. Bot. 50 ml. *otc.*
Use: Vitamin supplement.

Poly-Vi-Sol Tablets. (BM-Squibb) Vitamins A 2500 IU, E 15 IU, D 400 IU, C 60 mg, B_1 1.05 mg, B_2 1.2 mg, B_3 13.5 mg, B_6 1.05 mg, B_{12} 4.5 mcg, folic acid 0.3 mg/Chew. Tab. Bot. 100s. **With Iron:** Above formula plus iron 12 mg, zinc 8 mg/Tab. Bot. 100s. Circus shape Tab. Bot. 100s. *otc.*
Use: Vitamin/mineral supplement.

Poly-Vi-Sol w/Iron Drops. (BM-Squibb) Vitamins A 1500 IU, D 400 IU, E 5 IU, C 35 mg, B_1 0.5 mg, B_2 0.6 mg, B_3 8 mg, B_6 0.4 mg, iron 10 mg/ml. Bot. 50 ml. *otc.*
Use: Vitamin/mineral supplement.

Poly-Vi-Sol w/Iron Tablets, Chewable. (BM-Squibb) Iron 12 mg, vitamins A 2500 IU, D 400 IU, E 15 mg, B_1 1.05 mg, B_2 1.2 mg, B_3 13.5 mg, B_6 1.05 mg, B_{12} 4.5 mcg, C 60 mg, folic acid 0.3

mg, Cu, zinc 8 mg, sugar/Tab. Bot. 100s. *otc.*
Use: Vitamin/mineral supplement.

Poly-Vi-Sol w/Minerals. (Bristol-Myers) Iron 12 mg, vitamins A 2500 IU, D 400 IU, E 15 mg, B_1 1.05 mg, B_2 1.2 mg, B_3 13.5 mg, B_6 1.06 mg, B_{12} 4.5 mcg, C 60 mg, folic acid 0.3 mg, Cu, zinc 8 mg/Chew. tab. Bot. 60s, 100s. *otc.*
Use: Vitamin/mineral supplement.

poly-vitamin drops. (Schein) Vitamins A 1500 IU, D 400 IU, E 5 IU, B_1 0.5 mg, B_2 0.6 mg, B_3 8 mg, B_6 0.4 mg, B_{12} 1.5 mcg, C 35 mg/ml. Drop. Bot. 50 ml. *otc.*
Use: Vitamin supplement.

Polyvitamin Drops with Iron. (Various Mfr.) Iron 10 mg, vitamins A 1500 IU, D 400 IU, E 5 mg, B_1 0.5 mg, B_2 0.6 mg, B_3 8 mg, B_6 0.4 mg, C 35 mg/ml. Bot. 50 ml. *otc.*
Use: Vitamin/mineral supplement.

polyvitamin drops w/iron and fluoride. (Various Mfr.) Fluoride 0.25 mg, vitamins A 1500 IU, D 400 IU, E 5 IU, B_1 0.5 mg, B_2 0.6 mg, B_3 8 mg, B_6 0.4 mg, C 35 mg, iron 10 mg. Bot. 50 ml. *Rx.*
Use: Vitamin/mineral supplement; dental caries preventative.

polyvitamin fluoride. (Various Mfr.) Fluoride 0.25 mg, Vitamins A 1500 IU, D 400 IU, E 5 IU, B_1 0.5 mg, B_2 0.6 mg, B_3 8 mg, B_6 0.4 mg, B_{12} 2 mcg, C 35 mg/ml. Drop. Bot. 50 ml. *Rx.*
Use: Vitamin/mineral supplement; dental caries preventative.

poly-vitamins w/fluoride 0.5 mg. (Various Mfr.) **Drops:** Fluoride 0.5 mg, vitamins A 1500 IU, D 400 IU, E 5 IU, B_1 0.5 mg, B_2 0.6 mg, B_3 8 mg, B_6 0.4 mg, B_{12} 2 mcg, C 35 mg/ml. Bot. 50 ml. **Tab.:** Fluoride 0.5 mg, vitamins A 2500 IU, D 400 IU, E 15 mg, B_1 1 mg, B_2 1.2 mg, B_3 13.5 mg, B_6 1 mg, B_{12} 4.5 mcg, C 60 mg, folic acid 0.3 mg/Tab. Bot. 100s, 1000s. *Rx.*
Use: Vitamin/mineral supplement, dental caries preventative.

poly-vitamins w/fluoride tablets chewable. (Various Mfr.) Fluoride 1 mg, vitamins A 2500 IU, D 400 IU, E 15 mg, B_1 1.05 mg, B_2 1.2 mg, B_3 13.5 mg, B_6 1.05 mg, B_{12} 4.5 mcg, C 60 mg, folic acid 0.3 mg. Bot. 100s, 1000s. *Rx.*
Use: Vitamin/mineral supplement, dental caries preventative.

Polyvitamin Fluoride w/Iron. (Various Mfr.) Fluoride 1 mg, vitamins A 2500 IU, D 400 IU, E 15 mg, B_1 1.05 mg, B_2 1.2 mg, B_3 13.5 mg, B_6 1.05 mg, B_{12}

4.5 mcg, C 60 mg, folic acid 0.3 mg, iron 12 mg, Cu, zinc 10 mg/Tab. Bot. 100s, 1000s. *Rx.*
Use: Vitamin/mineral supplement, dental caries preventative.

Polyvitamin w/Fluoride. (Rugby) Fluoride 0.5 mg, vitamins A 1500 IU, D 400 IU, E 5 mg, B_1 0.5 mg, B_2 0.6 mg, B_3 8 mg, B_6 0.4 mg, B_{12} 2 mcg, C 35 mg/ml. Dropper bot. 50 ml. *Rx.*
Use: Vitamin/mineral supplement, dental caries preventative.

polyvitamins w/fluoride 0.5 mg and iron. (Rugby) Fluoride 0.5 mg, vitamins A 2500 IU, D 400 IU, E 15 IU, B_1 1.05 mg, B_2 1.2 mg, B_3 13.5 mg, B_6 1.05 mg, B_{12} 4.5 mcg, C 60 mg, folic acid 0.3 mg, Cu, iron 12 mg, zinc 10 mg, sucrose/Tab. Bot. 100s. *Rx.*
Use: Vitamin/mineral supplement; dental caries preventative.

Polyvite with Fluoride. (Geneva Generics) Fluoride 0.25 mg, vitamins A 1500 IU, D 400 IU, E 5 mg, B_1 0.5 mg, B_2 0.6 mg, B_3 8 mg, B_6 0.4 mg, B_{12} 2 mcg, C 35 mg/ml. Dropper bot. 50 ml. *Rx.*
Use: Vitamin/mineral supplement, dental caries preventative.

•**ponalrestat.** (poe-NAHL-ress-TAT) USAN.
Use: Aldose reductase inhibitor.

Ponaris. (Jamol) Nasal emollient of mucosal lubricating and moisturizing botanical oils. Cajeput, eucalyptus, peppermint in iodized cottonseed oil. Bot. 1 oz w/dropper. *otc.*
Use: Nasal moisturizer.

Pondimin. (Robins) Fenfluramine HCl 20 mg/Tab. Bot. 100s, 500s. *c-iv.*
Use: Anorexiant.

Ponstel Kapseals. (Parke-Davis) Mefenamic acid 250 mg/Cap. Bot. 100s. *Rx.*
Use: Nonsteroidal anti-inflammatory, analgesic.

Pontocaine. (Sanofi Winthrop) **Cream:** Tetracaine HCl 1%, glycerin, light mineral oil, methylparaben, sodium metabisulfite. Tube 28.35 g. **Oint.:** Tetracaine 0.5%, menthol, white petrolatum. Tube 28.35 g. *otc.*
Use: Topical anesthetic.

Pontocaine Hydrochloride. (Sanofi Winthrop) Tetracaine HCl. **Inj. 0.2%:** Dextrose 6%. Amp 2 ml. **0.3%:** Dextrose 6%. Amp 5 ml. **1%:** Acetone sodium bisulfite. Amp 2 ml. **Powd. for reconstitution:** Niphanoid (instantly soluble) amps 20 mg. *Rx.*
Use: Local anesthetic.

Pontocaine Hydrochloride 0.5% Solution for Ophthalmology. (Sanofi Winthrop) Tetracaine HCl 0.5%. Bot. 15 ml, 59 ml. *Rx.*
Use: Local anesthetic.

Pontocaine Hydrochloride in Dextrose (Hyperbaric). (Sanofi Winthrop) **0.2%:** Tetracaine HCl 2 mg/ml in a sterile solution containing dextrose 6%. Amp. 2 ml, 10s. **0.3%:** Tetracaine HCl 3 mg/ml in a sterile solution containing dextrose 6%. Amp. 5 ml, 10s. *Rx.*
Use: Local anesthetic.

Pontocaine Ointment. (Sanofi Winthrop) Tetracaine 0.5% and menthol in an ointment consisting of white petrolatum and white wax. Tube 1 oz. *Rx.*
Use: Local anesthetic.

Pontocaine 2% Aqueous Solution. (Sanofi Winthrop) Tetracaine HCl 20 mg, chlorobutanol 4 mg/ml of 2% soln. Bot. 30 ml, Box 12s. Bot. 118 ml, Box 6s. *Rx.*
Use: Local anesthetic. ,

Po-Pon-S. (Shionogi) Vitamins A 2000 IU, D 100 IU, E 5 mg, B_1 5 mg, B_2 3 mg, B_3 35 mg, B_5 15 mg, B_6 4 mg, B_{12} 6 mcg, C 100 mg, Ca, P/Tab. Bot. 60s, 240s. *otc.*
Use: Vitamin/mineral supplement.

poppy-seed oil, The ethyl ester of the fatty acids of the poppy w/iodine.
See: Lipiodol, Ascendant & Lafay, Amps., Vial (Savage).

Porcelana Skin Bleaching Agent. (DEP Corp.) **Regular:** Hydroquinone 2%. Jar 2 oz, 4 oz. **Sunscreen:** Hydroquinone 2%, octyl dimethyl PABA 2.5%. Jar 4 oz. *Rx.*
Use: Skin bleaching agent.

porcine islet preparation, encapsulated.
Use: For Type I diabetic patients already on immunosuppression. [Orphan drug]

•**porfimer sodium.** USAN.
Use: Antineoplastic. [Orphan drug]
See: Photofrin, Inj. (QLT Photo).

•**porfiromycin.** (par-FIH-row-MY-sin) USAN.
Use: Antibacterial, antineoplastic.

Pork NPH Iletin II. (Lilly) Purified pork insulin 100 units/ml in isophane insulin suspension (insulin w/ protamine and zinc). Inj. Bot. 10 ml.
Use: Antidiabetic.

Pork Regular Iletin II. (Lilly) Insulin 100 units/ml. Purified pork. Inj. Vial 10 ml.
Use: Antidiabetic.

pork thyroid, defatted.
See: Tuloidin, Tab. (Solvay).

•**porofocon a.** (PAR-oh-FOE-kahn A) USAN.
Use: Contact lens material (hydrophobic).

•**porofocon b.** (PAR-oh-FOE-kahn B) USAN.
Use: Contact lens material (hydrophobic).

Portabiday. (Washington Ethical) Concentrated soln. of alkylamine lauryl sulfate, a mild detergent with pH approx. 6 for use with Portabiday Vaginal Cleansing Kit. Bot. 3 oz. *otc.*
Use: Vaginal preparation.

Portagen. (Bristol-Myers) A nutritionally complete dietary powder containing as a % of the calories protein 14% as caseinate, fat 41% (medium chain triglycerides 86%, corn oil 14%), carbohydrate 45% as corn syrup solids and sucrose, vitamins A 5000 IU, D 500 IU, E 20 IU, C 52 mg, B_1 1 mg, B_2 1.2 mg, B_6 1.4 mg, B_{12} 4 mcg, niacin 13 mg, folic acid 0.1 mg, choline 83 mg, biotin 0.05 mg, calcium 600 mg, phosphorus 450 mg, magnesium 133 mg, iron 12 mg, iodine 47 mcg, copper 1 mg, zinc 6 mg, manganese 0.8 mg, chloride 550 mg, sodium 300 mg, potassium 800 mg, pantothenic acid 6.7 mg, K-1 0.1 mg/ Qt. 20 Kcal/fl oz. Can 1 lb. *otc.*
Use: Enteral nutritional supplement.

porton asparaginase.
See: Erwinia asparaginase.

positive and negative hcg urine controls. (Wampole) Positive and negative human urine controls for Wampole urine pregnancy tests. 1 set, 1 vial each.
Use: Diagnostic aid.

Poslam Psoriasis Ointment. (Last) Sulfur 5%, salicylic acid 2%. Jar 1 oz.
Use: Antipsoriatic.

postafene.
See: Bonamine, Tab. (Pfizer).

posterior pituitary hormones.
See: Pituitrin (S) (Parke-Davis).
Pitressin Synthetic (Parke-Davis).
Pitressin Tannate in Oil (Parke-Davis).
Diapid (Sandoz).
Concentraid (Ferring Labs).
DDAVP (Rhone-Poulenc Rorer).

posterior pituitary injection.
Use: Hormone (antidiuretic).

postlobin-o.
See: Pituitary, Posterior, Hormone (b).

postlobin-v.

See: Pituitary, Posterior, Hormone (a).

Posture. (Wyeth-Ayerst) Calcium phosphate 300 mg or 600 mg/Tab. Bot. 60s. *otc.*
Use: Calcium supplement.

Posture D 600. (Wyeth-Ayerst) Calcium phosphate 600 mg, vitamin D 125 IU/Tab. Bot. 60s. *otc.*
Use: Calcium/mineral supplement.

Potaba. (Glenwood) Potassium p-aminobenzoate. **Cap.:** 0.5 g. Bot. 250s, 1000s. **Pow.:** 100 g. 1 lb. **Tab.:** 0.5 g. Bot. 100s, 1000s. **Envule:** 2 g. Box 50s. *Rx.*
Use: Para-aminobenzoic acid supplement.

Potable Aqua Kit. (Wisconsin) Tetraglycine hydroperiodide 16.7% (6.68% titrable iodine). Tab. Bot. 50s with collapsible gallon container. *otc.*
Use: Water purification.

Potachlor 10%. (Rosemont) Potassium and chloride 20 mEq/15 ml. With alcohol 5%. Bot. pt, gal. With alcohol 3.8%. Bot. pt, gal, UD 15 ml and 30 ml. *Rx.*
Use: Potassium supplement.

Potachlor 20%. (Rosemont) Potassium and chloride 40 mEq/15 ml, alcohol free. Liq. Bot. pt, gal. *Rx.*
Use: Potassium supplement.

•**potash, sulfurated,** U.S.P. 23.
Use: Source of sulfide.

potassic saline lactated injection.
Use: Fluid and electrolyte replenisher.

•**potassium acetate,** U.S.P. 23. Acetic acid, potassium salt.
Use: Electrolyte replenisher; to avoid Cl when high concentration of potassium is needed.

potassium acetate. (Various Mfr.) **Inj.:**40 mEq, 20 ml in 50 ml Vial.
Use: Electrolyte replenisher; to avoid Cl when high concentration of potassium is needed.

potassium acid phosphate.
See: K-Phos, Tab. (Beach).
Uro-K, Tab. (Star).

potassium acid phosphate/sodium acid phosphate.
Use: Urinary tract product.
See: K-Phos M.F. (Beach).
K-Phos No. 2 (Beach.

•**potassium aspartate and magnesium aspartate.** (poe-TASS-ee-uhm ass-PAR-tates and mag-NEE-zee-uhm ass-PAR-tate) USAN.
Use: Nutrient.

•**potassium benzoate,** N.F. 18.
Use: Pharmaceutic aid (preservative).

•**potassium bicarbonate,** U.S.P. 23.
Use: Pharmaceutic necessity; electrolyte replenisher.

potassium bicarbonate effervescent tablets for oral solution.
Use: Potassium supplement.

potassium bicarbonate and potassium chloride for effervescent oral solution.
Use: Potassium supplement.

potassium bicarbonate and potassium chloride effervescent tablets for oral solution.
Use: Potassium supplement.

potassium bicarbonate and sodium bicarbonate and citric acid effervescent tablets for oral solution.
Use: Potassium supplement.

•**potassium bitartrate,** U.S.P. 23.
Use: Cathartic.

•**potassium carbonate,** U.S.P. 23.
Use: Potassium therapy; pharmaceutic aid (alkalizing agent).

•**potassium chloride,** U.S.P. 23.
Use: Electrolyte replenisher, potassium deficiency, hypopotassemia.

potassium chloride. (Abbott) **Ampules:** 20 mEq, 10 ml; 40 mEq, 20 ml. **Pintop Vials:** 10 mEq, 5 ml in 10 ml; 20 mEq, 10 ml in 20 ml; 30 mEq, 12.5 ml in 30 ml; 40 mEq, 12.5 ml in 30 ml. **Flip-top Vials:** 20 mEq, 10 ml in 20 ml; 40 mEq, 20 ml in 50 ml. **Univ. Add. Syr.:** 5 mEq/5 ml, 20 mEq/10 ml, 30 mEq/20 ml, 40 mEq/20 ml (Lilly) Amp. (40 mEq) 20 ml, 6s, 25s.
Capsules:
See: K-Norm, Cap. (Medeva). Micro-K Extencaps, Cap. (Robins). **Liquid:**
See: Cena-K, Liq. (Century). Choice 10 and 20, Soln. (Whiteworth Towne). Kaochlor, Preps. (Pharmacia & Upjohn).
Kaon-C1 20%, Liq. (Pharmacia & Upjohn).
Kay Ciel, Elix. (Berlex).
Klor-Con, Liq. (Upsher-Smith).
Klotrix, Tab. (Bristol-Myers).
Klowess (Sandoz).
K-Lyte/C1, Tab. (Bristol-Myers).
Pan-Kloride, Liq. (U.S. Products).
Potassine, Liq. (Recsei).
Taside, Liq. (Solvay).
Powder:
See: Kaochlor-Eff, Gran. (Pharmacia & Upjohn).
Kato, Pow. (Ingram).
Kay Ciel, Pow. (Berlex).
K-Lor, Pow. (Abbott).
K-Lyte/Cl, Pow. (Bristol-Myers).

Potage, Pow. (Lemmon).
Tablets:
See: K+8, ER Tab. (Alra).
Kaon, Tab. (Pharmacia & Upjohn).
Kaon Controlled Release Tab. (Pharmacia & Upjohn).
Klorvess Effervescent Tab. (Sandoz).
K-Lyte/Cl 50, Tab. (Bristol-Myers).
K-Tab, Tab. (Abbott).
Micro-K Extencap (Robins).
Slow-K, Tab. (Novartis).
Ten-K, Cap. (Novartis).

potassium chloride. (Roxane) **Oral soln.:** Potassium Cl, sugar free. 40 mEq/30 ml. Bot. 6 oz, 500 ml, 1 L, 5 L 20%. 80 mEq/30 ml. Bot. 500 ml, 1 L, 5 L. **Pow.:** 20 mEq/4 g. Pkt. 30s, 100s. *Rx.*
Use: Potassium supplement.

potassium chloride in dextrose and sodium chloride injection.
Use: Potassium supplement.

potassium chloride in lactated ringer's and dextrose injection.
Use: Potassium supplement.

potassium chloride in sodium chloride injection.
Use: Potassium supplement.

•**potassium chloride K 42.** USAN.
Use: Radioactive agent.

potassium chloride with potassium gluconate.
See: Kolyum, Prods. (Medeva).

potassium chloride, potassium bicarbonate, and potassium citrate effervescent tablets for oral solution.

potassium chloride solution, (Lederle) Potassium Cl 10% or 20%. Sugar free. Bot. 16 oz, gal. *Rx.*
Use: Potassium supplement.

•**potassium citrate,** U.S.P. 23. Tripotassium Citrate.
Use: Alkalizer. [Orphan drug]
See: Urocit-K, Tab. (Mission).
W/Sodium citrate.
See: Bicitra, Liq. (Baker Norton).
W/Sodium citrate, citric acid.
See: Polycitra-K, Crystals, Liq. (Baker Norton).
Polycitra-LC, Liq. (Baker Norton).

potassium citrate and citric acid oral solution.
Use: Systemic alkalizer.

potassium clavulanate/amoxicillin.
Use: Anti-infective, penicillin.
See: Amoxicillin and Potassium Clavulanate.

potassium clavulanate/ticarcillin.
Use: Anti-infective, penicillin.

See: Ticarcillin and Clavulanate Potassium.

potassium estrone sulfate.
W/Micro crystalline estrone.
See: Estrones Duo-Action, Vial (Med. Chem.).

•**potassium glucaldrate.** (poe-TASS-ee-uhm glue-KAL-drate) USAN.
Use: Antacid.

•**potassium gluconate,** U.S.P. 23.
Use: Electrolyte replenisher.
See: Kalinate, Elix. (Bock).
Kaon, Elixir, Tab. (Warren-Teed).

potassium gluconate and potassium chloride oral solution.
Use: Replacement therapy.

potassium gluconate and potassium chloride for oral solution.
Use: Replacement therapy.

potassium gluconate elixir. (Various Mfr.) Potassium 40 mEq provided by potassium gluconate 9.36 g/30 ml, alcohol 5%. Bot. pt, Patient-Cup 15 ml. *Rx.*
Use: Potassium supplement.

potassium gluconate, potassium citrate, and ammonium chloride oral solution.
Use: Potassium supplement.

potassium gluconate and potassium citrate oral solution.
Use: Potassium supplement.

potassium glutamate. The monopotassium salt of l-glutamic acid.

potassium G penicillin.
See: Penicillin G Potassium, U.S.P. 23.

•**potassium guaiacolsulfonate,** U.S.P. 23. Sulfoguaiacol. Potassium Hydroxymethoxybenzenesulfonate. Used in many cough preps.
Use: Expectorant.
See: Conex, Liq. (Westerfield).
Pinex Regular, Syr. (Pinex).

potassium guaiacolsulfonate w/combinations.
See: Cherralex, Syr. (Barre).
Guahist, Vial (Hickam).
Partuss, Liq. (Parmed).
Tusquelin, Syr. (Circle).

potassium hetacillin.
See: Versapen K, Inj., Cap. (Bristol-Myers).

•**potassium hydroxide,** N.F. 18.
Use: Pharmaceutic aid (alkalinizing agent).

potassium in sodium chloride. (Various Mfr.) Potassium Cl 0.15%, 0.22% or 0.3% in sodium Cl 0.9%. Soln. for Inj. 1000 ml. *Rx.*
Use: Intravenous replenishment solu-

tion, nutritional therapy.

•**potassium iodide,** U.S.P. 23.
Use: Expectorant, antifungal, supplement (iodine).
See: Pima, Syr., Expectorant (Fleming).
SSKI, Liq. (Upsher-Smith).

potassium iodide w/combinations.
See: Diastix, Reagent Strips (Bayer).
Elixophyllin-KI, Elix. (Berlex).
Iodo-Niacin, Tab. (Cole).
KIE, Syr., Tab. (Laser).
Mudrane, Tab. (ECR Pharm).
Mudrane-2, Tab. (ECR Pharm).
Quadrinal, Tab., Susp. (Knoll).

potassium iodide and niacinamide.
See: Iodo-Niacin, Tab. (Cole).

•**potassium metabisulfite,** N.F. 18.
Use: Pharmaceutic aid (antioxidant).

•**potassium metaphosphate,** N.F. 18.
Use: Pharmaceutic aid (buffering agent).

•**potassium nitrate,** U.S.P. 23.

potassium p-aminobenzoate.
See: Potaba, Preps. (Glenwood).
W/Potassium salicylate.
See: Pabalate-SF, Tab. (Robins).
W/Pyridoxine.
See: Potaba Plus 6, Cap., Tab. (Glenwood).

potassium p-aminosalicylate.
See: Paskalium, Preps. (Glenwood).

potassium penicillin G.
Use: Anti-infective, penicillin.
See: Penicillin G, Potassium U.S.P. 23.

potassium penicillin V.
Use: Anti-infective, penicillin.
See: Phenoxymethyl Penicillin Potassium, U.S.P. 23.

potassium perchlorate.
Use: Radiopaque agent.
See: Perchloracap (Mallinckrodt).

potassium phenethicillin. Phenethicillin Potassium, U.S.P. 23.
Use: Anti-infective.

potassium phenoxymethyl penicillin.
Use: Antibiotic.
See: Penicillin V Potassium, U.S.P. 23.

•**potassium phosphate, dibasic,** U.S.P. 23.
Use: Calcium regulator.

•**potassium phosphate, monobasic,** N.F. 18. Dipotassium hydrogen phosphate.
Use: Pharmaceutic aid (buffering agent), source of potassium.

potassium phosphate, monobasic.
(Abbott) 15 mM, 5 ml in 10 ml Vial; 45 mM, 15 ml in 20 ml/Inj. Vial.
Use: Pharmaceutic aid (buffering agent), source of potassium.

potassium reagent strips. (Bayer) Quantitative dry reagent strip test for potassium in serum or plasma. Bot. 50s.
Use: Diagnostic aid.

potassium-removing resins.
See: Sodium Polystyrene Sulfonate (Various Mfr.).
SPS (Carolina Medical Products Co.).
Kayexalate (Sanofi Winthrop.)

potassium rhodanate.
See: Potassium Thiocyanate.

potassium salicylate.
See: Neocylate, Tab. (Schwarz Pharma).
W/Mephenesin, colchicine alkaloid.
W/Potassium bromide, methapyrilene HCl, vitamins.
See: Alva-Tranquil, Cap., Tab., T.D. Tab. (Alva/Amco).
W/Potassium p-aminobenzoate.
See: Pabalate-SF, Tab. (Robins).

potassium salt.
See: Potassium Sorbate, N.F. 18.

•**potassium sodium tartrate,** U.S.P. 23.
Use: Laxative.

•**potassium sorbate,** N.F. 18.
Use: Pharmaceutic aid (antimicrobial).

potassium sulfocyanate. Potassium Rhodanate.
See: Potassium Thiocyanate (Various Mfr.).

potassium thiocyanate. Potassium sulfocyanate, Potassium Rhodanate.

potassium thiphencillin. (poe-TASS-ee-uhm thigh-FEN-sill-in)
Use: Anti-infective.

potassium troclosene. (poe-TASS-ee-uhm TROE-kloe-seen) (Monsanto) Potassium dichloroisocyanurate.
Use: Anti-infective.

•**povidone,** (POE-vih-dohn) U.S.P. 23.
Formerly Polyvidone, Polyvinylpyrrolidone.
Use: Pharmaceutic aid (dispersing and suspending agent).

•**povidone I 125.** (POE-vih-dohn) USAN.
Use: Radioactive agent.

•**povidone I 131.** (POE-vih-dohn) USAN.
Use: Radioactive agent.

•**povidone-iodine,** (POE-vih-dohn-EYE-uh-dine) U.S.P. 23.
Use: Anti-infective, topical.
See: Betadine, Preps. (Purdue-Fredrick).

Efo-Dine (Fougera).
Isodine, Preps. (Blair).
Massengill Medicated, Liq. (SK-
Beecham).
povidone-iodine complex.
See: Betadine, Preps. (Purdue-Freder-
ick).
Isodine, Preps. (Blair).
PowerMate. (Green Turtle Bay) Vitamins
A 5000 IU, E 100 IU, B_3 12.5 mg, C 250
mg, zinc 2.5 mg, Se, n-acetyl-L-cys-
teine/Tab. Bot. 50s. otc.
Use: Vitamin/mineral supplement.
PowerVites. (Green Turtle Bay) Vitamin
A 2500 IU, D 150 IU, E 12.5 IU, C 125
mg, B_1 6.3 mg, B_2 6.3 mg, B_3 25 mg,
B_5 25 mg, B_6 12.5 mg, B_{12} 6.3 mcg, bio-
tin, folic acid 0.15 mg, B, Ca, Mg, Cu,
Zn 2.5 mg, Cr, Mn, K, Se, betaine, hes-
peridin/Tab. Bot. 40s, 100s, 200s. otc.
Use: Vitamin/mineral supplement.
Poyaliver Stronger. (Forest Pharm) Liver
inj. (equivalent to 10 mcg B_{12}), vitamin
B_{12} 100 mcg, folic acid 10 mcg, niac-
inamide 1%/ml. Vial 10 ml. Rx.
Use: Parenteral nutritional supplement.
Poyamin Jel Injection. (Forest Pharm)
Cyanocobalamin 1000 mcg/ml. Vial 10
ml.
Use: Parenteral nutritional supplement.
Poyaplex. (Forest Pharm) Vitamins B_1
100 mg, niacinamide 100 mg, B_6 10
mg, B_2 1 mg, panthenol 10 mg, B_{12} 5
mcg/ml. Vial 10 ml, 30 ml. Rx.
Use: Parenteral nutritional supplement.
P.P.D. tuberculin.
See: Tuberculin, Purified Protein De-
rivative, U.S.P. (Various Mfr.).
P.P. factor (pellagra preventive factor).
See: Nicotinic Acid, Preps. (Various
Mfr.)
ppg-15 stearyl ether. (PPG-15 STEE-rill
EE-ther)
Use: Pharmaceutic aid (surfactant).
PPI-002. Rx.
Use: Malignant mesothelioma. [Orphan
drug]
PR-122 (redox-phenytoin). (Pharmatec)
Rx.
Use: Anticonvulsant. [Orphan drug]
PR-225 (redox-acyclovir). (Pharmatec)
Rx.
Use: Treatment of Herpes simplex en-
cephalitis in AIDS. [Orphan drug]
PR-239 (redox-penicillin g). (Phar-
matec) Rx.
Use: Treatment of AIDS-associated
neurosyphilis. [Orphan drug]
PR-320 (molecusol-carbamazepine).

(Pharmatec) Rx.
Use: Anticonvulsant. [Orphan drug]
•**practolol.** (PRAK-toe-lole) USAN.
Use: Antiadrenergic (β-receptor).
•**pralidoxime chloride.** (pra-lih-DOCK-
seem) U.S.P. 23.
Use: Cholinesterase reactivator.
See: Protopam Chloride, Tab., Inj. (Wyeth-Ayerst).
pralidoxime chloride. (Survival Technology) 600 mg. Benzyl alcohol, aminocaproic acid. Inj. Vial 2 ml. Rx.
Use: Antidote.
•**pralidoxime iodide.** USAN.
Use: Cholinesterase reactivator.
See: Protopam Iodide (Wyeth-Ayerst).
•**pralidoxime mesylate.** (pral-ih-DOX-
eem) USAN.
Use: Cholinesterase reactivator.
pralidoxime methiodide.
See: Pralidoxime Iodide (Various Mfr.).
Pramegel. (GenDerm) Pramoxine HCl
1%, menthol 0.5% in base w/benzyl
alcohol. Gel. Bot. 118 g. otc.
Use: Local anesthetic, topical.
Pramilet FA. (Ross) Vitamins A 4000 IU,
B_1 3 mg, B_2 2 mg, B_6 3 mg, B_{12} 3 mcg,
C 60 mg, D 400 IU, B_5 1 mg, B_3 10
mg, calcium 250 mg, Cu, I, iron 40 mg,
Mg, zinc, folic acid 1 mg/Filmtab. Bot.
100s. Rx.
Use: Vitamin/mineral supplement.
•**pramipexole.** (pram-ih-PEX-ole) USAN.
(Pharmacia & Upjohn).
Use: Antiparkinsonian, antischizophrenic, antidepressant (dopamine
agonist).
•**pramiracetam hydrochloride.** (PRAM-
ih-RASS-eh-tam) USAN. Formerly Am-
acetam Hydrochloride.
Use: Cognition adjuvant.
•**pramiracetam sulfate.** (PRAM-ih-RASS-
eh-tam) USAN. Formerly Amacetam
Sulfate.
Use: Cognition adjuvant.
•**pramlintide.** USAN.
Use: Antidiabetic.
Pramosone Cream 0.5%. (Ferndale)
Hydrocortisone acetate 0.5%, pramox-
ine HCl 1% in cream base. Tube 1 oz,
4 oz. Jar 4 oz, lb.
Use: Corticosteroid, local anesthetic.
Pramosone Cream 1%. (Ferndale)
Hydrocortisone acetate 1%, pramoxine
HCl 1% in cream base. Tube 1 oz, 4
oz. Jar 4 oz, lb. Rx.
Use: Corticosteroid, local anesthetic,
topical.
Pramosone Cream 2.5%. (Ferndale)

Hydrocortisone acetate 2.5%, pramoxine HCl 1% in cream base. Tube 1 oz, 4 oz. Jar lb. *Rx.*
Use: Corticosteroid, local anesthetic, topical.

Pramosone Lotion 0.5%. (Ferndale) Hydrocortisone acetate 0.5%, pramoxine HCl 1% in lotion base. Bot. 1 oz, 4 oz, 8 oz. *Rx.*
Use: Corticosteroid, local anesthetic, topical.

Pramosone Lotion 1%. (Ferndale) Hydrocortisone acetate 1%, pramoxine HCl 1% in lotion base. Bot. 2 oz, 4 oz, 8 oz. *Rx.*
Use: Corticosteroid, local anesthetic, topical.

Pramosone Lotion 2.5%. (Ferndale) Hydrocortisone acetate 2.5%, pramoxine HCl 1% in lotion base. Bot 2 oz, gal. *Rx.*
Use: Corticosteroid, local anesthetic, topical.

Pramosone Ointment 1%. (Ferndale) Hydrocortisone acetate 1%, pramoxine HCl 1% in ointment base. Tube 1 oz, 4 oz. Jar 4 oz, lb. *Rx.*
Use: Corticosteroid, local anesthetic, topical.

Pramoxine HC. (Rugby) Pramoxine HCl 1%, hydrocortisone acetate 1%. Aerosol foam. 10 g w/applicator. *Rx.*
Use: Anorectal preparation.

•**pramoxine hydrochloride,** U.S.P. 23.
Use: Anesthetic, topical.
See: Itch-X, Gel, Spray (B. F. Ascher & Co.).
Prax, Cream, Lot. (Ferndale).
Proctofoam, Aerosol (Reed & Carnrick).
Tronothane HCl, Cream, Jel (Abbott).

pramoxine hydrochloride w/combinations.
See: Anti-Itch, Lot. (Towne).
Dermarex, Cream (Hyrex).
Gentz, Jelly, Wipes (Philips Roxane).
1 + 1 Creme (Dunhall).
1 + 1-F Creme (Dunhall).
Otocalm-H Ear Drops (Parmed).
Perifoam, Aerosol (Rowell Labs.).
Proctofoam-HC, Aerosol (Reed-Carnrick).
Sherform-HC, Oint. (Sheryl).
Steraform Creme (Mayrand).
Steramine Otic, Drops (Mayrand).

•**pranolium chloride.** (pray-NO-lee-uhm) USAN.
Use: Cardiac depressant (antiarrhythmic).

Pravachol. (Bristol-Myers) Pravastatin sodium **10 mg or 20 mg:** Tab. Bot. 100s, UD 100s; **40 mg:** Tab. Bot. 100s. *Rx.*
Use: Antihyperlipidemic.

•**pravadoline maleate.** (pray-AH-doe-leen) USAN.
Use: Analgesic.

•**pravastatin sodium.** (PRUH-vuh-stuh-tin) USAN.
Use: Antihyperlipidemic.
See: Pravachol (Bristol-Myers).

Prax. (Ferndale) Pramoxine HCl 1%.
Cream: Glycerin, cetyl alcohol, white petrolatum. Jar 13.4 g. **Lot.:** Potassium sorbate, sorbic acid, mineral oil, cetyl alcohol, glycerin, lanolin. Bot. 15 ml, 120 ml, 240 ml. *otc.*
Use: Topical anesthetic.

•**prazepam,** (PRAY-zeh-pam) U.S.P. 23.
Use: Sedative, hypnotic.

prazepam. (Various Mfr.) **Cap.:** 5 mg or 10 mg. Bot. 100s, 500s. **Tab.:** 5 mg or 10 mg. Bot. 100s, 500s. *c-iv.*
Use: Sedative, hypnotic.

•**prazosin hydrochloride,** (PRAY-zoe-sin) U.S.P. 23.
Use: Antihypertensive.
See: Minipress, Cap. (Pfizer Laboratories).

prazosin hydrochloride. (Various Mfr.) 1 mg, 2 mg, 5 mg. Cap. Bot. 30s, 60s, 90s, 100s, 120s, 250s, 500s, 1000s, UD 100s.
Use: Antihypertensive.

Pre-Attain Liquid. (Sherwood) Sodium caseinate, maltodextrin, corn oil, soy lecithin, vitamins A, B_1, B_2, B_3, B_5, B_6, B_{12}, C, D, E, K, folic acid, Ca, Cl, Cu, Fe, I, Mg, Mn, P, Zn. Can 250 ml, closed system 1000 ml. *otc.*
Use: Nutritional supplement.

Precef for Injection. (Bristol-Myers) Ceforanide 500 mg or 1 g/Vial or piggyback. *Rx.*
Use: Anti-infective, cephalosporin.

Precision High Nitrogen Diet. (Sandoz Nutrition) Vanilla flavor: Maltodextrin, pasteurized egg white solids, sucrose, natural and artificial flavors, medium chain triglycerides, partially hydrogenated soybean oil, polysorbate 80, mono and diglycerides, vitamins, minerals. Pow. Packet 2.93 oz. *otc.*
Use: Nutritional supplement.

Precision LR Diet. (Sandoz Nutrition) Orange flavor: Maltodextrin, pasteurized egg white solids, sucrose, medium chain triglycerides, partially hydroge-

nated soybean oil with BHA, citric acid, natural and artificial flavors, mono- and diglycerides, polysorbate 80, FD & C Yellow No. 5 and No. 6, vitamins, minerals. Pow. Packet 3 oz. *otc.*
Use: Nutritional supplement.

Precose. (Bayer) Acarbose 50 mg or 100 mg/Tab. Bot. 100s, UD 100s. *Rx.*
Use: Treatment for hyperglycemia.

Predaject-50. (Mayrand) Prednisolone acetate 50 mg/ml. Vial 10 ml. *Rx.*
Use: Corticosteroid.

Predalone 50. (Forest) Prednisolone acetate 50 mg/ml. Vial 10 ml. *Rx.*
Use: Corticosteroid.

Predamide Ophthalmic. (Maurry) Sodium sulfacetamide 10%, prednisolone acetate 0.5%, hydroxyethyl cellulose, polysorbate 80, sodium thiosulfate, benzalkonium Cl 0.025%. Bot. 5 ml, 15 ml. *Rx.*
Use: Anti-infective, corticosteroid, ophthalmic.

Predcor-50 Injection. (Roberts) Prednisolone acetate 50 mg/ml. Vial 10 ml. *Rx.*
Use: Corticosteroid.

Pred-Forte. (Allergan) Prednisolone acetate 1%. Susp. Bot. 1 ml, 5 ml, 10 ml, 15 ml. *Rx.*
Use: Corticosteroid, ophthalmic.

Pred-G. (Allergan) Prednisolone acetate 1%, gentamicin sulfate 0.3%. Bot. 2 ml, 5 ml, 10 ml. *Rx.*
Use: Corticosteroid, anti-infective, ophthalmic.

Pred-G S.O.P. (Allergan) Prednisolone acetate 0.6%, gentamicin sulfate 0.3%, chlorobutanol 0.5%. Oint. Tube 3.5 g. *Rx.*
Use: Antibiotic, corticosteroid, ophthalmic.

Predicort-AP. (Dunhall) Prednisolone sodium phosphate 20 mg, prednisolone acetate 80 mg/ml. Vial 10 ml. *Rx.*
Use: Corticosteroid.

Predicort-RP. (Dunhall) Prednisolone sodium phosphate equivalent to prednisolone phosphate 20 mg, niacinamide 25 mg/ml. Vial 10 ml. *Rx.*
Use: Corticosteroid.

Pred Mild. (Allergan) Prednisolone acetate 0.12%. Susp. Bot. 5 ml, 10 ml. *Rx.*
Use: Corticosteroid, ophthalmic.

•**prednazate.** (PRED-nah-zate) USAN.
Use: Anti-inflammatory.

•**prednicarbate.** (PRED-nih-CAR-bate) USAN.
Use: Glucocorticoid.

See: Dermatop, Cream (Hoechst Marion Roussel).

Prednicen-M. (Schwarz Pharma) Prednisone 5 mg/Tab. Bot. 100s, 1000s. *Rx.*
Use: Corticosteroid.

•**prednimustine.** (PRED-nih-MUSS-teen) USAN.
Use: Antineoplastic. [Orphan drug]

•**prednisolone,** (pred-NISS-oh-lone) U.S.P. 23. Metacortandralone.
Use: Glucocorticoid.
See: Cordrol, Tab. (Vita Elixir).
Delta-Cortef, Tab. (Pharmacia & Upjohn).
Fernisolone, Tab., Inj. (Ferndale).
Orasone, Tab. (Solvay).
Orasone 50, Tab. (Solvay).
Prednis, Tab. (Rhone-Poulenc Rorer).
W/Aluminum hydroxide gel, dried.
See: Predoxide, Tab. (Roberts).
W/Aspirin.
See: Sarogesic, Tab. (Saron).
W/Chloramphenicol.
See: Chloroptic-P, Ophthalmic Oint. (Allergan).
W/Neomycin sulfate.
Neo-Deltef, Drops (Pharmacia & Upjohn).
W/Sulfacetamide sodium, methylcellulose.
See: Isopto Cetapred, Susp. (Alcon).
W/Sulfacetamide sodium.
See: Cetapred Ophthalmic Oint. (Alcon).

•**prednisolone acetate,** U.S.P. 23.
Use: Glucocorticoid.
See: Econopred, Susp. (Alcon).
Key-Pred, Inj. (Hyrex).
Nisolone, Vial (Ascher).
Predicort, Amp. (Dunhall).
Pred, Preps. (Allergan).
Pred-Forte, Ophthalmic Susp. (Allergan).
Savacort-50, 100, Vial (Savage).
Sigpred, Inj. (Sig).
Steraject, Vial (Mayrand).
Sterane, Inj. (Pfizer Laboratories).

prednisolone acetate. (Various Mfr.) 1% Susp. Bot. 5 ml, 10 ml.
Use: Glucocorticoid.

prednisolone acetate w/combinations.
See: Blephamide Liquifilm, Soln. (Allergan).
Blephamide S.O.P., Ophthalmic, Oint. (Allergan).
Cetapred Opthalmic Oint. (Alcon).
Dua-Pred, Inj. (Solvay).
Isopto Cetapred Susp. (Alcon).
Metimyd, Ophthalmic Susp., Oint. (Schering-Plough).

Neo-Delta-Cortef, Preps. (Pharmacia & Upjohn).
Panacort R-P, Vial (Ferndale).
Prednefrin, Mild, Susp. (Allergan).
Sulphrin Ophth. Oint. (Bausch & Lomb).
Tri-Ophtho, Ophthalmic (Maurry).
Vasocidin, Preps. (Novartis).

prednisolone acetate and prednisolone sodium phosphate. (Various Mfr.) Prednisolone acetate 80 mg, prednisolone sodium phosphate 20 mg/ml. Inj. Susp. Vial 10 ml. *Rx.*
Use: Corticosteroid.

prednisolone acetate ophthalmic suspension.
See: Prednisolone Acetate.

prednisolone butylacetate. 1,4-Pregnadiene-3,20-dione-11β,17α,21-triol-tert-butyl-acetate.
Use: Corticosteroid.
See: Hydeltra-T.B.A., Vial (Merck).

prednisolone cyclopentylpropionate.
Use: Corticosteroid.

•**prednisolone hemisuccinate,** U.S.P. 23.
Use: Glucocorticoid.

•**prednisolone sodium phosphate,** U.S.P. 23.
Use: Glucocorticoid.
See: AK-Pred, Soln. (Akorn).
Alto-Pred Soluble, Vial (Alto).
Hydeltrasol, Inj. (Merck).
Inflamase Forte, Ophthalmic Soln. (Novartis).
Inflamase, Ophthalmic Soln. (Novartis).
Key-Pred SP, Inj. (Hyrex).
Liquid Pred, Inj. (Muro).
Metreton, Ophthalmic Soln. Sterile (Schering-Plough).
Pediapred, Liq. (Medeva).
P.S.P. IV (Four), Inj. (Solvay).
Savacort-S, Inj. (Savage).
W/Neomycin sulfate.
See: Neo-Hydeltrasol, Ophthalmic Soln., Ophthalmic Oint. (Merck).
W/Niacinamide, disodium edetate, sodium bisulfite, phenol.
See: P.S.P. IV, Inj. (Solvay).
W/Prednisolone acetate.
See: Panacort R-P, Vial (Ferndale).
W/Sodium Sulfacetamide.
See: Optimyd, Soln. (Schering-Plough).
Vasocidin, Liq. (Novartis).

prednisolone sodium phosphate. (Various Mfr.) 0.125%, 1% Soln. Bot. 5 ml, 10 ml, 15 ml.
Use: Glucocorticoid.

•**prednisolone sodium succinate for injection,** U.S.P. 23.

Use: Glucocorticoid.

prednisolone tertiary-butylacetate.
See: Prednisolone Tebutate, U.S.P. 23.

Prednisol T.B.A. (Pasadena Research) Prednisolone tebutate 20 mg/ml. Vial 10 ml. *Rx.*
Use: Corticosteroid.

•**prednisolone tebutate,** U.S.P. 23.
Use: Glucocorticoid.
See: Hydeltra-T.B.A., Vial (Merck).
Metalone, Vial (Foy).

•**prednisone,** (PRED-nih-sone) U.S.P. 23.
Use: Glucocorticoid.
See: Delta-Dome, Tab. (Bayer).
Deltasone, Tab. (Pharmacia & Upjohn).
Keysone, Tab. (Hyrex).
Meticorten, Tab. (Schering-Plough).
Maso-Pred, Tab. (Mason).
Orasone, Tab. (Solvay).
Sterapred, Tab. (Mayrand).
W/Chlorpheniramine maleate.
See: Histone, Tab. (Blaine).
W/Phenylephrine HCl.
See: Prednefrin-S, Soln. (Allergan).

prednisone. (Various Mfr.) 1 mg, 5 mg, 20 mg/Tab. Bot. 100s, 1000s, UD 100s.
Use: Glucocorticoid.

Prednisone Intensol Oral Solution. (Roxane) Prednisone concentrated oral solution 5 mg/ml. Bot. 30 ml w/calibrated dropper. *Rx.*
Use: Corticosteroid.

•**prednival.** (PRED-nih-val) USAN.
Use: Glucocorticoid.

Predsulfair. (Bausch & Lomb) **Drops:** Prednisolone acetate 0.5%, sodium sulfacetamide 10%, hydroxypropyl methylcellulose, polysorbate 80 0.5%, sodium thiosulfate, benzalkonium Cl 0.01%. Bot. 5 ml, 15 ml. **Oint.:** Prednisolone acetate 0.5%, sodium sulfacetamide 10%, mineral oil, white petrolatum, lanolin, parabens. In 3.5 g. *Rx.*
Use: Corticosteroid, anti-infective, ophthalmic.

Preflex Daily Cleaning Especially for Sensitive Eyes. (Alcon) Isotonic, aqueous solution of sorbic acid, sodium phosphates, sodium Cl, tyloxapol, hydroxyethyl cellulose, polyvinyl alcohol, EDTA. Bot. 30 ml. *otc.*
Use: Soft contact lens care.

Prefrin Liquifilm. (Allergan) Phenylephrine HCl 0.12%. Bot. 20 ml. *otc.*
Use: Ophthalmic vasoconstrictor, mydriatic.

Pregestimil. (Bristol-Myers) Protein hy-

drolysate formula supplies 640 calories/ qt. protein 18 g, fat 26 g, carbohydrate 86 g, vitamins A 2000 IU, D 400 IU, E 15 IU, C 52 mg, folic acid 100 mcg, thiamine 0.5 mg, riboflavin 0.6 mg, niacin 8 mg, B_6 0.4 mg, B_{12} 2 mcg, biotin 0.05 mg, pantothenic acid 3 mg, K-1 100 mcg, choline 85 mg, inositol 30 mg, calcium 600 mg, phosphorus 400 mg, iodine 45 mcg, iron 12 mg, magnesium 70 mg, copper 0.6 mg, zinc 4 mg, manganese 0.2 mg, chloride 550 mg, potassium 700 mg, sodium 300 mg/Qt. (20 Kcal/fl oz.). Pow. Can lb. *otc.*
Use: Enteral nutritional supplement.

Pregnaslide Latex hCG Test with Fast Trak Slides. (Wampole) Latex agglutination slide test for the qualitative detection of human chorionic gonadotropin in urine. Test 24s. Test kit 96s.
Use: Diagnostic aid.

pregneninolone.
See: Ethisterone.

•**pregnenolone.** (preg-NEN-oh-lone) F.D.A.
Use: Treatment of rheumatoid arthritis.

•**pregnenolone succinate.** (PREG-nehno-lone) USAN.
Use: Non-hormonal sterol derivative.

Pregnosis Slide Test. (Roche Diagnostics) Latex agglutination inhibition slide test. 50s, 200s.
Use: Diagnostic aid.

Pregnyl. (Organon) Human chorionic gonadotropin 10,000 IU/Vial w/diluent 10 ml, mannitol, benzyl alcohol. Vial 10 ml. *Rx.*
Use: Chorionic gonadotropin.

Pre-Hist-D. (Marnel) Phenylephrine HCl 20 mg, chlorpheniramine maleate 8 mg, methscopolamine nitrate 2.5 mg/ S.R. Tab. or Capl. Bot. 100s. *Rx.*
Use: Decongestant, antihistamine, anticholinergic.

Preject Preinjection Topical Anesthetic. (Colgate Oral) Benzocaine 20% in polyethylene glycol base. Jar 2 oz. *otc.*
Use: Local anesthetic, topical.

Prelestrin. (Pasadena Research) Conjugated estrogens 0.625 mg or 1.25 mg/ Tab. Bot. 100s, 1000s. *Rx.*
Use: Estrogen.

Prelone Syrup. (Muro) Prednisolone 15 mg/5 ml, alcohol 5%, saccharin. Cherry flavor. 240 ml. *Rx.*
Use: Corticosteroid.

Prelu-2. (Boehringer Ingelheim) Phendimetrazine tartrate 105 mg/Cap. Bot. 100s. *c-III.*
Use: Anorexiant.

Premarin. (Wyeth-Ayerst) Conjugated estrogens tablets. Water-soluble conjugated estrogens derived from natural sources. Sucrose. 0.3 mg, 0.625 mg, 0.9 mg, 1.25 mg or 2.5 mg/Tab.: Bot. 100s, 1000s. 0.625 mg or 1.25 mg: 5000s, UD 100s. Cycle packs 25s. *Rx.*
Use: Estrogen.

Premarin Intravenous. (Wyeth-Ayerst) Conjugated Estrogens U.S.P., for Injection. Vial 25 mg/5 ml w/diluent. (Vial also contains lactose 200 mg, sodium citrate 12.5 mg, simethicone 0.2 mg). Diluent contains benzyl alcohol 2%, Water for Injection, U.S.P. *Rx.*
Use: Estrogen.

Premarin Vaginal Cream. (Wyeth-Ayerst) Conjugated Estrogens, U.S.P. 0.625 mg/1 g w/cetyl esters wax, cetyl alcohol, white wax, glyceryl monostearate, propylene glycol monostearate, methyl stearate, phenylethyl alcohol, sodium lauryl sulfate, glycerin, mineral oil. Tube w/applicator 1.5 oz. (42.5 g). Tube refill. *Rx.*
Use: Estrogen, vaginal.

Premarin w/Meprobamate.
See: PMB 200 and 400, Tab. (Wyeth-Ayerst).

Premarin w/Methyltestosterone. (Wyeth-Ayerst) Premarin (Conjugated Estrogens, U.S.P.) 1.25 mg, methyltestosterone 10 mg/Yellow Tab. Premarin 0.625 mg, methyltestosterone 5 mg/ Red Tab. Bot. 100s. *Rx.*
Use: Estrogen, androgen combination.

W/Methyltestosterone, methamphetamine HCl, vitamins.
See: Mediatric, Cap., Liq., Tab. (Wyeth-Ayerst).

Premate-200. (Major) Meprobamate 200 mg, tridihexethyl Cl 25 mg/Tab. Bot. 100s. *Rx.*
Use: Antianxiety, anticholinergic.

Premate-400. (Major) Meprobamate 400 mg, tridihexethyl Cl 25 mg/Tab. Bot. 100s. *Rx.*
Use: Antianxiety, anticholinergic.

Premphase. (Wyeth-Ayerst) Conjugated estrogens 0.625 mg/Tab. Medroxyprogesterone acetate 5 mg/Tab. Blister-card 28s (14 of each). *Rx.*
Use: Estrogen and progestin, combined.

Prempro. (Wyeth-Ayerst) Conjugated estrogen 0.625 mg, medroxyprogesterone acetate 2.5 mg, lactose, sucrose/ Tab. Blister-card 14s (2s). *Rx.*
Use: Estrogen and progestin, combined.

Premsyn PMS Caplets. (Chattem) Acetaminophen 500 mg, pamabrom 25 mg, pyrilamine maleate 15 mg/Capl. Bot. 20s, 40s. *otc.*
Use: Analgesic, diuretic, antihistamine.
•**prenalterol hydrochloride.** (PREE-NAL-teh-role) USAN.
Use: Adrenergic.

Prenatal Folic Acid + Iron. (Everett) Vitamins, minerals, folic acid 1 mg/Tab. Bot. 100s. *Rx.*
Use: Vitamin/mineral supplement.

Prenatal MR 90. (Ethex) Calcium 250 mg, iron 90 mg, vitamin A 4000 IU, D 400 IU, E 30 mg, B_1 3 mg, B_2 3.4 mg, B_3 20 mg, B_6 20 mg, B_{12} 12 mcg, C 120 mg, folic acid 1 mg, Zn 25 mg, I, Cu, DSS. Tab. Bot. 100s. *Rx.*
Use: Vitamin/mineral supplement.

Prenatal-S. (Goldline) Calcium 200 mg, iron 60 mg, vitamins A 4000 IU, D 400 IU, E 11 mg, B_1 1.5 mg, B_2 1.7 mg, B_3 18 mg, B_6 2.6 mg, B_{12} 4 mcg, C 100 mg, folic acid 0.8 mg, zinc 25 mg/Tab. Bot. UD 100s. *otc.*
Use: Vitamin/mineral supplement.

Prenatal with Folic Acid. (Geneva) Calcium 200 mg, iron 60 mg, vitamins A 4000 IU, D 400 IU, E 11 mg, B_1 1.5 mg, B_2 1.7 mg, B_3 18 mg, B_6 2.6 mg, B_{12} 4 mcg, C 100 mg, folic acid 0.8 mg, Zn 25 mg/Tab. Bot. 100s. *otc.*
Use: Vitamin/mineral supplement.

Prenatal with Folic Acid. (Eon Labs) Vitamins A 6000 IU, D 400 IU, E 30 IU, folic acid 1 mg, C 60 mg, B_1 1.1 mg, B_2 1.8 mg, B_6 2.5 mg, B_{12} 5 mcg, niacin 15 mg, calcium 125 mg, iron 65 mg/Tab. Bot. 100s, 1000s. *Rx.*
Use: Vitamin/mineral supplement.

Prenatal Maternal. (Ethex) Ca 250 mg, iron 60 mg, vitamins A 5000 IU, D 400 IU, E 30 mg, B_1 2.9 mg, B_2 3.4 mg, B_3 20 mg, B_5 10 mg, B_6 12.2 mg, B_{12} 12 mcg, C 100 mg, folic acid 1 mg, Cr, Cu, I, Mg, Mn, Mo, zinc 25 mg, biotin 30 mcg/Tab. Bot. 100s. *Rx.*
Use: Vitamin/mineral supplement.

Prenatal-1 + Iron. (Various Mfr.) Ca 200 mg, iron 65 mg, vitamins A 4000 IU, D 400 IU, E 11 mg, B_1 1.5 mg, B_2 3 mg, B_3 20 mg, B_6 10 mg, B_{12} 12 mcg, C 120 mg, folic acid 1 mg, Cu, zinc 25 mg/Tab. Bot. 100s, 500s. *Rx.*
Use: Vitamin/mineral supplement.

Prenatal Plus. (Goldline) Vitamin A (as acetate and carotene) 4000 IU, D IU 400, E 22 mg, C 120 mg, folic acid 1 mg, B_1 1.84 mg, B_2 3 mg, B_3 20 mg, B_6 10 mg, B_{12} 12 mcg, calcium 200 mg,

Fe 65 mg, Cu 2 mg, Zn 25 mg/Tab. Bot. 100s. *Rx.*
Use: Vitamin/mineral supplement.

Prenatal Plus with Beta Carotene. (Rugby) Ca 200 mg, iron 65 mg, vitamins A 4000 IU, D 400 IU, E 11 mg, B_1 1.84 mg, B_2 3 mg, B_3 20 mg, B_6 10 mg, B_{12} 12 mcg, C 120 mg, folic acid 1 mg, Cu, zinc 25 mg/Tab. Bot. 100s, 500s. *Rx.*
Use: Vitamin/mineral supplement.

Prenatal Plus-Improved. (Rugby) Ca 200 mg, iron 65 mg, vitamins A 4000 IU, D 400 IU, E 11 mg, B_1 1.5 mg, B_2 3 mg, B_3 20 mg, B_6 10 mg, B_{12} 12 mcg, C 120 mg, folic acid 1 mg, Cu, zinc 25 mg/Tab. Bot. 100s. *Rx.*
Use: Vitamin/mineral supplement.

Prenatal Rx with Beta Carotene. (Various Mfr.) Ca 200 mg, iron 60 mg, vitamins A 4000 IU, D 400 IU, E 15 mg, B_1 1.5 mg, B_2 1.6 mg, B_3 17 mg, B_5 7 mg, B_6 4 mg, B_{12} 2.5 mcg, C 80 mg, folic acid 1 mg, biotin 30 mcg, Cu, Mg, zinc 25 mg/Tab. Bot. 100s, 500s. *Rx.*
Use: Vitamin/mineral supplement.

Prenatal Z. (Ethex) Ca 300 mg, iron 65 mg, vitamins A 5000 IU, D 400 IU, E 30 mg, B_1 3 mg, B_2 3 mg, B_3 20 mg, B_6 12.2 mg, B_{12} 12 mcg, C 80 mg, folic acid 1 mg, zinc 20 mg, I, Mg/Tab. Bot. 100s. *Rx.*
Use: Vitamin/mineral supplement.

Prenate 90 Tablets. (Bock) Vitamins A 4000 IU, D 400 IU, E 30 mg, C 120 mg, folic acid 1 mg, B_1 3 mg, B_2 3.4 mg, B_6 20 mg, B_{12} 12 mcg, B_3 20 mg, DSS, calcium 250 mg, iodine, iron 90 mg, Cu, zinc 20 mg/FC Tab. Bot. 100s, 1000s. *Rx.*
Use: Vitamin/mineral supplement.

Prenavite. (Rugby) Ca 200 mg, iron 60 mg, vitamins A 4000 IU, D 400 IU, E 11 mg, B_1 1.5 mg, B_2 1.7 mg, B_3 18 mg, B_6 2.6 mg, B_{12} 4 mcg, C 100 mg, folic acic 0.8 mg, zinc 25 mg/Tab. Bot. 100s, 500s. *otc.*
Use: Vitamin/mineral supplement.

•**prenylamine.** (PREH-nill-ah-meen) USAN. Segontin; Synadrin lactate.
Use: Coronary vasodilator.

Preparation H. (Whitehall Robins) Shark liver oil 3%, cocoa butter 79%, corn oil, EDTA, parabens, tocopherol. Supp. 12s, 24s, 36s, 48s. *otc.*
Use: Anorectal preparation.

Preparation H Cleansing Tissues. (Whitehall Robins) Propylene glycol, phenoxyethanol, parabens, citric acid, alcohol free. In 15s, 40s. *otc.*

Use: Anorectal preparation.

Preparation H Cream. (Whitehall Robins) Petrolatum 78%, glycerin 12%, shark liver oil 3%, phenylephrine HCl 0.25%, cetyl and stearyl alcohol, EDTA, parabens, lanolin, tocopherol. Tube 27 g, 54 g. *otc.*
Use: Anorectal preparation.

Preparation H Ointment. (Whitehall Robins) Petrolatum 71.9%, mineral oil 14%, shark liver oil 3%, phenylephrine HCl 0.25%, corn oil, glycerin, lanolin, lanolin alcohol, parabens, tocopherol. Oint. 30 g, 60 g. *otc.*
Use: Anorectal preparation.

Prepcat. (Lafayette) Barium sulfate 1.2% w/w suspension. Bot. 480 ml, Case Bot. 24s.
Use: Radiopaque agent.

Prepcat 2000. (Lafayette) Barium sulfate 1.2% w/w suspension. Bot. 2000 ml, Case Bot. 4s.
Use: Radiopaque agent.

Prepcort Cream. (Whitehall Robins) Hydrocortisone 0.5%. Tube 0.5 oz, 1 oz.
Use: Corticosteroid.

Pre-Pen. (Kremers-Urban) Benzylpenicilloyl-polylysine 0.25 ml/Amp.
Use: Diagnostic aid.

Pre-Pen/MDM. (Kremers-Urban)
See: Benzylpenicillin, Benzylpenicilloic, Benzylpenilloic Acid.

Prepidil. (Pharmacia & Upjohn) Dinoprostone 0.5 mg/Gel. Syringes (with 2 shielded catheters 10 and 20 mm tip) 3 g. *Rx.*
Use: Agent for cervical ripening.

Prepodyne. (West) Titratable iodine. **Soln.:** 1%. Bot. pt, gal. **Scrub:** 0.75%. Bot. 6 oz, gal. **Swabs:** Saturated with soln. Pkt. 1s, Box 100s. **Swabsticks:** Saturated with soln. Pkt. 1s, Box 50s. Pkt. 3s, Box 75s.
Use: Topical antiseptic.

Presalin. (Roberts) Aspirin 260 mg, salicylamide 120 mg, acetaminophen 120 mg, aluminum hydroxide 100 mg/Tab. Bot. 50s. *otc.*
Use: Analgesic combination, antacid.

Prescription Strength Desenex. (Novartis) **Spray Liquid:** Miconazole nitrate 2%. 105 ml. **Spray Powder:** Miconazole nitrate 2%. 90 ml. **Cream:** Clotrimazole 1%. Tube 15 g. *otc.*
Use: Topical antifungal.

pressor agents.
See: Sympathomimetic agents.

Pressorol. (Baxter) Metaraminol bitartrate. Vial 10 ml (10 mg/ml). *Rx.*

Use: Vasopressor.

Presun 4 Creamy. (Bristol-Myers) Padimate O 1.4%, alcohol, titanium dioxide. Waterproof lotion. Bot. 4 oz. *otc.*
Use: Sunscreen.

Presun 8 Creamy. (Bristol-Myers) Padimate O 5%, oxybenzone 2%. Waterproof. Bot. 4 oz. *otc.*
Use: Sunscreen.

Presun 8 Lotion. (Bristol-Myers) Padimate O 7.3%, oxybenzone 2.3%, SD alcohol 40 60%. Bot. 4 oz. *otc.*
Use: Sunscreen.

Presun 15 Creamy. (Bristol-Myers) Padimate O 8%, oxybenzone 3%, benzyl alcohol. Waterproof. Bot. 4 oz. *otc.*
Use: Sunscreen.

Presun 15 Facial Sunscreen. (Bristol-Myers) Padimate O (Octyl dimethyl PABA) 8%, oxybenzone 3%. Bot. 2 oz. *otc.*
Use: Sunscreen.

Presun 15 Facial Sunscreen Stick. (Bristol-Myers) Octyl dimethyl PABA 8%, oxybenzone 3%. Stick 0.42 oz. *otc.*
Use: Sunscreen.

Presun 15 Lip Protector. (Bristol-Myers) Padimate O 8%, oxybenzone 3%. Stick 4.5 g. *otc.*
Use: Sunscreen.

Presun 15 Lotion. (Bristol-Myers) Padimate O 5%, PABA 5%, oxybenzone 3%, SD alcohol 40 58%. Bot. 4 oz. *otc.*
Use: Sunscreen.

Presun 15 Sensitive Skin Sunscreen. (Bristol-Myers) Octyl methoxycinnamate, oxybenzone, octyl salicylate, cetyl alcohol, PABA free, waterproof, SPF 15. Cream. Bot. 120 ml. *otc.*
Use: Sunscreen.

Presun 23. (Bristol-Myers) Padimate O, octyl methoxycinnamate, oxybenzone, octyl salicylate, SD alcohol 40 19%, waterproof. Spray mist. Bot. 105 ml. *otc.*
Use: Sunscreen.

Presun 29 Sensitive Skin Sunscreen. (Bristol-Myers) Octyl methoxycinnamate, oxybenzone, octyl salicylate. SPF 29. Waterproof. Bot. 4 oz. *otc.*
Use: Sunscreen.

Presun 39 Creamy Sunscreen. (Bristol-Myers) Padimate O, oxybenzone, cetyl alcohol, waterproof. Cream. Bot. 120 ml. *otc.*
Use: Sunscreen.

Presun Active. (Bristol-Myers) Octyl methoxycinnamate, oxybenzone, octyl salicylate, 69% SD alcohol 40. PABA free. Waterproof. SPF 15, 30. Gel. 120 g. *otc.*

Use: Sunscreen.

Presun for Kids Cream. (Bristol-Myers) Octyl methoxycinnamate, oxybenzone, octyl salicylate, cetyl alcohol, PABA free, waterproof SFP 29. Cream. Bot. 120 ml. *otc.*
Use: Sunscreen.

Presun for Kids Spray. (Bristol-Myers) Padimate O, octyl methoxycinnamate, oxybenzone, octyl salicylate, SD alcohol 40 19%, waterproof, SPF 23. Spray Bot. 105 ml. *otc.*
Use: Sunscreen.

Presun Moisturizing. (Bristol-Myers) Octyl dimethyl PABA, oxybenzone, cetyl alcohol, diazolidinyl urea. SPF 46. Lot. Bot. 120 ml. *otc.*
Use: Sunscreen.

Presun Moisturizing Sunscreen with Keri, SPF 15. (Bristol-Myers) Octyl dimethyl PABA, oxybenzone, cetyl alcohol, diazolidinyl urea. Waterproof. Lot. 120 ml. *otc.*
Use: Sunscreen.

Presun Moisturizing Sunscreen with Keri, SPF 25. (Bristol-Myers) Octyl methoxycinnamate, oxybenzone, octyl salicylate, petrolatum, cetyl alcohol, diazolidinyl urea. Waterproof. Lot. 120 ml. *otc.*
Use: Sunscreen.

Presun Spray Mist. (Bristol-Myers) Octyl dimethyl PABA, octyl methoxycinnamate, oxybenzone, octyl salicylate, 19% SD alcohol 40, C12-15 alcohols benzoate. Waterproof. SPF 23. 120 ml. *otc.*
Use: Sunscreen.

Pretend-U-Ate. (Vitalax) Enriched candy-appetite pacifier. Pkg. 20s. *otc.*
Use: Diet aid.

prethcamide. Mixture of crotethamide and cropropamide.
See: Micoren (Novartis).

Prett's Diet Aid. (MiLance) Alginic acid 200 mg, sodium carboxymethylcellulose 100 mg, sodium bicarbonate 70 mg/Chew. Tab. Bot. 60s. *otc.*
Use: Nonprescription diet aid.

Pretty Feet & Hands. (Menley & James) Paraffin, triethanolamine, parabens. Cream 90 g. *otc.*
Use: Emollient.

Pretz-Pak. (Parnell) Benzyl alcohol 3.5%, polyethylene glycols, carboxymethylcellulose, urea, poloxamer, *Mucoprotective Factor* yerba santa, allantoin, aluminum chlorhydroxy allantoin. Oint. Tube 15 g. *otc.*

Use: Operative and postoperative care in intranasal and endoscopic surgery; local anesthetic.

Prevacid. (TAP Pharm) Lansoprazole 15 mg or 30 mg/SR Cap. Bot. 30s, 100s, UD 100s. *Rx.*
Use: Proton pump inhibitor.

Prevalite. (Upsher-Smith) Cholestyramine 4 g, phenylalanine 14.1 mg/dose/Pow. Box. 5.5 g single dose packets. 60s. *Rx.*
Use: Antihyperlipidemic agent.

PreviDent Disclosing Drops. (Colgate Oral) Erythrosine sodium 1%. Bot. 1 oz.
Use: Disclosing dental plaque.

PreviDent Disclosing Tablet. (Colgate Oral) Erythrosine sodium 1%/Tab. UD strip 1000s.
Use: Disclosing dental plaque.

PreviDent Prophylaxis Paste. (Colgate Oral) Sodium fluoride containing 1.2% fluoride ion w/pumice and alumina abrasives. Cup 2 g, Box 200s. Jar 9 oz. *Rx.*
Use: Dental caries preventative.

PreviDent Rinse. (Colgate Oral) Neutral sodium fluoride 0.2%, alcohol 6%. Sol. Bot. 250 ml, gal (w/pump dispenser). *Rx.*
Use: Dental caries prevention.

Preview. (Lafayette) Barium sulfate 60% w/v suspension. Bot. 355 ml, Case 24 bot.
Use: Radiopaque agent.

Preview 2000. Barium sulfate 60% w/v suspension. Bot. 2000 ml, Case 4 Bot.
Use: Radiopaque agent.

Prevision. Mestranol, U.S.P. 23.

Prexonate Tablets. (Tennessee Pharm) Vitamins A acetate 5000 IU, D 500 IU, B_6 2 mg, B_1 5 mg, B_2 2 mg, C 100 mg, B_{12} 2.5 mcg, calcium pantothenate 1 mg, niacinamide 15 mg, folic acid 1 mg, iron 45 mg, calcium 500 mg, intrinsic factor 3 mg/Tab. Bot. 100s, 1000s. *Rx.*
Use: Vitamin/mineral supplement.

•**prezatide copper acetate.** (PREH-zat-IDE KAH-per) USAN.
Use: Immunomodulator.

Prid Salve. (Walker Pharmacal) Ichthammol, Phenol, Lead Oleate, Rosin, Beeswax, Lard. Tin 20 g. *otc.*
Use: Drawing salve.

•**pridefine hydrochloride.** (PRIH-deh-FEEN) USAN.
Use: Antidepressant.

•**prifelone.** (PRIH-feh-LONE) USAN.

Use: Anti-inflammatory (dermatologic).

•**priliximab.** (prih-LICK-sih-mab) USAN.
Use: Monoclonal antibody (autoimmune lymphoproliferative diseases, organ transplantation).

prilocaine and epinephrine injection.
Use: Local anesthetic.

•**prilocaine hydrochloride,** (PRILL-oh-cane) U.S.P. 23.
Use: Local anesthetic.
See: Citanest Hydrochloride, Vial, Amp. (Astra).

Prilosec. (Astra-Merck) Omeprazole 10 mg or 20 mg, lactose/DR Cap. **10 mg:** Bot. 30s, 100s, UD 100s. **20 mg:** Bot. 30s, 1000s, UD 100s. *Rx.*
Use: Duodenal ulcer, gastroesophageal reflux disease, hypersecretory conditions.

primacaine.
Use: Local anesthetic.

Primacor. (Sanofi Winthrop) Milrinone lactate. **Inj.:** 1 mg/ml. Single-dose vial 10 ml, 20 ml; Carpuject units 5 ml. **Inj., Premixed:** 200 mcg/ml in dextrose 5%. Vial 100 ml. *Rx.*
Use: Cardiotonic agent.
See: Milrinone.

•**primaquine phosphate,** (PRIM-uh-kween) U.S.P. 23.
Use: Antimalarial.

primaquine phosphate. (PRIM-uh-kween) (Sanofi Winthrop). 26.3 mg/Tab. Bot. 100s.
Use: Antimalarial.

primaquine phosphate. (PRIM-uh-kween) (Sterling Winthrop) *Rx.*
Use: Treatment of PCP associated with AIDS. [Orphan drug]

Primatene. (Whitehall Robins) Theophylline 130 mg, ephedrine HCl 24 mg, phenobarbital 7.5 mg/Tab. Bot. 24s. *otc.*
Use: Antiasthmatic combination.

Primatene Dual Action. (Whitehall Robins) Theophylline 60 mg, ephedrine HCl 12.5 mg, guaifenesin 100 mg/Tab. Bot. 24s. *otc.*
Use: Antiasthmatic combination.

Primatene Mist Solution. (Whitehall Robins) Epinephrine 0.2 mg, alcohol 34%. Bot. 0.5 oz. Spray. *otc.*
Use: Bronchodilator.

Primatene Mist Suspension. (Whitehall Robins) Epinephrine bitartrate 0.3 mg. Bot. 10 ml w/mouthpiece. Spray. *otc.*
Use: Bronchodilator.

Primatene M. Tablets. (Whitehall Robins) Theophylline 118 mg, ephedrine HCl 24 mg, pyrilamine maleate 16.6 mg/Tab. Bot. 24s, 60s. *otc.*
Use: Bronchodilator, antihistamine.

Primatene P Tablets. (Whitehall Robins) Theophylline 118 mg, ephedrine HCl 24 mg, phenobarbital 8 mg/Tab. Bot. 24s, 60s. *otc.*
Use: Bronchodilator, sedative, hypnotic.

Primatuss Cough Mixture 4 Liquid. (Rugby) Doxylamine succinate 3.75 mg, dextromethorphan HBr 7.5 mg/5 ml, alcohol 10% Liq. Bot. 180 ml. *otc.*
Use: Antihistamine, antitussive.

Primatuss Cough Mixture 4D Liquid. (Rugby) Pseudoephedrine HCl 20 mg, dextromethorphan HBr 10 mg, guaifenesin 67 mg/5 ml, alcohol 10%. Liq. Bot. 120 ml. *otc.*
Use: Decongestant, antitussive, expectorant.

Primaxin. (Merck) Imipenem (anhydrous equivalent), cilastatin w/sodium bicarbonate buffer. **250-250:** ADD-Vantage Vial, Tray 10s, 25s. Tray 10 infusion bottles. **500-500:** ADD-Vantage Vial, Tray 10s, 25s. Tray 10 infusion bottles. *Rx.*
Use: Anti-infective.

Primaxin I.M. (Merck) Imipenem (anhydrous equivalent), cilastatin w/ sodium bicarbonate buffer. Pow. for Inj. Vials 500 mg/500 mg, 750 mg/750 mg. *Rx.*
Use: Anti-infective.

Primaxin I.V. (Merck) Imipenem (anhydrous equivalent), cilastatin w/ sodium bicarbonate buffer. Pow. for Inj. Vials, infusion bot., ADD-Vantage vials 250 mg/250 mg, 500 mg/500 mg. *Rx.*
Use: Anti-infective.

•**primidolol.** (prih-MID-oh-lahl) USAN.
Use: Antihypertensive, antianginal, cardiac depressant (antiarrhythmic).

•**primidone,** (PRIM-ih-dohn) U.S.P. 23.
Use: Anticonvulsant.

primidone. (Various Mfr.) 250 mg. Tab. Bot. 100s, 500s, 1000s, UD 100s.
Use: Anticonvulsant.

primostrum. A prep. of primiparous colostrum.

Principen "125" for Oral Suspension. (Squibb) Ampicillin trihydrate 125 mg/ 5 ml, saccharin. Reconstitution to 80 ml, 100 ml, 150 ml, 200 ml, UD 5 ml 100s. *Rx.*
Use: Anti-infective, penicillin.

Principen "250" Capsules. (Squibb) Ampicillin 250 mg/Cap. Bot. 100s, 500s, UD 100s. *Rx.*
Use: Anti-infective, penicillin.

Principen "250" for Oral Suspension.

(Squibb) Ampicillin trihydrate 250 mg/5 ml, saccharin. Reconstitution to 80 ml, 100 ml, 150 ml, 200 ml, UD 5 ml 100s. *Rx.*
Use: Anti-infective, penicillin.

Principen "500" Capsules. (Squibb) Ampicillin trihydrate 500 mg/Cap. 100s, 500s, UD 100s. *Rx.*
Use: Anti-infective, penicillin.

Principen with Probenecid. (Squibb) Ampicillin (as trihydrate) 3.5 g, probenecid 1 g/regimen. Single dose bot., 9s. *Rx.*
Use: Anti-infective, penicillin.

Prinivil. (Merck) Lisinopril **2.5 mg/Tab.:** Bot. 30s, 100s, UD 100s. **5 mg/Tab.:** Bot. 1000s, Unit-of-Use 90s, 100s, UD 100s. **10 mg or 20 mg/Tab.:** Bot. 1000s, Unit-of-Use 30s, 90s, 100s, UD 100s. **40 mg/Tab.:** Bot. 100s. *Rx.*
Use: Antihypertensive.

•**prinomide tromethamine.** (PRIH-no-MIDE troe-METH-ah-meen) USAN.
Use: Antirheumatic.

•**prinoxodan.** (prin-OX-oh-dan) USAN.
Use: Cardiotonic.

Prinzide. (Merck) Lisinopril 10 or 20 mg, hydrochlorothiazide 12.5 mg/Tab or lisinopril 20 mg, hydrochlorothiazide 25 mg/Tab. Bot. 30s, 100s. *Rx.*
Use: Antihypertensive.

Priscoline. (Novartis) Tolazoline HCl 25 mg/ml, tartaric acid 0.65%, hydrous sodium citrate 0.65%. Vial 4 ml. *Rx.*
Use: Antihypertensive.

prisilidene hydrochloride.
See: Alphaprodine HCl (Various Mfr.).

privadorn.
See: Bromisovalum (Various Mfr.).

Privine. (Novartis) Naphazoline HCl. **Nasal Soln.:** 0.05%. Bot. 20 ml w/dropper. **Nasal Spray:** 0.05%. Bot. 15 ml. *otc.*
Use: Decongestant.

•**prizidilol hydrochloride.** (PRIH-zie-DILL-ole) USAN.
Use: Antihypertensive.

Pro-50. (Dunhall) Promethazine HCl 50 mg/ml. Vial 10 ml. *Rx.*
Use: Antihistamine, antiemetic.

Pro-Acet Douche Concentrate. (Pro-Acet) Lactic, citric, and acetic acids, sodium lauryl sulfate, lactose, dextrose and sodium acetate. Pkg. polyethylene envelope 10 ml. Contents of 1 envelope to be diluted with 2 quarts of water. Douche 6 oz, 12 oz. Travel Packet 10 ml. *otc.*
Use: Vaginal preparation.

•**proadifen hydrochloride.** (pro-AD-ih-fen) USAN.
Use: Synergist (non-specific).

ProAmatine. (Roberts) Midodrine HCl 2.5 mg and 5 mg/Tab. Bot. 100s. *Rx.*
Use: Antiemetic, antivertigo.

Probampacin Suspension. (Goldline) Ampicillin 3.5 g, probenecid 1 g. Bot. 60 ml. *Rx.*
Use: Anti-infective, penicillin.

Pro-Banthine. (Schiapparelli Searle) Propantheline bromide **7.5 mg/Tab.:** Bot. 100s. **15 mg/Tab.:** Bot. 100s, 500s, UD 100s.
Use: Anticholinergic, antispasmodic.

Probarbital Sodium. 5-Ethyl-5-isopropyl-barbiturate sodium.

Probax. (Fischer) Propolis 2%, petrolatum, mineral oil, lanolin. Gel. Tube 3.5 g. *otc.*
Use: Mouth and throat preparation.

Probec-T. (Roberts) Vitamins B₁ 12.2 mg, B₂ 10 mg, B₃ 100 mg, B₅ 18.4, B₆ 4.1 mg, B₁₂ 5 mcg, C 600 mg/Tab. Bot. 60s. *otc.*
Use: Vitamin/mineral supplement.

Proben-C. (Rugby) Probenecid 500 mg, colchicine 0.5 mg/Tab. Bot. 100s, 1000s. *Rx.*
Use: Agent for gout.

•**probenecid,** (pro-BEN-uh-sid) U.S.P. 23.
Use: Uricosuric.
See: Benemid, Tab. (Merck).
W/Ampicillin.
See: Amcill-GC, Oral Susp. (Parke-Davis).
Polycillin-PRB, Liq. (Bristol-Myers).
Principen w/Probenecid, Cap. (Squibb).
W/Ampicillin trihydrate.
See: Probampacin (Biocraft).

probenecid and colchicine. (Various Mfr.) Probenecid 500 mg, colchine 0.5 mg/Tab. Bot. 100s, 1000s. *Rx.*
Use: Uricosuric combination for chronic gouty arthritis.
See: Colbenemid, Tab. (Merck).

probenzamide. 0-Propoxybenzamide. (Warner-Lambert).

•**probicromil calcium.** (pro-BYE-KROE-mill) USAN.
Use: Antiallergic (prophylactic).

Pro-Bionate. (Natren) *Lactobacillus acidophilus* strain NAS 2 billion units/g. **Pow.** 52.5 g, 90 g. **Cap.** Bot. 30s, 60s. *otc.*
Use: Antidiarrheal, nutritional supplement.

•**probucol,** U.S.P. 23.

Use: Antihyperlipidemic.
See: Lorelco, Tab. (Hoechst Marion Roussel).

•**procainamide hydrochloride,** (pro-CANE-uh-mide) U.S.P. 23.
Use: Cardiac depressant (antiarrhythmic).
See: Procamide SR, Tab. (Solvay).
Procan SR, Tab. (Parke-Davis).
Pronestyl, Cap., Vial (Bristol-Myers).

procaine base.
W/Benzyl alcohol, propyl-p-aminobenzoate.
Use: Local anesthetic.
See: Rectocaine, Vial (Moore-Kirk).
W/Butyl-p-aminobenzoate, benzyl alcohol, in sweet almond oil.
See: Anucaine, Amp. (Calvin).

procaine butyrate. p-Aminobenzoyl-diethylaminoethanol butyrate.

•**procaine hydrochloride,** U.S.P. 23. Bernocaine, Chlorocaine, Ethocaine, Irocaine, Kerocaine, Syncaine.
Use: Local anesthetic.
See: Novocain, Inj. (Sanofi Winthrop).

procaine hydrochloride. (Abbott) 1% or 2% solution. Multiple-dose Vial 30 ml.
Use: Local anesthetic.

procaine hydrochloride and epinephrine injection.
Use: Local anesthetic.

procaine hydrochloride and levonordefrin injection.
Use: Local anesthetic.

procaine penicillin g suspension, sterile.
Use: Anti-infective, penicillin.
See: Crysticillin, Vial (Squibb).
Penicillin G, Procaine (Various Mfr.).
Pfizerpen For Injection (Pfipharmecs).

procaine, penicillin g w/aluminum stearate suspension, sterile.
Use: Anti-infective, penicillin.
See: Penicillin G Procaine with Aluminum Stearate, Sterile, U.S.P. 23.

procaine and phenylephrine hydrochlorides injection.
Use: Local anesthetic (dental).

procaine and tetracaine hydrochlorides and levonordefrin injection.
Use: Local anesthetic (dental).

procaine, tetracaine and nordefrin hydrochlorides injection.
Use: Local anesthetic.

procaine, tetracaine and phenylephrine hydrochlorides injection.
Use: Anesthetic.

Procalamine Injection. (McGaw) Injection of amino acid 3%, glycerin 3%,

electrolytes. Bot. 1000 ml. *Rx.*
Use: Parenteral nutritional supplement.

Pro-Cal-Sof. (Vangard) Docusate calcium 240 mg/Cap. Bot. 100s, 1000s, UD 100s. *otc.*
Use: Laxative.

Procanbid. (Parke-Davis) Procainamide 500 mg or 1000 mg/ER Tab. Bot. 60s, UD 100s. *Rx.*
Use: Antiarrhythmic.

•**procarbazine hydrochloride,** (pro-CAR-buh-ZEEN) U.S.P. 23. (Roche) Natulan.
Use: Cytostatic, antineoplastic.
See: Matulane, Cap. (Roche).

Procardia. (Pfizer) Nifedipine 10 mg or 20 mg/Cap. Bot. 100s, 300s, UD 100s. *Rx.*
Use: Calcium channel blocker.

Procardia XL. (Pfizer) Nifedipine 30 mg, 60 mg or 90 mg/SR Tab. **30 mg or 60 mg:** Bot. 100s, 300s, 5000s, UD 100s. **90 mg:** Bot 100s. *Rx.*
Use: Calcium channel blocker.

•**procaterol hydrochloride.** (PRO-CAT-ehr-ole) USAN.
Use: Bronchodilator.

Proception Sperm Nutrient Douche. (Milex) Ringer type glucose douche. Bot. ample for 10 douches. *otc.*
Use: Vaginal preparation.

•**prochlorperazine,** (pro-klor-PURR-uh-zeen) U.S.P. 23.
Use: Antiemetic.
See: Compazine, Preps. (SK-Beecham).
W/Isopropamide.
See: Iso-Perazine, Cap. (Lemmon).

prochlorperazine. (G & W Labs) Prochlorperazine 25 mg, coconut oil, palm kernel oil. Supp. 12s. *Rx.*
Use: Antiemetic.

•**prochlorperazine edisylate,** U.S.P. 23.
Use: Antipsychotic, antiemetic.
See: Compazine, Preps. (SK-Beecham).

prochlorperazine ethanedisulfonate. Prochlorperazine Edisylate, U.S.P. 23.
Use: Tranquilizer.

prochlorperazine/isopropamide. (Various Mfr.) Isopropamide iodide 5 mg, prochlorperazine maleate 10 mg/Cap. Bot. 100s, 500s, 1000s, UD 100s. *Rx.*
Use: Anticholinergic, antispasmodic, antiemetic, antivertigo.

•**prochlorperazine maleate,** U.S.P. 23.
Use: Antiemetic, antipsychotic.
See: Compazine, Preps. (SK-Beecham).

• **procinonide.** (pro-SIN-oh-nide) USAN.
Use: Adrenocortical steroid.

• **proclonol.** (PRO-klah-nole) USAN. Under study.
Use: Anthelmintic, antifungal.

Pro Comfort Athlete's Foot Spray.
(Scholl) Tolnaftate 1%. Aerosol Can 4 oz. *otc.*
Use: Antifungal, topical.

Pro Comfort Jock Itch Spray Powder.
(Scholl) Tolnaftate 1%. Aerosol can 3.5 oz. *otc.*
Use: Antifungal, topical.

Procort. (Roberts) Hydrocortisone 1%.
Cream: Tube. 30 g. **Spray:** Can. 45 ml. *otc.*
Use: Corticosteroid, topical.

Procrit. (Ortho Biotech) Epoetin alfa 2000, 3000, 4000 or 10,000 units. Inj. Vial. 1 ml. *Rx.*
Use: Recombinant human erythropoietin.

Proctocort. (Monarch Pharmaceuticals) Hydrocortisone 1%. Cream 30 g w/rectal applicator. *Rx.*
Use: Corticosteroid.

Proctocream-HC. (Schwarz Pharma) Hydrocortisone acetate 1% or 2.5%, pramoxine HCl 1%. Cream 30 g. *Rx.*
Use: Corticosteroid, local anesthetic.

Proctofoam. (Scwarz Pharma) Pramoxine HCl 1% in an anesthetic mucoadhesive foam base. Foam. Can. 15 g. *otc.*
Use: Anorectal preparation.

Proctofoam-HC. (Schwarz Pharma) Hydrocortisone acetate 1%, pramoxine HCl 1% in hydrophilic foam base. Bot. aerosol container, Aerosol foam 10 g w/ applicator. *Rx.*
Use: Corticosteroid, local anesthetic.

Proctofoam NS. (Schwarz Pharma) Pramoxine HCl 1%. Aerosol Bot. 15 g w/applicator. *otc.*
Use: Local anesthetic.

Pro-Cute Cream. (Ferndale) Silicone, hexachlorophene, lanolin. 2 oz, lb. *otc.*
Use: Emollient.

Pro-Cute Lotion. (Ferndale) Hexachlorophene, silicone, lanolin. Bot. 8 oz. *otc.*
Use: Emollient.

ProCycle Gold. (Cyclin Pharm) Vitamins A 833.3 IU, D 66.7 IU, E 66.7 IU, C 30 mg, B_1 1.7 mg, B_2 1.7 mg, B_3 3.3 mg, B_5 1.7 mg, B_6 3.3 mg, B_{12} 21 mcg, folic acid 66.7 mg, Ca 166.7 mg, iron 3 mg, zinc 2.5 mg, B, Cu, Cr, I, Mg, Mn, Se, PABA, inositol, rutin, biotin, hesperidin, pancreatin, betaine/Tab. Sugar free. Bot. 100s. *otc.*
Use: Vitamin/mineral supplement.

• **procyclidine hydrochloride,** (pro-SIGH-klih-deen) U.S.P. 23.
Use: Skeletal muscle relaxant; antiparkinsonian.
See: Kemadrin, Tab. (Glaxo Wellcome).

Procysteine. (Free Radical Sciences)
See: L_2-Oxothiazolidine$_4$-carboxylic acid.

Proderm Topical Dressing. (Hickam) Castor oil 650 mg, peruvian balsam 72.5 mg/0.82 cc. Aerosol 4 oz. *otc.*
Use: Prevention of decubiti.

• **prodilidine hydrochloride.** (pro-DIH-lih-deen) USAN.
Use: Analgesic.

Prodium. (Breckenridge) Phenazopyramide HCl 90 mg/Tab. Pkg. 12s, Bot. 30s. *otc.*
Use: Analgesic.

• **prodolic acid.** (PRO-dole-ik Acid) USAN.
Use: Anti-inflammatory.

Pro-Est. (Burgin-Arden) Progesterone 25 mg, estrogenic substance 25,000 IU, sodium carboxymethylcellulose 1 mg, sodium Cl 0.9%, benzalkonium Cl 1:10,000, sodium phosphate dibasic 0.1% in water. *Rx.*
Use: Progestin, estrogen combination.

• **profadol hydrochloride.** (PRO-fah-dahl) USAN.
Use: Analgesic.

profamina.
See: Amphetamine (Various Mfr.).

Profasi. (Serono Labs) Chorionic gonadotropin 5000 units or 10,000 units/Vial. Vial 10 ml. *Rx.*
Use: Chorionic gonadotropin.

Profenal. (Alcon) Suprofen 1% soln. Drop-Tainer 2.5 ml. *Rx.*
Use: Nonsteroidal anti-inflammatory, ophthalmic.

Profen LA. (Wakefield) Phenylpropanolamine HCl 75 mg, guaifenesin 600 mg/ TR Tab. Dye free. Bot. 100s. *Rx.*
Use: Decongestant, expectorant.

Profen II. (Wakefield) Phenylpropanolamine HCl 37.5 mg, guaifenesin 600 mg/TR Tab. Dye free. Bot. 100s. *Rx.*
Use: Decongestant, expectorant.

Professional Care Lotion, Extra Strength. (Walgreen) Zinc oxide 0.25% in a lotion base. Bot. 16 oz. *otc.*
Use: Astringent, antiseptic, skin protectant.

Profiber Liquid. (Sherwood) Sodium caseinate, dietary fiber from soy, calcium caseinate, hydrolyzed cornstarch,

corn oil, soy lecithin, vitamins A, B_1, B_2, B_3, B_5, B_6, B_{12}, C, D, E, K, folic acid, biotin, choline, Ca, Cl, Cr, Cu, Fe, I, Mg, Mn, Mo, P, Se, Zn. Can 250 ml, closed system 1000 ml. *otc.*
Use: Nutritional supplement.

Profilate HP. (Alpha Therapeutics) A stable freeze-dried concentrate of Antihemophilic Factor VIII: C (Human) suspended in heptane and heated. Inj. Vial. 10, 25 ml. *Rx.*
Use: Antihemophilic.

Profilinine Heat-Treated. (Alpha Therapeutics) Dried plasma fraction of coagulation factors II, VII, IX and X. Heparin free. Vial, single dose with diluent. *Rx.*
Use: Antihemophilic.

Profilnine SD. (Alpha Therapeutics) Dried plasma fraction of coagulation factors II, VII, IX and X. Heparin free. Solvent detergent treated. Inj. Single dose vials with diluent. *Rx.*
Use: Antihemophilic.

proflavine.
Use: Topical, antiseptic.

proflavine dihydrochloride. 3,6-Diaminoacridine dihydrochloride.

proflavine sulfate. 3,6-Diaminoacridine sulfate.

Profree/GP Weekly Enzymatic Cleaner. (Allergan) Papain, sodium Cl, sodium borate, sodium carbonate, edetate disodium. Kit 16s or 24s with vials. *otc.*
Use: Rigid gas permeable contact lens care.

•**progabide.** (pro-GAB-ide) USAN.
Use: Anticonvulsant, muscle relaxant.

Progens Tabs. (Major) Conjugated estrogens. **0.625 mg/Tab.:** Bot. 100s, 1000s; **1.25 mg/Tab.:** Bot. 1000s; **2.5 mg/ Tab.:** Bot. 100s, 1000s. *Rx.*
Use: Estrogen.

Pro-Gesic. (Nastech) Trolamine salicylate 10%, propylene glycol, methylparahydroxybenzoic acid, propyl parahydroxybenzoic acid, EDTA. Liq. Bot. 75 ml. *otc.*
Use: Rub/liniment.

Progestasert. (Alza) T-shaped intrauterine device (IUD) unit containing a reservoir of progesterone 38 mg with barium sulfate dispersed in medical grade silicone fluid. In 6s w/inserter. *Rx.*
Use: Contraceptive, progestin.

•**progesterone,** (pro-JESS-ter-ohn) U.S.P. 23. Flavolutan, Luteogan, Luteosan, Lutren.
Use: Progestin. [Orphan drug]

W/Aqueous. Susp.
See: Prorone, Inj. (Sig).
W/In Oil
See: Femotrone, Inj. (Bluco).
Lipo-Lutin, Amp. (Parke-Davis).
Progestin, Vial (Various Mfr.).
Prorone, Inj. (Sig).
W/Estradiol, testosterone, procaine HCl, procaine base.
See: Hormo-Triad, Vial (Bell).
W/Estrogenic substance.
See: Profoygen Aqueous (Foy).
Progex, Inj. (Pasadena Research).

progesterone. (Various Mfr.) Pow. 1 g, 10 g, 25 g, 100 g.
Use: Progestin.

progesterone in oil. (Various Mfr.) 50 mg/ml. In sesame or peanut oil with benzyl alcohol. Inj. Vial 10 ml. *Rx.*
Use: Progestin.

progesterone intrauterine contraceptive system.
Use: Contraceptive.

progestin. Progesterone (Various Mfr.).
See: Hydroxyprogesterone.
Medroxyprogesterone.
Megestrol.
Norethindrone.

•**proglumide.** (pro-GLUE-mid) USAN. (Wallace).
Use: Anticholinergic.

Proglycem. (Baker Norton) **Cap.:** Diazoxide 50 mg/Cap. Bot. 100s. **Oral Susp.:** Diazoxide 50 mg/ml. Bot. 30 ml w/calibrated dropper. *Rx.*
Use: Glucose elevating agent.

Prograf. (Fujisawa) **Cap.:** Tacrolimus 1 mg or 5 mg. Bot. 100s; **Inj.:** Tacrolimus 5 mg/ml. In 1 ml amps (10s). *Rx.*
Use: Immunosuppressant.

proguanil hydrochloride.
See: Chloroguanide Hydrochloride.
Paludrine, Tab. (Wyeth-Ayerst).

ProHance. (Bracco) Gadoteridol 279.3 mg, calteridol calcium 0.23 mg, tromethamine 1.21 mg/ml. Inj. Vials. 15 ml, 30 ml. *Rx.*
Use: Radiopaque agent.

ProHIBIT. (Pasteur-Merieux-Connaught) Purified capsular polysaccharide of *Haemophilus influenzae* type b 25 mcg, conjugated diphtheria toxoid protein 18 mcg/0.5 ml dose. Also called PRP-D. Inj. Vial 0.5 ml, 2.5 ml, 5 ml. Syr. 0.5 ml. *Rx.*
Use: Agent for immunization.

•**proinsulin human.** (PRO-in-suh-LIN HYOO-muhn) USAN.
Use: Antidiabetic.

Prolactin RIA. (Abbott Diagnostics) Quantitative measurement of total circulating human prolactin. Test unit 50s, 100s.
Use: Diagnostic aid.

Prolactin RIAbead. (Abbott Diagnostics) Radioimmunoassay for the quantitative measurement of prolactin in human serum and plasma.
Use: Diagnostic aid.

proladyl. Pyrrobutamine. 1-Pyrrolidyl-3-phenyl-4-(p-chlorophenyl)-2-butene phosphate.
Use: Antihistamine.

prolase. Proteolytic enzyme from *Carica papaya*.
See: Papain.

Prolastin. (Bayer) Alpha$_1$-proteinase inhibitor ≥ 20 mg alpha$_1$-PI/ml when reconstituted. W/polyethylene glycol, sucrose and small amounts of other plasma proteins. Inj. Vial, single dose. *Rx.*
Use: Alpha$_1$-proteinase inhibitor.

Proleukin. (Chiron) Aldesleukin, interleukin-2. Pow. for Inj. 22 million IU (1.3 mg)/vial.
Use: Cancer therapy.

•**proline,** (PRO-leen) U.S.P. 23.
Use: Amino acid.

•**prolintane hydrochloride.** (pro-LIN-tane) USAN.
Use: Antidepressant.

Prolixin. (Bristol-Myers) Fluphenazine HCl. **Tab.:** 1 mg. Bot. 50s, 500s; 2.5 mg. w/tartrazine. Bot. 50s, 500s; 5 mg. w/tartrazine. Bot. 500s, UD 100s; 10 mg. w/tartrazine. Bot. 50s, 500s. **Elixir:** 0.5 mg/ml, alcohol 14%. Dropper Bot. 60 ml. Bot. pt. **Inj.:** 2.5 mg/ml. Vial 10 ml w/methyl and propyl parabens. Unimatic syringe 1 ml, Single dose syringe 25 mg/ml. 10s. *Rx.*
Use: Antipsychotic.

Prolixin Concentrate. (Bristol-Myers) Fluphenazine HCl 5 mg/ml, alcohol 14%. Bot. 120 ml w/dropper. *Rx.*
Use: Antipsychotic.

Prolixin Decanoate. (Bristol-Myers) Fluphenazine decanoate 25 mg/ml (in sesame oil with benzyl alcohol). Unimatic syringe 1 ml. Vial 5 ml. *Rx.*
Use: Antipsychotic.

Prolixin Enanthate. (Bristol-Myers) Fluphenazine enanthate 25 mg/ml (in sesame oil with benzyl alcohol). Vial 5 ml. *Rx.*
Use: Antipsychotic.

Proloprim. (Glaxo Wellcome) Trimethoprim 100 mg/Tab. Bot. 100s, UD 100s (in sesame oil with benzyl alcohol). *Rx.*
Use: Urinary anti-infective.

Promachlor. (Geneva Pharm) Chlorpromazine HCl 10 mg, 25 mg, 50 mg, 100 mg or 200 mg/Tab. Bot. 100s, 1000s. *Rx.*
Use: Antiemetic, antivertigo, antipsychotic.

•**promazine hydrochloride,** U.S.P. 23.
Use: Antipsychotic, ataraxic, anticholinergic.
See: Sparine, Tab., Inj. (Wyeth-Ayerst).

Promega. (Parke-Davis) Omega-3 (N-3) polyunsaturated fatty acids 1000 mg, containing EPA 350 mg, DHA 150 mg, vitamins E (3% RDA), A, B$_1$, B$_2$, B$_3$, Ca, Fe (< 2% RDA)/Cap., cholesterol and sodium free. Bot. 30s. *otc.*
Use: Vitamin/mineral supplement.

Promega Pearls. (Parke-Davis) EPA 168 mg, DHA 72 mg, < cholesterol 2 mg, E 1 IU, < 2% RDA of A, B$_1$, B$_2$, B$_3$, Fe, Ca. Cap. Bot. 60s, 90s. *otc.*
Use: Fish oil.

Prometa. (Muro) Metaproterenol sulfate 10 mg/5 ml, with saccharin and sorbitol, strawberry flavor. Syr. Bot. 480 ml. *Rx.*
Use: Bronchodilator.

Promethazine DM. (Various Mfr.) Promethazine HCl 6.25 mg, dextromethorphan HBr 15 mg/5 ml. Syr. Bot. 120 ml, pt, gal. *Rx.*
Use: Antitussive, antihistamine.

Prometh VC Plain Liquid. (Various Mfr.) Phenylephrine HCl 5 mg, promethazine HCl 6.25 mgm/5 ml. Liq. Bot. 120 ml, 473 ml, gal. *Rx.*
Use: Decongestant, antihistamine.

promethazine. (pro-METH-uh-zeen)
Use: Antihistamine; antiemetic, sedative.

promethazine hydrochloride with codeine. (pro-METH-uh-zeen) (Various Mfr.) Promethazine HCl 6.25 mg, codeine phosphate 10 mg/5 ml, alcohol 7%. Syr. Bot. 120 ml, pt, gal. *c-v.*
Use: Antihistamine, antitussive.

•**promethazine hydrochloride,** (pro-METH-uh-zeen) U.S.P. 23.
Use: Antihistamine, antiemetic.
See: Pentazine, Expectorant, Vial (Century).
Phenergan, Preps. (Wyeth-Ayerst).
Phenerject, Vial (Mayrand).
Prorex, Vial, Amp. (Hyrex).
Provigan, Inj. (Solvay).
Remsed, Tab. (DuPont).
Sigazine, Inj. (Sig).

promethazine hydrochloride w/combinations. (pro-METH-uh-zeen)
Use: Antihistamine, antiemetic, antivertigo.
See: Mepergan, Vial, Cap. (Wyeth-Ayerst).
Phenergan-D, Tab. (Wyeth-Ayerst).
Phenergan VC Expectorant (Wyeth-Ayerst).
Promethazine VC. (Rosemont) Promethazine HCl 6.25 mg, phenylephrine HCl 5 mg/5 ml. 120 ml, 240 ml, 473 ml, gal. *Rx.*
Use: Antihistamine, decongestant.
Promethazine VC with Codeine. (Rosemont) Promethazine HCl 6.25 mg, phenylephrine HCl 5 mg, codeine 10 mg/5 ml, alcohol 7%. Bot. 4 oz, pt, gal. *c-v.*
Use: Antihistamine, decongestant, antitussive.
Promethazine VC Plain. (Goldline) Phenylephrine HCl 5 mg, promethazine HCl 6.25 mg/5 ml. Syr. Bot. 473 ml. *Rx.*
Use: Decongestant, antihistamine.
promethestrol dipropionate.
Use: Estrogen.
See: Meprane Dipropionate, Tab. (Reed & Carnrick).
W/Phenobarbital.
See: Meprane-Phenobarbital, Tab. (Reed & Carnrick).
Prometol. (Viobin) Concentrated wheat germ oil. **3 min/Cap.:** Bot. 100s, 250s. **10 min/Cap.:** Bot. 100s. *otc.*
Use: Supplement.
prominal.
See: Mephobarbital.
Prominol. (MCR American Pharm) Butalbital 50 mg, acetaminophen 650 mg/Tab. Bot. 100s. *Rx.*
Use: Analgesic.
Promine. (Major) Procainamide 250 mg, 375 mg or 500 mg/Cap. Bot. 100s, 250s, 1000s, UD 100s (375 mg/Cap. w/500s instead of 250s). *Rx.*
Use: Antiarrhythmic.
Promine S.R. (Major) Procainamide. **SR Tab.:** 250 mg. Bot. 100s, 250s; 500 mg. Bot. 100s, 250s, 1000s; 750 mg. Bot. 100s, 250s. **SR Cap.:** 250 mg, 375 mg or 500 mg. *Rx.*
Use: Antiarrhythmic.
Promist HD. (Whitby) Hydrocodone bitartrate 2.5 mg, pseudoephedrine HCl 30 mg, chlorpheniramine maleate 2 mg/5 ml, alcohol 5%, menthol, saccharin, sorbitol. Bot. pt. *c-iii.*
Use: Antitussive, decongestant, antihistamine.

Promist LA. (Whitby) Pseudoephedrine HCl 120 mg, guaifenesin 500 mg/Tab. Bot. 100s. *Rx.*
Use: Decongestant, expectorant.
Promit. (Pharmacia & Upjohn) Dextran 1 150 mg/ml Inj. Vial 20 ml. *Rx.*
Use: Prevention of dextran allergic reactions.
Pro-Mix R.D.P. (Navaco) Protein 15 g (from whey protein), fat 0.8 g, carbohydrate 1 g, sodium 46 mg, potassium 165 mg, chloride 46 mg, calcium 73.6 mg, phosphorus 64.4 mg, iron 0.3 mg, Cr, Cu, Mg, Mn, Mo, Se, Zn, 72 Cal./5 Tbsp. (20 g). Pow. Packet 20 g, can 300 g. *otc.*
Use: Nutritional supplement.
Promod. (Ross) Protein supplement. Nine scoops provides protein 45 g, 100% U.S. RDA. Pow. Can 9.7 oz. *otc.*
Use: Nutritional supplement.
Promylin Enteric Coated Microzymes. (Shear/Kershman) Enteric coated pancrelipase. Lipase 4000 units, amylase 20,000 units, protease 25,000 units. *Rx.*
Use: Digestive enzymes.
Pro-Nasyl. (Progonasyl Co.) o-iodobenzoic acid 0.5%, triethanolamine 5.5% in a special neutral hydrophilic base compounded from oleic acid, mineral oil, vegetable oil. Bot. 15 ml, 60 ml.
Use: Treatment of sinusitis.
Pronemia Hematinic. (Lederle) Iron 115 mg, B_{12} 15 mcg, IFC 75 mg, C 150 mg, folic acid 1 mcg. Cap. Bot. 30s. *Rx.*
Use: Iron w/B_{12} and intrinsic factor.
Pronestyl. (Bristol-Myers) Procainamide. **Cap.:** 250 mg. Bot. 100s, 1000s; 375 mg. Bot. 100s; 500 mg. Bot. 100s, 1000s. **Inj.:** 100 mg/ml w/benzyl alcohol 0.9%, sodium bisulfite 0.09%. Vial 10 ml; 500 mg/ml w/methylparaben 0.1%, sodium bisulfite 0.2%. Vial 2 ml. **Tab.:** 250 mg. Bot. 100s, 1000s, Unimatic 100s; 375 mg. Bot. 100s; 500 mg. Bot. 100s, 1000s, Unimatic 100s. *Rx.*
Use: Antiarrhythmic.
Pronestyl-SR. (Bristol-Myers) Procainamide 500 mg/Tab. Bot. UD 100s. *Rx.*
Use: Antiarrhythmic.
pronethelol. (Zeneca) Adrenergic beta-receptor antagonist; pending release.
Pronto Concentrate Lice Killing Shampoo Kit. (Del Pharm) Pyrethrins 0.33%, piperonyl butoxide technical 4%. Bot. 2 oz, 4 oz. *otc.*
Use: Pediculicide.
Pronto Lice Killing Spray. (Del Pharm) Spray cans 5 oz. *otc.*

Use: Pediculicide for inanimate objects.

Propac. (Biosearch) Protein 3 g (from whey protein), carbohydrate 0.2 g, fat 0.3 g, chloride 3 mg, potassium 20 mg, sodium 9 mg, calcium 24 mg, phosphorus 12 mg, 16 Cal./Tbsp. (4 g). Pow. Packet 19.5 g, Can 350 g. *otc.*
Use: Nutritional supplement.

Propacet 100. (Lemmon) Propoxyphene napsylate 100 mg, acetaminophen 650 mg/Tab. Bot. 100s, 500s. *c-iv.*
Use: Narcotic analgesic combination.

propaesin. Propyl p-Aminobenzoate. (Various Mfr.).

•**propafenone hydrochloride,** (pro-pah-FEN-ohn) U.S.P. 23.
Use: Cardiac depressant (antiarrhythmic).
See: Rythmol, Tab. (Knoll).

Propagest Tablets. (Schwarz Pharma) Phenylpropanolamine HCl 25 mg/Tab. Bot. 100s. *otc.*
Use: Decongestant.

Propagon-S. (Spanner) Estrone 2 mg or 5 mg/ml. Vial 10 ml. *Rx.*
Use: Estrogen.

Propain HC. (Springbok) Acetaminophen 500 mg, hydrocodone bitartrate 5 mg/Cap. Bot. 100s, 500s. *c-iii.*
Use: Narcotic analgesic combination.

propamidine isethionate 0.1% ophthalmic soln. *Rx.*
Use: Acanthamoeba keratitis. [Orphan drug]

•**propane,** N.F. 18.
Use: Aerosol propellant.

propanediol diacetate, 1,2.
See: VoSol, Liq. (Wampole).

1,2,3-propanetriol, trinitrate. Nitroglycerin Tab., U.S.P. 23.

•**propanidid.** (pro-PAN-ih-did) USAN.
Use: Anesthetic (intravenous).

propanolol. Propranolol.

•**propantheline bromide,** (pro-PAN-thuh-leen) U.S.P. 23.
Use: Anticholinergic.
See: Pro-Banthine, Preps. (Searle).
W/Phenobarbital.
See: Probital, Tab. (Searle).
W/Thiopropazate dihydrochloride.
See: Pro-Banthine W/Dartal, Tab. (Searle).

PROPApH Cleansing Lotion for Normal/Combination Skin. (Del Pharm) Salicylic acid 0.5%, SD alcohol 40, EDTA. Lot. Bot. 180 ml. Pads. 45s. *otc.*
Use: Antiacne.

PROPApH Cleansing for Oily Skin. (Del Pharm) Salicylic acid 0.6%, SD alcohol 40, EDTA, menthol. Lot. Bot. 180 ml. *otc.*
Use: Antiacne.

PROPApH Cleansing for Sensitive Skin. (Del Pharm) Salicylic acid 0.5%, SD alcohol 40, aloe vera gel, EDTA, menthol. Pads. In 45s. *otc.*
Use: Antiacne.

PROPApH Cleansing Maximum Strength. (Del Pharm) Salicylic acid 2%, SD alcohol 40, aloe vera gel, EDTA, propylene glycol, menthol. Pads. In 45s. *otc.*
Use: Antiacne.

PROPApH Cleansing Pads. (Del Pharm) Salicylic acid 0.5%, SD alcohol 40, EDTA, menthol. Pads. 45s. *otc.*
Use: Antiacne.

PROPApH Foaming Face Wash. (Del Pharm.) Salicylic acid 2%, aloe vera gel, EDTA, menthol. Alcohol, oil and soap free. Liq. Bot. 180 ml. *otc.*
Use: Antiacne.

PROPApH Maximum Strength Acne Cream. (Del Pharm) Salicylic acid 2%, acetylated lanolin alcohol, cetearyl alcohol, stearyl alcohol, EDTA, menthol. Cream. Tube 19.5 g. *otc.*
Use: Antiacne.

PROPApH Medicated Acne Cream with Aloe. (Del Pharm) Salicylic acid 2%. Tube 1 oz. *otc.*
Use: Antiacne.

PROPApH Medicated Acne Stick with Aloe. (Del Pharm) Salicylic acid 2%. Stick 0.05 oz. *otc.*
Use: Antiacne.

PROPApH Medicated Cleansing Pads with Aloe. (Del Pharm) Salicylic acid 0.5%, SD alcohol 40 25%, aloe. Jar containing 45 pads. *otc.*
Use: Antiacne.

PROPApH Peel-Off Acne Mask. (Del Pharm) Salicylic acid 2%, tartrazine, parabens, polyvinyl alcohol, vitamin E acetate, SD alcohol 40. In 60 ml. *otc.*
Use: Antiacne.

PROPApH Skin Cleanser with Aloe. (Del Pharm) Salicylic acid USP 0.5%, SD alcohol 40 25%. Bot. 6 oz, 10 oz. *otc.*
Use: Antiacne.

•**proparacaine hydrochloride,** U.S.P. 23.
Use: Anesthetic (topical, ophthalmic).
See: Alcaine Ophthalmic Soln. (Alcon).
AK-Taine, Soln. (Akorn).
Fluoracaine, Soln. (Akorn).
Ophthaine HCl, Soln. (Squibb Mark).
Ophthetic, Ophthalmic Soln. (Allergan).

proparacaine hydrochloride. (Various Mfr.) 0.5% Soln. Bot. 2 ml, 15 ml, UD 1 ml.
Use: Anesthetic (topical, ophthalmic).
proparacaine hydrochloride & fluorescein sodium. (Pasadena) Proparacaine HCl 0.5%, fluorescein sodium 0.25%, thimerosal 0.01%, EDTA. Soln. Bot. 5 ml. Rx.
Use: Anesthetic (local, ophthalmic).
proparacaine hydrochloride/procaine hydrochloride.
Use: Anesthetic.
See: Ravocaine and novocain w/Levophed (Cook-Waite).
Ravocaine and novocain w/neocobefrin (Cook-Waite).
•propatyl nitrate. (PRO-pah-till) USAN. Investigational drug in U.S. but available in England.
Use: Coronary vasodilator.
propazolamide. (Lilly).
•propenzolate hydrochloride. (pro-PEN-zoe-late) USAN.
Use: Anticholinergic.
propesin. Name used for Risocaine.
Prophene 65. (Halsey) Propoxyphene HCl 65 mg/Cap. Bot. 100s, 500s, 1000s. c-iv.
Use: Narcotic analgesic.
prophenpyridamine.
See: Pheniramine (Various Mfr.).
prophenpyridamine maleate.
See: Pheniramine Maleate.
prophenpyridamine maleate w/combinations.
See: Panadyl, Tab., Cap. (Misemer).
Polyectin, Liq. (Amid).
Trimahist Elix., Liq. (Tennessee).
Vasotus, Liq. (Sheryl).
Pro-Phree. (Ross) Fat 31 g, carbohydrate 60 g, linoleic acid 2250 mg, Fe 11.9 mg, Na 250 mg, K 875 mg, with appropriate vitamins and minerals, 520 Cal/100 g. Protein free. Pow. Can 350 g. otc.
Use: Nutritional supplement.
Prophyllin. (Rystan) Sodium propionate 5%, chlorophyll derivatives 0.0125%. Tube 1 oz. Rx.
Use: Anti-infective, topical.
•propikacin. (PRO-pih-KAY-sin) USAN.
Use: Antibacterial.
Propimex-1. (Ross) Protein 15 g, fat 23.9 g, carbohydrate 46.3 g, linoleic acid 1800 mg, Fe 9 mg, Na 190 mg, K 675 mg, with appropriate vitamins and minerals, 480 Cal/100 g. Methionine and valine free. Pow. Can 350 g. otc.

Use: Nutritional supplement.
Propimex-2. (Ross) Protein 30 g, fat 15.5 g, carbohydrate 30 g, Fe 13 mg, Na 880 mg, K 1370 mg, with appropriate vitamins and minerals, 410 Cal/100 g. Methionine and valine free. Pow. Can 325 g. otc.
Use: Nutritional supplement for propionic or methylmalonic acidemia.
Propine Sterile Ophthalmic Solution. (Allergan) Dipivefrin HCl 0.1%. Soln. Bot. 5 ml, 10 ml, 15 ml. Rx.
Use: Agent for glaucoma.
propiodal.
See: Entodon.
•propiolactone. (PRO-pee-oh-LACK-tone) USAN.
Use: Disinfectant, sterilization of vaccines and tissue grafts.
•propiomazine. (PRO-pee-oh-MAY-zeen) USAN.
Dorevane; Indorm.
Use: Sedative (pre-anesthetic).
See: Largon, Amp. (Wyeth-Ayerst).
propiomazine. (PRO-pee-oh-MAY-zeen) USAN.
Use: Sedative.
See: Largon, Inj. (Wyeth-Ayerst).
propiomazine hydrochloride. (PRO-pee-oh-MAY-zeen)
Use: Sedative.
See: Largon, Inj. (Wyeth-Ayerst). Propion Gel (Wyeth-Ayerst).
•propionic acid, N.F. 18.
Use: Antimicrobial; pharmaceutic aid (acidifying agent).
W/Sodium propionate, docusate sodium, salicylic acid.
See: Prosal, Liq. (Gordon).
Propionate-Caprylate Mixtures.
propionyl erythromycin lauryl sulfate.
See: Erythromycin Propionate Lauryl Sulfate.
•propiram fumarate. (PRO-pih-ram) USAN.
Use: Analgesic.
propisamine.
See: Amphetamine (Various Mfr.).
propitocaine. Prilocaine.
See: Citanest, Soln., Vial, Amp. (Astra).
Proplex. (Baxter) Factor IX Complex (Human), clotting Factor II (prothrombin), VII (proconvertin), IX (PTC, antihemophilic factor B) and X (Stuart-Prower factor) all dried and concentrated. Vial 30 ml w/Diluent. Rx.
Use: Antihemophilic.
Proplex T. (Baxter) Factor IX complex, heat treated. W/Factors II, VII, IX and

X. W/heparin. Dried concentrate. Vial w/ diluent. *Rx.*
Use: Antihemophilic.

•**propofol.** (PRO-puh-FOLE) USAN.
Use: Anesthetic (intravenous).
See: Diprivan, Inj. (Zeneca).

Proponade Capsules. (Halsey) Chlorpheniramine maleate 8 mg, phenylpropanolamine HCl 50 mg, isopropamide 2.5 mg/Cap. Bot. 100s. *Rx.*
Use: Antihistamine, decongestant.

Propoquin. Amopyroquin HCl.
Use: Antimalarial.

propoxamide.

•**propoxycaine hydrochloride,** U.S.P. 23.
Use: Local anesthetic.

propoxycaine and procaine hydrochlorides and levonordefrin injection.
Use: Local anesthetic (dental).

propoxycaine and procaine hydrochlorides and norepinephrine bitartrate injection.
Use: Local anesthetic (dental).
See: Ravocaine and Novocain w/levophed, Inj. (Cook-Waite).

propoxychlorinol. Toloxychlorinol.

•**propoxyphene hydrochloride,** (pro-POX-ih-feen) U.S.P. 23.
Use: Analgesic.
See: Darvon, Pulvules (Lilly).
Dolene, Cap. (Lederle).
Progesic, Cap. (Ulmer).
SK-65, Cap. (SK-Beecham).

propoxyphene hydrochloride w/combinations.
Use: Analgesic.
See: Darvon Compound, Pulvule (Lilly).
Darvon Compound-65, Cap. (Lilly).
Darvon With A.S.A., Cap. (Lilly).
Dolene, AP-65, Tab. (Lederle).
Dolene Compound-65, Cap. (Lederle).
Wygesic, Tab. (Wyeth-Ayerst).

propoxyphene hydrochloride and acetaminophen tablets. (pro-POX-eefeen HIGH-droe-KLOR-ide & ass-cet-ah-MEE-noe-fen tablets)
Use: Analgesic.

propoxyphene hydrochloride and acetaminophen tablets. (Various Mfr.) Propoxyphene HCl 65 mg, acetaminophen 650 mg/Tab. Bot. 500s. *c-iv.*
Use: Analgesic.

propoxyphene hydrochloride and APC capsules.
Use: Analgesic.

propoxyphene hydrochloride, aspirin and caffeine capsules.
Use: Analgesic.

propoxyphene hydrochloride compound capsules. (Various Mfr.) Propoxyphene HCl 65 mg, aspirin 389 mg, caffeine 32.4/Cap. Bot. 100s, 500s. *c-iv.*
Use: Analgesic.

•**propoxyphene napsylate,** (pro-POX-ihfeen NAP-sill-ate) U.S.P. 23.
Use: Analgesic.
See: Darvocet-N (Lilly).
Darvon-N, Tab. (Lilly).
W/Acetaminophen.
See: Darvocet-N, Tab. (Lilly).

propoxyphene napsylate and acetaminophen tablets. (Various Mfr.) Propoxyphene napsylate 50 mg, acetaminophen 325 mg/Tab. Bot. 100s, 500s, 550s, 1000s, UD 100s. Propoxyphene napsylate 100 mg, acetaminophen 650 mg/Tab. Bot. 30s, 50s, 100s, 500s, 1000s, UD 100s. *c-iv.*
Use: Analgesic.

propoxyphene napsylate and aspirin tablets.
Use: Analgesic.

•**propranolol hydrochloride,** (pro-PRAN-oh-lahl) U.S.P. 23.
Use: Cardiac depressant (antiarrhythmic) antiadrenergic (beta-receptor).
See: Betachron E-R, Cap. (Inwood).
Inderal, Tab., Inj. (Wyeth-Ayerst).

propranolol hydrochloride. (Roxane) **Oral Soln.:** 20 mg or 40 mg/5 ml. Patient cups UD 5 ml (10s). **Concentrated Oral Soln.:** 80 mg/ml. Bot. 30 ml w/ calibrated dropper.
Use: Cardiac depressant (antiarrhythmic), antiadrenergic (β-receptor).

propranolol hydrochloride and hydrochlorothiazide tablets. (Various Mfr.) Propanolol HCl 40 mg or 80 mg, hydrochlorothiazide 25 mg/Tab. Bot. 100s, 1000s. *Rx.*
Use: Antihypertensive.
See: Inderide, Tab. (Wyeth-Ayerst).

Propranolol Hydrochloride Intensol. (Roxane) Propranolol HCl 80 mg/ml concentrated oral soln. Bot. 30 ml with dropper. *Rx.*
Use: Beta-adrenergic blocking agent.

Propulsid. (Janssen) Cisapride. **Tab.:** 10 mg or 20 mg, lactose. Bot. 100s, 500s (10 mg only). **Susp.:** 1 mg/ml, parabens, sorbitol. Bot. 450 ml. *Rx.*
Use: Treatment of heartburn.

propyl p-aminobenzoate. (Various Mfr.) Propaesin.
Use: Local anesthetic.
W/Procaine base, benzyl alcohol, phenol.

See: Rectocaine, Vial (Moore-Kirk).

- **propylene carbonate, N.F. 18.**
  Use: Pharmaceutic aid (gelling agent).
- **propylene glycol, U.S.P. 23.**
  Use: Pharmaceutic aid (humectant, solvent, suspending agent).
- **propylene glycol alginate, N.F. 18.**
  Use: Pharmaceutic aid (suspending, viscosity-increasing agent).
- **propylene glycol diacetate, N.F. 18.**
  Use: Pharmaceutic aid (solvent).
- **propylene glycol monostearate, N.F. 18.**
  Use: Pharmaceutic aid (emulsifying agent).
- **propyl gallate, N.F. 18.**
  Use: Pharmaceutic aid (antioxidant).
- **propylhexedrine, U.S.P. 23.**
  Use: Adrenergic (vasoconstrictor), appetite suppressant, antihistamine.
  See: Benzedrex, Inhalant (SK-Beecham Prods).
- **propyliodone, U.S.P. 23.**
  Use: Diagnostic aid (radiopaque medium).
  See: Dionosil Oily (Glaxo).
- **propylnoradrenaline-iso.**
  See: Isoproterenol.
- **propylparaben,** (pro-pill-PAR-ah-ben) N.F. 18. Propyl Chemosept (Chemo Puro).
  Use: Pharmaceutic aid (antifungal agent).
- **propylparaben sodium,** (pro-pill-PAR-ah-ben) N.F. 18.
  Use: Pharmaceutic aid (antimicrobial preservative).
- **propylthiouracil,** (pro-puhl-thigh-oh-YOU-rah-sill) U.S.P. 23.
  Use: Thyroid inhibitor.
- **propylthiouracil.** (Abbott) 50 mg/Tab. Bot. 100s, 1000s. (Lilly) 50 mg/Tab. Bot. 100s, 1000s. (Lederle) 50 mg/Tab. Bot. 100s, 1000s. 50 mg/Tab. Bot. 100s, 1000s, UD 100s.
  Use: Thyroid inhibitor.
- **proquazone.** (PRO-kwah-zone) USAN.
  Use: Anti-inflammatory.
- **prorenoate potassium.** (pro-REN-oh-ate) USAN.
  Use: Aldosterone antagonist.

Prorex. (Hyrex) promethazine HCl 25 mg or 50 mg/ml. Vial 10 ml. *Rx.*
  Use: Antihistamine, antiemetic/antivertigo.

Prorone. (Sig) Progesterone 25 mg/ml. Aqueous or oil susp. Vial 10 ml. *Rx.*
  Use: Progestin.

- **proroxan hydrochloride.** (pro-ROCK-san) USAN. *Formerly Pyrroxane, Pirrousan.*
  Use: Anti-adrenergic (α-receptor).

Proscar. (Merck) Finasteride 5 mg/Tab. Unit-of-use 30s, 100s, UD 100s. *Rx.*
  Use: Androgen inhibitor.

- **proscillaridin.** (pro-sih-LARE-ih-din) USAN. Talusin, Tradenal.
  Use: Cardiotonic.

Prosed/DS. (Star) Methenamine 81.6 mg, phenyl salicylate 36.2 mg, methylene blue 10.8 mg, benzoic acid 9 mg, atropine sulfate 0.06 mg, hyoscyamine sulfate 0.06 mg. Tab. Bot. 100s, 1000s. *Rx.*
  Use: Urinary anti-infective.

Pro Skin. (Marlyn) Vitamins A 6250 IU, E 100 IU, C 100 mg, B_5 10 mg, zinc 10 mg, Se/Cap. Bot, 60s. *otc.*
  Use: Vitamin/mineral supplement.

ProSobee. (Bristol-Myers) Milk free formula supplies 640 cal./qt, protein 19.2 g, fat 34 g, carbohydrate 64 g, vitamins A 2000 IU, D 400 IU, E 20 IU, C 52 mg, folic acid 100 mcg, B_1 0.5 mg, B_2 0.6 mg, niacin 8 mg, B_6 0.4 mg, B_{12} 2 mcg, biotin 50 mcg, pantothenic acid 3 mg, K-1 100 mcg, choline 50 mg, inositol 30 mg, calcium 600 mg, phosphorus 475 mg, iodine 65 mcg, iron 12 mg, magnesium 70 mg, copper 0.6 mg, zinc 5 mg, manganese 1.6 mg, chloride 530 mg, potassium 780 mg, sodium 230 mg/Qt. (20 Kcal/fl oz). Concentrated liq. can 13 fl oz; Ready-to-use liq. can 8 fl oz, 32 fl oz. Pow., can 14 oz. *otc.*
  Use: Nutritional supplement.

ProSobee Concentrate. (Bristol-Myers) P-soy protein isolate, l-methionine. CHO. corn syrup solids, soy and coconut oil, lecithin, mono- and diglycerides. Protein 20.3 g, CHO 65.4 g, fat 33.6 g, iron 12 mg, 640 cal./serving. Concentrate 390 ml. *otc.*
  Use: Nutritional supplement.

Pro-Sof Plus. (Vangard) Docusate sodium 100 mg, casanthranol 30 mg/Cap. Bot. 100s, 1000s, UD 32s, 100s. *otc.*
  Use: Laxative.

Pro-Sof w/Casanthranol SG. (Vangard) Casanthranol 30 mg, docusate sodium 100 mg/Cap. Bot. 100s, 1000s.
  Use: Laxative.

Prosom. (Abbott) Estazolam 1 mg or 2 mg/Tab. Bot. 100s, UD 100s. *c-iv.*
  Use: Sedative, hypnotic.

prostaglandins.
Use: Abortifacient, agent for impotence, agent for cervical ripening, patent ductus arteriosis.
See: Caverject, Inj. (Pharmacia & Upjohn).
Cervidil, Inj. (Forest).
Hemabate, Inj. (Pharmacia & Upjohn).
Prepidil , Gel. (Pharmacia & Upjohn).
Prostin E2, Supp. (Pharmacia & Upjohn).
Prostin VR Pediatric, Inj. (Pharmacia & Upjohn).

prostaglandin E₁.
See: Alprostadil.

prostaglandin E₂.
See: Dinoprostone.

•**prostalene.** (PRAHST-ah-leen) USAN.
Use: Prostaglandin.

Prostaphlin Capsules. (Bristol-Myers) Sodium oxacillin 250 mg or 500 mg/ Cap. Bot. 48s, 100s, Dosatrol Pack 100s. *Rx.*
Use: Anti-infective, penicillin.

Prostaphlin for Injection. (Bristol-Myers) Crystalline oxacillin sodium 250 mg, 500 mg, 1 g, 2 g or 4 g/dry filled Vial. Piggyback vial 1 g, 2 g, Bulk vial 10 g. *Rx.*
Use: Anti-infective, penicillin.

Prostaphlin Oral Solution. (Bristol-Myers) Sodium oxacillin reconstituted for oral soln. 250 mg/5 ml. Bot. 100 ml, Dosa-Trol Pack 25s. *Rx.*
Use: Anti-infective, penicillin.

ProstaScint. (Cytogen) Pendetide 0.5 mg for conjugation w/indium-111. Kit.
Use: Radioimmunoscintigraphy.

ProStep. (Lederle) Transdermal nicotine 11 or 22 mg/day. Patch 7s. *Rx.*
Use: Smoking deterrent.

Prostigmin. (Zeneca) Injectable neostigmine methylsulfate. **1:1000:** 1 mg/ml w/ phenol 0.45%. Vial 10 ml. Box 10s.
1:2000: 0.5 mg/ml. Amp. 1 ml w/methyl and propylparabens 0.2%. Box 10s.
Vial 10 ml w/phenol 0.45%. Box 10s.
1:4000: 0.25 mg/ml Amp. 1 ml w/methyl and propylparabens 0.2%. Box 10s.
Rx.
Use: Cholinergic muscle stimulant.

Prostigmin Bromide Tablets. (Zeneca) Neostigmine bromide 15 mg/Tab. Bot. 100s, 1000s. *Rx.*
Use: Cholinergic muscle stimulant.

Prostin E2. (Pharmacia & Upjohn) Dinoprost 20 mg. Supp. Containers of 1 each. *Rx.*
Use: Abortifacient.

Prostin VR Pediatric. (Pharmacia & Upjohn) Alprostadil 500 mcg/ml. Amp. 1 ml. *Rx.*
Use: Agent for patent ductus arteriosus.

Prostonic. (Seatrace) Thiamine HCl 10 mg, alanine 130 mg, glutamic acid 130 mg, amino-acetic acid 130 mg/Cap. Bot. 100s. *Rx.*
Use: Palliative relief of benign prostatic hypertrophy

Protabolin. (Pasadena Research) Methandriol dipropionate 50 mg/ml. Vial 10 ml. *Rx.*
Use: Hormone.

•**protamine sulfate,** (PRO-tuh-meen) U.S.P. 23.
Use: Antidote to heparin.

protamine sulfate. (Lilly) Amp. 1%, 5 ml; 1s, 25s; 25 ml 6s.
Use: Antidote to heparin.

Protar Protein. (Dermol) Coal tar 5%. Odor free. Shampoo. Bot. 120 ml. *otc.*
Use: Antiseborrheic.

protargin mild.
See: Silver Protein, Mild (Various Mfr.).

Protargol. (Sterwin) Strong silver protein. Pow. Bot. 25 g. *Rx.*
Use: Topical silver antiseptic.

protease.
W/Pancreatin, amylase.
See: Dizymes, Cap. (Recsei).
W/Vitamins B₁, B₁₂.
See: Arcoret, Tab. (Arco).
W/Vitamins B₁, B₁₂, iron.
See: Arcoret W/Iron, Tab. (Arco).

Protectol Medicated Powder. (Daniels) Calcium undecylenate 15%. Bot. 2 oz. *otc.*
Use: Diaper rash product.

Protegra Softgels. (Lederle) Vitamins E 200 IU, C 250 mg, beta carotene 3 mg, zinc 7.5 mg, copper, selenium, manganese. Cap. Bot. 50s. *otc.*
Use: Vitamin supplement.

proteinase inhibitor, alpha 1.
See: Prolastin (Bayer).

protein c concentrate. *Rx.*
Use: Protein C deficiency. [Orphan drug]

•**protein hydrolysate injection,** U.S.P. 23.
Use: Fluid and nutrient replenisher.
See: Amigen, Inj. (Baxter Lab.).
Aminogen, Amp., Vial (Christina).
Lacotein, Vial (Christina).
Travamin, Inj. (Baxter).
Virex, Inj. (Burgin-Arden).

protein hydrolysates oral.

Use: Enteral nutritional supplement.
See: Lofenalac, Pow. (Bristol-Myers).
Nutramigen, Pow. (Bristol-Myers).
Pregestimil, Pow. (Bristol-Myers).
Stuart Amino Acids, Pow. (Stuart).
W/Vitamin B_{12}.
See: Stuart Amino Acids and B_{12}, Tab. (Stuart).
Protenate. (Baxter) Plasma protein fraction (Human) 5%. Inj. Vial 250 ml, 500 ml w/administration set. *Rx.*
Use: Plasma protein fraction.
proteolytic enzymes.
See: Papase, Tab. (Parke-Davis).
Vardase, Prods. (Lederle). W/Amylolytic enzyme, cellulolytic enzyme, lipolytic enzyme.
See: Arco-Lase, Tab. (Arco).
Kutrase, Cap. (Kremers-Urban).
Kuzyme, Cap. (Kremers-Urban).
Zymme, Cap. (Scrip). W/Amylolytic enzyme, lipolytic enzyme, cellulolytic enzyme, belladonna extract.
See: Mallenzyme, Tab. (Roberts).
W/Amylolytic, cellulolytic enzymes, lipase, phenobarbital, hyoscyamine sulfate, atropine sulfate.
See: Arco-Lipase Plus, Tab. (Arco).
W/Amylolytic enzyme, homatropine methylbromide, d-sorbitol. (Papain).
See: Converzyme, Liq. (Ascher).
W/Calcium carbonate, glycine, amylolytic and cellulolytic enzymes.
See: Co-Gel, Tab. (Arco).
W/Neomycin palmitrate, hydrocortisone acetate, water-miscible base.
See: Biozyme, Oint. (Centeon).
Prothers. (ICN) Soap Free. White petrolatum, disodium cocamido MIPA-sulfosuccinate, pentane, ammonium laureth sulfate, PEG-150 distearate, hydroxypropyl methylcellulose, imidazolidinyl urea, parabens, propylene glycol stearate, hydrogenated soy glyceride, sodium stearyl lactylate. Liq. Bot. 180 ml. *otc.*
Use: Skin cleanser.
prothipendyl hydrochloride.
Use: Sedative.
Proticuleen. (Spanner) Vitamin B_{12} activity 10 mcg, folic acid 10 mg, B_{12} crystalline 50 mcg, niacinamide 75 mg/ml. Multiple dose vial 10 ml. I.M. inj. *Rx.*
Use: Parenteral nutritional supplement.
•**protirelin.** (PRO-tie-reh-lin) USAN. *Formerly Lopremone.*
Use: Prothyrotropin.
See: Thypinone, Inj. (Abbott).
protirelin. (Whitby) *Rx.*
Use: Prevention of infant respiratory distress syndrome. [Orphan drug]
Protopam Chloride. (Wyeth-Ayerst)
Hospital package: Six 20 ml vials of 1 g each of sterile Protopam Cl powder, without diluent or syringe. *Rx.*
Use: Antidote.
Protosan. (Recsei) Protein 87.5%, lactose 0.5%, fat 1.3%, ash 3.5%, sodium 0.02%. Jar 1 lb, 5 lb. *otc.*
Use: Nutritional supplement.
Prot-O-Sea. (Barth's) Protein 90%, containing amino acids and minerals. Bot. 100s, 500s. *otc.*
Use: Nutritional supplement.
Protostat. (Ortho) Metronidazole 250 mg or 500 mg/Tab. **250 mg:** Bot. 100s. **500 mg:** Bot. 50s. *Rx.*
Use: Anti-infective.
protoveratrine A.
See: Pro-Amid, Tab. (Amid).
protoveratrines a & b maleate.
Protran Plus. (Vangard) Meprobamate 150 mg, ethoheptazine citrate 75 mg, aspirin 250 mg/ Tab. Bot. 100s. 500s. *Rx.*
Use: Antianxiety, analgesic combination.
•**protriptyline hydrochloride,** (pro-TRIP-tih-leen) U.S.P. 23.
Use: Antidepressant.
See: Vivactil, Tab. (Merck).
Protropin. (Genentech) Somatrem. Vial 5 mg (13 IU), 10 mg (26 IU). Contains 2 vials somatrem and 2 10 ml vials diluent. *Rx.*
Use: Growth hormone.
Protuss. (Horizon) Hydrocodone bitartrate 5 mg, potassium guaiacolsulfonate 300 mg/5 ml, saccharin, sorbitol. Alcohol free. Liq. Bot. 20 ml, 120 ml, 480 ml. *c-III.*
Use: Antitussive, expectorant.
Protuss-D. (Horizon) Hydrocodone bitartrate 5 mg, pseudoephedrine HCl 30 mg, potassium guaiacolsulfonate 300 mg/5 ml. Alcohol free, dye free. Liq. Bot. 120 ml, 480 ml. *c-III.*
Use: Antitussive, decongestant, expectorant.
Proval #3. (Solvay) Acetaminophen 325 mg, codeine phosphate 30 mg/Tab. Bot. 100s, 500s. *c-III.*
Use: Narcotic analgesic combination.
Proventil. (Schering-Plough) Albuterol sulfate 2 mg or 4 mg/Tab. Bot. 100s, 500s. *Rx.*
Use: Bronchodilator.
Proventil HFA. (Key) Albuterol 90 mcg per actuation/Aerosol. Can. 6.7 g/200 inhalations). *Rx.*

Use: Bronchodilator.

Proventil Inhaler. (Schering-Plough) Metered dose aerosol unit containing albuterol in propellants. Each actuation delivers 90 mcg of albuterol. Canister 17 g with oral adapter. Box 1s. *Rx.*
Use: Bronchodilator.

Proventil Repetabs. (Schering-Plough) Albuterol 4 mg, lactose/Tab. Bot. 100s, 500s. *Rx.*
Use: Bronchodilator.

Proventil Solution. (Schering-Plough) Albuterol sulfate solution. **0.5%:** Albuterol sulfate 6 mg/ml. Bot. 20 ml. Box 1s. **0.083%:** Albuterol sulfate 0.83 mg/ml. Bot. 3 ml. Box 100s. *Rx.*
Use: Bronchodilator.

Proventil Syrup. (Schering-Plough) Albuterol sulfate 2 mg/5 ml. Bot. 16 oz. *Rx.*
Use: Bronchodilator.

Provera. (Pharmacia & Upjohn) Medroxyprogesterone acetate 2.5 mg, 5 mg or 10 mg/Tab. **2.5 mg:** Bot. 25s. **5 mg:** Bot. 25s, 100s. **10 mg:** Bot. 25s, 100s, Dosepak 10s. *Rx.*
Use: Progestin.

Provocholine. (Roche) Methacholine Cl for inhalation 100 mg/5 ml for reconstitution. Vial 5 ml. *Rx.*
Use: Diagnostic aid.

Prox/APAP. (UAD Labs) Propoxyphene HCl 65 mg, acetaminophen 650 mg/Tab. Bot. 100s, 500s. *c-IV.*
Use: Narcotic analgesic combination.

•**proxazole.** (PROX-ah-zole) USAN.
Use: Smooth muscle relaxant, analgesic, anti-inflammatory.

•**proxazole citrate.** (PROX-ah-zole) USAN.
Use: Relaxant (smooth muscle), analgesic, anti-inflammatory.

•**proxicromil.** (prox-ih-KROE-mill) USAN.
Use: Antiallergic.

Proxigel. (Reed & Carnrick) Carbamide peroxide 10% in a water free gel base. Tube 34 g w/applicator. *otc.*
Use: Antiseptic, cleanser.

•**proxorphan tartrate.** (PROX-ahr-fan TAR-trate) USAN.
Use: Analgesic; antitussive.

Proxy 65. (Parmed) Propoxyphene HCl 65 mg, acetaminophen 650 mg/Tab. Bot. 100s, 500s. *c-IV.*
Use: Narcotic analgesic combination.

Prozac. (Dista) Fluoxetine HCl **Pulvules:** 10 mg or 20 mg Bot. 100s. **Liq.:** 20 mg/5 ml Bot. 120 ml. *Rx.*
Use: Antidepressant.

Prozine-50. (Roberts) Promazine HCl 50 mg/ml. Vial 10 ml.
Use: Antipsychotic.

Prudents. (Bariatric) Acetylphenylisatin 5 mg/Tab. Bot. 30s, 100s. Chewable protein and amino acid. *otc.*
Use: Laxative.

Prulet. (Mission) White phenolphthalein 60 mg/Tab. Strips 12s, 40s. *otc.*
Use: Laxative.

prune concentrate. W/cascarin.
See: Prucara, Tab. (ICN).

prune powder concentrated dehydrated.
See: Diacetyldihydroxyphenylisatin.
W/Cascara fluidextract aromatic and psyllium husk powder.
See: Casyllium, Pow. (Pharmacia & Upjohn).

Prurilo. (Whorton) Menthol 0.25%, phenol 0.25%, calamine lotion in special lubricating base. Bot. 4 oz, 8 oz. *otc.*
Use: Minor skin irritations.

Pseudo-Car DM. (Geneva Generics) Pseudoephedrine HCl 60 mg, carbinoxamine maleate 4 mg, dextromethorphan HBr 15 mg/5 ml, alcohol < 0.6%. Bot. pt, gal. *Rx.*
Use: Decongestant, antihistamine, antitussive.

Pseudo-Chlor. (Various Mfr.) Pseudoephedrine HCl 120 mg, chlorpheniramine maleate 8 mg/Cap. Bot. 100s, 250s. *Rx.*
Use: Decongestant, antihistamine.

•**pseudoephedrine hydrochloride,** (SUE-doe-eh-FED-rin) U.S.P. 23.
Use: Adrenergic (vasoconstrictor).
See: Cenafed, Tab., Syr. (Century).
D-Feda, Cap., Syr. (Dooner).
Novafed, Cap., Liq. (Hoechst Marion Roussel).
Sinufed, Cap. (Roberts).
Sudafed, Tab., Syr. (Glaxo Wellcome).
Sudafed S.A., Cap. (Glaxo Wellcome).
Ursinus, Inlay Tab. (Sandoz Consumer).

pseudoephedrine hydrochloride w/ combinations.
See: Actifed, Tab., Syr. (Glaxo Wellcome).
Actifed Allergy, Cap. (Glaxo Wellcome).
Ambenyl-D, Liq. (Hoechst Marion Roussel).
Anatuss DM, Syr., Tab. (Mayrand).
Atridine, Tab. (Interstate).
Banophen, Cap. (Major).
Brexin, Cap., Liq. (Savage).

Congestac, Tab. (SK-Beecham Prods).

CoTylenol, Tab. (McNeil).

CoTylenol Liquid Cold Formula (Mc-Neil).

Deconamine, Cap., Tab., Elix., Syr. (Berlex).

Dimacol, Cap., Liq. (Robins).

Dorcol, Prods. (Sandoz Consumer).

Fedrazil, Tab. (Glaxo Wellcome).

Isoclor, Preps. (DuPont Merck).

Kronofed-A, Cap. (Ferndale).

Mapap Cold Formula, Tab. (Major).

Maximum Strength Tylenol Flu, Tab. (McNeil-CPC).

Novafed A, Liq., Cap. (Hoechst Marion Roussel).

Novahistine Sinus, Tab. (Hoechst Marion Roussel).

Phenergan-D, Tab. (Wyeth-Ayerst).

Robitussin Cold & Cough, Cap. (Robins).

Robitussin-DAC, Liq. (Robins).

Robitussin-PE, Liq. (Robins).

Robitussin Severe Congestion, Cap. (Robins).

Rondec D, Drops; C, Tab.; S, Syr.; T, Filmtab (Ross).

Rondec DM, Drops, Syr. (Ross).

Sine-Aid IB, Cap. (McNeil-CPC).

Sine-Off, Prods. (SK-Beecham Prods).

Sudafed Plus, Tab., Syr. (Glaxo Wellcome).

Triphed, Tab. (Lemmon).

Tussafed Expectorant Liq. (Cavital).

Tylenol Cold Night Time, Liq. (McNeil-CPC).

Tyrodone, Liq. (Major).

pseudoephedrine hydrochloride and triprolidine hydrochloride. (Various Mfr.) Pseudoephedrine HCl 60 mg, triprolidine HCl 2.5 mg/Tab. Bot. 100s, 1000s, UD 100s. *Rx.*
Use: Decongestant, antihistamine.

•**pseudoephedrine polistirex.** (sue-doe-ee-FED-rin pahl-ee-STIE-rex) USAN.
Use: Nasal decongestant.

•**pseudoephedrine sulfate,** (sue-do-eh-FED-rin) U.S.P. 23.
Use: Bronchodilator.
See: Afrinol Repetabs (Schering-Plough).
W/Chlorpheniramine maleate.
See: Chlor-trimeton Decongestant, Tab. (Schering-Plough).
W/Dexbrompheniramine.
See: Disophrol Chronotabs, Tab. (Schering-Plough).
Drixoral S.A., Tab. (Schering-Plough).

W/Dexchlorpheniramine.
See: Polaramine Expectorant (Schering-Plough).

Pseudogest. (Major) Pseudoephedrine HCl 30 mg or 60 mg/Tab. Bot. 24s, 100s. *otc.*
Use: Decongestant.

Pseudogest Plus. (Major) Pseudoephedrine HCl 60 mg, chlorpheniramine maleate 4 mg/Tab. In 24s, 100s, 200s. *otc.*
Use: Decongestant, antihistamine.

Pseudo-Hist. (Holloway) Pseudoephedrine HCl 30 mg, chlorpheniramine maleate 10 mg/Cap. Bot. 100s. *otc.*
Use: Decongestant, antihistamine.

Pseudo-Hist Expectorant. (Holloway) Pseudoephedrine 15 mg, hydrocodone bitartrate 2.5 mg, guaifenesin 100 mg, alcohol 5%. Bot. 480 ml. *c-III.*
Use: Decongestant, antitussive, expectorant.

pseudomonas hyperimmune globulin (mucoid exopolysaccharide). *Rx.*
Use: Pulmonary infection in cystic fibrosis. [Orphan drug]

pseudomonas test.
Use: Urine test.
See: Isocult for *Pseudomonas aeruginosa* (SK-Beecham Diagnostics).

pseudomonic acid A.
Use: Topical anti-infective.
See: Bactroban (SK-Beecham).

Pseudo-Phedrine. (Whiteworth Towne) Pseudoephedrine HCl 30 mg/Tab. Bot. 100s, 1000s. *otc.*
Use: Decongestant.

Pseudo Plus. (Weeks & Leo) Pseudoephedrine HCl 60 mg, chlorpheniramine maleate 4 mg/Tab. Bot. 40s. *otc.*
Use: Decongestant, antihistamine.

Pseudo Syrup. (Major) Pseudoephedrine 30 mg/5 ml. Liq. Bot. 120 ml, pt, gal. *otc.*
Use: Decongestant.

psoralens.
See: Methoxsalen.
Trioxsalen.

Psor-A-Set. (Hogil) Salicylic acid 2%. Soap. Bar 97.5 g. *otc.*
Use: Keratolytic.

Psorcon. (Dermik) Diflorasone diacetate (0.05%) 0.5 mg/g. **Oint.:** Tube 15 g, 30 g, 60 g. **Cream:** Tube 15 g, 30 g, 60 g. *Rx.*
Use: Corticosteroid, topical.

Psorigel. (Galderma) Coal tar soln. 7.5%, alcohol 33% in hydroalcoholic gel vehicle. Tube 4 oz. *otc.*

Use: Tar-containing preparation.

Psorinail. (Summers) Coal tar solution w/ isopropyl alcohol 2.5%, 3-butylene glycol I, acetyl mandelic acid. Liq. Bot. 30 ml. *otc.*
Use: Antipsoriatic, topical.

Psorion Cream. (ICN) Betamethasone dipropionate 0.05%, mineral oil, white petrolatum, propylene glycol. Cream. Tube 15 g, 45 g. *Rx.*
Use: Topical corticosteroid.

psychotherapeutic agents.
See: Ataraxic Agents.
Tranquilizers.

psyllium granules.
Use: Laxative.
See: Perdiem Fiber, Gran. (Rhone-Poulenc Rorer Consumer).
W/Dextrose.
See: Muci-lax, Granules (Shionogi).
W/Senna.
See: Perdiem, Granules (Rhone-Poulenc Rorer Consumer).

•**psyllium husk,** U.S.P. 23.
Use: Laxative.
W/Cascara fluidextract aromatic, prune powder.
Use: Cathartic.
See: Casyllium, Pow. (Pharmacia & Upjohn).

psyllium hydrocolloid.
Use: Laxative.
See: Effersyllium, Pow. (Stuart).

psyllium hydrophilic mucilloid for oral suspension.
Use: Laxative.
See: Konsyl, Pow. (Lafayette).
Modane Versabran, Pow. (Pharmacia & Upjohn).
Mucillium, Pow. (Whiteworth Towne).
Mylanta Natural Fiber Supplement, Pow. (J & J-Merck).
Restore (Inagra).
W/Dextrose.
See: Hydrocil Plain (Solvay).
Konsyl-D Pow. (Lafayette).
V-lax, Pow. (Century).
W/Dextrose, casanthranol.
See: Hydrocil Fortified (Solvay).
W/Oxyphenisatin acetate.
See: Plova, Pow. (WEL).
W/Standardized senna concentrate.
See: Senokot w/Psyllium, Pow. (Purdue Frederick).

psyllium seed gel.
Use: Laxative.
W/Planta Ovata, gum Karaya, Brewer's yeast.
See: Plantamucin, Granules (ICN Pharm).

P.T.E.-4. (Fujisawa) Zinc 1 mg, copper 0.1 mg, chromium 1 mcg, manganese 25 mcg/ml. Vial 3 ml. *Rx.*
Use: Mineral supplement.

P.T.E.-5. (Fujisawa) Zinc 1 mg, copper 0.1 mg, chromium 1 mcg, manganese 25 mcg, selenium 15 mcg/ml. Vial 3 ml, 10 ml. *Rx.*
Use: Mineral supplement.

pteroic acid. The compound formed by the linkage of carbon 6 of 2-amine-4-hydroxypteridine by means of a methylene group with the nitrogen of p-aminobenzoic acid.

pteroylglutamic acid.
See: Folic Acid, Preps. (Various Mfr.).

pteroylmonoglutamic acid. Pteroylglutamic acid.
See: Folic Acid, Preps. (Various Mfr.).

PTFE. (Ethicon) Polytef.

PTU.
See: Propylthiouracil.

Pulmocare. (Ross) High-fat, low-carbohydrate liquid diet for pulmonary patients containing 1500 calories/Liter; 1420 calories provides 100% U.S. RDA vitamins and minerals. Calorie:Nitrogen ratio is 150:1. Osmolarity: 490 mosm/Kg water. Can 8 fl oz. *otc.*
Use: Nutritional supplement.

pulmonary surfactant replacement. (Scios Nova) *Rx.*
Use: Prevention & treatment of infant respiratory distress syndrome. [Orphan drug]

pulmonary surfactant replacement, porcine. *Rx.*
Use: Prevention/treatment of respiratory distress syndrome in premature infants. [Orphan drug]
See: Curosurf.

Pulmosin. (Spanner) Guaiacol 0.1 g, eucalyptol 0.08 g, camphor 0.05 g, iodoform 0.02 g/2 ml. Multiple dose vial 30 ml. Inj. I.M. *Rx.*

Pulmozyme. (Genentech) Dornase alfa 1 mg, calcium chloride dihydrate 0.15 mg, NaCl 8.77 mg/ml. Soln. for inhalation. Amps. Single-use 2.5 ml. *Rx.*
Use: Anti-infective.

•**pumice,** U.S.P. 23.
Use: Abrasive (dental).

punctum plug. (Eagle Vision) Silicone plug. 0.5 mm, 0.6 mm, 0.7 mm or 0.8 mm. Pkg. 2 plugs, one inserter tool. *Rx.*
Use: Punctal plug.

Pura. (D'Franssia) High potency vitamin E cream.
Use: Emollient.

Puralube. (Fougera) White petrolatum, light mineral oil. Oint. Tube 3.5 g. *otc.*
Use: Ophthalmic lubricant.

Puralube Tears. (Fougera) Polyvinyl alcohol 1%, polyethylene glycol 400 1%, EDTA, benzalkonium Cl. Soln. Bot. 15 ml. *otc.*
Use: Ophthalmic lubricant.

Purebrom Compound Elixir. (Purepac) Brompheniramine maleate 4 mg/5 ml, phenylephrine HCl, phenylpropanolamine HCl, alcohol. Bot. pt, gal. *Rx.*
Use: Antihistamine, decongestant.

Puresept Murine Saline. (Ross) **Disinfecting soln.:** Sterile hydrogen peroxide solution 3%, sodium stannate, sodium nitrate, phosphate buffers, thimerosal free. 237 ml. **Murine Saline Soln.:** Buffered isotonic solution w/borate buffers, NaCl, sorbic acid 0.1%, EDTA 0.1%. 60, 237, 355 ml. Includes cups and lens holder. *otc.*
Use: Soft contact lens care.

Purge Evacuant. (Fleming) Castor oil 95%. Bot. 1 oz, 2 oz. *otc.*
Use: Laxative.

Puri-Clens. (Sween) UD 2 oz. Bot. 8 oz.
Use: Wound deodorizer, cleanser.

purified oxgall.
See: Bile Extract, Ox (Various Mfr.).

purified protein derivative of tuberculin.
Use: Mantoux TB test.
See: Aplisol, Vial (Parke-Davis).
Aplitest, Jar (Parke-Davis).
Tubersol, Vial (Pasteur-Merieux-Connaught).

purified type II collagen.
Use: Juvenile rheumatoid arthritis. [Orphan drug]

Purinethol. (Glaxo Wellcome) Mercaptopurine 50 mg/Tab. Bot. 25s, 250s. *Rx.*
Use: Antineoplastic.

•**puromycin.** (PURE-oh-MY-sin) USAN.
Use: Antineoplastic; antiprotozoal (trypanosoma).

•**puromycin hydrochloride.** (PURE-oh-MY-sin) USAN.
Use: Antineoplastic; antiprotozoal (trypanosoma).

purple foxglove.
See: Digitalis, Preps. (Various Mfr.).

Purpose Shampoo. (Ortho Derm) Water, amphoteric-19, PEG-44 sorbitan laurate, PEG-150 distearate, sorbitan laurate, boric acid, fragrance, benzyl alcohol. Bot. 8 oz. *otc.*
Use: Shampoo.

Purpose Soap. (Johnson & Johnson) Sodium tallowate, sodium cocoate, glycerin, NaCl, BHT, EDTA. Bar 108 g, 180 g. *otc.*
Use: Skin cleanser.

Pursettes Premenstrual Tablets. (DEP Corp.) Acetaminophen 500 mg, pamabrom 25 mg, pyrilamine maleate 15 mg/Tab. Bot. 24s. *otc.*
Use: Analgesic, diuretic, antihistamine.

P.V. Carpine Liquifilm. (Allergan) Pilocarpine nitrate 1%, 2% or 4%, polyvinyl alcohol 1.4%, sodium acetate, sodium Cl, citric acid, menthol, camphor, phenol, eucalyptol, chlorobutanol 0.5%, purified water. Dropper bot. 15 ml. *Rx.*
Use: Agent for glaucoma.

PVP-I Ointment. (Day-Baldwin) Povidone-iodine. Tube 1 oz, Jar lb, Foilpac 1.5 g. *otc.*
Use: Antiseborrheic, antiseptic.

P-V-Tussin. (Solvay) Hydrocodone bitartrate 2.5 mg, pseudoephedrine HCl 30 mg, chlorpheniramine maleate 2 mg, alcohol 5%. Syrup. Bot. pt, gal. *c-III.*
Use: Antitussive, decongestant, antihistamine.

P-V-Tussin Tablets. (Solvay) Hydrocodone bitartrate 5 mg, phenindamine tartrate 25 mg, guaifenesin 200 mg/Tab. Bot. 100s. *c-III.*
Use: Antitussive, antihistamine, expectorant.

Py-Co-Pay Tooth Powder. (Block) Sodium Cl, sodium bicarbonate, calcium carbonate, magnesium carbonate, tricalcium phosphate, eugenol, methyl salicylate. Can 7 oz. *otc.*
Use: Dentifrice.

9-[3-pydidylmethyl]-9-deazaguanine. (Briocryst Pharm) *Rx.*
Use: Antineoplastic. [Orphan drug]

Pyma. (Forest Pharm) **TR Cap.:** Pyrilamine maleate 50 mg, chlorpheniramine maleate 6 mg, pheniramine maleate 20 mg, phenylephrine HCl 15 mg. Bot. 30s, 100s, 1000s. **Inj.:** Chlorpheniramine maleate 5 mg, phenylpropanolamine HCl 12.5 mg, atropine sulfate 0.2 mg/ml. Vial 10 ml. *Rx.*
Use: Antihistamine, decongestant, anticholinergic, antispasmodic.

Pyocidin-Otic Solution. (Forest) Hydrocortisone 5 mg, polymyxin B sulfate 10,000 USP units/ml in a vehicle containing water and propylene glycol. Bot. 10 ml w/sterile dropper. *Rx.*
Use: Corticosteroid, anti-infective otic.

•**pyrabrom.** USAN.
Use: Antihistamine.

Pyracol. (Davis & Sly) Pyrathyn HCl 0.08 g, ammonium Cl 0.778 g, citric acid 0.52 g, menthol 0.006 g/fl oz. Bot. pt.

pyradone.
See: Aminopyrine (Various Mfr.).

pyraminyl.
See: Pyrilamine Maleate (Various Mfr.).

pyranilamine maleate.
See: Pyrilamine Maleate, Preps. (Various Mfr.).

pyranisamine bromotheophyllinate.
See: Pyrabrom (Various Mfr.).

pyranisamine maleate.
See: Pyrilamine Maleate, Preps. (Various Mfr.).

•**pyrantel pamoate,** (pie-RAN-tell PAM-oh-ate) U.S.P. 23.
Use: Anthelmintic.
See: Antiminth, Oral Susp. (Pfizer Laboratories).
Pin-Rid, Cap., Liq. (Apothecary).
Pin-X, Liq. (Effcon).

•**pyrantel tartrate.** (pie-RAN-tell) USAN.
Use: Anthelmintic.

pyrathiazine hydrochloride.

•**pyrazinamide,** (peer-uh-ZIN-uh-mide) U.S.P. 23. Aldinamide, Zinamide.
Use: Antibacterial (tuberculostatic).

pyrazinamide. (Lederle) 500 mg/Tab. Bot. 500s.
Use: Antibacterial (tuberculostatic).

pyrazinecarboxamide. Pyrazinamide, U.S.P. 23.

•**pyrazofurin.** (pihr-AZZ-oh-FYOO-rin) USAN.
Use: Antineoplastic.

pyrazoline.
See: Antipyrine (Various Mfr.).

pyrbenzindole.
See: Benzindopyrine Hydrochloride (Various Mfr.).

•**pyrethrum extract,** U.S.P. 23.
Use: Pediculicide.

pyribenzamine.
See: PBZ, Prods. (Novartis).

pyricardyl.
See: Nikethamide, Inj. (Various Mfr.).

Pyridamole Tabs. (Major) Dipyridamole 25 mg, 50 mg or 75 mg/Tab. **25 mg:** Bot. 1000s, 2500s; **50 mg or 75 mg:** 100s, 1000s. Rx.
Use: Antianginal, antiplatelet.

Pyridate Tabs. (Major) Phenazopyridine 100 mg or 200 mg/Tab. Bot. 1000s. Rx.
Use: Urinary analgesic, anti-infective.

Pyridene. (Approved) Phenylazodiaminopyridine HCl 100 mg/Tab. Bot. 24s, 100s, 1000s. Rx.

Use: Urinary analgesic.

Pyridiate. (Rugby) Phenazopyridine HCl 100 mg/Tab. Bot. 100s. Rx.
Use: Urinary tract product.

pyridine-beta-carboxylic acid diethyl amide.
See: Nikethamide, Inj. (Various Mfr.).

Pyridium. (Parke-Davis) Phenazopyridine HCl 100 mg or 200 mg/Tab. Bot. 100s, 1000s, UD 100s. Rx.
Use: Urinary analgesic, anti-infective.
W/Hyoscyamine HBr, butabarbital.
See: Pyridium Plus, Tab. (Parke-Davis).

•**pyridostigmine bromide,** U.S.P. 23.
Use: Cholinergic.
See: Mestinon, Tab., Syr., Amp. (Roche).
Regonal (Organon).

Pyridox. (Oxford) **No. 1:** Pyridoxine HCl 100 mg/Tab. otc. **No. 2:** Pyridoxine HCl 200 mg/Tab. Bot. 100s. otc.
Use: Vitamin B_6 supplement.

pyridoxal. Vitamin B_6. otc.
Use: Vitamin B_6 supplement.

pyridoxamine. Vitamin B_6. otc.
Use: Vitamin B_6 supplement.
See: Pyridoxine.

•**pyridoxine hydrochloride,** (peer-ih-DOX-een) U.S.P. 23.
Use: Enzyme co-factor vitamin.
See: Hexa Betalin, Amp., Tab., Vial (Lilly).
Hexavibex, Vial (Parke-Davis).
Pan B_6, Tab. (Panray).

pyridoxol.
See: Pyridoxine, Vitamin B_6.

pyrilamine bromotheophyllinate.
See: Pyrabrom.
W/2-amino-2-methyl-1-propanol.
See: Bromaleate.

•**pyrilamine maleate,** U.S.P. 23.
Use: Antihistamine.

•**pyrimethamine,** U.S.P. 23.
Use: Antimalarial.
See: Daraprim, Tab. (Glaxo Wellcome).
W/Sulfadoxine.
See: Fansidar, Tab. (Roche).

Pyrinex Pediculicide. (Ambix) Pyrethrins 0.2%, piperonyl butoxide technical 2%, deodorized kerosene 0.8%. Shampoo. Bot. 118 ml. otc.
Use: Pediculicide.

•**pyrinoline.** (PIHR-ih-NO-leen) USAN.
Use: Cardiac depressant (antiarrhythmic).

pyrinyl. (Various Mfr.) Pyrethrins 0.2%, piperonyl butoxide technical 2%, deodorized kerosene 0.8%. Liq. Bot. 60, 120 ml. otc.

Use: Pediculicide.

Pyristan. (Arcum) Phenylephrine HCl 8 mg, phenylpropanolamine HCl 15 mg, chlorpheniramine maleate 3 mg, pyrilamine maleate 10 mg/Cap. Bot. 50s, 500s. Elix. Bot. 4 oz, pt, gal. *otc.*
Use: Decongestant, antihistamine.

pyrithen.
See: Chlorothen Citrate (Various Mfr.).

•**pyrithione sodium.** (PEER-ih-THIGH-ohn) USAN.
Use: Antimicrobial (topical).

•**pyrithione zinc.** (PEER-ih-THIGH-ohn) USAN. Zinc Omadine.
Use: Antibacterial, antifungal, antiseborrheic.
See: Danex Shampoo (Allergan Herbert).
Zincon Shampoo (Lederle).

Pyrogallic Acid Ointment. (Gordon) Pyrogallic acid 25%, chlorobutanol. Jar 1 oz, 1 lb.
Use: Verruca therapy.

pyrogallol. Pyrogallic acid.

Pyrohep Tabs. (Major) Cyproheptadine HCl 4 mg/Tab. Bot. 250s, 500s. *Rx.*
Use: Antihistamine.

pyrophenindane. (Bristol-Myers).

•**pyrovalerone hydrochloride.** (PIE-row-val-EH-rone) USAN.
Use: Central stimulant.

•**pyroxamine maleate.** (pihr-OX-ah-meen) USAN.
Use: Antihistamine.

•**pyroxylin,** U.S.P. 23. Soluble guncotton. Cellulose nitrate.
Use: Pharmaceutic necessity for Collodion.

pyrrobutamine phosphate, U.S.P. XXI.
Use: Antihistamine.
W/Clopane HCl, Histadyl.
See: Co-Pyronil, Preps. (Lilly).

•**pyrrocaine.** (PIHR-oh-cane) USAN.
Use: Local anesthetic.

pyrrocaine hydrochloride.
Use: Local anesthetic (dental).

pyrrocaine hydrochloride and epinephrine inj.
Use: Local anesthetic (dental).

•**pyrroliphene hydrochloride.** (pihr-OLE-ih-feen) USAN.
Use: Analgesic.

•**pyrrolnitrin.** (pihr-OLE-nye-trin) USAN. Under study.
Use: Antifungal.

Pyrroxate. (Roberts) Chlorpheniramine maleate 4 mg, phenylpropanolamine HCl 25 mg, acetaminophen 650 mg/Cap. Blister pkg. 24s. Bot. 500s. *otc.*
Use: Antihistamine, decongestant, analgesic.

•**pyrvinium pamoate,** U.S.P. 23.
Use: Anthelmintic.

Q

QB Liquid. (Major) Theophylline 150 mg, guaifenesin 90 mg. Bot. pt, gal. *Rx.*
Use: Bronchodilator, expectorant.

QT Quick Tanning Suntan by Coppertone. (Schering Plough) Ethylhexyl p-methoxycinnamate, dihydroxyacetone. SPF 2. Lot. Bot. 120 ml. *otc.*
Use: Sunscreen, artificial tanner.

Qua-Bid. (Quaker City Pharmacal) Papaverine HCl 150 mg. TR Cap. Bot. 100s, 1000s. *otc.*
Use: Peripheral vasodilator.

•**quadazocine mesylate.** (kwad-AZE-oh-SEEN) USAN.
Use: Antagonist (opioid).

Quadrinal. (Knoll) Ephedrine HCl 24 mg, phenobarbital 24 mg, theophylline calcium salicylate 130 mg, potassium iodide 320 mg. Tab. Bot. 100s. *Rx.*
Use: Bronchodilator, sedative, hypnotic, expectorant.

quadrodide.
See: Quadrinal, Susp., Tab. (Knoll).

quadruple sulfonamides.
See: Sulfonamide.

Quarzan. (Roche) Clidinium bromide 2.5 mg or 5 mg. Cap. Bot. 100s. *Rx.*
Use: Anticholinergic, antispasmodic.

•**quazepam.** (KWAY-zuh-pam) USAN.
Use: Sedative, hypnotic.
See: Doral (Baker Cummins).

•**quazinone.** (KWAY-zih-NOHN) USAN.
Use: Cardiotonic.

•**quazodine.** (KWAY-zoe-deen) USAN.
Use: Cardiotonic, bronchodilator.

•**quazolast.** (KWAY-ZOLE-ast) USAN.
Use: Antiasthmatic mediator release inhibitor.

Quelicin. (Abbott Hospital Prods) Succinylcholine Cl. **20 mg/ml:** Fliptop vial 10 ml, Abboject Syringe 5 ml; **50 mg/ml:** Amp. 10 ml; **100 mg/ml:** Amp. 10 ml; **Quelicin-500:** 5 ml in Pintop vial 10 ml; **Quelicin-1000:** 10 ml in Pintop vial 20 ml. *Rx.*
Use: Muscle relaxant.

Quelidrine Cough Syrup. (Abbott) Dextromethorphan HBr 10 mg, chlorpheniramine maleate 2 mg, ephedrine HCl 5 mg, phenylephrine HCl 5 mg, ammonium Cl 40 mg, ipecac fluidextract 0.005 ml, ethyl alcohol 2%/5 ml. Bot. 4 oz. *Rx.*
Use: Antitussive, antihistamine, bronchodilator, decongestant, expectorant.

Quercetin. Active constituent of rutin. Quertine.

Quertine.
Use: Bioflavonoid supplement.

Questran. (Bristol-Myers) Cholestyramine resin 4 g active ingredient/9 g Powder Packet. Box packet 60s. Can 378 g (42 dose). *Rx.*
Use: Antihyperlipidemic, antipruritic.

Questran Light. (Bristol-Myers) Anhydrous cholestyramine 4 g/Packet or scoopful. Pow. for Oral Susp. Can 210 g (42 doses), carton packet 5 g (60s). *Rx.*
Use: Antihyperlipidemic.

•**quetiapine fumarate.** (cue-TIE-ah-peen) USAN.
Use: Antipsychotic.

Quiagel. (Rugby) Kaolin 6 g, pectin 142.8 mg, hyoscyamine sulfate 0.1037 mg, atropine sulfate 0.0194 mg, scopolamine HBr 0.0065 mg/30 ml. Susp. Bot. pt, gal. *Rx.*
Use: Antidiarrheal.

quetiapine hydrochloride. (cue-TIE-ah-peen)
Use: Antipsychotic.

Quibron. (Roberts) Theophylline (anhydrous) 150 mg, guaifenesin 90 mg. Cap. Bot. 100s, 1000s, UD 100s. *Rx.*
Use: Bronchodilator, expectorant.

Quibron-300. (Roberts) Theophylline (anhydrous) 300 mg, guaifenesin 180 mg. Cap. Bot. 100s. *Rx.*
Use: Bronchodilator, expectorant.

Quibron Plus. (Bristol-Myers) Ephedrine HCl 25 mg, theophylline (anhydrous) 150 mg, butabarbital 20 mg, guaifenesin 100 mg. Tab. Bot. 100s. *Rx.*
Use: Antiasthmatic combination.

Quibron Plus Elixir. (Bristol-Myers) Theophylline 150 mg, ephedrine HCl 25 mg, guaifenesin 100 mg, butabarbital 20 mg, alcohol 15%. Elix. Bot. Pt. *Rx.*
Use: Antiasthmatic combination.

Quibron-T Dividose Tablets. (Roberts) Theophylline anhydrous 300 mg. Tab. Dividose design breakable into 100, 150 or 200 mg portions. Immediate release. Bot. 100s. *Rx.*
Use: Bronchodilator.

Quibron-T/SR Dividose Tablets. (Roberts) Theophylline anhydrous 300 mg. Tab. Dividose design breakable into 100 mg, 150 mg or 200 mg portions. Sustained release. Bot. 100s. *Rx.*
Use: Bronchodilator.

Quick CARE. (Novartis) **Disinfecting solution:** Isopropanol, sodium Cl, polyoxypropylenepolyoxyethylene block copolymer, disodium lauroamphodiac-

etate. Bot. 15 ml. **Rinse and neutralizer:** Sodium borate, boric acid, sodium perborate (generating up to 0.006% hydrogen peroxide), phophoric acid. Bot. 360 ml. *otc.*
Use: Contact lens care.

Quick-K. (Western Research) Potassium bicarbonate 650 mg (6.5 mEq) potassium. Tab. Bot. 30s, 100s. *Rx.*
Use: Potassium supplement.

Quick Pep. (Thompson) Caffeine 150 mg, dextrose 300 mg. Tab. Bot. 32s. *otc.*
Use: CNS stimulant.

Quiebar. (Nevin) Butabarbital sodium. **Spantab:** 1.5 gr. TR Spantab. Bot. 50s, 500s. **Elix.:** 30 mg/5 ml. Bot. pt, gal. **Tab.:** 15 mg. Bot. 100s, 1000s; 30 mg. Bot. 1000s. **A.C. Cap.:** Bot. 100s, 500s. *c-III.*
Use: Sedative, hypnotic.

Quiebel. (Nevin) Butabarbital sodium 15 mg, belladonna extract 15 mg. Cap. Bot. 100s, 1000s. Elix. pt, gal. *c-III.*
Use: Sedative, hypnotic, anticholinergic, antispasmodic.

Quiecof. (Nevin) Dextromethorphan HBr 7.5 mg, chlorpheniramine maleate 0.75 mg, guaiacol glyceryl ether 25 mg. Bot. 4 oz, pt, gal. *otc.*
Use: Antitussive, antihistamine, expectorant.

Quiess. (Forest) Hydroxyzine HCl 25 mg/ml. Vial 10 ml. *Rx.*
Use: Antianxiety agent, antihistamine.

Quiet Night. (Rosemont) Pseudoephedrine HCl 10 mg, doxylamine succinate 1.25 mg, dextromethorphan HBr 5 mg, acetaminophen 167 mg/5 ml. Liq. Bot. 180 ml, 300 ml. *otc.*
Use: Decongestant, antihistamine, antitussive, analgesic.

Quiet Time. (Whiteworth Towne) Acetaminophen 600 mg, ephedrine sulfate 8 mg, dextromethorphan HBr 15 mg, doxylamine succinate 7.5 mg, alcohol 25 mg/30 ml. Bot. 180 ml. *otc.*
Use: Analgesic, decongestant, antitussive, antihistamine.

Quiet World. (Whitehall Robins) Acetaminophen 2.5 gr, aspirin 3.5 gr, pyrilamine maleate 25 mg. Tab. Bot. 12s, 30s. *otc.*
Use: Analgesic combination, antihistamine.

•**quiflapon sodium.** (KWIH-flap-ahn) USAN.
Use: Antiasthmatic, inflammatory bowel disease suppressant.

Quik-Cept. (Laboratory Diagnostics) Slide test for pregnancy, rapid latex inhibition test. Kit 25s, 50s, 100s.
Use: Diagnostic aid.

Quik-Cult. (Laboratory Diagnostics) Slide test for fecal occult blood. Kit 150s, 200s, 300s and tape test.
Use: Diagnostic aid.

•**quilostigmine.** USAN.
Use: Cholinergic (cholinesterase inhibitor); treatment of Alzheimer's disease.

Quinaglute Dura-Tabs. (Berlex) Quinidine gluconate 324 mg. Tab. Bot. 100s, 250s, 500s, UD 100s. Unit-of-use 90s, 120s. *Rx.*
Use: Antiarrhythmic.

•**quinaldine blue.** (kwin-AL-deen) USAN.
Use: Diagnostic agent (obstetrics).

•**quinapril hydrochloride.** (KWIN-uh-PRILL) USAN.
Use: Antihypertensive, enzyme inhibitor (angiotensin-converting)
See: Accupril, Tab. (Parke-Davis).

•**quinaprilat.** (KWIN-ah-PRILL-at) USAN.
Use: Antihypertensive, enzyme inhibitor (angiotensin-converting).

•**quinazosin hydrochloride.** (kwin-AZZ-oh-sin) USAN.
Use: Antihypertensive.

•**quinbolone.** (KWIN-bole-ohn) USAN.
Use: Anabolic.

•**quindecamine acetate.** (kwin-DECK-ah-meen) USAN.
Use: Antibacterial.

•**quindonium bromide.** (kwin-DOE-nee-uhn) USAN.
Use: Cardiac depressant (antiarrhythmic).

•**quinelorane hydrochloride.** (kwih-NELL-oh-RANE) USAN.
Use: Antihypertensive, antiparkinsonian.

•**quinestrol.** USAN. U.S.P. XXII.
Use: Estrogen.

quinethazone, U.S.P. XXII.
Use: Diuretic.
See: Hydromox, Tab. (Lederle).
W/Reserpine.
See: Hydromox R, Tab. (Lederle).

•**quinetolate.** USAN.
Use: Smooth muscle relaxant.

•**quinfamide.** (KWIN-fah-mide) USAN.
Use: Antiamebic.

•**quingestanol acetate.** (kwin-JESS-tan-ahl) USAN.
Use: Progestin.

•**quingestrone.** (kwin-JESS-trone) USAN.
Use: Progestin.

Quinidex Extentabs. (Robins) Quinidine sulfate 300 mg. Tab. Bot. 100s, 250s. Dis-co pack 100s. *Rx.*
Use: Antiarrhythmic.

Quinidex L-A.
See: Quinidex Extentabs (Robins).

●**quinidine gluconate,** U.S.P. 23.
Use: Cardiac depressant (antiarrhythmic).
See: Duraquin, Tab. (Parke-Davis).
Quinaglute, Dura-Tab. (Berlex).

quinidine polygalacturonate.
See: Cardioquin Tab. (Purdue Frederick).

●**quinidine sulfate,** (KWIN-ih-deen) U.S.P. 23.
Use: Cardiac depressant (antiarrhythmic).
See: Quinidex Extentabs (Robins).
Quinora, Tab. (Key).

quinidine sulfate. (Various, eg, Copley) 300 mg. Tab. Bot. 100s, 250s, 1000s *Rx.*
Use: Cardiac depressant.

●**quinine ascorbate.** (KWIE-nine ass-CORE-bate) USAN. *Formerly quinine biascorbate.*
Use: Deterrent (smoking).

quinine bisulfate. (KWIE-nine)
Use: Analgesic, antipyretic, antimalarial.

quinine dihydrochloride. (KWIE-nine)
Use: Antimalarial.

quinine ethylcarbonate.
See: Euquinine (Various Mfr.).

quinine glycerophosphate. Quinine compound with glycerol phosphate.

●**quinine sulfate,** (KWIE-nine) U.S.P. 23.
Use: Antimalarial.
See: Quinamm, Tab. (Hoechst Marion Roussel).
W/Aminophylline.
See: Strema, Cap. (Foy).
W/Atropine sulfate, emetine HCl, aconitine, camphor monobromate.
See: Coryza, Tab. (Jones Medical).
W/Niacin, vitamin E.
See: Myodyne, Tab. (Paddock).

quinine and urea hydrochloride.
Use: Sclerosing agent.

quinisocaine.

See: Dimethisoquin HCl, USAN.

quinophan.
See: Cinchophen (Various Mfr.).

Quinora. (Key) Quinidine sulfate 300 mg. Tab. Bot. 100s, 1000s, UD 100s. *Rx.*
Use: Antiarrhythmic.

quinoxyl.
See: Chiniofon

●**quinpirole hydrochloride.** (KWIN-pihrole) USAN.
Use: Antihypertensive.

quinprenaline. Quinterenol Sulfate.

Quin-Release. (Major) Quinidine gluconate 324 mg. SR Tab. Bot. 100s, 250s, 500s, UD 100s. *Rx.*
Use: Antiarrhythmic.

Quinsana Plus. (Mennen) Undecylenic acid 2%, zinc undecylenate 20%. Pow. 81 g, 165 g. *otc.*
Use: Antifungal, topical.

Quintabs. (Freeda) Vitamins A 10,000 IU, D 400 IU, E 29 mg, B_1 25 mg, B_2 25 mg, B_3 100 mg, B_5 25 mg, B_6 25 mg, B_{12} 25 mcg, C 300 mg, folic acid 0.1 mg, inositol, PABA/Tab. Bot. 100s, 250s. *otc.*
Use: Vitamin supplement.

Quintabs-M. (Freeda) Iron 15 mg, Vitamins A 10,000 IU, D 400 IU, E 50 mg, B_1 30 mg, B_2 30 mg, B_3 150 mg, B_5 30 mg, B_6 30 mg, B_{12} 30 mcg, C 300 mg, folic acid 0.4 mg, Ca, Cu, K, Mg, Mn, Se, Zn 30 mg., PABA./Tab. Bot. 100s, 250s, 500s. *otc.*
Use: Vitamin/mineral supplement.

●**quinterenol sulfate.** (kwin-TER-en-ahl) USAN.
Use: Bronchodilator.

●**quinuclium bromide.** (kwih-NEW-klee-uhm) USAN.
Use: Antihypertensive.

●**quinupristin.** (kwih-NEW-priss-tin) USAN.
Use: Antibacterial.

●**quipazine maleate.** (KWIP-ah-zeen) USAN.
Use: Antidepressant, oxytocic.

quipenyl naphthoate.
See: Pamaquine naphthoate.
Plasmochin naphthoate.

R

R-3 Screen Test. (Wampole) A three-minute latex-eosin slide test for the qualitative detection of rheumatoid factor activity in serum. Kit 100s.
Use: Diagnostic aid.

•**rabeprazole sodium.** (rab-EH-pray-zahl) USAN.
Use: Antiulcerative; gastric acid pump inhibitor.

•**rabies immune globulin,** (RAY-beez-ih-MYOON GLAB-byoo-lin) U.S.P. 23.
Use: Immunizing agent (passive).
See: Bayrab (Bayer).
Hyperab (Cutter).
Imogam Rabies (Pasteur-Merieux-Connaught).

rabies immune globulin (RIG), human.
See: rabies immune globulin.

•**rabies vaccine,** (RAY-beez vaccine) U.S.P. 23.
Use: Immunizing agent (active).
See: Imovax Rabies, Syr. (Connaught).
rabies vaccine adsorbed, vial (Michigan Department of Public Health).

rabies vaccine (adsorbed). (Michigan Department of Public Health) Challenge virus standard (CVS) Kissling/MDPH Strain. Inj. Vial 1 ml. *Rx.*
Use: Immunizing agent, active.

•**racemethionine.** (RAY-see-meh-THIGH-oh-neen) USAN. *Formerly Methionine.*
Use: Acidifier (urinary).
See: Amurex, Cap. (Solvay).
Pedameth. Cap., Liq. (Forest).

racemethionine w/combinations.
See: Aminomin, Vial (Pharmex).
Aminovit, Vial (Hickam).
Ardiatric, Tab. (Burgin-Arden).
Limvic, Tab. (Briar).
Lipo-K, Cap. (Marcen).
Lychol-B, Inj. (Burgin-Arden).
Minoplex, Vial (Savage).
Vio-Geric, Tab. (Solvay).
Vio-Geric-H, Tab. (Solvay).

racemic amphetamine sulfate.
See: Amphetamine sulfate.

racemic calcium pantothenate.
See: Calcium Pantothenate, Racemic.

racemic desoxy-nor-ephedrine.
See: Amphetamine (Various Mfr.).

racemic ephedrine hydrochloride. Racephedrine HCl.

racemic pantothenic acid.
See: Vitamin, Preps.

•**racephedrine hydrochloride.** USAN.
Use: Vasoconstrictor, nasal decongestant.

See: Ephedrine Combinations W/Aminophylline, phenobarbital.
See: Amodrine, Tab. (Searle).
W/Theophylline sodium glycinate, phenobarbital.
See: Synophedal, Tab. (Central).

racephedrine hydrochloride. (Pharmacia & Upjohn) **Cap.:** ⅜ gr. Bot. 40s, 250s, 1000s. **Soln.:** 1%. Bot. 1 fl oz, pt, gal.
Use: Vasoconstrictor, nasal decongestant.

•**racephenicol.** (ray-see-FEN-ih-KAHL) USAN.
Use: Antibacterial.

•**racepinephrine hydrochloride,** U.S.P. 23
Use: Bronchodilator.

radioactive isotopes.
See: Aggregated Radioiodinated Albumin, Human I-131.
Chlormerodrin Hg-197, Inj.
Chlormerodrin Hg-203, Inj.
Cyanocobalamin Co-57, Cap.
Cyanocobalamin Co-60, Cap.
Gold Au-198, Inj.
Medotope, Prods. (Squibb).
Radio-Gold, Soln.
Radio-Iodinated Serum Albumin (Human).
Sodium Radio-Chromate, Inj.
Sodium Radio-Iodide, Soln.
Sodium Radio Phosphate, Soln.
Radiodinated Serum Albumin, Human I-125.
Radiodinated Serum Albuminia, Human I-131.
Selenomethionine Se-75, Inj.
Sodium Chromate Cr-51, Inj.
Sodium Iodide I-125, Soln., Cap.
Sodium Iodide I-131, Soln., Cap.
Sodium Phosphate P-32, Cap., Inj.
Sodium Rose Bengal I-131, Inj.
Strontium Nitrate Sr-85, Inj.
Technetium Tc-99m, Kit, Inj.
Triolein I-131, Cap., Soln.
Xenon Xe-133, Inj.

radiogold (^{198}Au), solution. Gold Au-198 Injection, U.S.P. 23.
Use: Irradiation therapy.
See: Auretope, Vial (Squibb).

radio-iodide (^{131}I), sodium.
Use: Radioactive isotope.
See: Iodotope (Squibb).
Radiocaps (Abbott).

radio-iodinated (^{131}I) serum albumin. (Human), Iodinated I-131 Albumin Injection, U.S.P. 23.

radio-iodinated serum albumin (human), (^{125}I).

See: Albumotope (^{125}I) (Squibb).

radiopaque polyvinyl chloride.
Use: GI contrast agent.
See: Sitzmarks (Lafayette Pharm).

radio-phosphate (^{32}P), sodium.
Use: Radioactive isotopes.

radioselenomethionine 75 Se. Selenomethionine Se 75.

radiotolpovidone I-131. Tolpovidone I-
131.
See: Raovin (Abbott).

•**rafoxanide.** (ray-FOX-ah-nide) USAN.
Use: Anthelmintic.

Ragus. (Miller) Magnesium 27 mg, vitamins C 100 mg, calcium 580 mg, phosphorus 450 mg, l-lysine 25 mg, dl-methionine 50 mg, A 5000 IU, D 400 IU, E
10 mg, B$_1$ 20 mg, B$_2$ 3 mg, B$_6$ 5 mg, B$_{12}$
9 mcg, niacinamide 80 mg, pantothenic
acid 5 mg, iron 20 mg, copper 1 mg,
manganese 2 mg, potassium 10 mg,
zinc 2 mg, iodine 0.1 mg/3 Tab. Bot.
100s. *otc.*
Use: Vitamin/mineral supplement.

•**ralitoline.** (rah-LIT-oh-leen) USAN.
Use: Anticonvulsant.

R A Lotion. (Medco Lab) Resorcinol 3%,
alcohol 43%. Plastic Bot. 120 ml, 240
ml, 480 ml.
Use: Antiacne.

•**raloxifene hydrochloride.** (ral-OX-ih-
FEEN) USAN.
Use: Antiestrogen.

•**raltitrexed.** USAN. (ral-tih-TREX-ehd)
Use: Advanced colorectal cancer treatment (thymidylate synthase inhibitor),
antineoplastic.

•**raluridine.** (ral-YOUR-ih-deen) USAN.
Use: Antiviral.

•**ramipril.** (ruh-MIH-prill) USAN.
Use: Antihypertensive, enzyme inhibi-
tor (angiotensin-converting); conges-
tive heart failure.
See: Altace, Cap. (Hoechst Marion
Roussel/Pharmacia & Upjohn).

•**ramoplanin.** (ram-oh-PLAN-in) USAN.
Use: Antibacterial.

Ramses. (Schmid) Nonoxynol 9 5%.
Vaginal jelly. 150 g. *otc.*
Use: Spermicide.

Ramses Bendex. (Schmid) Flexible
cushioned diaphragm; arcing spring.
65-90 mm. Pkg. w/Ramses Vaginal
Jelly Tube 1 oz, 3 oz. *Rx.*
Use: Contraceptive.

Ramses Diaphragm. (Schmid) Flexible
cushioned diaphragm 50-95 mm. Pkg.
diaphragm, tube of Ramses Vaginal
Jelly. Pkg. diaphragm alone. *Rx.*

Use: Contraceptive.

Ramses Extra. (Schmid) Condom with
nonoxynol 9 15%. In 3s, 12s, 24s, 36s.
otc.
Use: Contraceptive.

Ramses Jelly. (Schmid) Nonoxynol 9
5%. Tube w/applicator 150 g. *otc.*
Use: Contraceptive.

Randolectil. (Farbenfabriken Bayer) Butaperazine. *Rx.*
Use: Psychotropic.

ranestol. Triclofenol piperazine.
Use: Anthelmintic.

•**ranimycin.** (ran-ih-MY-sin) USAN.
Use: Antibacterial.

•**ranitidine.** (ran-EYE-tih-DEEN) USAN.
Use: Histamine H$_2$ receptor antago-
nist.
See: Zantac, Tab., Inj., Syr. (Glaxo and
Roche).

•**ranitidine bismuth citrate.** (ran-EYE-tih-
DEEN) USAN.
Use: Antiulcer agent (histamine H$_2$ re-
ceptor antagonist).
See: Tritec, Tab. (Glaxo Wellcome).

•**ranitidine hydrochloride,** U.S.P. 23.
(UDL) 15 mg/ml. Syr. Bot. UD 10 ml.
Use: Histamine H$_2$ receptor antagonist.
See: Zantac, Inj., Tab., Syr. (Glaxo
Pharm.).

ranitidine hydrochloride. (UDL) 15 mg/
ml. Syr. Bot. UD 10 ml.
Use: Histamine H$_2$ receptor antagonist.

**ranitidine hydrochloride in sodium
chloride injection.**
Use: Histamine H$_2$ antagonist.
See: Zantac Inj. Premixed (Glaxo
Pharm.).

•**ranolazine hydrochloride.** (RAY-no-lah-
ZEEN) USAN.
Use: Antianginal.

Rapid Test Strep. (SmithKline Diagnostics) Latex slide agglutination test for
identification of group A Streptococci. In
25s, 100s.
Use: Diagnostic aid.

•**rasagiline mesylate.** (rass-AH-jih-leen
MEH-sih-late) USAN.
Use: Antiparkinsonian.

rastinon. Tolbutamide, U.S.P. 23.
Use: Antidiabetic.

rattlesnake bite therapy.
See: Antivenin, (crotalidae) (Wyeth-
Ayerst).

Rauneed. (Hanlon) Rauwolfia 50 mg or
100 mg/Tab. Bot. 100s. *Rx.*
Use: Antihypertensive.

Raunescine. (Penick) An alkaloid of Rauwolfia serpentina. Under study.

Use: Antihypertensive.

Raunormine. (Penick) 11-Desmethoxy reserpine. *Rx.*

Raurine. (Westerfield) Reserpine. **Tab.:** 0.1 mg. Bot. 100s. **Delayed Action Cap.:** 0.5 mg. Bot. 100s. *Rx.*
Use: Antihypertensive.

Rauserfia. (New Eng. Phr. Co.) Rauwolfia serpentina 50 mg or 100 mg/Tab. Bot. 100s. *Rx.*
Use: Antihypertensive.

Rautina. (Fellows) Rauwolfia serpentina whole root 50 mg or 100 mg/Tab. Bot. 1000s. *Rx.*
Use: Antihypertensive.

Rauval. (Pal-Pak) Rauwolfia whole root 50 mg or 100 mg/Tab. Bot. 100s, 500s, 1000s. *Rx.*
Use: Antihypertensive.

rauwolfia/bendroflumethiazide. (Various Mfr.) Bendroflumethiazide 4 mg, powdered rauwolfia serpentina 50 mg/ Tab. Bot. 100s. *Rx.*
Use: Antihypertensive.
See: Rauzide, Tab. (B-M Squibb).

rauwolfia canescens alkaloid.
See: Harmonyl, Tab. (Abbott).

rauwolfia serpentina active principles (alkaloids). Deserpidine, Rescinnamine.
See: Reserpine, Inj. (Various Mfr.).

rauwolfia serpentina alkaloidal extract.
See: Alseroxylon (Various Mfr.).

• **rauwolfia serpentina,** U.S.P. 23.
Use: Antihypertensive.
See: Raudixin, Tab. (Bristol-Myers).
Rauja, Tab. (Table Rock).
Raumason, Tab. (Mason).
Rauneed, Tab. (Hanlon).
Rauval, Tab. (Pal-Pak).
Rawfola, Tab. (Foy).
Serfia, Tab. (Westerfield).
Serfolia, Tab. (Roberts).
T-Rau, Tab. (Tennessee Pharm).
Wolfina, Tab. (Westerfield).
W/Bendroflumethiazide.
See: Rautrax-N, Tab. (Bristol-Myers).
Rauzide, Tab. (Bristol-Myers).
W/Bendroflumethiazide, potassium Cl (400).
See: Rautrax, Tab. (Bristol-Myers).
W/Mannitol hexanitrate, rutin.
See: Maxitate W/Rauwolfia, Tab. (Fisons).

rauwolscine. An alkaloid of *Rauwolfia canescens.* Under study.
Use: Antihypertensive.

Rauzide. (B-M Squibb) Rauwolfia serpentina pow. 50 mg, bendroflumethia-zide 4 mg, tartrazine/Tab. Bot. 100s. *Rx.*
Use: Antihypertensive.

Ravocaine. (Cook-Waite) Propoxycaine HCl 4 mg, procaine 20 mg, norepinephrine bitartrate equivalent to 0.033 mg levophed base, sodium Cl 3 mg, acetone sodium bisulfite not more than 2 mg. Cartridge 1.8 ml. *Rx.*
Use: Local anesthetic.

Ravocaine and Novocain with Levophed. (Cook-Waite) Propoxycaine HCl 7.2 mg, procaine 36 mg, norepinephrine 0.12 mg, acetone sodium bisulfite 1.8 ml. Inj. Dental Cartridge. *Rx.*
Use: Local anesthetic.

Rawfola. (Foy) Rauwolfia serpentina 50 mg/Tab. Bot. 1000s. *Rx.*
Use: Antihypertensive.

Rawl Vite. (Rawl) Vitamins A 10,000 IU, D 500 IU, B_1 10 mg, B_2 5 mg, B_6 1 mg, calcium pantothenate 5 mg, nicotinamide 50 mg, C 125 mg, E 2.5 IU/Tab. Bot. 100s. *otc.*
Use: Vitamin/mineral supplement.

Rawl Whole Liver Vitamin B Complex. (Rawl) Whole liver 500 mg, amino acids found in the whole liver, vitamins B_1 1 mg, B_2 2 mg, niacinamide 5 mg, choline Cl 12 mg, B_6 0.2 mg, calcium pantothenate 0.2 mg, inositol 5 mg, biotin 0.6 mcg, B_{12} 0.3 mcg/Cap. Bot. 100s, 500s.
Use: Vitamin/mineral supplement.

Ray Block. (Del-Ray) Octyl dimethyl PABA 5%, benzophenone-3 3%, SD alcohol. Lot. Bot. 118.3 ml. *otc.*
Use: Sunscreen.

Ray-D. (Nion) Vitamin D 400 IU, thiamine mononitrate 1 mg, riboflavin 2 mg, niacin 10 mg, iodine 0.1 mg, calcium 375 mg, phosphorus 300 mg/6 Tab. In base of brewer's yeast. Bot. 100s, 500s. *otc.*
Use: Vitamin/mineral supplement.

Rayderm Ointment. (Velvet Pharmacal) Euphorbia extract, phenyl salicylate, neatsfoot oil, olive oil, lanolin in emulsion base preserved with methyl and propylparabens. Tube 1.5 oz, Jar lb. *otc.*
Use: Burn preparation.

• **rayon, purified,** (RAY-ahn) U.S.P. 23.
Use: Surgical aid.

raythesin. (Raymer).
See: Propyl p-Aminobenzoate.

Razepam. (Major) Temazepam 15 mg or 30 mg/Cap. Bot. 100s. *c-iv.*
Use: Sedative, hypnotic.

RCF. (Ross) Carbohydrate free low iron

soy protein formula base. Carbohydrate and water must be added. For infants unable to tolerate the amount or type of carbohydrate in conventional formulas. Can 14 fl oz. (Concentrated liq.). *otc.*
Use: Nutritional supplement.

R & C Shampoo. (Reed & Carnrick) Pyrethrin shampoo. Bot. 2 oz, 4 oz. *otc.*
Use: Pediculicide.

R & C Spray III. (Reed & Carnrick) Spray containing pyrethroid (sumethrin) 0.382%, other isomers 0.018%, petroleum distillate 4.255%. Aerosol Container 5 oz. *otc.*
Use: Pediculicide.

Reabilan. (Elan) Protein 31.5 g, fat 39 g, carbohydrates 131.5 g, Na 702 mg, K 1.252 g/L, lactose free. With appropriate vitamins and minerals. Liq. Bot. 375 ml. *otc.*
Use: Nutritional supplement.

Reabilan HN. (Elan) Protein 58.2 g, fat 52 g, carbohydrates 158 g, Na 1000 mg, K 1661 mg/L, lactose free. With appropriate vitamins and minerals. Liq. Bot. 375 ml. *otc.*
Use: Nutritional supplement.

Rea-Lo. (Whorton) Urea in water soluble moisturizing oil base. **Lot.:** 15%. Bot. 4 oz, pt. **Cream:** 30%. Jar 2 oz, 16 oz. *otc.*
Use: Emollient.

•**recainam hydrochloride.** (reh-CANE-am) USAN.
Use: Cardiac depressant (antiarrhythmic).

•**recainam tosylate.** (reh-CANE-am TAH-sill-ate) USAN.
Use: Cardiac depressant (antiarrhythmic).

•**reclazepam.** (reh-CLAY-zeh-pam) USAN.
Use: Sedative, hypnotic.

Reclomide. (Major) Metoclopramide HCl 10 mg/Tab. Bot. 100s, 500s, 1000s, UD 100s. *Rx.*
Use: GI stimulant, antiemetic.

recombinant human insulin-like growth factor I.
Use: Antibody-mediated growth hormone resistance. [Orphan drug]

recombinant tissue plasminogen activator. *Rx.*
See: Activase (Genetech).

recombinant vaccinia (human papillomavirus).
Use: Cervical cancer. [Orphan drug]

Recombinate. (Hyland) Concentrated recombinant antihemophilic factor, con-

tains albumin (human) 12.5 mg/ml, polyethylene glycol 1.5 mg, sodium 180 mEq/L, histidine 55 mm, polysorbate-80 1.5 mcg/AHF IU, calcium 0.2 mg/ml. Pow. for inj. Single dose bot. 250 IU, 500 IU, 1000 IU. *Rx.*
Use: Antihemophilic agent.

Recombivax-HB. (Merck) Hepatitis B vaccine recombinant. **Pediatric:** 2.5 mcg/0.5 ml. Single dose vials 0.5 ml and 3 ml. **Adolescent/High Risk Infant:** 5 mcg/0.5 ml. single dose vials 0.5 ml. **Adult:** 10 mcg/ml. Vials 1 ml, 3 ml. Box 5s (syringes), 10s (multidose vials). **Dialysis:** 40 mcg/ml. Vial 1 ml. *Rx.*
Use: Agent for immunization.

Recortex 10X in Oil. (Forest Pharm) 1000 mcg/ml. Vial 10 ml. *Rx.*

Recover. (Del Pharm) Bot. 2.25 oz. *otc.*
Use: Skin discoloration cover-up cream.

Rectagene. (Pfeiffer) Live yeast cell derivative supplying 2000 units Skin Respiratory Factor/oz, shark liver oil in a cocoa butter base. Supp. 12s. *otc.*
Use: Anorectal preparation.

Rectagene II. (Pfeiffer) Bismuth subgallate 2.25%, bismuth resorcin compound 1.75%, benzyl benzoate 1.2%, peruvian balsam 1.8%, zinc oxide 11%, bismuth subiodide, calcium phosphate in a hydrogenated vegetable oil base. Pkg, 12s. *Rx.*
Use: Anorectal preparation.

Rectagene Medicated Rectal Balm. (Pfeiffer) Live yeast cell derivative that supplies 2000 units Skin Respiratory Factor/30 g, refined shark liver oil 3%, white petrolatum, lanolin, thyme oil, 1:10,000 phenyl mercuric nitrate. Oint. 56.7 g. *otc.*
Use: Anorectal preparation.

Rectal Medicone. (Medicone) Benzocaine 2 gr, balsam peru 1 gr, hydroxyquinoline sulfate 0.25 gr, menthol ⅐ gr, zinc oxide 3 gr/Supp. Box 12s, 24s. *otc.*
Use: Antiseptic, local anesthetic, rectal.

Rectal Medicone Unguent. (Medicone) Benzocaine 20 mg, oxyquinoline sulfate 5 mg, menthol 4 mg, zinc oxide 100 mg, balsam peru 12.5 mg, petrolatum 625 mg, lanolin 210 mg/g. Tube 1.5 oz. *otc.*
Use: Anorectal preparation.

Rectules. (Forest Pharm) Chloral hydrate 10 or 20 gr in water-soluble base. Supp. Pkg. 12s.
Use: Sedative/hypnotic.

red blood cells. Human red blood cells given by IV infusion.
Use: Blood replenisher.

red cell tagging solution.
See: A-C-D Solution (Squibb).

Red Cross Toothache Kit. (Mentholatum) Eugenol 85%, sesame oil. Drops. Bot. 3.7 ml w/cotton pellets and tweezers. *otc.*
Use: Local anesthetic.

red ferric oxide.
Use: Pharmaceutic aid (color).

red mercuric iodide.
See: Auralcaine, Liq. (Truett).

Reditemp-C. (Wyeth-Ayerst) Ammonium nitrate, water and special additives. Pkg. large and small sizes. 4 × 10s.
Use: For short-term topical cold application.

Reducto, Improved. (Arcum) Phendimetrazine bitartrate 35 mg/Tab. Bot. 100s, 1000s. *c-iii.*
Use: Anorexiant.

Redutemp. (Inter. Ethical Labs.) Acetaminophen 500 mg/Tab. Bot. 60s. *otc.*
Use: Analgesic.

Redux. (Wyeth-Ayerst) Dexfenfluramine HCl 15 mg/Cap, lactose. Bot. 60s. *c-iv.*
Use: Anorexiant.

Reese's Pinworm. (Reese) Pyrantel pamoate 144 mg. Liq. 30 ml. *otc.*
Use: Anthelmintic.

Refresh. (Allergan) Polyvinyl alcohol 1.4%, povidone 0.6%, sodium Cl. UD 30s or 50s (0.3 ml single dose container). *otc.*
Use: Artificial tear solution.

Refresh Plus. (Allergan) Carboxymethylcellulose sodium 0.5%, KCl, NaCl. Preservative free. Soln. 0.3 ml/single use container. In 30s, 50s. *otc.*
Use: Artificial tear solution.

Refresh PM. (Allergan) White petrolatum 56.8%, mineral oil 41.5%, lanolin alcohol, sodium Cl. Tube 3.5 g. *otc.*
Use: Ocular lubricant.

Regain. (NCI) Protein 15 g, carbohydrates 52 g, fat 7 g, sodium 45 mg, K 75 mg, Ca 200 mg, P 100 mg, Ca, Fe, vitamin B_{12}, Mg, folic acid, fructose. With dietary fiber. 300 calories. Lactose free. Vanilla, strawberry and malt flavors. Bar 85 g. *otc.*
Use: Nutritional supplement for patients with impaired renal function.

Regitine. (Novartis) Phentolamine mesylate 5 mg/Vial (w/mannitol 25 mg in lyophilized form). Pkg. 2s, 6s.
Use: Diagnostic aid.

Reglan. (Robins) Metoclopramide HCl. **Inj.: 10 mg/2 ml:** Amp. 2 ml, 10 ml; **5 mg/ml:** Vial 2 ml, 10 ml, 30 ml. **Syr.:** 5 mg (as monohydrochloride monohydrate)/5 ml. Bot. pt, Dis-Co Pack 10×10s. **Tab.: 5 mg:** Bot. 100s. **10 mg:** Bot. 100s, 500s, Dis-co Pak 100s. *Rx.*
Use: Antiemetic, GI stimulant.

Regonol. (Organon) Pyridostigmine bromide 5 mg/ml. Amp 2 ml, Vial 5 ml. *Rx.*
Use: Cholinergic muscle stimulant.

•**regramostim.** (reh-GRAH-moe-STIM) USAN.
Use: Biological response modifier; antineoplastic adjunct; antineutropenic; hematopoietic stimulant.

Regroton. (Rhone-Poulenc Rorer) Chlorthalidone 50 mg, reserpine 0.25 mg/Tab. Bot. 100s. *Rx.*
Use: Antihypertensive.

Regroton Demi. (Rhone-Poulenc Rorer) Chlorthalidone 25 mg, reserpine 0.125 mg/Tab. Bot. 100s, 1000s. *Rx.*
Use: Antihypertensive.

Regular Iletin I. (Lilly) Insulin 100 units/ml. Beef and pork. Inj. Bot. 10 ml. *otc.*
Use: Antidiabetic agent.

regular insulin. (Novo Nordisk) Insulin 100 units/ml. Pork. Inj. Vial. 10 ml. *otc.*
Use: Antidiabetic agent.

regular purified pork insulin. (Novo Nordisk) Insulin 100 units/ml. Purified pork. Inj. Vial. 10 ml. *otc.*
Use: Antidiabetic agent.

Regular Strength Bayer Enteric Coated Caplets. (Bayer) Aspirin 325 mg. Bot. 50s, 100s. *otc.*
Use: Salicylate, analgesic.

Regular Strength Midol Multisymptom. (Bayer) Acetaminophen 325 mg, pyrilamine maleate 12.5 mg. Tab. Bot. 30s. *otc.*
Use: Analgesic combination.

Reguloid, Orange. (Rugby) Psyllium mucilloid 3.4 g, sucrose 70%/rounded tsp. Pow. 420 g, 630 g. *otc.*
Use: Laxative.

Reguloid Sugar Free. (Rugby) Psyllium hydrophilic mucilloid 3.4 g, sodium ≤ 0.01 g, aspartame, phenylalanine 6 mg. Pow. 222, 333 g. *otc.*
Use: Laxative.

Regutol. (Schering-Plough) Docusate sodium 100 mg/Tab. Box 30s, 60s, 90s. *otc.*
Use: Laxative.

Rehydralyte. (Ross) Sodium 75 mEq, potassium 20 mEq, chloride 65 mEq, citrate 30 mEq, dextrose 25 g/L, 100

calories/L. Ready-to-use Bot. 8 oz. *Rx.*
Use: Fluid/electrolyte replacement.

Relafen. (SK Beecham) Nabumetone 500 mg/Tab. Bot. 100s, 500s, UD 100s. Nabumetone 750 mg/Tab. Bot. 100s, 500s, UD 100s. *Rx.*
Use: Nonsteroidal anti-inflammatory, analgesic.

relaxin. A purified ovarian hormone of pregnancy (obtained from sows) responsible for pubic relaxation or separation of the symphysis pubis in mammals.
See: Lutrexin, Tab. (Becton Dickinson).

Relief Eye Drops. (Allergan) Phenylephrine HCl 0.12%, antipyrine 0.1%, polyvinyl alcohol 1.4%, edetate disodium. Bot. UD 0.3 ml. *otc.*
Use: Decongestant, ophthalmic.

relief solution. (Allergan) Phenylephrine HCl 0.12%, antipyrine 0.1%. soln. Bot. 20 ml. *otc.*
Use: Ophthalmic decongestant combination.

• **relomycin.** (REE-low-MY-sin) USAN. A macrolide antibiotic produced by a variant strain of *Streptomyces hygroscopicus.*
Use: Antibacterial.

• **remacemide hydrochloride.** (rem-ASS-eh-MIDE) USAN.
Use: Anticonvulsant (neuroprotective).

Rem Cough Medicine. (Last) Dextromethorphan HBr 5 mg/5 ml. Bot. 3 oz, 6 oz. *otc.*
Use: Antitussive.

Remegel Soft Chewable Antacid Tablets. (Warner-Lambert) Aluminum hydroxide-magnesium carbonate 476.4 mg/Chew. Tab. Pkg. 8s, 24s. *otc.*
Use: Antacid.

Remeron. (Organon) Mirtazapine 15 mg, 30 mg, lactose/Tab. Bot. 30s, 100s. *Rx.*
Use: Treatment of depression.

• **remifentanil hydrochloride.** (reh-mih-FEN-tah-nill) USAN.
Use: Analgesic.
See: Ultiva, Pow. for inj. (Glaxo Wellcome).

• **remiprostol.** (reh-mih-PROSTE-ole) USAN.
Use: Antiulcerative.

Remivox. (Janssen) Lorcainide HCl. *Rx.*
Use: Antiarrhythmic.

• **remoxipride.** (reh-MOX-ih-PRIDE) USAN.
Use: Antipsychotic.

• **remoxipride hydrochloride.** (reh-MOX-ih-PRIDE) USAN.

Use: Antipsychotic.

Remular-S. (Inter. Ethical Labs.) Chloroxazone 250 mg/Tab. Bot. 100s. *Rx.*
Use: Skeletal muscle relaxants.

Renacidin. (Guardian) The composition of this powder, as manufactured, is in terms of 156 to 171 g citric acid (anhydrous) and 21 to 30 g d-gluconic acid (as the lactone) w/purified magnesium hydroxycarbonate 75 to 87 g, magnesium acid citrate 9 to 15 g, calcium (as carbonate) 2 to 6 g, water 17 to 21 g per 300 g. Bot. 25 g 6s; 150 g, 300 g. *Rx.*
Use: Genitourinary irrigant.

Renaltabs-S.C. (Forest Pharm) Methenamine 40.8 mg, benzoic acid 4.5 mg, phenyl salicylate 18.1 mg, hyoscyamine sulfate $\frac{1}{2000}$ gr, atropine sulfate 0.03 mg, methylene blue 5.4 mg, gelsemium 6.1 mg/Tab. Bot. 1000s. *Rx.*
Use: Urinary anti-infective.

Renamin. (Clintec) Sterile hypertonic soln. of essential and non-essential amino acids. Bot. 250 ml, 500 ml. *Rx.*
Use: Parenteral nutritional supplement.

renanolone. *Rx.*
Use: Steroid anesthetic.

Renbu. (Wren) Butabarbital sodium 32.4 mg/Tab. Bot. 100s, 1000s. *c-III.*
Use: Sedative/hypnotic.

Renese. (Pfizer) Polythiazide 1 mg, 2 mg or 4 mg/Tab. Bot. 100s, 1000s. *Rx.*
Use: Diuretic, antihypertensive.

Renese-R Tablets. (Pfizer) Polythiazide 2 mg, reserpine 0.25 mg/Tab. Bot. 100s, 1000s. *Rx.*
Use: Antihypertensive.

Rengasil. (Geigy) Pirprofen. Investigational drug.
Use: Anti-inflammatory.

renoform.
See: Epinephrine, Preps. (Various Mfr.).

Renografin-60, -76. (Bracco DXS) **-60:** Diatrizoate meglumine 52%, sodium diatrizoate 8%, iodine 29.2%. Vial 10 ml, 100 ml, 10s; 30 ml, 50 ml, 25s. **-76:** Diatrizoate meglumine 66%, sodium diatrizoate 10%, iodine 37%. Vial 20 ml, 50 ml, 25s; 100 ml, 200 ml, 10s.
Use: Radiopaque agent.

Reno-M-Dip. (Bracco DXS) Diatrizoate meglumine, iodine 14.1%. 30% for drip infusion pyelography. Inj. Bot. 300 ml. Also w/soln. admin. sets. (Formerly Renografin-Dip).
Use: Radiopaque agent.

Reno-M-30. (Bracco DXS) Diatrizoate meglumine 30%, iodine 14.1%. Vial 50

ml, 100 ml, Box 25s.
Use: Radiopaque agent.

Reno-M-60. (Bracco DXS) Diatrizoate meglumine 60%, iodine 28%. Vial 10 ml, 30 ml, 50 ml, 100 ml.
Use: Radiopaque agent.

Renormax. (Sandoz) Spirapril 3 mg, 6 mg, 12 mg or 24 mg/Tab. *Rx.*
Use: ACE inhibitor.

Reno-Sed. (Vita Elixir) Methenamine 2 gr, salol 0.5 gr, methylene blue $^1/_{10}$ gr, benzoic acid $^1/_8$ gr, atropine sulfate $^1/_{1000}$ gr, hyoscyamine sulfate $^1/_{2000}$ gr/Tab. *Rx.*
Use: Urinary anti-infective.

Renova. (Ortho) Tretinoin 0.05%, water in oil emulsion. Cream 40 g, 60 g. *Rx.*
Use: Dermatologic preparation.

Renovist Inj. (Bracco DXS) Diatrizoate methylglucamine 34.3%, diatrizoate sodium 35%, iodine 37%. Vial 50 ml, Box 25s.
Use: Radiopaque agent.

Renovist II. (Bracco DXS) Diatrizoate sodium 29.1%, meglumine diatrizoate 28.5%, iodine 31%. Inj. Vial 30 ml, 60 ml, Box 25s.
Use: Radiopaque agent.

Renovue-65. (Bracco DXS) Iodamide meglumide 65%, organically bound iodine 30%, edetate disodium. Vial 50 ml.
Use: Radiopaque agent.

Renovue-Dip. (Bracco DXS) Iodamide meglumide 24%, iodine 11.1%. Infusion Bot. 300 ml.
Use: Radiopaque agent.

Renpap. (Wren) Acetaminophen 4 gr, salicylamide 3 gr, caffeine $^2/_3$ gr, allylisobutylbarbituric acid gr/Tab. Bot. 100s, 1000s. *otc.*
Use: Salicylate analgesic.

Rentamine Pediatric. (Major) Phenylephrine tannate 5 mg, chlorpheniramine tannate 4 mg, carbetapentane tannate, saccharin, sucrose. Pt.
Use: Decongestant, antihistamine, antitussive.

Renu Effervescent Enzymatic Cleaner. (Bausch & Lomb) Subtilisin, polyethylene glycol, sodium carbonate, sodium Cl, tartaric acid. Tab. In 10s, 20s, 30s. *otc.*
Use: Soft contact lens care.

Renu Liquid. (Biosearch) P-Ca and Na caseinates, CHO-maltodextrin sucrose, F-partially hydrogenated soy oil, mono and diglycerides, soy lecithin, protein 35 g, CHO 125 g, fat 40 g, sodium 500

mg, potassium 1250 mg/L, 1 Cal/ml, 300 mOsm/kg, H_2O. In 250 ml ready to use. *otc.*
Use: Nutritional supplement.

Renu Multi-Purpose. (Bausch & Lomb) Isotonic soln. w/sodium Cl, sodium borate, boric acid, poloxamine, polyaminopropyl biguanide 0.00005%, EDTA. Soln. Bot. 118 ml, 237 ml, 355 ml. *otc.*
Use: Soft contact lens care.

Renu Saline. (Bausch & Lomb) Isotonic buffered soln. of sodium Cl, boric acid, polyaminopropyl biguanide 0.00003%, EDTA. Soln. Bot. 355 ml. *otc.*
Use: Soft contact lens care.

Renu Thermal Enzymatic Cleaner. (Bausch & Lomb) Subtilisin, sodium carbonate, sodium Cl, boric acid. Tab. 16s. *otc.*
Use: Soft contact lens care.

ReoPro. (Lilly) Abciximab 2 mg/ml. Inj. Vial 5 ml. *Rx.*
Use: Antiplatelet, monoclonal antibody (antithrombotic).

Repan. (Everett) Butalbital 50 mg, caffeine 40 mg, acetaminophen 325 mg/Tab. or Cap. Bot. 100s. *Rx.*
Use: Analgesic, sedative, hypnotic.

Repan CF. (Everett) Acetaminophen 650 mg, butalbital 50 mg/Tab. Bot. 100s. *Rx.*
Use: Analgesic combination.

•**repirinast.** (reh-PIRE-ih-nast) USAN.
Use: Antiallergic; antiasthmatic.

Replens. (Warner-Lambert) Purified water, glycerin, mineral oil, methylparaben. Gel. Appl. 3, 8 pre-filled. *otc.*
Use: Vaginal preparation.

Replete Liquid. (Clintec Nutrition) K caseinate, Ca caseinate, maltodextrin, sucrose, corn oil, lecithin, vitamins A, B_1, B_2, B_3, B_5, B_6, B_{12}, C, D, E, K, folic acid, biotin, choline, Ca, Cl, Cu, Fe, I, Mg, Mn, P, Zn. In 250 ml. *otc.*
Use: Nutritional supplement.

Reposans-10. (Wesley) Chlordiazepoxide HCl 10 mg/Cap. Bot. 1000s. *c-iv.*
Use: Antianxiety agent.

Reprieve. (Mayer) Caffeine 32 mg, salicylamide 225 mg, vitamin B_1 50 mg, homatropine methylbromide 0.5 mg/Tab. Bot. 8s, 16s. *Rx.*
Use: Analgesic combination.

•**repromicin.** (rep-ROW-MY-sin) USAN.
Use: Antibacterial.

•**reproterol hydrochloride.** (rep-ROW-TEE-role) USAN.
Use: Bronchodilator.

Reptilase-R. (Abbott Diagnostics) Diag-

nostic for the investigation of fibrin formation and disturbances in fibrin formation due to causes other than thrombin inhibition.
Use: Diagnostic aid.

Requa's Charcoal Tablets. (Requa) Wood charcoal 10 gr/Tab. Pkg. 50s. Can 125s. *otc.*
Use: Antiflatulent.

Resa. (Vita Elixir) Reserpine 0.25 mg/Tab. *Rx.*
Use: Antihypertensive.

Resaid. (Geneva Pharm) Phenylpropanolamine HCl 75 mg, chlorpheniramine maleate 12 mg/Cap. Bot. 100s, 1000s. *Rx.*
Use: Decongestant, antihistamine.

Resaid S.R. (Geneva Pharm) Phenylpropanolamine HCl 75 mg, chlorpheniramine maleate 12 mg/SR Cap. Bot. 100s, 1000s. *Rx.*
Use: Decongestant, antihistamine.

Rescaps-D S.R. (Geneva Pharm) Phenylpropanolamine HCl 75 mg, caramiphen edisylate 40 mg/Cap. Bot. 100s. *Rx.*
Use: Decongestant, antitussive.

Rescon Capsules. (ION) Pseudoephedrine 120 mg, chlorpheniramine maleate 12 mg/TR Cap. Bot. 100s. *Rx.*
Use: Decongestant, antihistamine.

Rescon-DM. (ION) Dextromethorphan HBr 10 mg, pseudoephedrine HCl 30 mg, chlorpheniramine maleate 2 mg, sugar free. Liq. Bot. 120 ml. *otc.*
Use: Antitussive, decongestant, antihistamine.

Rescon-ED. (ION) Chlorpheniramine maleate 8 mg, pseudoephedrine HCl 120 mg/Cap. Bot. 100s. *Rx.*
Use: Antihistamine, decongestant.

Rescon-GG Capsules. (ION) Pseudoephedrine HCl 120 mg, chlorpheniramine maleate 8 mg/Cap. Bot. 100s. *otc.*
Use: Decongestant, antihistamine.

Rescon-GG Liquid. (ION) Phenylephrine HCl 5 mg, guaifenesin 100 mg/5 ml Bot. 4 oz. *otc.*
Use: Decongestant, expectorant.

Rescon Jr. (ION) Pseudoephedrine HCl 60 mg, chlorpheniramine maleate 4 mg/SR Cap. Bot. 100s. *Rx.*
Use: Decongestant, antihistamine.

Rescon Liquid. (ION) Phenylpropanolamine HCl 12.5 mg, chlorpheniramine maleate 2 mg/5 ml. Bot. 120 ml, 473 ml. *otc.*
Use: Decongestant, antihistamine.

Resectisol. (McGaw) Mannitol soln. 5 g/1000 ml in distilled water (275 mOsm/L.). In 2000 ml. *Rx.*
Use: Genitourinary irrigant.

Reserpaneed. (Hanlon) Reserpine 0.25 mg/Tab. Bot. 100s, 1000s. *Rx.*
Use: Antihypertensive.

•**reserpine, U.S.P. 23.**
Use: Antihypertensive.
See: Arcum R-S, Tab. (Arcum).
 Broserpine, Tab. (Brothers).
 De Serpa, Tab. (De Leon).
 Elserpine, Tab. (Canright).
 Maso-Serpine, Tab. (Mason).
 Rauloydin, Tab. (Solvay).
 Raurine, Tab. (Westerfield).
 Reserpaneed, Tab. (Hanlon).
 Serpasil Preps. (Novartis).
 Sertabs, Tab. (Table Rock).
 T-Serp, Tab. (Tennessee).
 Vio-Serpine, Tab. (Solvay).
 Zepine, Tab. (Foy).

reserpine w/combinations.
See: Demi-Regroton, Tab. (Rhone-Poulenc Rorer).
 Diupres, Tab. (Merck).
 Harbolin, Tab. (Arcum).
 Hydromox R, Tab. (Lederle).
 Hydropres-25 or -50, Tab. (Merck).
 Hydroserp, Tab. (Zenith).
 Hydroserpine, Tab. (Geneva Pharm).
 Hydrotensin-50, Tab. (Mayrand).
 Mallopress, Tab. (Roberts).
 Metatensin, Tab. (Hoechst Marion Roussel).
 Naquival, Tab. (Schering-Plough).
 Regroton, Tab. (Rhone-Poulenc Rorer).
 Renese-R, Tab. (Pfizer Laboratories).
 Salutensin, Tab. (Bristol-Myers).
 Ser-Ap-Es, Tab. (Novartis).
 Serpasil-Apresoline, Tab. (Novartis).
 Serpasil-Esidrix, Tab. (Novartis).
 Unipres, Tab. (Solvay).

reserpine and chlorothiazide tablets.
Use: Antihypertensive.

reserpine and hydrochlorothiazide tablets. (Various Mfr.) Hydrochlorothiazide 25 mg or 50 mg, reserpine 0.125 mg/Tab. Bot. 100s, 1000s. *Rx.*
Use: Antihypertensive.

reserpine, hydralazine hydrochloride and hydrochlorothiazide.
Use: Antihypertensive.

Resinol Medicinal Ointment. (Mentholatum) Zinc oxide 12%, calamine 6%, resorcinol 2% in a lanolin and petrolatum base. Jar 3.5 oz, 1.25 oz. *otc.*
Use: Skin protectant.

resin uptake kit with liothyronine i-125 buffer solution.
See: Thyrostat-3 (Squibb).
resins, antacid.
See: Polyamine methylene Resins.
•resocortol butyrate. (reh-so-CORE-tole BYOO-tih-rate) USAN.
Use: Corticosteroid; anti-inflammatory (topical).
Resol. (Wyeth-Ayerst) Sodium 50 mEq, potassium 20 mEq, Cl 50 mEq, citrate 34 mEq, calcium 4 mEq, magnesium 4 mEq, phosphate 5 mEq, glucose 20 g/L. Contains 80 calories/L. Ctn. 32 fl oz. *Rx.*
Use: Fluid/electrolyte replacement.
Resolve/GP Daily Cleaner. (Allergan) Buffered solution with cocoamphocarboxyglycinate, sodium lauryl sulfate, hexylene glycol, alkyl ether sulfate, fatty acid amide surfactant cleaning agents, preservative free. Soln. Bot. 30 ml. *otc.*
Use: Contact lens product.
Resonium-A. (Sanofi Winthrop) Sodium polystyrene sulfonate. *Rx.*
Use: Potassium removing resin.
resorcin.
See: Resorcinol (Various Mfr.).
•resorcinol, U.S.P. 23.
Use: Keratolytic.
resorcinol and sulfur lotion.
Use: Scabicide, parasiticide, antifungal.
resorcinol w/combinations.
See: Acnomel, Cake, Cream. (SK-Beecham).
Bicozene, Cream (Ex-Lax).
Black and White Ointment (Schering-Plough).
Clearasil, Stick (Procter & Gamble).
Lanacane Creme (Combe).
Mazon, Oint. (SK-Beecham).
RA Lot. (Medco).
Rezamid Lot. (Dermick).
•resorcinol monoacetate, U.S.P. 23.
Use: Antiseborrheic, keratolytic.
See: Euresol, Liq. (Knoll).
W/Salicylic acid, ethyl alcohol, castor oil.
See: Resorcitate w/oil, Lot. (Almay).
W/Salicylic acid, LCD, betanaphthol, castor oil, isopropyl alcohol.
See: Neomark, Liq. (C & M Pharm).
resorcinolphthalein sodium.
See: Fluorescein Sodium, U.S.P. 23. (Various Mfr.).
W/Oil. Resorcinol monoacetate 1.5%, salicylic acid 1.5%, castor oil 1.5%, ethyl alcohol 81%. Bot. 8 fl oz.
Use: Topical antiseborrheic.
Resource. (Sandoz Nutrition) Ca and Na caseinates, soy protein isolate 37 g, sugar, hydrolyzed cornstarch 140 g, corn oil, soy lecithin 37 g, Na 890 mg, K 1600 mg, A, B_1, B_2, B_3, B_5, B_6, B_{12}, C, D, E, K, Ca, P, I, Fe, Mg, Cu, Zn, Mn, Cl, gluten free, vanilla, chocolate, strawberry flavor. Liq. Bot. 237 ml. *otc.*
Use: Nutritional therapy.
Resource Instant Crystals. (Sandoz Nutrition) Vanilla flavor: maltodextrin, sucrose, hydrogenated soy oil, sodium caseinate, calcium caseinate, soy protein isolate, potassium citrate, polyglycerol esters of fatty acids, artificial flavors, vitamins and minerals. Instant Crystals 1.5 oz. or 2 oz. packets. *otc.*
Use: Nutritional supplement.
Resource Plus. (Sandoz Nutrition) Ca and Na caseinates, soy protein isolate 54.9 g, maltodextrin, sucrose 200 g, corn oil, lecithin 53.3 g, Na 899 mg, K 1740 mg, A, B_1, B_2, B_3, B_5, B_6, B_{12}, C, D, E, K, biotin, choline, Ca, P, I, Fe, Mg, Cu, Zn, Cl, Mn, gluten free, vanilla, chocolate, strawberry flavor. Liq. Bot. 8 oz. *otc.*
Use: Nutritional therapy.
Respa-1st. (Respa) Pseudoephedrine HCl 60 mg, guaifenesin 600 mg. SR Tab. Bot. 100s. *Rx.*
Use: Decongestant, expectorant.
Respa-DM. (Respa) Dextromethorphan HBr 30 mg, guaifenesin 600 mg. SR Tab. Bot. 100s. *Rx.*
Use: Antitussive, expectorant.
Respa-GF. (Respa) Guaifenesin 600 mg, lactose. SR Tab. Bot. 100s. *Rx.*
Use: Expectorant.
Respahist. (Respa). Pseudoephedrine HCl 60 mg, brompheniramine maleate 6 mg/SR Cap. Bot 100s. *Rx.*
Use: Decongenstant, antihistamine.
Respaire-60 SR. (Laser) Pseudoephedrine HCl 60 mg, guaifenesin 200 mg/S.R. Cap. Bot. 100s, 1000s. *Rx.*
Use: Decongestant, expectorant.
Respaire-120 SR. (Laser) Pseudoephedrine HCl 120 mg, guaifenesin 250 mg/SR Cap. Bot. 100s, 1000s. *Rx.*
Use: Decongestant, expectorant.
Respalor. (Bristol-Myers) Protein 75 g, carbohyrate 146 g, fat 70 g, Na 1248 mg, K 1456 mg, Fe 12.5 mg, cal/L 1498. Lactose free. Vanilla flavor. With appropriate vitamins and minerals. Liq. Bot. 237 ml. *otc.*
Use: Nutritional support.
Respbid. (Boehringer Ingelheim) Theophylline 250 mg or 500 mg/Tab. Bot. 100s. *Rx.*

Use: Bronchodilator.

RespiGam. (MedImmune) RSV immunoglobulin (human) 2500 mg, sucrose 5%, albumin (human) 1% w/sodium 1 to 1.5 mEq/50 ml. Preservative free. I.V. Vial 2500 mg/50 ml. *Rx.*
Use: Passive immunization.

Respihaler Decadron Phosphate. (Merck).
See: Decadron phosphate, respihaler (Merc).

Respiracult. (Orion Diagnostica) Culture test for group A beta-hemolytic streptococci. In 10s.
Use: Diagnostic aid.

Respiralex. (Orion Diagnostica) Latex agglutination test to detect group A streptococci in throat and nasopharynx. Kit 1s.
Use: Diagnostic aid.

respiratory syncytial virus immune globulin (human) (RSV-IG).
Use: Prophylaxis against respiratory tract infection. [Orphan drug]
See: RespiGam, Inj. (MedImmune).

respiratory syncytial virus immune globulin intravenous (human) (RSV-IVIG).
Use: Respiratory syncytial virus immune serum.
See: RespiGam (MedImmune).

Rest Easy. (Walgreen) Acetaminophen 1000 mg, pseudoephedrine HCl 60 mg, dextromethorphan HBr 30 mg, doxylamine succinate 7.5 mg/30 ml. Bot. 6 oz, 16 oz. *otc.*
Use: Analgesic, decongestant, antitussive, antihistamine.

Restore. (Inagra) Psyllium hydrophilic mucilloid fiber 3.4 g/12 g dose, orange flavor, saccharin, sucrose. Pow. 390 g, 538 g. Also available sugar free with aspartame, phenylalanine 30 mg/tsp, saccharin. Pow. 300 g, 425 g. *otc.*
Use: Laxative.

Restoril. (Sandoz) Temazepam 7.5 mg, lactose. Cap. Bot. 100s. ControlPak 25s, UD 100s. *c-iv.*
Use: Sedative, hypnotic.

Retavase. (Boehringer Mannheim) Reteplase 10.8 IU (18.8 mg)/Pow. for inj. Kit. *Rx.*
Use: Managment of acute myocardial infarction.

reteplase.
Use: Management of acute myocardial infarction.
See: Retavase, Pow. for inj. (Boehringer Mannheim).

Retin-A Cream. (Ortho) Tretinoin 0.1%, 0.05% or 0.025%. Tube 20 g, 45 g. *Rx.*
Use: Antiacne.

Retin-A Gel. (Ortho) Tretinoin 0.01% or 0.025%, alcohol 90%. Tube 15 g, 45 g. *Rx.*
Use: Antiacne.

Retin-A Liquid. (Ortho) Tretinoin (retinoic acid, Vitamin A acid) 0.05%, polyethylene glycol 400, butylated hydroxytoluene and alcohol 55%. Bot. 28 ml. *Rx.*
Use: Antiacne.

retinoic acid. Tretinoin, U.S.P. 23.
Use: Keratolytic.
See: Retin A Prods. (Ortho).

retinoic acid, 9-cis. *Rx.*
Use: Acute promyelocytic leukemia. [Orphan drug]

retinoin.
Use: Squamous metaplasia of the ocular surface epithelia with mucus defiency and keratinization. [Orphan drug]

Retinol. (NBTY) Vitamin A 100,000 IU, glycol stearate, mineral oil, propylene glycol, lanolin oil, propylene glycol stearate SE, lanolin alcohol, retinol, parabens, EDTA. Cream. Tube 60 g. *otc.*
Use: Emollient.

Retinol-A. (Young Again Products) Vitamin A palmitate 300,000 IU/30 g. Cream. 60 g. *otc.*
Use: Emollient.

Retrovir. (Glaxo Wellcome) Zidovudine **Tab.:** 300 mg. Bot. 60s. **Cap:** 100 mg/Cap. Bot. 100s. **Syrup:** 50 mg/5 ml. Bot. 240 ml. **Inj:** 10 mg/ml. Vial 20 ml. *Rx.*
Use: Antiviral.

Reversol. (Organon) Edrophonium chloride 10 mg/ml. Inj. Vial. 10 ml. *Rx.*
Use: Cholinergic muscle stimulant.

Revex. (Ohmeda) Nalmefene 100 mcg/ml or 1 mg/ml. Inj. **100 mcg/ml:** Amp 1 ml; **1 mg/ml:** Amp 2 ml. *Rx.*
Use: Narcotic antagonist, antidote.

Rēv-Eyes. (Storz/Lederle) Dapiprazole HCl 25 mg. Pow. Vial. 5 ml. *Rx.*
Use: Alpha-adrenergic blocking agent, ophthalmic.

ReVia. (DuPont Merck) Naltrexone HCl 50 mg/Tab. Bot. 50s. *Rx.*
Use: Narcotic antagonist.

Revs Caffeine T.D. Capsules. (Eon Labs) Caffeine 250 mg/Cap. Bot. 100s, 1000s. *otc.*
Use: CNS stimulant.

Rexahistine. (Econo Med) Phenyl-

ephrine HCl 5 mg, chlorpheniramine maleate 1 mg, menthol 1 mg, sodium bisulfite 0.1%, alcohol 5%/5 ml. Bot. Gal. *otc.*
Use: Decongestant, antihistamine.

Rexahistine DH. (Econo-Rx) Codeine phosphate 10 mg, phenylephrine HCl 10 mg, chlorpheniramine maleate 2 mg, menthol 1 mg, alcohol 5%/5 ml. Bot. gal. *c-v.*
Use: Antitussive, decongestant, antihistamine.

Rexahistine Expectorant. (Econo-Rx) Codeine phosphate 10 mg, phenylephrine HCl 10 mg, chlorpheniramine maleate 2 mg, guaifenesin 100 mg, menthol 1 mg, alcohol 5%/5 ml. Bot. Gal. *c-v.*
Use: Antitussive, decongestant, antihistamine, expectorant.

Rexigen. (ION) Phendimetrazine tartrate 35 mg/Tab. Bot. 100s. *c-iii.*
Use: Anorexiant.

Rexigen Forte Capsules. (ION) Phendimetrazine tartrate 105 mg/SR Cap. Bot. 100s. *c-iii.*
Use: Anorexiant.

Rezamid Lotion. (Summers) Sulfur 5%, resorcinol 2%, SD-40 alcohol 28%. Lot. 56.7 ml. *otc.*
Use: Antiacne.

Rezulin. (Parke-Davis) Troglitazone 200 mg, 400 mg/Tab. Bot. 30s, 90s, UD 100s. *Rx.*
Use: Treatment of diabetes.

Rezine. (Marnel) Hydroxyzine HCl 10 mg or 25 mg. Tab. Bot. 100s. *Rx.*
Use: Antianxiety agent.

RF Latex Test. (Laboratory Diagnostics) Rapid latex agglutination test for the qualitative screening and semi-quantitative determination of rheumatoid factor. Kit 100s.
Use: Diagnostic aid.

R-Frone. (Serono)
See: Interferon Beta (Recombinant).

R-Gel. (Healthline Labs) Capsaicin 0.025%, EDTA. Gel. Tube 15 ml, 30 ml. *otc.*
Use: Analgesic, topical.

R-Gen. (Galderma) Purified water, amphoteric 2, hydrolyzed animal protein, lauramine oxide, methylparaben, benzalkonium Cl, tetrasodium, EDTA, propylparaben, fragrance. Bot. 8 oz. *otc.*
Use: Protein shampoo.

R-Gen. (Goldline) Iodinated glycerol 60 mg/5 ml, alcohol 21.75%. Elixir. Bot. pt.

Use: Expectorant.

R-Gene 10. (Pharmacia & Upjohn) Arginine HCl 10% (950 mOsm/L) with Cl ion 47.5 mEq/100 ml. Inj. 300 ml. *Rx.*
Use: Diagnostic aid, pituitary (growth hormone) function test.

R-HCTZ-H. (Lederle) Reserpine 0.1 mg, hydrochlorothiazide 15 mg, hydralazine HCl 25 mg/Tab. Bot. 100s, 500s. *Rx.*
Use: Antihypertensive.

Rheaban Maximum Strength. (Pfizer) Activated attapulgite 750 mg. Capl. Pkg. 12s. *otc.*
Use: Antidiarrheal.

Rheomacrodex. (Medisan) Dextran 40 10% in sodium Cl 0.9% or in dextrose 5%. Soln. Bot. 500 ml. *Rx.*
Use: Plasma expander.

Rheumatex. (Wampole) Latex agglutination test for the qualitative detection and quantitative determination of rheumatoid factor in serum. Kit 100s.
Use: Diagnostic aid.

rheumatoid factor tests.
See: Rheumanosticon Dri-Dot (Organon Teknika).

Rheumaton. (Wampole) Two-minute hemagglutination slide test for the qualitative and quantitative determination of rheumatoid factor in serum or synovial fluid. Test kit 20s, 50s, 150s.
Use: Diagnostic aid.

Rheumatrex Dose Pack. (Lederle) Methotrexate 2.5 mg. Tab. Pkg. 5, 7.5, 10, 12.5, 15 mg/week dose packs. *Rx.*
Use: Antipsoriatic.

Rhinall Drops. (Scherer) Phenylephrine HCl 0.25%, sodium bisulfite. Bot. oz. *otc.*
Use: Decongestant.

Rhinall Spray. (Scherer) Phenylephrine HCl 0.25%. Bot. oz. *otc.*
Use: Decongestant.

Rhinall 10. (Scherer) Phenylephrine HCl 0.2%. Drop. Bot. oz. *otc.*
Use: Decongestant.

Rhinatate. (Major) Phenylephrine tannate 25 mg, chlorpheniramine tannate 8 mg, pyrilamine tannate 25 mg/Tab. Bot. 100s, 250s. *Rx.*
Use: Decongestant, antihistamine.

Rhinocaps. (Ferndale) Aspirin 162 mg, acetaminophen 162 mg, phenylpropanolamine HCl 20 mg/Cap. Bot. 100s, 1000s. *otc.*
Use: Analgesic, decongestant.

Rhinocort. (Astra) Budesonide 32 mcg/actuation (200 sprays). Can 7 g. *Rx.*

Use: Intranasal steroid.

Rhinolar-EX. (McGregor) Phenylpropanolamine HCl 75 mg, chlorpheniramine maleate 8 mg/SR Cap. Dye free. Bot. 60s. *Rx.*
Use: Decongestant, antihistamine.

Rhinolar-EX 12. (McGregor) Phenylpropanolamine HCl 75 mg, chlorpheniramine maleate 12 mg/SR Cap. Dye free. Bot. 60s. *Rx.*
Use: Decongestant, antihistamine.

Rhinosyn. (Great Southern) Pseudoephedrine HCl 60 mg, chlorpheniramine maleate 4 mg, alcohol 0.45%, sucrose. Liq. Bot. 120 ml, 473 ml. *otc.*
Use: Decongestant, antihistamine.

Rhinosyn-DM Liquid. (Great Southern) Pseudoephedrine HCl 30 mg, chlorpheniramine maleate 2 mg, dextromethorphan HBr 15 mg, alcohol 1.4%, sucrose. Bot. 120 ml. *otc.*
Use: Decongestant, antihistamine, antitussive.

Rhinosyn-DMX Syrup. (Great Southern) Dextromethorphan HBr 15 mg, guaifenesin 100 mg, alcohol 1.4%. Bot. 120 ml. *otc.*
Use: Antitussive, expectorant.

Rhinosyn-PD Liquid. (Great Southern) Pseudoephedrine HCl 30 mg, chlorpheniramine maleate 2 mg. Liq. Bot. 120 ml. *otc.*
Use: Decongestant, antihistamine.

Rhinosyn-X Liquid. (Great Southern) Pseudoephedrine HCl 30 mg, dextromethorphan HBr 10 mg, guaifenesin 100 mg, alcohol 7.5%. Bot. 120 ml. *otc.*
Use: Decongestant, antitussive, expectorant.

rhodanate.
See: Potassium Thiocyanate.

rhodanide. More commonly Rhodanate, same as thiocyanate.
See: Potassium thiocyanate.

•**rh$_o$ (d) immune globulin,** (RH$_o$D ih-MYOON GLAB-byoo-lin) U.S.P. 23.
Formerly Rh$_o$ (D) Immune Globulin
Use: Immunizing agent (passive).
See: Gamulin Rh, Vial (Centeon).
   Mini-Gamulin Rh (Centeon).
   MICRh$_o$GAM (Ortho).
   BayRh$_o$D (Bayer).
   RhoGAM (Ortho).
   WinRho SD (Univax Biologics).

rh$_o$(d) immune globulin (intravenous).
Use: Immune thrombocytopenic purpura. [Orphan drug]
See: WinRho SD (Univax Biologics).

RhoGAM. (Ortho Diagnostic) Rh$_o$ (D) immune globulin (human). Single-dose vial Pkg. 5s; Prefilled syringe Pkg. 5s, 25s. *Rx.*
Use: Agent for immunization.

Rhuligel. (Rydelle) Phenylcarbinol 2%, menthol 0.3%, camphor 0.3%, SD alcohol 23A 31%. Gel 60 g. *otc.*
Use: Topical poison ivy product.

Rhulispray. (Rydelle) Phenylcarbinol 0.67%, calamine 4.7%, menthol 0.025%, camphor 0.25%, benzocaine 1.15%, alcohol 28.8%. Aerosol 120 g. *otc.*
Use: Topical poison ivy product.

Rhythmin. (Sidmak) Procainamide 250 mg or 500 mg/SR Tab. Bot. 100s, 500s, 1000s. *Rx.*
Use: Antiarrhythmic.

•**ribaminol.** (rye-BAM-ih-nahl) USAN.
Use: Memory adjuvant.

•**ribavirin,** (rye-buh-VIE-rin) U.S.P. 23.
Use: Antiviral. [Orphan drug]
See: Virazole, Inj. (ICN).

•**riboflavin,** (RYE-boh-FLAY-vin) U.S.P. 23.
Use: Vitamin (enzyme co-factor).
W/Nicotinamide. (Lilly) Riboflavin 5 mg, nicotinamide 200 mg/ml Amp. 1 ml, Box 100s.
Use: IM, IV; Vitamin B therapy.
W/Vitamins.
See: Vitamin Preparations.

•**riboflavin 5'-phosphate sodium,** U.S.P. 23.
Use: Vitamin.

•**riboprine.** (RYE-boe-PREEN) USAN.
Use: Antineoplastic.

Ribozyme Injection. (Fellows) Riboflavin-5-Phosphate Sodium 50 mg/ml Vial 10 ml. *Rx.*

ricin (blocked) conjugated murine mca. (Immunogen) *Rx.*
Use: Antineoplastic. [Orphan drug]

ricin (blocked) conjugated murine moab.
Use: Antineoplastic. [Orphan drug]

ricinoleate sodium.
See: Preceptin, Gel (Ortho).

Ricolon Solution. (Sanofi Winthrop) Ricolon concentrate. *Rx.*
Use: Leucocytotic preparation.

Rid. (Pfizer) Piperonyl butoxide 3%, pyrethrins 0.3%, petroleum distillate 1.2%, benzyl alcohol 2.4%. Bot. 2 oz, 4 oz. *otc.*
Use: Pediculicide.

Rid-a-Pain Gel. (Pfeiffer) Benzocaine 10%, menthol, eucalyptol, alcohol 7.5%. Tube. 10 g. *otc.*

Use: Local anesthetic, oral.

Ridaura. (SK-Beecham) Auranofin 3 mg/ Cap. Bot. 60s. *Rx.*
Use: Antirheumatic.

Ridenol. (R.I.D.) Acetaminophen 80 mg/ 5 ml. Syr. Bot. 120 ml. *otc.*
Use: Analgesic.

Rid Lice Control Spray. (Pfizer) Synthetic pyrethroids 0.5%, related compounds 0.065%, aromatic petroleum hydrocarbons 0.664%. Can 5 oz. *otc.*
Use: Pediculicide.

Rid Lice Elimination System. (Pfizer) Rid lice killing shampoo, nit removal comb, Rid lice control spray and instruction booklet/unit. *otc.*
Use: Pediculicide.

Rid Lice Shampoo-Kit. (Pfizer) Pyrethrins 0.3%, piperonyl butoxide 3%. Bot. 2 oz, 4 oz. *otc.*
Use: Pediculicide.

Ridaura Capsules. (SK-Beecham) Auranofin 3 mg/Cap. Bot. 60s. *Rx.*
Use: Antirheumatic.

•**ridogrel.** (RYE-doe-grell) USAN.
Use: Thromboxane synthetase inhibitor.

•**rifabutin,** (RIFF-uh-BYOO-tin) U.S.P. 23.
Use: Antibacterial (antimycobacterial); MAC disease [Orphan drug]
See: Mycobutin.

Rifadin. (Hoechst Marion Roussel) Rifampin. **150 mg/Cap.:** Bot. 30s. **300 mg/Cap.:** Bot. 30s, 60s, 100s. **600 mg/Inj.:** Vials. *Rx.*
Use: Antituberculous agent.

Rifamate. (Hoechst Marion Roussel) Rifampin 300 mg, isoniazid 150 mg/ Cap. Bot. 60s. *Rx.*
Use: Antituberculous agent.

•**rifametane.** (RIFF-ah-met-ane) USAN.
Use: Antibacterial.

•**rifamexil.** (riff-ah-MEX-ill) USAN.
Use: Antibacterial.

•**rifamide.** (RIFF-am-ide) USAN.
Use: Antibacterial.

•**rifampin,** (RIFF-am-pin) U.S.P. 23.
Use: Antibacterial.
See: Rifadin, Cap, Inj. (Hoechst Marion Roussel)
Rifomycin (Various Mfr.).
Rimactane, Cap. (Novartis).

rifampin and isoniazid capsules.
Use: Anti-infective (tuberculostatic).

rifampin, isoniazid, pyrazinamide.
Use: Anti-infective (tuberculostatic). [Orphan drug]

Rifapentin.
Use: Pulmonary tuberculosis; mycobacterium avium complex in AIDS patients. [Orphan drug]

•**rifapentine.** (RIFF-ah-pen-teen) USAN.
Use: Antibacterial.

Rifater. (Hoechst Marion Roussel) Rifampin 120 mg, isoniazid 50 mg, pyrazinamide 300 mg. Tab. 60s, UD 100s. *Rx.*
Use: Antituberculous agent.

•**rifaximin.** (riff-AX-ih-min) USAN.
Use: Antibacterial.

R-IFN-Beta. (Biogen)
See: Interferon Beta (Recombinant).

RIG.
Use: Rabies prophylaxis product.
See: Hyperab (Bayer).
Imogam (Merieux).

Rilutek. (Rhone-Poulenc Rorer) Riluzole 50 mg/Tab. *Rx.*
Use: ALS agent.

•**riluzole.** (RILL-you-zole) USAN.
Use: Treatment of amyotrophic lateral sclerosis. [Orphan drug]
See: Rilutek, Tab. (Rhone-Poulenc Rorer).

Rimactane. (Novartis) Rifampin 300 mg/ Cap. Bot. 30s, 60s, 100s. *Rx.*
Use: Antituberculous agent.

Rimadyl. (Roche) *Rx.*
Use: Nonsteroidal anti-inflammatory agent, analgesic.
See: Carprofen.

•**rimantadine hydrochloride.** (rih-MAN-tuh-deen) USAN.
Use: Antiviral.
See: Flumadine, Tab., Syr. (Forest).

•**rimcazole hydrochloride.** (RIM-kazz-OLE) USAN.
Use: Antipsychotic.

•**rimexolone.** USAN.
Use: Anti-inflammatory.
See: Vexol, Susp. (Alcon).

•**rimiterol hydrobromide.** (RIH-mih-TER-ole) USAN.
Use: Bronchodilator.

Rimso-50. (Research Industries) Dimethyl sulfoxide in a 50% aqueous soln. Bot. 50 ml. *Rx.*
Use: Interstitial cystitis, intravesical instillation.

Rinade. (Econo Med) Chlorpheniramine maleate 8 mg, phenylephrine HCl 20 mg, methscopolamine nitrate 2.5 mg/ Cap. Bot. 120s. *Rx.*
Use: Antihistamine, decongestant, anticholinergic.

Rinade-BID. (Econo Med) Chlorpheniramine maleate 8 mg, pseudoephedrine HCl 120 mg/SR Cap. Bot. 100s. *Rx.*
Use: Antihistamine, decongestant.

ringer's-dextrose injection. (Various Mfr.) Dextrose 50 g/l, Na 147, K 4, C 4.5, Cl 156. 500, 1000 ml. *Rx.*
Use: Parenteral nutritional supplement.

• **ringer's injection,** U.S.P. 23.
Use: Fluid and electrolyte replenisher, irrigating soln.
W/Dextrose. (Bayer) 5% soln. Bot. 1000 ml.

ringer's injection. (Abbott) 250 ml, 500 ml, 1000 ml; (Invenex) 250 ml, 500 ml, 1000 ml; Abbo-Vac glass or flexible containers, Vial 50 ml Pkg. 25s. (Lilly) Amp. 20 ml, Pkg. 6s. (Bayer) Bot. 500 ml, 1000 ml.
Use: Fluid and electrolyte replenisher, irrigating soln.

ringer's injection, lactated.
Use: Fluid and electrolyte replenisher.

ringer's irrigation. (Various Mfr.) Sodium chloride 0.86 g, potassium chloride 0.03 g, calcium chloride 0.033 g/ 100 ml. Bot. 1 L. *Rx.*
Use: Irrigation solution.

Riopan. (Whitehall) Magaldrate 540 mg, sodium 0.1 mg/5 ml. Bot. 6 oz, 12 oz. Individual Cup 30 ml each. *otc.*
Use: Antacid.

Riopan Plus Double Strength Suspension. (Whitehall) Magaldrate 1080 mg, simethicone 40 mg/5 ml. Bot. 360 ml. *otc.*
Use: Antacid, antiflatulent.

Riopan Plus Double Strength Tablets. (Whitehall) Magaldrate 1080 mg, simethicone 20 mg. Chew. Tab. Bot. 60s. *otc.*
Use: Antacid, antiflatulent.

Riopan Plus Suspension. (Whitehall) Magaldrate 540 mg, simethicone 40 mg/5 ml. Bot. 360 ml. *otc.*
Use: Antacid, antiflatulent.

Riopan Plus Tablets. (Whitehall) Magaldrate 480 mg, simethicone 20 mg. Chew. Tab. Bot. 50s, 100s. *otc.*
Use: Antacid, antiflatulent.

• **rioprostil.** (RYE-oh-PRAHS-till) USAN.
Use: Gastric antisecretory.

• **ripazepam.** (rip-AZE-eh-pam) USAN.
Use: Tranquilizer (minor).

• **risedronate sodium.** (riss-ED-row-nate) USAN.
Use: Regulator (calcium).

• **rismorelin porcine.** (riss-more-ELL-in PORE-sine) USAN.
Use: Growth hormone-releasing hormone.

• **risocaine.** (RIZZ-oh-cane) USAN.
Use: Anesthetic (local).

• **risotilide hydrochloride.** (rih-SO-tih-LIDE) USAN.
Use: Cardiac depressant (antiarrhythmic).

Risperdal. (Janssen) Risperidone 1 mg, 2 mg, 3 mg, 4 mg. Tab. Bot. 60s, blister pack 100s. Risperidone 1 mg/ml/ Oral Soln. Bot. 100 ml w/calibrated pipette. *Rx.*
Use: Antipsychotic.

• **risperidone.** (RISS-PURR-ih-dohn) USAN.
Use: Antipsychotic, neuroleptic.
See: Risperdal, Tab. (Janssen).

• **ristianol phosphate.** (riss-TIE-ah-NOLE) USAN.
Use: Immunoregulator.

Ritalin Hydrochloride. (Novartis) Methylphenidate HCl. 5 mg, 10 mg, 20 mg. Tab. Bot. 100s. *c-ii.*
Use: CNS stimulant.

Ritalin-SR. (Novartis) Methylphenidate HCl 20 mg/SR Tab. Bot. 100s. *c-ii.*
Use: CNS stimulant.

• **ritanserin.** (rih-TAN-ser-in) USAN.
Use: Serotonin antagonist.

• **ritodrine.** (RIH-toe-DREEN) USAN.
Use: Smooth muscle relaxant.
See: Yutopar, Inj. (Astra).

• **ritodrine hydrochloride,** (RIH-toe-dreen) U.S.P. 23.
Use: Relaxant (smooth muscle).

ritodrine hydrochloride. (Abbott) Ritodrine HCl 10 mg/ml, 15 mg/ml or 0.3 mg/ml. **10 mg/ml:** Amp. 5 ml. **15 mg/ ml:** Vial 10 ml. **0.3 mg/ml:** In 15% dextrose. LifeCare flexible container 500 ml. *Rx.*
Use: Uterine relaxant.

• **ritolukast.** (rih-tah-LOO-kast) USAN.
Use: Antiasthmatic (leukotriene antagonist).

• **ritonavir.** (rih-TON-a-veer) USAN.
Use: Antiviral.
See: Norvir, Cap., Susp. (Abbott).

• **rizatriptan benzoate.** (rye-zah-TRIP-tan BENZ-oh-ate) USAN.
Use: Antimigraine.

• **rizatriptan sulfate.** (rye-zah-TRIP-tan) USAN.
Use: Antimigraine.

RMS Suppositories. (Upsher-Smith) Morphine sulfate 5 mg, 10 mg, 20 mg or 30 mg/Supp. Box 12s. *c-ii.*
Use: Narcotic analgesic.

Robafen. (Major) Guaifenesin 100 mg/5 ml, alcohol 3.5%. Syr. Bot. 118 ml, 240 ml, pt, gal. *otc.*
Use: Expectorant.

Robafen AC Cough. (Major) Guaifenesin 100 mg, codeine phosphate 10 mg/5 ml, alcohol 3.5%, parabens. Syrup. Bot. 473 ml. *c-v.*
Use: Expectorant, narcotic antitussive.

Robafen-CF. (Major) Phenylpropanolamine HCl 12.5 mg, dextromethorphan HBr 10 mg, guaifenesin 100 mg, alcohol 4.75%. Bot. 118 ml. *otc.*
Use: Antitussive, expectorant, decongestant.

Robafen DAC. (Major) Pseudoephedrine 30 mg, codeine phosphate 10 mg, guaifenesin 100 mg, alcohol 1.4%. Bot. Pt. *c-v.*
Use: Decongestant, antitussive, expectorant.

Robafen DM. (Major) Dextromethorphan HBr 10 mg, guaifenesin 100 mg/5 ml, alcohol 1.4%. Syrup. Bot. 473 ml. *otc.*
Use: Antitussive, expectorant.

robanul.
See: Robinul, Preps. (Robins).

Robathol Bath Oil. (Pharmaceutical Specialties) Cottonseed oil, alkyl aryl polyether alcohol. Lanolin free. Bot. 240 ml, 480 ml, gal. *otc.*
Use: Bath dermatological.

Robaxin. (Robins) Methocarbamol. **Tab.:** 500 mg, Bot. 100s, 500s, UD 100s. **Inj.:** 1 g/10 ml of a 50% aqueous soln. of polyethylene glycol 300. Vial 10 ml. *Rx.*
Use: Skeletal muscle relaxant.

Robaxin-750. (Robins) Methocarbamol 750 mg/Tab. Bot. 100s, 500s, Dis-Co Pak 100s. *Rx.*
Use: Skeletal muscle relaxant.

Robaxisal. (Robins) Methocarbamol (Robaxin) 400 mg, aspirin 325 mg/Tab. Bot. 100s, 500s, Dis-Co pack 100s. *Rx.*
Use: Muscle relaxant, analgesic.

Robimycin. (Robins) Erythromycin 250 mg/Tab. Bot. 100s, 500s. *Rx.*
Use: Anti-infective, erythromycin.

Robinul. (Robins) Glycopyrrolate 1 mg/Tab. Bot. 100s, 500s. *Rx.*
Use: Anticholinergic.

Robinul Forte Tablets. (Robins) Glycopyrrolate 2 mg/Tab. Bot. 100s. *Rx.*
Use: Anticholinergic.

Robinul Injectable. (Robins) Glycopyrrolate 0.2 mg/ml, benzyl alcohol 0.9%. Vial 1 ml, 2 ml, 5 ml, 20 ml. *Rx.*
Use: Anticholinergic.

Robitet. (Robins) Tetracycline HCl. Cap. **250 mg:** Bot. 100s, 1000s; **500 mg:** Bot. 100s, 500s.
Use: Anti-infective, tetracycline.

Robitussin. (Robins) Guaifenesin 100 mg/5 ml, alcohol 3.5%. Bot 1 oz, 4 oz, 8 oz, 1 pt, gal. UD 5 ml, 10 ml, 15 ml. *otc.*
Use: Expectorant.

Robitussin A-C. (Robins) Guaifenesin 100 mg, codeine phosphate 10 mg/5 ml, alcohol 3.5%, saccharin, sorbitol. Bot. 2 oz, 4 oz, pt, gal. *c-v.*
Use: Expectorant, antitussive.

Robitussin-CF. (Robins) Guaifenesin 100 mg, phenylpropanolamine HCl 12.5 mg, dextromethorphan HBr 10 mg/10 ml, alcohol 4.75%, saccharin, sorbitol. Syr. Bot. 4 oz, 8 oz, 12 oz, pt. *otc.*
Use: Expectorant, decongestant, antitussive.

Robitussin Cold & Cough Liqui-Gels. (Robins) Guaifenesin 200 mg, pseudoephedrine HCl 30 mg, dextromethorphan HBr 10 mg, sorbitol. Cap. Bot. 20s. *otc.*
Use: Antitussive, expectorant, decongestant.

Robitussin Cough Calmers. (Robins) Dextromethorphan HBr 5 mg, corn syrup, sucrose, cherry flavor. Loz. Pkg. 16s. *otc.*
Use: Antitussive.

Robitussin Cough Drops. (Robins) Menthol 7.4 mg and 10 mg, eucalyptus oil, sucrose, corn syrup. Loz. Pkg. 9s, 25s, menthol 10 mg, eucalyptus oil, sucrose, corn syrup, honey-lemon flavor. Loz. Pkg. 9s, 25s. *otc.*
Use: Antitussive.

Robitussin-DAC. (Robins) Guaifenesin 100 mg, pseudoephedrine HCl 30 mg, codeine phosphate 10 mg/5 ml, alcohol 1.9%, saccharin, sorbitol. Syr. Bot. 4 oz, pt. *c-v.*
Use: Expectorant, decongestant, antitussive.

Robitussin Dis-Co. (Robins) Guaifenesin 100 mg, alcohol 3.5%/5 ml. Syr. UD pack 5 ml, 10 ml, 15 ml; (10 × 10s). *otc.*
Use: Expectorant.

Robitussin-DM. (Robins) Guaifenesin 100 mg, dextromethorphan HBr 10 mg/5 ml. Syr. Bot. 4 oz, 8 oz, pt, gal, UD 5 ml, 10 ml (100s). *otc.*
Use: Expectorant, antitussive.

Robitussin Liquid Center Cough Drops. (Robins) Menthol 10 mg, eucalyptus oil, corn syrup, honey, lemon oil, high fructose, parabens, sorbitol, sucrose. Loz. Pkg. 20s. *otc.*
Use: Mouth and throat products.

Robitussin Maximum Strength Cough & Cold Formula. (Robins) Dextro-

methorphan HBr 15 mg, pseudoephedrine HCl 30 mg, alcohol 1.4%, glucose. Liq. Bot. 240 ml. *otc.*
Use: Antitussive, decongestant.

Robitussin Night Relief. (Robins) Acetaminophen 108.3 mg, pseudoephedrine HCl 10 mg, pyrilamine maleate 8.3 mg, dextromethorphan HBr 5 mg, alcohol-free, saccharin, sorbitol. Bot. 300 ml. *otc.*
Use: Analgesic, decongestant, antihistamine, antitussive.

Robitussin-PE. (Robins) Guaifenesin 100 mg, pseudoephedrine HCl 30 mg/5 ml, alcohol 1.4%, saccharin. Syr. Bot. 4 oz, 8 oz, pt. *otc.*
Use: Expectorant, decongestant.

Robitussin Pediatric. (Robins) Dextromethorphan HBr 7.5 mg/5 ml, alcohol free, saccharin, sorbitol, cherry flavor. Liq. Bot. 120, 240 ml. *otc.*
Use: Antitussive.

Robitussin Pediatric Cough & Cold Formula. (Robins) Dextromethorphan HBr 7.5 mg, pseudoephedrine HCl 15 mg/5 ml. Liq. Bot. 120 ml. *otc.*
Use: Antitussive, decongestant.

Robitussin Severe Congestion Liqui-Gels. (Robins) Guaifenesin 200 mg, pseudoephedrine HCl 30 mg, sorbitol. Cap. Pkg. 24s. *otc.*
Use: Expectorant, decongestant.

Robomol/ASA Tabs. (Major) Methocarbamol w/ASA. Bot. 100s, 500s. *Rx.*
Use: Skeletal muscle relaxant, analgesic.

Rocaltrol. (Roche) Calcitriol 0.25 mcg or 0.5 mcg/Cap. **0.25 mcg:** Bot. 30s, 100s. **0.5 mcg:** Bot. 100s. *Rx.*
Use: Management of hypocalcemia in patients undergoing chronic renal dialysis.

• **rocastine hydrochloride.** (row-KASS-teen) USAN.
Use: Antihistamine.

Rocephin. (Roche) Ceftriaxone sodium 250 mg, 500 mg, 1 g, 2 g, or 10 g/ Vial. **250 mg, 500 mg:** Vial. **1 g, 2 g:** Vial, piggyback vial, ADD-Vantage vial. **10 g:** Bulk Containers. **1 g, 2 g, Frozen Premixed:** 50 ml plastic containers. *Rx.*
Use: Anti-infective, cephalosporin.

• **rocuronium bromide.** (row-kuhr-OH-nee-uhm) USAN.
Use: Neuromuscular blocking agent.
See: Zemuron, Inj. (Organon).

• **rodocaine.** (ROW-doe-cane) USAN.
Use: Local anesthetic.

roentgenography.
See: Iodine Products, Diagnostic.

Roferon-A. (Roche) Interferon alfa-2a, recombinant as 3 million, 6 million, 9 million, 18 million or 36 million IU/Vial in injectable soln. Available as Sterile Pow. yielding 18 million IU/3 ml when reconstituted. Subcutaneous or intramuscular Inj. 3 million IU/ml. 6 million IU/ml. 9 million IU/0.9 ml. 18 million IU/3 ml. 36 million IU/1 ml. Single-dose vial (3, 6 million IU/ml); multidose vial (9, 18, 36 million IU). *Rx.*
Use: Antineoplastic agent.

• **roflurane.** (row-FLEW-rane) USAN.
Use: Anesthetic (inhalation).

Rogaine. (Pharmacia & Upjohn) Minoxidil 2% Topical Soln. Bot. 60 ml w/applicator. *otc.*
Use: Male pattern baldness.

• **rogletimide.** (row-GLETT-ih-MIDE) USAN. Pyridoglutethimide.
Use: Antineoplastic (aromatase inhibitor).

Rolaids Calcium Rich. (Warner-Lambert) Calcium carbonate 412 mg, magnesium hydroxide 80 mg. Chew. Tab. 12s, 36s, 75s, 150s. *otc.*
Use: Antacid.

Rolatuss Expectorant Liquid. (Huckaby) Phenylephrine HCl 5 mg, chlorpheniramine maleate 2 mg, codeine phosphate 9.85 mg, ammonium Cl 33.3 mg, alcohol 5%. Bot. 480 ml. *c-v.*
Use: Decongestant, antitussive, antihistamine, expectorant.

Rolatuss w/Hydrocodone. (Major) Phenylpropanolamine HCl 3.3 mg, phenylephrine HCl 5 mg, pyrilamine maleate 3.3 mg, pheniramine maleate 3.3 mg, hydrocodone bitartrate 1.67 mg. Liq. Bot. 480 ml. *c-iii.*
Use: Decongestant, antitussive, antihistamine.

Rolatuss Plain Liquid. (Major) Phenylephrine HCl 5 mg, chlorpheniramine maleate 2 mg/5 ml. Liq. Bot. 473 ml. *otc.*
Use: Decongestant, antihistamine.

• **roletamide.** (row-LET-am-ide) USAN.
Use: Sedative, hypnotic.

• **rolgamidine.** (role-GAM-ih-deen) USAN.
Use: Antidiarrheal.

Rolicap. (Arcum) Vitamins A acetate 5000 IU, D_2 400 IU, B_1 3 mg, B_2 2.5 mg, B_6 10 mg, C 50 mg, niacinamide 20 mg, B_{12} 1 mcg/Chew. Tab. Bot. 100s, 1000s. *otc.*
Use: Vitamin supplement.

- **rolicyprine.** (ROW-lih-SIGH-preen) USAN.
  Use: Antidepressant.
- **rolipram.** (ROLE-ih-pram) USAN.
  Use: Tranquilizer.
- **rolitetracycline.** (ROW-lee-tet-rah-SIGH-kleen) USAN.
  Use: Antibacterial.
- **rolitetracycline nitrate.** (ROW-lee-tet-rah-SIGH-kleen) USAN. Tetrim.
  Use: Antibacterial.
- **rolodine.** (ROW-low-deen) USAN.
  Use: Muscle relaxant (skeletal).

Romach Antacid Tablets. (Last) Magnesium carbonate 400 mg, sodium bicarbonate 250 mg/Tab. Strip pack 60s, 500s. *otc.*
  Use: Antacid.

- **romazarit.** (row-MAZZ-ah-rit) USAN.
  Use: Anti-inflammatory, antirheumatic.

Romazicon. (Roche) Flumazenil 0.1 mg/ml, parabens, EDTA. Inj. vials 5 and 10 ml. *Rx.*
  Use: Antidotes.

Romex Cough & Cold Capsules. (APC) Guaifenesin 65 mg, dextromethorphan HBr 10 mg, chlorpheniramine maleate 1.5 mg, pyrilamine maleate 12.5 mg, phenylephrine HCl 5 mg, acetaminophen 160 mg/Cap. Bot. 21s. *otc.*
  Use: Expectorant, antitussive, antihistamine, decongestant.

Romex Cough & Cold Tablets. (APC) Dextromethorphan HBr 7.5 mg, phenylephrine HCl 2.5 mg, ascorbic acid 30 mg. Box 15s. *otc.*
  Use: Antitussive, decongestant.

Romex Troches & Liquid. (APC) **Troche:** Polymyxin B sulfate 1000 units, benzocaine 5 mg, cetalkonium Cl 2.5 mg, gramicidin 100 mcg, chlorpheniramine maleate 0.5 mg, tyrothricin 2 mg. Pkg. 10s. **Liq.:** Guaifenesin 200 mg, dextromethorphan HBr 60 mg, chlorpheniramine maleate 12 mg, phenylephrine HCl 30 mg/fl oz. Bot. 4 oz. *Rx.*
  Use: Anti-infective, antihistamine, expectorant, antitussive, decongestant.

Rondamine-DM. (Major) Pseudoephedrine 25 mg/ml, carbinoxamine maleate 2 mg/ml, dextromethorphan HBr 4 mg/ml. Drop. 30 ml. *Rx.*
  Use: Decongestant, antihistamine, antitussive.

Rondec-DM Oral Drops. (Dura) Carbinoxamine maleate 2 mg, pseudoephedrine HCl 25 mg, dextromethorphan HBr 4 mg/ml, alcohol 6%. Bot. 30 ml w/dropper. *Rx.*

  Use: Antihistamine, decongestant, antitussive.

Rondec-DM Syrup. (Dura) Carbinoxamine maleate 4 mg, pseudoephedrine HCl 60 mg, dextromethorphan HBr 15 mg/5 ml, alcohol 6%. Bot. 4 oz, pt. *Rx.*
  Use: Antihistamine, decongestant, antitussive.

Rondec Oral Drops. (Dura) Carbinoxamine maleate 2 mg, pseudoephedrine HCl 25 mg/ml. Bot. 30 ml. *Rx.*
  Use: Antihistamine, decongestant.

Rondec Syrup. (Dura) Carbinoxamine maleate 4 mg, pseudoephedrine HCl 60 mg/5 ml. Syr. Bot. 120 ml, 473 ml. *Rx.*
  Use: Antihistamine, decongestant.

Rondec Tablets. (Dura) Pseudoephedrine HCl 60 mg, carbinoxamine maleate 4 mg, lactose/Tab. Bot. 100s, 500s. *Rx.*
  Use: Decongestant, antihistamine.

Rondec-TR. (Dura) Carbinoxamine 8 mg, pseudoephedrine HCl 120 mg/SR Tab. Bot. 100s. *Rx.*
  Use: Antihistamine, decongestant.

- **ronidazole.** (row-NYE-dazz-OLE) USAN.
  Use: Antiprotozoal.
- **ronnel.** (RAHN-ell) USAN. Fenchlorphos.
  Use: Insecticide (systemic).
  See: Korlan (Dow).
    Trolene (Dow).

Ronvet. (Armenpharm) Erythromycin stearate 250 mg/Tab. Bot. 100s. *Rx.*
  Use: Anti-infective, erythromycin.

- **ropinirole hydrochloride.** (row-PIN-ih-role) USAN.
  Use: Antiparkinsonian (D_2 receptor agonist).
- **ropitoin hydrochloride.** (ROW-pih-toe-in) USAN.
  Use: Cardiac depressant (antiarrhythmic).

ropivacaine HCl.
  Use: Anesthetic.
  See: Naropin, Inj. (Astra USA).

- **ropizine.** (row-PIH-zeen) USAN.
  Use: Anticonvulsant.
- **roquinimex.** (row-KWIH-nih-mex) USAN.
  Use: Biological response modifier; immunomodulator; antineoplastic. [Orphan drug]
  See: Linomide.

rosa gallical.
  See: Estivin, Soln. (Alcon).

rosaniline dyes.
  See: Fuchsin, Basic (Various Mfr.).
    Methylrosaniline Cl, Soln., Inj. (Various Mfr.).

- **rosaramicin.** (row-ZAR-ah-MY-sin) USAN. *Formerly Rosamicin.*
  Use: Antibacterial.
- **rosaramicin butyrate.** (row-ZAR-ah-MY-sin BYOO-tih-rate) USAN. *Formerly Rosamicin Butyrate.*
  Use: Antibacterial.
- **rosaramicin propionate.** (row-ZAR-ah-MY-sin PRO-pee-oh-nate) USAN. *Formerly Rosamicin Propionate.*
  Use: Antibacterial.
- **rosaramicin sodium phosphate.** (row-ZAR-ah-MY-sin) USAN. *Formerly Rosamicin Sodium Phosphate.*
  Use: Antibacterial.
- **rosaramicin stearate.** (row-ZAR-ah-MY-sin STEE-ah-rate) USAN. *Formerly Rosamicin Stearate.*
  Use: Antibacterial.
- **rose bengal.** (Akorn) Rose bengal 1%. Bot. 5 ml.
  Use: Diagnostic for staining dead ocular tissue.
- **rose bengal sodium I 125.** USAN.
  Use: Radioactive agent.
- **rose bengal sodium I 131 injection,** U.S.P. 23.
  Use: Diagnostic aid (hepatic function), radioactive agent.
- **rose bengal strips.** (Pilkington Barnes Hind) Rose bengal 1.3 mg. Strip box 100s. *otc.*
  Use: Diagnostic aid.
- **Rose-C Liquid.** (Barth's) Vitamin C 300 mg, rose hip extract/Tsp. Dropper Bot. 2 oz, 8 oz. *otc.*
  Use: Vitamin C supplement.
- **rose hips.** (Burgin-Arden) Vitamin C 300 mg, in base of sorbitol. Bot. 4 oz, 8 oz. *otc.*
  Use: Vitamin C supplement.
- **rose hips vitamin C.** (Kirkman Sales) Vitamin C. **100 mg/Tab:** Bot. 100s, 250s. **250 mg or 500 mg/Tab:** Bot. 100s, 250s, 500s. *otc.*
  Use: Vitamin C supplement.
- **rose oil,** N.F. 18.
  Use: Pharmaceutic aid (perfume).
- **Rosets.** (Akorn) Rose bengal 1.3 mg/strip. Pkg. 100s. *Rx.*
  Use: Diagnostic agent, ophthalmic.
- **rose water, stronger,** N.F. 18.
  Use: Pharmaceutic aid (perfume).
- **rose water ointment.**
  Use: Emollient, ointment base.
- **rosin,** U.S.P. XXI.
  Use: Stiffening agent, pharmaceutical necessity.

- **rosoxacin.** (row-SOX-ah-sin) USAN.
  Use: Antibacterial.
  See: Rosoxacin, Pow. (Sanofi Winthrop).
- **Ross SLD.** (Ross) Low-residue nutritional supplement for patients restricted to a clear liquid feeding or with fat malabsorption disorders. Packet 1.35 oz. Ctn. 6s. Case 4 ctn. Can 13.5 oz. Case 6s. *otc.*
  Use: Nutritional supplement.
- **Rotalex Test.** (Orion Diagnostica) Latex slide agglutination test for detection of rotavirus in feces. Kit 1s.
  Use: Diagnostic aid.
- **Rotazyme II.** (Abbott Diagnostics) Enzyme immunoassay for detection of rotavirus antigen in feces. Test kit 50s.
  Use: Diagnostic aid.
- **rotoxamine.** (row-TOX-ah-meen) USAN.
  Use: Antihistamine.
- **Rowasa.** (Solvay) **Rectal Susp.:** Mesalamine 4 g/60 ml. In units of 7 disposable bot. **Supp.:** Mesalamine 500 mg. Box 12s, 24s. *Rx.*
  Use: Ulcerative colitis, proctosigmoiditis, proctitis.
- **roxadimate.** (rox-AD-ih-mate) USAN.
  Use: Sunscreen.
- **Roxanol Oral Solution.** (Roxane) Morphine sulfate concentrated oral soln, sugar-free and alcohol free. **20 mg/ml:** Bot. 30 ml or 120 ml w/calibrated dropper. **100 mg/5 ml:** Bot. 240 ml w/calibrated spoon. *c-II.*
  Use: Narcotic analgesic.
- **Roxanol Rectal.** (Roxane) Morphine sulfate 5, 10, 20, 30 mg. Supp. 12s. *c-II.*
  Use: Narcotic agonist analgesic.
- **Roxanol 100.** (Roxane) Morphine sulfate 100 mg/5 ml. Soln. Bot. 240 ml. *c-II.*
  Use: Narcotic agonist analgesic.
- **Roxanol Rescudose.** (Roxane) Morphine sulfate 10 mg/2.5 ml. Oral Soln. UD 2.5 ml. *c-II.*
  Use: Narcotic agonist analgesic.
- **Roxanol SR Tablets.** (Roxane) Morphine sulfate 30 mg/SR Tab. Bot. 50s, 250s, UD 100s. *c-II.*
  Use: Narcotic analgesic.
- **Roxandol UD.** (Roxane) Morphine sulfate 20 mg/5 ml. Soln. Bot. 100, 500 ml. *c-II.*
  Use: Narcotic agonist analgesic.
- **roxarsone.** (ROX-AHR-sone) USAN.
  Use: Antibacterial.
- **roxatidine acetate hydrochloride.** (ROX-ah-tih-DEEN) USAN.
  Use: Antiulcer.

Roxicet Oral Solution. (Roxane) Oxycodone HCl 5 mg, acetaminophen 325 mg/5 ml. Bot. UD 5 ml, 500 ml. *c-II*.
Use: Narcotic analgesic combination.

Roxicet 5/500. (Roxane) Oxycodone HCl 5 mg, acetaminophen 500 mg/Cap. Bot. 100s, UD 100s. *c-II*.
Use: Narcotic analgesic combination.

Roxicet Tablets. (Roxane) Oxycodone HCl 5 mg, acetaminophen 325 mg, 0.4% alcohol/Tab. Bot. 100s, 500s, UD 100s. *c-II*.
Use: Narcotic analgesic combination.

Roxicodone. (Roxane) **Liq.:** Oxycodone HCl 5 mg/5 ml. Bot. 500 ml. **Tab.:** Oxycodone HCl 5 mg. Bot. 100s, UD 4 × 25s. *c-II*.
Use: Narcotic analgesic.

Roxilox. (Roxane) Oxycodone HCl 5 mg, acetaminophen 500 mg/Cap. Bot. 100s. *c-II*.
Use: Narcotic analgesic combination.

Roxiprin Tablets. (Roxane) Oxycodone HCl 4.5 mg, oxycodone terephthalate 0.38 mg, aspirin 325 mg/Tab. Bot. 100s, 1000s, UD 100s. *c-II*.
Use: Narcotic analgesic combination.

• **roxithromycin.** (ROX-ith-row-MY-sin) USAN.
Use: Antibacterial.

R/S Lotion. (Summers) Sulfur 5%, resorcinol 2%, alcohol 28%. Lot. Bot. 56.7 ml. *otc*.
Use: Antiacne.

R-S Lotion. (Hill) No. 2: Sulfur 8%, resorcinol monoacetate 4%. Bot. 2 oz. *otc*.
Use: Topical drying medication.

R-Tannamine. (Qualitest) Phenylephrine tannate 25 mg, chlorpheniramine tannate 8 mg, pyrilamine tannate 25 mg/Tab. Bot. 100s. *Rx*.
Use: Decongestant, anithistamine.

R-Tannamine Pediatric. (Qualitest) Phenylephrine tannate 5 mg, chlorpheniramine tannate 2 mg, pyrilamine tannate 12.5 mg, 120 ml, 473 ml. *Rx*.
Use: Decongestant, antihistamine.

R-Tannate Tablets. (Various Mfr.) Phenylephrine tannate 25 mg, chlorpheniramine tannate 8 mg, pyrilamine tannate 25 mg. In 100s. *Rx*.
Use: Decongestant, antihistamine.

R-Tannate Pediatric Suspension. (Various Mfr.) Phenylephrine tannate 5 mg, chlorpheniramine tannate 2 mg, pyrilamine tannate 12.5 mg, saccharin. In 473 ml. *Rx*.
Use: Decongestant, antihistamine.

RII Retinamide.

Use: Myelodysplastic syndromes. [Orphan drug]

rt-PA.
Use: Tissue plasminogen.
See: Activase (Genetech).

RU 486.
Use: Antiprogesterone.
See: Mifepristone.

Rubacell. (Abbott Diagnostics) Passive hemagglutination (PHA) test for the detection of antibody to rubella virus in serum or recalcified plasma.
Use: Diagnostic aid.

Rubacell II. (Abbott) Passive hemagglutination (PHA) test to detect antibody to rubella in serum or recalcified plasma. In 100s, 1000s.
Use: Diagnostic aid.

Rubaquick Diagnostic Kit. (Abbott Diagnostics) Rapid passive hemagglutination (PHA) for the detection of antibodies to rubella virus in serum specimens.
Use: Diagnostic aid.

Ruba-Tect. (Abbott Diagnostics) Hemagglutination inhibition test for the detection and quantitation of rubella antibody in serum. In 100s.
Use: Diagnostic aid.

Rubazyme. (Abbott Diagnostics) Enzyme immunoassay for 1 gG antibody to rubella virus. Test kit 100s, 1000s.
Use: Diagnostic aid.

Rubazyme-M. (Abbott Diagnostics) Enzyme immunoassay for IgM antibody to rubella virus in serum. Test kit 50s.
Use: Diagnostic aid.

rubella & measles vaccine. (Merck) M-R-VAX II. Inj. Vial. *Rx*.
Use: Agent for immunization.

rubella & mumps virus vaccine, live.
Use: Active immunizing agent.
See: Biavax II, Inj. (Merck).

• **rubella virus vaccine, live,** U.S.P. 23.
Use: Active immunizing agent.
See: Meruvax II, Inj. (Merck).
W/Measles vaccine.
See: M-R-Vax II, Inj. (Merck).
W/Measles vaccine, mumps vaccine.
See: M-M-R Vax II, Inj. (Merck).

Rubex. (Bristol-Myers Oncology) Doxorubicin HCl 10 mg, 50 mg or 100 mg. **10 mg:** w/lactose 50 mg. **50 mg:** w/lactose 250 mg. **100 mg:** w/lactose 500 mg. Pow. for Inj. Vial. *Rx*.
Use: Antineoplastic.

• **rubidium chloride Rb 82 injection,** (roo-BIH-dee-uhm) U.S.P. 23.
Use: Diagnostic aid (radioactive, cardiac disease).

•**rubidium chloride Rb 86.** USAN.
Use: Radioactive agent.

Rubratope-57. (Squibb) Cyanocobalamin Co 57 Capsules; Soln U.S.P. *otc.*
Use: Vitamin supplement.

Ru-lets M 500. (Rugby) Vitamin C 500 mg, B_3 100 mg, B_5 20 mg, B_1 15 mg, B_2 10 mg, B_6 5 mg, A 10,000 IU, B_{12} 12 mcg, D 400 IU, E 30 mg, magnesium, iron 20 mg, copper, zinc 1.5 mg, manganese, iodine/Tab. Bot. 100s. *otc.*
Use: Vitamin/mineral supplement.

Rulox. (Rugby) **#1 Tab.:** Aluminum hydroxide 200 mg, magnesium hydroxide 200 mg. **#2 Tab.:** Aluminum hydroxide 400 mg, magnesium hydroxide 400 mg. Bot. 100s, 1000s. *otc.*
Use: Antacid.

Rulox Plus Suspension. (Rugby) Aluminum hydroxide 500 mg, magnesium hydroxide 450 mg, simethicone 40 mg/5 ml. Bot. 355 ml. *otc.*
Use: Antacid, antiflatulent.

Rulox Plus Tablets. (Rugby) Aluminum hydroxide 200 mg, magnesium hydroxide 200 mg, simethicone 25 mg. Chew. Tab. Bot. 50s. *otc.*
Use: Antacid, antiflatulent.

Rulox Suspension. (Rugby) Aluminum hydroxide 225 mg, magnesium hydroxide 200 mg/5 ml. Susp. Bot. 360 ml, 769 ml, gal. *otc.*
Use: Antacid.

Rum-K. (Fleming) Potassium Cl 10 mEq/5 ml in butter/rum flavored base. Bot. pt, gal. *Rx.*
Use: Potassium supplement.

rust inhibitor.
See: Anti-Rust, Tab. (Sanofi Winthrop). Sodium Nitrite, Tab. (Various Mfr.).

•**rutamycin.** (ROO-tah-MY-sin) USAN. From strain of *Streptomyces rutgersensis.* Under study.
Use: Antifungal.

rutgers 612.
See: Ethohexadiol. (Various Mfr.).

rutin. (Various Mfr.) 3-Rhamnoglucoside of 5,7,3',4-tetrahydroxyflavonol. Eldrin, globulariacitrin, myrticalorin, oxyritin, phytomelin, rutoside, sophorin. Tab. 20 mg, 50 mg, 60 mg, 100 mg. *Rx.*
Use: Vascular disorders.

rutin combinations.
See: Hexarutan, Tab. (Westerfield). Vio-Geric-H, Tab. (Solvay).

rutoside.
See: Rutin, Tab. (Various Mfr.).

Ru-Tuss DE. (Knoll Pharm) Pseudoephedrine HCl 120 mg, guaifenesin 600 mg/Tab. Bot. 100s. *Rx.*
Use: Decongestant, expectorant.

Ru-Tuss II. (Knoll Pharm) Phenylpropanolamine HCl 75 mg, chlorpheniramine maleate 12 mg/Cap. Bot. 100s. *Rx.*
Use: Decongestant, antihistamine.

Ru-Tuss Expectorant. (Knoll Pharm) Pseudoephedrine HCl 30 mg, dextromethorphan HBr 10 mg, guaifenesin 100 mg/5 ml, alcohol 10%. Bot. pt. *otc.*
Use: Decongestant, antitussive, expectorant.

Ru-Tuss Liquid. (Knoll Pharm) Phenylephrine HCl 5 mg, chlorpheniramine maleate 2 mg/5 ml, alcohol 5%. Bot. 473 ml. *otc.*
Use: Decongestant, antihistamine.

Ru-Tuss w/Hydrocodone. (Knoll Pharm) Hydrocodone bitartrate 1.67 mg, phenylephrine HCl 5 mg, phenylpropanolamine HCl 3.3 mg, pheniramine maleate 3.3 mg, pyrilamine maleate 3.3 mg/5 ml, alcohol 5%. Bot. 473 ml. *c-III.*
Use: Antitussive, decongestant, antihistamine.

Ru-Vert M. (Solvay) Meclizine HCl 25 mg/Tab. Bot. 100s. *Rx.*
Use: Antiemetic, antivertigo.

RVPaque. (ICN Pharm) Red petrolatum, zinc oxide, cinoxate, in water-resistant base. Tube 15 g, 37.5 g. *otc.*
Use: Sunscreen.

Rymed. (Edwards) Pseudoephedrine HCl 30 mg, guaifenesin 250 mg/Cap. Bot. 100s. *otc.*
Use: Decongestant, expectorant.

Rymed Liquid. (Edwards) Pseudoephedrine HC1 30 mg, guaifenesin 100 mg/5 ml, alcohol 1.4%. Bot. pt. *otc.*
Use: Decongestant, expectorant.

Rymed-TR. (Edwards) Phenylpropanolamine HCl 75 mg, guaifenesin 400 mg/Tab. Bot. 100s. *otc.*
Use: Decongestant, expectorant.

Ryna. (Wallace) Chlorpheniramine 2 mg, pseudoephedrine HCl 30 mg/5 ml. Bot. 118 ml, 473 ml. *otc.*
Use: Antihistamine, decongestant.

Ryna-C. (Wallace) Codeine phosphate 10 mg, pseudoephedrine HCl 30 mg, chlorpheniramine maleate 2 mg, saccharin, sorbitol/5 ml. Bot. 4 oz, pt. *c-v.*
Use: Antitussive, decongestant, antihistamine.

Ryna-CX. (Wallace) Guaifenesin 100 mg, pseudoephedrine HCl 30 mg, codeine phosphate 10 mg, alcohol 7.5%, saccharin, sorbitol/5 ml. Bot. 4 oz, pt. *c-v.*

Use: Expectorant, decongestant, antitussive.

Rynatan. (Wallace) **Tab.**: Phenylephrine tannate 25 mg, chlorpheniramine tannate 8 mg, pyrilamine tannate 25 mg. Bot. 100s, 500s, 2000s. **Pediatric Susp.**: Phenylephrine tannate 5 mg, chlorpheniramine tannate 2 mg, pyrilamine tannate 12.5 mg/5 ml. Bot. 473 ml. *Rx.*
Use: Decongestant, antihistamine.

Rynatan-S Pediatric Suspension. (Wallace) Phenylephrine tannate 5 mg, chlorpheniramine tannate 2 mg, pyrilamine tannate 12.5 mg/5 ml. Susp. Bot. 120 ml w/syringe. *Rx.*
Use: Decongestant, antihistamine.

Rynatuss. (Wallace) Carbetapentane tannate 60 mg, chlorpheniramine tannate 5 mg, ephedrine tannate 10 mg, phenylephrine tannate 10 mg/Tab. Bot. 100s. *Rx.*
Use: Decongestant, antihistamine, antitussive.

Rynatuss Pediatric Suspension. (Wallace) Carbetapentane tannate 30 mg, chlorpheniramine tannate 4 mg, ephedrine tannate 5 mg, phenylephrine tannate 5 mg, saccharin, tartrazine/5 ml. Susp. Bot. 8 oz, pt. *Rx.*
Use: Decongestant, antihistamine, antitussive.

Rythmol. (Knoll) Propafenone HCl 150 mg, 225 mg or 300 mg. Tab. **50 mg or 300 mg:** Bot. 100s, 500s. **225 mg:** Bot. 100s, UD 100s. *Rx.*
Use: Antiarrhythmic.

S

S-2 Inhalant & Nebulizers. (Nephron) Racemic epinephrine HCl 1.25%. Bot. 0.25 oz, 0.5 oz, 1 oz. *Rx.*
Use: Bronchodilator.

Saave+. (NeuroGenesis/Matrix) Vitamin D 40 mg, L-phenylalanine, L-glutamine 25 mg, vitamins A 333.3 IU, B₁ 2.417 mg, B₂ 0.85 mg, B₃ 33 mg, B₅ 15 mg, B₆ 3 mg, B₁₂ 5 mcg, folic acid 0.067 mg, C 100 mg, E 5 IU, biotin 0.05 mg, calcium 25 mg, chromium 0.01 mg, iron 1.5 mg, magnesium 25 mg, zinc 2.5 mg/ Cap. Yeast and preservative free. Bot. 42s, 180s. *otc.*
Use: Vitamin/mineral supplement.

• **sabeluzole.** (sah-BELL-you-zole) USAN.
Use: Anticonvulsant; antihypoxic.

sabin vaccine.
Use: Agent for immunization.
See: Orimune (Lederle).

Sac-500. (Western Research) Vitamin C 500 mg/Timed Release Cap. Bot. 1000s. *otc.*
Use: Vitamin C supplement.

sacarasa.
See: Sucrase (yeast-derived).

• **saccharin,** N.F. 18.
Use: Pharmaceutic aid (flavor).
See: Necta Sweet, Tab. (Procter & Gamble).

saccharin. (Merck) Pkg. 1 oz, 0.25 lb, 1 lb. (Squibb) Tabs. 0.25, 0.5 gr. Bot. 500s, 1000s; 1 gr. Bot. 1000s.
Use: Pharmaceutic aid (flavor).

• **saccharin calcium,** U.S.P. 23.
Use: Non-nutritive sweetener.

• **saccharin sodium,** U.S.P. 23.
Use: Sweetener (non-nutritive).
See: Crystallose, Crystals, Liq. (Jamieson).
Ril Sweet, Liq. (Schering-Plough).
Sweeta (Squibb Mark).

saccharin sodium. (Various Mfr.) Pow., Bot. 1 oz, 0.25 lb, 1 lb. Tab.
Use: Sweetener (non-nutritive).

saccharin soluble.
See: Saccharin Sodium, Tab., Pow. (Various Mfr.).

Saf-Clens. (Calgon Vestal) Meroxapol 105, NaCl, potassium sorbate NF, DMDM hydantoin/Spray. Bot. 177 ml. *otc.*
Use: Wound cleanser.

Safeskin. (C & M Pharmacal) A dermatologically acceptable detergent for patients who are sensitive to ordinary detergents. No whiteners, brighteners or other irritants. Bot. qt.
Use: Laundry detergent for sensitive skin.

Safe Suds. (Ar-Ex) Hypoallergenic, all-purpose detergent for patients whose hands or respiratory membranes are irritated by soaps or detergents. pH 6.8. No enzymes, phosphates, lanolin, fillers, bleaches. Bot. 22 oz.
Use: Laundry detergent for sensitive skin.

Safe Tussin 30. (Kramer) Guaifenesin 100 mg, dextromethorphan HBr 15 mg/ 5 ml. Liq. Bot. 120 ml. *otc.*
Use: Antitussive, expectorant.

Safety-Coated Arthritis Pain Formula. (Whitehall Robins) Enteric coated aspirin 500 mg/Tab. Bot. 24s, 60s. *otc.*
Use: Salicylate analgesic.

safflower oil.
Use: Nutritional supplement.
See: Microlipid (Sherwood).

• **safflower oil,** U.S.P. 23.
Use: Pharmaceutic aid (vehicle, oleaginous).
See: Safflower Oil Caps. (Various Mfr.).
W/Choline bitartrate, soybean lecithin, inositol, natural tocopherols, B₆, B₁₂, and panthenol.
See: Nutricol, Cap., Vial (Nutrition).

• **safingol.** (saff-IN-gole) USAN.
Use: Antineoplastic (adjunct); antipsoriatic.

• **safingol hydrochloride.** (saff-IN-gole) USAN.
Use: Antineoplastic (adjunct); antipsoriatic.

safrole.

SalAc Cleanser. (GenDerm) Salicylic acid 2%, benzyl alcohol, glyceryl cocoate. Liq. Bot. 177 ml. *otc.*
Use: Antiacne.

salacetin.
See: Acetylsalicylic Acid (Various Mfr.).

Sal-Acid. (Pedinol) Salicylic acid 40% in collodion-like vehicle. Plaster. Pkg. 14s. *otc.*
Use: Keratolytic.

Salacid 25%. (Gordon) Salicylic acid 25% in ointment base. Jar 2 oz, lb. *otc.*
Use: Keratolytic.

Salacid 60%. (Gordon) Salicylic acid 60% in ointment base. Jar 2 oz. *otc.*
Use: Keratolytic.

Salactic Film. (Pedinol) Salicylic acid 16.7% in flexible collodion w/color. Applicator bot. 0.5 oz. *otc.*
Use: Keratolytic.

Salagen. (SAL-an-tell) (MGI Pharma)

Pilocarpine HCl 5 mg. Tab. Bot. 100s. *Rx.*
Use: Mouth and throat product.

Salazide-Demi Tablets. (Major) Hydroflumethiazide 25 mg, reserpine 0.125 mg/Tab. Bot. 100s. *Rx.*
Use: Antihypertensive combination.

Salazide Tabs. (Major) Hydroflumethiazide 50 mg, reserpine 0.125 mg/Tab. Bot. 100s, 500s, 1000s. *Rx.*
Use: Antihypertensive combination.

salbutamol.
See: albuterol.

Salcegel. (Apco) Sodium salicylate 5 gr, calcium ascorbate 25 mg, calcium carbonate 1 gr, dried aluminum hydroxide gel 2 gr/Tab. Bot. 100s. *otc.*
Use: Analgesic.

Sal-Clens Acne Cleanser Gel. (C & M Pharm) Salicylic acid 2%. Gel. Tube 240 g. *otc.*
Use: Antiacne.

•**salcolex.** (SAL-koe-lex) USAN.
Use: Analgesic, anti-inflammatory, antipyretic.

•**salethamide maleate.** (sal-ETH-ah-MIDE) Under study.
Use: Analgesic.

saletin.
See: Acetylsalicylic Acid (Various Mfr.).

Saleto. (Roberts Med) Aspirin 210 mg, acetaminophen 115 mg, salicylamide 65 mg, caffeine anhydrous 16 mg/Tab. Bot. 50s, 100s, 1000s, Sani-Pak 1000s. *otc.*
Use: Analgesic.

Saleto-200. (Roberts Med) Ibuprofen 200 mg/Tab. Bot. 1000s, UD 50s. *otc.*
Use: Nonsteroidal anti-inflammatory, analgesic.

Saleto-400. (Roberts Med) Ibuprofen 400 mg/Tab. Bot. 100s, 500s. *Rx.*
Use: Nonsteroidal anti-inflammatory, analgesic.

Saleto-600. (Roberts Med) Ibuprofen 600 mg/Tab. Bot. 100s, 500s. *Rx.*
Use: Nonsteroidal anti-inflammatory, analgesic.

Saleto-800. (Roberts Med) Ibuprofen 800 mg/Tab. Bot. 100s, 500s. *Rx.*
Use: Nonsteroidal anti-inflammatory, analgesic.

Saleto CF. (Roberts Med) Phenylpropanolamine 12.5 mg, dextromethorphan HBr 10 mg, acetaminophen 325 mg/Tab. Bot. UD 8s, 1000s. *otc.*
Use: Decongestant, antitussive, analgesic.

Saleto D. (Roberts Med) Acetaminophen

240 mg, salicylamide 120 mg, caffeine 16 mg, phenylpropanolamine HCl 18 mg/Cap. Bot. 50s, 1000s, Sani-Pak 500s. *otc.*
Use: Analgesic, decongestant.

Salflex. (Carnrick Labs) Salsalate 500 mg or 750 mg/Tab. Bot. 100s. *Rx.*
Use: Analgesic.

•**salicyl alcohol.** (SAL-ih-sill AL-koe-hahl) USAN. *Formerly Saligenin, Saligenol, Salicain.*
Use: Local anesthetic.

•**salicylamide,** U.S.P. 23.
Use: Analgesic.

salicylamide w/combinations.
See: Anodynos, Tab. (Buffington).
Anodynos Forte, Tab. (Buffington).
Arthol, Tab. (Towne).
Cenaid, Tab. (Century).
Centuss, MLT Tab. (Century).
Dapco, Tab. (Mericon).
Decohist, Cap. (Towne).
Dengesic, Tab. (Scott-Alison).
Duoprin, Tab. (Dunhall).
Emersal, Liq. (Medco).
F.C.A.H., Cap. (Scherer).
Lobac, Cap. (Seatrace).
Myocalm, Tab. (Parmed).
Nokane, Tab. (Wren).
Partuss-A, Tab. (Parmed).
Partuss T.D., Tab. (Parmed).
P.M.P. Compound, Tab. (Mericon).
Presalin, Tab. (Roberts).
Renpap, Tab. (Wren).
Rhinex, Tab. (Lemmon).
S.A.C., Preps. (Towne).
Saleto, Preps. (Roberts).
Salipap, Tab. (Freeport).
Salocol, Tab. (Roberts).
Salphenyl, Liq., Cap. (Roberts).
Scotgesic, Cap., Elix. (Scott/Cord).
Sedalgesic, Tab. (Table Rock).
Sinulin, Tab. (Schwarz Pharma).
Sleep, Tab. (Towne).
Triaprin-DC, Cap. (Dunhall).

salicylanilide.
Use: Antifungal.

salicylated bile extract. Chologestin.

•**salicylate meglumine.** USAN.
Use: Antirheumatic, analgesic.

salicylazosulfapyridine.
See: Sulfasalazine, U.S.P. 23.

•**salicylic acid,** U.S.P. 23.
Use: Keratolytic.
See: Calicylic, Creme (Gordon).
Listrex Scrub, Liq. (Warner-Lambert).
Maximum Strength Wart Remover, Liq. (Stiefel).
OFF-Ezy Corn & Callous Remover, Kit (Del).

Sal-Acid, Plaster (Pedinol).
Salactic Film, Liq. (Pedinol).
Salicylic Acid Acne Treatment, Bar
(Stiefel)
Sal-Plant, Gel (Pedinol).
Sebulex, Cream (Westwood Squibb).
Trans-Plantar, Transdermal patch
(Tsumura Medical).
Wart-Off, Liq. (Pfizer).
Salicylic Acid Cleansing Bar. (Stiefel)
Salicylic acid 2%, EDTA. Cake 113 g.
otc.
Use: Antiseborrheic, keratolytic.
salicylic acid combinations.
See: Acnaveen, Bar (Rydelle).
Acno (Cummins).
Akne Drying Lotion, Liq. (Alto).
Clearasil, Preps (Procter & Gamble).
Cuticura (Purex).
Duofilm, Liq. (Stiefel).
Duo-WR, Soln. (Whorton).
Fostex, Cream, Liq. (Westwood
Squibb).
Ionax, Liq. (Galderma).
Ionil, Liq. (Galderma).
Ionil T, Liq. (Galderma).
Keralyt, Gel (Westwood Squibb).
Komed, Lot. (Pilkington Barnes Hind).
Neutrogena T/Sal, Shampoo (Neu-
trogena).
Occlusal HP, Liq. (GenDerm).
Oxy Clean Medicated Pads for Sensi-
tive Skin (SK-Beecham).
Oxy Night Watch, Lot. (SK-Beecham).
Pernox, Lot. (Westwood Squibb).
Pragmatar, Oint. (Menley & James).
Propa pH, Preps (Del Pharm).
Sal-Dex, Liq. (Scrip).
Salicylic Acid Soap (Stiefel).
Saligel, Gel (Stiefel).
Salsprin, Tab. (Seatrace).
Sebaveen, Shampoo (Rydelle).
Sebucare, Liq. (Westwood Squibb).
Sebucare Shampoo, Liq. (Westwood
Squibb).
Therac, Lot. (C & M Pharm).
Tinver, Lot. (Pilkington Barnes Hind).
Vanseb, Dandruff Shampoo (Aller-
gan Herbert).
Vanseb-T Tar Shampoo (Allergan Her-
bert).
Vericin, Oint. (Gordon).
Ver-Var, Soln. (Galderma).
Zemacol, Lot. (Procter & Gamble).
Salicylic Acid & Sulfur Soap. (Stiefel)
Salicylic acid 3%, sulfur 10%, EDTA.
Cake 116 g. *otc.*
Use: Antiseborrheic, keratolytic.
salicylic acid topical foam.
Use: Keratolytic.

salicylsalicylic acid. Salsalate. USAN.
Use: Analgesic.
See: Arcylate, Tab. (Roberts)
Disalcid, Tab. (3M).
W/Aspirin.
See: Duragesic, Tab. (Meyer).
Persistin, Tab. (Medeva).
salicylsulphonic acid. Sulfosalicylic
acid.
See: Dextrotest (Bayer).
Saligenin. (City Chem.) Salicyl alcohol.
Bot. 25 g, 100 g.
W/Merodicein.
See: Thantis, Loz. (Becton Dickinson).
Saline. (Bausch & Lomb) Buffered iso-
tonic. Thimerosal 0.001%, boric acid,
NaCl, EDTA. Soln. Bot. 355 ml. *otc.*
Use: Soft contact lens care.
Saline Solution. (Americal) Saline solu-
tion, isotonic, preserved. Bot. 12 oz.
otc.
Use: Soaking agent.
Saline Spray. (Americal) Isotonic nonpre-
served saline aerosol soln. Bot. 2 oz, 8
oz, 12 oz. *otc.*
Use: Soft contact lens care.
Salinex Nasal Drops. (Muro) Buffered
nasal isotonic saline drops. Bot. 15 ml
w/dropper. *otc.*
Use: Nasal moisturizer.
Salinex Nasal Mist. (Muro) Sodium Cl
0.4%. Drops 15 ml, spray 50 ml. *otc.*
Use: Nasal moisturizer.
Salipap. (Freeport) Salicylamide 5 gr,
acetaminophen 5 gr/Tab. Bot. 1000s.
otc.
Use: Analgesic.
Salithol Liquid. (Madland) Balm of
methyl salicylate, menthol, camphor.
Bot. pt, gal. Oint. Jar 1 lb, 5 lb. *otc.*
Use: Analgesic, topical.
Salivart. (Gebauer) Sodium carboxy-
methylcellulose 1%, sorbitol 3%, so-
dium Cl 0.084%, potassium Cl 0.12%,
calcium Cl 0.015%, magnesium Cl
0.005%, dibasic potassium phosphate
0.034% and nitrogen (as propellant).
Soln. Spray can 25 ml, 75 ml. *otc.*
Use: Mouth preparation.
Saliva Substitute. (Roxane) Sorbitol, sodium carboxymethylcellulose. Soln. 5
ml and 120 ml vials. *otc.*
Use: Mouth preparation.
Salix. (Scandinavian Natural Health and
Beauty) Sorbitol, dicalcium phosphate,
hydroxypropyl methylcellulose, carboxy
methylcellulose, malic acid, hydrogenated cottonseed oil, sodium citrate, citric acid, silicon dioxide. Loz. 100s. *otc.*

Use: Saliva substitute.

Salk vaccine.
See: poliovirus vaccine, inactivated.

•**salmeterol.** (sal-MEH-teh-role) USAN.
Use: Bronchodilator.

•**salmeterol xinafoate.** (sal-MEH-teh-role zin-AF-oh-ate) USAN.
Use: Bronchodilator.

•**salnacedin.** (sal-NAH-seh-din) USAN.
Use: Anti-inflammatory (topical).

Salocol. (Roberts) Acetaminophen 115 mg, aspirin 210 mg, salicylamide 65 mg, caffeine 16 mg/Tab. Bot. 1000s. *Rx.*
Use: Analgesic combination.

Sal-Oil-T. (Syosset) Coal tar 10%, salicylic acid 6%, allantoin vegetable oils. Soln. Bot. 60 ml. *Rx.*
Use: Antiseborrheic, keratolytic.

Salpaba w/Colchicine. (Madland) Sodium salicylate 0.25 g, para-aminobenzoic acid 0.25 g, vitamin C 20 mg, colchicine 0.25 mg/Tab. Bot. 100s, 1000s. *Rx.*
Use: Agent for gout.

Sal-Plant. (Pedinol) Salicylic acid 17% in flexible collodion vehicle. Gel. Tube 14 g. *otc.*
Use: Keratolytic.

•**salsalate,** (SAL-sah-late) U.S.P. 23.
Use: Analgesic; anti-inflammatory.

Salsitab. (Upsher-Smith) Salsalate 500 mg or 750 mg/Tab. Bot. 100s, 500s, UD 100s. *Rx.*
Use: Analgesic.

Salten. (Wren) Salicylamide 10 gr/Tab. Bot. 100s, 1000s. *otc.*
Use: Analgesic.

Sal-Tropine. (Hope Pharm) Atropine sulfate 0.4 mg. Tab. Bot. 100s. *Rx.*
Use: Anticholinergic.

salt replacement products.
See: Slo-Salt (Mission).
Slo-Salt-K (Mission).
Sodium Chloride (Various Mfr.).

•**salts, rehydration, oral.** U.S.P. 23.
Use: Electrolyte combination.

salt substitutes.
Use: Sodium-free seasoning agent.
See: Adolph's Salt Substitute (Adolph's).
Adolph's Seasoned Salt Substitute (Adolph's).
Morton Salt Substitute (Morton Salt).
Morton Seasoned Salt Substitute (Morton Salt).
NoSalt (SK-Beecham).
Nu-Salt (Cumberland Pkg.).

salt tablets. (Cross) Sodium Cl 650 mg/Tab. Dispenser 500s. *otc.*

Use: Salt replenisher.

Saluron. (Bristol-Myers) Hydroflumethiazide 50 mg/Tab. Bot. 100s. *Rx.*
Use: Diuretic.

Salutensin. (Roberts) Hydroflumethiazide 50 mg, reserpine 0.125 mg/Tab. Bot. 100s, 1000s. *Rx.*
Use: Antihypertensive combination.

Salutensin-Demi. (Bristol-Myers) Hydroflumethiazide 25 mg, reserpine 0.125 mg/Tab. Bot. 100s. *Rx.*
Use: Antihypertensive combination.

Salvarsan.
Use: Antisyphilitic.

Salvite-B. (Faraday) Sodium chloride 7 gr, dextrose 3 gr, vitamin B, 1 mg/Tab. Bot. 100s, 1000s. *otc.*

•**samarium Sm 153 lexidronam pentasodium.** (Sm 153 lex-IH-drah-nam pentah-SO-dee-uhm) USAN.
Use: Antineoplastic, radioactive agent.

Sancura. (Thompson) Benzocaine, chlorobutanol, chlorothymol, benzoic acid, salicylic acid, benzyl alcohol, cod liver oil, lanolin in a washable petrolatum base. Oint. 30 g, 90 g.
Use: Local anesthetic, topical.

•**sancycline.** (SAN-SIGH-kleen) USAN.
Use: Antibacterial.

Sandimmune. (Sandoz) Cyclosporine. **Oral soln.:** 100 mg/ml. Bot. 50 ml with graduated pipette. **Inj.:** 50 mg/ml Amp. 5 ml. **Cap.:** 50 mg/Cap. Bot. Sorbitol. UD 30s. *Rx.*
Use: Immunosuppressant.

Sandoglobulin. (Sandoz) Reconstitution fluid 1 g, 3 g, 6 g, 12g NaCl 0.9%/lyophilized pow. for inj. Vials or kits. Also available as bulk packs without diluent. *Rx.*
Use: Immune globulin.

sandoptal. Isobutyl allylbarbituric acid.
See: Butalbital.
W/Caffeine, aspirin, phenacetin.
See: Fiorinal, Tab., Cap. (Sandoz).
W/Caffeine, aspirin, phenacetin, codeine phosphate.
See: Fiorinal w/codeine, Cap. (Sandoz).

sandoptal sodium.
W/Sodium diethylbarbiturate, sodium phenylethylbarbiturate, scopolamine HBr, dihydroergotamine methanesulfonate.
See: Plexonal (Sandoz).

Sandostatin. (Sandoz) Octreotide acetate. **0.05 mg, 0.1 mg, 0.5 mg/ml:** Inj. Amp 1 ml. **0.2 mg, 1 mg/ml:** 5 ml multidose vials. *Rx.*

Use: Adjunctive treatment of certain tumors.

Sanestro. (Sandia) Estrone 0.7 mg, estradiol 0.35 mg, estriol 0.14 mg/Tab. Bot. 100s, 1000s. *Rx.*
Use: Estrogen.

•**sanfetrinem cilexitil.** (san-FEH-trih-nem sigh-LEX-eh-till) USAN.
Use: Antibacterial.

•**sanfetrinem sodium.** (san-FEH-trih-nem) USAN.
Use: Antibacterial.

•**sanguinarium chloride.** (san-gwih-NARE-ee-uhm) USAN. *Formerly Sanguinarine Chloride.*
Use: Antimicrobial, anti-inflammatory, antifungal.

Sanguis. (Sig) Liver 10 mcg, vitamin B_{12} 100 mcg, folic acid 1 mcg/ml. Vial 10 ml. *Rx.*
Use: Nutritional supplement.

Sanhist T.D. 5. (Sandia) Phenylpropanolamine HCl 50 mg, chlorpheniramine maleate 5 mg, ascorbic acid 100 mg/Tab. Bot. 100s, 1000s. *Rx.*
Use: Decongestant, antihistamine.

Sanhist T.D. 12. (Sandia) Phenylpropanolamine HCl 50 mg, chlorpheniramine maleate 12 mg, ascorbic acid 100 mg, methscopolamine nitrate 4 mg/Tab. Bot. 100s, 1000s. *Rx.*
Use: Decongestant, antihistamine combination.

Sani-Supp. (G & W Labs) Glycerin, sodium stearate. Supp. 10s, 12s, 24s, 25s, 48s, 50s, 100s, 1000s. *otc.*
Use: Laxative.

sanluol.
See: Arsphenamine (Various Mfr.).

Sanorex. (Sandoz) Mazindol 1 mg or 2 mg/Tab. Bot. 100s. *c-iv.*
Use: Anorexiant.

Sansert. (Sandoz) Methysergide maleate 2 mg/Tab. Bot. 100s. *Rx.*
Use: Agent for migraine.

Sanstress. (Sandia) Vitamins A 25,000 IU, D 400 IU, B_1 10 mg, B_2 5 mg, niacinamide 100 mg, B_6 1 mg, B_{12} 5 mcg, C 150 mg, calcium 103 mg, phosphorus 80 mg, iron 10 mg, copper 1 mg, iodine 0.1 mg, magnesium 5.5 mg, manganese 1 mg, potassium 5 mg, zinc 1.4 mg/Cap. Bot. 100s, 1000s. *otc.*
Use: Vitamin/mineral supplement.

Santiseptic Lotion. (Santiseptic) Menthol, phenol, benzocaine, zinc oxide, calamine. Bot. 4 oz. *otc.*
Use: Minor skin irritations.

Santyl. (Knoll) Proteolytic enzyme de-

rived from *Clostridium histolyticum.* 250 units/g Oint. Tube 15 g, 30 g. *Rx.*
Use: Topical enzyme preparation.

•**saperconazole.** (SAP-ehr-KOE-nah-zole) USAN.
Use: Antifungal.

saponated cresol solution.
See: Cresol (Various Mfr.).

saponins, water soluble.

•**saprisartan potassium.** (sap-rih-SAHR-tan) USAN.
Use: Antihypertensive.

•**saquinavir mesylate.** (sack-KWIN-uh-vihr) USAN.
Use: Antiviral.
See: Invirase, Cap. (Roche).

•**sarafloxacin hydrochloride.** USAN. (sa-rah-FLOX-ah-SIN)
Use: Anti-infective (DNA gyrase inhibitor).

•**saralasin acetate.** (sare-AL-ah-sin) USAN.
Use: Antihypertensive.

Saratoga. (Blair) Boric acid, zinc oxide, eucalyptol, white petrolatum. Oint. Tube 1 oz, 2 oz. *otc.*
Use: Minor skin irritations.

Sardo Bath Oil Concentrate. (Schering-Plough) Mineral oil, isopropyl palmitate. Bot. 3.75 oz, 7.75 oz. *otc.*
Use: Emollient.

Sardo Bath & Shower. (Schering-Plough) Mineral oil, tocopherol. Oil. Bot. 112.5 ml. *otc.*
Use: Emollient.

Sardoettes. (Schering-Plough) Mineral oil, tocopherol, beta carotene. Towelettes. Box 25s. *otc.*
Use: Emollient.

Sardoettes Moisturizing Towelettes. (Schering-Plough) Mineral oil, isopropyl palmitate, impregnated towelling material. Individual packets. Box 25s. *otc.*
Use: Emollient.

•**sargramostim.** (sar-GRUH-moe-STIM) USAN.
Use: Antineutropenic, hematopoietic stimulant, leukopoietic (granulocyte macrophage colony-stimulating factor). [Orphan drug]
See: Leukine (Immunex).

Sarisol No. 2. (Halsey) Butabarbital sodium 30 mg/Tab. Bot. 100s, 1000s. *c-iii.*
Use: Sedative, hypnotic.

•**sarmoxicillin.** (sar-MOX-ih-SILL-in) USAN.
Use: Antibacterial.

Sarna. (Stiefel) Camphor 0.5%, menthol 0.5%, phenol 0.5% in a soothing emollient base. Bot. 7.4 oz. *otc.*
Use: Emollient.

Sarna Anti-Itch. (Stiefel) Camphor 5%, menthol 5%, carbomer 940, cetyl alcohol, DM DM hydantoin. Foam. Bot. 105 ml. *otc.*
Use: Emollient.

•**sarpicillin.** (sahr-PIH-SILL-in) USAN.
Use: Antibacterial.

SAStid soap. (Stiefel) Precipitated sulfur 10%. Bar 116 g. *otc.*
Use: Antiacne.

satumomab pendetide. *Rx.*
Use: Detection of ovarian cancer. [Orphan drug]
See: Oncoscint CR/OV.

saxol.
See: Petrolatum Liquid (Various Mfr.).

Scabene Lotion. (Stiefel) Lindane 1% in lotion base. Bot. 2 oz, 16 oz. *Rx.*
Use: Pediculicide.

Scabene Shampoo. (Stiefel) Lindane 1% in shampoo base. Bot. 2 oz, 16 oz. *Rx.*
Use: Pediculicide.

scabicides.
See: Benzyl Benzoate (Various Mfr.).
Cuprex, Liq. (SK-Beecham).
Eurax, Cream, Lot. (Novartis).
Kwell, Lot., Cream, Shampoo (Schwarz Pharma).

Scadan Scalp Lotion. (Bayer) Cetyl trimethyl ammonium bromide (cetab) 1%, stearyl dimethyl benzyl ammonium Cl 0.1%. Bot. 4 oz. *otc.*
Use: Antiseborrheic.

Scalpicin. (Combe) Hydrocortisone 1%, menthol, SD alcohol 40. Liq. Bot. 45 ml, 75 ml, 120 ml. *otc.*
Use: Topical corticosteroid.

Scan. (Parker) Water soluble gel. Bot. 8 oz, gal.
Use: Ultrasound B scan procedures.

Scarlet Red Ointment Dressings. (Sherwood Medical) 5% scarlet red, lanolin, olive oil, petrolatum. Gauze. 5"×9" strips. *Rx.*
Use: Wound healing agent.

Schamberg's. (C & M Pharmacal) Menthol 0.15%, phenol 1%, zinc oxide, peanut oil, lime water. Bot. pt, gal. *otc.*
Use: Antipruritic, counterirritant.

•**schick test control,** U.S.P. 23. *Formerly Diphtheria Toxin, Inactivated Diagnostic.*
Use: Diagnostic aid (dermal reactivity indicator).

Schirmer Tear Test. (Various Mfr.) Sterile tear test strips. 250s. *otc.*
Use: Diagnostic aid, ophthalmic.

Schlesinger's Solution.
See: Morphine HCl (Various Mfr.).

Sclerex. (Miller) Inositol 2 g, magnesium complex 34 mg, vitamins C 100 mg, calcium succinate 25 mg, A 2500 IU, D 200 IU, E 100 IU, B$_1$ 5 mg, B$_2$ 5 mg, B$_6$ 5 mg, B$_{12}$ 5 mcg, niacin 10 mg, niacinamide 30 mg, pantothenic acid 7.5 mg, folic acid 0.1 mg, iron 10 mg, copper 1 mg, manganese 2 mg, zinc 9 mg, iodine 0.10 mg/3 Tab. Bot. 60s. *otc.*
Use: Vitamin/mineral supplement.

Scleromate. (Palisades Pharm) Morrhuate sodium 50 mg/ml. Inj. Vial 30 ml. *Rx.*
Use: Sclerosing agent.

sclerosing agents.
See: Morrhuate Sodium (Taylor).
Scleromate (Palisades Pharm).
Sotradecol (Elkins-Sinn).

•**scopafungin.** (SKOE-pah-FUN-jin) USAN.
Use: Antibacterial, antifungal.

Scope. (Procter & Gamble) Cetylpyridinium Cl, tartrazine, saccharin, SD alcohol 38F 67.9%. Liq. Bot. 90 ml, 180 ml, 360 ml, 720 ml, 1080 ml, 1440 ml. *otc.*
Use: Mouthwash.

scopolamine. (skoe-PAHL-uh-meen) Hyoscine, l-Scopolamine, Epoxytropine tropate.
See: Hyoscine, Preps. (Various Mfr.).

scopolamine aminoxide hydrobromide.
W/Acetylcarbromal and bromisovalum.
See: Tranquinal, Tab. (Pilkington Barnes Hind).

•**scopolamine hydrobromide,** (skoe-PAHL-uh-meen) U.S.P. 23. *Formerly Hyoscien Hydrobromide.*
Use: Sedative, hypnotic, anticholinergic (ophthalmic), mydriatic, cycloplegic.
W/Atropine and hyoscyamine.
See: Atropine sulfate tab.
Belladonna alkaloids.
W/Butabarbital, chlorpheniramine maleate.
See: Pedo-Sol, Elix., Tab. (Warren).
W/Hydroxypropyl methylcellulose.
See: Isopto HBr, Soln. (Alcon).
W/Hyoscyamine sulfate, atropine sulfate, phenobarbital.
See: Hyonal C.T., Tab. (Paddock).
Hytrona, Tab. (PolyMedica).
Nilspasm, Tab. (Parmed).
Sedamine, Tab. (Dunhall).
Sedapar, Tab. (Parmed).

Setamine, Tab. (Solvay).

Spasaid, Cap. (Century).

W/Pamabrom, pyrilamine maleate, homatropine methylbromide, hyoscyamine sulfate, methamphetamine HCl.
See: Aridol, Tab. (MPL).

scopolamine hydrobromide. (Invenex) Scopolamine HBr 0.3 mg/ml. Inj. Vial 1 ml. *Rx.*
Use: Pre-anesthetic sedation, obstetric amnesia, calming agent.

scopolamine hydrobromide. (Glaxo Wellcome) Scopolamine HBr 0.86 mg/ml. Inj. amp. 0.5 ml. *Rx.*
Use: Pre-anesthetic sedation, obstetric amnesia, calming agent.

scopolamine hydrobromide. (Various Mfr.) Scopolamine HBr 0.4 mg and 1 mg/ml. Inj. Amp., Vial 1 ml. *Rx.*
Use: Preanesthetic sedation, obstetric amnesia, calming agent.

scopolamine hydrobromide combinations.
See: Belladonna Products.
Hyoscine HBr. (Various Mfr.).

scopolamine methobromide.
See: Methscopolamine Bromide, Preps. (Various Mfr.).

scopolamine methyl nitrate.
See: Methscopolamine Nitrate, Prep. (Various Mfr.).

scopolamine salts.
See: Belladonna Products.
Hyoscine salts.

Scorbex/12. (Taylor) Vitamins B_1 20 mg, B_2 3 mg, B_3 75 mg, B_5 5 mg, B_6 5 mg, B_{12} 1000 mcg, C 100 mg/ml. Vial dual compartment 10 ml. *Rx.*
Use: Vitamin supplement.

Scotavite. (Scott/Cord) Vitamins A 25,000 IU, D 400 IU, B_1 10 mg, B_2 10 mg, B_6 5 mg, B_{12} 5 mcg, niacinamide 100 mg, calcium pantothenate 20 mg, C 200 mg, d-alpha tocopheryl 15 IU, acid succinate iodine 0.15 mg/Tab. Bot. 100s, 500s. *otc.*
Use: Vitamin/mineral supplement.

Scotcil. (Scott/Cord) **Tab.:** Potassium penicillin 400,000 units w/calcium carbonate/Tab. Bot. 100s, 500s. **Pow.:** 80 ml, 150 ml. *Rx.*
Use: Anti-infective; penicillin.

Scotcof. (Scott/Cord) Dextromethorphan HBr 6.85 mg, chlorpheniramine maleate 1.8 mg, phenylephrine HCl 4.4 mg, guaifenesin 66 mg, ammonium Cl 30 mg, chloroform 0.125 mg, alcohol 4.1%/5 ml. Bot. 4 oz, pt, gal. *otc.*
Use: Antitussive, antihistamine, decongestant, expectorant.

Scotnord. (Scott/Cord) Chlorpheniramine maleate 8 mg, phenylephrine HCl 20 mg, methscopolamine nitrate 2.5 mg/Cap. Bot. 100s, 500s. *Rx.*
Use: Antihistamine, decongestant, anticholinergic.

Scotonic. (Scott/Cord) Vitamins B_1 10 mg, B_2 5 mg, B_6 1 mg, niacinamide 50 mg, choline Cl 100 mg, inositol 100 mg, B_{12} 25 mcg, calcium 19 mg, iron 50 mg, folic acid 0.15 mg, alcohol 15%, sodium benzoate 0.1%/45 ml. Bot. pt, gal. *otc.*
Use: Vitamin/mineral supplement.

Scotrex. (Scott/Cord) Tetracycline 250 mg/Cap. or 5 ml. Cap. Bot. 16s, 100s, 500s. Syr. 2 oz, pt. *Rx.*
Use: Anti-infective, tetracycline.

Scott's Emulsion. (SK-Beecham) Vitamins A 1250 IU, D 1400 IU/4 tsp. Bot. 6.25 oz, 12.5 oz. *otc.*
Use: Vitamin A & D supplement.

Scot-Tussin Allergy. (Scot-Tussin) Diphenhydramine HCl 12.5 mg/5 ml, parabens, menthol. Liq. Dye free, sugar free. Bot. 120 ml. *otc.*
Use: Antihistamine.

Scot-Tussin DM Cough Chasers. (Scot-Tussin) Dextromethorphan HBr 2.5 mg, dye free, sorbitol. Loz. Pkg. 20s. *otc.*
Use: Antitussive.

Scot-Tussin DM Liquid. (Scot-Tussin) Dextromethorphan HBr 15 mg, chlorpheniramine maleate 2 mg/5 ml, alcohol 10%. Bot. 4 oz, 8 oz. Sugar free. *otc.*
Use: Antihistamine.

Scot-Tussin DM2 Syrup. (Scot-Tussin) Dextromethorphan HBr 15 mg, guaifenesin 100 mg, alcohol 1.4%/5 ml. Bot. 120 ml, 240 ml. *otc.*
Use: Antitussive, expectorant.

Scot-Tussin Expectorant. (Scot-Tussin) Guaifenesin 100 mg/5 ml, alcohol 3.5%, saccharin, menthol, sorbitol, dye free. Syr. Bot. pt, gal, 120 ml. *otc.*
Use: Expectorant.

Scot-Tussin Original 5-Action. (Scot-Tussin) Phenylephrine HCl 4.2 mg, pheniramine maleate 13.33 mg, sodium citrate 83.33 mg, sodium salicylate 83.33 mg, caffeine citrate 25 mg/5 ml, non-alcoholic. Bot. 118 ml, 473 ml, gal. *otc.*
Use: Decongestant, antihistamine, analgesic combination.

Scot-Tussin Original 5-Action Cold Formula. (Scot-Tussin) Phenylephrine

HCl 4.2 mg, pheniramine maleate 13.3 mg, sodium citrate 83.3 mg, sodium salicylate 83.3 mg, caffeine citrate 25 mg/5 ml, sugar. Alcohol free. Grape flavor. Syr. Bot. 118 ml, 473 ml, gal. *otc.*
Use: Decongestant, antihistamine, analgesic.

Scot-Tussin Senior Clear. (Scot-Tussin) Guaifenesin 200 mg, dextromethorphan HBr 15 mg per 5 ml, parabens, phenylalanine, menthol, aspartame/Liq. Alcohol and sugar free. Bot 118.3 ml. *otc.*
Use: Antitussive, expectorant.

Scot-Tussin Sugar-Free. (Scot-Tussin) Dextromethorphan HBr 15 mg, chlorpheniramine maleate 2 mg/5 ml. Bot. 4 oz, 8 oz, 16 oz, gal. *otc.*
Use: Antitussive, antihistamine.

Scot-Tussin Sugar Free Expectorant. (Scot-Tussin) Guaifenesin 100 mg/5 ml w/alcohol 3.5%. Dye free, sodium free, sugar free. *otc.*
Use: Expectorant.

Scot-Tussin with Sugar. (Scot-Tussin) Phenylephrine HCl 4.17 mg, pheniramine maleate 13.3 mg, sodium citrate 83.33 mg, sodium salicylate 83.33 mg, caffeine citrate 25 mg/5 ml. Bot. 4 oz, 8 oz, 16 oz, gal. *otc.*
Use: Decongestant, antihistamine, analgesic combination.

scurenaline.
See: Epinephrine, Prep. (Various Mfr.).

scuroforme.
See: Butyl Aminobenzoate (Various Mfr.).

S.D.M. #5. (Zeneca) Mannitol hexanitrate 7% in lactose. *Rx.*
Use: Vasodilator.

S.D.M. #17. (Zeneca) Nitroglycerin 10% in lactose. *Rx.*
Use: Vasodilator.

S.D.M. #23. (Zeneca) Pentaerythritol tetranitrate 20% in lactose. *Rx.*
Use: Vasodilator.

S.D.M. #27. (Zeneca) Nitroglycerin 10% in propylene glycol. *Rx.*
Use: Vasodilator.

S.D.M. #35. (Zeneca) Pentaerythritol tetranitrate 35% in mannitol. *Rx.*
Use: Vasodilator.

S.D.M. #37. (Zeneca) Nitroglycerin 10% in ethanol. *Rx.*
Use: Vasodilator.

S.D.M. #40. (Zeneca) Isosorbide dinitrate 25% in lactose. *Rx.*
Use: Vasodilator.

S.D.M. #50. (Zeneca) Isosorbide dinitrate 50% in lactose. *Rx.*

Use: Vasodilator.

SDZ MSL-109. (Sandoz)
Use: Antiparkinson. [Orphan drug]

Sea Greens. (Modern) Iodine 0.25 mg/Tab. Bot. 220s, 460s. *otc.*

Seale's Lotion-Modified. (C & M) Sulfur 6.4%. Bot. 60 ml, 480 ml. *otc.*
Use: Antiacne.

Sea Master. (Barth's) Vitamins A 10,000 units, D 400 units/Cap. Bot. 100s, 500s. *otc.*
Use: Vitamin supplement.

Sea-Omega 30. (Rugby) N-3 fat content (mg) EPA 180, DHA 140. 100s. *otc.*
Use: Nutritional supplement.

Sea-Omega 50. (Rugby) Omega-3 polyunsaturated fatty acid 1000 mg/Cap. containing EPA 300 mg, DHA 200 mg, vitamin E 1 IU Bot. 30s, 50s. *otc.*
Use: Nutritional supplement.

Sea & Ski Baby Lotion Formula. (Carter Products) Octyl-dimethyl PABA. SPF 2. Lot. Bot. 120 ml. *otc.*
Use: Sunscreen.

Sea & Ski Golden Tan. (Carter Products) Padimate O. SPF 4. Lot. Bot. 120 ml. *otc.*
Use: Sunscreen.

Seba-Lo. (Whorton) Acetone-alcohol cleanser. Bot. 4 oz. *otc.*
Use: Skin cleanser.

Sebana Shampoo. (Myers) Salicylic acid 2%. Bot. 4 oz, 8 oz, pt, qt, 0.5 gal. *otc.*
Use: Antiseborrheic.

Sebanatar Shampoo. (Myers) Salicylic acid 2%, liquor carbonis detergens 3%. Bot. 4 oz, 8 oz, pt, qt, 0.5 gal, gal. *otc.*
Use: Antiseborrheic.

Seba-Nil Cleansing Mask. (Galderma) Astringent face mask containing SD alcohol-40, sulfated castor oil, methylparaben. Tube 105 g. *otc.*
Use: Antiacne.

Seba-Nil Liquid. (Galderma) Alcohol 49.7%, acetone, polysorbate 20. Liq. Bot. 240 ml, pt. *otc.*
Use: Antiacne.

Seba-Nil Oily Skin Cleanser. (Galderma) SD alcohol, acetone. Liq. Bot. 240 ml, 473 ml. *otc.*
Use: Antiacne.

Sebasorb Lotion. (Summers) Activated attapulgite 10%, salicylic acid 2%. Bot. 45 ml. *otc.*
Use: Antiacne.

Sebex. (Rugby) Pyrithione zinc 2%. Shampoo. Bot. 120 ml. *otc.*
Use: Antiseborrheic.

Sebex-T. (Rugby) Coal tar soln. 5%, colloidal sulfur 2%, salicylic acid 2%. Shampoo. Bot. 120 ml. *otc.*
Use: Antiseborrheic.

Sebizon Lotion. (Schering) Sulfacetamide sodium 100 mg, methylparaben 1 mg w/trisodium edetate, sodium thiosulfate, propylene glycol, isopropyl myristate, propylene glycol monostearate, polyethylene glycol 400 monostearate, water. Tube 3 oz. *otc.*
Use: Antiseborrheic.

Sebucare Scalp Lotion. (Westwood Squibb) Laureth-4, salicylic acid 1.5%, alcohol 61%, water, PPG 40 butyl ether, dihydroabietyl alcohol, fragrance. Bot. 4 oz. *otc.*
Use: Antiseborrheic.

Sebulex Cream Shampoo. (Westwood Squibb) Same formula as Sebulex in a cream shampoo. Tube 4 oz. *otc.*
Use: Antiseborrheic.

Sebulex with Conditioners. (Westwood Squibb) Sulfur 2%, salicylic acid 2%. Bot. 4 oz, 8 oz. *otc.*
Use: Antiseborrheic.

Sebutone Cream Shampoo. (Westwood Squibb) Tar equivalent to coal tar U.S.P. 5%, sulfur 2%, salicylic acid 2%, in sebulytic type surface-active soapless cleansers, wetting agents. Tube 4 oz. *otc.*
Use: Antiseborrheic, antipsoriatic.

Sebutone Therapeutic Tar Shampoo. (Westwood Squibb) Tar equivalent to coal tar, U.S.P. 0.5%, sulfur 2%, salicylic acid 2%, in sebulytic-type surface-active soapless cleansers, wetting agents. Bot. 4 oz, 8 oz. *otc.*
Use: Antiseborrheic, antipsoriatic.

•**secalciferol.** (seh-kal-SIFF-eh-ROLE) USAN.
Use: Regulator (calcium); treatment of familial hypophosphatemic rickets. [Orphan drug]
See: Osteo-D (Tera, Israel).

•**seclazone.** (SEK-lah-zone) USAN.
Use: Anti-inflammatory; uricosuric.

•**secobarbital,** (see-koe-BAR-bih-tahl) U.S.P. 23.
Use: Sedative, hypnotic.

secobarbital combinations.
See: Efed, Syr., Tab. (Alto).
Monosyl, Tab. (Arcum).

secobarbital elixir.
See: Seconal Elix. (Lilly).

•**secobarbital sodium,** (see-koe-BAR-bih-tahl) U.S.P. 23.
Use: Sedative, hypnotic.

See: Seconal Sodium, Prep. (Lilly).

secobarbital sodium. (Wyeth-Ayerst) 50 mg/ml. Inj. Tubex 2 ml. *c-II.*
Use: Sedative, hypnotic.

secobarbital sodium and amobarbital sodium capsules.
Use: Hypnotic, sedative.
See: Tuinal, Cap. (Lilly).

Seconal Sodium Pulvules. (Lilly) Secobarbital sodium 100 mg. Cap. Bot. 100s, UD 100s. *c-II.*
Use: Sedative, hypnotic.

Secran Liquid. (Scherer) Vitamins B_1 10 mg, B_3 10 mg, B_{12} 25 mcg, alcohol 17%. Bot. 480 ml. *otc.*
Use: Vitamin B supplement.

Secretin Ferring Powder. (Ferring) Secretin 75 cu/10 ml Vial. 10 cu/ml when reconstituted with 7.5 ml.
Use: Diagnostic aid.

Sectral. (Wyeth-Ayerst) Acebutolol HCl 200 or 400 mg/ Cap. Bot. 100s, UD 100s. *Rx.*
Use: Antihypertensive.

sedaform.
See: Chlorobutanol (Various Mfr.).

Sedamine. (Approved) Phosphorated carbohydrate soln. Bot. 4 oz. *otc.*
Use: Antinauseant.

Sedamine. (Dunhall) Hyoscyamine sulfate 0.1037 mg, atropine sulfate 0.0194 mg, hyoscine HBr 0.0065 mg, phenobarbital 16.2 mg/Tab. Bot. 100s, 1000s. *Rx.*
Use: Antispasmodic, sedative.

Sedapap #3 Capsules. (Mayrand) Acetaminophen 500 mg, butalbital 50 mg, codeine phosphate 30 mg/Cap. Bot. 100s. *c-III.*
Use: Narcotic analgesic combination.

Sedapap-10 Tablets. (Mayrand) Acetaminophen 10 gr, butabarbital 50 mg/ Tab. Bot. 100s. *Rx.*
Use: Analgesic, sedative.

Sedapar. (Parmed) Atropine sulfate 0.0195 mg, hyoscine HBr 0.0065 mg, hyoscyamine sulfate 0.1040 mg, phenobarbital 0.25 gr/Tab. Bot. 1000s. *Rx.*
Use: Sedative, antispasmodic.

sedative/hypnotic agents.
See: Bromides (Various Mfr.).
Barbiturates (Various Mfr.).
Butisol Sodium (McNeil).
Carbamide (Urea) Compounds (Various Mfr.).
Chloral Hydrate, Preps. (Various Mfr.).
Chlorobutanol (Various Mfr.).
Dalmane, Cap. (Roche).
Intasedol, Elix. (Zeneca).

Largon, Inj. (Wyeth-Ayerst).
Lotusate, Cap. (Sanofi Winthrop).
Noludar, Tab., Cap. (Roche).
Paraldehyde, Preps. (Various Mfr.).
Phenergan HCl, Preps. (Wyeth-Ayerst).
Placidyl, Cap. (Abbott).
Plexonal, Tab. (Sandoz).
Restoril, Cap. (Sandoz).
Triazolam, Tab. (Various Mfr.).
Valmid, Tab. (Lilly).
Vingesic, Cap. (T.E. Williams).
sedeval.
See: Barbital (Various Mfr.).
●**sedoxantrone trihydrochloride.** (sed-OX-an-trone) USAN.
Use: Antineoplastic (DNA topoisomerase II inhibitor).
Sedral. (Vita Elixir) Phenobarbital ⅛ gr, theophylline 2 gr, ephedrine gr/Tab. *Rx.*
Use: Sedative, bronchodilator.
●**seglitide acetate.** (SEH-glih-TIDE) USAN.
Use: Antidiabetic.
Seldane. (Marion Merrill Dow) Terfenadine 60 mg/Tab. Bot. 100s, 500s. *Rx.*
Use: Antihistamine.
Seldane-D. (Hoechst Marion Roussel) Pseudoephedrine HCl 120 mg, terfenadine 60 mg/SR Tab. Lactose. Bot. 100s. *Rx.*
Use: Decongestant, antihistamine.
●**selegiline hydrochloride,** (seh-LEH-jih-leen) U.S.P. 23.
Use: Antidyskinetic, antiparkinsonian (in combination with levodopa/carbidopa). [Orphan drug]
See: Eldepryl (Somerset).
selegiline HCl. (Endo Labs) 5 mg/Tab. Bot. 60s, 500s. *Rx.*
Use: Antidyskinetic, antiparkinsonian.
Selenicel. (Taylor) Selenium yeast complex 200 mcg, vitamins C 100 mg, E 100 mg/Cap. Bot. 90s. *otc.*
Use: Vitamin supplement.
●**selenious acid,** U.S.P. 23.
Use: Supplement (trace mineral).
selenium. (Nion) Selenium 50 mcg/Tab. Bot. 100s. *Rx.*
Use: Parenteral nutritional supplement.
selenium disulfide.
See: Selenium Sulfide, Deterg., Susp. (Various Mfr.).
●**selenium sulfide,** U.SP. 23.
Use: Treatment of dandruff; antifungal, antiseborrheic.
See: Exsel Lotion (Allergan Herbert).
Iosel 250, Liq. (Galderma).
Selsun, Susp. (Abbott).

Selsun Gold for Women, Shampoo (Ross).
●**selenomethionine Se 75.** (seh-LEE-no-meh-THIGH-oh-neen Se 75) USAN. U.S.P. XXII.
Use: Diagnostic aid (pancreas function determination); radioactive agent.
See: Sethotope, Inj. (Squibb).
Sele-Pak. (SoloPak) Selenium 40 mcg/ml. Inj. Vial 10 ml, 30 ml. *Rx.*
Use: Parenteral nutritional supplement.
Selepen. (Fujisawa) Selenium 40 mcg/ml. Vial 3 ml, 10 ml. *Rx.*
Use: Parenteral nutritional supplement.
●**selfotel.** (SELL-fah-tell) USAN.
Use: NMDA antagonist.
Selora Powder. (Sanofi Winthrop) Potassium Cl. *otc.*
Use: Salt substitute.
Selsun Blue. (Ross) Selenium sulfide 1% in lotion base. Bot. 4 oz, 7 oz, 11 oz. Dry, oily, normal extra conditioning, and extra medicated (contains 0.5% menthol) formulas. *otc.*
Use: Antiseborrheic.
Selsun Gold for Women. (Ross) Selenium sulfide 1%. Shampoo. Bot. 120 ml, 210 ml, 330 ml. *otc.*
Use: Antiseborrheic.
Selsun Suspension. (Abbott) Selenium sulfide 2.5%. Bot. 4 fl oz. *Rx.*
Use: Antiseborrheic.
●**sematilide hydrochloride.** (SEH-may-tih-LIDE) USAN.
Use: Cardiac depressant (antiarrhythmic).
●**semduramicin.** (sem-DER-ah-MY-sin) USAN.
Use: Coccidiostat.
●**semduramicin sodium.** (sem-DER-ah-MY-sin) USAN.
Use: Coccidiostat.
Semicid. (Whitehall Robins) Nonoxynol-9 100 mg/Vag. Supp. Box 9s, 18s. *otc.*
Use: Contraceptive.
Semprex-D. (Glaxo Wellcome) Acrivastine 8 mg, pseudoephedrine HCl 60 mg. Cap. Bot. 100s. *Rx.*
Use: Decongestant.
●**semustine.** (SEH-muss-teen) USAN.
Use: Antineoplastic.
Senexon. (Rugby) Senna concentrate 5.6 mg/Tab. Sugar. Bot. 100s, 1000s. *otc.*
Use: Laxative.
Senilavite. (Defco) Vitamins A 5000 IU, C 100 mg, B_1 2.5 mg, B_2 2 mg, nicotinamide 10 mg, B_6 1 mg, calcium pantothenate 5 mg, B_{12} w/intrinsic factor

concentrate 0.133 IU, ferrous fumarate 150 mg, glutamic acid HCl 150 mg, docusate sodium 50 mg/Cap. Bot. 100s. *otc.*
Use: Nutritional supplement.

Senilezol. (Edwards) Vitamins B_1 0.42 mg, B_2 0.42 mg, B_3 1.67 mg, B_5 0.83 mg, B_6 0.17 mg, B_{12} 0.83 mcg, ferric pyrophosphate 3.3 mg, alcohol 15%. Bot. 473 ml. *otc.*
Use: Vitamin/mineral supplement.

•**senna,** (SEN-ah) U.S.P. 23.
Use: Laxative.
See: Senokot (Purdue Frederick).

senna conc., standardized.
Use: Cathartic.
See: Senokot, Gran., Tab., Supp. (Purdue Frederick).
X-Prep. Pow. (Gray).
W/Docusate sodium.
See: Gentlax S. Tab. (Blair).
Senokap-DSS, Cap. (Purdue Frederick).
Senokot S., Tab. (Purdue Frederick).
W/Guar gum.
See: Gentlax B Tab., Gran. (Blair).
W/Psyllium.
See: Perdiem, Gran. (Rhone-Poulenc Rorer Consumer).
Senokot W/Psyllium Pow. (Purdue Frederick).

senna fruit extract, standarized.
Use: Cathartic.
See: Senokot, Syr. (Purdue Frederick).
X-Prep, Liq. (Gray).

Senna-Gen. (Goldline) Senna concentrate 187 mg/Tab. Bot. 1000s. *otc.*
Use: Laxative.

•**sennosides,** U.S.P. 23.
Use: Laxative.
See: Gentle Nature (Sandoz).

sennosides a & b.
Use: Laxative.
See: Ex-Lax Gentle Nature (Sandoz).

Senokot Tablets and Granules. (Purdue Frederick) **Gran.:** Standardized senna concentrate. Canister 2 oz, 6 oz, 12 oz. **Tab.:** Bot. 50s, 100s, 1000s, Unit strip pack 100s, Box 20s. *otc.*
Use: Laxative.

Senokot S Tablets. (Purdue Frederick) Standardized senna concentrate w/ docusate sodium. Tab. Bot. 30s, 60s, 1000s. *otc.*
Use: Laxative.

Senokot Suppositories. (Purdue Frederick) Standardized senna concentrate. Pkg. 6s. *otc.*
Use: Laxative.

Senokot Syrup. (Purdue Frederick) Standardized extract senna fruit. Bot. 2 oz, 8 oz. *otc.*
Use: Laxative.

Senokotxtra. (Purdue Frederick) Senna concentrate 374 mg/Tab. Bot. 12s. *otc.*
Use: Laxative.

Senolax. (Schein) Senna concentrate 217 mg/Tab. Bot. 100s, 1000s. *otc.*
Use: Laxative.

Sensitive Eyes. (Bausch & Lomb) Sorbic acid 0.1%, EDTA 0.025%, sodium Cl, boric acid, sodium borate. Soln. Bot. 118 ml, 237 ml, 355 ml. *otc.*
Use: Soft contact lens care.

Sensitive Eyes Daily Cleaner. (Bausch & Lomb) Sorbic acid 0.25%, EDTA 0.5%, sodium Cl, hydroxypropyl methylcellulose, poloxamine, sodium borate. Soln. Bot. 20 ml. *otc.*
Use: Soft contact lens care.

Sensitive Eyes Drops. (Bausch & Lomb) Isotonic solution, sorbic acid 0.1%, EDTA 0.025%, sodium Cl, boric acid, sodium borate. Soln. Bot. 30 ml. *otc.*
Use: Soft contact lens care.

Sensitive Eyes Plus. (Bausch & Lomb) Boric acid, sodium borate, potassium chloride, sodium chloride, polyaminopropyl biguanide 0.00003%, EDTA 0.025%. Soln. Bot. 118 ml, 355 ml. *otc.*
Use: Soft contact lens care.

Sensitive Eyes Saline. (Bausch & Lomb) Sodium Cl, borate buffer, sorbic acid 0.1%, EDTA. Soln. Bot. 118 ml, 237 ml, 355 ml. *otc.*
Use: Soft contact lens care.

Sensitive Eyes Saline/Cleaning Solution. (Bausch & Lomb) Isotonic solution w/borate buffer, NaCl, poloxamine, sorbic acid 0.15%, sodium borate, boric acid, EDTA 0.1%. Soln. Bot. 237 ml. *otc.*
Use: Soft contact lens care.

Sensodyne Fresh Mint Toothpaste. (Block) Potassium nitrate 5%, sodium monofluorophosphate 0.76%, saccharin, sorbitol, mint flavor. Tube 2.4 oz, 4.6 oz. *otc.*
Use: Preparation for sensitive teeth.

Sensodyne-SC Toothpaste. (Block) Glycerin, sorbitol, sodium methyl cocoyltaurate, PEG-40 stearate, strontium Cl hexahydrate 10%, methyl and propylparabens, tint. Tube 2.1 oz, 4.0 oz. *otc.*
Use: Preparation for sensitive teeth.

SensoGARD. (Block) Benzocaine 20%. Gel. Parabens. Tube 0.5 g. *otc.*
Use: Local anesthetic.

Sensorcaine. (Astra) Bupivacaine HCl 0.25%: w/methylparaben. 50 ml. w/epinephrine 1:200,000 methylparaben. 50 ml. 0.5%: w/methylparaben. 50 ml. w/ epinephrine 1:200,000, methylparaben. 50 ml. 0.75%: 30 ml. Inj. *Rx.*
Use: Local anesthetic.

Sensorcaine MPF. (Astra) Bupivacaine HCl. 0.25%: 10 or 30 ml. w/epinephrine 1:200,000, sodium metabisulfite. 10 ml, 30 ml. 0.5%: 10 or 30 ml. w/epinephrine 1:200,000, sodium metabisulfite. 5, 10 or 30 ml. 0.75%: 10 or 30 ml. w/epinephrine 1:200,000, sodium metabisulfite. 10 or 30 ml. Inj. *Rx.*
Use: Local anesthetic.

Sensorcaine MPF Spinal. (Astra) Bupivacaine HCl 0.75%, dextrose 8.25%. Inj. 2 ml. *Rx.*
Use: Local anesthetic.

Sensorcaine MPF Spinal. (Astra) Bupivacaine HCl 0.75%, dextrose 8.25%/ Inj. Bot. 2ml. *Rx.*
Use: Local anesthetic.

•**sepazonium chloride.** (SEP-ah-ZOE-nee-uhm) USAN.
Use: Anti-infective, topical.

•**seperidol hydrochloride.** (seh-PURR-ih-dahl) USAN.
Use: Neuroleptic, antipsychotic.

•**seprilose.** (SEH-prih-LOHS) USAN.
Use: Antirheumatic.

•**seproxetine hydrochloride.** (sep-ROX-eh-teen) USAN.
Use: Antidepressant.

Septa. (Circle) Bacitracin 400 units, neomycin sulfate 5 mg, polymyxin B sulfate 5000 units/g in ointment base. Tube oz. *otc.*
Use: Anti-infective, topical.

Septi-Chek. (Roche Diagnostics) Blood culture and simultaneous sub-culture system with three media to support clinically significant pathogens. Quick and easy assembly forms a closed system to protect sub-cultures from contamination.
Use: Diagnostic aid.

Septiphene. (SEP-tih-feen) (Monsanto)
Use: Disinfectant.

Septi-Soft. (SK-Beecham) Hexachlorophene 0.25%. Liq. Bot. 240 ml, pt, gal. *otc.*
Use: Antiseptic, germicide.

Septisol. (SK-Beecham) **Soln.:** Hexachlorophene 0.25%. Bot. 240 ml, qt, gal. **Foam:** Hexachlorophene 0.23%, alcohol 46%. In 180 ml, 600 ml. *otc.*
Use: Antiseptic, germicide.

Septo. (Vita Elixir) Methylbenzethonium Cl, ethanol 2%, menthol. *otc.*
Use: Antiseptic, germicide.

Septra. (Glaxo Wellcome) Sulfamethoxazole 400 mg, trimethoprim 80 mg/Tab. Bot. 100s. *Rx.*
Use: Anti-infective.

Septra DS. (Glaxo Wellcome) Trimethoprim 160 mg, sulfamethoxazole 800 mg/Tab. Bot. 100s, 250s, UD 100s. *Rx.*
Use: Anti-infective.

Septra Grape Suspension. (Glaxo Wellcome) Trimethoprim 40 mg, sulfamethoxazole 200 mg/5 ml. Bot. 473 ml. *Rx.*
Use: Anti-infective.

Septra I.V. (Glaxo Wellcome) **80/400:** Trimethoprim 80 mg, sulfamethoxazole 400 mg/5 ml. Amp. 5 ml, Vial 10 ml, 20 ml, multidose vials 20 ml. *Rx.*
Use: Anti-infective.

Septra Suspension. (Glaxo Wellcome) Trimethoprim 40 mg, sulfamethoxazole 200 mg/5 ml. Bot. 20 ml, 100 ml, 150 ml, 200 ml, 473 ml. *Rx.*
Use: Anti-infective.

•**seractide acetate.** (seer-ACK-tide) USAN.
Use: Corticotrophic peptide, hormone (adrenocorticotropic).

Ser-A-Gen. (Goldline) Hydrochlorothiazide 15 mg, reserpine 0.1 mg, hydralazine HCl 25 mg/Tab. Bot. 100s, 1000s. *Rx.*
Use: Antihypertensive combination.

Seralyzer. (Bayer) A system for the measurement of enzymes, potassium levels, blood chemistries and therapeutic drug assays consisting of a reflectance photometer and a series of solid-phase reagent strips.
Use: Diagnostic aid.

Ser-Ap-Es. (Novartis) Reserpine 0.1 mg, hydralazine HCl 25 mg, hydrochlorothiazide 15 mg/Tab. Bot. 100s, 1000s. *Rx.*
Use: Antihypertensive combination.

•**seratrodast.** (seh-RAH-troe-dast) USAN.
Use: Anti-inflammatory (non-antihistaminic), antiasthmatic (thromboxane receptor antagonist).

Serax. (Wyeth-Ayerst) Oxazepam. **Cap.:** 10 mg, 15 mg, 30 mg. Bot. 100s, 500s, Redipak 25s, 100s. **Tab.:** 15 mg. Bot. 100s. *c-iv.*
Use: Antianxiety.

•**serazapine hydrochloride.** (ser-AZE-ah-PEEN) USAN.
Use: Antianxiety.

Sereen. (Foy) Chlordiazepoxide HCl 10 mg/Cap. Bot. 500s, 1000s. *c-iv.*
Use: Antianxiety.

Sereine Cleaning Solution. (Optikem) Cocoamphodiacetate and glycols, EDTA 0.1%, benzalkonium Cl 0.01%. Soln. Bot. 60 ml. *otc.*
Use: Contact lens care.

Sereine Wetting Solution. (Optikem) EDTA 0.1%, benzalkonium chloride 0.01%. Soln. Bot. 60 ml, 120 ml. *otc.*
Use: Hard contact lens care.

Sereine Wetting/Soaking Solution. (Optikem) EDTA 0.1%, benzalkonium Cl 0.01%. Soln. Bot. 120 ml. *otc.*
Use: Wetting/soaking solution, hard lenses.

Serene. (Approved) Salicylamide 2 gr, scopolamine aminoxide HBr 0.2 mg/Cap. Bot. 24s, 60s. *Rx.*
Use: Analgesic, sedative.

Serentil. (Boehringer Ingelheim) Mesoridazine besylate. **Inj.:** 25 mg/ml Amp. 1 ml **Tab.:** 10 mg, 25 mg, 50 mg, 100 mg. Bot. 100s. **Oral Conc.:** 25 mg/ml dropper. *Rx.*
Use: Antipsychotic.

Serevent. (Glaxo Wellcome) Salmeterol xinafoate 25 mcg from actuator/actuation. Aerosol. Canister 60 actuations, refills 120 actuations. *Rx.*
Use: Bronchodilator.

•**sergolexole maleate.** (SER-go-LEX-ole) USAN.
Use: Antimigraine.

sericinase. A proteolytic enzyme.

•**serine,** (SER-een) U.S.P. 23.
Use: Amino acid.

•**sermetacin.** (ser-MET-ah-sin) USAN.
Use: Anti-inflammatory.

•**sermorelin acetate.** (SER-moe-REH-lin) USAN.
Use: Growth hormone-releasing factor, diagnostic aid. [Orphan drug]

Seromycin. (Dura) Cycloserine 250 mg/Pulv. Bot. 40s. *Rx.*
Use: Antituberculous agent.

Serophene. (Serono) Clomiphene citrate 50 mg/Tab. Bot. 10s, 30s. *Rx.*
Use: Ovulation stimulant.

serotonin reuptake inhibitors, selective.
Use: Antidepressant.
See: Paxil, Tab. (SK-Beecham).
  Prozac, Liq., Pulv. (Dista).
  Zoloft, Tab. (Roerig).

Serpasil-Apresoline. (Novartis) **#1:** Reserpine 0.1 mg, hydralazine HCl 25 mg/Tab. Bot. 100s. **#2:** Reserpine 0.2

mg, hydralazine HCl 50 mg/Tab. Bot. 100s. *Rx.*
Use: Antihypertensive combination.

Serpasil-Esidrix. (Novartis) **#1:** Reserpine 0.1 mg, hydrochlorothiazide 25 mg/Tab. **#2:** Reserpine 0.1 mg, hydrochlorothiazide 50 mg/Tab. Bot. 100s, 1000s. *Rx.*
Use: Antihypertensive combination.

Serpazide Tablets. (Major) Reserpine 0.1 mg, hydralazine HCl 25 mg, hydrochlorothiazide 15 mg. Bot. 100s, 1000s. *Rx.*
Use: Antihypertensive combination.

serratia marcescens extract (polyribosomes). *Rx.*
Use: Primary brain malignancies. [Orphan drug]

Sertabs. (Table Rock) Reserpine 0.25 mg or 0.5 mg/Tab. Bot. 100s, 500s. *Rx.*
Use: Antihypertensive.

Sertina. (Fellows) Reserpine 0.25 mg/Tab. Bot. 1000s, 5000s. *Rx.*
Use: Antihypertensive.

•**sertindole.** (ser-TIN-dole) USAN.
Use: Antipsychotic; neuroleptic.

•**sertraline hydrochloride.** (SIR-truh-leen) USAN.
Use: Antidepressant.
See: Zoloft (Roerig)

serum, albumin, normal human.
See: Albumin Human, U.S.P. 23. (Various Mfr.).

serum, albumin, human, radioiodinated.
See: Iodinated. I-125
  Albumin Injection, U.S.P. 23

serum, globulin (human), immune.
See: immune globulin intramuscular or immune globulin intravenous.

Serutan. (SK-Beecham) Psyllium. **Gran.:** Pkg. 6 oz, 18 oz. **Pow.:** 7 oz, 14 oz, 21 oz. Fruit flavored: 6 oz, 12 oz, 18 oz. *otc.*
Use: Laxative.

Serzone. (Bristol-Myers Squibb) Nefazodone 100 mg, 150 mg, 200 mg or 250 mg/Tab. Bot. 60s, 100s (except 250 mg). *Rx.*
Use: Antidepressant.

Sesame Street Plus Extra C. (McNeil-CPC) Vitamins A 2750 IU, D 200 IU, E 10 IU, B$_1$ 0.75 mg, B$_2$ 0.85 mg, B$_3$ 10 mg, B$_5$ 5 mg, B$_6$ 0.7 mg, B$_{12}$ 3 mcg, C 80 mg, FA 0.2 mg/Tab. Bot. 50s. *otc.*
Use: Vitamin supplement.

•**sesame oil,** N.F. 18.
Use: Pharmaceutic aid (solvent; vehicle, oleaginous).

Sesame Street Complete. (McNeil-CPC) Ca 80 mg, iron 10 mg, vitamins A 2750 IU, D 200 IU, E 10 mg, B_1 0.75 mg, B_2 0.85 mg, B_3 10 mg, B_5 5 mg, B_6 0.7 mg, B_{12} 3 mcg, C 40 mg, folic acid 0.2 mg, biotin 15 mg, Cu, I, Mg, Zn 8 mg, lactose/Tab. Bot. 50s. *otc.*
Use: Vitamin/mineral supplement.

Sesame Street Plus Extra C. (McNeil) Vitamins A 2750 IU, D 200 IU, E 10 IU, B_1 0.75 mg, B_2 0.85 mg, B_3 10 mg, B_5 5 mg, B_6 0.7 mg, B_{12} 3 mcg, C 80 mg, folic acid 0.2 mg/Tab. Bot. 50s. *otc.*
Use: Vitamin supplement.

Sesame Street Plus Iron. (McNeil-CPC) Iron 10 mg, vitamins A 2750 IU, D 200 IU, E 10 IU, B_1 0.75 mg, B_2 0.85 mg, B_3 10 mg, B_5 5 mg, B_6 0.7 mg, B_{12} 3 mcg, C 40 mg, folic acid 0.2 mg/Chew. Tab. Bot. 50s *otc.*
Use: Vitamin/mineral supplement.

Sesame Street Vitamins. (McNeil-CPC) **For ages 4 and older:** Vitamins A 5000 IU, B_1 1.5 mg, B_{12} 6 mcg, C 60 mg, D 400 IU, E 30 IU, folic acid 400 mcg, biotin 300 mcg/Chew Tab. Bot. 60s. **For ages 2-3:** Vitamins A 2500 IU, B_1 0.7 mg, B_2 0.8 mg, B_3 9 mg, B_5 5 mg, B_6 0.7 mg, B_{12} 3 mcg, C 40 mg, D 400 IU, E 10 IU, folic acid 200 mcg, biotin 150 mcg/Chew Tab. Bot. 60s. *otc.*
Use: Vitamin supplement.

Sesame Street Vitamins and Minerals. (McNeil-CPC) **For ages 4 and older:** Vitamins A 5000 IU, B_1 1.5 mg, B_2 1.7 mg, B_3 20 mg, B_5 10 mg, B_6 2 mg, B_{12} 6 mcg, C 60 mg, D 400 IU, E 30 IU, folic acid 400 mcg, biotin 300 mcg, calcium 100 mg, iron 18 mg, iodine 150 mcg, zinc 15 mg, copper 2 mg/Chew Tab. Bot. 60s. **For ages 2-3:** Vitamins A 2500 IU, B_1 0.7 mg, B_{12} 3 mcg, C 40 mg, D 400 IU, E 10 IU, folic acid 200 mcg, biotin 150 mcg, calcium 80 mg, iron 10 mg, iodine 70 mcg, zinc 8 mg, copper 1 mg/Chew Tab. Bot. 60s. *otc.*
Use: Vitamin/mineral supplement.

sestron. (Smith, Miller & Patch).

Sethotope. (Squibb) Selenomethionine selenium 75; available as 0.25, 1 mCi.

• **setoperone.** (SEE-toe-per-OHN) USAN.
Use: Antipsychotic.

• **sevirumab.** (seh-VIE-roo-mab) USAN.
Use: Monoclonal antibody (antiviral).

• **sevoflurane.** (SEE-voe-FLEW-rane) USAN.
Use: Anesthetic (inhalation).
See: Ultane, Soln. for Inh. (Abbott).

• **sezolamide hydrochloride.** (seh-ZOLE-ah-MIDE) USAN.

Use: Carbonic anhydrase inhibitor.

SFC Lotion. (Stiefel) Soap free. Stearyl alcohol, PEG-75, sodium cocoyl isethionate, parabens. Bot. 237 ml, 480 ml. *otc.*
Use: Skin cleanser.

Shade. (Schering-Plough) SPF 15. Contains one or more of the following ingredients: Padimate O, oxybenzone, ethylhexyl-p-methoxycinnamate. Bot. 118 ml, 120 ml, 240 ml. *otc.*
Use: Sunscreen.

Shade Cream. (O'Leary) Jar 0.25 oz. *otc.*
Use: Contouring cream.

Shade Sunblock Gel, 15 SPF. (Schering-Plough) Ethylhexyl p-methoxycinnamate, octyl salicylate, oxybenzone, SD alcohol 40. PABA free. SPF 15. Waterproof. Gel. Bot. 120 g. *otc.*
Use: Sunscreen.

Shade Sunblock Gel, 25 SPF. (Schering-Plough) Ethylhexyl p-methoxycinnamate, octyl salicylate, homosalate, oxybenzone, SD alcohol 40. PABA free. Gel. Bot. 120 g. *otc.*
Use: Sunscreen.

Shade Sunblock Gel, 30 SPF. (Schering-Plough) Ethylhexyl p-methoxycinnamate, homosalate, oxybenzone, 73% SD alcohol 40. Bot. 120 g. *otc.*
Use: Sunscreen.

Shade Sunblock Lotion, 15 SPF. (Schering-Plough) Ethylhexyl p-methoxycinnamate, oxybenzone, benzyl alcohol, phenethyl alcohol. PABA free. Waterproof. Lot. Bot. 120 ml. *otc.*
Use: Sunscreen.

Shade Sunblock Lotion, 30 SPF. (Schering-Plough) Ethylhexyl p-methoxycinnamate, 2-ethylhexyl salicylate, homosalate, oxybenzone, benzyl alcohol, phenethyl alcohol. PABA free. Waterproof. Lot. Bot. 120 ml. *otc.*
Use: Sunscreen.

Shade Sunblock Lotion, 45 SPF. (Schering-Plough) Ethylhexyl p-methoxycinnamate, oxybenzone, 2-ethylhexyl salicylate, benzyl alcohol, phenethyl alcohol. PABA free. Waterproof. Lot. Bot. 120 ml. *otc.*
Use: Sunscreen.

Shade Sunblock Stick, 30 SPF. (Schering-Plough) Ethylhexyl p-methoxycinnamate, oxybenzone, 2-ethylhexyl salicylate, homosalate. PABA free. Waterproof. Stick. 18 g. *otc.*
Use: Sunscreen.

Shade Uvaguard. (Schering-Plough) Octyl methoxycinnamate 7.5%, avoben-

zone 3%, oxybenzone 3%. Waterproof.
SPF 15. Lot. 120 ml. *otc.*
Use: Sunscreen.

Sheik Elite. (Schmid) Condom with non-oxynol 9 15%. In 3s, 12s, 24s, 36s. *otc.*
Use: Contraceptive.

•**shellac,** N.F. 18.
Use: Pharmaceutic aid (tablet coating agent).

Shepard's Cream Lotion. (Dermik) Creamy lotion with no lanolin or mineral oil, for entire body. Scented or unscented. Bot. 8 oz, 16 oz. *otc.*
Use: Emollient.

Shepard's Skin Cream. (Dermik) Scented or unscented, w/no lanolin or mineral oil. Jar 4 oz. *otc.*
Use: Emollient.

Sherform-HC Creme. (Sheryl) Hydrocortisone 1%, pramoxine HCl 0.5%, clioquinol 3%. Oint. Tube 0.5 oz. *Rx.*
Use: Corticosteroid, local anesthetic, topical antifungal.

Sherhist. (Sheryl) Phenylephrine HCl, pyrilamine maleate/Tab. 100s. Liq. pt.
Use: Decongestant, antihistamine.

Shernatal Tablets. (Sheryl) Phosphorus free calcium, non-irritating iron, trace minerals and essential vitamins. Tab. 100s.
Use: Vitamin/mineral supplement.

Shertus Liquid. (Sheryl) Dextromethorphan HBr, chlorpheniramine maleate, phenylephrine HCl, ammonium Cl. Liq. pt.
Use: Antitussive, antihistamine, decongestant, expectorant.

Shohl's Solution. Sodium Citrate and Citric Acid Oral Soln, U.S.P. 23.
Use: Systemic alkalizer.

short chain fatty acid solution. *Rx.*
Use: Ulcerative colitis. [Orphan drug]

Shur-Clens. (SK-Beecham) Poloxamer 188 20%. Soln. Bot. UD 100, 200 ml. *otc.*
Use: Topical drug, miscellaneous.

Shur Seal Gel. (Milex) Nonoxynol-9 2%. In 24 UD gel paks. *otc.*
Use: Contraceptive jelly for use with diaphragm.

Sibelium. (Janssen) Flunarizine HCl. *Rx.*
Use: Vasodilator.

•**sibopirdine.** (sih-BOE-pihr-deen) USAN.
Use: Nootropic; cognition enhancer (Alzheimer's disease).

•**sibutramine hydrochloride.** (sih-BYOO-trah-meen) USAN.
Use: Antidepressant; anorexic.

sickle cell test.
Use: Diagnostic aid.
See: Sickledex Test (Ortho Diag.).

Sickledex. (Ortho Diag.) Test kit 12s, 100s.
Use: Diagnostic aid.

Sigamine. (Sig) Cyanocobalamin injection 1000 mcg/ml. Vial 10 ml, 30 ml. Also Sigamine L.A. Vial 10 ml. *Rx.*
Use: Vitamin B$_{12}$ supplement.

Sigazine. (Sig) Promethazine HCl 50 mg/ml. Vial 10 ml. *Rx.*
Use: Antihistamine.

Signa Creme. (Parker) Conductive cosmetic quality electrolyte cream. Bot. 5 oz, 2 L, 4 L.
Use: High conductive electrode cream for diagnostic electrocardiograms.

Signa Gel. (Parker) Conductive saline electrode gel. Tube 250 g.
Use: Defibrillation, ECG, EMG, electrosurgery.

Signa Pad. (Parker) Pre-moistened electrode pads.
Use: ECG procedures.

Signatal C. (Sig) Calcium 230 mg, iron 49.3 mg, vitamins A 4000 IU, D 400 IU, B$_1$ 2 mg, B$_2$ 2 mg, B$_6$ 1 mg, B$_{12}$ 2 mcg, folic acid 0.1 mg, niacinamide 10 mg, C 50 mg, iodine 0.15 mg/S.C. Tab. Bot. 100s, 1000s. *otc.*
Use: Vitamin/mineral supplement.

Signate. (Sig) Dimenhydrinate 50 mg, propylene glycol 50%, benzyl alcohol 5%/ml. Vial 10 ml. *Rx.*
Use: Antiemetic, antivertigo.

Signef "Supps". (Fellows) Hydrocortisone 15 mg/Supp. 12s. w or w/out appl. *Rx.*
Use: Corticosteroid, vaginal.

Sigpred. (Sig) Prednisolone acetate. Vial 10 ml. *Rx.*
Use: Corticosteroid.

Sigtab. (Roberts) Vitamins A 5000 IU, D 400 IU, B$_1$ 10.3 mg, B$_2$ 10 mg, C 333 mg, B$_3$ 100 mg, B$_6$ 6 mg, B$_5$ 20 mg, folic acid 0.4 mg, B$_{12}$ 18 mcg, E 15 mg/Tab. Bot. 90s, 500s. *otc.*
Use: Vitamin supplement.

Sigtab-M. (Roberts) Vitamins A 6000 IU, D$_3$ 400 IU, E 45 mg, C 100 mg, B$_3$ 25 mg, B$_1$ 5 mg, B$_2$ 5 mg, B$_6$ 3 mg, folic acid 400 mcg, B$_5$ 0.015 mg, biotin 45 mcg, Ca 200 mg, P, iron 18 mg, Mg, Cu, zinc 15 mg, Mn, K, Cl, Mo, Se, Cr, Ni, Sn, V, Si, B, vitamin K, I/Tab. Bot.100s. *otc.*
Use: Vitamin/mineral supplement.

Silace. (Silarx) Docusate sodium 20 mg/

5 ml. ≤ 1% alcohol. Syrup. Bot. 473 ml. *otc.*
Use: Laxative.

Silace-C. (Silarx) Docusate sodium 60 mg, casanthranol 30 mg/15 ml. 10% alcohol. Syrup. Bot. 473 ml. *otc.*
Use: Laxative combination.

Siladryl. (Silarx) Diphenhydramine HCl 12.5 mg/5 ml. 5.6% alcohol. Elixir. 118 ml. *otc.*
Use: Antihistamine.

Silafed. (Silarx) Pseudoephedrine HCl 30 mg, triprolidine HCl 1.25 mg/5 ml. Syrup. Bot. 120 ml, 240 ml, 473 ml, gal. *otc.*
Use: Decongestant, antihistamine.

•**silafilcon a.** (SIH-lah-FILL-kahn A) USAN.
Use: Contact lens material (hydrophilic).

•**silafocon a.** USAN.
Use: Contact lens material (hydrophobic).

Silaminic Cold. (Silarx) Phenylpropanolamine HCl 12.5 mg, chlorpheniramine maleate 2 mg/5 ml. 5% alcohol. Bot. 118 ml. *otc.*
Use: Decongestant, antihistamine.

Silaminic Expectorant. (Silarx) Phenylpropanolamine HCl 12.5 mg, guaifenesin 100 mg/5 ml. Liq. Bot. 118 ml. *otc.*
Use: Decongestant, expectorant.

•**silandrone.** (sil-AN-drone) USAN.
Use: Androgen.

Sildec-DM. (Silarx) **Drops, Pediatric:** Carbinoxamine maleate 2 mg, pseudoephedrine HCl 25 mg, dextromethorphan HBr 4 mg/ml. Alcohol and sugar free. Bot. 30 ml. **Syrup:** Carbinoxamine maleate 4 mg, pseudoephedrine HCl 60 mg, dextromethorphan HBr 15 mg/5 ml. Bot. 473 ml. *Rx.*
Use: Antihistamine, decongestant, antitussive.

Sildicon-E. (Silarx) Phenylpropanolamine HCl 6.25 mg, guaifenesin 30 mg. Pediatric drops. 0.6% alcohol. Bot. 30 ml. *otc.*
Use: Decongestant, expectorant.

•**silica, dental-type,** N.F. 18.
Use: Pharmaceutic aid.

•**siliceous earth, purified,** N.F. 18.
Use: Pharmaceutic aid (filtering medium).

•**silicon dioxide,** N.F. 18. *Formerly Silica Gel.*
Use: Pharmaceutic aid (dispersing and suspending agent).

•**silicon dioxide, colloidal,** N.F. 18.
Use: Pharmaceutic aid (tablet/capsule diluent, suspending and thickening agent).

Silicone. (Dow Chemicals) Dimethicone. Liq., Bot. oz. Bulk Pkg. Oint.
See also:
W/Nitro-Cellulose, castor oil.
See: Covicone, Cream (Abbott).
W/Triethylene glycol, mineral oil.
See: Allergex, Liq., Spray (Bayer).

silicone oil.
See: polydimethylsiloxane (silicone oil).

silicone ointment. Dimethicone Dimethyl polysiloxane.
See: Covicone Cream (Abbott).

Silicone Ointment No. 2. (C & M Pharmacal) High viscosity silicone 10% in a blend of petrolatum and hydrophobic starch. Jar 2 oz, lb. *otc.*
Use: Protective agent.

Silicone Powder. (Gordon) Talc with silicone. Pkg. 4 oz, 1 lb, 5 lb. *otc.*
Use: Dusting powder to prevent tape from adhering to clothing.

•**silodrate.** (SILL-oh-drate) USAN.
Use: Antacid.

Silphen Cough. (Silarx) Diphenhydramine HCl 12.5 mg/5 ml, alcohol 5%, menthol, sucrose. Syrup. Bot. 118 ml. *otc.*
Use: Antihistamine.

Silphen DM. (Silarx) Dextromethorphan HBr 10 mg/5 ml. Syrup. 5% alcohol. Bot. 118 ml. *otc.*
Use: Antitussive.

Siltapp with Dextromethorphan HBr Cold & Cough. (Silarx) Brompheniramine maleate 2 mg, phenylpropanolamine HCl 12.5 mg, dextromethorphan HBr 10 mg/5 ml. Elix. 2.3% alcohol, sorbitol, saccharin. Bot. 118 ml. *otc.*
Use: Antihistamine, decongestant, antitussive.

Sil-Tex. (Silarx) Phenylephrine HCl 5 mg, phenylpropanolamine HCl 20 mg, guaifenesin 100 mg/5 ml. Liq. 5% alcohol, saccharin, sorbitol, sucrose. In 473 ml. *Rx.*
Use: Expectorant.

Siltussin. (Silarx) Guaifenesin 100 mg/5 ml. Syrup. Saccharin, menthol, methylparaben. Alcohol and dye free. Bot. 473 ml. *otc.*
Use: Expectorant.

Siltussin-CF. (Silarx) Phenylpropanolamine HCl 12.5 mg, dextromethorphan HBr 10 mg, guaifenesin 100 mg/5 ml. Liq. 4.75% alcohol. Bot. 118 ml. *otc.*
Use: Decongestant, antitussive, expectorant.

Siltussin DM. (Silarx) Dextromethorphan HBr 10 mg, guaifenesin 100 mg/5 ml. Syrup. Alcohol free. Saccharin, sucrose. Bot. 118 ml. *otc.*
Use: Antitussive, expectorant.

Silvadene. (Hoechst Marion Roussel) Silver sulfadiazine (10 mg/Gm) 1%, base w/white petrolatum, stearyl alcohol, isopropyl myristate, sorbitan monooleate, polyoxyl 40 stearate, propylene glycol, water, methylparaben. Cream Jar 50 g, 85 g, 400 g, 1000 g. Tube 20 g. *Rx.*
Use: Antimicrobial, topical.

silver compounds.
See: Silver Iodide, Colloidal.
Silver Nitrate, Preps. (Various Mfr.).
Silver Protein, Mild (Various Mfr.).
Silver Protein, Strong (Various Mfr.).

• **silver nitrate,** U.S.P. 23.
Use: Anti-infective (topical).

silver nitrate ointment. (Gordon) Silver nitrate 1% in ointment base. Jar oz. *Rx.*
Use: Astringent, epithelial stimulant.

silver nitrate ophthalmic solution. *Rx.*
Use: Astringent, anti-infective.
Generic Products:
(Gordon)–Soln. 10%, 25%, 50%. Bot. oz.
(Lilly)–Amp. 1%, 100s.
(Parke-Davis)–Cap. 1%, 100s.

silver nitrate topical sticks. (Graham-Field) Silver nitrate, potassium nitrate 25%. Appl. 100s. *Rx.*
Use: Cauterizing agent.

• **silver nitrate, toughened,** U.S.P. 23.
Use: Caustic.

silver protein, mild. Argentum Vitellinum, Cargentos, Mucleinate Mild, Protargin Mild.
See: Argyrol Prods. (Ciba Vision).

silver protein, strong.
See: Protargol, Pow. (Sterling).

silver sulfadiazine. (SILL-ver SULL-fah-DIE-ah-zeen)
Use: Anti-infective, topical.
See: Silvadene, Cream (Hoechst Marion Roussel).
SSD Cream (Knoll Pharm).
SSD AF Cream (Knoll Pharm).
Thermazene, Cream (Sherwood).

Simaal Gel. (Schein) Aluminum hydroxide 200 mg, magnesium hydroxide 200 mg, simethicone 20 mg/5 ml. Liq. Bot. 360 ml. *otc.*
Use: Antacid, antiflatulant.

Simaal 2 Gel. (Schein) Aluminum hydroxide 500 mg, magnesium hydroxide 400 mg, simethicone 40 mg/5 ml. Liq. Bot. 360 ml. *otc.*

Use: Antacid, antiflatulant.

• **simethicone,** (sih-METH-ih-cone) U.S.P. 23. Mixture of liquid dimethyl polysiloxanes with silica aerogel.
Use: Antiflatulent.
See: Mylicon, Tab., Liq. (J & J Merck).
Mylicon-80, Tab. (J & J Merck).
Silain, Tab. (Robins).
Ingredients of:
Mylanta, Tab., Liq. (J & J Merck).
Phazyme, Tab. (Reed & Carnick).
W/Aluminum hydroxide, magnesium hydroxide.
See: Di-Gel, Liq., Tab. (Schering-Plough).
Mylanta, Mylanta II, Tab., Liq. (J & J Merck).
Silain-Gel, Liq. (Robins).
Simeco, Liq. (Wyeth-Ayerst).
Simethox, Liq. (Quality Generics).
W/Enzymes.
See: Phazyme, Tab. (Schwarz Pharma).
W/Hyoscyamine sulfate, atropine sulfate, hyoscine HBr, butabarbital sodium.
See: Sidonna, Tab. (Schwarz Pharma).
W/Hyoscyamine sulfate, atropine sulfate, scopolamine HBr, phenobarbital.
See: Kinesed, Chew. Tab. (J & J Merck).
W/Magnesium aluminum hydroxide.
See: Maalox Plus, Susp. (Rhone-Poulenc Rorer).
W/Magnesium carbonate.
See: Di-Gel, Tab., Liq. (Schering-Plough).
W/Magnesium hydroxide.
See: Laxsil, Liq. (Schwarz Pharma).
W/Magnesium hydroxide, dried aluminum hydroxide gel.
See: Maalox Plus, Tab. (Rhone-Poulenc Rorer).
W/Pancreatin.
See: Phazyme, Tab. (Schwarz Pharma).
Phazyme-95, Tab. (Reed & Carnrick).
W/Pancreatin, phenobarbital.
See: Phazyme-PB, Tab. (Schwarz Pharma).

Similac 13/Similac 13 with Iron. (Ross) Milk-based infant formula ready-to-feed containing 13 calories/fl oz, 1.8 mg iron/100 calories. Bot. 4 fl. oz. *otc.*
Use: Nutritional therapy for infants.

Similac 20/Similac with Iron 20. (Ross) Milk-based infant formula. Standard dilution (20 cal/fl oz). Similac with iron: iron 1.8 mg/100 cal. **Pow.:** Can lb. **Concentrated Liq.:** Can 13 fl oz. **Ready-to-feed:** Can 8 fl oz, 32 fl oz. Bot. 4 fl oz, 8 fl oz. *otc.*
Use: Nutritional therapy for infants.

Similac 24 LBW. (Ross) Low-iron infant formula, ready-to-feed, 24 calories/fl oz. Bot. 4 fl oz. *otc.*
Use: Nutritional therapy for infants.

Similac 24/Similac 24 with Iron. (Ross) Milk-based infant formula ready-to-feed (24 cal/fl oz), iron 1.8 mg/100 calories. Bot. 4 fl oz. *otc.*
Use: Nutritional therapy for infants.

Similac 27. (Ross) Milk-based ready-to-feed infant formula (27 cal/fl oz). Bot. 4 fl oz. *otc.*
Use: Nutritional therapy for infants.

Similac Low-Iron Liquid & Powder. (Ross) Protein 14.3 g, carbohydrates 72 g, fat 36 g, iron 1.5 mg, with appropriate vitamins and minerals. **Liq.:** 390 ml concentrate, 240 ml and 1 qt. ready-to-use, 120 ml and 240 ml nursettes. **Pow.:** 1 lb. *otc.*
Use: Nutritional therapy for infants.

Similac Natural Care Human Milk Fortifier. (Ross) Liquid fortifier designed to be mixed with human milk or fed alternately with human milk to low-birth-weight infants. Supplied as 24 cal/fl oz. Bot. 4 fl oz. *otc.*
Use: Nutritional therapy for infants.

Similac PM 60/40. (Ross) Milk-based formula ready-to-feed or powder with 60:40 whey to casein ratio (20 cal/fl oz). **Bot.:** Hospital use 4 fl oz. ready-to-feed. **Pow.:** Can lb. *otc.*
Use: Nutritional therapy for infants.

Similac Special Care 20. (Ross) Infant formula ready-to-feed (20 cal/fl oz). Bot. 4 fl oz. *otc.*
Use: Nutritional therapy for infants.

Similac Special Care 24. (Ross) Infant formula ready-to-feed (24 Cal/fl oz). Bot. 4 fl oz. *otc.*
Use: Nutritional therapy for infants.

Simplet. (Major) Pseudoephedrine HCl 60 mg, chlorpheniramine maleate 4 mg, acetaminophen 650 mg/Tab. Bot. 100s. *otc.*
Use: Decongestant, antihistamine, analgesic.

Simron. (SK-Beecham) Iron (supplied as ferrous gluconate) 10 mg/Cap. Bot. 100s. *otc.*
Use: Iron supplement.

Simron Plus. (SK-Beecham) Iron 10 mg, vitamins B$_{12}$ 3.33 mcg, C 50 mg, B$_6$ 1 mg, folic acid 0.1 mg/Cap. Parabens. Bot. 100s. *otc.*
Use: Iron supplement.

•**simtrazene.** (SIM-trah-seen) USAN.
Use: Antineoplastic.

•**simvastatin,** (SIM-vuh-STAT-in) U.S.P. 23. *Formerly Synvinolin.*
Use: Antihyperlipidemic.
See: Zocor (Merck).

Sinapils. (Pfeiffer) Phenylpropanolamine HCl 12.5 mg, chlorpheniramine maleate 2 mg, acetaminophen 325 mg, caffeine 32.5 mg/Tab. Bot. 36s. *otc.*
Use: Decongestant, antihistamine, analgesic.

Sinarest 12 Hour. (Novartis Consumer Health) Oxymetazoline HCl 0.05%. Spray Bot. 15 ml. *otc.*
Use: Decongestant.

Sinarest Decongestant Nasal Spray. (Novartis Consumer Health) Oxymetazoline HCl 0.05%. Bot. 0.5 oz. *otc.*
Use: Decongestant.

Sinarest, Extra-Strength. (Novartis Consumer Health) Acetaminophen 500 mg, chlorpheniramine maleate 2 mg, pseudoephedrine HCl 30 mg/Tab. 24s. *otc.*
Use: Analgesic, antihistamine, decongestant.

Sinarest, No Drowsiness. (Novartis Consumer Health) Pseudoephedrine HCl 30 mg, acetaminophen 500 mg/Tab. Pkg. 20s. *otc.*
Use: Decongestant, analgesic.

Sinarest Sinus. (Novartis Consumer Health) Acetaminophen 325 mg, chlorpheniramine maleate 2 mg, pseudoephedrine HCl 30 mg/Tab. Pkg. 20s, 40s, 80s. *otc.*
Use: Analgesic, antihistamine, decongestant.

•**sincalide.** (SIN-kah-lide) USAN.
Use: Choleretic.

Sine-Aid IB. (McNeil-CPC) Pseudoephedrine 30 mg, ibuprofen 200 mg. Capl. Pkg. 20s. *otc.*
Use: Decongestant, analgesic.

Sine-Aid Maximum Strength. (McNeil-CPC) Pseudoephedrine HCl 30 mg, acetaminophen 500 mg/Tab.or Cap. **Tab.:** Bot. 24s, 100s. **Cap.:** Bot. 24s, 50s. *otc.*
Use: Decongestant, analgesic.

Sine-Aid Sinus Headache Caplets, Extra Strength. (McNeil Prods) Acetaminophen 500 mg, pseudoephedrine HCl 30 mg/Capl. Bot. 24s, 50s. *otc.*
Use: Analgesic, decongestant.

Sine-Aid Sinus Headache Tablets. (McNeil Prods) Acetaminophen 325 mg, pseudoephedrine HCl 30 mg/Tab. Bot. 24s, 50s, 100s. *otc.*
Use: Analgesic, decongestant.

•**sinefungin.** (sih-neh-FUN-jin) USAN.

Use: Antifungal.

Sinemet CR. (DuPont Pharma) Carbidopa 25 or 50 mg, levodopa 100 or 200 mg/SR Tab. Bot. 100s, UD 100s. *Rx.*
Use: Antiparkinsonian.

Sinemet 10/100. (DuPont Merck) Carbidopa 10 mg, levodopa 100 mg/Tab. Bot. 100s, UD 100s. *Rx.*
Use: Antiparkinsonian.

Sinemet 25/100. (DuPont Merck) Carbidopa 25 mg, levodopa 100 mg/Tab. Bot. 100s, UD 100s. *Rx.*
Use: Antiparkinsonian.

Sinemet 25/250. (DuPont Merck) Carbidopa 25 mg, levodopa 250 mg/Tab. Bot. 100s, UD 100s. *Rx.*
Use: Antiparkinsonian.

Sine-Off Maximum Strength No Drowsiness Formula Caplets. (SK-Beecham) Pseudoephedrine HCl 30 mg, acetaminophen 500 mg/Cap. Pkg. 24s. *otc.*
Use: Decongestant, analgesic.

Sine-Off Sinus Medicine. (SK-Beecham) Chlorpheniramine maleate 2 mg, pseudoephedrine HCl 30 mg, acetaminophen 500 mg/Cap. Pkg. 24s. *otc.*
Use: Antihistamine, decongestant, analgesic.

Sine-Off Tablets. (SK-Beecham) Chlorpheniramine maleate 2 mg, phenylpropanolamine HCl 12.5 mg, aspirin 325 mg. Tab. Pkg. 24s, 48s, 100s. *otc.*
Use: Antihistamine, decongestant, analgesic.

Sinequan. (Roerig) Doxepin HCl. **Cap.:** 10 mg/Cap. Bot. 100s, 1000s, UD 100s; 25 mg or 50 mg/Cap. Bot. 90s, 100s, 1000s, UD 100s; 75 mg/Cap. Bot. 100s, 1000s, UD 100s; 100 mg/Cap. Bot. 100s, 1000s, UD 100s; 150 mg/Cap. Bot. 50s, 500s, UD 100s. **Oral Concentrate:** 10 mg/ml. Bot. 120 ml. *Rx.*
Use: Antidepressant.

Sinex. (Procter & Gamble) Phenylephrine HCl 0.5%, cetylpyridinium Cl 0.04% w/ thimerosal 0.001% preservative. Nasal spray. Bot. 0.5 oz, 1 oz. *otc.*
Use: Decongestant.

Singlet for Adults. (SK-Beecham) Pseudoephedrine HCl 60 mg, chlorpheniramine maleate 4 mg, acetaminophen 650 mg/Tab. Bot. 100s. *otc.*
Use: Decongestant, antihistamine, analgesic.

Sinocon TR. (Vangard) Phenylpropanol-

amine HCl 20 mg, phenylephrine HCl 5 mg, phenyltoloxamine citrate 7.5 mg, chlorpheniramine maleate 2.5 mg/Tab. Bot. 100s, 1000s. *Rx.*
Use: Decongestant, antihistamine.

Sino-Eze MLT. (Global Pharms) Salicylamide 3.5 gr, acetaminophen 100 mg, phenylephrine HCl 5 mg, chlorpheniramine maleate 2 mg/Tab. Bot. 1000s. *Rx.*
Use: Analgesic, decongestant, antihistamine.

Sinografin. (Squibb) Meglumine diatrizoate 52.7%, meglumine iodipamide 26.8%. Vial 10 ml.
Use: Diagnostic aid.

Sinucol. (Tennessee Pharm) Chlorpheniramine maleate 8 mg, phenylephrine HCl 20 mg, methscopolamine nitrate 2.5 mg/Cap. Bot. 100s, 500s. Inj. Vial 10 ml. *Rx.*
Use: Antihistamine, decongestant combination.

Sinufed Timecelle. (Roberts) Pseudoephedrine HCl 60 mg, guaifenesin 300 mg/Cap. Bot. 100s. *Rx.*
Use: Decongestant, expectorant.

Sinulin Tablets. (Carnrick) Phenylpropanolamine HCl 25 mg, chlorpheniramine maleate 4 mg, acetaminophen 650 mg/Tab. Bot. 20s, 100s. *otc.*
Use: Decongestant, antihistamine, analgesic.

Sinumist-SR. (Roberts) Guaifenesin 600 mg/Tab. Bot. 100s. *Rx.*
Use: Expectorant.

Sinupan. (ION) Phenylephrine HCl 40 mg, guaifenesin 200 mg/SR Cap. Bot. 100s. *Rx.*
Use: Decongestant, expectorant.

Sinuseze. (Amlab) Acetaminophen 325 mg, phenylpropanolamine HCl 25 mg, phenyltoloxamine citrate 22 mg/Tab. Bot. 36s. *otc.*
Use: Analgesic, decongestant, antihistamine.

Sinus Excedrin Extra Strength. (Bristol-Myers Squibb) Pseudoephedrine HCl 30 mg, acetaminophen 500 mg/Tab or Cap. Bot. 50s. *otc.*
Use: Decongestant, analgesic.

Sinus Headache & Congestion Tablets. (Rugby) Pseudoephedrine HCl 30 mg, chlorpheniramine maleate 2 mg, acetaminophen 500 mg/Tab. Bot. 100s, 1000s. *otc.*
Use: Decongestant, antihistamine, analgesic.

Sinus Pain Formula Allerest. (Medeva)

Pseudoephedrine HCl 30 mg, chlorpheniramine maleate 2 mg, acetaminophen 500 mg. **Cap.:** Bot. 24s, 50s. **Gelcap:** Bot. 20s, 40s. *otc.*
Use: Decongestant, antihistamine, analgesic.

Sinus Relief. (Major) Pseudoephedrine HCl 30 mg, acetaminophen 325 mg/Tab. Bot. 24s, 100s, 1000s. *otc.*
Use: Decongestant, analgesic.

Sinus Tablets. (Walgreen) Acetaminophen 325 mg, chlorpheniramine maleate 2 mg, pseudoephedrine HCl mg/Tab. Bot. 30s. *otc.*
Use: Analgesic, antihistamine, decongestant.

Sinutab Maximum Strength Sinus Allergy. (Warner Lambert) Acetaminophen 500 mg, pseudoephedrine HCl 30 mg, chlorpheniramine maleate 2 mg/Tab., Capl. Blister pack 24s. *otc.*
Use: Analgesic, decongestant, antihistamine.

Sinutab Non-Drying. (Warner Lambert) Pseudoephedrine HCl 30 mg, guaifenesin 200 mg/Cap.(Liq.) Pkg. 24s. *otc.*
Use: Decongestant, expectorant.

Sinutab Sinus Maximum Strength Without Drowsiness Formula. (Warner Lambert) Acetaminophen 500 mg, pseudoephedrine HCl 30 mg/Tab or Cap. Pack 24s. *otc.*
Use: Analgesic, decongestant.

Sinutab Sinus Regular Strength Without Drowsiness. (Warner Lambert) Pseudoephedrine HCl 30 mg, acetaminophen 325 mg/Tab. Bot. 24s. *otc.*
Use: Decongestant, analgesic.

Sinutrol. (Weeks & Leo) Phenylpropanolamine HCl 25 mg, phenyltoloxamine citrate 22 mg, acetaminophen 325 mg/Tab. Bot. 40s, 90s. *otc.*
Use: Decongestant, antihistamine, analgesic.

Sinuvent. (WE Pharm) Phenylpropanolamine 75 mg, guaifenesin 600 mg. LA Tab. Bot. 100s. *Rx.*
Use: Decongestant, expectorant.

Siroil. (Siroil) Mercuric oleate, cresol, vegetable and mineral oil. Emulsion, Bot. 8 oz. *otc.*
Use: Antiseptic.

sir-o-lene. (Siroil) Tube 4 oz.
Use: Emollient.

•**sirolimus.** (SER-oh-lih-muss) USAN.
Formerly Rapamycin.
Use: Immunosuppressant.

•**sisomicin.** (SIS-oh-MY-sin) USAN.
Use: Antibacterial.

•**sisomicin sulfate,** (SIS-oh-MY-sin) U.S.P. 23.
Use: Antibacterial.

Sitabs. (Canright) Lobeline sulfate 1.5 mg, benzocaine 2 mg, aluminum hydroxide–magnesium carbonate co-dried gel 150 mg/Loz. Bot. 100s. *otc.*
Use: Smoking deterrent.

•**sitogluside.** (SIGH-toe-GLUE-side) USAN.
Use: Antiprostatic hypertrophy.

Sitzmarks. (Konsyl Pharm) Radiopaque rings 20/Cap. Bot. 10s.
Use: GI contrast agent.

Sixameen. (Spanner) Vitamins B_1 100 mg, B_6 100 mg/ml. Vial 10 ml. *otc.*
Use: Vitamin B supplement.

Skeeter Stik. (Outdoor Recreation) Lidocaine 4%, phenol 2%, isopropyl alcohol 45.5% in a propylene glycol base. Stick 1s. *otc.*
Use: Local anesthetic.

Skelaxin. (Carnrick) Metaxalone 400 mg/Tab. Bot. 100s, 500s. *Rx.*
Use: Skeletal muscle relaxant.

skeletal muscle relaxants.
See: Anectine, Soln., Pow. (Glaxo Wellcome).
Flexeril, Tab. (Merck).
Mephenesin (Various Mfr.).
Metubine Iodide, Vial (Lilly).
Neostig, Tab. (Freeport).
Paraflex, Tab. (McNeil).
Parafon Forte, Tab. (McNeil).
Quelicin, Fliptop & Pintop Vials, Syringe w/lancet, Amp. (Abbott).
Rela, Tab. (Schering Plough).
Robaxin, Tab., Inj. (Robins).
Skelaxin, Tab. (Carnrick).
Soma, Preps. (Wallace).
Sucostrin, Vial, Amp. (Squibb).
Syncurine, Vial (Glaxo Wellcome).
Trancopal, Cap. (Sanofi Winthrop).
d-Tubocurarine Chloride (Various Mfr.).

Skelid. (Sanofi-Winthrop) Tiludronate sodium 240 mg/lactose/Tab. Box. 56s. *Rx.*
Use: Treatment of Paget's disease.

SK&F 110679. (SK-Beecham) *Rx.*
Use: Growth hormone. [Orphan drug]

Skin Degreaser. (Health & Medical Techniques) Freon 100%. Bot. 2 oz, 4 oz. *otc.*
Use: Presurgical skin degreaser.

Skin Shield. (Del) Dyclonine HCl 0.75%, benzethonium Cl 0.2%, acetone, castor oil, SD alcohol 40 10%. Waterproof. Liq. 13.3 ml. *otc.*
Use: Liquid skin protectant.

skin test antigen, multiple.
See: Multitest CMI (Pasteur-Merieux-Connaught).

Sleep II. (Walgreen) Diphenhydramine HCl 25 mg/Tab. Bot. 16s, 32s, 72s. *otc.*
Use: Nonprescription sleep aid.

Sleep Cap. (Weeks & Leo) Diphenhydramine HCl 50 mg/Cap. Bot. 25s, 50s. *otc.*
Use: Nonprescription sleep aid.

Sleep-Eze Tablets. (Whitehall Robins) Diphenhydramine HCl 25 mg/Tab. Pkg. 12s, 26s, 52s. *otc.*
Use: Nonprescription sleep aid.

Sleep-Eze 3. (Whitehall Robins) Diphenhydramine HCl 25 mg/Tab. Pkg. 12s, 24s. *otc.*
Use: Nonprescription sleep aid.

Sleep Tabs. (Towne) Scopolamine aminoxide HBr 0.2 mg, salicylamide 250 mg/Tab. Bot. 36s, 90s. *Rx.*
Use: Sleep aid.

Sleepwell 2-Nite. (Rugby) Diphenhydramine HCl 25 mg. Tab. Bot. 72s. *otc.*
Use: Nonprescription sleep aid.

Slender. (Carnation) Skim milk, vegetable oils, caseinates, vitamins, minerals. **Liq.:** 220 cal/ 10 oz. Can. **Pow.:** 173 or 200 cal mixed w/6 oz skim or low fat milk. Pkg oz. *otc.*
Use: Nonprescription diet aid.

Slender-X. (Progressive Drugs) Phenylpropanolamine, methylcellulose, caffeine, vitamins/Tab. Pkg. 21s, 42s, 84s. Gum 20s, 60s. *otc.*
Use: Nonprescription diet aid.

Slimettes. (Halsey) Phenylpropanolamine HCl 35 mg, caffeine 140 mg/Cap. Box 20s. *otc.*
Use: Nonprescription diet aid.

Slim-Fast. (Thompson Medical) Meal replacement powder mixed with milk to replace 1, 2 or 3 meals a day. *otc.*
Use: Nonprescription diet aid.

Slim-Line. (Thompson Medical) Benzocaine, dextrose/Chewing gum. Box 24s. *otc.*
Use: Nonprescription diet aid.

Slim-Mint. (Thompson) Benzocaine 6 mg, lecithin, tartrazine. Pkg. Gum. 24s. *otc.*
Use: Nonprescription diet aid.

Slim Plan Plus Without Caffeine. (Whiteworth Towne) Phenylpropanolamine HCl 75 mg/Tab. Box 40s. *otc.*
Use: Nonprescription diet aid.

Slim-Tabs. (Wesley) Phendimetrazine tartrate 35 mg/Tab. Bot. 1000s. *c-III.*

Use: Anorexiant.

Sloan's Liniment. (Warner-Lambert Prods) Capsicum oleoresin 0.62%, methyl salicylate 2.66%, oil of camphor 3.35%, turpentine oil 46.76%, oil of pine 6.74%. Bot. 2 oz, 7 oz. *otc.*
Use: Analgesic, topical.

Slo-Bid Gyrocaps. (Rhone-Poulenc Rorer) Theophylline anhydrous 50 mg, 75 mg, 100 mg, 125 mg, 200 mg or 300 mg/TR Cap. Bot. 100s, 1000s, UD 100s. *Rx.*
Use: Bronchodilator.

Slo-Niacin. (Upsher-Smith) Niacin **250 mg/Tab.** Bot. 100s, 1000s. **500 mg/Tab.** Bot. 100s, UD 100s. **750 mg/Tab.** Bot. 100s. *otc.*
Use: Vitamin supplement.

Slo-Phyllin 80 Syrup. (Rhone-Poulenc Rorer) Theophylline anhydrous 80 mg/15 ml. Nonalcoholic. Bot. 4 oz, pt, gal, UD 15 ml. *Rx.*
Use: Bronchodilator.

Slo-Phyllin GG. (Rhone-Poulenc Rorer) Theophylline anhydrous 150 mg, guaifenesin 90 mg/Cap. or 15 ml syr. **Cap.:** Bot. 100s. **Syr.:** Bot. 480 ml. *Rx.*
Use: Bronchodilator, expectorant.

Slo-Phyllin Gyrocaps. (Rhone-Poulenc Rorer) Theophylline anhydrous 60 mg, 125 mg, 250 mg/TR Cap. Bot. 100s, 1000s, UD 100s. *Rx.*
Use: Bronchodilator.

Slo-Phyllin Tablets. (Rhone-Poulenc Rorer) Theophylline anhydrous 100 mg, 200 mg/Tab. Bot. 100s, 1000s, UD 100s. *Rx.*
Use: Bronchodilator.

Slo-Salt-K. (Mission) Potassium Cl 150 mg, sodium Cl 410 mg/Tab. Bot. 1000s. Strip 100s. *otc.*
Use: Salt substitute.

Slow Fe. (Novartis) Dried ferrous sulfate 160 mg/Tab. Bot. 30s, 100s. *otc.*
Use: Iron supplement.

Slow Fe Slow Release Iron With Folic Acid. (Novartis) Iron 50 mg, folic acid 0.4 mg/SR Tab. Bot. 20s. *otc.*
Use: Iron supplement with folic acid.

Slow-K. (Novartis) Potassium Cl. Bot. 100s, 1000s, Accu-Pak units 100s. Consumer Pack 100s. *Rx.*
Use: Potassium supplement.

Slow-Mag. (Searle) Magnesium 64 mg/DR Tab. Bot. 60s. *otc.*
Use: Magnesium supplement.

SLT. (Western Research) Sodium levothyroxine 0.1 mg, 0.2 mg or 0.3 mg /Tab. Bot. 1000s.

Use: Thyroid hormone.

SLT Lotion. (C & M Pharmacal) Salicylic acid 3%, lactic acid 5%, coal tar soln. 2%. Bot. 4.3 oz. *otc.*
Use: Antiseborrheic.

S-M-A Formula. (Wyeth-Ayerst) *otc.*
A series of liquid feeding formulas:
Iron Fortified, Infant Formula-Powder.
Iron Fortified, Infant Formula-Ready to Feed.
Iron Fortified, Infant Formula-Liquid.
Use: Nutritional therapy for infants.

Small Fry Chewable Tabs. (Approved) Vitamins A 5000 IU, D 1000 IU, B_{12} 5 mcg, B_1 3 mg, B_2 2.5 mg, B_6 1 mg, C 50 mg, niacinamide 20 mg, calcium pantothenate 1 mg, E 1 IU, l-lysine 15 mg, biotin 10 mg/Tab. Bot. 100s, 250s, 365s. *otc.*
Use: Vitamin/mineral supplement.

•**smallpox vaccine,** U.S.P. 23.
Use: Agent for immunization (active).

smallpox vaccine. (Lederle) – Tube 1s, 5s, 10s, vaccinations. 1 vaccination and needle in glass capillary tube. (Wyeth-Lederle)–Tube 100 vaccinations.
Use: Agent for immunization (active).

SN-13, 272.
See: Primaquine Phosphate, U.S.P. 23. (Various Mfr.).

snakebite antivenins.
See: Antivenin (Crotalidae) (Wyeth-Ayerst).
Antivenin (Micurus fulvius) (Wyeth-Ayerst).

snake venom.
Use: SC, IM, orally; trypanosomiasis.

Snaplets-D. (Baker Cummins) Pseudoephedrine HCl 6.25 mg, chlorpheniramine maleate 1 mg, taste free. Granules 30s. *otc.*
Use: Decongestant, antihistamine.

Snaplets-DM. (Baker Cummins) Phenylpropanolamine HCl 6.25 mg, dextromethorphan HBr 5 mg, taste free. Granules. 30s. *otc.*
Use: Antitussive, decongestant.

Snaplets-EX. (Baker Cummins) Phenylpropanolamine HCl 6.25 mg, guaifenesin 50 mg, taste free. Granules 30s. *otc.*
Use: Expectorant, decongestant.

Snaplets-FR. (Baker Cummins) Acetaminophen 80 mg. Granules Pks. 32 premeasured. *otc.*
Use: Analgesic.

Snaplets-Multi. (Baker Cummins) Phenylpropanolamine HCl 6.25 mg, chlorpheniramine maleate 1 mg, dextro-

methorphan HBr 5 mg, taste free. Granules 30s. *otc.*
Use: Antitussive, decongestant.

Snootie by Sea & Ski. (Carter Products) Padimate O. SPF 10. Lot. Bot. 30 ml. *otc.*
Use: Sunscreen.

Sno-Strips. (Akorn) Sterile tear flow test strips, 100s. *otc.*
Use: Diagnostic aid, ophthalmic. *otc.*

Soac-Lens. (Alcon) Thimerosal 0.004%, EDTA 0.1%, wetting agents. Soln. Bot. 118 ml. *otc.*
Use: Contact lens care.

Soakare. (Allergan) Benzalkonium Cl 0.01%, edetate disodium, NaOH to adjust pH, purified water. Bot. 4 fl oz. *otc.*
Use: Hard contact lens care.

•**soap, green,** U.S.P. 23.
Use: Detergent.

soaps, germicidal.
See: Dial, Preps. (Centeon).
Fostex, Cake, Cream, Liq. (Westwood Squibb).
pHisoHex, Liq. (Sanofi Winthrop).
Thylox, Shampoo, Soap (Dent).

soap substitutes.
See: Acne-Dome, Cleanser (Bayer).
Domerine, Shampoo (Bayer).
Lowila, Cleanser (Westwood Squibb).
pHisoDerm, Preps. (Sanofi Winthrop).

•**soda lime,** N.F. 18.
Use: Carbon dioxide absorbant.

Soda Mint. (Jones Medical) Sodium bicarbonate 5 gr, peppermint oil q.s./Tab. Bot. 100s, 1000s. *otc.*
Use: Antacid.

Soda Mint. (Lilly) Sodium bicarbonate 5 gr, peppermint oil q.s./Tab. Bot. 100s. *otc.*
Use: Antacid.

Sodasone. (Fellows) Prednisolone sodium phosphate 20 mg, niacinamide 25 mg/ml. Vial 10 ml. *Rx.*
Use: Corticosteroid.

•**sodium acetate,** U.S.P. 23.
Use: Pharmaceutic aid (in dialysis solutions).

sodium acetate & theophylline.

•**sodium acetate c 11 injection,** U.S.P. 23.
Use: Radioactive agent.

sodium acetosulfone. (SO-dee-uhm ah-SEE-toe-sull-FONE)
Use: Leprostatic agent.
See: Promacetin, Tab. (Parke-Davis).

sodium acid phosphate.
See: Sodium Biphosphate (Various Mfr.).

sodium actinoquinol. (SO-dee-uhm
ack-TIH-no-kwin-OLE)
Use: Treatment of flash burns (ophthalmic).
See: Uviban.

•**sodium alginate,** N.F. 18.
Use: Pharmaceutic aid (suspending
agent).

sodium aminobenzoate.
Use: Dermatomyositis and scleroderma.

sodium aminopterin. Aminopterin sodium.

sodium aminosalicylate.
See: Aminosalicylate Sodium, U.S.P.
23.

sodium amobarbital. Amobarbital Sodium, U.S.P. 23.

•**sodium amylosulfate.** (SO-dee-uhm
AM-ill-oh-sull-fate) USAN.
Use: Enzyme inhibitor.

sodium anazolene. (SO-dee-uhm an-
AZE-oh-leen)
Use: Diagnostic aid.

sodium antimony gluconate. (Pentos-
tam)
Use: Anti-infective.

•**sodium arsenate As 74.** USAN.
Use: Radioactive agent.

•**sodium ascorbate,** U.S.P. 23. Monoso-
dium L-ascorbate.
Use: Vitamin (antiscorbutic).
See: Cenolate, Inj. (Abbott).
Sodascorbate, Tab. (Mosso).
Vitac Injection, Vial (Hickman).

sodium aurothiomalate.
See: Gold Sodium Thiosulfate, U.S.P.
23.

•**sodium benzoate,** (SO-dee-uhm BEN-
zoe-ate) N.F. 18.
Use: Pharmaceutic aid (antifungal, preservative); antihyperammonemic.

**sodium benzoate and sodium phenyl-
acetate.** *Rx.*
Use: For urea cycle enzymopathies.
[Orphan drug]
See: Ucephan (McGaw).

sodium benzylpenicillin. Penicillin G
Sodium, U.S.P. 23. Sodium Penicillin G.
Rx.
Use: Anti-infective, penicillin.

•**sodium bicarbonate,** (SO-dee-uhm by-
CAR-boe-nate) U.S.P. 23.
Use: Antacid, electrolyte replenisher,
systemic alkalizer.
W/Bismuth subcarbonate and Magnesia.
See: Anachloric A, Tab. (Pharmacia &
Upjohn).
W/Sodium Bitartrate.

See: Ceo-Two, Supp. (Beutlich).
W/Sodium carboxymethylcellulose, al-
ginic acid.
See: Pretts, Tab. (Hoechst Marion
Roussel).

sodium bicarbonate. (Abbott) Inj. **4.2%:**
(5 mEq) Infant 10 ml Syringe (21 G ×
1.5 in. needle). **7.5%:** (44.6 mEq) 50
ml Syringe (18 G × 1.5 in. needle) or 50
ml Amp. **8.4%:** (10 mEq) Pediatric 10
ml Syringe (21 G × 1.5 in. needle) or
(50 mEq) 50 ml Syringe (18 G × 1.5
in. needle) or 50 ml Vial.
Use: Antacid, electrolyte replenisher,
systemic alkalizer.

sodium biphosphate.
Use: Cathartic.
See: Sodium Phosphate Monobasic,
U.S.P. 23.

**sodium biphosphate/ammonium pho-
phate sodium acid.**
See: Ammonium biphosphate, sodium
biphosphate and sodium acid pyrophosphate.

sodium bismuth tartrate.
See: Bismuth Sodium Tartrate, Preps.

sodium bisulfite. Sulfurous acid, monosodium salt. Monosodium sulfite.
Use: Antioxidant.

•**sodium borate,** N.F. 18.
Use: Pharmaceutic aid (alkalizing
agent).

sodium butabarbital.
See: Butabarbital Sodium, U.S.P. 23.

sodium calcium edetate.
See: Calcium Disodium Versenate,
Amp., Tab. (3M).

•**sodium carbonate,** N.F. 18.
Use: Pharmaceutic aid (alkalizing
agent).

sodium carboxymethylcellulose.
Carboxymethylcellulose Sodium, U.S.P.
23. CMC. Cellulose Gum.

sodium cellulose glycolate.
See: Carboxymethylcellulose, sodium
(Various Mfr.).

sodium cephalothin. (SO-dee-uhm
SEFF-ah-low-thin) Cephalothin Sodium,
U.S.P. 23.
Use: Anti-infective.

•**sodium chloride,** U.S.P. 23.
Use: Pharmaceutic aid (tonicity agent).

sodium chloride and dextrose tablets.
Use: Electrolyte and nutrient replenisher.

sodium chloride injection. U.S.P. 23.
(Abbott) Normal saline 0.9% in 150 ml,
250 ml, 500 ml, 1,000 ml cont.; **Partial-fill:** 50 ml in 200 ml, 50 ml in 300 ml,

100 ml in 300 ml; **Fliptop vial:** 10 ml, 20 ml, 50 ml, 100 ml; **Bacteriostatic vial:** 10 ml, 20 ml, 30 ml; 50 mEq, 20 ml in 50 ml fliptop or pintop vial; 100 mEq, 40 ml in 50 ml fliptop vial; 50 mEq, 20 ml univ. add. syr.; sodium Cl 0.45%, 500 ml, 1,000 ml; sodium Cl 5%, 500 ml; sodium Cl irrigating solution, 250 ml, 500 ml, 1,000 ml, 3,000 ml; (Pharmacia & Upjohn) sodium Cl 9 mg/ml w/benzyl alcohol 9.45 mg. Vial 20 ml (Sanofi Winthrop) **Carpuject:** 2 ml fill cartridge, 22 gauge 1 1/4 inch needle or 25 gauge 5/8 inch needle.
Use: Fluid and irrigation, electrolyte replenisher, isotonic vehicle.
•**sodium chloride Na 22.** USAN.
Use: Radioactive agent.
sodium chloride substitutes.
See: Salt substitutes.
sodium chloride tablets. (Parke-Davis) Sodium Cl 15 1/2 gr/Tab. Bot. 1000s.
Use: Preparation of normal saline solution.
sodium chloride therapy.
See: Thermotabs., Tab. (SK-Beecham).
sodium chlorothiazide for injection. (SO-dee-uhm KLOR-oh-thigh-AZZ-ide) Chlorothiazide Sodium For Injection, U.S.P. 23.
Use: Diuretic.
•**sodium chromate Cr 51 injection,** U.S.P. 23.
Use: Diagnostic aid (blood volume determination); radioactive agent.
See: Radio Chromate Cr 51 Sodium.
•**sodium citrate,** U.S.P. 23.
Use: Alkalizer (systemic).
See: Anticoagulant Citrate Dextrose Solution, U.S.P. 23.
Anticoagulant Citrate Phosphate Dextrose Solution, U.S.P. 23.
sodium citrate and citric acid oral solution. Shohl's Solution.
Use: Systemic alkalinizer.
sodium cloxacillin. (SO-dee-uhm CLOX-ah-SILL-in)
See: Cloxacillin Sodium, U.S.P. 23.
sodium colistimethate. Colistimethane Sodium, Sterile, U.S.P. 23. Antibiotic produced by *Aerobacillus colistinus.*
sodium colistin methanesulfonate. Colistimethane Sodium, U.S.P. 23. The sodium methanesulfonate salt of an antibiotic substance elaborated by *Aerobacillus colistinus.*
Use: Anti-infective.
•**sodium dehydroacetate,** N.F. 18.
Use: Pharmaceutic aid (antimicrobial preservative).

sodium dextrothyroxine. (SO-dee-uhm DEX-troe-thigh-ROCK-seen) Sodium D-3,3',5,5-tetraiodothyronine. Sodium D-3-(4-(4-Hydroxy-3,5-diiodophenoxy)-3,5-diiodophenyl)-alanine.
Use: Anticholesteremic.
sodium diatrizoate. Diatrizoate Sodium, U.S.P. 23.
Use: Radiopaque medium.
sodium dichloroacetate.
Use: Treatment of lactic acidosis and familial hypercholesterolemia. [Orphan drug]
sodium dicloxacillin. (SO-dee-uhm die-KLOX-ass-IH-lin) Dicloxacillin Sodium, U.S.P. 23.
Use: Anti-infective.
sodium dicloxacillin monohydrate.
Use: Anti-infective.
See: Pathocil, Prep. (Wyeth-Ayerst).
sodium dihydrogen phosphate. Sodium Biphosphate, U.S.P. 23.
sodium dimethoxyphenyl penicillin.
See: Methicillin Sodium (Various Mfr.).
sodium dioctyl sulfosuccinate.
See: Docusate Sodium, U.S.P. 23.
sodium diphenylhydantoin. Phenytoin Sodium, U.S.P. 23. Diphenylhydantoin Sodium.
Use: Anticonvulsant.
sodium edetate, (SO-dee-uhm eh-deh-TATE) Edetate Disodium, U.S.P. 23. Tetrasodium ethylenediaminetetraacetate.
Use: Chelating agent.
See: Vagisec products (Julius Schmid).
sodium ethacrynate. (SO-dee-uhm ETH-ah-krih-nate) Ethacrynate Sodium for Injection, U.S.P. 23.
Use: Diuretic.
•**sodium ethasulfate.** (SO-dee-uhm ETH-ah-SULL-fate) USAN.
Use: Detergent.
sodium ethyl-mercuri-thio-salicylate.
See: Thimerosal (Various Mfr.).
Merthiolate, Preps. (Lilly).
sodium fluorescein. Fluorescein Sodium U.S.P. 23. Resorcinolphthalein sodium.
Use: Diagnostic aid (corneal trauma indicator).
•**sodium fluoride,** U.S.P. 23. Oral Soln., Tab, U.S.P. 23.
Use: Dental caries prophylactic.
See: Fluoride, Tab. (Kirkman Sales).
Fluoride Loz. (Kirkman Sales).
Flura Drops, Drops (Kirkman Sales).
Flura-Loz, Loz. (Kirkman Sales).
Karidium, Liq., Tab. (Young Dental).

Kari-Rinse, Liq. (Young Dental).
Luride, Tab. (Colgate Oral).
Mouthkote F/R, Rinse (Parnell).
NaFeen, Tab., Liq. (Pacemaker).
Pediaflor, Drops (Ross).
T-Fluoride, Tab. (Tennessee Pharm).
W/Vitamins.
 See: Fluorac, Tab. (Rhone-Poulenc
  Rorer).
 Mulvidren-F, Tab. (Zeneca).
 So-Flo, Tab., Drops (Professional
  Pharm).
W/Vitamins A, D, C.
 See: Tri-Vi-Flor, Drops, Tab. (Bristol-
  Myers).
**sodium fluoride and phosphoric acid
gel.**
 Use: Dental caries prophylactic.
**sodium fluoride and phosphoric acid
topical solution.**
 Use: Dental caries prophylactic.
•**sodium fluoride F 18,** Injection., U.S.P.
23.
 Use: Radioactive agent.
sodium folate. Monosodium folate.
 Use: Water-soluble, hematopoietic vita-
  min.
•**sodium formaldehyde sulfoxylate,** N.F.
18.
 Use: Pharmaceutic aid (preservative).
sodium-free salt.
 See: Co-Salt, Bot. (Rhone-Poulenc
  Rorer).
 Diasal, Prep. (Savage).
sodium gamma-hydroxybutyric acid.
 Under study. *Rx.*
 Use: Anesthetic adjuvant, sleep disor-
  ders. [Orphan drug]
sodium gentisate.
 See: Gentisate Sodium.
•**sodium gluconate,** U.S.P. 23.
 Use: Replenisher (electrolyte).
sodium glucosulfone inj.
 Use: Leprostatic.
sodium glutamate.
 See: Glutamate.
sodium glycerophosphate. Glycerol
 phosphate sodium salt.
 Use: Pharmaceutic necessity.
sodium glycocholate, a bile salt.
 See: Bile Salts.
W/Phenolphthalein, cascara sagrada ex-
 tract, sodium taurocholate, aloin.
 See: Oxiphen, Tab. (PolyMedica).
W/Sodium nitrite, blue flag.
 See: So-Nitri-Nacea, Cap. (Scrip).
W/Sodium taurocholate, sodium salicy-
 late, phenolphthalein, bile extract, cas-
 cara sagrada extract.

 See: Glycols, Tab. (Jones Medical).
sodium heparin. Heparin Sodium, U.S.P.
23.
 Use: Anticoagulant.
sodium hexacyclonate.
sodium hexobarbital.
 Use: Intravenous general anesthetic.
sodium hyaluronate.
 Use: Ophthalmic.
 See: Amo Vitrax (Allergan).
 Amvisc (Chiron).
 Amvisc Plus (Chiron).
 Healon (Pharmacia & Upjohn).
W/Chondroitin sulfate.
 See: Viscoat, Soln. (Alcon).
**Sodium Hyaluronate and Fluorescein
Sodium.**
 Use: Ophthalmic surgical aid.
 See: Healon Yellow (Pharmacia & Up-
  john).
sodium hydrogen citrate. (Various Mfr.).
•**sodium hydroxide,** N.F. 18.
 Use: Pharmaceutic aid (alkalizing
  agent).
sodium hydroxydione succinate. So-
 dium 21-hydroxypregnane-3,20-dione
 succinate.
•**sodium hypochlorite solution,** U.S.P.
23.
 Use: Local anti-infective, disinfectant.
 See: Antiformin.
 Dakin's Soln.
 Hyclorite.
sodium hypophosphite. Sodium phos-
 phinate.
 Use: Pharmaceutic necessity.
sodium hyposulfite.
 See: Sodium Thiosulfate (Various Mfr.).
W/Potassium guaiacolsufonate.
 See: Guaiadol Aqueous, Vial (Medical
  Chem.).
W/Potassium guaiacolsulfonate, chlorpheniramine maleate, sodium bisulfite.
 See: Gomahist, Inj. (Burgin-Arden).
W/Sulfur, sodium citrate, phenol, benzyl
 alcohol.
 See: Sulfo-Iodide, Inj. (Marcen).
•**sodium iodide,** U.S.P. 23.
 Use: Supplement (iodine).
•**sodium iodide I 123 capsules,** U.S.P.
23.
 Use: Diagnostic aid (thyroid function de-
  termination), radioactive agent.
•**sodium iodide I 125.** USAN.
 Use: Diagnostic aid (thyroid function determination); radioactive agent.
•**sodium iodide I 131 capsules,** U.S.P.
23.
 Use: Antineoplastic; diagnostic aid (thy-

roid function determination); radioactive agent.
See: Iodotope, Cap., Soln. (Squibb).

Sodium iodide I 131 (therapeutic). (Mallinckrodt) 0.75 to 100 mCi/Cap. 3.5 to 150 mCi/Vial. *Rx.*
Use: Antithyroid agent.

sodium iodipamide. Disodium 3,3'- (Adipoyl-diimino) bis-[2,4,6- tri-iodobenzoate].
Use: Radiopaque medium.

sodium iodomethamate.

sodium iodomethane sulfonate. Methiodal Sodium, U.S.P. 23.

sodium iothalamate. Iothalmate Sodium Inj., U.S.P. 23.
Use: Radiopaque medium.

sodium iothiouracil.

sodium ipodate. (SO-dee-uhm EYE-poe-date) Ipodate Sodium, U.S.P. 23.
Use: Radiopaque.
See: Biloptin.
Oragrafin Sodium, Cap. (Squibb).

sodium isoamylethylbarbiturate.
See: Amytal Sodium, Prep. (Lilly).

•**sodium lactate injection,** U.S.P. 23.
Use: Fluid and electrolyte replenisher.

sodium lactate injection. (Abbott) 1/6 Molar, 250 ml, 500 ml, 1,000 ml; 50 mEq, 10 ml in 20 ml fliptop vial.
Use: Electrolyte replenisher.

sodium lactate solution.
Use: Replenisher (electrolyte).

•**sodium lauryl sulfate,** N.F. 18. Sulfuric acid monododecyl ester sodium salt. Sodium monododecyl sulfate.
Use: Pharmaceutic aid (surfactant).
See: Duponol.
W/Hydrocortisone.
See: Nutracort, Cream, Lot. (Galderma).

sodium levothyroxine. Levothyroxine Sodium, U.S.P. 23.

sodium liothyronine. Liothyronine Sodium, U.S.P. 23.
Use: Thyroid hormone.

sodium lyapolate. (LIE-app-OLE-ate) Polyethylene sulfonate sodium. Peson (Hoechst Marion Roussel).
Use: Anticoagulant.

sodium malonylurea.
See: Barbital Sodium (Various Mfr.).

sodium mercaptomerin. Mercaptomerin Sodium, U.S.P. 23.
Use: Diuretic.

•**sodium metabisulfite,** N.F. 18.
Use: Pharmaceutic aid (antioxidant).

sodium methiodal. Methiodal Sodium, U.S.P. 23. Sodium monoiodomethanesulfonate. Sodium Iodomethanesulfonate, Inj.
Use: Radiopaque medium.

sodium methohexital for injection. Methohexital Sodium for Injection, U.S.P. 23.
Use: General anesthetic.
See: Brevital Sod., Pow. (Lilly).

sodium methoxycellulose. Mixture of methylcellulose and sodium.

•**sodium monofluorophosphate,** U.S.P. 23.
Use: Dental caries prophylactic.

sodium morrhuate, inj. Morrhuate Sodium Inj., U.S.P. 23.
Use: Sclerosing agent.

sodium nafcillin. (SO-dee-uhm naff-SILL-in) Nafcillin Sodium, U.S.P. 23.
Use: Anti-infective.

sodium nicotinate. (Various Mfr.). W/Adenosine 5 monophosphoric acid.
Use: IV nicotinic acid therapy.

•**sodium nitrite,** U.S.P. 23.
Use: Antidote to cyanide poisoning, antioxidant.
W/Sodium thiosulfate, amyl nitrite.
Use: Vasodilator and antidote to cyanide poisoning.
See: Cyanide Antidote Pkg. (Lilly).

sodium nitrite. (Various Mfr.) Gran., Bot. 0.25 lb, 1 lb.
Use: Antidote to cyanide poisoning.

sodium nitrate combinations.
See: Veraphen, Tab. (Davis and Sly).

•**sodium nitroprusside,** U.S.P. 23.
Use: Antihypertensive.
See: Keto-Diastix (Bayer).
Nipride, Vial (Roche).
Nitropress, Vial (Abbott).

sodium nitroprusside. (Elkins-Sinn) 50 mg/Pow. for Inj. 5 ml. *Rx.*
Use: Antihypertensive.

sodium novobiocin. Sodium salt of antibacterial substance produced by *Streptomyces niveus.* Novobiocin monosodium salt.
Use: Anti-infective.
See: Albamycin, Cap., Syr., Vial (Pharmacia & Upjohn).

sodium ortho-iodohippurate. Iodohippurate Sodium, I-131 Injection, U.S.P. 23.
See: Hipputope (Squibb).

•**sodium oxybate.** (SO-dee-uhm OX-ee-bate) USAN.
Use: Adjunct to anesthesia.

sodium pantothenate.
Use: Orally, dietary supplement.

sodium para-aminobenzoate.
See: p-Aminobenzoate, Sodium (Various Mfr.).

sodium para-aminohippurate injection.
Use: IV, to determine kidney tubular excretion function.

sodium para-aminosalicylate.
See: p-Aminosalicylate, Sodium (Various Mfr.).

sodium penicillin G. Penicillin G Sodium, Sterile, U.S.P. 23. Sodium benzylpenicillin.

sodium penicillin O.

sodium pentobarbital. Pentobarbital Sodium, U.S.P. 23.
Use: Hypnotic.

•**sodium perborate monohydrate.** USAN.

sodium peroxyborate.
See: Sodium Perborate. (Various Mfr.).

sodium peroxyhydrate.
See: Sodium Perborate. (Various Mfr.).

•**sodium pertechnetate Tc 99m injection,** U.S.P. 23. Pertechnetic acid, sodium salt.
Use: Radioactive agent.
See: Minitec (Squibb).

sodium phenobarbital. Phenobarbital Sodium, U.S.P. 23.
Use: Anticonvulsant, hypnotic.

•**sodium phenylacetate.** (FEN-ill-ASS-eh-tate) USAN.
Use: Antihyperammonemic.

•**sodium phenylbutyrate.** (fen-ill-BYOOT-ih-rate) USAN.
Use: Antihyperammonemic.
See: Buphenyl (Ucyclyd Pharma).

sodium phenylethylbarbiturate. Phenobarbital Sodium, U.S.P. 23.

sodium phosphate. Disodium hydrogen phosphate. (Abbott) 3 mM P and 4 mEq sodium. 15 ml in 30 ml fliptop vial.
Use: Cathartic, buffering agent, source of phosphate.
W/Gentamicin sulfate, monosodium phosphate, sodium Cl, benzalkonium Cl.
See: Garamycin Ophthalmic, Soln. (Schering Plough).
W/Sodium biphosphate.
See: Enemeez, Enema (Centeon).
Fleet Enema (Fleet).
Phospho-Soda, Liq. (Fleet).
Saf-tip, Enemas (Fuller).

sodium phosphate, dibasic.
Use: Laxative.

•**sodium phosphate, dried,** U.S.P. 23.
Use: Cathartic.

•**sodium phosphate, monobasic,** U.S.P. 23. Monosodium Phosphate. Sodium Acid Phosphate, Sodium Dihydrogen Phosphate, Sodium Biphosphate.
Use: Cathartic.
See: Travad, Enema (Knoll Pharm).
W/Gentamicin sulfate, disodium phosphate, sodium Cl, benzalkonium Cl.
See: Garamycin Ophthalmic Soln. (Schering Plough).
W/Methenamine.
See: Uro-Phosphate, Tab. (ECR Pharm).
W/Methenamine mandelate, levo-hyoscyamine sulfate.
See: Levo-Uroquid, Tab. (Beach).
W/Methenamine, phenyl salicylate, methylene blue, hyoscyamine, alkaloid.
See: Urostat Forte, Tab. (Zeneca).
W/Sodium acid pyrophos, sodium bicarbonate.
See: Vacuetts, Supp. (Sandoz).
W/Sodium phosphate.
See: Enemeez Enema (Centeon).
Fleet Enema (Fleet).
Phospho-Soda, Liq. (Fleet).
Saf-tip Enemas (Fuller).

sodium phosphates enema.
Use: Cathartic.

sodium phosphates oral solution.
Use: Cathartic.

•**sodium phosphate P 32 solution,** U.S.P. 23. Phosphoric -32P acid, disodium salt. Disodium phosphate -32P.
Use: Antineoplastic, antipolycythemic (neoplasm), radioactive agent.

sodium phosphate P 32. (Mallinckrodt) 0.67 mCi/ml. 5 mCi/Vial. Soln. for Inj. *Rx.*
Use: Antineoplastic.

sodium phytate. (FYE-tate) Nonasodium phytate: Sodium cyclohexanehexyl (hexaphosphate).
Use: Chelating agent.

•**sodium polyphosphate.** (pahl-ee-FOSS-fate) USAN.
Use: Pharmaceutic aid.

•**sodium polystyrene sulfonate,** (pah-lee-STYE-reen SULL-fuh-nate) U.S.P. 23. Benzene, ethenyl-, homopolymer, sulfonated, sodium salt. Styrene polymer, sulfonated, sodium salt.
Use: Ion exchange resin (potassium).
See: Kayexalate, Pow. (Sanofi Winthrop).

sodium polystyrene sulfonate. (Roxane) 15 g, sorbitol 14.1 g, alcohol 0.1%/60 ml. Susp. Bot. 60 ml, 120 ml, 200 ml, 500 ml. *Rx.*
Use: Ion exchange resin (potassium).

sodium polystyrene sulfonate.
(Crookes-Barnes) 5% Soln. Eye-drops.
Lacrivial 15 ml.
Use: Ion exchange resin (potassium).
•**sodium propionate, N.F. 18.**
Use: Pharmaceutic aid (preservative).
W/Chlorophyll "a"
See: Prophyllin, Pow., Oint. (Rystan).
W/Neomycin sulfate.
See: Otobiotic, Ear Drops (Schering Plough).
W/Propionic acid, docusate sodium, salicylic acid.
See: Prosal, Liq. (Gordon).
•**sodium propionate, N.F. 18.**
Use: Pharmaceutic aid (preservative).
sodium psylliate.
Use: Sclerosing agent.
•**sodium pyrophosphate.** (SO-dee-uhm pie-row-FOSS-fate) USAN.
Use: Pharmaceutic aid.
sodium radio chromate inj. Sodium Chromate Cr 51 Inj., U.S.P. 23.
sodium radio iodide solution. Sodium Iodide I-131 Solution, U.S.P. 23.
Use: Thyroid tumors, hyperthyroidism, cardiac dysfunction.
sodium radio-phosphate, P-32. Soln. Radio-Phosphate P32 Solution. Sodium phosphate P-32 Solution, U.S.P. 23.
sodium removing resins.
See: Resins.
sodium rhodanate.
See: Sodium Thiocyanate.
sodium rhodanide.
See: Sodium Thiocyanate.
sodium saccharin. Saccharin Sodium, U.S.P. 23.
Use: Noncaloric sweetener.
•**sodium salicylate, U.S.P. 23.**
Use: Analgesic.
W/Iodide (Various Mfr.).
Use: Intravenous injection.
W/Iodide and cholchicine. (Various Mfr.).
Use: I.V., gout.
sodium salicylate, natural.
Use: Analgesic.
See: Alysine, Elix. (Hoechst Marion Roussel).
sodium salicylate combinations.
See: Apcogesic, Tab. (Apco).
Bisalate, Tab. (Allison).
Bufosal, Gran. (Table Rock).
Corilin, Liq. (Schering Plough).
Nucorsal, Tab. (Westerfield).
Pabalate, Tab. (Robins).
pHisoDan, Liq. (Sanofi Winthrop).
sodium secobarbital. Secobarbital Sodium, U.S.P. 23.

Use: Hypnotic.
sodium secobarbital and sodium amobarbital capsules.
Use: Sedative.
See: Tuinal, Cap. (Lilly).
•**sodium starch glycolate, N.F. 18.**
Use: Pharmaceutic aid (tablet excipient).
•**sodium stearate, N.F. 18.** Octadecanoic acid, sodium salt.
Use: Pharmaceutic aid (emulsifying and stiffening agent).
•**sodium stearyl fumarate, N.F. 18.**
Use: Pharmaceutic aid (tablet/capsule lubricant).
sodium stibogluconate.
Use: CDC anti-infective agent.
sodium succinate.
Use: Alkalinize urine & awaken patients following barbiturate anesthesia.
Sodium Sulamyd Ophthalmic Oint. 10% Sterile. (Schering Plough) Sulfacetamide sodium 10%. Tube 3.5 g. *Rx.*
Use: Anti-infective, ophthalmic.
Sodium Sulamyd Ophthalmic Soln. 10% Sterile. (Schering Plough) Sulfacetamide sodium 10%. Bot. 5 ml, 15 ml. *Rx.*
Use: Anti-infective, ophthalmic.
Sodium Sulamyd Ophthalmic Soln. 30% Sterile. (Schering Plough) Sulfacetamide sodium 30%. Bot. 15 ml. Box 1s. *Rx.*
Use: Anti-infective, ophthalmic.
sodium sulfabromomethazine.
Use: Anti-infective.
sodium sulfacetamide.
See: Sulfacetamide Sodium Preps. (Various Mfr.).
sodium sulfadiazine.
See: Sulfadiazine Sodium Preps. (Various Mfr.).
sodium sulfamerazine.
See: Sulfamerazine Sodium Preps. (Various Mfr.).
sodium sulfapyridine.
See: Sulfapyridine Sodium Pow. (Pfaltz & Bauer).
•**sodium sulfate, U.S.P. 23.**
Use: Regulator (calcium).
•**sodium sulfate S 35.** USAN.
Use: Radioactive agent.
sodium sulfathiazole.
Use: Anti-infective.
See: Sulfathiazole Sodium, Inj. (Various Mfr.).
sodium sulfoacetate. W/Sodium alkyl aryl polyether sulfonate, docusate sodium, kerohydric, sulfur, salicylic acid, hexachlorophene.

See: Sebulex, Liq., Cream (Westwood Squibb).

sodium sulfobromophthalein. Sulfobromophthalein Sodium, U.S.P. XXII.
Use: Diagnostic aid (hepatic function determination).

sodium sulfocyanate.
See: Sodium Thiocyanate. (Various Mfr.).

sodium sulfoxone. Sulfoxone Sodium, U.S.P. 23. Disodium sulfonyl-bis(p-phenyleneimino)dimethanesulfonate.
See: Diasone Sodium, Tab. (Abbott).

sodium suramin.
See: Suramin Sodium.

sodium taurocholate, a bile salt.
See: Bile Salts.

W/Phenolphthalein, cascara sagrada extract, sodium glycocholate, aloin.
See: Oxiphen, Tab. (PolyMedica).

sodium tetradecyl sulfate. *Rx.*
Use: Bleeding esophageal varices. [Orphan drug]
See: Sotradecol, Inj. (Elkins-Sinn).

sodium tetraiodophenolphthalein.
See: Iodophthalein Sodium (Various Mfr.).

sodium thiacetphenarsamide. (Abbott).

sodium thiamylal for injection. Thiamylal Sodium For Injection, U.S.P. 23.
Use: General anesthetic.
See: Surital, Inj. (Parke-Davis).

sodium thiocyanate. Sodium Sulfocyanate. Sodium Rhodanide.

sodium thiopental.
See: Thiopental Sodium, U.S.P. 23.

sodium thiosalicylate.
See: Rexolate, Vial (Hyrex).
Thiolate (Hickam).
Th-Sal, Vial (Foy).

•**sodium thiosulfate,** U.S.P. 23. Sodium hyposulfite. "Hypo." Thiosulfuric acid, disodium salt, pentahydrate. Disodium thiosulfate pentahydrate. *Rx.*
Use: For argyria, cyanide and iodine poisoning, arsphenamine reactions; prevention of spread of ringworm of feet; antidote to cyanide poisoning.

W/Salicylic acid, hydrocortisone acetate, alcohol.
See: Komed HC, Lot. (Pilkington Barnes Hind).

W/Salicylic acid, isopropyl alcohol.
See: Tinver, Lot. (Pilkington Barnes Hind).

W/Salicylic acid, resorcinol, alcohol.
See: Mild Komed, Lot. (Pilkington Barnes Hind).
Komed, Lot. (Pilkington Barnes Hind).

W/Sodium nitrite, amyl nitrite.
See: Cyanide Antidote Pkg. (Lilly).

sodium thiosulfate. (Various Mfr.) 250 mg/ml. KCl 4.4 mg, boric acid 2.8 mg/ Inj. 50 ml. *Rx.*
Use: Antidote.

sodium l-thyroxine.
See: Letter, Tab. (Centeon).
Levoid, Inj., Tab. (Nutrition Control).
Roxstan, Tab. (Solvay).
Synthroid, Tab., Inj. (Knoll Pharm).

sodium tolbutamide. Tolbutamide Sodium, U.S.P. 23.
Use: Diagnostic aid (diabetes).

sodium triclofos. (SO-dee-uhm TRY-kloe-foss) Sodium trichloroethylphosphate.
Use: Sedative, hypnotic.

•**sodium trimetaphosphate.** (SO-dee-uhm try-met-AH-FOSS-fate) USAN.
Use: Pharmaceutic aid.

sodium valproate.
See: Valproate sodium.

sodium vinbarbital injection.
Use: Sedative.

sodium warfarin. Warfarin Sodium, U.S.P. 23.
Use: Anticoagulant.

Sod-Late 10. (Schlicksup) Sodium salicylate 10 gr/Tab. Bot. 1000s. *otc.*
Use: Analgesic.

Sodol Compound. (Major) Carisoprodol 200 mg, aspirin 325 mg/Tab. Bot. 100s, 500s. *Rx.*
Use: Skeletal muscle relaxant.

Sofcaps. (Alton) Docusate sodium 100 mg or 250 mg/Cap. Bot. 100s, 1000s. *otc.*
Use: Laxative.

Sofenol 5. (C & M Pharmacal) Moisturizing lotion formulation. Bot. 8 oz. *otc.*
Use: Emollient.

Soflens Enzymatic Contact Lens Cleaner. (Allergan) Papain, sodium Cl, sodium carbonate, sodium borate, edetate disodium/Tab. Vial 12s, 24s, 48s, Refill 24s, 36s. *otc.*
Use: Soft contact lens care.

Sof/Pro Clean SA. (Sherman) Hypertonic solution: salt buffers, copolymers of ethylene and propylene oxide, octylphenoxypolyethoxyethanol, lauryl sulfate salt of imidazoline, sodium bisulfite 0.1%, sorbic acid 0.1%, trisodium EDTA 0.25%, thimerosal free. Bot. 30 ml. *otc.*
Use: Soft contact lens care.

Sof/Pro-Clean. (Sherman) Buffered, hypertonic solution with thimerosal

0.004%, EDTA 0.1%, ethylene and propylene oxide, octylphenoxypolyethoxyethanol, lauryl sulfate salt of imidazoline. Bot. 30 ml. *otc.*
Use: Soft contact lens care.

Soft Mate Comfort Drops for Sensitive Eyes. (Pilkington Barnes Hind) Borate buffered, potassium sorbate 0.13%, EDTA 0.1%, sodium Cl, hydroxyethylcellulose, octylphenoxyethanol. Drop. Bot. 15 ml. *otc.*
Use: Soft contact lens care.

Soft Mate Consept 1. (Pilkington Barnes Hind) Hydrogen peroxide 3% w/ polyoxyl 40 stearate, sodium stannate, sodium nitrate, phosphate buffer. 240 ml. *otc.*
Use: Soft contact lens care.

Soft Mate Consept 2. (Pilkington Barnes Hind) **Soln:** Isotonic solution of sodium thiosulfate 0.5%, borate buffers, chlorhexidine gluconate 0.001%. Bot. 360 ml. **Spray:** Isotonic sodium thiosulfate 0.5%, borate buffers. Aerosol 360 ml. *otc.*
Use: Soft contact lens care.

Soft Mate Daily Cleaning for Sensitive Eyes. (Pilkington Barnes Hind) Isotonic solution w/NaCl, octylphenoxy (oxyethylene) ethanol hydroxyethylcellulose w/potassium sorbate 0.13%, EDTA 0.2%. Soln. Bot. 1 or 30 ml. *otc.*
Use: Soft contact lens care.

Soft Mate Daily Cleaning Solution. (Pilkington Barnes Hind) Sterile aqueous isotonic solution w/sodium Cl, octylphenoxy (oxyethylene) ethanol, hydroxyethylcellulose, thimerosal 0.004%, edetate disodium 0.2%. Bot. 30 ml. *otc.*
Use: Soft contact lens care.

Soft Mate Disinfecting Solution For Sensitive Eyes. (Pilkington Barnes Hind) Sterile, aqueous, isotonic solution w/sodium Cl, povidone, octylphenoxy (oxyethylene) ethanol, chlorhexidine gluconate 0.005%, borate buffer, edetate disodium 0.1%. Thimerosal free. Bot. 240 ml. *otc.*
Use: Soft contact lens care.

Soft Mate Disinfection and Storage Solution. (Pilkington Barnes Hind) Sterile aqueous isotonic solution w/sodium Cl, povidone, octylphenoxl (oxyethylene) ethanol with a borate buffer, thimerosal 0.001%, edetate disodium 0.1%, chlorhexidine gluconate 0.005%. Bot. 8 oz. *otc.*
Use: Soft contact lens care.

Soft Mate Enzyme Plus Cleaner. (Pilkington Barnes Hind) Subtilisin, poloxamer 338, povidone, citric acid, potassium bicarbonate, sodium carbonate, sodium benzoate. Tab. Pkg. 8s. *otc.*
Use: Soft contact lens care.

Soft Mate Lens Drops. (Pilkington Barnes Hind) Sterile aqueous isotonic solution w/sodium Cl, potassium sorbate 0.13%, edetate disodium 0.025%. Thimerosal free. Bot. 2 oz. *otc.*
Use: Soft contact lens care.

Soft Mate Preservative-Free Saline Solution. (Pilkington Barnes Hind) Sterile aqueous isotonic solution w/sodium Cl, borate buffer. Contains no preservatives. Bot. 0.5 oz, 30 single use. *otc.*
Use: Soft contact lens care.

Soft Mate PS Comfort Drops. (Pilkington Barnes Hind) Sterile aqueous isotonic solution w/potassium sorbate 0.13%, edetate disodium 0.1%. Bot. 15 ml. *otc.*
Use: Contact lens care.

Soft Mate PS Daily Cleaning Solution. (Pilkington Barnes Hind) Sterile aqueous isotonic solution w/sodium Cl, octylphenoxy (oxyethylene) ethanol, hydroxyethyl cellulose, potassium sorbate 0.13%, edetate disodium 0.2%. Bot. 30 ml. *otc.*
Use: Soft contact lens care.

Soft Mate PS Saline Solution. (Pilkington Barnes Hind) Sterile aqueous isotonic solution w/sodium Cl, potassium sorbate 0.13%, edetate disodium 0.025%. Bot. 8 oz, 12 oz. *otc.*
Use: Soft contact lens care.

Soft Mate Rinsing Solution. (Pilkington Barnes Hind) Sterile aqueous isotonic solution w/sodium Cl, thimerosal 0.001%, edetate disodium 0.1%, chlorhexidine gluconate 0.005%. Bot. 8 oz. *otc.*
Use: Soft contact lens care.

Soft Mate Saline for Sensitive Eyes. (Pilkington Barnes Hind) Isotonic, sorbic acid 0.1%, EDTA 0.1%, NaCl, borate buffer. Bot. 360 (2s) or 480 ml. *otc.*
Use: Soft contact lens care.

Soft Mate Saline Preservative-Free. (Pilkington Barnes Hind) Sodium Cl w/ borate buffer. Soln. Bot. 15 ml. *otc.*
Use: Soft contact lens care.

Soft Mate Saline Solution. (Pilkington Barnes Hind) Sterile aqueous isotonic solution of sodium Cl. Preservative free. Bot. 8 oz, 12 oz. *otc.*
Use: Soft contact lens care.

Soft Mate Soft Lens Cleaners. (Pilkington Barnes Hind) Kit containing: Soft Mate daily cleaning solution II (4 oz.); soft mate weekly cleaning solution (1.2 oz.); Hydra-Mat II cleaning and storage unit. *otc.*
Use: Soft contact lens care.

Soft'n Soothe. (Ascher) Benzocaine, menthol, moisturizers. Tube 50 g. *otc.*
Use: Local anesthetic, topical.

Soft Sense. (Bausch & Lomb) Lot.: Petrolatum, vitamin E, aloe, parabens. Non-greasy. 444 ml. Body Lot.: Petrolatum, vitamin E, parabens. Non-greasy. 444 ml. *otc.*
Use: Emollient.

SoftWear. (Ciba Vision) Isotonic, sodium Cl, boric acid, sodium borate, sodium perborate (generating up to 0.006% hydrogen peroxide stabilized with phosphoric acid). Soln. Bot. 120 ml, 240 ml, 360 ml. *otc.*
Use: Soft contact lens care.

Solaneed. (Hanlon) Vitamin A 25,000 units/Cap. Bot. 100s. *Rx.*
Use: Vitamin A supplement.

Solaquin. (Zeneca) Hydroquinone 2%, ethyl dihydroxypropyl PABA 5%, dioxybenzone 3%, oxybenzone 2%. Tube oz. *otc.*
Use: Skin bleaching agent with sunscreen.

Solaquin Forte Cream. (Zeneca) Hydroquinone 4%, ethyl dihydroxypropyl PABA 5%, dioxybenzone 3%, oxybenzone 2% in a vanishing cream base. Tube 0.5 oz, 1 oz. *otc.*
Use: Skin bleaching agent with sunscreen.

Solaquin Forte Gel. (Zeneca) Hydroquinone 4%, ethyl dihydroxypropyl PABA 5%, dioxybenzone 3%, oxybenzone 2%. Tube 0.5 oz, 1 oz. *Rx.*
Use: Skin bleaching agent with sunscreen.

Solarcaine. (Schering-Plough). **Lot.:** Benzocaine, triclosan, mineral oil, alcohol, aloe extract, tocoheryl acetate, menthol, camphor, parabens, EDTA. 120 ml. **Spray (aerosol):** Benzocaine 20%, triclosan 0.13%, SD alcohol 40 35%, tocopheryl acetate. 90 or 120 ml. *otc.*
Use: Local anesthetic, topical.

Solarcaine Aloe Extra Burn Relief. (Schering-Plough) Cream: Lidocaine 0.5%, aloe, EDTA, lanolin oil, lanolin, camphor, propylparaben, eucalyptus oil, menthol, tartrazine. 120 g. Gel: Lidocaine 0.5%, aloe vera gel, glycerin,

EDTA, isopropyl alcohol, menthol, diazolidinyl urea, tartrazine. 120 or 240 g. Spray: Lidocaine 0.5%, aloe vera gel, glycerin, EDTA, diazolidinyl urea, vitamin E, parabens. 135 ml. *otc.*
Use: Topical anesthetic.

Solar Cream. (Doak) PABA, titanium dioxide, magnesium stearate in a flesh-colored, water-repellent base. Tube oz. *otc.*
Use: Sunscreen.

solargentum.
See: Mild silver protein (Various Mfr.).

Solar Shield 15 SPF. (Akorn) Ethylhexyl-p-methoxy-cinnamate 7.5%, oxybenzone in a moisturizing base 5%, PABA free, waterproof. Lot. Bot. 120 ml. *otc.*
Use: Sunscreen.

Solar Shield 30 SPF. (Akorn) Ethylhexyl-p-methoxycinnamate 7.5%, oxybenzone 6%, 2-ethylhexyl salicylate 5%, 3-diphenylacrylate 7.5%, 2-ethylhexyl-2-cyano-3 in a moisturizing base, PABA free, waterproof. Lot. Bot. 120 ml. *otc.*
Use: Sunscreen.

Solbar PF Cream 50 SPF. (Person & Covey) Oxybenzone, octyl methoxycinnamate, octocrylene, PABA free, waterproof. Cream. 120 g. *otc.*
Use: Sunscreen.

Solbar PF Liquid. (Person & Covey) Octyl methoxycinnamate 7.5%, oxybenzone 6%, SD alcohol 40 76%, PABA free. SPF 30. Liq. 120 ml. *otc.*
Use: Sunscreen.

Solbar PF 15 Cream. (Person & Covey) Octyl methoxycinnamate 7.5%, oxybenzone 5%. Bot. 1 oz, 4 oz. *otc.*
Use: Sunscreen.

Solbar PF 50. (Person & Covey) Oxybenzone, octyl methoxycinnamate, octocrylene, PABA free. Waterproof. Cream 120 ml. *otc.*
Use: Sunscreen.

Solbar PF Paba Free 15. (Person & Covey) Oxybenzone 5%, octyl methoxycinnamate 7.5%. Sunscreen SPF 15. Tube 2.5 oz. *otc.*
Use: Sunscreen.

Solbar Plus 15. (Person & Covey) Padimate 6%, oxybenzone 4%, dioxybenzone 2%. Tube 1 oz, 4 oz. *otc.*
Use: Sunscreen.

Solex A15 Clear Lotion Sunscreen. (Dermol) SPF 15. Octyl dimethyl PABA 5%, benzophenone 33%, SD alcohol. Lot. Bot. 120 ml. *otc.*
Use: Sunscreen.

Solfoton. (ECR Pharm) Phenobarbital

16 mg/Tab. or Cap. Bot. 100s, 500s. *c-iv.*
Use: Sedative, hypnotic.

Solfoton S/C Tabs. (ECR Pharm) Phenobarbital 16 mg/SC Tab. Bot. 100s. *c-iv.*
Use: Sedative, hypnotic.

Solganal. (Schering Plough) Aurothioglucose 50 mg/ml. Vial 10 ml. *Rx.*
Use: IM, gold therapy, antiarthritic.

Soliwax. Docusate Sodium, U.S.P. 23. Docusate Sodium, Solasulfone (I.N.N.).

Soltice Quick-Rub. (Chattem) Methyl salicylate, camphor, menthol, eucalyptol. Cream. Bot. 1.33 oz, 3.75 oz. *otc.*
Use: Analgesic, topical.

Solu-Barb 0.25 Tablets. (Forest Pharm) Phenobarbital 0.25 gr/Tab. Bot. 24s. *c-iv.*
Use: Sedative, hypnotic.

soluble complement receptor (recombinant human) type 1.
Use: Prevention or reduction of adult respiratory distress syndrome. [Orphan drug]

Solu-Cortef. (Pharmacia & Upjohn) **100 mg:** Hydrocortisone sodium succinate, w/benzyl alcohol. Plain vial, 5s, 25s. 100 mg/2 ml Mix-O-Vial. **250 mg:** Hydrocortisone sodium succinate, benzyl alcohol. Mix-O-Vial 2 ml, 5s, 25s. 25-Pack, 25s, 50s, etc. **500 mg:** Hydrocortisone sodium succinate, benzyl alcohol. Mix-O-Vial, 5s, 25s. **1000 mg:** Hydrocortisone sodium succinate, benzyl alcohol. Mix-O-Vial, 5s, 25s. *Rx.*
Use: Corticosteroid.

Solu-Eze. (Forest) Hydroxyquinoline 0.12%, carbitol acetate 12.10%. Bot. 3 oz. *Rx.*
Use: Skin bleaching agent.

Solu-Medrol. (Pharmacia & Upjohn) **40 mg:** Methylprednisolone sodium succinate, benzyl alcohol. Univial 1 ml. **125 mg:** Methylprednisolone sodium succinate, benzyl alcohol. Act-O-Vial 2 ml, 5s, 25s. 25-Pack, 25s, 50s etc. **500 mg:** Methylprednisolone sodium succinate, benzyl alcohol. Vial 8 ml, vials w/diluent 8 ml. **1000 mg:** Methylprednisolone sodium succinate, benzyl alcohol. Vial 16 ml, vial w/diluent 16 ml. **2000 mg:** Methylprednisolone sodium succinate powder for injection, benzyl alcohol. Vial 30.6 ml, vial w/diluent 30.6 ml. *Rx.*
Use: Corticosteroid.

Solumol. (C & M Pharmacal) Petrolatum, mineral oil, cetyl-stearyl alcohol, sodium lauryl sulfate, glycerin, propylene glycol, sorbic acid, purified water. Jar lb. *otc.*

Use: Ointment base.

Solurex. (Hyrex) Dexamethasone sodium phosphate 4 mg/ml. W/methyl and propyl parabens, sodium bisulfite. Vial 5 ml, 10 ml, 30 ml. *Rx.*
Use: Corticosteroid.

Solurex L.A. (Hyrex) Dexamethasone acetate 8 mg/ml w/polysorbate 80, carboxymethylcellulose, sodium bisulfite, EDTA, benzyl alcohol. Susp. Vial 5 ml. *Rx.*
Use: Corticosteroid.

Soluvite CT. (Pharmics) Vitamins A 2500 IU, D 400 IU, B_1 1.05 mg, B_2 1.2 mg, B_6 1.05 mg, B_{12} 4.5 mcg, C 60 mg, B_3 13.5 mg, E 15 IU, fluoride 1 mg, folic acid 0.3 mg/Tab. Bot. 100s, 1000s. *Rx.*
Use: Vitamin/mineral supplement.

Soluvite-F Drops. (Pharmics) Vitamins A 1500 IU, D 400 IU, C 35 mg, fluoride 0.25 mg/0.6 ml. Bot. 57 ml. *Rx.*
Use: Vitamin/mineral supplement.

Solvent-G. (Syosset) Alcohol 47.5%, laureth-4, isopropyl alcohol 4%, propylene glycol. Lot. Bot. 50 ml. *otc.*
Use: Lotion base.

Solvisyn-A. (Towne) Water soluble vitamin A 10,000 units, 25,000 units or 50,000 units/Cap. Bot. 100s, 1000s. *otc, Rx.*
Use: Vitamin A supplement.

• **solypertine tartrate.** (SAHL-ee-PURR-teen) USAN.
Use: Antiadrenergic.

Soma. (Wallace) Carisoprodol 350 mg/Tab. Bot. 100s, 500s, UD 500s. *Rx.*
Use: Skeletal muscle relaxant.

Soma Compound Tabs. (Wallace) Carisoprodol 200 mg, aspirin 325 mg/Tab. Bot. 100s, 500s, UD 500s. *Rx.*
Use: Skeletal muscle relaxant combination.

Soma Compound w/Codeine. (Wallace) Carisoprodol 200 mg, aspirin 325 mg, codeine phosphate 16 mg/Tab. Sodium metabisulfite. Bot. 100s. *c-iii.*
Use: Skeletal relaxant combination.

Somagard. (Roberts Pharm)
See: Deslorelin.

• **somantadine hydrochoride.** (sah-MAN-tah-deen) USAN.
Use: Antiviral.

somatostatin. *Rx.*
Use: Digestive aid. [Orphan drug]
See: Zecnil.

• **somatrem.** (so-muh-TREM) USAN.
Use: Growth hormone.
See: Protropin, Inj. (Genentech).

• **somatropin.** (SO-muh-TROE-pin) USAN.

Growth hormone derived from the anterior pituitary gland.
Use: Growth hormone. [Orphan drug]
See: Humatrope, Inj. (Lilly).
Nutropin, Inj. (Genentech).

Sominex. (SK-Beecham) Diphenhydramine HCl 25 mg/Tab. Blister pack 16s, 32s, 72s. *otc.*
Use: Nonprescription sleep aid.

Sominex Caplets. (SK-Beecham) Diphenhydramine HCl 50 mg. Tab. Blister pack 8s, 16s, 32s. *otc.*
Use: Nonprescription sleep aid.

Sominex Pain Relief Formula. (SK-Beecham) Diphenhydramine HCl 25 mg, acetaminophen 500 mg/Tab. Blister pack 16s. Bot. 32s. *otc.*
Use: Nonprescription sleep aid, analgesic.

Sonacide. (Wyeth-Ayerst) Potentiated acid glutaraldehyde. Bot. 1 gal, 5 gal. *otc.*
Use: Sterilizing & disinfecting.

Sonekap. (Eastwood) Cap. Bot. 100s.
soneryl.
See: Butethal (Various Mfr.).

Soothaderm. (Pharmakon Labs) Pyrilamine maleate 2.07 mg, benzocaine 2.08 mg, zinc oxide 41.35 mg/ml, camphor, menthol. Lot. Bot. 118 ml. *otc.*
Use: Antihistamine, local anesthetic, topical.

Soothe. (Alcon) Tetrahydrozoline 0.05%, benzalkonium Cl 0.004%, adsorbobase. Bot. 15 ml. *otc.*
Use: Decongestant, ophthalmic.

Soothe. (Walgreen) Bismuth subsalicylate 100 mg/Tsp. Bot. 9 oz. *otc.*
Use: Antidiarrheal.

soquette. (Pilkington Barnes Hind) Polyvinyl alcohol w/benzalkonium Cl 0.01%, EDTA 0.2%. Bot. 4 fl oz. *otc.*
Use: Hard contact lens care.

Sorbase Cough Syrup. (Fort David) Dextromethorphan HBr 10 mg, guaifenesin 100 mg/5 ml in sorbitol base. Bot. 4 oz, pt, gal. *otc.*
Use: Antitussive, expectorant.

•**sorbic acid,** N.F. 18.
Use: Pharmaceutic aid (antimicrobial).

Sorbide T.D. (Mayrand) Isosorbide dinitrate 40 mg/TR Cap. Bot. 100s. *Rx.*
Use: Antianginal.

Sorbidon Hydrate. (Gordon) Water-in-oil ointment. Jar 2 oz, 0.5 oz, 1 lb, 5 lb. *otc.*
Use: Emollient.

sorbimacrogol oleate 300.
See: Polysorbate 80.

•**sorbinil.** (SORE-bih-nill) USAN.
Use: Enzyme inhibitor (aldose reductase).

•**sorbitan monolaurate,** (SORE-bih-tan MAHN-oh-LORE-ate) N.F. 18. Mixture of laurate esters of sorbitol and its anhydrides.
Use: Pharmaceutic aid (surfactant).
See: Span 20 (Zeneca).

•**sorbitan monooleate,** (SORE-bih-tan MAHN-oh-OH-lee-ate) N.F. 18. Mixture of oleate esters of sorbitol and its anhydrides.
Use: Pharmaceutic aid (surfactant).
See: Span 80 (Zeneca).

sorbitan monooleate polyoxyethylene derivatives.
See: Polysorbate 80, N.F. 18.

•**sorbitan monopalmitate,** (SORE-bih-tan MAHN-oh-PAL-mih-tate) N.F. 18. Mixture of palmitate esters of sorbitol and its anhydrides.
Use: Pharmaceutic aid (surfactant).
See: Span 40 (Zeneca).

•**sorbitan monostearate,** (SORE-bih-tan MAHN-oh-STEE-ah-rate) N.F. 18. Mixture of stearate esters of sorbitol and its anhydrides.
Use: Pharmaceutic aid (surfactant).
See: Span 60 (Zeneca).

•**sorbitan sesquioleate,** (SORE-bih-tan SESS-kwih-OH-lee-ate) N.F. 18. Sorbitan mono-oleate and sorbitan dioleate.
Use: Pharmaceutic aid (surfactant).
See: Arlacel C (Zeneca).

•**sorbitan trioleate,** (SORE-bih-tan TRY-OH-lee-ate) N.F. 18.
Use: Pharmaceutic aid (surfactant).
See: Span 85 (Zeneca).

•**sorbitan tristearate.** (SORE-bih-tan TRY-STEE-ah-rate) USAN.
See: Span 65 (Zeneca).
Use: Pharmaceutic aid (surfactant).

sorbitans.
See: Polysorbate 80, U.S.P.

•**sorbitol,** N.F. 18.
Use: Diuretic, dehydrating agent, humectant, pharmaceutic aid (sweetening agent, tablet excipient flavor).
See: Sorbo (Zeneca).

W/Homatropine methylbromide.
See: Probilagol Liq. (Purdue Frederick).

W/Mannitol.
See: Sorbitol-mannitol Irrigation (Abbott).

•**sorbitol solution,** U.S.P. 23.
Use: Pharmaceutic aid (flavor, tablet excipient).

Sorbitol-Mannitol. (Abbott) Mannitol 0.54 g, sorbitol/100 ml 2.7 g. 1500 ml, 3000 ml. *Rx.*
Use: Genitourinary irrigant.

Sorbitrate. (Zeneca) Isosorbide dinitrate. **Tab.:** 5 mg Bot. 100s, 500s, UD 100s; 10 mg Bot. 100s, 500s, UD 100s; 20 mg, 30 mg Bot. 100s, UD 100s. **SA Tab.:** 40 mg Bot. 100s, UD 100s; **Sublingual Tab.:** 2.5 mg, 5 mg, 10 mg Bot. 100s. **Chew. Tab.:** 5 mg Bot. 100s, 500s; 10 mg Bot. 100s. *Rx.*
Use: Antianginal.

Sorbitrate SA. (Zeneca) Isosorbide dinitrite, oral 40 mg/SR Tab. Bot. 100s, UD 100s. *Rx.*
Use: Antianginal agent.

Sorbo. (Zeneca) Sorbitol Solution, U.S.P. 23.

Sorbsan. (Dow B. Hickam) Calcium alginate fiber 2"×2", 3"×3", 4"×4", 4"×8". 1s. Wound packing fibers-calcium alginate fiber 1/4" × 12". 1s. *Rx.*
Use: Wound dressing.

sorethytan (20) mono-oleate.
See: Polysorbate 80 (Various Mfr.).

•**sorivudine.** (so-RIV-you-deen) USAN.
Use: Antiviral.

Sosegon Solution. (Sanofi Winthrop) Pentazocine. *c-iv.*
Use: Analgesic.

Sosegon Suspension. (Sanofi Winthrop) Pentazocine. *c-iv.*
Use: Analgesic.

Sosegon Tablets. (Sanofi Winthrop) Pentazocine. *c-iv.*
Use: Analgesic.

Soss-10. (Roberts) Sodium sulfacetamide 10%. Soln. Bot. 15 ml. *Rx.*
Use: Anti-infective, ophthalmic.

•**sotalol hydrochloride.** (SOTT-uh-lahl) USAN.
Use: Beta-adrenergic blocking agent.
See: Betapace (Berlex).

•**soterenol hydrochloride.** (so-TER-en-ole) USAN.
Use: Bronchodilator.

Sotradecol. (Elkins-Sinn) Sodium tetradecyl sulfate 1% or 3%. Inj. Dosette amp. 2 ml. *Rx.*
Use: Sclerosing agent.

Soxa-Forte. (Vita Elixir) Sulfisoxazole 0.5 g, phenazopyridine 50 mg/Tab. *Rx.*
Use: Anti-infective.

Soxa Tablets. (Vita Elixir) Sulfisoxazole 0.5 g/Tab. Bot. 100s, 1000s. *Rx.*
Use: Anti-infective.

Soyalac. (Mt. Vernon Foods) Infant formula based on an extract from whole soybeans containing all essential nutrients. **Ready to Serve Liq.:** Can 32 fl oz. **Double Strength Conc.:** Can 13 fl oz. **Pow.:** Can 14 oz. *otc.*
Use: Nutritional supplement.

Soyalac-I. (Mt. Vernon Foods) Soy protein isolate infant formula containing no corn derivatives and a negligible amount of soy carbohydrates. Contains all essential nutrients in various forms. **Ready to Serve Liq.:** Can 32 fl oz. **Double Strength Conc.:** Can 13 fl oz. *otc.*
Use: Nutritional supplement.

soya lecithin. Soybean extract. 100s.
Use: Phosphorus therapy.
See: Neo-Vadrin (Scherer).

soybean lecithin.
W/Safflower oil, choline bitartrate, whole liver, inositol, methionine, natural tocopherols, vitamins B_6, B_{12}, panthenol.
See: Nutricol, Cap., Vial (Nutrition Control).

•**soybean oil,** U.S.P. 23.
Use: Pharmaceutic necessity.

Spabelin No. 1. (Arcum) Phenobarbital 15 mg, belladonna powdered extract 1/8 gr/Tab. Bot. 100s, 1000s. *Rx.*
Use: Sedative, hypnotic.

Spabelin No. 2. (Arcum) Phenobarbital 30 mg, belladonna powdered extract 1/8 gr/Tab. Bot. 100s, 1000s. *Rx.*
Use: Sedative, hypnotic.

Spabelin Elixir. (Arcum) Hyoscyamine sulfate 81 mcg, atropine sulfate 15 mcg, scopolamine HBr 5 mcg, phenobarbital 16.2 mg/5 ml. Bot. 16 oz, gal. *Rx.*
Use: Anticholinergic, antispasmodic, sedative, hypnotic.

Span 20. (Zeneca) Sorbitan Monolaurate, N.F. 18.

Span 40. (Zeneca) Sorbitan Monopalmitate, N.F. 18.

Span 60. (Zeneca) Sorbitan Monostearate, N.F. 18.

Span 65. (Zeneca) Sorbitan tristearate. Mixture of stearate esters of sorbitol and its anhydrides.
Use: Surface active agent.

Span 80. (Zeneca) Sorbitan mono-oleate, N.F. 18.

Span 85. (Zeneca) Sorbitan trioleate. Mixture of oleate esters of sorbitol and its anhydrides.
Use: Surface-active agent.

Span C. (Freeda) Citrus bioflavonoids 300 mg, rutin 50 mg, vitamin C 200 mg/Tab. Bot. 100s, 250s, 500s. *otc.*

Use: Vitamin supplement.

Span FF. (Lexis) Ferrous fumarate 325 mg/Cap. Bot. 60s, 500s. *otc.*
Use: Iron supplement.

Span PD. (Lexis) Phentermine HCl 37.5 mg/Cap. Bot. 100s. *c-iv.*
Use: Anorexiant.

Span-RD. (Lexis) d-Methamphetamine HCl 12 mg, dl-methamphetamine HCl 6 mg, butabarbital 30 mg/Tab. Bot. 100s, 1000s. *c-iii.*
Use: Amphetamine, sedative, hypnotic.

•**sparfloxacin.** (spar-FLOX-ah-sin) USAN.
Use: Antibacterial.
See: Zagam, Tab. (Rhone-Poulenc Rorer)

•**sparfosate sodium.** (spar-FOSS-ate) USAN.
Use: Antineoplastic.

Sparine. (Wyeth-Ayerst) Promazine HCl 25 mg, 50 mg or 100 mg/Tab. Bot. 50s. *Rx.*
Use: Antipsychotic.

Sparkles Effervescent Granules. (Lafayette) Sodium bicarbonate 2000 mg, citric acid 1500 mg, simethicone. Bot. UD 50s. *otc.*
Use: Antacid.

Sparkles Granules. (Lafayette) Effervescent granules 4 g/Packet or 6 g/Packet. Each 6 g produces 500 ml of carbon dioxide gas. Ctn. 25 packets. Pkg. 2 Ctn.
Use: Carbon dioxide production as an aid during air contrast stomach examinations.

Sparkles Tablets. (Lafayette) Effervescent tablets. Each 4.3 g of tablets produces 250 ml of carbon dioxide gas. Tab. Bot. 43 g (10 doses).
Use: Carbon dioxide production as an aid during air contrast stomach examination.

•**sparsomycin.** (SPAR-so-MY-sin) USAN.
Use: Antineoplastic.

•**sparteine sulfate.** (SPAR-teh-een SULL-fate) USAN.
Use: Oxytocic.
W/Sodium Cl.
See: Tocosamine sulfate, Amp. (Trent).

Spasmatol. (Pharmed) Homatropine MBr 3 mg, pentobarbital 12 mg, mephobarbital 8 mg/Tab. Bot. 100s, 1000s. *Rx.*
Use: Anticholinergic, antispasmodic, sedative, hypnotic.

Spasmolin. (Global Pharms) Phenobarbital 16.2 mg, hyoscyamine sulfate 0.1037 mg, atropine sulfate 0.0194 mg, hyoscine HBr 0.0065 mg/Tab. Bot. 1000s. *Rx.*

Use: Sedative, hypnotic, anticholinergic, antispasmodic.

spasmolytic agents.
See: Antispasmodics.

Spasno-Lix. (Freeport) Phenobarbital 16.2 mg, hyoscyamine sulfate 0.1037 mg, atropine sulfate 0.0194 mg, hyoscine HBr 0.0065 mg, alcohol 21%-23%/5 ml. Bot. 4 oz. *Rx.*
Use: Sedative, hypnotic, anticholinergic, antispasmodic.

S.P.B. Tablet. (Sheryl) Therapeutic B complex formula with ascorbic acid 300 mg/Tab. Bot. 100s. *otc.*
Use: Vitamin supplement.

SPD. (A.P.C.) Methyl salicylate, methyl nicotinate, dipropylene glycol salicylate, oleoresin capsicum, camphor, menthol. Cream Bot. 4 oz, Tube 1.5 oz. *otc.*
Use: Analgesic, topical.

spearmint, N.F. XVI.
Use: Flavor.

spearmint oil, N.F. XVI.
Use: Flavor.

Special Shampoo. (Del-Ray) Non medicated shampoo. *otc.*
Use: Cleansing shampoo.

Spectazole. (Ortho) Econazole nitrate 1% in a water miscible base. Tube 15 g, 30 g, 85 g. *Rx.*
Use: Antifungal, topical.

spectinomycin. (speck-TIN-oh-MY-sin) Formerly Actinospectocin. An antibiotic isolated from broth cultures of *Streptomyces spectabilis. Rx.*
Use: Anti-infective.
See: Trobicin, Vial, Amp. (Pharmacia & Upjohn).

•**spectinomycin hydrochloride, sterile,** (speck-TIN-oh-MY-sin) U.S.P. 23. For Susp., U.S.P. 23. An antibiotic produced by *Streptomyces spectabilis.*
Use: Antibacterial.

Spectra 360. (Parker) Salt-free electrode gel. Tube 8 oz.
Use: T.E.N.S. application, ECG pediatric, and long-term procedures.

Spectrobid Powder for Oral Suspension. (Roerig) Bacampicillin powder 125 mg/5 ml. Bot. 70 ml, 100 ml, 140 ml, 200 ml. *Rx.*
Use: Anti-infective; penicillin.

Spectrobid Tablets. (Roerig) Bacampicillin HCl 400 mg/Tab. Bot. 100s. *Rx.*
Use: Anti-infective; penicillin.

Spectro-Biotic. (A.P.C.) Bacitracin 400 units, neomycin sulfate 5 mg, polymyxin B sulfate 5000 units/g Oint. 0.5 oz, 1 oz. *otc.*

Use: Anti-infective, topical.

Spectrocin Plus. (Numark Labs.) Polymyxin B sulfate 5000 units/g or ml, neomycin 3.5 mg/g or ml, bacitracin 400 units/g or ml, lidocaine 5 mg, mineral oil, white petrolatum. Oint. Tube 15 g, 30 g. *otc.*
Use: Topical anti-infectives.

Spectro-Jel. (Recsei) Soap free. Iodomethylcellulose, carboxypolymethylene, cetyl alcohol, sorbitan mono-oleate, fumed silica, triethanolamine stearate, glycol polysiloxane, propylene glycol, glycerin, isopropyl alcohol 5%. Bot. 127.5 ml, pts, gal. *otc.*
Use: Skin cleanser.

Spec-T Sore Throat Anesthetic Lozenges. (Apothecon) Benzocaine 10 mg/Loz. Box 10s. *otc.*
Use: Local anesthetic.

Spec-T Sore Throat/Cough Suppressant Lozenges. (Apothecon) Benzocaine 10 mg, dextromethorphan HBr 10 mg w/tartrazine. *otc.*
Use: Local anesthetic, antitussive.

Spec-T Sore Throat/Decongestant Lozenges. (Apothecon) Benzocaine 10 mg, phenylephrine HCl 5 mg, phenylpropanolamine HCl 10.5 mg w/tartrazine. Loz. Pkg. 10s. *otc.*
Use: Local anesthetic, decongestant.

spermaceti.
Use: Stiffening agent; pharmaceutic necessity for cold cream.

spermine. Diaminopropyltetramethylene.

Sperti Ointment. (Whitehall Robins) Live yeast cell derivative supplying 2000 units skin respiratory factor/g w/shark liver oil 3%, phenylmercuric nitrate 1:10,000. Tube oz. *otc.*
Use: Healing ointment.

Spherulin. (ALK Laboratories) Coccidioidin: 1:100 equivalent, vial 1 ml, 1:10 equivalent, Vial 0.5 ml.
Use: Skin test.

spider-bite antivenin.
See: Antivenin, Latrodectus Mactans (Merck).

Spider-Man Children's Chewable Vitamin. (NBTY) Vitamins A 2500 IU, D 400 IU, E 15 mg, B$_1$ 1.05 mg, B$_2$ 1.2 mg, B$_3$ 13.5 mg, B$_6$ 1.05 mg, B$_{12}$ 4.5 mcg, C 60 mg, folic acid 0.3 mg/Tab., xylitol, sorbitol. Bot. 75s, 130s. *otc.*
Use: Vitamin supplement.

•**spiperone.** (spih-per-OHN) USAN.
Use: Antipsychotic.

•**spiradoline mesylate.** (spy-RAH-doe-leen) USAN.

Use: Analgesic.

•**spiramycin.** (SPIH-rah-MY-sin) USAN. Antibiotic substance from cultures of *Streptomyces ambofaciens.*
Use: Antibacterial.

•**spirapril hydrochloride.** (SPY-rah-prill) USAN.
Use: ACE inhibitor.
See: Renormax, Tab. (Sandoz).

•**spiraprilat.** (SPY-rah-PRILL-at) USAN.
Use: ACE inhibitor.

spirobarbital sodium.

•**spirogermanium hydrochloride.** (SPY-row-JER-MAY-nee-uhm) USAN.
Use: Antineoplastic.

•**spiromustine.** (SPY-row-MUSS-teen) USAN. *Formerly spirohydantoin mustard.*
Use: Antineoplastic.

spironazide. (Schein) Spironolactone 25 mg, hydrochlorothiazide 25 mg/Tab. Bot. 100s, 1000s, UD 100s. *Rx.*
Use: Diuretic combination.

•**spironolactone,** (SPEER-oh-no-LAK-tone) U.S.P. 23.
Use: Diuretic; aldosterone antagonist.
See: Aldactone, Tab. (Searle).
W/Hydrochlorothiazide.
See: Aldactazide, Tab. (Searle).

spironolactone w/hydrochlorothiazide. (Various Mfr.) Spironolactone 25 mg, hydrochlorothiazide 25 mg. Tab. Bot. 30s, 60s, 100s, 250s, 500s, 1000s, UD 32s, 100s. *Rx.*
Use: Diuretic combination.

spiropitan. (SPY-row-PLAT-in) (Janssen) Spiperone. *Rx.*
Use: Antipsychotic.

•**spiroplatin.** (SPY-row-PLAT-in) USAN.
Use: Antineoplastic.

spirotriazine hydrochloride.
Use: Anthelmintic.

•**spiroxasone.** (spy-ROX-ah-sone) USAN.
Use: Diuretic.

Spirozide. (Rugby) Spironolactone 25 mg, hydrochlorothiazide 25 mg/Tab. Bot. 100s, 500s, 1000s. *Rx.*
Use: Diuretic combination.

SPL-Serologic Types I and III. (Delmont Labs) Staphylococcus aureus 120 to 180 million units, staphylococcus bacteriophage plaque forming units 100 to 1000 million/ml. Inj. Amp. 1 ml, Vial 10 ml. *Rx.*
Use: Anti-infective.

Sporanox. (Janssen) Itraconazole 100 mg, sucrose. Cap. Sugar. Bot. 30s, UD 30s. *Rx.*
Use: Antifungal.

Sportscreme. (Thompson) Triethanolamine salicylate 10% in a nongreasy base. Cream. 37.5 g, 90 g. *otc.*
Use: Analgesic, topical.

Sports Spray Extra Strength. (Mentholatum) Methyl salicylate 35%, menthol 10%, camphor 5%, alcohol 58%, isobutane. Spray. 90 ml. *otc.*
Use: Analgesic, topical.

Spray Skin Protectant. (Morton) Isopropyl alcohol, polyvinylpyrolidone, vinyl alcohol, plasticizer & propellant. Aerosol can 6 oz. *otc.*
Use: Protective skin coating.

Spray-U-Thin. (Caprice Greystoke) Phenylpropanolamine HCl 6.58 mg, sorbitol, saccharin. Spray. Bot. 44 ml. *otc.*
Use: Nonprescription diet aid.

spreading factor.
See: Hyaluronidase (Various Mfr.).

•**sprodiamide.** (sprah-DIE-ah-mide) USAN.
Use: Diagnostic aid (paramagnetic).

SPRX-105. (Reid-Provident) Phendimetrazine tartrate 105 mg/Cap. S.R. Bot. 28s, 500s. *c-iii.*
Use: Anorexiant.

SPS. (Carolina Medical Prod. Co.) Sodium polystyrene sulfonate 15 g, sorbitol solution 21.5 ml, alcohol 0.3%/60 ml. Susp. Bot. 120 ml, 480 ml, UD 60 ml. *Rx.*
Use: Potassium-removing resin.

S-P-T. (Fleming) Pork thyroid, desiccated 1 gr, 2 gr, 3 gr, 5 gr/Cap. Bot. 100s, 1000s. *Rx.*
Use: Hypothyroidism.

•**squalane,** N.F. 18.
Use: Pharmaceutic aid (vehicle, oleaginous).

SRC Expectorant. (Edwards) Hydrocodone bitartrate 5 mg, pseudoephedrine HCl 60 mg, guaifenesin 200 mg w/alcohol 12.5%. Bot. pt. *c-iii.*
Use: Antitussive, decongestant, expectorant.

SSD AF. (Knoll Pharm) Silver sulfadiazine 1% in a cream base containing white petrolatum, stearyl alcohol, isopropyl myristate, sorbitan mono-oleate, polyoxyl 40 stearate, sodium hydroxide, propylene glycol, methylparaben 3%. Cream. 50 g, 400 g, 1000 g. *Rx.*
Use: Burn preparation.

SSD Cream. (Knoll Pharm) Silver sulfadiazine cream 1%. Jar 50 g, 85 g, 400 g, 1000 g. Tube 25 g. *Rx.*
Use: Burn preparation.

SSKI. (Upsher-Smith) Potassium iodide 300 mg/0.3 ml. Soln. Dropper Bot. 1 oz, 8 oz.
Use: Expectorant.

S-Spas. (Southern States) Pentobarbital 16.2 mg, atropine sulfate 0.0194 mg, hyoscyamine sulfate 0.1037 mg, hyoscine HBr 0.0065 mg/Tab. or 5 ml **Liq.:** Bot. pt. **Tab.:** Bot. 100s, 1000s. *Rx.*
Use: Sedative, hypnotic, anticholinergic, antispasmodic.

Stadol. (Bristol) Butorphanol tartrate 1 mg/ml; Vial 1 ml. 2 mg/ml; Vial 1 ml, 2 ml, 10 ml. *Rx.*
Use: Analgesic.

Staftabs. (Modern) Fine bone flour containing calcium, phosphorus, iron, iodine, vitamin D, magnesium/Tab. Bot. 85s, 160s. *otc.*
Use: Vitamin/mineral supplement.

Stagesic. (Huckaby) Hydrocodone bitartrate 5 mg, acetaminophen 500 mg/ Cap. Bot. 100s. *c-iii.*
Use: Narcotic analgesic combination.

Stahist. (Huckaby) Phenylpropanolamine HCl 50 mg, phenylephrine HCl 25 mg, chlorpheniramine maleate 8 mg, hyoscyamine sulfate 0.19 mg, atropine sulfate 0.04 mg, scopolamine HBr 0.01 mg/SR Tab. Bot. 100s *Rx.*
Use: Decongestant, antihistamine, anticholinergic.

stainless iodized ointment. (Day-Baldwin) Jar lb.

stainless iodized ointment with methyl salicylate 5%. (Day-Baldwin) Jar lb.

•**stallimycin hydrochloride.** (stal-IH-MY-sin) USAN.
Use: Antibacterial.

Stamoist E. (Huckaby) Pseudoephedrine HCl 120 mg, guaifenesin 500 mg. SR Tab. Bot. 100s. *Rx.*
Use: Decongestant, expectorant.

Stamoist LA. (Huckaby) Phenylpropanolamine HCl 75 mg, guaifenesin 400 mg. SR Tab. Bot. 100s. *Rx.*
Use: Decongestant, expectorant.

Stamyl Tablets. (Sanofi Winthrop) Pancreatin.
Use: Digestive aid.

•**stannous chloride.** (STAN-uhs KLOR-ide) USAN.
Use: Pharmaceutic aid.

•**stannous fluoride,** (STAN-uhs) U.S.P. 23.
Use: Dental caries prophylactic.

•**stannous pyrophosphate.** (STAN-uhs PIE-row-FOSS-fate) USAN.
Use: Diagnostic aid (skeletal imaging).

•**stannous sulfur colloid.** (STAN-uhs SULL-fer KAHL-oyd) USAN.
Use: Diagnostic aid (bone, liver, and spleen imaging).

•**stanozolol,** (STAN-oh-zole-ahl) U.S.P. 23. *Formerly Androstanazole.*
Use: Androgen.
See: Stromba.
Winstrol Tab. (Sanofi Winthrop).

staphage lysate (SPL). (Delmont) Phage-lysed staphylococci 120-180 million/ml Amp. 1 ml, package 10s for Inj.; multidose Vial 10 ml for other methods of administration. *Rx.*
Use: Anti-infective.

Staphcillin. (Bristol) Methicillin sodium w/ 3 mEq sodium/Gm, 1 g/Vial. Vial 1 g, 4 g, 6 g; Piggyback Vial. 1 g, 4 g. *Rx.*
Use: Anti-infective; penicillin.

staphylococcus bacteriophage lysate.
See: Staphage Lysate (Delmont).

staphylococcus test.
See: Isocult for Staphylococcus Aureus (Smith Kline Diagnostics).

•**starch,** N.F. 18.
Use: Dusting powder; pharmaceutic aid.

starch glycerite.
Use: Emollient.

•**starch, pregelatinized,** N.F. 18.
Use: Pharmaceutic aid (tablet excipient).

•**starch, topical,** U.S.P. 23.
Use: Dusting powder.

Star-Otic. (Star) Burrows soln. 10%, acetic acid 1%, boric acid 1%. Drop bot. 15 ml. *otc.*
Use: Otic preparation.

Staticin. (Westwood Squibb) Erythromycin 1.5%, alcohol 55%. Soln. Bot. 60 ml. *Rx.*
Use: Anti-acne.

•**statolon.** (STAY-toe-lone) USAN. Antiviral agent derived from *Penicillium stoloniferum.*
Use: Antiviral.

Statomin Maleate II. (Jones Medical) Chlorpheniramine maleate 2 mg, acetaminophen 324 mg, caffeine 32 mg/Tab. Bot. 1000s. *Rx.*
Use: Antihistamine, analgesic.

Statuss Expectorant. (Huckaby) Phenylpropanolamine HCl 12.5 mg, codeine phosphate 10 mg, guaifenesin 100 mg, alcohol 5%, menthol, saccharin, sorbitol/5 ml. Dye free. Liq. Bot. 473 ml. *c-v.*
Use: Decongestant, antitussive, expectorant.

Statuss Green. (Huckaby) Phenylpropanolamine HCl 3.3 mg, phenylephrine HCl 5 mg, pheniramine maleate 3.3 mg, pyrilamine maleate 3.3 mg, hydrocodone bitartrate 1.67 mg/5 ml, alcohol 5%, saccharin, parabens, sorbitol, glucose. Liq. Bot. 480 ml. *c-iii.*
Use: Decongestant, antihistamine, antitussive.

•**stavudine.** (STAHV-you-deen) USAN.
Use: Antiviral.
See: Zerit, Cap. (Bristol-Myers Squibb).

Sta-Wake Dextabs. (Approved) Caffeine 1.5 gr, dextrose 3 gr/Tab. Bot. 36s, 1000s. *otc.*
Use: CNS stimulant.

Stay Awake Capsules. (Whiteworth Towne) Caffeine 250 mg/Cap. Bot. 30s. *otc.*
Use: CNS Stimulant.

Stay-Brite. (Sherman) EDTA 0.25%, benzalkonium Cl 0.01%. Spray 30 ml. *otc.*
Use: Hard contact lens care.

Stay Moist Lip Conditioner. Padimate O, oxybenzone, aloe vera, vitamin E, tropical fruit flavor. SPF 15. Lip Balm: 48 g. *otc.*
Use: Emollient.

Stay Trim. (Schering-Plough) Phenylpropanolamine. **Gum:** 8.33 mg. Pkg. 20s. **Mints:** 12.5 mg. Pkg. 36s. *otc.*
Use: Nonprescription diet aid.

Stay-Wet. (Sherman) Polyvinyl alcohol, hydroxyethylcellulose, povidone, sodium Cl, potassium Cl, sodium carbonate, benzalkonium Cl 0.01%, EDTA 0.025%. Soln. Bot. 30 ml. *otc.*
Use: Hard contact lens care.

Stay-Wet 3. (Sherman) Sodium and potassium Cl salts containing polyvinyl pyrrolidone, polyvinyl alcohol, hydroxyethylcellulose, sodium bisulfite 0.02%, benzyl alcohol 0.1%, sorbic acid 0.05%, EDTA 0.1%. Soln. 30 ml. *otc.*
Use: Ophthalmic lubricant.

Stay Wet 4. (Sherman) Benzyl alcohol 0.15%, EDTA 0.1%, NaCl, KCl, polyvinyl alcohol, hydroxyethyl cellulose. Thimerosol free. Soln. 30 ml. *otc.*
Use: Disinfecting/wetting/soaking (RGP lenses).

Stay-Wet Rewetting. (Sherman) Polyvinyl alcohol, hydroxyethylcellulose, povidone, NaCl, KCL, sodium carbonate, benzalkonium Cl 0.01%, EDTA 0.025%. *otc.*
Use: Ophthalmic lubricant.

Stay-Wet 3 Wetting. (Sherman) Polyvinyl alcohol, hydroxyethylcellulose, povidone, sodium Cl, potassium Cl, so-

dium carbonate, benzalkonium Cl 0.01%, EDTA 0.025%. Soln. 30 ml. *otc.*
Use: Ophthalmic lubricant.

Staze. (Del Pharm) Karaya gum. Tube 1.75 oz, 3.5 oz. *otc.*
Use: Denture adhesive.

S-T Cort Cream. (Scot-Tussin) Hydrocortisone 0.5%, water-washable base, parabens. 120 g. *Rx.*
Use: Corticosteroid, topical.

S-T Cort lotion. (Scot-Tussin) Hydrocortisone 0.5%, water-washable, lanolin alcohol, mineral oil base. 60 ml, 120 ml. *Rx.*
Use: Corticosteroid, topical.

steapsin.
W/Oxidized bile acids, ox bile, homatropine methylbromide.
See: Oxacholin, Tab. (Philips Roxane).

•**stearic acid,** N.F. 18. Octadecanoic acid.
Use: Pharmaceutic aid (emulsion adjunct, tablet/capsule lubricant).

•**stearyl alcohol,** (STEE-rill AL-koe-hahl) N.F. 18.
Use: Pharmaceutic aid (emulsion adjunct).

•**steffimycin.** (steh-fih-MY-sin) USAN.
Use: Antibacterial, antiviral.

Stelazine. (SK-Beecham) Trifluoperazine HCl. **Tab.:** 1 mg, 2 mg, 5 mg, 10 mg. Bot. 100s, 1000s, UD 100s. **Vial:** 10 ml (2 mg/ml) Box 1s, 20s. **Oral Conc.:** (10 mg/ml) Bot. 2 fl oz. Ctn. 12s. *Rx.*
Use: Antipsychotic.

•**stenbolone acetate.** (STEEN-bow-lone) USAN.
Use: Anabolic.

Step 2. (GenDerm) Benzyl alcohol, cetyl alcohol, formic acid 8%, glyceryl stearate, PEG-100 stearate, polyquaternium-10. Creme rinse. 60 ml. *otc.*
Use: Nit removal system.

Steraject. (Mayrand) Prednisolone acetate 25 mg or 50 mg/ml. Vial 10 ml. *Rx.*
Use: Corticosteroid.

Sterapred DS. (Mayrand) Prednisone 10 mg/Tab. Uni-pak 21s. *Rx.*
Use: Corticosteroid.

Sterapred-Unipak. (Mayrand) Prednisone 5 mg/Tab. Dosepak 21 tab. *Rx.*
Use: Corticosteroid.

Sterculia Gum.
See: Karaya Gum (Various Mfr.).
W/Vitamin B₁.
See: Imbicoll W/Vitamin B₁ (Pharmacia & Upjohn).

Stericol. (Alton) Isopropyl alcohol 91%. Bot. 16 oz, 32 oz, gal. *otc.*
Use: Anti-infective, topical.

sterile aurothioglucose suspension.
Authothioglucose Injection. Gold thioglucose.
Use: Antirheumatic.
See: Solganal, Vial (Schering Plough).

sterile erythromycin gluceptate.
Erythromycin monoglucoheptonate (salt). Erythromycin glucoheptonate (1:1) (salt).
Use: Anti-infective.

Sterile Lens Lubricant. (Blairex) Isotonic w/borate buffer system, sodium Cl, hydroxypropyl methylcellulose, glycerin, sorbic acid 0.25%, EDTA 0.1%, thimerosol free. Soln. 15 ml. *otc.*
Use: Ophthalmic lubricant.

Sterile Saline. (Bausch & Lomb) Sodium Cl, borate buffer, EDTA, thimerosal free. Soln. 60 ml. *otc.*
Use: Ophthalmic lubricant.

sterile thiopental sodium. Thiopental sodium, U.S.P. 23.
See: Pentothal Sodium, Amp. (Abbott).

sterile water for irrigation. (Various Mfr.) 0.45% or 0.9%. Soln. Bot. 150 ml, 250 ml, 500 ml, 1000 ml, 1500 ml, 2000 ml, 4000 ml. *Rx.*
Use: Genitourinary irrigant.

Sterinail. (Dr. Nordyke's Labs) Undecylenic acid, tolnaftate, propylene glycol, acetone, acetic acid, propionic acid, benzyl alcohol, eucalyptol and benzyl acetate, *Steri-Scrub* (mineral oil, glyceryl stearate, propylene glycol, lanolin alcohol, calcium carbonate, propylene glycol monostearate, triethanolamine, sodium hypochlorite, parabens, DMDM hydantoin, diazolidinyl urea). *Steri-Brush* included. *otc.*
Use: Antifungal.

Steri-Unna Boot. (Pedinol) Glycerin, gum acacia, zinc oxide, white petrolatum, amylum in an oil base. 10 yds. × 3.5 in. sterilized bandage.
Use: Treatment of leg ulcers, varicosities, sprains, strains & to reduce swelling after surgery.

S-T Forte 2 Liquid. (Scot-Tussin) Chlorpheniramine maleate 2 mg, hydrocodone bitartrate 2.5 mg, 99.7% glycerin, menthol, parabens. Alcohol and dye free. Bot. Pt. or gal. *c-III.*
Use: Antihistamine, antitussive.

S-T Forte Sugar Free Liquid. (Scot-Tussin) Hydrocodone bitartrate 2.5 mg, phenylephrine HCl 5 mg, phenylpropanolamine HCl 5 mg, pheniramine maleate 13.33 mg, guaifenesin 80 mg/5 ml w/alcohol 5%. Bot. 4 oz, 8 oz, pt, gal. *c-III.*

Use: Antitussive, decongestant, antihistamine, expectorant.

S-T Forte Syrup. (Scot-Tussin) Hydrocodone bitartrate 2.5 mg, phenylephrine HCl 5 mg, phenylpropanolamine HCl 5 mg, pheniramine maleate 13.33 mg, guaifenesin 80 mg/5 ml, w/alcohol 5%. Bot. 4 oz, 8 oz, pt. gal. *c-III.*
Use: Antitussive, decongestant, antihistamine, expectorant.

stilbamidine isethionate. 2-Hydroxyethane-sulfonic acid compound with 4, 4'-stilbenedicarboxamidine.
Use: Antiprotozoal.

• **stilbazium iodide.** (still-BAY-zee-uhm EYE-oh-dide) USAN.
Use: Anthelmintic.

stilbestrol.
See: Diethylstilbestrol, U.S.P. 23. (Various Mfr.).

stilbestronate.
See: Diethylstilbestrol Dipropionate (Various Mfr.).

stilboestrol.
See: Diethylstilbestrol (Various Mfr.).

Stilboestrol DP.
See: Diethylstilbestrol Dipropionate (Various Mfr.).

stillman's. (Stillman) Cream Jar. 7/8 oz, oz, Cream Bella Aurora oz.

• **stilonium iodide.** (STILL-oh-nee-uhm EYE-oh-dide) USAN.
Use: Antispasmodic.

Stilphostrol. (Bayer) Diethylstilbestrol diphosphate. Amp. (250 mg/5 ml as sodium salt) 5 ml. Box 20s. Tab. 50 mg, Bot. 50s. *Rx.*
Use: Antineoplastic.

Stilronate.
See: Diethylstilbestrol Dipropionate (Various Mfr.).

Stimate. (centeon) Desmopressin acetate 1.5 mg, chlorobutanol 5 mg, sodium Cl 9 mg/ml. Nasal spray. Vial 2.5 ml. *Rx.*
Use: Posterior pituitary hormone.

Sting-Eze. (Wisconsin) Diphenhydramine HCl, camphor, phenol, benzocaine, eucalyptol. Bot. 15 ml. *otc.*
Use: Antihistamine, topical.

Sting-Kill. (MiLance) Benzocaine 18.9%, menthol 0.9%. Swab 14 ml, 0.5 ml (5s). *otc.*
Use: Local anesthetic, topical.

• **stiripentol.** (STY-rih-PEN-tole) USAN.
Use: Anticonvulsant.

St. Joseph Adult Chewable Aspirin. (Schering-Plough) Aspirin 81 mg, saccharin. Chew. Tab. Bot. 36s.

Use: Salicylate analgesic.

St. Joseph Aspirin for Adults. (Schering-Plough) Aspirin 5 gr/Tab. Bot. 36s, 100s, 200s. *otc.*
Use: Salicylate analgesic.

St. Joseph Aspirin-Free Cold for Children. (Schering-Plough) Phenylpropanolamine HCl 3.125 mg, acetaminophen 80 mg, fruit flavor. Chew. Tab. Bot. 30s. *otc.*
Use: Pediatric decongestant combination.

St. Joseph Aspirin-Free Elixir for Children. (Schering-Plough) Acetaminophen 160 mg/5 ml. Alcohol Free. Bot. 2 oz, 4 oz. *otc.*
Use: Analgesic.

St. Joseph Aspirin-Free for Children Chewable. (Schering-Plough) Acetaminophen 80 mg, fruit flavor. Tab. Bot. 30s. *otc.*
Use: Analgesic.

St. Joseph Aspirin-Free Infant Drops. (Schering-Plough) Acetaminophen 100 mg/ml/0.8 ml dropper. Aspirin and sugar free. Bot. 0.5 oz. *otc.*
Use: Analgesic.

St. Joseph Aspirin-Free Tablets for Children. (Schering-Plough) Acetaminophen 80 mg/Tab. Bot. 30s. *otc.*
Use: Analgesic.

St. Joseph Cold Tablets for Children. (Schering-Plough) Aspirin 80 mg, phenylpropanolamine HCl 3.125 mg/Tab. Bot. 30s. *otc.*
Use: Analgesic, decongestant.

St. Joseph Cough Suppressant. (Schering-Plough) Dextromethorphan HBr 7.5 mg/5 ml, alcohol free, sucrose, cherry flavor. Liq. Bot. 60 ml, 120 ml. *otc.*
Use: Antitussive.

St. Joseph Cough Syrup for Children. (Schering-Plough) Dextromethorphan HBr 7.5 mg/5 ml. Bot. 2 oz, 4 oz. *otc.*
Use: Antitussive.

Stomal. (Foy) Phenobarbital 16.2 mg, hyoscyamine sulfate 0.1037 mg, atropine sulfate 0.0194 mg, scopolamine HBr 0.0065 mg/Tab. Bot. 1000s. *Rx.*
Use: Sedative, hypnotic, anticholinergic, antispasmodic.

ST1-RTA immunotoxin (SR44163). *Rx.*
Use: Leukemia, graft-v-host disease in bone marrow transplants. [Orphan drug]

Stool Softener. (Amlab) Docusate sodium 100 mg, 250 mg/Cap. Bot. 100s. *otc.*

Use: Laxative.

Stool Softener. (Weeks & Leo) Docusate sodium 100 mg, 250 mg/Cap. Bot. 30s, 100s. Calcium docusate 240 mg/Cap. Bot. 100s. *otc.*
Use: Laxative.

Stop. (Oral-B) Stannous fluoride 0.4%. Tube 2 oz. *Rx.*
Use: Dental caries preventative.

Stopayne Capsules. (Springbok) Co- · deine phosphate 30 mg, acetaminophen 357 mg/Cap. Bot. 100s, 500s, UD 100s. *c-III.*
Use: Antitussive, analgesic.

Stopayne Syrup. (Springbok) Acetaminophen 120 mg, codeine phosphate 12 mg/5 ml. Bot. 4 oz, 16 oz. *c-v.*
Use: Analgesic, antitussive.

Stop-Zit. (Purepac) Denatonium benzoate in a clear nail polish base. Bot. 0.75 oz. *otc.*
Use: Thumbsucking-nail biting deterrent.

•**storax,** U.S.P. 23.
Use: Pharmaceutic necessity for Benzoin Tincture compound.

Stovarsol.
Use: Trichomonas vaginalis vaginitis, amebiasis, Vincent's angina.
See: Acetarsone, Tab.

Strema. (Foy) Quinine sulfate 260 mg/Cap. Bot. 100s, 500s, 1000s.
Use: Antimalarial.

Stren-Tab. (Barth's) Vitamins C 300 mg, B_1 10 mg, B_2 10 mg, niacin 33 mg, B_6 2 mg, pantothenic acid 20 mg, B_{12} 4 mcg/Tab. Bot. 100s, 300s, 500s. *otc.*
Use: Vitamin supplement.

Streptase. (Astra) Streptokinase IV infusion. Ctn. Vial 10s. 250,000 IU/Vial 6.5 ml; 750,000 IU/Vial 6.5 ml. *Rx.*
Use: Thrombolytic enzyme.

streptococcus immune globulin group B. *Rx.*
Use: Immunization in neonates. [Orphan drug]

streptokinase.
Use: Thrombolytic enzyme.
See: Kabikinase (SKF).
Streptase (Hoechst-Roussell).

Streptolysin O Test. (Laboratory Diagnostics) Reagent 6 × 10 ml, buffer 6 × 40 ml, Control Serum, 6 × 10 ml or Kit.
Use: Diagnosis of "Group A" Streptococcal infections.

streptomycin calcium chloride. Streptomycin Calcium Chloride Complex.

streptomycin isoniazid.

See: Streptohydrazid.

•**streptomycin sulfate injection,** U.S.P. 23.
Use: Antibacterial (antituberculostatic). W/Dihydrostreptomycin sulfate.
See: Streptoduocin, Inj. (Various Mfr.).

streptomycylidene isonicotinyl hydrazine sulfate.
See: Streptohydrazid.

Streptonase B. (Wampole) Tube test for determination of streptococcal infection by serum DNase-B antibodies. Kit 1.
Use: In vitro diagnostic aid.

•**streptonicozid.** (STREP-toe-nih-KOE-zid) USAN. Streptomycylidene isonicotinyl hydrazine sulfate.
Use: Antibacterial.
See: Streptohydrazid.

•**streptonigrin.** (strep-toe-NYE-grin) USAN. Antibiotic isolated from both filtrates of *Streptomyces flocculus.*
Use: Antineoplastic.
See: Nigrin (Pfizer).

streptovaricin. An antibiotic composed of several related components derived from cultures of *Streptomyces variabilis.* Dalacin (Pharmacia & Upjohn).

•**streptozocin.** (STREP-toe-ZOE-sin) USAN.
Use: Antineoplastic.
See: Zanosar, Powder (Pharmacia & Upjohn).

Streptozyme. (Wampole) Rapid hemagglutination slide test for the qualitative detection and quantitative determination of streptococcal extracellular antigens in serum, plasma and peripheral blood. Kit 15s, 50s, 150s.
Use: An aid in the diagnosis of *Streptococcal A* sequelae.

Stress "1000". (NBTY) Vitamins E 22 mg, B_1 15 mg, B_2 15 mg, B_3 100 mg, B_5 20 mg, B_6 5 mg, B_{12} 12 mcg, C 1000 mg/Tab. Bot. 60s. *otc.*
Use: Vitamin supplement.

Stress B-Complex. (Moore) Vitamins E 30 IU, B_1 15 mg, B_2 15 mg, B_3 100 mg, B_5 20 mg, B_6 20 mg, B_{12} 12 mcg, C 500 mg, folic acid 0.4 mg, Zn 23.9 mg, Cu, biotin 45 mcg/Tab. Bot. 60s. *otc.*
Use: Vitamin/mineral supplement.

Stress B Complex with Vitamin C. (Mission) Vitamins B_1 13.8 mg, B_2 10 mg, B_3 50 mg, B_6 4.1 mg, C 300 mg, Zn 15 mg/Tab. Bot. 60s. *otc.*
Use: Vitamin/mineral supplement.

Stress-Bee Capsules. (Rugby) Vitamins B_1 10 mg, B_2 10 mg, B_3 100 mg, B_5 20 mg, B_6 2 mg, B_{12} 6 mcg, C 300 mg/

Cap. Bot. 100s. *otc.*
Use: Vitamin supplement.
Stressform "605" With Iron. (NBTY)
Iron 27 mg, vitamins E 30 mg, B_1 15
mg, B_2 15 mg, B_3 100 mg, B_5 20 mg, B_6
5 mg, B_{12} 12 mcg, C 605 mg, folic acid
0.4 mg, biotin 45 mg/Tab. Bot. 60s.
otc.
Use: Vitamin supplement.
Stress Formula. (Various Mfr.) Vitamins
E 30 mg, B_1 15 mg, B_2 15 mg, B_3 100
mg, B_5 20 mg, B_6 5 mg, B_{12} 12 mcg,
C 600 mg, folic acid 0.4 mg, biotin 45
mcg/Cap., Tab. **Cap.:** Bot. 60s, 100s,
1000s. **Tab.:** Bot. 30s, 60s, 100s, 250s,
300s, 400s, 1000s, UD 100s. *otc.*
Use: Vitamin supplement.
Stress Formula 600. (Vanguard). Vitamins E 30 IU, B_1 15 mg, B_2 10 mg, B_3
100 mg, B_5 20 mg, B_6 5 mg, B_{12} 12
mcg, C 500 mg, folic acid 0.4 mg, biotin 45 mcg/Tab. Bot. UD 100s. *otc.*
Use: Vitamin supplement.
Stress Formula 600 w/Iron. (Halsey).
Use: Vitamin supplement.
Stress Formula 600 Plus Iron. (Schein)
Iron 27 mg, vitamins E 30 IU, B_1 15 mg,
B_2 15 mg, B_3 100 mg, B_5 20 mg, B_6 5
mg, B_{12} 12 mcg, C 600 mg, folic acid
0.4 mg, biotin 45 mcg/Tab. Bot. 60s,
250s. *otc.*
Use: Vitamin/mineral supplement.
Stress Formula 600 Plus Zinc. (Schein)
Vitamins E 30 mg, B_1 20 mg, B_2 10 mg,
B_3 100 mg, B_5 25 mg, B_6 5 mg, B_{12} 12
mcg, C 600 mg, folic acid 0.4 mg, zinc
23.9 mg, Cu, Mg, biotin 45 mcg/Tab.
Bot. 60s, 250s. *otc.*
Use: Vitamin/mineral supplement.
Stress Formula 600 w/Zinc. (Halsey).
Use: Dietary supplement.
Stress Formula "605". (NBTY) Vitamins
E 30 mg, B_1 15 mg, B_2 15 mg, B_3 100
mg, B_5 20 mg, B_6 5 mg, B_{12} 12 mcg,
C 605 mg, folic acid 0.4 mg, biotin 45
mg/Tab. Bot. 60s. *otc.*
Use: Vitamin supplement.
Stress Formula "605" with Zinc.
(NBTY) Vitamins E 30 mg, B_1 20 mg,
B_2 10 mg, B_3 100 mg, B_5 25 mg, B_6 5
mg, B_{12} 12 mcg, C 605 mg, folic acid
0.4 mg, zinc 23.9 mg, copper, biotin 45
mcg/Tab. Bot. 60s. *otc.*
Use: Vitamin/mineral supplement.
Stress Formula Vitamins. (Various Mfr.)
Vitamins E 30 mg, B_1 10 mg, B_2 10 mg,
B_3 100 mg, B_5 20 mg, B_6 5 mg, B_{12} 12
mcg, C 500 mg, folic acid 0.4 mg, biotin 45 mcg. Cap. Bot. 100s/Tab. Bot.
60s. *otc.*

Use: Vitamin supplement.
Stress Formula with Iron. (NBTY) Vitamins C 500 mg, B_1 10 mg, B_2 10 mg,
B_3 100 mg, B_5 20 mg, B_6 5 mg, B_{12} 12
mcg, E 30 IU, iron 27 mg, folic acid
0.4 mg, biotin 45 mcg. Tab. Bot. 60s.
otc.
Use: Vitamin/mineral supplement.
Stress Formula w/Zinc. (Various Mfr.)
Vitamins E 30 IU, B_1 10 mg, B_2 10
mg, B_3 100 mg, B_5 20 mg, B_6 5 mg, B_{12}
12 mcg, C 500 mg, folic acid 0.4 mg,
biotin 45 mcg, zinc 23.9 mg, Cu/Tab.
Bot. 60s. *otc.*
Use: Vitamin/mineral supplement.
Stress Formula with Zinc. (Towne) Vitamins E 45 IU, C 600 mg, folic acid 400
mcg, B_1 20 mg, B_2 10 mg, niacinamide
100 mg, B_6 10 mg, B_{12} 25 mcg, biotin
40 mcg, pantothenic acid 25 mg, copper
3 mg, zinc 23.9 mg/Tab. Bot. 60s. *otc.*
Use: Vitamin/mineral supplement.
Stress 600 w/Zinc. (Nion) Vitamins E 45
IU, B_1 20 mg, B_2 10 mg, B_3 100 mg,
B_5 25 mg, B_6 10 mg, B_{12} 25 mcg, C 600
mg, folic acid 0.4 mg, Zn 5.5 mg, Cu,
biotin 45 mcg/Tab. Bot. 60s. *otc.*
Use: Vitamin/mineral supplement.
Stresstabs. (Lederle) Vitamins E 30 mg,
B_1 10 mg, B_2 10 mg, B_3 100 mg, B_5 20
mg, B_6 5 mg, B_{12} 12 mcg, C 500 mg,
folic acid 0.4 mg, biotin 45 mcg/Tab.
Bot. 60s. *otc.*
Use: Vitamin supplement.
Stresstabs + Iron. (Lederle) Iron 18 mg,
E 30 IU, B_1 10 mg, B_2 10 mg, B_3 100
mg, B_5 20 mg, B_6 5 mg, B_{12} 12 mcg, C
500 mg, folic acid 0.4 mg, biotin 45
mcg/Tab. Bot. 60s. *otc.*
Use: Vitamin/mineral supplement.
Stresstabs + Zinc. (Lederle) Vitamins E
30 mg, B_1 10 mg, B_2 10 mg, B_3 100
mg, B_5 20 mg, B_6 5 mg, B_{12} 12 mcg, C
500 mg, folic acid 0.4 mg, zinc 23.9
mg, copper, biotin 45 mcg/Tab. Bot. 60s.
otc.
Use: Vitamin/mineral supplement.
Stresstabs 600. (Lederle) Vitamins B_1
15 mg, B_2 10 mg, B_6 5 mg, B_{12} 12
mcg, C 600 mg, niacinamide 100 mg,
vitamin E 30 IU, biotin 45 mcg, folic acid
400 mcg, calcium pantothenate 20 mg/
Tab. Bot. 30s, 60s. UD 10 × 10s. *otc.*
Use: Vitamin supplement.
Stresstabs 600 with Iron Tablets. (Lederle) Ferrous fumarate 27 mg, vitamins
E 30 IU, B_1 15 mg, B_2 15 mg, B_3 100
mg, B_5 20 mg, B_6 5 mg, B_{12} 12 mcg, C
600 mg, folic acid 0.4 mg, biotin 45
mcg/Tab. Bot. 30s, 60s. *otc.*

Use: Vitamin/mineral supplement.

Stresstabs 600 with Zinc. (Lederle) Vitamins B_1 15 mg, B_2 10 mg, B_3 100 mg, B_5 20 mg, B_6 5 mg, B_{12} 12 mcg, C 600 mg, E 30 IU, folic acid 0.4 mg, biotin 45 mcg, Cu, zinc 23.9 mg/Tab. Bot. 30s, 60s. *otc.*
Use: Vitamin/mineral supplement.

Stresstein. (Sandoz Nutrition) Maltodextrin, medium chain triglycerides, l-leucine, soybean oil, l-isoleucine, l-valine, l-glutamic acid, l-arginine, l-lysine acetate, l-alanine, l-threonine, l-phenylalanine, l-asparticacid, l-histidine, l-methionine, glycine, polyglycerol esters of fatty acids, l-serine, l-proline, sodium Cl, l-tryptophan, l-cysteine, sodium citrate, vitamins and minerals. Powder 3.4 oz. packets. *otc.*
Use: Highprotein, branched chain enriched tube feeding.

Stri-Dex Antibacterial Cleansing. (Bayer) Triclosan 1%, acetylated lanolin alcohol, EDTA. Bar. 105 g. *otc.*
Use: Antiacne.

Stri-Dex B.P. (Bayer) Benzoyl peroxide 10%. in greaseless, vanishing cream base. *otc.*
Use: Antiacne.

Stri-Dex Clear. (Bayer) Salicylic acid 2%, SD alcohol 9.3%, EDTA. Gel: 30 g. *otc.*
Use: Antiacne.

Stridex Face Wash. (Bayer) Triclosan 1%, glycerin, EDTA, alcohol free. Soln.: 237 ml. *otc.*
Use: Antiacne.

Stri-Dex Lotion. (Bayer) Salicylic acid 0.5%, alcohol 28%, sulfonated alkyl benzenes, citric acid, sodium carbonate, simethicone, water. Bot. 4 oz. *otc.*
Use: Antiacne.

Stri-Dex Maximum Strength Pads. (Bayer) Salicylic acid 2%, SD alcohol 44%, citric acid, menthol. In pads 55s, 90s, dual-textured 32s. *otc.*
Use: Anti-acne.

Stri-Dex Oil Fighting Formula Pads. (Bayer) Salicylic acid 2%, citric acid, menthol, SD alcohol 54%. Super Scrub Pads 55s. *otc.*
Use: Antiacne.

Stri-Dex Regular Strength Pads. (Bayer) Salicylic acid 0.5%, SD alcohol 28%, citric acid, menthol. In 55s. *otc.*
Use: Antiacne.

Stri-Dex Sensitive Skin Pads. (Bayer) Salicylic acid 0.5%, citric acid, aloe vera gel, menthol, SD alcohol 28%. In 50s, 90s. *otc.*

Use: Antiacne.

Stromba Ampules. (Sanofi Winthrop) Stanozolol. *c-iii.*
Use: Anabolic steroid.

strong iodine tincture. (Various Mfr.) Iodine 7%, potassium iodide 5%, alcohol 83%. Soln. Bot. 500 ml, 4000 ml. *otc.*
Use: Antiseptic and germicide.

strontium bromide. Cryst. or Granule, Bot. 0.25 lb, 1 lb. Amp. 1 g/10 ml. *Rx.*
Use: Sedative, antiepileptic.

• **strontium chloride SR 85.** (STRAHN-shee-uhm) USAN.
Use: Radioactive agent.

• **strontium chloride SR 89 injection,** U.S.P. 23.
Use: Antineoplastic; radioactive agent.
See: Metastron, Inj. (Amersham).

strontium lactate trihydrate.

• **strontium nitrate Sr 85.** USAN.
Use: Radioactive agent.

strontium SR 85 injection.
Use: Diagnostic aid (bone scanning).

strophanthin. K-strophanthin.

Strovite Plus. (Everett) Vitamins A 5000 IU, E 30 mg, B_1 20 mg, B_2 20 mg, B_3 100 mg, B_5 25 mg, B_6 25 mg, B_{12} 50 mcg, C 500 mg, iron 9 mg, folic acid 0.8 mg, zinc 22.5 mg, biotin 150 mcg, Cr, Cu, Mg, Mn. Bot. 100s. *otc.*
Use: Vitamin/mineral supplement.

Strovite Tablets. (Everett) Vitamins B_1 15 mg, B_2 15 mg, B_3 100 mg, B_5 18 mg, B_6 4 mg, B_{12} 5 mcg, C 500 mg, folic acid 0.5 mg. Bot. 100s. *otc.*
Use: Vitamin/mineral supplement.

S.T. 37. (SK-Beecham) Hexylresorcinol 0.1% in glycerin aqueous soln. Bot. 5.5 oz, 12 oz. *otc.*
Use: Antiseptic, topical.

Stuart Formula. (J & J Merck) Vitamins A 5000 IU, B_1 1.5 mg, B_2 1.7 mg, B_3 20 mg, B_6 1 mg, B_{12} 2 mcg, C 50 mg, D 400 IU, E 10 IU, iron 5 mg, Cu, folic acid 0.4 mg, Ca, I, P/Tab. Bot. 100s. *otc.*
Use: Vitamin/mineral supplement.

Stuartnatal Plus. (Wyeth-Ayerst) Vitamins A 4000 IU, D 400 IU, E 22 mg, C 120 mg, B_1 1.84 mg, B_2 3 mg, B_3 20 mg, B_6 10 mg, B_{12} 12 mcg, calcium 200 mg, folic acid 1 mg, iron 65 mg, zinc 25 mg, Cu 2 mg. Tab. Bot. 100s. *Rx.*
Use: Vitamin/mineral supplement.

Stuart Prenatal. (Wyeth-Ayerst) Vitamins A 4000 IU, B_1 1.8 mg, B_2 1.7 mg, B_6 2.6 mg, B_{12} 4 mcg, C 100 mg, D 400 IU, E 11 mg, B_3 18 mg, iron 60 mg, calcium 200 mg, copper 2 mg, zinc 25

mg, folic acid 0.8 mg/Tab. Bot. 100s. *otc.*
Use: Vitamin/mineral supplement.

Stulex. (Jones Medical) Docusate sodium 250 mg/Tab. Bot. 100s, 1000s. *otc.*
Use: Fecal softener.

Stye. (Del) White petrolatum 55%, mineral oil 32%, boric acid, wheat germ oil, stearic acid. Oint. Bot. 3.5 g. *otc.*
Use: Ocular lubricant.

Stypt-Aid. (Pharmakon Labs) Benzocaine 28.71 mg, methylbenzethonium HCl 9.95 mg, aluminum Cl hexahydrate 55.43 mg, ethyl alcohol 70.97%/ml in a glycerine, menthol base. Spray. In 60 ml. *otc.*
Use: Topical local anesthetic.

styptirenal.
See: Epinephrine (Various Mfr.).

Stypto-Caine Solution. (Pedinol) Hydroxyquinoline sulfate, tetracaine HCl, aluminum Cl, aqueous glycol base. Bot. 2 oz. *Rx.*
Use: Hemostatic solution.

styrene polymer, sulfonated, sodium salt. Sodium Polystyrene Sulfonate, U.S.P. 23.

styronate resins. Ammonium and potassium salts of sulfonated styrene polymers.
Use: Conditions requiring sodium restriction.

Sublimaze. (Janssen) Fentanyl 0.05 mg as citrate/ml. Amp. 2 ml, 5 ml, 10 ml, 20 ml. *c-II.*
Use: Analgesic, anesthetic agent.

Sublingual B Total Liquid. (Pharmaceutical Lab) Vitamins B_2 1.7 mg, B_3 20 mg, B_5 30 mg, B_6 2 mg, B_{12} 1000 mcg, C 60 mg. Liq. Bot. 30 ml. *otc.*
Use: Vitamin supplement.

Suby's Solution G. (Various Mfr.) Citric acid 3.24 g, sodium carbonate 0.43 g, magnesium oxide 0.38 g/100 ml. Soln. Bot. 1000 ml. *Rx.*
Use: Genitourinary irrigant.

•**succimer.** (SUX-ih-mer) USAN.
Use: Diagnostic aid; cystine kidney stones, mercury and lead poisoning [Orphan drug]
See: Chemet (McNeil-CPC).

succinchlorimide. N-Chlorosuccinimide.

succinic acid.
See: Cenasert, Tab. (Schwarz Pharma).

•**succinylcholine chloride,** U.S.P. 23.
Use: Neuromuscular blocking agent.
See: Anectine Cl, Amp. (Glaxo Wellcome).

Quelicin, Amp., Additive Syringes, Fliptop & Pintop Vials (Abbott).
Sucostrin, Amp., Vial (Squibb Marsam).

succinylsulfathiazole.
Use: Intestinal anti-infective.

Succus Cineraria Maritima. (Walker Corp.) Aqueous and glycerin solution of senecio compositae, hamamelis water and boric acid. Soln. Bot. 7 ml. *Rx.*
Use: Ophthalmic.

Sucostrin. (Apothecon) Succinylcholine Cl 20 mg/ml Inj. Vial 10 ml. *Rx.*
Use: Depolarizing neuromuscular blocking agent.

Sucostrin Chloride. (Squibb-Marsam) Succinylcholine Cl 20 mg/ml w/methylparaben 0.1%, propylparaben 0.01%. Vial 10 ml; High potency 100 mg/ml. Vial 10 ml. *Rx.*
Use: Muscle relaxant.

•**sucralfate,** (sue-KRAL-fate) U.S.P. 23.
Use: Antiulcer (gastrointestinal); oral complications of chemotherapy [Orphan drug]
See: Carafate, Tab., Susp. (Hoechst Marion Roussel).

sucralfate. (Biocraft) Sucralfate 1 g/Tab. Bot. 30s, 100s and 500s. *Rx.*
Use: Anti-ulcer agent (gastrointestinal).

sucrase (yeast-derived). *Rx.*
Use: Treatment of congenital sucrase-isomaltase deficiency. [Orphan drug]
See: Sacarasa.

Sucrets Children's Sore Throat Lozenges. (SK-Beecham) Dyclonine HCl 1.2 mg/lozenge. Corn syrup, sucrose, cherry flavor. Tin 24s. *otc.*
Use: Sore throat treatment for children 3 years and over.

Sucrets Cold Decongestant Lozenge. (SK-Beecham) Phenylpropanolamine HCl 25 mg/lozenge. Box 24s. *otc.*
Use: Decongestant.

Sucrets Cough Control Lozenge. (SK-Beecham) Dextromethorphan HBr 5 mg/lozenge. Tin 24s. *otc.*
Use: Antitussive.

Sucrets 4-Hour Cough. (SK-Beecham) Dextromethorphan 15 mg/lozenge. Menthol, sucrose, corn syrup. Pkg. 20s. *otc.*
Use: Antitussive.

Sucrets Maximum Strength. (SK-Beecham) Dyclonine HCl 3 mg/lozenge. Corn syrup, menthol, sucrose. Tin 24s, 48s, 55s. *otc.*
Use: Temporary relief of minor sore throat, pain and mouth irritation.

Sucrets Sore Throat Lozenge. (SK-Beecham) Hexylresorcinol 2.4 mg/loz. Tin 24s. *otc.*
Use: Minor throat, pain and mouth irritation.

Sucrets Sore Throat Spray. (SK-Beecham) Dyclonine HCl 0.1%, alcohol 10%, sorbitol spray. Bot. 90 ml, 120 ml. *otc.*
Use: Temporary relief of minor sore throat pain and mouth irritation.

Sucrets Wintergreen. (SK-Beecham) Dyclonine HCl 0.1%, alcohol 10%, sorbitol. Spray bot. 90 ml. *otc.*
Use: Temporary relief of minor sore throat pain and mouth irritation.

•**sucrose,** N.F. 18.
Use: IV; diuretic & dehydrating agent; pharmaceutic aid (flavor, tablet excipient).

•**sucrose octaacetate,** N.F. 18.
Use: Pharmaceutic aid (alcohol denaturant).

•**sucrosofate potassium.** (sue-KROE-so-FATE) USAN.
Use: Antiulcerative.

Sudafed 12 Hour Capsules. (Warner Lambert) Pseudoephedrine HCl 120 mg/Sustained Action Cap. Box 10s, 20s, 40s. *otc.*
Use: Decongestant.

Sudafed Cold & Cough Liquid Caps. (Warner Lambert) Dextromethorphan HBr 10 mg, pseudoephedrine HCl 30 mg, acetaminophen 250 mg, guaifenesin 100 mg. Pkg. 10s, 20s. *otc.*
Use: Analgesic, decongestant, antitussive, expectorant.

Sudafed Plus. (Warner Lambert) **Tab.:** Pseudoephedrine HCl 60 mg, chlorpheniramine maleate 4 mg/Tab. Box 24s, 48s. *otc.*
Use: Decongestant, antihistamine.

Sudafed, Severe Cold. (Warner Lambert) Pseudoephedrine HCl 30 mg, dextromethorphan HBr 15 mg, acetaminophen 500 mg/Tab. Pkg. 10s, 20s. *otc.*
Use: Decongestant, antitussive, analgesic.

Sudafed Sinus Maximum Strength. (Warner Lambert) Pseudoephedrine HCl 30 mg, acetaminophen 500 mg. Caplets: In 24s. *otc.*
Use: Decongestant, analgesic.

Sudafed Tablets. (Warner Lambert) Pseudoephedrine HCL 30 mg or 60 mg/Tab. **30 mg:** Box 24s, 48s. Bot. 100s, 1000s. **60 mg:** Bot. 100s, 1000s. *otc.*

Use: Decongestant.

Sudanyl. (Dover) Pseudoephedrine HCl/Tab. Sugar, lactose and salt free. UD Box 500s.
Use: Decongestant.

Sudden Tan Lotion. (Schering-Plough) Padimate O, dihydroxyacetone, Bot. 4 oz. *otc.*
Use: Artificial tanning agent, ultraviolet sunscreen, moisturizer.

Sudex. (Atley) Pseudoephedrine HCl 120 mg, guaifenesin 600 mg. 100s. *Rx.*
Use: Expectorant.

Sudex. (Roberts) Pseudophedrine HCl 30 mg/Tab. UD 8s, 100s. *otc.*
Use: Decongestant, expectorant.

•**sudoxicam.** (sue-DOX-ih-kam) USAN.
Use: Anti-inflammatory.

Sudrin. (Jones Medical) Pseudoephedrine HCl 30 mg/Tab. Bot. 100s, 1000s. *otc.*
Use: Decongestant.

Sufenta. (Janssen) Sufentanil citrate 50 mcg/ml. Amps. 1 ml, 2 ml, 5 ml. *c-II.*
Use: Analgesic, anesthetic agent.

•**sufentanil.** (sue-FEN-tuh-nill) USAN.
Use: Analgesic.

•**sufentanil citrate,** (sue-FEN-tuh-nill SIH-trate) U.S.P. 23.
Use: Narcotic analgesic.
See: Sufenta (Janssen).

sufentanil citrate. (ESI Lederle) 50 mcg/ml. Inj. 1, 2, 5 ml. *c-II.*
Use: Narcotic analgesic.

•**sufotidine.** (sue-FOE-tih-DEEN) USAN.
Use: Antagonist (to histamine H_2 receptors).

Sufrex. (Janssen) Ketanserin tartrate. *Rx.*
Use: Serotonin antagonist.

•**sugar, compressible,** N.F. 18.
Use: Pharmaceutic aid (flavor; tablet excipient).

•**sugar, confectioner's,** N.F. 18.
Use: Pharmaceutic aid (flavor; tablet excipient).

•**sugar, invert, injection.** U.S.P. 23.
Use: Replenisher (fluid and nutrient).

•**sugar spheres,** N.F. 18.
Use: Pharmaceutic aid (vehicle, solid carrier).

Sulamyd Sodium.
Use: Ophthalmic sulfonamide.
See: Sodium Sulamyd, Ophth. Soln. (Schering Plough).

Sular. (Zeneca) 10, 20, 30, 40 mg nisoldipine, lactose/E.R. Tab. 100s, UD 100s. *Rx.*
Use: Calcium channel blocker.

• **sulazepam.** (sull-AZE-eh-pam) USAN.
Use: Tranquilizer (minor).

Sulazo. (Freeport) Sulfisoxazole 500 mg, phenylazodiaminopyridine HCl 50 mg/ Tab. Bot. 1000s. *Rx.*
Use: Anti-infective, analgesic.

• **sulbactam benzathine.** (sull-BACK-tam BENZ-ah-theen) USAN.
Use: Synergistic (penicillin/cephalosporin), inhibitor (β-lactamase).

• **sulbactam pivoxil.** (sull-BACK-tam pihv-OX-ill) USAN.
Use: Inhibitor (β-lactamase), synergist (penicillin/cephalosporin).

• **sulbactam sodium sterile,** (sull-BACK-tam) U.S.P. 23.
Use: Inhibitor (β-lactamase), synergist (penicillin/cephalosporin).

sulbactam sodium/ampicillin sodium.
Use: Anti-infective, penicillin.
See: Unasyn (Roerig).

• **sulconazole nitrate,** (SULL-CONE-ah-zole) U.S.P. 23.
Use: Antifungal.
See: Exelderm (Syntex).

• **sulesomab.** (sue-LEH-so-mab) USAN.
Use: Monoclonal antibody (diagnostic aid for detection of infectious diseases).

Sulf-10. (Ciba Vision) Sodium sulfacetamide 10%. Bot. 15 ml; Dropperette 1 ml. *Rx.*
Use: Anti-infective, ophthalmic.

Sulf-15. (Ciba Vision) Sodium sulfacetamide 15%. Soln. Bot. 5 ml, 15 ml. *Rx.*
Use: Anti-infective, ophthalmic.

Sulfa-10 Ophthalmic. (Maurry) Sodium sulfacetamide 10%, hydroxyethylcellulose, sodium borate, boric acid, disodium edetate, sodium metabisulfite, sodium thiosulfate 0.2%, chlorobutanol 0.2%, methyl paraben 0.015%. Bot. 15 ml. *Rx.*
Use: Anti-infective, ophthalmic.

• **sulfabenz.** (SULL-fah-benz) USAN.
Use: Antibacterial.

• **sulfabenzamide,** (SULL-fah-BENZ-ah-mid) U.S.P. 23.
Use: Antibacterial.
See: Sultrin, Vag. Tab., Cream (Ortho).

sulfabromethazine sodium.
Use: Anti-infective.

Sulfacet. (Dermik).
See: Sulfacetamide.

Sulfacet-R. (Dermik) Sulfur 5%, sulfacetamide sodium 10%, parabens. Lot. Bot. 25 ml. *Rx.*
Use: Antiacne.

• **sulfacetamide,** U.S.P. 23.
Use: Antibacterial.

sulfacetamide w/combinations.
See: Acet-Dia-Mer Sulfonamides.
Cetapred, Oint. (Alcon).
Chero-Trisulfa (V), Susp. (Vita Elixir).
Sulf-10, Ophth. Soln. (Ciba Vision).
Sultrin, Tab., Cream (Ortho).
Triurisul, Tab. (Sheryl).

• **sulfacetamide sodium,** U.S.P. 23.
Use: Antibacterial.
See: AK-Sulf, Preps. (Akorn).
Bleph 10, Liquifilm (Allergan).
Cetamide, Ophth. Oint. (Alcon).
Isopto Cetamide, Ophth. Soln. (Alcon).
Ocusulf-10, Ophth. Soln. (Optopics).
Sebizon Lotion (Schering Plough).
Sodium Sulamyd Ophthalmic Ointment 30% (Schering Plough).
Sulf-10, Drops (Maurry).
Sulf-10, Soln., Drops (Ciba Vision).
Sulf-15, Ophth. Soln. (Ciba Vision).
W/Fluorometholone.
See: FML-S Susp. (Allergan).
W/Methylcellulose.
See: Sodium Sulamyd Ophth. Soln. 10% (Schering Plough).
W/Phenylephrine HCl, methylparaben, propylparaben.
See: Vasosulf, Liq. (Ciba Vision).
W/Prednisolone.
See: Cetapred Ophthalmic Ointment (Alcon).
Vasocidin, Soln. (Ciba Vision).
W/Prednisolone acetate.
See: Blephamide S.O.P., Ophth. Oint. and Susp. (Allergan).
Metimyd, Ophth. Oint. and Susp. (Schering Plough).
W/Prednisolone, methylcellulose.
See: Isopto Cetapred, Susp. (Alcon).
W/Prednisolone acetate, phenylephrine.
See: Blephamide Liquifilm, Ophth. Susp. (Allergan).
Tri-Ophtho, Ophth. Drops (Maurry).
W/Prednisolone phosphate.
See: Optimyd Soln., Sterile (Schering Plough).
W/Prednisolone sodium phosphate, phenylephrine, sulfacetamide sodium.
Vasocidin, Ophth. Soln. (Ciba Vision).
W/Sulfur.
See: Novacet, Lot. (Genderm).
Sulfacet-R, Lot. (Dermik).

sulfacetamide sodium. (Various Mfr.)
Soln.: 10% or 30%: Bot. 15 ml; **Oint.:** 10% Tube 3.5 g.
Use: Antibacterial.

sulfacetamide sodium and predniso-

lone acetate ophthalmic ointment.
Use: Anti-infective, anti-inflammatory.
See: AK-Cide (Akorn).
  Blephamide S.O.P. (Allergan).
  Cetapred (Alcon).
  Metimyd (Schering Plough).
  Predsulfair (Bausch & Lomb).
  Sulphrin (Bausch & Lomb).
  Vasocidin (Ciba Vision).
**sulfacetamide sodium and predniso-
lone sodium phosphate.** (Schein)
Sulfacetamide sodium 10%, predniso-
lone sodium phosphate 0.25%. Soln. 5
ml, 10 ml. *Rx.*
Use: Anti-infective, ophthalmic.
**Sulfacetamide Sodium 10% and Sulfur
5%.** (Glades) Sulfur 5%, sodium sulfa-
cetamide 10%, cetyl alcohol, benzyl
alcohol, EDTA. Bot. 25 ml. Tube 30 ml.
Rx.
Use: Antiacne.
**sulfacetamide, sulfadiazine, & sulfa-
merazine oral suspension.**
See: Acet-Dia-Mer-Sulfonamides.
Sulfacet-R Lotion. (Dermik) Sodium sulfacetamide 10%, sulfur 5%, in flesh-
tinted base. Bot. 25 g. *Rx.*
Use: Treatment of acne and seborrheic
  dermatitis.
•**sulfacytine.** (SULL-fah-SIGH-teen)
USAN.
Use: Antibacterial.
sulfadiasulfone sodium. Acetosulfone
sodium.
•**sulfadiazine,** (SULL-fah-DIE-ah-zeen)
U.S.P. 23.
Use: Antibacterial. [Orphan drug]
sulfadiazine. (Stanley Pharm) 500 mg.
Use: Antibacterial.
sulfadiazine combinations. (SULL-fah-
DIE-ah-zeen)
See: Acet-Dia-Mer-Sulfonamides. (Vari-
  ous Mfr.).
  Chemozine, Tab., Susp. (Tennessee
    Pharmaceutic).
  Chero-Trisulfa, Susp. (Vita Elixir).
  Dia-Mer-Sulfonamides (Various Mfr.).
  Dia-Mer-Thia-Sulfonamide (Various
    Mfr.).
  Meth-Dia-Mer-Sulfonamides (Various
    Mfr.).
  Silvadene (Hoechst Marion Roussel).
  Terfonyl, Liq., Tab. (Squibb).
  Triple Sulfa, Tab. (Various Mfr.).
sulfadiazine and sulfamerazine. Citra-
sulfas.
See: Dia-Mer-Sulfonamides.
•**sulfadiazine, silver,** U.S.P. 23.
Use: Anti-infective (topical).

•**sulfadiazine sodium,** (SULL-fah-DIE-ah-
zeen) U.S.P. 23.
Use: Antibacterial.
W/Sod. bicarbonate.
  (Pitman-Moore)–Tab. 5 gr, Bot. 1000s;
    2.5 gr, Bot. 100s, 500s, 1000s.
**sulfadiazine, sulfamerazine & sulfa-
cetamide suspension.**
See: Acet-Dia-Mer-Sulfonamides.
  Coco Diazine (Lilly).
sulfadimetine. (Novartis).
sulfadimidine.
See: Sulfamethazine.
sulfadine.
See: Sulfadimidine.
  Sulfamethazine.
  Sulfapyridine, Tab. (Various Mfr.).
•**sulfadoxine,** (SULL-fah-DOX-een)
U.S.P. 23.
Use: Antibacterial.
W/Pyrimethamine.
See: Fansidar, Tab. (Roche).
**sulfadoxine and pyrimethamine tab-
lets.**
Use: Anti-infective, antimalarial.
sulfaethylthiadiazole.
See: Sulfaethidole.
sulfaguanidine.
Use: GI tract infections.
W/Sulfamethazine, sulfamerazine & sul-
fadiazine.
See: Quadetts, Tab. (Zeneca).
  Quad-Ramoid, Susp. (Zeneca).
Sulfair 15. (Bausch & Lomb) Sodium sul-
facetamide 15%. Soln. Bot. 15 ml. *Rx.*
Use: Anti-infective, ophthalmic.
Sulfalax Calcium. (Major) Docusate cal-
cium 240 mg/Cap. Bot. 500s. *otc.*
Use: Laxative.
•**sulfalene.** (SULL-fah-leen) USAN.
Use: Antibacterial.
•**sulfamerazine,** U.S.P. 23.
Use: Antibacterial.
sulfamerazine combinations.
Use: Anti-infective.
See: Chemozine Tab., Susp. (Tennes-
  see Pharmaceutic).
  Chero-Trisulfa-V, Susp. (Vita Elixir).
  Terfonyl, Liq., Tab. (Squibb).
  Triple Sulfa, Tab. (Various Mfr.).
sulfamerazine sodium.
Use: Anti-infective.
sulfamerazine & sulfadiazine.
See: Dia-Mer-Sulfonamides.
**sulfamerazine, sulfadiazine & sulfa-
methazine.**
Use: Anti-infective.
See: Meth-Dia-Mer-Sulfonamides.

sulfamerazine, sulfadiazine & sulfathiazole.
Use: Anti-infective.
See: Dia-Mer-Thia-Sulfonamides.
• **sulfameter.** (SULL-fam-EE-ter) USAN.
Use: Antibacterial.
• **sulfamethazine,** U.S.P. 23.
Use: Antibacterial.
See: Neotrizine, Susp., Tab. (Lilly).
W/Sulfacetamide, sulfadiazine, sulfamerazine.
See: Sulfa-Plex, Vaginal Cream (Solvay).
W/Sulfadiazine, sulfamerazine.
See: Sulfaloid, Susp. (Westerfield).
Terfonyl, Liq., Tab. (Squibb).
Triple Sulfa, Tab. (Various Mfr.).
• **sulfamethizole,** U.S.P. 23.
Use: Antibacterial.
See: Bursul, Tab. (Burlington).
Microsul, Tab. (Star).
Proklar-M, Liq., Tab. (Westerfield).
Sulfasol, Tab. (Hyrex-Key).
Sulfurine, Tab. (Table Rock).
Thiosulfil, Forte, Tab. (Wyeth-Ayerst).
Urifon, Tab. (T.E. Williams).
sulfamethizole w/combinations.
Use: Anti-infective.
See: Microsul-A, Tab. (Star).
Thiosulfil-A, Tab. (Wyeth-Ayerst).
Thiosulfil-A Forte, Tab. (Wyeth-Ayerst).
Triurisul, Tab. (Sheryl).
Urobiotic, Cap. (Pfizer).
Urotrol, Tab. (Mills).
sulfamethoprim. (Par Pharm) Sulfamethoxazole 400 mg, trimethoprim 80 mg/Tab. Bot. 100s, 500s. *Rx.*
Use: Anti-infective.
• **sulfamethoxazole,** (sull-fah-meth-OX-ah-zole) U.S.P. 23.
Use: Antibacterial.
See: Gantanol, Prep. (Roche).
W/Trimethoprim.
See: Bactrim, Prods. (Roche).
Septra, Tab. (Glaxo Wellcome).
Septra DS, Tab. (Glaxo Wellcome).
sulfamethoxazole and phenazopyridine hydrochloride.
Use: Urinary anti-infective.
See: Azo-Gantanol, Tab. (Roche).
sulfamethoxazole and trimethoprim for injection concentrate. (SULL-fah-meth-OX-ah-zole and try-METH-oh-prim)
Use: Urinary anti-infective.
sulfamethoxazole and trimethoprim oral suspension. (Various Mfr.) Trimethoprim 40 mg, sulfamethoxazole 200 mg/5 ml. Bot. 150 ml, 200 ml, 480 ml. *Rx.*

Use: Urinary anti-infective.
sulfamethoxazole and trimethoprim tablets. (Various Mfr.) Trimethoprim 80 mg, sulfamethoxazole 400 mg/Tab. Bot. 100s, 500s. *Rx.*
Use: Urinary anti-infective.
sulfamethoxazole/trimethoprim DS. (Various Mfr.) Trimethoprim 160 mg, sulfamethoxazole 800 mg. Tab, double strength. Bot. 100s, 500s. *Rx.*
Use: Anti-infective.
sulfamethoxydiazine. Sulfameter.
Use: Anti-infective.
sulfamethoxypyridazine acetyl.
Use: Anti-infective.
sulfamethylthiadiazole.
Use: Anti-infective.
See: Sulfamethizole Preps.
sulfametin. N^1-(5-Methoxy-2-pyrimidinyl) sulfanilamide. (Formerly sulfamethoxydiazine).
Use: Anti-infective.
sulfamezanthene.
Use: Anti-infective.
See: Sulfamethazine.
Sulfamide Suspension. (Rugby) Prednisolone acetate 0.5%, sodium sulfacetamide, hydroxypropyl methylcellulose, polysorbate 80, sodium thiosulfate, benzalkonium Cl 0.01%. Susp. Bot. 5 and 15 ml. *Rx.*
Use: Anti-infective, ophthalmic.
• **sulfamonomethoxine.** (SULL-fah-mahn-oh-meh-THOCK-seen) USAN.
Use: Antibacterial.
• **sulfamoxole.** (sull-fah-MOX-ole) USAN.
Use: Antibacterial.
p-sulfamoylbenzylamine hydrochloride. Sulfbenzamide.
Sulfamylon Cream. (Dow B. Hickam) Mafenide acetate equivalent to 85 mg of base/g. w/cetyl alcohol, stearyl alcohol, cetyl esters wax, polyoxyl 40 stearate, polyoxyl 8 stearate, glycerin, water w/methylparaben and propylparaben, sodium metabisulfite, edetate disodium. Tube 2 oz, 4 oz. Can 14.5 oz. *Rx.*
Use: Adjunctive therapy in second and third-degree burns.
sulfanilamide. p-Aminobenzene sulfonamide.
Use: Anti-infective.
sulfanilamide. (Various Mfr.) Sulfanilamide 15%. Vaginal Cream. Tube 120 g with applicator. *Rx.*
Use: Anti-infective, vaginal.
sulfanilamide combinations.
Use: Anti-infective.

See: AVC/Dienestrol Cream, Supp. (Hoechst Marion Roussel).
AVC, Cream, Supp. (Hoechst Marion Roussel).
Par Cream (Parmed).
Vagacreme, Cream (Delta).
Vagisan Creme (Sandia).
Vagisul, Creme (Sheryl).
Vagitrol, Cream, Supp. (Lemmon).
2-sulfanilamidopyridine. Sulfadiazine, U.S.P. 23.
Use: Anti-infective.
•**sulfanilate zinc.** USAN.
Use: Antibacterial.
n-sulfanilylacetamide.
Use: Anti-infective.
See: Sulfacetamide, Tab. (Various Mfr.).
sulfanilylbenzamide.
Use: Anti-infective.
See: Sulfabenzamide.
•**sulfanitran.** (SULL-fah-NYE-tran) USAN.
Use: Antibacterial.
•**sulfapyridine,** U.S.P. 23.
Use: Dermatitic herpetiformis suppressant. [Orphan drug]
sulfarsphenamine.
•**sulfasalazine,** (SULL-fuh-SAL-uh-zeen) U.S.P. 23. *Formerly Salicylazosulfapyridine.*
Use: Antibacterial.
See: Azulfidine, Tab., Susp. (Pharmacia & Upjohn).
Salazopyrin.
Salicylazosulfapyridine.
Salazopyrin.
S.A.S.-50, Tab. (Solvay).
S.A.S.P., Tab. (Zenith).
Sulcolon, Tab. (Lederle).
Sulfapyridine (I.N.N.).
sulfasalazine. (Lederle) 0.5 g/Tab. Bot. 500s.
Use: Antibacterial.
•**sulfasomizole.** (SULL-fah-SAHM-ih-zole) USAN.
Use: Anti-infective, sulfonamide.
See: Bidizole.
sulfasymasine.
Use: Anti-infective sulfonamide.
Sulfa-Ter-Tablets. (A.P.C.) Trisulfapyrimidines, U.S.P. Bot. 1000s.
•**sulfathiazole,** U.S.P. 23.
Use: Antibacterial.
W/Chlorophyllin.
sulfathiazole combinations.
See: Sultrin, Tab. & Cream (Ortho).
sulfathiazole carbamide.
See: Otosmosan, Liq. (Wyeth-Ayerst).
sulfathiazole, sulfacetamide, and sulfabenzamide vaginal cream.

See: Dayto Sulf (Dayton).
Triple Sulfa Vaginal Cream.
sulfathiazole, sulfacetamide, and sulfabenzamide vaginal tablets.
See: Triple Sulfa Vaginal Tablets.
Sulfatrim. (Various Mfr.) Trimethoprim 40 mg, sulfamethoxazole 200 mg/5 ml Susp. Bot. 473 ml. *Rx.*
Use: Anti-infective.
Sulfatrim DS Tabs. (Goldline) Trimethoprim 800 mg, sulfamethoxazole 160 mg/Tab. Bot. 100s, 500s. *Rx.*
Use: Anti-infective.
Sulfatrim SS Tabs. (Goldline) Trimethoprim 400 mg, sulfamethoxazole 80 mg/Tab. Bot. 100s. *Rx.*
Use: Anti-infective.
Sulfa-Trip. (Major) Sulfathiazole 3.42%, sulfacetamide 2.86%, sulfabenzamide 3.7%, urea 0.64%. Cream. In 82.5 g. *Rx.*
Use: Anti-infective, vaginal.
Sulfa Triple No. 2. (Global Pharms) Sulfadiazine 162 mg, sulfamerizine 162 mg, sulfamethazine 162 mg/Tab. Bot. 1000s. *Rx.*
Use: Anti-infective.
•**sulfazamet.** (sull-FAZE-ah-MET) USAN.
Use: Antibacterial.
See: Vesulong (Novartis).
sulfhydryl ion.
See: Hydrosulphosol (Lientz).
•**sulfinalol hydrochloride.** (SULL-FIN-ah-lahl) USAN.
Use: Antihypertensive.
•**sulfinpyrazone,** (sull-fin-PEER-uh-zone) U.S.P. 23.
Use: Uricosuric.
See: Anturane, Tab., Cap. (Novartis).
•**sulfisoxazole,** (sull-fih-SOX-uh-zole) U.S.P. 23.
Use: Antibacterial.
See: Gantrisin Preps. (Roche).
Soxa, Tab. (Vita Elixir).
Sulfisoxazole, Tab. (Purepac).
Sulfium, Ophthalmic, Soln., Oint. (Alcon).
Sulfizin, Tab. (Solvay).
W/Aminoacridine HCl, allantoin.
See: Vagilia, Cream (Lemmon).
W/Phenazopyridine.
See: Azo-Gantrisin, Tab. (Roche).
Azo-Soxazole, Tab. (Quality Generics).
Azo-Sulfisoxazole, Tab. (Global Pharms; Century).
W/Phenylazodiaminopyridine HCl.
See: Azo-Sulfizin (Solvay).
•**sulfisoxazole, acetyl,** (sull-fih-SOX-uh-

zole, ASS-eh-till) U.S.P. 23.
Use: Antibacterial.
W/Erythromycin Ethylsuccinate.
See: Pediazol, Susp. (Ross).

sulfisoxazole diethanolamine. Sulfisoxazole Diolamine.

• **sulfisoxazole diolamine,** (sull-fin-SOX-azz-ole die-OLE-ah-meen) U.S.P. 23.
Use: Antibacterial.
See: Gantrisin, Ophth. Soln. & Oint. (Roche).

Sulfoam Medicated Antidandruff Shampoo. (Kenwood/Bradley) Sulfur 2% with cleansers & conditioners. Bot. 4 oz, 8 oz, 15.5 oz. *otc.*
Use: Control dandruff.

sulfobromophthalein sodium, U.S.P. XXII.
Use: Liver function test.

sulfocarbolates. Salts of Phenolsulfonic Acid, Usually Ca, Na, K, Cu, Zn.

sulfocyanate.
See: Potassium Thiocyanate.

Sulfo-Ganic. (Marcen) Thioglycerol 20 mg, sodium citrate 5 mg, phenol 0.5%, benzyl alcohol 0.5%/ml. Vial 10 ml, 30 ml.
Use: IM, adjunctive treatment in arthritides due to sulfur metabolism disorders or deficiencies.

sulfoguaiacol.
See: Pot. Guaiacolsulfonate.

Sulfoil. (C & M Pharmacal) Sulfonated castor oil, water. Bot. pt, Gal. *otc.*
Use: Soap free cleanser for skin and hair.

Sulfolax Calcium. (Major) Docusate calcium 240 mg/Cap. Bot. 100s. *otc.*
Use: Laxative.

Sulfo-Lo. (Whorton) Sublimed sulfur, freshly precipitated polysulfides of zinc, potassium, sulfate, and calamine in aqueous-alcoholic suspension. **Lotion:** Bot. 4 oz, 8 oz, **Soap:** 3 oz. *otc.*
Use: Antiacne.

• **sulfomyxin.** (SULL-foe-MIX-in) USAN.
Use: Antibacterial.

sulfonamide, doubles.
See: Dia-Mer-Sulfonamides.

sulfonamide preps.
See: Acet-Dia-Mer (Various Mfr.).
Dayto Sulf, Vag. cream (Dayton).
Dia-Mer Sulfonamides (Various Mfr.).
Dia-Mer-Thia (Various Mfr.).
Gyne-Sulf, Vag. cream (G & W).
Meth-Dia-Mer, Preps. (Various Mfr.).
Sultrin Triple Sulfa, Vag. cream, Tab. (Ortho).
Triple Sulfa, Vag. cream (Various Mfr.).

Trysul, Vag. cream (Savage).
V.V.S., Vag. cream (Econo Med).

sulfonamides, quadruple.
See: Quadetts, Tab. (Zeneca).
Quad-Ramoid, Susp. (Zeneca).

sulfonamides, triple.
See: Acet-Dia-Mer Sulfonamides.
Dia-Mer-Thia Sulfonamides.
Meth-Dia-Mer Sulfonamides.

sulfones.
See: Avlosulfon, Tab. (Wyeth-Ayerst).
Dapsone.
Diasone, Enterabs (Abbott).
Glucosulfone Sodium.
Promacetin, Tab. (Parke-Davis).

sulfonethylmethane. 2,2-Bis-(ethylsulfonyl)butane.

sulfonithocholylglycine.
See: S.L.C.G., Kit (Abbott).

sulfonmethane.

sulfonphthal.
See: Phenolsulfonphthalein, Prep. (Various Mfr.).

• **sulfonterol hydrochloride.** (sull-FAHN-teer-ole) USAN.
Use: Bronchodilator.

sulfonylureas.
See: DiaBeta (Hoechst Marion Roussel).
Diabinese, Tab. (Pfizer).
Dymelor, Tab. (Lilly).
Glucotrol (Roerig).
Glynase PresTab (Pharmacia & Upjohn).
Micronase (Pharmacia & Upjohn).
Orinase, Tab., Vial (Pharmacia & Upjohn).
Tolinase, Tab. (Pharmacia & Upjohn).

Sulforcin Lotion. (Galderma) Sulfur 5%, resorcinol 2%, SD alcohol 40 11.65%, methylparaben. Bot. 120 ml. *otc.*
Use: For acne, seborrheic dermatitis & oily skin conditions.

sulformethoxine. Name used for Sulfadoxine.

sulforthomidine. Name used for Sulfadoxine.

sulfosalicylate w/methenamine.
See: Hexalet, Tab. (PolyMedica).

sulfosalicylic acid. Salicylsulphonic acid.

sulfoxone sodium, U.S.P. XXII.

sulfoxyl regular. (Stiefel) Benzoyl peroxide 5%, sulfur 2% Bot. 60 ml. *Rx.*
Use: Antiacne.

sulfoxyl strong. (Stiefel) Benzoyl peroxide 10%, sulfur 5% Bot. 60 ml. *Rx.*
Use: Antiacne.

Sulfur-8 Hair & Scalp Conditioner.
(Schering-Plough) Sulfur 2%, menthol
1%, triclosan 0.1%. Jar 2 oz, 4 oz, 8 oz.
otc.
Use: Antiseborrheic.
**Sulfur-8 Light Formula Hair & Scalp
Conditioner.** (Schering-Plough) Sul-
fur, triclosan, menthol. Jar 2 oz, 4 oz.
otc.
Use: Antiseborrheic.
Sulfur-8 Shampoo. (Schering-Plough)
Triclosan 0.2%. Bot. 6.85 oz, 10.85
oz. *otc.*
Use: Antiseborrheic.
sulfur, antiarthritic.
See: Thiocyl, Amp. (Torigian).
sulfurated lime topical solution. Vlem-
inckx Lotion.
Use: Scabicide, parasiticide.
sulfur combinations.
See: Acnaveen, Bar (Rydelle).
Acne-Aid, Cream, Lot. (Stiefel).
Akne Oral Kapsulets, Cap. (Alto).
Acnomel, Cake, Cream (SK-
Beecham).
Acno, Soln., Lot. (Cummins).
Acnotex, Liq. (C & M Pharmaceutic).
Akne, Drying Lot. (Alto).
Antrocol, Tab., Cap. (ECR Pharm).
Aracain Rectal Oint. (Del Pharm).
Bensulfoid, Cream (ECR Pharm).
Clearasil, Stick (Procter & Gamble).
Epi-clear, Lotion (Squibb).
Exzit, Preps. (Bayer).
Fomac, Cream (Dermik).
Fostex, Liq. Cream, Bar (Westwood
Squibb).
Fostex, Cream, Liq. (Westwood
Squibb).
Fostex CM, Cream (Westwood
Squibb).
Fostril, Cream (Westwood Squibb).
Hydro Surco, Lot. (Almo).
Klaron, Lot. (Dermik).
Liquimat, Liq. (Galderma).
Lotio-P (Alto).
Neutrogena Disposables (Neutro-
gena).
Pernox, Lot. (Westwood Squibb).
pHisoDan, Liq. (Sanofi Winthrop).
Postacne, Lot. (Dermik).
Pragmatar, Oint. (Menley & James).
Proseca, Liq. (Westwood Squibb).
Rezamid, Lot. (Summers).
Sastid Soap (Stiefel).
Sebaveen, Shampoo (Rydelle).
Sebulex Shampoo, Liq. (Westwood
Squibb).
Sulfacet-R, Lot. (Dermik).
Sulfo-lo, Lot. (Wharton).

Sulforcin, Pow., Lot. (Galderma).
Sulfur-8, Prods. (Schering-Plough).
Sulpho-Lac, Cream (Kenwood/Brad-
ley).
Teenac, Cream (Zeneca).
Vanseb, Cream (Allergan Herbert).
Vanseb-T Tar Shampoo (Allergan Her-
bert).
Xerac, Oint. (Person & Covey).
•**sulfur dioxide,** N.F. 18.
Use: Pharmaceutic aid (antioxidant).
sulfur ointment.
Use: Scabicide, parasiticide.
•**sulfur, precipitated,** U.S.P. 23.
Use: Scabicide, parasiticide.
See: Bensulfoid, Pow., Lot. (ECR
Pharm).
Epi-Clear, Lot. (Squibb).
Ramsdell's Sulfur Cream (Fougera).
SAStid Soap, Bar (Stiefel).
Sulfur Soap (Steifel Labs).
sulfur, salicyl diasporal. (Doak).
See: Diasporal, Cream (Doak).
sulfur soap. (Stiefel) Precipitated sulfur
10%, EDTA. Cake 116 g. *otc.*
Use: Antiacne.
•**sulfur, sublimed,** U.S.P. 23. Flowers of
Sulfur.
Use: Parasiticide, scabicide.
sulfur, topical.
See: Thylox, Liq., Soap (Dent).
•**sulfuric acid,** N.F. 18.
Use: Pharmaceutic aid (acidifying
agent).
Sulfurine. (Table Rock) Sulfamethizole
0.5 g/Tab. Bot. 100s & 500s. *Rx.*
Use: Urinary anti-infective.
•**sulindac,** (sull-IN-dak) U.S.P. 23.
Use: Anti-inflammatory.
See: Clinoril Tab. (Merck).
•**sulisobenzone.** (sul-EYE-so-BEN-zone)
USAN.
Use: Ultraviolet screen.
See: Uval Lotion (Sandoz).
Uvinul MS-40 (General Aniline &
Film).
•**sulmarin.** (SULL-mah-rin) USAN.
Use: Hemostatic.
Sulmasque. (C & M) Sulfur 6.4%, isopro-
pyl alcohol 15%, methylparaben. Mask
150 g. *otc.*
Use: Antiacne.
Sulnac. (NMC Labs) Sulfathiazol 3.42%,
sulfacetamide 2.86%, sulfabenzamide
3.7%, urea 0.64% in cream base. Tube
2.75 oz. *Rx.*
Use: Anti-infective.
•**sulnidazole.** (sull-NIH-dah-zole) USAN.
Use: Antiprotozoal (trichomonas).

sulocarbilate. 2-Hydroxyethyl-p-sulfamylcarbanilate.

•**suloctidil.** (sull-OCK-tih-dill) USAN.
Use: Vasodilator (peripheral).

•**sulofenur.** (SUE-low-FEN-ehr) USAN.
Use: Antineoplastic.

•**sulopenem.** (sue-LOW-PEN-em) USAN.
Use: Antibacterial.

•**sulotroban.** (suh-LOW-troe-ban) USAN.
Use: Treatment of glomerulonephritis.

•**suloxifen oxalate.** USAN.
Use: Bronchodilator.

suloxybenzone. (Lederle).

sulphabenzide.
See: Sulfabenzamide.

Sulpho-Lac Acne Medication. (Doak Dermatologics) Sulfur 5%, zinc sulfate 27%, Vleminckx's Soln. 53%. Cream. Tube 28.35 g, 50 g. *otc.*
Use: Antiacne.

Sulpho-Lac Soap. (Doak Dermatologics) Sulfur 5%, a coconut and tallow oil soap base. Bar 85 g. *otc.*
Use: Antiacne.

sulphomyxin. Penta-(N-sulphomethyl) polymyxin B.

•**sulpiride.** (SULL-pih-ride) USAN.
Use: Antidepressant.

•**sulprostone.** (sull-PRAHST-ohn) USAN.
Use: Prostaglandin.

Sul-Ray Acne Cream. (Last) Sulfur 2% in cream base. Jars 1.75 oz, 6.75 oz, 20 oz. *otc.*
Use: Antiacne.

Sul-Ray Aloe Vera Analgesic Rub. (Last) Camphor 3.1%, menthol 1.25%. Bot. 4 oz, 8 oz. *otc.*
Use: Analgesic, topical.

Sul-Ray Aloe Vera Skin Protectant Cream. (Last) Zinc oxide 1%, allantoin 0.5%. Jar 1 oz. *otc.*
Use: Skin protectant cream.

Sul-Ray Shampoo. (Last) Sulfur shampoo 2%. Bot. 8 oz. *otc.*
Use: Medicated shampoo for dandruff.

Sul-Ray Soap. (Last) Sulfur soap. Bar 3 oz. *otc.*
Use: Antiacne.

Sulster. (Akorn) Sulfacetamide sodium 1%, prednisolone sodium phosphate 0.25%. Soln. 5 and 10 ml. *Rx.*
Use: Anti-infective.

•**sultamicillin.** (SULL-TAM-ih-sill-in) USAN.
Use: Antibacterial.

•**sulthiame.** (sull-THIGH-aim) USAN.
Use: Anticonvulsant.

Sultrin Triple Sulfa Vaginal Tablets. (Ortho) Sulfathiazole 172.5 mg, sulfacetamide 143.75 mg, sulfabenzamide 184 mg/Vag. Tab. Pkg. 20s w/appl. *Rx.*
Use: Treatment of *H. vaginalis* (Gardnerella) vaginitis.

Sultrin Triple Sulfa Cream. (Ortho) Sulfathiazole 3.42%, sulfacetamide 2.86%, sulfabenzamide 3.7%, urea 0.64%. Tube 78 g. with measured dose applicator. *Rx.*
Use: Treatment of *H. vaginalis* (Gardnerella) vaginitis.

•**sulukast.** (suh-LOO-kast) USAN.
Use: Antiasthmatic (leukotriene antagonist).

Sumacal Powder. (Biosearch) CHO 95 g, 380 Cal., Na 100 mg, Chloride 210 mg, K < 39 mg, Ca 20 mg/100 g. Pwd. In 100 g. *otc.*
Use: Glucose polymer.

•**sumarotene.** (sue-MAHR-oh-teen) USAN.
Use: Keratolytic.

•**sumatriptan succinate.** (SUE-muh-TRIP-tan SOOS-in-ate) USAN.
Use: Antimigraine; treatment of cluster headaches.
See: Imitrex.

Summer's Eve Disposable Douche. (Fleet) **Soln.:** Vinegar. 135 ml (1s, 2s). **Soln. Reg.:** Citric acid, sodium benzoate. **Soln. Scented:** Citric acid, sodium benzoate, octoxynol 9, EDTA. 135 ml (1s, 2s, 4s). *otc.*
Use: Douche.

Summer's Eve Disposable Douche Extra Cleansing. (Fleet) Vinegar, sodium Cl, benzoic acid. Soln. 135 ml (1s, 2s, 4s). *otc.*
Use: Douche.

Summer's Eve Medicated Disposable Douche. (Fleet) Contains povidone-iodide 0.3%. Single or twin 135 ml disposable units. *otc.*
Use: Temporary relief of minor vaginal irritation and itching.

Summer's Eve Post-Menstrual Disposable Douche. (Fleet) Sodium lauryl sulfate, parabens, monosodium and disodium phosphates, EDTA. Soln. 135 ml (2s). *otc.*
Use: Douche.

Sumycin. (Apothecon) Tetracycline HCl. **Cap.** 250 mg/Cap. Bot. 100s, 1000s, Unimatic 100s; 500 mg/Cap. Bot. 100s, 500s, Unimatic 100s. **Tab.** 250 mg/Tab. Bot. 100s, 1000s; 500 mg/Tab. Bot. 100s, 500s. *Rx.*
Use: Anti-infective, tetracycline.

•**suncillin sodium.** (SUN-SILL-in SO-dee-uhm) USAN.
Use: Antibacterial.

Sundown. (Johnson & Johnson) A series of products marketed under the Sundown name including: **Moderate** (SPF 4) Padimate O, oxybenzone. **Extra** (SPF 6) Oxybenzone, Padimate O. **Maximal** (SPF 8) Oxybenzone, Padimate O. **Ultra** (SPF 15, 30) oxybenzone, Padimate O, Octyl Methoxycinnamate. *otc.*
Use: Sunscreen.

Sundown Sport Sunblock. (Johnson & Johnson) Titanium dioxide, zinc oxide. Waterproof. PABA free. SPF 15. Lot. 90 ml. *otc.*
Use: Sunscreen.

Sundown Sunblock Cream Ultra SPF 24. (Johnson & Johnson) Padimate O, oxybenzone. *otc.*
Use: Sunscreen.

Sundown Sunblock Stick SPF 15. (Johnson & Johnson) Octyl dimethyl PABA, oxybenzone. Stick 0.35 oz. *otc.*
Use: Sunscreen.

Sundown Sunblock Stick SPF 20. (Johnson & Johnson) Octyl dimethyl PABA, octyl methoxycinnamate, oxybenzone and titanium dioxide. *otc.*
Use: Sunscreen.

Sundown Sunblock Ultra Lotion 30 SPF. (Johnson & Johnson) Octyl methoxycinnamate, octyl salicylate, oxybenzone, titanium dioxide, cetyl alcohol, PABA free, waterproof. Lot. Bot. 120 ml. *otc.*
Use: Sunscreen.

Sundown Sunblock Ultra SPF 20. (Johnson & Johnson) Octyl dimethyl PABA, octyl methoxycinnamate, oxybenzone, titanium dioxide. *otc.*
Use: Sunscreen.

Sundown Sunscreen Stick SPF 8. (Johnson & Johnson) Octyl Dimethyl PABA, oxybenzone. Stick 0.35 oz. *otc.*
Use: Sunscreen.

Sundown Sunscreen Ultra. (Johnson & Johnson) Octyl methoxycinnamate, octyl salicylate, oxybenzone, titanium dioxide, stearyl alcohol, cetyl alcohol, PABA free, waterproof. SPF 15. Cream. Tube 60 g. *otc.*
Use: Sunscreen.

Sunice. (Citroleum) Allantoin 0.25%, menthol 0.25%, methyl salicylate 10%/ Cream. 3 oz. *otc.*
Use: Burn remedy.

SunKist Multivitamins Complete, Children's. (Novartis) Iron 18 mg, vitamin A 5000 IU, D_3 400 IU, E 30 IU, B_1 1.5 mg, B_2 1.7 mg, B_3 20 mg, B_5 10 mg, B_6 2 mg, B_{12} 6 mcg, C 60 mg, folic acid 400 mcg, Ca 100 mg, Cu, I, K, Mg, Mn, P, zinc 10 mg, biotin 40 mcg, K_1 10 mcg, sorbitol, aspartame, phenylalanine, tartrazine. Chew. Tab. Bot. 60s. *otc.*
Use: Vitamin/mineral supplement.

SunKist Multivitamins + Extra C, Children's. (Novartis) Vitamin A 2500 IU, E 15 IU, D_3 400 IU, B_1 1.05 mg, B_2 1.2 mg, B_3 13.5 mg, B_6 1.05 mg, B_{12} 4.5 mcg, C 250 mg, folic acid 0.3 mg, vitamin K 5 mcg, sorbitol, aspartame, phenylalanine/Chew. Tab. Bot. 60s. *otc.*
Use: Vitamin supplement.

SunKist Multivitamins + Iron, Children's. (Novartis) Iron 15 mg, vitamin A 2500 IU, E 15 IU, D_3 400 IU, E 30 IU, B_1 1.05 mg, B_2 1.2 mg, B_3 13.5 mg, B_6 1.05 mg, B_{12} 4.5 mcg, C 60 mg, folic acid 0.3 mg, K_1 5 mcg, sorbitol, aspartame, phenylalanine, tartrazine. Chew. Tab. Bot. 60s. *otc.*
Use: Vitamin/mineral supplement.

SunKist Vitamin C. (Novartis) Vitamin C (as ascorbic acid) 500 mg. Capl. Bot. 60s. *otc.*
Use: Vitamin C supplement.

SunKist Vitamin C. (Novartis) Vitamin C (as ascorbic acid) 60 mg, sorbitol, sucrose, lactose. Chew. Tab. Pkg. 11s. *otc.*
Use: Vitamin C supplement.

SunKist Vitamin C. (Novartis) Vitamin C (as sodium ascorbate and ascorbic acid) 250 mg or 500 mg, fructose, sorbitol, sucrose, lactose. Chew. Tab. Bot. 60s. *otc.*
Use: Vitamin C supplement.

SUNPRuF 15. (C & M) SPF 15. Octyl methoxycinnamate 7.5%, benzopherone-3 5%. PABA free. Waterproof. Lot. Bot. 240 ml. *otc.*
Use: Sunscreen.

SUNPRuF 17. (C & M) SPF 17. Octyl methoxycinnamate 7.8%, octyl salicylate 5.2%, oil-free, water-resistant. Lot. Bot. 120 g. *otc.*
Use: Sunscreen.

Sunshine Chewable Tablets. (Fibertone) Iron 5 mg, vitamins A 5000 IU, D 400 IU, E 67 mg, B_1 15 mg, B_2 15 mg, B_3 25 mg, B_5 20 mg, B_6 15 mg, B_{12} 15 mcg, C 150 mg, folic acid 0.1 mg, Ca, Cu, Mn, Zn, K, iodide, biotin, betaine, PABA, choline bitartrate, inositol, lecithin, hesperidin, rutin, bioflavonoids,

sorbitol, aspartame, citrus flavor/Tab. Bot. 60s. *otc.*
Use: Vitamin/mineral supplement.

Sunstick. (Rydelle) Lip and face protectant containing digalloyl trioleate 2.5% in emollient base. Plas. swivel container 0.14 oz. *otc.*
Use: Prevention & relief of chapping and sunburning of lips.

SU-101.
Use: Malignant glioma. [Orphan drug]

Supac. (Mission) Acetaminophen 160 mg, aspirin 230 mg, caffeine 33 mg, calcium gluconate 60 mg/Tab. Bot. 100s. *otc.*
Use: Analgesic.

Super Aytinal Tablets. (Walgreen) Vitamins A 7000 IU, B_1 5 mg, B_2 5 mg, B_5 10 mg, B_6 3 mg, B_{12} 9 mcg, C 90 mg, pantothenic acid 10 mg, D 400 IU, E 30 IU, niacin 30 mg, biotin 55 mcg, folic acid 0.4 mg, iron 30 mg, calcium 162 mg, P 125 mg, iodine 150 mcg, copper 3 mg, manganese 7.5 mg, magnesium 100 mg, potassium 7.7 mg, zinc 24 mg, Cl 7 mg, chromium 15 mcg, selenium 15 mcg, choline bitartrate 1000 mcg, inositol 1000 mcg, PABA 1000 mcg, rutin 1000 mcg, yeast 12 mg. Bot. 50s, 100s, 365s. *otc.*
Use: Vitamin/mineral supplement.

Super-B. (Towne) Vitamins B_1 50 mg, B_2 20 mg, B_6 5 mg, B_{12} 15 mcg, C 300 mg, liver dessic. 100 mg, dried yeast 100 mg, niacinamide 25 mg, Ca pantothenate 5 mg, iron 10 mg/Captab. Bot. 50s, 100s, 150s, 250s. *otc.*
Use: Vitamin/mineral supplement.

Super Calicaps M-Z. (Nion) Calcium 1200 mg, magnesium 400 mg, zinc 15 mg, Vitamins A 5000 IU, Vitamins D 400 IU, selenium 15 mcg/3 Tabs. Bot. 90s. *otc.*
Use: Vitamin/mineral supplement.

Super Calcium 1200. (Schiff) Calcium carbonate 1512 mg (600 mg calcium)/Cap. Bot. 60s, 120s. *otc.*
Use: Calcium supplement.

Super Citro Cee. (Marlyn) Lemon bioflavonoids 500 mg, rutin 50 mg, ascorbic acid 500 mg, rosehips powder. 500 mg. Tab. Bot. 50s, 100s, 200s. *otc.*
Use: Vitamin supplement.

Super Complex C-500. (Approved Pharmaceutic) Citrus hesperidin complex 25 mg, citrus bioflavonoid complex 100 mg, rutin 50 mg, ascorbic acid 500 mg, rose hips 100 mg, acerola, green pepper & black currant concentrate, sodium free. Tab. Bot. 100s. *otc.*

Use: Vitamin supplement.

Super D. (Pharmacia & Upjohn) Vitamins A 10,000 IU, D 400 IU/Perle. Bot. 100s. *otc.*
Use: Vitamin supplement.

Superdophilus. (Natren) *Lactobacillus acidophilus* strain DDS-1.2 billion/Gm Pow. 37.5 g, 75 g, 135 g. *otc.*
Use: Antidiarrheal, nutritional supplement.

Super D Perles. (Pharmacia & Upjohn) Vitamins A 10,000 IU, D 400 IU/Cap. Bot. 100s. *otc.*
Use: Vitamins A and D.

Super EPA. (Advanced Nutritional Tech.) Omega-3 polyunsaturated fatty acids 1200 mg/Cap. containing EPA 360 mg, DHA 240 mg. Bot. 60s, 90s. *otc.*
Use: Nutritional supplement.

Superepa 2000. (Advanced Nutritional) EPA 563 mg, DHA 312 mg, vitamin E 20 IU. Cap. Bot. 30s, 60s, 90s. *otc.*
Use: Fish oil.

Supere-Pect. (Barth's) Alpha tocopherol 400 IU, apple pectin 100 mg/Cap. Bot. 50s, 100s, 250s. *otc.*
Use: Nutritional supplement.

Super Hi Potency. (Nion) Vitamins A 10,000 IU, D 400 IU, E 150 IU, B_1 75 mg, B_2 75 mg, B_3 75 mg, B_5 75 mg, B_6 75 mg, B_{12} 75 mcg, C 250 mg, folic acid 0.4 mg, Zn 15 mg, betaine, biotin 75 mcg, Ca, Fe, hesperidin, I, K, Mg, Mn, Se/Tab. Bot. 100s. *otc.*
Use: Vitamin/mineral supplement.

Super Hydramin Protein Powder. (Nion) Protein 41%, carbohydrate 21.8%, fat 1% in powder form. Cans 1 lb. *otc.*
Use: Nutritional supplement.

superinone. Tyloxapol.
See: Triton WR-1339 (Rohm & Haas).

Super Nutri-Vites. (Faraday) Vitamins A 36,000 IU, D 400 IU, B_1 25 mg, B_2 25 mg, B_6 50 mg, B_{12} 50 mcg, niacinamide 50 mg, Ca pantothenate 12.5 mg, choline bitartrate 150 mg, inositol 150 mg, betaine HCl 25 mg, PABA 15 mg, glutamic acid 25 mg, dessic. liver 50 mg, C 150 mg, E 12.5 IU, Mn gluconate 6.15 mg, bone meal 162 mg, Fe gluconate 50 mg, Cu gluconate 0.25 mg, Zn gluconate 2.2 mg, K iodide 0.1 mg, Ca 53.3 mg, P 24.3 mg, Mg gluconate 7.2 mg/Protein Coated Tab. Bot. 60s, 100s. *otc.*
Use: Vitamin/mineral supplement.

superoxide dismutase (human, recombinant human).
Use: Protection of donor organ tissue. [Orphan drug]

Super Plenamins Multiple Vitamins and Minerals. (Rexall) Vitamins A 8000 IU, D_2 400 IU, Vitamins B_1 2.5 mg, B_2 2.5 mg, C 75 mg, niacinamide 20 mg, B_6 1 mg, B_{12} 3 mcg, biotin 20 mcg, E 10 IU, pantothenic acid 3 mg, liver conc. 100 mg, iron 30 mg, calcium 75 mg, phosphorus 58 mg, iodine 0.15 mg, copper 0.75 mg, manganese 1.25 mg, magnesium 10 mg, zinc 1 mg/Tab. Bot. 36s, 72s, 144s, 288s, 365s. *otc.*
Use: Vitamin/mineral supplement.

Superplex T. (Major) Vitamins B_1 15 mg, B_2 10 mg, B_3 100 mg, B_5 20 mg, B_6 5 mg, B_{12} 10 mcg, C 500 mg/Tab. Bot. 100s. *otc.*
Use: Vitamin supplement.

Super Poli-Grip/Wernet's Cream. (Block) Carboxymethylcellulose gum, ethylene oxide polymer, petrolatum-mineral oil base. Tube 0.7, 1.4, 2.4 oz. *otc.*
Use: Denture adhesive cream.

Super Quints-50. (Freeda) Vitamins B_1 50 mg, B_2 50 mg, B_3 50 mg, B_5 50 mg, B_6 50 mg, B_{12} 50 mcg, folic acid 0.4 mg, PABA 30 mg, d-biotin 50 mcg, inositol 50 mg. Tab. Bot. 100s, 250s, 500s. *otc.*
Use: Vitamin supplement.

Super Shade SPF-25. (Schering-Plough) Ethylhexyl p-methoxycinnamate, padimate O oxybenzone, SPF-25. Bot. 4 fl. oz. *otc.*
Use: Sunscreen.

Super Shade Sunblock Stick SPF-25. (Schering-Plough) Ethylhexyl p-methoxycinnamate, oxybenzone, padimate O in stick, SPF-25. Tube 0.43 oz. *otc.*
Use: Sunscreen.

Super Stress. (Towne) Vitamins C 600 mg, E 30 IU B_1 15 mg, B_2 15 mg, niacin 100 mg, B_6 5 mg, B_{12} 12 mcg, pantothenic acid 20 mg/Tab. Bot. 60s. *otc.*
Use: Vitamin supplement.

Super Thera 46. (Faraday) Vitamin A 36,000 IU, essential vitamins, minerals, amino acids w/nutrient factors, digestive enzymes, B_{12} 25 mcg/Tab. Bot. 100s.

Super Troche. (Weeks & Leo) Benzocaine 5 mg, cetalkonium Cl 1 mg/lozenge. Bot. 15s, 30s. *otc.*
Use: Relief of minor sore throat & irritation.

Super Troche Plus. (Weeks & Leo) Benzocaine 10 mg, cetalkonium Cl. 2 mg/loz. Bot. 12s. *otc.*
Use: Relief of minor sore throat & irritation.

Super-T with Zinc. (Towne) Vitamins A 10,000 IU, D 400 IU, E 15 IU, C 200 mg, B_1 10 mg, B_2 10 mg, B_6 5 mg, B_{12} 6 mcg, niacinamide 50 mg, iron 18 mg, iodine 0.1 mg, copper 2 mg, manganese 1 mg, zinc 15 mg/Cap. Bot. 130s. *otc.*
Use: Vitamin/mineral supplement.

Supervim Tablets. (U.S. Ethicals) Vitamins and minerals. Bot. 100s.
Use: Multiple vitamin/mineral supplement.

Super Wernet's Powder. (Block) Carboxymethylcellulose gum, ethylene oxide polymer. Bot. 0.63, 1.75, 3.55 oz. *otc.*
Use: Denture adhesive.

Suplena. (Ross) A vanilla flavored liquid containing 29.6 g protein, 252.5 g carbohydrates, 95 g fat per liter. With appropriate vitamins and minerals. Cans 240 ml. *otc.*
Use: Nutritional therapy for people with renal conditions.

Suplical. (Parke-Davis Prods) Calcium 600 mg/Square. Bot. 30s, 60s. *otc.*
Use: Calcium supplement.

Suppap-120. (Raway) Acetaminophen 120 mg/Supp. 12s, 50s, 100s, 500s, 1000s. *otc.*
Use: Analgesic.

Suppap-650. (Raway) Acetaminophen 650 mg/Supp. 50s, 100s, 500s, 1000s. *otc.*
Use: Analgesic.

Supprelin. (Roberts) Histrelin acetate 200 mcg, 300 mcg or 600 mcg/ml. Vials 0.6 ml. *Rx.*
Use: Precocious puberty.

Suppress. (Ferndale) Dextromethorphan HBr 7.5 mg/loz. 1000s. *otc.*
Use: Antitussive.

Supra Min. (Towne) Vitamins A 10,000 IU, D 400 IU, E 30 IU, C 250 mg, folic acid 0.4 mg, B_1 10 mg, B_2 10 mg, niacin 100 mg, B_6 5 mg, B_{12} 6 mcg, pantothenic acid 20 mg, iodine 150 mcg, iron 100 mg, magnesium 2 mg, copper 20 mg, manganese 1.25 mg/Tab. Bot. 130s. *otc.*
Use: Vitamin/mineral supplement.

Suprane. (Ohmeda) Desflurane. 240 ml. Bot. *Rx.*
Use: General anesthetic.

Suprarenal. Dried, partially defatted and powdered adrenal gland of cattle, sheep or swine.

Suprax. (Lederle) Cefixime **Tab.:** 200 mg, Bot. 100s or 400 mg, 50s, 100s. **Pow.:**

(strawberry flavor) 100 mg/5 ml. 50 ml, 100 ml. *Rx.*
Use: Anti-infective, cephalosporin.

Suprazine Tabs. (Major) Trifluoperazine 1 mg/Tab. Bot. 100s, 250s, 1000s; 2 mg/Tab. Bot. 100s, 250s, 1000s, UD 100s; 5 mg/Tab. Bot. 100s, 250s, 1000s; 10 mg/Tab. Bot. 100s, 250s, 1000s. *Rx.*
Use: Tranquilizer.

Suprins. (Towne) Vitamins A palmitate 10,000 IU, D 400 IU, B_1 10 mg, B_2 10 mg, B_6 5 mg, B_{12} 6 mcg, C 250 mg, calcium pantothenate 20 mg, niacinamide 100 mg, biotin 25 mcg, vitamins E 15 IU, calcium 103 mg, phosphorus 80 mg, iron 10 mg, iodine 0.1 mg, copper 1.0 mg, zinc 20 mg, manganese 1.25 mg/Captab. Bot. 100s. *otc.*
Use: Vitamin/mineral supplement.

•**suproclone.** (SUH-pro-klone) USAN.
Use: Sedative, hypnotic.

•**suprofen,** (sue-PRO-fen) U.S.P. 23.
Use: Anti-inflammatory.
See: Profenal (Alcon).

Suramin Sodium.

Surbex Filmtab. (Abbott) B_1 6 mg, B_2 6 mg, B_3 30 mg, B_6 2.5 mg, B_5 10 mg, B_{12} 5 mcg/Filmtab. Bot. 100s. *otc.*
Use: Vitamin/mineral supplement.
W/Vitamins C. (Abbott) Same as Surbex Filmtab, except vitamins C 250 mg/Filmtab. Bot. 100s, 500s.

Surbex-T Filmtab. (Abbott) Vitamins B_1 15 mg, B_2 10 mg, B_3 100 mg, B_6 5 mg, B_{12} 10 mcg, B_5 20 mg, C 500 mg/Filmtab. Bot. 100s. *otc.*
Use: Vitamin/mineral supplement.

Surbex with C Filmtabs. (Abbott) Vitamins B_1 6 mg, B_2 6 mg, B_3 30 mg, B_5 10 mg, B_6 2.5 mg, B_{12} 5 mg, C 500 mg/Film coated. Tab. Bot. 100s. *otc.*
Use: Vitamin supplement.

Surbex-750 with Iron. (Abbott) Vitamins B_1 15 mg, B_2 15 mg, B_6 25 mg, B_{12} 12 mcg, C 750 mg, B_5 20 mg, E 30 IU, B_3 100 mg, iron 27 mg, folic acid 0.4 mg/Tab. Bot. 50s. *otc.*
Use: Vitamin/mineral supplement.

Surbex-750 with Zinc. (Abbott) B_1 15 mg, B_2 15 mg, B_6 20 mg, B_{12} 12 mcg, C 750 mg, E 30 IU, B_5 20 mg, niacin 100 mg, folic acid 0.4 mg, zinc 22.5 mg/Tab. Bot. 50s. *otc.*
Use: Vitamin/mineral supplement.

Surbu-Gen-T. (Goldline) Vitamins B_1 15 mg, B_2 10 mg, B_3 100 mg, B_5 20 mg, B_6 5 mg, B_{12} 10 mcg, C 500 mg/Tab. Bot. 100s. *otc.*

Use: Vitamin supplement.

Surecell Chlamydia Test. (Kodak) Monoclonal antibody-based ELISA (enzyme linked immunosorbent assay) to detect lipopolysaccharide antigen from the cell wall of *Chlamydia trachomatis psittaci.* Kit 10s, 25s, 100s.
Use: Diagnostic aid.

Surecell HCG-Urine Test. (Kodak) Polyclonal/monoclonal antibody sandwich-based ELISA to detect human chorionic gonadotropin in urine. Kit 10s, 25s, 100s.
Use: Diagnostic aid.

Surecell Herpes (HSV) Test. (Kodak) Monoclonal antibody-based ELISA to detect HSV 1 & 2 antigens from lesions. Kit 10s, 25s.
Use: Diagnostic aid.

Surecell Strep A Test. (Kodak) ELISA to detect Group A streptococci. Kit 10s, 25s, 100s.
Use: Diagnostic aid.

Surelac. (Caraco) 3000 FCC lactase units, sorbitol or mannitol. Chew. Tab. Bot. 60s. *otc.*
Use: Nutritional supplement.

surface active extract of saline lavage of bovine lungs. *Rx.*
Use: Respiratory failure in preterm infants. [Orphan drug]

surfactant, natural lung.
Use: Surfactant replacement therapy in neonatal respiratory distress syndrome.
See: Survanta (Ross Laboratories).

surfactant, synthetic lung.
Use: Surfactant replacement therapy in neonatal respiratory distress syndrome.
See: Exosurf Neonatal (Glaxo Wellcome).

Surfak. (Pharmacia & Upjohn) Docusate calcium. 50 mg: 30s, 100s. 240 mg: 30s, 100s, 500s, UD 100s. Cap. *otc.*
Use: Laxative.

•**surfilcon a.** (SER-FILL-kahn A) USAN.
Use: Hydrophilic contact lens material.

Surfol Post Immersion Bath Oil. (Stiefel) Mineral oil, isopropyl myristate, isostearic acid, PEG-40, sorbitan peroleate. Bot. 8 oz. *otc.*
Use: Post-immersion bath oil for dry skin.

•**surfomer.** (SER-foe-mer) USAN.
Use: Hypolipidemic.

Surgasoap. (Wade) Castile vegetable oils. Bot. qt., gal. *otc.*

Use: Surgical soap.

Surgel. (Ulmer) Propylene glycol, glycerin. Gel. 120 ml, 240 ml, 480 ml, gal. *otc.*
Use: Lubricant.

Surgel Liquid. (Ulmer) Patient lubricant fluid. Bot. 4 oz, 8 oz, gal.
Use: Lubricant.

•**surgibone.** (SER-jih-bone) USAN. Bone and cartilage obtained from bovine embryos and young calves.
Use: Prosthetic aid (internal bone splint).
See: Unilab Surgibone (Unilab).

Surgical Simplex P. (Howmedica) Methyl methacrylate 20 ml poly 6.7 g, methyl methacrylate-styrene copolymer 33.3 g. **Pow.** 40 g. **Liq.** 20 ml.
Use: Bone cement.

Surgical Simplex P Radiopaque. (Howmedica) Methyl methacrylate 20 ml, poly 6 g, methyl methacrylate-styrene copolymer 30 g. **Pow.** 40 g. **Liq.** 20 ml.
Use: Bone cement.

Surgicel. (Johnson & Johnson) Sterile absorbable knitted fabric prepared by controlled oxidation of regenerated cellulose. Sterile strips 2"×14", 4"×8", 2"×3", 0.5"×2". Surgical Nu-knit: 1"×1", 3"×4", 6"×9". 1s.
Use: Absorbable hemostat.

Surgidine. (Continental) Iodine 0.8% in iodine complex. Germicide. Bot. 8 oz, gal. Foot operated dispenser 8 oz, gal. *otc.*
Use: Antiseptic.

Surgi-Kleen. (Sween) Bot. 2 oz, 8 oz, 16 oz, 21 oz, gal., 5 gal., 30 gal., 55 gal.
Use: Skin cleanser and shampoo.

Surgilube. (Day-Baldwin) Sterile-bacteriostatic. Foilpac: 3 g, 5 g, Tube: 5 g, 2 oz, 4.5 oz.
Use: Surgical lubricant.

Surgilube. (Fougera) Sterile surgical lubricant. Foilpac: 3 g, 5 g; Tube 5 g, 2 oz, 4.25 oz.
Use: Sterile surgical lubricant.

•**suricainide maleate.** (ser-ih-CANE-ide) USAN.
Use: Cardiac depressant (antiarrhythmic).

•**suritozole.** (suh-RIH-tah-ZOLE) USAN.
Use: Antidepressant.

Surmontil. (Wyeth-Ayerst) Trimipramine maleate 25 mg, 50 mg or 100 mg/Cap. Bot. 100s. Redipaks. *Rx.*
Use: Antidepressant.

surofene. Hexachlorophene.

•**suronacrine maleate.** (SUE-row-NAH-kreen) USAN.
Use: Cholinergic, cholinesterase inhibitor.

Survanta. (Ross) Beractant 25 mg/ml. Inj. Vial 8 ml. *Rx.*
Use: Lung surfactant.

Susano Elixir. (Halsey) Phenobarbital 0.25 gr, hyoscyamine sulfate 0.1037 mg, atropine sulfate 0.0194 mg, scopolamine HBr 0.0065 mg/5 ml. 23% alcohol, tartrazine. Bot. 16 oz, gal. *Rx.*
Use: Sedative, antispasmodic.

Suspen. (Circle) Penicillin V potassium 250 mg/5 ml. Bot. 100 ml. *Rx.*
Use: Anti-infective, penicillin.

Sus-Phrine Injection. (Forest) Epinephrine 1:200 Amp. 0.3 ml, 12s, 25s. Multiple Dose Vial 5 ml, 1s. *Rx.*
Use: Bronchial asthma.

sus scrofa linne var domesticus. W/Proteolytic enzyme, autolyzed.
See: Saromide Injection, Vial (Saron).

Sustacal Basic. (Bristol-Myers) A vanilla, strawberry or chocolate flavored liquid containing 36.6 g protein, 34.6 g fat, 145.8 g carbohydrate, 833 mg Na, 1583 mg K/L. 1.04 Cal/ml, with appropriate vitamin and mineral levels to meet 100% of the US RDAs. Liq. Can 240 ml. *otc.*
Use: Nutritional supplement.

Sustacal HC. (Bristol-Myers) High calorie nutritionally complete food. Protein 16%, fat 34%, carbohydrate 50%. Cans 8 oz. Vanilla, chocolate or eggnog. *otc.*
Use: Nutritional supplement.

Sustacal Plus. (Bristol-Myers) A vanilla, eggnog or chocolate flavored liquid containing 61 g protein, 58 g fat, 190 g carbohydrate, 15.2 mg Fe, 850 mg Na, 1480 mg K, 1520 cal/L, with appropriate vitamin and mineral levels to meet 100% of the US RDAs. Liq. Bot. 237 ml, 960 ml. *otc.*
Use: Nutritional supplement.

Sustacal Powder. (Bristol-Myers) Caloric distribution and nutritional value when added to milk are similar to that of Sustacal liquid except lactose. Contains vanilla: Pow. 1.9 oz. packets 4's, 1 lb. can; Chocolate 1.9 oz. packets 4s. *otc.*
Use: Nutritional supplement.

Sustacal Pudding. (Bristol-Myers) Ready-to-eat fortified pudding containing at least 15% of the US RDAs for protein, vitamins and minerals, in a 240 calorie serving. As a % of the calories, protein 11%, fat 36%, carbohydrate

53%. Flavors: chocolate, vanilla, and butterscotch. Tins, 5 oz, 110 oz. *otc.*
Use: Nutritional supplement.

Sustagen. (Bristol-Myers) High-calorie, high-protein supplement containing as a % of the calories, 24% protein, 8% fat, 68% carbohydrate. Contains all known essential vitamins and minerals. Prepared from nonfat milk, corn syrup solids, powdered whole milk, calcium caseinate, and dextrose. Vanilla: Can 1 lb, 5 lb. Chocolate: Can 1 lb. *otc.*
Use: Nutritional supplement.

Sustaire. (Pfizer Laboratories) Theophylline 100 mg, 300 mg/Sust. Released Tab. Bot. 100s. *Rx.*
Use: Long-acting relief of reversible bronchospasm.

•**sutilains,** U.S.P. 23.
Use: Enzyme (proteolytic).

•**suture, absorbable surgical,** U.S.P. 23.
Use: Surgical aid.

•**suture, nonabsorbable surgical,** U.S.P. 23.
Use: Surgical aid.

Suvaplex Tablet. (Tennessee Pharmaceutic) Vitamins A 5000 IU, D 500 IU, B_1 2.5 mg, B_2 2.5 mg, B_6 0.5 mg, B_{12} 1 mcg, C 37.5 mg, Ca pantothenate 5 mg, niacinamide 20 mg, folic acid 0.1 mg/Tab. Bot. 100s. *otc.*
Use: Vitamin/mineral supplement.

•**suxemerid sulfate.** (sux-EM-er-rid) USAN.
Use: Antitussive.

swamp root. Compound of various organic roots in an alcohol base.
Use: Diuretic to the kidney.

Sween-A-Peel. (Sween) Wafer 4×4. Box 5s, 20s; Sheets 1212. Box 2s, 12s.
Use: Wafer skin protectant.

Sween Cream. (Sween) Vitamin A and D cream. Tube 0.5 oz, 2 oz, 5 oz. Jar 2 oz, 9 oz. *otc.*
Use: Skin treatment.

Sween Kind Lotion. (Sween) Bot. 21 oz, gal.
Use: Lotion skin cleaner.

Sween Prep. (Sween) Box wipes 54s. Dab-o-matic 2 oz. Spray top 4 oz.
Use: Medicated skin barrier.

Sween Soft Touch. (Sween) Bot. 2 oz, 16 oz, 21 oz, 32 oz, 1 gal., 5 gal.
Use: Medicated, antimicrobial lotion skin cleanser.

Sweeta. (Squibb Mark) Saccharin sodium and sorbitol. Bot. 24 ml, 2 oz, 4 oz. *otc.*
Use: Sweetening Agent.

Sweetaste. (Purepac) Saccharin 0.25 g, 0.5 g, 1 g/Tab. w/Sodium bicarbonate. Bot. 1000s. *otc.*
Use: Sugar substitute.

sweetening agents.
See: Ril-Sweet (Schering-Plough).
Saccharin, Preps. (Various Mfr.).
Sucaryl, Preps. (Abbott).
Sweetaste, Tab. (Purepac).

Sweet'n Fresh Clotrimazole-7. (Nutra-Max Products) **Cream:** Clotrimazole 1%, benzyl and cetostearyl alcohol. 45 g. **Vaginal inserts:** Clotrimazole 100 mg. 7s. *otc.*
Use: Antifungal agent, vaginal.

Swim Ear. (Fougera) 2.75% boric acid in isopropyl alcohol. Bot. 1 oz. *otc.*
Use: Prevention of external otitis.

Swiss Kriss. (Modern) Senna leaves, herbs. Coarse cut mixture. Can 1.5 oz, 3.25 oz, Tab. 24s, 120s, 250s. *otc.*
Use: Laxative.

Syllact. (Wallace) Psyllium seed husks 3.3 g/tsp., saccharin. Pow. Bot. 11 oz. *otc.*
Use: Laxative.

Syllamalt. (Wallace) Malt soup extract 4 g, psyllium seed husks 3 g, calories/rounded tsp 13. Pow. 300 g. *otc.*
Use: Laxative.

•**symclosene.** (SIM-kloe-seen) USAN. Trichloroisocyanuric acid.
Use: Anti-infective, topical.

•**symetine hydrochloride.** (SIM-eh-teen) USAN.
Use: Antiamebic.

Symmetrel. (DuPont Merck) Amantadine HCl. 50 mg/5 ml. Syr. Bot. pt. *Rx.*
Use: Antiviral agent, treatment of Parkinson's disease, treatment of drug-induced extrapyramidal symptoms.

sympatholytic agents.
See: Adrenergic-Blocking Agents.
D.H.E. 45, Amp. (Sandoz).
Dibenzyline, Cap. (SK-Beecham).
Dihydroergotamine.
Ergotamine Tartrate.
Gynergen, Amp., Tab. (Sandoz).

sympathomimetic agents.
See: Adrenalin (Parke-Davis).
Adrenergic agents.
Aerolate Sr. & Jr., Cap. (Fleming).
Aerolone Cpd. (Lilly).
Afrin, Preps. (Schering Plough).
Miles Diagnosticec, Enseal, Pulvule (Lilly).
Aramine, Amp., Vial (Merck).
Arlidin HCl, Tab. (Rhone-Poulenc Rorer).

Brethine, Amp., Tab (Novartis).
Bronkephrine, Amp., (Sanofi Winthrop).
Bronkometer (Sanofi Winthrop).
Bronkosol Soln. (Sanofi Winthrop).
Delcobese, Tab. (Delco).
Demazin, Tab., Syr. (Schering Plough).
Desoxyn, Gradumet, Tab. (Abbott).
Dexamyl Tab. (SK-Beecham).
Dexedrine, Elix., Spansule, Tab. (SK-Beecham).
D-Feda, Cap., Liq. (Dooner).
Didrex, Liq., Tab. (Pharmacia & Upjohn).
Dipivefrin HCl, Soln. (Schein).
Duovent, Tab. (3M).
Ectasule Minus Sr. & Jr., Cap. (Fleming).
Ectasule III, Cap. (Fleming).
Ephedrine preps.
Epinephrine salts.
Extendryl, Cap., Syr., Tab. (Fleming).
Fedrazil, Tab. (Glaxo Wellcome).
Fiogesic, Tab. (Sandoz).
Histabid, Cap. (Glaxo).
Isoephedrine HCl.
Isuprel HCl, Preps. (Sanofi Winthrop).
Levophed Bitartrate, Amp. (Sanofi Winthrop).
Metaproterenol Sulfate (Various Mfr.).
Napril, Cap. (Hoechst Marion Roussel).
Neo-Synephrine HCl, Preps. (Sanofi Winthrop).
Nolamine, Tab. (Carnrick).
Norisodrine Sulfate, Soln. (Abbott).
Obedrin-LA, Tab. (SK-Beecham).
Obetrol, Tab. (Obetrol).
Orthoxine, Orthoxine & Aminophylline (Pharmacia & Upjohn).
Orthoxine HCl, Tab., Syr. (Pharmacia & Upjohn).
Otrivin, Soln., Spray (Novartis).
Phenylephrine HCl, Preps.
Phenylpropanolamine HCl.
Pseudoephedrine HCl, Syr., Tab.
Rondec DSC & T (Ross).
Slo-Fedrin & Slo-Fedrin A (Dooner).
Sudafed, Tab., Syr. (Glaxo Wellcome).
Triaminic, Prep. (Sandoz).
Triaminicol, Syr. (Sandoz).
Tussagesic, Susp., Tab. (Sandoz).
Tussaminic, Tab. (Sandoz).
Ursinus, Tab. (Sandoz).
Vasoxyl HCl, Amp., Vial (Glaxo Wellcome).
Wyamine Sulfate, Amp., Vial (Wyeth-Ayerst).
Syna-Clear. (Pruvo) Decongestant plus Vitamins C. 25 mg/Tab. Bot. 12s, 30s.

Use: Decongestant.
Synacol CF. (Roberts) Dextromethorphan HBr 15 mg, guiafenesin 200 mg/Tab. Bot. UD 8s, 500s. *otc.*
Use: Antitussive, expectorant.
Synacort. (Syntex) Hydrocortisone cream. **1%:** Tube 15 g, 30 g, 60 g. **2.5%:** Tube 30 g. *Rx.*
Use: Corticosteroid, topical.
Synalar. (Syntex) Fluocinolone acetonide. **Cream: 0.01%** Tube 15 g, 30 g, 45 g, 60 g, 120 g. Jar 425 g. **0.025%** Tube 15 g, 30 g, 60 g, 120 g. Jar 425 g. **Oint.: 0.025%:** Tube 15 g, 30 g, 60 g, 120 g. Jar 425 g. **Soln. 0.01%:** Bot. 20 ml, 60 ml. *Rx.*
Use: Corticosteroid, topical.
Synalar-HP Cream. (Syntex) Fluocinolone acetonide 0.2% in water-washable aqueous base. Tube 12 g. *Rx.*
Use: Corticosteroid, topical.
Synalgos-DC Capsules. (Wyeth-Ayerst) Dihydrocodeine bitartrate 16 mg, aspirin 356.4 mg, caffeine 30 mg/Cap. Bot. 100s, 500s. *c-III.*
Use: Analgesic, relaxant.
Synapp-R. (Halsey) Acetaminophen 325 mg, phenylpropanolamine HCl 25 mg, phenyltoloxamine citrate 22 mg/Tab. Bot. 40s. *otc.*
Use: Analgesic, decongestant.
Synarel. (Syntex) Nafarelin acetate 2 mg/ml (as nafarelin base). Nasal solution. Bottle 10 ml with metered pump spray. *Rx.*
Use: Treatment of endometriosis.
Synatuss-One. (Freeport) Guaifenesin 100 mg, dextromethorphan HBr. 15 mg, alcohol 1.4%/5 ml. Bot. 4 oz. *otc.*
Use: Antitussive.
Syncaine.
See: Procaine Hydrochloride, Inj., Tab. (Various Mfr.).
Syncort.
See: Desoxycorticosterone Acetate, Inj., Pellets (Various Mfr.).
Syncortyl.
See: Desoxycorticosterone Acetate, Inj., Pellets (Various Mfr.).
Syndolor Capsules. (Knight) Bot. 100s, 1000s.
Use: Analgesic.
Synemol. (Syntex) Fluocinolone acetonide 0.025% in water-washable aqueous emollient base. Tube 15 g, 30 g, 60 g, 120 g. *Rx.*
Use: Corticosteroid, topical.
synkonin.
See: Hydrocodone (Various Mfr.).

Synophylate. (Schwarz Pharma) Theophylline sodium glycinate. **Elix.:** Theophylline 165 mg/15 ml w/alcohol 20%. Bot. pt, gal. **Tab.:** Theophylline 165 mg/Tab. Bot. 100s, 1000s. *Rx.*
Use: Bronchodilator.

Synophylate-GG. (Schwarz Pharma) Theophylline sodium glycinate 300 mg, guaifenesin 100 mg. **Syr.** 10% alcohol, pt, gal.
Use: Bronchodilator.

Syn-Rx. (Adams) **AM:** Pseudoephedrine HCl 60 mg, guiafenesin 600 mg/CR Tab. Bot. 28s. **PM:** Guiafenesin 600 mg/CR Tab. Bot. 28s. In 14-day treatment regimen of 56 tablets. *Rx.*
Use: Decongestant, expectorant.

Synsorb PK.
Use: Verocytotoxogenic *E. coli* infections. [Orphan drug]

Synthaloids. (Buffington) Benzocaine, calcium-iodine complex/lozenge. Salt free. Bot. 100s, 1000s. Unit boxes 8s, 16s. Box 24s. Dispens-A-Kit 500s. Aidpaks 100s. Medipaks 200s. *otc.*
Use: Sore throat relief.

synthetic lung surfactant.
See: Exosurf Neonatal (Glaxo Wellcome).

synthoestrin.
See: Diethylstilbestrol, Preps. (Various Mfr.).

Synthroid. (Knoll) Sodium levothyroxine 25 mcg, 50 mcg, 75 mcg, 88 mcg, 100 mcg, 112 mcg, 125 mcg, 137 mcg, 150 mcg, 200 mcg, 300 mcg/Tab. Bot. 100s (all), 1000s (except 88 mcg, 200 mcg), UD 100s (except 25 mcg, 88 mcg, 200 mcg). *Rx.*
Use: Thyroid hormone.

Synthroid Injection. (Knoll Pharm) Lyophilized sodium levothyroxine 200 mcg or 500 mcg/vial. (100 mcg/ml when reconstituted.) Vial 10 ml. *Rx.*
Use: Thyroid hormone; myxedema coma.

Syntocinon Ampuls. (Sandoz) A sterile aqueous sol. of synthetic oxytocin w/ chlorobutanol 0.5%, alcohol 0.61%. Amp. (10 IU/ml) 1 ml. *Rx.*
Use: Induction, stimulation or management of labor and for prevention and control of postpartum hemorrhage.

Syntocinon Nasal Spray. (Sandoz) Syn. oxytocin 40 IU/ml w/exsic. sodium phosphate, citric acid, sodium Cl, glycerine, sorbitol, methyl & propylparaben, chlorobutanol 0.05% and Purified Water U.S.P. q.s. Squeeze bottle 2 ml & 5 ml. *Rx.*
Use: Initial milk let-down.

Syphilis (FTA-ABS) Fluoro Kit. (Clinical Sciences).
Use: Test for syphilis.

Syprine. (Merck) Trientine HCl 250 mg/Cap. Bot. 100s. *Rx.*
Use: Chelating agent.

Syracol. (Roberts) Phenylpropanolamine HCl 12.5 mg, dextromethorphan 7.5 mg Liq. 60 and 120 ml. *otc.*
Use: Decongestant, antitussive.

Syracol CF. (Roberts Med) Dextromethorphan HBr 15 mg, guaifenesin 200 mg/Tab. Bot. 500s. *otc.*
Use: Antitussive, expectorant.

Syroxine Tabs. (Major) Sodium levothyroxine 0.1 mg, 0.2 mg, or 0.3 mg/Tab. Bot. 100s, 250s, 1000s, UD 100s. (3 mg 1000s.). *Rx.*
Use: Thyroid hormone.

Syrpalta. (Emerson) Syr. containing comb. of fruit flavors. Bot. 1 pt, 1 gal.
Use: Vehicle for masking drug taste.

•**syrup,** N.F. 18.
Use: Pharmaceutic aid (flavor).

Syrvite. (Various Mfr.) Vitamins A 2500 IU, D 400 IU, E 15 mg, B_1 1.05 mg, B_2 1.2 mg, B_3 13.5 mg, B_6 1.05 mg, B_{12} 4.5 mcg, C 60 mg/5 ml Liq. Bot. 480 ml. *otc.*
Use: Vitamin supplement.

T

T-3 RIAbead. (Abbott Diagnostics) Test kit 50s, 100s.
Use: Radioimmunoassay for qualitative measurement of total circulating serum liothyronine.

T4.
See: levothyroxine sodium.

t4 endonuclease v, liposome encapsulated. *Rx.*
Use: Xeroderma pigmentosum. [Orphan drug]

T-4 RIA (PEG). (Abbott Diagnostics) Diagnostic kit 50s, 100s, 500s.
Use: For quantitative measurement of total circulating serum thyroxine.

t4, soluble, human recombinant. (Biogen) Phase I/II HIV.
Use: Antiviral.

TA. (Wampole-Zeus) Antithyroid antibodies by IFA. Test 48s.
Use: A useful tool in identifying two thyroid autoantibodies in a single test.

Tabasyn. (Freeport) Chlorpheniramine maleate 2 mg, phenylephrine HCl 10 mg, acetaminophen 5 gr, salicylamide 5 gr/Tab. Bot. 1000s. *Rx.*
Use: Antihistamine, decongestant, analgesic.

Tab-A-Vite. (Major) Vitamins A 5000 IU, D 400 IU, E 30 IU, B_1 1.5 mg, B_2 1.7 mg, B_3 20 mg, B_5 10 mg, B_6 2 mg, B_{12} 6 mcg, C 60 mg, FA 0.4 mg/Tab. Bot. 30s, 100s, 250s, 1000s, UD 100s. *otc.*
Use: Vitamin/mineral supplement.

Tab-A-Vite + Iron. (Major) Iron 18 mg, vitamins A 5000 IU, D 400 IU, E 30 IU, B_1 1.5 mg, B_2 1.7 mg, B_3 20 mg, B_5 10 mg, B_6 2 mg, B_{12} 6 mcg, C 60 mg, FA 0.4 mg, tartrazine/Tab. Bot. 100s. *otc.*
Use: Vitamin/mineral supplement.

TAC-3. (Allergan Herbert). Triamcinolone acetonide 3 mg/ml. Susp. Vial 5 ml. *Rx.*
Use: Corticosteroid.

TAC-40. (Parnell) Triamcinolone acetonide 40 mg/ml. Inj. Susp. Vial 5 ml. *Rx.*
Use: Corticosteroid.

Tacaryl. (Westwood Squibb) Methdilazine HCl **Tab.:** 8 mg/Tab. Bot. 100s. **Syr.:** 4 mg/5 ml. Bot. 16 oz. *Rx.*
Use: Antipruritic.

Tacaryl Chewable Tab. (Westwood Squibb) Methdilazine 3.6 mg/Tab. Bot. 100s. *Rx.*
Use: Antipruritic.

Tace. (Hoechst Marion Roussel) Chlorotrianisene 12 mg, 25 mg, 72 mg, tartra-

zine/Cap. (12 mg) Bot. 28s, 100s, 500s; (25 mg) Bot. 60s. (72 mg) Pkg. 48s. *Rx.*
Use: Estrogen therapy.

tachysterol.
See: Dihydrotachysterol, Tab. (Philips Roxane).

Tacitin. (Novartis) Under study. Benzoctamine, B.A.N.

•**taclamine hydrochloride.** (TACK-lah-meen) USAN.
Use: Tranquilizer (minor).

TA Cream. (C & M Pharmacal) Triamcinolone acetonide 0.025% or 0.05%. Jar 2 oz., 8 oz., 1 lb. *Rx.*
Use: Corticosteroid, topical.

•**tacrine hydrochloride.** (TACK-reen) USAN.
Use: Cognition adjuvant.
See: Cognex (Parke-Davis).

•**tacrolimus.** (tack-CROW-lih-muss) USAN.
Use: Immunosuppressant.
See: Prograf (Fujisawa).

Tagamet. (SK-Beecham) Cimetidine **FC Tab.: 200 mg** Bot. 100s. **300 mg** Bot. 100s, UD 100s. **400 mg** Bot. 60s, UD 100s. **800 mg** Bot. 30s, UD 100s. **Liq.:** 300 mg (as HCl)/5 ml 2.8% alcohol. Bot. 240 ml, UD 5 ml (10s). **Inj.: 300 mg** (as HCl)/2 ml with phenol in an aqueous solution. Single-dose vials, disp. syringes, ADD-Vantage vials and 8 ml vials. **300 mg** (as HCl) in 50 ml 0.9% sodium chloride. Single-dose container. *Rx.*
Use: Histamine H_2 antagonist.

Tagamet HB. (SmithKline Beecham) Cimetidine 100 mg/Tab. Bot. 16s, 32s, 64s. *otc.*
Use: Histamine H_2 antagonist.

Talacen. (Sanofi Winthrop) Pentazocine HCl 25 mg, acetaminophen 650 mg/Caplet. Bot. 100s. UD 250s. (10 × 25s). *c-iv.*
Use: Narcotic analgesic combination.

•**talampicillin hydrochloride.** (TAL-AM-pih-sill-in) USAN.
Use: Antibacterial.

•**talc,** U.S.P. 23. A native hydrous magnesium silicate.
Use: Dusting powder, pharmaceutic aid (tablet/capsule lubricant).

•**taleranol.** (TAL-ehr-ah-nole) USAN.
Use: Enzyme inhibitor (gonadotropin).

•**talisomycin.** (tal-EYE-so-MY-sin) USAN.
Formerly Tallysomycin A.
Use: Antineoplastic.

•**talmetacin.** (TAL-MET-ah-sin) USAN.

Use: Analgesic, antipyretic, anti-inflammatory.

• **talniflumate.** (tal-NYE-FLEW-mate) USAN.
Use: Anti-inflammatory, analgesic.

Taloin. (Pharmacia & Upjohn) Methylbenzethonium chloride, zinc oxide, calamine, eucalyptol in a water-repellent base. Oint.: Tube 2 oz.
Use: Skin protectant & antiseptic.

• **talopram hydrochloride.** (TAY-lowpram) USAN.
Use: Potentiator (catecholamine).

• **talosalate.** (TAL-oh-SAL-ate) USAN.
Use: Analgesic, anti-inflammatory.

• **talsaclidine fumarate.** (tale-SACK-lihdeen) USAN.
Use: Alzheimer's disease treatment (muscarinic M₁-agonist).

Talwin Compound. (Sanofi Winthrop) Pentazocine HCl 12.5 mg, asprin 325 mg/Tab. Bot. 100s. *c-iv.*
Use: Narcotic analgesic.

Talwin Injection. (Sanofi Winthrop) Pentazocine lactate injection. 30 mg/ml. **Vials:** 10 ml. **Uni-Amps:** 1, 1.5, 2 ml. **Uni-Nest amps:** 1 ml, 2 ml. **Carpujects:** 1, 1.5, 2 ml. *c-iv.*
Use: Narcotic analgesic.

Talwin NX. (Sanofi Winthrop) Pentazocine HCl 50 mg, naloxone 0.5 mg/Tab. Bot. 100s. UD 250s. *c-iv.*
Use: Narcotic analgesic.

Tambocor. (3M) Flecainide acetate 50 mg, 100 mg or 150 mg/Tab. Bot. 100s, UD 100s. *Rx.*
Use: Antiarrhythmic agent.

• **tametraline hydrochloride.** (tah-METrah-leen) USAN.
Use: Antidepressant.

Tamine S.R. (Geneva Pharm) Phenylpropanolamine HCl 15 mg, phenylephrine HCl 15 mg, brompheniramine maleate 12 mg. Sugar coated. Tab. Bot. 100s, 1000s. *Rx.*
Use: Antihistamine, decongestant.

tamoxifen. (Barr) Tamoxifen citrate 10 mg. Tab. Bot. 60s, 250s. *Rx.*
Use: Antineoplastic agent, antiestrogen.

• **tamoxifen citrate,** (ta-MOX-ih-fen) U.S.P. 23.
Use: Treatment of mammary carcinoma, antiestrogen.
See: Nolvadex, Tab. (Zeneca).
Tamoxifen, Tab. (Barr).

• **tampramine fumarate.** (TAM-prah-MEEN) USAN.
Use: Antidepressant.

Tamp-R-Tel. (Wyeth-Ayerst) A tamper-resistant package for narcotic drugs which includes the following:
Codeine phosphate 30 mg, 60 mg/1 ml.
Hydromorphone HCl 1 mg, 2 mg, 3 mg, 4 mg/Tubex.
Meperidine HCl 25 mg/ml and **Promethazine HCl** 25 mg/ml 2 ml.
Meperidine HCl 25 mg/1 ml, 50 mg/1 ml, 75 mg/1 ml, 100 mg/1 ml.
Morphine Sulfate 2 mg, 4 mg, 8 mg, 10 mg, 15 mg/1 ml.
Pentobarbital, Sodium 100 mg/2 ml.
Phenobarbital, Sodium 30 mg, 60 mg, 130 mg/1 ml.
Secobarbital, Sodium 100 mg/2 ml.

• **tamsulosin hydrochoride.** USAN.
Use: Benign prostatic hyperplasia therapy.

Tanac Gel. (Del Pharm) Dyclonine HCl 1%, allantoin 0.5%, petrolatum, lanolin. Tube. 9.45 g. *otc.*
Use: Cold sores, fever blisters, cracked lips.

Tanac Liquid. (Del Pharm) Benzalkonium Cl 0.12%, benzocaine 10%, tannic acid 6%. Saccharin. Bot. 13 ml. *otc.*
Use: Mouth sores, cold sores, fever blisters.

Tanac Roll-On. (Del Pharm) Tannic acid 6%, benzalkonium Cl 0.12%, benzocaine 5%. Bot. 8.8 ml. *otc.*
Use: Cold sores, fever blister, cracked lips.

Tanac Stick. (Del Pharm) Benzocaine 7.5%, tannic acid 6%, octyl dimethyl PABA 0.75%, allantoin 0.2%, benzalkonium Cl. 7.5%. Saccharin. Stick 0.1 oz. *otc.*
Use: Cold sores, fever blisters, dry lips.

Tanadex. (Del Pharm) Tannic acid 2.86%, phenol 1.05%, benzocaine 0.47%. Bot. 3 oz. *otc.*
Use: Throat gargle.

Tan-a-Dyne. (Archer-Taylor) Tannic acid compound w/iodine. Bot. 4 oz., pt., gal. *otc.*
Use: Swab and gargle concentrate.

Tanafed. (Horizon) Chlorpheniramine tannate 4.5 mg, pseudoephedrine tannate > 5 mg/5 ml. Susp. Bot. 20 ml, 118 ml, 473 ml. *Rx.*
Use: Decongestant, antihistamine.

tanbismuth.
See: Bismuth Tannate.

• **tandamine hydrochloride.** (TAN-dah-meen) USAN.
Use: Antidepressant.

● **tandospirone citrate.** (tan-DOE-spy-rone) USAN.
Use: Antianxiety.

● **tannic acid.** U.S.P. 23. Gallotannic acid. Glycerite. Tannin.
Use: Astringent.
See: Amertan, Oint. (Lilly).
 Zilactin Medicated, Gel (Zila Pharm).
W/Benzocaine, phenol, thymol iodide, ephedrine HCl, zinc oxide, peru balsam.
See: Hemocaine, Oint. (Roberts).
W/Bisacodyl.
See: Clysodrast, Packet (Pilkington Barnes Hind).
W/Boric acid, salicylic acid, isopropyl alcohol.
See: Sal Dex Boro, Liq. (Scrip).
W/Chlorobutanol, isopropyl alcohol.
See: Outgro, Soln. (Whitehall Robins).
W/Cyanocobalamin, zinc acetate, glutathione, phenol.
See: Depinar, Amp. (Centeon).
W/Merthiolate.
See: Amertan, Oint. (Lilly).
W/Salicylic acid, boric acid.
See: Tan-Bor-Sal, Liq. (Gordon).

Tannic Spray. (Gebauer) Tannic acid 4.5%, chlorobutanol 1.3%, menthol < 1%, benzocaine < 1%, propylene glycol 33%, ethanol 60%. Bot. 2 oz. & 4 oz. *otc.*
Use: Relief of sunburn and other minor burns.

Tanoral. (Pharmed) Phenylepherine tannate 25 mg, chlorpheniramine tannate 8 mg, pyrilamine tannate 25 mg/Tab. Bot. 100s. *Rx.*
Use: Decongestant, antihistamine.

tanphetamin.
See: Dextroamphetamine tannate.

Tao. (Roerig) Troleandomycin equivalent to 250 mg oleandomycin/Cap. Bot. 100s. *Rx.*
Use: Anti-infective.

Tapar Tablets. (Warner-Chilcott) Acetaminophen 325 mg/Tab. Bot. 100s. *otc.*
Use: Analgesic.

Tapazole. (Lilly) Methimazole. 1-methyl-2-mercaptoimidazole. 5 mg or 10 mg/Tab. Bot. 100s. *Rx.*
Use: Hyperthyroidism.

● **tape, adhesive,** U.S.P. 23.
Use: Surgical aid.

Ta-Poff. (Ulmer) Adhesive tape remover. Bot. 1 pt. Aerosol. Can 6 oz.

Tapuline. (Wesley) Activated attapulgite 600 mg, pectin 60 mg, homatropine methylbromide 0.5 mg/Chew. Tab. Bot. 100s, 1000s. *otc.*
Use: Antidiarrheal.

tar.
See: Coal Tar, Preps.

Tar Distillate. (Doak) Decolorized fractional distillate of crude coal tar. Each ml equiv. to 1 g whole crude coal tar. Bot. 2 oz., 16 oz.
Use: Active ingredient for dermatologic preparations.

Tarka. (Knoll) Trandolapril maleate 2 mg, verapamil HCl 180 mg or trandolapril 1 mg, verapamil HCl 240 or trandolapril 2 mg, verapamil 240 mg or trandolapril 4 mg, verapamil 240 mg/Tab. Bot. 30s. *Rx.*
Use: Antihypertensive.

Tarlene Lotion. (Medco Lab) Refined crude coal tar, salicylic acid, propylene glycol. Plastic Applicator Bot. 2 oz. *otc.*
Use: Seborrheic dermatitis.

Tarnphilic. (Medco Lab) Coal tar 1%, polysorbate 0.5% in aquaphilic base. Jar 16 oz. *otc.*
Use: Treatment of psoriasis, eczema, contact dermatitis.

Tarpaste. (Doak) Coal tar distilled 5% in zinc paste. Tube 1 oz, Jar 4 oz, w/ Hydrocortisone 0.5%. Tube 1 oz. *otc.*
Use: Dermatitis.

Tarsum Shampoo/Gel. (Summers) Coal tar 10%, salicylic acid 5% in shampoo base. Bot. 4 oz. *otc.*
Use: Dermatologic, shampoo for treatment of psoriasis, seborrheic dermatitis, chronic eczema and dermatitis of scalp.

tartar emetic.
See: Antimony Potassium Tartrate, U.S.P.

● **tartaric acid,** N.F. 18.
Use: Pharmaceutic aid (buffering agent).

Tashan, Skin Cream. (Block) Vitamin A palmitate, D_2, D-panthenol, Vit. E. Tube 1 oz. *otc.*
Use: Emollient.

● **tasosartan.** (tass-OH-sahr-tan) USAN.
Use: Antihypertensive.

Taste Function Test, Accusens T. (Westport Pharmaceuticals) Tastant 60 ml. Kit. 15 Bot.
Use: In vitro diagnostic aid.

taurocholic acid.
W/Pancreatin, pepsin.
See: Enzymet, Tabs. (Westerfield).

Ta-Verm. (Table Rock) Piperazine citrate 100 mg/ml Syr. Bot. 1 pt., 1 gal. Tabs. 500 mg Bot. 100s, 500s. *Rx.*
Use: Anthelmintic.

Tavilen Plus. (Table Rock) Liver solution 1 g, ferric pyrophosphate soluble 500 mg, vitamins B_1 6 mg, B_2 7.2 mg, B_6 3 mg, B_{12} 24 mcg, panthenol 3 mg, niacinamide 60 mg, l-lysine HCl 300 mg, 5% alcohol/ml. Bot. 16 oz., 1 gal. *otc.*
Use: Hematinic.

Tavist. (Sandoz) Clemastine fumarate 2.68 mg/Tab. Bot. 100s. *Rx.*
Use: Antihistamine.

Tavist Syrup. (Sandoz) Clemastine fumarate 0.67 mg/5 ml. Bot. 4 oz. *Rx.*
Use: Antihistamine.

Tavist-1 Tablets. (Sandoz) Clemastine fumarate 1.34 mg/Tab. Bot. 100s. *otc.*
Use: Antihistamine.

Tavist-D. (Sandoz) Clemastine fumarate 1.34 mg, phenylpropanolamine HCl 75 mg/SR Tab. Pkg. 8s, 16s. *otc.*
Use: Antihistamine, decongestant.

Taxol. (Bristol-Myers Squibb) Paclitaxel. 30 mg/5 ml. Inj. Single-dose vial. *Rx.*
Use: Antineoplastic.

Taxotere. (Rhone-Poulenc Rorer) 20 mg/0.5 ml single-dose vial. 80 mg/2 ml single-dose vial. Inj. with diluent.
Use: Antineoplastic (breast cancer).

•**tazadolene succinate.** (TAZZ-ah-DOE-leen) USAN.
Use: Analgesic.

•**tazarotene.** (tazz-AHR-oh-teen) USAN.
Use: Keratolytic.

Tazicef Injection. (Abbott) Ceftazidime. Vial: 1 g/20 ml, 2 g/60 ml or 6 g/100 ml. Piggyback: 1 g/100 ml or 2 g/100 ml. IM or IV Pharmacy Bulk: 6 g/100 ml. *Rx.*
Use: Anti-infective; cephalosporin.

Tazidime. (Lilly) Ceftazidime dry powder. 500 mg/10 ml Traypak 25s; 1 g/20 ml Traypak 10s; 1 g/100 ml; 2 g/50 ml Traypack 10s; 2 g/100 ml Traypack 10s; 6 g/100 ml Traypak 6s. ADD-Vantage Vials 1 g or 2 g Traypak 10s. *Rx.*
Use: Anti-infective, cephalosporin.

•**tazifylline hydrochloride.** (TAY-zih-FIH-lin) USAN.
Use: Antihistamine.

•**tazobactam.** (TAZZ-oh-BACK-tam) USAN.
Use: Inhibitor (beta-lactamase).

•**tazobactam sodium.** (TAZZ-oh-BACK-tam) USAN.
Use: Inhibitor (beta-lactamase).

tazobactam sodium/piperacillin sodium.
See: piperacillin sodium, sterile w/tazobactam.

•**tazofelone.** (TAY-zah-feh-lone) USAN.

Use: Suppressant (inflammatory bowel disease).

•**tazolol hydrochloride.** (TAY-zoe-lole) USAN.
Use: Cardiotonic.

TBA-Pred. (Keene) Prednisolone tebutate 10 mg/ml Susp. Vial 10 ml. *Rx.*
Use: Corticosteroid.

TC Suspension. (Rhone-Poulenc Rorer) Aluminum hydroxide 600 mg, magnesium hydroxide 300 mg/5 ml, sorbitol, sodium 0.8 mg Liq. In UD 15 ml, 30 ml (100s). *otc.*
Use: Antacid.

T/Derm Tar Emollient. (Neutrogena) Neutar solubilized coal tar extract 5% in oil base. Bot. 4 oz. *otc.*
Use: Antipsoriatic; antipruritic.

T-Dry. (Jones Medical) Pseudoephedrine HCl 120 mg, chlorpheniramine maleate 12 mg/Cap. S.R. Bot. 100s. *Rx.*
Use: Antihistamine, decongestant.

T-Dry Jr. (Jones Medical) Pseudoephedrine HCl 60 mg, chlorpheniramine maleate 4 mg/Cap. S.R. Bot. 100s. *otc.*
Use: Antihistamine, decongestant.

TDX Cortisol. (Abbott Diagnostics) Fluorescence polarization immunoassay for the quantitative determination of cortisol in serum, plasma or urine.
Use: Diagnostic aid.

TDX Thyroxine. (Abbott Diagnostics) Automated assay for quantitation of unsaturated thyroxine binding sites in serum or plasma.
Use: Diagnostic aid.

TDX Total Estriol. (Abbott Diagnostics) Fluorescence polarization immunoassay for the quantitative determination of total estriol in serum, plasma or urine.
Use: Diagnostic aid.

TDX Total T3. (Abbott Diagnostics) Automated assay for quantitation of total circulating triiodothyronine (T3) in serum or plasma.
Use: Diagnostic aid.

TDX T-Uptake. (Abbott Diagnostics) Automated assay for the determination of thyroxine binding capacity in serum or plasma.
Use: Diagnostic aid.

Te Anatoxal Berna. (Berna Products) Tetanus toxoid adsorbed, 10 Lf units/0.5 ml. Vial 5 ml, Syr. 0.5 ml. *Rx.*
Use: Agent for immunization.

Tear Drop. (Parmed) Benzalkonium Cl 0.01%, polyvinyl alcohol, NaCl, EDTA. Soln. Drop. bot. 15 ml. *otc.*
Use: Artificial tears.

TearGard. (KM Lee) Hydroxyethylcellulose, sorbic acid 0.25%, EDTA 0.1%. Soln. Bot. 15 ml. *otc.*
Use: Ophthalmic lubricant.

Teargen. (Goldline) Benzalkonium Cl 0.01%, EDTA, NaCl, polyvinyl alcohol. Soln. Bot. 15 ml. *otc.*
Use: Artificial tears.

Teargen II. (Goldline) Hydroxypropyl methylcellulose 0.3%, dextran 70 0.1%, benzalkonium Cl 0.01%, EDTA 0.05%. Bot. 15 ml. *otc.*
Use: Artificial tears.

Tearisol. (Ciba Vision) Hydroxypropyl methylcellulose 0.5%, edetate disodium, benzalkonium chloride 0.01%, boric acid, potassium chloride. Bot. 15 ml. *otc.*
Use: Artificial tears.

Tears Naturale. (Alcon) Dextran 70 0.1%, benzalkonium Cl 0.01%, hydroxypropyl methylcellulose 0.3%, sodium Cl, EDTA, hydrochloric acid, sodium HCl, potassium Cl. Bot. 15 ml, 30 ml. *otc.*
Use: Artificial tear, lubricant.

Tears Naturale II. (Alcon) Dextran 70 0.1%, hydroxypropyl methylcellulose 2910 0.3%, polyquaternium-1 0.001%, sodium Cl, potassium Cl, sodium borate. Droptainer 15 ml, 30 ml. *otc.*
Use: Artificial tears, lubricant.

Tears Naturale Free. (Alcon) Hydroxypropyl methylcellulose 2910 0.3%, dextran 70 0.1%, NaCl, KCl, sodium borate. Soln. Single-use containers 0.6 ml. *otc.*
Use: Artificial tears.

Tears Plus. (Allergan) Polyvinyl alcohol 1.4%, NaCl, povidone 0.6%, chlorobutanol 0.5%. *otc.*
Use: Artificial tears.

Tears Renewed Ointment. (Akorn) White petrolatum, light mineral oil. Ophth. Tube 3.5 g. *otc.*
Use: Ophthalmic lubricant.

Tears Renewed Solution. (Akorn) Dextran 70 0.1%, sodium chloride, hydroxypropyl methylcellulose 2906, benzalkonium chloride 0.01%, EDTA. Soln. Bot. 2 ml, 15 ml, 30 ml. *otc.*
Use: Artificial tears.

tea tree oil. (Metabolic Prod.) Australian oil of Melaleuca alternifolia 100% pure. Bot. 1 oz, 4 oz, 8 oz, 16 oz. **Cream** Bot. 8 oz. **Oint.** Tube 1 oz, 3 oz. *otc.*
Use: Antiseptic, antifungal, topical.

Tebamide. (G & W) Trimethobenzamide HCl 100 mg/Supp. In 10s. *Rx.*
Use: Antiemetic, antivertigo.

•**tebufelone.** (teh-BYOO-feh-LONE) USAN.
Use: Analgesic, anti-inflammatory.

•**tebuquine.** (TEH-buh-KWIN) USAN.
Use: Antimalarial.

T.E.C. (Invenex) Zinc 1 mg, copper 0.4 mg, chromium 4 mcg, manganese 0.1 mg. Vial 10 ml. *Rx.*
Use: Trace element additives for TPN therapy.

•**teceleukin.** (teh-see-LOO-kin) USAN.
Use: Immunostimulant.

Technescan MAA. (Mallinckrodt Medical). Aggregated albumin (human).
Use: Preparation of Tc 99m Aggregated Albumin (Human).

Techneplex. (Squibb) Technetium Tc 99m penetate kit. 10 vials/kit.
Use: Radiodiagnostic.

•**technetium Tc 99m albumin aggregated injection,** (tek-NEE-shee-uhm Tc 99m al-BYOO-min AGG-reh-GAY-tuhd) U.S.P. 23.
Use: Diagnostic aid (lung imaging), radioactive agent.

•**technetium Tc 99m albumin colloid injection,** (tek-NEE-shee-uhm) U.S.P. 23.
Use: Radioactive agent.

•**technetium Tc 99m albumin injection,** (tek-NEE-shee-uhm Tc 99m al-BYOO-min) U.S.P. 23.
Use: Radioactive agent.

•**technetium Tc 99m albumin microaggregated.** (tek-NEE-shee-uhm) USAN.
Use: Radioactive agent.

technetium Tc 99m antimelanoma murine monoclonal antibody. (tek-NEE-shee-uhm)
Use: Diagnostic aid. [Orphan drug]

•**technetium Tc 99m antimony trisulfide colloid.** (tek-NEE-shee-uhm) USAN.
Use: Radioactive agent.

•**technetium Tc 99m bicisate.** (tek-NEE-shee-uhm Tc 99m bye-SIS-ate) USAN.
Use: Diagnostic aid (brain imaging), radioactive agent.

•**technetium Tc 99m disofenin injection,** (tek-NEE-shee-uhm) U.S.P. 23.
Use: Radioactive agent; diagnostic aid (hepatobiliary function determination).

•**technetium Tc 99m etidronate injection,** (tek-NEE-shee-uhm) U.S.P. 23.
Use: Radioactive agent.

•**technetium Tc 99m exametazime.** (tek-NEE-shee-uhm) USAN.
Use: Radioactive agent.

technetium Tc 99m ferpentetate injection, (tek-NEE-shee-uhm) U.S.P. XXII.
Use: Radioactive agent.

•**technetium Tc 99m furifosmin.** (tek-NEE-shee-uhm Tc 99m fyoor-ih-FOSS-min) USAN.
Use: Diagnostic aid (radioactive, cardiac disease), radioactive agent.

technetium Tc 99m generator solution. (tek-NEE-shee-uhm) (New England Nuclear) Pertechnetate sodium Tc 99 m.
Use: Radiodiagnostic.

•**technetium Tc 99m glucepate injection,** (tek-NEE-shee-uhm) U.S.P. 23.
Formerly Technetium Tc 99m Sodium Gluceptate.
Use: Radioactive agent.

•**technetium Tc 99m lidofenin injection,** (tek-NEE-shee-uhm) U.S.P. 23.
Use: Radioactive agent.

•**technetium Tc 99m mebrofenin injection,** (tek-NEE-shee-uhm) U.S.P. 23.
Use: Radioactive agent.

•**technetium Tc 99m medronate injection,** (tek-NEE-shee-uhm) U.S.P. 23.
Use: Diagnostic aid (skeletal imaging), radioactive agent.
See: Macrotec, Inj. (Squibb).

•**technetium Tc 99m medronate disodium.** (tek-NEE-shee-uhm) USAN.
Use: Radioactive agent.

•**technetium Tc 99m mertiatide,** (tek-NEE-shee-uhm Tc 99m MEER-TIE-ahtide) U.S.P. 23.
Use: Diagnostic aid (renal function); radioactive agent.

technetium Tc 99m murine monoclonal antibody to hCG. (tek-NEE-shee-uhm)
Use: Diagnostic aid. [Orphan drug]

technetium Tc 99m murine monoclonal antibody to human afp. (tek-NEE-shee-uhm)
Use: Diagnostic aid. [Orphan drug]

technetium Tc 99m murine monoclonal antibody (IgG2a) to BCE.
Use: Diagnostic aid. [Orphan drug]

•**technetium Tc 99m oxidronate injection,** (tek-NEE-shee-uhm) U.S.P. 23.
Use: Diagnostic aid (skeletal imaging), radioactive agent.

•**technetium Tc 99m pentetate injection,** (tek-NEE-shee-uhm) U.S.P. 23.
Formerly Technetium Tc 99m Pentetate Sodium.
Use: Radioactive agent.

•**technetium Tc 99m pentetate calcium trisodium.** (tek-NEE-shee-uhm) USAN.
Use: Radioactive agent.

•**technetium Tc 99m pyrophosphate injection,** (tek-NEE-shee-uhm) U.S.P. 23.
Use: Radioactive agent.

•**technetium Tc 99m (pyro- and trimetra-) phosphates injection,** (tek-NEE-shee-uhm) U.S.P. 23.
Use: Radioactive agent.

•**technetium Tc 99m red blood cells injection,** (tek-NEE-shee-uhm) U.S.P. 23.
Use: Radioactive agent.

•**technetium Tc 99m sestamibi,** (tek-NEE-shee-uhm Tc 99 m SESS-tah-MIH-bih) U.S.P. 23.
Use: Diagnostic aid (radiopaque medium, cardiac perfusion); radioactive agent.

•**technetium Tc 99m siboroxime.** (tek-NEE-shee-uhm Tc 99m sih-boe-ROX-eem) USAN.
Use: Diagnostic aid (brain imaging), radioactive agent.

•**technetium Tc 99m succimer injection,** (tek-NEE-shee-uhm) U.S.P. 23.
Use: Radioactive agent, diagnostic aid (renal function determination).

technetium Tc 99m sulfur colloid kit. (tek-NEE-shee-uhm)
Use: Radioactive agent.
See: Tesuloid (Squibb).

•**technetium Tc 99m sulfur colloid injection,** (tek-NEE-shee-uhm) U.S.P. 23.
Use: Radioactive agent.

•**technetium Tc 99m teboroxime.** (tek-NEE-shee-uhm Tc 99m teh-boe-ROX-eem) USAN.
Use: Diagnostic aid (radiopaque medium, cardiac perfusion), radioactive agent.

teclosine. Under study.
Use: Amebicide.

•**teclozan.** (TEH-kloe-zan) USAN.
Use: Antiamebic.
See: Falmonox (Sanofi Winthrop).

Tecnu Poison Oak-n-Ivy. (Tec Labs) Deodorized mineral spirits, propylene glycol, polyethylene glycol, octylphenoxypolyethoxyethanol, mixed fatty acid soap. Liq. Bot. 118.3 ml, 355 ml. *otc.*
Use: Topical poison ivy treatment.

•**tecogalan sodium.** USAN.
Use: Antineoplastic adjunct.

Teczem. (Hoechst Marion Roussel) Enalapril maleate 5 mg, diltiazem maleate 180 mg, sucrose/ER Tab. Bot. 100s. *Rx.*
Use: combinations.

Tedral. (Parke-Davis) **Tab.:** Theophylline 118 mg, ephedrine HCl 24 mg, phenobarbital 8 mg/Tab. Bot. 24s, 100s, 1000s. UD 100s. **Susp. (Pediatric):**

Theophylline 65 mg, ephedrine HCl 12 mg, phenobarbital 4 mg/5 ml. Bot. 8 oz. *Rx.*
Use: Antiasthmatic.

Tedral Elixir. (Parke-Davis) Theophylline 32.5 mg, ephedrine HCl 6 mg, phenobarbital 2 mg/5 ml. Alcohol 15%. Pediatric. Bot. pt. *Rx.*
Use: Antiasthmatic.

Tedral-SA. (Parke-Davis) Theophylline 180 mg, ephedrine HCl 48 mg, phenobarbital 25 mg/S.A. Tab. Bot. 100s, 1000s. *Rx.*
Use: Antiasthmatic.

Tedrigen. (Goldline) Theophylline 120 mg, ephedrine HCl 22.5 mg, phenobarbital 7.5 mg/Tab. Bot. 100s, 1000s. *otc.*
Use: Antiasthmatic.

Teebacin. (CMC) Sod. p-aminosalicylate **Tab.** 0.5 g Bot. 1000s. **Pow.** Bot. lb. *Rx.*
Use: Antituberculosis agent.

Teebaconin. (CMC) Isoniazid 50, 100, 300 mg/Tab. Bot. 100s, 1000s. *Rx.*
Use: Antituberculosis agent.

Teebaconin w/Vitamin B$_6$. (CMC) Isoniazid 100 mg, 10 mg pyridoxine HCl/Tab. Bot. 100s, 500s, 1000s. Isoniazid 300 mg, 30 mg pyridoxine HCl/Tab. Bot. 100s and 1000s. *Rx.*
Use: Antituberculosis agent.

Teen Midol. (Bayer) Acetaminophen 400 mg, pamabrom 25 mg. Cap. Bot. 16s. *otc.*
Use: Analgesic combination.

Teev. (Keene) Estradiol valerate 4 mg, testosterone enanthate 90 mg/ml Inj. Vial 10 ml. *Rx.*
Use: Estrogen/androgen.

• **teflurane.** (TEH-flew-rane) USAN.
Use: Inhalation anesthetic.

tegacid.
See: Glyceryl monostearate.

• **tegafur.** (TEH-gah-fer) USAN.
Use: Antineoplastic.

Tegamide. (G & W) Trimethobenzamide HCl 100 mg, or 200 mg/ Supp. Boxes 10s, 50s.
Use: Antiemetic.

Tegison. (Roche) Etretinate 10 mg or 25 mg/Cap. Prescription Paks 30s. *Rx.*
Use: Antipsoriatic.

Tegopen. (Bristol-Myers) Cloxacillin sodium 250 mg/Cap. Bot. 100s. 500 mg/Cap. Bot. 100s. Granules for Soln. 125 mg/5 ml. Bot. 100 ml, 200 ml. *Rx.*
Use: Anti-infective; penicillin.

Tegretol. (Novartis) Carbamazepine **Tab.:** 200 mg. Bot. 100s, 1000s. UD

100s. **Chew. Tab.:** 100 mg/Tab. Bot. 100s. UD 100s; **Susp.:** 100 mg/5 ml, sorbitol. Sucrose. Bot. 450 ml. *Rx.*
Use: Anticonvulsant.

Tegretol-XR. (Novartis) Carbamazepine 100 mg, 200 mg and 400 mg, mannitol/Tabs, extended release. Bot. 100s, UD 100s. *Rx.*
Use: Anticonvulsant.

Tegrin Cream. (Block) Allantoin 2%, coal tar ext. 5% in cream base. Tube 2 oz., 4.4 oz.
Use: Antipsoriatic.

Tegrin-LT. (Block) Pyrethrins 0.33%, piperonyl butoxide (technical) 3.15%. Shampoo/Conditioner. Bot. 118 ml available w/wo 142 g insecticide spray. *otc.*
Use: Pediculicide.

Tegrin Medicated. (Block) **Lot.:** Crude coal tar 5%, allantoin 1.7%. Lot. 180 ml. **Shampoo:** Crude coal tar 7%, sodium lauryl sulfate, ammonium lauryl sulfate, alcohol 6.4%. Cream 110 ml. *otc.*
Use: Antiseborrheic.

Tegrin Medicated Extra Conditioning. (Block) Coal tar solution 7%, alcohol 6.4%. Shampoo. Bot. 110 ml, 198 ml. *otc.*
Use: Antiseborrheic.

T.E.H. Compound. (Various Mfr.) Theophylline 130 mg, ephedrine sulfate 25 mg, hydroxyzine HCl 10 mg/Tab. Bot. 100s, 500s. *Rx.*
Use: Antiasthmatic.

• **teicoplanin.** (teh-kah-PLAN-in) USAN.
Use: Antibacterial.

Telachlor. (Major) Chlorpheniramine maleate 8 or 12 mg/S.R. Cap. Bot. 100s, 250s, 1000s. *Rx.*
Use: Antihistamine.

Telachlor TD Caps. (Major) Chlorpheniramine maleate 8 mg or 12 mg/T.D. Tab. Bot. 1000s. *Rx.*
Use: Antihistamine.

Teldrin Maximum Strength Capsules. (SK-Beecham) Chlorpheniramine maleate 12 mg/Spansule. Pkg. 12s, 24s, 48s. *otc.*
Use: Antihistamine.

Teldrin Tablets. (SK-Beecham) Chlorpheniramine maleate 4 mg/Tab. *otc.*
Use: Antihistamine.

Teldrin 12-Hour Allergy Relief. (SK-Beecham) Chlorpheniramine maleate 8 mg, pseudoephedrine HCl 75 mg/Cap. Pkg. 12s, 24s. Bot. 48s. *otc.*
Use: Antihistamine, decongestant.

Telepaque. (Sanofi Winthrop) Iopanoic acid. 0.5 g/Tab. Bot. 30s and 150s.
Use: Radiopaque agent.

●**telinavir.** (teh-LIN-ah-veer) USAN.
Use: Antiviral.

Telodron. (Norden) Chlorpheniramine maleate.
Use: Antihistamine.

●**teloxantrone hydrochloride.** (teh-LOX-an-trone) USAN.
Use: Antineoplastic.

●**teludipine hydrochloride.** (teh-LOO-dih-peen) USAN.
Use: Antihypertensive; calcium channel antagonist.

●**temafloxcin hydrochloride.** (teh-mah-FLOX-ah-SIN) USAN.
Use: Antibacterial (microbial DNA topoisomerase inhibitor).

●**tematropium methylsulfate.** (teh-mah-TROE-pee-UHM METH-ill-SULL-fate) USAN.
Use: Anticholinergic.

●**temazepam,** (tem-AZE-uh-pam) U.S.P. 23.
Use: Minor tranquilizer.
See: Restoril, Cap. (Sandoz).

temazepam. (Various Mfr.) 7.5 mg/Cap. 100s, UD 100s. *c-iv.*
Use: Sedative, hypnotic.

●**temelastine.** (teh-mell-ASS-teen) USAN.
Use: Antihistamine.

Temetan. (Nevin) Acetaminophen 324 mg/Tab. Bot. 100s, 500s. Elixir (324 mg/5 ml) Bot. pt. *otc.*
Use: Analgesic.

●**temocapril hydrochloride.** (teh-MOE-cap-RILL) USAN.
Use: Antihypertensive.

●**temocillin.** (TEE-moe-SIH-lin) USAN.
Use: Antibacterial.

●**temoporfin.** (teh-moe-PORE-fin) USAN.
Use: Antineoplastic.

Temovate Cream. (Glaxo Wellcome) Clobetasol propionate 0.05%. Tube 15 g, 30 g, 45 g. *Rx.*
Use: Corticosteroid, topical.

Temovate Emollient. (Glaxo Wellcome) Clobetasol propionate 0.05%. Cream. 15 g, 30 g, 60 g. *Rx.*
Use: Corticosteroid, topical.

Temovate Gel. (Glaxo Wellcome) Clobetasol propionate 0.05%/Gel. 15, 30, 60 g. *Rx.*
Use: Corticosteroid, topical.

Temovate Ointment. (Glaxo Wellcome) Clobetasol propionate 0.05%. Tube 15 g, 30 g; 45 g. *Rx.*
Use: Corticosteroid, topical.

Temovate Scalp. (Glaxo Wellcome)
Oint.: Clobetasol propionate 0.05%, white petro base. 15 g, 30 g, 45 g.
Cream: Clobetasol propionate 0.03%, 15 g, 30 g, 45 g. **Scalp application:** Clobetasol propionate 0.05%, carbomer 934 P. 25 ml, 50 ml. *Rx.*
Use: Corticosteroid, topical.

Tempo. (Thompson Medical) Calcium carbonate 414 mg, aluminum hydroxide 133 mg, magnesium hydroxide 81 mg, simethicone 20 mg. Chew. Tab. Bot. 10s, 30s, 60s. *otc.*
Use: Antacid, antiflatulent.

Temporary Punctal/Canalicular Collagen Implant. (Eagle Vision) In 0.2 mm, 0.3 mm, 0.4 mm, 0.5 mm, 0.6 mm. Box 72s. *Rx.*
Use: Collagen implant, ophthalmic.

Tempra. (Bristol-Myers) Acetaminophen.
Drops: Grape flavor. 80 mg/0.8 ml. Bot. w/dropper 15 ml. **Red syrup:** Cherry flavor. 160 mg/5 ml. Bot. 4 oz. **Tab.:** 80 mg/Chewable Grape flavor Tab. Bot 30s. 160 mg/Chewable Grape flavor Tab. Bot. 30s. *otc.*
Use: Analgesic.

●**temurtide.** (teh-MER-TIDE) USAN.
Use: Vaccine adjuvant.

Tencet Capsules. (Hauck) Acetaminophen 500 mg, butalbital 50 mg, caffeine 40 mg. Cap. Bot. 100s, UD 1000s. *Rx.*
Use: Analgesic, sedative, hypnotic.

Tencon. (Inter. Ethical Labs) Acetaminophen 650 mg, butalbital 50 mg. Cap. Bot. 100s. *Rx.*
Use: Analgesic, sedative, hypnotic.

Tenex. (Robins) Guanfacine HCl 1 mg, 2 mg/Tab. Bot. 100s, 500s (1 mg only), UD 100s (1 mg only). *Rx.*
Use: Antihypertensive.

●**tenidap.** (TEH-nih-DAP) USAN.
Use: Anti-inflammatory (osteoarthritis and rheumatoid arthritis).

●**tenidap sodium.** (TEH-nig-DAP) USAN.
Use: Anti-inflammatory (osteoarthritis and rheumatoid arthritis).

●**teniposide.** (TEN-ih-POE-side) USAN.
Use: Antineoplastic. [Orphan drug]
See: Vumon (Bristol-Myers Oncology)

Ten-K. (Novartis) Potassium Cl 750 mg (10 mEq)/Controlled Release Cap. Bot. 100s, 500s. UD, blister pak 100s. *Rx.*
Use: Potassium supplement.

Tenol. (Vortech) Acetaminophen 325 mg/ Tab. Bot. 1000s. *otc.*
Use: Analgesic.

Tenol Liquid. (Vortech) Acetaminophen

120 mg, NAPA alcohol 7%/5 ml. Bot. 3 oz., 4 oz., Gal. *otc.*
Use: Analgesic.

Tenol-Plus. (Vortech) Acetaminophen 250 mg, aspirin 250 mg, caffeine 65 mg/ Tab. Bot. 1000s. *otc.*
Use: Analgesic.

Tenoretic Tablets. (Zeneca) **50 mg:** Atenolol 50 mg, Chlorthalidone 25 mg/ Tab. Bot. 100s. **100 mg:** Atenolol 100 mg, Chlorthalidone 25 mg/Tab Bot. 100s. *Rx.*
Use: Antihypertensive, diuretic.

Tenormin. (Zeneca) **Oral:** Atenolol 50 mg or 100 mg/Tab. Bot. 100s. UD 100s. **Parenteral:** 5 mg/10 ml. Amp. 10 ml. *Rx.*
Use: .

•**tenoxicam.** (ten-OX-ih-kam) USAN.
Use: Anti-inflammatory.

Tensilon. (Zeneca) Edrophonium chloride. **Vial:** 10 mg/ml, w/phenol 0.45%, sodium sulfite 0.2% 10 ml. **Amp.** 10 mg/ ml, w/sodium sulfite 0.2%. 1 ml.
Use: Differential diagnosis of myasthenia gravis.

Tensive Conductive Adhesive Gel. (Parker) Non-flammable conductive adhesive electrode gel, eliminates tape and tape irritation. Tube 60 g.
Use: For TENS, EMS, EMG, EEG and other electromedical procedures.

Tensocaine Tablets. (Sanofi Winthrop) Acetaminophen. *otc.*
Use: Analgesic.

Tensolate. (Apco) Phenobarbital 0.25 gr, hyoscyamine sulfate 0.1037 mg, atropine sulfate 0.0194 mg, hyoscine HBr 0.0065 mg/Tab. Bot. 100s. *Rx.*
Use: Antispasmodic sedative, for visceral spasm.

Tensolax Tablets. (Sanofi Winthrop) Chlormezanone. *Rx.*
Use: Muscle relaxant.

Tensopin. (Apco) Phenobarbital 0.25 gr, homatropine methylbromide 2.5 mg/ Tab. Bot. 100s. *Rx.*
Use: Antispasmodic.

Tenuate. (Hoescht Marion Roussel) Diethylpropion HCl 25 mg/Tab. Bot. 100s. *c-iv.*
Use: Anorexiant.

Tenuate Dospan. (Hoescht Marion Roussel) Diethylpropion HCl 75 mg/SR Tab. Bot. UD 100s, 250s. *c-v.*
Use: Anorexiant.

T.E.P. (Geneva Pharm) Phenobarbital 8 mg, theophylline 130 mg, ephedrine HCl 24 mg/Tab. Bot. 100s. *Rx.*

Use: Antiasthmatic combination.

Tepanil. (3M) Diethylpropion HCl. Tab. 25 mg Bot. 100s. *c-iv.*
Use: Anorexiant.

Tepanil Ten-Tab. (3M) Diethylpropion 75 mg/Tab. Bot. 30s, 100s, 250s. *c-iv.*
Use: Anorexiant.

•**tepoxalin.** (teh-POX-ah-lin) USAN.
Use: Antipsoriatic.

•**teprotide.** (TEH-pro-tide) USAN.
Use: Enzyme-inhibitor (angiotensin-converting).

tequinol sodium. Name used for Actino-quinol Sodium.

Terak Ointment. (Akorn) Polymyxin B sulfate 10,000 units/g or ml, oxytetracycline HCl 5 mg/g. Tube 3.5 g. *Rx.*
Use: Antibiotic, ophthalmic.

teralase. W/Pancreatin, polysorbate-80.
See: Digolase, Cap. (Boyle).

Terazol 3. (Ortho) **Cream, Vaginal:** Terconazole 0.8%. Tube 20 g with applicator. **Vaginal Supp.:** Terconazole 80 mg. Pks. 3s with applicator. *Rx.*
Use: Vaginal antifungal.

Terazol 7. (Ortho) Terconazole 0.4% Cream. In 45 g. *Rx.*
Use: Vaginal antifungal.

•**terazosin hydrochloride.** (ter-AZE-oh-sin) USAN.
Use: Antihypertensive.
See: Hytrin, Tab. (Abbott and Glaxo Wellcome).

•**terbinafine.** (TER-bin-ah-feen) USAN.
Use: Antifungal.
See: Lamisil (Sandoz).

•**terbutaline sulfate,** (ter-BYOO-tuh-leen) U.S.P. 23.
Use: Bronchodilator.
See: Brethine, Amp., Tab. (Novartis).

Tercodryl. (Approved) Codeine phos. ¾ gr, pyrilamine maleate 25 mg/fl. oz. Bot. 4 oz. *c-v.*
Use: Antihistamine, antitussive.

•**terconazole.** (ter-CONE-uh-zole) USAN. *Formerly Triaconazole.*
Use: Antifungal.
See: Terazol 3, Vag. Cream, Supp. (Ortho).
Terazol 7, Vag. Cream. (Ortho).

•**terfenadine,** (ter-FEN-uh-deen) U.S.P. 23.
Use: Antihistamine.
See: Seldane, Tab. (Hoechst Marion Roussel).

Terfenadine. (Goldline) 60 mg/Tab. Bot. 30s, 100s, 500s. *Rx.*
Use: Antihistamine.

Terg-a-Zyme. (Alconox) Alconox with enzyme action. Box 4 lb. Ctn. 9×4 lb., 25 lb., 50 lb., 100 lb., 300 lb. *otc.*
Use: Biodegradable detergent and wetting agent.

Teridol Jr. (Approved) Terpin hydrate, cocillana, potassium guaiacolsulfonate, ammonium chloride. Bot. 3 oz. *otc.*
Use: Expectorant.

• **teriparatide.** USAN.
Use: Bone resorption inhibitor, osteoporosis therapy adjunct, diagnostic aid, thyroid function. [Orphan drug]
See: Parathar.

• **teriparatide acetate.** (TEH-rih-PAR-ah-TIDE) USAN.
Use: Diagnostic aid (hypocalcemia).

• **terlakiren.** (ter-lah-KIE-ren) USAN.
Use: Antihypertensive.

terlipressin.
Use: Treatment of bleeding esophageal varices. [Orphan drug]
See: Glypressin.

• **terodiline hydrochloride.** (TEH-row-DIE-leen) USAN.
Use: Vasodilator (coronary).

• **teroxalene hydrochloride.** (ter-OX-ah-leen) USAN.
Use: Antischistosomal.

• **teroxirone.** (TER-OX-ih-rone) USAN.
Use: Antineoplastic.

Terpex Jr. (Approved) d-Methorphan 25 mg, terpin hydrate, pot. guaiacolsulfonate, cocillana, ammonium chloride. Bot. 4 oz. *otc.*
Use: Expectorant.

Terphan Elixir. (Pal-Pak) Terpin hydrate 85 mg, dextromethorphan hydrobromide 10 mg/5 ml w/alcohol 40% Bot. Gal. *otc.*
Use: Expectorant, antitussive.

• **terpin hydrate,** U.S.P. 23.
Use: Expectorant for chronic cough.
See: Terp, Liq. (Scrip).

terpin hydrate w/combinations.
See: Histogesic, Tab. (Century).
Prunicodeine, Liq. (Lilly).
W/Dextromethorphan, phenylpropanolamine HCl, pheniramine maleate, pyrilamine maleate.
See: Tussaminic, Tab. (Sandoz).
W/Dextromethorphan, phenylpropanolamine HCl, pheniramine maleate, pyrilamine maleate, acetaminophen.
See: Chexit, Tab. (Sandoz).
Tussagesic, Tab., Liq. (Sandoz).

terpin hydrate and dextromethorphan hydrobromide elixir.
Use: Expectorant, antitussive.

Terra-Cortril. (Roerig) Hydrocortisone 1.5%, oxytetracycline HCl 0.5%. Ophth. Susp. Bot. 5 ml. *Rx.*
Use: Corticosteroid, anti-infective, ophthalmic.

Terramycin. (Pfizer Laboratories) Oxytetracycline. **Cap.:** HCl salt 250 mg. Bot. 100s, 500s. **Oint., Ophth.:** Ocytetracycline HCl 5 mg, polymyxin B sulfate 1 mg/g. Tube 3.75 g. **Oint., Topical:** Oxytetracycline HCl 100 mg, polymyxin B sulfate 10,000 units/g. Tube 0.5 oz., 1 oz. **Pow. Topical:** Oxytetracycline HCl 30 mg, polymyxin B sulfate 10,000 units/g Bot. 28.4 g. **Tab., Oral:** Oxytetracycline HCl 250 mg/Tab. Bot. 100s. **Tab., Vaginal:** Oxytetracycline HCl 100 mg, polymyxin B sulfate 100,000 units/Tab. Box 10s. *Rx.*
Use: Anti-infective.

Terramycin Capsules. (Pfizer Laboratories) Oxytetracycline HCl 250 mg/Cap. Bot. 100s, 500s. *Rx.*
Use: Anti-infective.

Terramycin Topical Ointment. (Pfizer) Oxytetracycline HCl 30 mg, polymyxin B sulfate 10,000 units/g. Tube 0.5 oz, 1 oz. Ctn. 12s. *Rx.*
Use: Anti-infective, topical.

Terramycin w/Polymyxin B Ointment. (Roerig) Polymyxin B sulfate 10,000 units/g or ml, oxytetracycline HCl 5 mg/g. Oint. Tube 3.5 g. *Rx.*
Use: Anti-infective.

Terramycin Topical Powder with Polymyxin B Sulfate. (Pfizer) Oxytetracycline HCl 30 mg, polymyxin B sulfate 10,000 units/g. Bot. oz. *Rx.*
Use: Anti-infective, topical.

Tersaseptic. (Doak) DEA-lauryl sulfate, lauramide DEA, propylene glycol, ethoxydiglycol, PEG-12 distearate, EDTA, triclosan, citric acid/Shampoo/cleanser. Soapless. 473 ml. *otc.*
Use: Treatment of acne.

tersavid.
Use: Monoamine oxidase inhibitor.

tertiary amyl alcohol.
See: Amylene Hydrate. (Various Mfr.).

Tesamone. (Dunhall) Testosterone aqueous suspension. 25 mg/ml, 50 mg/ml or 100 mg/ml. Amp. 10 ml. *c-III.*
Use: Androgen therapy.

• **tesicam.** (TESS-ih-kam) USAN.
Use: Anti-inflammatory.

• **tesimide.** (TESS-ih-mide) USAN.
Use: Anti-inflammatory.

Teslac. (Squibb Mark) Testolactone 50 mg, lactose/Tab. Bot. 100s. *c-III.*

Use: Antineoplastic, androgen.

Tesogen. (Sig) Testosterone 25 mg, estrone 2mg/ml. Vial 10 ml. *c-III.*
Use: Androgen.

Tesogen L.A. (Sig) Testosterone enanthate 180 mg, 90 mg, 50 mg, estradiol valerate 8 mg, 4 mg and 2 mg respectively/ml. Vial 10 ml. *Rx.*
Use: Androgen, estrogen.

Tesone. (Sig) Testosterone 25 mg, 50 mg, 100 mg/ml. Vial 10 ml. *c-III.*
Use: Androgen hormonal.

Tesone L.A. (Sig) Testosterone enanthate 200 mg/ml. Vial 10 ml. *c-III.*
Use: Androgen.

tespa.
Use: Alkylating agent.
See: Thiotepa (Lederle).

Tessalon Perles. (Forest Pharm) Benzonatate 100 mg/Cap. Bot. 100s. *Rx.*
Use: Antitussive.

Testamone. (Dunhall) Testosterone 100 mg/ml. Inj. Vial 10 ml. *c-III.*
Use: Androgen.

Test-Estro Cypionates. (Rugby) Estradiol cypionate 2 mg, testosterone cypionate 50 mg/ml. Inj. Vial 10 ml. *Rx.*
Use: Estrogen/androgen.

Testex. (Taylor Pharmaceuticals) Testosterone propionate in sesame oil 50 mg, 100 mg/ml. Vial 10 ml. *c-III.*
Use: Androgen.

Testoderm. (Alza) Testosterone 10 mg or 15 mg per 40 or 60 cm², respectively. Transdermal system. Box 30s. *c-III.*
Use: Treatment of hypogonadism, androgen.

Testoject. (Mayrand) Testosterone cypionate 100 mg/ml. Vial 10 ml. *c-III.*
Use: Androgen.

Testoject-50. (Mayrand) Testosterone 50 mg/ml. Vial 10 ml. *c-III.*
Use: Androgen.

Testoject-LA. (Mayrand) Testosterone cypionate 200 mg/ml in oil. Vial 10 ml. *c-III.*
Use: Androgen.

• **testolactone,** (TESS-toe-LAK-tone) U.S.P. 23.
Use: Antineoplastic.
See: Teslac, Vial, Tab. (Squibb Mark).

Testolin. (Taylor Pharmaceuticals) Testosterone suspension 25 mg, 50 mg, 100 mg/ml. Vial 10 ml 25 mg/ml. Vial 30 ml. *c-III.*
Use: Androgen.

Testopel. (Bartor Pharmacal) Testosterone 75 mg, stearic acid 0.2 mg, polyvinylpyrrolidone 2 mg/pellet. 1 pellet/vial. *c-III.*
Use: Androgen.

• **testosterone,** (tess-TAHS-ter-ohn) U.S.P. 23.
Use: Androgen.
See: Androderm, Transderm. Patch (SK-Beecham).
Android-T, Vial (Zeneca).
Andronaq, Aq. Susp., Vial (Central).
Depotest, Vial (Hyrex).
Homogene-S, Inj., Vial (Spanner).
Malotrone Aqueous Injection (Bluco).
Neo-Hombreol-F, Aq. Susp., Vial (Organon).
Tesone, Inj. (Sig).
Testoderm, Transdermal patch (Alza).
Testolin, Vial (Taylor Pharmaceuticals).
Testopel (Bartor Pharmacal).

testosterone aqueous. (Various Mfr.) Testosterone (in aqueous suspension) 25 mg, 50 mg or 100 per ml/Inj. Vial 10 ml, 30 ml.
Use: Androgen, parenteral.
See: Histerone 100, Inj. (Roberts/ Hauck).
Tesamone, Inj. (Dunhall).

testosterone w/combinations.
See: Andesterone, Vial (Lincoln).
Angen, Vial (Davis & Sly).
Depo-Testadiol, Vial (Pharmacia & Upjohn).
Glutest, Vial (Zeneca).
Terogen, Vial (Taylor Pharmaceuticals).
Tesogen, Inj. (Sig).

testosterone cyclopentane propionate.
Testosterone Cypionate, U.S.P. 23.

• **testosterone cypionate,** U.S.P. 23.
Use: Androgen.
See: Andro-Cyp 100, Inj. (Keene).
Andro-Cyp 200, Inj. (Keene).
depAndro, Inj. (Forest).
Depo-Testosterone, Inj. (Pharmacia & Upjohn).
Dep-Test, Inj. (Sig).
Depotest, Vial (Hyrex).
D-Test 100, 200, Inj. (Burgin-Arden).
Durandro, Inj. (Ascher).
Duratest, Inj. (Roberts Hauck).
Testoject, Vial (Mayrand).
W/Combinations.
See: D-Diol, Inj. (Burgin-Arden).
Depotestogen, Vial (Hyrex).
Depo-Testadiol, Soln. (Pharmacia & Upjohn).
Duo-Cyp (Keene).

Duracrine, Inj. (Ascher).
Menoject-L.A. Vial (Kay).
T.E. Ionate P.A., Inj. (Solvay).
Testadiate-Depo, Vial (Kay).
testosterone cypionate. (Various Mfr.)
100 mg/ml or 200 mg/ml. Inj. Vial 10
ml.
Use: Androgen.
**testosterone cypionate/estradiol
cypionate.**
See: Estradiol cypionate w/testoster-
one cypionate.
**testosterone cypionate and estradiol
cypionate.** (Schein) Testosterone
cypionate 50 mg, estradiol cypionate 2
mg/ml. Vials 10 ml. *Rx.*
Use: Androgen, estrogen therapy.
• **testosterone enanthate,** U.S.P. 23.
Use: Androgen.
See: Andryl, Inj. (Keene).
Andropository-200, Inj. (Rugby).
Arderone 100, 200, Inj. (Burgin-
Arden).
Delatest, Inj. (Dunhall).
Delatestryl, Inj., Vial (Squibb).
Everone 200 mg, Vial (Hyrex).
Tesone L. A., Inj. (Sig).
Testate, Inj. (Savage).
Testrin-P.A., Inj. (Taylor Pharmaceuti-
cals).
W/Chlorobutanol.
See: Anthatest, Vial (Kay).
Andro L.A. 200, Inj. (Forest).
Delatestryl, Inj. (Gynex).
Durathate-200, Inj. (Roberts Hauck).
Everone 200, Inj. (Hyrex).
W/Estradiol valerate.
See: Valertest No. 1, Amp., Vial (Hy-
rex).
testosterone enanthate. (Various Mfr.)
100 mg/ml or 200 mg/ml. Inj. Vial 10
ml.
Use: Androgen.
testosterone heptanoate.
Use: Androgen.
See: Testosterone enanthate.
• **testosterone ketolaurate.** (tess-TAHS-
ter-ohn KEY-toe-LORE-ate) USAN.
Testosterone 3-oxododecanoate.
Use: Androgen.
testosterone ointment 2%. *Rx.*
Use: Vulvar dystrophies. [Orphan drug]
• **testosterone phenylacetate.** (tess-
TAHS-ter-ohn fen-ill-ASS-ah-tate)
USAN. Perandren phenylacetate.
Use: Androgen.
• **testosterone propionate,** U.S.P. 23.
Use: Androgen.
testosterone propionate. (Various Mfr.)

Testosterone propionate (in oil) 100 mg
per ml. Inj. Vial 10 ml.
Use: Androgen.
testosterone sublingual. *Rx.*
Use: Delay of growth and puberty in
boys. [Orphan drug]
Testred. (ICN) Methyltestosterone 10 mg/
Cap. Bot. 100s. *c-III.*
Use: Androgen.
Testred Cypionate.
Use: Androgen hormone inhibitor.
See: Proscar (Merck).
Testred Cypionate 200. (Zeneca) Testo-
sterone cypionate 200 mg/ml. Vial 10
ml. *c-III.*
Use: Androgen.
Testrin-P.A. (Taylor Pharmaceuticals)
Testosterone enanthate 200 mg, in
sesame oil with chlorobutanol/ml. Vial
10 ml. *c-III.*
Use: Androgen.
Testuria. (Wyeth-Ayerst) Combination kit
containing 5 × 20 sterile dip strips and
5 × 20 culture trays of trypticase soy
agar.
Use: Diagnostic aid.
Tesuloid. (Squibb) Technetium Tc 99m
sulfur colloid. 5 vials/kit.
Use: Radiodiagnostic.
**tetanus and diphtheria toxoids ad-
sorbed for adult use,** (TET-ah-nus and
diff-THEER-ee-uh toxoids) U.S.P. 23.
Use: Active immunizing agent for persons over 7 yrs. old.
Generic Products:
(Pasteur-Merieux-Connaught) Vial 5
ml for IM use.
(Wyeth-Lederle) Vial 5 ml.
• **tetanus antitoxin,** U.S.P. 23.
Use: Immunizing agent (passive).
**tetanus-diphtheria toxoids, aluminum
phosphate adsorbed.** (Wyeth-Lederle)
Vial 5 ml, Tubex 0.5 ml. *Rx.*
Use: Agent for immunization.
**tetanus, diphtheria & pertussis vac-
cine.**
Use: Vaccine toxoid.
See: Acel-Immune, Vial (Wyeth-Led-
erle)
Diphtheria and Tetanus Toxoids and
Whole Cell Pertussis Vaccine, Vial
(Pasteur-Merieux-Connaught).
Tri-Immunol, Vial (Wyeth-Lederle).
Tripedia, Vial (Pasteur-Merieux-Con-
naught).
**tetanus and diphtheria toxoids ad-
sorbed purogenated.** (Wyeth-Lederle)
Adult Lederject disposable syringe 10
× 0.5 ml. Vial 5 ml New package. *Rx.*

Use: Agent for immunization.

• **tetanus immune globulin,** (TET-ah-nus ih-MYOON GLAH-byoo-lin) U.S.P. 23. *Formerly Tetanus Immune Human Globulin.* Gamma globulin fraction of the plasma of persons who have been hyperimmunized with tetanus toxoid, 16.5%. Vial 250 units.
Use: Prophylaxis of injured, against tetanus (passive immunizing agent).
See: Hyper-Tet Injection Vial, 250 u. (Bayer).

tetanus immune globulin, human. 250 units/Tubex, 1 ml Dissolved in glycine 0.3 M; contains thimerosal 0.01%. *Rx.*
Use: Agent for active immunization.

• **tetanus toxoid,** U.S.P. 23.
Use: Immunizing agent (active).

• **tetanus toxoid, adsorbed.** U.S.P. 23.
Use: Immunizing agent (active).
See: Te Anatoxal Becna, Vial, Syr. (Berna).

tetanus toxoid, adsorbed. 20 Lf purified tetanus toxoid, 0.01% thimerosal as preservative/ml. Box 2 ampuls of 0.5 ml. Vial 5 ml, 7.5 ml, 0.5 ml. Amp. for booster injection. (Biocine Sclavo) Vial 0.5 ml, 5 ml. (Pasteur-Merieux-Connaught) Vial 5 ml for IM use. (Wyeth-Lederle) Vial 5 ml, disp. syringes 0.5 ml. *Rx.*
Use: Active immunizing agent against tetanus.

tetanus toxoid adsorbed purogenated. (Wyeth-Lederle) Vial 5 ml. Lederject disposable syringe 0.5 ml. Box 10s, 100s. *Rx.*
Use: Agent for immunization.

tetanus toxoid, aluminum phosphate adsorbed.
Use: Active immunizing agent.
See: (Wyeth-Lederle) Vial 5 ml 10s. Lederject Disp. Syr. 10 0.5 ml.

tetanus toxoid fluid. (Pasteur-Merieux-Connaught) Vial 7.5 ml for IM or SC use. (Wyeth-Lederle) Vial 7.5 ml, Tubex 0.5 ml.
Use: Active immunizing agent against tetanus.

tetanus toxoid, fluid purogenated. (Wyeth-Lederle) Vial 7.5 ml Lederject disposable syringe. 0.5 ml. Box 10s, 100s. *Rx.*
Use: Agent for immunization.

tetanus toxoid purified, fluid. (Wyeth-Lederle) Vial 7.5 ml, Tubex 0.5 ml. *Rx.*
Use: Agent for immunization.

tetiothalein sodium.
See: Iodophthalein Sodium. (Var. Mfr.).

Tetrabead. (Abbott Diagnostics) Solid phase radioimmunoassay for the quantitative measurement of total circulating serum thyroxine.

Tetrabead-125. (Abbott Diagnostics) T-3 uptake radioassay for the measurement of thyroid function by indirectly determining the degree of saturation of serum thyroxine binding globulin (TBG).

• **tetracaine,** U.S.P. 23.
Use: Anesthetic (topical).
See: Pontocaine, Oint., Cream (Sanofi Winthrop).

tetracaine and menthol ointment.
Use: Local anesthetic, topical.

• **tetracaine hydrochloride,** U.S.P. 23.
Use: Local, topical, spinal anesthetic.
See: Bristacycline, Cap. (Bristol-Myers). Pontocaine Hydrochloride Inj., Pow. (Sanofi Winthrop).
W/Benzocaine, butyl aminobenzoate.
See: Cetacaine, Liq., Oint., Spray (Cetylite).
W/Hexachlorophene, dimethyl polysiloxane, methyl salicylate, pyrilamine maleate, zinc oxide.
W/Isocaine, benzalkonium Cl.
See: Isotraine Oint. (Philips Roxane).

tetracaine hydrochloride 0.5%. (Alcon) 0.5%/1 ml Drop-Tainer, Ophth. 15 ml Steri-Unit, 2 ml (Ciba Vision) Dropperettes 1 ml in 10s. *Rx.*
Use: Local anesthetic, ophthalmic.

Tetracap. (Circle) Tetracycline HCl 250 mg/Cap. Bot. 100s. *Rx.*
Use: Anti-infective; tetracycline.

tetrachlorethylene, U.S.P. XXI. Perchlorethylene, tetrachlorethylene.
Use: Anthelmintic (hookworms and some trematodes).

Tetracon. (Professional Pharmacal) Tetrahydrozoline HCl 0.5 mg, disodium edetate 1 mg, boric acid 12 mg, benzalkonium Cl 0.1 mg, sodium Cl 2.2 mg, sodium borate 0.5 mg/ml w/water. Liq. Bot. 15 ml. *otc.*
Use: Minor eye irritation.

• **tetracycline,** (teh-truh-SIGH-kleen) U.S.P. 23.
Use: Antiamebic, antibacterial, antirickettsial.
See: Sumycin, Syrup (Squibb).
W/N-acetyl-para-amino-phenol, phenyltoloxamine citrate.
Use: Anti-infective; tetracycline.
See: Paltet, Cap. (Roberts).
Tetrex, Bid Cap., Cap., Vial (Bristol-Myers).

tetracycline and amphotericin B, U.S.P. XXI.

•**tetracycline hydrochloride,** U.S.P. 23.
Use: Antibacterial, antiamebic, antirickettsial.
See: Achromycin, Preps. (Storz/Lederle).
  Bicycline, Caps. (Knight).
  Centet 250, Tab. (Central).
  Cyclopar, Cap. (Parke-Davis).
  G-Mycin, Cap. & Syr. (Coast).
  Maso-Cycline, Cap. (Mason).
  Panmycin, Cap. (Pharmacia & Upjohn).
  Scotrex, Caps. (Scott/Cord).
  Sumycin, Cap., Tab., Syr. (Squibb Mark).
  Tetracap 250, Cap. (Circle).
  Tetracyn, Cap. (Pfizer Laboratories).
  Tetram, Cap., Syr. (Dunhall).
  Tetramax, Cap. (Rand).
  Topicycline, Liq. (Proctor & Gamble).
W/Citric Acid.
See: Achromycin V, Cap., Drop, Susp., Syr. (Lederle).
W/Nystatin.
See: Comycin, Cap. (Pharmacia & Upjohn).

tetracycline hydrochloride fiber.
Use: Anti-infective, tetracycline.
See: Actisite (Alza).

tetracycline hydrochloride and nystatin capsules.
Use: Anti-infective, tetracycline.
See: Comycin, Cap. (Pharmacia & Upjohn)

tetracycline oral suspension.
Use: Anti-infective, tetracycline.
See: Brand names under Tetracycline.

•**tetracycline phosphate complex,** U.S.P. 23.
Use: Antibacterial.

Tetracyn. (Pfizer Laboratories) Tetracycline HCl. 250 mg or 500 mg/Cap.
250 mg: Cap. Bot. 1000s. **500 mg:** Bot. 100s. *Rx.*
Use: Anti-infective, tetracycline.

tetradecyl sulfate, sodium.
Use: Sclerosing agent.
See: Sotradecol (Elkins-Sinn).

tetraethylammonium bromide (teab).
Use: Diagnostic & therapeutic agent in peripheral vascular disorders. Diagnostic in hypertension.

tetraethylammonium chloride.
Use: Ganglionic blocking agent.

tetraethylthiuram disulfide.
See: Disulfiram.

•**tetrafilcon a.** USAN.
Use: Contact lens material (hydrophilic).

tetrahydroaminoacridine.
Use: A cholinergic agent for Alzheimer's disease.
See: Cognex (Warner-Lambert).

tetrahydrophenobarbital calcium.
See: Cyclobarbital Calcium, Prep.

tetrahydroxyquinone. Name used for Tetroquinone.

•**tetrahydrozoline hydrochloride,** U.S.P. 23.
Use: Adrenergic (vasoconstrictor).
See: Collyrium Fresh Eye Drops (Wyeth-Ayerst).
  Eysine, Soln., (Akorn).
  Geneye Extra, Drops (Goldline).
  Mallazine Eye Drops (Roberts Hauck).
  Murine Plus (Abbott).
  Optigene 3, Soln. (Pfeiffer).
  Soothe, Soln., (Alcon).
  Tetrasine, Soln., (Optopics).
  Tyzine, Soln. (Key).
  Visine, Soln. (Pfizer).

tetraiodophenolphthalein sodium.
See: Iodophthalein Sodium.

tetraiodophthalein sodium.
See: Iodophthalein Sodium.

tetramethylene dimethanesulfonate.
See: Busulfan, U.S.P. 23.

tetramethylthiuram disulfide. Thiram.
Use: Anti-infective, antifungal.
See: Rezifilm, Aerosol (Squibb).

•**tetramisole hydrochloride.** (teh-TRAM-ih-sole) USAN.
Use: Anthelmintic.
See: Ripercol (American Cyanamid).

Tetramune. (Wyeth-Lederle) 12.5 Lf units of tetanus toxoid, 5 Lf units of diphtheria toxoid, 4 units of pertussis vaccine and 10 mcg *Haemophilus influenzae* type b oligosaccharide, each per 0.5 ml. Vial, 5 ml. *Rx.*
Use: Vaccine.

Tetraneed. (Hanlon) Pentaerythritol tetranitrate 80 mg/Time Cap. Bot. 100s. *Rx.*
Use: Antianginal.

tetrantoin.
Use: Anticonvulsant.

Tetrasine. (Optopics) Tetrahydrozoline HCl 0.05%. Bot. 15 ml, 22.5 ml. *otc.*
Use: Ophthalmic vasoconstrictor/mydriatic.

Tetrasine Extra. (Optopics) Polyethylene glycol 400 1%, tetrahydrozoline HCl 0.05%. Bot. 15 ml. *otc.*
Use: Ophthalmic vasoconstrictor/mydriatic.

Tetratab. (Freeport) Pentaerythritol tetranitrate 10 mg/Tab. Bot. 1000s. *Rx.*
Use: Management, prophylaxis and

treatment of angina attacks.

Tetratab No. 1. (Freeport) Pentaerythritol tetranitrate 20 mg/Tab. Bot. 1000s. *Rx.*
Use: Management, prophylaxis and treatment of angina attacks.

•**tetrazolast meglumine.** (teh-TRAZZ-oh-last meh-GLUE-meen) USAN.
Use: Antiallergic; antiasthmatic.

Tetrazyme. (Abbott Diagnostics) Test kit 100s, 500s.
Use: Enzyme immunoassay for quantitative measurement of total circulating serum thyroxine (free and protein bound).

•**tetrofosmin.** (teh-troe-FOSS-min) USAN.
Use: Diagnostic aid.

•**tetroquinone.** (TEH-troe-kwih-NOHN) USAN.
Use: Treat keloids, keratolytic (systemic).
See: Kelox (Zeneca).

•**tetroxoprim.** (tet-ROX-oh-prim) USAN.
Use: Antibacterial.

•**tetrydamine.** (teh-TRID-ah-meen) USAN.
Use: Analgesic, anti-inflammatory.

Tetterine. (Shuptrine) **Oint.:** Antifungal agents in green petrolatum base. Tin oz.; Antifungal agents in white petroleum base. Tube oz. **Powder:** Fungicide, germicide formula powder for heat and diaper rash. Can 2.25 oz. **Soap:** Bar 3.25 oz.
Use: Treatment ringworm, athlete's foot, diaper rash and other skin conditions.

Texacort Scalp Lotion. (GenDerm Co.) Hydrocortisone 1%, alcohol 33%. Lipid free. Dropper Bot. 1 fl. oz. *Rx.*
Use: Corticosteroid.

T-Fluoride. (Tennessee) Sodium fluoride 2.21 mg/Tab. Bot. 100s, 1000s. *Rx.*
Use: Dental caries preventative.

TG.
Use: Antineoplastic.
See: Thioguanine (Glaxo Wellcome).

T/Gel Scalp Solution. (Neutrogena) Neutar coal tar extract 2%, salicyclic acid 2%. Bot. 2 oz. *otc.*
Use: Antipsoriatic, antiseborrheic.

T/Gel Therapeutic Conditioner. (Neutrogena) Neutar coal tar extract 1.5% in oil free conditioner base. Bot. 1.4 oz. *otc.*
Use: Antipsoriatic, antiseborrheic.

T/Gel Therapeutic Shampoo. (Neutrogena) Neutar coal tar extract 2% in mild shampoo base. Bot. 4.4 oz., 8.5 oz. *otc.*

Use: Antipsoriatic, antiseborrheic.

T-Gen Suppositories. (Goldline) Trimethobenzamide HCl 100 mg/Pediatric Supp. or 200 mg/Adult Supp. Box 10s, 50s. *Rx.*
Use: Antiemetic.

T-Gesic Capsule. (T.E. Williams) Hydrocodone bitartrate 5 mg, acetaminophen 500 mg/Cap. Bot. 100s. *c-III.*
Use: Narcotic analgesic combination, sedative, hypnotic.

•**thalidomide.** (the-LID-oh-mide) USAN.
Use: Hypnotic, sedative, anti-infective. [Orphan drug]

Thalitone. (Horus Therapeutics) Chlorthalidone 15 or 25 mg, lactose/Tab. Bot. 100s. *Rx.*
Use: Diuretic.

•**thallous chloride Tl 201 injection,** (THAL-uhs) U.S.P. 23.
Use: Diagnostic aid (radiopaque medium), radioactive agent.

Tham-E. (Abbott) Tromethamine 36 g, sodium Cl. 30 mEq/L, potassium Cl. 5 mEq/L, chloride 35 mEq/L. Total osmolarity 367 mOsm/L. Single dose container 150 ml. *Rx.*
Use: Nutritional supplement.

Tham Solution. (Abbott) Tromethamine 18 g, acetic acid 2.5 g single-dose container. *Rx.*
Use: Nutritional supplement.

THC.
Use: Antiemetic, antivertigo.
See: Marinol (Roxane).

theamin. Monoethanolamine salt of theophylline.
See: Monotheamin, Supp. (Lilly).
W/Amobarbital.
See: Monotheamin and Amytal, Pulvule (Lilly).

thenalidine tartrate.
Use: Antihistamine; antipruritic.

thenyldiamine hydrochloride.
Use: Antihistamine.

thenylpyramine.
See: Methapyrilene Hydrochloride, Preps.

Theo-24. (Whitby) Theophylline anhydrous 100 mg, 200 mg, or 300 mg/Controlled Release Cap. 100 mg Bot. 100s. UD 100s; 200 mg Bot. 100s, 500s. UD 100s; 300 mg Bot. 100s, 500s. UD 100s. *Rx.*
Use: Bronchodilator, antiasthmatic.

Theobid Duracap. (Ross) Theophylline anhydrous 260 mg/TR Cap. Bot. 60s, 500s. *Rx.*
Use: Bronchodilator, antiasthmatic.

Theobid Jr Duracap. (Ross) Anhydrous theophylline 130 mg/TR Cap. Bot 60s. *Rx.*
Use: Bronchodilator, antiasthmatic.

theobroma oil. Cocoa Butter, N.F. 18.
Use: Suppository base.

theobromine with phenobarbital combinations.
See: Harbolin, Tab. (Arcum).
Theocardone, Tab. (Lemmon).
T.P. KI, Tab. (Wendt-Bristol).

theobromine calcium gluconate.
(Bates) Tab., Bot. 100s, 1000s. Also available w/phenobarbital. (Grant) Tab., Bot. 100s, 500s, 1000s.

theobromine sodium acetate. Theobromine calcium salt mixture with calcium salicylate.
Use: Diuretic; smooth muscle relaxant.

theobromine sodium salicylate.
See: Doan's Pills (Purex).
W/Cal. lactate, Phenobarbital.
See: Theolaphen, Tab. (Zeneca).

Theochron. (Various Mfr.) Theophylline anhydrous 100 mg, 200 mg, 300 mg. ER Tab. 100s, 500s, 1000s. *Rx.*
Use: Bronchodilator.

Theochron. (Forest Labs) Theophylline 200 mg/Tab. T.R. Bot. 100s, 500s, 1000s. 300 mg/Tab. T.R. Bot. 100s, 500s. *Rx.*
Use: Bronchodilator.

Theoclear 80 Syrup. (Central) Theophylline 80 mg/15 ml. Bot. Pt., Gal. *Rx.*
Use: Bronchodilator.

Theoclear L.A.-130. (Central) Theophylline 130 mg/Cenule. Bot. 100s. *Rx.*
Use: Bronchodilator.

Theoclear L.A.-260. (Central) Theophylline 260 mg/Cenule Bot. 100s, 1000s. *Rx.*
Use: Bronchodilator.

Theocolate. (Rosemont) Theophylline 150 mg, guaifenesin 90 mg/15 ml Liq. Bot. pt., gal. *Rx.*
Use: Antiasthmatic.

Theodrine. (Rugby) Theophylline 120 mg, ephedrine HCl 22.5 mg/Tab. Bot. 1000s. *otc.*
Use: Antiasthmatic.

Theo-Dur. (Schering-Plough) Theophylline 450 mg/Tab. S.R. Bot. 100s, UD 100s. *Rx.*
Use: Bronchodilator.

Theo-Dur Tablets. (Key) Theophylline 100 mg, 200 mg or 300 mg/SA Tab. Bot. 100s, 500s, 1000s, 5000s. UD 100s. *Rx.*
Use: Bronchodilator.

•**theofibrate.** (THEE-oh-FIH-brate) USAN.
Use: Antihyperlipoproteinemic.

Theogen. (Sig) Conjugated estrogens 2 mg/ml. Vial 10 ml, 30 ml. *Rx.*
Use: Estrogen.

Theogen I.P. (Sig) Estrone 2 mg, potassium estrone sulfate 1 mg/ml. Vial 10 ml. *Rx.*
Use: Estrogen.

Theolair. (3M) Theophylline 125, 250 mg/Tab. Box 100s, 250s as foil strip 10s. Bot. 100s. *Rx.*
Use: Bronchodilator.

Theolair Liquid. (3M) Theophylline 80 mg/15 ml. Bot. pt. *Rx.*
Use: Bronchodilator.

Theolair-SR 200. (3M) Theophylline 200 mg/Tab. (slow release). Bot. 100s. Box 100s as foil strip 10s. *Rx.*
Use: Bronchodilator.

Theolair-SR 250. (3M) Theophylline 250 mg/Tab. (slow release). Bot. 100s, 250s. *Rx.*
Use: Bronchodilator.

Theolair-SR 300. (3M) Theophylline 300 mg/Tab. (slow release). Bot. 100s. Box 100s as foil strip 10s. *Rx.*
Use: Bronchodilator.

Theolair-SR 500. (3M) Theophylline 500 mg/Tab. (slow release). Bot. 100s, 250s. *Rx.*
Use: Bronchodilator.

Theolate Liquid. (Various Mfr.) Theophylline 150 mg, guaifenesin 90 mg/15 ml. Liq. Bot. 118 ml, pt, gal. *Rx.*
Use: Antiasthmatic.

Theomax DF Syrup. (Various Mfr.) Theophylline 97.5 mg, ephedrine sulfate 18.75 mg, alcohol 5%, hydroxyzine HCl 7.5 mg/15 ml. Bot. pt. gal. *Rx.*
Use: Antiasthmatic.

Theo-Organidin. (Wallace) Theophylline anhydrous 120 mg, iodinated glycerol 30 mg/15 ml w/alcohol 15%, saccharin. Bot. pt., gal. *Rx.*
Use: Antiasthmatic.

Theophenyllin. (H.L. Moore) Theophylline 130 mg, ephedrine HCl 24 mg, phenobarbital 8 mg/Tab. Bot. 1000s. *Rx.*
Use: Antiasthmatic.

Theophyl-SR. (McNeil Pharm) Theophylline 125 mg. Bot. 100s. *Rx.*
Use: Bronchodilator.

•**theophylline,** (thee-AHF-ih-lin) U.S.P. 23.
Use: Bronchodilator; coronary vasodilator, diuretic; pharmaceutic necessity for Aminophylline Injection.
See: Accurbron, Liq. (Hoechst Marion Roussel).

Aerolate, Cap., Elix. (Fleming).
Aquaphyllin, Syr. (Ferndale).
Bronkodyl, Cap. (Sanofi Winthrop).
Duraphyl, Tab. (McNeil Pharm).
Elixicon, Susp. (Berlex).
Elixophyllin, Elix., Cap. (Berlex).
Elixophyllin SR, Cap. (Berlex).
Lodrane, Cap. (ECR Pharm).
Optiphyllin, Elix. (Fougera).
Oralphyllin, Liq. (Consol. Midland).
Quibron-T Dividose, Tab. (Bristol-Myers).
Quibron-T/SR Dividose, Tab. (Bristol-Myers).
Slo-bid, Caps. (Rhone-Poulenc Rorer).
Slo-Phyllin, Cap., Syr., Tab. (Dooner).
Somophyllin, Cap. (Medeva).
Sustaire, Tab. (Pfizer Laboratories)
Theo-II, Elix. (Fleming).
Theobid, Cap. (Ross).
Theobid Jr, Cap. (Ross).
Theochron, ER Tab. (Various Mfr.)
Theoclear 80, Liq. (Central).
Theoclear L.A., Cenule (Central).
Theo-Dur, Tab. (Key).
Theophylline Extended Release, ER Tab. (Sidmark).
Theolair, Tab., Liq. (3M).
Theolair SR, Tab. (3M).
Theospan, Cap. (Laser).
Theostat, Prods. (Laser).
Theovent Long-Acting, Cap. (Schering-Plough).
Theo-X, CR Tab. (Schwarz Pharma).
theophylline. (Various Mfr.) 100 mg, 125 mg, 200 mg, 300 mg/ER Cap. Bot. 100s. *Rx.*
Use: Bronchodilator.
theophylline, 8-chloro, diphenhydramine. Dimenhydrinate, U.S.P. 23.
See: Dramamine, Prep. (Searle).
theophylline aminoisobutanol. Theophylline w/2-amino-2-methyl-1-propanol.
See: Butaphyllamine (Var. Mfr.).
theophylline-calcium salicylate.
W/Ephedrine HCl, phenobarbital, pot. iodide.
See: Quadrinal, Tab., Susp. (Knoll).
W/Phenobarbital, ephedrine HCl, guaifenesin.
See: Verequad, Tab., Susp. (Knoll).
W/Potassium iodide.
See: Theokin, Tab., Elix. (Knoll).
theophylline choline salt.
See: Choledyl, Tab., Elix. (Parke-Davis).
Theophylline and 5% Dextrose. (Abbott and Baxter) Inj. 200 mg/Cont.: 50 ml and 100 ml. 400 mg/Cont.: 100 ml,

250 ml, 500 ml and 1000 ml. 800 mg/Cont.: 250 ml, 500 ml and 1000 ml.
Use: Bronchodilator.
theophylline, ephedrine hydrochloride, and phenobarbital tablets.
Use: Bronchodilator, sedative.
theophylline ethylenediamine.
See: Aminophylline, Prep., (Var. Mfr.).
theophylline extended-release. (Sidmak) Theophylline anhydrous 450 mg, lactose (SL 518). Tab. Bot. 100s, 250s, 500s. *Rx.*
Use: Bronchodilator.
theophylline extended-release capsules.
Use: Bronchodilator.
theophylline w/combinations.
See: Asma-lief, Tab., Susp. (Quality Generics).
B.A. Prods. (Federal).
Bronkaid, Tab. (Brew).
Co-Xan, Liq. (Central).
Elixophyllin-Kl, Elix. (Berlex).
Liquophylline, Liq. (Paddock).
Marax DF, Syr. (Roerig).
Quibron, Cap., Liq. (Bristol-Myers).
Quibron-300, Cap. (Bristol-Myers).
Quibron Plus, Cap. (Bristol-Myers).
Slo-Phyllin Gg, Cap., Syr. (Dooner).
Synophylate, Liq. (Central).
Tedral SA, Tab. (Parke-Davis).
Theocol, Cap., Liq. (Quality Generics).
Theofenal, Tab. (Cumberland).
Theolair Plus, Tab., Liq. (3M).
Theo-Organidin, Elix. (Wampole).
theophylline and guaifenesin capsules.
Use: Smooth muscle relaxant, expectorant.
theophylline and guaifenesin oral solution.
Use: Smooth muscle relaxant, expectorant.
theophylline KI. (Various Mfr.) Theophylline 80 mg, potassium iodide 130 mg/15 ml. Elix. 480 ml, gal. *Rx.*
Use: Antiasthmatic combination.
theophylline olamine. Theophylline compound with 2-amino-ethanol (1:1).
Use: Smooth muscle relaxant.
theophylline with phenobarbital combinations.
See: Asma-Lief, Tab., Susp. (Quality Generics).
Bronkolixir, Elix. (Sanofi Winthrop).
Bronkotab, Tab. (Sanofi Winthrop).
Ceepa, Tab. (Geneva Pharm).
theophylline reagent strips. (Bayer)

Seralyzer reagent strip. Bot. 25s.
Use: A quantitative strip test for theophylline in serum or plasma.

• **theophylline sodium glycinate,** U.S.P. 23.
Use: Smooth muscle relaxant.
See: Synophylate, Elix., Tab. (Central).
Theofort, Elix. (Federal Pharm).
W/Guaifenesin.
See: Asbron G, Tab., Elix. (Sandoz).
Synophylate-GG, Tab., Syr. (Central).
W/Phenobarbital.
See: Synophylate w/Phenobarbital, Tab. (Central).
W/Potassium iodide.
See: TSG-KI, Elix. (Zeneca).
W/Potassium iodide, ephedrine HCl, codeine phosphate.
See: TSG Croup Liquid. (Zeneca).
W/Racephedrine & phenobarbital.
See: Synophedal, Tab. (Central).

Theo-Sav. (Savage) Theophylline 100 mg/Tab. Bot. 100s. 200 mg or 300 mg/Tab. Bot. 100s, 500s, 1000s. *Rx.*
Use: Bronchodilator.

Theospan-SR 130. (Laser) Theophylline anhydrous 130 mg/Cap. Bot. 100s, 1000s. *Rx.*
Use: Bronchodilator.

Theospan-SR 260. (Laser) Theophylline anhydrous 260 mg/Cap. Bot. 100s, 1000s. *Rx.*
Use: Bronchodilator.

Theostat 80 Syrup. (Laser) Theophylline anhydrous 80 mg/15 ml. Bot. Pt., Gal. *Rx.*
Use: Bronchodilator.

Theotal. (Major) Theophylline 125 mg, ephedrine HCl 25 mg, phenobarbital 8 mg, lactose. Tab. Bot. 1000s. *Rx.*
Use: Antiasthmatic combination.

Theo-Time. (Major) Theophylline 100 mg, 200 mg and 300 mg/Tab. T.R. Bot. 100s, 500s. *Rx.*
Use: Bronchodilator.

Theo-Time SR Tabs. (Major) Theophylline 100 mg, 200 mg, or 300 mg/S.R. Tab. Bot. 100s, 500s.
Use: Bronchodilator.

Theovent Long-Acting. (Schering-Plough) Theophylline anhydrous 125 mg or 250 mg/Cap. Bot. 100s. *Rx.*
Use: Bronchodilator.

Theo-X. (Schwarz Pharma) Theophylline anhydrous 100 mg, 200 mg or 300 mg/Tab. Dye free, lactose. Bot. 100s, 500s, 1000s. *Rx.*
Use: Bronchodilator.

Thera Bath. (Walgreen) Mineral oil 90%. Bot. 16 oz. *otc.*

Use: Emollient.

Thera Bath with Vitamin E. (Walgreen) Mineral oil 91%, Vit E 2000 IU/16 oz. *otc.*
Use: Emollient.

Therabid. (Mission) Vitamins C 500 mg, B_1 15 mg, B_2 10 mg, B_3 100 mg, B_5 20 mg, B_6 10 mg, B_{12} 5 mcg, A 5000 IU, D 200 IU, E 30 mg/Tab. Bot. 60s. *otc.*
Use: Vitamin/mineral supplement.

Therabloat. (Norden) Poloxalene.

Therabrand. (Approved) Vitamins A 25,000 IU, D 1000 IU, B_1 10 mg, B_2 10 mg, niacinamide 100 mg, C 200 mg, B_6 5 mg, calcium pantothenate 20 mg, B_{12} 5 mcg/Cap. Bot. 100s, 1000s. *otc.*
Use: Vitamin/mineral supplement.

Therabrand-M. (Approved) Vitamins A 25,000 IU, D 1000 IU, C 200 mg, B_1 10 mg, B_2 10 mg, B_6 5 mg, niacinamide 100 mg, calcium pantothenate 20 mg, E 5 IU, B_{12} 5 mcg, iodine 0.15 mg, iron 15 mg, copper 1 mg, calcium 125 mg, manganese 1 mg, magnesium 6 mg, zinc 1.5 mg/Cap. Bot. 100s, 1000s. *otc.*
Use: Vitamin/mineral supplement.

Therac. (C & M) Colloidal sulfur 4% in lotion base. Bot. 60 ml. *otc.*
Use: Antiacne.

Theracap. (Arcum) Vitamins A 10,000 IU, D 400 IU, B_1 10 mg, B_2 5 mg, niacinamide 150 mg, C 150 mg/Cap. Bot. 100s, 1000s. *otc.*
Use: Vitamin supplement.

Thera-Combex H-P. (Parke-Davis Prods) Vitamins C 500 mg, B_1 25 mg, B_2 15 mg, B_{12} 5 mcg, niacinamide 100 mg, panthenol 20 mg/Cap. Bot. 100s. *otc.*
Use: Vitamin supplement.

TheraCys. (Pasteur-Merieux-Connaught) 81 mg dry weight per vial, 1.7 to 19.2 $\times 10^8$ CFU per vial. Vial with 3 ml vial of diluent; 50 ml vials of phosphate-buffered sodium chloride are available for use as final diluent. *Rx.*
Use: Antineoplastic.

TheraFlu, Flu and Cold Medicine. (Sandoz) Pseudoephedrine HCl 60 mg, chlorpheniramine maleate 4 mg, acetaminophen 650 mg, sucrose, lemon flavor. Pow. Pks. 6, 12. *otc.*
Use: Decongestant, antihistamine, analgesic.

TheraFlu, Flu Cold & Cough Medicine. (Sandoz) Pseudoephedrine HCl 60 mg, chlorpheniramine maleate 4 mg, dextromethorphan HBr 20 mg, acetaminophen 650 mg. Pow. Pks. 6s. *otc.*
Use: Decongestant, antihistamine, antitussive, analgesic.

Thera-Flu Non-Drowsy Flu, Cold & Cough Maximum Strength. (Sandoz) Pseudoephedrine HCl 60 mg, dextromethorphan HBr 30 mg, acetaminophen 1000 mg. Pow. 6s, 12s. *otc.*
Use: Decongestant, antitussive, analgesic.

Thera-Flu Non-Drowsy Formula, Maximum Strength. (Sandoz) Pseudoephedrine HCl 30 mg, dextromethorphan HBr 15 mg, acetaminophen 500 mg. Capl. Pkg. 24s. *otc.*
Use: Decongestant, antitussive.

Thera-Flur. (Colgate Oral) Fluoride 0.5% (from sod. fluoride 1.1%). pH 4.5. Gel-Drops. Bot. 24 and 60 ml. *Rx.*
Use: Dental caries preventative.

Thera-Flur-N. (Colgate Oral) Neutral sodium fluoride 1.1% Bot. 24 ml, 60 ml. *Rx.*
Use: Dental caries preventative.

Therafortis. (General Vitamin) Vitamins A 12,500 IU, D 1000 IU, B₁ 5 mg, B₂ 5 mg, B₆ 1 mg, B₁₂ 3 mcg, niacinamide 50 mg, pantothenic acid salt 10 mg, C 150 mg, folic acid 0.5 mg/Cap. Bot. 100s, 1000s. *otc.*
Use: Vitamin supplement.

Theragenerix. (Goldline) Vitamins A 5500 IU, D 400 IU, E 30 mg, B₁ 3 mg, B₂ 3.4 mg, B₃ 30 mg, B₅ 10 mg, B₆ 3 mg, B₁₂ 9 mcg, C 120 mg, folic acid 0.4 mg, biotin 15 mcg, betacarotene 2500 IU. Tab. Bot. 130s, 1000s. *otc.*
Use: Vitamin/mineral supplement.

Theragenerix-H. (Goldline) Iron 66.7 mg, vitamins A 8333 IU, D 133 IU, E 5 IU, B₁ 3.3 mg, B₂ 3.3 mg, B₃ 33.3 mg, B₅ 11.7 mg, B₆ 3.3 mg, B₁₂ 50 mcg, C 100 mg, folic acid 0.33 mg, Cu, Mg/Tab. Bot. 100s, 1000s. *otc.*
Use: Vitamin/mineral supplement.

Theragenerix-M. (Goldline) Iron 27 mg, vitamins A 5000 IU, D 400 IU, E 30 mg, B₁ 3 mg, B₂ 3.4 mg, B₃ 30 mg, B₅ 10 mg, B₆ 3 mg, B₁₂ 9 mcg, C 120 mg, folic acid 0.4 mg, Ca, Cl, Cr, Cu, I, K, biotin 15 mcg, Mg, Mn, Mo, P, Se, zinc 15 mg, beta carotene 2500 IU. Tab. Bot. 130s, 1000s. *otc.*
Use: Vitamin/mineral supplement.

Thera-Gesic. (Mission) Methylsalicylate, menthol. Balm. In 90 g, 150 g. *otc.*
Use: Analgesic, topical.

Theragran. (B-M Squibb) Vitamins A 5000 IU, D 400 IU, E 30 IU, B₁ 3 mg, B₂ 3.4 mg, B₃ 20 mg, B₅ 10 mg, B₆ 3 mg, B₁₂ 9 mcg, C 90 mg, folic acid 0.4 mg, biotin 30 mcg/Capl. Bot. 100s. *otc.*
Use: Vitamin supplement.

Theragran AntiOxident. (Bristol-Myers Squibb) Vitamins A 5000 IU, C 250 mg, E 200 IU, Mn, Cu, Zn, Se/Softgel Cap. Bot. 50s. *otc.*
Use: Vitamin/mineral supplement.

Theragran Jr. with Iron. (Squibb) Iron 18 mg, vitamins A 5000 IU, D 400 IU, E 30 mg, B₁ 1.5 mg, B₂ 1.7 mg, B₃ 20 mg, B₆ 2 mg, B₁₂ 6 mcg, C 60 mg, folic acid 0.4 mg w/tartrazine/Tab. Bot. 75s. *otc.*
Use: Vitamin/mineral supplement.

Theragran Hematinic. (Apothecon) Iron 66.7 IU, vitamins A 1400 IU, D 400 IU, E 5 IU, B₁ 3.3 mg, B₂ 3.3 mg, B₃ 33.3 mg, B₅ 11.7 mg, B₆ 3.3 mg, B₁₂ 50 mcg, C 100 mg, folic acid 0.33 mg, Ca, Cu, Mg/Tab. Bot. 90s. *Rx.*
Use: Vitamin/mineral supplement.

Theragran Liquid. (BM-Squibb) Vitamins A 5000 IU, D 400 IU, B₁ 10 mg, B₂ 10 mg, B₃ 100 mg, B₅ 21.4 mg, B₆ 4.1 mg, B₁₂ 5 mcg, C 200 mg/5 ml. Liq. Bot. 120 ml. *otc.*
Use: Vitamin supplement.

Theragran-M. (BM-Squibb) Ca 40 mg, iron 27 mg, vitamins A 5000 IU, D 400 IU, E 30 mg, B₁ 3 mg, B₂ 3.4 mg, B₃ 20 mg, B₅ 10 mg, B₆ 3 mg, B₁₂ 9 mcg, C 90 mg, folic acid 0.4 mg, Cl, Cr, Cu, I, K, Mg, Mn, Mo, P, Se, Zn 15 mg, biotin 30 mcg, lactose, sucrose/Capl. Bot. 90s, 130s, 180s, 200s. *otc.*
Use: Vitamin/mineral supplement.

Theragran Stress Formula. (BM-Squibb) Iron 27 mg, vitamins E 30 IU, B₁ 15 mg, B₂ 15 mg, B₃ 100 mg, B₅ 20 mg, B₆ 25 mg, B₁₂ 12 mcg, C 600 mg, folic acid 0.4 mg, biotin 45 mcg/Tab. Bot. 75s. *otc.*
Use: Vitamin/mineral supplement.

Thera Hematinic. (Major) Iron 66.7 mg, A 8333 IU, D 133 IU, E 5 IU, B₁ 3.3 mg, B₂ 3.3 mg, B₃ 33.3 mg, B₅ 11.7 mg, B₆ 3.3 mg, B₁₂ 50 mcg, C 100 mg, folic acid 0.33 mg, Cu, Mg/Tab. Bot. 250s, 1000s. *otc.*
Use: Iron with vitamin supplements.

Thera-Hist. (Major) Pseudoephedrine HCl 60 mg, chlorpheniramine maleate 4 mg, acetaminophen 500 mg, sucrose. Pow. Pks. 6. *otc.*
Use: Decongestant, antihistamine, analgesic.

Thera-Hist Syrup. (Major) Phenylpropanolamine HCl 12.5 mg, chlorpheniramine maleate 2 mg/5 ml. Syr. Bot. 120 ml. *otc.*
Use: Decongestant, antihistamine.

Thera H Tabs. (Major) Bot. 100s, 250s.
Use: Vitamin/mineral supplement.

Thera-M. (Various Mfr.) Vitamins A 5000 IU, B_1 3 mg, B_2 3.4 mg, B_3 20 mg, B_5 10 mg, B_6 3 mg, B_{12} 9 mcg, C 90 mg, D 400 IU, E 30 IU, iron 27 mg, folic acid 0.4 mg, biotin 30 mcg, P, Ca, Cu, Cr, Se, Mo, K, Cl, I, Mg, Mn, zinc 15 mg. Tab. Bot. 130s, 1000s. *otc.*
Use: Vitamin/mineral supplement.

Theramin. (Arcum) Vit. A 10,000 IU, D 400 IU, B_1 10 mg, B_2 5 mg, niacinamide 100 mg, B_6 5 mg, B_{12} 10 mcg, C 150 mg, cal. pantothenate 15 mg, calcium 103.6 mg, iodine 0.1 mg, iron 15 mg, potassium 80 mg, magnesium 6 mg/Tab. Bot. 30s, 100s, 1000s.
Use: Vitamin/mineral supplement.

Thera Multi-Vitamin. (Major) Vitamins A 10,000 IU, D 400 IU, B_1 10 mg, B_2 10 mg, B_3 100 mg, B_5 21.4 mg, B_6 4.1 mg, B_{12} 5 mcg, C 200 mg/5 ml. Liq. Bot. 118 ml. *otc.*
Use: Vitamin supplement.

Theramycin Z. (Medicis) Erythromycin 2%, SD alcohol 40-B 81%. Topical Soln. 60 ml. *Rx.*
Use: Antiacne.

Theraneed. (Hanlon) Vitamins A 16,000 IU, B_1 10 mg, B_2 10 mg, B_6 2 mg, C 300 mg, calcium pantothenate 10 mg, niacinamide 10 mg, B_{12} 10 mcg/Cap. Bot. 100s. *otc.*
Use: Vitamin/mineral supplement.

Therapals. (Faraday) Vitamins A 25,000 IU, D 400 IU, B_1 10 mg, B_2 5 mg, niacinamide 150 mg, B_6 0.5 mg, E 5 IU, C 150 mg, B_{12} 10 mcg, calcium 103 mg, cobalt 0.1 mg, copper 1 mg, potassium 0.15 mg, magnesium 6 mg, manganese 1 mg, molybdenum 0.2 mg, phosphorus 80 mg, potassium 5 mg, zinc 1.2 mg/Tab. Bot. 100s, 250s, 1000s. *otc.*
Use: Vitamin/mineral supplement.

Therapeutic B Complex with Vitamin C. (Upsher-Smith) Vitamins B_1 15 mg, B_2 10.2 mg, B_3 50 mg, B_5 10 mg, B_6 5 mg, C 300 mg/Cap. Bot. UD 100s. *otc.*
Use: Vitamin supplement.

Therapeutic-H. (Goldline) Iron 66.7 mg, A 8333 IU, D 133 IU, E 5 IU, B_1 3.3 mg, B_2 3.3 mg, B_3 33.3 mg, B_5 11.7 mg, B_6 3.3 mg, B_{12} 50 mcg, C 100 mg, folic acid 0.33 mg, Cu, Mg/Tab. Bot. 100s. *otc.*
Use: Iron with vitamin supplement.

Therapeutic-M. (Goldline) Iron 27 mg, vitamins A 5000 IU, D 400 IU, E 30 IU, B_1 3 mg, B_2 3.4 mg, B_3 20 mg, B_5 10 mg, B_6 3 mg, B_{12} 9 mcg, C 90 mg, folic acid 0.4 mg, Ca, Cl, Cr, Cu, I, K, Mg, Mn, Mo, P, Se, Zn 15 mg, biotin 30 mcg/Tab. Bot. 1000s. *otc.*
Use: Vitamin/mineral supplement.

Therapeutic Mineral Ice. (Bristol-Myers) Menthol 2%, ammonium hydroxide, carbomer 934, cupric sulfate, isopropyl alcohol, magnesium sulfate, thymol. Gel. Tube 105 g, 240 g, 480 g. *otc.*
Use: Rub/liniment.

Therapeutic Tablets. (Goldline) Vitamins A 5000 IU, D 400 IU, E 30 IU, B_1 3 mg, B_2 3.4 mg, B_3 20 mg, B_5 10 mg, B_6 3 mg, B_{12} 9 mcg, C 90 mg, folic acid 0.4 mg, d-biotin 30 mcg/Tab. Bot. 100s, 130s. *otc.*
Use: Vitamin supplement.

Therapeutic V & M. (Whiteworth Towne) Vitamins A 10,000 IU, D 400 IU, B_1 10 mg, B_2 10 mg, B_6 5 mg, B_{12} 5 mcg, niacinamide 100 mg, calcium pantothenate 20 mg, C 200 mg, E 15 IU, iodine 0.15 mg, iron 12 mg, copper 2 mg, manganese 1 mg, magnesium 60 mg, zinc 1.5 mg/Tab. *otc.*
Use: Vitamin/mineral supplement.

Therapeutic Vitamin Formula w/Minerals. (Towne) Vitamins A palmitate 10,000 IU, D 400 IU, B_1 15 mg, B_2 10 mg, B_6 5 mg, B_{12} 12 mcg, C 200 mg, niacinamide 100 mg, calcium pantothenate 20 mg, E 15 IU, calcium 103 mg, iron 10 mg, manganese 1 mg, potassium 5 mg, zinc 1.5 mg, magnesium 6 mg/Cap. Bot. 30s, 60s, 100s, 250s. *otc.*
Use: Vitamin/mineral supplement.

Therapeutic Vitamin Formula w/Minerals. (Towne) Vitamins A palmitate 25,000 IU, D 1000 IU, B_1 10 mg, B_2 5 mg, B_6 1 mg, B_{12} 5 mcg, C 150 mg, niacinamide 100 mg, calcium 103 mg, phosphorus 80 mg, iron 10 mg, iodine 0.1 mg, manganese 1 mg, potassium 5 mg, copper 1 mg, zinc 1.4 mg, magnesium 5.5 mg/Cap. Bot. 100s, 1000s. *otc.*
Use: Vitamin/mineral supplement.

Theraphon. (Approved) Vitamins A 25,000 IU, D 1000 IU, B_1 10 mg, B_2 5 mg, C 150 mg, niacinamide 150 mg/Cap. Bot. 100s, 1000s. *otc.*
Use: Vitamin supplement.

Theraplex T. (Medicis) Coal tar 1%, benzyl alcohol. Shampoo. Bot. 240 ml. *otc.*
Use: Antiseborrheic.

Theraplex Z. (Medicis) Pyrithione zinc 1%. Shampoo. Bot. 240 ml. *otc.*
Use: Antiseborrheic.

Theravee Hematinic Vitamin. (Vangard) Iron 66.7 mg, A 8333 IU, D 133 IU, E 5 IU, B_1 3.3 mg, B_2 3.3 mg, B_3 33.3 mg, B_5 11.7 mg, B_6 3.3 mg, B_{12} 50 mcg, C 100 mg, folic acid 0.33 mg, Cu, Mg/Tab. Bot. UD 100s. *otc.*
Use: Vitamin/mineral supplement.

Theravee M. (Vangard) Iron 27 mg, vitamin A 5000 IU, D 400 IU, E 30 IU, B_1 3 mg, B_2 3.4 mg, B_3 30 mg, B_5 10 mg, B_6 3 mg, B_{12} 9 mcg, C 120 mg, folic acid 0.4 mg, Ca, Cl, Cr, Cu, K, I, Mg, Mn, Mo, Se, Zn 15 mcg, biotin 15 mcg, beta carotene 2500 IU/Tab. Bot. 100s, 1000s. UD 100s. *otc.*
Use: Vitamin/mineral supplement.

Theravee Vitamin. (Vangard) Vitamins A 5500 IU, D 400 IU, E 30 IU, B_1 3 mg, B_2 3.4 mg, B_3 30 mg, B_5 10 mg, B_6 3 mg, B_{12} 9 mcg, C 120 mg, folic acid 0.4 mg, biotin 15 mcg/Tab. Bot. 100s. UD 100s. *otc.*
Use: Vitamin supplement.

Theravim. (NBTY) Vitamins A 5000 IU, D 400 IU, E 30 IU, B_1 3 mg, B_2 3.4 mg, B_3 30 mg, B_5 10 mg, B_6 3 mg, B_{12} 9 mcg, C 90 mg, folic acid 0.4 mg, beta carotene 1250 IU, biotin 35 mcg/Tab. Bot. 130s. *otc.*
Use: Vitamin supplement.

Theravim M. (NBTY) Iron 27 mg, vitamins A 5000 IU, D 400 IU, E 30 mg, B_1 3 mg, B_2 3.4 mg, B_3 20 mg, B_5 10 mg, B_6 3 mg, B_{12} 9 mcg, C 90 mg, folic acid 0.4 mg, Ca, Cl, Cr, Cu, I, K, Mg, Mn, Mo, P, Se, zinc 15 mg, biotin 30 mcg/Tab. Bot. 130s. *otc.*
Use: Vitamin/mineral supplement.

Theravite. (Barre-National) Vitamins A 10,000 IU, D 400 IU, B_1 10 mg, B_2 10 mg, B_3 100 mg, B_5 21.4 mg, B_6 4.1 mg, B_{12} 5 mcg, C 200 mg/5 ml. Liq. Bot. 118 ml. *otc.*
Use: Vitamin supplement.

Therems. (Rugby) Vitamins A 5000 IU, D 400 IU, E 30 mg, B_1 3 mg, B_2 3.4 mg, B_3 30 mg, B_5 10 mg, B_6 3 mg, B_{12} 9 mcg, C 120 mg, folic acid 0.4 mg, beta carotene 1250 IU, biotin 15 mcg/Tab. Bot. 130s, 1000s. *otc.*
Use: Vitamin supplement.

Therems-M. (Rugby) Iron 27 mg, vitamins A 5500 IU, D 400 IU, E 30 mg, B_1 3 mg, B_2 3.4 mg, B_3 20 mg, B_5 10 mg, B_6 3 mg, B_{12} 9 mcg, C 90 mg, folic acid 0.4 mg, Ca, Cl, Cr, Cu, I, K, Mg, Mn, Mo, P, Se, zinc 15 mg, biotin 30 mcg/Tab. Bot. 90s, 100s, 1000s. *otc.*
Use: Vitamin/mineral supplement.

Therevac. (Jones Medical) Docusate potassium 283 mg, benzocaine 20 mg/Tube capsule w/soft soap in PEG 400 and glycerin base. Unit 4 ml, packages 4s, 12s, 50s. *otc.*
Use: Disposable enema.

Therevac Plus. (Jones Medical) Docusate sodium 283 mg, benzocaine 20 mg in a base of soft soap, PEG 400, glycerin/Cap. 3.9 g Jar 30s. Disposable enema. *otc.*
Use: Laxative.

Therevac-SB. (Jones Medical) Docusate sodium 283 mg in a base of soft soap, PEG 400, glycerin/Cap. 3.9 g Bot. 30s. Disposable enema. *otc.*
Use: Laxative.

Therex No. 1. (Halsey) Vit A 10,000 IU, D 400 IU, E 15 IU, C 200 mg, B_1 10 mg, B_2 10 mg, niacinamide 100 mg, B_6 5 mg, B_{12} 5 mcg, calcium pantothenate 20 mg/Tab. Bot. 100s. *otc.*
Use: Vitamin/mineral supplement.

Therex and Zinc. (Halsey)
Use: Dietary supplement.

Therex-M. (Halsey) Vitamins A 10,000 IU, D 400 IU, E 15 IU, C 200 mg, B_1 10 mg, B_2 10 mg, niacinamide 100 mg, B_6 5 mg, B_{12} 5 mcg, calcium pantothenate 20 mg, iodine 150 mcg, iron 12 mg, Mg 65 mg, Cu 2 mg, zinc 1.5 mg, Mn 1 mg/Tab. Bot. 100s. *otc.*
Use: Vitamin/mineral supplement.

Therex-Z. (Halsey) Vitamins A 10,000 IU, D 400 IU, E 15 IU, C 200 mg, B_1 10 mg, B_2 10 mg, niacinamide 100 mg, B_{12} 5 mcg, B_6 5 mg, Ca pantothenate 20 mg, iodine 150 mcg, Cu 2 mg, iron 12 mg, Zn 22.5 mg/Tab. Bot. 100s. *otc.*
Use: Vitamin/mineral supplement.

Therma-Kool. (Nortech) Compresses in following sizes: 3"×5", 4"×9", 8.5"×10.5".
Use: Cold or hot compress.

Thermazene. (Sherwood) Silver sulfadiazine 1% in white pet. Cream. In 50, 400 and 1000 g. *Rx.*
Use: Treatment of second, third degree burns.

Thermodent. (Mentholatum) Strontium Cl. 10%. Tubes. *otc.*
Use: Toothpaste for sensitive teeth.

Theroal. (Vangard) Theophylline 24 mg, ephedrine HCl 24 mg, phenobarbital 8 mg/Tab. Bot. 100s, 1000s. *Rx.*
Use: Antiasthmatic combination.

Theroxide Wash. (Medicis) Benzoyl peroxide 10%. Liq. 120 ml. *Rx.*
Use: Antiacne.

Thex Forte. (KM Lee) Vitamins B_1 25 mg, B_2 15 mg, B_3 100 mg, B_5 10 mg, B_6 5 mg, C 500 mg/Cap. Bot. 75s. *otc.*
Use: Vitamin supplement.

Thia. (Sig) Thiamine HCl 100 mg/ml. Vial 30 ml. *Rx.*
Use: Thiamine supplement.

•**thiabendazole,** (THIGH-uh-BEND-uhzole) U.S.P. 23.
Use: Anthelmintic.
See: Mintezol, Tab., Susp. (Merck).

thiacetarsamide sodium. Sodium mercaptoacetate S,S-diester with p-carbamoyldithiobenzenearsonous acid.
Use: Antitrichomonal.

Thia-Dia-Mer-Sulfonamides. Sulfadiazine w/sulfamerazine & sulfathiazole.
See: Trionamide, Tab. (O'Neal).

thialbarbital.
See: Kemithal.

•**thiamine hydrochloride,** (THIGH-uhmin) U.S.P. 23.
Use: Enzyme co-factor vitamin.
See: Apatate (Kenwood).
Betalin S, Amp., Elixir, Tab. (Lilly).
Thia, Vial (Sig).

•**thiamine mononitrate,** U.S.P. 23.
Use: Enzyme co-factor vitamin.
W/Sodium salicylate, colchicine.
See: Sodsylate, Tab. (Durst).

•**thiamiprine.** (thigh-AM-ih-preen) USAN.
Use: Antineoplastic.

•**thiamphenicol.** (THIGH-am-FEN-ih-kahl) USAN.
Use: Antibacterial.

•**thiamylal,** U.S.P. 23.
Use: Anesthetic (intravenous)

•**thiamylal sodium, for injection,** U.S.P. 23.
Use: Anesthetic (intravenous).
See: Surital Sodium, Prep. (Parke-Davis).

thiazesim.
Use: Antidepressant.

•**thiazesim hydrochloride.** (thigh-AZE-eh-sim) USAN.
Use: Antidepressant.

•**thiazinamium chloride.** (THIGH-ah-ZINam-ee-uhm)
Use: Antiallergic.

thiethylene thiophosphoramide.
See: Thiotepa.

•**thiethylperazine.** (THIGH-eth-ill-PURRah-zeem) USAN.
Use: Central nervous system depressant; antiemetic.
See: Torecan.

•**thiethylperazine malate,** (THIGH-eth-ill-PURR-ah-zeen MAL-ate) U.S.P. 23.
Use: Antiemetic.

•**thiethylperazine maleate,** U.S.P. 23.
Use: Antiemetic.
See: Norzine, Inj., Supp., Tab. (Purdue Frederick).
Torecan, Amp., Supp., Tab. (Boehringer Ingelheim).

thihexinol methylbromide.
Use: Anticholinergic.

•**thimerfonate sodium.** USAN.
Use: Topical anti-infective.

•**thimerosal,** U.S.P. 23.
Use: Topical anti-infective; pharmaceutic aid (preservative).
See: Aeroaid, Aerosol (Aeroceuticals).
Merphol Tincture 1:1000, Liq. (Jones Medical).
Mersol, Liq. (Century).
Merthiolate, Prep. (Lilly).

thiocarbanidin. Under study.
Use: Tuberculosis.

thiocyanate sodium. Sodium thiocyanate.
Use: Hypotensive.

thiodinone. Name used for Nifuratel.

thiodiphenylamine.
See: Phenothiazine.

thiofuradene.

thioglycerol.
W/Sod. citrate, phenol, benzyl alcohol.
See: Sulfo-ganic, Vial (Marcen).

•**thioguanine,** (THIGH-oh-GWAHN-een) U.S.P. 23.
Use: Antineoplastic.
See: Tabloid (Glaxo Wellcome).

thiohexamide. N-(p-Methyl-mercaptophenylsulfonyl)N'-cyclohexylurea.
Use: Blood sugar-lowering compound.

thioisonicotinamide. Under study.
Use: Antituberculosis drug.

Thiola. (Mission). Tiopronin 100 mg. Tablets: In 100s. *Rx.*
Use: Kidney stone preventative.

•**thiopental sodium,** (thigh-oh-PEN-tahl) U.S.P. 23.
Use: Anesthetic (intravenous), anticonvulsant.
See: Pentothal Sodium, Amp. (Abbott).

thiopental sodium. (IMS) Thiopental sodium 20 mg/ml or 25 mg/ml. Pow. for Inj. **20 mg/ml:** 400 mg *Min-I-Mix* vial w/ injector; **25 mg/ml:** 250 or 500 mg *Min-I-Mix* vials w/ injector; 500 mg, 1 g, 2.5 g, 5 g, 10 g kits. *Rx.*
Use: General anesthetic.

thiophosphoramide.
See: ThioTepa, Vial (Lederle).

Thioplex. (Immunex) Thiotepa 15 mg. Powd. for Inj. Vials. *Rx.*

Use: Alkylating agent.

thiopropazate hydrochloride.
Use: Tranquilizer.

thioproperazine mesylate.
Use: Central depressant; antiemetic.

●**thioridazine,** (THIGH-oh-RID-uh-zeen) U.S.P. 23.
Use: Antipsychotic, sedative, hypnotic.
See: Mellaril, Susp. (Sandoz).

●**thioridazine hydrochloride,** (THIGH-oh-RID-ah-zeen) U.S.P. 23.
Use: Antipsychotic, sedative, hypnotic.
See: Mellaril, Tabs., Soln. (Sandoz).

thioridazine hydrochloride concentrate. (Various Mfr.) Thioridazine HCl **30 mg/ml.** Bot. 120 ml. **100 mg/ml.** Bot 120 ml, 3.4 ml (UD 100s). *Rx.*
Use: Antipsychotic.

thioridazine hydrochloride intensol oral solution. (Roxane) Thioridazine HCl oral concentrated soln. 30 mg/ml or 100 mg/ml. Bot. 120 ml w/calibrated dropper. *Rx.*
Use: Antipsychotic.

●**thiosalan.** (THIGH-oh-sal-AN) USAN.
Use: Disinfectant.

thiosalicylic acid salt.

●**thiotepa,** (thigh-oh-TEP-uh) U.S.P. 23.
Use: Antineoplastic.

thiotepa. (thigh-oh-TEP-uh) (Lederle) Powder for reconstitution: Thiotepa powder 15 mg, sodium chloride 80 mg, sodium bicarbonate 50 mg/Vial. Vial 15 mg. *Rx.*
Use: Antineoplastic.
See: Thioplex, Powd. (Immunex).

●**thiothixene,** (THIGH-oh-THIX-een) U.S.P. 23.
Use: Antipsychotic.
See: Navane, Cap., Vial (Roerig).
Navane Concentrate Solution (Roerig).

●**thiothixene hydrochloride,** (THIGH-oh-THIX-een) U.S.P. 23.
Use: Antipsychotic.
See: Navane Hydrochloride (Pfizer).

thiothixene hydrochloride intensol. (Roxane) Thiothixene HCl 5 mg/ml, EDTA. Alcohol free. Soln. Bot. 30 ml, 120 ml with dropper. *Rx.*
Use: Antipsychotic.

thiouracil. 2-Thiouracil.
Use: Treatment of hyperthyroidism, angina pectoris, congestive heart failure.

thioxanthenes.
See: Chlorprothixine (Taractan Roche). Navane (Roerig). Thiothixine (Various Mfr.).

thioxanthene derivative.
See: Taractan, Prep. (Roche).

thiphenamil. F.D.A. S-[2-(Diethylamino)-ethyl]-diphenylthioacetate.

●**thiphenamil hydrochloride.** (thigh-FEN-ah-mill) USAN.
Use: Smooth muscle relaxant.

●**thiphencillin potassium.** USAN.
Use: Antibacterial.

Thipyri-12. (Sig) Vitamins B_1 1000 mg, B_6 1000 mg, cyanocobalamin (B_{12}) 10,000 mcg, sod. chloride 0.5%, sod. bisulfite 0.1%, benzyl alcohol (as preservative) 0.9%. Univial 10 ml. *Rx.*
Use: Vitamin supplement.

●**thiram.** (THIGH-ram) USAN.
Use: Antifungal.

Thixo-Flur Topical Gel. (Colgate Oral) Acidulated phosphate sodium fluoride in gel base 1.2%. Bot. 32 oz. 8 oz., 4 oz.
Use: Dental caries prevention.

●**thonzonium bromide.** (thahn-ZOE-nee-uhm) USAN. U.S.P. XXII.
Use: Detergent.
W/Colistin base, neomycin base, hydrocortisone acetate, polysorbate 80, acetic acid, sodium acetate.
See: Coly-Mycin-S, Otic, Liq. (Warner-Chilcott).
W/Isoproterenol.
See: Nebair, Aerosol (Warner-Chilcott).
W/Neomycin sulfate, gramicidin, thonzylamine HCl, phenylephrine HCl.
See: Biomydrin, Spray, Drops (Warner-Chilcott).

●**thonzylamine hydrochloride.** USAN.
Use: Antihistamine.

Thorazine. (SK-Beecham) Chlorpromazine HCl, **Tab.:** (10, 25, 50, 100, 200 mg) Bot. 100s, 1000s. Single unit pkg. 100s. *Rx.*
Amp.: (25 mg w/ascorbic acid 2 mg, sodium bisulfite 1 mg, sodium sulfite 1 mg, NaCl 6 mg/1 ml), 1 ml, 2 ml. Box 10s, 100s, 500s. Vial: 10 ml. Box 1s, 20s, 100s.
Spansule: 30, 75, 150 & 200 mg Bot. 50s, 100s (S.U.P.), 500s. 300 mg Bot. 50s, 100s (S.U.P.).
Syr.: (10 mg/5 ml) Bot. 4 oz.
Supp.: Chlorpromazine base, w/glycerin, glyceryl monopalmitate, glyceryl monostearate, hydrogenated coconut oil fatty acids, hydrogenated palm kernel oil fatty acids. (25, 100 mg) Box 12. **Conc.:** (30 mg/ml) Bot. 4 oz. in Ctn. 36s., 1 gal. (100 mg/ml) Bot. 8 oz.
Use: Antiemetic, antipsychotic.

Thorets. (Buffington) Benzocaine lozenge. Dispens-A-Kits 500s. Sugar, lactose and salt free. *otc.*
Use: Sore throat relief.

Thor-Prom Tabs. (Major) Chlorpromazine 10 mg, 25 mg, 50 mg, or 100 mg Tab. Bot. 100s, 1000s; 200 mg/Tab. Bot. 250s, 1000s.
Use: Antiemetic, antipsychotic.

Thor Syrup. (Towne) Dextromethorphan HBr 90 mg, pyrilamine maleate 22.5 mg, phenylephrine HCl 10 mg, ephedrine sulfate 15 mg, sod. citrate 325 mg, ammon. chloride 650 mg, guaifenesin 50 mg/fl. oz. Bot. 4 oz. *otc.*
Use: Antitussive, antihistamine, decongestant, expectorant.

•**thozalinone.** (thoe-ZAL-ah-nohn) USAN.
Use: Antidepressant.
See: Stimsen (Lederle).

Threamine DM. (Various Mfr.) Phenylpropanolamine HCl 12.5 mg, chlorpheniramine maleate 2 mg, dextromethorphan HBr 10 mg/5 ml Syr. Bot. pt., gal. *otc.*
Use: Antihistamine, decongestant, antitussive.

Three-Amine TD. (Eon Labs) Phenylpropanolamine HBr 50 mg, pheniramine maleate 25 mg, pyrilamine maleate 25 mg/Time Rel. Cap. *otc.*
Use: Antihistamine, decongestant.

3 mg, Biotin Forte. (Vitaline) Vitamins B$_1$ 10 mg, B$_2$ 10 mg, B$_3$ 40 mg, B$_5$ 10 mg, B$_6$ 25 mg, B$_{12}$ 10 mcg, C 200 mg, biotin 3 mg, folic acid 800 mcg, Zn 30 mg/Tab. Bot. 60s, 1000s. *otc.*
Use: Vitamin/mineral supplement.

•**threonine,** (THREE-oh-neen) U.S.P. 23.
Use: Amino acid, antispasmodic. [Orphan drug]
See: Threostat.

threonine. (Various Mfr.) Threonine 500 mg. **Capsules:** In 60s and 100s. **Tablets:** In 100s and 250s. *otc.*
Use: Nutritional supplement.

threostat. (Tyson) *Rx.*
Use: Antispasmodic.
See: Threonine.

Throat Discs. (SK-Beecham) Capsicum, peppermint, mineral oil, sucrose. Box 60s. *otc.*
Use: Minor throat irritations.

Throat-Eze. (Faraday) Cetylpyridinium chloride 1:3000, cetyl dimethyl benzyl ammonium chloride 1:3000, benzocaine 10 mg/Wafer. Loz., foil wrapped. Vial 15. *otc.*
Use: Anesthetic lozenge.

Thrombate III.
See: Antithrombin III Human.

•**thrombin,** U.S.P. 23. Thrombin, topical, mammalian origin.
Use: Local hemostatic.
See: Thrombinar, Pow. (Jones Medical).
Thrombin-JMI, Pow. (Jones Medical).
Thrombogen, Pow. (Johnson & Johnson).
Thrombostat, Pow. (Parke-Davis).

Thrombinar. (Jones Medical) Thrombin topical. 1000 units: 50% mannitol, 45% sodium chloride. 5000 units: 50% mannitol, 45% sodium chloride, sterile water for injection. 50,000 units: 50% mannitol, 45% sodium chloride. Pow. Vials. Preservative free. *Rx.*
Use: Hemostat, topical.

Thrombin-JMI. (Jones Medical) Pow. 10,000, 20,000 or 50,000 units. *Rx.*
Use: Hemostatic, topical.

Thrombogen. (Johnson & Johnson) Thrombin 1000 units. 5000 units: With isotonic saline diluent and transfer needle. 10,000 units or 20,000 units: With isotonic saline diluent, benzethonium chloride and transfer needle. *Rx.*
Use: Hemostatic, topical.

thrombolytic enzymes.
See: Abbokinase (Abbott).
Abbokinase Open-Cath (Abbott).
Eminase (SK-Beecham).
Kabikinase (Pharmacia & Upjohn).
Streptase (Astra).

thromboplastin.
Use: Diagnostic aid (prothrombin estimation).

Thrombostat. (Parke-Davis) Prothrombin is activated by tissue thromboplastin in the presence of calcium chloride. **1000 U.S. (N.I.H.) units:** Vial 10 ml: **5000 U.S. units:** Vial 10 ml and 5 ml diluent. **10,000 U.S. units:** Vial 20 ml and 10 ml diluent. **20,000 U.S. units:** Vial 30 ml and 20 ml diluent. *Rx.*
Use: Local hemostatic.

Thylox. (C.S. Dent) Medicated bar soap w/absorbable sulfur. Bar 3.4 oz. *otc.*
Use: Cleansing aid.

•**thymalfasin.** USAN. *Formerly Thymosin 9.*
Use: Antineoplastic; vaccine enhancement; hepatitis, infectious disease treatment.

•**thymol,** N.F. 18.
Use: Antifungal, anti-infective, local anesthetic, antitussive, decongestant, pharmaceutic aid (stabilizer).
See: Vicks Regular & Wild Cherry Medi-

cated Cough Drops (Procter & Gamble).

Vicks Vaporub, Oint. (Procter & Gamble).

W/Combinations.

See: Listerine Antiseptic, Soln. (Warner-Lambert).

thymol. (Various Mfr.) 0.25 lb, 1 lb.

Use:

Use: Antifungal, anti-infective, local anesthetic, antitussive, decongestant, pharmaceutic aid (stabilizer).

thymol iodide.

Use: Antifungal; anti-infective.

•**thymopentin.** (THIGH-moe-PEN-tin) USAN. *Formerly Thymopoietin.*

Use: Immunoregulator.

thymosin alpha-1. *Rx.*

Use: Adjunctive treatment of hepatitis B. [Orphan drug]

thyodatil. Name used for Nifuratel.

Thypinone. (Abbott Diagnostics) Protirelin 500 mcg/1 ml Amp.

Use: Adjunctive agent in the diagnostic assessment of thyroid function.

Thyrar. (Rhone-Poulenc Rorer) Bovine thyroid preparation 0.5 gr, 1 gr, 2 gr/Tab. Bot. 100s. *Rx.*

Use: Hypothyroid states.

Thyrel-TRH. (Ferring) Protirelin 0.5 mg/ml/Inj. 1 ml. *Rx.*

Use: Diagnostic aid.

Thyro-Block. (Wallace) Potassium iodide 130 mg/Tab. In 14s. *Rx.*

Use: Antithyroid.

•**thyroid,** U.S.P. 23.

Use: Thyroid hormone.

See: Arco Thyroid, Tab. (Arco).

Armour Thyroid, Tab. (Rhone-Poulenc Rorer).

Delcoid, Tab. (Delco).

Marion Thyroid, Tab. (Hoechst Marion Roussel).

S-P-T., Cap. (Fleming).

Thyrocrine, Tab. (Lemmon).

thyroid combinations.

See: Henydin, Prep. (Arcum).

thyroid desiccated. (THIGH-royd DESS-ih-KATE-uhd)

Use: Thyroid hormone.

See: Armour Thyroid (Rhone-Poulenc Rorer).

S-P-T (Fleming).

Thyrar (Rhone-Poulenc Rorer).

Thyroid Strong (Jones Medical).

Thyroid USP (Various Mfr.).

thyroid diagnostic aids.

Use: In vivo diagnostic aid.

See: Relefact TRH (Hoechst Marion Roussel).

Sodium Iodide I 123 (Mallinckrodt Diagnostics).

Thypinone (Abbott).

Thytropar (Centeon).

thyroid hormones.

See: Liothyronine Sod.

Thyroxin (Various Mfr.).

thyroid preparations.

See: Proloid, Tab. (Parke-Davis).

Thyrar, Tab. (Rhone-Poulenc Rorer).

Thyroxin, Prep. (Var. Mfr.).

thyroid stimulating hormone (TSH). *Rx.*

Use: Adjunct in diagnosis of thyroid cancer. [Orphan drug]

Thyroid Strong. (Jones Medical) Thyroid desiccated 30 mg, 60 mg, 120 mg/Tab. Bot. 100s, 1000s; 30 mg, 120 mg, 180 mg Tab. Bot. 100s; 60 mg/sugar coated. Tab. Bot. 100s, 1000s. *Rx.*

Use: Thyroid hormone.

Thyrolar. (Forest) Liotrix. 0.25 gr/Tab. Bot. 100s; 0.5 gr, 1 gr, 2 gr, 3 gr/Tab. Bot. 100s, 1000s. *Rx.*

Use: Thyroid hormone.

•**thyromedan hydrochloride.** (thigh-ROW-meh-dan) USAN.

Use: Thyromimetic.

thyropropic acid. 4-(4-Hydroxy-3-iodophenoxy)-3,5-diio-dohydrocinnamic acid. Triopron (Warner Chilcott).

Use: Anticholesteremic.

thyrotropic hormone. *Rx.*

Use: In vivo diagnostic aid.

See: Thytropar (Centeon).

thyrotropic principle of bovine anterior pituitary glands.

See: Thytropar, Vial (Centeon Labs.).

thyrotropin.

Use: In vivo diagnostic aid.

See: Thytropar (Centeon).

thyrotropin-releasing hormone.

Use: In vivo diagnostic aid.

See: Relefact TRH (Hoechst Marion Roussell).

Thypinone (Abbott).

•**thyroxine I 125.** USAN.

Use: Radioactive agent.

•**thyroxine I 131.** USAN.

Use: Radioactive agent.

thyrozyme-II A. (Abbott Diagnostics) T-4 diagnostic kit. 100 & 500 test units.

Use: Quantitative measurement of unsaturated thyroxine binding globulin in serum.

Thytropar. (Centeon) Thyrotropin from bovine anterior pituitary glands. Thyrotropin. Vial 10 IU.

Use: Thyroid myxedema due to pituitary insufficiency.

•**tiacrilast.** (TIE-ah-KRILL-ast) USAN.
Use: Antiallergic.

•**tiacrilast sodium.** (TIE-ah-KRILL-ast) USAN.
Use: Antiallergic.

Tiagabine. (Abbott/Novo Nordisk)
Use: Antiepileptic.

•**tiagabine hydrochloride.** USAN.
Use: Anticonvulsant.

Tiamate. (Hoechst Marion Roussel) Diltiazem maleate 120 mg, 180 mg, 240 mg, sucrose/ER Tab. Bot. UD 30s. *Rx.*
Use: Calcium channel blocker.

•**tiamenidine.** (TIE-ah-MEN-ih-DEEN) USAN.
Use: Antihypertensive.

•**tiamenidine hydrochloride.** USAN.
Use: Antihypertensive.

•**tiapamil hydrochloride.** (tie-APP-ah-mill) USAN.
Use: Antagonist (to calcium).

•**tiaramide hydrochloride.** (TIE-ar-ah-MIDE) USAN.
Use: Antiasthmatic.

Tiazac. (Forest) Diltiazem HCl 120, 180, 240, 300 or 360 mg/ER Cap. *Rx.*
Use: Calcium channel blocker.

•**tiazofurin.** (TIE-AZE-oh-few-rin) USAN.
Use: Antineoplastic.

Ti-Baby Natural. (Fischer) Titanium dioxide 5%. SPF 16. Lot. Bot. 120 ml. *otc.*
Use: Sunscreen.

•**tibenelast sodium.** (TIE-ben-ell-ast) USAN.
Use: Antiasthmatic; bronchodilator.

•**tibolone.** (TIH-bole-ohn) USAN.
Use: Menopausal symptoms suppressant.

•**tibric acid.** (TIE-brick) USAN.
Use: Antihyperlipoproteinemic.

•**tibrofan.** (TIE-broe-fan) USAN.
Use: Disinfectant.

•**ticabesone propionate.** (tie-CAB-eh-sone) USAN.
Use: Glucocorticoid.

Ticar. (SK-Beecham) Ticarcillin disodium. 1 g, 3 g, 6 g/Vial in 10s. Piggyback Vials 3 g in 10s. Bulk Pharmacy Pkg. 20 g in 10s. Bulk Pharmacy Pkg. 30 g/Vial, 10s. ADD-Vantage 3 g Pkg. 10s. *Rx.*
Use: Anti-infective.

•**ticarbodine,** (tie-CAR-boe-deen) USAN.
Use: Anthelmintic.

ticarcillin and clavulanate potassium.
Use: Penicillin.
See: Timentin (SK-Beecham Labs).

•**ticarcillin cresyl sodium.** (tie-CAR-SIH-lin KREH-sill) USAN.

Use: Antibacterial.

•**ticarcillin disodium, sterile,** (tie-CAR-SIH-lin) U.S.P. 23.
Use: Antibacterial.
See: Ticar, inj. (SK-Beecham).

ticarcillin disodium and clavulanate potassium, sterile.
Use: Anti-infective, inhibitor (β-lactamase).
See: Timentin, Inj. (SK-Beecham).

•**ticarcillin monosodium,** U.S.P. 23.
Use: Antibacterial.

TICE BCG Vaccine. (Organon) BCG. Intravesical 50 mg/2 ml amps. Freeze-dried suspension for reconstitution.
Use: Antineoplastic.

•**ticlatone.** (TIE-klah-tone) USAN.
Use: Antibacterial, antifungal.

Ticlid. (Syntex) Ticlopidine 250 mg/Tab. Bot. 30s, UD 100s. *Rx.*
Use: Antiplatelet.

•**ticlopidine hydrochloride.** (tie-KLOE-pih-DEEN) USAN.
Use: Inhibitor (platelet).
See: Ticlid, Tab. (Syntex).

•**ticolubant.** USAN.
Use: Antipsoriatic.

Ticon. (Roberts) Trimethobenzamide HCl 100 mg per ml/Inj. Vial 20 ml. *Rx.*
Use: Antiemetic, antivertigo.

ticonazole.
Use: Vaginal antifungal.
See: Vagistat-1, Oint. (Bristol-Myers Squibb).

•**ticrynafen.** USAN.
Use: Diuretic, uricosuric, antihypertensive.

Tidex. (Allison) Dextroamphetamine sulfate, 5 mg/Tab. Bot. 100s, 1000s. *c-ii.*
Use: Obesity control.

Tidexsol Tablets. (Sanofi Winthrop) Acetaminophen. *otc.*
Use: Analgesic.

•**tifurac sodium.** (TIE-fyoor-ak) USAN.
Use: Analgesic.

Tigan. (Roberts) Trimethobenzamide hydrochloride. **Cap.** 100 mg Bot. 100s, 250 mg Bot. 100s. **Amp:** (100 mg/ml) 2 ml. Box 10s. Vial 20 ml **Supp:** 200 mg Box 10s, 50s. **Pediatric Supp:** 100 mg Box 10s. *Rx.*
Use: Antiemetic.

•**tigemonam dicholine.** (TIE-jem-OH-nam die-KOE-leen) USAN.
Use: Antimicrobial.

•**tigestol.** (tie-JESS-tole) USAN.
Use: Progestin.

Tigo. (Burlington) Polymyxin B sulfate 5000 units, zinc bacitracin 400 units,

neomycin sulfate 5 mg/g Oint. Tube 0.5 oz. *otc.*
Use: Anti-infective, topical.

Tihist-DP. (Vita Elixir) d-methorphan HBr 10 mg, pyrilamine maleate 16 mg, sodium citrate 3.3 gr/5 ml. *otc.*
Use: Antitussive, antihistamine.

Tihist Nasal Drops. (Vita Elixir) Pyrilamine maleate 0.1%, phenylephrine HCl 0.25%, sodium bisulfite 0.2%, methylparaben 0.02%, propylparaben 0.01%/30 ml. *otc.*
Use: Decongestant, antihistamine.

Tija Tablets. (Vita Elixir) Oxytetracycline HCl 250 mg/Tab. *Rx.*
Use: Anti-infective, tetracycline.

Tija Syrup. (Vita Elixir) Oxytetracycline HCl 125 mg/5 ml. *Rx.*
Use: Anti-infective, tetracycline.

Tilade. (Medeva) Nedocromil sodium. 1.75 mg per actuation. Aerosol/Can. 16.2 g with mouthpiece. *Rx.*
Use: Respiratory inhalant (anti-inflammatory).

• **tiletamine hydrochloride,** (tie-LET-ah-meen) USAN.
Use: Anesthetic; anticonvulsant.

• **tilidine hydrochloride.** (TIH-lih-DEEN) USAN.
Use: Analgesic.

Ti-Lite. (Fischer) Ethylhexyl p-methoxycinnamate 7.5%, titanium dioxide 2%, cetyl alcohol, phenethyl alcohol, parabens, EDTA. Cream 60 g. *otc.*
Use: Sunscreen.

• **tilomisole.** (TILL-oh-mih-sahl) USAN.
Use: Immunoregulator.

• **tilorone hydrochloride.** (TIE-lore-ohn) USAN.
Use: Antiviral.

• **tiludronate disodium.** (tie-LOO-droe-nate) USAN.
Use: Paget's disease, osteoporosis.
See: SKelid, Tab. (Sanofi-Winthrop).

Timed Reducing Aids-Caffeine Free. (Weeks & Leo) Phenylpropanolamine HCl 75 mg/T.R. Cap. Bot. 28s, 56s. *otc.*
Use: Reducing aid.

• **timefurone.** (tie-MEH-fyoor-OHN) USAN.
Use: Antiatherosclerotic.

Timentin. (SK-Beecham) Ticarcillin disodium 3 g, clavulanic acid (as potassium salt) 0.1 g. Vials 3.1 g, Box 10s. Piggyback Vials 3.1 g, Box 10s. *Rx.*
Use: Anti-infective.

• **timobesone acetate.** (tie-MOE-beh-sone) USAN.
Use: Adrenocortical steroid (topical).

Timolide 10-25. (Merck) Timolol maleate 10 mg, hydrochlorothiazide 25 mg/Tab. Bot. 100s. *Rx.*
Use: Antihypertensive.

• **timolol.** (TI-moe-lahl) USAN.
Use: Antiadrenergic (β-receptor).

• **timolol maleate,** (TI-moe-lahl) U.S.P. 23.
Use: Treatment of chronic open angle, aphakic and secondary glaucoma, antihypertensive, prevention of recurrent MI; antiadrenergic (β-receptor).
See: Blocadren, Tab. (Merck) Timoptic, Oph. (Merck).
Timoptic In Ocudose, Oph. (Merck).

timolol maleate. (TI-moe-lahl) (Various Mfr.) 0.25% or 0.5%. Ophth. Soln. Bot. 5 ml, 10 ml, 15 ml.
Use: Treatment of chronic open angle, aphakic and secondary glaucoma, antihypertensive, prevention of recurrent MI; antiadrenergic (β-receptor).

timolol maleate and hydrochlorothiazide tablets.
Use: Antihypertensive combination.
See: Timolide,Tab. (Merck).

Timolol Maleate Ophthalmic Solution. (Various) Timolol maleate 3.4 mg/0.25 ml and 6.8 mg/0.5 ml/Soln. Bot. 2.5 ml, 5 ml, 10 ml, 15 ml. *Rx.*
Use: Treatment of glaucoma.

Timoptic. (Merck) Timolol maleate 0.25% and 0.5% solution. Ocumeter Ophthalmic Dispenser 2.5 ml, 5 ml, 10 ml, 15 ml. *Rx.*
Use: Agent for glaucoma.

Timoptic in Ocudose. (Merck) Timolol maleate 0.25% or 0.5%. Preservative free in sterile ocudose ophthalmic UD 60s. *Rx.*
Use: Agent for glaucoma.

Timoptic-XE. (Merck) Timolol maleate 0.25% or 0.5%. Gel. Tube 2.5 ml, 5 ml. *Rx.*
Use: Agent for glaucoma.

• **tinabinol.** (tie-NAB-ih-NOLE) USAN.
Use: Antihypertensive.

Tinactin. (Schering-Plough) **Soln. 1%:** Tolnaftate (10 mg/ml) w/butylated hydroxytoluene, in nonaqueous homogeneous PEG 400. Plastic squeeze bot. 10 ml. **Cream 1%:** Tolnaftate (10 mg/g) in homogeneous, nonaqueous vehicle of PEG-400, propylene glycol, carboxypolymethylene, monoamylamine, titanium dioxide and butylated hydroxytoluene. Tube 15 g, 30 g, UD 0.7 g. **Powder 1%:** Tolnaftate w/corn starch, talc. Plastic container 45 g, 90 g. **Powd. Aerosol 1%:** Tolnaftate w/butylated hydroxytoluene, talc, polyethylene-poly-

propylene glycol monobutyl ether, denatured alcohol and inert propellant of isobutane. Spray can 100 g. **Liq. Aerosol 1%:** Tolnaftate w/butylated hydroxytoluene, polyethylene-polyproplyene glycol monobutyl ether, 36% alcohol, and inert propellant of isobutane. Spray can 120 ml. *otc.*
Use: Antifungal.

Tinastat. (Vita Elixir) Sodium hyposulfite, benzethonium Cl/2 oz. *otc.*
Use: Keratolytic lotion.

Tinaval Powder. (Pal-Pak) Tolnaftate 1%. Bot. 45 g. *otc.*
Use: Antifungal for jock itch, athlete's foot.

tine test, old tuberculin. (Wyeth-Lederle). Box of 25, 100 or 250 test applicators.
See: Tuberculin Tine Test (Lederle).

tine test, purified protein derivative. (Wyeth-Lederle). Box of 25 or 100 test applicators.
See: Tuberculin Tine Test (Lederle).

tin fluoride. Stannous Fluoride, U.S.P. 23.

Ting. (Novartis) **Cream:** Benzoic acid, boric acid, zinc oxide, zinc stearate, alcohol 18.7%. Tube 0.9 oz., 1.8 oz. **Powder:** Boric acid, benzoic acid, zinc stearate, zinc oxide. Can 2.5 oz. **Spray Powder:** Total undecylenate 19% as undecylenic acid and zinc undecylenate. Can 2.5 oz. *otc.*
Use: Fungal infections, athlete's foot.

• **tinidazole.** USAN.
Use: Antiprotozoal.
See: Fasigyn (Pfizer).
Simplotan (Pfizer).

Tinset. (Janssen) Oxatomide.
Use: Antiallergenic, antiasthmatic.

Tinver Lotion. (Pilkington Barnes Hind) Sodium thiosulfate 25%, salicylic acid 1%, isopropyl alcohol 10%, propylene glycol, menthol, disodium edetate, colloidal alumina. Bot. 4 oz., 6 oz. *Rx.*
Use: Specific for tinea versicolor.

• **tinzaparin sodium.** USAN.
Use: Anticoagulant; antithrombotic.

• **tioconazole,** (TIE-oh-KOE-nah-zole) U.S.P. 23.
Use: Antifungal.
See: Vagistat (Fujisawa SmithKline)

• **tiodazosin.** (TIE-oh-DAY-zoe-sin) USAN.
Use: Antihypertensive.

• **tiodonium chloride.** (TIE-oh-doe-nee-uhm) USAN.
Use: Antibacterial.

• **tioperidone hydrochloride.** (tie-oh-

PURR-ih-dohn) USAN.
Use: Antipsychotic.

• **tiopinac.** (tie-OH-pin-ACK) USAN.
Use: Anti-inflammatory, analgesic, antipyretic.

tiopronin. *Rx.*
Use: Homozygous cystinuria. [Orphan drug]
See: Thiola (Mission).

• **tiospirone hydrochloride.** (tie-OH-spih-rone) USAN.
Use: Antipsychotic.

• **tiotidine.** (TIE-OH-tih-deen) USAN.
Use: Antagonist to histamine H_2 receptor.

• **tioxidazole.** (tie-OX-ih-DAH-zole) USAN.
Use: Anthelmintic.

• **tipentosin hydrochloride.** (TIE-pin-toe-SIN) USAN.
Use: Antihypertensive.

Tipramine Tabs. (Major) Imipramine 10 mg/Tab. Bot. 250s; 25 mg or 50 mg/Tab. Bot. 250s, 1000s. *Rx.*
Use: Antidepressant.

• **tipredane.** (tie-PRED-ANE) USAN.
Use: Adrenocortical steroid (topical).

• **tiprenolol hydrochloride.** (tie-PREH-no-lole) USAN.
Use: Antiadrenergic (β-receptor).

• **tiprinast meglumine.** (TIE-prih-nast meh-GLUE-meen) USAN. A BM-Squibb investigative drug.
Use: Antiallergic.

• **tipropidil hydrochloride.** (TIE-PRO-pih-dill) USAN.
Use: Vasodilator.

• **tiqueside.** (TIE-kweh-side) USAN.
Use: Antihyperlipidemic.

• **tiquinamide hydrochloride.** (tie-KWIN-ah-mide) USAN.
Use: Anticholinergic (gastric).

• **tirapazamine.** (tie-rah-PAZZ-ah-meen) USAN.
Use: Antineoplastic.

tiratricol. *Rx.*
Use: Antineoplastic. [Orphan drug]

Tirend. (SK-Beecham) Caffeine 100 mg/Tab. Bot. 12s, 25s, 50s. *otc.*
Use: CNS stimulant.

• **tirilazad mesylate.** (tie-RIH-lah-zad MEH-sih-late) USAN.
Use: Inhibitor (lipid peroxidation).
See: Freedox (Pharmacia & Upjohn).

• **tirofiban hydrochloride.** (tie-rah-FIE-ban) USAN.
Use: Treatment of unstable angina.

TI-Screen. (Pedinol) **Gel:** SPF 20+, ethylhexyl p-methoxycinnamate 7.5%, oxy-

benzone 5%, 2-ethylhexyl salicylate 5%, SD alcohol 40 71%. 120 g; **Lip Balm:** SPF 8+, ethylhexyl p-methoxycinnamate 7.5%, oxybenzone 5%, petrolatum. 4.5 g; **Lot.: SPF 8:** Ethylhexyl p-methoxycinnamate 6%, oxybenzone 2%. Bot. 120 ml; **SPF 15:** Ethylhexyl p-methoxycinnamate 7.5%, oxybenzone 5%. Bot. 120 ml; **SPF 30:** Octyl methoxycinnamate 7.5%, octyl salicylate 5%, oxybenzone 6%, octocrylene 7.5%. Bot. 120 ml. *otc.*
Use: Sunscreen.

TI-Screen Natural. (Pedinol) Titanium dioxide 5%. Lot. Bot. 120 ml. *otc.*
Use: Sunscreen.

•**tisilfocon a.** USAN.
Use: Contact lens material (hydrophobic).

Tisit. (Pfeiffer) Pyrethrins 0.3%, piperonyl butoxide technical 3%, petroleum distillate 1.2%, benzyl alcohol 2.4%. Shampoo. Bot. 118 ml. *otc.*
Use: Treatment of lice.

TiSol. (Parnell) Benzyl alcohol 1%, menthol 0.04%, isotonic sodium chloride 0.9%, sorbitol, EDTA. Soln. Bot. 237 ml. *otc.*
Use: Temporary relief of minor sore throat pain and irritation.

tissue fixative and wash solution. (Wampole-Zeus) A modified Michel's tissue fixative and buffered wash solution.
Use: To facilitate the transport and processing of fresh tissue biopsies.

tissue plasminogen activator, recombinant.
See: Activase (Gentech).

tissue respiratory factor (trf). (International Hormone) RSF, SRF, LYCD, PCO, Procytoxid marketed as 2000 units. Supplied as bulk liquid concentrate. *Rx.*
Use: Promotion of cellular oxidation.

Tis-U-Sol. (Baxter) Pentalyte irrigation containing NaCl 800 mg, KCl 40 mg, magnesium sulfate 20 mg, sodium phosphate 8.75 mg, and 6.25 mg monobasic potassium phosphate per 100 ml. Bot. 250 ml, 1000 ml. *Rx.*
Use: Physiologic irrigating solution.

Titan. (Pilkington Barnes Hind) EDTA 2%, nonionic cleaner buffers, potasssium sorbate 0.13%. Soln. Bot. 30 ml. *otc.*
Use: Hard contact lens cleaning solution.

•**titanium dioxide,** U.S.P. 23.
Use: Solar ray protectant (topical).

titicum ripens.
W/Oxyquinoline sulfate, charcoal.
See: Triticoll, Tabs. (Western Research).

Titralac. (3M Pharm) Calcium carbonate 420 mg, saccharin, sodium 0.3 mg. Chew. Tab. Bot. 40s, 100s, 1000s. *otc.*
Use: Antacid.

Titralac Extra Strength Tablets. (3M Pharm) Calcium carbonate 750 mg, saccharin, sodium 0.6 mg. Chew. Tab. Bot. 100s. *otc.*
Use: Antacid.

Titralac Plus Liquid. (3M Personal Health Care) Calcium carbonate 500 mg, simethicone 20 mg, saccharin, sorbitol, sodium 0.15 mg. Bot. 360 ml. *otc.*
Use: Antacid.

Titralac Plus Tablets. (3M Pharm) Calcium carbonate 420 mg, simethicone 21 mg, saccharin, sodium 1.1 mg. Chew. Tab. Bot. 100s. *otc.*
Use: Antacid.

•**tixanox.** (TIX-ah-nox) USAN.
Use: Antiallergic.

•**tixocortol pivalate.** (tix-OH-kahr-tole PIH-vah-late) USAN.
Use: Anti-inflammatory (topical).

tizanidine hydrochloride. (tie-ZAN-ih-deen)
Use: Antispasmodic.
See: Zanaflex.

•**tizanidine hydrochloride.** USAN.
Use: Antispasmodic. [Orphan drug]

T-Koff. (T.E. Williams) Phenylpropanolamine HCl 20 mg, phenylephrine HCl 20 mg, chlorpheniramine maleate 5 mg, codeine phosphate 10 mg/5 ml Syr. Bot. 480 ml Grape flavor. *c-v.*
Use: Antihistamine, decongestant, antitussive.

t-lymphotropic virus type III gp 160 antigens. *Rx.*
Use: Treatment for AIDS. [Orphan drug]
See: Vaxsyn HIV-1.

TMP-SMZ. *Rx.*
Use: Anti-infective.
See: Proloprim (Glaxo Wellcome).
Trimethoprim (Various Mfr.).
Trimpex (Roche).

Tobrades Suspension. (Alcon) Dexamethasone 0.1%, tobramycin 0.3%, thimerisol 0.001%, alcohol 0.5%, propylene glycol, polyoxyethylene, polyoxypropylene. 2.5 ml, 5 ml. *Rx.*
Use: Anti-infective, corticosteroid.

TobraDex. (Alcon). 0.3% tobramycin and 0.1% dexamethasone. Susp. Bot. 2.5 ml or 5 ml. *Rx.*

Use: Corticosteroid, anti-infective, ophthalmic.

TobraDex, Ointment. (Alcon Labs) Dexamethasone 0.1%, tobramycin 0.3%, chlorobutanol 0.5%, mineral oil, white petrolatum. Ophthalmic 3.5 g. *Rx.*
Use: Corticosteroid anti-infective, ophthalmic.

●**tobramycin,** (TOE-bruh-MY-sin) U.S.P. 23. An antibiotic obtained from cultures of *Streptomyces tenebrarius.*
Use: Antibacterial, ophthalmic. [Orphan drug]
See: Tobrex, Soln., Oint. (Alcon).

tobramycin. (TOE-bruh-MY-sin) (Bausch & Lomb) Tobramycin 0.3%, benzalkonium Cl 0.01%, boric acid. Soln. 5 ml. *Rx.*
Use: Anti-infective, ophthalmic.

tobramycin and dexamethasone ophthalmic ointment.
Use: Anti-infective, ophthalmic.

tobramycin sulfate. (Various Mfr.) Tobramycin sulfate 40 mg/ml. Inj. Syringes: 1.5 ml, 2 ml. Vial 2 ml. Pediatric inj. 10 mg/ml. Vial 2 ml. *Rx.*
Use: Aminoglycoside, anti-infective.

●**tobramycin sulfate,** U.S.P. 23.
Use: Antibacterial, aminoglycoside.
See: Nebcin, Amp., Hyporet. (Lilly).

Tobrex Ophthalmic Ointment. (Alcon) Tobramycin 0.3% in sterile ointment base. Tube 3.5 g. *Rx.*
Use: Anti-infective, ophthalmic.

Tobrex Solution. (Alcon) Tobramycin 0.3%. ophthalmic solution. Bot. 5 ml Drop-Tainer. *Rx.*
Use: Anti-infective, ophthalmic.

●**tocainide.** (TOE-cane-ide) USAN.
Use: Antiarrhythmic, cardiac depressant.
See: Tonocard, Tab. (Merck).

●**tocainide hydrochloride,** U.S.P. 23.
Use: Antiarrhythmic, cardiac depressant.

●**tocamphyl.** (toe-KAM-fill) USAN.
Use: Choleretic.
See: Gallogen, Tab. (SK-Beecham).

tocopherol-dl-alpha. Vitamin E, U.S.P. 23.
   Cap. & Tab.:
   Denamone, Cap. (3 min., 10 min.) wheat germ oil (Vio-Bin).
   Ecofrol, Cap. (O'Neal).
   Eprolin, Gelseal (Lilly).
   Epsilan M, Cap. (Warren-Teed).
   Oint.:
   Myopone (Drug Prods.).
   Sol.:

Aquasol E, Soln. (Rhone-Poulenc Rorer).

●**tocopherols excipient,** N.F. 18.
Use: Pharmaceutic aid (antioxidant).

●**tocophersolan.** (toe-KAHF-ehr-SO-lan) USAN.
Use: Vitamin E supplement.

tocopheryl acetate-d-alpha. Vitamin E, U.S.P. 23.
See: Aquasol E, Prods. (Rhone-Poulenc Rorer).
   Epsilan-M, Cap. (Warren-Teed).
   Tocopher, Cap. (Quality Generics).
   Tokols, Cap. (Ulmer).
   Vitamins E. (Var. Mfr.).

tocopheryl acetates, conc. d-alpha. Vitamin E, U.S.P. 23.
Use: Treatment of habitual & threatened abortion.

tocopheryl acid succinated d-alpha. Vitamin E, U.S.P. 23.
See: E-Ferol Succinate, Tab., Cap. (Forest).
   Vitamins E (Various Mfr.).

Tocosamine. (Trent) Sparteine sulfate 150 mg, sod. chl. 4.5 mg/ml. Amps. 1 ml. Box 12s, 100s. *Rx.*
Use: Oxytocic.

Today Vaginal Contraceptive Sponge. (VLI) Nonoxynol-9, citric, sorbic, benzoic acid, sodium dihydrogen, citrate, sodium metabisulfite, polyurethane foam sponge. 3s, 6s, and 12s.
Use: Contraceptive.

●**tofenacin hydrochloride.** (tah-FEN-ah-sin) USAN.
Use: Anticholinergic.

tofranazine. (Novartis) Combination of imipramine and promazine. Pending release.

Tofranil. (Novartis) Imipramine HCl. **Tab.** 10 mg Bot. 100s, 1000s; 25 mg & 50 mg. Bot. 100s, 1000s. UD 100s. Gy-Pak 100s, 1 unit (12×100); 6 units (72100). **Amps.** 25 mg/2 ml w/ascorbic acid 2 mg, sod. bisulfite 1 mg, sod. sulfite 1 mg and 2 ml amps. *Rx.*
Use: Antidepressant, antienuretic.

Tofranil-PM. (Novartis) Imipramine pamoate 75 mg, 100 mg, 125 mg or 150 mg/Cap. Bot. 30s, 100s. 75 mg/Cap. Bot. 1000s. UD 75 mg and 150 mg in 100s. *Rx.*
Use: Antidepressant.

Tolamide Tabs. (Major) Tolazamide 100 mg/Tab. Bot. 100s, 250s; 250 mg/Tab. 200s, 500s; 500 mg/Tab. Bot. 100s, 500s. *Rx.*
Use: Antidiabetic.

•**tolamolol.** (tahl-AIM-oh-lahl) USAN.
Use: Beta-adrenergic receptor blocking agent, coronary vasodilator, cardiac depressant (antiarrhythmic).

•**tolazamide,** (tole-AZE-uh-mid) U.S.P. 23.
Use: Hypoglycemic, antidiabetic.
See: Tolinase, Tab. (Pharmacia & Upjohn).

tolazamide. (Various Mfr.) 100, 250 or 500 mg/Tab. 100s, 200s, 250s, 500s, 1000s, UD 100s. *Rx.*
Use: Antidiabetic.

•**tolazoline hydrochloride,** U.S.P. 23.
Use: Antiadrenergic, antihypertensive, vasodilator (peripheral).
See: Priscoline, Inj. (Novartis).

•**tolbutamide,** (tole-BYOO-tuh-mide) U.S.P. 23.
Use: Hypoglycemic; antidiabetic.
See: Orinase, Tab. (Pharmacia & Upjohn).

tolbutamide. (Various Mfr.) 500 mg/Tab. 100s, 500s, 1000s, UD 100s. *Rx.*
Use: Antidiabetic.

•**tolbutamide sodium, sterile,** (tole-BYOO-tuh-mide) U.S.P. 23.
Use: Diagnostic aid (diabetes).
See: Orinase Diagnostic (Pharmacia & Upjohn).

•**tolcapone.** (TOLE-kah-pone) USAN. [Investigational]
Use: Antiparkinsonian.

•**tolciclate.** USAN.
Use: Antifungal.

Tolectin 200. (McNeil Pharm) Tolmetin sodium 200 mg/Tab. Bot. 100s. *Rx.*
Use: Nonsteroidal anti-inflammatory, analgesic.

Tolectin 600. (McNeil Pharm) Tolmetin sodium 600 mg/Tab. Bot. 100s. *Rx.*
Use: Nonsteroidal anti-inflammatory, analgesic.

Tolectin DS. (McNeil Pharm) Tolmetin sodium 400 mg/Cap Bot. 100s, 500s, UD 100s. *Rx.*
Use: Nonsteroidal anti-inflammatory, analgesic.

Tolerex. (Procter & Gamble) Protein 20.6 g, carbohydrate 226.3 g, fat 1.45 g, sodium 468 mg, potassium 1172 mg, mOsm/Kg H_2O 550, cal/ml 1, vitamins A, B_1, B_2, B_3, B_5, B_6, B_{12}, C, D, E, K, folic acid, biotin, choline, Ca, P, I, Fe, Mg, Cu, Zn, Mn, Se, Mo, Cr. Assorted flavors Pow. Pkts. 80 g. *otc.*
Use: Vitamin/mineral supplement.

•**tolfamide.** (TAHL-fah-MIDE) USAN.
Use: Enzyme inhibitor (urease).

Tolfrinic. (Ascher) Ferrous fumarate 200 mg, Vitamins B_{12} 25 mcg, Vitamins C 100 mg/Tab. Bot. 100s. *otc.*
Use: Vitamin/mineral supplement.

•**tolgabide.** (TOLE-gah-bide) USAN.
Use: Antiepileptic (control of abnormal movements).

•**tolimidone.** (TAHL-IH-mih-dohn) USAN.
Use: Antiulcerative.

Tolinase. (Pharmacia & Upjohn) Tolazamide 100 mg (unit-of-use 100s), 250 mg (200s, 1000s, UD 100s, unit-of-use 100s), 500 mg (unit-of-use 100s)/Tab. *Rx.*
Use: Antidiabetic.

•**tolindate.** (TOLE-in-DATE) USAN.
Use: Antifungal.
See: Dalnate (Rhone-Poulenc Rorer).

•**tolmetin.** (TOLE-meh-tin) USAN.
Use: Anti-inflammatory.

•**tolmetin sodium,** (TOLE-mee-tin) U.S.P. 23.
Use: Anti-inflammatory.
See: Tolectin, Tab. (McNeil).
Tolectin DS, Cap. (McNeil).

•**tolnaftate,** (tahl-NAFF-tate) U.S.P. 23.
Use: Antifungal.
See: Absorbine Antifungal, Cream (W.F. Young).
Aftate, Prods. (Schering-Plough).
Tinactin, Soln., Cream, Pow., Pow. Aer. (Schering-Plough).

•**tolofocon a.** (TOE-low-FOE-kahn A) USAN.
Use: Contact lens material (hydrophobic).

tolonium chloride.

toloxychlorinal.
Use: Sedative.

•**tolpovidone I 131.** (tahl-POE-vih-dohn I 131) USAN.
Use: Diagnostic aid (hypoalbuminemia), radioactive agent.
See: Raovin (Abbott).

•**tolpyrramide.** (tahl-PIHR-ah-mid) USAN.
Use: Oral hypoglycemic; antidiabetic.

•**tolrestat.** (TOLE-ress-TAT) USAN.
Use: Inhibitor (aldose reductase).
See: Alredase (Wyeth-Ayerst).

•**tolu balsam,** U.S.P. 23. N.F. XVII.
Use: Pharmaceutic necessity for Compound Benzoin Tincture, expectorant.
See: Vicks Regular & Wild Cherry Medicated Cough Drops (Procter & Gamble).

tolu balsam syrup, N.F. XVII. (Lilly) Bot. 16 fl. oz.
Use: Vehicle.

tolu balsam tincture, N.F. XVII.
Use: Flavor.

toluidine blue o chloride.
See: Blutene Chloride.

Tolu-Sed (No Sugar). (Scherer) Codeine phosphate 10 mg, guaifenesin 100 mg/5 ml w/alcohol 10%. Bot. 4 oz., pt. c-v.
Use: Antitussive, expectorant.

Tolu-Sed DM (No Sugar). (Scherer) Dextromethorphan HBr 10 mg, guaifenesin 100 mg/5 ml w/alcohol 10%. Bot. 4 oz., pt. otc.
Use: Antitussive, expectorant.

•**tomelukast.** (tah-MELL-you-KAST) USAN.
Use: Antiasthmatic (leukotriene antagonist).

Tomocat. (Lafayette) CT barium sulfate 1.5% w/v. Case of 24 Bot.
Use: Mark alimentary tract during CT scans.

Tomocat 1000. (Lafayette) Barium sulfate suspension concentrate 5% w/v/Bot. for dilution to 1.5% w/v at time of use. Bot. 225 ml w/1000 ml dilution Bot. Case 24 Bot. and 2 Dilution Bot.
Use: Radiopaque medium used to mark the GI tract during CT scans.

•**tomoxetine hydrochloride.** (TOE-MOX-eh-teen) USAN.
Use: Antidepressant.

Tonavite-M Elixir. (Goldline) Bot. 12 oz., pt., gal.
Use: Dietary supplement.

•**tonazocine mesylate.** (tone-AZE-oh-SEEN) USAN.
Use: Analgesic.

Tono-B Pediatric. (Pal-Pak) Iron 5 mg, thiamine HCl 0.167 mg, riboflavin 0.133 mg/Tab. Bot. 1000s. otc.
Use: Vitamin/mineral supplement.

Tonocard. (Astra Merck) Tocainide HCl 400 mg and 600 mg/Tab. Bot. 100s. UD 100s. Rx.
Use: Antiarrhythmic.

Tonojug 2000. (Lafayette) Barium sulfate powder 1200 g for suspension to make 2000 ml. Bot. 2000 g Case: 8 Bot.
Use: Radiopaque contrast medium for use during x-ray examination of the GI tract.

Tonopaque Oral Barium. (Lafayette) Barium sulfate powder 180 g for suspension. Bot. 180 g Case 24s.
Use: Radiopaque contrast medium for use during x-ray examination of the GI tract.

Toothache Gel. (Roberts Med) Benzocaine, oil of cloves, benzyl alcohol, propylene glycol. Tube 15 g. otc.
Use: Local anesthetic.

Toothache Relief-3 in 1. (C.S. Dent) Toothache gum, toothache drops, benzocaine lotion. otc.
Use: Treatment of toothache.

Topamax. (McNeil) Topiramate 25 mg, 100 mg, 200 mg, lactose/Tab. Bot. 60s. Rx.
Use: Anticonvulsant.

Top Brass ZP-11. (Revlon) Zinc pyrithione 0.5% in cream base.
Use: Antidandruff hairdress.

Top-Form. (Colgate Oral) Topical formfitting gel applicators. Disposable trays for topical fluoride office treatments, plus permanent trays for topical fluoride home self-treatments. Box 100s. Rx.
Use: Topical fluoride applications in home or office.

Topic. (Syntex) 5% benzyl alcohol in greaseless gel base containing camphor, menthol, w/30% isopropyl alcohol. Tube 2 oz. otc.
Use: Antipruritic.

topical anesthetics, miscellaneous.
See: Ethyl Chloride (Gebauer).
Flouri-Methane (Gebauer).
Fluro-Ethyl (Gebauer).

Topical Fluoride. (Pacemaker). Acidulated phosphate fluoride. Flavors: Orange, bubblegum, lime, raspberry, grape, cinnamon. Liq. Bot. 4 oz., pt.
Use: Corticosteroid, topical.

Topicort Cream. (Hoechst Marion Roussel) Desoximetasone 0.25% emollient cream consisting of isopropyl myristate, cetyl stearyl alcohol, white petrolatum, mineral oil, lanolin alcohol and purified water. Tubes 15 g, 60 g, 120 g. Rx.
Use: Corticosteroid, topical.

Topicort Gel. (Hoechst Marion Roussel) Desoximetasone 0.05% in gel base. 20% alcohol. Tube 15 g, 60 g. Rx.
Use: Corticosteroid, topical.

Topicort LP Cream. (Hoechst Marion Roussel) Desoximetasone 0.05%. Tubes 15 g, 60 g. Rx.
Use: Corticosteroid, topical.

Topicort Ointment. (Hoechst Marion Roussel) Desoximetasone 0.25% in ointment base. Tube 15 g, 60 g. Rx.
Use: Corticosteroid, topical.

Topicycline. (Roberts) Tetracycline HCl 2.2 mg/ml w/sodium bisulfite, ethanol 40%. Bot. 70 ml w/diluent. Rx.
Use: Antiacne.

•**topiramate.** (toe-PIRE-ah-MATE) USAN.
Use: Anticonvulsant.
See: Topamax, Tab. (McNeil).

topocaine.

See: Surfacaine (Lilly).

Toposar. (Pharmacia & Upjohn) Etoposide 20 mg, benzyl alcohol 30 mg, alcohol 30.5%/ml. Inj. 5 ml, 10 ml, 25 ml. *Rx.*
Use: Mitotic inhibitor.

• **topotecan hydrochloride.** (toe-poe-TEE-kan) USAN.
Use: Antineoplastic (DNA topoisomerase I inhibitor).
See: Hycamtin, Pow. for inj. (SK-Beecham).

Toprol XL. (Astra) Metoprolol succinate 47.5 mg, 95 mg or 190 mg/ER Tab. Bot. 100s. *Rx.*
Use: Antihypertensive.

• **topterone.** (TOP-ter-ohn) USAN.
Use: Antiandrogen.

TOPV.
Use: Vaccine, viral.
See: Orimune (Lederle).

• **toquizine.** (TOE-kwih-zeen) USAN.
Use: Anticholinergic.

Toradol. (Syntex) Ketorolac tromethamine 15 mg/ml and 30 mg/ ml. Injection. 15 mg/ml in 1 ml Tubex syringes, 30 mg/ml in 1 ml and 2 ml Tubex syringes. *Rx.*
Use: Nonsteroidal anti-inflammatory, analgesic.

Toradol Tablets. (Syntex) Ketorolac tromethamine 10 mg/Tab. Bot. 100s, UD 100s. *Rx.*
Use: Nonsteroidal anti-inflammatory.

Torecan. (Boehringer Ingelheim) Thiethylperazine. **Tab.** 10 mg w/tartrazine. Bot. 100s. **Amp.** 10 mg/2 ml (w/sod. metabisulfite 0.5 mg, ascorbic acid 2 mg, sorbitol 40 mg, q.s. carbon dioxide). **Supp.** 10 mg (w/cocoa butter) Box 12s. *Rx.*
Use: Antiemetic, antinauseant.

toremifene. (TORE-EM-ih-feen SIH-trate) *Rx.*
Use: Antineoplastic. [Orphan drug]
See: Estrinex.

• **toremifene citrate.** USAN.
Use: Antiestrogen; antineoplastic.

Tornalate. (Dura) Bitolterol mesylate 0.2%, alcohol 25%, propylene glycol. Soln. for inhalation. Bot. 10 ml, 30 ml, 60 ml. *Rx.*
Use: Bronchodilator for bronchial asthma and reversible bronchospasms.

Tornalate Inhaler. (Dura) Bitolterol mesylate metered inhaler. Bot. 16.4 g w/ oral inhaler. Refill 16.4 g. *Rx.*
Use: Bronchodilator for bronchial asthma and reversible bronchospasms.

Tornalate Tablets. (Sanofi Winthrop) Bitolterol mesylate. *Rx.*
Use: Bronchodilator.

• **torsemide.** (TORE-suh-MIDE) USAN.
Use: Diuretic.
See: Demadex, Tab., Inj. (Boehringer Mannheim)

torula yeast, dried, Obtained by growing *Candida (torulopsis) utilis* yeast on wood pulp wastes (Nutritional Labs.) Conc. 100 lb. drums.
Use: Natural source of protein and Vitamin B-complex vitamins.

• **tosifen.** USAN.
Use: Antianginal.

• **tosufloxacin.** (toe-SUE-FLOX-ah-sin) USAN.
Use: Antibacterial.

Totacillin. (SK-Beecham) Ampicillin trihydrate equivalent to: **Cap.** 250 mg/Cap. Bot. 500s. 500 mg/Cap. Bot. 500s. **Susp.:** 125 mg/5 ml. Bot. 100 ml, 150 ml, 200 ml; 250 mg/5 ml. Bot. 100 ml, 200 ml. *Rx.*
Use: Anti-infective, penicillin.

Totacillin-N. (SK-Beecham) Ampicillin sodium 250 mg, 500 mg, 1 g, 2 g/Vial in 10s; Piggyback Vials 500 mg, 1 g, 2 g, in 25s; Bulk Pharm pkg. 10 g in 25s. *Rx.*
Use: Anti-infective, penicillin.

Total. (Allergan) Polyvinyl alcohol, edetate disodium and benzalkonium chloride in a sterile, buffered, isotonic solution. Soln. Bot. 60 ml, 120 ml. *otc.*
Use: Hard contact lens all purpose solution.

Total Eclipse Cooling Alcohol. (Sandoz) Padimate O, oxybenzone, glyceryl PABA, alcohol 77%. SPF 15. Lot. Bot. 120 ml. *otc.*
Use: Sunscreen.

Total Eclipse Moisturizing. (Sandoz) Padimate O, oxybenzone, octyl salicylate. Moisturizing base. SPF 15. Lot. Bot. 120 ml. *otc.*
Use: Sunscreen.

Total Eclipse Oil & Acne Prone Skin Sunscreen. (Eclipse) Padimate O, oxybenzone, glyceryl PABA, alcohol 77%. SPF 15. Lot. Bot. 120 ml. *otc.*
Use: Sunscreen.

Total Formula. (Vitaline) Iron 20 mg, vitamins A 10,000 IU, D 400 IU, E 30 IU, B_1 15 mg, B_2 15 mg, B_3 25 mg, B_5 25 mg, B_6 25 mg, B_{12} 25 mcg, C 100 mg, folic acid 0.4 mg, Ca, Cr, Cu, I, K, Mg,

Mn, Mo, P, Se, Si, V, vitamin K, biotin 300 mcg, Zn 30 mg, choline, bioflavonoids, hesperidin, inositol, PABA, rutin/Tab. Bot. 90s, 100s. *otc.*
Use: Vitamin/mineral supplement.

Total Formula-2. (Vitaline) Iron 20 mg, vitamins A 10,000 IU, D 400 IU, E 30 IU, B_1 15 mg, B_2 15 mg, B_3 25 mg, B_5 25 mg, B_6 25 mg, B_{12} 25 mcg, C 100 mg, folic acid 0.4 mg, Ca, Cr, Cu, I, K, Mg, Mn, Mo, P, Se, Si, V, vitamin K, biotin 300 mcg, Zn 30 mg, choline, bioflavonoids, hesperidin, inositol, PABA, rutin/Tab. with boron. Bot. 60s. *otc.*
Use: Vitamin/mineral supplement.

Total Solution. (Allergan) Isotonic, buffered soln. of polyvinyl alcohol, benzalkonium chloride, EDTA. Soln. Bot. 60 ml, 120 ml. *otc.*
Use: Ophthalmic.

totaquine. Alkaloids from Cinchona bark, 7% to 12% quinine anhydrous, 70% to 80% total alkaloids (cinchonidine, cinchonine, quinidine & quinine).

totomycin hydrochloride. Tetracycline, U.S.P. 23.

Touro A & D. (Dartmouth Pharm) Chlorpheniramine maleate 4 mg, phenyltoloxamine citrate 50 mg, phenylephrine HCl 20 mg/SR Cap. Bot. 100s. *Rx.*
Use: Antihistamine, decongestant.

Touro EX. (Dartmouth Pharm) Guaifenesin 600 mg. SR Capl. Bot. 100s. *Rx.*
Use: Expectorant.

Touro LA. (Dartmouth) Pseudoephedrine HCl 120 mg, guaifenesin 500 mg/Cap. Bot. 100s. *Rx.*
Use: Decongestant, expectorant.

Toxo. (Wampole-Zeus) *Toxoplasma* antibody test system. Tests 120s.
Use: An IFA test system for the detection of antibodies to *Toxoplasma gondii.*

toxoid, diphtheria.
Use: Immunizing agent (active).
See: Acel-Immune, Vial (Wyeth-Lederle).
ActHIB/DTP, Set of DTwP vial plus Hib Pow. for Inj. (Pasteur-Merieux-Connaught).
diphtheria and tetanus toxoids (pediatric strength).
diphtheria and tetanus toxoids with pertussis vaccine, Vial (Various Mfr.).
tetanus and diphteria toxoids (adult strength), Vial.
Tetramune, Vial (Wyeth-Lederle).
Tri-Immunol, Vial (Wyeth-Lederle).
Tripedia, Vial (Pasteur-Merieux-Connaught).

toxoid, tetanus adsorbed.
Use: Immunizing agent (active).

toxoid, tetanus. *Rx.*
Use: Agent for immunization.
See: Acel-Immune, Vial (Wyeth-Lederle).
ActHIB/DTP, Set of DTwP vial plus Hib Pow. for Inj. (Pasteur-Merieux-Connaught).
diphtheria and tetanus toxoids (pediatric strength).
diphtheria and tetanus toxoids with pertussis vaccine, Vial (Various Mfr.).
tetanus and diphteria toxoids (adult strength), Vial.
Tetramune, Vial (Wyeth-Lederle).
Tri-Immunol, Vial (Wyeth-Lederle).
Tripedia, Vial (Pasteur-Merieux-Connaught).

toxoplasmosis test.
Use: In vitro diagnostic aid.
See: TPM Test (Wampole).

t-PA.
Use: Tissue plasminogen activator.
See: Activase (Genentech).

T-Phyl. (Purdue Frederick) Theophylline 200 mg/Tab. Bot. 100s. *Rx.*
Use: Bronchodilator.

TPM-Test. (Wampole) Indirect hemagglutination test for the qualitative and quantitative determination of antibodies to *Toxoplasma gondii* in serum. Kit 120s,
Use: An aid in the diagnosis of toxoplasmosis.

TPN Electrolytes. (Abbott Hospital Prods) Multiple electrolyte additive: 321 mg sodium chloride, 331 mg calcium chloride, 1491 mg potassium chloride, 508 mg magnesium chloride, 2420 mg sodium acetate; 20 ml in 50 ml fliptop or pintop vial or 20 ml Univ. Add. syr. *Rx.*
Use: Provides electrolytes during total parenteral nutrition.

TPN Electrolytes II. (Abbott) Na 15 mEq/L, K 18 mEq/L, Ca 4.5 mEq/L, Mg 5 mEq/L, Cl 35 mEq/L, acetate 7.5 mEq/L. In 20 ml fill in 50 ml fliptop and pintop vials and 20 ml fill syringes. *Rx.*
Use: Parenteral nutritional therapy.

TPN Electrolytes III. (Abbott) Na 25 Eq/L, K 40.6 mEq/L, Ca 5 mEq/L, Mg 5 mEq/L, Cl 33.5 mEq/L, acetate 40.6 mEq/L, gluconate 5 mEq/L. In 20 ml fill in 50 ml fliptop and pintop vials and 20 ml fill syringes. *Rx.*
Use: Parenteral nutritional therapy

• **tracazolate.** (track-AZE-oh-late) USAN.
Use: Sedative, hypnotic.

Trace. (Young Dental Manufacturing) Erythrosine conc. soln. Squeeze Bot. 30 ml, 60 ml Dispenser Packets 200s. *otc.*
Use: Diagnostic aid to disclose dental plaque.

Trace 28 Liquid. (Young Dental Manufacturing) D & C Red No. 28 in Aqueous Soln. Bot. 30 ml, 60 ml. *otc.*
Use: Diagnostic aid to disclose dental plaque.

Trace 28 Tablets. (Young Dental Manufacturing) D & C Red No. 28. Tablets. Box 30s, 180s, 700s. *otc.*
Use: Diagnostic aid to disclose dental plaque.

Tracelyte. (Fujisawa) A combination of electrolytes and trace elements additive. Vial 20 ml. *Rx.*
Use: Electrolyte and trace element replenishment.

Tracelyte-II. (Fujisawa) A combination of electrolytes and trace elements additive. Vial 20 ml. *Rx.*
Use: Electrolyte and trace element replenishment.

Tracelyte-II with Double Electrolytes. (Fujisawa) Combination of electrolytes and trace elements additive. Vial 40 ml. *Rx.*
Use: Electrolyte and trace element replenisher.

Tracelyte with Double Electrolytes. (Fujisawa) A combination of electrolytes and trace elements additive. Vial 40 ml. *Rx.*
Use: Electrolyte and trace element replenisher.

Traceplex. (Enzyme Process) Iron 30 mg, iodine 0.1 mg, copper 0.5 mg, magnesium 40 mg, zinc 10 mg, B_{12} 5 mcg/4 Tabs. Bot. 100s, 250s. *otc.*
Use: Mineral supplement.

Tracer bG. (Boehringer Mannheim) Reagent strips. Kit. 25s, 50s.
Use: In vitro diagnostic aid.

Tracrium Injection. (Glaxo Wellcome) Atracurium besylate 10 mg/ml Amp. 5 ml. Box 10s; 10 ml MDV. Box 10s. *Rx.*
Use: Surgical muscle relaxant.

Trac Tabs 2X. (Hyrex) Atropine sulfate 0.06 mg, hyoscyamine sulfate 0.03 mg, methenamine 120 mg, methylene blue 6 mg, phenyl salicylate 30 mg, benzoic acid 7.5 mg/Tab. Bot. 100s, 1000s. *Rx.*
Use: Urinary tract infections.

•**tragacanth,** N.F. 18.
Use: Pharmaceutic aid (suspending agent).

•**tralonide.** (TRAY-low-nide) USAN.

Use: Glucocorticoid.

•**tramadol hydrochloride.** (TRAM-uh-dole) USAN.
Use: Analgesic.
See: Ultram, Tab. (Ortho-McNeil).

•**tramazoline hydrochloride,** (tram-AZE-oh-leen) USAN.
Use: Adrenergic.

trancin. Fluphenazine.
Use: To treat anxiety and tension.

Trancopal. (Sanofi Winthrop) Chlormezanone 100 mg w/saccharin/Cap. Bot. 100s. 200 mg/Cap. Bot. 100s, 1000s. *Rx.*
Use: Relaxant and tranquilizer for mild anxiety and tension states.

Trandate Hydrochlorothiazide. (Allen & Hanburys) **Tablets:** Labetalol 100 mg, 200 mg or 300 mg, all w/25 mg hydrochlorothiazide. In 100s. *Rx.*
Use: Antihypertensive combination.

Trandate Injection. (Allen & Hanburys) Labetalol HCl 5 mg/ml Amp. 1 ml. Box 1s. Vial 20 ml, 40 ml. Box 1s. Prefilled Syringes 4 ml, 8 ml. *Rx.*
Use: Antihypertensive.

Trandate Tablets. (Allen & Hanburys) Labetalol HCl 100 mg, 200 mg or 300 mg/Tab. Bot. 100s, 500s. UD 100s. *Rx.*
Use: Antihypertensive.

Trandolapril.
Use: Antihypertensive.
See: Mavik, Tab. (Knoll).

•**tranexamic acid.** (tran-ex-AM-ik) USAN.
Use: Hemostatic. [Orphan drug]
See: Cyclokapron, Tab., Inj. (Pharmacia & Upjohn).

•**tranilast.** (TRAN-ill-ast) USAN.
Use: Antiasthmatic.

tranquilizers.
See: A-poxide, Cap. (Abbott).
Atarax, Prep. (Roerig).
Centrax, Cap. (Parke-Davis).
Compazine, Prep. (SK-Beecham).
Equanil, Tab. (Wyeth-Ayerst).
Fenarol, Tab. (Sanofi Winthrop).
Haldol, Tab., Inj., Conc. Soln. (McNeil).
Harmonyl, Tab. (Abbott).
Librium, Cap., Inj. (Roche).
Loxitane, Prod. (Lederle).
Mellaril, Tab., Soln. (Sandoz).
Meprobamate (Various Mfr.).
Miltown, Prep. (Wallace).
Permitil, Prep. (Schering-Plough).
Proketazine Maleate, Prep. (Wyeth-Ayerst).
Prolixin, Prep. (Squibb).
Sparine HCl, Prep. (Wyeth-Ayerst).

Stelazine, Prep. (SK-Beecham).
Taractan, Prep. (Roche).
Thorazine HCl, Prep. (SK-Beecham).
Tindal, Tab. (Schering-Plough).
Trancopal, Cap. (Sanofi Winthrop).
Tranxene, Cap. (Abbott).
Trilafon, Prep. (Schering-Plough).
Ultran, Prep. (Lilly).
Valium, Prep. (Roche).
Vesprin, Prep. (Squibb).
Vistaril, Prep. (Pfizer).

Tranquils Capsules. (Halsey) Pyrilamine maleate 25 mg/Cap. Bot. 30s. *otc.*
Use: Nonprescription sleep aid.

Tranquils Tablets. (Halsey) Acetaminophen 300 mg, pyrilamine maleate 25 mg/Tab. Bot. 30s. *otc.*
Use: Analgesic, nonprescription sleep aid.

•**transcainide.** (trans-CANE-ide) USAN.
Use: Antiarrhythmic, cardiac depressant.

Transclomiphene.

Transderm-Nitro. (Summit) Nitroglycerin 12.5 mg, 25 mg, 50 mg, 75 mg or 100 mg/patch. **12.5 mg, 25 mg, 50 mg:** Box 30s, UD 30s, 100s. **75 mg:** Box 30s. **100 mg:** Box 30s, UD 30s. *Rx.*
Use: Prevention and treatment of angina pectoris due to coronary artery disease.

Transderm-Scop. (Novartis) Scopolamine 0.5 mg per 2-unit blister pkg. (programmed delivery over 3-day period).
Use: Antiemetic, antivertigo.

transforming growth factor-beta 2. (Celtrix) *Rx.*
Use: Treatment of macular holes. [Orphan drug]

Transthyretin EIA. (Abbott Diagnostics) Test kits 100s.
Use: Enzyme immunoassay for the quantitative determination of transthyretin in human serum or plasma.

Trans-Ver-Sal Adult-Patch. (Doak Dermatologics) Salicylic acid 15%/Transdermal patch. 6 mm., 12 mm. In 40s. Securing tape and cleaning file. *otc.*
Use: Keratolytic.

Trans-Ver-Sal Pedia-Patch. (Doak Dermatologics) Salicylic acid 15%/Transdermal patch. 6 mm. In 20s. Securing tape and cleaning file. *otc.*
Use: Keratolytic.

Trans-Ver-Sal Plantar-Patch. (Doak Dermatologics) Salicylic acid 15%, 20 mm patches, 25s. Securing tapes, cleaning file. *otc.*

Use: Treatment of verruca plantaris.

Tranxene Capsules. (Abbott) Clorazepate dipotassium 3.75 mg, 7.5 mg or 15 mg/Cap. UD 100s. *c-iv.*
Use: Minor tranquilizer.

Tranxene-SD. (Abbott) Clorazepate dipotassium 11.25 mg or 22.5 mg/Tab. Bot. 100s. *c-iv.*
Use: Minor tranquilizer.

Tranxene-SD Half Strength Tablets. (Abbott) Clorazepate dipotassium 11.25 mg/Tab. Bot. 100s. *c-iv.*
Use: Minor tranquilizer.

Tranxene T Tablets. (Abbott) Clorazepate dipotassium 3.75 mg, 7.5 mg or 15 mg/Tab. Bot. 100s, 500s, UD 100s. *c-iv.*
Use: Minor tranquilizer.

tranylcypromine sulfate, (tran-ill-SIP-row-meen) U.S.P. XXI..
Use: Antidepressant.
See: Parnate, Tab. (SK-Beecham).

Trasicor. (Novartis) Oxprenolol HCl, B.A.N.

Trasylol. (Bayer) Aprotinin 1.4 mg/ml. Inj. Vial 100 ml, 200 ml. *Rx.*
Use: Antihemophilic.

Traumacal. (Bristol-Myers) Nutritionally complete formula for traumatized patients. Cans 8 oz. Vanilla flavor. *otc.*
Use: Specific for nitrogen and energy needs in a limited volume for multiple trauma and major burns.

T-Rau Tablet. (Tennessee Pharm) Rauwolfia serpentina 50 mg or 100 mg/Tab. Bot. 100s, 1000s. *Rx.*
Use: Hypotensive, tranquilizer.

Travamulsion 10% Intravenous Fat Emulsion. 1.1 kcal/ml 270 mOsm/L. Bot. 500 ml. *Rx.*
Use: Parenteral nutrition supplement.

Travamulsion 20% Intravenous Fat Emulsion. (Baxter) 2 kcal/ml 300 mOsm/L. Bot. 500 ml. *Rx.*
Use: Parenteral nutrition supplement.

Travasol. (Baxter) Crystalline L-amino acids injection 5.5%, 8.5% (with or without electrolytes). IV Bot. 500 ml, 1000 ml, 2000 ml. *Rx.*
Use: Parenteral nutrition supplement.

Travasol 3.5% M Injection with Electrolyte #45. (Baxter) Crystalline L-amino acids 3.5% Soln. Bot. IV 500 ml, 1000 ml. *Rx.*
Use: Parenteral nutrition supplement.

Travasol 3.5% w/Electrolytes. (Clintec) Amino acid concentration 3.5%, nitrogen 0.591 g/100 ml, 500 ml, 1000 ml. *Rx.*

Use: Parenteral nutritional supplement.

Travasol 10%. (Baxter) Crystalline L-amino acids injection 10%. Bot. 200 ml, 500 ml, 1000 ml, 2000 ml. *Rx.*
Use: Parenteral nutrition supplement.

Travasorb HN Peptide Diet. (Baxter) High-nitrogen defined peptide 333 kcal/Pkt. 6 pkt/Carton. *otc.*
Use: Nutrition supplement.

Travsorb MCT Liquid Diet. (Baxter) Digestible protein medium-chain triglyceride diet. 89 g packets. *otc.*
Use: Nutrition supplement.

Travasorb MCT Powder Diet. (Baxter) Digestible protein medium-chain triglyceride diet 400 kcal/Pkt. 6 pkt./Carton. *otc.*
Use: Nutrition supplement.

Travasorb Renal Diet. (Baxter) 467 kcal/Pkt. 6 pkt/Carton. 112 g packets. *otc.*
Use: Nutritional supplement.

Travasorb Standard Diet. (Baxter) Defined peptide diet, 333 kcal/pkt. 6 packets/Carton. *otc.*
Use: Nutritional supplement.

Travasorb STD. (Clintec Nutrition) Enzymatically hydrolyzed lactalbumin 10 g, glucose oligosaccharides 63.3 g, MCT (fractioned coconut oil) 4.5 g, sunflower oil 4.5 g, sodium 307 mg, potassium 390 mg, mOsm/560 Kg, H_2O, cal 333.3/ml, vitamins A, B_1, B_2, B_3, B_5, B_6, B_{12}, C, D, E, K, Ca, Cl, Cu, Fe, I, Mg, Mn, P, Zn. Gluten free. Pow. Pkts. 83.3 g. *otc.*
Use: Nutritional supplement.

Travasorb Whole Protein Liquid Diet. (Baxter) Lactose free complete nutrition 250 kcal/Can. Cans 8 oz. *otc.*
Use: Nutritional supplement.

Travel Aids. (Faraday) Dimenhydrinate 50 mg/Tab. Bot. 30s. *otc.*
Use: Antiemetic, antivertigo.

Travel-Eze. (Approved) Pyrilamine maleate 25 mg, hyoscine hydrobromide 0.325 mg/Tab. Pkg. 20s. *otc.*
Use: Antiemetic, antivertigo.

Travel Sickness. (Walgreen) Dimenhydrinate 50 mg/Tab. Bot. 24s. *otc.*
Use: Antiemetic, antivertigo.

Traveltabs. (Armenpharm) Dimenhydrinate 50 mg/Tab. Bot. 100s. *otc.*
Use: Antiemetic, antivertigo.

Travert. (Baxter) Invert sugar injection. 10% in water or saline. Plastic Bot. 500 ml, 1000 ml. *Rx.*
W/electrolyte No. 2 Bot. 500 ml, 1000 ml,
W/electrolyte No. 4 Bot. 250, 500 ml Soln. (10%).

Use: Fluid/electrolyte replacement.

5% Travert and Electrolyte No. 2. (Baxter) Invert sugar 50 g/L, calories 196 Cal/L, sodium 56 mEq/L, potassium 25 mEq/L, magnesium 6 mEq/L, chloride 56 mEq/L, phosphate 12.5 mEq/L, lactate 25 mEq/L, osmolarity 449 mOsm/L. 1000 ml. *Rx.*
Use: Parenteral nutritional supplement.

10% Travert and Electrolyte No. 2. (Baxter) Invert sugar 100 g/L, calories 384 Cal/L, sodium 56 mEq/L, potassium 25 mEq/L, magnesium 6 mEq/L, chloride 56 mEq/L, phosphate 12.5 mEq/L, lactate 25 mEq/L, osmolarity 726 mOsm/L. 1000 ml. *Rx.*
Use: Parenteral nutritional supplement.

•**trazodone hydrochloride,** (TRAY-zoe-dohn) U.S.P. 23.
Use: Antidepressant.
See: Desyrel, Tab. (Bristol-Myers).

•**trebenzomine hydrochloride.** (TRAY-BEN-zoe-meen) USAN.
Use: Antidepressant.

Trecator S.C. (Wyeth-Ayerst) Ethionamide. 2-Ethyl thioisonicotinamide. 250 mg/Tab. Bot. 100s. *Rx.*
Use: Antitubercular agent.

•**trefentanil hydrochloride.** (treh-FEN-tah-nill) USAN.
Use: Analgesic.

•**treloxinate.** (trell-OX-ih-nate) USAN.
Use: Antihyperlipoproteinemic.

Trental Tablets. (Hoechst Marion Roussel) Pentoxifylline 400 mg/Controlled Release Tab. Bot. 100s. UD 100s. *Rx.*
Use: Oral hemorrheologic agent for peripheral vascular disease.

Treo. (Biopharm Labs) *otc.* **SPF 8:** Octocrylene, octyl methoxycinnamate, benzophenone-3, octyl salicylate, isostearyl alcohol, diazolidinyl urea, propylparabens, citronella oil 0.05% (as insect repellant). Lot. Bot. 118 ml. **SPF 15:** Octocrylene, octyl methoxycinnamate, benzophenone-3, octyl salicylate, isostearyl alcohol, diazolidinyl urea, propylparabens, citronella oil 0.05% (as insect repellant). Lot. Bot. 118 ml. **SPF 30:** Octocrylene, octyl methoxycinnamate, benzophenone-3, octyl salicylate, isostearyl alcohol, diazolidinyl urea, propylparabens, citronella oil 0.05% (as insect repellant). Lot. Bot. 118 ml.
Use: Sunscreen.

treosulfan. *Rx.*
Use: Antineoplastic. [Orphan drug]
See: Ovastat.

•**trepipam maleate.** (TREH-pih-pam MAL-

ee-ate) USAN. *Formerly Trimopam Maleate.*
Use: Sedative, hypnotic.

• **trestolone acetate.** (TRESS-toe-lone) USAN.
Use: Antineoplastic, androgen.

trethocanoic acid.
Use: Anticholesteremic.

• **tretinoin,** (TREH-tih-NO-in) U.S.P. 23.
Use: Keratolytic. [Orphan drug]
See: Retin-A, Cream, Gel, Soln. (Ortho).
Renova, Cream (Ortho).
Vesanoid, Cap. (Hoffman-LaRoche).

tretinoin If, iv. (Argus) *Rx.*
Use: Antineoplastic. [Orphan drug]

Trexan Cablets. (DuPont Merck) Naltrexone HCl 50 mg/Tab. Bot. 50s. *Rx.*
Use: Opioid antagonist.

Triac. (Eon Labs) Triprolidine HCl 2.5 mg, pseudoephedrine HCl 60 mg/Tab. Bot. 100s, 1000s. *Rx.*
Use: Antihistamine, decongestant.

Triacet Cream. (Lemmon) Triamcinolone acetonide 0.1%. Tube 15 g, 80 g. *Rx.*
Use: Corticosteroid, topical.

• **triacetin,** U.S.P. 23. *Formerly glyceryl triacetate.*
Use: Topical antifungal.
See: Enzactin, Preps. (Wyeth-Ayerst).
Fungacetin, Oint. (Blair).

triacetyloleandomycin. (try-ASS-eh-till-oh-lee-AN-do-MY-sin) Troleandomycin. *Rx.*
Use: Anti-infective.

Triacin C. (Various Mfr.) Pseudoephedrine HCl 30 mg, triprolidine HCl 1.25 mg, codeine phosphate 10 mg/5 ml, alcohol 4.3%. Syr. Bot. pt., gal. *c-v.*
Use: Antihistamine, decongestant, antitussive.

Triact Liquid. (Sanofi Winthrop) Aluminum, magnesium hydroxide, simethicone. *otc.*
Use: Antacid, antiflatulent.

Triact Tablets. (Sanofi Winthrop) Aluminum, magnesium hydroxide, simethicone. *otc.*
Use: Antacid, antiflatulent.

Triad. (UAD) Butalbital 50 mg, acetaminophen 325 mg, caffeine 40 mg. Cap. Bot. 100s. *Rx.*
Use: Analgesic, sedative, hypnotic.

Triafed with Codeine Syrup. (Schein) Pseudoephedrine HCl 30 mg, triprolidine HCl 1.25 mg, codeine phosphate 10 mg. Bot. 473 ml. *c-v.*
Use: Decongestant, antihistamine, antitussive.

• **triafungin.** (TRY-ah-FUN-jin) USAN.
Use: Antifungal.

Triam-A. (Hyrex) Triamcinolone acetonide 40 mg/ml. Inj. Vial 5 ml. *Rx.*
Use: Corticosteroid.

• **triamcinolone,** (TRY-am-SIN-oh-lone) U.S.P. 23.
Use: Glucocorticoid.
See: Aristocort, Tab., Syr. (Lederle).
Aristoderm, Foam (Lederle).
Aristospan, Parenteral (Lederle).
Kenacort, Tab., Syr. (Squibb Mark).
SK-Triamcinolone, Tab. (SK-Beecham).

• **triamcinolone acetonide,** (TRY-am-SIN-oh-lone ah-SEE-toe-nide) U.S.P. 23.
Use: Glucocorticoid, topical anti-inflammatory.
See: Aristocort, Cream, Oint (Fujisawa).
Aristoderm Foam (Lederle).
Aristogel, Gel (Lederle).
Delta-Tritex, Cream, Oint. (Dermol).
Flutex, Cream, Oint. (Syosset).
Kenalog Preps. (Westwood Squibb).
Kenonel, Cream (Marnel).
Triacet, Cream (Lemmon).
Tramacin, Cream (Johnson & Johnson).
Triderm, Cream (Del-Ray).
Tri-Kort, Inj. (Keene).
W/Neomycin, gramicidin, Nystatin.
See: Mycolog, Preps. (Squibb).

triamcinolone acetonide. (Various Mfr.)
Cream: 0.025%, 0.1%: Tube 15 g, 80 g, 454 g; **0.5%:** 15 g. **Lot.:** 0.025% or 0.1%. Bot. 60 ml. **Oint.: 0.025%, 0.1%:** Tube 15 g, 80 g, 454 g; **0.5%:** Tube 15 g. **Paste:** 0.1%.
Use: Glucocorticoid, topical anti-inflammatory.

• **triamcinolone acetonide sodium phosphate.** (TRY-am-SIN-oh-lone ah-SEE-toe-nie) USAN.
Use: Glucocorticoid.

• **triamcinolone diacetate,** (try-am-SIN-oh-lone try-ASS-ah-tate) U.S.P. 23. Sterile Susp., Syrup, U.S.P. 23.
Use: Glucocorticoid.
See: Amcort, Inj. (Keene).
Aristocort Diacetate Forte (Lederle).
Aristocort Diacetate Intralesional, Inj. (Lederle).
Kenacort, Syr. (Squibb Mark).
Tracilon, Susp. (Savage).
Triam-Forte, Inj. (Hyrex).

• **triamcinolone hexacetonide,** (TRY-am-SIN-ole-ohn HEX-ah-SEE-tone-ide) U.S.P. 23.
Use: Glucocorticoid.
See: Aristospan, Prep. (Lederle).

Triam-Forte. (Hyrex) Triamcinolone diacetate 40 mg/ml. Vial 5 ml. *Rx.*
Use: Adrenocortical steroid therapy.

Triaminic. (Sandoz) Pyrilamine maleate 25 mg, pheniramine maleate 25 mg, phenylpropanolamine HCl 50 mg/ Timed-release Tab. Bot. 100s, 250s. *otc.*
Use: Antihistamine, decongestant.
W/Dormethan, terpin hydrate.
See: Tussaminic, Tab. (Sandoz).

Triaminic-12 Tablets. (Sandoz) Phenylpropanolamine HCl 75 mg, chlorpheniramine maleate 12 mg/S.R. Tab. Pkg. 20s. *otc.*
Use: Decongestant, antihistamine.

Triaminic Allergy Tablets. (Sandoz) Phenylpropanolamine HCl 25 mg, chlorpheniramine maleate 4 mg/Tab. Blister pk. 24s. *otc.*
Use: Decongestant, antihistamine.

Triaminic AM Decongestant Formula. (Sandoz) Pseudoephedrine HCl 15 mg/ 5 ml, sorbitol, sucrose, orange flavor, alcohol and dye free. Syr. 118 ml, 237 ml. *otc.*
Use: Decongestant.

Triaminic AM Cough and Decongestant Formula. (Sandoz) Pseudoephedrine HCl 15 mg, dextromethorphan HBr 7.5 mg/5 ml, sorbitol, sucrose, orange flavor. Alcohol and dye free. Liq. 118 ml, 237 ml. *otc.*
Use: Decongestant, antitussive.

Triaminic Chewable Tablets. (Sandoz Consumer) Phenylpropanolamine HCl 6.25 mg, chlorpheniramine maleate 0.5 mg/Tab. Blister pkg. 24s. *otc.*
Use: Decongestant, antihistamine.

Triaminic Cold Syrup. (Sandoz) Phenylpropanolamine HCl 12.5 mg, chlorpheniramine maleate 2 mg/5 ml. Bot. 4 oz., 8 oz. W/sorbitol. *otc.*
Use: Decongestant, antihistamine.

Triaminic Cold Tablets. (Sandoz) Phenylpropanolamine HCl 12.5 mg, chlorpheniramine maleate 2 mg/Tab. Blister pkg. 24s. *otc.*
Use: Decongestant, antihistamine.

Triaminic-DM Syrup. (Sandoz) Phenylpropanolamine HCl 6.25 mg, dextromethorphan HBr 5 mg, sorbitol, sucrose. Alcohol free. Bot. 120 ml, 240 ml. *otc.*
Use: Decongestant, antitussive.

Triaminic Expectorant. (Sandoz) Phenylpropanolamine HCl 12.5 mg, guaifenesin 100 mg/5 ml w/alcohol 5%, saccharin, sorbitol. Bot. 4 oz., 8 oz. *otc.*

Use: Decongestant, expectorant.

Triaminic Expectorant w/Codeine. (Sandoz) Phenylpropanolamine HCl 12.5 mg, codeine phosphate 10 mg, guaifenesin 100 mg/5 ml w/alcohol 5%, saccharin, sorbitol. Liq. Bot. pt. *otc.*
Use: Decongestant, antitussive, expectorant.

Triaminic Expectorant DH. (Sandoz) Guaifenesin 100 mg, phenylpropanolamine HCl 12.5 mg, pheniramine maleate 6.25 mg, pyrilamine maleate 6.25 mg, hydrocodone bitartrate 1.67 mg/10 ml w/alcohol 5%, saccharin, sorbitol. Bot. pt. *c-III.*
Use: Expectorant, decongestant, antihistamine, antitussive.

Triaminic Nite Light Liquid. (Sandoz). 15 mg pseudoephedrine, 1 mg chlorpheniramine maleate, 7.5 mg dextromethorphan HBr. 120 and 240 ml. *otc.*
Use: Decongestant, antihistamine, antitussive.

Triaminic Oral Infant Drops. (Sandoz) Phenylpropanolamine HCl 20 mg, pheniramine maleate 10 mg, pyrilamine maleate 10 mg/ml. Dropper bot. 15 ml. *Rx.*
Use: Decongestant, antihistamine.

Triaminic Sore Throat Formula Liquid. (Sandoz) Pseudoephedrine HCl 15 mg, dextromethorphan HBr 7.5 mg, acetaminophen 160 mg, EDTA, sucrose, alcohol free. Bot. 240 ml. *otc.*
Use: Decongestant, antitussive, analgesic.

Triaminic Syrup. (Sandoz) Phenylpropanolamine HCl 6.25 mg, chlorpheniramine maleate 1 mg, sorbitol, sucrose, alcohol free. Bot. 120 ml, 240 ml. *otc.*
Use: Decongestant, antihistamine.

Triaminic TR Tablets. (Sandoz) Phenylpropanolamine HCl 50 mg, pheniramine maleate 25 mg, pyrilamine maleate 25 mg/T.R. Tab. 100s, 250s. *otc.*
Use: Decongestant, antihistamine.

Triaminicin Cold, Allergy, Sinus Tablets. (Sandoz Consumer) Phenylpropanolamine HCl 25 mg, acetaminophen 650 mg, chlorpheniramine maleate 4 mg/Tab. Pkg. 12s. *otc.*
Use: Decongestant, analgesic, antihistamine.

Triaminicol Multi Symptom Cold Syrup. (Sandoz) Phenylpropanolamine HCl 12.5 mg, chlorpheniramine maleate 2 mg, dextromethorphan HBr 10 mg/5 ml. *otc.*
Use: Decongestant, antihistamine, antitussive.

Triaminicol Multi-Symptom Cough and Cold Tablet. (Sandoz) Phenylpropanolamine HCl 12.5 mg, chlorpheniramine maleate 2 mg, dextromethorphan HBr 10 mg/Tab. Blister pkg. 24s. *otc.*
Use: Decongestant, antitussive, antihistamine.

Triaminicol Multi-Symptom Relief. (Sandoz) Phenylpropanolamine HCl 6.25 mg, chlorpheniramine maleate 1 mg, dextromethorphan HBr 5 mg/5 ml. Liq. Bot. 120 ml. *otc.*
Use: Pediatric antitussive, decongestant, antihistamine.

triaminilone-16,17-acetonide.
See: Triamcinolone acetonide.

Triamolone 40. (Forest) Triamcinolone diacetate 40 mg/ml. Vial 5 ml. *Rx.*
Use: Corticosteroid.

Triamonide 40. (Forest) Triamcinolone acetonide 40 mg/ml. Vial 5 ml. *Rx.*
Use: Corticosteroid.

•**triampyzine sulfate.** (TRY-AM-pih-zeen SULL-fate) USAN.
Use: Anticholinergic.

•**triamterene,** (try-AM-tur-een) U.S.P. 23.
Use: Diuretic.
See: Dyrenium, Cap. (SK-Beecham).

triamterene/hydrochlorothiazide. (Various Mfr.) **Cap.:** Triamterene 50 mg, hydrochlorothiazide 25 mg. Bot. 100s, 1000s. **Tab.:** Triamterene 37.5 mg, hydrochlorothiazide 25 mg. Bot. 100s, 500s, 1000s; Triamterene 75 mg, hydrochlorothiazide 50 mg. Bot. 100s, 250s, 500s, 1000s. *Rx.*
Use: Diuretic combination.

triamterene and hydrochlorothiazide capsules.
Use: Diuretic.
See: Dyazide, Cap. (SK-Beecham).

Trianide. (Seatrace) Triamcinolone acetonide 40 mg/ml. Vial 5 ml. *Rx.*
Use: Corticosteroid.

Triaprin. (Dunhall) Acetaminophen 325 mg, butalbital 50 mg/Caps. Bot. 100s, 500s. *Rx.*
Use: Analgesic, sedative, hypnotic.

Tri-Aqua. (Pfeiffer) Caffeine 100 mg, extracts of buchu, uva ursi, zea, triticum/Tab. Bot. 50s, 100s. *otc.*
Use: Diuretic.

Triavil. (Merck) Perphenazine 4 mg, amitriptyline HCl 10 mg/salmon-colored Tab.; perphenazine 2 mg, amitriptyline HCl 25 mg/orange Tab.; perphenazine 4 mg, amitriptyline 25 mg/yellow Tab.; perphenazine 2 mg, amitriptyline HCl 10 mg/blue Tab. Bot. 100s, 500s. UD 100s. Perphenazine 4 mg, amitryptyline 50 mg/orange Tab. Bot. 60s, 100s. UD 100s. *Rx.*
Use: Tranquilizer, antidepressant.

Tri-A-Vite F. (Major) F 0.5 mg, Vitamins A 1500 IU, D 400 IU, C 35 mg/ml Drops. Bot. 50 ml. *Rx.*
Use: Vitamin supplement.

•**triazolam,** (try-AZE-oh-lam) U.S.P. 23.
Use: Sedative, hypnotic.
See: Halcion, Tab. (Pharmacia & Upjohn).

Triazolam. (Various Mfr.) 0.125 mg, 0.25 mg. Tab. Bot. 500s, UD 100s, unit-of-use 100s. *c-iv.*
Use: Sedative.

Triban. (Great Southern) Trimethobenzamide HCl 200 mg, benzocaine 2%. Supp. Pkg. 10s, 50s. *Rx.*
Use: Antiemetic.

Triban, Pediatric. (Great Southern) Trimethobenzamide HCl 100 mg, benzocaine 2%. Supp. Pkg. 10s. *Rx.*
Use: Antiemetic.

•**tribenoside.** (try-BEN-oh-SIDE) USAN. Not available in U.S.
Use: Sclerosing agent.

Tri-Biocin. (Approved) Bacitracin 400 units, polymyxin B sulfate 5000 units, neomycin 5 mg/g Tube 0.5 oz. *otc.*
Use: Topical antibiotic.

Tribiotic Plus. (Thompson) Polymyxin B sulfate 5000 units, neomycin sulfate (equivalent to 3.5 mg neomycin base), bacitracin 500 units, lidocaine 40 mg/g, lanolin, light mineral oil, petrolatum. Oint. Tube 28.35 g. *otc.*
Use: Topical anti-infective.

tribromoethanol.
Use: Anesthetic (inhalation).

tribromomethane. Bromoform.

•**tribromsalan.** (try-BROME-sah-lan) USAN.
Use: Disinfectant.
See: Diaphene (or ASC-4) (Stecker). Tuasol 100 (Hoechst Marion Roussel).

tricalcium phosphate.
Use: Minerals and electrolytes, oral.
See: Posture (Whitehall Robins).

•**tricetamide.** (TRY-see-tam-id) USAN.
Use: Sedative, hypnotic.

Tri-Chlor. (Gordon) Trichloracetic acid 80%. Bot. 15 ml. *Rx.*
Use: Topical, as a caustic verruca cauterant.

trichloran.
See: Trichloroethylene.

• **trichlormethiazide,** U.S.P. 23.
Use: Diuretic; antihypertensive.
See: Metahydrin, Tab. (Hoechst Marion Roussel).
Naqua, Tab. (Schering-Plough).
W/Reserpine.
See: Metatensin, Tab. (Hoechst Marion Roussel).
Naquival, Tab. (Schering-Plough).

trichloroacetic acid, U.S.P. XXI. Acetic acid, trichloro.
Use: Topical, as a caustic.

trichlorobutyl alcohol.
See: Chlorobutanol.

trichlorocarbanilide. W/Salicylic acid, sulfur.

• **trichloromonofluoromethane,** N.F. 18.
Use: Pharmaceutic aid (aerosol propellant).

tricholine citrate.
See: Choline citrate.

trichomonas test.
See: Isocult for *Trichomonas vaginalis.* (SmithKline Diagnostics).

Trichotine. (Schwarz Pharma) **Pow.:** Sodium lauryl sulf., sod. perborate, monohydrate silica. Pkg. 150 g, 360 g. **Liq.:** Sodium lauryl sulfate, sodium borate, SD alcohol 40 8%, SD alcohol 23-A, EDTA. Bot. 120 ml, 240 ml. *otc.*
Use: Vaginal douche.

• **triciribine phosphate.** (TRY-SIH-bean FOSS-fate) USAN. *Formerly Phosphate Salt of Tricyclic Nucleoside.*
Use: Antineoplastic.

• **tricitrates oral solution,** U.S.P. 23.
Use: Alkalizer (systemic, urinary); antiurolithic (cystine calculi, uric acid calculi); buffer (neutralizing).

triclobisonium. Triburon, Oint. (Roche).

triclobisonium chloride.
Use: Topical anti-infective.

• **triclocarban.** (TRY-kloe-CAR-ban) USAN.
Use: Disinfectant.
See: Artra Beauty Ban (Schering-Plough).
W/Clofulcarban.
See: Safeguard Bar Soap, (P & G).

• **triclofenol piperazine.** (TRY-kloe-FEE-nole pih-PURR-ah-zeen) USAN.
Use: Anthelmintic.

• **triclofos sodium.** (TRY-kloe-foss) USAN.
Use: Sedative, hypnotic.

• **triclonide.** (TRY-kloe-nide) USAN.
Use: Anti-inflammatory.

• **triclosan.** (TRY-kloe-san) USAN.
Use: Anti-infective; disinfectant.

See: Ambi 10, Bar (Kiwi Brands).
Clearasil Daily Face Wash (Procter & Gamble).
Clearasil Soap (Procter & Gamble).
Oxy ResiDon't, Liq. (SK-Beecham).

Tricodene Cough and Cold. (Pfeiffer) Pyrilamine maleate 12.5 mg, codeine phosphate 8.2 mg, menthol, honey, glucose, sucrose. Liq. Bot. 120 ml. *c-v.*
Use: Antitussive, antihistamine.

Tricodene Forte. (Pfeiffer) Phenylpropanolamine HCl 12.5 mg, chlorpheniramine maleate 2 mg, dextromethorphan HBr 10 mg/5 ml Liq. Bot. 120 ml. *otc.*
Use: Antihistamine, decongestant, antitussive.

Tricodene Liquid. (Pfeiffer) Chlorpheniramine maleate 0.5 mg, dextromethorphan HBr 10 mg, ammonium Cl 90 mg, sodium citrate, sorbitol, mannitol/5 ml Liq. Bot. 120 ml. *otc.*
Use: Antihistamine, antitussive, expectorant.

Tricodene NN. (Pfeiffer) Phenylpropanolamine HCl 12.5 mg, chlorpheniramine maleate 2 mg, dextromethorphan HBr 10 mg/5 ml. Syr. Bot. 120 ml. *otc.*
Use: Antihistamine, decongestant, antitussive.

Tricodene Pediatric Cough & Cold Liquid. (Pfeiffer) Phenylpropanolamine HCl 12.5 mg, Dextromethorphan HBr 10 mg/5 ml Liq. 120 ml. *otc.*
Use: Decongestant, antitussive.

Tricodene Sugar Free. (Pfeiffer) Chlorpheniramine maleate, dextromethorphan HBr 10 mg, menthol, saccharin, sorbitol, alcohol free. Liq. 120 ml. *otc.*
Use: Antihistamine, antitussive.

Tricodene Syrup. (Pfeiffer) Pyrilamine maleate 4.17 mg, codeine phosphate 8.1 mg, terpin hydrate, menthol/5 ml Syr. Bot. 120 ml. *c-v.*
Use: Antihistamine, antitussive.

Tricomine. (Major) Pseudoephedrine HCl 60 mg, carbinoxamine maleate 4 mg, dextromethorphan HBr 15 mg/5 ml, alcohol 5%. Expec. Bot. 120 ml. *otc.*
Use: Antihistamine, decongestant, antitussive.

Tricosal. (Invamed) Choline magnesium trisalicylate 500 mg, 750 mg, 1000 mg/ Tab. Bot. 100s, 500s. *Rx.*
Use: Salicylate.

tricylatate hydrochloride.

Triderm Cream. (Del-Ray) Triamcinolone acetonide 0.1%. Tube 30 g, 90 g. *Rx.*

Use: Glucocorticoid, topical.

Tridesilon Cream. (Bayer) Desonide 0.05% in vehicle buffered to the pH range of normal skin w/glycerin, methyl paraben, sodium lauryl sulfate, aluminum sulfate, calcium acetate, cetyl stearyl alcohol, synthetic bees wax, white petrolatum, mineral oil. Tube 15 g, 60 g. *Rx.*
Use: Corticosteroid.

Tridesilon Otic. (Bayer) Desonide 0.05%, acetic acid 2% in vehicle. Bot. 10 ml. *Rx.*
Use: Otic preparation.

Tridex Tab., Timed Tridex Cap., Timed Tridex Jr. Cap. (Fellows) Changed to Daro Tab., Daro Timed Cap., Daro Jr. Timed Cap.

tridihexethyl chloride, U.S.P. XXII.
Use: Anticholinergic.
W/Phenobarbital.
See: Pathilon w/Phenobarbital Tab., Cap. (Lederle).

Tridil 0.5 mg/ml. (Faulding) Nitroglycerin 0.5 mg/ml w/alcohol 10%, water for injection, buffered with sodium phosphate. Amp. 10 ml. Box 20s. *Rx.*
Use: Vasodilator; antianginal, hypotensive.

Tridil 5 mg/ml. (Faulding) Nitroglycerin 5 mg/ml w/alcohol 30%, propylene glycol 30%, water for injection. Amp. 5 ml, 10 ml. Vial 5 ml, 10 ml, 20 ml. Box 20s. Special administration set w/10 ml Amp. *Rx.*
Use: Vasodilator; antianginal, hypotensive.

Tridione. (Abbott) Trimethadione. (Troxidone). Cap. 300 mg, Bot. 100s. Dulcet Tab. 150 mg, Bot. 100s. *Rx.*
Use: Anticonvulsant.

Tridrate Bowel Evacuant Kit. (Mallinckrodt) Magnesium citrate soln. 300 ml, bisacodyl 5 mg/Tab. (3s), bisacodyl 10 mg/Supp. (1). Kit. *otc.*
Use: Laxative.

•**trientine hydrochloride,** (TRY-en-TEEN) U.S.P. 23.
Use: Chelating agent; Wilson's disease therapy adjunct. [Orphan drug]
See: Cuprid, Cap, (Merck).

triethanolamine,
See: Trolamine, N.F. 18.

triethanolamine polypeptide oleate condensate.
See: Cerumenex, Drops (Purdue Frederick).

triethanolamine salicylate.
See: Aspercreme, Cream (Thompson).

Aspergel, Oint. (LaCrosse).
Myoflex, Cream (Warren-Teed).

triethanolamine trinitrate biphosphate.
Trolnitrate Phosphate.

•**triethyl citrate,** N.F. 18.
Use: Pharmaceutic aid (plasticizer).

triethylenemelamine. Tretamine TEM. 2,4,6-Tris(1-aziridinyl)-5-triazine.
Use: Antineoplastic.

triethylenethiophosphoramide.
See: Thiotepa (Lederle).

Trifed-C. (Geneva Pharm) Pseudoephedrine HCl 30 mg, triprolidine HCl 1.25 mg, codeine phosphate 10 mg/5 ml, alcohol 4.3%. Syr. Bot. pt., gal. *c-v.*
Use: Antihistamine, decongestant, antitussive.

•**trifenagrel.** (try-FEN-ah-GRELL) USAN.
Use: Antithrombotic.

•**triflocin.** (try-FLOW-sin) USAN.
Use: Diuretic.

Tri-Flor-Vite with Fluoride. (Everett) Fluoride 0.25 mg, vitamin A 1500 IU, D 400 IU, C 35 mg/ml/Drop. 50 ml. *Rx.*
Use: Vitamin/fluoride supplement.

•**triflubazam.** (try-FLEW-bah-zam) USAN.
Use: Tranquilizer (minor).

•**triflumidate.** (try-FLEW-mih-DATE) USAN.
Use: Anti-inflammatory.

•**trifluoperazine hydrochloride,** (try-flew-oh-PURR-uh-zeen) U.S.P. 23.
Use: Tranquilizer, antipsychotic, sedative, hypnotic.
See: Stelazine Inj., Liq., Tab. (SK-Beecham).

n-trifluoroacetyladriamycin-14-valerate. (Anthra Pharm) *Rx.*
Use: Antineoplastic. [Orphan drug]

trifluorothymidine. *Rx.*
Use: Ophthalmic.
See: Viroptic (Glaxo Wellcome).

•**trifluperidol.** (TRY-flew-PURR-ih-dahl) USAN.
Use: Antipsychotic.

•**triflupromazine,** U.S.P. 23.
Use: Tranquilizer, antipsychotic.

•**triflupromazine hydrochloride,** U.S.P. 23.
Use: Tranquilizer, antipsychotic.
See: Vesprin Prods. (Bristol-Myers).

•**trifluridine.** (try-FLEW-RIH-deen) USAN.
Use: Antiviral used to treat herpes simplex eye infections.
See: Viroptic Ophthalmic Soln., (Glaxo Wellcome).

triglycerides, medium chain.
Use: Nutritional therapy.
See: MCT (Bristol-Myers).

triglyceride reagent strip. (Bayer) Sera-lyzer reagent strip. Bot. 25s.
Use: A quantitative strip test for triglyc-erides in serum or plasma.

Trihemic-600. (Lederle) Vitamins C 600 mg, B_{12} 25 mcg, intrinsic factor conc. 75 mg, folic acid 1 mg, Vitamins E 30 IU, ferrous fumarate 115 mg, dioctyl sod. succinate 50 mg/Tab. Bot. 30s, 500s. *Rx.*
Use: Vitamin/mineral supplement.

Trihexane. (Rugby) Trihexyphenidyl 2 mg/Tab. Bot. 100s, 1000s. *Rx.*
Use: Anticholinergic, antiparkinsonian.

Trihexidyl. (Schein) Trihexyphenidyl 2 mg/Tab. Bot. 100s, 1000s. *Rx.*
Use: Anticholinergic, antiparkinsonian.

Trihexy-2. (Geneva Pharm) Trihexy-phenidyl 2 mg/Tab. Bot. 100s, 1000s. *Rx.*
Use: Anticholinergic, antiparkinsonian.

Trihexy-5. (Geneva Pharm) Trihexy-phenidyl 5 mg/Tab. Bot. 100s, 1000s. *Rx.*
Use: Anticholinergic, antiparkinsonian.

• **trihexyphenidyl hydrochloride,** (try-hex-ee-FEN-in-dill) U.S.P. 23.
Use: Anticholinergic, antiparkinsonian.
See: Artane, Elixir & Tab. (Lederle).

TriHIBIT. (Pasteur-Merieux-Connaught) Package containing lyophilized vials of ActHIB brand of Hib vaccine and vi-als of Tripedia brand of DTaP vaccine. *Rx.*
Use: Vaccine.
See: ActHIB (Pasteur-Merieux-Con-naught).
Tripedia (Pasteur-Merieux-Con-naught).

Tri-Histin. (Recsei) **25 mg Tab.:** Pyril-amine maleate 10 mg, chlorphenir-amine maleate 1 mg. **50 mg Tab.:** Pyrilamine maleate 20 mg, methapyril-ene HCl 15 mg, chlorpheniramine ma-leate 2 mg. **100 mg S.A. Cap.:** Pyril-amine maleate 40 mg, pheniramine maleate 25 mg. **Expectorant:** Pyril-amine maleate 5 mg, chlorpheniramine maleate 0.5 mg, guaifenesin 20 mg, phenylpropanolamine 7.5 mg, phenyl-ephrine HCl 2.5 mg, sod. citrate 100 mg/5 ml. Bot. pt. gal. **Liquid:** Pyrilamine maleate 5 mg, chlorpheniramine male-ate 0.5 mg/5 ml. Bot. pt. gal. **Tab.:** Bot. 100s, 500s, 1000s. 50 mg Bot. 1000s. **Cap.:** Bot. 100s, 500s, 1000s. *otc, Rx.*
Use: Triple antihistamine therapy.
W/Benzyl alcohol, chlorobutanol and iso-propyl alcohol.
See: Derma-Pax, Liq. (Recsei).

W/Codeine phosphate, guaifenesin, phenylpropanolamine, phenylephrine HCl, sodium citrate.
See: Trihista-Cod., Liq. (Recsei).

W/Ephedrine HCl, aminophylline, mepho-barbital.
See: Asmasan, Tab. (Recsei).

Tri-Hydroserpine. (Rugby) Hydrochloro-thiazide 15 mg, reserpine 0.1 mg, hy-dralazine HCl 25 mg. Tab. Bot. 100s, 1000s. *Rx.*
Use: Antihypertensive combination.

Trihydroxyestrine. Trihydroxyestrin.

Trihydroxyethylamine. Triethanolamine.

Tri-Immunol. (Wyeth-Lederle) 12.5 LF units diphtheria, 5 LF units tetanus tox-oids and 4 units pertussis vaccine combined, aluminum phosphate ad-sorbed purogenated. Vial 7.5 ml. *Rx.*
Use: Agent for immunization.

triiodomethane.
See: Iodoform. (Various Mfr.).

Tri-K. (Century) Potassium acetate 0.5 g, potassium bicarbonate 0.5 g, po-tassium citrate 0.5 g/fl. oz. Saccharin. Bot. pt., gal. *Rx.*
Use: Potassium supplement.

• **trikates oral solution,** U.S.P. 23.
Use: Replenisher (electrolyte).

Tri-Kort. (Keene) Triamcinalone aceto-nide suspension 40 mg/ml. Vial 5 ml. *Rx.*
Use: Corticosteroid, topical.

Trilafon. (Schering-Plough) Perphen-azine. **Tab.:** 2, 4, 8 & 16 mg. Bot. 100s, 500s. **Inj.:** 5 mg/ml, w/disodium citrate 24.6 mg, sod. bisulfite 2 mg, and wa-ter for injection/ml. Amp. 1 ml **Repetabs:** 8 mg. Bot. 100s. **Concen-trate:** 16 mg/5 ml. Bot. 4 oz. w/dropper. *Rx.*
Use: Tranquilizer.

Tri-Levlen 21 Tablets. (Berlex). *Rx.*
Group 1: Levonorgestrel 0.05 mg, ethinyl estradiol 0.03 mg/Tab.
Group 2: Levonorgestrel 0.075 mg, ethinyl estradiol 0.04 mg/Tab.
Group 3: Levonorgestrel 0.125 mg, ethinyl estradiol 0.03 mg/Tab. Slide-case 21s. Box 3s.
Use: Oral contraceptive.

Tri-Levlen 28 Tablets. (Berlex). *Rx.*
Group 1: Levonorgestrel 0.05 mg, ethinyl estradiol 0.03 mg/Tab.
Group 2: Levonorgestrel 0.075 mg, ethinyl estradiol 0.04 mg/Tab.
Group 3: Levonorgestrel 0.125 mg, ethinyl estradiol 0.03 mg/Tab.
Group 4: Inert tablets. Slidecase 28s. Box 3s.

Use: Oral contraceptive.

Trilisate Liquid. (Purdue Frederick) Choline magnesium trisalicylate from choline salicylate 293 mg, magnesium salicylate 362 mg/ tsp. to provide 500 mg salicylate/tsp. Bot. 8 oz. *Rx.*
Use: Nonsteroidal anti-inflammatory, antiarthritic, analgesic.

Trilisate Tablets. (Purdue Frederick) Choline magnesium trisalicylate. **500 mg/Tab.** of salicylate from choline salicylate 293 mg, magnesium salicylate 362 mg/Tab. Bot. 100s. **750 mg/Tab.** of salicylate from choline salicylate 400 mg and magnesium salicylate 544 mg Bot. 100s. 1000 mg/Tab. of salicylate from choline salicylate 587 mg, magnesium salicylate 725 mg Bot. 60s. *Rx.*
Use: Nonsteroidal anti-inflammatory, antiarthritic, analgesic.

Trilog. (Roberts) Triamcinolone acetonide 40 mg/ml. Vial 5 ml. *Rx.*
Use: Corticosteroid.

Trilone. (Century) Triamcinalone diacetate susp. Amp. 10 ml. *Rx.*
Use: Corticosteroid.

Trilone. (Roberts) Triamcinolone diacetate 40 mg/ml. Vial 5 ml. *Rx.*
Use: Corticosteroid.

•**trilostane.** USAN.
Use: Adrenocortical suppressant.

Trimahist Elixir. (Tennessee Pharm) Phenylephrine HCl 5 mg, prophenpyridamine maleate 12.5 mg, l-menthol 1 mg, alcohol 5%/5 ml. Bot. pt., gal. *Rx.*
Use: Antihistamine, decongestant .

Trimax Gel. (Sanofi Winthrop) Aluminum, magnesium hydroxide, simethicone. *otc.*
Use: Antacid, antiflatulent.

Trimax Tablet. (Sanofi Winthrop) Aluminum, magnesium hydroxide, simethicone. *otc.*
Use: Antacid, antiflatulent.

Trimazide. (Major) **Capsules:** Trimethobenazamide 250 mg/Cap. Bot. 100s. **Suppositories:** 100 mg and 200 mg/ Supp. 10s. *Rx.*
Use: Antiemetic.

trimazinol.
Use: Anti-inflammatory agent.

•**trimazosin hydrochloride.** (try-MAY-zoe-sin) USAN.
Use: Antihypertensive.

•**trimegestone.** USAN.
Use: Progestin (hormone deficiency in postmenopausal women).

trimetamide. Trimethamide.

•**trimethadione,** U.S.P. 23.

Use: Anticonvulsant.
See: Tridione, Prep. (Abbott).

trimethamide.
Use: Antihypertensive.

•**trimethaphan camsylate,** U.S.P. 23.
Use: Antihypertensive.

•**trimethobenzamide hydrochloride,** (trymeth-oh-BEN-zuh-mide) U.S.P. 23.
Use: Antiemetic.
See: Tegamide, Suppos. (G & W).
Tigan, Preps. (SK-Beecham).

trimethobenzamide hydrochloride and benzocaine suppositories.
Use: Antiemetic.
See: Pediatric Triban (Great Southern).
Triban (Great Southern).

•**trimethoprim,** (try-METH-oh-prim) U.S.P. 23.
Use: Antibacterial.
See: Proloprim, Tab. (Glaxo Wellcome).
Trimpex, Tab. (Roche).
W/Polymyxin B Sulfate.
See: Polytrim Ophth. Soln. (Allergan).
W/Sulfamethoxazole.
See: Bactrim, Oral Susp., Ped. Susp., Tab. (Roche).
Septra, Tab. (Glaxo Wellcome).
Septra DS, Tab. (Glaxo Wellcome).

trimethoprim and sulfamethoxazole. (try-METH-oh-prim and suhl-fuh-meth-OX-uh-zole) (Various Mfr.) **Tab:** Trimethoprim 80 mg, sulfamethoxazole 400 mg/Tab. Bot. 100s, 500s. **Susp.:** Trimethoprim 40 mg, sulfamethoxazole 200 mg/5 ml. Bot. 150 ml, 200 ml, 480 ml. **Inj.:** Sulfamethoxazole 80 mg/ml, trimethoprim 16 mg/ml. 5 ml. *Rx.*
Use: Anti-infective combination.

trimethoprim and sulfamethoxazole DS. (Various Mfr.) Trimethoprim 160 mg, sulfamethoxazole 800 mg/Tab. Bot. 100s, 500s. *Rx.*
Use: Anti-infective combination.

•**trimethoprim sulfate.** USAN.
Use: Antibacterial.

trimethylene. Cyclopropane, U.S.P. 23.

•**trimetozine.** (try-MET-oh-zeen) USAN.
Use: Sedative, hypnotic.

•**trimetrexate.** (TRY-meh-TREK-sate) USAN.
Use: Antineoplastic.
See: Neutrexin, Vial (US Bioscience).

•**trimetrexate glucuronate.** (TRY-meh-TREK-sate glue-CURE-uh-nate) USAN.
Use: Antineoplastic. [Orphan drug]

Triminol. (Rugby) Phenylpropanolamine HCl 12.5 mg, chlorpheniramine maleate 2 mg, dextromethorphan HBr 10

mg/5 ml Syr. Bot. 120 ml. *otc.*
Use: Antihistamine, decongestant, antitussive.

•**trimipramine.** (TRY-MIH-prah-meen) USAN.
Use: Antidepressant.

•**trimipramine maleate.** (TRY-MIH-prah-meen) USAN.
Use: Antidepressant.
See: Surmontil (Wyeth-Ayerst).

trimipramine maleate. (Various Mfr.) 25 mg, 50 mg or 100 mg. Cap. Bot. 100s, UD 100s.
Use: Antidepressant.

Trimixin. (Hance) Bacitracin 200 units, polymyxin B sulfate 4000 units, neomycin sulfate 3 mg/g Oint., Tube 0.5 oz. *otc.*
Use: Anti-infective, topical.

•**trimoprostil.** (TRY-moe-PRAHS-till) USAN.
Use: Gastric antisecretory.

Trimo-San. (Milex) Oxyquinoline sulfate 0.025%, boric acid 1%, sodium borate 0.7%, sodium lauryl sulfate 0.1%, glycerin, methylparaben. Jelly. 120 g w/ applicator, 120 g refill. *otc.*
Use: Vaginal preparation.

Trimox. (Squibb Mark) **Cap.:** Amoxicillin trihydrate 250 mg/Cap. Bot. 100s, 500s; 500 mg/Cap. Bot. 50s, 500s. UD 100s. **Oral Susp.:** 125 mg/5 ml. Bot. 80 ml, 100 ml, 150 ml, Unimatic Bot. 5 ml, Ctn. 4 × 25s; 250 mg/5 ml. Bot. 80 ml, 100 ml, 150 ml, Unimatic Bot. 5 ml, Ctn. 4 25s. *Rx.*
Use: Anti-infective, penicillin.

•**trimoxamine hydrochloride.** (TRY-MOX-am-een) USAN.
Use: Antihypertensive.

Trimpex. (Roche) Trimethoprim 100 mg/ Tab. Bot. 100s; Tel-E-Dose 100s. *Rx.*
Use: Urinary anti-infective.

Trim-Qwik. (Columbia) Powder-based meal food supplement. Can 10 oz. *otc.*
Use: Meal replacement.

Trimstat. (Laser) Phendimetrazine tartrate 35 mg/Tab. Bot. 100s, 1000s. *c-III.*
Use: Anorexiant.

Trim Sulf D/S. (Lexis) Sulfamethoxazole 800 mg, trimethoprim 160 mg/Tab. Bot. 100s, 500s. *Rx.*
Use: Anti-infective.

Trim Sulf S/S. (Lexis) Sulfamethoxazole 400 mg, trimethoprim 80 mg/Tab. Bot. 100s, 500s. *Rx.*
Use: Anti-infective.

Trim-Sulfa. *Rx.*

Use: Anti-infective.
See: Proloprim (Glaxo Wellcome).
Trimethoprim (Various Mfr.).
Trimpex (Roche).

Trinalin Repetabs. (Key) Azatadine maleate 1 mg, pseudoephedrine sulfate 120 mg/Tab. Bot 100s. *Rx.*
Use: Antihistamine, decongestant.

Trind. (Bristol-Myers) Phenylpropanolamine HCl 12.5 mg, chlorpheniramine maleate 2 mg/5 ml w/alcohol 5%, sorbitol. Bot. 5 oz. *otc.*
Use: Decongestant, antihistamine.

Tri-Nefrin Extra Strength. (Pfeiffer) Phenylpropanolamine HCl 25 mg, chlorpheniramine maleate 4 mg/Tab. in 24s. *otc.*
Use: Antihistamine, decongestant.

trinitrin tablets.
See: Nitroglycerin Tablets, U.S.P. 23.

trinitrophenol.
See: Picric Acid (Various Mfr.).

Tri-Norinyl. (Syntex) Norethindrone 1 mg with ethinyl estradiol 0.035 mg/Tab. Norethindrone 0.5 mg with ethinyl estradiol 0.035 mg/Tab. 21 and 28 day. (7 inert tabs) Wallette. *Rx.*
Use: Oral contraceptive.

Trinotic. (Forest Pharm) Secobarbital 65 mg, amobarbital 40 mg, phenobarbital 25 mg/Tab. Bot. 1000s. *c-II.*
Use: Hypnotic.

Trinsicon. (Whitby) Liver-stomach concentrate 240 mg, iron 110 mg, vitamin C 75 mg, folic acid 0.5 mg, B_{12} 15 mcg. Cap. Bot. 60s, 500s, UD 100s. *Rx.*
Use: Nutritional supplement.

Trinsicon M. (Whitby) Formerly listed by Russ.

Triobead-125. (Abbott Diagnostics) T3 diagnostic kit. Test units 50s, 100s, 500s.
Use: T3 uptake radioassay for the measurement of thyroid function by indirectly determining the degree of saturation of serum thyroxine binding globulin (TBG).

triocil.
See: Hexetidine.

Triofed Syrup. (Barre-National) Pseudoephedrine HCl 30 mg, triprolidine HCl 1.25 mg/5 ml Syr. Bot. 118 ml, 473 ml. *otc.*
Use: Antihistamine, decongestant.

•**triolein I 125.** USAN.
Use: Radioactive agent.

•**triolein I 131.** USAN.
Use: Radioactive agent.

Triostat. (SK-Beecham) Liothyronine 10

mcg/ml, w/ammonia 2.19 mg/ml, alcohol 6.8%. Vial 1 ml. *Rx.*
Use: Treatment of myxedema coma/precoma.

Triosulfon DMM. (CMC) Tab. Bot. 100s, 250s, 1000s.

Triotann. (Various Mfr.) Phenylephrine tannate 25 mg, chlorpheniramine tannate 8 mg, pyrilamine tannate 25 mg/Tab. Bot. 100s, 500s. *Rx.*
Use: Decongestant, antihistamine.

Triotann Pediatric. (Various Mfr.) Phenylephrine tannate 5 mg, chlorpheniramine tannate 2 mg, pyrilamine tannate 12.5 mg, saccharin, sucrose. Susp. pt. *Rx.*
Use: Decongestant, antihistamine.

Tri-Otic. (Pharmics) Chloroxylenol 1 mg, pramoxine HCl 10 mg, hydrocortisone 10 mg/ml. Drops. Vial 10 ml. *Rx.*
Use: Otic preparation.

trioxane.
See: Trioxymethylene (Various Mfr.).

•**trioxifene mesylate.** (TRY-OX-ih-feen) USAN.
Use: Antiestrogen.

•**trioxsalen,** (TRI-OX-sale-en) U.S.P. 23.
Use: Pigmenting and phototherapeutic agent.
See: Trisoralen, Tab. (Zeneca).

trioxymethylene. Name is incorrectly used to denote paraformaldehyde in some pharmaceuticals.
See: Paraformaldehyde (Various Mfr.).
W/Sod. oleate, triethanolamine, docusate sodium, stearic acid & aluminum silicate.
See: Cooper Creme (Whittaker).

Tri-Pain. (Ferndale) Acetaminophen 162 mg, aspirin 162 mg, salicylamide 162 mg, caffeine 16.2 mg/Tab. Bot. 100s. *otc.*
Use: Analgesic combination.

•**tripamide.** (TRIP-ah-mide) USAN.
Use: Antihypertensive, diuretic.

Tripedia. (Pasteur-Merieux-Connaught) Diphtheria 6.7 Lf units, tetanus 5 Lf units and pertussis antigens 46.8 mcg/0.5 ml, aluminum potassium sulfate (alum), thimerosal, gelatin, polysorbate 80/Inj. 7.5 ml. *Rx.*
Use: Agent for immunization.

•**tripelennamine citrate,** U.S.P. 23.
Use: Antihistamine.

•**tripelennamine hydrochloride,** U.S.P. 23.
Use: Antihistamine.
See: Pyribenzamine hydrochloride, Preps. (Novartis).

Triphasil-21. (Wyeth-Ayerst) Three drug phases in 21 day cycle: **Phase I:** 6 brown tab. Levonorgestrel 0.05 mg, ethinyl estradiol 0.03 mg/Tab. **Phase II:** 5 white tab. Levonorgestrel 0.075 mg, ethinyl estradiol 0.04 mg/Tab. **Phase III:** 10 yellow tab. Levonorgestrel 0.125 mg, ethinyl estradiol 0.03 mg/Tab. *Rx.*
Use: Oral contraceptive.

Triphasil-28. (Wyeth-Ayerst) Three drug phases and one inert phase in 28 day cycle: **Phase I:** 6 brown tab. Levonorgestrel 0.05 mg, ethinyl estradiol 0.03 mg/Tab. **Phase II:** 5 white tab. Levonorgestrel 0.075/mg, ethinyl estradiol 0.04 mg Tab. **Phase III:** 10 yellow tab. Levonorgestrel 0.125 mg, ethinyl estradiol 0.03 mg/Tab. **Phase IV:** 7 inert green tablets. *Rx.*
Use: Oral contraceptive.

Tri-Phen-Chlor. (Rugby) Phenylpropanolamine HCl 20 mg, phenylephrine HCl 5 mg, chlorpheniramine maleate 2.5 mg, phenyltoloxamine citrate 7.5 mg/5 ml Syr. Bot. 473 ml. *Rx.*
Use: Antihistamine, decongestant.

Tri-Phen-Chlor Tabs, Timed Released. (Rugby) Phenylpropanolamine HCl 40 mg, phenylephrine HCl 10 mg, chlorpheniramine maleate 5 mg, phenyltoloxamine citrate 15 mg. 100s. *Rx.*
Use: Upper respiratory combination.

Tri-Phen-Chlor Pediatric Drops. (Rugby) Phenylpropanolamine HCl 5 mg, phenylephrine HCl 1.25 mg, chlorpheniramine maleate 0.5 mg, phenyltoloxamine citrate 2 mg. Bot. w/drop 30 ml. *Rx.*
Use: Upper respiratory combination.

Tri-Phen-Chlor Pediatric Syrup. (Rugby) Phenylpropanolamine HCl 5 mg, phenylephrine HCl 1.25 mg, chlorpheniramine maleate 0.5 mg, phenyltoloxamine citrate 2 mg/5 ml. Syr. Bot. 118 ml, 473 ml, gal. *Rx.*
Use: Decongestant, antihistamine.

Tri-Phen-Mine Pediatric Drops. (Goldline) Phenylpropanolamine HCl 5 mg, phenylephrine HCl 1.25 mg, chlorpheniramine maleate 0.5 mg, phenyltoloxamine citrate 2 mg/ml. Drop. Bot. 30 ml. *Rx.*
Use: Decongestant, antihistamine.

Tri-Phen-Mine Pediatric Syrup. (Goldline) Phenylpropanolamine HCl 5 mg, phenylephrine HCl 1.25 mg, chlorpheniramine maleate 0.5 mg, phenyltoloxamine citrate 2 mg/5 ml. Syr. Bot. 473 ml. *Rx.*
Use: Decongestant, antihistamine.

Tri-Phen-Mine S.R. (Goldline) Chlorpheniramine maleate 5 mg, pyrilamine maleate 15 mg, phenylpropanolamine HCl 40 mg, phenylephrine HCl 10 mg/ SR Tab. Bot. 100s. *Rx.*
Use: Antihistamine, decongestant.

Triphenyl. (Rugby) Phenylpropanolamine HCl 12.5 mg, Chlorpheniramine maleate 2 mg/5 ml, alcohol free. Syr. Bot. 118 ml. *otc.*
Use: Antihistamine, decongestant.

Triphenyl Expectorant. (Rugby) Phenylpropanolamine HCl 12.5 mg, guaifenesin 100 mg/5 ml, alcohol 5%. Expec. Bot. 120 ml, pt., gal. *otc.*
Use: Decongestant, expectorant.

triphenylmethane dyes.
See: Fuchsin.
Methylrosaniline Chloride.

Triphenyl T.D. (Rugby) Phenylpropanolamine HCl 50 mg, pyrilamine maleate 25 mg, pheniramine maleate 25 mg/ Tab. Bot. 100s, 1000s. *Rx.*
Use: Antihistamine, decongestant.

triphenyltetrazolium chloride. TTC.
See: Uroscreen (Pfizer).

tripiperazine dicititrate, hydrous.
See: Piperazine Citrate, U.S.P. 23.

triple antibiotic ophthalmics. (Various Mfr.) Polymyxin B sulfate 10,000 units/ g or ml, neomycin sulfate 3.5 mg/g or ml, bacitracin 400 units. Oint. 3.5 g. *Rx.*
Use: Anti-infective, ophthalmic.

triple antibiotic w/HC. (Various Mfr.) Hydrocortisone 1%, neomycin sulfate = neomycin base 0.35%, bacitracin zinc 400 units, polymyxin B sulfate/g 10,000.
Use: Anti-infective, corticosteroid, ophthalmic.

triple barbiturate elixir. (CMC) Phenobarbital 0.25 gr, butabarbital ⅛ gr, pentobarbital gr/5 ml. Bot. pt., gal. *c-II.*
Use: Sedative.

triple bromides, effervescent tablets. W/Phenobarbital.
See: Palagren, Liq. (Westerfield).

Triple Dye. (Kerr) Gentian violet, proflavine, hemisulfate, brilliant green in water. Dispensing Bot. 15 ml. Single Use Dispos-A-Swab 0.65 ml. Box 10s. Case 10×50 Box.
Use: Umbilical area antiseptic.

Triple Dye. (Xttrium) Brilliant green 2.29 mg, proflavine hemisulfate 1.14 mg, gentian violet 2.29 mg/ml. Bot. 30 ml.
Use: Umbilical area disinfectant.

Triple-Gen Suspension. (Goldline) Hydrocortisone 1%, neomycin sulfate 0.35%, polymyxin B sulfate 10,000

units/ml, benzalkonium chloride, cetyl alcohol, glyceryl monostearate, polyoxyl 40 stearate, propylene glycol, mineral oil. Bot. 7.5 ml. *Rx.*
Use: Ophthalmic corticosteroid, anti-infective.

Triplen. (Interstate) Tripelennamine HCl 50 mg/Tab. Bot. 100s, 1000s. *Rx.*
Use: Antihistamine.

triple sulfa tablets. (Century; Stanlabs) Sulfadiazine 2.5 gr, sulfamerazine 2.5 gr, sulfamethazine 2.5 gr/Tab. Bot. 100s, 1000s. *Rx.*
Use: Anti-infective, sulfonamide.

•**triple sulfa vaginal cream,** U.S.P. 23.
Use: Anti-infective, vaginal.

triple sulfa vaginal tablets.
Use: Anti-infective, vaginal.

Triple Sulfoid. (Pal-Pak) Sulfadiazine 167 mg, sulfamerazine 167 mg, sulfamethazine 167 mg/5 ml or Tab. **Liq.:** Bot. pt., 2 oz. 12s. **Tab.:** Bot. 100s, 1000s. *Rx.*
Use: Anti-infective, sulfonamide.

triple sulfonamide. Dia-Mer-Thia Sulfonamides. Meth-Dia-Mer Sulfonamides.
Use: Anti-infective, sulfonamide.

Triple Vita. (Rosemont) Vitamins A 1500 IU, D 400 IU, C 35 mg/ml, alcohol free. Drops. Bot. 50 ml. *otc.*
Use: Vitamin supplement.

Triple Vita-Flor. (Rosemont) Fluoride 0.5 mg, vitamins A 1500 IU, D 400 IU, C 35 mg/ml, alcohol free. Drops. Bot. 50 ml. *Rx.*
Use: Dental caries preventative, vitamin supplement.

Triple Vitamin ADC w/Fluoride. (Nilor Pharm) Fluoride 0.5 mg, vitamins A 1500 IU, D 400 IU, C 35 mg/ml. Drops. Bot. 50 ml. *Rx.*
Use: Vitamin/mineral supplement; dental caries preventative.

Triple Vitamins w/Fluoride. (Major) Vitamin A 2500 IU, D 400 IU, C 60 mg, fluoride 1 mg, dextrose, sucrose/Chew. Tab. Bot. 100s. *Rx.*
Use: Vitamin supplement, dental caries preventative.

Triplevite w/Fluoride. (Geneva Pharm) Fluoride 0.25 mg/ml, vitamins A 1500 IU, D 400 IU, C 35 mg, alcohol free. Drop. Bot. 50 ml. *Rx.*
Use: Dental caries preventative, vitamin supplement.

Triplevite w/Fluoride. (Geneva Pharm) Fluoride 0.5 mg/ml, vitamins A 1500 IU, D 400 IU, C 35 mg/ml, alcohol free, cherry flavor. Drop. Bot. 50 ml. *Rx.*

Use: Dental caries preventative, vitamin supplement.

Triple X. (Schmid) Pyrethrins 0.3%, piperonyl butoxide 3.0%, petroleum distillate 1.2%, benzyl alcohol 2.4%. Bot. 2 oz, 4 oz. *otc.*
Use: Pediculicide.

Tripodrine. (Schein) Pseudoephedrine HCl 60 mg, triprolidine HCl 2.5 mg/Tab. Bot. 100s, UD 100s. *Rx.*
Use: Decongestant, antihistamine.

Triposed Syrup. (Halsey) Triprolidine HCl 1.25 mg, pseudoephedrine HCl 30 mg/5 ml. Bot. 120 ml, 240 ml, 473 ml, gal. *otc.*
Use: Antihistamine, decongestant.

Triposed Tablets. (Halsey) Triprolidine HCl 2.5 mg, pseudoephedrine HCl 60 mg/Tab. Bot. 100s, 1000s. *otc.*
Use: Antihistamine, decongestant.

tripotassium citrate.
See: Potassium Citrate, U.S.P. 23.

•**triprolidine hydrochloride,** (try-PRO-lih-deen) U.S.P. 23.
Use: Antihistamine.
See: Actidil, Syr. (Glaxo Wellcome).
W/Codeine phosphate, pseudoephedrine HCl, guaifenesin.
See: Actifed-C Syr. (Glaxo Wellcome).

triprolidine hydrochloride and pseudoephedrine hydrochloride syrup. (Various Mfr.) Triprolidine HCl 1.25 mg, pseudoephedrine HCl 30 mg/5 ml. Syr. Bot. 118 ml, 237 ml. *Rx.*
Use: Antihistamine, decongestant.
See: Actifed, Syr. (Glaxo Wellcome).

triprolidine hydrochloride and pseudoephedrine hydrochloride tablets, U.S.P. 23.
Use: Antihistamine, decongestant.
See: Actifed, Tab., (Glaxo Wellcome).
Atridine, Tab. (Interstate).
Sudahist, Tab. (Upsher-Smith).
Suda-Prol, Tab., Cap. (Quality Generics).
Triphed, Tab. (Lemmon).
Triphedrine, Tab. (Redford).

Triptifed. (Weeks & Leo) Triprolidine HCl 2.5 mg, pseudoephedrine HCl 60 mg/Tab. Bot. 36s, 100s. *Rx.*
Use: Antihistamine, decongestant.

Triptone Caplets. (Del Pharm) Dimenhydrinate 50 mg/Tab. Bot. 12s. *otc.*
Use: Antiemetic, antivertigo.

•**triptorelin.** (TRIP-toe-RELL-in) USAN.
Use: Antineoplastic.

triptorelin pamoate.
Use: Treatment of advanced ovarian carcinoma. [Orphan drug]

See: Decapeptyl Injection (Organon).

trisaccharides a and b. *Rx.*
Use: Hemolytic disease of the newborn. [Orphan drug]

trisodium citrate concentration.
Use: Leukapheresis procedures. [Orphan drug]

Trisol. (Buffington) Borax, sodium Cl, boric acid. Irrigator Bot. oz, 4 oz. *otc.*
Use: Artificial tears.

Trisoralen. (Zeneca) Trioxsalen 5 mg/Tab. Tartrazine. Bot. 28s, 100s. *Rx.*
Use: Psoralen.

Tri-Statin. (Rugby) Triamcinolone acetonide 0.1%, neomycin sulfate 0.25%, gramicidin 0.25 mg, nystatin 100,000 units/g Cream. In 15, 30, 60, 120 and 480 g. *Rx.*
Use: Topical corticosteroid, anti-infective.

Tri-Statin II. (Rugby) Triamcinolone acetonide 0.1%, 100,000 units nystatin per g, white petrolatum, parabens. Cream. Tube 15 g, 30 g, 60 g, 120 g, 480 g. *Rx.*
Use: Corticosteroid, antifungal, topical.

Tristoject. (Mayrand) Triamcinolone diacetate 40 mg/ml. Vial 5 ml. *Rx.*
Use: Corticosteroid.

trisulfapyridmines.
Use: Anti-infective, sulfonamide.
See: Triple Sulfa No. 2 (Rugby).

•**trisulfapyrimidines oral susp.,** U.S.P. 23.
Use: Antibacterial.
See: Meth-Dia-Mer Sulfonamides (Various Mfr.).
Neotrizine, Prep. (Lilly).
Terfonyl, Liq., Tab. (Squibb Mark).

Tritan. (Eon) Phenylephrine tannate 25 mg, chlorpheniramine tannate 8 mg, pyrilamine tannate 25 mg/Tab. Bot. 100s, 250s, 1000s. *Rx.*
Use: Decongestant, antihistamine.

Tritane. (Econo Med) Brompheniramine maleate 2 mg, guaifenesin 100 mg, phenylephrine HCl 5 mg, phenylpropanolamine HCl 5 mg, alcohol 3.5%/5 ml. Bot. Gal. *Rx.*
Use: Antihistamine, expectorant, decongestant.

Tritane DC. (Econo Med) Brompheniramine maleate 2 mg, guaifenesin 100 mg, phenylephrine HCl 5 mg, phenylpropanolamine HCl 5 mg, alcohol 3.5%, codeine phosphate 10 mg/5 ml. Bot. Gal. *c-v.*
Use: Antihistamine, expectorant, decongestant, antitussive.

Tri-Tannate. (Rugby) Phenylephrine tannate 25 mg, chlorpheniramine tannate 8 mg, pyrilamine tannate 25 mg. Tab. Bot. 100s, 250s. *Rx.*
Use: Decongestant, antihistamine.

Tri-Tannate Pediatric. (Rugby) Phenylephrine tannate 5 mg, chlorpheniramine tannate 2 mg, pyrilamine tannate 12.5 mg. Susp. Bot. 473 ml. *Rx.*
Use: Decongestant, antihistamine.

Tri-Tannate Plus Pediatric Suspension. (Rugby) Phenylephrine tannate 5 mg, ephedrine tannate 5 mg, chlorpheniramine tannate 4 mg, carbetapentane tannate 30 mg/5 ml. Bot. 480 ml. *Rx.*
Use: Decongestant, antitussive, antihistamine.

Tritec. (Glaxo Wellcome) Ranitidine bismuth citrate 400 mg/Tab. Bot. 100s, UD 100s. *Rx.*
Use: In combination with clarithromycin to treat active duodenal ulcer associated with *H. pylori.*

• **tritiated water.** USAN.
Use: Radioactive agent.
See: Tritiotope (Squibb).

Tri-Tinic. (Vortech) Liver desic. 75 mg, stomach 75 mg, Vitamins B_{12} 15 mcg, Fe 110 mg, folic acid 1 mg, ascorbic acid 75 mg/Cap. Bot. 100s. *Rx.*
Use: Vitamin/mineral supplement.

Tritussin Cough Syrup. (Towne) Pyrilamine maleate 40 mg, pheniramine maleate 20 mg, citric acid 100 mg, codeine phosphate 58 mg/fl. oz. w/menthol and glycerin in flavored base. Bot. 4 oz. *c-v.*
Use: Antihistamine, expectorant, antitussive.

Triurisul. (Sheryl) Sulfacetamide 250 mg, sulfamethizole 250 mg, phenazopyridine HCl 50 mg/Tab. Bot. 100s. *Rx.*
Use: Urinary anti-infective, analgesic.

Triva Douche Powder. (Boyle) Alkyl aryl sulfonate 35%, sod. sulfate 53%, oxyquinoline sulfate 2%, lactose 9.67%, EDTA 0.33%. Packet 3 g, 24s. *otc.*
Use: Douche for trichomonal and monilial infections.

Tri-Vert. (T.E. Williams) Dimenhydrinate 25 mg, niacin 50 mg, pentylenetetrazol 25 mg/Cap. Bot. 100s. *otc.*
Use: Motion sickness treatment.

Tri-Vi-Flor 0.25 mg Drops. (BM-Squibb) Fluoride 0.25 mg, Vitamins A 1500 IU, D 400 IU, C 35 mg/1 ml Drop. Bot. 50 ml. *Rx.*
Use: Caries prophylaxis, dietary supplement.

Tri-Vi-Flor 0.25 mg with Iron Drops. (BM-Squibb) Fluoride 0.25 mg, Vitamins A 1500 IU, D 400 IU, C 35 mg, iron 10 mg/1 ml Drop. Bot. 50 ml. *Rx.*
Use: Caries prophylaxis, dietary supplement with iron.

Tri-Vi-Flor 0.5 mg Drops. (BM-Squibb) Fluoride 0.5 mg, Vitamins A 1500 IU, D 400 IU, C 35 mg/1 ml. Bot. 50 ml. *Rx.*
Use: Caries prophylaxis, dietary supplementation.

Tri-Vi-Flor 1.0 mg Tablets. (BM-Squibb) Fluoride 1 mg, Vitamins A 2500 IU, D 400 IU, Vitamins C 60 mg, sucrose/Tab. Bot. 100s, 1000s. *Rx.*
Use: Caries prophylaxis, dietary supplementation.

Tri-Vi-Sol Drops. (BM-Squibb) Vitamin A 1500 IU, D 400 IU, C 35 mg/1 ml Drops. Bot. 50 ml with calibrated "Safti-dropper." *otc.*
Use: Vitamin supplement.

Tri-Vi-Sol with Iron Drops. (BM-Squibb) Vitamins A 1500 IU, C 35 mg, D 400 IU, iron 10 mg/ml. Bot. 50 ml. *otc.*
Use: Vitamin/mineral supplement.

Trivitamin Fluoride. (Schein) Drops: Fluoride 0.25 mg or 0.5 mg, vitamins A 1500 IU, D 400 IU, C 35 mg/ml. Bot. 50 ml. Chew. Tab.: Fluoride 0.5 mg, vitamins A 2500 IU, D 400 IU, C 60 mg, sucrose. Bot. 100s. *Rx.*
Use: Vitamin with fluoride supplement; dental caries preventative.

Tri-Vitamin with Fluoride. (Rugby) Fluoride 0.5 mg, Vitamins A 1500 IU, D 400 IU, C 35 mg/ml Drops. Bot. 50 ml. *Rx.*
Use: Vitamin/mineral supplement.

Tri Vit w/Fluoride 0.25 mg. (Barre-National) Fluoride 0.25 mg, vitamins A 1500 IU, D 400 IU, C 35 mg/ml. Drops. Bot. 50 ml. *Rx.*
Use: Vitamin/mineral supplement; dental caries preventative.

Tri Vit w/Fluoride 0.5 mg. (Barre-National) Fluoride 0.5 mg, vitamins A 1500 IU, D 400 IU, C 35 mg/ml. Drops. Bot. 50 ml. *Rx.*
Use: Vitamin/mineral supplement; dental caries preventative.

Tri-Vite. (Foy) Thiamine HCl 100 mg, pyridoxine HCl 100 mg, cyanocobalamine 1000 mcg/ml. Vial 10 ml. *Rx.*
Use: Vitamin B supplement.

Trobicin. (Pharmacia & Upjohn) Spectinomycin HCl equivalent to spectinomycin activity: **2 g/Vial** w/ampule of diluent containing bacteriostatic water for injection 3.2 ml, benzyl alcohol 0.945% in ampule. **4 g/Vial** w/ampule

of diluent containing bacteriostatic water for injection 6.2 ml, benzyl alcohol 0.945%. *Rx.*
Use: Treatment of gonorrhea.

Trocaine. (Roberts) Benzocaine 10 mg. Lozenges. UD 4s, 500s. *otc.*
Use: Diet aid.

Trocal. (Roberts Med) Dextromethorphan HBr 7.5 mg, guaifenesin 50 mg/Loz. In 500s. *otc.*
Use: Antitussive, expectorant.

•**troclosene potassium.** USAN.
Use: Topical anti-infective.

•**troglitazone.** (TROE-glih-tazz-ohn) USAN.
Use: Antidiabetic.
See: Rezulin, Tab. (Parke-Davis).

•**trolamine,** N.F. 18. *Formerly Triethanolamine.*
Use: Pharmaceutic aid (alkalizing agent), analgesic.
W/Ortho-iodobenzoic.
See: Progonasyl (Saron).

•**troleandomycin,** (troe-lee-AN-doe-MY-sin) U.S.P. 23. *Formerly Triacetyloleandomycin.*
Use: Antibacterial; steroid-requiring asthma [Orphan drug]
See: Tao (Roerig).

tromal.
Use: Analgesic, antidepressant agent.

•**tromethamine,** (TROE-meth-ah-meen) U.S.P. 23.
Use: Alkalizer.

Tronolane Cream. (Ross) Pramoxine HCl 1% in cream base. Tubes 30 g, 60 g. *otc.*
Use: Anorectal preparation.

Tronolane Suppositories. (Ross) Zinc oxide 11%, hard fat 95%. Pkg. 10s, 20s. *otc.*
Use: Anorectal preparation.

Tronothane HCl. (Abbott) Pramoxine HCl 1%, cetyl alcohol, glycerin, parabens. Cream. 28.4 g. *otc.*
Use: Topical anesthetic.

Tropamine +. (NeuroGenesis/Matrix) Vitamins D 250 mg, l-phenylalanine, l-tyrosine 150 mg, l-glutamine 50 mg, B_1 1.67 mg, B_2 2.5 mg, B_3 16.7 mg, B_5 15 mg, B_6 3.3 mg, B_{12} 5 mcg, folic acid 0.067 mg, C 100 mg, calcium 25 mg, chromium 0.01 mg, iron 1.5 mg, magnesium 25 mg, zinc 5 mg, yeast and preservative free. Cap. Bot. 42s, 180s. *otc.*
Use: Oral nutritional supplement.

•**tropanserin hydrochloride.** (trope-ANE-ser-IN) USAN.

Use: Seratonin receptor antagonist (specific in migraine).

Trophamine Injection. (McGaw) Nitrogen 4.65 g, amino acids 30 g, protein 29 g/500 ml. Bot 500 ml IV infusion. *otc.*
Use: Nutritional supplement.

Troph-Iron. (SK-Beecham) Vitamins B_{12} 25 mcg, B_1 10 mg, iron 20 mg/5 ml. Saccharin. Bot. 4 fl. oz. *otc.*
Use: Vitamin/mineral supplement.

Trophite & Iron. (Menley & James) Iron 60 mg, B_1 30 mg, B_{12} 75 mcg. Liq. Bot. 120 ml. *otc.*
Use: Vitamin/mineral supplement.

Tropicacyl. (Akorn) Tropicamide solution 0.5%. In 15 ml. 1% tropicamide. 2 ml, 15 ml. *Rx.*
Use: Mydriatic, cycloplegic.

Tropical Blend. (Schering-Plough) A series of products is marketed under the Tropical Blend name including: Hawaii Blend Oil SPF 2 (Bot. 8 oz.); Hawaii Blend Lotion SPF 2 (Bot. 8 oz.); Rio Blend Oil SPF 2 (Bot. 8 oz.); Rio Blend Lotion SPF 2 (Bot. 8 oz.); Jamaica Blend Oil SPF 2 (Bot. 8 oz.); Jamaica Blend SPF 2 (Bot. 8 oz.). All contain homosalate in various oil and lotion bases. *otc.*
Use: Sunscreen.

Tropical Blend Dark Tanning. (Schering-Plough) **SPF 2:** Homosalate. **Oil:** Bot. 180 ml, 240 ml; **Lot.:** Bot. 240 ml. **SPF 4:** Ethylhexyl p-methoxycinnamate, oxybenzone. Bot. 240 ml; **Oil:** Padimate O, oxybenzone. Bot. 240 ml. *otc.*
Use: Sunscreen.

Tropical Blend Dry Oil. (Schering-Plough) Homosalate, oxybenzone. Oil Bot. 180 ml. *otc.*
Use: Sunscreen.

Tropical Blend Tan Magnifier. (Schering-Plough) Triethanolmine salicylate. Oil Bot. 240 ml. *otc.*
Use: Sunscreen.

Tropical Gold Dark Tanning Lotion. (Goldline) SPF 4. Ethylhexyl p-methoxycinnamate, oxybenzone, benzyl alcohol, parabens, aloe extract, jojoba oil, vitamin E, EDTA. PABA free. Waterproof. Lot. Bot. 240 ml. *otc.*
Use: Sunscreen.

Tropical Gold Dark Tanning Oil. (Goldline) SPF 2. Ethylhexyl p-methoxycinnamate, octyldimethyl PABA, mineral oil, coconut oil, cocoa butter, aloe, lanolin, eucalyptus oil, oils of plumeria, manako (mango), kuawa (guava), mikara (papaya), liliko (passion fruit), taro,

kukui. Oil. Bot. 240 ml. *otc.*
Use: Sunscreen.

Tropical Gold Sport Sunblock. (Goldline) SPF 15. Ethylhexyl p-methoxycinnamate, oxybenzone, diazolidinyl urea, parabens, aloe extract, jojoba oil, vitamin E, EDTA. PABA free. Perspiration proof. Lot. Bot. 180 ml. *otc.*
Use: Sunblock.

Tropical Gold Sunblock. (Goldline) **SPF 15:** Ethylhexyl p-methoxycinnamate, oxybenzone, vegetable oil, benzyl alcohol, parabens, imidazolidinyl urea, vitamin E, aloe extract, jojoba oil, EDTA. PABA free. Waterproof. Lot. Bot. 118 ml. **SPF 17:** Ethylhexyl p-methoxycinnamate, 2-ethylhexyl salicylate, homosalate, oxybenzone, aloe extract, vitamin E, vegetable and jojoba oils, benzyl alcohol, imidazolidinyl urea, parabens, EDTA. PAPA free. Waterproof. Lot. Bot. 118 ml. **SPF 30:** Ethylhexyl p-methoxycinnamate, 2-ethylhexyl salicylate, homosalate, oxybenzone, aloe extract, vitamin E, vegetable and jojoba oils, benzyl alcohol, imidizolidinyl urea, parabens, EDTA. PABA free. Waterproof. 118 ml. *otc.*
Use: Sunblock.

Tropical Gold Sunscreen. (Goldline) SPF 8. Ethylhexyl p-methoxycinnamate, oxybenzone, benzyl alcohol, parabens, aloe extract, jojoba oil, vitamin E, EDTA. PABA free. Waterproof. Lot. Bot. 118 ml. *otc.*
Use: Sunscreen.

•**tropicamide,** (TROP-ik-ah-mid) U.S.P. 23.
Use: Anticholinergic (ophthalmic).
See: Mydriacyl, Drops. (Alcon).
 Opticyl, Soln. (Optopics).
 Tropicacyl, Soln. (Akorn).

tropicamide. (Various Mfr.) 0.5%, 1%. Soln. Bot. 2 ml (0.5%), 15 ml.
Use: Anticholinergic (ophthalmic).

tropine benzohydryl ester methanesulfonate. (also named benztropine methane-sulfonate).

•**trospectomycin sulfate.** (TROE-specktoe-MY-sin) USAN.
Use: Antibacterial.

•**trovafloxacin mesylate.** (TROE-vah-FLOX-ah-sin) USAN.
Use: Antibacterial.

Trovit. (Sig) Vitamins B_2 0.3 mg, B_6 1 mg, choline Cl 25 mg, panthenol 2 mg, dl-methionine 10 mg, inositol 20 mg, niacinamide 50 mg, Vitamins B_{12} 10 mcg/ml. Vial 30 ml. *Rx.*
Use: Vitamin B supplement.

T.R.U.E. Test. (Glaxo Dermatology) Allergens incluse nickel sulfate, wool alcohols (lanolin), neomycin sulfate, potassium dichromate (chromium), caine mix (benzocaine, dibucaine, tetracaine), fragrance mix, colophony, epoxy resin, quinoline mix, balsam of peru, ethylenediamine, cobalt, p-tert-butylphenol formaldehyde, paraben mix, carba mix, black rubber mix, chlorormethyl isothiazolinone, Quaternium-15, mercaptobenzothiazole, p-phenylenediamine, formaldehyde, mercapto mix, thimerosal and thiuram mix. Test in multipak cartons (5s). *Rx.*
Use: For diagnosis of allergic contact dermatitis.

Truphylline. (G & W) Aminophylline 250 mg/Supp. (equiv. to theophylline 198 mg) In UD 10s, 25s. *Rx.*
Use: Bronchodilator.

TruSopt. (Merck) Dorzolamide HCl 2%. Soln. Bot. 5 ml, 10 ml. *Rx.*
Use: Agent for glaucoma.

Trynisin Cold Syrup. (Halsey) Bot. 4 oz., 8 oz.
Use: Antihistamine.

tryparsamide.

•**trypsin, crystallized,** U.S.P. 23.
Use: Proteolytic enzyme.
W/Castor oil.
See: Granulex (Hickam).
W/Chymotrypsin.
See: Chymolase, Tab. (Warren-Teed).
 Orenzyme, Tab. (Hoechst Marion Roussel).

tryptizol hydrochloride. Amitriptyline HCl. U.S.P 23.

•**tryptophan,** (TRIP-toe-FAN) U.S.P. 23.
Use: Amino acid.

Trysul. (Savage) Sulfathiazole 3.42%, sulfacetamide 2.86%, sulfabenzamide 3.7%, urea 0.64%. Tube 78 g. *Rx.*
Use: Anti-infective, vaginal.

T/Scalp. (Neutrogena) Hydrocortisone 1%. Liq. Greaseless. Bot. 60 ml, 105 ml. *otc.*
Use: Topical corticosteroid, antipruritic.

T-Serp Tablet. (Tennessee) Reserpine alkaloid 0.25 mg/Tab. Bot. 100s, 1000s. *Rx.*
Use: Antihypertensive.

TSPA.
Use: Antineoplastic.
See: Thiotepa (Lederle).

T-Stat. (Westwood Squibb) Erythromycin 2% w/alcohol 71.2%. Bot. 60 ml; Pads, disposable premoistened 60s. *Rx.*
Use: Antiacne.

TTC. Triphenyltetrazolium Chloride.
See: Uroscreen, Tube (Pfizer).
tuaminoheptane sulfate, U.S.P. XX.
Use: Adrenergic.
• **tuberculin.** (too-BURR-kyoo-lin) U.S.P.
23.
Use: Diagnostic aid (dermal reactivity
indicator).
See: Aplisol (Parke-Davis) Aplitest
(Parke-Davis).
Tuberculin, Mono-Vacc Test. (Lincoln)
Mono-Vacc test is a sterile, disposable
multiple puncture scarifier with liquid
Old Tuberculin on the points. Box 25
tests.
Use: Diagnostic aid.
Tuberculin, Old Monovacc Test. (Led-
erle) 5 TU activity test. Soln. of Old
Tuberculin containing acacia 7%, lac-
tose 8.5%. Test. Kits 25s, 100s, 250s.
Use: Diagnostic aid.
Tuberculin, Old Tine Test. (Lederle) 5
TY activity per test. Soln. of Old Tuber-
culin, containing acacia 7%, lactose
8.5%. Test. Kits 25s, 100s, 250s.
Use: Diagnostic aid.
tuberculin purified protein derivative.
(Squibb) (Pasteur-Merieux-Connaught)
A concentrated solution for multiple
puncture testing. Vial 1 ml.
Use: For screening tuberculin activity.
tuberculin tests.
Use: Diagnostic aid.
See: Aplisol (Parke-Davis).
Aplitest (Parke-Davis).
Sclavo Test-PPD (Sclavo).
Tine Test PPD (Lederle).
Tuberculin, Old Mono Vacc Test (Pasteur-Merieux-Connaught).
Tuberculin, Old, Tine Test (Lederle).
Tubersol (Squibb) (Pasteur-Merieux-
Connaught).
tuberculin tine test. (Lederle) **Old
Tuberculin (OT):** Each disposable test
unit consists of a stainless steel disc,
with four tines (or prongs) 2 millimeters
long, attached to a plastic handle. The
tines have been dip-dried with antigenic
material. The entire unit is sterilized by
ethylene oxide gas. The test has been
standardized by comparative studies,
utilizing 0.05 mg US Standard Old
Tuberculin (5 International Units) or
0.0001 mg US Standard (5 International
Units) by the Mantoux technique. The
reliability appears to be comparable to
the standard Mantoux. Tests in a jar
25s. Package 100s. Bin Package 250s.
Purified Protein Derivative (PPD):
Equivalent to or more potent than 5 TU

PPD Mantoux test. Tests in a jar 25s.
Package 100s.
Use: Diagnostic aid.
tuberculosis vaccine.
Use: Vaccine, bacterial.
See: TICE BCG (Organon).
Tuberlate. (Heun) Sod. p-aminosalicy-
late 12 gr, succinic acid 4 gr/Tab. Bot.
500s.
Use: Tuberculosis treatment.
Tubersol. (Pasteur-Merieux-Connaught)
Tuberculin purified protein derivative
(Mantoux) 1 TU/0.1 ml: Vial 1 ml. 5 TU/
0.1 ml: Vial 1 ml, 5 ml. 250 TU/0.1 ml:
Vial 1 ml.
Use: For the detection of tuberculosis
infection.
Tubex. (Wyeth-Ayerst, Wyeth-Lederle)
The following drugs are available in
various Tubex sizes:
Ativan
Bicillin C-R
Bicillin C-R 900/300
Bicillin Long-Acting
Codeine Phosphate
Cyanocobalamin
Digoxin
Dimenhydrinate
Diphenhydramine HCl
Diphtheria and Tetanus Toxoids Ad-
sorbed
(Pediatric)
Epinephrine
Furosemide
Heparin Flush Kits
Heparin Lock Flush
Heparin Sodium Solution
Hydromorphone HCl
Hydroxyzine HCl
Influenza Virus Vaccine, Trivalent
Mepergan
Meperidine HCl
Morphine Sulfate
Naloxone Injection
Naloxone Injection, Neonatal
Oxytocin
Pentobarbital Sodium
Phenergan
Phenobarbital Sodium
Prochlorperazine Edisylate
Secobarbital Sodium
Sodium Chloride, Bacteriostatic
Sparine HCl
Tetanus and Diphtheria Toxoids Ad-
sorbed (Adult)
Tetanus Immune Globulin (Human).
Tetanus Toxoid Alum. Phos. Ad.
Tetanus Toxoid, Fluid
Thiamine Hydrochloride
Wycillin

•**tubocurarine chloride,** U.S.P. 23.
Use: Neuromuscular blocking agent.
tubocurarine chloride. (Lilly) 3 mg/ml.
Amp. 10 ml. (Abbott) 3 mg/ml in 10 ml
fliptop vials; 15 mg in 5 ml Abboject Syringe.
Use: Neuromuscular blocking agent.
tubocurarine chloride, dimethyl. Dimethyl ether of d-tubocurarine chloride.
tubocurarine chloride hydrochloride
pentahydrate. Tubocurarine Chloride,
U.S.P. 23.
tubocurarine iodide, dimethyl. Dimethyl
ether of d-tubocurarine iodide.
Use: Skeletal muscle relaxant.
See: Metubine, Vial (Lilly).
•**tubulozole hydrochloride.** (too-BYOO-
lah-ZAHL) USAN.
Use: Antineoplastic (microtubule inhibitor).
Tucks. (Parke-Davis Prods) Pads saturated with solution of witch hazel 50%,
glycerin 10%, benzalkonium Cl 0.003%.
Jar 40s, 100s. *otc.*
Use: Proctologic & dermatologic disorders.
Tucks Clear Gel. (Warner Lambert Con-
sumer Health Products) Hamamelis wa-
ter 50%, glycerin 10%, benzyl alco-
hol, EDTA. Gel. Tube 19.8 g. *otc.*
Use: Anorectal preparation.
Tucks Take-Alongs. (Parke-Davis
Prods) Non-woven wipes saturated with
solution of witch hazel 50%, glycerine
10%, benzalkonium chloride 0.003%.
Box 12s. *otc.*
Use: Anorectal preparation.
Tuinal. (Lilly) Equal parts Seconal Sod.
& Amytal Sod. Pulvule **100 mg** Bot.
100s; **200 mg** Bot. 100s. *c-II.*
Use: Sedative, hypnotic.
tumor necrosis factor-binding protein
I and II. (Serono) *Rx.*
Use: Treatment of AIDS. [Orphan drug]
Tums. (SK-Beecham) Calcium carbo-
nate 500 mg/Tab. Available in pepper-
mint and assorted flavors in various
package sizes. Rolls of 12 singles, 3-
roll wraps. Bot. 75s, 150s. *otc.*
Use: Antacid.
Tums 500. (SK-Beecham) Calcium
carbonate 1250 mg (500 mg calcium),
sucrose, sodium < 4 mg. Chew. tab.
Bot. 60s. *otc.*
Use: Calcium supplement.
Tums E-X Extra Strength. (SK-
Beecham) Calcium carbonate 750 mg,
wintergreen or fruit flavors. 12s, 48s,
96s. *otc.*

Use: Antacid.
Tums Plus. (SK-Beecham) Calcium
carbonate 500 mg, (elemental calcium
200 mg), simethicone 20 mg, sucrose,
sodium ≤ 2 mg, assorted fruit and mint
flavors. Tab. Bot. 48s. *otc.*
Use: Antacid.
Tums Ultra. (SK-Beecham) Calcium
carbonate 1000 mg. Chew. tab. Bot.
36s, 72s. *otc.*
Use: Calcium supplement.
Tur-Bi-Kal Nasal Drops. (Emerson)
Phenylephrine HCl in a saline solution.
Dropper Bot. oz., 12s. *otc.*
Use: Decongestant.
Turbilixir. (Burlington) Chlorpheniramine
maleate 2 mg, phenylephrine HCl 5 mg,
phenylpropanolamine HCl 5 mg/5 ml.
Bot. Pts., gal. *otc.*
Use: Antihistamine, decongestant.
Turbinaire.
See: Decadron Phosphate, Preps.
(Merck).
Turbinaire Decadron Phosphate.
(Merck) Each metered spray delivers
dexamethasone sodium phosphate
equivalent to ≈ dexamethasone 84 mcg
(170 sprays per cartridge), alcohol 2%.
Aerosol. 12.6 g w/adapter or 12.6 g
refill. *Rx.*
Use: Intranasal steroid.
Turbispan Leisurecaps. (Burlington)
Chlorpheniramine maleate 12 mg, 1-
phenylephrine HCl 15 mg, phenylpro-
panolamine HCl 15 mg/Sus. Rel. Cap.
Bot. 30s. *otc.*
Use: Antihistamine, decongestant.
Turgasept Aerosol. (Wyeth-Ayerst) Ethyl
alcohol 44.25%, essential oils 0.9%, n-
alkyl (50% C-14, 40% C-12, 10% C-
16) dimethyl benzylammonium Cl
0.33%, o-phenylphenol 0.25% w/pro-
pellant. Spray can 11.5 oz. in bouquet,
fresh lemon, leather, citrus blossom
scents.
Use: Spray disinfectant, air deodorant.
turpentine oil w/combinations.
See: Sloan's Liniment, Liq. (Warner-
Lambert).
Tusibron. (Kenwood/Bradley) Guaifenesin 100 mg/5 ml. 3.5% alcohol. Liq. Bot.
118 ml. *otc.*
Use: Expectorant.
Tusibron-DM. (Kenwood/Bradley) Guaifenesin 100 mg, dextromethorphan 15
mg/5 ml. Liq. Bot. 118 ml. *otc.*
Use: Expectorant, antitussive.
tusilan. Dextromethorphan HBr.
Tusquelin. (Circle) Dextromethorphan

HBr 15 mg, chlorpheniramine maleate 2 mg, phenylpropanolamine 5 mg, phenylephrine HCl 5 mg, fl. ext. ipecac 0.17 min., potassium guaiacolsulfonate 44 mg/5 ml. Alcohol 5%. Syrup, pt. *Rx.*
Use: Antitussive, expectorant, antihistamine, decongestant.

Tussabar. (Tennessee) Acetaminophen 400 mg, salicylamide 500 mg, potassium guaiacolsulfonate 120 mg, pyrilamine maleate 30 mg, ammonium chloride 500 mg, sodium citrate 500 mg, phenylephrine HCl 30 mg/oz. Bot. pt., gal. *Rx.*
Use: Analgesic, decongestant, expectorant, antihistamine.

Tussabid. (ION) Guaifenesin 200 mg, dextromethorphan HBr 30 mg/Cap. Bot. 24s, 100s. *otc.*
Use: Antihistamine, expectorant.

Tussafed Drops. (Everett) Carbinoxamine maleate 2 mg, pseudoephedrine HCl 25 mg, dextromethorphan HBr 4 mg/1 ml. Bot. 30 ml with calibrated dropper. *Rx.*
Use: Antihistamine, decongestant, antitussive.

Tussafed Syrup. (Everett) Dextromethorphan HBr 15 mg, pseudoephedrine HCl 60 mg, carbinoxamine maleate 4 mg/ 5 ml. Bot. 4 oz., 16 oz. *Rx.*
Use: Antitussive, decongestant, antihistamine.

Tussahist. (Defco) Codeine phosphate 10 mg, phenylpropanolamine HCl 12.5 mg, chlorpheniramine maleate 2 mg, pyrilamine maleate 7.5 mg, guaifenesin 100 mg/5 ml. Bot. 4 oz. pt, gal. *c-v.*
Use: Antitussive, decongestant, antihistamine, expectorant.

Tuss Allergine Modified T.D. (Rugby) Phenylpropanolamine HCl 75 mg, caramiphen edisylate 40 mg/Cap. T.R. Bot. 100s. *Rx.*
Use: Decongestant, antitussive.

Tussafin Expectorant Liquid. (Rugby) Pseudoephedrine HCl 60 mg, hydrocodone bitartrate 5 mg, guaifenesin 200 mg, alcohol 2.5%. Bot. 480 ml. *c-iii.*
Use: Decongestant, antitussive, expectorant.

Tussanil DH. (Misemer) Phenylpropanolamine HCl 25 mg, guaifenesin 100 mg, hydrocodone bitartrate 1.66 mg, salicylamide 300 mg/Tab. In 100s. *c-iii.*
Use: Decongestant, expectorant, antitussive, analgesic.

Tussanil DH Syrup. (Misemer) Phenylephrine HCl 10 mg, chlorpheniramine maleate 4 mg, hydrocodone bitartrate 2.5 mg/5 ml w/alcohol 5%. Bot. pt. *c-iii.*
Use: Decongestant, antihistamine, antitussive.

Tussanil Expectorant Syrup. (Misemer) Hydrocodone bitartrate 2.5 mg, phenylephrine HCl 10 mg, guaifenesin 100 mg/5 ml w/alcohol 5%. Bot. pt. *c-iii.*
Use: Antitussive, decongestant, expectorant.

Tussanol. (Tyler) Pyrilamine maleate ¾ gr, codeine phosphate 1 gr, ammonium chloride 7.5 gr, sodium citrate 5 gr, menthol gr/fl. oz. Bot. 4 fl. oz, pt, gal. *c-v.*
Use: Antihistamine, antitussive, expectorant.

Tussanol with Ephedrine. (Tyler) Ephedrine sulfate 2 gr, pyrilamine maleate ¾ gr, codeine phosphate 1 gr, ammonium chloride 7.5 gr, sodium citrate 5 gr, menthol gr/30 ml. Bot. 16 fl. oz. *c-v.*
Use: Bronchodilator, antihistamine, antitussive, expectorant.

Tussar-2 Syrup. (Rhone-Poulenc Rorer) Codeine phosphate 10 mg, guaifenesin 100 mg, pseudoephedrine HCl 30 mg/5 ml, alcohol 2.5%. Bot. 473 ml. *c-v.*
Use: Antitussive, expectorant, decongestant.

Tussar DM. (Rhone-Poulenc Rorer) Dextromethorphan HBr 15 mg, chlorpheniramine maleate 2 mg, phenylephrine HCl 5 mg/5 ml w/methylparaben 0.1% Bot. 4 oz., pt. *Rx.*
Use: Antitussive, antihistamine, expectorant.

Tussar SF. (Rhone-Poulenc Rorer) Codeine phosphate 10 mg, guaifenesin 100 mg, pseudoephedrine HCl 30 mg/ 5 ml, alcohol 2.5%. Bot. 120 ml, 473 ml. *c-v.*
Use: Antitussive, decongestant, expectorant.

Tuss-DM. (Hyrex) Dextromethorphan HBr (10 mg), guaifenesin 200 mg, dye free. Tab. Bot. 100s, 1000s. *Rx.*
Use: Antitussive, expectorant.

Tussend. (Monarch) Hydrocodone bitartrate 2.5 mg, chlorpheniramine maleate 2 mg/5 ml. 5% alcohol/Syrup. Bot. 480 ml, banana flavor. *c-iii.*
Use: Antitussive and expectorant combination.

Tussex Cough. (Various Mfr.) Phenylephrine HCl 5 mg, dextromethorphan HBr 10 mg, guaifenesin 100 mg/5 ml Syr. Bot. 120 ml, gal. *Rx.*
Use: Decongestant, antitussive, expectorant.

Tuss-Genade Modified Caps. (Goldline) Phenylpropanolamine HCl 75 mg, caramiphen edisylate 40 mg. Bot. 100s, 1000s. *Rx.*
Use: Decongestant, antitussive.

Tussgen Expectorant. (Goldline) Bot. pt, gal.
Use: Expectorant.

Tussgen Liquid. (Goldline) Pseudoephedrine HCl 60 mg, hydrocodone bitartrate 5 mg/5 ml. Bot. 100s, 1000s. *c-III.*
Use: Decongestant, antitussive.

Tussidram. (Dram) Dextromethorphan 10 mg, phenylpropanolamine 12.5 mg, guaifenesin 50 mg, chlorpheniramine maleate 2 mg/5 ml. Bot. pt. *Rx.*
Use: Antitussive, decongestant, expectorant, antihistamine.

Tussigon. (Daniels) Hydrocodone bitartrate 5 mg, homatropine methylbromide 1.5 mg/Tab. Bot. 100s, 500s. *c-III.*
Use: Antitussive, anticholinergic, antispasmodic.

Tussionex. (Medeva) Hydrocodone (as polistirex) 10 mg, chlorpheniramine 8 mg. Liq. Bot. 473 ml and 900 ml. *c-III.*
Use: Antitussive, antihistamine.

Tussi-Organidin DM NR. (Wallace) Dextromethorphan HBr 10 mg, guaifenesin 100 mg/5 ml. Saccharin, sorbitol. Liq. Bot. 120 ml, pt, gal. *c-v.*
Use: Antitussive, expectorant.

Tussi-Organidin NR. (Wallace) Codeine phosphate 10 mg, guaifenesin 100 mg/5 ml. Saccharin, sorbitol. Bot. 120 ml, pt, gal. *c-v.*
Use: Antitussive, expectorant.

Tussirex. (Scot-Tussin) Phenylephrine HCl 4.2 mg, pheniramine maleate 13.3 mg, codeine phosphate 10 mg, sodium citrate 83.3 mg, sodium salicylate 83.3 mg, caffeine citrate 25 mg/5 ml Syr. Bot. 120 and 240 ml, pt, gal. *c-v.*
Use: Decongestant, antihistamine, antitussive, expectorant.

Tussirex Sugar Free Liquid. (Scot-Tussin) Codeine phosphate 10 mg, pheniramine maleate 13.33 mg, phenylephrine HCl 4.17 mg, sodium citrate 83.33 mg, sodium salicylate 83.33 mg, caffeine citrate 25 mg/5 ml. Bot. 120 ml, pt. gal. *c-v.*
Use: Antitussive, antihistamine, decongestant, expectorant, salicylate analgesic.

Tuss-LA. (Hyrex) Pseudoephedrine HCl 120 mg, guaifenesin 500 mg/L.A. Tab. Bot. 100s. *Rx.*
Use: Decongestant, expectorant.

Tusso-DM. (Everett) Dextromethorphan HBr 10 mg, iodianted glycerol 30 mg, alcohol free. Liq. Bot. 473 ml.
Use: Cough preparation.

Tussogest. (Major) Phenylpropanolamine HCl 75 mg, caramiphen edisylate 40 mg/Cap. T.R. Bot. 100s, 500s, 1000s. *Rx.*
Use: Decongestant, antitussive.

Tusstat Expectorant. (Century) Diphenhydramine HCl 80 mg, ammonium chloride 12 gr, sodium citrate 5 gr, menthol $\frac{1}{10}$ gr, alcohol 5%/oz. Bot. 4 fl. oz, pt, gal. *Rx.*
Use: Antihistamine, expectorant.

•**tuvirumab.** (tuh-VIE-roo-mab) USAN.
Use: Monoclonal antibody (antiviral).

TVC-2 Dandruff Shampoo. (Dermol) Zinc pyrithione 2%. Bot. 120 ml. *otc.*
Use: Antiseborrheic.

T-Vites. (Freeda) Vitamins B_1 25 mg, B_2 25 mg, B_3 150 mg, B_5 25 mg, B_6 25 mg, C 100 mg, biotin 30 mcg, PABA, K, Mg, Mn carbonate 2 mg, Zn gluconate 20 mg/Tab. Bot. 100s. *otc.*
Use: Vitamin/mineral supplement.

tween 20, 40, 60, 80. (Zeneca) Polysorbates, N.F. 18.
Use: Surface active agents.

12-Hour Antihistamine Nasal Decongestant. (URL) Pseudoephedrine sulfate 120 mg, dexbrompheniramine maleate 6 mg, sugar, sucrose. SR Tab. Bot. 10s. *otc.*
Use: Decongestant.

12-Hour Cold Tablets. (Goldline) Dexbrompheniramine maleate 6 mg, pseudoephedrine sulfate 120 mg/SR Tab. Pkg. 10s, 20s. *otc.*
Use: Antihistamine, decongestant.

Twice-a-Day. (Major). Oxymetazoline 0.05%. Solution: In 15 and 30 ml. *otc.*
Use: Decongestant.

Twilite. (Pfeiffer) Diphenhydramine HCl 50 mg. Tab. 20s. *otc.*
Use: Nonprescription sleep aid.

Twin-K Liquid. (Knoll Pharm) Potassium ions 20 mEq./15 ml. Bot. pt. *Rx.*
Use: Treatment of hypokalemia.

2-Tone Disclosing Solution. (Young Dental Manufacturing) Dropper Bot. 2 oz.
Use: Disclosing solution.

2-24. (Walgreen) Belladonna alkaloids 0.2 mg, phenylpropanolamine HCl 50 mg, chlorpheniramine maleate 4 mg/Cap. Bot. 10s. *otc.*
Use: Anticholinergic, antispasmodic, decongestant, antihistamine.

Two-Cal HN High Nitrogen Liquid Nutrition. (Ross) High-nitrogen liquid nutrition (2 calories/ml). 1900 calories (1 quart) provide 100% US RDA for vitamins and minerals for adults and children over 4 yrs. Can 8 fl. oz. *otc.*
Use: Nutritional supplement.

Two-Dyne Capsules. (Hyrex) Butalbital 50 mg, caffeine 40 mg, acetaminophen 325 mg/Cap. Bot. 100s, 1000s. *Rx.*
Use: Sedative, hypnotic, analgesic.

● **tybamate.** USAN.
Use: Tranquilizer (minor).

Ty-Caplets. (Major) Acetaminophen 500 mg/Tab. Bot. 100s. *otc.*
Use: Analgesic.

Ty-Caps. (Major) Acetaminophen 500 mg/Cap. Bot. 100s, 1000s, UD 100s. *otc.*
Use: Analgesic.

Tycodene Sugar Free. (Pfeiffer) Chlorpheniramine maleate 2 mg, dextromethorphan HBr 10 mg, menthol, saccharin, sorbitol, alcohol free. Liq. Bot. 120 ml. *otc.*
Use: Antihistamine, antitussive.

Ty-Cold Tablets. (Major) 30 mg pseudoephedrine, 2 mg chlorpheniramine maleate, 15 mg dextromethorphan HBr, 325 mg acetaminophen. 24s. *otc.*
Use: Decongestant, antihistamine, antitussive, analgesic.

Tylenol Children's. (McNeil-CPC) Acetaminophen 160 mg/5 ml. Butylparaben, corn syrup, sorbitol. Alcohol free. Susp. Bot. 60 ml. *otc.*
Use: Analgesic.

Tylenol Children's Chewable Tablets. (McNeil-CPC) Acetaminophen 80 mg/Tab. Bot. 30s, 48s. Blisters 2s. Hospital pack 250 × 1. *otc.*
Use: Analgesic.

Tylenol Children's Elixir. (McNeil-CPC) Acetaminophen 160 mg/5 ml. Bot. 2 oz., 4 oz., pt. UD 100 × 5 ml, 100 × 10 ml. *otc.*
Use: Analgesic.

Tylenol Cold. (McNeil-CPC) Pseudoephedrine HCl 30 mg, chlorpheniramine maleate 2 mg, dextromethorphan HBr 15 mg, acetaminophen 325 mg, Tab. Cap. Bot. 24s, 50s. *otc.*
Use: Decongestant, antihistamine, antitussive, analgesic.

Tylenol Cold & Flu Medication. (McNeil-CPC) Pseudoephedrine HCl 60 mg, chlorpheniramine maleate 4 mg, dextromethorphan HBr, acetaminophen 650 mg, aspartame, sucrose, phenylalanine 11 mg, lemon flavor. Pow. Pks. 6s, 12s. *otc.*
Use: Decongestant, antihistamine, analgesic.

Tylenol Cold & Flu No Drowsiness. (McNeil-CPC) Acetaminophen 650 mg, pseudoephedrine HCl 60 mg, dextromethorphan HBr per packet 30 mg, aspartame (as phenylalanine 11 mg), sucrose, lemon flavor. Pow. 6s, 12s. *otc.*
Use: Decongestant, antihistamine, analgesic.

Tylenol Cold Liquid, Children's. (McNeil-CPC) Pseudoephedrine 15 mg, chlorpheniramine maleate 1 mg, acetaminophen 160 mg, sorbitol, sucrose, alcohol free, grape flavor. Liq. Bot. 120 ml. *otc.*
Use: Decongestant, antihistamine, analgesic.

Tylenol Cold Multisymptom Plus Cough, Children's. (McNeil-CPC) Acetaminophen 160 mg, dextromorphan HBr 5 mg, chlorpheniramine maleate 1 mg, pseudoephedrine 15 mg/ 5 ml. Liq. Bot. 120 ml. *otc.*
Use: Decongestant, antihistamine, antitussive.

Tylenol Cold Night Time. (McNeil-CPC) Pseudoephedrine HCl 10 mg, diphenhydramine HCl 8.3 mg, acetaminophen 108.3 mg/5 ml, alcohol 10%, sucrose, cherry flavor. Liq. Bot. 150 ml. *otc.*
Use: Decongestant, antihistamine, analgesic.

Tylenol Cold No Drowsiness Caplets & Gelcaps. (McNeil-CPC) Pseudoephedrine HCl 30 mg, dextromethorphan HBr 15 mg, acetaminophen 325 mg/Tab. **Capl.:** Bot. 24s, 50s. **Gel.:** 20s, 40s. *otc.*
Use: Decongestant, antitussive, analgesic.

Tylenol Cold Tablets, Children's. (McNeil-CPC) Pseudoephedrine HCl 7.5 mg, chlorpheniramine maleate 0.5 mg, acetaminophen 80 mg, aspartame, sucrose, phenylalanine 4 mg. Grape flavor. Chew. Tab. Bot. 24s. *otc.*
Use: Decongestant, antihistamine, analgesic.

Tylenol Cough. (McNeil-CPC) Dextromethorphan HBr, acetaminophen 250 mg, saccharin, sorbitol, sucrose. Liq. Bot. 120 ml. *otc.*
Use: Antitussive, analgesic.

Tylenol Cough w/Decongestant. (McNeil-CPC) Pseudoephedrine HCl 15 mg, dextromethorphan HBr 7.5 mg, acetaminophen 250 mg, alcohol 10%,

saccharin, sobitol, sucrose. Liq. Bot. 120 ml, 240 ml. *otc.*
Use: Decongestant, antitussive, analgesic.

Tylenol Elixir, Children's. (McNeil-CPC) Acetaminophen 160 mg/5 ml. Elix. Bot. 60 mg, 120 ml. *otc.*
Use: Analgesic.

Tylenol Extended Relief. (McNeil-CPC) Acetaminophen 650 mg/ER Capl. 100s. *otc.*
Use: Analgesic.

Tylenol Extra-Strength. (McNeil Prods) Acetaminophen 500 mg/Tab. or Caplet. **Tab.:** Bot. 30s, 60s, 100s, 200s. **Caplets:** Bot. 24s, 50s, 100s, 175s. *otc.*
Use: Analgesic.

Tylenol Extra-Strength Adult Liquid. (McNeil Prods) Acetaminophen 1000 mg/30 ml w/alcohol 8.5%. Bot. 8 oz. Hosp. 8 oz. *otc.*
Use: Analgesic.

Tylenol Extra Strength Caplets. (McNeil-CPC) Acetaminophen 500 mg/Capl. Bot. 24s, 50s, 100s, 175s. *otc.*
Use: Anaglesic.

Tylenol Extra Strength Gel-Cap. (McNeil-CPC) Acetaminophen 500 mg/Gelcap. Bot. 24s, 50s, 100s. *otc.*
Use: Analgesic.

Tylenol Extra Strength Geltabs. (McNeil-CPC) Acetaminophen 500 mg, parabens. Tab. Bot. 24s, 50s, 100s. *otc.*
Use: Analgesic.

Tylenol Flu Maximum Strength. (McNeil-CPC) Pseudoephedrine HCl 30 mg, dextromethorphan HBr 15 mg, acetaminophen 500 mg/Gelcap. Pkg. 10s, 20s. *otc.*
Use: Decongestant, antitussive, analgesic.

Tylenol Infants' Drops. (McNeil-CPC) Acetaminophen 80 mg/0.8 ml. Butylparaben, corn syrup, sorbitol. Alcohol free. Bot. w/dropper 7.5 ml, 15 ml. *otc.*
Use: Analgesic.

Tylenol Junior Strength. (McNeil-CPC) Acetaminophen 160 mg, aspartame (6 mg phenylalanine)/Chew. tab. 24s. *otc.*
Use: Analgesic.

Tylenol Junior Strength Swallowable Tablets. (McNeil-CPC) 160 mg/Tab. Box. 30s. Hosp. 250 × 1. *otc.*
Use: Analgesic.

Tylenol Maximum-Strength Allergy Sinus. (McNeil-CPC) Pseudoephedrine HCl 30 mg, chlorpheniramine maleate 2 mg, acetaminophen 500 mg, Capl. Bot. 24s, 50s. Gelcap. Bot. 20s, 40s. *otc.*
Use: Decongestant, antihistamine, analgesic.

Tylenol Maximum Strength Sinus Medication. (McNeil-CPC) Acetaminophen 500 mg, pseudoephedrine HCl 30 mg/Tab. or Caplet. **Tab.:** Bot. 24s, 50s. **Caplet:** Bot. 24s, 50s. *otc.*
Use: Analgesic, decongestant.

Tylenol Multi-Symptom Hot Medication. (McNeil-CPC) Pseudoephedrine HCl 60 mg, chlorpheniramine maleate 4 mg, dextromethorphan HBr 30 mg, acetaminophen 650 mg. Powd. 6s. *otc.*
Use: Decongestant, antihistamine, antitussive, analgesic.

Tylenol No Drowsiness Cold. (McNeil-CPC) Pseudoephedrine HCl 30 g, dextromethorphan HBr 15 mg, acetaminophen 325 mg. Cap. Bot. 24s, 50s. *otc.*
Use: Decongestant, antitussive, analgesic.

Tylenol PM, Extra Strength. (McNeil-CPC) Acetaminophen 500 mg, diphenhydramine 25 mg. Tab. Cap. Bot. 24s, 50s. *otc.*
Use: Analgesic, antitussive.

Tylenol Regular Strength. (McNeil-CPC) Acetaminophen 325 mg/Tab. or Caplet. **Tab.:** Tin 12s. Vial 12s. Bot. 24s, 50s, 100s, 200s. **Caplet:** Bot. 24s, 50s. *otc.*
Use: Analgesic.

Tylenol Severe Allergy. (McNeil-CPC) Diphenhydramine HCl 12.5 mg, acetaminophen 500 mg/Capl. Pkg. 12s, 24s. *otc.*
Use: Antihistamine, analgesic.

Tylenol with Codeine. (McNeil Pharm) **Tab.:** Acetaminophen 300 mg with codeine phosphate. **No. 2:** codeine phosphate 15 mg. Bot. 100s, 500s. **No. 3:** Codeine phosphate 30 mg. Bot. 100s, 500s, 1000s, UD 100s. **No. 4:** Codeine phosphate 60 mg. Bot. 100s, 500s, UD 500s. *c-III.*
Use: Narcotic analgesic combination.

Tylenol with Codeine Elixir. (McNeil Pharm) Acetaminophen 120 mg, codeine phosphate 12 mg/5 ml w/alcohol 7%. Bot. 480 ml. *c-v.*
Use: Narcotic analgesic combination.

Tylosterone. (Lilly) Diethylstilbestrol 0.25 mg, methyltestosterone 5 mg/Tab. Bot. 100s. *Rx.*
Use: Estrogen, androgen.

Tylox. (McNeil) Oxycodone HCl 5 mg, acetaminophen 500 mg/Cap. Bot. 100s UD 100s. *c-II.*
Use: Narcotic analgesic combination.

•**tyloxapol,** (till-OX-ah-pahl) U.S.P. 23.
Use: Detergent, ophthalmic; cystic fibrosis. [Orphan drug].
See: Enuclene (Alcon).

Tympagesic. (Pharmacia & Upjohn) Phenylephrine HCl 0.25%, antipyrine 5%, benzocaine 5%, in propylene glycol. Liq. Bot. w/dropper 13 ml. *Rx.*
Use: Antihistamine, otic.

Ty-Pap. (Major) **Elix.:** Acetaminophen 160 mg/5 ml. Bot. pt., gal. **Supp.:** Acetaminophen 120 mg, 650 mg In 12s. *otc.*
Use: Analgesic.

Typhim Vi. (Pasteur-Merieux-Connaught) Typhoid Vi polysaccharide vaccine 0.5 ml. Inj. Single-dose syringes and 25 ml, 50 ml vials. *Rx.*
Use: Typhoid vaccine, active immunizing agent.

•**typhoid vaccine,** U.S.P. 23.
Use: Active immunizing agent.

typhoid vaccine. (Wyeth-Lederle) 8 units per ml (not > 1 billion organisms per ml). Heat-phenol treated vaccine. Vial 5 ml, 10 ml, 20 ml. Acetone-killed and dried vaccine. Pow. for Inj. 50-dose vial.
Use: Active immunizing agent.

typhoid vaccine capsule. *Rx.*
Use: Agent for immnization.
See: Vivotif Berna (Berna Products).

typhoid vaccine polysaccharide. *Rx.*
Use: Agent for immunization.
See: Typhim Vi (Pasteur-Merieux-Connaught).

Tyrex-2. (Ross) Protein 30 g, fat 15.5 g, carbohydrates 30 g, Fe 13 mg, Na 880 mg, K 1370 mg, Cal 410/100 g. With appropriate vitamins and minerals. Phenylalanine and tyrosine free. Pow. Can 325 g. *otc.*
Use: Nutritional supplement.

Tyrodone. (Major) Hydrocodone bitartrate 5 mg, chlorpheniramine maleate 2 mg, pseudoephedrine HCl 60 mg/5 ml, alcohol 5%. Liq. Bot. 473 ml. *c-III.*
Use: Decongestant, antitussive.

Tyromex-1. (Ross) Protein 15 g, fat 23.9 g, carbohydrates 46.3 g, linoleic acid

1800 mg, Fe 9 mg, Na 190 mg, K 675 mg, Cal 480/100 g. With appropriate vitamins and minerals. Phenylalanine, tyrosine and methionine free. Pow. Can 350 g. *otc.*
Use: Nutritional supplement.

•**tyropanoate sodium,** (TIE-row-PAN-oh-ate) U.S.P. 23.
Use: Diagnostic aid (radiopaque medium, cholecystographic).
See: Bilopaque (Sanofi Winthrop).

tyropaque caps. (Sanofi Winthrop) Tyropanoate sodium. *Rx.*
Use: Oral cholecystographic medium.

•**tyrosine,** (TIE-row-SEEN) U.S.P. 23. L-Tyrosine.
Use: Amino acid.

tyrosine hydroxylase inhibitor.
Use: Antihypertensive.
See: Demser (Merck).

Tyrosum Skin Cleanser. (Summers) Isopropanol 50%, polysorbate 80 2%, and acetone 10%. Bot. 120 ml, pt. Towelettes 24s, 50s. *otc.*
Use: Skin cleaner for acne and oily skin.

•**tyrothricin,** U.S.P. 23. An antibiotic from *Bacillus brevis.* Tyrodac; Tyroderm.
Use: Antibacterial.

Ty-Tabs. (Major) Acetaminophen with codeine #2, #3, #4. Bot. 100s, 500s, 1000s. *c-III.*
Use: Narcotic analgesic combination.

Ty-Tabs, Children's . (Major) Acetaminophen 80 mg/Tab. Bot. 30s, 100s. *otc.*
Use: Analgesic.

Ty-Tabs Extra Strength. (Major) Acetaminophen 500 mg/Tab. Bot. 100s, 1000s. *otc.*
Use: Analgesic.

Tyzine Nasal Solution. (Key) Tetrahydrozoline HCl 0.1%. Bot. pt., oz. *otc.*
Use: Decongestant.

Tyzine Nasal Spray. (Key) Tetrahydrozoline HCl 0.1%. Bot. 0.5 oz. *otc.*
Use: Decongestant.

Tyzine Pediatric Nasal Drops. (Key) Tetrahydrozoline HCl 0.05%. Bot. 0.5 oz. *otc.*
Use: Decongestant.

U

UAA. (Econo Med) Methenamine 40.8 mg, phenyl salicylate 18.1 mg, methylene blue 5.4 mg, benzoic acid 4.5 mg, atropine sulfate 0.03 mg, hyoscyamine 0.03 mg/Tab. Bot. 100s, 1000s. *Rx.*
Use: Urinary anti-infective.

UAD Cream. (UAD) Clioquinol 3%, hydrocortisone 1%, ceresin, glyceryl oleate, propylene glycol, parabens, mineral oil, pramoxine HCl. 15 g. *Rx.*
Use: Corticosteroid; local anesthetic, topical.

UAD Lotion. (UAD) Clioquinol 0.75%, hydrocortisone 0.25%, cetyl alcohol, glyceryl stearate, lanolin, parabens, mineral oil, pramoxine HCl, propylene glycol. 20 ml. *Rx.*
Use: Corticosteroid; local anesthetic, topical.

UAD Otic, (UAD) Hydrocortisone 1%, neomycin sulfate 5 mg, polymyxin B sulfate 10,000 units per ml, thimersol 0.01%, cetyl alcohol, propylene glycol, polysorbate 80. Susp. 10 ml w/dropper. *Rx.*
Use: Otic preparation.

UBT. (Biomerica) For detection of blood in the urine.
Use: Diagnostic aid.

Ucephan. (McGaw) Sodium benzoate 10%, sodium phenylacetate 10% (10 g/100 ml). Liq. Bot. 100 ml. *Rx.*
Use: For urea cycle enzymopathies.

UCG-Beta Slide Monoclonal II. (Wampole) Two-minute latex agglutination inhibition slide test for the qualitative detection of B-hCG/hCG (sensitivity 0.5 IU hCG/ml) in urine. Kit 50s, 100s, 300s.
Use: Diagnostic aid.

UCG-Beta Stat. (Wampole) One-hour passive hemagglutination inhibition tube test for the qualitative detection and quantitative determination of B-hCG/hCG (sensitivity 0.2 IU hCG/ml) in urine. Kit 50s, 300s.
Use: Diagnostic aid.

UCG-Lyphotest. (Wampole) One-hour passive hemagglutination inhibition tube test for the qualitative or quantitative determination of human chorionic gonadotropin (sensitivity 0.5-1 IU hCG/ml) in urine. Kit 10s, 50s, 300s.
Use: Diagnostic aid.

UCG-Slide Test. (Wampole) Rapid latex agglutination inhibition slide test for the qualitative detection of human chorionic gonadotropin (Sensitivity: 2 IU hCG/ml) in urine. Kit 30s, 100s, 300s, 1000s.
Use: Diagnostic aid.

UCG-Test. (Wampole) Two-hour hemagglutination inhibition tube test for the determination of human chorionic gonadotropin (sensitivity 0.5 IU hCG/ml undiluted specimen. 1.5 IU hCG/ml 1:3 diluted specimen) in urine and serum. Kit 10s, 25s, 100s, 300s.
Use: Diagnostic aid.

UCG-Titration Set. (Wampole) A two-hour hemagglutination inhibition tube test for the determination of human chorionic gonadotropin (Sensitivity 1 IU hCG/ml) in urine or serum. Kit 45s.
Use: Diagnostic aid.

Ulcerease. (Med Derm) Liquified phenol 0.6%, glycerin, sugar free/Liq. 180 ml. *otc.*
Use: Anesthetic mouth rinse.

Ulcerin P Tablets. (Sanofi Winthrop) Aluminum hydroxide. *otc.*
Use: Antacid.

Ulcerin Tablets. (Sanofi Winthrop) Aluminum hydroxide. *otc.*
Use: Antacid.

•**uldazepam.** (uhl-DAY-zeh-pam) USAN.
Use: Sedative, hypnotic.

Ulpax. (Hoffman-LaRoche). Ablukast sodium.
Use: Antiasthmatic (leukotriene antagonist).

ULR-LA. (Geneva Pharm) Phenylpropanolamine HCl 75 mg, guaifenesin 400 mg. Tab. Bot. 100s. *Rx.*
Use: Decongestant, expectorant.

Ultane. (Abbott) Volatile liquid for inhalation: sevoflurane. Bot. 250 ml. *Rx.*
Use: General anesthetic.

Ultiva. (Glaxo Wellcome) Remifentanil HCl/Pow. for injection. Vial. 3 ml, 5 ml, 10 ml. *Rx.*
Use: Narcotic agonist analgesic.

Ultra B50. (NBTT) Vitamins B_1 50 mg, B_2 50 mg, B_3 50 mg, B_5 50 mg, B_6 50 mg, B_{12} 50 mcg, folic acid 0.1 mg, PABA 50 mg, inositol 50 mg, biotin 50 mcg, choline 50 mg, lecithin 50 mg/Tab. Bot. 60s, 180s. *otc.*
Use: Vitamin supplement.

Ultra B100. (NBTY) Vitamins B_1 100 mg, B_2 100 mg, B_3 100 mg, B_5 100 mg, B_6 100 mg, B_{12} 100 mcg, folic acid 0.1 mg, PABA 100 mg, inositol 100 mg, biotin 100 mcg, choline bitartrate 100 mg/TR Tab. Bot. 50s. *otc.*
Use: Vitamin supplement.

Ultrabex. (Approved) Vitamins B_1 20 mg,

C 50 mg, B_2 2 mg, B_6 0.5 mg, niacinamide 35 mg, calcium pantothenate 0.5 mg, wheat germ oil 30 mg, B_{12} 20 mcg, liver desiccated 150 mg, iron 11.58 mg, calcium 29 mg, phosphorus 23 mg, dicalcium phosphate 100 mg, magnesium 1.11 mg, manganese 1.3 mg, potassium 2.24 mg, zinc 0.68 mg, choline 25 mg, inositol 25 mg, pepsin 32.5 mg, diastase 32.5 mg, hesperidin 25 mg, biotin 20 mcg, hydrolyzed yeast 81.25 mg, protein digest 47.04 mg, amino acids 34.21 mg/Cap. Bot. 50s, 100s, 1000s. *otc.*
Use: Vitamin/mineral supplement.

ULTRAbrom. (WE Pharm) Brompheniramine maleate 12 mg, pseudoephedrine HCl 120 mg/SR Cap. Bot. 100s. *Rx.*
Use: Antihistamine, decongestant.

ULTRAbrom-PD. (WE Pharm) Brompheniramine maleate 6 mg, pseudoephedrine 60 mg/SR Cap. Bot. 100s. *Rx.*
Use: Antihistamine, decongestant.

Ultracal. (Bristol-Myers) Protein 44 g, carbohydrate 123 g, fat 45 g, Na 930 mg, K 1610 mg, mOsm 310 kg H_2O, cal. 1.06/ml, vitamins A, B_1, B_2, B_3, B_5, B_6, B_{12}, C, D, E, K, folic acid, choline, biotin, Ca, P, I, Fe, Mg, Cu, Zn, Mn, Cl, Se, Cr, Mo. Liq. Can. 8 oz. *otc.*
Use: Nutritional therapy.

Ultra Cap. (Weeks & Leo) Acetaminophen 300 mg, guaifenesin 100 mg, chlorpheniramine maleate 4 mg, phenylephrine HCl 10 mg, dextromethorphan HBr 6 mg/Cap. Vial 18s. *Rx.*
Use: Analgesic, expectorant, antihistamine, decongestant, antitussive.

Ultra-Care. (Allergan) **Disinfecting Soln.:** Hydrogen peroxide 3%, sodium stannate, sodium nitrate, phosphate buffer. Bot. 120 ml, 360 ml; **Neutralizer Tab.:** Catalase, hydroxypropyl methylcellulose, buffering agents. Pkg. 12s, 36s w/ cup. *otc.*
Use: Soft contact lens care.

Ultracortinol. (Novartis) Agent to suppress overactive adrenal glands. Pending release.

Ultra-Derm Bath Oil. (Baker/Cummins) Bot. 8 oz. *otc.*
Use: Emollient.

Ultra-Derm Moisturizer. (Baker/Cummins) Bot. 8 oz. *otc.*
Use: Emollient.

Ultra-Freeda. (Freeda) Vitamins A 4166 IU, D 133 IU, E 66.7 mg, B_1 16.7 mg, B_2 16.7 mg, B_3 33 mg, B_5 33 mg, B_6 16.7 mg, B_{12} 33 mcg, C 333 mg, folic

acid 0.27 mg, iron 2 mg, calcium 27 mg, zinc 1.1 mg, choline, inositol, bioflavonoids, PABA, biotin 100 mcg, Cr, I, K, Mg, Mn, Mo, Se. Tab. Bot. 90s, 180s, 270s. *otc.*
Use: Vitamin/mineral supplement.

Ultra-Freeda Iron Free. (Freeda) Vitamins A 4166 IU, D 133 IU, E 66.7_2 mg, B_1 16.7 mg, B_2 16.7 mg, B_3 33 mg, B_5 33 ng, B_6 16.7 mg, B_{12} 33 mcg, C 333 mg, FA 0.27 mg, Ca 27 mg, Zn 1.1 mg, choline, inositol, bioflavonoids, PABA, biotin 100 mcg, Cr, I, K, Mg, Mn, Mo, Se. Tab. Bot. 90s, 180s, 270s. *otc.*
Use: Vitamin/mineral supplement.

Ultragesic. (Stewart-Jackson) Acetaminophen 500 mg, hydrocodone bitartrate 5 mg/Cap. Bot. 100s. *c-III.*
Use: Narcotic analgesic combination.

Ultralan. (Elan) Protein 60 g, fat 50 g, carbohydrates 202 g, Na 1.035 g, K 1.755 g/L. Lactose free. With appropriate vitamins and minerals. Liq. In 1000 ml New Pak systems with and without ColorCheck. *otc.*
Use: Nutritional supplement.

ultralente insulin.
See: Iletin (Lilly).

Ultram. (Ortho-McNeil) Tramadol HCl 50 mg/Tab. Bot. 100s, UD 100s. *Rx.*
Use: Central analgesic.

Ultra Mide 25. (Baker/Cummins) Bot. 8 oz. *otc.*
Use: Emollient.

Ultrapred. (Horizon) Prednisolone acetate 1%. Susp. Bot. 5 ml. *Rx.*
Use: Corticosteroid, ophthalmic.

Ultrasone. (Gordon) Ultrasonic contact cream. Bot. qt, gal. Plastic Bot. 8 oz.
Use: Ultrasonic contact cream.

Ultra Tears. (Alcon) Hydroxypropyl methylcellulose 2910 1%, benzalkonium Cl 0.01%, NaCl. Bot. 15 ml. *otc.*
Use: Artificial tears.

Ultravate. (Westwood Squibb) Halobetasol propionate. *Rx.*
Use: Corticosteroid, topical.

Ultravist. (Berlex) Iopromide. 150 mg (311.7 mg iopromide), 240 mg (498.72 mg iopromide), 300 mg (623.4 mg iopromide), 370 mg (768.86 mg iopromide). Tromethamine 2.42 mg, EDTA 0.1 mg/ml, iodine 48.12%. 50 ml, 100 ml (except 150 mg), 250 ml (240 mg, 370 mg), 150 ml (300 mg). Inj. *Rx.*
Use: Diagnostic aid.

Ultra Vitamin A & D. (NBTY) Vitamins A 25,000 IU, D 1000 IU. Tab. Bot. 100s. *otc.*

Use: Vitamin A & D combination.

Ultra Vita Time. (NBTY) Iron 6 mg, vitamins A 10,000 IU, D 400 IU, E 13 IU, B$_1$ 25 mg, B$_2$ 25 mg, B$_3$ 50 mg, B$_5$ 12.5 mg, B$_6$ 15 mg, B$_{12}$ 50 mcg, C 150 mg, folic acid 0.4 mg, B, Ca, Cr, Cu, I, K, Mg, Mn, Mo, P, Se, Zn 5 mg, biotin 1 mg, bioflavonoids, bone meal, PABA, choline bitartrate, betaine, inositol, lecithin, desiccated liver, rutin/Tab. Bot. 100s. *otc.*
Use: Vitamin/mineral supplement.

Ultrazyme Enzymatic Cleaner. (Allergan) Subtilisin A, effervescing, buffering and tableting agents for dilution in hydrogen peroxide 3%. Tab. Pkg. 5s, 10s, 15s, 20s. *otc.*
Use: Soft contact lens care.

Ultrum. (Towne) Vitamins A 5000 IU, E 30 IU, C 90 mg, folic acid 400 mcg, B$_1$ 2.25 mg, B$_2$ 2.6 mg, niacinamide 20 mg, B$_6$ 3 mg, B$_{12}$ 9 mcg, biotin 45 mcg, D 400 IU, pantothenic acid 10 mg, calcium 162 mg, phosphorus 125 mg, iodine 150 mcg, iron 27 mg, magnesium 100 mg, copper 3 mg, manganese 7.5 mg, potassium 7.5 mg, zinc 22.5 mg/Tab. Bot. 100s. *otc.*
Use: Vitamin/mineral supplement.

Ultrum with Selenium. (Towne) Vitamins A 5000 IU, E 30 IU, C 90 mg, folic acid 2.25 mg, B$_1$ 2.25 mg, B$_2$ 2.6 mg, niacinamide 20 mg, B$_6$ 3 mg, B$_{12}$ 9 mcg, D 400 IU, biotin 45 mcg, pantothenic acid 10 mg, calcium 162 mg, phosphorus 125 mg, iodine 150 mcg, iron 27 mg, magnesium 100 mg, copper 3 mg, manganese 7.5 mg, potassium 7.7 mg, chloride 7 mg, molybdenum 15 mcg, selenium 15 mcg, zinc 22.5 mg/Tab. Bot. 130s. *Rx.*
Use: Vitamin/mineral supplement.

Unasyn. (Roerig) Ampicillin sodium 1 g, sulbactam sodium 0.5 g, ampicillin sodium 2 g, sulbactam sodium 1 g. Pow. for inj. Vial, piggyback vial. *Rx.*
Use: Anti-infective, penicillin.

10-undecenoic acid. Undecylenic Acid, U.S.P. 23.
Use: Antifungal, topical.

10-undecenoic acid, zinc (2+) salt. Zinc Undecylenate, U.S.P. 23.
Use: Antifungal, topical.

undecoylium chloride-iodine. Virac, Preps. (Ruson).
Use: Anti-infective, topical.

•**undecylenic acid,** U.S.P. 23.
Use: Antifungal, topical.
See: Desenex, Preps (Novartis).
W/Benzethonium Cl, benzalkonium Cl,

tannic acid, isopropyl alcohol.
See: Tulvex, Liq. (Del Pharm).
W/Dichlorophene.
See: Fungicidal Talc (Gordon).
Onychomycetin, Liq. (Gordon).
W/Salicylic acid.
See: Sal-Dex, Liq. (Scrip).
W/Salicylic acid, benzoic acid, sulfur, dichlorophene.
See: Fungicidal, Oint. (Gordon).
W/Sodium propionate, sodium caprylate, propionic acid, salicylic acid, copper undecylenate.
See: Verdefam, Soln. (Texas).
W/Zinc undecylenate.
See: Cruex Cream, Spray Pow. (Novartis) Desenex, Preps. (Novartis).
Ting, Aerosol (Novartis).

undecylenic acid salts. Calcium, copper, zinc.

Undelenic Ointment. (Gordon) Undecylenic acid 5%, zinc undecylenate 20%. Jar oz, lb. *otc.*
Use: Antifungal, topical.

Undelenic Tincture. (Gordon) Undecylenic acid 10%, chloroxylenol 0.5%. Brush Bot. oz. Bot. pt. *otc.*
Use: Antifungal, topical.

undulant fever diagnosis. Brucella Abortus Antigen. Brucellergen.

Unguentine Ointment "Original Formula". (Mentholatum) Phenol 1% in ointment base. Tube oz. *otc.*
Use: Minor skin irritations.

Unguentine Plus First Aid Cream. (Mentholatum) Parachlorometaxylenol 2%, lidocaine HCl 2%, phenol 0.5% in a moisturizing cream base. Tube ½ oz, 1 oz, 2 oz. *otc.*
Use: Minor skin irritations.

Unguentum Bossi. (Doak) Ammoniated mercury 5%, methamine sulfosalicylate 2%, tar distillate "Doak" 5%, Doak oil 40%, petrolatum, sorbitol sesquioleate, cholesterol derivatives, beeswax. Cream. Tube 60 g, 480 g. *Rx.*
Use: Antipsoriatic.

Uni-Ace. (URL) Acetaminophen 100 mg per ml. Alcohol free. Liq. Bot. 15 ml with dropper. *otc.*
Use: Analgesic.

Unibase. (Parke-Davis) Water-absorbing oint. base. Jar lb. *Rx.*
Use: Ointment base.

Uni-Bent Cough. (URL) Diphenhydramine HCl 12.5 mg/5 ml, alcohol 5%. Syr. Bot 118 ml. *Rx.*
Use: Antihistamine.

Unicap Capsules. (Pharmacia & Up-

john) Vitamins A 5000 IU, D 400 IU, E 30 IU, B_1 1.5 mg, B_2 1.7 mg, B_3 20 mg, B_6 2 mg, B_{12} 6 mcg, C 60 mg, FA 0.4 mg/Cap. Bot. 120s. *otc.*
Use: Vitamin supplement.

Unicap Junior Chewable. (Pharmacia & Upjohn) Vitamins A 5000 IU, D 400 IU, E 15 IU, C 60 mg, folic acid 400 mcg, B_1 1.5 mg, B_2 1.7 mg, B_3 20 mg, B_6 2 mg, B_{12} 6 mcg/Tab. Bot. 120s. *otc.*
Use: Vitamin supplement.

Unicap M. (Pharmacia & Upjohn) Iron 18 mg, vitamins A 5000 IU, D 400 IU, E 30 IU, B_1 1.5 mg, B_2 1.7 mg, B_3 20 mg, B_5 10 mg, B_6 2 mg, B_{12} 6 mcg, C 60 mg, folic acid 0.4 mg, Ca, Cu, I, K, Mn, P, Zn 15 mg, tartrazine/Tab. Bot. 120s. *otc.*
Use: Vitamin/mineral supplement.

Unicap Plus Iron. (Pharmacia & Upjohn) Vitamins A 5000 IU, D 400 IU, E 30 IU, C 60 mg, folic acid 0.4 mg, B_1 1.5 mg, B_2 1.7 mg, B_3 20 mg, B_5 10 mg, B_6 2 mg, B_{12} 6 mcg, iron 22.5 mg, Ca/Tab. Bot. 120s. *otc.*
Use: Vitamin/mineral supplement.

Unicap Senior. (Pharmacia & Upjohn) Iron 10 mg, vitamins A 5000 IU, D 200 IU, E 15 IU, B_1 1.2 mg, B_2 1.4 mg, B_3 16 mg, B_5 10 mg, B_6 2.2 mg, B_{12} 3 mcg, C 60 mg, folic acid 0.4 mg, Ca, Cu, I, K, Mg, Mn, P, Zn 15 mg/Tab. Bot. 120s. *otc.*
Use: Vitamin/mineral supplement.

Unicap T. (Pharmacia & Upjohn) Iron 18 mg, vitamins A 5000 IU, D 400 IU, E 30 IU, B_1 10 mg, B_2 20 mg, B_3 100 mg, B_5 25 mg, B_6 6 mg, B_{12} 18 mcg, C 500 mg, folic acid 0.4 mg, Cu, I, K, Mn, Se, Zn 15 mg, tartrazine/Tab. Bot. 60s. *otc.*
Use: Vitamin/mineral supplement.

Unicap Tablets. (Pharmacia & Upjohn) Vitamins A 5000 IU, D 400 IU, E 15 IU, B_1 1.5 mg, B_2 1.7 mg, B_3 20 mg, B_6 2 mg, B_{12} 6 mcg, C 60 mg, FA 0.4 mg/Tab. Bot. 120s. *otc.*
Use: Vitamin supplement.

Unicomplex-M. (Rugby) Iron 18 mg, vitamins A 5000 IU, D 400 IU, E 15 IU, B_1 1.5 mg, B_2 1.7 mg, B_3 20 mg, B_5 10 mg, B_6 2 mg, B_{12} 6 mcg, C 60 mg, folic acid 0.4 mg, Ca, Cu, I, K, Mn, Zn/Tab. Bot. 90s, 1000s. *otc.*
Use: Vitamin/mineral supplement.

Unicomplex-T with Minerals. (Rugby) Iron 10 mg, vitamins A 5000 IU, D 400 IU, E 15 mg, B_1 10 mg, B_2 10 mg, B_3 100 mg, B_5 20 mg, B_6 2 mg, B_{12} 4 mcg, C 300 mg, folic acid 0.4 mg, Ca,

Cu, I, K, Mg, Mn/Tab. Bot. 60s. *otc.*
Use: Vitamin/mineral supplement.

Unicomplex - T & M. (Rugby) Iron 18 mg, vitamins A 5000 IU, D 400 IU, E 30 mg, B_1 10 mg, B_2 10 mg, B_3 100 mg, B_5 25 mg, B_6 6 mg, B_{12} 18 mcg, C 500 mg, FA 0.4 mg, Ca, Cu, I, K, Mn, Zn 15 mg/Tab. Bot. 60s. *otc.*
Use: Vitamin/mineral supplement.

Uni-Decon. (URL) Phenylpropanolamine HCl 40 mg, phenylephrine HCl 10 mg, chlorpheniramine maleate 5 mg, phenyltoloxamine citrate 15 mg/Tab. Bot. 100s, 500s and 1000s. *Rx.*
Use: Decongestant, antihistamine.

Uni-Dur. (Key) Theophylline 400 mg or 600 mg, sugar free, lactose/ER Tab. Bot. 100s. *Rx.*
Use: Bronchodilator.

Unifiber. (Dow B. Hickam) Powdered cellulose 3 g per tbsp. < 4 calories per serving. Corn syrup solids, xanthan gum. Pow. Bot. 454 g. *otc.*
Use: Laxative.

•**unifocon a.** (you-nih-FOE-kahn A) USAN.
Use: Contact lens material (hydrophic).

Unilax. (B.F. Ascher) Docusate 230 mg, phenolphthalein 130 mg. Sorbitol. Cap. Bot. 15s, 20s, 60s. *otc.*
Use: Laxative.

Unipen. (Wyeth-Ayerst) Sodium nafcillin. **Cap.:** 250 mg. Bot. 100s, Redipak 100s. **Tab.:** 500 mg. Bot. 50s. Cap. and Tab. buffered w/calcium carbonate. **Vial:** Vial 2 g, Piggyback Vial 2 g, Bulk vial 10 g. **Oral Soln.:** 250 mg/5 ml w/ alcohol 2%. Bot. to make 100 ml. *Rx.*
Use: Anti-infective, penicillin.

Uniphyl Tablets. (Purdue Frederick) Theophylline 200 mg, 400 mg, 600 mg/ Controlled-release Tab. **200 mg:** Bot. 60s, 100s, UD 100s. **400 mg:** Bot. 60s, 100s, 500s, UD 100s. **600 mg:** Bot. 100s. *Rx.*
Use: Bronchodilator.

Unisol. (Alcon) Buffered isotonic solution with sodium Cl, boric acid, sodium borate. Bot. 15 ml (25s), 120 ml (2s, 3s). *otc.*
Use: Soft contact lens care.

Unisol 4 Sterile Saline. (Alcon) Buffered isotonic solution with sodium Cl, boric acid, sodium borate. Bot. 120 ml. *otc.*
Use: Soft contact lens care.

Unisol Plus. (Alcon) Buffered isotonic solution w/ NaCl, boric acid, sodium borate. Aerosol 240 ml or 360 ml. *otc.*

Use: Soft contact lens care.

Unisom Nighttime Sleep-Aid. (Pfizer) Doxylamine succcinate 25 mg/Tab. Blister 8s, 16s, 32s, 48s.
Use: Nonprescription sleep aid.

Unisom with Pain Relief. (Pfizer) Acetaminophen 650 mg, diphenhydramine HCl 50 mg/Tab. Blister 16s. *otc.*
Use: Analgesic, nonprescription sleep aid.

Unituss HC. (URL) Hydrocodone bitartrate 2.5 mg, phenylephrine HCl 5 mg, chlorpheniramine maleate 2 mg/5 ml. Saccharin, sorbitol, sugar free. Syrup. Bot. 473 ml. *c-III.*
Use: Antitussive, decongestant, antihistamine.

Uni-Tussin DM. (URL) Dextromethorphan HBr 10 mg, guaifenesin 100 mg/5 ml. Syr. Bot. 118 ml. *otc.*
Use: Antitussive, expectorant.

Uni-Tussin Syrup. (United Research Laboratories) Dextromethorphan HBr 15 mg, guaifenesin 100 mg, alcohol 1.4%. Bot. 120 ml. *otc.*
Use: Antitussive, expectorant.

Univasc. (Schwarz Pharma) Moexipril HCl 7.5 mg or 15 mg, lactose/Tab. Bot. 100s, UD 90s. *Rx.*
Use: Antihypertensive.

unna's boot.
See: Zinc Gelatin, U.S.P. 23.

Unproco Capsules. (Solvay) Dextromethorphan HBr 30 mg, guaifenesin 200 mg/Cap. Bot. 100s. *otc.*
Use: Antitussive, expectorant.

Uplex. (Arcum) Vitamins A 5000 IU, D 400 IU, B_1 3 mg, B_2 3 mg, B_6 1 mg, B_{12} 2.5 mcg, nicotinamide 20 mg, calcium pantothenate 5 mg, C 50 mg/Cap. Bot. 100s, 1000s. *otc.*
Use: Vitamin/mineral supplement.

Uplex No. 2. (Arcum) Vitamins A palmitate 10,000 IU, D 400 IU, B_1 5 mg, B_2 5 mg, C 100 mg, B_6 2 mg, B_{12} 3 mcg, E 2.5 IU, niacinamide 25 mg, calcium pantothenate 5 mg/Cap. Bot. 100s, 1000s. *otc.*
Use: Vitamin/mineral supplement.

Urabeth Tabs. (Major) Bethanechol 5 mg, 10 mg, 25 mg or 50 mg/Tab. **5 mg:** Bot. 100s. **10 mg:** Bot. 250s. **25 mg:** Bot. 250s, 1000s. **50 mg:** Bot. 100s, UD 100s. *Rx.*
Use: Urinary tract product.

Uracid. (Wesley) dl-Methionine 0.2 g/Cap. Bot. 100s, 1000s. *Rx.*
Use: Diaper rash product.

•**uracil mustard.** (YOU-ruh-sill) USAN. U.S.P. XXII.

Use: Antineoplastic.

uracil mustard. (Pharmacia & Upjohn) 1 mg/Cap. Bot. 50s.
Use: Antineoplastic.

uradal.
See: Carbromal (Various Mfr.)

•**urea,** U.S.P. 23.
Use: Topically for dry skin; diuretic.
See: Aquacare, Cream, Lot. (Allergan Herbert).
Aquacare-HP, Cream, Lot. (Allergan Herbert).
Artra Ashy Skin, Cream (Schering-Plough).
Calmurid, Cream (Pharmacia & Upjohn).
Carmol, Cream (Ingram).
Carmol Ten, Lot. (Ingram).
Elaqua 10% or 20%, Cream (ICN Pharm).
Gormel, Cream (Gordon).
Nutraplus, Cream, Lot. (Galderma).
Rea-lo, Lot. (Whorton).
W/Benzocaine, benzyl alcohol, p-chloro-m-xylenol, propyleneglycol.
See: 20-Cain Burn Relief (Alto).
W/Hydrocortisone acetate.
See: Carmol-HC, Cream (Ingram).
W/Glycerin.
See: Kerid Ear Drops, Liq. (Blair).
W/Sulfur colloidal, red mercuric sulfide.
See: Teenac, Cream, Oint. (ICN Pharm).
W/Zinc oxide, sulfur, salicylic acid, benzalkonium Cl, isopropyl alcohol.
See: Akne Drying Lotion

urea peroxide.
See: Cankaid (Becton Dickinson).
Gly-Oxide Liquid (Hoechst Marion Roussel).
Oragel Brace-aid Rinse (Del Pharm).
Proxigel (Reed & Carnrick).

Ureacin-10 Lotion. (Pedinol) Urea 10%. Bot. 8 oz. *otc.*
Use: Emollient.

Ureacin-20 Creme. (Pedinol) Urea 20%. Jar 2.5 oz. *otc.*
Use: Emollient.

Ureaphil. (Abbott Hospital Prods) Sterile urea 40 g, citric acid 1 mg/150 ml. Bot. 150 ml. *Rx.*
Use: Osmotic diuretic.

Urecholine. (Merck) Bethanechol Cl. **Inj.:** 5 mg/ml Vial 1 ml, 6s. **Tab.:** 5 mg, 10 mg, 25 mg or 50 mg. Bot. 100s, UD 100s. *Rx.*
Use: Urinary tract product.

•**uredepa.** (YOU-ree-DEH-pah) USAN.
Use: Antineoplastic.
See: Avinar (Centeon).

p-ureidobenzenearsonic acid.
See: Carbarsone, U.S.P. 23.

Urelief. (Rocky Mtn.) Methenamine 2 gr, salol 0.5 gr, methylene blue 1/10 gr, benzoic acid gr, hyoscyamine sulfate gr, atropine sulfate gr/Tab. Bot. 100s. *Rx.*
Use: Urinary anti-infective.

Urese. (Roerig)
See: Benzthiazide.

urethan. Ethyl Carbamate, Ethyl Urethan, Urethane.
Use: Antineoplastic.

Urex Tablets. (3M Pharmaceuticals) Methenamine hippurate 1 g/Tab. Bot. 100s. *Rx.*
Use: Urinary anti-infective.

U.R.I. (Sig) Atropine sulfate 0.2 mg, chlorpheniramine maleate 5 mg, phenylpropanolamine HCl 12.5 mg/ml. Vial 10 ml. *Rx.*
Use: Anticholinergic, antispasmodic, antihistamine, decongestant.

Uric Acid Reagent Strips. (Bayer) Seralyzer reagent strip. For uric acid in serum or plasma. Bot. 25s.
Use: Diagnostic aid.

uricosuric agents.
See: Anturane, Tab., Cap. (Geigy).
Benemid, Tab. (Merck).
ColBenemid, Tab. (Merck).

Uricult. (Orion Diagnostica) Urine culture test to detect bacteria and identify uropathogens. Bot. 10s.
Use: Diagnostic aid.

uridine, 2-deoxy-5-iodo-. Idoxuridine, U.S.P. 23.

Uridium. (Ferndale) Phenylazodiamine pyridine HCl 75 mg, sulfacetamide 250 mg/Tab. Bot. 30s, 100s, 1000s. (Ferndale) 100s.
Use: Urinary anti-infective.

Uridon Modified. (Rugby) Methenamine 40.8 mg, phenyl salicylate 18.1 mg, atropine sulfate 0.03 mg, hyoscyamine 0.03 mg, benzoic acid 4.5 mg, methylene blue 5.4 mg/Tab. Bot. 100s, 1000s. *Rx.*
Use: Urinary anti-infective.

Urifon-Forte. (T.E. Williams) Sulfamethizole 450 mg, phenazopyridine HCl 50 mg/Cap. Bot. 100s, 1000s. *Rx.*
Use: Urinary anti-infective.

Urigen. (Fellows) Calcium mandelate 0.2 g, methenamine 0.2 g, phenazopyridine HCl 50 mg, sodium phosphate 80 mg/Cap. Bot. 100s, 1000s. *Rx.*
Use: Urinary anti-infective.

Urimar-T. (Marnel) Methenamine 81.6 mg, sodium biphosphate 40.8 mg, phenyl salicylate 36.2 mg, methylene blue 10.8 mg, hyoscyamine sulfate 0.12 mg. Tab. Bot. 100s. *Rx.*
Use: Urinary anti-infective.

Urinary Antiseptic #2. (Various Mfr.) Atropine sulfate 0.03 mg, hyoscyamine 0.03 mg, methenamine 40.8 mg, methylene blue 5.4 mg, phenyl salicylate 18.1 mg, benzoic acid 4.5 mg/Tab. Bot. 100s, 1000s. *Rx.*
Use: Urinary anti-infective.

Urinary Antiseptic #2 S.C.T. (Lemmon) Atropine sulfate 0.03 mg, hyoscyamine sulfate 0.03 mg, methenamine 40.8 mg, methylene blue 5.4 mg, phenyl salicylate 18.1 mg, benzoic acid 4.5 mg/Tab. Bot. 100s, 1000s. *Rx.*
Use: Urinary anti-infective.

Urinary Antiseptic #3 S.C.T.. (Lemmon) Atropine sulfate 0.06 mg, hyoscyamine sulfate 0.03 mg, methenamine 120 mg, methylene blue 6 mg, phenyl salicylate 30 mg, benzoic acid 7.5 mg/Tab. Bot. 100s, 1000s. *Rx.*
Use: Urinary anti-infective.

urine.
See: Diagnostic agents.

urine glucose tests.
See: Biotel Diabetes (Biotel).
Clinitest Tablets (Bayer).
Chemstrip uG Strips (Boehringer Mannheim).
Clinistix Strips (Bayer).
Dialstix Strips (Bayer).
Test Tape (Lilly).

urine sugar test.
See: Clinistix (Bayer).

urine tests misc.
See: Nitrazine Paper (Apothecon).
Phenistix Reagent Strips (Bayer).

Urin-Tek. (Bayer) Tubes, plastic caps, adhesive labels, collection cups, and disposable tube holder. Package 100×5.

Urisan-P. (Sandia) Atropine sulfate 0.03 mg, hyoscyamine 0.03 mg, gelsemium 6.1 mg, methenamine 40.8 mg, salol 18.1 mg, benzoic acid 4.5 mg, methylene blue 5.4 mg, phenylazodiaminopyridine HCl 100 mg/Tab. Bot. 100s, 1000s. *Rx.*
Use: Urinary anti-infective.

Urised. (PolyMedica) Atropine sulfate 0.03 mg, hyoscyamine 0.03 mg, methenamine 40.8 mg, methylene blue 5.4 mg, benzoic acid 4.5 mg, phenyl salicylate 18.1 mg/Tab. Bot. 100s, 500s. *Rx.*
Use: Urinary anti-infective.

Urisedamine. (PolyMedica) Methenamine mandelate 500 mg, l-hyoscy-

amine 0.15 mg/Tab. Bot. 100s. *Rx.*
Use: Urinary anti-infective.

Urispas. (SK-Beecham) Flavoxate HCl 100 mg/Tab. Bot. 100s, UD 100s. *Rx.*
Use: Urinary antispasmodic.

uristix. (Bayer) Urine test for glucose, protein and blood. Test. 100s.
Use: Diagnostic aid.

Uristix 4 Reagent Strips. (Bayer) Urinalysis reagent strip test for glucose, protein, nitrite, leukocytes. Bot. 100s.
Use: Diagnostic aid.

Uristix Reagent Strips. (Bayer) Urinalysis reagent strip test for protein and glucose. Bot. 100s.
Use: Diagnostic aid.

Uritin. (Global Pharms) Methenamine 40.8 mg, atropine sulfate 0.03 mg, hyoscyamine sulfate 0.03 mg, salol 18.1 mg, benzoic acid 4.5 mg, methylene blue 5.4 mg, gelsemium 6.1 mg/Tab. Bot. 1000s. *Rx.*
Use: Urinary anti-infective.

Uritin Formula. (Various Mfr.) Atropine sulfate 0.03 mg, hyoscyamine 0.03 mg, methenamine 40.8 mg, methylene blue 5.4 mg, phenyl salicylate 18.1 mg, benzoic acid 4.5 mg/Tab. Bot. 1000s. *Rx.*
Use: Urinary anti-infective.

Urobak. (Shionogi) Sulfamethoxazole 500 mg/Tab. Bot. 100s, 1000s. *Rx.*
Use: Anti-infective, sulfonamide.

Urobiotic. (Roerig) Oxytetracycline as the HCl equivalent to oxytetracycline 250 mg, sulfamethizole 250 mg, phenazopyridine HCl 50 mg/Cap. Bot. 50s, UD pack Box 100s. *Rx.*
Use: Urinary anti-infective.

Urobiotic-250. (Pfizer) Oxytetracycline (as HCl) 250 mg, sulfamethizole 250 mg, phenazopyridine HCl 50 mg/Cap. Bot. 50s. *Rx.*
Use: Urinary anti-infective.

Urocit-K. (Mission) Potassium citrate **540 mg:** Tab. Bot. 100s; **10 mEq:** Tab. Bot. 100s. *Rx.*
Use: Urinary tract product.

•**urofollitropin.** (YOUR-oh-fahl-ih-TROE-pin) USAN.
Use: Hormone (follicle-stimulating). Induction of ovulation in patients with polycystic ovary disease. [Orphan drug]
See: Metrodin, Inj. (Serono).

urogastrone. *Rx.*
Use: Corneal transplant surgery. [Orphan drug]

Urogesic. (Edwards) Phenazopyridine

HCl 100 mg, hyoscyamine HBr 0.12 mg, atropine sulfate 0.08 mg, scopolamine HBr 0.003 mg/Tab. Bot. 100s, 500s. *Rx.*
Use: Urinary analgesic.

Urogesic Blue. (Edwards) Methenamine 81.6 mg, sodium biphosphate 40.8 mg, phenyl salicylate 36.2 mg, methylene blue 10.8 mg, hyoscyamine (as sulfate) 0.12 mg. Tab. Bot. 100s. *Rx.*
Use: Urinary anti-infective.

urography agents.
See: Diodrast.
Iodohippurate Sodium, Inj.
Iodopyracet.
Iodopyracet Compound.
Methiodal, Inj.
Renografin (Squibb).
Renovist (Squibb).
Renovue (Squibb).
Sodium Acetrizoate, Inj.
Sodium Iodomethamate, Inj.

•**urokinase.** (YUR-oh-KIN-ace) USAN. Plasminogen activator isolated from human kidney tissue.
Use: Plasminogen activator.

Uro-KP-Neutral. (Star) Sodium (as dibasic sodium phosphate) 1361 mg, potassium 298.6 mg, phosphorus (as dibasic potassium phosphate) 1037 mg/6 Tab. Bot. 100s. *Rx.*
Use: Phosphorus supplement.

Urolene Blue. (Star) Methylene blue 65 mg/Tab. Bot. 100s, 1000s. *Rx.*
Use: Urinary anti-infective.

Urologic Sol G. (Abbott Hospital Prods) Bot. 1000 ml.
Use: Irrigating solution.
See: Thiosulfil, Preps. (Wyeth-Ayerst).

Uro-Mag. (Blaine) Magnesium oxide 140 mg/Cap. Bot. 100s, 1000s. *otc.*
Use: Antacid.

uronal.
See: Barbital (Various Mfr.).

Uro-Phosphate. (ECR Pharm) Sodium biphosphate 434.78 mg, methenamine 300 mg/Film Coated Tab. Bot. 100s. *Rx.*
Use: Urinary anti-infective.

Uroplus DS. (Shionogi) Trimethoprim 160 mg, sulfamethoxazole 800 mg/Tab. Bot. 100s, 500s. *Rx.*
Use: Anti-infective.

Uroplus SS. (Shionogi) Trimethoprim 80 mg, sulfamethoxazole 800 mg/Tab. Bot. 100s, 500s. *Rx.*
Use: Anti-infective.

Uroquid-Acid No. 2. (Beach) Methenamine mandelate 500 mg, sodium acid

phosphate monohydrate 500 mg/Tab. Bot. 100s. *Rx.*
Use: Urinary anti-infective.

urotropin new. Methenamine Anhydromethylene Citrate (Various Mfr.).

Urovist Cysto. (Berlex) Diatrizoate meglumine 300 mg, edetate calcium disodium 0.05 mg/ml. Dilution Bot. 500 ml w/300 ml Soln.
Use: Radiopaque agent.

Urovist Cysto Pediatric. (Berlex) Diatrizoate meglumine 300 mg, edetate calcium disodium 0.1 mg/ml. Dilution bot. 300 ml w/100 ml soln.
Use: Radiopaque agent.

Urovist Meglumine DIU/CT. (Berlex) Diatrizoate meglumine 300 mg, edetate calcium disodium 0.05 mg/ml. Bot. 300 ml, Ctn. 10s.
Use: Radiopaque agent.

Urovist Sodium 300. (Berlex) Diatrizoate sodium 500 mg, edetate calcium disodium 0.1 mg/ml. Vial 50 ml, Box 10s.
Use: Radiopaque agent.

Ursinus Inlay-Tabs. (Sandoz) Pseudoephedrine HCl 30 mg, aspirin 325 mg/Tab. Bot. 24s. *otc.*
Use: Decongestant, salicylate analgesic.

ursodeoxycholic acid. *Rx.*
Use: Primary biliary cirrhosis. [Orphan drug]

•**ursodiol,** (ERR-so-DIE-ole) U.S.P. 23. Ursodeoxycholic acid.
Use: Anticholelithogenic. Gallstone solubilizing agent; management of primary biliary cirrhosis. [Orphan drug]
See: Actigall (Novartis).

uterine relaxant.
See: Ritodrine HCl, Inj. (Abbott). Yutopar, Inj. (Astra).

Utimox. (Parke-Davis) Amoxicillin trihydrate. **Cap.:** 250 mg Bot. 100s, 500s, UD 100s; 500 mg Bot. 100s, UD 100s; **Oral susp.:** 125 mg or 250 mg/5 ml Bot. 80 ml, 100 ml, 150 ml, 200 ml. *Rx.*
Use: Anti-infective, penicillin.

U-Tran. (Scruggs) Atropine sulfate 0.03 mg, hyoscyamine 0.03 mg, methenamine 40.8 mg, benzoic acid 4.5 mg, salol 18.1 mg, methylene blue 5.4 mg/Tab. Bot. 100s, 1000s. *Rx.*
Use: Urinary anti-infective.

U-Tri Special Formula Ointment. (U-Tri) Oint. Jar 4 oz, 7 oz.
Use: Analgesic, topical.

Uvadex. (Therakos, Inc.)
See: 8-Methoxsalen.

uvaleral.
See: Bromisovalum.

Uvasal Powder. (Sanofi Winthrop) Sodium bicarbonate, tartaric acid. *otc.*
Use: Antacid.

uva ursi. Leaves. (Sherwood Labs.) Fluid extract. Bot. pt, gal.

Uviban. Sodium Actinoquinol.
Use: Treatment of flash burns (ophthalmic).

Uvinul MS-40. (General Aniline & Film)
See: Sulisobenzone.

V

vaccine, adenovirus. *Rx.*
Use: Agent for immunization.
See: adenovirus vaccine (Wyeth-Lederle).

vaccine, anthrax. *Rx.*
Use: Agent for immunization.
See: anthrax vaccine (Michigan Department of Public Health).

vaccine, BCG. *Rx.*
Use: Agent for immunization.
See: TheraCys (Pasteur-Merieux-Connaught).
Tice BCG, Amp (Organon).

vaccine, cholera. *Rx.*
Use: Agent for immunization.
See: cholera vaccine, Vial (Wyeth Lederle).

vaccine, Haemophilus influenzae type b. *Rx.*
Use: Agent for immunization.
See: ActHIB/DTP, Set of DTwP vial plus Hib Pow. for Inj. (Pasteur-Merieux-Connaught).
HibTITER, Vial (Wyeth Lederle).
OmniHIB, Pow. for Inj. (SK-Beecham).
PedVaxHIB, Pow. for Inj. (Merck).
ProHIBIT, Vial, Syr. (Pasteur-Merieux-Connaught).
Tetramune, Vial (Wyeth Lederle).

vaccine, hepatitis A. *Rx.*
Use: Agent for immunization.
See: Havrix (SK-Beecham).

vaccine, hepatitis B. *Rx.*
Use: Agent for immunization.
See: Engerix-B (SK-Beecham).
Recombivax-HB (Merck).

vaccine, influenza A&B. *Rx.*
Use: Agent for immunization.
See: Fluogen (Parke-Davis).
Flu-Shield (Wyeth Lederle).
Fluvirin (Adams).
Fluzone (Connaught).

vaccine, Japanese encephalitis. *Rx.*
Use: Agent for immunization.
See: JE-Vax (Pasteur-Merieux-Connaught).

vaccine, measles. *Rx.*
Use: Agent for immunization.
See: Attenuvax (Merck).
W/rubella vaccine.
See: M-R II (Merck).
W/mumps and rubella vaccines.
See: M-M-R II (Merck).

vaccine, meningococcal. *Rx.*
Use: Agent for immunization.
See: Menomune A/C/Y/W-135, Pow. for Inj. (Pasteur-Merieux-Connaught).

vaccine, mumps. Mumps Virus Vaccine Live, U.S.P. 23.
Use: Agent for immunization.
See: Mumpsvax (Merck).

vaccine, pertussis. Pertussis Vaccine.
Use: Active immunizing agent.
See: Acel-Imune, Vial (Wyeth Lederle).
ActHIB/DTP, Set of DTwP vial plus Hib Pow. for Inj. (Pasteur-Merieux-Connaught).
diphtheria and tetanus toxoids with pertussis vaccine (Various Mfr.).
Tetramune, Vial (Wyeth Lederle).
Tri-Immunol, Vial (Wyeth Lederle).
Tripedia, Vial (Pasteur-Merieux-Connaught).

vaccine, plague. *Rx.*
Use: Agent for immunization.
See: plague vaccine (Greer).

vaccine, pneumococcal. *Rx.*
Use: Agent for immunization.
See: Pneumovax-23 (Merck).
Pnu-Imune 23 (Wyeth Lederle).

vaccine, poliomyelitis. *Rx.*
Use: Agent for immunization.
See: IPOL (Pasteur-Merieux-Connaught).
Orimune (Wyeth Lederle).
Poliovirus vaccine, U.S.P. 23.

vaccine, rabies. Rabies Vaccine.
Use: Active immunizing agent.
See: Imovax Rabies (Pasteur-Merieux-Connaught).
Rabies vaccine adsorbed (Michigan Department of Public Health).

vaccine, smallpox. Smallpox Vaccine.
Use: Active immunizing agent.

vaccine, typhoid. *Rx.*
Use: Agent for immunization.
See: Typhim Vi (Pasteur-Merieux-Connaught).
Typhoid vaccine (Wyeth Lederle).
Vivotif Berna (Berna Products).

vaccine, varicella. *Rx.*
Use: Agent for immunization.
See: Varivax (Merck).

vaccine, whooping cough. Pertussis Vaccine, U.S.P. 23.
Use: Active immunizing agent.
See: Acel-Imune, Vial (Wyeth Lederle).
ActHIB/DTP, Set of DTwP vial plus Hib Pow. for Inj. (Pasteur-Merieux-Connaught).
diphtheria and tetanus toxoids with pertussis vaccine (Various Mfr.).
Tetramune, Vial (Wyeth Lederle).
Tri-Immunol, Vial (Wyeth Lederle).
Tripedia, Vial (Pasteur-Merieux-Connaught).

vaccine, yellow fever. *Rx.*
Use: Agent for immunization.
See: YF-Vax (Pasteur-Merieux-Connaught).

• **vaccinia immune globulin,** U.S.P. 23. *Formerly Vaccinia Immune Human Globulin.*
Use: Prevention or modification of smallpox or vaccinia infections; passive immunizing agent.

vaccinia immune globulin. (Baxter) Gamma globulin fraction of serum of healthy adults recently immunized w/ vaccinia virus 16.5%. Vial 5 ml.
Use: Prevention or modification of smallpox or vaccinia infections, passive immunizing agent.

vacocin. Under study.
Use: Anti-infective.

Vademin-Z. (Roberts) Vitamin A 12,500 IU, D 50 IU, E 50 mg, B_1 10 mg, B_2 5 mg, B_3 25 mg, B_5 10 mg, B_6 2 mg, C 150 mg, zinc 2.6 mg, Mg, Mn/Cap. Bot. 60s. *otc.*
Use: Vitamin/mineral supplement.

Vaginex Creme. (Schmid) Tripelennamine HCl. In 30 g. *otc.*
Use: Vaginal preparation.

Vagisec. (Schmid) Polyoxyethylene nonyl phenol, EDTA. Soln. Bot. 120 ml. *Rx.*
Use: Vaginal preparation.

Vagisec Plus Suppositories. (Schmid) Polyoxyethylene nonyl phenol 5.25 mg, sodium edetate 0.66 mg, docusate sodium 0.07 mg, aminoacridine HCl 6 mg. Box 28s. *Rx.*
Use: Vaginal preparation.

Vagisil. (Combe) Benzocaine and resorcin with lanolin alcohol, parabens, trisodium HEDTA, mineral oil and sodium sulfite. Creme. 30, 60 g. *otc.*
Use: Vaginal preparation.

Vagisil Powder. (Combe) Cornstarch, aloe, mineral oil, benzethonium chloride. Pow. 198 g, 312 g. *otc.*
Use: Vaginal preparation.

Vagistat-1. (Bristol-Myers Squibb) Tioconazole 6.5%. Vaginal oint. Prefilled applicator 4.6 g. *otc.*
Use: Antifungal, vaginal.

Valacet. (Pal-Pak) Hyoscyamus 10.8 mg, aspirin 259.2 mg, caffeine anhydrous 16.2 mg, gelsemium extract 0.6 mg/Tab. or Cap. Bot. 100s, 1000s, 5000s. *Rx.*
Use: Anticholinergic, antispasmodic, salicylate analgesic.

• **valacyclovir hydrochlordide.** (val-lay-SIGH-kloe-vihr) USAN.

Use: Antiviral.
See: Valtrex, Tab. (Glaxo Wellcome).

Valergen. (Hyrex) Estradiol valerate 10 mg, 20 mg or 40 mg/ml. Vial 10 ml. *Rx.*
Use: Estrogen.

Valerian. (Lilly) Tincture, alcohol 68%. Bot. 4 fl oz, 16 fl oz.
W/Phenobarbital, passiflora, hyoscyamus.
See: Aluro, Tab. (Foy).

Valertest. (Hyrex) **No. 1:** Estradiol valerate 4 mg, testosterone enanthate 90 mg/ml. Vial 10 ml. **No. 2:** Double strength. Vial 10 ml. Amp. 2 ml, 10s. *Rx.*
Use: Estrogen, androgen.

valethamate bromide.
Use: Anticholinergic.

• **valine,** (VAY-leen) U.S.P. 23.
Use: Amino acid.

Valisone. (Schering Plough) Betamethasone valerate. **Cream:** 1 mg/g Hydrophilic cream of water, mineral oil, petrolatum, polyethylene glycol 1000 monocetyl ether, cetostearyl alcohol, monobasic sodium phosphate, phosphoric acid, 4-chloro-m-cresol as preservative. Tube 15 g, 45 g, 110 g. Jar 430 g. **Oint.:** 1 mg/g base of liquid and white petrolatum and hydrogenated lanolin. Tube 15 g, 45 g. **Lot.:** 1 mg/g w/isopropyl alcohol 47.5%, water slightly thickened w/carboxy vinyl polymer, pH adjusted w/sodium hydroxide. Bot. 20 ml, 60 ml. **Reduced Strength Cream 0.01%:** Hydrophilic cream of water, mineral oil, petrolatum, polyethylene glycol 1000 monocetyl ether, cetostearyl alcohol, monobasic sodium phosphate, phosphoric acid, 4-chloro-m-cresol as preservative. Tube 15 g, 60 g. *Rx.*
Use: Corticosteroid, topical.

Valium Injectable. (Roche) Diazepam 5 mg/ml, propylene glycol 40%, ethyl alcohol 10%, sodium benzoate, benzoic acid 5%, benzyl alcohol 1.5%. Amp. 2 ml, 10s and Vial 10 ml. Tel-E-Ject (Disposable syringe) 2 ml. *c-iv.*
Use: Antianxiety.

Valium Tablets. (Roche) Diazepam 2 mg, 5 mg or 10 mg/Tab. Bot. 100s, 500s. UD 100s. *c-iv.*
Use: Antianxiety.

vallergine.
See: Promethazine HCl, U.S.P. 23.

Valnac Cream. (NMC Labs) Betamethasone valerate 0.1%. Cream Tube 15 g, 45 g. *Rx.*

Use: Corticosteroid, topical.

Valnac Ointment. (NMC Labs) Beta-methasone valerate 0.1%. Oint. Tube 15 g, 45 g. *Rx.*
Use: Corticosteroid, topical.

•**valnoctamide.** (val-NOCK-tah-mid) USAN.
Use: Tranquilizer.

valpipamate methylsulfate.
See: Pentapiperide Methylsulfate.

•**valproate sodium.** (VAL-pro-ate) USAN.
Use: Anticonvulsant.

•**valproic acid,** (VAL-pro-ik acid) U.S.P. 23
Use: Anticonvulsant, antimigraine.
See: Depakene, Cap., Liq. (Abbott).
Depakote (Abbott).
Myproic Acid Syr. (Rosemont).
valproic acid (Various Mfr.).

valproic acid. (Various Mfr.) **Cap.:** Val-proic acid 250 mg. Bot. 100s, 250s, 500s. **Syrup:** 250 mg/5 ml. Cups. 50 ml, 480 ml, UD 5 ml. *Rx.*
Use: Anticonvulsant.

•**valsartan.** (VAL-sahr-tan) USAN.
Use: Antihypertensive.
See: Diovan, Cap. (Novartis).

Valtrex. (Glaxo Wellcome) Valacyclovir HCl 500 mg/Capl. Bot. 42s, 60s, UD 100s. *Rx.*
Use: Antiviral.

Valuphed. (H.L. Moore) Pseudo-ephedrine HCl 60 mg, triprolidine HCl 2.5 mg/Tab. Pkg. 24s. *otc.*
Use: Decongestant, antihistamine.

Vamate. (Major) Hydroxyzine pamoate 50 mg/Cap. Bot. 100s, 250s, 500s, UD 100s. *Rx.*
Use: Antianxiety.

Vanadryx TR. (Vangard) Dexbromphenir-amine maleate 6 mg, psuedoephedrine sulfate 120 mg/Tab. Bot. 100s, 500s. *Rx.*
Use: Antihistamine, decongestant.

Vancenase AQ Nasal. (Schering Plough) Beclomethasone dipropionate monohy-drate 0.042%, 0.084%. Bot. 25 g with metering atomizing pump and nasal adapter (0.042%), 19 g with metered pump (0.084%). *Rx.*
Use: Intranasal steroid.

Vancenase Nasal Inhaler. (Schering Plough) Metered-dose aerosol unit containing beclomethasone dipropio-nate in propellants. Each actuation de-livers 42 mcg. Canister 16.8 g w/na-sal adapter. *Rx.*
Use: Intranasal steroid.

Vanceril Inhaler. (Schering Plough) Me-tered-dose aerosol unit beclometha-sone dipropionate in propellants. Each actuation delivers 42 mcg of beclo-methasone dipropionate. Canister 16.8 g w/oral adapter. Box 1s. *Rx.*
Use: Corticosteroid.

Vancocin IV. (Lilly) Vancomycin HCl 500 mg/vial. 1s; 1 g/vial. 10s; ADD-Vantage 500 mg or 1 g/vial. 1s. *Rx.*
Use: Anti-infective.

Vancocin Capsules. (Lilly) Vancomycin HCl 125 mg or 250 mg/Pulvule. Bot. 10s, 20s. *Rx.*
Use: Anti-infective.

Vancocin Oral. (Lilly) Vancomycin HCl for oral soln. Traypak 1 g, Container 10 g. *Rx.*
Use: Anti-infective.

Vancoled Injection. (Lederle) Vanco-mycin HCl equivalent to vancomycin 500 mg/10 ml reconstituted soln. Vial 10 ml. *Rx.*
Use: Anti-infective.

•**vancomycin,** (van-koe-MY-sin) U.S.P. 23.
Use: Antibacterial.

•**vancomycin hydrochloride,** U.S.P. 23. An antibiotic from *Streptomyces orien-talis.*
Use: (IV) Gram-positive (staph.) infec-tion; antibacterial.
See: Vancocin, Prods. (Lilly).
Vancoled, Vial (Lederle).

vancomycin hydrochloride. (ESI Led-erle) Vancomycin (after reconstitution) 250 mg/ml/Pow. for oral soln. Bot. 1 g. *Rx.*
Use: Antibacterial.

Vancor Intravenous. (Pharmacia & Up-john) Vancomycin HCl 500 mg or 1 g. Pow. for inj. Vials.
Use: Anti-infective.

Vanex Expectorant Liquid. (Jones Medi-cal) Pseudoephedrine HCl 30 mg, hydrocodone bitartrate 2.5 mg, guai-fenesin 100 mg, alcohol 5%, glucose, saccharin, sorbitol, sucrose, tartrazine. Tropical fruit punch flavor. Liq. Bot. 473 ml. *c-III.*
Use: Decongestant, antitussive, expec-torant.

Vanex-Forte. (Jones Medical) Phenyl-propanolamine HCl 50 mg, phenyleph-rine HCl 10 mg, chlorpheniramine ma-leate 4 mg, pyrilamine maleate 25 mg, lactose, sugar. Cap. Bot. 100s. *Rx.*
Use: Decongestant, antihistamine.

Vanex-HD. (Jones Medical) Phenyl-ephrine HCl 5 mg, chlorpheniramine

maleate 2 mg, hydrocodone bitartrate 1.67 mg. Liq. Bot. Pt. gal. *c-III*.
Use: Decongestant, antitussive.

Vanex-LA. (Jones Medical) Phenylpropanolamine HCl 75 mg, guaifenesin 400 mg. Tab. Bot. 100s, 500s. *Rx.*
Use: Decongestant, expectorant.

Vanicream. (Pharmaceutical Specialties) Oil in water vanishing cream containing white petrolatum, cetearyl alcohol, ceteareth-20, sorbitol, propylene glycol, simethicone, glyceryl monostearate, polyethylene glycol monostearate, sorbic acid. Oint. lb. *otc.*
Use: Ointment base.

vanilla, N.F. XVII.
Use: Pharmaceutic aid (flavor).

vanillal.
See: Ethyl Vanillin.

•**vanillin,** N.F. 18. 4-Hydroxy-3-methoxybenzaldehyde.
Use: Pharmaceutic aid (flavor).

vanirome.
See: Ethyl Vanillin.

Vanoxide. (Dermik) Benzoyl peroxide 5%, cetyl alcohol, lanolin alcohol, parabens, EDTA, calcium phosphate 64%, silica 1%, mineral oil. Bot. 25 ml, 50 ml. *otc.*
Use: Antiacne.

Vanoxide-HC. (Dermik) Hydrocortisone alcohol 0.5%, benzoyl peroxide 5%/25 g in lotion w/same ingredients as Vanoxide. Bot. 25 g. *Rx.*
Use: Antiacne.

Vanquish. (Bayer) Aspirin 227 mg, acetaminophen 194 mg, caffeine 33 mg, dried aluminum hydroxide gel 25 mg, magnesium hydroxide 50 mg/Tab. Capsule shaped tablets. Bot. 30s, 60s, 100s. *otc.*
Use: Analgesic combination, antacid.

Vansil. (Pfizer Laboratories) Oxaminiquine 250 mg/Cap. Bot. 24s. *Rx.*
Use: Anthelmintic.

Vantin. (Pharmacia & Upjohn) Cefpodoxime proxetil, lactose. **Tab.:** 100, 200 mg/Bot. 20s, 100s, UD 100s; **Gran. for Susp.:** 50 mg/ml, 100 mg/ml. Bot. 100 ml. Sucrose. *Rx.*
Use: Anti-infective.

•**vapiprost hydrochloride.** (VAP-ihprahst) USAN.
Use: Antagonist (thromboxane A_2).

Vapocet Tablets. (Major) Hydrocodone 5 mg, acetaminophen 500 mg/Tab. Bot. 100s. *c-III.*
Use: Narcotic analgesic combination.

Vaponefrin Solution. (Medeva) A 2.25% solution of bioassayed racemic epinephrine as HCl, chlorobutanol 0.5%. Vial 7.5 ml, 15 ml, 30 ml. *otc.*
Use: Bronchodilator.

Vaporizer in a Bottle. (Columbia) Wick dispensed medicated vapors.
Use: Cough, cold, sinus, hayfever treatment.

Vapor Lemon Sucrets. (SK-Beecham) Dyclonine HCl 2 mg, corn syrup sucrose. Loz. Pkg. 18s. *otc.*
Use: Mouth and throat product.

Vaporub. (Procter & Gamble).
See: Vicks Vaporub (Procter & Gamble).

Vaposteam. (Procter & Gamble).
See: Vicks Vaposteam (Procter & Gamble).

•**vapreotide.** (vap-REE-oh-tide) USAN.
Use: Antineoplastic.

VAQTA. (Merck) **Adult:** Hepatitis A antigen 50 U/ml, sodium chloride 0.9%/Inj. Vial. 1 ml single use (1s and 5s). Syringe 1 ml single-use (1s and 5s). **Pediatric/Adolescent:** Hepatitis A antigen 25 U/0.5 ml, sodium chloride 0.9%/Inj. Vial. 0.5 ml single use (1s and 5s). Syringe. 0.5 ml single use (1s and 5s). *Rx.*
Use: Hepatitis A vaccine.

varicella virus vaccine.
Use: Agent for immunization.
Use: Varivax, Inj. (Merck).

varicella-zoster IgG IFA test system. (Wampole-Zeus) Test for the qualitative or semi-qualitative detection of VZ IgG antibody in human serum. Test kit 100s.
Use: Diagnostic aid.

•**varicella-zoster immune globulin,** U.S.P. 23.
Use: Passive immunizing agent.

varicella-zoster immune globulin, human. (Massachusetts Public Health Biologic Labs) Varicella-zoster virus antibody 125 units ≤ 2.5 ml. Vial, single dose.
Use: Immune serum.

Vari-Flavors. (Ross) Flavor packets to provide flavor variety for patients on liquid diets. Dextrose, artificial flavor, artificial color. Packet 1 g, Ctn. 24s. *Rx.*
Use: Liquid nutrition flavoring aid.

Variplex-C. (NBTY) Vitamins B_1 15 mg, B_2 10 mg, B_3 100 mg, B_5 20 mg, B_6 5 mg, B_{12} 10 mcg, C 500 mg/Tab. Bot. 100s. *otc.*
Use: Vitamin supplement.

Varivax. (Merck) Varicella virus vaccine.

1350 PFU of Oka/Merck varicella virus (live). Inj. Single-dose vials (1s, 10s). *Rx.*
Use: Agent for immunization.

Vascor. (McNeil) Bepridil HCl, 200 mg, 300 mg or 400 mg/Tab. Bot. 90s, UD 100s. *Rx.*
Use: Antianginal.

Vascoray. (Mallinckrodt) Iothalamate meglumine 52%, iothalamate sodium 26% (40% iodine). Vial 50 ml. Bot. 100 ml, 150 ml, 200 ml.
Use: Radiopaque agent.

Vascunitol. (Apco) Mannitol hexanitrate 0.5 gr/Tab. Bot. 100s. *Rx.*
Use: Vasodilator.

Vascused. (Apco) Mannitol hexanitrate 0.5 gr, phenobarbital 0.25 gr/Tab. Bot. 100s. *Rx.*
Use: Vasodilator.

Vaseline Dermatology Formula Cream. (Chesebrough-Pond's) Petrolatum, mineral oil, dimethicone. Jar 3 oz, 5.25 oz. *otc.*
Use: Emollient.

Vaseline Dermatology Formula Lotion. (Chesebrough-Pond's) Petrolatum, mineral oil, dimethicone. Bot. 5.5 oz, 11 oz, 16 oz. *otc.*
Use: Emollient.

Vaseline First Aid Carbolated Petroleum Jelly. (Chesebrough-Pond's) Petrolatum, chloroxylenol. Plastic Jar 1.75 oz, 3.75 oz. Plastic Tube 1 oz, 2.5 oz. *otc.*
Use: Medicated anti-infective.

Vaseline Intensive Care Active Sport. (Chesebrough-Pond's) Ethylhexyl p-methoxycinnamate, oxybenzone. PABA free. **SPF 8:** Lot. Bot. 120 ml; **SPF 15:** Lot. Bot. 120 ml. *otc.*
Use: Sunscreen.

Vaseline Intensive Care Baby SPF 15. (Chesebrough-Pond's) Titanium dioxide. PABA free. Waterproof. Lot. Bot. 120 ml. *otc.*
Use: Sunscreen.

Vaseline Intensive Care Baby SPF 30. (Chesebrough-Pond's) Ethylhexyl p-methoxycinnamate, oxybenzone, 2-ethylhexyl salicylate, titanium dioxide, C12-15 alkyl benzoate, glycerin, aloe vera gel, vitamin E, cetyl alcohol, parabens, EDTA. Lot. Bot. 118 ml. *otc.*
Use: Sunscreen.

Vaseline Intensive Care Blockout SPF 30. (Chesebrough-Pond's) Ethylhexyl p-methoxycinnamate, oxybenzone, 2-ethylhexyl salicylate, titanium dioxide.

Waterproof. Lot. Bot. 120 ml. *otc.*
Use: Sunscreen.

Vaseline Intensive Care Blockout SPF 40+. (Chesebrough-Pond's) Padimate O, ethylhexyl p-methoxycinnamate, oxybenzone, 2-ethylhexyl salicylate, titanium dioxide. Waterproof. Lot. Bot. 120 ml. *otc.*
Use: Sunscreen.

Vaseline Intensive Care Moisturizing Sunscreen. (Chesebrough-Pond's) Ethylhexyl p-methoxycinnamate, oxybenzone, C12-15 alkyl octanoate, glycerin, aloe vera gel, cetyl alcohol, petrolatum, vitamin E, parabens, EDTA. **SPF8, SPF4:** Lot. Bot. 117 ml. *otc.*
Use: Sunscreen.

Vaseline Intensive Care No Burn No Bite SPF 8, 15. (Chesebrough-Pond's) Ethylhexyl p-methoxycinnamate, oxybenzone. PABA free. Waterproof. Lot. Bot. 180 ml. *otc.*
Use: Sunscreen.

Vaseline Intensive Care Sport Sunblock. (Chesebrough-Pond's) Ethylhexyl p-methoxycinnamate, oxybenzone, C12-15 alkyl benzoate, aloe vera gel, vitamin E, EDTA. Lot. Bot. 118 ml. *otc.*
Use: Sunscreen.

Vaseline Intensive Care Sunblock. (Chesebrough-Pond's) Ethylhexyl p-methoxycinnamate, oxybenzone, 2-ethylhexyl salicylate. PABA free. Waterproof. **SPF 4:** Lot. Bot. 180 ml; **SPF 8:** Lot. Bot. 120 ml, 180 ml; **SPF 15:** Lot. Bot. 120 ml, 180 ml; **SPF 25:** Lot. Bot. 120 ml, 180 ml. *otc.*
Use: Sunscreen.

Vaseline Intensive Care Ultra Violet Daily Defense. (Chesebrough-Pond's) Ethylhexyl p-methoxycinnamate, oxybenzone, vitamin E, cetyl alcohol, acetylated lanolin, alcohol, parabens, EDTA. **SPF 15.** Lot. Bot. 118 ml. *otc.*
Use: Sunscreen.

Vaseline Pure Petroleum Jelly Skin Protectant. (Chesebrough-Pond's) White petrolatum. Tube 1 oz, 2.5 oz. Jar 1.75 oz, 3.75 oz, 7.75 oz, 13 oz. *otc.*
Use: Protectant for minor skin irritations.

Vaseretic. (Merck) Enalapril maleate 5 mg: Hydrochlorothiazide 12.5 mg, lactose. Unit-of-use 100s. 10 mg: Hydrochlorothiazide 25 mg/Tab. Bot. 100s. *Rx.*
Use: Antihypertensive.

Vasimid.
See: Tolazoline HCl, U.S.P. 23.

vasoactive intestinal polypeptide. (Research Triangle) *Rx.*
Use: Treatment of acute esophageal food impaction. [Orphan drug]

Vasocidin Ophthalmic Ointment. (Ciba Vision) Prednisolone acetate 0.5%, sulfacetamide sodium 10%. Tube 3.5 g. *Rx.*
Use: Corticosteroid, anti-infective, ophthalmic.

Vasocidin Ophthalmic Solution. (Ciba Vision) Prednisolone sodium phosphate 0.25%, sulfacetamide sodium 10%. Bot. 5 ml, 10 ml. *Rx.*
Use: Corticosteroid, anti-infective, ophthalmic.

VasoClear. (Ciba Vision) Naphazoline HCl 0.02%. Bot. 15 ml. *otc.*
Use: Vasoconstrictor, mydriatic, ophthalmic.

VasoClear A. (Ciba Vision) Naphazoline HCl 0.02%. Bot. 15 ml. *otc.*
Use: Vasoconstrictor, mydriatic, ophthalmic.

Vasocon-A Ophthalmic Solution. (Ciba Vision) Naphazoline HCl 0.05%, antazoline phosphate 0.5%. Bot. 15 ml. *Rx.*
Use: Vasoconstrictor, mydriatic, ophthalmic.

Vasocon Regular. (Ciba Vision) Naphazoline HCl 0.1%. Bot. 15 ml. *Rx.*
Use: Vasoconstrictor, mydriatic, ophthalmic.

Vasoderm. (Taro) Fluocinonide 0.05%, anhydrous glycerin base. Cream. Tube 15 g, 30 g, 60 g. *Rx.*
Use: Topical corticosteroid.

Vasoderm-E. (Taro) Fluocinonide 0.05%, emollient mineral oil and white petrolatum base. Cream. Tube 15 g, 30 g, 60 g, 120 g. *Rx.*
Use: Topical corticosteroid.

Vasodilan. (Bristol-Myers) Isoxsuprine HCl 10 mg or 20 mg/Tab. **10 mg:** Bot. 100s, 1000s, UD 100s. **20 mg:** Bot. 100s, 500s, 1000s, UD 100s. *Rx.*
Use: Peripheral vasodilator.

vasodilators.
See: Amyl Nitrite.
Apresoline, Tab., Amp. (Novartis).
Arlidin, Tab. (Rhone-Poulenc Rorer).
Cardilate, Tab. (Glaxo Wellcome).
Cyclospasmol, Tab., Cap. (Wyeth).
Erythrityl Tetranitrate, Tab.
Glyceryl Trinitrate Preps.
Isordil, Tab. (Wyeth).
Kortrate, Cap. (T.E. Williams).
Mannitol Hexanitrate.
Metamine, Tab. (Pfizer).

Nisane, Elix. (T.E. Williams).
Nitroglycerin.
Pentritol, Cap., Tempule (Centeon).
Peritrate, Tab. (Parke-Davis).
Sodium Nitrate.
Sorbitrate, Tab. (Stuart).
Vasodilan, Tab., Amp. (Bristol-Myers).

vasodilators, coronary.
See: Glyceryl Trinitrate, Preps. (Various Mfr.).
Isordil, Tab. (Wyeth).
Khellin (Various Mfr.).
Papaverine, Inj., Tab. (Various Mfr.).
Pentaerythritol Tetranitrate, Tab.
Peritrate, Tab. (Parke-Davis).
Roniacol Elix., Tab. (Roche).
Sorbitrate, Tab. (Stuart).

Vasoflo. (Roberts) Papaverine HCl 150 mg/Cap. Bot. 100s. *Rx.*
Use: Peripheral vasodilator.

Vasolate. (Parmed) Pentaerythritol tetranitrate 30 mg/Cap. Bot. 100s, 1000s. *Rx.*
Use: Antianginal.

Vasolate-80. (Parmed) Pentaerythritol tetranitrate 80 mg/Cap. Bot. 100s, 1000s. *Rx.*
Use: Antianginal.

•**vasopressin,** (VAY-so-PRESS-in) U.S.P. 23. Beta-hypophamine. Posterior pituitary pressor hormone.
Use: Hormone (antidiuretic).
See: Pitressin, Amp. (Parke-Davis).

vasopressin. (American Regent) 20 pressor units/ml, chlorobutanol/Inj. Vial. 0.5 ml, 1 ml, 10 ml. *Rx.*
Use: Posterior pituitary hormone.

Vasosulf. (Ciba Vision) Sulfacetamide sodium 15%, phenylephrine HCl 0.125%. Bot. 5 ml, 15 ml. *Rx.*
Use: Anti-infective, decongestant (ophthalmic).

Vasotec. (Merck) Enalapril maleate 2.5 mg, 5 mg, 10 mg or 20 mg/Tab. **2.5 mg:** Bot. 100s, 1000s, 10,000s, UD 100s, unit-of-dose 90s, 100s. **5 mg; 10 mg:** 100s, 1000s, 4000s, 10,000s, UD 100s, unit-of-dose 90s, 180s. **20 mg:** 100s, 1000s, 10,000s, UD 100s, unit-of-dose 90s. *Rx.*
Use: Antihypertensive.

Vasotec I.V. (Merck) Enalaprilat 1.25 mg/ml. Inj. Vial 1 ml, 2 ml. *Rx.*
Use: Antihypertensive.

Vasotus Liquid. (Sheryl) Codeine phosphate ⅛ gr, phenylephrine HCl, prophenpyridamine maleate. Liq. Bot. pt. *c-v.*
Use: Antitussive, decongestant, antihistamine.

Vasoxyl. (Glaxo Wellcome) Methoxamine HCl 0.1%. Inj. 20 mg/ml. *Rx.*
Use: Vasopressor used in shock.

Vaxsyn HIV-1. (Microgenesys)
See: T-Lymphotropic Virtus Type III GP 160 Antigen.

Vazosan. (Sandia) Papaverine HCl 150 mg/Tab. Bot. 100s, 1000s. *Rx.*
Use: Peripheral vasodilator.

VCF. (Apothecus) Contraceptive film: nonoxynol-9 28%, glycerin and polyvinyl alcohol. Pkg. 3s, 6s, 12s. *otc.*
Use: Spermicide.

V-Cillin-K. (Lilly) Penicillin V potassium 125 mg, 250 mg or 500 mg/Tab. **125 mg:** Bot. 100s. **250 mg:** Bot. 100s, 500s. **500 mg:** Bot. 24s, 100s, 500s. *Rx.*
Use: Anti-infective, penicillin.

V-Cillin-K for Oral Solution. (Lilly) Penicillin V potassium 125 mg or 250 mg/5 ml. **125 mg:** Bot. 100 ml, 150 ml, 200 ml, UD 5 ml. **250 mg:** Bot. 100 ml, 150 ml, 200 ml. *Rx.*
Use: Anti-infective, penicillin.

V-Dec-M. (Seatrace) Pseudoephedrine HCl 120 mg, guaifenesin 500 mg/SR Tab. Bot. 100s. *Rx.*
Use: Decongestant, expectorant.

VDRL Antigen. (Laboratory Diagnostics) VDRL antigen with buffered saline. Blood test in diagnosis of syphillis. **Vial:** Sufficient for 500 tests. **Amp.:** 10 × 0.5 ml sufficient for 500 tests.
Use: Diagnostic aid.

VDRL Slide Test. (Laboratory Diagnostics) VDRL antigen. Slide flocculation and spinal fluid test for syphilis. Vial 5 ml Complete kit, reactive control, nonreactive control, 5 ml.
Use: Diagnostic aid.

VE-400. (Western Research) Vitamin E 400 IU/Cap. Bot. 1008s. *otc.*
Use: Vitamin E supplement.

•**vecuronium bromide.** (veh-CUE-row-nee-uhm) USAN.
Use: Blocking agent (neuromuscular).

Veetids. (Squibb) Penicillin-V potassium. **Soln.:** 125 mg or 250 mg/5 ml Bot. 100 ml, 200 ml. **Tab.:** 250 mg or 500 mg. Bot. 100s, 1000s, Unimatic 100s. *Rx.*
Use: Anti-infective, penicillin.

Veetids '500'. (Squibb) Penicillin V potassium 500 mg/Tab. Bot. 100s, 1000s, UD 100s. *Rx.*
Use: Anti-infective, penicillin.

•**vegetable oil, hydrogenated,** N.F. 18.
Use: Pharmaceutic aid (tablet/capsule lubricant).

vehicle/n and vehicle/n mild. (Neutrogena) Topical vehicle system for compounding. Appliderm Applicator Bot. oz. *otc.*
Use: Extemporaneous compounding.

velacycline. N-Pyrrolidinomethyl tetracycline. *Rx.*
Use: Anti-infective, tetracycline.

Velban. (Lilly) Extract from Vinca rosea Linn. Vinblastine sulfate, lyophilized. Vial 10 mg. *Rx.*
Use: Antineoplastic.

•**velnacrine maleate.** (VELL-NAH-kreen) USAN.
Use: Inhibitor (cholinesterase).
See: Mentane (Hoecsht Marion Roussel).

Velosef. (Squibb) Cephradine. **Oral Susp.:** 125 mg or 250 mg/5 ml. Bot. 100 ml, 200 ml. **Cap.:** 250 mg or 500 mg Bot. 24s, 100s, UD Unimatic 100s. **Inj.:** (w/anhydrous sodium carbonate. Sodium equivalent to 136 mg/g cephradine) 250 mg, 500 mg, 1 g or 2 g/vial. 2 g vial is sodium free for infusion. Bot. 200 ml. *Rx.*
Use: Anti-infective, cephalosporin.

Velosulin Human. (Novo Nordisk) Human insulin injection 100 IU/ml, Vial 10 ml. *otc.*
Use: Antidiabetic.

Velvachol. (Galderma) Hydrophilic ointment base petrolatum, mineral oil, cetyl alcohol, cholesterol, parabens, stearyl alcohol, purified water, sodium lauryl sulfate. Jar lb. *otc.*
Use: Hydrophilic ointment base.

venesetic.
See: Amobarbital Sodium, Preps. (Various Mfr.).

venethene. No mfr. listed.

venlafaxine.
Use: Antidepressant.
See: Effexor, Tab. (Wyeth-Ayerst).

•**venlafaxine hydrochloride.** (VEN-lah-fax-EEN) USAN.
Use: Antidepressant.

Venoglobulin-I. (Alpha Therapeutics) Immune globulin IV (IGIV). Pow. for Inj. 500 mg. Vial 2.5 g, 5 g, 10 g. *Rx.*
Use: Immune globulin.

Venoglobulin-S. (Alpha Therapeutics) Immune globulin IV (human) 5%: Vial. 2.5 g, 5 g, 10 g. 10%: Vial 5 g, 10 g, 20 g. Solvent detergent treated. Inj. 50, 100, 200 ml w/sterile IV administration set. *Rx.*
Use: Immune globulin.

Venomil. (Bayer) Freeze-dried venom or

venom protein. Vials of 12 mcg or 120 mcg for honey bee, white-faced hornet, yellow hornet, yellow jacket or wasp. Vials of 36 mcg or 360 mcg for mixed vespids (white-faced hornet, yellow hornet, yellow jacket). Diagnostic 1 mcg/ml, Maintenance 100 mcg/ml. Individual patient kit. *Rx.*
Use: Hymenoptera venom.

Venstat. (Seatrace) Brompheniramine maleate 10 mg/ml. Vial 10 ml. *Rx.*
Use: Antihistamine.

Ventolin Inhalation Aerosol. (Glaxo Wellcome) Albuterol 90 mcg/actuation. Aerosol canister 17 g containing 200 metered inhalations. Canister 17 g w/ oral adapter. Refill canister 17 g. *Rx.*
Use: Bronchodilator.

Ventolin Inhalation Solution. (Glaxo Wellcome) Albuterol sulfate 5 mg/ml. Bot. 20 ml w/calibrated dropper. *Rx.*
Use: Bronchodilator.

Ventolin Nebules. (Glaxo Wellcome) Albuterol sulfate 0.083%, sulfuric acid. Soln. for inhalation. In 3 ml unit dose nebules. *Rx.*
Use: Bronchodilator.

Ventolin Rotacaps. (Glaxo Wellcome) Microfine albuterol 200 mg. Cap. for inhalation. Bot. UD 96s, Hosp. UD 24s. For use with the Rotahaler inhalation device. *Rx.*
Use: Bronchodilator.

Ventolin Syrup. (Glaxo Wellcome) Albuterol sulfate 2 mg/5 ml. Bot. pt. *Rx.*
Use: Bronchodilator.

Ventolin Tablets. (Glaxo Wellcome) Albuterol sulfate 2 mg or 4 mg/Tab. Bot. 100s, 500s. *Rx.*
Use: Bronchodilator.

VePesid. (Bristol-Myers/Bristol Oncology) Etoposide. **Vial:** 100 mg/Vial. **Cap.:** 50 mg/Cap. Bot. 20s. *Rx.*
Use: Antineoplastic.

Veracolate. (Numark) Phenolphthalein 0.5 gr, capsicum oleoresin 0.05 min, cascara extract 1 gr/Tab. Bot. 100s. *otc.*
Use: Laxative.

•**veradoline hydrochloride.** (VEER-aid-OLE-een) USAN.
Use: Analgesic.

•**verapamil.** (veh-RAP-ah-mill) USAN.
Use: Vasodilator (coronary).

•**verapamil hydrochloride,** (veh-RAP-ah-mill) U.S.P. 23.
Use: Antianginal, cardiac depressant (antiarrhythmic).
See: Calan, Tab. (Searle).
  Calan SR, Capl. (Searle).

Isoptin, Tab. Inj. (Knoll).
  Verelan, SR Cap. (Lederle).

verapamil hydrochloride. (Various Mfr.) Verapamil HCl **40 mg/Tab.:** Bot. 100s. **80 mg, 120 mg/Tab.:** 100s, 250s, 500s, 1000s, UD 100s. **180 mg, 240 mg/SR Tab.:** 100s and 500s. **5 mg/2 ml/Inj.:** 2 ml, 4 ml vials, amps and syringes and 4 ml fill in 5 ml vials. *Rx.*
Use: Calcium channel blocker.
See: Calan, Tab. (Searle).
  Calan SR, Tab. (Searle).
  Isopfin, Tab., Inj. (Knoll).
  Verelan, SR Cap. (Lederle).

veratrum alba.
See: Protoveratrines A and B (Various Mfr.).

Verazeptol. (Femco) Chlorothymol, eucalyptol, menthol, phenol, boric acid, zinc sulfate. Pow. Bot. 3 oz, 6 oz, 10 oz. *otc.*
Use: Vaginal preparation.

Verazinc. (Forest) Zinc sulfate 220 mg/ Cap. Bot. 100s, 1000s. *otc.*
Use: Zinc supplement.

Verelan. (Lederle) Verapamil HCl 120, 180, 240, 360 mg/SR Cap. Bot. 100s. *Rx.*
Use: Calcium channel blocker.

Vergo Oint. (Daywell) Calcium pantothenate 8%, ascorbic acid 2%, starch. Tube 0.5 oz. *Rx.*
Use: Keratolytic.

Vergon. (Marnel) Meclizine HCl 30 mg. Cap. Bot. 100s. *otc.*
Use: Antiemetic, antivertigo.

•**verilopam hydrochloride.** (veh-RILL-OH-pam) USAN.
Use: Analgesic.

Verin. (Roberts) Aspirin (Acetylsalicylic Acid; ASA) 650 mg/TR Tab. Bot. 100s.
Use: Salicylate analgesic.

•**verlukast.** (ver-LOO-kast) USAN.
Use: Antiasthmatic (leukotriene antagonist).

Verluma. (NeoRx, DuPont Merck) Nofetumomab merpentan 10 mg for conjugation w/technetium-99m. Kit.
Use: Radioimmunoscintigraphy.

Vermox. (Janssen) Mebendazole 100 mg/Tab. Box 12s. *Rx.*
Use: Anthelmintic.

vernamycins. Under study.
Use: Anti-infective.

vernolepin. A sesquiterpene dilactone. Under study.
Use: Against Walker carcinosarcoma 256.

•**verofylline.** (VER-OH-fill-in) USAN.

Use: Bronchodilator, antiasthmatic.

veronal sodium.
See: Barbital Sodium (Various Mfr.).

Verr-Canth. (C & M Pharmacal) Cantharidin 0.7%, penederm 0.5%. Bot. 7.5 ml. *Rx.*
Use: Keratolytic.

Verrex. (C & M Pharmacal) Salicylic acid 30%, podophyllin 10%. Bot. 7.5 ml w/ applicator tip. *Rx.*
Use: Keratolytic.

Versacaps. (Seatrace) Pseudoephedrine HCl 60 mg, guaifenesin 300 mg/Cap. Bot. 100s. *Rx.*
Use: Decongestant, expectorant.

Versal. (Suppositoria) Bismuth subgallate, balsam peru, zinc oxide, benzyl benzoate/Supp. Box 12s, 100s, 1000s. *otc.*
Use: Anorectal preparation.

Versa-Quat. (Ulmer) Quaternary ammonium one-step cleaner-disinfectant-sanitizer-fungicide-virucide for general housekeeping. Bot. gal.
Use: Cleanser, disinfectant.

Versed. (Roche) Midazolam HCl 1 mg or 5 mg/ml, sodium Cl 0.8%, disodium edetate 0.01%, benzyl alcohol 1%. **1 mg/ml:** Vial 2 ml, 5 ml, 10 ml. Box 10s. **5 mg/ml:** Vial 1 ml, 2 ml, 5 ml, 10 ml. Box 10s. Disposable Syringe 2 ml Box 10s. *c-iv.*
Use: General anesthetic.

versenate, calcium disodium.
See: Calcium Disodium Versenate, Amp. (3M).

versenate disodium.
See: Disodium Versenate, Amp. (3M).

•**versetamide.** (ver-SET-ah-mide) USAN.
Use: Pharmaceutic aid.

Versiclear. (Hope Pharmaceuticals) Sodium thiosulfate 25%, salicylic acid 1%, isopropyl alcohol 10%, menthol, EDTA. Lot. 120 ml. *Rx.*
Use: Anti-infective, topical.

versidyne.
Use: Analgesic.

Verstran. (Parke-Davis) Prazepam.
Use: Antianxiety.
See: Centrax, Tab. (Parke-Davis).

Vertab. (UAD) Dimenhydrinate 50 mg. Tab. Bot. 100s.
Use: Anticholinergic.

•**verteporfin.** USAN.
Use: Antineoplastic.

Verukan-20. (Syosset) Salicylic acid 16.7%, lactic acid in flexible collodion 16.7%. Bot. 15 ml. *otc.*
Use: Keratolytic.

Verv Alertness Capsules. (APC) Caffeine 200 mg/Cap. Vial 15s. *otc.*
Use: CNS stimulant.

Vesanoid. (Hoffmann-LaRoche) Tretinoin 10 mg. Cap. Bot. 100s. *Rx.*
Use: Antineoplastic.

•**vesnarinone.** (VESS-nah-rih-NOHN) USAN.
Use: Cardiotonic.

Vetuss HC. (Cypress) Hydrocodone bitartrate 1.7 mg, phenylephrine HCl 5 mg, phenylpropanolamine HCl 3.3 mg, pyrilamine maleate 3.3 mg, pheniramine maleate 3.3 mg/5 ml, alcohol 5%/Syrup. Bot. 1 pt. *c-iii.*
Use: Antitussive combination.

Vexol. (Alcon) Rimexolone 1%. Susp. Ophthalmic. Drop-Tainers. 5 ml, 10 ml. *Rx.*
Use: Corticosteroid, ophthalmic.

Viacaps. (Manne) Vitamins A (soluble) 45,000 IU, C 500 mg/Cap. Bot. 60s, 120s, 1000s. *otc.*
Use: Vitamin supplement.

Vi antigen. *Rx.*
Use: Agent for immunization.
See: Typhim Vi (Pasteur-Merieux-Connaught).

vibesate. Polvinate 9.3%, molrosinol 3.1% with propellant.

Vibramycin. (Pfizer Laboratories) Doxycycline. **Cap.:** 50 mg Bot. 50s, UD pak 100s, X-Pack (10 Cap.) 5s; 100 mg Bot. 50s, 500s; UD pak 100s, V-Pak (5 Cap) 5s, Nine-Pak 10s. **Pediatric Oral Susp.:** 25 mg/5 ml. Bot. 2 oz. **Syr.:** 50 mg/5 ml. Bot. oz, pt. *Rx.*
Use: Anti-infective, tetracycline.

Vibramycin IV. (Roerig) Doxycycline (as hyclate) 200 mg. Powder for Inj. Vial. *Rx.*
Use: Anti-infective, tetracycline.

Vibra-Tabs. (Pfizer Laboratories) Doxycycline hyclate 100 mg/Tab. Bot. 50s, 500s, UD Pack 100s. *Rx.*
Use: Anti-infective, tetracycline.

Vicam IV. (Keene) Vitamins B_1 50 mg, B_2 5 mg, B_{12} 1000 mcg, B_6 5 mg, dexpanthenol 6 mg, niacinamide 125 mg, C 50 mg/ml, benzyl alcohol 1% as preservative in water for injection. Vial multiple dose. *Rx.*
Use: Parenteral nutritional supplement.

Vicam Injection. (Keene) Vitamins B_1 50 mg, B_2 5 mg, B_3 125 mg, B_5 6 mg, B_6 5 mg, B_{12} 1000 mcg, C 50 mg/ml. Inj. Vial 10 ml. *Rx.*
Use: Vitamin supplement.

Vicks Children's Chloraseptic Loz-

enges. (Procter & Gamble) Benzocaine 5 mg, corn syrup, sucrose. Grape flavor. Loz. Pkg. 18s. *otc.*

Vicks Children's Chloraseptic Spray. (Procter & Gamble) Phenol 0.5%, saccharin, sorbitol. Alcohol free. Spray. Bot. 177 ml. *otc.*
Use: Antiseptic, anesthetic.

Vicks Children's NyQuil Nighttime Cold/Cough Liquid. (Procter & Gamble) Pseudoephedrine HCl 10 mg, dextromethorphan HBr 5 mg, chlorpheniramine maleate 0.67 mg/5 ml, alcohol free. Bot. 120 ml, 240 ml. *otc.*
Use: Decongestant, antihistamine, antitussive.

Vicks Chloraseptic Mouthrinse/Gargle. (Procter & Gamble) Phenol 1.4%, saccharin. Alcohol free. Liq. 355 ml. *otc.*
Use: Antiseptic.

Vicks Chloraseptic Sore Throat. (Procter & Gamble) Benzocaine 6 mg, menthol 10 mg. Loz. Pkg. 18s. *otc.*
Use: Anesthetic.

Vicks Cough Drops. (Procter & Gamble) Menthol. **Menthol flavor:** Benzyl alcohol, camphor, eucalyptus oil, tolu balsam, corn syrup, sucrose, thymol. **Cherry flavor:** Corn syrup, sucrose, citric acid. Box 14. Bag 40. *otc.*
Use: Mouth and throat preparation.

Vicks DayQuil Allergy Relief 4 Hour. (Procter & Gamble) Phenylpropanolamine HCl 25 mg, brompheniramine maleate 4 mg. Tab. Pkg. 24s. *otc.*
Use: Decongestant, antitussive.

Vicks DayQuil Allergy Relief 12 Hour. (Procter & Gamble) Phenylpropanolamine HCl 75 mg, brompheniramine maleate 12 mg/SR Tab. Pkg. 12s, 24s. *otc.*
Use: Decongestant, antitussive.

Vicks DayQuil Liquicaps. (Procter & Gamble) Dextromethorphan HBr 10 mg, pseudoephedrine HCl 30 mg, acetaminophen 250 mg, guaifenesin 100 mg. Softgel Cap. Pkg. 12s, 20s. *otc.*
Use: Analgesic, decongestant, antitussive, expectorant.

Vicks DayQuil Liquid. (Procter & Gamble) Pseudoephedrine HCl 60 mg, guaifenesin 200 mg, acetaminophen 650 mg, dextromethorphan HBr 20 mg/ 30 ml. Bot. 6 oz. *otc.*
Use: Decongestant, expectorant, analgesic, antitussive.

Vicks DayQuil Sinus Pressure & Congestion Relief. (Procter & Gamble) Phenylpropanolamine HCl 25 mg, guaifenesin 200 mg. Cap. Pkg. 12s, 24s. *otc.*

Use: Decongestant, expectorant.

Vicks DayQuil Sinus Pressure & Pain Relief. (Procter & Gamble) Pseudoephedrine HCl 30 mg, acetaminophen 500 mg. Cap. Pkg. 24s. *otc. otc.*
Use: Decongestant, analgesic.

Vicks Dry Hacking Cough. (Procter & Gamble) Dextromethorphan HBr 30 mg/10 ml, alcohol 10%, invert sugar. Liq. Bot. 4 oz, 8 oz w/Vicks AccuTip Dispenser. *otc.*
Use: Antitussive.

Vicks 44 Non-Drowsy Cold & Cough liquicaps. (Procter & Gamble) Dextromethorphan HBr 30 mg, pseudoephedrine HCl 60 mg. Cap. Pkg. 10s. *otc.*
Use: Decongestant, antitussive.

Vicks 44D Cough & Decongestant Liquid. (Procter & Gamble) Pseudoephedrine HCl 20 mg, dextromethorphan HBr 10 mg/5 ml, alcohol 10%, saccharin, sucrose. Bot. 120 ml, 240 ml. *otc.*
Use: Decongestant, antitussive.

Vicks 44D Cough & Head Congestion. (Procter & Gamble) Dextromethorphan 10 mg, pseudoephedrine HCl 20 mg/ Liq. Bot. 5 ml. *otc.*
Use: Decongestant, antitussive.

Vicks 44d Dry Hacking-Cough and Head Congestion, Pediatric. (Procter & Gamble) Dextromethorphan HBr 15 mg/15 ml, pseudephedrine HCl 3 mg, alcohol free, sorbitol, sucrose, cherry flavor. Liq. Bot. 120 ml with Vicks AccuTip Dispenser. *otc.*
Use: Decongestant, antitussive.

Vicks 44d Pediatric Cough & Decongestant Liquid. (Procter & Gamble) Pseudoephedrine HCl 10 mg, dextromethorphan HBr 5 mg/5 ml, alcohol free. Bot. 120 ml. *otc.*
Use: Decongestant, antitussive.

Vicks 44E Liquid. (Procter & Gamble) Dextromethorphan HBr 20 mg, guaifenesin 200 mg. Bot. 118 ml, 236 ml. *otc.*
Use: Antitussive, expectorant.

Vicks 44e Pediatric Liquid. (Procter & Gamble) Dextromethorphan HBr 10 mg, guaifenesin 100 mg, sorbitol, sucrose. Alcohol free. Bot. 120 ml w/Vicks AccuTip Dispenser. *otc.*
Use: Antitussive, expectorant.

Vicks 44M Cough, Cold and Flu Liquid. (Procter & Gamble) Dextromethorphan HBr 30 mg, pseudoephedrine HCl 60 mg, chlorpheniramine maleate 4 mg, acetaminophen 650 mg/20 ml, alcohol 10%. Bot. 4 oz, 8 oz, with Vicks

AccuTip Dispenser. *otc.*
Use: Antitussive, decongestant, antihistamine, analgesic.

Vicks 44M Cold, Flu & Cough Liquicaps. (Procter & Gamble) Dextromethorphan HBr 10 mg, pseudoephedrine HCl 30 mg, chlorpheniramine maleate 2 mg, acetaminophen 250 mg. Cap. Pkg. 12s. *otc.*
Use: Decongestant, antitussive, antihistamine, analgesic.

Vicks NyQuil Liquicaps. (Procter & Gamble) Acetaminophan 250 mg, pseudoephedrine HCl 30 mg, dextromethorphan HBr 10 mg, doxylamine succinate 6.25 mg. Pkg. 12s, 20s. *otc.*
Use: Analgesic, decongestant, antitussive, antihistamine.

Vicks NyQuil Liquid Multi-Symptom Cold Flu Relief. (Procter & Gamble) Acetaminophen 1000 mg, doxylamine succinate 12.5 mg, pseudoephedrine HCl 60 mg, dextromethorphan HBr 30 mg/30 ml, alcohol 10%. Regular and cherry flavors. Regular contains FD&C Yellow No. 6. Bot. 6 oz, 10 oz, 14 oz. *otc.*
Use: Analgesic, antihistamine, decongestant, antitussive.

Vicks NyQuil Multi-Symptom Cold Flu Relief. (Procter & Gamble) Pseudoephedrine HCl 10 mg, doxylamine succinate 2.1 mg, dextromethorphan HBr 5 mg, acetaminophen 167 mg/5 ml. Liq. Alcohol 10%, sucrose. 180, 300 and 420 ml *otc.*
Use: Analgesic, antihistamine, decongestant, antitussive.

Vicks Sinex. (Procter & Gamble) Phenylephrine HCl 0.5%, camphor, menthol, eucalyptol, disodium EDTA. Nasal Spray. Plastic Squeeze Bot. 0.5 oz, 1 oz. *otc.*
Use: Decongestant.

Vicks Sinex 12-Hour. (Procter & Gamble) Oxymetazoline HCl 0.05%, camphor, menthol, eucalyptol, disodium EDTA. Nasal Spray. Plastic Squeeze Bot. 1 oz, 0.5 oz. *otc.*
Use: Decongestant.

Vicks Vapor Inhaler. (Procter & Gamble) l-Desoxyephedrine 50 mg, Special Vicks Vapors (menthol, camphor, bornyl acetate, lavender oil). Inhaler 0.007 oz (198 mg). *otc.*
Use: Decongestant.

Vicks Vaporub. (Procter & Gamble) Camphor 4.7%, menthol 2.6%, eucalyptus oil 1.2%, cedarleaf oil, nutmeg oil. **Ointment:** Mineral oil, petrolatum.

Cream: Isopropyl palmitate, EDTA, glycerin, imidazolidinyl urea, cetyl alcohol, parabens, stearyl alcohol, titanium dioxide. Cream. Jar 56.7 g. *otc.*
Use: Decongestant vaporizing ointment.

Vicks Vaposteam. (Procter & Gamble) Eucalyptus oil 1.5%, camphor 6.2%, menthol 3.2%, alcohol 74%, cedarleaf oil, nutmeg oil. Bot. 4 oz, 8 oz. *otc.*
Use: Steam medication, decongestant, antitussive.

Vicks Vitamin C Drops. (Procter & Gamble) Vitamin C 60 mg as sodium ascorbate and ascorbic acid. Orange flavor. Bag. 14s, 30s. *otc.*
Use: Vitamin C supplement.

Vicodin. (Knoll) Hydrocodone bitartrate 5 mg, acetaminophen 500 mg/Tab. Bot. 100s, 500s, UD 100s. *c-III.*
Use: Narcotic analgesic combination.

Vicodin ES. (Knoll) Hydrocodone bitartrate 7.5 mg, acetaminophen 750 mg/Tab. Bot. 100s, UD 100s. *c-III.*
Use: Narcotic analgesic combination.

Vicodin HP. (Knoll) Hydrocodone bitartrate 10 mg, acetaminophen 660 mg/Tab. Bot. 100s.
Use: Narcotic analgesic combination.

Vicodin Tuss. (Knoll) Hydrocodone bitartrate 5 mg, guaifenesin 100 mg/5 ml, sugar free. Syrup. Bot. 480 ml. *c-III.*
Use: Narcotic antitussive, expectorant.

Vicon-C. (Whitby) Vitamins B_1 20 mg, B_2 10 mg, B_3 100 mg, B_5 20 mg, B_6 5 mg, C 300 mg, Mg, zinc sulfate 80 mg/Cap. Bot. 60s, UD 100s. *otc.*
Use: Vitamin/mineral supplement.

Vicon Forte. (Whitby) Vitamins A 8000 IU, E 50 IU, C 150 mg, B_3 25 mg, B_1 10 mg, B_5 10 mg, B_2 5 mg, B_6 2 mg, B_{12} 10 mcg, folic acid 1 mg, zinc sulfate 18 mg, Mg, Mn, lactose/Cap. Bot. 60s, 500s, UD 100s. *Rx.*
Use: Vitamin/mineral supplement.

Vicon Plus. (Whitby) Vitamins A 4000 IU, E 50 IU, C 150 mg, B_3 25 mg, B_1 10 mg, B_5 10 mg, B_2 5 mg, zinc sulfate 18 mg, Mg, Mn, lactose, B_6 2 mg/Cap. Bot. 60s. *otc.*
Use: Vitamin/mineral supplement.

Victors. (Procter & Gamble) Special Vicks Medication (menthol, eucalyptus oil) in a soothing Vicks sugar base. Regular or Cherry flavor drops. Stick-Pack 10s, Bag 40s. *otc.*
Use: Local anesthetic.

Victor's Vapor Cough. (Procter & Gamble) Menthol, eucalyptus oil. Loz. Pkg. 10s. *otc.*

Use: Local anesthetic.

• **vidarabine,** (vih-DAR-ah-BEAN) U.S.P. 23.
Use: Antiviral.

• **vidarabine phosphate.** (vih-DAR-ah-BEAN) USAN.
Use: Antiviral.

• **vidarabine sodium phosphate.** (vih-DAR-ah-BEAN) USAN.
Use: Antiviral.

Vi-Daylin ADC Drops. (Ross) Vitamins A 1500 IU, C 35 mg, D 400 IU/ml. Bot. 30 ml, 50 ml. Bot. 50 ml w/dropper. *otc.*
Use: Vitamin supplement.

Vi-Daylin ADC Vitamin + Iron Drops. (Ross) Vitamins A 1500 IU, C 35 mg, D 400 IU, iron 10 mg/ml, methylparaben. Bot. 50 ml. *otc.*
Use: Vitamin/mineral supplement.

Vi-Daylin Chewable. (Ross) Vitamins A 2500 IU, D 400 IU, E 15 IU, C 60 mg, folic acid 0.3 mg, B$_1$ 1.05 mg, B$_2$ 1.2 mg, niacin 13.5 mg, B$_6$ 1.05 mg, B$_{12}$ 4.5 mcg/Tab. Bot. 100s. *otc.*
Use: Vitamin supplement.

Vi-Daylin/F Chewable Multivitamin. (Ross) Fluoride 1 mg, vitamins A 2500 IU, D 400 IU, E 15 mg, B$_1$ 1.05 mg, B$_2$ 1.2 mg, B$_3$ 13.5 mg, B$_6$ 1.05 mg, B$_{12}$ 4.5 mcg, C 60 mg, folic acid 0.3 mg, sucrose, cherry flavor. Tab. Bot. 100s. *Rx.*
Use: Dental caries preventative, vitamin/mineral supplement.

Vi-Daylin Chewable w/Fluoride. (Ross) Fluoride 1 mg, vitamins B$_1$ 1.05 mg, B$_2$ 1.2 mg, niacinamide 13.5 mg, B$_6$ 1.05 mg, C 60 mg, A 2500 IU, B$_{12}$ 4.5 mcg, E 15 IU, folic acid 0.3 mg, D 400 IU/Tab. Bot. 100s. *Rx.*
Use: Dental caries preventative, vitamin/mineral supplement.

Vi-Daylin Drops. (Ross) Vitamins A 1500 IU, D 400 IU, E 5 IU, C 35 mg, B$_1$ 0.5 mg, B$_2$ 0.6 mg, niacin 8 mg, B$_6$ 0.4 mg, B$_{12}$ 1.5 mcg/ml. Bot. 50 ml. *otc.*
Use: Vitamin supplement.

Vi-Daylin/F ADC Vitamins Drops. (Ross) Vitamins A 1500 IU, D 400 IU, C 35 mg, fluoride 0.25 mg/ml. Alcohol ≈ 0.3%, parabens. Bot. 50 ml. *Rx.*
Use: Vitamin supplement, dental caries preventative.

Vi-Daylin/F ADC + Iron Drops. (Ross) Vitamins A 1500 IU, C 35 mg, D 400 IU, iron 10 mg, fluoride 0.25 mg/ml, methylparaben. Bot. 50 ml. *Rx.*
Use: Vitamin/mineral supplement, dental caries preventative.

Vi-Daylin/F Drops. (Ross) Vitamins A 1500 IU, D 400 IU, E 5 IU, C 35 mg, B$_1$ 0.5 mg, B$_2$ 0.6 mg, B$_3$ 8 mg, B$_6$ 0.4 mg, fluoride 0.25 mg/ml, methylparaben. Bot. 50 ml. *Rx.*
Use: Vitamin supplement, dental caries preventative.

Vi-Daylin/F Multivitamin + Iron. (Ross) **Drops:** Fluoride 0.25 mg, vitamins A 1500 IU, D 400 IU, E 4.1 mg, B$_1$ 0.5 mg, B$_2$ 0.6 mg, B$_3$ 8 mg, B$_6$ 0.4 mg, C 35 mg, iron 10 mg/ml, alcohol < 0.1%, methylparaben. Bot. 50 ml. **Chew. Tab.:** Fluoride 1 mg, vitamins A 2500 IU, D 400 IU, E 15 mg, B$_1$ 1.05 mg, B$_2$ 1.2 mg, B$_3$ 13.5 mg, B$_6$ 1.05 mg, B$_{12}$ 4.5 mcg, C 60 mg, folic acid 0.3 mg, iron 12 mg. Bot. 100s. *Rx.*
Use: Dental caries preventative, vitamin/mineral supplement.

Vi-Daylin Liquid. (Ross) Vitamins A 2500 IU, B$_1$ 1.05 mg, B$_2$ 1.2 mg, B$_6$ 1.05 mg, B$_{12}$ 4.5 mcg, C 60 mg, D 400 IU, E 20.4 mg (as d-alpha tocopheryl acetate), niacin 13.5 mg/5 ml. Bot. 8 oz, pt. *otc.*
Use: Vitamin supplement.

Vi-Daylin Multivitamin Drops. (Ross) Vitamins A 1500 IU, D 400 IU, E 5 mg, B$_1$ 0.5 mg, B$_2$ 0.6 mg, B$_3$ 8 mg, B$_6$ 0.4 mg, B$_{12}$ 1.5 mcg, C 35 mg/ml, < 0.5% alcohol. Bot. 50 ml. *otc.*
Use: Vitamin supplement.

Vi-Daylin Multivitamin Liquid. (Ross) Vitamins A 2500 IU, D 400 IU, E 15 mg, B$_1$ 1.05 mg, B$_2$ 1.2 mg, B$_3$ 13.5 mg, B$_6$ 1.05 mg, B$_{12}$ 4.5 mcg, C 60 mg/5 ml, ≤ 0.5% alcohol. Bot. 240, 480 ml. *otc.*
Use: Vitamin supplement.

Vi-Daylin Multivitamin + Iron Drops. (Ross) Iron 10 mg, vitamins A 1500 IU, D 400 IU, E 5 mg, B$_1$ 0.5 mg, B$_2$ 0.6 mg, B$_3$ 8 mg, B$_6$ 0.4 mg, C 35 mg, < 0.5% alcohol, methylparaben. Bot. 50 ml. *otc.*
Use: Vitamin/mineral supplement.

Vi-Daylin Multivitamin Plus Iron Chewable. (Ross) Vitamins A 2500 IU, D 400 IU, E 15 IU, C 60 mg, folic acid 0.3 mg, B$_1$ 1.05 mg, B$_2$ 1.2 mg, B$_3$ 13.5 mg, B$_6$ 1.05 mg, B$_{12}$ 4.5 mcg, iron 12 mg/Tab. Bot. 100s. *otc.*
Use: Vitamin/mineral supplement.

Vi-Daylin Multivitamin Plus Iron Liquid. (Ross) Vitamins A 2500 IU, D 400 IU, C 60 mg, E 15 IU, B$_1$ 1.05 mg, B$_2$ 1.2 mg, B$_3$ 13.5 mg, B$_6$ 1.05 mg, B$_{12}$ 4.5 mcg, iron 10 mg/tsp. ≤ 0.5% alcohol, glucose, sucrose, parabens. In 237 ml, 473 ml. *otc.*

Use: Vitamin/mineral supplement.

Videcon. (Vita Elixir) Vitamin D 50,000 units/Cap. *Rx.*
Use: Vitamin D supplement.

Vi-Derm Soap. (Arthrins) Extract of Amaryllis 10%. Pkg. cake 1s. Bar 3.5 oz. *otc.*
Use: Skin cleanser.

• **vifilcon a.** (vie-FILL-kahn A) USAN.
Use: Contact lens material (hydrophilic).

• **vifilcon b.** (vie-FILL-kahn B) USAN.
Use: Contact lens material (hydrophilic).

Vifluorineed. (Hanlon) Vitamins A 5000 IU, D 400 IU, C 75 mg, B_1 2 mg, B_2 3 mg, niacinamide 20 mg, fluoride 1 mg/ Chew. Tab. Bot. 100s. *Rx.*
Use: Vitamin/mineral supplement.

• **vigabatrin.** (vie-GAB-at RIN) USAN.
Use: Anticonvulsant (tardive dyskinesia).

Vigomar Forte. (Marlop Pharm) Iron 12 mg, vitamins A 10,000 IU, D 400 IU, E 15 IU, B_1 10 mg, B_2 10 mg, B_3 100 mg, B_5 20 mg, B_6 5 mg, B_{12} 5 mcg, C 200 mg, I, Mg, Mn, Cu, Zn 1.5 mg/ Tab. Bot. 100s. *otc.*
Use: Vitamin/mineral supplement.

Vigortol. (Rugby) Vitamins B_1 0.8 mg, B_2 0.4 mg, B_3 8.3 mg, B_5 1.7 mg, B_6 0.2 mg, B_{12} 0.2 mcg, iron 0.3 mg, Zn 0.3 mg, choline, I, Mg, Mn, alcohol 18%, sugar, methylparaben. Liq. Bot. 473 ml. *otc.*
Use: Vitamin/mineral supplement.

Vilex. (Dunhall) Vitamin B_1 100 mg, riboflavin phosphate sodium 1 mg, B_6 10 mg, panthenol 5 mg, niacinamide 100 mg/ml. Amp. 30 ml. *Rx.*
Use: Vitamin supplement.

Viliva. (Vita Elixir) Ferrous fumarate 3 gr. *otc.*
Use: Iron supplement.

• **viloxazine hydrochloride.** (vih-LOX-ah-zeen) USAN.
Use: Antidepressant.
See: Catatrol (Zeneca).

Viminate. (Various Mfr.) Vitamins B_1 2.5 mg, B_2 1.25 mg, B_3 25 mg, B_5 5 mg, B_6 0.5 mg, B_{12} 0.5 mcg, iron 7.5 mg, zinc 1 mg, choline, I, Mg, Mn/5 ml, alcohol 18%. Liq. Bot. 480. *otc.*
Use: Vitamin/mineral supplement.

Vi-Min-for-All. (Barth's) Vitamins A 3 mg, D 10 mcg, C 120 mg, B_1 35 mg, B_{12} 15 mcg, biotin, niacin 2.33 mg, E 30 IU, B_6, pantothenic acid, calcium 375 mg, phosphorus 180 mg, iron 20 mg, iodine 0.1 mg, rutin 10 mg, hesperidin-lemon bioflavonoid complex 10 mg, choline,

inositol 2.4 mg, copper 10 mcg, manganese 2 mg, zinc 110 mcg, silicone 210 mcg/Tab. Bot. 100s, 500s. *otc.*
Use: Vitamin/mineral supplement.

Vimms-38. (Approved) Vitamins A 12,500 IU, D 1200 IU, B_1 15 mg, B_2 10 mg, C 75 mg, niacinamide 30 mg, calcium pantothenate 2 mg, B_6 0.5 mg, E 5 IU, Brewer's yeast 10 mg, B_{12} 15 mcg, iron 11.58 mg, desiccated liver 15 mg, choline bitartrate 30 mg, inositol 30 mg, calcium 59 mg, phosphorus 45 mg, zinc 0.68 mg, dicalcium phosphate 200 mg, manganese 1.11 mg, magnesium 1 mg, potassium 0.68 mg, pepsin 16.5 mg, diastase 16.5 mg, yeast 40.63 mg, protein digest 23.52 mg, amino acids 34.22 mg/Cap. Bot. 50s, 100s, 1000s. *otc.*
Use: Vitamin/mineral supplement.

Vinactane Sulfate. (Novartis) Viomycin Sulfate.

• **vinafocon a.** (VIE-nah-FOE-kahn A) USAN.
Use: Contact lens material (hydrophobic).

vinbarbital.
Use: Sedative, hypnotic.

vinbarbital sodium.
Use: Sedative, hypnotic.

• **vinblastine sulfate,** (vin-BLAST-een) U.S.P. 23. Vincaleukoblastine. Alkaloid extracted from *Vinca rosea* Linn.
Use: Antineoplastic.
See: Velban, Vial (Lilly).

vinblastine sulfate. (Various Mfr.) Vinblastine sulfate 10 mg. Pow. for Inj. *Rx.*
Use: Mitotic inhibitor.

vinblastine sulfate. (Fujisawa) Vinblastine sulfate 1 mg/ml, 0.9% benzyl alcohol. Pow. for Inj. 10 ml. *Rx.*
Use: Antineoplastic.

vincaleukoblastine, 22-oxo-sulfate (1:1) (salt). Vincristine Sulfate, U.S.P. 23.

Vincasar PFS. (Pharmacia & Upjohn) Vincristine sulfate 1 mg/ml. Vial 1 ml. *Rx.*
Use: Antineoplastic.

• **vincofos.** (VIN-koe-foss) USAN.
Use: Anthelmintic.

• **vincristine sulfate,** (vin-KRISS-teen) U.S.P. 23.
Use: Antineoplastic.
See: Oncovin, Amp. (Lilly).
Vincasar PFS, Vial (Pharmacia & Upjohn).

• **vindesine.** (VIN-deh-seen) USAN.

Use: Antineoplastic.

●**vindesine sulfate.** (VIN-deh-seen) USAN.
Use: Antineoplastic.

●**vinepidine sulfate.** (VIN-eh-pih-DEEN) USAN.
Use: Antineoplastic.

●**vinglycinate sulfate.** (vin-GLIE-sin-ate) USAN.
Use: Antineoplastic.

●**vinleurosine sulfate.** (vin-LOO-row-seen) USAN. Sulfate salt of an alkaloid extracted from *Vinca rosea* Linn. Also see Vinblastine.
Use: Antineoplastic.

●**vinorelbine tartrate.** (vih-NORE-ell-bean) USAN. Sulfate salt of an alkaloid extracted from *Vinca Rosea* Linn.
Use: Antineoplastic.
See: Navelbine, Inj. (Glaxo Wellcome).

●**vinpocetine.** (VIN-poe-SEH-teen) USAN.
Use: Antineoplastic.

●**vinrosidine sulfate.** (vin-ROW-sih-deen) USAN. Sulfate salt of an alkaloid extracted from *Vinca rosea* Linn.
See: Vinblastine.
Use: Antineoplastic.

vinylacetate-polyvinylpyrrolidone.
See: Ivy-Rid Spray (Mallard).

vinyl ether, U.S.P. XXI.
Use: General anesthetic (inhalation).
See: Vinethene, Liq.

vinyzene. Bromchlorenone.
Use: Fungicide.

●**vinzolidine sulfate.** (VIN-ZOLE-ih-deen) USAN.
Use: Antineoplastic.

Vio-Bec. (Solvay) Vitamins B₁ 25 mg, B₂ 25 mg, niacinamide 100 mg, calcium pantothenate 40 mg, B₆ 25 mg, C 500 mg/Cap. Bot. 100s. *otc.*
Use: Vitamin/mineral supplement.

Viodo HC. (NMC Labs) Iodochlor-hydroxyquin 3%, hydrocortisone 1% in cream base. Tube 20 g. *otc.*
Use: Corticosteroid, antifungal, topical.

Vioform. (Novartis) Clioquinol. **Cream:** 3%. Tube oz. **Oint.:** 3% in petrolatum base. Tube oz. *otc.*
Use: Antifungal, topical.

Viogen-C. (Goldine) Vitamins B₁ 20 mg, B₂ 10 mg, B₃ 100 mg, B₅ 20 mg, B₆ 5 mg, C 300 mg, Mg, zinc sulfate 50 mg, tartrazine/Cap. Bot. 100s. *otc.*
Use: Vitamin/mineral supplement.

Viokase. (Robins) **Tab.:** Lipase 8000 units, protease 30,000 units, amylase 30,000 units/Tab. Bot. 100s, 500s. **Pow.:** Lipase 16,800 units, protease

70,000 units, amylase 70,000 units/0.7 g (0.25 tsp.). *Rx.*
Use: Digestive enzymes.

Viosterol w/Halibut Liver Oil. Vitamins A 50,000 IU, D 10,000 IU/g. (Abbott) Bot. 5 ml, 20 ml, 50 ml. Cap.: Vitamins A 5000 IU, D 1000 IU (Ives) Cap.: Vitamins A 5000 IU, D 1700 IU. *otc.*
Use: Vitamin supplement.

●**viprostol.** (vie-PRAHST-ole) USAN.
Use: Hypotensive, vasodilator.

Viquin Forte. (Zeneca) Hydrochloroquine 4%, padimate O 80 mg, dioxybenzone 30 mg, oxybenzone/g 20 mg, stearyl alcohol, cetearyl alcohol, EDTA, sodium metabisulfite/Cream. Tube 28.4 g. SPF 19. PABA-free. *Rx.*
Use: Temporary bleaching of hyperpigmented skin.

Vira-A Ophthalmic. (Parke-Davis) Vidarabine 3%. Tube 3.5 g. *Rx.*
Use: Antiviral, ophthalmic.

Virac. (Ruson) Undecoylium Cl⁻iodine. Iodine complexed with a cationic detergent. Surgical soln. Bot. 2 oz, 8 oz, 1 gal. *otc.*
Use: Antiseptic.

Viracil. (Approved) Phenylephrine HCl 5 mg, hesperidin 50 mg, thenylene HCl 12.5 mg, pyrilamine maleate 12.5 mg, vitamin C 50 mg, salicylamide 2.5 gr, caffeine 0.5 gr, sodium salicylate 1.25 gr/Cap. Bot. 16s, 36s. *otc.*
Use: Decongestant, vitamin supplement, antihistamine, analgesic.

Viramisol. (Seatrace) Adenosine phosphate 25 mg/ml. Vial 10 ml. *otc.*
Use: Relief of varicose vein complications.

Viramune. (Roxane) Nevirapine 200 mg/ Tab. Bot. *Rx.*
Use: Antiviral.

Viranol. (American Dermal) Salycylic acid in collodion gel w/lactic acid, camphor, pyroxylin, ethyl alcohol, ethyl acetate. Gel 8 g. *otc.*
Use: Treatment and removal of plantar and other common warts.

Virazole. (Zeneca) Ribavirin 6 g/Vial. *Rx.*
Use: Antiviral.

●**virginiamycin.** (vihr-JIH-nee-ah-MY-sin) USAN. An antibiotic produced by *Streptomyces virginie.*
Use: Antibacterial.

Viridium. (Vita Elixir) Phenylazodiamino-pyridine HCl 100 mg/Tab.
Use: Urinary tract product.

●**viridofulvin.** (vih-RID-oh-FULL-vin) USAN.

Use: Antifungal.

Virilon. (Star) Methyltestosterone 10 mg/ SR Cap. Bot. 100s, 1000s. *c-III.*
Use: Androgen.

Virogen Herpes Slide Test. (Wampole) Latex agglutination slide test for the detection of herpes simplex virus antigens directly from lesions or cell culture. Test kit 100s.
Use: Diagnostic aid.

Virogen Rotatest. (Wampole) Latex agglutination slide test for the qualitative detection of rotavirus in fecal specimens. Test kit 50s.
Use: Diagnostic aid.

Virogen Rubella Microlatex Test. (Wampole) Latex agglutination microlatex test for the detection of rubella virus antibody in serum. Test kit 500s, 5000s.
Use: Diagnostic aid.

Virogen Rubella Slide Test. (Wampole) Latex agglutination slide test for the detection of rubella virus antibody in serum. Test kit 100s, 500s, 5000s.
Use: Diagnostic aid.

Virogen Rubella Slide Test with Fast Trak Slides. (Wampole) Latex agglutination slide test for the detection of rubella virus antibody in serum.
Use: Diagnostic aid.

Viro-Med Tablets. (Whitehall Robins) Acetaminophen 500 mg, chlorpheniramine maleate 2 mg, pseudoephedrine HCl 30 mg, dextromethorphan HBr 15 mg/Tab. Bot. 20s, 48s. *otc.*
Use: Analgesic, antihistamine, decongestant, antitussive.

Viroptic Ophthalmic Solution. (Glaxo Wellcome) Trifluridine 1%. Bot. 7.5 ml. *Rx.*
Use: Antiviral, ophthalmic.

• **viroxime.** (vie-ROX-eem) USAN.
Use: Antiviral.

Virozyme Injection. (Marcen) Sodium nucleate 2.5%, phenol 0.5%, protein hydrolysate 2.5%, benzyl alcohol 0.2%. Vial 5 ml, 10 ml. *Rx.*
Use: Promote leukocytosis and phagocytosis.

Virugon. Under study. Anhydro bis-(beta-hydroxyethyl) biguanide derivative.
Use: Treatment of influenza, mumps, measles, chicken pox and shingles.

viscarin w/iodine, boric acid, phenol, chlorophyll.
See: Triophyll, Liq. (Schaffer).

Viscoat Solution. (Alcon) Sodium chondroitin sulfate 40 mg, sodium hyaluro-

nate 30 mg, sodium dihydrogen phosphate hydrate 0.45 mg, disodium hydrogen phosphate 2 mg, sodium Cl 4.3 mg/ml. Syringe disposable 0.5 ml. *Rx.*
Use: Viscoelastic solution.

viscum album, extract. Visnico.
Use: Vasodilator.

Visine Allergy Relief. (Pfizer) Tetrahydrozoline HCl 0.05%. Bot. 15 ml, 30 ml. *otc.*
Use: Vasoconstrictor, mydriatic (ophthalmic).

Visine Moisturizing. (Pfizer) Polyethylene glycol 400 1%, tetrahydrozoline HCl 0.05%. Drop Bot. 15 ml, 30 ml. *otc.*
Use: Ophthalmic vasoconstrictor, mydriatic.

Visine L.R. (Pfizer) Oxymetazoline HCl 0.025%. Soln. Bot. 15, 30 ml. *otc.*
Use: Ophthalmic vasoconstrictor, mydriatic.

Vision Care Enzymatic Cleaner. (Alcon) Highly purified pork pancreatin to be diluted in saline solution. Tab. Pkg. 24s. *otc.*
Use: Soft contact lens care.

Visipaque (Nycomed) iodixanol. Iodixanol 270 mg. In 50 ml vials, 100 ml and 200 ml bottles, 150 fill/200 ml bottles, and 100 ml, 150 ml, 200 ml flexible containers. 320 mg iodixanol and 50 ml vials, 100 ml, 200 ml bottles, 150 ml/ fill bottles 100 ml, 150 ml, 200 ml flexible containers.
Use: Diagnostic aid.

Visken. (Sandoz) Pindolol 5 mg or 10 mg/ Tab. Bot. 100s. *Rx.*
Use: Antihypertensive.

Vistacon. (Roberts) Hydroxyzine HCl 50 mg/ml. Vial 10 ml. *Rx.*
Use: Antianxiety.

Vistaquel 50. (Taylor) Hydroxyzine HCl 50 mg/ml. Vial 10 ml. *Rx.*
Use: Antianxiety.

Vistaril. (Pfizer Laboratories) Hydroxyzine pamoate equivalent to hydroxyzine HCl. **Cap.:** 25 mg, 50 mg or 100 mg. Bot. 100s, 500s, UD 100s. **Oral Susp.:** 25 mg/5 ml. Bot. 120 ml, pt. *Rx.*
Use: Antianxiety.

Vistaril I.M. (Roerig) Hydroxyzine HCl. **25 mg/ml:** Vial 10 ml, Box 1s. **50 mg/ ml:** Vial 10 ml, Box 1s.; Vial 1 ml, UD 25s. **100 mg/2 ml:** Vial 2 ml, UD 25s. *Rx.*
Use: Antianxiety.

Vistaril Isoject I.M. (Roerig) Hydroxyzine HCl 50 mg/ml or 100 mg/2 ml Amp. 1 ml, 2 ml. *Rx.*

Use: Antianxiety.

Vistazine 50. (Keene) Hydroxyzine HCl 50 mg/ml. Vial 10 mg/ml. *Rx.*
Use: Antianxiety.

Vistide. (Gilead Sciences) Cidofovir 75 mg/ml/Inj. Amp. 5 ml. *Rx.*
Use: Antiviral.

Visual Eyes. (Optopics) Sodium Cl, sodium phosphate mono- and dibasic, benzalkonium Cl, EDTA. Soln. Bot. 120 ml. *otc.*
Use: Ophthalmic irrigation solution.

Vita-Bee with C Caplets. (Rugby) Vitamins B_1 15 mg, B_2 10.2 mg, B_3 50 mg, B_5 10 mg, B_6 5 mg, C 300 mg/TR Cap. Bot. 100s, 1000s. *otc.*
Use: Vitamin supplement.

Vitabix. (Spanner) Vitamins B_1 100 mg, B_2 2 mg, B_6 5 mg, B_{12} 30 mcg, niacinamide 100 mg, panthenol 10 mg/ml. Vial 10 ml. Multiple dose vial 30 ml. *Rx.*
Use: Vitamin supplement.

Vita-Bob Softgel Capsules. (Scot-Tussin) Vitamins A 5000 IU, D 400 IU, E 30 mg, B_1 1.5 mg, B_2 1.7 mg, B_3 20 mg, B_6 2 mg, B_{12} 6 mcg, C 60 mg, folic acid 0.4 mg/Cap. Bot. 100s. *otc.*
Use: Vitamin supplement.

Vita-C. (Freeda) Ascorbic acid 4 g/tsp. Crystals 100 g, 500 g, 1000 g. *otc.*
Use: Vitamin C supplement.

Vitacarn. (McGaw) L-carnitine 1 g/10 ml. UD Box 50s, 100s. *Rx.*
Use: L-carnitine supplement.

Vit-A-Drops. (Vision Pharm) Vitamin A 5000 IU, polysorbate 80. Bot. 10 ml, 15 ml. *otc.*
Use: Ocular lubricant.

Vitadye. (Zeneca) FD&C yellow No. 5, FD&C red No. 40, FD&C blue No. 1 dyes and dihydroxyacetone 5%. Bot. 0.5 oz, 2 oz. *otc.*
Use: Cosmetic cover for hypopigmented skin.

Vita-Feron. (Vitaline) Iron 150 mg, folic acid 800 mcg, B_{12} 6 mcg. Tab. Bot. 90s. *otc.*
Use: Vitamin/mineral supplement.

Vitafol. (Everett) Iron 90 mg, B_3 39.9 mg, B_6 6 mg, B_{12} 25.02 mcg, folic acid 0.75 mg. Syr. Bot. 473 ml. *Rx.*
Use: Vitamin/mineral supplement.

Vitafol Caplets. (Everett) Iron 65 mg, vitamins A 6000 IU, D 400 IU, E 30 mg, B_1 1.1 mg, B_2 1.8 mg, B_3 15 mg, B_6 2.5 mg, B_{12} 5 mcg, C 60 mg, folic acid 1 mg, calcium/Tab. Bot. 100s, 1000s. *Rx.*
Use: Vitamin/mineral supplement.

Vita-Iron Formula. (Barth's) Iron 120 mg, vitamins B_1 5 mg, B_2 10 mg, C 20 mg, niacin 2 mg, B_{12} 25 mcg, lysine, desiccated liver 200 mg, bromelain/Tab. Bot. 100s, 500s. *otc.*
Use: Vitamin/mineral supplement.

Vita-Kaps Filmtabs. (Abbott) Vitamins A 5000 IU, D 400 IU, B_1 3 mg, B_2 2.5 mg, nicotinamide 20 mg, B_6 1 mg, C 50 mg, B_{12} 3 mcg/Filmtab. Bot. 100s, 1000s. *otc.*
Use: Vitamin supplement.

Vitakaps-M. (Abbott) Vitamins A 5000 IU, D 400 IU, B_1 3 mg, B_2 2.5 mg, nicotinamide 20 mg, B_6 1 mg, B_{12} 3 mcg, C 50 mg, iron 10 mg, copper 1 mg, iodine 0.15 mg, manganese 1 mg, zinc 7.5 mg/Filmtab. Bot. 100s. *otc.*
Use: Vitamin/mineral supplement.

Vita-Kid Chewable Wafers. (Solgar) Vitamins A 10,000 IU, D 400 IU, E 10 mg, B_1 2 mg, B_2 2 mg, B_3 10 mg, B_6 2 mg, B_{12} 5 mcg, C 100 mg, FA 0.3 mg, orange flavor. Tab. Bot. 50s, 100s. *otc.*
Use: Vitamin Supplement.

Vitalax. (Vitalax) Candy base, gumdrop flavored. Pkg. 20s. *otc.*
Use: Laxative.

Vital B-50. (Goldline) Vitamins B_1 50 mg, B_2 50 mg, B_3 50 mg, B_5 50 mg, B_6 50 mg, B_{12} 50 mcg, folic acid 0.1 mg, biotin 50 mcg, PABA, choline bitartrate, inositol/TR Tab. Bot 60s. *otc.*
Use: Vitamin supplement.

Vitalets Tablets. (Freeda) Iron 10 mg, vitamins A 5000 IU, D 400 IU, E 5 mg, B_1 2.5 mg, B_2 0.9 mg, B_3 20 mg, B_5 3 mg, B_6 2 mg, B_{12} 5 mcg, C 60 mg, biotin 25 mcg, Mn, Ca. Chew. Tab. Bot 100s, 250s. *otc.*
Use: Vitamin/mineral supplement.

VitalEyes. (Allergan) Vitamin A 10,000 IU, C 200 mg, E 100 IU, Zn 40 mg, Cu, Se, Mn/Cap. Bot. 60s. *otc.*
Use: Vitamin/mineral supplement.

Vital High Nitrogen. (Ross) Amino acids, partially hydrolyzed whey, meat and soy, hydrolyzed cornstarch, sucrose, safflower oil, MCT mono and diglycerides, soy lecithin, vitamins A, B_1, B_2, B_3, B_5, B_6, B_{12}, C, D, E, K, folic acid, biotin, choline, Ca, P, Mg, Fe, Cu, Zn, Mn, I, Cl. Packet 80 g. *otc.*
Use: Nutritional supplement.

Vitalize SF. (Scot-Tussin) Iron 66 mg, B_1 30 mg, B_6 15 mg, B_{12} 75 mcg, L-lysine 300 mg. Liq. Bot. 120 ml. *otc.*
Use: Iron with vitamin supplement.

Vitamel with Iron. (Eastwood) Drops 50 ml. Chew. Tab. Bot. 100s.

Use: Vitamin/mineral supplement.

•**vitamin A, U.S.P. 23.** Oleovitamin A.
Use: Antixerophthalmic vitamin, emollient.
See: Aquasol A, Drops, Cap., Inj. (Astra USA).
Del-Vi-A, Cap. (Del-Ray).
Palmitate-A 5000, Tab. (Akorn).

vitamin A. (Various Mfr.) Cap. 10,000 IU: 100s, 250s and 1000s. otc.
25,000 IU: 100s, 250s, 500s and 1000s. Rx.
50,000 IU: 100s, 250s, 500s and 1000s. Rx.
Use: Antixerophthalmic vitamin, emollient.

vitamin A acid.
See: tretinoin.

vitamin A, alphalin. (Lilly) Vitamin A 50,000 IU/Gelseal. Bot. 100s. Rx.
Use: Vitamin A supplement.

vitamin A, water miscible, or soluble.
Water-miscible vitamin A.
Use: Vitamin A supplement.

vitamin Bc.
See: Folic Acid (Various Mfr.).

vitamin B₁. Thiamine HCl, U.S.P. 23.
Use: Vitamin B₁ supplement.

vitamin B₁ mononitrate. Thiamine mononitrate.
Use: Vitamin B₁ supplement.

vitamin B₁ w/pancreatin, ox bile extract pepsin, glutamic acid HCl.
See: Maso-Gestive, Tab. (Mason).

vitamin B₁ w/thyroid.
See: T & T, Tab. (Mason).

vitamin B₂. Riboflavin.
Use: Vitamin B₂ supplement.

vitamin B₃. Niacinamide, Nicotinamide.
Use: Vitamin B₃ supplement.

vitamin B₅. Calcium Pantothenate.
Use: Vitamin B₅ supplement.

vitamin B₆. Pyridoxine HCl.
Use: Vitamin B₆ supplement.
See: Hexa-Betalin, Tab. (Lilly).
Hexavibex, Vial (Parke-Davis).

vitamin B₈.
See: Adenosine phosphate.

vitamin B₁₂. Cyanocobalamin. Cobalamine.
See:
Cap., Tab.:
Redisol (Merck).
Vial, Amp.: Bedoce (Lincoln).
Berubigen (Pharmacia & Upjohn).
Betalin-12 (Lilly).
Cabadon-M (Solvay).
Cobadoce Forte (Solvay).
Crysto-Gel (Solvay).

Cyano-Gel, Liq. (Maurry).
Dodex (Organon).
Redisol (Merck).
Rubramin (Squibb).
Ruvite 1000 (Savage).
Sigamine (Sig).
Sytobex-H (Parke-Davis).
Vi-Twel, Inj. (Berlex).
W/Ferrous sulfate, ascorbic acid, folic acid.
See: Intrin, Cap. (Merit).
W/Folic acid, niacinamide, liver.
See: Hepfomin 500, Inj. (Keene Pharm).
W/Thiamine.
See: Cobalin, Vial (Ulmer).
Cyamine, Vial (Keene).
W/Thiamine, vitamin B₆.
See: Orexin, Tab. (Stuart).

vitamin B₁₂. (Various Mfr.) Cyanocobalamin crystalline 100 mcg/ml or 1000 mcg/ml. **100 mcg/ml:** Vials 30 ml.
1000 mcg/ml: Multidose vials 10 ml or 30 ml. Rx.
Use: Vitamin supplement.

vitamin B₁₂. (Goldline) Cyanocobalamin crystalline 500 mcg or 1000 mcg. Tab. Bot. 100s. otc.
Use: Vitamin supplement.

vitamin B₁₂ a & b.
See: Hydroxocobalamin (Various Mfr.).

vitamin B₁₅.
Use: Alleged to increase oxygen supply in blood. Not approved by FDA as a vitamin or drug. Illegal to sell Vitamin B₁₅.

vitamin B complex. Concentrated extract of dried brewer's yeast and extract of corn processed w/Clostridium acetobutylicum.
See: Becotin, Pulvules (Lilly).
Betalin Complex, Amp. (Lilly).
Savaplex, Vial (Savage).

Vitamin B complex 100. (McGuff) Vitamin B₁ 100 mg, B₂ 2 mg, B₃ 100 mg, B₅ 2 mg, B₆ 2 mg/ml/Inj. Vial 10 ml, 30 ml. Rx.
Use: Vitamin supplement.

Vitamin B Complex No. 104. (Century) Vitamins B₁ 100 mg, B₂ 2 mg, B₆ 2 mg, d-panthenol 10 mg, niacinamide 125 mg, benzyl alcohol 1%, gentisic acid ethanolamide 2.5%/Vial 30 ml. Rx.
Use: Vitamin supplement.

Vitamin B Complex, Betalin Complex, Elixir. (Lilly) Vitamins B₁ 2.7 mg, B₂ 1.35 mg, B₁₂ 3 mcg, B₆ 0.555 mg, pantothenic acid 2.7 mg, niacinamide 6.75 mg, liver fraction 500 mg/5 ml, alcohol 17%. Bot. 16 oz. otc.
Use: Vitamin supplement.

Vitamin B Complex w/Vitamin C. (Century) Vitamins B_1 25 mg, B_2 5 mg, B_6 5 mg, niacinamide 50 mg, panthenol 5 mg, calcium 50 mg, propethylene glycol 300 10%, gentisic acid ethanolamide 2.5%, benzyl alcohol 2%/Vial 30 ml. *Rx.*
Use: Vitamin/mineral supplement.

Vitamin B Complex, Betalin Complex Capsules. (Lilly) Vitamins B_1 1 mg, B_2 2 mg, B_6 0.4 mg, pantothenic acid 3.333 mg, niacinamide 10 mg, B_{12} 1 mcg/Pulvule. Bot. 100s. *otc.*
Use: Vitamin supplement.

vitamin C.
See: Ascorbic Acid Preps.

vitamin C, cevalin. (Lilly) Ascorbic acid 250 mg or 500 mg/Tab. Bot. 100s. *otc.*
Use: Vitamin C supplement.

vitamin C w/combinations.
See: Allbee C-800, Prods. (Robins).
Allbee with C, Cap. (Robins).
Allbee-T, Tab. (Robins).
Antiox, Cap. (Mayrand).
Anti-therm, Tab. (Scrip).
Bejectal w/Vitamin C (Abbott).
Colrex, Cap. (Solvay).
Nialexo-C, Tab. (Mallard).
Protegra Softgels, Cap. (Lederle).
Thex, Cap. (Ingram).
Thex Forte, Cap. (Ingram).
Vicon-C, Cap. (Glaxo).
Vicon Forte, Cap. (Glaxo).
Vicon Plus, Cap. (Glaxo).
Vi-Zac, Cap. (Glaxo).
Z-BEC, Tab. (Robins).

vitamin D. Cholecalciferol.
Use: Vitamin D supplement.

vitamin D, deltalin. (Lilly) Vitamin D-2 50,000 units (1.25 mg)/Gelseal. Bot. 100s. *Rx.*
Use: Vitamin D supplement.

vitamin D, synthetic.
See: Activated 7-Dehydro-cholesterol Calciferol.

vitamin D-1.
See: Dihydrotachysterol.

vitamin D-2. Activated ergasterol, Ergocalciferol.
See: Calciferol, Preps. (Various Mfr.).
Drisdol, Liq. (Winthrop Pharm).
Viosterol (Various Mfr.).

vitamin D-3.
See: Activated 7-dehydrocholesterol. Calciferol Prep. for related activity.

vitamin D-3-cholesterol. Compound of crystalline vitamin D-3 and cholesterol.

vitamin D-4.
See: Dihydrotachysterol, Preps. (Various Mfr.).

• **vitamin E,** U.S.P. 23.
Use: Vitamin E supplement.
See: Aquasol E (Rhone-Poulenc Rorer).
Eprolin, Gelseal (Lilly).
E-Vites, Cap. (Quality Generics).
Lactinol-E Creme (Pedinol).
Tocopher, Prod. (Quality Generics).
Tocopherol, Preps. (Various Mfr.).
Wheat Germ Oil (Various Mfr.).

vitamin E, eprolin. (Lilly) Alpha-tocopherol 100 units/Gelseal. Bot. 100s.
Use: Vitamin E supplement.

vitamin E w/quinine sulfate, niacin.
See: Myodyne, Tab. (Paddock).

vitamin F.
See: Fats, Unsaturated.
Fatty Acids, Unsaturated.

vitamin G.
See: Riboflavin.

vitamin K.
See: Hykinone, Amp. (Abbott).
Menadiol, Sodium Diphosphate, Preps. (Various Mfr.).
Menadione, Preps. (Various Mfr.).
Menadione Sodium Bisulfite, Preps. (Various Mfr.).

vitamin K-1.
See: Phytonadione, U.S.P. 23.

vitamin K-3.
See: Menadione, U.S.P. 23.

vitamin K oxide. Not available, but usually K-1 is desired.

vitamin M.
See: Folic Acid, U.S.P. 23.

vitamin-mineral-supplement liquid.
(Pennex) Vitamins B_1 0.83 mg, B_2 0.42 mg, B_3 8.3 mg, B_5 1.67 mg, B_6 0.17 mg, B_{12} 0.17 mcg, I, Fe 2.5 mg, Mg, Zn 0.3 mg, Mn, choline, alcohol 18%. Liq. 473 ml. *otc.*
Use: Vitamin/mineral supplement.

vitamin P. Citrin.
See: Bio-Flavonoid Compounds (Various Mfr.).
Hesperidin Preps. (Various Mfr.).
Quercetin (Various Mfr.).
Rutin, Preps. (Various Mfr.).

vitamin T. Sesame seed factor, termite factor.
Use: Claimed to aid proper blood coagulation and promote formation of blood platelets. Not approved by FDA as an active vitamin.

vitamin U. Present in cabbage juice.

vitamin, maintenance formula.
See: Stuart Formula, Tab., Liq. (Stuart).
Vi-Magna, Cap. (Lederle).

vitamins: stress formula.

See: Cebefortis, Tab. (Pharmacia & Upjohn).
Folbesyn, Tab., Vial (Lederle).
Probec-T, Tab. (Stuart).
Stresscaps, Cap. (Lederle).
Stresscaps With Iron (Lederle).
Stresscaps With Zinc (Lederle).
StressForm "605" w/ Iron, Tab. (NBTY).
Stress Formula with Iron, Tab. (NBTY).
Stresstabs-600 (Lederle).
Thera-combex Kap. (Parke-Davis).

vitamins w/antiobesity agents.
See: Fetamin, Tab. (Mission).
Obedrin, Cap. or Tab. (Massengill).

vitamins w/liver & lipotropic agents.
See: Heptuna, Cap. (Roerig).
Lederplex, Preps. (Lederle).
Livitamin, Preps. (SK-Beecham).
Metheponex, Cap. (Rawl).
Methischol, Cap. (Rhone-Poulenc Rorer).

Vita Natal. (Scot-Tussin) Folic acid 1 mg/ Tab. Bot. 100s. *Rx.*
Use: Folic acid supplement.

Vitaneed. (Biosearch) P-beef, Ca and Na caseinates, CHO-maltodextrin. F-partially hydrogenated soy oil, mono and diglycerides, soy lecithin. Protein 35 g, CHO 125 g, fat 40 g, sodium 500 mg, potassium 1250 mg/L, 1 Cal/ml, 375 mOsm/kg H_20. Liq. Ready-to-use 250 ml. *otc.*
Use: Nutritional supplement.

Vitaon. (Vita Elixir) Vitamin B_{12} 25 mcg, thiamine HCl 10 mg, ferric pyrophosphate 250 mg/5 ml. *otc.*
Use: Vitamin supplement.

Vita-Plus B12. (Scot-Tussin) Vitamin B_{12} 1000 mcg/ml. Inj. *Rx.*
Use: Vitamin B_{12} supplement.

Vita-Plus E. (Scot-Tussin) Vitamin E 294 mg as d-alpha tocopheryl acetate/Cap. *otc.*
Use: Vitamin E supplement.

Vita-Plus G Softgel. (Scot-Tussin) Vitamins A 5000 IU, D 400 IU, E 10 IU, B_1 5 mg, B_2 5 mg, B_3 15 mg, B_5 5 mg, B_6 1 mg, B_{12} 1 mcg, C 50 mg, iron 3.3 mg, Ca 145 mg, Zn 0.5 mg, K, Mg, Mn, P, I, Cu, choline, l-lysine, inositol/Cap. Bot. 100s. *otc.*
Use: Vitamin/mineral supplement.

Vita-Plus H Softgel. (Scot-Tussin) Iron 13.4 mg, vitamins A 5000 IU, D 400 IU, E 3 IU, B_1 3 mg, B_2 2.5 mg, B_3 20 mg, B_5 5 mg, B_6 1.5 mg, B_{12} 2.5 mcg, C 50 mg, Ca, K, Mg, Mn, P, Zn 1.4 mg/ Cap. Bot. 100s. *otc.*

Use: Vitamin/mineral supplement.

Vita-Plus H Liquid Sugar Free. (Scot-Tussin) Vitamins B_1 30 mg, l-lysine monohydrochloride 300 mg, B_{12} 75 mcg, B_6 15 mg, iron pyrophosphate soluble 100 mg/5 ml. Bot. 4 oz, 8 oz, pt, gal. *otc.*
Use: Vitamin/mineral supplement.

Vita-PMS. (Bajamar) Vitamins A 2083 IU, E 16.7 IU, D_3 16.7 IU, folic acid 33 mcg, B_1 4.2 mg, B_2 4.2 mg, B_3 4.2 mg, B_5 4.2 mg, B_6 50 mg, B_{12} 10.4 mcg, biotin, C 250 mg, Ca, Mg, I, Fe, Cu, Zn 4.2 mg, Mn, K, Se, Cr, betaine/Tab. Bot. 100s. *otc.*
Use: Vitamin/mineral supplement.

Vita-PMS Plus. (Bajamar) Vitamins A 667 IU, E 16.7 IU, D_3 16.7 IU, folic acid 33 mcg, B_1 4.2 mg, B_2 4.2 mg, B_3 4.2 mg, B_5 4.2 mg, B_6 16.7 mg, B_{12} 10.4 mcg, biotin, C 250 mg, Mg, I, Ca, Fe, Cu, Zn 4.2 mg, Mn, K, Se, Cr, betaine/ Tab. Bot. 100s. *otc.*
Use: Vitamin/mineral supplement.

Vita-Ray Creme. (Gordon) Vitamins E 3000 IU, A 200,000 IU/oz w/aloe 10%. Jar 0.5 oz, 2.5 oz. *otc.*
Use: Emollient.

Vitarex. (Taylor) Vitamins A 10,000 IU, D 200 IU, B_1 15 mg, B_2 10 mg, B_6 5 mg, B_{12} 5 mcg, C 250 mg, B_3 100 mg, B_5 20 mg, E 15 mg, iron 15 mg, Ca, Cu, I, K, Mg, Mn, P, Zn 10 mg/Tab. Bot. 100s. *otc.*
Use: Vitamin/mineral supplement.

Vitazin. (Mesemer) Ascorbic acid 300 mg, niacinamide 100 mg, thiamine mononitrate 20 mg, d-calcium pantothenate 20 mg, riboflavin 10 mg, pyridoxine HCl 5 mg, magnesium sulfate 70 mg, zinc 25 mg/Cap. Bot. 100s. *otc.*
Use: Vitamin/mineral supplement.

Vita-Zoo. (Towne) Vitamins A 2500 IU, D 400 IU, E 15 IU, C 60 mg, folic acid 0.3 mg, B_1 1.05 mg, B_2 1.2 mg, niacin 13.5 mg, B_6 1.05 mg, B_{12} 4.5 mcg/Tab. Bot. 100s. *otc.*
Use: Vitamin supplement.

Vita-Zoo Plus Iron. (Towne) Vitamins A 2500 IU, D 400 IU, E 15 IU, C 60 mg, folic acid 0.3 mg, B_1 1.05 mg, B_2 1.2 mg, niacin 13.5 mg, B_6 1.05 mg, B_{12} 4.5 mcg, iron 15 mg/Tab. Bot. 100s. *otc.*
Use: Vitamin/mineral supplement.

Vitec. (Pharmaceutical Specialties) Dl-alpha tocopheryl acetate in a vanishing cream base. Cream. 120 g. *otc.*
Use: Emollient.

Vitormains. (Roberts) Tab. Bot. 100s.
Use: Vitamin supplement.

Vitrasert. (Chiron Vision) Ganciclovir 4.5 mg (released over 5 to 8 months)/Intravitreal implant. Box. 1. *Rx.*
Use: To treat CMV retinitis in AIDS patients.

Vitron-C. (Novartis) Ferrous fumarate 200 mg, ascorbic acid 125 mg/Tab. Bot. 100s, 1000s. *otc.*
Use: Vitamin/mineral supplement.

Vitron-C Plus Tablets. (Novartis) Ferrous fumarate 400 mg, vitamin C 250 mg/Tab. Bot. 30s, 100s, 500s. *otc.*
Use: Vitamin/mineral supplement.

Vivactil. (Merck) Protriptyline HCl 5 mg or 10 mg/Tab. **5 mg:** Bot. 100s. **10 mg:** Bot. 100s, UD 100s. *Rx.*
Use: Antidepressant.

Viva-Drops. (Vision Pharm) Polysorbate 80, sodium Cl, EDTA, retinyl palmitate, mannitol, sodium citrate, pyruvate. Soln. Bot. 10 ml, 15 ml. *otc.*
Use: Artificial tears.

Vivarin. (SK-Beecham) Caffeine alkaloid 200 mg/Tab. Blister Pk. 16s, 40s, 80s. *otc.*
Use: CNS stimulant.

Vivikon. (Zeneca) Vitamins B_1 5 mg, B_2 2 mg, B_6 10 mg, d-panthenol 5 mg, niacinamide 10 mg, procaine HCl 2%/ml. 100 ml. *otc.*
Use: Vitamin supplement.

Vivonex Flavor Packets. (Procter & Gamble) Non-nutritive flavoring for Vivonex diets when consumed orally. Orange-pineapple, lemon-lime, strawberry and vanilla. Pkg. 60s. *otc.*
Use: Flavoring.

Vivonex, Standard. (Procter & Gamble) Free amino acid/complete enteral nutrition. Six packets provide kilocalories 1800, available nitrogen 5.88 g as amino acids 37 g, fat 2.61 g, carbohydrate 407 g, and full day's balanced nutrition. Calorie:nitrogen ratio is 300:1. Unflavored pow. Packet 80 g, Pkg. 6s. *otc.*
Use: Nutritional supplement.

Vivonex T.E.N. (Procter & Gamble) Free amino acid, high nitrogen/high branched chain amino acid complete enteral nutrition. Ten packets provide kilocalories 3000, available nitrogen 17 g, amino acids 115 g, fat 8.33 g, carbohydrate 617 g and full day's balanced nutrition. Calorie:nitrogen ratio is 175:1. Unflavored pow. Packet 80 g, Pkg. 10s. *otc.*
Use: Nutritional supplement.

Vivotif Berna. (Berna) Typhoid vaccine (oral). *S. typhi* Ty21a (viable) 2 to 6 × 10⁹ colony forming units and *S. typhi* Ty21a² (non-viable) 5 to 50 × 10⁹ colony forming units/Cap. Single foil blister with 4 doses. *Rx.*
Use: Agent for immunization.

Vi-Zac. (Whitby) Vitamins A 5000 IU, E 50 IU, C 500 mg, Zn 18 mg, lactose. Bot. 60s. *otc.*
Use: Vitamin/mineral supplement.

V-Lax. (Century) Psyllium mucilloid (hydrophilic) 50%, dextrose 50%. Pow. 0.25 lb, 1 lb. *otc.*
Use: Laxative.

Vlemasque. (Dermik) Sulfurated lime topical solution 6% (Vleminck's Soln.), alcohol 7% in drying clay mask. Jar 4 oz. *otc.*
Use: Antiacne.

VM. (Last) Vitamins B_1 6 mg, B_2 4 mg, niacinamide 40 mg, iron 100 mg, calcium 188 mg, phosphorus 188 mg, manganese 4 mg, alcohol 12%. Bot. 16 oz. *otc.*
Use: Vitamin/mineral supplement.

V-M Capsules. (Pal-Pak) Vitamins A, D, B_1, B_2, B_6, C, niacinamide, Ca, Fe, calcium pantothenate, Mg, Mn, K, Zn, P/Tab. Bot. 100s, 1000s. *otc.*
Use: Vitamin/mineral supplement.

•**volazocine.** (voe-LAY-zoe-SEEN) USAN.
Under study.
Use: Analgesic.

Volidan. (British Drug House) Megestrol acetate. *Rx.*
Use: Hormone.

Volitane. (Trent) Parethoxycaine 0.2%, hexachlorophene 0.025%, dichlorophene 0.025%. Aerosol spray can 3 oz. *otc.*
Use: Counterirritant, antiseptic.

Volmax tablets. (Muro) Albuterol sufate 4 mg or 8 mg. ER Tab. Bot. UD 60s. *Rx.*
Use: Bronchodilator.

Voltaren. (Novartis) Diclofenac sodium 25 mg, 50 mg, 75 mg. Tab. **25 mg:** Bot. 60s, 100s, UD 100s; **50 mg, 75 mg:** Bot. 60s, 100s, 1000s, UD 100s. *Rx.*
Use: Nonsteroidal anti-inflammatory, analgesic.

Voltaren-XR. (Novartis) Diclofenac sodium 100 mg, sucrose/E.R. Tab. 100s, UD 100s. *Rx.*
Use: Nonsteroidal anti-inflammatory, analgesic.

Voltaren, Ophthalmic Solution. (Ciba Vision) Diclofenac sodium. 0.1%. Soln. Bot. 2.5, 5 ml w/dropper. *Rx.*

Use: Nonsteroidal anti-inflammatory, ophthalmic.

vonedrine hydrochloride. Vonedrine (phenylpropylmethylamine) HCl. *otc.*
Use: Decongestant.

Vontrol. (SK-Beecham) Diphenidol 25 mg as HCl/Tab. Bot. 100s. *Rx.*
Use: Antiemetic, antivertigo.

•**vorozole.** (VORE-oh-zole) USAN.
Use: Antineoplastic.

Vortel. Clorprenaline HCl.
Use: Bronchodilator.

Vosol HC Otic Solution. (Wallace) Propylene glycol diacetate 3%, acetic acid 2%, benzethonium Cl 0.02%, hydrocortisone 1%. Bot. 10 ml. *Rx.*
Use: Otic preparation.

Vosol Otic Solution. (Wallace) Propylene glycol diacetate 3%, acetic acid 2%, benzethonium Cl 0.02%, sodium acetate 0.015%. Bot. 15 ml, 30 ml. *Rx.*
Use: Otic preparation.

•**votumumab.** (vah-TOOM-uh-mab) USAN.
Use: Monoclonal antibody.

Voxsuprine Tabs. (Major) Isoxsuprine HCl 10 mg or 20 mg/Tab. Bot. 100s, 250s, 1000s, UD 100s. *Rx.*
Use: Vasodilator.

V-Tuss Expectorant. (Vangard) Hydrocodone bitartrate 5 mg, pseudoephedrine HCl 60 mg, guaifenesin 200 mg/5 ml, alcohol 12.5%. *c-III.*
Use: Antitussive, decongestant, expectorant.

Vumon. (Bristol-Myers Oncology) Teniposide 10 mg/ml. Amp. 5 ml. *Rx.*
Use: Antineoplastic.

V.V.S. (Econo Med) Sulfathiazole 3.42%, sulfacetamide 2.86%, sulfabenzamide 3.7%, urea 0.64%. Cream. Tube 90 g w/applicator. *Rx.*
Use: Vaginal preparation, anti-infective.

Vytone Cream. (Dermik) Hydrocortisone 1%, iodoquinol 1%, greaseless base. Cream. Bot. 30 g. *Rx.*
Use: Corticosteroid, anti-infective, topical.

VZIG. (Varicella-Zoster Immune Globulin) Human (American Red Cross, Northeast Region; Massachusetts Public Health Biologic Laboratories) Globulin fraction of human plasma, primarily 1 G/10% to 18% in single dose vials containing 125 units varicella-zoster virus antibody in 2.5 mg or less. Inj.
Use: Immune serum.

W

Wade Gesic Balm. (Wade) Menthol 3%, methyl salicylate 12%, petrolatum base. Tube oz, Jar lb. *otc.*
Use: Analgesic, topical.

Wade's Drops. Compound Benzoin Tincture.

Wakespan. (Weeks & Leo) Caffeine 250 mg/TR Cap. Vial 15s. *Rx.*
Use: CNS stimulant.

Wal-Finate Allergy Tabs. (Walgreen) Chlorpheniramine maleate 4 mg/Tab. Bot. 50s. *otc.*
Use: Antihistamine.

Wal-Finate Decongestant Tabs. (Walgreen) Chlorpheniramine maleate 4 mg, pseudoephedrine sulfate 60 mg/Tab. Bot. 50s. *otc.*
Use: Antihistamine, decongestant.

Wal-Formula Cough Syrup with D-Methorphan. (Walgreen) Dextromethorphan HBr 15 mg, doxylamine succinate 7.5 mg, sodium citrate 500 mg/10 ml. Bot. 6 oz, 8 oz. *otc.*
Use: Antitussive, antihistamine, expectorant.

Wal-Formula D Cough Syrup. (Walgreen) Dextromethorphan HBr 20 mg, phenylpropanolamine HCl 25 mg, guaifenesin 100 mg/10 ml, alcohol 10%. Bot. 6 oz, 8 oz. *otc.*
Use: Antitussive, decongestant, expectorant.

Wal-Formula M Cough Syrup. (Walgreen) Dextromethorphan HBr 30 mg, pseudoephedrine HCl 60 mg, guaifenesin 200 mg, acetaminophen 500 mg/20 ml Bot. 8 oz. *otc.*
Use: Antitussive, decongestant, expectorant, analgesic.

Wal-Frin Nasal Mist. (Walgreen) Phenylephrine HCl 0.5%, pheniramine maleate 0.2% Bot. 0.5 oz. *otc.*
Use: Decongestant, antihistamine.

Walgreen Artificial Tears. (Walgreen) Hydroxypropyl methylcellulose 0.5%. Bot. 0.5 oz. *otc.*
Use: Artificial tear solution.

Walgreen's Finest Iron Tablets. (Walgreen) Iron 30 mg/Tab. Bot. 100s. *otc.*
Use: Iron supplement.

Walgreen's Finest Vit B$_6$. (Walgreen) Pyridoxine HCl 50 mg/Tab. Bot. 100s. *otc.*
Use: Vitamin B$_6$ supplement.

Walgreen Soda Mints. (Walgreen) Sodium bicarbonate 300 mg/Tab. Bot. 100s, 200s. *otc.*
Use: Antacid.

Wal-Minic. (Walgreen) Phenylpropanolamine HCl 12.5 mg, guaifenesin 100 mg/5 ml, alcohol 5%. Bot. 6 oz, 8 oz. *otc.*
Use: Decongestant, expectorant.

Wal-Minic Cold Relief Medicine. (Walgreen) Phenylpropanolamine HCl 12.5 mg, chlorpheniramine maleate 2 mg/5 ml Bot. 6 oz, 8 oz. *otc.*
Use: Decongestant, antihistamine.

Wal-Minic DM. (Walgreen) Phenylpropanolamine HCl 12.5 mg, dextromethorphan HBr 10 mg/5 ml Bot. 6 oz, 8 oz. *otc.*
Use: Decongestant, antitussive.

Wal-Phed Plus. (Walgreen) Pseudoephedrine HCl 60 mg, chlorpheniramine maleate 4 mg/Tab. Bot. 50s. *otc.*
Use: Decongestant, antihistamine.

Wal-Phed Syrup. (Walgreen) Pseudoephedrine HCl 30 mg/5 ml. Bot. 4 oz. *otc.*
Use: Decongestant.

Wal-Phed Tablets. (Walgreen) Pseudoephedrine HCl 30 mg/Tab. Bot. 50s, 100s. *otc.*
Use: Decongestant.

Wal-Tap Elixir. (Walgreen) Brompheniramine maleate 2 mg, phenylpropanolamine HCl 12.5 mg/5 ml. Bot. 4 oz. *otc.*
Use: Antihistamine, decongestant.

Wal-Tussin. (Walgreen) Guaifenesin 100 mg/5 ml. Bot. 4 oz. *otc.*
Use: Expectorant.

Wal-Tussin DM. (Walgreen) Guaifenesin 100 mg, dextromethorphan HBr 15 ml/5 ml. Bot. 4 oz, 8 oz. *otc.*
Use: Expectorant, antitussive.

Wampole One-Step hCG. (Wampole) For in vitro detection of human chorionic gonadotropin in serum and urine. Test. In 3, 24, 96, 500 test kits.
Use: Pregnancy test.

•**warfarin sodium,** (WORE-fuh-rin) U.S.P. 23.
Use: Anticoagulant.
See: Coumadin Sodium, Tab., Inj. (DuPont Merck).
Panwarfin, Tab. (Abbott).

Wart Fix. (Last) Castor oil 100%. Bot. 0.3 fl oz. *otc.*
Use: Wart removal.

Wart-Off. (Pfizer) Salicylic acid 17% in flexible collodion, alcohol 20.5%, ether 54.2%. Bot. 0.5 oz. *otc.*
Use: Keratolytic.

wasp vemon. *Rx.*
Use: Agent for immunization.

See: Albay (Bayer).
Pharmalgen (ALK Laboratories).
Venomil (Bayer).

•**water for injection,** U.S.P. 23.
Use: Pharmaceutic aid (solvent).

•**water O 15,** Inj., U.S.P. 23.
Use: Diagnostic aid (radioactive, vascular disorders), radioactive agent.

Water Babies Little Licks by Coppertone. (Schering-Plough) SPF 30, ethylhexyl p-methoxycinnamate, oxybenzone, 2-ethylhexyl salicylate, cherry flavor. Tube 4.8 g. *otc.*
Use: Sunscreen.

Water Babies Sunblock Cream. (Schering-Plough) SPF 25, ethylhexyl p-methoxycinnamate, 2-ethylhexyl salicylate, homosalate, oxybenzone, benzyl alcohol. PABA free, waterproof. Cream. Bot. 90 g. *otc.*
Use: Sunscreen.

Water Babies UVA/UVB Sunblock Lotion. (Schering-Plough) SPF 30 ethylhexyl p-methoxycinnamate, 2-ethylhexyl salicylate, homosalate, oxybenzone, benzyl alcohol. PABA free, waterproof. Lot. Bot. 120 ml, 240 ml. *otc.*
Use: Sunscreen.

Water Babies UVA/UVB Sunblock Lotion. (Schering-Plough) SPF 45, ethylhexyl p-methoxycinnamate, 2-ethylhexyl salicylate, otocrylene oxybenzone, benzyl alcohol. PABA free, waterproof. Lot. Bot. 120 ml. *otc.*
Use: Sunscreen.

Water Babies UVA/UVB Sunblock Lotion. (Schering-Plough) Ethylhexyl-p-methoxycinnamate, oxybenzone in lotion base, SPF-15. Bot. 120 ml. *otc.*
Use: Sunscreen.

watermelon seed extract. Citrin (Table Rock).

watermelon seed extract. W/Phenobarbital, theobromine. Cithal (Table Rock).

•**water, purified,** U.S.P. 23.
Use: Pharmaceutic aid (solvent).

•**wax, carnauba,** N.F. 18.
Use: Pharmaceutic aid (tablet coating agent).

•**wax, emulsifying,** N.F. 18.
Use: Pharmaceutic aid (emulsifying, stiffening agent).

•**wax, microcrystalline,** N.F. 18.
Use: Pharmaceutic aid (stiffening, tablet coating agent).

•**wax, white,** N.F. 18.
Use: Pharmaceutic aid (stiffening agent).

•**wax, yellow,** N.F. 18.
Use: Pharmaceutic aid (stiffening agent).

Waxsol. Docusate Sodium, U.S.P. 23.

Wayds. (Wayne) Docusate sodium 100 mg/Cap. Bot. 100s. *otc.*
Use: Laxative.

Wayds-Plus Capsules. (Wayne) Docusate w/casanthranol. Bot. 50s. *otc.*
Use: Laxative.

Wayne-E Capsules. (Wayne) Vitamin E 100 IU or 200 IU/Cap.: Bot. 1000s. 400 IU/Cap.: Bot. 100s. *otc.*
Use: Vitamin E supplement.

Wehless. (Roberts) Phendimetrazine tartrate 35 mg/Cap. Bot. 100s. *c-III.*
Use: Anorexiant.

Wehless-105 Timecelles. (Roberts) Phendimetrazine tartrate 105 mg/SA Cap. Bot. 100s. *c-III.*
Use: Anorexiant.

Wehydryl. (Roberts) Diphenhydramine HCl 50 mg/ml. Vial 10 ml. *Rx.*
Use: Antihistamine.

Welders Eye Lotion. (Weber) Tetracaine, potassium Cl, boric acid, camphor, glycerin, disodium edetate, benzalkonium Cl as preservatives. Bot. oz. *otc.*
Use: Burn preparation.

Wellbutrin. (Glaxo Wellcome) Bupropion 75 mg or 100 mg/Tab. Bot. 100s. *Rx.*
Use: Antidepressant.

Wellbutrin SR. (Glaxo Wellcome) Bupropion HCl 100 mg/ER Tab. Bot. 60s.
Use: Antidepressant.

Wellcovorin. (Glaxo Wellcome) Leucovorin 5 mg or 25 mg as calcium. **Tab.: 5 mg:** Bot. 20s, 100s, UD 50s. **25 mg:** Bot. 25s, UD 10s. **Pow. for Inj.:** 100 mg/vial as calcium. *Rx.*
Use: Prophylaxis and treatment of the undesired hematopoietic effects of folic acid antagonists.

Wernet's Adhesive Cream. (Block) Carboxymethylcellulose gum, ethylene oxide polymer, petrolatum in mineral oil base. Cream. Tube 1.5 oz. *otc.*
Use: Denture adhesive.

Wernet's Powder. (Block) Karaya gum, ethylene oxide polymer. Bot. 0.63 oz, 1.75 oz, 3.55 oz. *otc.*
Use: Denture adhesive.

Wes-B/C. (Western Research) Vitamins B_1 15 mg, B_2 10 mg, B_6 5 mg, niacinamide 50 mg, calcium pantothenate 10 mg, C 300 mg/Cap. Bot. 1000s. *otc.*
Use: Vitamin/mineral supplement.

Wesmatic Forte Tablets. (Wesley) Phenobarbital ⅛ gr, ephedrine sulfate 0.25 gr, chlorpheniramine maleate 2

mg, guaifenesin 100 mg/Tab. Bot. 100s, 1000s. *Rx.*
Use: Sedative, hypnotic, decongestant, antihistamine, expectorant.

Westcort Cream. (Westwood-Squibb) Hydrocortisone valerate 0.2% in a hydrophilic base with white petrolatum. Tube 15 g, 45 g, 60 g, 120 g. *Rx.*
Use: Corticosteroid, topical.

Westcort Ointment. (Westwood-Squibb) Hydrocortisone valerate 0.2% in hydrophilic base with white petrolatum, mineral oil. Tube 15 g, 45 g, 60 g. *Rx.*
Use: Corticosteroid, topical.

Westhroid. (Western Research) Thyroid 0.5 gr, 1 gr, 2 gr, 3 gr or 4 gr/Tab.; 5 gr/ SC Tab. Handicount 28s (36 bags of 28s). *Rx.*
Use: Thyroid hormone.

Westrim. (Western Research) Phenylpropanolamine HCl 37.5 mg/Tab. Bot. 100s. *otc.*
Use: Nonprescription diet aid, decongestant.

Westrim-LA 50. (Western Research) Phenylpropanolamine HCl 50 mg/TR Cap. Bot. 1000s. *otc.*
Use: Nonprescription diet aid, decongestant.

Westrim-LA 75. (Western Research) Phenylpropanolamine HCl 75 mg/TR Cap. Bot. 1000s. *otc.*
Use: Nonprescription diet aid, decongestant.

Wesvite. (Western Research) Vitamins B₁ 10 mg, B₂ 5 mg, B₆ 2 mg, pantothenic acid 10 mg, niacinamide 30 mg, B₁₂ 3 mcg, C 100 mg, E 5 IU, A 10,000 IU, D 400 IU, iron 15 mg, copper 1 mg, iodine 0.15 mg, manganese 1 mg, zinc 1.5 mg/Tab. Bot. 1000s. *otc.*
Use: Vitamin/mineral supplement.

Wet-n-Soak. (Allergan) Borate buffered. WSCP 0.006%, hydroxyethylcellulose. Soln. Bot. 15 ml. *otc.*
Use: Hard contact lens care.

Wet-n-Soak Plus. (Allergan). Polyvinyl alcohol, edetate disodium, benzalkonium Cl 0.003%. Soln. Bot. 120 ml, 180 ml. *otc.*
Use: Contact lens care.

Wetting Solution. (Pilkington Barnes Hind) Polyvinyl alcohol, benzalkonium Cl 0.004%, EDTA 0.02%. Soln. Bot. 60 ml. *otc.*
Use: Hard contact lens care.

Wetting and Soaking. (Pilkington Barnes Hind) Buffered, isotonic. Chlorhexidine gluconate 0.005%, EDTA 0.02%,

NaCl, octylphenoxy (oxyethylene) ethanol, povidone, polyvinyl alcohol, propylene glycol, hydroxyethylcellulose. Soln. Bot. 120 ml. *otc.*
Use: Hard contact lens care.

Wetting and Soaking Solution. (Bausch & Lomb) Chlorhexidine gluconate 0.006%, EDTA 0.05%, cationic cellulose derivative polymer. Bot. 118 ml. *otc.*
Use: Disinfecting, wetting, soaking solution.

wheat germ oil. (Viobin) **Liq.:** Bot. 4 oz, 8 oz, pt, qt. **Cap.: 3 min.** Bot. 100s, 400s; **6 min.** Bot. 100s, 225s, 400s; **20 min.** Bot. 100s. *otc.*
Use: Vitamin E supplement.

wheat germ oil. (Various Mfr.).
See: Natural Wheat Germ Oil, Cap., Oint. (Spirt).
Natural Viobin Wheat Germ Oil, Liq. (Spirt).
Tocopherol Preps. (Various Mfr.).
Use: Vitamin E supplement.

Wheat Germ Oil Concentrate. (Thurston) Perles. 6 min. Bot. 100s. *otc.*
Use: Heart disorders, heart muscle fatigue.

whey protein concentrate (bovine).
See: bovine whey protein concentrate.

Whirl-Sol. (Sween) Moisturizing bath additive. Bot. 2 oz, 8 oz, 16 oz, 21 oz, gal, 5 gal, 30 gal, 55 gal. *otc.*
Use: Emollient.

white-faced hornet venom. *Rx.*
Use: Agent for immunization.
See: Albay (Bayer).
Pharmalgen (ALK Laboratories).
Venomil (Bayer).

•**white lotion,** U.S.P. 23. Lotio Alba.
Use: Astringent, topical protectant.
See: Lotioblanc, Lot. (Arnar-Stone).

white precipitate.
See: Ammoniated Mercury, U.S.P. 23.

Whitfield's Ointment. (Various Mfr.) Benzoic acid 6%, salicylic acid 3%. *otc.*
Use: Anti-infective, topical.

whooping cough vaccine.
See: Acel-Imune, Vial (Wyeth Lederle).
ActHIB/DTP, Set of DTwP vial plus Hib Pow. for Inj. (Connaught).
diphtheria and tetanus toxoids with pertussis vaccine (Various Mfr.).
Pertussis Vaccine, U.S.P. 23.
Tetramune, Vial (Wyeth Lederle).
Tri-Immunol, Vial (Wyeth Lederle).
Tripedia, Vial (Connaught).

Whorton's Calamine Lotion. (Whorton) Calamine, zinc oxide, glycerin (U.S.P. strength) in carboxymethylcellulose lo-

tion vehicle. Bot. 4 oz, gal. *otc.*
Use: Minor skin irritations.

Wibi Lotion. (Galderma) Purified water, SD alcohol 40, glycerin, PEG-4, PEG-6-32 stearate, PEG-6-32, glycol stearate, carbomer 940, PEG-75, methylparaben, propylparaben, triethanolamine, menthol, fragrance. Bot. 8 oz, 16 oz. *otc.*
Use: Emollient.

widow spider species antivenin (latrodectus mactans). (Merck) Antivenin, Lactrodectus mactans, U.S.P. 23.
Use: Passive immunizing agent.

Wigraine. (Organon) Ergotamine tartrate 1 mg, caffeine 100 mg/Tab. or Supp. **Tab.:** Box 20s, 100s. **Supp.:** Box 12s. *Rx.*
Use: Agent for migraine.

wild cherry.
Use: Flavored vehicle.

Wilpowr. (Foy) Phentermine HCl 30 mg/Cap. Bot. 100s, 500s, 1000s.
Use: Anorexiant.

Wilpor-Clear. (Foy) Phentermine HCl 30 mg/Cap. Bot. 1000s. *c-iv.*
Use: Anorexiant.

WinRho SD. (Univax) RHo(D) immune globulin IV human. 600 IU or 1500 IU. Vial 2.5 ml (10s). *Rx.*
Use: Prevention of Rh isoimmunization; immune thrombocytopenic purpura.

Winstrol. (Sanofi Winthrop) Stanozolol 2 mg/Tab. Bot. 100s. *c-iii.*
Use: Anabolic steroid.

Wintergreen Sucrets. (SK-Beecham) Dyclonine HCl 0.1%, alcohol 10%, sorbitol. Spray. Bot. 90 ml. *otc.*
Use: Mouth and throat product.

•**witch hazel,** U.S.P. 23.
Use: Astringent.

witch hazel. (Various Mfr.) Hamamelis water (Witch Hazel). Bot. 120 ml, 240 ml, 280 ml, 480 ml, 960 ml, gal.
Use: Astringent.

Within. (Bayer) Vitamins A 5000 IU, E 30 IU, C 60 mg, folic acid 0.4 mg, B_1 1.5 mg, B_2 1.7 mg, niacin 20 mg, B_6 2 mg, B_{12} 6 mcg, pantothenic acid 10 mg, D 400 IU, iron 27 mg, calcium 450 mg, zinc 15 mg/Tab. Bot. 60s, 100s. *otc.*
Use: Vitamin/mineral supplement.

WNS Suppositories. (Sanofi Winthrop) Sulfamylon HCl. *Rx.*
Use: Anorectal preparation.

Wonderful Dream Salve. (Kondon) Phenylmercuric nitrate 1:5000, oils of tar, turpentine, olive and linseed oil, rosin, burgundy pitch, camphor.

Wonder Ice. (Pedinol) Menthol in a specially formulated base. Gel. Tube 113 g. *otc.*
Use: Liniment.

Wondra. (Procter & Gamble) Petrolatum, lanolin acid, glycerin, stearyl alcohol, cyclomethicone, EDTA, hydrogenated vegetable glycerides phosphate, cetyl alcohol, isopropyl palmitate, stearic acid, PEG-100 stearate, carbomer-934, dimethicone, titanium dioxide, imidazolidinyl urea, parabens. Lot. Bot. 180 ml, 300 ml, 450 ml. *otc.*
Use: Emollient.

wood charcoal tablets. (Cowley) 5 gr or 10 gr/Tab. Bot. 1000s. *otc.*

wood creosote.
See: Creosote (Various Mfr.).

wool fat. Lanolin, Anhydrous.

Wyamine Sulfate Injection. (Wyeth-Ayerst) Mephentermine sulfate 15 mg or 30 mg, methylparaben 1.8 mg, propylparaben 0.2 mg/ml. Vial 10 ml. Amp. 2 ml. *Rx.*
Use: Vasopressor.

Wyanoids Relief Factor. (Wyeth-Ayerst) Cocoa butter 79%, shark liver oil 3%, corn oil, EDTA, parabens, tocopherol. Supp. 12s. *otc.*
Use: Anorectal preparation.

Wydase Lyophilized. (Wyeth-Ayerst) Hyaluronidase. Vial 150 units/ml or 1500 units/10 ml with lactose and thimerosal. *Rx.*
Use: Hyaluronidase.

Wydase Stabilized Solution. (Wyeth-Ayerst) Hyaluronidase 150 units in sterile saline soln. with sodium Cl, EDTA, thimerosal. Vial 1 ml, 10 ml. *Rx.*
Use: Hyaluronidase.

Wygesic. (Wyeth-Ayerst) Propoxyphene HCl 65 mg, acetaminophen 650 mg/Tab. Bot. 100s, 500s, Redipak 100s. *c-iv.*
Use: Narcotic analgesic combination.

Wymox. (Wyeth-Ayerst) Amoxicillin as trihydrate. **Cap.:** 250 mg Bot. 100s, 500s; 500 mg Bot. 50s, 500s. **Oral Susp.:** 125 mg/5 ml Bot. to make 80 ml, 100 ml, 150 ml; 250 mg/5 ml Bot. to make 80 ml, 100 ml, 150 ml. *Rx.*
Use: Anti-infective, penicillin.

Wytensin. (Wyeth-Ayerst) Guanabenz acetate. **4 mg/Tab.:** Bot. 100s, 500s, Redipak 100s. **8 mg/Tab.:** Bot. 100s. **16 mg/Tab.:** Bot. 100s. *Rx.*
Use: Antihypertensive.

X

- **xamoterol.** (ZAM-oh-ter-ole) USAN.
  Use: Cardiac stimulant.
- **xamoterol fumarate.** (ZAM-oh-ter-ole) USAN.
  Use: Cardiac stimulant.

Xanax. (Pharmacia & Upjohn) Alprazolam 0.25 mg, 0.5 mg, 1 mg or 2 mg. Tab. **0.25 mg, 0.5 mg, 2 mg:** 100s, 500s, UD 100s. Visipack 4 × 25s. **1 mg:** 30s, 90s, 100s, 500s, UD 100s. *c-IV.*
  Use: Antianxiety.

- **xanomeline.** (zah-NO-meh-leen) USAN.
  Use: Cholinergic agonist (for Alzheimer's disease).
- **xanomeline tartrate.** (zah-NO-meh-leen) USAN.
  Use: Cholinergic agonist (for Alzheimer's disease).
- **xanoxate sodium.** (ZAN-ox-ate) USAN.
  Use: Bronchodilator.
- **xanthan gum,** N.F. 18.
  Use: Pharmaceutic aid, suspending agent.

xanthine derivatives.
  See: Caffeine.
  Theobromine.
  Theophylline.

- **xanthinol niacinate.** (ZAN-thih-nahl NYE-ah-SIN-ate) USAN.
  Use: Vasodilator (peripheral).
  See: Complamin (3M Pharm).

xanthiol hydrochloride.
  Use: Antinauseant.
  See: Daxid (Roerig).

xanthotoxin. Methoxsalen.

- **xemilofiban hydrochloride.** USAN.
  Use: Treatment of unstable angina, prevention of post-recanalization reocclusion of coronary vessels.
- **xenalipin.** (ZEN-ah-LIH-pin) USAN.
  Use: Hypolipidemic.
- **xenbucin.** (ZEN-BYOO-sin) USAN.
  Use: Antihyperlipidemic.
- **xenon Xe 127,** U.S.P. 23.
  Use: Diagnostic aid; medicinal gas; radioactive agent.
- **xenon Xe 133,** U.S.P. 23.
  Use: Radioactive agent.

xenthiorate hydrochloride.

Xerac AC. (Person & Covey) Aluminum Cl hexahydrate 6.25% in anhydrous ethanol 96%. Bot 35 ml, 60 ml. *Rx.*
  Use: Antiacne.

Xeroderm Lotion. (Dermol Pharm.) Mineral oil, acetylate lanolin alcohol, cetyl alcohol, glycerin, triethanolamine, parabens, imidazolidinyl urea. 267 ml. *otc.*
  Use: Emollient.

Xeroform Ointment 3%. (City, Consolidated) Pow. 0.25 lb, 1 lb. Jar 1 lb, 5 lb.

Xero-Lube. (Scherer) Monobasic potassium phosphate, dibasic potassium phosphate, magnesium Cl, potassium Cl, calcium Cl, sodium Cl, sodium fluoride, sorbitol soln., sodium carboxymethylcellulose, methylparaben. Bot. 6 oz. *otc.*
  Use: Mouth and throat product.

- **xilobam.** (ZIE-low-bam) USAN.
  Use: Relaxant (muscle).
- **xipamide.** (ZIP-ah-mide) USAN.
  Use: Antihypertensive, diuretic.
- **xorphanol mesylate.** (ZAHR-fan-ahl) USAN.
  Use: Analgesic.

X-Prep Bowel Evacuant Kit-1. (Purdue Frederick) Kit contains Senokot S tab., X-Prep liquid, Rectolax supp. *otc.*
  Use: Laxative.

X-Prep Bowel Evacuant Kit-2. (Purdue Frederick) Kit contains citralax granules, X-Prep liquid, Rectolax supp. *otc.*
  Use: Laxative.

X-Prep Liquid. (Gray) Senna extract with alcohol 7%, sucrose 50 g. Bot. 2.5 oz. *otc.*
  Use: Laxative.

X-Ray Contrast Media.
  See: Iodine Products, Diagnostic.

X-Seb Plus. (Baker Cummins) Pyrithionic zinc 1%, salicylic acid 2%. Shampoo. Bot. 120 ml. *otc.*
  Use: Antiseborrheic combination.

X-Seb Shampoo. (Baker/Cummins) Salicylic acid 4%, coal tar soln. 10% in a blend of surface-active agents. Bot. 4 oz. *otc.*
  Use: Antiseborrheic.

X-Seb T. (Baker/Cummins) Coal tar soln. 10%, salicylic acid 4%. Bot. 4 oz. *otc.*
  Use: Antiseborrheic.

X-Sep T Plus. (Baker Cummins) Coal tar solution 10%, salicylic acid, menthol 1%. Shampoo. Bot. 120 ml. *otc.*
  Use: Antiseborrheic combination.

Xtracare. (Sween) Bot. 2 oz, 4 oz, 8 oz, 21 oz, gal. *otc.*
  Use: Emollient.

Xtra-Vites. (Barth's) Vitamins A 10,000 IU, D 400 IU, C 150 mg, B_1 5 mg, B_2 1 mg, niacin 3.33 mg, pantothenic acid 183 mcg, B_6 250 mcg, B_{12} 215 mcg, E 15 IU, rutin 20 mg, citrus bioflavonoid complex 15 mg, choline 6.67 mg, ino-

sitol 10 mg, folic acid 50 mcg, biotin, aminobenzoic acid/Tab. Bot. 30s, 90s, 180s, 360s. *otc.*
Use: Vitamin supplement.

X-Trozine Capsules. (Rexar) Phendimetrazine tartrate 35 mg/Cap. Bot. 1000s. *c-III.*
Use: Anorexiant.

X-Trozine S.R. Capsules. (Rexar) Phendimetrazine tartrate 105 mg/SR Cap. Bot. 100s, 200s, 1000s. *c-III.*
Use: Anorexiant.

X-Trozine Tablets. (Rexar) Phendimetrazine tartrate 35 mg/Tab. Bot. 1000s. *c-III.*
Use: Anorexiant.

• **xylamidine tosylate.** (zie-LAM-ih-deen TAH-sill-ate) USAN.
Use: Serotonin inhibitor.

• **xylazine hydrochloride.** (ZIE-lih-zeen HIGH-droe-KLOR-ide) USAN.
Use: Analgesic, relaxant (muscle).

• **xylitol,** N.F. 18.
Use: Pharmaceutic aid (vehicle, sweetened).

Xylocaine Hydrochloride. (Astra) Lidocaine HCl. **Amp.:** (1%): 2 ml, 5 ml, 30 ml; w/epinephrine 1:200,000 30 ml. (1.5%): 20 ml; w/epinephrine 1:200,000 30 ml. (2%): 2 ml, 10 ml; w/epinephrine 1:200,000 20 ml. (4%): 5 ml. **Multidose Vial:** (0.5%): 50 ml; w/epinephrine 1:200,000 50 ml. (1%): 20 ml, 50 ml; w/epinephrine 1:100,000 20 ml, 50 ml. (2%): 20 ml, 50 ml; w/epinephrine 1:100,000 20 ml, 50 ml. **Single-dose Vial:** (1%): 30 ml. (1.5%) 20 ml; w/ epinephrine 1:200,000 10 ml, 30 ml. (2%) w/epinephrine 1:200,000 20 ml. *Rx.*
Use: Local anesthetic.

Xylocaine Hydrochloride for Cardiac Arrhythmia. (Astra) **Intravenous:** Lidocaine 2%. Amp 5 ml, disp. syringe 5 ml. Continuous infusion 1 g/25 ml Vial; 2 g/50 ml Vial. Prefilled syringe 100 mg/5 ml, 12s. Continuous infusion prefilled syringe 1 g, 2 g. **Intramuscular:** Amp. 10%, 5 ml. *Rx.*
Use: Local anesthetic.

Xylocaine Hydrochloride 4% Solution. (Astra) Topical use. Bot. 50 ml. *Rx.*
Use: Local anesthetic, topical.

Xylocaine Hydrochloride for Spinal Anesthesia. (Astra) Lidocaine HCl 1.5% or 5%, glucose 7.5%, sodium hydroxide to adjust pH. Specific gravity 1.028-1.034. Amp. 2 ml. Box 10s. *Rx.*
Use: Local anesthetic.

Xylocaine Hydrochloride w/Dextrose. (Astra) Lidocaine HCl 1.5%, dextrose 7.5%. Inj. Amps. 2 ml. *Rx.*
Use: Local anesthetic.

Xylocaine Hydrochloride w/Epinephrine. (Astra) Lidocaine HCl 2% w/epinephrine 1:200,000. Amps w/sodium metabisulfite 20 ml. Inj. Single dose vials w/sodium metabisulfite. 20 ml. *Rx.*
Use: Local anesthetic.

Xylocaine Hydrochloride w/Glucose. (Astra) Lidocaine HCl 5%, glucose 7.5%. Inj. Amp. 2 ml. *Rx.*
Use: Local anesthetic.

Xylocaine Jelly. (Astra) Lidocaine HCl 2% in sodium carboxymethylcellulose with parabens. Tube 5 ml and 30 ml. *Rx.*
Use: Local anesthetic, topical.

Xylocaine Ointment. (Astra) Lidocaine 2.5%, water soluble carbowaxes. 35 g *otc.*
Use: Topical anesthetic.

Xylocaine MPF Injection. (Astra) Lidocaine HCl. **0.5%** 50 ml. **1%** 2, 5, or 30 ml. **1.5%** 10 or 20 ml. **2%** 2, 5 or 10 ml. **4%** 5 ml. **1%** w/ epinephrine 1:200,000, sodium bisulfite. 5, 10 or 30 ml. **2%**w/ epinephrine, sodium bisulfite. 5, 10 or 20 ml. **5%**w/ glucose 7.5%. 2 ml. *Rx.*
Use: Local anesthetic.

Xylocaine Viscous. (Astra) Lidocaine HCl 2%, sodium carboxymethylcellulose, parabens. Bot. 20 ml (25s), 100 ml, 450 ml and UD 20 ml. *Rx.*
Use: Local anesthetic.

• **xylofilcon a.** (ZILE-oh-FILL-kahn A) USAN.
Use: Contact lens material (hydrophilic).

• **xylometazoline hydrochloride,** U.S.P. 23.
Use: Adrenergic (vasoconstrictor).
See: Isohalent L.A., Liq. (Zeneca).
Long Acting Neo-Synephrine, Prods. (Winthrop Consumer Products).
Otrivin Spray (Novartis).
Rhinall L.A., Liq. (First Texas).
Sine-Off, Spray (Menley & James).
Vicks Sinex Long Acting, Nasal Spray (Procter & Gamble).

Xylo-Pfan. (Pharmacia & Upjohn) Xylose 25 g/Bot.
Use: Diagnostic aid.

Xylophan D-Xylose Tolerance Test. (Pfanstiehl) D-xylose 25 g/UD bot.
Use: Diagnostic aid.

• **xylose,** U.S.P. 23.
Use: Diagnostic aid (intestinal function determination).

Y

Yager's Liniment. (Yager) Oil of turpentine and camphor w/clove oil fragrance, emulsifier, emollient, ammonium oleate (less than 0.5% free ammonia) penetrant base. *otc.*
Use: Rubefacient.

yatren.
See: Chiniofon, Tab.

YDP Lice Spray. (Youngs Drug) Synthetic pyrethroid in aerosol. Can 5 oz. *otc.*
Use: Pediculicide for inanimate objects.

yeast adenylic acid. An isomer of adenosine 5-monophosphate, has been found inactive.
See: Adenosine 5-Monophosphate, Preps. for active compounds.

yeast, dried.
Use: Protein and vitamin B Complex source.

yeast tablets, dried.
Use: Supplementary source of B complex vitamins.
See: Brewer's Yeast, Tab.

Yeast-Gard. (Lake) Pulsatilla 28x, **Candida parapsilosis:** 28x, **Candida albicans:** 28x. Supp. 10s, 15s w/applicator. *otc.*
Use: Vaginal preparation.

Yeast-Gard Maximum Strength. (Lake) Benzocaine 20%, resorcinol 3%, methylparaben, sodium sulfite, EDTA, mineral oil. Cream. Tube 28.35 g. *otc.*
Use: Vaginal preparation.

Yeast-Gard Medicated Disposable Douche. (Lake Pharm) Povidone-iodine 0.3% when reconstituted. Soln. 180 ml twin-pack w/two 5.4 ml medicated douche concentrate packets. *otc.*
Use: Douche.

Yeast-Gard Medicated Disposable Douche Premix. (Lake Pharm) Octoxynol-9, lactic acid, sodium lactate, sodium benzoate, aloe vera. Soln. 180 ml twin-pack. *otc.*
Use: Douche.

Yeast-Gard Medicated Douche. (Lake Pharm) Povidone-iodine 10%. Soln. Concentrate. 240 ml. *otc.*
Use: Douche.

Yeast-Gard Sensitive Formula. (Lake Pharm.) Benzocaine 5%, resorcinol 2%, methylparaben, sodium sulfite, EDTA, mineral oil. Cream. Tube 28.35 g. *otc.*
Use: Vaginal preparation.

yeast, torula.

See: Torula Yeast.

yeast w/iron.
See: Natural Super Iron Yeast Powder (Spirt) Bot. 200s.

Yeast-X. (C.B. Fleet) **Supp.:** Pulsatilla 28x. Pkg. 12s; **Pow.:** Cornstarch, zinc oxide, benzethonium chloride. 196 g. *otc.*
Use: Vaginal preparation.

Yelets. (Freeda) Iron 20 mg, vitamins A 10,000 IU, D 400 IU, E 10 IU, B_1 10 mg, B_2 10 mg, B_3 25 mg, B_5 10 mg, B_6 10 mg, B_{12} 10 mcg, C 100 mg, folic acid 0.1 mg, PABA, lysine, glutamic acid, Ca, I, Mg, Mn, Se, Zn 4 mg/Tab. Bot. 100s, 250s. *otc.*
Use: Vitamin/mineral supplement.

yellow enzyme.
See: Riboflavin (Various Mfr.).

•**yellow fever vaccine,** U.S.P. 23.
Use: Active immunizing agent.
See: YF-Vax, Inj. (Pasteur-Merieux-Connaught).

yellow hornet venom.
See: Albay (Bayer).
Pharmalgen (ALK Labs).
Venomil (Bayer).
Use: Immunizing agent.

yellow jacket venom.
See: Albay (Bayer).
Pharmalgen (ALK Labs).
Venomil (Bayer).
Use: Immunizing agent.

yellow mercuric oxide 1%. (Various Mfr.) Oint. Tube 3.5, 3.75, 30 g. *otc.*
Use: Antiseptic.

yellow mercuric oxide 2%. (Various Mfr.) Oint. Tube 3.5, 3.75, 30 g. *otc.*
Use: Antiseptic.
See: Stye, Oint. (Del Pharm).

yellow ointment.
Use: Pharmaceutic aid (ointment base).

yellow wax.
Use: Pharmaceutic aid (stiffening agent).

YF-Vax. (Pasteur-Merieux-Connaught) Yellow fever vaccine. Inj. Vial 1 dose, 5 dose, 20 dose with diluent. *Rx.*
Use: Agent for immunization.

Yocon. (Palisades) Yohimbine HCl 5.4 mg/Tab. Bot. 100s, 1000s. *Rx.*
Use: Impotence.

Yodora Deodorant Cream. (SK-Beecham) Jar 2 oz. *otc.*
Use: Deodorant.

Yodoxin. (Glenwood) Iodoquinol 210 mg or 650 mg/Tab. Bot. 100s, 1000s. Pow. Bot. 25 g. *Rx.*
Use: Amebicide.

yohimbine hydrochloride. Indolalkylamine alkaloid. (Various Mfr.) 5.4 mg/Tab. Bot. 100s, 500s. *Rx.*
Note: Yohimbine has no FDA sanctioned indications.
W/Methyltestosterone, nux vomica extract.
See: Climactic, Tab. (Burgin-Arden)

Yohimex. (Kramer) Yohimbine HCl 5.4 mg/Tab. Bot. 100s. *Rx.*
Use: Impotence.

Your Choice Non-Preserved Saline Solution. (Amcon) Buffered, isotonic soln. w/ NaCl, boric acid, sodium borate. Bot. 360 ml. *otc.*

Use: Soft contact lens care.

Your Choice Sterile Preserved Saline Solution. (Amcon) Isotonic. Sorbic acid 0.1%, EDTA, NaCl, boric buffer. Bot. 60 ml or 360 ml. *otc.*
Use: Soft contact lens care.

ytterbium Yb 169 pentetate injection, U.S.P. XXII.
Use: Radioactive agent.

Yutopar. (Astra) Ritodrine HCl 10 mg/ml, Amp. 5 ml; 15 mg/ml, vial 10 ml, inj. syringe 10 ml. *Rx.*
Use: Uterine relaxant.

Z

• **zacopride hydrochloride.** (ZAK-oh-pride) USAN.
Use: Antiemetic, stimulant (peristaltic).

• **zafirlukast.** (zah-FEER-loo-kast) USAN.
Use: Antiasthmatic (leukotriene antagonist).
See: Accolate, Tab. (Zeneca).

Zagam. (Rhone-Poulenc Rorer) Sparfloxacin 200 mg/Tab. Bot. *Rx.*
Use: Fluoroquinolone.

• **zalcitabine.** (zal-SITE-ah-BEAN) USAN.
Use: Antiviral, AIDS. [Orphan drug]

• **zaleplon.** USAN.
Use: Sedative, hypnotic.

• **zalospirone hydrochloride.** USAN.
Use: Antianxiety.

• **zaltidine hydrochloride.** (ZAHL-tih-deen) USAN.
Use: Antagonist to histamine H_2 receptors.

zanaflex. (Athena)
See: tizanidine hydrochloride.

• **zankiren hydrochloride.** USAN.
Use: Antihypertensive.

Zanosar. (Pharmacia & Upjohn) Streptozocin sterile pow. 100 mg/ml. Vial 1 g. *Rx.*
Use: Antineoplastic.

• **zanoterone.** zan-OH-ter-ohn) USAN.
Use: Antiandrogen.

Zantac EFFERdose Effervescent Granules and Tablets. (Glaxo) Ranitidine HCl 150 mg. **Granules:** 1.44 g packets (30s, 60s); **Tab:** Bot. 30s, 60s. *Rx.*
Use: Histamine H_2 antagonist.

Zantac GELdose. (Glaxo) Ranitidine HCl 150 mg or 300 mg/Cap. **150 mg:** Bot. 60s, UD 60s; **300 mg:** Bot. 30s, UD 30s. *Rx.*
Use: Histamine H_2 antagonist.

Zantac Injection. (Glaxo) Ranitidine 25 mg HCl/ml. Vial 2 ml, 10 ml, 40 ml, syringe 2 ml. *Rx.*
Use: Histamine H_2 antagonist.

Zantac Injection Premixed. (Glaxo) Ranitidine 0.5 mg as HCl/ml. 100 ml single-dose plastic container. *Rx.*
Use: Histamine H_2 antagonist.

Zantac Syrup. (Glaxo) Ranitidine 15 mg as HCl/ml, alcohol 7.5%. Bot. 480 ml. *Rx.*
Use: Histamine H_2 antagonist.

Zantac Tablets. (Glaxo) Ranitidine 150 mg or 300 mg as HCl/Tab. **150 mg:** Bot. 60s, 500s, UD 100s. **300 mg:** Bot. 30s, 250s, UD 100s. *Rx.*
Use: Histamine H_2 antagonist.

Zantine. (Lexis) Dipyridamole 25 mg, 50 mg or 75 mg/Tab. Bot. 1000s. *Rx.*
Use: Coronary vasodilator.

Zantryl. (ION) Phentermine HCl 30 mg/SR Cap. Bot. 100s. *c-iv.*
Use: Anorexiant.

Zarontin. (Parke-Davis) Ethosuximide. **Cap.:** 250 mg. Bot. 100s. **Syr.:** 250 mg/5 ml. Bot. pt. *Rx.*
Use: Anticonvulsant.

Zaroxolyn. (Medeva) Metolazone 2.5 mg, 5 mg or 10 mg/Tab. Bot. 100s, 500s, 1000s, UD 100s. *Rx.*
Use: Diuretic.

Zartan. (Dartmouth) Cephalexin monohydrate 500 mg. Cap. Bot. 100s. *Rx.*
Use: Anti-infective, cephalosporin.

• **zatosetron maleate.** (ZAt-oh-SEH-trahn) USAN.
Use: Antimigraine.

Z-Bec. (Robins) Vitamins E 45 mg, C 600 mg, B_1 15 mg, B_2 10.2 mg, B_3 100 mg, B_6 10 mg, B_{12} 6 mcg, pantothenic acid 25 mg, zinc 22.5 mg/Tab. Bot. 60s, 100s, 500s. *otc.*
Use: Vitamin/mineral supplement.

ZBT Baby. (Glenwood) Talc, mineral oil, magnesium stearate, propylene glycol, BHT. Pow. 120 g. *otc.*
Use: Diaper rash product.

Zeasorb-AF Powder. (Stiefel) Miconazole nitrate 2%. Can 2.5 oz. *otc.*
Use: Antifungal, topical.

Zeasorb Powder. (Stiefel) Talc, microporous cellulose, supersorb carbohydrate acrylic copolymer. Sifter-top Can 2.5 oz, 8 oz. *otc.*
Use: Moisture absorbent.

Zebeta. (Lederle) Bisoprolol fumarate. **5 mg:** Tab/Bot. 14s, 30s, 100s, 500s, 1000s, UD 10s, **10 mg:** Tab/Bot. 14s, 30s, 100s, 500s, 1000s, UD 10s. *Rx.*
Use: Beta-adrenergic blocker.

Zecaps. (Everett) Vitamin E 200 mg, zinc 9.6 mg as gluconate/Cap. Bot. 60s. *otc.*
Use: Vitamin/mineral supplement.

Zefazone. (Pharmacia & Upjohn) Cefmetazole sodium 1 g or 2 g/vial. Pow. for inj. *Rx.*
Use: Anti-infective.

• **zein,** N.F. 18.
Use: Pharmaceutic aid (coating agent).

Zemalo. (Barre) Sulfur, zinc oxide, camphor, titanium oxide. Bot. 4 oz, pt, gal. *otc.*
Use: Minor skin irritations.

Zenate. (Solvay) Vitamins A 5000 IU, D 400 IU, E 30 mg, C 80 mg, folic acid 1 mg, thiamine 3 mg, riboflavin 3 mg,

niacin 20 mg, B$_6$ 10 mg, B$_{12}$ 12 mcg, calcium 300 mg, iodine 175 mcg, iron 65 mg, magnesium 100 mg, zinc 20 mg/Tab. Bot. 100s. *Rx.*
Use: Vitamin/mineral supplement.

● **zenazocine mesylate.** USAN.
Use: Analgesic.

Zendium. (Oral-B) Sodium fluoride 0.22%. Tube 0.9 oz, 2.3 oz.
Use: Dental caries preventative.

● **zeniplatin.** (zen-ih-PLAT-in) USAN.
Use: Antineoplastic.

Zentel. (SK Beecham) Albendazole.
Use: Anthelmintic.

Zephiran. (Winthrop Pharm) **Aqueous soln.:** Benzalkonium Cl 1:750. Bot. 240 ml, gal. **Disinfectant concentrate:** 17% in 120 ml, gal. **Tincture:** 1:750 in gal. **Tincture spray:** 1:750 in 30 g, 180 g, gal. *otc.*
Use: Antiseptic, germicide.

Zephiran Towelettes. (Winthrop Pharm) Moist paper towels with soln. of zephiran Cl 1:750. Box 20s, 100s, 1000s. *otc.*
Use: Antiseptic, germicide.

Zephrex Tablets. (Bock) Pseudo-ephedrine HCl 60 mg, guaifenesin 400 mg/SR Tab. Bot. 100s. *Rx.*
Use: Decongestant, expectorant.

Zephrex-LA Tablets. (Bock) Pseudo-ephedrine HCl 120 mg, guaifenesin 600 mg/Tab. Bot. 100s. *Rx.*
Use: Decongestant, expectorant.

Zepine. (Foy) Reserpine alkaloid 0.25 mg/Tab. Bot. 100s, 500s, 1000s. *Rx.*
Use: Antihypertensive.

● **zeranol.** (ZER-ah-nole) USAN.
Use: Anabolic.

Zerit. (Bristol-Myers Squibb) Stavudine 15 mg, 20 mg, 30 mg, 40 mg/Cap. Bot. 60s. Stavudine 1 mg 1 ml/Pow. for oral solution. Bot. 200 ml. *Rx.*
Use: Antiviral.

Zestoretic. (Zeneca) Lisinopril 10 mg, hydrochlorothiazide 12.5 mg or lisinopril 20 mg, hydrochlorothiazide 12.5 mg or lisinopril 20 mg, hydrochlorothiazide 25 mg/Tab. Bot. 100s. *Rx.*
Use: Antihypertensive combination.

Zestril. (Zeneca) Lisinopril 5 mg, 10 mg, 20 mg, or 40 mg/Tab. Bot. 100s, UD 100s. *Rx.*
Use: Antihypertensive.

Zetar Emulsion. (Dermik) Colloidal whole coal tar 30% (300 mg/ml) in polysorbates. Bot. 6 oz. *otc.*
Use: Antiseborrheic.

Zetar Shampoo. (Dermik) Colloidal

whole coal tar 1% in a shampoo. Bot. 6 oz. *otc.*
Use: Antiseborrheic.

Z-Gen. (Goldline) Vitamins E 45 mg, B$_1$ 15 mg, B$_2$ 10.2 mg, B$_3$ 100 mg, B$_5$ 25 mg, B$_6$ 10 mg, B$_{12}$ 6 mcg, C 600 mg, zinc 22.5 mg/Tab. Bot. 60s, 100s. *otc.*
Use: Vitamin/mineral supplement.

Ziac. (Lederle) Bisoprolol fumarate 2.5 mg, 5 mg or 10 mg; hydrochloro-thiazide 6.25 mg. Tab. **2.5 mg or 5 mg:** Bot. 30s, 100s. **10 mg:** Bot. 30s. *Rx.*
Use: Antihypertensive.

● **zidometacin.** USAN.
Use: Anti-inflammatory.

● **zidovudine.** (zie-DOE-view-DEEN) USAN. *Formerly azidothymidine, AZT.*
Use: Antiviral for management of certain AIDS and other serious HIV infections. [Orphan drug]
See: Retrovir, Cap. (Glaxo Wellcome).

● **zifrosilone.** USAN.
Use: Acetylcholinesterase inhibitor.

Zilactin-B Medicated. (Zila Inc.) Benzo-caine 10%, alcohol 76%. Gel. Tube 7.5 g. *otc.*
Use: Local anesthetic, oral.

Zilactin-L. (Zila) Lidocaine 2.5%, alcohol 79.3%. Liq. Bot. 7.5 ml. *otc.*
Use: Local anesthetic, topical.

Zilactin Medicated Gel. (Zila) Tannic acid 7%, suspended in alcohol 80.8%. Tube 0.25 oz. *otc.*
Use: Treatment of cold sores.

Ziladent. (Zila) Benzocaine 6%, alcohol 74.9%. Gel. Tube. 7.5 g and single packs. *otc.*
Use: Local anesthetic, topical.

● **zilantel.** (ZILL-an-tell) USAN.
Use: Anthelmintic.

● **zileuton.** (ZIE-loo-tone) USAN.
Use: Inhibitor (5-lipoxygenase).
See: Zyflo, Tab. (Abbott).

zimco. (Sterwin) Vanillin.

● **zimeldine hydrochloride.** (zie-MELL-ih-deen) USAN. *Formerly Zimelidine Hy-drochloride.*
Use: Antidepressant.

Zinacef. (Glaxo Pharmaceuticals) Cefur-oxime 750 mg, 1.5 g or 7.5 g as so-dium. **750 mg, 1.5 g:** Vials and infu-sion pack. **7.5 g:** Pharmacy bulk Pkg. **750 mg, 1.5 g, premixed:** Bot. 50 ml. *Rx.*
Use: Anti-infective, cefalosporin.

Zinc-220. (Alto) Zinc sulfate 220 mg/Cap. Bot. 100s, 1000s, UD 100s. *otc.*
Use: Zinc supplement.

•**zinc acetate,** U.S.P. 23. Acetic acid, zinc salt, dihydrate.
Use: Pharmaceutic necessity for Zinc-Eugenol Cement; Wilson's disease [Orphan drug]

Zinca-Pak. (SoloPak) Zinc 1 mg or 5 mg/ml. Inj. **1 mg:** Vial 10 ml, 30 ml. **5 mg:** Vial 5 ml. *Rx.*
Use: Parenteral nutritional supplement.

Zincate. (Paddock) Zinc sulfate 220 mg (elemental zinc 50 mg)/Cap. Bot. 100s, 1000s. *otc.*
Use: Zinc supplement.

zinc bacitracin. Bacitracin Zinc, U.S.P. 23.
Use: Anti-infective.

•**zinc carbonate,** U.S.P. 23.
Use: Antiseptic, topical; astrigent.

•**zinc chloride,** U.S.P. 23.
Use: Astringent, dentin desensitizer.
W/Formaldehyde.
See: Forma Zincol Concentrate (Ingram).

•**zinc chloride Zn 65.** USAN.
Use: Radioactive agent.

zinc-eugenol cement, U.S.P. XXI.
Use: Dental protectant.

Zincfrin. (Alcon) Zinc sulfate 0.25%, phenylephrine HCl 0.12%. Soln. Droptainer 15 ml, 30 ml. *otc.*
Use: Astringent, decongestant, ophthalmic.

zinc gelatin, U.S.P. XXI. Impregnated gauge, U.S.P. 23.
Use: Topical protectant.

Zinc-Glenwood. (Glenwood) Zinc Sulfate 220 mg/Cap. Bot. 100s. *otc.*
Use: Zinc supplement.

•**zinc gluconate,** U.S.P. 23.
Use: Supplement (trace mineral).

zinchlorundesal. Zincundesal.

zinc insulin.
See: Insulin Zinc, Preps. (Various Mfr.).

Zincon Shampoo. (Lederle) Pyrithione zinc 1%, sodium methyl cocoyltaurate, sodium Cl, magnesium aluminum silicate, sodium cocoyl isethionate, glutaral, water w/pH adjusted. Bot. 4 oz, 8 oz. *otc.*
Use: Antiseborrheic.

Zinc Lozenges. (Goldline) Zinc citrate 23 mg, zinc gluconate, fructose/Lozenge. Bot. 30s. *otc.*
Use: Mineral supplement.

•**zinc oxide,** U.S.P. 23. Flowers of zinc.
Use: Astringent, topical protectant).
See: Calamine Preps.
W/Combinations.
See: Akne, Drying Lot. (Alto).

Almophen, Oint. (Jones Medical).
Anocaine, Supp. (Mallard).
Anugesic, Oint., Supp. (Parke-Davis).
Anusol, Oint., Supp. (Parke-Davis).
Anusol-HC, Supp. (Parke-Davis).
Aracain Rectal Oint., Supp. (Del Pharm.).
Bonate, Supp. (Suppositoria).
Calamatum, Preps. (Blair).
Cala-Zinc-Ol, Liq. (Emerson).
Caldesene, Oint. (Novartis).
Caleate HC Cream, Oint. (Zeneca).
Caloxol, Oint. (Jones Medical).
CZO, Lot. (Zeneca).
Dereq Medicone HC, Supp. (Medicone).
Dermatrol, Oint. (Gordon).
Desitin, Oint. (Pfizer).
Diaprex, Oint. (Moss, Belle).
Doctient, Supp. (Suppositoria).
Elder Diaper Rash Oint. (Zeneca).
Epinephricaine, Oint. (Pharmacia & Upjohn).
Ergophene, Oint. (Pharmacia & Upjohn).
Hemocaine, Oint. (Mallard).
Hemorrhoidal Oint. (Towne).
Hydro Surco, Lot. (Alma).
Ladd's Paste (Paddock).
Lasan, Oint. (Stiefel).
Medicated Powder (Johnson & Johnson).
Medicated Foot Powder (Pharmacia & Upjohn).
Mexsana, Pow. (Schering-Plough).
Nullo Foot Cream (DePree).
Pazo, Oint., Supp. (Bristol-Myers).
Petrozin Compound Oint. (Jones Medical).
PZM Oint. (Wendt-Bristol).
Rectal Medicone HC, Supp. (Medicone).
RVPaque, Oint. (Zeneca).
Saratoga, Oint. (Blair).
Schamberg, Lot. (Paddock).
Sebasorb, Lot. (Summer).
Supertah, Oint. (Purdue Frederick).
Taloin, Tube (Warren-Teed).
Ting, Cream, Pow. (Novartis).
Unguentine Oint. "Original Formula" (Procter & Gamble).
Versal, Supp. (Suppositoria).
Wyanoids, Preps. (Wyeth-Ayerst).
Xylocaine Supp. (Astra).
Zinc Boric Lotion, Liq. (Emerson).

zinc phenolsulfonate.
Use: Astringent.
W/Belladonna leaf extract, kaolin, pectin, sodium carboxymethylcellulose.
See: Gelcomul, Liq. (Del Pharm.).
W/Bismuth subgallate, kaolin, pectin, opium pow.

See: Diastay,Tab. (Zeneca).
W/Bismuth subsalicylate, salol, methyl salicylate.
See: Pepto-Bismol, Liq. (Procter & Gamble).
W/Kaolin, pectin.
See: Pectocel, Liq. (Lilly).
W/Opium pow., bismuth subgallate, pectin, kaolin.
See: Bismuth, Pectin & Paregoric (Lemmon).

zinc pyrithione.
Use: Bactericide, fungicide, antiseborrheic.
See: Breck One, Shampoo (Breck).
TVC-2 Dandruff Shampoo (Dermol).
Zincon, Shampoo (Lederle).
ZP-11, Liq. (Revlon).

•**zinc stearate,** U.S.P. 23. Octadecanoic acid, zinc salt.
Use: Dusting powder; pharmaceutic aid (tablet/capsule lubricant).
W/Combinations.
See: Ting, Cream, Pow. (Novartis).

zinc sulfanilate. Zinc sulfanilate tetrahydrate. Nizin, Op-Isophrin-Z, Op-Isophrin-Z-M (Broemmel).
Use: Anti-infective.

•**zinc sulfate,** U.S.P. 23. Sulfuric acid, zinc salt (1:1), heptahydrate.
Use: Astringent (ophthalmic).
See: Eye-Sed, Soln. (Scherer).
Op-Thal-Zin Ophth. (Alcon).
Scrip-Zinc, Cap. (Scrip).
Zinc-Glenwood, Cap. (Glenwood).
Zin-Cora, Cap. (Zeneca).
W/Boric acid, phenylephrine HCl.
See: Phenylzin Drops, Ophth. Soln. (Smith, Miller & Patch).
W/Calcium lactate.
See: Zinc-220, Cap. (Alto).
W/Menthol, methyl salicylate, alum, boric acid, oxyquinoline citrate.
See: Maso pH Powder (Mason).
W/Phenylephrine HCl, polyvinyl alcohol.
See: Prefrin-Z, Liquifilm (Allergan).
W/Piperocaine HCl, boric acid, potassium Cl.
See: M-Z Drops (Smith, Miller & Patch).
W/Sodium Cl.
See: Bromidrosis Crystals (Gordon).
W/Vitamins.
See: Neovicaps TR, Cap. (Scherer).
Vicon-C, Cap. (Glaxo).
Vicon Forte, Cap. (Glaxo).
Vicon Plus, Cap. (Glaxo).
Vi-Zac, Cap. (Glaxo).
Z-Bec, Tab. (Robins).
zinc sulfate. (Various Mfr.) Zinc 5 mg/ml (as sulfate 21.95 mg). Inj. Vial 5, 10 ml.

Use: Parenteral nutritional supplement.
zinc sulfate. (Various Mfr.) Zinc 1 mg/ml (as sulfate 4.39 mg). Inj. Vial 10, 30 ml. *Rx.*
Use: Parenteral nutritional supplement.
zinc sulfocarbolate.
W/Aluminum hydroxide, pectin, kaolin, bismuth subsalicylate, salol.
See: Wescola Antidiarrheal-Stomach Upset (Western Research).
zinc trace metal additive. (IMS) Zinc 4 mg/ml. Inj. Vial. 10 ml. *Rx.*
Use: Parenteral nutritional supplement.
zincundesal.
See: Zinchlorundesal.
zinc-10-undecenoate.
See: Zinc Undecylenate, U.S.P. 23.
•**zinc undecylenate,** U.S.P. 23.(Various Mfr.).
Use: Antifungal.
W/Benzocaine, hexachlorophene.
See: Fung-O-Spray (Scrip).
W/Benzocaine, undecylenic acid, menthol.
See: Decyl-Cream LBS (Scrip).
W/Caprylic acid, sodium propionate.
See: Deso-Cream (Quality Generics).
Deso-Talc, Foot Pow. (Quality Generics).
W/Undecylenic acid.
See: Cruex Cream, Spray Pow. (Novartis).
Desenex, Prods. (Novartis).
Ting, Aerosol (Novartis).
Quinsana, Med. Oint. (Mennen).
Zincvit. (Kenwood) Vitamin A 5000 IU, D_3 50 IU, E 50 IU, B_1 10 mg, B_2 5 mg, B_6 2 mg, C 300 mcg, B_3 25 mg, Zn 40 mg, Mg 9.7 mg, Mn 1.3 mg, folic acid 1 mg/Cap. Bot. 60s. *Rx.*
Use: Vitamin/mineral supplement.
Zinecard. (Pharmacia & Upjohn) Dexrazoxane 250 mg or 500 mg. Powd. for Inj. Lyophilized. Vial 25 ml (250 mg) or 50 ml (500 mg) of 0.167 Molar Sodium Lactate Injection. *Rx.*
Use: Antidote.
•**zindotrine.** USAN.
Use: Bronchodilator.
•**zinoconazole hydrochloride.** (zih-no-KOE-nah-zole) USAN.
Use: Antifungal.
•**zinostatin.** (ZEE-no-STAT-in) USAN. *Formerly* neocarzinostatin.
Use: Antineoplastic.
•**zinterol hydrochloride.** USAN.
Use: Bronchodilator.
•**zinviroxime.** (zin-VIE-rox-eem) USAN.
Use: Antiviral.

• **ziprasidone hydrochloride.** (zih-PRAY-sih-dohn) USAN.
Use: Antipsychotic.

Ziradryl Lotion. (Parke-Davis Prods) Benadryl HCl 2%, zinc oxide 2%, alcohol 2%. Bot. 6 oz. *otc.*
Use: Anesthetic, local.

zirconium carbonate or oxide.
See: Dermaneed, Lot. (Hanlon).
W/Benzocaine, menthol, camphor.
See: Rhulicream, Oint. (Lederle).
W/Benzocaine, menthol, camphor, calamine, pyrilamine maleate.
See: Ivarest, Cream (Carbisulphoil).
W/Benzocaine, menthol, camphor, calamine, isopropyl alcohol.
See: Rhulispray, Aerosol (Lederle).
W/Parethoxycaine, calamine.
See: Zotox, Spray, Oint. (Del Pharm.).

Zithromax. (Pfizer) Azithromycin (as dihydrate) 250 mg, lactose. Cap. Bot. 50s, UD 50s, Z-Pak 6s. *Rx.*
Use: Anti-infective, macrolide.

ZNG. (Western Research) Zinc gluconate 35 mg/Tab. Handicount 28s (36 bags of 28 tab.). *otc.*
Use: Zinc supplement.

ZNP Bar. (Stiefel) Zinc pyrithione 2%. Bar 4.2 oz. *otc.*
Use: Antiseborrheic.

ZN-Plus Protein. (Miller) Zinc in a zinc-protein complex made with isolated soy protein 15 mg/Tab. Bot. 100s. *otc.*
Use: Zinc supplement.

Zocor. (Merck) Simvastatin w/lactose **5 mg Tab.** Bot. 60s, 90s, UD 100s. **10 mg Tab.** Bot. 60s, 90s, UD 100s, 1000s, 10,000s. **20 mg Tab.** Bot. 60s, 1000s, 10,000s. **40 mg Tab.** Bot. 60s. *Rx.*
Use: Antihyperlipidemic.

Zodeac-100. (Econo Med) Iron 60 mg, vitamins A 8000 IU, D 400 IU, E 30 IU, B_1 1.7 mg, B_2 2 mg, B_3 20 mg, B_5 11 mg, B_6 4 mg, B_{12} 8 mcg, C 120 mg, folic acid 1 mg, biotin 300 mcg, Ca, Cu, I, Mg, Zn 15 mg/Tab. Bot. 100s. *Rx.*
Use: Vitamin/mineral supplement.

• **zofenopril calcium.** (zoe-FEN-oh-PRILL) USAN.
Use: Enzyme inhibitor (angiotensin-converting).

• **zofenoprilat arginine.** (zoe-FEN-oh-PRILL-at) USAN.
Use: Antihypertensive.

Zofran. (Cerenex) Ondansetron HCl **Tab.:** 4 mg, 8 mg Bot. 30s, UD 100s, 1 x 3 UD pack. **Inj.:** 2 mg/ml in 2 ml, 20 ml vials, or 32 mg/50 ml (premixed) in 50 ml containers (6s). *Rx.*
Use: Antiemetic.

Zoladex. (Zeneca) Goserelin acetate 3.6 mg. Implant. Syringes. *Rx.*
Use: LHRH agonist.

• **zolamine hydrochloride.** (zoe-lah-meen) USAN.
Use: Antihistamine; anesthetic, topical.
W/Eucupin dihydrochloride.
See: Otodyne, Soln. (Schering-Plough).

• **zolazepam hydrochloride.** (zole-AZE-eh-pam) USAN.
Use: Sedative, hypnotic.

• **zoledronate disodium.** (ZOE-leh-droe-nate) USAN.
Use: Bone resorption inhibitor; osteoporosis treatment and prevention.

• **zoledronate trisodium.** (ZOE-leh-droe-nate) USAN.
Use: Bone resorption inhibitor; osteoporosis treatment and prevention.

• **zoledronic acid.** (ZOE-leh-drah-nik) USAN.
Use: Calcium regulator; osteoporosis treatment and prevention.

• **zolertine hydrochloride.** (ZOE-ler-teen) USAN.
Use: Antiadrenergic, vasodilator.

Zolicef. (Apothecon) Cefazolin 500 mg. Pow. for inj. Vial 10 ml. *Rx.*
Use: Anti-infective, cephalosporin.

• **zolimomab aritox.** (zah-LIM-ah-mab a-rih-TOX) USAN.
Use: Monoclonal antibody (antithrombotic).

Zoloft. (Roerig) Sertraline 25 mg, 50 mg, 100 mg/Tab. Bot. 50s. *Rx.*
Use: Antidepressant.

• **zolpidem tartrate.** (ZOLE-pih-dem) USAN.
Use: Sedative, hypnotic.
See: Ambien.

• **zomepirac sodium.** (ZOE-mih-PEER-ack) USAN. U.S.P. XXI.
Use: Analgesic, anti-inflammatory.

• **zometapine.** (zoe-MET-ah-peen) USAN.
Use: Antidepressant.

Zone-A Forte. (UAD) Hydrocortisone 2.5%, pramoxine HCl in a hydrophilic base containing stearic acid 1%, forlan-L, glycerin, triethanolamine, polyoxyl-40-stearate, diisopropyl adipate, povidone, silicone fluid-200. Paraben free. Lot. Bot. 60 ml. *Rx.*
Use: Corticosteroid; local anesthetic, topical.

Zone-A Lotion. (UAD Labs) Hydrocortisone acetate 1%, pramoxine HCl 1%. Bot. 2 oz. *Rx.*

Use: Corticosteroid; local anesthetic, topical.

•**zoniclezole hydrochloride.** (zoe-NIH-klih-ZOLE) USAN.
Use: Anticonvulsant.

•**zonisamide.** (zoe-NISS-ah-MIDE) USAN.
Use: Anticonvulsant.

Zonite Liquid Douche Concentrate. (Menley & James) Benzalkonium Cl 0.1%, menthol, thymol, EDTA in buffered soln. Bot. 240 ml, 360 ml. *otc.*
Use: Vaginal preparation.

•**zopolrestat.** (zoe-PAHL-reh-STAT) USAN.
Use: Antidiabetic, aldose reductase inhibitor.

•**zorbamycin.** (ZAHR-bah-MY-sin) USAN.
Use: Antibacterial.

ZORprin. (Knoll Pharm.) Aspirin 800 mg/SR Tab. Bot. 100s. *Rx.*
Use: Salicylate analgesic.

•**zorubicin hydrochloride.** (zoe-ROO-bih-sin) USAN.
Use: Antineoplastic.

Zostrix. (GenDerm) Capsaicin 0.025%. Cream 45 g. *Rx.*
Use: Analgesic, topical.

Zostrix-HP. (GenDerm) Formerly called Axsain, formerly marketed by Galen.

Zosyn. (Lederle) Piperacillin sodium/tazobactam sodium 2 g/0.25 g, 3 g/0.375 g, 4 g/0.5 g vials. *Rx.*
Use: Anti-infective, penicillins.

Zoto HC. (Horizon) Chloroxylenol 1 mg, pramoxine HCl 10 mg, hydrocortisone 10 mg/ml in non-aqueous vehicle with 3% propylene glycol diacetate. Drops, otic. Vial 10 ml. *Rx.*
Use: Otic preparation.

Zovirax Capsules. (Glaxo Wellcome) Acyclovir 200 mg/Cap. Bot. 100s, UD 100s. *Rx.*
Use: Antiviral.

Zovirax Ointment 5%. (Glaxo Wellcome) Acyclovir 50 mg/Gm. Tube 15 g. *Rx.*
Use: Antiviral, topical.

Zovirax Powder. (Glaxo Wellcome) Acyclovir sodium 500 mg/vial or 1000 mg/vial. **500 mg:** Vial 10 ml. **1000 mg:** Vial 20 ml. *Rx.*
Use: Antiviral.

Zovirax Suspension. (Glaxo Wellcome) Acyclovir 200 mg/5 ml. Susp. Bot. 473 ml. *Rx.*
Use: Antiviral.

Zovirax Tablets. (Glaxo Wellcome) Acyclovir 400 mg or 800 mg/Tab. **400 mg:** Bot. 100s. **800 mg:** Bot. 100s, UD 100s, Shingles Relief Pak 35s. *Rx.*
Use: Antiviral.

Z-Pro-C. (Person & Covey) Zinc sulfate 200 mg (elemental zinc 45 mg), ascorbic acid 100 mg/Tab. Bot. 100s. *otc.*
Use: Vitamin/mineral supplement.

Z-Tec. (Seatrace) Iron equivalent 50 mg/ml from iron dextran complex. Vial 10 ml. *Rx.*
Use: Iron supplement.

•**zucapsaicin.** USAN.
Use: Analgesic, topical.

•**zuclomiphene.** USAN. *Formerly transclomiphene.*

Zurinol. (Major) Allopurinol. **100 mg/Tab.:** Bot. 100s, 500s, 1000s, UD 100s. **300 mg/Tab.:** Bot. 100s, 500s, UD 100s. *Rx.*
Use: Agent for gout.

Zyderm I. (Collagen Corp.) Highly purified bovine dermal collagen 35 mg/ml implant. Sterile syringe 0.1 ml, 0.5 ml, 1 ml, 2 ml.
Use: Collagen implant.

Zyderm II. (Collagen Corp.) Highly purified bovine dermal collagen 65 mg/ml implant. Syringe 0.75 ml.
Use: Collagen implant.

Zydone. (DuPont Merck) Hydrocodone bitartrate 5 mg, acetaminophen 500 mg/Cap. Bot. 100s. *c-III.*
Use: Narcotic analgesic combination.

Zyflo. (Abbott) Zileuton 600 mg/Tab. Bot. 120s. *Rx.*
Use: Treatment of asthma.

Zyloprim. (Glaxo Wellcome) Allopurinol. **100 mg/Tab.:** Bot. 100s, 1000s, UD 100s; **300 mg/Tab.:** Bot. 30s, 100s, 500s, UD 100s. *Rx.*
Use: Agent for gout.

Zymacap. (Pharmacia & Upjohn) Vitamins A 5000 IU, D 400 IU, E 15 mg, C 90 mg, folic acid 400 mcg, B_1 2.25 mg, B_2 2.6 mg, niacin 30 mg, B_6 3 mg, B_{12} 9 mcg, pantothenic acid 15 mg/Cap. Bot. 90s, 240s. *otc.*
Use: Vitamin supplement.

Zymase. (Organon) Lipase 12,000 units, protease 24,000 units, amylase 24,000 units. Cap. Bot. 100s. *Rx.*
Use: Digestive enzyme.

Zyprexa. (Eli Lilly & Co.) Olanzapine 5 mg, 7.5 mg, 10 mg/Tab. Bot. 60s, 100s. *Rx.*
Use: Antipsychotic.

Zyrtec. (Pfizer) Cetirizine 5 mg, 10 mg/Tab. Bot. 100s. Cetirizine 5 mg/ml/Syrup. Bot. 120 ml. *Rx.*
Use: Antihistamine.

Reference
Information

Common Abbreviations

Word	Abbreviation	Meaning
ana	$\overline{aa}$, aa	of each
ante cibum	a.c.	before meals or food
ad	ad.	to, up to
aurio dextra	a.d.	right ear
ad libitum	ad lib	at pleasure
aurio laeva	a.l.	left ear
ante meridiem	A.M.	morning
aqua	aq.	water
aqua destillata	aq.dest	distilled water
aurio sinister	a.s.	left ear
aures utrae	a.u.	each ear
bis in die	b.i.d.	twice daily
bowel movement	b.m.	bowel movement
blood pressure	b.p.	blood pressure
cong	c.	a gallon
cum	$\bar{c}$	with
capsula	caps	capsule
cubic centimeter	cc	cubic centimeter
compositus	comp	compound
dies	d.	day
dilue	dil.	dilute
dispensa	disp.	dispense
divide	div	divide
dentur tales doses	d.t.d.	give of such a dose
elixir	el.	elixir
as directed	e.m.p.	as directed
et	et	and
in water	ex aq	in water
fac, fiat, fiant	f., ft.	make, let be made
Food and Drug Administration	FDA	Food and Drug Administration
gramma	Gm., g.	gram
granum	gr	grain
gutta	gtt.	a drop
hora	h.	hour
hora somni	h.s., hor. som.	at bedtime
intramuscular	i.m., I.M.	intramuscular
intravenous	i.v.	intravenous
liquor	liq.	a liquor, solution
microgram	mcg	microgram
milligram	mg	milligram
milliliter	ml.	milliliter
misce	M.	mix
more dictor	m. dict.	as directed
mixtura	mixt.	a mixture
National Formulary	N.F.	National Formulary
numerus	no.	number
nocturnal	noc.	in the night
non repetatur	non. rep.	do not repeat, no refills
octarius	O, Oct.	a pint
oculus dexter	o.d.	right eye
oculus laevus	o.l.	left eye
oculus sinister	o.s.	left eye
oculo uterque	o.u.	each eye

Word	Abbreviation	Meaning
post cibos	p.c., post. cib.	after meals
post meridiem	P.M.	afternoon or evening
per os	p.o.	by mouth
pro re nata	p.r.n.	as needed
pulvis	pulv.	a powder
quoque alternis die	q.a.d.	every other day
every day	q.d.	every day
quiaque hora	q.h.	every hour
quater in die	q.i.d.	four times a day
every other day	q.o.d.	every other day
quantum sufficiat	q.s.	a sufficient quantity
a sufficient quantity to make	q.s. ad.	a sufficient quantity to make
quam volueris	q.v.	as much as you wish
recipe	Rx	take, a recipe
repetatur	rep	let it be repeated
sine	s̄, s.	without
secundum artem	s.a.	according to art
sataratus	sat.	saturated
signa	Sig.	label, or let it be printed
solutio	sol.	solution
dissolve	solv.	dissolve
semis	s̄s, ss	one-half
si opus sit	s.o.s.	if there is need
statim	stat.	at once, immediately
suppositorium	supp.	suppository
syrupus	syr.	syrup
tabella	tab.	tablet
such	tal.	such
such doses	tal. dos.	such doses
ter in die	t.i.d.	three times a day
tincture	tr., tinct.	tincture
tritura	.trit	triturate
teaspoonful	tsp	teaspoonful
unguentum	ung.	ointment
United States Adopted Names	USAN.	official adopted names
United States Pharmacopeia	U.S.P.	United States Pharmacopeia
ut dictum	ut. dict.	as directed
while awake	.w.a.	while awake

NOTE: The listing of commonly used abbreviations is included as an aid in interpreting medical orders.

Common Systems of Weights and Measures*

METRIC SYSTEM

Metric Weight

1 microgram†	µg (mcg)	=	0.000001	g
1 milligram	mg	=	0.001	g
1 centigram	cg	=	0.01	g
1 decigram	dg	=	0.1	g
1 gram	g	=	1.0	g
1 dekagram	Dg	=	10.0	g
1 hectogram	Hg	=	100.0	g
1 kilogram	Kg	=	1000.0	g

Metric Liquid Measure

1 microliter	µl	=	0.000001	L
1 milliliter	ml	=	0.001	L
1 centiliter	cl	=	0.01	L
1 deciliter	dl	=	0.1	L
1 liter	L	=	1.0	L
1 dekaliter	Dl	=	10.0	L
1 hectoliter	Hl	=	100.0	L
1 kiloliter	Kl	=	1000.0	L

APOTHECARY SYSTEM

Apothecary Weight

1 grain‡	gr	=	1 gr			
1 scruple	+	=	20 gr			
1 dram	/	=	60 gr	=	3+	
1 ounce	0	=	480 gr	=	8/	
1 pound	G	=	5760 gr	=	12o	

Apothecary Liquid Measure

1 minim	.	=	1.			
1 fluidram	f/	=	60.			
1 fluidounce	f0	=	480.	=	8 f/	
1 pint	pt	=	7680.	=	16 f0	
1 quart	qt	=	15630.	=	32 f0	
1 gallon	gal	=	61440.	=	8 pt0	

AVOIRDUPOIS SYSTEM

Avoirdupois Weight

1 ounce	= 1 oz	= 437.5 grains (gr)	
1 pound	= 1 lb	= 16 ounces (oz)	= 7000 grains (gr)

* The listing of common systems of weights and measures is included to aid the practitioner in calculating dosages.

† The abbreviation µg or mcg is used for microgram in pharmacy rather than gamma (γ) as in biology.

‡ The grain in each of the above systems has the same value, and thus serves as a basis for the interconversion of the other units.

Approximate
Practical Equivalents*

Weight Equivalents

1 grain	=	1 gr	=	64.8	milligrams
1 gram	=	1 Gm or g	=	15.432	grains
1 kilogram	=	1 Kg	=	2.20	pounds avoirdupois (G)
1 ounce avoirdupois	=	1 oz	=	28.35	grams
1 ounce apothecary	=	1 0	=	31.1	grams
1 pound avoirdupois	=	1 G	=	454.0	grams

Measure Equivalents

1 milliliter	=	1 ml	=	16.23	minims (.)
1 fluidram†	=	1 f/	=	3.4	ml
1 teaspoonful†	=	1 tsp	=	5.0	ml
1 tablespoonful	=	1 tbs or tbsp	=	15.0	ml
1 fluidounce	=	1 f0	=	29.57	ml
1 wineglassful	=	2 f0	=	60.0	ml
1 teacupful	=	4 f0	=	120.0	ml
1 tumblerful	=	8 f0	=	240.0	ml
1 pint	=	1 pt or O or Oct	=	473.0	ml
1 liter	=	1 L	=	33.8	fluidounces (f0)
1 gallon	=	1 gal or C or Cong	=	3785.0	ml

* The listing of approximate practical equivalents is included to aid the practitioner in calculating and converting dosages among the various systems.

† On prescription a fluidram is assumed to contain a teaspoonful which is 5 ml.

International System of Units

The *Système international d'unités* (International System of Units) or *SI* is a modernized version of the metric system. The primary goal of the conversion to SI units is to revise the present confused measurement system and to improve test-result communications. The SI has 7 basic units from which other units are derived:

Base Units of SI		
Physical quantity	Base unit	SI symbol
length	meter	m
mass	kilogram	kg
time	second	s
amount of substance	mole	mol
thermodynamic temperature	kelvin	K
electric current	ampere	A
luminous intensity	candela	cd

Combinations of these base units can express any property although, for simplicity, special names are given to some of these derived units.

Representative Derived Units		
Derived unit	Name and symbol	Derivation from base units
area	square meter	m^2
volume	cubic meter	m^3
force	newton (N)	$kg \cdot m \cdot s^{-2}$
pressure	pascal (Pa)	$kg \cdot m^{-1} \cdot s^{-2}$ (N/m^2)
work, energy	joule (J)	$kg \cdot m^2 \cdot s^{-2}$ (N·m)
mass density	kilogram per cubic meter	kg/m^3
frequency	hertz (Hz)	s^{-1}
temperature degree	Celsius (°C)	$°C = °K - 273.15$
concentration		
mass	kilogram/liter	kg/L
substance	mole/liter	mol/L
molality	mole/kilogram	mol/kg
density	kilogram/liter	kg/L

Prefixes to the base unit are used in this system to form decimal multiples and submultiples. The preferred multiples and submultiples listed below change the quantity by increments of 10^3 or 10^{-3}. The exceptions to these recommended factors are within the middle rectangle.

Prefixes and Symbols for Decimal Multiples and Submultiples		
Factor	Prefix	Symbol
10^{18}	exa	E
10^{15}	peta	P
10^{12}	tera	T
10^{9}	giga	G
10^{6}	mega	M
10^{3}	kilo	k
10^{2}	hecto	h
10^{1}	deka	da
10^{-1}	deci	d
10^{-2}	centi	c
10^{-3}	milli	m
10^{-6}	micro	μ
10^{-9}	nano	n
10^{-12}	pico	p
10^{-15}	femto	f
10^{-18}	atto	a

To convert drug concentrations to or from SI units:

$$\text{Conversion factor (CF)} = \frac{1000}{\text{mol wt}}$$

Conversion *to* SI units: $\mu g/ml \times CF = \mu mol/L$

Conversion *from* SI units: $\mu mol/L \div CF = \mu g/ml$

Normal Laboratory Values

In the following tables, normal reference values for commonly requested laboratory tests are listed in traditional units and in SI units. The tables are a guideline only. Values are method dependent and "normal values" may vary between laboratories.

Blood, Plasma or Serum		
	Reference Value	
Determination	Conventional Units	SI Units
Ammonia (NH_3)	10-80 mcg/dl	5-50 mcmol/L
Amylase	≤ 130 U/L	≤ 130 U/L
Antinuclear antibodies	negative at 1:10 dilution of serum	negative at 1:10 dilution of serum
Antithrombin III (AT III)	18-30 mg/dl	18-30 g/L
Bilirubin: conjugated	≤ 0.2 mg/dl	≤ 4 mcmol/L
total	0.1-1 mg/dl	2-18 mcmol/L
Calcitonin	< 100 pg/ml	< 100 ng/L
Calcium: female < 50 years old	8.8-10 mg/dl	2.2-2.5 mmol/L
female > 50 years old	8.8-10.2 mg/dl	2.2-2.56 mmol/L
male	8.8-10.3 mg/dl	2.2-2.58 mmol/L
all populations	4.4-5.1 mEq/L	2.2-2.56 mmol/L
Carbon dioxide content	22-28 mEq/L	22-28 mmol/L
Carcinoembryonic antigen	< 3 ng/ml	< 3 mcg/L
Chloride	95-105 mEq/L	95-105 mmol/L
Coagulation screen:		
Bleeding time	2-9 min	60-540 sec
Prothrombin time	10-12 sec	10-12 sec
Partial thromboplastin time (activated)	35-45 sec	35-45 sec
Protein C	0.4 mg/dl	0.4 g/L
Protein S	2.3 mg/dl	2.3 g/L
Copper, total	70-140 mcg/dl	11-22 mcmol/L
Corticotropin (ACTH adrenocorticotropic hormone)	20-100 pg/ml	4-22 pmol/L
Cortisol: 0800 hr	4-19 mcg/dl	110-520 nmol/L
1800 hr	2-15 mcg/dl	50-410 nmol/L
2400 hr	< 5 mcg/dl	< 140 nmol/L
Creatine phosphokinase, total (CK, CPK)	≤ 150 U/L	≤ 150 U/L
Creatine kinase isoenzymes, MB fraction	> 5% in MI	> 0.05 fraction of 1
Creatinine	0.6-1.2 mg/dl	50-110 mcmol/L
Fibrinogen (coagulation factor I)	150-350 mg/dl	1.5-3.5 g/L
Follicle stimulating hormone (FSH):		
female	2-15 mIU/ml	2-15 IU/L
peak production	20-50 mIU/ml	20-50 IU/L
male	1-10 mIU/ml	1-10 IU/L
Glucose, fasting	70-110 mg/dl	3.9-6.1 mmol/L
Haptoglobin	50-220 mg/dl	0.5-2.2 g/L
Hematologic tests:		
Hematocrit (Hct), female	33%-43%	0.33-0.43 fraction of 1
male	39%-49%	0.39-0.49 fraction of 1
Hemoglobin (Hb), female	11.5-15.5 g/dl	115-155 g/L
male	14-18 g/dl	140-180 g/L
Leukocyte count (WBC)	3200-9800/mm^3	3.2-9.8 x 10^9/L
Erythrocyte count (RBC), female	3.5-5 × 10^6/mm^3	3.5-5 x 10^{12}/L
male	4.3-5.9 × 10^6/mm^3	4.3-5.9 x 10^{12}/L
Mean corpuscular volume (MCV)	76-100 mcm^3	76-100 fL
Mean corpuscular hemoglobin (MCH)	27-33 pg	27-33 pg

Blood, Plasma or Serum		
	Reference Value	
Determination	Conventional Units	SI Units
Mean corpuscular hemoglobin concentration (MCHC)	33-37 g/dl	330-370 g/L
Erythrocyte sedimentation rate (sedrate, ESR): female	≤ 30 mm/hr	≤ 30 mm/hr
male	≤ 20 mm/hr	≤ 20 mm/hr
Ferritin	18-300 ng/ml	18-300 mcg/L
Folic acid: normal	> 3.8 ng/ml	8.4 nmol/L
Platelet count	130-400 × 10^3/mm^3	130-400 x 10^9/L
Vitamin B$_{12}$	200-1000 pg/ml	150-750 pmol/L
Iron		
female	60-160 mcg/dl	11-29 mcmol/L
male	80-180 mcg/dl	14-32 mcmol/L
Iron binding capacity	250-460 mcg/dl	45-82 mcmol/L
Lactic acid (lactate)	0.5-2 mEq/L	0.5-2 mmol/L
Lactic dehydrogenase	50-150 U/L	50-150 U/L
Lead (toxic levels)	> 60 mcg/dl	> 2.9 mcmol/L
Lipids:		
Triglycerides		
Desirable	< 250 mg/dl	< 2.82 mmol/L
Borderline	250-500 mg/dl	2.82-5.65 mmol/L
High	> 500 mg/dl	> 5.65 mmol/L
LDL Cholesterol		
Desirable	< 130 mg/dl	< 3.36 mmol/L
Borderline	130-159 mg/dl	3.36-4.11 mmol/L
High	> 159 mg/dl	> 4.11 mmol/L
HDL Cholesterol		
low	< 35 mg/dl	< 0.91 mmol/L
Total Cholesterol		
Desirable	< 200 mg/dl	5.17 mmol/L
Borderline	200-239 mg/dl	5.17-6.18 mmol/L
High	> 239 mg/dl	> 6.18 mmol/L
Magnesium	1.6-2.4 mEq/L	0.8-1.2 mmol/L
Osmolality	280-300 mOsm/kg	280-300 mmol/kg
Oxygen saturation (arterial)	96%-100%	0.96-1 fraction of 1
PCO$_2$, arterial	35-45 mmHg	4.7-6 kPa
pH, arterial	7.35-7.45	7.35-7.45
PO$_2$, arterial: Breathing room air	75-100 mmHg	10-13.3 kPa
Phosphatase (acid)	2-11 IU/L	3-183 mckat/L
Phosphatase alkaline (ALP)	25-100 IU/L	4-1.7 mckat/L
Phosphorus, inorganic (phosphate)	2.5-5 mg/dl	0.8-1.6 mmol/L
Potassium	3.5-5 mEq/L	3.5-5 mmol/L
Progesterone		
Follicular phase	< 2 ng/ml	< 6 nmol/L
Luteal phase	2-20 ng/ml	6-64 nmol/L
Prolactin	< 20 ng/ml	< 20 mcg/L

Blood, Plasma or Serum		
	Reference Value	
Determination	Conventional Units	SI Units
Protein: Total	5.5-9 g/dl	55-90 g/L
Albumin	3.5-5 g/dl	35-50 g/L
Globulin	2-3 g/dl	20-30 g/L
Rheumatoid factor	< 80 IU/ml	< 80 kIU/L
Sodium	135-147 mEq/L	135-147 mmol/L
Testosterone: female	< 0.6 ng/ml	< 2 nmol/L
male	4-8 ng/ml	14-28 nmol/L
Thyroid Hormone Function Tests:		
Thyroid-stimulating hormone (TSH)	2-11 mcU/ml	2-11 mU/L
Thyroxine-binding globulin capacity	12-28 mcg/dl	150-360 nmol/L
Total triiodothyronine (T_3)	75-220 ng/dl	1.2-3.4 nmol/L
Total thyroxine (T_4)	4-11 mcg/dl	51-142 nmol/L
T_3 uptake	25%-35%	0.25-0.35 fraction of 1
Transaminase, AST (aspartate aminotrans-ferase, SGOT)	≤ 35 U/L	≤ 35 U/L
Transaminase, ALT (alanine aminotrans-ferase, SGPT)	≤ 35 U/L	≤ 35 U/L
Urea nitrogen (BUN)	8-18 mg/dl	3-6.5 mmol/L
Uric acid	2-7 mg/dl	120-420 mcmol/L
Vitamin A (retinol)	10-50 mcg/dl	0.35-1.75 mcmol/L
Zinc	75-120 mcg/dl	11.5-18.5 mcmol/L

Urine				
	Reference Value			
Determination	Conventional Units		SI Units	
Catecholamines: Epinephrine	< 10 mcg/day		< 55 nmol/day	
Norepinephrine	< 100 mcg/day		< 590 nmol/day	
Creatinine: female	14-22 mg/kg/24 h		0.12-0.19 mmol/kg/day	
male	20-26 mg/kg/24 h		0.18-0.23 mmol/kg/day	
Potassium (diet-dependent)	25-100 mEq/day		25-100 mmol/day	
Protein, quantitative	< 150 mg/day		< 0.15 g/day	
Steroids:	(mg/day)		(mcmol/day)	
Age (yrs)	male	female	male	female
17-Ketosteroids 10	1-4	1-4	3-14	3-14
20	6-21	4-16	21-73	14-56
30	8-26	4-14	28-90	14-49
50	5-18	3-9	17-62	10-31
70	2-10	1-7	7-35	3-24
17-Hydroxycorticosteroids (as cortisol):				
female	2-8 mg/day		5-25 mcmol/day	
male	3-10 mg/day		10-30 mcmol/day	

Drug Levels†		
	Reference Value	
Drug Determination	Conventional Units	SI Units
Aminoglycosides (peak levels)		
Amikacin	16-32 µg/ml	nd
Gentamicin	4-8 µg/ml	nd
Kanamycin	15-40 µg/ml	nd
Netilmicin	6-10 µg/ml	nd
Streptomycin	20-30 µg/ml	nd
Tobramycin	4-8 µg/ml	nd
Antiarrhythmics		
Amiodarone	0.5-2.5 µg/ml	nd
Bretylium	0.5-1.5 µg/ml	nd
Digitoxin	9-25 µg/L	11.8-32.8 nmol/L
Digoxin	0.5-2.2 ng/ml	0.6-2.8 nmol/L
Disopyramide	2-8 µg/ml	6-18 µmol/L
Flecainide	0.2-1 µg/ml	nd
Lidocaine	1.5-6 µg/ml	4.5-21.5 µmol/L
Mexiletine	0.5-2 µg/ml	nd
Procainamide	4-8 µg/ml	17-34 µmol/ml
Propranolol	50-200 ng/ml	190-770 nmol/L
Quinidine	2-6 µg/ml	4.6-9.2 µmol/L
Tocainide	4-10 µg/ml	nd
Verapamil	0.08-0.3 µg/ml	nd
Anticonvulsants		
Carbamazepine	4-12 µg/ml	17-51 µmol/L
Phenobarbital	15-40 µg/ml	65-172 µmol/L
Phenytoin	10-20 µg/ml	40-80 µmol/L
Primidone	5-12 µg/ml	25-46 µmol/L
Valproic acid	50-100 µg/ml	350-700 µmol/L
Antidepressants		
Amitriptyline	110-250 ng/ml	nd
Amoxapine	200-500 ng/ml	nd
Bupropion	25-100 ng/ml	nd
Clomipramine	80-100 ng/ml	nd
Desipramine	125-300 ng/ml	nd
Doxepin	100-200 ng/ml	nd
Imipramine	200-350 ng/ml	nd
Maprotiline	200-300 ng/ml	nd
Nortriptyline	50-150 ng/ml	nd
Protriptyline	100-200 ng/ml	nd
Trazodone	800-1600 ng/ml	nd
Antipsychotics		
Chlorpromazine	30-500 ng/ml	nd
Fluphenazine	0.13-2.8 ng/ml	nd
Haloperidol	5-20 ng/ml	nd
Perphenazine	0.8-1.2 ng/ml	nd
Thiothixene	2-57 ng/ml	nd
Miscellaneous		
Amantadine	300 ng/ml	nd
Amrinone	3.7 µg/ml	nd
Chloramphenicol	10-20 µg/ml	31-62 µmol/L
Cyclosporine[1]	250-800 ng/ml (whole blood, RIA)	nd
	50-300 ng/ml (plasma, RIA)	nd
Ethanol[2]	0 mg/dl	0 mmol/L
Hydralazine	100 ng/ml	nd
Lithium	0.5-1.5 mEq/L	0.5-1.5 mmol/L
Salicylate	100-200 mg/L	724-1448 µmol/L
Sulfonamide	5-15 mg/dl	nd
Terbutaline	0.5-4.1 ng/ml	nd
Theophylline	10-20 µg/ml	55-110 µmol/L
Vancomycin (peak)	30-40 ng/ml	nd

† The values given are generally accepted as desirable for achieving therapeutic effect without toxicity for most patients. However, exceptions are not uncommon.
[1] 24 hour trough values. [2] Toxic: 50-100 mg/dl (10.9-21.7 mmol/L).   nd – No data available.

Trademark Glossary

Many companies use trademarks to identify specific dosage forms or unique packaging materials. The following list is provided as a guide to the interpretation of these descriptions.

Abbo-Pac (Abbott)
Unit dose package

Accu-Pak (Novartis)
Unit dose blister pack

Act-O-Vial (Pharmacia & Upjohn)
Vial system

ADD-Vantage (Abbott)
Sterile dissolution system for admixture

ADT (Pharmacia & Upjohn)
Alternate day therapy

Arm-A-Med (Centeon)
Single-dose plastic vial

Arm-A-Vial (Centeon)
Single-dose plastic vial

Aspirol (Lilly)
Crushable ampule for inhalation

Back-Pack (Merck & Co.)
Unit-of-use package

bidCAP (B-M Squibb)
Double strength capsule

Bristoject (B-M Squibb)
Unit dose syringe

Caplet, Captab (Various)
Capsule shaped tablet

Carpuject (Sanofi Winthrop)
Cartridge needle unit

Carpuject Smartpak (Sanofi Winthrop)
Cartridge needle unit package

Chronotab (Schering-Plough)
Sustained action tablet

Clinipak (Wyeth-Ayerst)
Unit dose package

ControlPak (Sandoz)
Unit dose rolls, tamper resistant

Delcap (Ortho McNeil)
Unit dispensing cap

Detecto-Seal (Sanofi Winthrop)
Tamper resistant parenteral package

Dialpak (Ortho)
Compliance package

Dis-Co Pack (Robins)
Unit dose package

Disket (Lilly)
Dispersible tablet

Dispenserpak (Glaxo Wellcome)
Unit-of-use package

Dispertab (Abbott)
Particles in tablet

Dispette (Lederle)
Disposable pipette

Divide-Tab (Abbott)
Scored tablet

Dividose (B-M Squibb)
Tablet, bisected/trisected

Dosa-Trol Pack (B-M Squibb)
Unit-dose box packaging

Dosepak (Pharmacia & Upjohn)
Unit-of-use package

Dosette (Elkins-Sinn)
Single dose ampule or vial

Drop Dose (Glaxo Wellcome)
Ophthalmic dropper dispenser

Drop-Tainer (Alcon)
Ophthalmic dropper dispenser

Dulcet (Abbott)
Chewable tablet

Dura-Tab (Berlex)
Sustained release tablet

Enduret (Boehringer Ingelheim)
Prolonged action tablet

Enseal (Lilly)
Enteric coated tablet

EN-tabs (Pharmacia & Upjohn)
Enteric coated tablet

Expidet (Wyeth-Ayerst)
Fast-dissolving doseform

Extencap (Robins)
Controlled release capsule

Extentab (Robins)
Continuous release tablet

Fast-Trak (Wyeth-Ayerst)
Quick-loading hypodermic syringe

Filmlok (B-M Squibb)
Veneer coated tablet

Filmseal (Parke-Davis)
Film coated tablet

Filmtab (Abbott)
Film coated tablet

Flo-Pack (Glaxo Wellcome)
Vial for preparation of IV drips

Gelseal (Lilly)
Soft gelatin capsule

Gradumet (Abbott)
Controlled release tablet

Gy-Pak (Novartis)
Unit-of-issue package

Gyrocap (Rhone-Poulenc Rorer)
Timed release capsule

Hyporet (Lilly)
Unit dose syringe

Identi-Dose (Lilly)
Unit dose package

Infatab (Parke-Davis)
Chewable pediatric tablet

Inject-all (B-M Squibb)
Prefilled disposable dilution syringe

Inlay-Tabs (Sandoz)
Inlaid tablets

Isoject (Pfizer)
Unit dose syringe

Kapseal (Parke-Davis)
Banded (sealed) capsule

Kronocap (Ferndale)
Sustained release capsule

Lederject (Lederle)
Disposable syringe

Liquitab (Mission)
Chewable tablet

Memorette (Syntex)
Compliance package

Mix-O-Vial (Pharmacia & Upjohn)
Two compartment vial

Mono-Drop (Sanofi Winthrop)
Ophthalmic plastic dropper

Ocumeter (Merck & Co.)
Ophthalmic dropper dispenser

Perle (Forest)
Soft gelatin capsule

Pilpak (Wyeth-Ayerst)
Compliance pack

Plateau CAP (Hoechst Marion Roussel)
Controlled release capsule

Pulvule (Lilly)
Bullet-shaped capsule

Rediject (Organon)
Unit dose syringe

Redipak (Wyeth-Ayerst)
Unit dose or unit-of-issue package

Redi Vial (Lilly)
Dual compartment vial

Repetabs (Schering-Plough)
Extended release tablet

Rescue Pak (Glaxo Wellcome)
Unit dose packaging

Respihaler (Merck & Co.)
Aerosol for inhalation

Robicap (Robins)
Capsule

Robitab (Robins)
Tablet

SandoPak (Sandoz)
Unit dose blister package

Sani-Pak (Roberts)
Sanitary dispensing box

Secule (Wyeth-Ayerst)
Single dose vial

Sequels (Lederle)
Sustained release capsule or tablet

SigPak (Sandoz)
Unit-of-use package

Snap Tabs (Sandoz)
Tablet with facilitated bisect

Solvet (Lilly)
Soluble tablet

Spansule (SmithKline Beecham)
Sustained release capsule

Stat-Pak (Pharmacia & Upjohn)
Unit dose package

Steri-Dose (Parke-Davis)
Unit dose syringe

Steri-Vial (Parke-Davis)
Ampule

Supprette (PolyMedica)
Suppository

Tabloid (Glaxo Wellcome)
Branded tablet (with raised lettering)

Tamp-R-Tel (Wyeth-Ayerst)
Tubex, tamper resistant

Tel-E-Amp (Roche)
Single dose amp

Tel-E-Dose (Roche)
Unit dose strip package

Tel-E-Ject (Roche)
Unit dose syringe

Tel-E-Pack (Roche)
Packaging system

Tel-E-Vial (Roche)
Single dose vial

Tembids (Wyeth-Ayerst)
Sustained action capsule

Tempule (Centeon)
Timed release capsule or tablet

Thera-Ject (SmithKline Beecham)
Unit dose syringe

Tiltab (SmithKline Beecham)
Tablet shape

Timecap (Schwarz Pharma)
Sustained release capsule

Timecelle (Roberts)
Timed release capsule

Timespan (Roche)
Timed release tablet

Titradose (Wyeth-Ayerst)
Scored tablet

Traypak (Lilly)
Multivial carton

Tubex (Wyeth-Ayerst)
Cartridge-needle unit

Turbinaire (Merck & Co.)
Aerosol for nasal inhalation

UDIP (Hoechst Marion Roussel)
Unit dose indentification pack

U-Ject (Pharmacia & Upjohn)
Disposable syringe

Uni-Amp (Sanofi Winthrop)
Single dose ampule

Unimatic (B-M Squibb)
Unit dose syringe

Uni-nest (Sanofi Winthrop)
Ampule

UNI-Rx (Hoechst Marion Roussel)
Unit dose packages and containers

Unisert (Upsher-Smith)
Suppository

Vaporole (Glaxo Wellcome)
Crushable ampule for inhalation

Visipak (Pharmacia & Upjohn)
Reverse numbered pack

Wyseals (Wyeth-Ayerst)
Film coated tablet

Medical Terminology Glossary

Abduction – the act of drawing away from a center.

Abstergent – a cleansing application or medicine.

Acaricide – an agent lethal to mites.

Achlorhydria – the absence of hydrochloric acid from gastric secretions.

Acidifier, systemic – a drug used to lower internal body pH in patients with systemic alkalosis.

Acidifier, urinary – a drug used to lower the pH of the urine.

Acidosis – an accumulation of acid in the body.

Acne – an inflammatory disease of the skin accompanied by the eruption of papules or pustules.

Addison's Disease – a condition caused by adrenal gland destruction.

Adduction – the act of drawing toward a center.

Adenitis – a gland or lymph node inflammation.

Adjuvant – an ingredient added to a prescription which complements or accentuates the action of the primary agent.

Adrenergic – a sypathomimetic drug that activates organs innervated by the sympathetic branch of the autonomic nervous system.

Adrenocorticotropic Hormone – an anterior pituitary hormone that stimulates and regulates secretion of the adrenocortical steroids.

Adrenocortical steroid, anti-inflammatory – an adrenal cortex hormone that participates in regulation of organic metabolism and inhibits the inflammatory response to stress; a glucocorticoid.

Adrenocortical steroid, salt regulating – an adrenal cortex hormone that maintains sodium-potassium electrolyte balance by stimulating and regulating sodium retention and potassium excretion by the kidneys.

Adsorbent – an agent that binds chemicals to its surface; it is useful in reducing the free availability of toxic chemicals.

Alkalizer, systemic – a drug that raises internal body pH in patients with systemic acidosis.

Allergen – a specific substance that causes an unwanted reaction in the body.

Amblyopia – pertaining to a dimness of vision.

Amebiasis – an infection with a pathogenic amoeba.

Amenorrhea – an abnormal discontinuation of the menses.

Amphiarthrosis – a joint in which the surfaces are connected by discs of fibrocartilage.

Anabolic – an agent that promotes conversion of simple substance into more complex compounds; a constructive process for the organism.

Analeptic – a potent central nervous system stimulant used to maintain vital functions during severe central nervous system depression.

Analgesic – a drug that selectively suppresses pain perception without inducing unconsciousness.

Ancyclostomiasis – the presence of hookworms in the intestine.

Androgen – a hormone that stimulates and maintains male secondary sex characteristics.

Anemia – a deficiency of red blood cells.

Anesthetic, general – a drug that eliminates pain perception by inducing unconsciousness.

Anesthetic, local – a drug that eliminates pain perception in a limited area by local action on sensory nerves; a topical anesthetic.

Angina pectoris – a sharp chest pain starting in the heart, often spreading down the left arm. A symptom of coronary disease.

Angiography – an X-ray of the blood vessels.

Anhydrotic – a drug that checks perspiration flow systemically; an antidiaphoretic.

Anodyne – a drug which acts on the sensory nervous system, either centrally or peripherally, to produce relief from pain.

Anorexiant – a drug that suppresses appetite, usually secondary to central stimulation of mood.

Anorexigenic – an agent promoting a dislike or aversion to food.

Antacid – a drug that neutralizes excess gastric acid locally.

Anthelmintic – a drug that kills or inhibits worm infestations such as pinworms and tapeworms (nematodes, cestodes, trematodes).

Antiadrenergic – a drug that prevents response to sympathetic nervous system stimulation and adrenergic drugs; a sympatholytic or sympathoplegic drug.

Antiamebic – a drug that kills or inhibits the pathogenic protozoan *Entamoeba histolytica,* the causative agent of amebic dysentery.

Antianemic – a drug that stimulates the production of erythrocytes in normal size, number and hemoglobin content; useful in treating anemias.

Antiasthmatic – an agent that relieves the symptoms of asthma.

Antibacterial – a drug that kills or inhibits pathogenic bacteria, the causative agents of many systemic gastrointestinal and superficial infections.

Antibiotic – an agent produced by or derived from living cells of molds, bacteria or other plants, which destroy or inhibit the growth of microbes.

Anticholesteremic – a drug that lowers blood cholesterol levels.

Anticholinergic – a drug that prevents response to parasympathetic nervous system stimulation and cholinergic drugs; a parasympatholytic or parasympathoplegic drug.

Anticoagulant – a drug that inhibits clotting of circulating blood or prevents clotting of collected blood.

Anticonvulsant – a drug that selectively prevents epileptic seizures; a central depressant used to arrest convulsions by inducing unconsciousness.

Antidepressant – a psychotherapeutic drug that induces mood elevation, useful in treating depressive neuroses and psychoses.

Antidiabetic – a drug used to prevent the development of diabetes.

Antidote – a drug that prevents or counteracts the effects of poisons or drug overdoses, by adsorption in the gastrointestinal tract (general antidotes) or by specific systemic action (specific antidotes).

Antieczematic – a topical drug that aids in the control of exudative inflammatory skin lesions.

Antiemetic – a drug that prevents vomiting, especially that of systemic origin.

Antifibrinolytic – an agent (drug) that inhibits liquifaction of fibrin.

Antifilarial – a drug that kills or inhibits pathogenic filarial worms of the superfamily *Filarioidea*, the causative agents of diseases such as loaiasis.

Antiflatulant – an agent inhibiting the excessive formation of gas in the stomach or intestines.

Antifungal – a drug that kills or inhibits pathogenic fungi, the causative agents of systemic, gastrointestinal and superficial infections.

Antihemophilic – a blood derivative containing the clotting factors absent in the hereditary disease hemophilia.

Antihistaminic – a drug that prevents response to histamine, including histamine released by allergic reactions.

Antihypercholesterolemic – a drug that lowers blood cholesterol levels, especially elevated levels sometimes associated with cardiovascular disease.

Antihypertensive – a drug that lowers blood pressure, especially diastolic blood pressure in hypertensive patients.

Antiinfective, local – a drug that kills a variety of pathogenic microorganisms and is suitable for sterilizing the skin or wounds.

Anti-inflammatory – a drug which counteracts or suppresses inflammation, and produces suppression of the pain, heat, redness and swelling of inflammation.

Antileishmanial – a drug that kills or inhibits pathogenic protozoa of the genus *Leishmania*, the causative agents of diseases such as kala-azar.

Antileprotic – an agent which fights leprosy, a generally chronic skin disease.

Antilipemic – an agent reducing the amount of circulating lipids.

Antimalarial – a drug that kills or inhibits the causative agents of malaria.

Antimetabolite – a substance that competes with or replaces a certain metabolite.

Antimethemoglobinemic – a drug that reduces nonfunctional methemoglobin (Fe^{+++}) to normal hemoglobin (Fe^{++}).

Antimycotic – an agent inhibiting the growth of fungi.

Antinauseant – a drug that suppresses nausea, especially that due to motion sickness.

Antineoplastic – a drug that is selectively toxic to rapidly multiplying cells and is useful in destroying malignant tumors.

Antioxidant – an agent used to reduce decay or transformation of a material from oxidation.

Antiperiodic – a drug that modifies or prevents the return of malarial fever; an antimalarial.

Antiperistaltic – a drug that inhibits intestinal motility, especially for the treatment of diarrhea.

Antipruritic – a drug that prevents or relieves itching.

Antipyretic – a drug employed to reduce fever temperature of the body; a febrifuge.

Antirheumatic – a drug that alleviates inflammatory symptoms of arthritis and related connective tissue diseases.

Antirickettsial – a drug that kills or inhibits pathogenic microorganisms of the genus *Rickettsia*, the causative agents of diseases such as typhus (e.g. Chloramphenicol USP).

Antischistosomal – a drug that kills or inhibits pathogenic flukes of the genus *Schistosoma*, the causative agents of schistosomiasis.

Antiseborrheic – a drug that aids in the control of seborrheic dermatitis ("dandruff").

Antiseptic – a substance that will inhibit the growth and development of microorganisms without necessarily destroying them.

Antisialagogue – a drug which diminishes the flow of saliva.

Antispasmodic – an agent used to quiet the spasms of voluntary and involuntary muscles; calmative or antihysteric.

Antisyphilitic – a remedy used in the treatment of syphilis.

Antitoxin – a biological drug containing antibodies against the toxic principles of a pathogenic microorganism, used for passive immunization against the associated disease.

Antitrichomonal – a drug that kills or inhibits the pathogenic protozoan *Trichomonas vaginalis*, the causative agent of trichomonal vaginitis.

Antitrypanosomal – a drug that kills or inhibits pathogenic protozoa of the genus *Trypanosoma*, the causative agents of diseases such as West African trypanosomiasis.

Antitussive – a drug that suppresses coughing.

Antivenin – a biological drug containing antibodies against the venom of a poisonous animal; an antidote for a venomous bite.

Anxiety – a feeling of apprehension, uncertainty and fear.

Aperient – a mild laxative.

Aphasia – the inability to use or understand written and spoken words, due to damage of cortical speech centers.

Aphonia – a whisper voice due to disease of the larynx or its innervation.

Apnea – the absence of breathing.

Areola – a pigmented ring on the skin.

Arsenical – having to do with arsenic.

Arteriosclerosis – a hardening of the arteries.

Arthritis – an inflammation of a joint.

Ascariasis – a condition caused by roundworms in the intestine.

Ascaricide – an agent that kills roundworms of the genus *Ascaris*.

Aspergillus – a fungi genus including many types of molds.

Astasia – the inability to stand up without help.

Asthma – a disease characterized by recurring breathing difficulty due to bronchial muscle constriction.

Astringent – a mild protein precipitant suitable for local application to toughen, shrink, blanch, wrinkle and harden tissue; diminish secretions and coagulate blood.

Ataractic – an agent having a quieting, tranquilizing effect.

Ataxia – incoordination, especially of gait.

Atheroma – a fatty granular degeneration of an artery wall.

Atrophy – a wasting away.

Avitaminosis – a disease caused by lack of one or more vitamins in the diet.

Axilla – armpit.

Bacteriostatic – an agent that inhibits the growth of bacteria.

Basedow's disease – a form of hyperthyroidism, also known as Grave's disease and Parry's disease.

Biliary Colic – a sharp pain in the upper right side of the abdomen due to a gallstone impaction.

Bilirubin – a bile pigment.

Biliuria – the presence of bile in the urine.

Blood Calcium Regulator – a drug that maintains the blood level of ionic calcium, especially by regulating its metabolic disposition elsewhere.

Blood Volume Supporter – an intravenous solution whose solutes are retained in the vascular system to supplement the osmotic activity of plasma proteins.

Bradycardia – a slow heart rate.

Bright's Disease – a disease of the kidneys, including the presence of edema and excessive urine protein formation.

Bromidrosis – foul smelling perspiration.

Bronchitis – an inflammation of the bronchi.

Bronchodilator – a drug which can dilate the lumina of air passages of the lungs.

Bruit – an arterial sound audible with a stethoscope.

Buerger's Disease – a thromboanglitis obliterans inflammation of the walls and surrounding rise of the veins and arteries.

Bursitis – an inflammation of the bursa.

Callus – a hard bonelike material developing around a fractured bone.

Calmative – a sedative.

Candidiasis – an infection by the yeastlike organism *Candida albicans*.

Carbonic Anhydrase Inhibitor – an enzyme inhibitor, the therapeutic effects of which are diuresis and reduced formation of intraocular fluid.

Carcinoma – a malignant growth.

Cardiac Depressant – a drug that depresses myocardial function so as to supress rhythmic irregularities characterized by fast rate; an antiarrhythmic.

Cardiac Stimulant – a drug that increases the contractile force of the myocardium, especially in weakened conditions such as congestive heart failure; a cardiotonic.

Cardiopathy – a disease of the heart.

Caries – decay of the teeth.

Carminative – an aromatic or pungent drug that mildly irritates the gastrointestinal tract and is useful in the treatment of flatulence and colic. Peppermint Water is a common carminative.

Caruncle – a small fleshy projection on the skin.

Cathartic – a drug that promotes defecation, usually by enhancing peristalsis or by softening and lubricating the feces.

Caudal – pertains to the distal end or tail.

Caustic – a topical drug that destroys tissue on contact and is suitable for removal of abnormal skin growths.

Central Depressant – a drug that reduces the functional state of the central nervous system and with increasing dosage induces sedation, hypnosis and general anesthesia; respiration is depressed.

Central Stimulant – a drug that increases the functional state of the central nervous system and with increasing dosage induces restlessness, insomnia, disorientation and convulsions; respiration is stimulated.

Cerebral – pertaining to the brain.

Cerumen – earwax.

Chloasma – skin discoloration.

Cholagogue – a drug that stimulates the emptying of the gallbladder and the flow of bile into the duodenum.

Cholecystitis – an inflammation of the gallbladder.

Cholecystokinetic – an agent that promotes emptying of the gallbladder.

Cholelithiasis – the presence of calculi (stones) in the gallbladder.

Choleretic – a drug that increases the production and secretion of dilute bile by the liver.

Chorea – a disorder, usually of childhood, characterized by uncontrolled spasmotic muscle movements; sometimes referred to as St. Vitus' dance.

Chymotrypsin – a proteinase in the gastrointestinal tract; its proposed use has been the treatment of edema and inflammation.

Claudication – limping.

Climacteric – a time period in women just preceding termination of the reproductive processes.

Clonus – a spasm in which rigidity and relaxation succeed each other.

Coagulant – a drug that replaces a deficient blood factor necessary for coagulation; clotting factor.

Coccidiostat – a drug used in the treatment of coccidal (protozoal) infections in animals, especially birds; used in veterinary medicine.

Colitis – an inflammation of the colon.

Colloid – a disperse system of particles larger than those of true solutions but smaller than those of suspensions (1 to 100 millimicrons in size).

Collyrium – an eyewash.

Colostomy – the surgical formation of a more or less permanent opening into the colon.

Corticoid – a term applied to hormones of the adrenal cortex or any substance, natural or synthetic, having similar activity.

Corticosteroid – a steroid produced by the adrenal cortex.

Coryza – a headcold.

Counterirritant – an agent (irritant) which causes irritation of the part to which it is applied, and draws blood away from a deep seated area.

Cranial – pertaining to the skull.

Crepitation – the grating of a joint.

Cryptitis – an inflammation of a follicle or glandular tubule, usually in the rectum.

Cryptococcus – a genus of fungi which does not produce spores, but reproduces by budding.

Cryptorchidism – the failure of one or both testes to descend.

Cutaneous – pertaining to the skin.

Cyanosis – a blue or purple skin discoloration due to oxygen deficiency.

Cycloplegia – the loss of accommodation.

Cyclopegic – a drug which paralyzes accommodation of the eye.

Cystitis – an inflammation of the bladder.

Cystourethography – the examination by x-ray of the bladder and urethra.

Cytostasis – a slowing of the movement of blood cells at an inflamed area, sometimes causing capillary blockage.

Debridement – the cutting away of dead or excess skin from a wound.

Decongestant – a drug which reduces congestion caused by an accumulation of blood.

Decubitus – the patient's position in bed; the act of lying down.

Demulcent – an agent used generally internally to sooth and protect mucous membranes.

Dermatitis – an inflammation of the skin.

Dermatomycosis – lesions or eruptions caused by fungi on the skin.

Detergent – an emulsifying agent useful for cleansing wounds and ulcers as well as the skin.

Dextrocardia – when the heart is located on the right side of the chest.

Diagnostic Aid – a drug used to determine the functional state of a body organ or the presence of a disease.

Diaphoretic – a drug used to increase perspiration; a hydroticorsudorfice.

Diarrhea – an abnormal frequency and fluidity of stools.

Digestive Enzyme – an enzyme that promotes digestion by supplementing the naturally occurring counterpart.

Digitalization – the administration of digitalis to obtain a desired tissue level of drug.

Diplopia – double vision.

Disinfectant – an agent that destroys pathogenic microorganisms on contact and is suitable for sterilizing inanimate objects.

Distal – farthest from a point of reference.

Diuretic – a drug that promotes renal excretion of electrolytes and water, thereby increasing urine volume.

Dysarthria – difficulty in speech articulation.

Dysmenorrhea – pertaining to painful menstruation.

Dysphagia – difficulty in swallowing.

Dyspnea – difficult breathing.

Ecbolic – a drug used to stimulate the gravid uterus to the expulsion of the fetus, or to cause uterine contraction; an oxytocic.

Eclampsia – a toxic disorder occurring late in pregnancy involving hypertension, weight gain, edema and renal dysfunction.

Ectasia – pertaining to distension or stretching.

Ectopic – out of place; not in normal position.

Eczema – an inflammatory disease of the skin with infiltrations, watery discharge, scales and crust.

Effervescent – bubbling; sparkling; giving off gas bubbles.

Embolus – a blood clot in the blood stream lodged in a vessel, thus obstructing circulation.

Emetic – a drug that induces vomiting, either locally by gastrointestinal irritation or systemically by stimulation of receptors in the central nervous system.

Emollient – a topical drug, especially an oil or fat, used to soften the skin and make it more pliable.

Endometrium – the uterine mucous membrane.

Enteralgia – an intestinal pain.

Enterobiasis – a pinworm infestation.

Enuresis – involuntary urination, as in bedwetting.

Epidermis – the outermost layer of the skin.

Episiotomy – a surgical incision of the vulva when deemed necessary during childbirth.

Epistaxis – a nosebleed.

Erythema – redness.

Erythrocyte – a red blood cell.

Escharotic – corrosive.

Estrogen – a hormone that stimulates and maintains female secondary sex characteristics and functions in the menstrual cycle to promote uterine gland proliferation.

Etiology – the cause of a disease.

Euphoria – an exaggerated feeling of well being.

Eutonic – having normal muscular tone.

Exfoliation – a scaling of the skin.

Exophthalmos – a protrusion of the eyeballs.

Expectorant – a drug that increases secretion of respiratory tract fluid, thereby lowering its viscosity and cough-inducing irritancy and promoting its ejection.

Extension – the movement of a joint to move two body parts away from each other.

Exteroceptors – receptors on the exterior of the body.

Fasciculations – the visible twitching movements of muscle bundles.

Fibroid – a tumor of fibrous tissue, resembling fibers.

Filariasis – the condition of having round worm parasites reproducing in the body tissues.

Fistula – an abnormal opening leading from a body cavity to the outside of the body or to another cavity.

Flexion – the movement of a joint in which two moveable parts are brought toward each other.

Fungistatic – inhibiting the growth of fungi.

Furunculosis – a condition marked by the presence of boils.

Gallop Rhythm – a heart condition where three separate beats are heard instead of two.

Gastralgia – a stomach pain.

Gastritis – inflammation of the stomach lining.

Gastrocele – a hernial protrusion of the stomach.

Gastrodynia – pain in the stomach, a stomach ache.

Geriatrics – a branch of medicine which treats problems peculiar to old age.

Germicidal – an agent that is destructive to pathogenic microorganisms.

Gingivitis – an inflammation of the gums.

Glaucoma – a disease of the eye evidenced by an increase in intraocular pressure and resulting in hardness of the eye, atrophy of the retina and eventual blindness.

Glossitis – an inflammation of the tongue.

Glucocorticoid – a corticoid which increases gluconeogenesis, thereby raising the concentration of liver glycogen and blood sugar.

Glycosuria – an abnormal quantity of glucose in the urine.

Gout – a disorder which is characterized by a high uric acid level and sudden onset of recurrent arthritis.

Granulation – the formation of small round fleshy granules on a wound in the healing process.

Hematemesis – the vomiting of blood.

Hematinic – a drug that promotes hemoglobin formation by supplying a factor essential for its synthesis.

Hemiplegia – a condition in which one side of the body is paralyzed.

Hematopoietic – a drug that stimulates formation of blood cells, especially by supplying deficient vitamins.

Hemoptysis – expectoration of blood.

Histoplasmosis – a lung infection caused by the inhalation of fungus spores, often resulting in pneumonitis.

Hodgkin's Disease – a disease marked by chronic lymph enlargement sometimes including spleen and liver enlargement.

Hydrocholeresis – puffing out a thinner, more watery bile.

Hypercholesterolemia – the condition of having an abnormally large amount of cholesterol in the body cells.

Hemorrhage – copious bleeding.

Hemostatic – a locally acting drug that arrests hemorrhage by promoting clot formation or by serving as a mechanical matrix for a clot.

Hepatitis – an inflammation of the liver.

Hyperemia – an excess of blood in any part of the body.

Hyperesthesia – an increase in sensations.

Hyperglycemic – a drug that elevates blood glucose level, especially for the treatment of hypoglycemic states.

Hypertension – blood pressure above the normally accepted limits, high blood pressure.

Hypertriglyceridemia – an increased level of triglycerides in the blood.

Hypnotic – a central depressant which, with suitable dosage, induces sleep.

Hypodermoclysis – a subcutaneous injection with a solution.

Hypoesthesia – a diminished sensation of touch.

Hypoglycemic – a drug that promotes glucose metabolism and lowers blood glucose level, useful in the control of diabetes mellitus.

Hypokalemia – an abnormally small concentration of potassium ions in the blood.

Hyposensitize – to reduce the sensitivity to an agent, referring to allergies.

Hypotensive – a drug which diminishes tension or pressure, to lower blood pressure.

Ichthyosis – an inherited skin disease characterized by dryness and scales.

Idiopathic – denoting a disease of unknown cause.

Ileostomy – the establishment of an opening from the ileum to the outside of the body.

Immune Serum – a biological drug containing antibodies for a pathogenic microorganism, useful for passive immunization against the associated disease.

Immunizing Agent, active – an antigenic preparation (toxoid or vaccine) used to induce formation of specific antibodies against a pathogenic microorganism, which provides delayed but permanent protection against the associated disease.

Immunizing Agent, passive – a biological preparation (antitoxin, antivenin or immune serum) containing specific antibodies against a pathogenic microorganism, which provides immediate but temporary protection against the associated disease.

Impetigo – an inflammatory skin infection with isolated pustules.

Insulin – one of the hormones that regulate carbohydrate metabolism, used as replacement therapy in diabetes mellitus.

Inversion – a turning inward.

Irrigating solution – a solution for washing body surfaces or various body cavities.

Isoniazid – a compound effective in tuberculosis treatment.

Keratitis – an inflammation of the cornea.

Keratolytic – a topical drug that softens the superficial keratin-containing layer of the skin to promote exfoliation.

Lacrimal – pertaining to tears.

Laxative – a gentle purgative medicine; a mild cathartic.

Leishmaniasis – a number of types of infections transmitted by sand flies.

Leucocytopenia – a decrease in the number of white cells.

Leucocytosis – an increased white cell count.

Leukoderma – an absence of pigment from the skin.

Libido – sexual desire or creative energy.

Leucocyte – a white blood cell.

Lipoma – a fatty tumor.

Lipotropic – a drug, especially one supplementing a dietary factor, that prevents the abnormal accumulation of fat in the liver.

Lochia – a vaginal discharge of mucus, blood and tissue after childbirth.

Lues – a plague; specifically syphilis.

Macrocyte – a large red blood cell.

Malaise – a general feeling of illness.

Melasma – a darkening of the skin.

Melena – black feces or black vomit from altered blood in the higher GI tract.

Meninges – the membranes covering the brain and spinal cord.

Metastasis – the shifting of a disease or its symptoms from one part of the body to another.

Mastitis – an inflammation of the breast.

Miotics – agents which constrict the pupil of the eye; a myotic.

Moniliasis – an infection with any of the species of monilia types of fungi *(Candida)*.

Mucolytic – an agent that can destroy or dissolve mucous membrane secretions.

Myalgia – a pain in the muscles.

Myasthenia Gravis – a chronic progressive muscular weakness caused by myoneural conduction, usually spreading from the face and throat.

Myelocyte – an immature white blood cell in the bone marrow.

Myelogenous – originating in bone marrow.

Myoclonus – involuntary, sudden and rapid unpredictable jerks; faster than chorea.

Mydriatic – a drug that dilates the pupil of the eye, usually by anticholinergic or adrenergic mechanism.

Myoneural – pertaining to muscle and nerve.

Myopia – nearsightedness.

Narcotic – a drug that produces insensibility or stupor, a class of drug regulated by law.

Neonatal – pertaining to the first four weeks of life.

Neoplasm – an abnormal tissue growing more rapidly than usual showing a lack of structural organization.

Nephritis – an inflammation of the kidney.

Nephrosclerosis – a hardening of the kidney tissue.

Neuralgia – a pain extending along the course of one or more of the nerves.

Neurasthenia – nervous prostration.

Neuroglia – the supporting elements of the nervous system.

Neuroleptic – a substance that acts on the nervous system.

Neurosis – a functional disorder of the nervous system.

Nocturia – urination at night.

Normocytic – pertaining to anemia due to some defect in the blood-forming tissues.

Nuchal – the nape of the neck.

Nystagmus – a rhythmic oscillation of the eyes.

Oleaginous – oily or greasy.

Omphalitis – an inflammation of the navel in a newborn.

Onychomycosis – a ringworm or fungus infection of the nails.

Ophthalmic – pertaining to the eye.

Oral – pertaining to the mouth.

Orthopnea – a discomfort in breathing in any but the upright sitting or standing positions.

Ossification – a formation of, or conversion to, bone.

Osteomyelitis – an inflammation of the marrow of the bone.

Osteoporosis – a reduction in bone quantity; skeletal atrophy.

Otalgia – pain in the ear; an earache.

Otitis – inflammation of the ear.

Otomycosis – an ear infection caused by fungus.

Otorrhea – a discharge from the ear.

Oxytocic – a drug that selectively stimulates uterine motility and is useful in obstetrics, especially in the control of postpartum hemorrhage.

Palpitations – an awareness of one's heart action.

Paget's Disease – a disease characterized by lesions around the nipple and areola found in elderly women.

Pallor – the lack of the normal red color imparted to the skin by the blood of the superficial vessels.

Parasympatholytic – See Anticholinergic.

Parasympathomimetic – See Cholinergic.

Parenteral – pertaining to the administration of a drug by means other than through the alimentary canal; subcutaneous, intramuscular or intravenous administration of drug.

Parkinsonism – a group of neurological disorders marked by hypokinesia, tremor, and muscular rigidity.

Paroxysm – a sudden recurrence or intensification of symptoms.

Pathogenic – giving origin to disease.

Pediatric – pertaining to children's diseases.

Pediculicide – an insecticide suitable for erradicating louse infestations in humans (pediculosis).

Pediculosis – an infestation with lice.

Pellagra – characterized by GI disturbances, mental disorders, and skin redness and scaling due to niacin deficiency.

Pernicious – particularly dangerous or harmful.

Phlebitis – an inflammation of a vein.

Pleurisy – an inflammation of the membrane surrounding the lungs and the thoracic cavity.

Pneumonia – an infection of the lungs.

Poikilocytosis – a condition in which pointed or irregularly shaped red blood cells are found in the blood.

Polydipsia – excessive thirst.

Posology – the science of dosage.

Posterior Pituitary Hormone(s) – a multifunctional hormone with oxytocic-milk ejection, and antidiuretic-vasopressor fractions.

Progestin – a hormone that functions in the menstrual cycle and during pregnancy to promote uterine gland secretion and to reduce uterine motility.

Pronation – the act of turning the palm downward or backward.

Prophylactic – a remedy that tends to prevent disease.

Protectant – a topical drug that remains on the skin and serves as a physical barrier to the environment.

Proteolytic Enzyme – an enzyme used to liquefy fibrinous or purulent exudates.

Psoriasis – an inflammatory skin disease accompanied with itching.

Psychotherapeutic – a drug that selectively affects the central nervous system to alter emotional state. See Antidepressant; Tranquilizer.

Ptosis – a drooping or sagging of the muscle.

Pulmonary – pertaining to the lungs.

Purulent – containing or forming pus.

Pyelitis – a local inflammation of renal and pelvic cells due to bacterial infection.

Pylorospasm – a spasmodic muscle contraction of the pyloric portion of the stomach.

Pyoderma – any skin discharge characterized by pus formation.

Radiopaque Medium – a diagnostic drug, opaque to X-rays, whose retention in a body organ or cavity makes X-ray visualization possible.

Raynaud's Phenomenon – spasms of the digital arteries with blanching and numbness of the fingers, usually with another disease.

Reflex Stimulant – a mild irritant suitable for application to the nasopharynx to induce reflex respiratory stimulation.

Rheumatoid – a condition resembling rheumatism.

Rhinitis – an inflammation of the mucous membrane of the nose.

Rubefacient – a topical drug that induces mild skin irritation with erythema, sometimes used to relieve the discomfort of deep-seated inflammation.

Rubeola – a synonym popularly used for both measles and rubella.

Saprophytic – getting nourishment from dead material.

Sarcoma – a malignant tumor derived from connective tissue.

Scabicide – an insecticide suitable for the erradication of itch mite infestations in humans (scabies).

Schistosomacide – an agent which destroys schistosomes; destructive to the trematodic parasites or flukes.

Schistosomiasis – an infection with *Schistosoma haematobium* involving the urinary tract and causing cystitis and hematuria.

Scintillation – a visual sensation manifested by an emission of sparks.

Sclerosing Agent – an irritant suitable for injection into varicose veins to induce their fibrosis and obliteration.

Scotomata – an area of varying size and shape within the visual field in which vision is absent or depressed.

Seborrhea – a condition arising from an excess secretion of sebum.

Sebum – the fatty secretions of sebaceous glands.

Sedative – a central depressant which, in suitable dosage, induces mild relaxation useful in treating tension.

Sinusitis – an inflammation of a sinus.

Skeletal Muscle Relaxant – a drug that inhibits contraction of voluntary muscles, usually by interfering with their innervation.

Smooth Muscle Relaxant – a drug that inhibits contraction of involuntary (eg, visceral) muscles, usually by action upon their contractile elements.

Sociopath – a psychopathic person who, due to his unaccepted attitudes, is badly adjusted to society.

Spasmolytic – an agent that relieves spasms and involuntary contraction of a muscle; an antispasmodic.

Sputum – mucous spit from the mouth.

Stenosis – the narrowing of the lumen of a blood vessel.

Stomachic – a drug which is used to stimulate the appetite and gastric secretion.

Stomatitis – an inflammation of the mouth.

Subcutaneous – under the skin.

Sudorific – causing perspiration.

Superacidity – an increase of the normal acidity of the gastric secretion; hyperacidity.

Supination – the act of turning the palm forward or upward.

Suppressant – a drug useful in the control, rather than the cure, of a disease.

Surfactant – a surface active agent that decreases the surface tension between two miscible liquids; used to prepare emulsions, act as a cleansing agent, etc.

Synarthrosis (fibrous joint) – a joint in which the bony elements are united by continuous fibrous tissue.

Syncope – fainting.

Synovia – clear fluid which lubricates the joints; joint oil.

Systole – the ventricular contraction phase of a heartbeat.

Tachycardia – a rapid contraction rate of the heart.

Taeniacide – an agent used to kill tapeworms.

Taeniafuge – agent to expel tapeworms.

Therapeutic – a treatment of disease.

Thoracic – pertaining to the chest.

Thyroid Hormone – a drug containing one or more of the iodinated amino acids that stimulate and regulate the metabolic rate and functional state of body tissues.

Thyroid Inhibitor – drug that reduces excessive thyroid hormone production, usually by blocking hormone synthesis.

Tics – a repetitive twitching of muscles, often in the face and upper trunk.

Tinea – a fungal infection of the skin.

Tonic – an agent used to stimulate the restoration of tone to muscle tissue.

Tonometry – the measurement of tension in some part of the body.

Topical – the local external application of a drug to a particular place.

Toxoid – a modified bacterial toxin, less toxic than the original form, used to induce active immunity to bacterial pathogens.

Tranquilizer – a psychotherapeutic drug that induces emotional repose without significant sedation, useful in treating certain neuroses and psychoses.

Tremors – involuntary rhythmic tremulous movements.

Trichomoniasis – an infestation with parasitic flagellate protozoa of the genus *Trichomonas*.

Trypanosomiasis – a disease caused by protozoan flagellates in the blood.

Uricosuric – drug that promotes renal uric acid excretion; used to treat gout.

Urolithiasis – a condition marked by the formation of stones in the urinary tract.

Urticaria – a rash of hives generally of systemic origin.

Vaccine – preparation of live attenuated or dead pathogenic microorganisms, used to induce active immunity.

Vasoconstrictor – an adrenergic drug used locally in the nose to constrict blood vessels and reduce tissue congestion.

Vasodilator – a drug that relaxes vascular smooth muscles, expecially for the purpose of improving peripheral or coronary blood flow.

Vasopressor – an adrenergic drug used systemically to constrict blood vessels and raise blood pressure.

Verruca – a wart.

Vertigo – illusion of movement.

Vesicant – an agent which, when applied to the skin causes blistering and the formation of vesicles, an epispastic.

Visceral – pertaining to the internal organs.

Vitamin – an organic chemical essential in small amounts for normal body metabolism, used therapeutically to supplement the naturally occurring counterpart in foods.

Container Requirements for U.S.P. 23 Drugs

The listing of container and storage requirements for U.S.P. drugs is included as an aid to the practitioner in storing and dispensing.

Legend:

WC	=	Well Closed Container		In	=	Inert Atmosphere
T	=	Tight Container		U	=	Unit Dose
LR	=	Light Resistant Container		S	=	Separate Ingredient Packaging Before Mixing
+	=	Controlled Temperature		A	=	Pressurized Container
P	=	Plastic Specified		OT	=	Ophthalmic Tube
G	=	Glass Specified		SC	=	Radioactive Shielding
C	=	Collapsible Tubes		R	=	Remote from Fire
S/M	=	Single Dose/Multi Dose		F	=	Avoid Freezing
H	=	Reduced Moisture		Ox	=	Protect from Oxidation
SP	=	Special Consideration		CD	=	Cool, Dry Place
WP	=	Well Filled Container		He	=	Protect from Excessive Heat
Sy	=	Syringes		Co	=	Cold Place
TP	=	Tamper-Proof				

a	=	Tablets	i	=	Suppository	r	=	Inhalation	y	= Emulsion
b	=	Capsules	j	=	Suspension	s	=	Nasal	z	= Tincture
c	=	Solution	k	=	Ophthalmic	t	=	Gel/Jelly	*	= Effervescent
d	=	Syrup	l	=	Aerosol	u	=	Granules	§	= Sterile if Required
e	=	Elixir	m	=	Vaginal	v	=	Otic		
f	=	Cream	n	=	Lozenges	w	=	Intraocular Solution		
g	=	Ointment	o	=	Powder	x	=	Veterinary Use		
h	=	Lotion	p	=	Enema					

Drugs (Dosage Form)	WC	T	LR
Acebutolol HCl		X^o	
Acepromazine Maleate	X^{oa}		X^{oa}
Acetaminophen	X^{it}	X^{abo}	X^o
Acetaminophen Oral		X^{ej*}	
Acetaminophen and Aspirin (tab)		X	
Acetaminophen, Aspirin and Caffeine	X^a	X^b	
Acetaminophen and Caffeine		X^{ab}	
Acetaminophen and Codeine Phosphate		X^{ab}	X^{ab}
Acetaminophen and Codeine Phosphate Oral		X^{cj}	X^{cj}
Acetaminophen and Diphenhydramine Citrate (tab)		X	
Acetaminophen for Effervescent Oral Soln.		X	
Acetaminophen and Pseudoephedrine HCl		X^a	
Acetohydroxamic Acid		X^{ao+}	
Acetazolamide	X^{ao}		

Drugs (Dosage Form)	WC	T	LR
Acetic Acid Otic Soln.		X	
Acetohexamide	X^{ao}		
Acetohydroxamic Acid		X^{ao+}	
Acetylcysteine (Soln.)		S/M(In)	
Acyclovir		X^o	
Adenine	X^o		
Medical Air			
Alanine	X^o		
Albendazole	X^o		
Albendazole, Oral		X^{j+}	
Albuterol	X^{oa}		X^{oa}
Albuterol Sulfate	X^o		X^o
Alclometasone Dipropionate		X^{o}C^{fg}	
Alcohol		R	
Dehydrated Alcohol		R	
Rubbing Alcohol		R	
Allopurinol	X^{ao}		
Aloe	X		
Alprazolam	X^o	X^a	X^a
Alprostadil			X$^+$
Alteplase	SP$^+$		

Drugs (Dosage Form)	WC	T	LR
Alum	X		
Ammonium Alum	X		
Potassium Alum	X		
Alumina & Magnesia	X^a		
Alumina & Magnesia Oral			X^{j+}
Alumina & Magnesium Carbonate Oral	X^a		F^{j+}
Alumina, Magnesia and Calcium Carbonate Oral	X^a	F	
Alumina & Magnesium Carbonate and Magnesium Oxide (tab)		X	
Alumina & Magnesium Trisilicate Oral		X^{j+a}	
Alumina, Magnesia, Calcium Carbonate, & Simethicone (tabs)	X		
Alumina, Magnesia & Simethicone Oral		F^{j+}	
Aluminum Acetate Topical Soln.		X	
Aluminum Chloride		X^o	
Aluminum Chlorhydrate	X^{oc}		
Aluminum Chlorhydrex Polyethylene Glycol	X		
Aluminum Dichlorhydrate	X^{oc}		
Aluminum Dichlorhydrex Polyethylene Glycol	X		
Aluminum Hydroxide Gel	X^{ab}	X^{j+}	
Dried Aluminum Hydroxide Gel	X^{ab}	X^o	
Aluminum Phosphate Gel	F^a	F^{j+}	
Aluminum Sesquichlorhydrate	X^{oc}		
Aluminum Sesquichlorhydrex Polyethylene Glycol	X		
Aluminum Subacetate Topical Soln.		X	
Aluminum Sulfate	X^o		
Aluminum Sulfate and Calcium Acetate for Topical Solution		He^a	
Aluminum Zirconium Octachlorohydrate	X^{oc}		
Aluminum Zirconium Octachlorhydrex Gly	X^{oc}		
Aluminum Zirconium Pentachlorohydrate	X^{oc}		
Aluminum Zirconium Pentachlorohydrex Gly	X^{oc}		

Drugs (Dosage Form)	WC	T	LR
Aluminum Zirconium Tetrachlorohydrate	X^{oc}		
Aluminum Zirconium Tetrachlorohydrex Gly	X^{oc}		
Aluminum Zirconium Trichlorohydrate	X^{oc}		
Aluminum Zirconium Trichlorohydrex Gly	X^{oc}		
Amantadine HCl	X^o	X^{bd}	
Amcinonide	X^o	X^{fg}	
Amdinocillin		X^o	
Amikacin	X^o		
Amikacin Sulfate	X^o		
Amiloride HCl	X^{ao}		
Amiloride HCl & Hydrochlorothiazide (tab)	X		
Aminobenzoic Acid		X^{tc}	X^{tc}
Aminobenzoic Acid Topical		X^c	X^c
Aminobenzoate Potassium	X^{ba}	X^c	
Aminobenzoate Potassium Oral		X^c	
Aminobenzoate Sodium	X^o		
Aminocaproic Acid		X^{ad}	
Aminoglutethimide	X^o	X^a	X^a
Aminophylline	X^{i+}	X^a	
Aminophylline, Oral		X^c	
Aminosalicylate Sodium		X^{ao+}	X^{ao+}
Aminosalicylic Acid		X^{ao+}	X^{ao+}
Amitriptyline HCl	X^{ao}		
Aromatic Ammonia Spirit		X$^+$	X$^+$
Ammonium Chloride	X^o		
Ammonium Chloride Delayed Release (tab)		X	
Amobarbital Sodium		X^o	
Ammonium Molybdate		X^o	
Amodiaquine		X	
Amodiaquine HCl		X^{oa}	
Amoxapine	X^a	X^o	
Amoxicillin		X$^{abo+§}$	
Amoxicillin Intramammary Infusion		SY^{x+}	
Amoxicillin Oral Susp.	M^{x+}		
Amoxicillin for Oral Susp.		X$^+$	
Amoxicillin & Clavulanate Potassium		X^{h+a}	
Amoxicillin & Clavulanate Potassium for Oral Susp.		X$^+$	
Amphetamine Sulfate		X^{ao}	
Amphotericin Ba	C^{fgh}		
Ampicillin (all dosage forms)		X	

Drugs (Dosage Form)	WC	T	LR
Ampicillin Boluses		X^x	
Ampicillin Soluble Powder		X^x	
Ampicillin Sodium		X^o§	
Ampicillin & Probenecid (cap)		X	
Ampicillin and Probenecid for Oral Susp.		U	
Amprolium (all dosage forms)		X	
Amrinone	X		X
Amyl Nitrite (inhalant)		UG^+	UG^+
Anileridine HCl		X^ao	X^ao
Antazoline Phosphate		X^o	
Anthralin		X^fg+	X^fg+
Antimony Potassium Tartrate	X^o		
Antimony Sodium Tartrate		X	
Antipyrine	X^o		
Antipyrine & Benzocaine Otic Soln.		X	X
Antipyrine, Benzocaine and Phenylephrine HCl Otic Soln.		X	X
Apomorphine HCl		X^ao	X^oa
Apraclonidine HCl		X^o	X^o
Apraclonidine Ophthalmic		X^c	X^c
Arginine	X^o		
Arginine HCl	X^o		
Arsanilic Acid	X^o		
Ascorbic Acid (tab)		X	X
Ascorbic Acid Oral		X^c	X^c
Calcium Ascorbate		X^o	X^o
Aspirin	X^i+	X^abo	
Aspirin Boluses	X		
Aspirin, Buffered		X^a	
Aspirin, Delayed Release		X^ab	
Aspirin Effervescent Tablets for Oral Soln.		X	
Aspirin Extended-Release (tab)		X	
Aspirin, Alumina and Magnesia (tab)		X	
Aspirin, Alumina, and Magnesium Oxide (tab)		X	
Aspirin, Caffeine and Dihydrocodeine Bitartrate (cap)		X	
Aspirin and Codeine Phosphate (tab)	X		X
Aspirin, Codeine Phosphate, Alumina and Magnesia (tab)	X		X
Aspirin, Codeine Phosphate and Caffeine	X^ab		
Atenolol	X^oa		
Atenolol and Chlorthalidone	X^a		
Atropine		X^o	X^o
Atropine Sulfate	X^ao		
Atropine Sulfate Ophthalmic	C^g	X^c	
Attapulgite Activated	X		
Colloidal Activated Attapulgite	X		
Azaperone	X^o		
Azatadine Maleate	X^ao		
Azathioprine		X^a	X^ao
Azithromycin	X^b	X^o	
Azrithromycin for Oral		X^j	
Azlocillin Sodium		X^o§	
Azathioprine (tab)			X
Aztreonam		X^o	
Bacampicillin HCl		X^ao	
Bacampicillin HCl for Oral Susp.	X		
Bacitracin		X^o+	
Bacitracin (ointment)	X^g+	COT^k+	
Bacitracin and Polymixin B Sulfate Topical		A^l+	
Bacitracin Methylene Disalicylate, Soluble	X^x	X^ox	
Bacitracin Zinc Soluble Powder		X^x	
Bacitracin Zinc	X^g+	X^o+	
Bacitracin Zinc & Polymixin B Sulfate (ointment)	X	COT^k	X
Baclofen	X^a	X^o	
Adhesive Bandage	SP		
Gauze Bandage	SP		
Barium Hydroxide Lime		X^o	
Barium Sulfate	X^o		
Barium Sulfate for Suspension	X		
Beclomethasone Dipropionate	X		
Belladonna Extract		X^ao	X^ao
Belladonna Leaf	X^o		X^o
Belladonna Tincture		X^+	X^+
Bendroflumethiazide		X^ao	
Benoxinate HCl	X^o		
Benoxinate HCl Ophthalmic Soln.		X	

Drugs (Dosage Form)	WC	T	LR
Benzethonium Chloride (Tincture)		X	X
Benzethonium Chloride Topical	X^c	X^c	
Benzocaine	X^{tn}	X^{fg+}	X^{fg+}
Benzocaine Otic Soln.		X$^+$	X$^+$
Benzocaine Topical		X^{cl+}	X^{c+}
Benzocaine, Butamben, and Tetracaine HCl Topical	A^{l+}	F^{c+}	
Benzocaine, Butamben, and Tetracaine HCl		F^{gt}	
Benzocaine and Menthol Topical		AH^e	
Benzoic Acid	X^o		
Benzoic & Salicylic Acid (ointment)	X$^+$		
Benzoin (Resin)	X		
Benzoin Tincture Compound		X$^+$	X$^+$
Benzonatate		X^{bo}	X^{bo}
Hydrous Benzoyl Peroxide	SP		
Benzoyl Peroxide		X^{ht}	
Benzthiazide		X^{ao}	
Benztropine Mesylate	X^a	X^o	
Benzyl Benzoate		X^{ho}	WP^{o+}
Benzylpenicilloyl Polylysine Concentrate		X	
Beta Carotene		X^{ob}	X^{ob}
Betaine HCl	X		
Betamethasone	X^{ad}	C^f	
Betamethasone Acetate		X^o	
Betamethasone Benzoate		X^{ko}C^k	
Betamethasone Dipropionate	XC^g	X^{hi}	C^f
Betamethasone Dipropionate Topical		A^{l+}	
Betamethasone Sodium Phosphate		X^o	
Betamethasone Valerate	C^{fg}	X^{fgo}	X^h
Betaxolol HCl		X^{oa}	
Betaxolol HCl Ophthalmic		X^c	
Bethanechol Chloride		X^{oa}	
Biotin		X^o	
Biperiden	X^o		X^o
Biperiden HCl	X^o	X^a	X^o
Bisacodyl	X^{aio+}		
Milk of Bismuth	X$^+$		
Bismuth Subcarbonate	X^o		X^o
Bismuth Subgallate		X^o	X^o

Drugs (Dosage Form)	WC	T	LR
Bismuth Subnitrate	X^o		
Bismuth Subsalicylate		X^o	X^o
Bleomycin Sulfate		X^o	
Bretylium Tosylate	X^o		
Bromocriptine Mesylate		X^{ao+}	X^{ao+}
Bromodiphenhydramine HCl		X^{bo}	X^e
Brompheniramine Maleate	X^e	X^{ao}	X^{eo}
Brompheniramine Maleate and Pseudo-ephedrine Sulfate Syr.	X		X
Bumetanide		X^{ao}	X^{ao}
Buprenorphine HCl		X^o	X^o
Buspirone HCl		X^{oa+}	X^{oa+}
Busulfan	X^a	X^o	
Butabarbital		X^o	
Butabarbital Sodium	X^{ab}	X^{eo}	
Butalbital	X^o		
Butalbital, Acetaminophen, and Caffeine		X^{ab}	
Butabital and Aspirin (tab)		X	
Butabital, Aspirin & Caffeine		X^{ab}	
Butalbital, Aspirin, Caffeine and Codeine Phosphate		X^b	X^b
Butamben	X		
Butoconazole Nitrate	X^o	C^{f+}	X^o
Butorphanol Tartrate		X^o	
Caffeine, hydrous		X^o	
Caffeine, anhydrous	X^o		
Calamine	X^o	X^h	
Calamine, Phenolated		X^h	
Calciferol		X^{bo+}	X^{bo+}
Calcium Acetate		X	
Calcium Ascorbate		X^o	X^o
Calcium Carbonate	X^{aon}		
Calcium Carbonate Oral		F^j	
Calcium Carbonate & Magnesia (tab)	X		
Calcium & Magnesium Carbonates (tab)	X		
Calcium Carbonate, Magnesia & Simethicone (tab)	X		
Calcium Chloride		X^o	
Calcium Citrate	X^o		
Calcium Glubionate		X^{d+}	
Calcium Gluceptate	X^o		
Calcium Gluconate	X^{ao}		
Calcium Hydroxide Topical Soln.		X	

Drugs (Dosage Form)	WC	T	LR
Calcium Lactate	X^a	X^o	
Calcium Lactobionate	X^o		
Calcium Levulinate	X^o		
Calcium Pantothenate		X^{ao}	
Racemic Calcium Pantothenate		X^o	
Calcium Phosphate, dibasic	X^{ao}		
Calcium Polycarbophil		X^o	
Calcium Saccharate	X^o		
Calcium Undecylenate	X^o		
Camphor		X^o	
Camphor Spirit		X	
Candicidin	XT^{g+}	X^{m+}	
Capreomycin Sulfate		X^o	
Capsaicin		CD	CD
Captopril		X^{oa}	
Captopril and Hydrochlorithiazide		X^a	
Carbachol		X^o	
Carbachol Soln.		X^{kw+}	
Carbamazepine		X^oGH^a	
Carbamazepine Oral		F^{j+}	F^{j+}
Carbamide Peroxide		X^{o+}	X^{o+}
Carbamide Peroxide Topical Soln.		X^+	X^+
Carbenicillin Disodium		X^o	
Carbenicillin Indanyl Sodium		X^{ao+}	
Carbidopa	X^o		
Carbidopa & Levodopa	X^a		X^a
Carbinoxamine Maleate		X^{ao}	X^{ao}
Carbol-Fuchsin Topical Soln.		X	X
Carbon Dioxide	A		
Carbon Monoxide C-11	$(S/M)A^+$		
Carboprost Tromethamine	X^{o+}		
Carboxymethylcellulose Sodium Paste	X^+		
Carboxymethylcellulose Sodium		X^{ao}	
Carisoprodol	X^a	X^o	
Carisoprodol and Aspirin (tab)	X		
Carisoprodol, Aspirin & Codeine Phosphate (tab)	X		
Carteolol HCl	X^o	X^a	
Carteolol HCl Soln.	X^k		
Casanthranol		X^{o+}	X^{o+}
Cascara Sagrada Extract		X^+	X^+

Drugs (Dosage Form)	WC	T	LR
Cascara Sagrada Fluid extract		X^+	X^+
Cascara (tab)		X	
Cascara, Aromatic Fluid extract		X^+	X^+
Castor Oil		X^{by+}	
Castor Oil, Aromatic		X	
Cefaclor		X^{bo}	
Cefaclor for Oral Susp.		X	
Cefadroxil		X^{abo}	
Cefadroxil for Oral Susp.		X	
Cefazolin		X^o	
Cefazolin Sodium		X^o	
Cefixime for Oral Susp.		X^j	
Cefixime		X^{ao}	
Cefmenoxime HCl		$X^{o§}$	
Cefonicid Sodium		$X^{o§}$	
Cefoperazone Sodium		$X^{o§}$	
Ceforanide		$X^{o§}$	
Cefotaxime Sodium		$X^{o§}$	
Cefotetan		$X^{o§}$	
Cefotetan Disodium		$X^{o§}$	
Cefotiam HCl		$X^{o§}$	
Cefoxitin Sodium		X^o	
Cefpiramide		$X^{o§}$	
Cefprozil		X^{oa}	
Cefprozil for Oral Susp.		X^j	
Ceftazidime		$X^{o§}$	
Ceftizoxime Sodium		$X^{o§}$	
Ceftriaxone Sodium		$X^{o§}$	
Cefuroxime Axetil	X^a	X^o	
Cefuroxime Sodium		$X^{o§}$	
Cellulose Sodium Phosphate	X		
Cephalexin		X^{abo}	
Cephalexin for Oral Susp.	X		
Cephalexin HCl		X^o	
Cephalothin Sodium		$X^{o§}$	
Cephapirin Benzathine	X^o		
Cephapirin Benzathine Intramammary Infusion	S^{y+}		
Cephapirin Sod.		$X^{o§}$	
Cephapirin Sodium Intramammary Infusion	S^{y+}		
Cephradine		$X^{ab§}$	
Cephradine for Oral Susp.		X^j	
Cetylpyridinium Chloride	X^{no}		
Cetylpyridinium Chloride Topical Soln.		X^j	

Drugs (Dosage Form)	WC	T	LR
Charcoal, Activated	X		
Chloral Hydrate		X^{bo}	X^d
Chlorambucil	X^a	X^o	X^{ao}
Chloramphenicol (all dosage forms)		X	
Chloramphenicol Ophthalmic		CTP^{cg+}	
Chloramphenicol Palmitate		X^o	
Chloramphenicol Palmitate Oral Susp.		X	X
Chloramphenicol and Hydrocortisone Acetate for Ophthalmic Susp.		X	
Chloramphenicol and Polymixin B Sulfate Ophthalmic Oint.		COT	
Chloramphenicol, Polymixin B Sulfate & Hydrocortisone Acetate Ophthalmic Oint.		COT	
Chloramphenicol & Polymixin B Sulfate Ophthalmic Oint.		COT	
Chloramphenicol & Prednisolone Ophthalmic Oint.		COT	
Chlordiazepoxide		X^{ao}	X^{ao}
Chlordiazepoxide & Amitriptyline HCl (tab)	X	X	
Chlordiazepoxide HCl		X^{bo}	X^{bo}
Chlordiazepoxide HCl and Clidinium Bromide (cap)		X	X
Chlorphyllin Copper Complex Sodium		X^o	X^o
Chloroprocaine HCl	X^o		
Chloroquine	X^o		
Chloroquine Phosphate	X^{ao}		
Chlorothiazide	X^{ao}		
Chlorothiazide Oral Susp.		X	
Chloroxylenol	X^o		
Chlorpheniramine Maleate		X^{ado}	X^{do}
Chlorpheniramine Maleate Extended Release (cap)		X	
Chlorpromazine	X^i	X^o	X^{oi}
Chlorpromazine HCl	X^a	X^{do}	X^{ao}
Chlorpromazine HCl Oral Concentrate		X	X
Chlorpromazine HCl (supp)	X$^+$		X$^+$

Drugs (Dosage Form)	WC	T	LR
Chlorpropamide	X^{ao}		
Chlorprothixene	X^{ao}		X^{ao}
Chlorprothixene Oral Susp.		X	X
Chlortetracycline Bisulfate		X^o	X^o
Chlortetracycline HCl	C^g	X^{ba}	C^{g}X^{ba}
Chlortetracycline and Sulfamethazine Bisulfates Soluble Pwd.		X^x	X^x
Chlortetracycline HCl Soluble Pwd.		X^x	X^x
Chlortetracycline HCl Ophthalmic Oint.		COT	
Chlorthalidone	X^{ao}		
Chlorzoxazone		X^{ao}	
Cholecalciferol		In^{o+}	In^{o+}
Cholestyramine Resin		X^o	
Cholestyramine for Oral Susp.		X	
Chromic Chloride		X^o	
Chymotrypsin		X^{o+}	
Chymotrypsin for Ophthalmic Soln.		UG$^+$	
Ciclopirox Olamine	X^{o}C^{f+}		
Ciclopirox Olamine Topical		X^j	
Cimetidine		X^{ao+}	X^{ao+}
Cinoxacin	X^b	X^o	
Cinoxate		X^{ho+}	X^{ho+}
Ciprofloxacin	X^a	X^o	X^o
Ciprofloxacin HCl	X^a	X^o	X^o
Ciprofloxacin Soln.		RT^k	X^k
Ciprofloxacin Ophth.		X^{c+}	X^{c+}
Cisplatin		X^o	X^o
Citric Acid		X^o	
Clarithromycin		X^{ao}	
Clavulanate Potassium		X	
Clemastine Fumarate	X^a	X^{o+}	X^{o+}
Clidinium Bromide		X^{bo}	X^{bo}
Clindamycin HCl		X^{bo}	
Clindamycin Palmitate HCl		X^o	
Clindamycin Palmitate HCl for Oral Soln.		X	
Clindamycin Phosphate		X^{ot}	
Clindamycin Phosphate Cream	X^m		
Clindamycin Phosphate Topical		X^{cj}	
Clioquinol	X^o	C^{fg}	C^{fg}
Compound Clioquinol Topical		X^o	

Drugs (Dosage Form)	WC	T	LR
Clioquinol and Hydrocortisone		XC^fg	X^fg
Clocortolone Pivalate		X°C^f	X°C^f
Clofazimine	X^b	X^o+	X^o+
Clofibrate	X^b	X°	X^bo
Clomiphene Citrate	X^ao		X^a
Clonazepam		X^ao+	X^ao+
Clonidine HCl	X^ao		
Clonidine HCl & Chlorthalidone (tabs)	X		
Clorazepate Dipotassium		In°	In°
Clorsulon	X°		
Clotrimazole	X^mo+	X^h+	X^+
Clotrimazole Topical		X^ct	
Clotrimazole (cream)		C^+	
Clotrimazole and Betamethasone Dipropionate (cream)		XC	
Cloxacillin Benzathine		X^ox	
Cloxacillin Sodium		X^bo+	
Cloxacillin Sodium for Oral Soln.		X	
Coal Tar		X^g	
Coal Tar Topical		X^c	
Cyanocobalamin Co-57	X^b	X^c	X^bc
Cocaine		X°	X°
Cocaine HCl		X°	X°
Cocaine HCl Tablets for Topical Soln.	X		
Cod Liver Oil		In	
Codeine		X°	X°
Codeine Phosphate	X^a	X°	X^ao
Codeine Sulfate	X^a	X°	X°
Colchicine	X^a	X°	X^ao
Colestipol HCl		X°	
Colestipol HCl for Oral Susp.		XU	
Colistin Sulfate		X°	
Colistin Sulfate for Oral Susp.		X	X
Colistin & Neomycin Sulfates & Hydrocortisone Acetate Otic Susp.		X	
Collodion		X	
Collodion, Flexible		X^+	
Colloidal Oatmeal	X		
Copper Gluconate	X°		
Cortisone Acetate	X^ao		
Purified Cotton	SP		
Cromolyn Sodium		X°	
Cromolyn Sodium Inhalation		S/M	

Drugs (Dosage Form)	WC	T	LR
Cromolyn Sodium for Inhalation		X^+	X^+
Cromolyn Sodium Soln.	X^s		X^s
Cromolyn Sodium Ophthalmic		S/M^c	S/M^c
Crotamiton		X°C^f	C^fX°
Cupric Chloride		X°	
Cupric Sulfate		X°	
Cyanocobalamin		X°	X°
Cyclacillin		X^ao	
Cyclacillin for Oral Susp.	X		
Cyclizine HCl		X^ao	X^ao
Cyclobenzaprine HCl	X^ao		
Cyclopentolate HCl		X^+	
Cyclopentolate HCl Ophthalmic Soln.		X^+	
Cyclophosphamide		X^ao+	
Cyclopropane		A	
Cycloserine		X^bo	
Cyclosporine		X^bo	X°
Cyclosporine Oral Soln.		X	
Cyproheptadine HCl	X^ao	X^d	
Cysteine HCl	X°		
Cytarabine		X°	X°
Dacarbazine		X^o+	X^o+
Dactinomycin		X^o+	X^o+
Danazol	X^b	X°	X°
Dapsone	X^ao		X^ao
Daunorubicin HCl		X^o+	X^o+
Decoquinate	PM^x	X°	
Deferoxamine Mesylate		X°	
Dehydrocholic Acid	X^ao		
Demecarium Bromide		X°	X°
Demecarium Bromide Ophthalmic Soln.		X	X
Demeclocycline		X°	X°
Demeclocycline Oral Susp.		X	X
Demeclocycline HCl		X^abo	X^abo
Demeclocycline HCl & Nystatin		X^ab	X^ab
Desipramine HCl		X^ab	
Deslanoside		X°	X°
Desoximetasone	C^ftg+	C^ft+	C^f
Desoxycortisone Acetate	X°		X°
Dexamethasone	X^ao	X°C^t+	
Dexamethasone Topical	A^l+		
Dexamethasone Ophth.		X^j	
Dexamethasone Acetate	X°		
Dexamethasone Sodium Phosphate		C^fX^rt	C^k
Dexamethasone Sodium Phosphate Inhalation	A^l+		

Drugs (Dosage Form)	WC	T	LR
Dexamethasone Sodium Phosphate Ophth.	C^k	X^c	X^c
Dexbrompheniramine Maleate		X^o	X^o
Dexchlorpheniramine Maleate		X^{ado}	X^{do}
Dexpanthenol		X^o	
Dexpanthenol Preparation		X	
Dextroamphetamine Sulfate	X^{ao}	X^{eb}	X^e
Dextromethorphan		X^o	
Dextromethorphan HBr		X^{ao}	X^a
Dextrose	X^o		
Diatrizoate Meglumine	X^o		
Diatrizoate Meglumine & Diatrizoate Sodium Solution		X	X
Diatrizoate Sodium	X^o		
Diatrizoate Sodium Soln.		X	X
Diatrizoic Acid	X^o		
Diazepam		X^{abo}	X^{abo}
Diazepam Extended-Release (cap)		X	X
Diazoxide	X^{bo}		
Diazoxide Oral Susp.		X	X
Dibucaine		X^{o}C^{fg}	X^{o}C^{fg}
Dibucaine HCl		X^o	X^o
Dichloralphenazone	X^o		
Dichlorphenamide	X^{ao}		
Diclofenac Sodium		X	X
Diclofenac Sod. Delayed Release		X^a	X^a
Dicloxacillin Sodium		X^{bo}	
Dicloxacillin Sodium for Oral Susp.		X	
Dicyclomine HCl	X^{abo}	X^d	
Dienestrol	X^o	C^f	
Diethylcarbamazine Citrate		X^{ao}	
Diethylpropion HCl	X^{ao}		X^o
Diethylstilbestrol	X^a	X^o	X^o
Diethylstilbestrol Diphosphate		X$^+$	
Diethyltoluamide		X^o	
Diethyltoluamide Topical Soln.		X	
Diflorasone Diacetate		X^{o}C^{fg+}	C^{fg+}
Diflunisal	X^{ao}		
Digitalis		X^{ab}	X^o
Digitoxin	X^a	X^o	
Digoxin		X^{aeo+}	
Dihydrocodeine Bitartrate		X^o	
Dihydrostreptomycin Sulfate Boluses		X^x	
Dihydroergotamine Mesylate		X^o	X^o
Dihydrotachysterol	X^{ba}	In^o	X^{ba}
Dihydrotachysterol Oral Soln.		X	X
Dihydroxyaluminum Aminoacetate	X^{abo}		
Dihydroxyaluminum Aminoacetate Magma	F$^+$		
Dihydroxyaluminum Sodium Carbonate	X^a	X^o	
Diltiazem HCl		X^{ao}	X^{ab}
Diltiazem HCl Extended Release	X^{ab}		
Dimenhydrinate	X^{ao}	X^d	
Dimercaprol		X$^+$	
Dimethyl Sulfoxide		X$^+$	X$^+$
Dinoprost Tromethamine		X^o	
Diphenhydramine Citrate		X^o	X^o
Diphenhydramine HCl		X^{bo}	X^{eo}
Diphenhydramine and Pseudoephedrine (cap)		X	
Diphenoxylate HCl	X^o		
Diphenoxylate HCl & Atropine Sulfate (tab)	X		X
Diphenoxylate HCl and Atropine Sulfate Oral Soln.		X	X
Dipivefrin HCl		X^o	X^o
Dipivefrin HCl Ophth		X^c	X^c
Dipyridamole		X^{ao}	X^{ao}
Disopyramide Phosphate	X^b	X^o	X^o
Disopyramide Phosphate Extended-Release	X^b		
Disulfiram		X^{ao}	X^{ao}
Dobutamine HCl		X^{o+}	
Docusate Calcium	X^o	X^{b+}	
Docusate Potassium	X^o	X^{b+}	
Docusate Sodium	X^{ao}	X^{b+dc}	X^d
Dopamine HCl		X^o	
Doxapram		X^o	
Doxepin HCl	X^{bo}		
Doxepin HCl Oral Soln.		X	X
Doxorubicin HCl		X^o	
Doxycycline		X^{ob}	X^b
Doxycycline for Oral Susp.		X	X
Doxycycline Calcium Oral Susp.		X	X

Drugs (Dosage Form)	WC	T	LR
Doxycycline Hyclate		X^abo	X^abo
Doxycycline Hyclate De-layed-Release (cap)		X	X
Doxylamine Succinate	X^ao	X^d	X^ado
Dronabinol	X^b+	In^o+	In^bo+
Droperidol		In^o+	In^o+
Dusting Powder, Absorb-able	X		
Dyclonine HCl Topical Soln.		X	X
Dyclonine HCl (gel)		P/G	G
Dydrogestrone	X^ao		
Dydrogesterone (tab)	X		
Dyphylline		X^aeo	
Dyphylline and Guai-fenesin		X^ac	
Echothiophate Iodide		X^o	X^o
Echothiophate Iodide for Ophthalmic Soln.		G^+	
Econazole Nitrate	X^o		X^o
Edetate Calcium Di-sodium		X^o	
Edrophonium Chloride	X^o		
Elm	CD^o		
Emetine HCl		X^o	X^o
Enalapril Maleate	X^ao		
Enalaprilat	X^o		
Enflurane		X^o+	X^o+
Ephedrine		X^o+	X^o+
Ephedrine HCl	X^o		X^o
Ephedrine Sulfate	X^a	X^bd	X^bd
Ephedrine Sulfate Nasal		X^c	X^c
Ephedrine Sulfate & Phenobarbital (cap)	X		
Epinephrine		X^o	X^o
Epinephrine Soln.		X^krs	X^krs
Epinephrine Inhalation Aerosol		X	X
Epinephrine Bitartrate	X^o	X^k	X^k
Epinephrine Bitartrate In-halation Aerosol	X	X	
Epinephryl Borate Oph-thalmic Soln.		X	X
Epitetracycline HCl		X^o	X^o
Equilin		X^o	X^o
Ergocalciferol		In^oX^ab	In^oX^ab
Ergocalciferol Oral Soln.		X	X
Ergoloid Mesylates Oral Soln.		X^+	X^+
Ergoloid Mesylates		X^abo+	X^abo+
Ergonovine Maleate	X^a	X^o	X^o
Ergotamine Tartrate	X^ao		X^o

Drugs (Dosage Form)	WC	T	LR
Ergotamine Tartrate In-halation Aerosol		A	A
Ergotamine Tartrate & Caffeine	X^a	X^i+	X^a
Diluted Erythrityl Tetra-nitrate		X^+	
Erythrityl Tetranitrate (tab)		X^+	
Erythromycin		X^ao	
Erythromycin Delayed-Release		X^ab	
Erythromycin (oint)		CX^+	
Erythromycin Ophthal-mic		COT^g	
Erythromycin Pledgets		X	
Erythromycin Topical		X^ct	
Erythromycin and Ben-zoyl Peroxide Topical		SX^t	
Erythromycin Estolate		X^abjo	
Erythromycin Estolate Oral Susp.		X^+	
Erythromycin Estolate for Oral Soln.		X	
Erythromycin Estolate & Sulfisoxazole Acetyl Oral		X^j	
Erythromycin Ethylsuc-cinate		X^ao	
Erythromycin Ethylsuc-cinate Oral Susp.	X		
Erythromycin Ethylsuc-cinate for Oral Susp.		X	
Erythromycin Ethylsuc-cinate & Sulfisoxazole Acetyl for Oral Susp.	X		
Erythromycin Stearate		X^ao	
Estradiol		X^ao	X^ao
Estradiol, Cream		C^m	
Estradiol Cypionate		X^o	X^o
Estradiol Valerate		X^o	X^o
Estriol		X^o	
Estrogens, Conjugated	X^ao		
Estrogens, Esterified	X^a	X^o	
Estrone		X^o	X^o
Estropipate	X^a	C^mfX^o	
Ethacrynic Acid	X^ao		
Ethambutol HCl	X^ao		
Ethchlorvynol		X^bap^o	X^bao
Ether		R^+	R^+
Ethinyl Estradiol	X^a	X^o	X^o
Ethionamide		X^ao	
Ethopropazine HCl	X^a	X^o	X^ao
Ethosuximide		X^bo	
Ethotoin		X^ao	

Drugs (Dosage Form)	WC	T	LR
Ethyl Chloride		R⁺	
Ethylene Diamine		WP,G	
Ethynodiol Diacetate	Xº		
Ethynodiol Diacetate & Ethinyl Estradiol (tab)	X		
Ethynodiol Diacetate & Mestranol (tab)	X		
Etidronate Disodium		Xᵃº	
Etoposide		Xᵇº	Xᵇº
Eucatropine HCl		Xº	Xº
Eucatropine HCl Ophthalmic Soln.		X	
Eugenol	X	X	
Factor 1X Complex		X⁺	
Famotidine	Xᵃº		Xᵃº
Fenoprofen Calcium	Xᵃᵇº		
Fentanyl Citrate		Xº	
Ferrous Fumarate		Xº	Xᵃ
Ferrous Fumarate & Docusate Sodium Extended-Release (tabs)	X		
Ferrous Gluconate		Xᵃᵇᵉº	Xᵉ
Ferrous Sulfate		Xᵃᶜᵈº	Xᶜ
Ferrous Sulfate, Dried	Xº		
Flecainide Acetate	Xᵃº		Xᵃ
Floxuridine		Xº	Xº
Flucytosine		Xᵇº	Xᵇº
Fluhydrocortisone Acetate	Xᵃº		Xº
Flumethasone Pivalate		XºCᶠ	Xº
Flunisolide Nasal Soln.	X⁺	X⁺	
Flunixin Meglumine	Xᵒᵘᵍ		
Fluocinolone Acetonide	Xº	Cᶠᵍ	
Fluocinolone Acetate Topical Soln.		X	
Fluocinonide	XºCᶠᵍᵗ		
Fluocinonide Topical		Xᶜ	
Fluorescein		Xº	
Fluorescein Sodium		Xº	
Fluorescein Sodium and Benoxinate HCl Ophthalmic		Xᶜ	Xᶜ
Fluorescein Sodium & Proparacaine HCl Ophthalmic		G+	G⁺
Fluorometholone		XºCᶠ	Xº
Fluorometholone Ophthalmic Susp.		X	
Fluorouracil		Xᵒᶠ⁺	Xº
Fluorouracil Topical		Xᶜ⁺	
Fluoxymesterone	Xᵃº		Xᵃº
Fluphenazine Decanoate	Xº	Xº	
Fluphenazine Enanthate	Xº	Xº	

Drugs (Dosage Form)	WC	T	LR
Fluphenazine HCl Oral Soln.		X	X
Fluphenazine HCl		Xᵃᵉº	Xᵉᵃº
Flurandrenolide		Xᶠᵍʰ	Xᶠᵍʰ
Flurandrenolide tape	X⁺		
Flurazepam HCl		Xᵇº	Xᵇº
Flurbiprofen	Xᵃ	Xº	
Flurbiprofen Sodium		Xº	
Flurbiprofen Sodium Ophthalmic Soln.		X	
Flutamide		Xº	Xº
Folic Acid	Xᵃº		Xº
Formaldehyde Soln.		X⁺	
Fructose		Xº	
Basic Fuchsin	Xº		
Furazolidone		Xʲ⁺º	Xʲ⁺º
Furosemide	Xᵃ	Xᵒ⁺	Xᵃᵒ⁺
Gallamine Triethiodide		Xº	Xº
Gauze (all)	X		
Gemfibrozil		Xᵃᵇ	
Gentamicin Sulfate		XᵈºCᶠᵍ	
Gentamicin Sulfate Ophthalmic	Xᶜ⁺	COTᵍ	
Gentamicin Sulfate and Betamethasone Acetate Soln.		Xᵏ	
Gentamicin Sulfate and Betamethasone Valerate		CT	
Gentamicin Sulfate and Betamethasone Valerate Topical		Xᶜᵛ	
Gentamicin and Prednisolone Acetate Ophthalmic	OTᵍ⁺	Xʲ	
Gentian Violet		XᶜCᶠᵗ	
Gentian Violet Topical		Xᶜ	
Glipizide		Xº	
Glucagon		InG⁺	
Gluconolactone	Xº		
Glucose Enzymatic Test Strip	SP⁺		
Glutaral Concentrate		X⁺	X⁺
Glutethimide	Xᵃᵇº		
Glyburide	Xᵃ	Xº	
Glycerin		X	
Glycerin Oral Soln.		X	
Glycerin Suppository	X⁺		
Glycerin Ophthalmic Soln.		TPG/P	X
Glycopyrrolate		Xᵃº	
Gold Sodium Thiomalate	Xº	Xº	
Chorionic Gonadotropin	G⁺		
Gramicidin		Xº	

Drugs (Dosage Form)	WC	T	LR
Green Soap Tincture		X	
Griseofulvin		X^abo	
Griseofulvin Oral Susp.		X	
Griseofulvin, Ultramicro-size (tab)		X	
Guaifenesin		X^abdo	
Guaifenesin & Codeine Phosphate Syrup		X^+	X^+
Guaifenesin and Pseu-doephedrin HCl		X^b	X^b
Guaifenesin, Pseudo-ephedrine HCl and Dextromethorphan HBr		X^b	X^b
Guanabenz Acetate		X^ao	X^ao
Guanadrel Sulfate	X°	X^a	X^a
Guanfacine HCl		X^oa	X^oa
Gutta Percha	X°		X°
Halazone		X°	X°
Halazone Tablets for So-lution		X	X
Halcinonide	X^afgo		
Haloperidol		X^ao	X^ao
Haloperidol Oral Soln.		X	X
Haloprogin		X^+fo	X^fo
Haloprogin Topical Soln.		X^+	X
Halothane		G^+	X^+
Helium		A	
Heparin Calcium		X°	
Heparin Sodium		X^o+	
Hetacillin Potassium	X^ao		
Hetacillin Potassium Oral Susp.		X	
Hexachlorophen		X°	X°
Hexachlorophene Cleansing Emulsion		X	X
Hexachlorophene Liquid Soap		X	X
Hexylresorcinol		X^no	X°
Histamine Phosphate		X°	X°
Histidine	X°		
Homatropine HBr		X°	X°
Homatropine Hydrobro-mide Ophthalmic Soln.		X	
Homatropine Methylbro-mide		X^ao	X^ao
Hydralazine HCl		X^ao	X^a
Hyrochlorothiazide	X^ao		
Hydrocodone Bitartrate		X^ao	X^ao
Hydrocodone Bitartrate and Acetaminophen		X^a	X^a
Hydrocortisone	X^ag	X^fhpt	
Hydrocortisone Acetate	X^fg	X^h	

Drugs (Dosage Form)	WC	T	LR
Hydrocortisone Acetate Ophthalmic		X^gk	
Hydrocortisone and Ace-tic Acid Otic Soln.		X	X
Hydrocortisone Butyrate	X^fo		
Hydrocortisone Hemis-uccinate		X°	
Hydrocortisone Sodium Phosphate		X°	
Hydrocortisone Sodium Succinate		X°	X°
Hydrocortisone Valerate	X^fo		
Hydroflumethiazide		X^ao	
Hydrogen Peroxide Con-centrate	SP^+		
Hydrogen Peroxide Topi-cal Soln.		X^+	X^+
Hydromorphone HCl		X^ao	X^ao
Hydroquinone	X^f	X°	X^+o
Hydroquinone Topical Soln.		X	X
Hydroxocobalamin		X°	X°
Hydroxyamphetamine HBr	X°		X°
Hydroxyamphetamine HBr Ophthalmic Solu-tion		X	X
Hydroxychloroquine Sulfate	X°	X^a	X^ao
Hydroxyprogesterone Caproate	X°		X°
Hydroxypropyl Cellulose Ocular System		U^+	
Hydroxypropyl Methyl-cellulose (all grades)	X°		
Hydroxypropyl Methyl-cellulose Ophthalmic Soln.		X	
Hydroxyurea		X^bo	
Hydroxyzine HCl		X^ado	X^d
Hydroxyzine Pamoate	X^b	X°	
Hydroxyzine Pamoate Oral Susp.		X	X
Hyoscyamine	X^a	X°	X^ao
Hyoscyamine HBr		X°	X°
Hyoscyamine Sulfate		X^aeo+	X^aeo+
Hyoscyamine Sulfate Oral Soln.		X^+	X^+
Ibuprofen	X^a	X°	
Ibuprofen Oral	X^i+		
Ibuprofen and Pseudo-ephedrine HCl		X^a	
Ichthammol	X	C^g+	
Idarubicin HCl		X°	

Drugs (Dosage Form)	WC	T	LR
Idoxuridine		X°	X°
Idoxuridine Ophthalmic	C^gt	X^c	X^c
Ifosfamide		X^o+§	
Imipramine HCl		X^ao	
Indapamide	X^oa		
Indigotindisulfonate Sodium		X°	X°
Indium In 111 Oxyquinoline		U^c+	
Indocyanine Green	X^o§		
Indomethacin	X^bi+o		
Indomethacin Extended-Release (cap)	X		
Indomethacin Oral		X^j	X^j
Indomethacin Sodium	X^o§		X°
Insulin		X^+	X
Insulin Human		X^+	X
Inulin	X°		
Iocetamic Acid	X°	X^a	
Iodine (all Soln. & Tinct.)		X^+	X^+
Iodide, Sodium, 1-123, 1-131	X^bc		
Iodipamide	X°		
Iodoquinol	X^ao		
Iohexol	X°		X°
Iopamidol	X°		X°
Iopanoic Acid		X^ao	X^ao
Iophendylate		X	X
Iothalamic Acid	X°		
Ioversol	X		
Ioxaglic Acid	X°		
Ipecac		X^d+o	
Ipodate Calcium		X°	
Ipodate Calcium for Oral Susp.	X		
Ipodate Sodium		X^ao	
Isocarboxazid	X^ao		X^a
Isoetharine Inhalation Soln.		WF	Ox
Isoetharine HCl		X°	
Isoetharine Mesylate		X°	
Isoetharine Mesylate Inhalation Aerosol			X
Isoflurane		X°	X°
Isoflurophate		G^+	
Isoflurophate Ophthalmic		C^g	
Isoleucine	X°		
Isometheptene Mucate	X°		
Isometheptene Mucate Dichloralphenazone, and Acetaminophen	X^b		
Isoniazid	X^a	X^do	X^ado

Drugs (Dosage Form)	WC	T	LR
Isopropamide Iodide	X^ao		X°
Isopropyl Alcohol (all)		X^+	
Isoproterenol Inhalation Soln.		WF	Ox
Isoproterenol HCl	X^a	X^arlo	X^arlo
Isoproterenol HCl Inhalation		A^l	
Isoproterenol HCl & Phenylephrine Bitartrate Inhalation Aerosol		X	X
Isoproterenol Sulfate		X°	X°
Isoproterenol Sulfate Inhalation		WF^cl	Ox^cl
Isosorbide Concentrate		X	X
Isosorbide Oral Soln.	X		
Diluted Isosorbide Dinitrate		X	
Isosorbide Dinitrate (tab)	X		
Isosorbide Dinitrate Chewable (tab)	X		
Isosorbide Dinitrate Extended Release	X^ab		
Isosorbide Dinitrate Sublingual (tab)	X		
Isotretinoin		In^mo	X°
Isoxsuprine HCl	X^ao		
Juniper Tar		X^+	X^+
Kanamycin Sulfate		X^bo	
Kaolin	X°		
Ketamine HCl	X°		
Ketoconazole	X^ao		
Ketoprofen		X°	
Ketorolac Tromethamine	X°H^a+		X°H^a+
Krypton Ke 81m		SP^+	
Labetalol HCl		X^oat	X^oat
Lactic Acid	X		
Lactulose (soln/conc)	X^+		
Lanolin	X^+		
Modified Lanolin		X^+(Rust proof)	
Leucine	X°		
Leucovorin Calcium	X^a+o		X^a+o
Levamisole HCl	X^ao		X°
Levmetamfetamine		X	X
Levobunolol HCl	X°		
Levobunolol HCl Oph thalmic Soln.		X	
Levocarnitine		X^ao	
Levocarnitine Oral Soln.	X		
Levodopa		X^abo+	X^abo+
Levonordefrin	X°		
Levonorgestrel	X^ao		X^ao

Drugs (Dosage Form)	WC	T	LR
Levonorgestrel and Ethinyl Estradiol (tab)	X		
Levorphanol Tartrate	X^{ao}		
Levothyroxine Sodium		X^{ao}	X^{ao}
Levothyroxine Sodium Oral		X^{o}	X^{o}
Lidocaine	X^{o}	X^{gl}	
Lidocaine Topical		A^{l}	
Lidocaine Oral Topical Soln.		X	
Lidocaine HCl Oral Topical Soln.		X	
Lidocaine Topical Soln.		X	
Lidocaine HCl	X^{o}	X^{t}	
Lime		X	
Lincomycin HCl		X^{bdo§}	
Lindane		X^{fho}	
Lindane Shampoo		X	
Liothyronine Sodium		X^{ao}	
Liotrix (tab)		X	
Lisinopril	X^{oa}		
Lithium Carbonate	X^{abo}		
Lithium Carbonate Extended-Release (tab)	X		
Lithium Citrate		X^{do}	
Lithium Hydroxide		X^{o}	
Loperamide HCl	X^{bao}		
Loracarbef	X^{b}	X^{o}	
Loracarbef for Oral Susp.		X	
Lorazepam		X^{ao}	X^{ao}
Lorazepam Oral Conc.	X		X
Lovastatin	X^{a+}	In^{o+}	X^{a+}
Loxapine Succinate		X^{o}	
Loxapine		X^{bo}	
Lypressin Nasal Soln.		P	
Lysine Acetate	X^{o}		
Lysine HCl	X^{o}		
Mafenide Acetate		X^{f+o}	X^{f+o}
Magaldrate	X^{ao}		
Magaldrate Oral Susp.		X	
Magaldrate & Simethicone (tab)	X		
Magaldrate & Simethicone Oral Susp.		X^{+}	
Milk of Magnesia		F^{+}	
Magnesia (tab)	X		
Magnesium Carbonate	X^{o}		
Magnesium Carbonate & Sodium Bicarbonate for Oral Susp.		X	
Magnesium Chloride		X^{o}	
Magnesium Citrate		X	

Drugs (Dosage Form)	WC	T	LR
Magnesium Citrate Oral Soln.		SP^{+}	
Magnesium Gluconate	X^{ao}		
Magnesium Hydroxide		X^{o}	
Magnesium Hydroxide Paste		X	
Magnesium Oxide	X^{abo}		
Magnesium Salicylate		X^{ao}	
Magnesium Sulfate	X^{o}		
Magnesium Trisilicate	X^{ao}		
Malathion		X^{o}G^{h}	X^{o}
Manganese Chloride		X^{o}	
Manganese Gluconate	X^{o}		
Manganese Sulfate		X^{o}	
Mannitol	X^{o}		
Maprotiline HCl	X^{a}	X^{o}	
Mazindol		X^{ao+}	
Mebendazole	X^{ao}		
Mebrofenin		X^{o}	
Mecamylamine HCl	X^{a}	X^{o}	
Mechlorethamine HCl		X	X
Meclizine HCl	X^{a}	X^{o}	
Meclocycline Sulfosalicylate		X^{fo+}	X^{fo+}
Meclofenamate Sodium		X^{bo+}	X^{bo+}
Medroxyprogesterone Acetate	X^{aj}	X^{o}	X^{o}
Mefenamic Acid		X^{ob}	X^{o}
Megestrol Acetate	X^{ao}		X^{o}
Meglumine	X^{o}		
Melphalon	X^{a}	G^{o}	G^{o}
Menadiol Sodium Diphosphate	X^{a}	X^{o+}	X^{ao+}
Menadione	X^{o}		X^{o}
Menotropins		G^{o+}	
Menthol		X^{+}	
Meperidine HCl	X^{a}	X^{d}	X^{ad}
Mephentermine Sulfate	X^{o}		X^{o}
Mephenytoin	X^{ao}		
Mephobarbital	X^{ao}		
Mepivacaine HCl	X^{o}		
Meprednisone		X^{+}	X^{+}
Meprobamate	X^{a}	X^{o}	
Meprobamate Oral Susp.		X	
Mercaptopurine	X^{ao}		
Ammoniated Mercury	X^{o}		X^{o}
Mercury, Ammoniated (ointment)		C^{k}	
Mesoridazine Besylate	SP^{a}X^{o}		X^{ao}
Mesoridazine Besylate Oral Soln.		X^{+}	X^{+}
Mestranol	X^{o}		X^{o}
Metacresol		X^{o}	X^{o}

Drugs (Dosage Form)	WC	T	LR
Metaproterenol Sulfate	X^a	X^{od}	X^{oda}
Metaproterenol Sulfate Soln.	A^r	WF^l	Ox^l
Metaraminol Bitartrate	X^o		
Methacholine Chloride		X^o	
Methacycline HCl		X^{ao}	X^{ao}
Methacycline HCl Oral Susp.		X	X
Methadone HCl	X^a	X^o	X^o
Methadone HCl Oral Soln.		X^+	X^+
Methadone HCl Oral Concentrate		X^+	X^+
Methamphetamine HCl	X^a	X^o	X^{oa}
Methazolamide	X^{ao}		
Methdilazine		X^{ao}	X^{ao}
Methdilazine HCl		X^{ado}	X^{ado}
Methenamine	X^{ao}	X^e	
Methenamine & Monobasic Sodium Phosphate (tab)		X	
Methenamine Mandelate (tab)	X		
Methenamine Mandelate for Oral Soln.	X^c	X^j	
Methicillin Sodium		$X^{+§}$	
Methimazole	X^{ao}		X^{ao}
Methionine	X^o		
Methocarbamol		X^{ao}	
Methohexital		X^o	
Methotrexate	U^a	X^o	X^o
Methoxsalen	X^o	X^b	X^{bo}
Methotrimeprazine	X^o		X^o
Methoxsalen Topical Solution		X	X
Methoxyflurane		X^{o+}	X^{o+}
Methsuximide		X^{bo+}	
Methylclothiazide	X^{ao}		
Methylbenzethonium Chloride	X^e	$X^{bo}C^g$	
Methylbenzethonium Chloride Topical		X^o	
Methylcellulose	X^{ao}		
Methylcellulose Ophth Soln.		X	
Methylcellulose Oral Soln.		X^+	X^+
Methyldopa	X^{ao}		X^o
Methyldopa Oral Susp.		X^+	X^+
Methyldopa and Chlorothiazide (tab)	X		
Methyldopa & Hydrochlorothiazide (tab)	X		
Methyldopate HCl	X^o		
Methylene Blue	X^o		
Methylergonovine Maleate		X^{ao+}	X^{ao+}
Methylphenidate HCl	X^o	X^a	
Methylphenidate HCl Extended-Release		X^a	
Methylprednisolone		X^{ao}	X^{ao}
Methylprednisolone Acetate	X^p	X^oC^f	X^{fo}
Methylprednisolone Hemisuccinate		X^o	
Methylprednisolone Sodium Succinate		X^o	X^o
Methyltestosterone	X^{abo}		X^o
Methysergide Maleate		X^{ao}	X^o
Metoclopramide Oral Soln.		F^+	F^+
Metoclopramide HCl		X^{oa}	X^{oa}
Metocurine Iodide		X^o	
Metolazone		X^{oa}	X^{oa}
Metoprolol Fumarate		X^o	X^o
Metoprolol Tartrate		X^{oa}	X^{oa}
Metoprolol Tartrate & Hydrochorothiazide (tab)		X	X
Metronidazole	X^{ao}	CP^{t+}	X^{ao}
Metyrapone		X^{ao+}	X^{ao+}
Metyrosine (cap)	X		
Mezlocillin Sodium		$X^§$	
Mexiletine HCl		X^{bo}	
Miconazole	X^o		X^o
Miconazole Nitrate		$X^{mi}C^f$	
Miconazole Nitrate Topical	X^o		
Miconazole Nitrate Vaginal (Supp)		X^+	
Mineral Oil		X^{py}	
Mineral Oil, Light, Topical		X	
Minocycline HCl		$X^{abo§}$	X^{abo}
Minocycline HCl Oral Susp.		X	X
Minoxidil	X^o	X^a	
Mitomycin		X^o	X^o
Mitotane		X^{ao}	X^{ao}
Mitoxantrone HCl		X^o	
Molindone HCl		X^{ao}	X^{ao}
Monobenzone		X^{fo+}	X^{o+}
Morphine Sulfate		X^o	X^o
Mupirocin	XC^g	X^o	
Nadolol	X^o	X^a	
Nadolol and Bendroflumethiazide (tab)		X	
Nafcillin Sodium		X^{bao}	X^a

Drugs (Dosage Form)	WC	T	LR
Nafcillin Sodium for Oral Soln.		X	
Nalidixic Acid		X^{ao}	
Nalidixic Acid Oral Susp.		X	
Nalorphine HCl		X°	X°
Naloxone HCl		X°	X°
Nandrolone Decanoate		X°	X°
Nandrolone Phenpropionate		X°	X°
Naphazoline HCl		X°	X°
Naphazoline HCl Soln.		X^{ks}	X^{ks}
Naproxen	X°	X°	
Naproxen Oral		X^{i+}	X^{i+}
Naproxen Sodium	X^a	X°	
Natamycin		X°	X°
Natamycin Ophthalmic Susp.		TP	
Neomycin Sulfate	X^{gf+}	X^{ao}	X°
Neomycin Sulfate Ophthalmic Oint.		COT+	
Neomycin Sulfate Oral Soln.		X+	X+
Neomycin Sulfate & Bacitracin		X^{g+}	X^{g+}
Neomycin Sulfate & Bacitracin Zinc	XC^g		
Neomycin Sulfate & Dexamethasone Sodium Phosphate		X^f	
Neomycin Sulfate & Dexamethasone Sodium Phosphate Ophthalmic	X^{c+}	COT^g	X^{c+}
Neomycin Sulfate & Fluocinolone Acetonide		XC^f	
Neomycin Sulfate & Fluorometholone	CX^g		
Neomycin Sulfate & Flurandrenolide		CX^{fgh}	X^{fgh}
Neomycin Sulfate & Gramicidin	CX^g		
Neomycin Sulfate & Hydrocortisone	CX^{fg}		
Neomycin Sulfate & Hydrocortisone Otic Susp.	X	X	
Neomycin Sulfate & Hydrocortisone Acetate	CX^{fgh}		
Neomycin Sulfate & Hydrocortisone Acetate Ophthalmic		X^{i}COT^g	
Neomycin Sulfate & Methylprednisolone Acetate		CX^f	X^f
Neomycin Sulfate & Prednisolone Acetate Ophthalmic		COTX^j	
Neomycin Sulfate & Prednisolone Sodium Phosphate Ophthalmic Oint.		COT	
Neomycin Sulfate, Sulfacetamide Sodium and Prednisolone Acetate Ophthalmic		COT^g	
Neomycin Sulfate & Triamcinolone Acetonide		XCT^f	
Neomycin Sulfate & Triamcinolone Acetonide Ophthalmic Oint.		COT	
Neomycin & Polymixin B Sulfates	X^{g+}		
Neomycin & Polymixin B Sulfates Ophthalmic	COT^{g+}		X^{c+}
Neomycin & Polymixin B Sulfate & Bacitracin Zinc	CX^g	CX^g	X^{g+}
Neomycin & Polymixin B Sulfate & Bacitracin Zinc & Hydrocortisone Acetate Ophthalmic Oint.		COT	
Neomycin & Polymixin B Sulfate & Bacitracin Zinc & Hydrocortisone Acetate Oint.	CX+		
Neomycin and Polymixin B Sulfates, Bacitracin and Lidocaine	X^{g+}		
Neomycin & Polymixin B Sulfates, Bacitracin Zinc & Hydrocortisone Acetate Ointment	X^{gk+}		
Neomycin & Polymixin B Sulfate & Hydrocortisone Otic Soln.		X	X
Neomycin & Polymixin B Sulfates & Dexamethasone Ophthalmic	COT^{g}X^j	X^j	
Neomycin & Polymixin B Sulfate & Gramicidin	CX^f		
Neomycin & Polymixin B Sulfate & Gramicidin Ophthalmic Soln.		X	

Drugs (Dosage Form)	WC	T	LR
Neomycin & Polymyxin B Sulfates, Gramicidin & Hydrocortisone Acetate Cream	X		
Neomycin & Polymyxin B Sulfates & Hydrocortisone Susp.		TP^{kv}	X^{kv}
Neomycin & Polymyxin B Sulfate & Hydrocortisone Soln.		TP^{kv}	X^{kv}
Neomycin & Polymyxin B Sulfates & Hydrocortisone Acetate Ophthalmic Susp.		X	
Neomycin & Polymyxin B Sulfates & Prednisolone Acetate Ophthalmic Susp.		X	
Neostigmine Bromide		X^{ao}	
Neostigmine Methylsalicylate		X^o	
Netilmicin Sulfate		X^o	
Niacin	X^{ao}		
Niacinamide		X^{ao}	
Nicotine	InH$^+$		H$^+$
Nicotine Transdermal System	SPU		SPU
Nicotine Polacrilex		X	
Nicotine Polacrilex Gum	SPU		SPU
Nifedipine		X^{bo+}	X^{bo+}
Nitrofurantoin		X^{abo}	X^{abo}
Nitrofurantoin Oral Susp.	X		X
Nitrofurazone		X^{fgo}	X^{fgo}
Nitrofurazone Topical Soln.	X		X
Nitroglycerin, Diluted		X$^+$	X$^+$
Nitroglycerin		G^{a+}	X^g
Nitromersol		X^o	X^o
Nitromersol Topical Solution	X		X
Nitrous Oxide		A$^+$	
Nizatidine		X^{ob+}	X^{ob+}
Nonoxynol 9		X^o	
Norepinephrine Bitartrate		X^o	X^o
Norethindrone	X^{ao}		
Norethindrone & Ethinyl Estradiol (tab)	X		
Norethindrone & Mestranol (tab)	X		
Norethindrone Acetate	X^{ao}		
Norethindrone Acetate & Ethinyl Estradiol (tab)	X		
Norethynodrel	X^o		

Drugs (Dosage Form)	WC	T	LR
Norfloxacin	X^a	X^o	X^o
Norgestrel	X^{ao}		
Norgestrel & Ethinyl Estradiol (tab)	X		
Nortriptyline HCl		X^{ao}	X^o
Nortryptyline HCl Oral		X^c	X^c
Noscapine	X^o		
Novobiocin Sod		X^{bo}	X^b
Nystatin	X^{g+}	X^{ah+n}	X^{ah+n}
Nystatin Cream		XC$^+$	
Nystatin Vaginal		X^{ai+}	X^{ai+}
Nystatin Oral Susp.		X	X
Nystatin for Oral Susp.		X	
Nystatin, Neomycin Sulfate, Gramicidin & Triamcinolone Acetonide		X^{fg}	
Nystatin, Neomycin Sulfate, Thiostrepton, and Triamcinolone Acetonide		X^{fg}	
Nystatin & Triamcinolone Acetonide		X^{fg}	
Ofloxacin	X^o		X^o
Ointment, White or Yellow	X		
Hydrophilic Ointment		X	
Oleovitamin A & D		X^{b}ln	X^{b}ln
Omeprazole	COH^o		
Bland Lubricating Ophthalmic	OT^g		
Opium Powder	X		
Opium Tincture		X$^+$	X$^+$
Orphenadrine Citrate		X^o	X^o
Oxacillin Sodium		X$^{bo+\S}$	
Oxacillin Sodium for Oral Soln.		X$^+$	
Oxamniquine	X^o	X^b	
Oxandrolone	X^o	X^a	X^{ao}
Oxazepam	X^{abo}		
Oxprenolol HCl	X^o	X^a	X^a
Oxprenolol HCl Extended Release (tab)		X	X
Oxtriphylline	X^o		
Oxtriphylline Oral		X^c	
Oxtriphylline Delayed Release (tab)		X	
Oxtriphylline Extended Release (tab)		X	
Oxybenzone		X^o	X^o
Oxybutynin Chloride	X^o	X^{ad}	X^{ad}
Oxycodone and Acetaminophen		X^{ab}	X^{ab}
Oxycodone and Aspirin (tab)		X	X

Drugs (Dosage Form)	WC	T	LR
Oxycodone HCl		X^{oa}	X^{a}
Oxycodone HCl Oral Soln.		X	X
Oxycodone Terephthalate		X^{o}	
Oxygen 93 Percent		A^{+}	
Oxymetazoline HCl		X^{o}	
Oxymetazoline HCl Soln.		X^{ks}	
Oxymetholone	X^{ao}		
Oxymorphone HCl	X^{l+}	X^{o}	X^{o}
Oxyphenbutazone		X^{ao}	
Oxytetracycline		X^{ao§}	X^{ao}
Oxytetracycline Calcium	X^{o}	X^{o}	
Oxytetracycline Calcium Oral Susp.		X	X
Oxytetracycline HCl		X^{bo}	X^{bo}
Oxytetracycline & Nystatin (cap)		X	X
Oxytetracycline and Nystatin for Oral Susp.		X^{+}	X^{+}
Oxytetracycline HCl & Hydrocortisone Ointment	X		X
Oxytetracycline HCl & Hydrocortisone Acetate Ophthalmic Susp.		X	X
Oxytetracycline & Phenazopyridine Hydrochlorides & Sulfamethizole (cap)		X	X
Oxytetracycline HCl & Polymixin B Sulfate	X^{gom}		X^{g}
Oxytetracycline HCl & Polymixin B Ophthalmic Oint.		COT	
Oxtriphylline		X^{a}	
Oxytocin Nasal Soln	SP		
Padimate O		X^{ho}	X^{ho}
Pancreatin		X^{ab+}	
Pancrelipase		X^{abo+}	
Pancrelipase Delayed-Release		X^{b+}	
Panthenol		X^{o}	
Papain		X^{o}	X^{o}
Papain Tablets for Topical Soln.		X^{+}	X^{+}
Papaverine HCl		X^{ao}	X^{o}
Parachlorophenol		X^{o}	X^{o}
Parachlorophenol, Camphorated		X	X
Paraldehyde		G,WF^{+}	WF^{+}
Paramethasone Acetate	X^{a}	X^{o}	
Paregoric		X^{+}	X^{+}
Paromomycin Sulfate		X^{bdo}	

Drugs (Dosage Form)	WC	T	LR
Pectin	X		
Penbutolol Sulfate	X^{a}	X^{oa}	X^{oa}
Penicillamine		X^{abo}	
Penicillin G Benzathine	X^{ao§}		
Penicillin G Benzathine Oral Susp.		X	
Penicillin G Potassium		X^{ao§}	
Penicillin G Potassium Tablets for Oral Soln.		X	
Penicillin G Procaine, Neomycin & Polymixin B Sulfates & Hydrocortisone Acetate Topical Susp.	X		
Penicillin V		X^{ao}	
Penicillin V for Oral Susp.		X	
Penicillin V Benzathine		X	
Penicillin V Benzathine Oral Susp.		X^{+}	
Penicillin V Potassium		X^{ao}	
Penicillin V Potassium for Oral Soln.		X	
Pentaerythritol Tetranitrate		X^{ao+}	
Pentazocine		X^{o}	X^{o}
Pentazocine HCl		X^{ao}	X^{ao}
Pentazocine HCl & Aspirin (tab)		X	X
Pentazocine and Naloxone HCl (tab)		X	X
Pentetic Acid	X^{o}		
Pentobarbital		X^{aeo}	
Pentobarbital Sodium		X^{bo}	
Peppermint Spirit		X	
Perflubron		X^{o}	X^{o}
Perphenazine	X^{d}	X^{ao}	X^{dao}
Perphenazine Oral Soln.	X		X
Perphenazine & Amitriptyline HCl (tab)	X		
Petrolatum (all)	X		
Hydrophilic Petrolatum	X		
Phenacemide	X^{a}	X^{o}	
Phenazopyridine HCl		X^{ao}	
Phendimetrazine Tartrate	X^{a}	X^{bo}	
Phenelzine Sulfate		X^{ao+}	X^{ao+}
Phenmetrazine HCl		X^{ao}	
Phenobarbital	X^{ao}	X^{e}	X^{e}
Phenol		X	X
Phenol, Liquefied		X	X
Phenolphthalein (all)	X^{o}	X^{a}	
Phenoxybenzamine HCl	X^{ob}		
Phentermine HCl		X^{bao}	

Drugs (Dosage Form)	WC	T	LR
Phentolamine Mesylate	X°		X°
Phenylalanine	X°		
Phenylbutazone		X^abo	
Phenylbutazone Boluses	X^x		
Phenylephrine HCl		X°	X°
Phenylephrine HCl Soln.		X^ks	X^ks
Phenylephrine HCl Nasal Jelly	X		
Phenylethyl Alcohol		X^+	X^+
Phenylpropanolamine HCl		X°	X°
Phenylpropanolamine HCl Extended-Release		X^ba	X^ba
Phenytoin	X^a	X°	
Phenytoin Oral Susp.		X^+	
Phenytoin Sodium		X°	
Phenytoin Sodium, Extended (cap)		X	
Phenytoin Sodium, Prompt (cap)		X	
Physostigmine		X°	X°
Physostigmine Salicylate		X°	X°
Physostigmine Salicylate Ophthalmic Solution		X	X
Physostigmine Sulfate		X°	X°
Physostigmine Sulfate Ophthalmic Ointment		COT	
Phytonadione	X^a	X°	X^ao
Pilocarpine		X°	X°
Pilocarpine HCl		X°	X°
Pilocarpine HCl Ophthalmic Soln.		X	
Pilocarpine Nitrate		X°	X°
Pilocarpine Nitrate Ophthalmic		X	X
Pimozide		X^oa	X^ao
Pindolol	X^ao		X^ao
Piperacillin	X^o§		
Piperacillin Sodium		X°	
Piperazine		X	X
Piperazine Citrate	X°	X^ad	
Piroxicam		X^bo	X^bo
Plantago Seed	X		
Plicamycin		X	X
Podophyllum Resin		X°	X°
Podophyllum Resin Topical Soln.		X	X
Polycarbophil		X°	
PEG 3350 and Electrolytes for Oral Soln.		X	
Polymyxin B Sulfate		X°	X°
Polymyxin B Sulfate & Bacitracin Zinc Topical	X°	A^lt	

Drugs (Dosage Form)	WC	T	LR
Polymyxin B Sulfate & Hydrocortisone Otic Soln.		X	X
Polythiazide		X^ao	X^ao
Polyvinyl Alcohol	X°		
Sulfurated Potash		SP	
Potassium Acetate		X°	
Potassium Bicarbonate	X°		
Potassium Bicarbonate Effervescent Tabs for Oral Soln.		X^+	
Potassium Bicarbonate & Potassium Chloride for Effervescent Oral Soln.		X^+oa	
Potassium and Sodium Bicarbonate and Citric Acid Effervescent for Oral Solution (tab)		X	X
Potassium Bitartrate		X°	
Potassium Carbonate	X°		
Potassium Chloride	X°		
Potassium Chloride Oral Soln.		X	
Potassium Chloride for Oral Soln.		X	
Potassium Chloride Extended Release		X^ab+	
Potassium Chloride, Potassium Bicarbonate, and Potassium Citrate Effervescent Tablets for Oral Soln.		X^+	
Potassium Citrate		X°	
Potassium Citrate Extended-Release (tabs)		X	
Potassium Citrate & Citric Acid Oral Solution		X	
Potassium Gluconate		X^aeo	X^e
Potassium Gluconate & Potassium Chloride for Oral Soln.	X		
Potassium Gluconate & Potassium Chloride Oral		X	
Potassium Gluconate & Potassium Citrate Oral Soln.	X		
Potassium Gluconate, Potassium Citrate, & Ammonium Chloride Oral Soln.		X	
Potassium Guaiacolsulfonate	X°		X°
Potassium Iodide		X°	X^a

Drugs (Dosage Form)	WC	T	LR
Potassium Iodide Oral Soln.		X	X
Potassium Nitrate		X^{oc}	
Potassium Permanganate	X^{o}		
Dibasic Potassium Phosphate	X^{o}		
Potassium Sodium Tartrate		X^{o}	
Povidone		X^{o}	
Povidone-Iodine		X	
Povidone-Iodine Topical Soln.		X^{+}	
Povidone-Iodine Topical Aerosol Solution		A^{+}	
Povidone-Iodine Oint.		X	
Povidone-Iodine Cleansing Soln.		X	
Pralidoxime Chloride	X^{ao}		
Pramoxine HCl		X$^{ftC^{t}}$	
Prazepam		X^{abo}	X^{abo}
Praziquantel	X^{o}	X^{a}	X^{o}
Prazosin HCl	X^{b}	X^{o}	X^{bo}
Prednisolone	X^{ao}	X^{cfd}	X^{d}
Prednisolone Acetate	X^{o}		
Prednisolone Acetate Ophthalmic Susp.		X	
Prednisolone Hemisuccinate		X^{o}	
Prednisolone Sodium Phosphate		X^{o}	
Prednisolone Sodium Phosphate Ophthalmic Solution		X	X
Prednisolone Tebutate		In^{+}	
Prednisone	X^{ao}	X^{d}	
Prednisone Oral Soln.		X	
Prilocaine HCl	X^{o}		
Primaquine Phosphate	X^{ao}		X^{ao}
Primadone	X^{a}		
Primadone Oral Susp.		X	X
Probenecid	X^{ao}		
Probenecid & Colchicine (tab)	X		X
Probucol	X^{ao}		X^{ao}
Procaine HCl	X^{o}		
Procainamide HCl		X^{abo}	
Procainamide HCl Extended Release (tab)		X	
Procarbazine HCl		X^{bo}	X^{bo}
Prochlorperazine		X^{co}	X^{o}
Prochlorperazine Oral		X^{c}	X^{c}
Prochlorperazine Edisylate		X^{o}	X^{o}
Prochlorperazine Edisylate Oral Soln.		X	X
Prochlorperazine Maleate	X^{a}	X^{o}	X^{ao}
Procyclidine HCl		X^{ao+}	X^{o+}
Progesterone		X^{o}	X^{o}
Promazine HCl		X^{ado}	X^{ado}
Proline	X^{o}		
Promazine HCl Oral Soln		X	X
Promethazine HCl		X^{adi+}	X^{adi+}
Propafenone HCl		X^{o}	X^{o}
Propantheline Bromide	X^{ao}		
Proparacaine HCl	X^{o}		
Proparacaine HCl Ophthaimic Soln.		X	X
Propoxycaine HCl	X^{o}		X^{o}
Propoxyphene HCl		X^{bo}	
Propoxyphene HCl & Acetaminophen (tab)		X	
Propoxyphene HCl, Aspirin, & Caffeine (cap)		X^{+}	
Propoxyphene Napsylate		X^{ao}	
Propoxyphene Napsylate Oral Susp.		X	X
Propoxyphene Napsylate & Acetaminophen (tab)		X^{+}	
Propoxyphene Napsylate & Aspirin (tab)		X	
Propranolol HCl	X^{ao}		
Propranolol HCl Extended-Release (cap)	X		
Propranolol HCl and Hydrochlorothiazide (tab)	X		
Propranolol HCl and Hydrochlorothiazide Extended-Release (cap)	X		
Propylene Glycol		X	
Propylhexedrine		X	
Propylhexedrine Inhalant		X^{+}	
Propylthiouracil	X^{ao}		
Protamine Sulfate		X^{+}	X^{+}
Protriptyline HCl	X^{o}	X^{a}	
Pseudoephedrine HCl		X^{ado}	X^{do}
Psyllium Hydrophilic Mucilloid for Oral Susp.		X	
Pumice	X^{o}		
Pyrantel Pamoate	X^{o}		X^{o}
Pyrantel Pamoate Oral Suspension		X	X
Pyrazinamide	X^{ao}		

Drugs (Dosage Form)	WC	T	LR
Pyrethrum Extract		X	X
Pyridostigmine Bromide		X^ado	X^d
Pyridoxine HCl	X^a	X^o	X^ao
Pyrilamine Maleate	X^a	X^o	X^o
Pyrimethamine		X^ao	X^ao
Pyroxylin			SP
Pyrvinium Pamoate		X^ao	X^ao
Pyrvinium Pamoate Oral Susp.		X	X
Quinidine Gluconate	X^o		X^o
Quinidine Gluconate Extended-Release	X^a		X^a
Quinidine Sulfate	X^ao	X^b	X^abo
Quinidine Sulfate Extended Release (tab)	X		X
Quinine Sulfate	X^ao	X^b	X^o
Racepinephrine		X^o	X^o
Racepinephrine Soln.		X^r+	X^r+
Racepinephrine HCl		X^o	X^o
Ranitidine HCl		X^ao	X^ao
Ranitidine Oral Soln.		X^+	X^+
Rauwolfia Serpentina	SP	X^a	X^a
Purified Rayon	SP		
Oral Rehydration Salts		SX^a+	
Reserpine		X^aeo	X^aeo
Reserpine & Chlorothiazide (tab)		X	X
Reserpine, Hydralazine HCl & Hydrochlorothiazide (tab)		X	X
Reserpine & Hydrochlorothiazide (tab)		X	X
Resorcinol	X^o		X^o
Resorcinol, Compound Ointment		X^+	
Resorcinol & Sulfur Lotion	X		
Resorcinol Monoacetate		X	X
Ribavirin		X^o	
Ribavirin for Inhalation Soln.		H^+	
Riboflavin		X^ao	X^ao
Riboflavin 5'-Phosphate Sodium		X^o	X^o
Rifampin		X^bo+	X^bo+
Rifampin & Isoniazid (cap)		X^+	X^+
Ritodrine HCl		X^ao+	
Rose Water Ointment		X	X
Saccharin Calcium	X^o		
Saccharin Sodium	X^ao		
Saccharin Sodium Oral Solution		X	
Safflower Oil		X	X

Drugs (Dosage Form)	WC	T	LR
Salicylamide	X^o		
Salicylic Acid	X^o		
Salicylic Acid Collodion		X^+	
Salicylic Acid Gel		XC^+	
Salicylic Acid Plaster	X^+		
Salicylic Acid Topical Foam		X	
Salsalate		X^oab	
Scopolamine HBr		X^ao	X^ao
Scopolamine HBr Ophthalmic		X^cC^g	
Secobarbital		X^o	
Secobarbital Elixir		X	
Secobarbital Sodium		X^bo	
Secobarbital Sodium and Amobarbital Sodium	X^b		
Selegiline HCl	X^oa	X	X^a
Selenious Acid		X^o	
Selenium Sulfide	X^o		
Selenium Sulfide Lotion		X	
Senna Fluid extract		X^+	X^+
Senna Syrup		X^+	
Sennosides	X^ao		
Serine	X^o		
Silver Nitrate		X^o	X^o
Silver Nitrate Ophthalmic Soln.		X	X
Toughened Silver Nitrate		X	X
Simethicone	X^a	X^yo	
Simethicone Oral Susp.		X	X
Simvastatin	In^o		
Sisomicin Sulfate		X^o	
Sodium Acetate		X^o	
Sodium Acetate Soln.		X	
Sodium Ascorbate		X^o	X^o
Sodium Bicarbonate	X^ao		
Sodium Bicarbonate Oral Powder	X^o		
Sodium Chloride	X^ao		
Sodium Chloride Ophthalmic		X^cC^k	
Sodium Chloride Inhalation Soln.	S^r		
Sodium Chloride Tablet for Soln.	X		
Sodium Chloride & Dextrose (tab)	X		
Sodium Citrate & Citric Acid Oral Soln.		X	
Sodium Fluoride	X^o	X^a	
Sodium Fluoride Oral Soln.		XP	

Drugs (Dosage Form)	WC	T	LR
Sodium Fluoride & Phosphoric Acid		Pᵗ	
Sodium Fluoride and Phosphoric Acid Topical Soln.		P	
Sodium Gluconate	X°		
Sodium Hypochlorite Soln.		X⁺	X⁺
Sodium Iodide		X°	
Sodium Lactate Soln.		X	
Sodium Monofluorophosphate	X°		
Sodium Nitrate		X°	
Sodium Nitroprusside		X°	X°
Dibasic Sodium Phosphate		X°	
Monobasic Sodium Phosphate	X°		
Sodium Phosphate	Xᴾ		
Sodium Phosphates Oral Soln.		X	
Sodium Polystyrene Sulfonate	X°		
Sodium Polystyrene Sulfonate Susp.	X⁺		
Sodium Salicylate	Xᵃᵒ		X°
Sodium Sulfate Inj.		X⁺	
Sodium Thiosulfate		X°	
Sorbitol Soln.		X	
Soybean Oil		X⁺	X⁺
Spironolactone (tab)	X°	Xᵃ	Xᵃ
Spironolactone and Hydrochlorothiazide		Xᵃ	X°
Stannous Fluoride	X°		
Stannous Fluoride Gel	X		
Stanozolol		Xᵃᵒ	Xᵃᵒ
Topical Starch	X		
Storax	X°		
Succinyl Chloride	X°		
Sucralfate		Xᵃᵒ	
Sufentanil Citrate	X°		
Sulbactam Sodium		X§	
Sulconazole Nitrate	X°		X°
Triple Sulfa Vaginal	XᵃCᶠ		XᵃCᶠ
Sulfabenzamide	X°		X°
Sulfacetamide	X°		X°
Sulfacetamide Sodium		X°	X°
Sulfacetamide Sodium Ophthalmic	COTᵍ	Xᶜ⁺	Xᶜ⁺
Sulfacetamide Sodium & Prednisolone Acetate Ophthalmic		TPʲ CTPᵍ	
Sulfachlorpyridazine	X°	X°	
Sulfadiazine	Xᵃᵒ	Xᵃᵒ	

Drugs (Dosage Form)	WC	T	LR
Silver Sulfadiazine	X°	Cᶠ	Xᶠᵒ
Sulfadoxine	X°		X°
Sulfadoxine & Pyrimethamine (tab)	X		X
Sulfamerazine	Xᵃᵒ		X°
Sulfamethizole	Xᵃᵒ		X°
Sulfamethazine	X°		X°
Sulfamethazine Granulated	Xˣ		
Sulfamethizole Oral Susp.		X	X
Sulfamethoxazole	Xᵃᵒ		Xᵃᵒ
Sulfamethoxazole Oral Susp.		X	X
Sulfamethoxazole & Trimethoprim	Xᵃ		Xᵃ
Sulfamethoxazole and Trimethoprim Oral Susp.		X	X
Sulfapyridine	Xᵃᵒ		Xᵃᵒ
Sulfaquinoxaline	X°		X°
Sulfasalazine	Xᵃ	X°	X°
Sulfathiazole	X°		X°
Sulfinpyrazone	Xᵃᵇ		
Sulfisoxazole (tab)	X		X
Sulfisoxazole Diolamine		X°	X°
Sulfisoxazole Acetyl Oral Suspension		X	X
Sulfisoxazole Diolamine Ophthalmic		CᵍXᶜ	Xᶜ
Precipitated Sulfur	X°		
Sulfur Ointment	X⁺		
Sublimed Sulfur	X°		
Sulindac	Xᵃᵒ		
Suprofen	X°		
Suprofen Ophthalmic		Xᶜ	
Sutilains		X⁺	
Sutilains Ointment		CX⁺	
Absorbable Surgical Suture	SP		
Nonabsorbable Surgical Suture	SP		
Talc	X		
Tamoxifen Citrate	Xᵃᵒ		Xᵃᵒ
Tannic Acid		X°	X°
Tape, Adhesive	X⁺		
Temazepam	Xᵇᵒ		Xᵇᵒ
Terbutaline Sulfate	X°⁺	X⁺	X°⁺
Terbutaline Sulfate Inhalation		Aⁱ⁺	Aⁱ⁺
Terfenadine		Xᵒᵃ	Xᵒᵃ
Terpin Hydrate	X°		
Terpin Hydrate Elixir		X	

Drugs (Dosage Form)	WC	T	LR
Terpin Hydrate & Codeine Elixir		X	
Terpin Hydrate & Dextromethorphan HBr Elixir		X	
Testolactone	X^{ao}		
Testosterone	X°		
Testosterone Cypionate	X°		X°
Testosterone Enanthate	X^{o+}		
Testosterone Propionate	X°		X°
Tetracaine Ophthalmic Oint.		C	
Tetracaine		X°C^f	X°
Tetracaine & Menthol Oint.		C	
Tetracaine HCl		X°C^f	X°
Tetracaine HCl Topical Soln.		X	X
Tetracaine HCl Ophthalmic Soln.		X	X
Tetracycline		X°	X°
Tetracycline Boluses		X^x	
Tetracycline Oral Suspension		X	X
Tetracycline HCl (tablet/capsule/ophthalmic/suspension/topical/ solution)		X	X
Tetracycline HCl Ophthalmic	COT^g		
Tetracycline HCl Soluble Pwd.		X^x	
Tetracycline HCl for Topical Soln.		X	X
Tetracycline HCl and Novobiocin Sodium (tab)		X^x	
Tetracycline Phosphate Complex and Novobiocin Sodium (cap)		X^x	
Tetracycline HCl & Nystatin (cap)		X	X
Tetracycline Phosphate Complex		X^{bo}	X^{bo}
Tetrahydrozoline HCl		X°	
Tetrahydrozoline HCl Soln.		X^{ks}	
Theophylline	X^{abo}		
Theophylline Extended Release (cap)	X		
Theophylline, Ephedrine HCl & Phenobarbital (tab)	X		
Theophylline & Guaifenesin		X^b	

Drugs (Dosage Form)	WC	T	LR
Theophylline Guaifenesin Oral Soln.	X		
Theophylline Sodium Glycinate	X^a	X^e	
Thiabendazole	X°	X^a	
Thiabendazole Oral Susp.		X	
Thiamine HCl		X^{aeo}	X^{aeo}
Thiamine Mononitrate		X^{eo}	X^{eo}
Thiamylal	X°		
Thiethylperazine Maleate		X^{aio+}	X^{aio+}
Thimerosal		X°	X°
Thimerosal Topical		X^{cl+}	X^{cl+}
Thimerosal Tincture		X$^+$	X$^+$
Thioguanine		X^{ao}	
Thiopental Sodium		X°	
Thioridazine	X°		X°
Thioridazine Oral Susp.		X	X
Thioridazine HCl		X^{ao}	X^{ao}
Thioridazine HCl Oral Soln.		X$^+$	X$^+$
Thiostrepton		X°	
Thiotepa		X°	X°
Thiothixene	X^b	X°	X^{bo}
Thiothixine HCl		X°	X°
Thiothixene HCl Oral Solution		X	X
Threonine	X°		
Thyroid		X^{ao}	
Ticarcillin Monosodium		X°	
Timolol Maleate Ophthalmic Soln.		X	
Timolol Maleate	X^{ao}		X^a
Timolol Maleate & Hydrochlorothiazide (tab)	X		X
Tioconazole		X^{oaf}	
Titanium Dioxide	X°		
Tobramycin		X°	
Tobramycin Ophthalmic		X^{c}COT^g	
Tobramycin and Dexamethasone Ophthalmic		X^{l}C^g	
Tobramycin and Fluorometholone Acetate Ophthalmic		X^c	
Tobramycin Sulfate		X°	
Tocainide HCl	X^{oa}		
Tolazamide	X°	X^a	
Tolbutamide	X^{ao}		
Tolmetin Sodium	X^{ao}	X^b	
Tolnaftate		X^{fto}	
Tolnaftate Topical		X^{lco+}	

Drugs (Dosage Form)	WC	T	LR
Tolu Balsam		X+	
Trazodone HCl		Xoa	Xoa
Tretinoin		CfXc	Xcft
Triacetin		X	
Triamcinolone	Xao		
Triamcinolone Acetonide	Xgo	Xfh	
Triamcinolone Acetonide Topical		Xi+	
Triamcinolone Acetonide Dental Paste		X	
Triamcinolone Diacetate	Xo	Xd	Xd
Triamcinolone Hexaceto-nide	X		
Triamterene		Xbo	Xbo
Triamterene and Hydro-chlorothiazide		Xab	Xab
Triazolam		Xao	Xao
Trichlorfon	X+		
Trichlormethiazide	Xo	Xa	
Tricitrates Oral Soln.		X	
Trientine HCl		Xao+	Ino
Trifluoperazine HCl	Xa	Xdo	Xado
Triflupromazine		Xo	Xo
Triflupromazine Oral Suspension		X	X
Triflupromazine HCl (tab)	X		X
Trihexyphenidyl HCl		Xaeo	
Trihexyphenidyl HCl Ex-tended-Release (cap)		X	
Trikates Oral Soln.		X	X
Trimeprazine Tartrate	Xa	Xdo	Xado
Trimethadione		Xabco+	
Trimethaphan Camsy-late		X+	
Trimethobenzamide HCl	Xbo		
Trimethoprim		Xao	Xao
Trioxsalen	Xao		Xao
Tripelennamine Citrate	Xa	Xe	Xee
Tripelennamine HCl	Xao		Xo
Triprolidine HCl		Xado	Xado
Triprolidine & Pseudo-ephedrine Hydrochlo-rides		Xad	Xad
Trisulfapyrimidines (tab)	X		
Trisulfapyrimidines Oral Susp.		X+	
Tromethamine		Xo	
Tropicamide		Xo	Xo
Tropicamide Ophthalmic Soln.		X+	

Drugs (Dosage Form)	WC	T	LR
Trypsin, Crystallized		X+	
Tryptophan	Xo		
Tubocurarine Chloride		Xo	
Tyloxapol		Xo	
Tyropanoate Sodium		Xbo	Xbo
Tyrosine	Xo		
Tyrothricin		Xo	
Undecylenic Acid		Xo	Xo
Undecylenic Acid, Com-pound Ointment		X+	
Urea	Xo		
Valine	Xo		
Valproic Acid		GPoXbd+	
Vancomycin	Xo		
Vancomycin HCl		Xbo	
Vancomycin HCl for Oral Soln.	X		
Verapamil HCl		Xao	Xao
Verapamil HCl Extended Release		Xa	Xa
Vidarabine Ophthalmic Ointment		COT+	
Vinblastine Sulfate		X+	X+
Vincristine Sulfate		X+	X+
Vitamin A		Xbo+	Xbo+
Vitamin E		InoX	X
Vitamin E Preparation		In	X
Oil-Soluble Vitamins		Xab	Xab
Warfarin Sodium	Xo	Xa	Xao
Purified Water		X	
Sterile Purified Water		X	
White Lotion		X	
Witch Hazel		X	
Xylometazoline HCl		Xo	Xo
Xylometazoline HCl Nasal Soln.		X	X
Xylose		X+	
Zinc Acetate		Xo	
Zinc Carbonate		Xo	
Zinc Chloride		Xo	
Zinc Gluconate	Xoa		
Zinc Oxide	Xo		
Zinc Oxide (oint/paste)	X+		
Zinc Oxide and Salicylic Acid Paste	X		
Zinc Stearate	Xo		
Zinc Sulfate		Xo	
Zinc Sulfate Ophthalmic Solution		X	
Zinc Undecylenate	Xo		

Provided by Dr. Kenneth S. Alexander, Professor of Pharmacy, College of Pharmacy, University of Toledo.
The listing of container and storage requirements for Compendial drugs is included as an aid to the practitioner in stor-ing and dispensing.

Container and Storage Requirements for Sterile U.S.P. 23 Drugs

The listing of container and storage requirements for U.S.P. drugs is included as an aid to the practitioner in storing and dispensing.

Legend:

I	=	Containers for Sterile Solids as Described Under Injections	D	=	Type II or III Glass Depending on Final Soln. pH
N	=	Intact Flexible Container Meeting the General Requirements	In	=	Inert Atmosphere
S	=	Single Dose	M	=	Protect from Moisture
M	=	Multiple Dose	LR	=	Light Resistant
U	=	Unspecified	L	=	Protect from Light
P	=	Plastic	R	=	Refrigerator (2°-8°C)
A	=	Type I Glass	F	=	Freezer (-4°C)
B	=	Type II Glass	H	=	Protect From Heat
C	=	Type III Glass	RT	=	Controlled Room Temperature
Sy	=	Syringe	TP	=	Tamper-Proof
O	=	Original Package	W	=	Transparent
T	=	Avoid Toxic Substances	SC	=	Radioactive Shielding
SS	=	Stated Size Limitation	Tr	=	Treated to Prevent Adsorption
CV	=	Controlled Volume	WC	=	Well Closed
X	=	Colorless	PA	=	Does not adversely affect performance

Drugs	Container	Glass Type	Storage Conditions
Acepromazine Maleate Inj.	S,M	A	L
Acetazolamide for Inj.	I	C	
Acetic Acid Irrigation	S,P	A,B	
Acetylcholine for Ophthalmic Soln.	I		
Acetylcysteine Solution	S,M	A,P	O_2 excluded
Acetylcysteine and Isoproterenol HCl Inhal. Soln.	S,M	A	WC
Albumin, Human	S	U	RT
Dehydrated Alcohol Inj.	S	A	In (head space)
Alcohol in Dextrose Inj.	S	A,B	
Alphaprodine HCl Inj.	S,M	A	
Alprostadil Inj.	S	A	R
Alteplase for Inj.			R-RT/L
Amdinocillin for Inj.	I		
Amikacin Sulfate Inj.	S,M	A,C	
Aminoacetic Acid Irrigation	S	A,B	
Aminocaproic Acid Inj.	S,M	A	
Aminohippurate Sodium Inj.	S,M	A	
Aminophylline Inj.	S	A	CO_2 excluded
Amitriptyline HCl Inj.	S,M	A	
Ammonium Chloride Inj.	S,M	A,B	
Ammonium Molybdate Inj.	S,M	A,B	
Amobarbital Sodium for Inj.	I	D	
Amoxicillin for Injectable Suspension	I	I	
Amphotericin B for Inj.	I		R,L
Ampicillin for Inj.	I		
Ampicillin for Injectable Oil Suspension	S,M	A	
Ampicillin for Injectable Suspension	I		

Drugs	Container	Glass Type	Storage Conditions
Ampicillin and Sulbactam for Inj.	I		
Amrinone Inj.	S	A	L,RT
Anileridine Inj.	S,M	A	L
Anticoagulant Citrate Dextrose Solution	S,P	A,B	
Anticoagulant Citrate Phosphate Dextrose Adenine Solution	S,P	A,B	X,W
Anticoagulant Sodium Citrate Soln.	S	A,B	
Anticoagulant Heparin Soln.	S,P	A,B	
Antihemophilic Factor			R
Cryoprecipitated Antihemophilic Factor			F (-18°C)
Antirabies Serum	U		R
Antivenin (Crotalidae) Polyvalent	S		H
Antivenin (Latrodectus mactans)	S		H
Antivenin (Micrurusfulvius)	S		H
Arginine HCl Inj.	S	B	
Ascorbic Acid Inj.	S	A,B	LR
Atenolol Inj.	S,M	A	LR (Do not freeze)
Atropine Sulfate Inj.	S,M	A	
Sterile Aurothioglucose Suspension	I		
Aurothioglucose Injectable Oil Suspension	S,M	A	L
Azaperone Inj.	S,M	A	L
Azathioprine Sodium for Inj.	I	C	RT
Azlocillin for Inj.	I		
Aztreonam	I		
Aztreonam for Inj.	I		F
Sterile Bacitracin	I	D	R
Sterile Bacitracin Zinc	I		R (cool place)
BCG Vaccine	U	A	R
Benztropine Mesylate Inj.	S,M	A	
Benzylpenicilloyl-Polylysine Inj.	S,M	A	R
Betamethasone Sodium Phosphate Inj.	S,M	A	
Betamethasone Sodium Phosphate & Betamethasone Acetate Injectable Suspension	M	A	
Bethanechol Chloride Inj.	S	A	
Biological Indicator for Dry Heat Sterilization, Paper Strip	O		L,H,M,PA
Biological Indicator for Ethylene Oxide Sterilization, Paper Strip	O		L,H,M,PA
Biological Indicator for Steam Sterilization, Paper Strip	O		L,H,M,PA
Biological Indicative for Steam Sterilzation, Self-contained	O		L,H,M,PA
Biperiden Lactate Inj.	S	A	L
Bleomycin for Inj.	I	B	
Blood Grouping Serums (All)	U		R
Botulism Antitoxin	S		R
Bretylium Tosylate Injection	S	A	
Bretylium Tosylate in Dextrose Inj.	S,M	A,B,P	
Brompheniramine Maleate Inj.	S,M	A	L
Bumetanide Inj.	S,M	A	L
Bupivacaine HCl Inj.	S,M	A	
Bupivacaine & Epinephrine Inj.	S,M	A	L

Drugs	Container	Glass Type	Storage Conditions
Bupivacaine in Dextrose Inj.	S	A	
Butorphanol Tartrate Inj.	S,M	A	L
Caffeine & Sodium Benzoate Inj.	S	A	
Calcium Chloride Inj.	S	A	
Calcium Gluceptate Inj.	S	A,B	
Calcium Gluconate Inj.	S	A	
Calcium Levulinate Inj.	S	A	
Capreomycin for Inj.	I	B	R
Carbenicillin for Inj.	I	D	
Carboprost Tromethamine Inj.	S,M	A	R
Cefamandole Nafate for Inj.	I	D	
Sterile Cefamandole Nafate	I		
Sterile Cefamandole Sodium	I		
Cefamandole Sodium for Inj.	I		
Cefazolin Inj.	I		F
Cefmenoxime for Inj.	I		
Sterile Cefmetazole Sodium	I		
Cefoperazone Inj.	I		F
Cefoperazone for Inj.	I		
Cefoperazone Inj.	I		F
Ceforanide for Inj.	I		
Sterile Cefotaxime Sodium	I	B	
Cefotaxime Sodium Inj.	S,M		F
Cefotetan Injection	I		F
Cefotetan for Injection	I		
Cefotetan Disodium	I		
Cefotiam for Inj.	I	C	
Sterile Cefoxitin Sodium	I	B	
Cefoxitin Sodium Inj.	I		F
Cefpiramide for Inj.	I		
Ceftazidime Inj.	I		F
Ceftazidime for Inj.	I		L
Sterile Ceftazidime	I		L
Ceftizoxime for Inj.	I		
Ceftizoxime Inj.	I		F
Ceftriaxone Inj.	I		F
Ceftriaxone for Inj.	I		F
Cefuroxime Inj.	I		F
Cefuroxime for Inj.	I		
Cellulose Oxidized (all)	I		L,R
Cephalothin Inj.	I		F
Cephalothin for Inj.	I		
Cephapirin for Inj.	I		
Cephradine for Inj.	I		
Chloramphenicol Inj.	S,M		
Sterile Chloramphenicol	I		
Sterile Chloramphenicol Sodium Succinate	I	B	
Sterile Chlordiazepoxide HCI	I	B	L
Chloroprocaine HCI Inj.	S,M	A	
Chloroquine HCI Inj.	S	A	
Chlorothiazide Sodium for Inj.	I	C	

Drugs	Container	Glass Type	Storage Conditions
Chlorphenamine Maleate Inj.	S,M	A	L
Chlorpromazine HCl Inj.	S,M	A	L
Chlorprothixene Inj.	S		L
Sterile Chlortetracycline HCl	I		L
Cholera Vaccine	U		R
Sodium Chromate Cr51 Inj.	S,M		
Chromic Chloride Inj.	S,M	A,B	
Sterile Cilastatin Sod.	I	C	R
Ciprofloxacin Inj.	S,M	A	R,L
Cisplatin for inj.	I		
Citric Acid, Magnesium Oxide Sodium Carbonate Irrigation	S	A,B	
Sterile Clavulanate Potassium	I		
Clindamycin for Inj.	I		
Clindamycin Inj.	S,M	A,P	
Sterile Cloxacillin Benzathine	U (tight)		
Cloxacilllin Benzathine Intramammary Infusion	Sy		
Sterile Cloxacillin Sodium	U (tight)		
Cloxacillin Sodium Intramammary Infusion	Sy		TP
Coccidioidin			R
Codeine Phosphate Inj.	S,M	A	L
Colchicine Inj.	S	A	L
Colistimethate Sodium	I		
Colistimethate for Inj.	I		
Corticotropin Inj.	S,M	A	R
Corticotropin for Inj.	I	B	
Repository Corticotropin Inj.	S,M	A	
Corticotropin Zinc Hydroxide Injectable Suspension	S,M	A	RT
Cortisone Acetate Injectable Suspension	S,M	A	
Cromolyn Sodium Inhalation	S (double ended Ampul)	A,B,P	
Cupric Chloride Inj.	S,M	A,B	
Cupric Sulfate Inj.	S,M	A,B	
Cyanocobalamin Inj.	S,M	A	LR
Cyclizine Lactate Inj.	S	A	
Cyclophosphamide for Inj.	I		RT
Cyclosporine Concentrate for Inj.	S,M		
Cysteine HCl Inj.	S,M	A	
Cytarabine	I		
Cytarabine for Inj.	I		
Dacarbazine for Inj.	S,M or I	A	L
Dactinomycin for Inj.	I	B	LR
Daunorubicin HCl for Inj.	I	B	LR
Deferoxamine Mesylate for Inj.	S,M	A	
Deslanoside Inj.	S	A	
Desoxycorticosterone Acetate Inj.	S,M	A,C	Lh.
Desoxycorticosterone Acetate Pellets	U (tight)		
Dexamethasone Acetate Injectable Suspension	S,M	A	
Dextrose Inj.	S	A,B,P	
Dextrose & Sodium Chloride Inj.	S	A,B,P	
Diatrizoate Meglumine Inj.	S,M	A,C	L

Drugs	Container	Glass Type	Storage Conditions
Diatrizoate Meglumine & Diatrizoate Sodium Inj.	S	A,C	L
Diatrizoate Sodium Inj.	S. M	A,C	L
Diazepam Inj.	S,M	A	L
Diazoxide Inj.	S	A	L
Dibucaine HCl Inj.	S,M	A	L
Dicyclomine HCl Inj.	S,M	A	
Diethylstilbestrol Inj.	S,M	A	LR
Diethylstilbestrol Diphosphate Inj.	S,M		
Digitoxin Inj.	S,M	A	L
Digoxin Inj.	S	A	LR, H
Dihydroergotamine Mesylate Inj.	S	A	Avoid heat
Dihydrostreptomycin Inj.	S,M		
Dimenhydrinate Inj.	S,M	A,C	
Dimercaprol Inj.	S,M	A,C	
Dimethyl Sulfoxide Irrigation	S		RT,L
Dinoprost Tromethamine Inj.	S,M	A	
Diphenhydramine HCl Inj.	S,M	A	L
Diphtheria Antitoxin	U		R
Diphtheria Toxin for Schick Test	U		R
Diphtheria Toxoid	U		R
Diptheria Toxoid Adsorbed	U		R
Diphtheria and Tetanus Toxoids	U		R
Diphtheria & Tetanus Toxoids/Adsorbed	U		R
Diphtheria and Tetanus Toxoids and Pertussis Vaccine	U		R
Diphtheria & Tetanus Toxoids & Pertussis Vaccine Adsorbed	U		R
Dobutamine Inj.	S,M	A	
Dobutamine for Inj.	I	B	RT
Dopamine HCl Inj.	S	A	
Dopamine HCl & Dextrose Inj.	S	A,B	
Doxapram HCl Inj.	S,M	A	
Doxorubicin HCl Inj.	S,M	A	LR,R (not to exceed 100 ml if multidose)
Doxorubicin HCl for Inj.	I	B	(not to exceed 250 ml if multidose)
Doxycycline Hyclate for Inj.	I	B	L
Sterile Doxycycline Hyclate	I		L
Droperidol Inj.	S,M	A	L
Dyphylline Inj.	S,M	A	RT,L
Edetate Calcium Disodium Inj.	S	A	
Edetate Disodium Inj.	S	A	
Edrophonium Chloride Inj.	S,M	A	
Multiple Electrolytes Inj. (Type 1)	S	A,B,P	
Multiple Electrolytes Inj. (Type 2)	S	A,B,P	
Multiple Electrolytes and Dextrose Inj. (Type 1)	S	A,B,P	
Multiple Electrolytes and Dextrose Inj. (Type 2)	S	A,B,P	
Multiple Electrolytes and Dextrose Inj. (Type 3)	S	A,B,P	
Multiple Electrolytes and Dextrose Inj. (Type 4)	S	A,B,P	
Multiple Electrolytes and Invert Sugar Inj. (Type 1)	S	A,B,P	
Multiple Electrolytes and Invert Sugar Inj. (Type 2)	S	A,B,P	

Drugs	Container	Glass Type	Storage Conditions
Multiple Electrolytes and Invert Sugar Inj. (Type 3)	S	A,B,P	
Trace Elements Inj.	S,M	A,B	
Emetine HCl Inj.	S	A	LR
Ephedrine Sulfate Inj.	S,M	A	LR
Epinephrine Inj.	S,M	A	LR
Epinephrine Injectable Oil Susp.	S	A,C	LR
Epinephrine Bitartrate for Ophthalmic Solution	I		
Ergonovine Maleate Inj.	S	A	LR,R
Ergotamine Tartrate Inj.	S	A	LR
Erythromycin Ethylsuccinate Inj.	S,M	A	
Sterile Erythromycin Ethylsuccinate	I		
Sterile Erythromycin Gluceptate	I	D	
Sterile Erythromycin Lactobionate	I		
Erythromycin Lactobionate for Inj.	I	D	
Estradiol Pellets	U		
Estradiol Injectable Suspension	S,M	A	
Estradiol Cypionate Inj.	S,M	A	LR
Estradiol Valerate Inj.	S,M	A,C	LR
Estrone Inj.	S,M	A	
Estrone Injectable Suspension	S,M	A	
Ethacrynate Sodium for Inj.	I	D	
Ethiodized Oil Inj.	S,M		LR
Fentanyl Citrate Inj.	S	A	L
Ferrous Citrate Fe 59 Inj.	S,M		
Sterile Floxuridine	M	A	L (discard after 2 wks when reconstituted)
Fludeoxyglucose F 18 Inj.	S,M		SC
Flunixin Meglumine Injection	M		RT
Fluorescein Inj.	S	A	
Fluorescein Sodium Ophth. Strips	S,SS,U		
Sodium Fluoride F 18 Inj.	S,M		SC
Fluorescein Inj.	S	A	
Fluorodopa F 18 Inj.	S,M		SC
Fluorouracil Inj.	S	A	RT,L
Fluphenazine Decanoate Inj.	S,M	A	L
Fluphenazine Enanthate Inj.	S,M	A,C	L
Fluphenazine HCl Inj.	S,M	A	L
Folic Acid Inj.	S,M	A	
Fructose Inj.	S	A,B	
Fructose & Sodium Chloride Inj.	S	A,B	
Furosemide Inj.	S,M	A	LR
Gadopentetate Dimeglumine Inj.	S	A	LR,RT
Gallamine Triethiodide Inj.	S,M	A	L
Gallium Citrate Ga 67 Inj.	S,M		
Absorbable Gelatin Film	U		
Absorbable Gelatin Sponge	U		
Gentamicin Sulfate Inj.	S,M	A	
Sterile Gentamicin Sulfate	I		
Immune Globulin	U		R
Rho(D) Immune Globulin	U		R
Anti-Human Globulin Serum	U		R

Drugs	Container	Glass Type	Storage Conditions
Glucagon for Inj.	I/S,M w/solvent		
Glycine Irrigation	S	A,B	
Glycopyrrolate Inj.	S,M	A	
Gold Sodium Thiomalate Inj.	S,M	A	L
Chorionic Gonadotropin for Inj.	I	D	
Haloperidol Inj.	S,M	A	L
Heparin Calcium Inj.	S,M	A	R
Heparin Lock Flush Solution	S,M	A	
Heparin Sodium Inj.	S,M	A	
Hepatitis B Immune Globulin	U		R
Hepatitis B Virus Vaccine Inactivated	U		R
Hetacillin Potassium Intramammary Infusion	Sy		
Histamine Phosphate Inj.	S,M	A	L
Histoplasmin	U		R
Hyaluronidase Inj.	S,M	A	R
Hyaluronidase for Inj.	I	A,C	RT
Hydralazine HCl Inj.	S,M	A	
Hydrocortisone Injectable Suspension	S,M	A	
Hydrocortisone Acetate Injectable Suspension	S,M	A	
Hydrocortisone Sodium Phosphate Inj.	I	C	
Hydrocortisone Sodium Succinate for Inj.	I	C	
Hydromorphone HCl Inj.	S,M	A	L
Hydroxocobalamin Inj.	S,M	A	L
Hydroxyprogesterone Caproate Inj.	S,M	A,C	
Hydroxyzine HCl Inj.	S,M		L
Hyoscyamine Sulfate Inj.	S,M	A	
Idarubicin HCl for Inj.	I		
Ifosfamide for Inj.	I		RT
Imipenem & Cilastatin Sodium for Inj.	I		RT
Sterile Imipenem & Cilastatin Sodium	I		RT
Sterile Imipenem	I		RT
Imipramine HCl Inj.	S	A	LR
Indigotindisulfonate Sodium Inj.	S	A	LR
Indium In 111 Chloride Solution	S		RT
Indium In 111 Pentetate Inj.	S		
Indocyanine Green for Inj.	I		
Indomethacin Sodium for Inj.	I		
Influenza Virus Vaccine	U		R
Insulin Inj.	M		R
Insulin Zinc Suspension	M		R
Isophane Insulin Suspension	M		R
Extended Insulin Zinc Suspension	M		R
Prompt Insulin Zinc Suspension	M		R
Insulin Human Inj.	M		R
Inulin & Sodium Chloride Inj.	S	A,B	
Iobenguane I 123 Injection	S,M		SC,F
Iodinated I 125 Albumin Inj.	S,M		R
Iodinated I131 Albumin Inj.	U		
Iodinated I 131 Albumin Aggreg. Inj.	S,M		R
Iodipamide Meglumine Inj.	S	A,C	
Iodohippurate Sodium I123 Inj.	S,M		SC

Drugs	Container	Glass Type	Storage Conditions
Iodohippurate Sodium I 131 Inj.	S,M		
Iohexol Inj. (Intravascular/Intrathecal)	S	A	L
Iopamidol Inj. (Intravascular/Intrathecal)	S	A	L
Iophendylate Inj.	S	A	LR
Iothalamate Meglumine Inj.	S	A	L
Iothalamate Meglumine & Sodium Iothalamate Inj.	S	A	L
Iothalamate Sodium I-125 Inj.	S	A	L
Ioversol Inj.	S	A	L
Ioxaglate Meglumine & Ioxaglate Sodium Inj.	S	A	LR
Iron Dextran Inj.	S,M	A,B	
Iron Sorbitex Inj.	S	A	
Isoniazid Inj.	S,M	A	L
Isoproterenol HCl Inj.	S	A	L
Isoxsuprine HCl Inj.	S,M	A	
Kanamycin Inj.	S,M	A,C	
Ketamine HCl Inj.	S,M	A	L,H
Ketorolac Tromethamine Inj.	S	A	LR,RT
Labetalol HCl Inj.	S,M (60 ml max)	A	R,RT,L
Leucovorin Calcium Inj.	S	A	LR
Levorphanol Tartrate Inj.	S,M	A	
Sterile Lidocaine HCl	I		
Lidocaine HCl Inj.	S,M	A	
Lidocaine HCl & Dextrose Inj.	S	A,B	
Lidocaine & Epinephrine Inj.	S,M	A	LR
Lincomycin Inj.	S,M	A	
Lorazepam Inj.	S,M	A	L
Magnesium Sulfate Inj.	S,M	A	
Magnesium Sulfate in Dextrose Injection	S	A,G,P	
Manganese Chloride Inj.	S,M	A,B	
Manganese Sulfate Inj.	S,M	A,B	
Mannitol Inj.	S	A,B,P	
Mannitol & Sodium Chloride Inj.	U	D	LR
Measles Virus Vaccine Live	S,M		R
Measles & Mumps Virus Vaccine Live	S,M		LR,R
Measles, Mumps & Rubella Virus Vaccine Live	S,M		LR,R
Measles & Rubella Virus Vaccine Live	S,M		LR,R
Mechlorethamine HCl for Inj	I	B	
Sterile Medroxyprogesterone Acetate Susp.	S,M	A	
Menadiol Sodium Diphosphate Inj.	S	A	LR
Menadione Inj.	S,M	A	
Meningococcal Polysaccharide Vaccine (Group A)	M		R
Meningococcal Polysaccharide Vaccine (Group C)	M		R
Meningococcal Polysaccharide Vaccine (Groups A & C combined)	M		R
Menotropins for Inj.	S,M	A	
Meperidine HCl Inj.	S,M	A	
Mephentermine Sulfate Inj.	S,M	A	
Mepivacaine HCl Inj.	S,M	A	
Mepivacaine HCl & Levonordefrin Inj.	S,M	A	
Meprobamate Inj.	S	A	
Mesoridazine Besylate Inj.	S	A	L

Drugs	Container	Glass Type	Storage Conditions
Metaraminol Bitartrate Inj.	S,M	A	L
Methadone HCl Inj.	S,M	A	LR
Methicillin for Inj.	I		L,RT
Methionine C II Inj.	S,M		SC
Methocarbamol Inj.	S	A	
Methohexital Sodium for Inj.	I	C	
Methotrexate for Inj.	I		L
Methotrexate Inj.	S,M	A	L
Methotrimeprazine Inj.	S,M	A	L
Methyldopate HCl Inj.	S	A	
Methylene Blue Inj.	S	A	
Methylergonovine Maleate Inj.	S	A	LR
Methylprednisolone Acetate Injectable Suspension	S,M	A	
Methylprednisolone Sodium Succinate for Inj.	I	C	
Metoclopramide Inj.	S,M	A	LR (no antioxidant)
Metocurine Iodide Inj.	S,M	A	
Metoprolol Tartrate Inj.	S	A,B	L
Metronidazole Inj.	S,P	A,B	L
Mezlocillin for Inj.	I		
Miconazole Inj.	S	A	RT
Minocycline HCl for Inj.	I		L
Mitomycin for Inj.	I	D	L
Mitoxantrone for Inj. Conc.	S	A	
Morphine Sulfate Inj.	S,M	A	L
Morphine Sulfate Inj. (Preservative Free)	S	A	L
Morrhuate Sodium Inj.	S,M	A	
Moxalactam Disodium for Inj.	I		
Mumps Skin Test Antigen	U		R
Mumps Virus Vaccine Live	S,M		LR,R
Sterile Nafcillin Sodium	I		
Nafcillin Sodium Inj.	I		F
Nafcillin Sodium for Inj.	I	D	
Nalorphine HCl Inj.	S,M	A	
Naloxone HCl Inj.	S,M	A	L
Nandrolone Decanoate Inj.	S,M	A	L
Nandrolone Phenpropionate Inj.	S,M	A	L
Sterile Neomycin Sulfate	I		
Neomycin & Polymyxin B Sulfates Soln. for Irrigation	U		
Neostigmine Methylsulfate Inj.	S,M		L
Netilmicin Sulfate Inj.	S,M	A	
Niacin Inj.	S,M	A	
Niacinamide Inj.	S,M	A	
Ammonia N 13 Inj.	S,M		SC
Nitroglycerin Inj.	S,M	A,B	
Norepinephrine Bitartrate Inj.	S	A	LR
Novobiocin Sod. Intramammary Infusion	Sy		WC
Orphenadrine Citrate Inj.	S,M	A	L
Oxacillin Inj.	I		F
Oxacillin for Inj.	I		RT
Oxacillin Sodium	I		

Drugs	Container	Glass Type	Storage Conditions
Water 0-15 Inj.	S		SC
Oxymorphone HCl Inj.	S,M	A	L
Oxytetracycline	I		L
Oxytetracycline Inj.	S,M		L
Oxytetracycline for Inj.	I		L
Oxytetracycline HCl	I		L
Oxytocin Inj.	S,M	A	(do not freeze)
Papaverine HCl Inj.	S,M	A	
Penicillin G Benzathine	I		
Penicillin G Benzathine Injectable Susp.	S,M	A,B	R
Penicillin G Benzathine & Penicillin G Procaine Injectable Susp.	S,M	A,C	
Penicillin G Potassium for Inj.	I	D	
Penicillin G Potassium Inj.	S		F
Penicillin G Procaine	I		
Penicillin G Procaine for Injectable Susp.	S,M	A,C	
Penicillin G Procaine Injectable Susp.	S,M	A,C	R
Penicillin G Procaine Intramammary Infusion	Sy (well closed)		
Penicillin G Procaine w/Aluminum Stearate Injectable Oil Suspension	S,M	A,C	
Penicillin G Procaine and Dihydrostreptomycin Sulfate Injectable Suspension	S,M (tight)		
Penicillin G Procaine Dihydrostreptomycin Sulfate Intramammary Infusion	Sy (well closed)		
Penicillin G Procaine, Dihydrostreptomycin Sulfate & Prednisolone Injectable Susp.	S,M (tight)		
Penicillin G Procaine, Dihydrostreptomycin Sulfate, Chlorpheniramine Maleate, and Dexamethasone Injectable Suspension	S,M (tight)		R
Penicillin G Procaine, Dihydrostreptomycin Sulfate and Prednisolone Injectable Suspension	S,M (tight)		
Penicillin G Sodium for Inj.	I		
Pentazocine Lactate Inj.	S,M	A	
Pentobarbital Sodium Inj.	S,M	A	
Perphenazine Inj.	S,M	A	L
Pertussis Immune Globulin	U		R
Pertussis Vaccine	U		R
Pertussis Vaccine Adsorbed	U		R
Sterile Phenobarbital Sodium	I	D	
Phenobarbital Sodium Inj.	I	D	
Phentolamine Mesylate for Inj.	I	B	
Phenylbutazone Injection	S,M (vet, use)	A	L,R
Phenylephrine HCl Inj.	S,M	A	L
Phenytoin Sodium Inj.	S,M	A	RT
Chromic Phosphate P 32 Susp.	S,M		
Sodium Phosphate P 32 Soln.	S,M	Tr	
Physostigmine Salicylate Inj.	S	A	L
Phytonadione Inj.	S,M	A	L
Pilocarpine Ocular System	S		R
Piperacillin for Inj.	I		
Posterior Pituitary Inj.	S,M	A	
Plague Vaccine	U		R

Drugs	Container	Glass Type	Storage Conditions
Plasma Protein Fraction	U		(as labeled)
Platelet Concentrate	U	A,B	(as labeled)
Plicamycin for Inj.	I	D	L
Poliovirus Vaccine Inactivated	U		R
Poliovirus Vaccine Live Oral	S,M		F,R
Sterile Polymyxin B Sulfate	I	D	L
Potassium Acetate Inj.	S,M	A,B	
Potassium Chloride for Inj. Conc.	S,M	A,B	
Potassium Chloride in Dextrose Inj.	S	A,B,P	
Potassium Chloride in Dextrose and Sodium Chloride Inj.	S	A,B,P	
Potassium Chloride in Lactated Ringer's and Dextrose Inj.	S	A,B,P	
Potassium Chloride in Sodium Chloride Inj.	S	A,B,P	
Potassium Phosphates Inj.	S	A	
Sterile Pralidoxime Chloride	I	B	
Prednisolone Acetate Injectable Susp.	S,M	A	
Prednisolone Sodium Phosphate Inj.	S,M	A	L
Prednisolone Sodium Succinate for Inj.	I	D	
Prednisolone Tebutate Injectable Susp.	S,M	A	
Prilocaine HCl Inj.	S,M	A	
Prilocaine & Epinephrine Inj.	S,M	A	L
Procainamide HCl Inj.	S,M	A	
Procaine HCl Inj.	S,M	A,B	
Sterile Procaine HCl	I	D	
Procaine HCl & Epinephrine Inj.	S,M	A,B	LR
Procaine & Phenylephrine HCl Inj.	S,M	A	
Procaine & Tetracycline Hydrochlorides & Levonordefrin Inj.	S,M	A	
Prochlorperazine Edisylate Inj.	S,M	A	L
Progesterone Inj.	S,M	A,C	
Progesterone Injectable Susp.	S,M	A	
Progesterone Intrauterine Contraceptive Sys.	S		
Promazine HCl Inj.	S,M	A	L
Promethazine HCl Inj.	S,M	A	L
Sterile Propantheline Bromide	S	D	
Propoxycaine & Procaine Hydrochlorides & Levonordefrin Inj.	S	A	
Propoxycaine & Procaine Hydrochlorides & Norepinephrine Bitartrate Inj.	S,M	A	
Propranolol HCl Inj.	S	A	LR
Propyliodone Injectable Oil Susp.	S		LR
Protamine Sulfate Inj.	S	A	R
Protamine Sulfate for Inj.	I	D	
Protein Hydrolysate Inj.	S	A,B	H
Pyridostigmine Bromide Inj.	S	A	L
Pyridoxine HCl Inj	S,M	A	L
Quinidine Gluconate Inj.	S,M	A	
Rabies Immune Globulin	U		R
Rabies Vaccine	U		R
Raclopeide C II Inj.	S,M		SC
Ranitidine Inj.	S,M	I	LR,RT

Drugs	Container	Glass Type	Storage Conditions
Ranitidine in Sodium Chloride Inj.	N		LR,R/RT
Reserpine Inj.	S	A	LR
Riboflavin Inj.	S,M	A	LR
Rifampin for Inj.	I		
Ringer's Inj.	S	A,B,P	
Ringer's and Dextrose Inj.	S	A,B,P	
Lactated Ringer's Inj.	S	A,B,P	
Lactated Ringer's and Dextrose Inj.	S	A,B,P	
Half-Strength Lactated Ringer's and Dextrose Inj.	S	A,B,P	
Modified Lactated Ringer's and Dextrose Inj.	S	A,B,P	
Ringer's Irrigation	S,SS	A,B,P	
Ritodrine HCl Inj.	S	A	RT
Rose Bengal Sodium I 131 Inj.	S,M		
Rubella Virus Vaccine Live	S,M		LR,R
Rubella & Mumps Virus Vaccine Live	S,M		LR,R
Rubidium Chloride Rb 82 Inj.			NA
Schick Test Control			R
Scopolamine Hydrobromide Inj.	S,M	A	LR
Secobarbital Sodium Inj.	S,M	A	L,R
Sterile Secobarbital Sodium	I	D	
Selenious Acid Inj.	S,M	A,B	
Sisomicin Sulfate Inj.	S,M	A	
Smallpox Vaccine	U		R
Sodium Acetate Inj.	S	A	
Sodium Acetate C II Inj.	S,M		SC
Sodium Bicarbonate Inj.	S	A	
Sodium Chloride Inhalation Soln.	S		
Sodium Chloride Inj.	S	A,B	
Sodium Chloride Irrigation	S,SS	A,B,P	
Bacteriostatic Sodium Chloride Inj.	S,M	A,B	
Sodium Lactate Inj.	S	A,B	
Sodium Nitrite Inj.	S	A	
Sterile Sodium Nitroprusside	I	D	L
Sodium Pertechnetate Tc 99m Inj.	S,M		R
Sodium Phosphates Inj.	S,M	A	
Sodium Sulfate Inj.	S	A	
Sodium Thiosulfate Inj.	S	A	
Sterile Spectinomycin HCl	I		
Spectinomycin for Injectable Suspension	I		
Streptomycin Sulfate Inj.	S,M	A	
Sterile Streptomycin Sulfate	I	D	
Sterile Succinylcholine Chloride	I	D	
Succinylcholine Chloride Inj.	S,M	A,B	R
Sufentanil Citrate Inj.	S,M	A	
Invert Sugar Inj.	S,P	A,B	
Sulfadiazine Sodium Inj.	S	A	LR
Sulfamethoxazole & Trimethoprim for Inj. Concentrate	S,M	A	L
Sulfisoxazole Diolamine Inj.	S,M	A	L
Technetium Tc 99m Albumin Inj.	S,M		R
Technetium Tc 99m Albumin Aggregated Inj.	S,M		R

Drugs	Container	Glass Type	Storage Conditions
Technetium Tc 99m Albumin Colloid Inj.	S,M		R
Technetium Tc 99m Disofenin Inj.	S,M		In
Technetium Tc 99m Etidronate Inj.	S,M		
Technetium Tc 99m Exametazine Inj.	S,M		RT
Technetium Tc 99m Gluceptate Inj.	S,M		R
Technetium Tc 99m Lidofenin Inj.	S,M		R
Technetium Tc 99m Medronate Inj.	S,M		
Technetium Tc 99m Oxidronate Inj.	S,M		
Technetium Tc 99m Pentetate Inj.	S,M		R
Technetium Tc 99m Pyrophos. Inj.	S,M		R
Technetium Tc 99m (Pyro- & Trimeta-) Phosphates Inj.	U		D
Technetium Tc 99m Succimer Inj.	S		RT,L
Technetium Tc 99m Sulfur Colloid Inj.	S,M		
Terbutaline Sulfate Inj.	S	A	L,RT
Testosterone Injectable Susp.	S,M	A	
Testosterone Cypionate Inj.	S,M	A	L
Testosterone Enanthate Inj.	S,M	A	
Testosterone Propionate Inj.	S,M	A	
Tetanus Antitoxin	U		R
Tetanus Immune Globulin	U		R
Tetanus Toxoid	U		R
Tetanus Toxoid Adsorbed	U		R
Tetanus and Diphtheria Toxoids Adsorbed (for adult use)	U		R
Sterile Tetracaine HCl	I	A	
Tetracaine HCl Inj.	S,M	A	R,L
Tetracaine HCl in Dextrose Inj.	S,M (up to 100 ml)	A	R,L,RT (tray for 12 months)
Sterile Tetracycline HCl	I		L
Tetracycline HCl for Inj.	I	B	L
Tetracycline Phosphate Complex for Inj.	I	B	L
Sterile Tetracycline Phosphate Complex	I		L
Thallous Chloride Tl 201 Inj.	S,M		
Theophylline in Dextrose Inj.	S	A,B,P	
Thiamine HCl Inj.	S,M	A	L
Thiamylal Sodium for Inj.	I	C	
Thiethylperazine Malate Inj.	S	A	L
Thiopental Sodium for Inj.	I	C	
Thiotepa for Inj.	I	D	R,L
Thiothixene HCl Inj.	S	A	L
Thiothixene HCl for Inj.	I		LR
Thrombin			R
Sterile Ticarcillin Disodium	I	D	
Sterile Ticarcillin Disodium & Clavulanate Potassium	I		
Ticarcillin Disodium and Clavulanate Potassium Inj.	I		F
Tilmicosin Injection	I		
Sterile Tobramycin Sulfate	I		
Tobramycin Sulfate Inj.	S,M	A,P	
Sterile Tolbutamide Sodium	I	D	

Drugs	Container	Glass Type	Storage Conditions
Triamcinolone Acetonide Injectable Susp.	S,M	A	L
Triamcinolone Diacetate Injectable Susp.	S,M	A	
Triamcinolone Hexacetonide Injectable Susp.	S,M	A	
Trifluoperazone HCl Inj.	M	A	L
Triflupromazine HCl Inj.	S,M	A	L
Trimethaphan Camsylate Inj.	S,M	A	R
Trimethobenzamide HCl Inj.	S,M	A	
Tromethamine for Inj.	S,M	A	C
Crystallized Trypsin for Inhalation Aerosol	S	A	RT
Tuberculin			R
Tubocurarine Chloride	S,M		
Typhoid Vaccine	U		R
Sterile Urea	I	D	
Vaccinia Immune Globulin	U		R
Vancomycin HCl for Inj.	I		
Varicella-Zoster Immune Globulin	U		R
Vasopressin Inj.	S,M	A	
Verapamil HCl Inj.	S	A	LR
Vidarabine Concentrate for Inj.	S,M	A	
Vinblastine Sulfate for Inj.	I	D	R
Vincristine Sulfate Inj.	U	U	L,R
Vincristine Sulfate for Inj.	U		L,R
Warfarin Sodium for Inj.	I	D	LR
Water for Inj.	SP		
Sterile Bacteriostatic Water for Inj.	S,M, CV	A,B,P	
Sterile Water for Inhalation	S		
Sterile Water for Inj.	S	A,B,P	SS
Sterile Water for Irrigation	S	A,B	
Sterile Purified Water	WC	U	
Xenon Xe 127	S (leakproof stoppers)		RT,SC
Xenon Xe 133	S (leakproof stoppers)		RT,SC
Xenon X3 133 Inj.	S (totally filled)		RT,SC
Yellow Fever Vaccine	U (nitrogen filled ampules)		R
Zinc Chloride Inj.	S,M	A,B	
Zinc Sulfate Inj.	S,M		

Provided by Dr. Kenneth S. Alexander, Professor of Pharmacy, College of Pharmacy, University of Toledo.

Oral Dosage Forms That Should
Not Be Crushed or Chewed

This listing is included to alert the healthcare practitioner about oral dosage forms that should not be crushed or chewed and to serve as an aid in consulting with patients. Refer to the end of the table for a complete explanation of all alphabetical references.

Drug Product	Manufacturer	Dosage Form	Reason/Comments
Accutane	Roche	Capsule	Mucous membrane irritant
Actifed 12 Hour	Warner Lambert Consumer Health Products	Capsule	Slow release (i)
Acutrim	Novartis Consumer Health	Tablet	Slow release
Aerolate SR, JR, III	Fleming & Co.	Capsule	Slow release*(i)
Afrinol Repetabs	Schering-Plough	Tablet	Slow release
Allerest 12 Hour	Novartis Consumer Health	Caplet	Slow release
Artane Sequels	Lederle	Capsule	Slow release*(i)
Arthritis Bayer TR	Bayer	Capsule	Slow release
ASA Enseals	Lilly	Tablet	Enteric-coated
Asbron G Inlay	Sandoz	Tablet	Multiple compressed tablet (i)
Atrohist Plus	Adams	Tablet	Slow release
Atrohist Sprinkle	Adams	Capsule	Slow release*
Azulfidine Entabs	Pharmacia & Upjohn	Tablet	Enteric-coated
Baros	Lafayette	Tablet	Effervescent tab (d)
Bayer Extra Strength Enteric 500	Bayer	Tablet	Slow release
Bayer Low Adult 81 mg Strength	Bayer	Tablet	Enteric-coated
Bayer Regular Strength 325 mg Caplet	Bayer	Tablet	Enteric-coated
Betachron E-R	Inwood	Capsule	Slow release
Betapen-VK	Apothecon	Tablet	Taste (c)
Biohist-LA	Wakefield	Tablet	Slow release (h)
Bisacodyl	(Various Mfr.)	Tablet	Enteric-coated (a)
Bisco-Lax	Raway	Tablet	Enteric-coated (a)
Bontril-SR	Carnrick	Capsule	Slow release
Breonesin	Sanofi Winthrop	Capsule	Liquid filled (b)
Brexin LA	Savage	Capsule	Slow release (i)
Bromfed	Muro	Capsule	Slow release (i)
Bromfed-PD	Muro	Capsule	Slow release (i)
Calan SR	Searle	Tablet	Slow release (h)
Cama Arthritis Pain Reliever	Sandoz Consumer	Tablet	Multiple compressed tablet
Carbiset-TR	Nutripharm	Tablet	Slow release
Cardizem	Hoechst Marion Roussel	Tablet	Slow release
Cardizem CD	Hoechst Marion Roussel	Capsule	Slow release*
Cardizem SR	Hoechst Marion Roussel	Capsule	Slow release*
Carter's Little Pills	Carter-Wallace	Tablet	Enteric-coated

Drug Product	Manufacturer	Dosage Form	Reason/Comments
Cefal Filmtab	Abbott	Tablet	Enteric-coated
Ceftin	Glaxo Wellcome	Tablet	Taste (c) Use suspension for children
Charcoal Plus	Kramer	Tablet	Enteric-coated
Chloral Hydrate	(Various Mfr.)	Capsule	Liquid in capsule (i)
Chlorpheniramine Maleate Time Release	(Various Mfr.)	Capsule	Slow release
Chlor-Trimeton Repetab	Schering-Plough	Tablet	Slow release (i)
Choledyl SA	Parke-Davis	Tablet	Slow release (i)
Cipro	Bayer	Tablet	Taste (c)
Claritin-D	Schering-Plough	Tablet	Slow release
Codimal LA	Schwarz Pharma	Capsule	Slow release
Codimal LA Half	Schwarz Pharma	Capsule	Slow release
Colace	Roberts	Capsule	Taste (c)
Comhist LA	Roberts	Capsule	Slow release*
Compazine Spansule	SmithKline Beecham	Capsule	Slow release (i)
Congess SR, JR	Fleming & Co.	Capsule	Slow release
Constant T	Novartis	Tablet	Slow release*
Contac	SmithKline Beecham	Capsule	Slow release*
Cotazym-S	Organon	Capsule	Enteric-coated*
Covera-HS	Searle	Tablet	Slow release
Creon 10, 20	Solvay	Capsule	Enteric-coated*
Cystospaz-M	Schwarz Pharma	Capsule	Slow release
Cytoxan	Bristol-Myers	Tablet	May be crushed but maker recommends injection.
Dallergy	Laser	Capsule	Slow release
Dallergy-D	Laser	Capsule	Slow release
Dallergy-JR	Laser	Capsule	Slow release
Deconamine SR	Berlex	Capsule	Slow release (i)
Deconsal II	Adams	Tablet	Slow release
Deconsal Sprinkle	Adams	Capsule	Slow release*
Defen-LA	Horizon	Tablet	Slow release (h)
Demazin Repetabs	Schering-Plough	Tablet	Slow release (i)
Depakene	Abbott	Capsule	Slow release, mucous membrane irritant (i)
Depakote	Abbott	Capsule	Enteric-coated
Desoxyn Gradumets	Abbott	Tablet	Slow release
Desyrel	Apothecon	Tablet	Taste (c)
Dexatrim, Max. Strength	Thompson Medical	Tablet	Slow release
Dexedrine Spansule	SmithKline Beecham	Capsule	Slow release
Diamox Sequels	Lederle	Capsule	Slow release
Dilatrate SR	Schwarz Pharma	Capsule	Slow release
Dimetane Extentab	Robins	Tablet	Slow release (i)
Disobrom	Geneva Pharm.	Tablet	Slow release
Disophrol Chronotab	Schering-Plough	Tablet	Slow release
Ital	UAD	Capsule	Slow release
Donnatal Extentab	Robins	Tablet	Slow release (i)
Donnazyme	Robins	Tablet	Enteric-coated
Drisdol	Sanofi Winthrop	Capsule	Liquid filled (b)

Drug Product	Manufacturer	Dosage Form	Reason/Comments
Drixoral	Schering-Plough	Tablet	Slow release (i)
Drixoral Plus	Schering-Plough	Tablet	Slow release
Dulcolax	Boehringer Ingelheim	Tablet	Enteric-coated (a)
Dynabac	Bock Pharmacal	Tablet	Enteric-coated
Easprin	Parke-Davis	Tablet	Enteric-coated
Ecotrin	SmithKline Beecham	Tablet	Enteric-coated
Efidac 24	Novartis Consumer Health	Tablet	Slow release
Elixophyllin SR	Forest	Capsule	Slow release* (i)
E.E.S. 400	(Various Mfr.)	Tablet	Enteric-coated (i)
E-Mycin	Knoll Pharm.	Tablet	Enteric-coated
Endafed	UAD	Capsule	Slow release
Entex LA	Dura	Tablet	Slow release (i)
Entozyme	Robins	Tablet	Enteric-coated
Equanil	Wyeth-Ayerst	Tablet	Taste (c)
Ergostat	Parke-Davis	Tablet	Sublingual form (g)
Eryc	Parke-Davis	Capsule	Enteric-coated*
Ery-tab	Abbott	Tablet	Enteric-coated
Erythrocin Stearate	(Various Mfr.)	Tablet	Enteric-coated
Erythromycin Base	(Various Mfr.)	Tablet	Enteric-coated
Eskalith CR	SmithKline Beecham	Tablet	Slow release
Exgest LA	Carnrick	Tablet	Slow release
Fedahist Timecaps	Schwarz Pharma	Capsule	Slow release (i)
Feldene	Pfizer	Capsule	Mucous membrane irritant
Feocyte	Dunhall	Tablet	Slow release
Feosol	SmithKline Beecham	Tablet	Enteric-coated (i)
Feosol Spansule	SmithKline Beecham	Capsule	Slow release*(i)
Feratab	Upsher-Smith	Tablet	Enteric-coated (i)
Fergon	Sanofi Winthrop	Capsule	Slow release*
Fero-Grad-500	Abbott	Tablet	Slow release
Fero-Gradumet	Abbott	Tablet	Slow release
Ferralet SR	Mission	Tablet	Slow release
Festal 11	Hoechst Marion Roussel	Tablet	Enteric-coated
Feverall Sprinkle Caps	Upsher-Smith	Capsule	Taste*(j)
Fumatinic	Laser	Capsule	Slow release
Gastrocrom	Medeva	Capsule	Dissolve in water (k)
Geocillin	Roerig	Tablet	Taste
Glucotrol XL	Pratt	Tablet	Slow release
Gris-PEG	Allergan	Tablet	Crushing may precipitate (l)
Guaifed	Muro	Capsule	Slow release
Guaifed-PD	Muro	Capsule	Slow release
Guaifenex LA	Ethex	Tablet	Slow release (h)
Guaifenex PSE 120	Ethex	Tablet	Slow release (h)
Guaimax-D	Schwarz Pharma	Tablet	Slow release
Humibid DM	Adams	Tablet	Slow release
Humibid DM Sprinkle	Adams	Capsule	Slow release*
Humibid LA	Adams	Tablet	Slow release

Drug Product	Manufacturer	Dosage Form	Reason/Comments
Humibid Sprinkle	Adams	Capsule	Slow release*
Hydergine LC	Sandoz	Capsule	Liquid in capsule (i)
Hydergine Sublingual	Sandoz	Tablet	Sublingual route (i)
Hytakerol	Sanofi Winthrop	Capsule	Liquid filled (b)(i)
Iberet	Abbott	Tablet	Slow release (i)
Iberet 500	Abbott	Tablet	Slow release (i)
ICaps Plus	LaHaye Labs	Tablet	Slow release
ICaps Time Release	LaHaye Labs	Tablet	Slow release
Ilotycin	Dista	Tablet	Enteric-coated
Imdur	Key	Tablet	Slow release (h)
Inderal LA	Wyeth-Ayerst	Capsule	Slow release
Inderide LA	Wyeth-Ayerst	Capsule	Slow release
Indocin SR	Merck	Capsule	Slow release*(i)
Ionamin	Medeva	Capsule	Slow release
Isoclor Timesule	Medeva	Capsule	Slow release (i)
Isoptin SR	Knoll Pharm.	Tablet	Slow release
Isordil Sublingual	Wyeth-Ayerst	Tablet	Sublingual form (g)
Isordil Tembid	Wyeth-Ayerst	Tablet	Slow release
Isosorbide Dinitrate Sublingual	(Various Mfr.)	Tablet	Sublingual form (g)
Isosorbide Dinitrate SR	(Various Mfr.)	Tablet	Slow release
Isuprel Glossets	Sanofi Winthrop	Tablet	Sublingual form (g)
K + 8	Alra	Tablet	Slow release (i)
K + 10	Alra	Tablet	Slow release (i)
Kaon CL 8 mEq	Savage	Tablet	Slow release (i)
Kaon-Cl-10	Savage	Tablet	Slow release (i)
K + Care	Alra	Tablet	Effervescent tablet (d)(i)
Klor-Con	Upsher-Smith	Tablet	Slow release (i)
Klor-Con/EF	Upsher-Smith	Tablet	Effervescent tablet (d)(i)
Klorvess	Sandoz	Tablet	Effervescent tablet (d)(i)
Klotrix	Apothecon	Tablet	Slow release (i)
K-Lyte	Apothecon	Tablet	Effervescent tablet (d)
K-Lyte/Cl 50	Apothecon	Tablet	Effervescent tablet (d)
K-Tab	Abbott	Tablet	Slow release (i)
Levsinex Timecaps	Schwarz Pharma	Capsule	Slow release
Lexxel	Astra Merck	Tablet	Slow release
Lithobid	Novartis	Tablet	Slow release (i)
Lodrane LD	ECR Pharmaceutical	Capsule	Slow release*
Mag-Tab SR	Niche	Tablet	Slow release
Meprospan	Wallace	Capsule	Slow release*
Mestinon Timespan	ICN	Tablet	Slow release (i)
Mi-Cebrin	Dista	Tablet	Enteric-coated
Mi-Cebrin T	Dista	Tablet	Enteric-coated
Micro K	Robins	Capsule	Slow release*(i)
Monafed	Monarch	Tablet	Slow release
Monafed DM	Monarch	Tablet	Slow release
Motrin	Pharmacia & Upjohn	Tablet	Taste (c)
MS Contin	Purdue Frederick	Tablet	Slow release (i)

Drug Product	Manufacturer	Dosage Form	Reason/Comments
MSC Triaminic	Sandoz	Tablet	Enteric-coated
Muco-Fen-LA	Wakefield	Tablet	Slow release (h)
Naldecon	Bristol	Tablet	Slow release (i)
Naprelan	Wyeth-Ayerst	Tablet	Slow release
Nasatab LA	ECR Pharmaceutical	Tablet	Slow release (h)
Nico-400	Jones Medical	Capsule	Slow release
Nicobid	Rhone-Poulenc Rorer	Capsule	Slow release
Nitro Bid	Hoechst Marion Roussel	Capsule	Slow release*
Nitrocine Timecaps	Schwarz Pharma	Capsule	Slow release
Nitroglyn	Kenwood	Capsule	Slow release*
Nitrong	Rhone-Poulenc Rorer	Tablet	Sublingual route (g)
Nitrostat	Parke-Davis	Tablet	Sublingual route (g)
Nitro-Time	Time-Cap Labs	Capsule	Slow release
Noctec	Apothecon	Capsule	Liquid in capsule (i)
Nolamine	Carnrick	Tablet	Slow release
Nolex LA	Carnrick	Tablet	Slow release
Norflex	3M Pharmaceuticals	Tablet	Slow release
Norpace CR	Searle	Capsule	Slow release
Novafed	Hoechst Marion Roussel	Capsule	Slow release
Novafed A	Hoechst Marion Roussel	Capsule	Slow release
Ondrox	Unimed	Tablet	Slow release
Optilets-500 Filmtab	Abbott	Tablet	Enteric-coated
Optilets-M-500 Filmtab	Abbott	Tablet	Enteric-coated
Oragrafin	Bracco DXS	Capsule	Liquid in capsule
Oramorph SR	Roxane	Tablet	Slow release (i)
Ornade Spansule	SmithKline Beecham	Capsule	Slow release
Oxycontin	Purdue Pharma	Tablet	Slow release
Pabalate	Robins	Tablet	Enteric-coated
Pabalate SF	Robins	Tablet	Enteric-coated
Pancrease	Ortho McNeil	Capsule	Enteric-coated*
Pancrease MT	Ortho McNeil	Capsule	Enteric-coated*
Panmycin	Pharmacia & Upjohn	Capsule	Taste
Papaverine Sustained Action	(Various Mfr.)	Capsule	Slow release
Pathilon Sequeles	Lederle	Capsule	Slow release*
Pavabid Plateau	Hoechst Marion Roussel	Capsule	Slow release*
PBZ-SR	Novartis	Tablet	Slow release (i)
Pentasa	Hoechst Marion Roussel	Tablet	Slow release
Perdiem	Rhone-Poulenc Rorer	Granules	Wax coated
Peritrate SA	Parke-Davis	Tablet	Slow release (h)
Permitil Chronotab	Schering	Tablet	Slow release (i)
Phazyme	Schwarz Pharma	Tablet	Slow release
Phazyme 95	Schwarz Pharma	Tablet	Slow release
Phenergan	Wyeth-Ayerst	Tablet	Taste (c)(i)
Phyllocontin	Purdue Frederick	Tablet	Slow release

Drug Product	Manufacturer	Dosage Form	Reason/Comments
Plendil	Astra Merck	Tablet	Slow release
Pneumomist	ECR Pharmaceutical	Tablet	Slow release (h)
Polaramine Repetabs	Schering-Plough	Tablet	Slow release (i)
Prelu-2	Boehringer Ingelheim	Capsule	Slow release
Prevacid	TAP Pharmaceutical	Capsule	Slow release
Prilosec	Astra Merck	Capsule	Slow release
Pro-Banthine	Roberts	Tablet	Taste
Procainamide HCL SR	(Various Mfr.)	Tablet	Slow release
Procan SR	Parke-Davis	Tablet	Slow release
Procanbid	Parke-Davis	Tablet	Slow release
Procardia	Pfizer	Capsule	Delays absorption (b)(e)
Procardia XL	Pfizer	Tablet	Slow release, AUC is unaffected
Profen II	Wakefield	Tablet	Slow release (h)
Profen-LA	Wakefield	Tablet	Slow release (h)
Pronestyl SR	Bristol-Myers Squibb	Tablet	Slow release
Proscar	Merck	Tablet	See handling instructions (m)
Proventil Repetabs	Schering-Plough	Tablet	Slow release (i)
Prozac	Dista	Capsule	Slow release*
Quadra Hist	Schein	Tablet	Slow release
Quibron-T/SR	Bristol-Myers Squibb	Tablet	Slow release (i)
Quinaglute DuraTabs	Berlex	Tablet	Slow release
Quinalan Lanatabs	Lannett	Tablet	Slow release
Quinalan SR	Lannett	Tablet	Slow release
Quinidex Extentabs	Robins	Tablet	Slow release
Quin-Release	Major	Tablet	Slow release
Respa-1st	Respa	Tablet	Slow release (h)
Respa-DM	Respa	Tablet	Slow release (h)
Respa-GF	Respa	Tablet	Slow release (h)
Respahist	Respa	Capsule	Slow release*
Respaire SR	Laser	Capsule	Slow release
Respbid	Boehringer Ingelheim	Tablet	Slow release
Ritalin-SR	Novartis	Tablet	Slow release
Robimycin Robitab	Robins	Tablet	Enteric-coated
Rondec TR	Dura	Tablet	Slow release (i)
Roxanol SR	Roxane	Tablet	Slow release (i)
Ru-Tuss DE	Knoll Pharm.	Tablet	Slow release
Sinemet CR	DuPont Pharm	Tablet	Slow release (h)
Singlet	SmithKline Beecham	Tablet	Slow release
Slo-Bid Gyrocaps	Rhone-Poulenc Rorer	Capsule	Slow release*
Slo-Niacin	Upsher Smith	Tablet	Slow release (h)
Slo-Phyllin GG	Rhone-Poulenc Rorer	Capsule	Slow release (i)
Slo-Phyllin Gyrocaps	Rhone-Poulenc Rorer	Capsule	Slow release*(i)
Slow FE	Novartis Consumer Health	Tablet	Slow release (i)
Slow FE with Folic Acid	Novartis Consumer Health	Tablet	Slow release
Slow-K	Summit	Tablet	Slow release (i)

Drug Product	Manufacturer	Dosage Form	Reason/Comments
Slow-Mag	Searle	Tablet	Slow release
Sorbitrate SA	Zeneca	Tablet	Slow release
Sorbitrate Sublingual	Zeneca	Tablet	Sublingual route
Sparine	Wyeth-Ayerst	Tablet	Taste (c)
S-P-T	Fleming	Capsule	Liquid gelatin thyroid suspension
Sudafed 12 hour	Warner Lambert Consumer Health Products	Capsule	Slow release (i)
Sudex	Atley	Tablet	Slow release (h)
Sustaire	Pfizer	Tablet	Slow release (i)
Syn-RX	Adams Lab	Tablet	Slow release
Syn-Rx DM	Adams Lab	Tablet	Slow release
Tavist-D	Sandoz	Tablet	Multiple compressed tablet
Tedral SA	Parke-Davis	Tablet	Slow release
Tegretol-XR	Novartis	Tablet	Slow release
Teldrin	SmithKline Beecham	Capsule	Slow release*
Tepanil Ten-Tab	3M Pharmaceuticals	Tablet	Slow release
Tessalon Perles	Forest	Capsule	Slow release
Theo-24	UCB Pharma	Tablet	Slow release (i)
Theobid	UCB Pharma	Capsule	Slow release*(i)
Theochron	(Various Mfr.)	Tablet	Slow release
Theoclear LA	Schwarz Pharma	Capsule	Slow release (i)
Theo-Dur	Key	Tablet	Slow release (i)
Theo-Dur Sprinkle	Key	Capsule	Slow release* (i)
Theolair SR	3M Pharmaceuticals	Tablet	Slow release (i)
Theo-Sav	Savage	Tablet	Slow release (h)
Theovent	Schering-Plough	Capsule	Slow release (i)
Theo-X	Carnrick	Tablet	Slow release
Therapy Bayer	Glenbrook	Caplet	Enteric-coated
Thorazine Spansule	SmithKline Beecham	Capsule	Slow release
Touro A & H	Dartmouth	Capsule	Slow release
Touro DM	Dartmouth	Tablet	Slow release
Touro EX	Dartmouth	Tablet	Slow release
Touro LA	Dartmouth	Tablet	Slow release
Toprol XL	Astra	Tablet	Slow release (h)
T-Phyl	Purdue Frederick	Tablet	Slow release
Trental	Hoechst Marion Roussel	Tablet	Slow release
Triaminic	Sandoz	Tablet	Enteric-coated (i)
Triaminic-12	Sandoz	Tablet	Slow release (i)
Triaminic TR	Sandoz	Tablet	Multiple compressed tablet (i)
Trilafon Repetabs	Schering-Plough	Tablet	Slow release (i)
Tri-Phen-Chlor Time Release	Rugby	Tablet	Slow release
Tri-Phen-Mine SR	Goldline	Tablet	Slow release
Triptone Caplets	Del Pharm	Tablet	Slow release
Tuss-LA	Hyrex	Tablet	Slow release
Tuss Ornade Spansule	SmithKline Beecham	Capsule	Slow release
Tylenol Extended Relief	Ortho McNeil	Capsule	Slow release

Drug Product	Manufacturer	Dosage Form	Reason/Comments
ULR-LA	Geneva Pharm	Tablet	Slow release
Uniphyl	Purdue Frederick	Tablet	Slow release
Valrelease	Roche	Capsule	Slow release
Verelan	Lederle	Capsule	Slow release*
Volmax	Muro	Tablet	Slow release
Wellbutrin	Glaxo Wellcome	Tablet	Anesthetize mucous membrane
Wyamycin S	Wyeth Ayerst	Tablet	Slow release
Wygesic	Wyeth-Ayerst	Tablet	Taste
ZORprin	Knoll Pharm.	Tablet	Slow release
Zyban	Glaxo Wellcome	Tablet	Slow release
Zymase	Organon	Capsule	Enteric-coated

Revised by John F. Mitchell, PharmD, FASHP, from an article originally appearing in *Hospital Pharmacy*, 31:27-37, 1996.

* Capsule may be opened and the contents taken without crushing or chewing; soft food such as applesauce or pudding may facilitate administration; contents may generally be administered via nasogastric tube using an appropriate fluid provided entire contents are washed down the tube.

(a) Antacids or milk may prematurely dissolve the coating of the tablet.

(b) Capsule may be opened and the liquid contents removed for administration.

(c) The taste of this product in a liquid form would likely be unacceptable to the patient; administration via nasogastric tube should be acceptable.

(d) Effervescent tablets must be dissolved in the amount of diluent recommended by the manufacturer.

(e) If the liquid capsule is crushed or the contents expressed, the active ingredient will be, in part, absorbed sublingually.

(f) Acid contents of the stomach may prematurely activate the ingredients.

(g) Tablets are made to disintegrate under the tongue.

(h) Tablet is scored and may be broken in half without affecting release characteristics.

(i) Liquid dosage forms of the product are available; however, dose, frequency of administration, and manufacturers may differ from that of the solid dosage form.

(j) Capsule contents intended to be placed in a teaspoonful of water or soft food.

(k) Contents may be dissolved in water for administration.

(l) Crushing may result in precipitation of larger particles.

(m) Crushed tablet should not be handled by women who are pregnant or who may become pregnant.

Drug Names That Look
Alike and Sound Alike

Dispensing errors can be caused by drug names that look alike and sound alike. The list below contains several such combinations. Some similarities sound dangerously close while others may appear more obviously different. In both circumstances good communications skills are vital when dealing with these drugs.

This list has been prepared to sensitize health professionals and their support personnel for the need to properly communicate when writing, speaking, reading and hearing drug names.

Trade names are capitalized whereas other names are in lower case letters.

"Look-Alike, Sound-Alike Drugs" was originated and developed by Benjamin Teplitsky, retired Chief Pharmacist of Veterans Administration Hospitals in Albany, NY and Brooklyn, NY.

A

abciximab	arcitumomab
acetazolamide	acetohexamide
acetohexamide	acetazolamide
acetylcholine	acetylcysteine
acetylcysteine	acetylcholine
Acthar	Acthrel
Acthar	Acular
Acthrel	Acthar
Acular	Acthar
Adderall	Inderal
Adeflor M	Aldoclor
Adriamycin	Idamycin
Afrin	aspirin
Akineton	Ecotrin
Albutein	albuterol
albuterol	atenolol
albuterol	Albutein
Alcaine	Alcare
Alcare	Alcaine
Aldactazide	Aldactone
Aldactone	Aldactazide
Aldoclor	Aldoril
Aldoclor	Adeflor M
Aldomet	Aldoril
Aldoril	Aldoclor
Aldoril	Aldomet
Alfenta	Sufenta
alfentanil	Anafranil
alfentanil	fentanyl
alfentanil	sufentanil
Alkeran	Leukeran
alprazolam	lorazepam
alprazolam	alprostadil
alprostadil	alprazolam

Altace	alteplase
Altace	Artane
alteplase	anistreplase
alteplase	Altace
Alupent	Atrovent
Ambenyl	Aventyl
Ambien	Amen
Amen	Ambien
Amicar	Amikin
Amikin	Amicar
amiloride	amiodarone
amiloride	amlodipine
aminophylline	amitriptyline
aminophylline	ampicillin
amiodarone	amiloride
amiodarone	amrinone
Amipaque	Omnipaque
amitriptyline	nortriptyline
amitriptyline	aminophylline
amlodipine	amiloride
amoxapine	amoxicillin
amoxicillin	amoxapine
ampicillin	aminophylline
amrinone	amiodarone
Anafranil	enalapril
Anafranil	nafarelin
Anafranil	alfentanil
Anaprox	Anaspaz
Anaspaz	Anaprox
Ancobon	Oncovin
anisindione	anisotropine
anisotropine	anisindione
anistreplase	alteplase
Antabuse	Anturane
Anturane	Artane

Anturane	Antabuse
Anusol	Aplisol
Anusol	Aquasol
Aplisol	Aplitest
Aplisol	Anusol
Aplisol	Atropisol
Aplitest	Aplisol
Apresazide	Apresoline
Apresoline	Apresazide
Aquasol	Anusol
arcitumomab	abciximab
Aricept	Ascriptin
Artane	Altace
Artane	Anturane
Asacol	Os-Cal
Ascriptin	Aricept
Asendin	aspirin
aspirin	Asendin
aspirin	Afrin
Atarax	Ativan
Atarax	Marax
atenolol	timolol
atenolol	albuterol
Ativan	Avitene
Ativan	Atarax
Atropisol	Aplisol
Atrovent	Alupent
Aventyl	Ambenyl
Aventyl	Bentyl
Aventyl	Serentil
Avitene	Ativan
azatadine	azathioprine
azathioprine	azidothymidine
azathioprine	Azulfidine
azathioprine	azatadine
azidothymidine	azathioprine
Azulfidine	azathioprine

B

bacitracin	Bactrim
bacitracin	Bactroban
baclofen	Bactroban
baclofen	Beclovent
Bactine	Bactrim
Bactine	Banthine
Bactrim	bacitracin
Bactrim	Bactine
Bactroban	bacitracin
Bactroban	baclofen

Banthine	Brethine
Banthine	Bactine
Beclovent	baclofen
Beminal	Benemid
Benadryl	Bentyl
Benadryl	Benylin
Benadryl	benazepril
benazepril	Benadryl
Benemid	Beminal
Benoxyl	PerOxyl
Benoxyl	Brevoxyl
Bentyl	Aventyl
Bentyl	Benadryl
Benylin	Ventolin
Benylin	Benadryl
benztropine	bromocriptine
Bepridil	Prepidil
Betadine	betaine
Betagan	Betagen
Betagen	Betagan
betaine	Betadine
Betoptic	Betoptic S
Betoptic S	Betoptic
Bicillin	V-Cillin
Bicillin	Wycillin
Bontril	Vontrol
Brethaire	Brethine
Brethaire	Bretylol
Brethine	Banthine
Brethine	Brethaire
Bretylol	Brevital
Bretylol	Brethaire
Brevital	Bretylol
Brevoxyl	Benoxyl
brimonidine	bromocriptine
bromocriptine	benztropine
bromocriptine	brimonidine
Bronkodyl	Bronkosol
Bronkosol	Bronkodyl
Bumex	Buprenex
bupivacaine	mepivacaine
Buprenex	Bumex
bupropion	buspirone
buspirone	bupropion
butabarbital	Butalbital
Butalbital	butabarbital

C

Cafergot	Carafate

Caladryl	calamine
calamine	Caladryl
calcifediol	calcitriol
calciferol	calcitriol
calcitonin	calcitriol
calcitriol	calcifediol
calcitriol	calciferol
calcitriol	calcitonin
calcium glubionate	calcium gluconate
calcium gluconate	calcium glubionate
Capastat	Cepastat
Capitrol	Captopril
Captopril	Capitrol
Carafate	Cafergot
Carbex	Surbex
Carboplatin	Cisplatin
Cardene	Cardura
Cardene	codeine
Cardene SR	Cardizem SR
Cardizem SR	Cardene SR
Cardura	Coumadin
Cardura	K-Dur
Cardura	Cardene
Cardura	Cordarone
Catapres	Catarase
Catapres	Cetapred
Catapres	Combipres
Catarase	Catapres
cefamandole	cefmetazole
cefazolin	cephalothin
cefazolin	cefprozil
cefmetazole	cefamandole
Cefobid	cefonicid
cefonicid	Cefobid
Cefotan	Ceftin
cefotaxime	cefoxitin
cefotaxime	cefuroxime
cefotetan	cefoxitin
cefoxitin	Cytoxan
cefoxitin	cefotaxime
cefoxitin	cefotetan
cefprozil	cefazolin
ceftazidime	ceftizoxime
Ceftin	Cefotan
ceftizoxime	ceftazidime
cefuroxime	cefotaxime
cefuroxime	deferoxamine
Cefzil	Kefzol
Cepastat	Capastat
cephalexin	cephalothin
cephalothin	cefazolin
cephalothin	cephalexin
cephapirin	cephradine
cephradine	cephapirin
Cerebyx	Cerezyme
Ceredase	Cerezyme
Cerezyme	Cerebyx
Cerezyme	Ceredase
Cetaphil	Cetapred
Cetapred	Cetaphil
Cetapred	Catapres
Chenix	Cystex
chlorambucil	Chloromycetin
Chloromycetin	chlorambucil
chloroxine	Choloxin
chlorpromazine	chlorpropamide
chlorpromazine	clomipramine
chlorpropamide	chlorpromazine
Choloxin	chloroxine
Chorex	Chymex
Chymex	Chorex
Cidex	Lidex
Ciloxan	Cytoxan
Ciloxan	cinoxacin
cimetidine	simethicone
cinoxacin	Ciloxan
Cisplatin	Carboplatin
Citracal	Citrucel
Citrucel	Citracal
Clinoril	Clozaril
clofazimine	clozapine
clofibrate	clorazepate
clomiphene	clomipramine
clomiphene	clonidine
clomipramine	chlorpromazine
clomipramine	clomiphene
clonidine	quinidine
clonidine	clomiphene
clorazepate	clofibrate
clotrimazole	co-trimoxazole
Cloxapen	clozapine
clozapine	clofazimine
clozapine	Cloxapen
Clozaril	Clinoril
co-trimoxazole	clotrimazole
codeine	Cardene
codeine	Lodine

codeine . . . . .Cordran
Combipres . . . . .Catapres
Compazine . . . . .Copaxone
Copaxone . . . . .Compazine
Cordarone . . . . .Cardura
Cordarone . . . . .Cordran
Cordran . . . . .codeine
Cordran . . . . .Cordarone
Cort-Dome . . . . .Cortone
Cortone . . . . .Cort-Dome
Cortrosyn . . . . .Cotazym
Cotazym . . . . .Cortrosyn
Coumadin . . . . .Kemadrin
Coumadin . . . . .Cardura
Cozaar . . . . .Zocor
cyclobenzaprine . . . . .cycloserine
cyclobenzaprine . . . . .cyproheptadine
cyclophosphamide . . . . .cyclosporine
cycloserine . . . . .cyclosporine
cycloserine . . . . .cyclobenzaprine
cyclosporin . . . . .Cyklokapron
cyclosporine . . . . .cyclo-
phosphamide
cyclosporine . . . . .cycloserine
Cyklokapron . . . . .cyclosporin
cyproheptadine . . . . .cyclobenzaprine
Cystex . . . . .Chenix
Cytadren . . . . .cytarabine
cytarabine . . . . .vidarabine
cytarabine . . . . .Cytadren
CytoGam . . . . .Cytoxan
Cytosar U . . . . .Cytovene
Cytosar U . . . . .Cytoxan
Cytotec . . . . .Cytoxan
Cytovene . . . . .Cytosar U
Cytoxan . . . . .Cytotec
Cytoxan . . . . .Cytosar U
Cytoxan . . . . .CytoGam
Cytoxan . . . . .cefoxitin
Cytoxan . . . . .Ciloxan

D

dacarbazine . . . . .Dicarbosil
dacarbazine . . . . .procarbazine
Dacriose . . . . .Danocrine
dactinomycin . . . . .daunorubicin
dactinomycin . . . . .doxorubicin
Dalmane . . . . .Dialume
Dalmane . . . . .Demulen
Danocrine . . . . .Dacriose

Dantrium . . . . .Daraprim
dapsone . . . . .Diprosone
Daranide . . . . .Daraprim
Daraprim . . . . .Dantrium
Daraprim . . . . .Daranide
Daricon . . . . .Darvon
Darvocet-N . . . . .Darvon-N
Darvon . . . . .Daricon
Darvon-N . . . . .Darvocet-N
daunorubicin . . . . .doxorubicin
daunorubicin . . . . .dactinomycin
deferoxamine . . . . .cefuroxime
Delsym . . . . .Desyrel
Demerol . . . . .Demulen
Demerol . . . . .Dymelor
Demulen . . . . .Dalmane
Demulen . . . . .Demerol
Depo-Estradiol . . . . .Depo-Testadiol
Depo-Medrol . . . . .Solu-Medrol
Depo-Testadiol . . . . .Depo-Estradiol
Dermatop . . . . .Dimetapp
Desferal . . . . .Disophrol
desipramine . . . . .disopyramide
desipramine . . . . .imipramine
desoximetasone . . . . .dexamethasone
Desoxyn . . . . .digitoxin
Desoxyn . . . . .digoxin
Desyrel . . . . .Zestril
Desyrel . . . . .Delsym
dexamethasone . . . . .desoximetasone
Dexedrine . . . . .dextran
Dexedrine . . . . .Excedrin
dextran . . . . .Dexedrine
DiaBeta . . . . .Zebeta
Dialume . . . . .Dalmane
Diamox . . . . .Trimox
diazepam . . . . .diazoxide
diazepam . . . . .Ditropan
diazoxide . . . . .Dyazide
diazoxide . . . . .diazepam
Dicarbosil . . . . .dacarbazine
dichloroacetic acid . . . . .trichloroacetic acid
diclofenac . . . . .Diflucan
diclofenac . . . . .Duphalac
dicyclomine . . . . .dyclonine
dicyclomine . . . . .doxycycline
Diflucan . . . . .diclofenac
digitoxin . . . . .digoxin
digitoxin . . . . .Desoxyn

digoxin . . . . .doxepin

digoxin . . . . .Desoxyn

digoxin . . . . .digitoxin

Dilantin . . . . .Dilaudid

Dilaudid . . . . .Dilantin

dimenhydrinate . . . . .diphenhydramine

Dimetane . . . . .Dimetapp

Dimetapp . . . . .Dermatop

Dimetapp . . . . .Dimetane

diphenhydramine . . . . .dimenhydrinate

Diprosone . . . . .dapsone

dipyridamole . . . . .disopyramide

Disophrol . . . . .Desferal

disopyramide . . . . .desipramine

disopyramide . . . . .dipyridamole

dithranol . . . . .Ditropan

Ditropan . . . . .diazepam

Ditropan . . . . .dithranol

dobutamine . . . . .dopamine

Donnagel . . . . .Donnatal

Donnatal . . . . .Donnagel

dopamine . . . . .Dopram

dopamine . . . . .dobutamine

Dopar . . . . .Dopram

Dopram . . . . .dopamine

Dopram . . . . .Dopar

doxacurium . . . . .doxapram

doxacurium . . . . .doxorubicin

doxapram . . . . .doxepin

doxapram . . . . .doxacurium

doxapram . . . . .doxazosin

doxapram . . . . .doxorubicin

doxazosin . . . . .doxapram

doxazosin . . . . .doxorubicin

doxazosin . . . . .doxepin

doxepin . . . . .doxazosin

doxepin . . . . .digoxin

doxepin . . . . .doxapram

doxepin . . . . .Doxidan

Doxil . . . . .Paxil

doxorubicin . . . . .doxapram

doxorubicin . . . . .dactinomycin

doxorubicin . . . . .daunorubicin

doxorubicin . . . . .doxacurium

doxorubicin . . . . .doxazosin

doxycycline . . . . .doxylamine

doxycycline . . . . .dicyclomine

doxylamine . . . . .doxycycline

dronabinol . . . . .droperidol

droperidol . . . . .dronabinol

Duphalac . . . . .diclofenac

Dyazide . . . . .diazoxide

dyclonine . . . . .dicyclomine

Dymelor . . . . .Demerol

Dynacin . . . . .DynaCirc

DynaCirc . . . . .Dynacin

E

Ecotrin . . . . .Edecrin

Ecotrin . . . . .Akineton

Edecrin . . . . .Ecotrin

Elavil . . . . .Equanil

Elavil . . . . .Mellaril

Eldepryl . . . . .enalapril

Emcyt . . . . .Eryc

enalapril . . . . .Anafranil

enalapril . . . . .Eldepryl

encainide . . . . .flecainide

Enduronyl Forte . . . . .Inderal 40 mg

enflurane . . . . .isoflurane

Entex . . . . .Tenex

ephedrine . . . . .epinephrine

epinephrine . . . . .ephedrine

Epogen . . . . .Neupogen

Equagesic . . . . .EquiGesic
                       (Veterinary)

Equanil . . . . .Elavil

EquiGesic (Veterinary) . . . . .Equagesic

Eryc . . . . .Emcyt

Erythrocin . . . . .Ethmozine

Esimil . . . . .Estinyl

Esimil . . . . .Ismelin

Estinyl . . . . .Esimil

Estraderm . . . . .Testoderm

Ethmozine . . . . .Erythrocin

ethosuximide . . . . .methsuximide

etidocaine . . . . .etidronate

etidronate . . . . .etretinate

etidronate . . . . .etidocaine

etidronate . . . . .etomidate

etomidate . . . . .etidronate

etretinate . . . . .etidronate

Eurax . . . . .Serax

Eurax . . . . .Urex

Excedrin . . . . .Dexedrine

F

Factrel . . . . .Sectral

Feldene . . . . .Seldane

fentanyl	alfentanil
Feosol	Fer-in-Sol
Fer-in-Sol	Feosol
Feridex	Fertinex
Ferralyn	Verelan
Fertinex	Feridex
Fioricet	Fiorinal
Fiorinal	Florinef
Fiorinal	Fioricet
flecainide	encainide
Flexeril	Floxin
Flexon	Floxin
Florinef	Fiorinal
Florvite	Folvite
Floxin	Flexeril
Floxin	Flexon
Fludara	FUDR
Flumadine	flunisolide
Flumadine	flutamide
flunisolide	fluocinonide
flunisolide	Flumadine
fluocinolone	fluocinonide
fluocinonide	flunisolide
fluocinonide	fluocinolone
fluoxetine	fluvastatin
flutamide	Flumadine
fluvastatin	fluoxetine
folic acid	folinic acid
folinic acid	folic acid
Folvite	Florvite
fosinopril	lisinopril
FUDR	Fludara
Fulvicin	Furacin
Furacin	Fulvicin
furosemide	Torsemide

G

Gantanol	Gantrisin
Gantrisin	Gantanol
Glaucon	glucagon
glimepiride	glipizide
glipizide	glyburide
glipizide	glimepiride
glucagon	Glaucon
Glucotrol	glyburide
glutethimide	guanethidine
glyburide	glipizide
glyburide	Glucotrol
GoLYTELY	NuLytely

gonadorelin	gonadotropin
gonadorelin	guanadrel
gonadotropin	gonadorelin
guaifenesin	guanfacine
guanabenz	guanadrel
guanabenz	guanfacine
guanadrel	gonadorelin
guanadrel	guanabenz
guanethidine	guanidine
guanethidine	glutethimide
guanfacine	guanidine
guanfacine	guaifenesin
guanfacine	guanabenz
guanidine	guanethidine
guanidine	guanfacine

H

halcinonide	Halcion
Halcion	Haldol
Halcion	Healon
Halcion	halcinonide
Haldol	Halog
Haldol	Halcion
Halog	Haldol
Halotestin	Halotex
Halotestin	halothane
Halotex	Halotestin
halothane	Halotestin
Healon	Halcion
Heparin	Hespan
Hespan	Heparin
Humalog	Humulin
Humulin	Humalog
Hycodan	Hycomine
Hycodan	Vicodin
Hycomine	Hycodan
hydralazine	hydroxyzine
hydrochloro- thiazide	hydroflumethia- zide
hydrocortisone	hydroxychloro- quine
hydroflumethia- zide	hydrochloro- thiazide
hydromorphone	morphine
hydroxychloroquine	hydrocortisone
hydroxyproges- terone	medroxyproges- terone
hydroxyurea	hydroxyzine
hydroxyzine	hydralazine
hydroxyzine	hydroxyurea

Hygroton . . . . .Regroton
HyperHep . . . . .Hyperstat
Hyperstat . . . . .Nitrostat
Hyperstat . . . . .HyperHep
Hytone . . . . .Vytone

I

Idamycin . . . . .Adriamycin
Iletin .Lente
Imipenem . . . . .Omnipen
imipramine . . . . .desipramine
Imodium . . . . .Ionamin
Imuran . . . . .Inderal
indapamide . . . . .Iopidine
indapamide . . . . .iodamide
indapamide . . . . .iopamidol
Inderal . . . . .Inderide
Inderal . . . . .Isordil
Inderal . . . . .Adderall
Inderal . . . . .Imuran
Inderal 40 mg . . . . .Enduronyl Forte
Inderide . . . . .Inderal
interferon 2 . . . . .interleukin 2
interferon alfa 2a . . . . .interferon alfa 2b
interferon alfa 2b . . . . .interferon alfa 2a
interleukin 2 . . . . .interferon 2
Intropin . . . . .Isoptin
iodamide . . . . .indapamide
iodine . . . . .Iopidine
iodine. . . . . .Lodine
iodapamide . . . . .Iopidine
Ionamin . . . . .Imodium
iopamidol . . . . .indapamide
Iopidine . . . . .Lodine
Iopidine . . . . .indapamide
Iopidine . . . . .iodine
Iopidine . . . . .iodapamide
Ismelin . . . . .Isuprel
Ismelin . . . . .Esimil
isoflurane . . . . .enflurane
Isoptin . . . . .Intropin
Isopto Carbachol . . . . .Isopto Carpine
Isopto Carpine . . . . .Isopto Carbachol
Isordil . . . . .Isuprel
Isordil . . . . .Inderal
Isuprel . . . . .Ismelin
Isuprel . . . . .Isordil

K

K-Dur . . . . .Cardura

K-Lor .Kaochlor
K-Phos Neutral . . . . .Neutra-Phos-K
Kaochlor . . . . .K-Lor
Keflex . . . . .Keflin
Keflin . . . . .Keflex
Kefzol . . . . .Cefzil
Kemadrin . . . . .Coumadin
Klaron . . . . .Klor-Con
Klor-Con . . . . .Klaron

L

lactose . . . . .lactulose
lactulose . . . . .lactose
Lamictal . . . . .Lomotil
Lamictal . . . . .Lamisil
Lamisil . . . . .Lamictal
lamivudine . . . . .lamotrigine
lamotrigine . . . . .lamivudine
Lanoxin . . . . .Levsinex
Lasix . . . . .Lidex
Lasix . . . . .Luvox
Lente . . . . .Iletin
Leukeran . . . . .Leukine
Leukeran . . . . .Alkeran
Leukine . . . . .Leukeran
Leustatin . . . . .lovastatin
Levatol . . . . .Lipitor
Levbid . . . . .Lithobid
levothyroxine . . . . .liothyronine
Levsinex . . . . .Lanoxin
Librax . . . . .Librium
Librium . . . . .Librax
Lidex . . . . .Cidex
Lidex . . . . .Lasix
Lioresal . . . . .lisinopril
liothyronine . . . . .levothyroxine
Lipitor . . . . .Levatol
lisinopril . . . . .fosinopril
lisinopril . . . . .Lioresal
Lithobid . . . . .Lithostat
Lithobid . . . . .Lithotabs
Lithobid . . . . .Levbid
Lithonate . . . . .Lithostat
Lithostat . . . . .Lithobid
Lithostat . . . . .Lithonate
Lithostat . . . . .Lithotabs
Lithotabs . . . . .Lithostat
Lithotabs . . . . .Lithobid
Livostin . . . . .lovastatin

Lodine	codeine
Lodine	iodine
Lodine	Iopidine
Lomotil	Lamictal
Loniten	Lotensin
Lopressor	Lopurin
Lopurin	Lopressor
Lopurin	Lupron
Lorabid	Lortab
lorazepam	alprazolam
Lortab	Lorabid
Lotensin	Loniten
Lotensin	lovastatin
lovastatin	Lotensin
lovastatin	Leustatin
lovastatin	Livostin
Luminal	Tuinal
Lupron	Nuprin
Lupron	Lopurin
Luvox	Lasix

M

Maalox	Maolate
Maalox	Marax
magnesium sulfate	manganese sulfate
manganese sulfate	magnesium sulfate
Maolate	Maalox
Marax	Atarax
Marax	Maalox
Maxidex	Maxzide
Maxzide	Maxidex
Mazicon	Mivacron
Mebaral	Medrol
Mebaral	Mellaril
mecamylamine	mesalamine
Medrol	Mebaral
medroxyproges- terone	methyltestoster- one
medroxyproges- terone	hydroxyproges- terone
medroxyproges- terone	methylpred- nisolone
Mellaril	Elavil
Mellaril	Mebaral
melphalan	Mephyton
Mephenytoin	Mephyton
Mephenytoin	phenytoin
mephobarbital	methocarbamol
Mephyton	melphalan

Mephyton	Mephenytoin
mepivacaine	bupivacaine
mesalamine	mecamylamine
Mesantoin	Mestinon
Mestinon	Mesantoin
Mestinon	Metatensin
metaproterenol	metoprolol
metaproterenol	metipranolol
Metatensin	Mestinon
methazolamide	metolazone
methenamine	methionine
methicillin	mezlocillin
methionine	methenamine
methocarbamol	mephobarbital
methsuximide	ethosuximide
methylpred- nisolone	medroxyproges- terone
methyltestos- terone	medroxyproges- terone
metipranolol	metaproterenol
metolazone	metoprolol
metolazone	methazolamide
metoprolol	metaproterenol
metoprolol	metolazone
metyrapone	metyrosine
metyrosine	metyrapone
Mevacor	Mivacron
mezlocillin	methicillin
miconazole	Micronase
miconazole	Micronor
Micro-K	Micronase
Micronase	Micronor
Micronase	Micro-K
Micronase	miconazole
Micronor	miconazole
Micronor	Micronase
Midrin	Mydfrin
Milontin	Miltown
Milontin	Mylanta
Miltown	Milontin
Minocin	Mithracin
Minocin	niacin
Mithracin	Minocin
mithramycin	mitomycin
mitomycin	mithramycin
Mivacron	Mazicon
Mivacron	Mevacor
Moban	Mobidin
Mobidin	Moban
Modane	Mudrane

Monopril . . . . .Monurol
Monurol . . . . .Monopril
morphine . . . . .hydromorphone
Mudrane . . . . .Modane
Myambutol . . . . .Nembutal
Mycelex . . . . .Myoflex
Myciguent . . . . .Mycitracin
Mycitracin . . . . .Myciguent
Mydfrin . . . . .Midrin
Mylanta . . . . .Mynatal
Mylanta . . . . .Milontin
Myleran . . . . .Mylicon
Mylicon . . . . .Myleran
Mynatal . . . . .Mylanta
Myoflex . . . . .Mycelex

N

nafarelin . . . . .Anafranil
Naldecon . . . . .Nalfon
Nalfon . . . . .Naldecon
naloxone . . . . .naltrexone
naltrexone . . . . .naloxone
Narcan . . . . .Norcuron
Navane . . . . .Nubain
Navane . . . . .Norvasc
Nembutal . . . . .Myambutol
Nephro-Calci . . . . .Nephrocaps
Nephrocaps . . . . .Nephro-Calci
Neupogen . . . . .Nutramigen
Neupogen . . . . .Epogen
Neutra-Phos-K . . . . .K-Phos Neutral
niacin . . . . .Minocin
nicardipine . . . . .nifedipine
Nicobid . . . . .Nitro-Bid
Nicoderm . . . . .Nitroderm
Nicorette . . . . .Nordette
nifedipine . . . . .nimodipine
nifedipine . . . . .nicardipine
Nilstat . . . . .Nitrostat
Nilstat . . . . .Nystatin
nimodipine . . . . .nifedipine
Nitro-Bid . . . . .Nicobid
Nitroderm . . . . .Nicoderm
nitroglycerin n. . . . . .itroprusside
nitroprussid . . . . .nitroglycerin
Nitrostat . . . . .Nystatin
Nitrostat . . . . .Hyperstat
Nitrostat . . . . .Nilstat
Norcuron . . . . .Narcan

Nordette . . . . .Nicorette
Norflex . . . . .Noroxin
Norgesic #40 . . . . .Norgesic Forte
Norgesic Forte . . . . .Norgesic #40
Noroxin . . . . .Norflex
nortriptyline . . . . .amitriptyline
Norvasc . . . . .Navane
Nubain . . . . .Navane
NuLytely . . . . .GoLYTELY
Nuprin . . . . .Lupron
Nutramigen . . . . .Neupogen
Nystatin . . . . .Nilstat
Nystatin . . . . .Nitrostat

O

OctreoScan . . . . .OncoScint
Ocufen . . . . .Ocuflox
Ocuflox . . . . .Ocufen
olanzapine . . . . .olsalazine
olsalazine . . . . .olanzapine
Omnipaque . . . . .Amipaque
Omnipen . . . . .Unipen
Omnipen . . . . .Imipenem
OncoScint . . . . .OctreoScan
Oncovin . . . . .Ancobon
Ophthaine . . . . .Ophthetic
Ophthetic . . . . .Ophthaine
Oretic . . . . .Oreton
Oreton . . . . .Oretic
Orexin . . . . .Ornex
Orinase . . . . .Ornade
Orinase . . . . .Ornex
Ornade . . . . .Orinase
Ornex . . . . .Orexin
Ornex . . . . .Orinase
Os-Cal . . . . .Asacol
Otobiotic . . . . .Urobiotic
oxaprozin . . . . .oxazepam
oxazepam . . . . .oxaprozin
oxymetazoline . . . . .oxymetholone
oxymetholone . . . . .oxymetazoline
oxymetholone . . . . .oxymorphone
oxymorphone . . . . .oxymetholone

P

paclitaxel . . . . .paroxetine
paclitaxel . . . . .Paxil
Pamine . . . . .Pelamine
Panadol . . . . .pindolol
pancuronium . . . . .pipecuronium

Paraplatin	Platinol
paregoric	Percogesic
Parlodel	pindolol
paroxetine	paclitaxel
Patanol	Platinol
Pathilon	Pathocil
Pathocil	Placidyl
Pathocil	Pathilon
Pavabid	Pavatine
Pavatine	Pavabid
Pavulon	Peptavlon
Paxil	Doxil
Paxil	paclitaxel
Paxil	Taxol
Pediapred	PediaProfen
Pediapred	Pediazole
PediaProfen	Pediapred
Pediazole	Pediapred
Pelamine	pemoline
Pelamine	Pamine
pemoline	Pelamine
Penetrex	Pentrax
penicillamine	penicillin
penicillin	Polycillin
penicillin	penicillamine
pentobarbital	phenobarbital
pentosan	pentostatin
pentostatin	pentosan
Pentrax	Permax
Pentrax	Penetrex
Peptavlon	Pavulon
Percocet	Percodan
Percodan	Percogesic
Percodan	Periactin
Percodan	Percocet
Percogesic	paregoric
Percogesic	Percodan
Periactin	Persantine
Periactin	Percodan
Permax	Pentrax
Permax	Pernox
Pernox	Permax
PerOxyl	Benoxyl
Persantine	Periactin
phenobarbital	pentobarbital
phentermine	phentolamine
phentolamine	phentermine
phenytoin	Mephenytoin
Phos-Flur	PhosLo

PhosChol	PhosLo
PhosChol	Phosphocol P32
PhosLo	Phos-Flur
PhosLo	PhosChol
Phosphocol P32	PhosChol
Phrenilin	Trinalin
physostigmine	Prostigmin
physostigmine	pyridostigmine
pindolol	Parlodel
pindolol	Panadol
pindolol	Plendil
pipecuronium	pancuronium
Pitocin	Pitressin
Pitressin	Pitocin
Placidyl	Pathocil
Platinol	Paraplatin
Platinol	Patanol
Plendil	pindolol
Polocaine	prilocaine
Polycillin	penicillin
Ponstel	Pronestyl
pralidoxime	Pramoxine
pralidoxime	pyridoxine
Pramoxine	pralidoxime
Pravachol	Prevacid
Pravachol	propranolol
prednimustine	prednisone
prednisolone	prednisone
prednisone	primidone
prednisone	prednimustine
prednisone	prednisolone
Premarin	Primaxin
Prepidil	Bepridil
Prevacid	Pravachol
Prilocaine	Prilosec
prilocaine	Polocaine
Prilosec	Prozac
Prilosec	Prilocaine
Prilosec	Prinivil
Primaxin	Premarin
primidone	prednisone
Prinivil	Proventil
Prinivil	Prilosec
ProAmatine	protamine
Probenecid	Procanbid
Procanbid	Probenecid
procarbazine	dacarbazine
Proloprim	Protropin
promazine	promethazine

promethazine	promazine
Pronestyl	Ponstel
propranolol	Pravachol
Proscar	Psorcon
Proscar	ProSom
Proscar	Prozac
ProSom	Proscar
ProSom	Prozac
ProSom	Psorcon
Prostigmin	physostigmine
protamine	Protopam
protamine	Protropin
protamine	ProAmatine
Protopam	protamine
Protopam	Protropin
Protropin	Protopam
Protropin	Proloprim
Protropin	protamine
Proventil	Prinivil
Prozac	Proscar
Prozac	Prilosec
Prozac	ProSom
Psorcon	Proscar
Psorcon	ProSom
Pyridium	pyridoxine
pyridostigmine	physostigmine
pyridoxine	pralidoxime
pyridoxine	Pyridium

Q

Quarzan	quazepam
Quarzan	Questran
quazepam	Quarzan
Questran	Quarzan
quinidine	quinine
quinidine	Quinora
quinidine	clonidine
quinine	quinidine
Quinora	quinidine

R

ranitidine	ritodrine
ranitidine	rimantadine
Reglan	Regonol
Regonol	Reglan
Regonol	Regroton
Regroton	Regonol
Regroton	Hygroton
reserpine	Risperidone
Restoril	Vistaril

Retrovir	ritonavir
Revex	ReVia
ReVia	Revex
Ribavirin	riboflavin
riboflavin	Ribavirin
rifabutin	rifampin
Rifadin	Ritalin
Rifamate	rifampin
rifampin	rifabutin
rifampin	Rifamate
rimantadine	ranitidine
Risperidone	reserpine
Ritalin	Rifadin
ritodrine	ranitidine
ritonavir	Retrovir
Roxanol	Roxicet
Roxicet	Roxanol

S

salsalate	sucralfate
salsalate	sulfasalazine
Sandimmune	Sandoglobulin
Sandimmune	Sandostatin
Sandoglobulin	Sandostatin
Sandoglobulin	Sandimmune
Sandostatin	Sandimmune
Sandostatin	Sandoglobulin
saquinavir	Sinequan
Sectral	Factrel
Sectral	Septra
Seldane	Feldene
selegiline	Stelazine
Septa	Septra
Septra	Sectral
Septra	Septa
Serax	Xerac
Serax	Eurax
Serentil	Serevent
Serentil	Aventyl
Serevent	Serentil
simethicone	cimetidine
Sinequan	saquinavir
Slow FE	Slow-K
Slow-K	Slow FE
Solu-Medrol	Depo-Medrol
somatrem	somatropin
somatropin	sumatriptan
somatropin	somatrem
sotalol	Stadol

Stadol . . . . .sotalol
Stelazine . . . . .selegiline
sucralfate . . . . .salsalate
Sufenta . . . . .Alfenta
Sufenta . . . . .Survanta
sufentanil . . . . .alfentanil
sulfadiazine . . . . .sulfasalazine
sulfamethizole . . . . .sulfameth-
                                                          oxazole
sulfamethoxazole . . . . .sulfamethizole
sulfasalazine . . . . .sulfisoxazole
sulfasalazine . . . . .salsalate
sulfasalazine . . . . .sulfadiazine
sulfisoxazole . . . . .sulfasalazine
sumatriptan . . . . .somatropin
Surbex . . . . .Surfak
Surbex . . . . .Carbex
Surfak . . . . .Surbex
Survanta . . . . .Sufenta

T

Taxol .Paxil
Tazicef . . . . .Tazidime
Tazidime . . . . .Tazicef
Tegopen . . . . .Tegretol
Tegopen . . . . .Tegrin
Tegretol . . . . .Toradol
Tegretol . . . . .Tegopen
Tegrin . . . . .Tegopen
Ten-K . . . . .Tenex
Tenex . . . . .Xanax
Tenex . . . . .Entex
Tenex . . . . .Ten-K
terbinafine . . . . .terfenadine
terbinafine . . . . .terbutaline
terbutaline . . . . .tolbutamide
terbutaline . . . . .terbinafine
terconazole . . . . .tioconazole
terfenadine . . . . .terbinafine
Testoderm . . . . .Estraderm
testolactone . . . . .testosterone
testosterone . . . . .testolactone
Theolair . . . . .Thyrolar
Thera-Flur . . . . .TheraFlu
TheraFlu . . . . .Thera-Flur
thiamine . . . . .Thorazine
thioridazine . . . . .Thorazine
Thorazine . . . . .thiamine
Thorazine . . . . .thioridazine
Thyrar . . . . .Thyrolar

Thyrolar . . . . .Theolair
Thyrolar . . . . .Thyrar
Ticar .Tigan
Tigan .Ticar
timolol . . . . .atenolol
Timoptic . . . . .Viroptic
tioconazole . . . . .terconazole
TobraDex . . . . .Tobrex
tobramycin . . . . .Trobicin
Tobrex . . . . .TobraDex
tolazamide . . . . .tolbutamide
tolbutamide . . . . .terbutaline
tolbutamide . . . . .tolazamide
tolnaftate . . . . .Tornalate
Topic .Topicort
Topicort . . . . .Topic
Toradol . . . . .Tegretol
Tornalate . . . . .tolnaftate
Torsemide . . . . .furosemide
Trandate . . . . .Trental
Trandate . . . . .Tridrate
Trental . . . . .Trandate
tretinoin . . . . .trientine
triamcinolone . . . . .Triaminicin
triamcinolone . . . . .Triaminicol
Triaminic . . . . .TriHemic
Triaminic . . . . .Triaminicin
Triaminicin . . . . .Triaminic
Triaminicin . . . . .triamcinolone
Triaminicol . . . . .triamcinolone
triamterene . . . . .trimipramine
trichloracetic   dichloroacetic
  acid . . . . acid
Tridrate . . . . .Trandate
trientine . . . . .tretinoin
trifluoperazine . . . . .triflupromazine
triflupromazine . . . . .trifluoperazine
TriHemic . . . . .Triaminic
trimipramine . . . . .triamterene
Trimox . . . . .Tylox
Trimox . . . . .Diamox
Trinalin . . . . .Phrenilin
Trobicin . . . . .tobramycin
Tronolane . . . . .Tronothane
Tronothane . . . . .Tronolane
Tuinal . . . . .Tylenol
Tuinal . . . . .Luminal
Tylenol . . . . .Tylox
Tylenol . . . . .Tuinal

Tylox	Trimox
Tylox	Tylenol

U

Unicap	Unipen
Unipen	Urispas
Unipen	Omnipen
Unipen	Unicap
Urex	Eurax
Urised	Urispas
Urispas	Urised
Urispas	Unipen
Urobiotic	Otobiotic

V

V-Cillin	Bicillin
Vancenase	Vanceril
Vanceril	Vansil
Vanceril	Vancenase
Vansil	Vanceril
Vantin	Ventolin
Vasocidin	Vasodilan
Vasodilan	Vasocidin
Vasosulf	Velosef
Velosef	Vasosulf
Ventolin	Benylin
Ventolin	Vantin
VePesid	Versed
Verelan	Vivarin
Verelan	Voltaren
Verelan	Ferralyn
Verelan	Virilon
Versed	VePesid
Vexol	VoSol
Vicodin	Hycodan
vidarabine	cytarabine
vinblastine	vincristine
vinblastine	vinorelbine
vincristine	vinblastine
vinorelbine	vinblastine
Virilon	Verelan
Viroptic	Timoptic
Visine	Visken
Visken	Visine

Vistaril	Restoril
Vivarin	Verelan
Voltaren	Vontrol
Voltaren	Verelan
Vontrol	Bontril
Vontrol	Voltaren
VoSol	Vexol
Vytone	Hytone

W

Wellbutrin	Wellcovorin
Wellbutrin	Wellferon
Wellcovorin	Wellferon
Wellcovorin	Wellbutrin
Wellferon	Wellbutrin
Wellferon	Wellcovorin
Wyamine	Wydase
Wycillin	Bicillin
Wydase	Wyamine

X

Xanax	Zantac
Xanax	Tenex
Xerac	Serax

Z

Zantac	Zofran
Zantac	Xanax
Zarontin	Zaroxolyn
Zaroxolyn	Zarontin
Zebeta	DiaBeta
Zestril	Zostrix
Zestril	Desyrel
Zocor	Cozaar
Zofran	Zantac
Zofran	Zosyn
ZORprin	Zyloprim
Zostrix	Zovirax
Zostrix	Zestril
Zosyn	Zofran
Zovirax	Zostrix
Zyloprim	ZORprin
Zyprexa	Zyrtec
Zyrtec	Zyprexa

This list was compiled by Neil M. Davis MS, Pharm D, FASHP, President, Safe Medication Practices Consulting, Inc., 1143 Wright Drive, Huntingdon Valley, PA, 19006.

Recommended Childhood Immunization Schedule

In January 1995, the recommended childhood immunization schedule was published in *MMWR* following issuance by the Advisory Committee on Immunization Practices (ACIP), the American Academy of Pediatrics, and the American Academy of Family Physicians (*1*). This schedule was the first unified schedule developed through a collaborative process among the recommending groups, the pharmaceutical manufacturing industry, and the Food and Drug Administration. This collaborative process should assist in maintaining a common childhood vaccination schedule and enabling further simplification of the schedule.

OPV remains the recommended vaccine for routine polio vaccination in the United States. IPV is recommended for persons with compromised immune systems and their household contacts and is an acceptable alternative for other persons. ACIP is developing recommendations for expanded use of IPV in the United States.

Vaccine Recommendations Changes: *Hepatitis B, infant.* Because of the availability of different formulations of hepatitis B vaccine, doses are presented in micrograms rather than volumes. In addition, the footnote includes recommendations for vaccination of infants born to mothers whose hepatitis B surface antigen status is unknown.

Hepatitis, B adolescent. The three-dose series of hepatitis B vaccine should be initiated or completed for adolescents ages 11-12 years who have not previously received three doses of hepatitis B vaccine.

Poliovirus. Although oral poliovirus vaccine (OPV) is recommended for routine vaccination, inactivated poliovirus vaccine (IPV) is indicated for certain persons (ie, those with a compromised immune system and their household contacts) and continues to be an acceptable alternative for other persons. The schedule for IPV is included in the footnote.

Measles-mumps-rubella vaccine. The second dose of measles-mumps-rubella vaccine is routinely administered at age 4-6 years or at age 11-12 years; however, it may be administered at any visit if at least 1 month has elapsed since receipt of the first dose.

Var. Var was licensed in March 1995 and has been added to the schedule. This vaccine is recommended for all children at age 12-18 months. It may be adminstered to susceptible persons any time after age 12 months, and should be given at age 11-12 years to previously unvaccinated persons lacking a reliable history of chickenpox.

References

1. ACIP. Recommended childhood immunization schedule — United States, 1997. *MMWR* 1997; 46:35-40.

Recommended Childhood Vaccination Schedule* United States, July-December 1996										
	Age/Range of Acceptable Ages for Vaccination									
Vaccine	Birth	1 Mo.	2 Mos.	4 Mos.	6 Mos.	12 Mos.	15 Mos.	18 Mos.	4-6 Yrs.	11-12 Yrs.	14-16 Yrs.
Hepatitis B†	Hep B-1									
		Hep B-2			Hep B-3					Hep B§
Diphtheria and tetanus toxoids and pertussis vaccine¶			DTaP or DTwP	DTaP or DTwP	DTaP or DTwP		DTaP or DTwP		DTwP or DTaP	Td
Haemophilus influenzae type b**			Hib	Hib	Hib	Hib				
Poliovirus††			OPV	OPV		OPV			OPV	
Measles-mumps-rubella§§						MMR			MMR¹	
Varicella zoster virus¶¶						Var			Var***	

¹ The second dose of measles-mumps-rubella vaccine should be administered either at 4 to 6 years or at 11 to 12 years.

* Vaccines are listed under the routinely recommended ages.

† **Infants born to hepatitis B surface antigen (HBsAg)-negative mothers** should receive 2.5 µg of Recombivax HB® (Merck & Co.) or 10 µg of Engerix-B® (SmithKline Beecham). The second dose should be administered > 1 month after the first dose. **Infants born to HBsAg-positive mothers** should receive 0.5 ml hepatitis B immune globulin (HBIG) within 12 hours of birth, and either 5 µg of Recombivax HB® or 10 µg of Engerix-B® at a separate site. The second dose is recommended at age 1-2 months and the third dose at age 6 months. **Infants born to mothers whose HBsAg status is unknown** should receive either 5 µg of Recombivax HB® or 10 µg of Engerix-B® within 12 hours of birth. The second dose of vaccine is recommended at age 1 month and the third dose at age 6 months. Blood should be drawn at the time of delivery to determine the mother's HBsAg status; if it is positive, the infant should receive HBIG as soon as possible (by age 1 week). The dosage and timing of subsequent vaccine doses should be based on the mother's HBsAg status.

§ Children and adolescents who have not been vaccinated against hepatitis B during infancy may begin the series during any childhood visit. Those who have not received three doses of hepatitis B vaccine should initiate or complete the series at age 11-12 years. The second dose should be administered ≥ 1 month after the first dose, and the third dose should be administered ≥ 4 months after the first dose and ≥ 2 months after the second dose.

¶ DTaP is the preferred vaccine for all doses in the vaccination series, including completion of the series in children who have received one or more doses of DTwP. Whole-cell DTP is an acceptable alternative to DTaP. The fourth dose of DTaP may be administered as early as 12 months of age provided 6 months have elapsed since the third dose and if the child is considered unlikely to return at age 15 to 18 months. Tetanus and diphtheria toxoids (Td), adsorbed, for adult use, is recommended at age 11 to 12 years if ≥ 5 years have elapsed since the last dose of DTwP, DTaP or diphtheria and tetanus toxoids. Subsequent routine Td boosters are recommended every 10 years.

** Three *Haemophilus influenzae* type b (Hib) conjugate vaccines are licensed for infant use. If PedvaxHIB® (Merck) is administered at ages 2 and 4 months, a dose at 6 months is not required. After completing the primary series, any Hib conjugate vaccine may be used as a booster.

†† Two poliovirus vaccines are currently licensed in the US: Inactivated poliovirus vaccine (IPV) and oral poliovirus vaccine (OPV). The following schedules are all acceptable by ACIP, AAP and AAFP, and parents and providers may choose among them: (1) IPV at ages 2 and 4 months and OPV at age 12 to 18 months and at age 4 to 6 years; (2) PV at ages 2, 4 and 12 to 18 months and at age 4 to 6 years; and (3) OPV at ages 2, 4, and 6 to 18 months and at age 4 to 6 years. ACIP routinely recommends schedule 1. IPV is the only poliovirus vaccine recommended for immunocompromised people and their household contacts.

§§ The second dose of measles-mumps-rubella vaccine (MMR) is routinely recommended at age 4-6 years or at age 11-12 years but may be administered at any visit provided ≥ 1 month has elapsed since receipt of the first dose and that both doses are administered at or after age 12 months.

¶¶ Susceptible children may receive varicella vaccine (Var) during any visit after the first birthday, and unvaccinated people who lack a reliable history of chickenpox should be vaccinated at age 11 to 12 years. Susceptible people aged ≥ 13 years should receive two doses ≥ 1 month apart.

*** "Catch-Up" Vaccination. Unvaccinated children who lack a reliable history of chickenpox should be vaccinated at age 11-12 years.

Use of trade names and commercial sources is for identification only and does not imply endorsement by the Public Health Service or the U.S. Department of Health and Human Services.

Source: Advisory Committee on Immunization Practices, American Academy of Pediatrics, and American Academy of Family Physicians.

Radio-Contrast Media

Generic Name	Dose Form	Trade Name	Manufacturer
Barium sulfate	Powder	Baroflave	Lannett
Barium sulfate	Powder	various	various
Barium sulfate	Suspension	E-Z-CAT	E-Z-EM
Barium sulfate	Suspension	E-Z-Paque	E-Z-EM
Barium sulfate	Suspension	Intropaque	Lafayette
Barium sulfate	Suspension	Novopaque	Picker
Barium sulfate	Suspension	Polibar-Plus	E-Z-EM
Barium sulfate	Suspension	Preview	Lafayette
Barium sulfate	Suspension	Redi-CAT	E-Z-Em
Barium sulfate	Suspension	Sol-O-Pake	E-Z-EM
Barium sulfate 1.5%	Suspension	Baro-Cat	Lafayette
Barium sulfate 1.5%	Suspension	PrepCat	Lafayette
Barium sulfate 46%	Granules	Baros	Lafayette
Barium sulfate 5%	Suspension	EneCat	Lafayette
Barium sulfate 5%	Suspension	TomoCat	Lafayette
Barium sulfate 50%	Suspension	Entrobar	Lafayette
Barium sulfate 60%	Suspension	Barosperse Liq.	Lafayette
Barium sulfate 85%	Suspension	HD 85	Lafayette
Barium sulfate 91%	Powder	Intropaque	Lafayette
Barium sulfate 92.5%	Powder	Barotrast	Armour
Barium sulfate 92%	Powder	Micropaque	Picker
Barium sulfate 95%	Powder	Barosperse	Lafayette
Barium sulfate 95%	Powder	E-Z-Paque	E-Z-EM
Barium sulfate 95%	Powder	Tonopaque	Lafayette
Barium sulfate 95%	Powder	Ultra-R	E-Z-EM
Barium sulfate 96%	Powder	Baroloid	Lafayette
Barium sulfate 96%	Powder	Mixture III	Picker
Barium sulfate 96%	Powder	Polibar	E-Z-EM
Barium sulfate 97%	Powder	Barodense	Lafayette
Barium sulfate 97%	Powder	Sol-O-Pake	E-Z-EM
Barium sulfate 97%	Suspension	Barobag	Lafayette
Barium sulfate 98%	Powder	Baricon	Lafayette
Barium sulfate 98%	Powder	HD 200 Plus	Lafayette
Barium sulfate 100%	Paste	Anatrast	Lafayette
Barium sulfate 100%	Suspension	Flo-Coat	Lafayette
Barium sulfate 100%	Suspension	Liquipake	Lafayette
Barium sulfate 150%	Suspension	Epi-C	Lafayette
Diatrizoate meglumine	Injection	Angiovist 282	Berlex
Diatrizoate meglumine	Injection	Cystografin	Squibb
Diatrizoate meglumine	Injection	Hypaque Meglumine 30%	Nycomed
Diatrizoate meglumine	Injection	Hypaque Meglumine 60%	Nycomed
Diatrizoate meglumine	Injection	Hypaque-Cysto	Nycomed
Diatrizoate meglumine	Injection	Hypaque-M 18%	Nycomed

Generic Name	Dose Form	Trade Name	Manufacturer
Diatrizoate meglumine	Injection	Hypaque-M 30%	Nycomed
Diatrizoate meglumine	Injection	Hypaque-M 60%	Nycomed
Diatrizoate meglumine	Injection	Reno-Dip	Squibb
Diatrizoate meglumine	Injection	Reno-M-60	Squibb
Diatrizoate meglumine	Injection	Urovist Cysto	Berlex
Diatrizoate meglumine	Injection	Urovist Meglumine DIU/CT	Berlex
Diatrizoate meglumine & Iodipamide meglu.	Injection	Sinografin	Squibb
Diatrizoate meglumine & sodium	Injection	Angiovist 292	Berlex
Diatrizoate meglumine & sodium	Injection	Angiovist 370	Berlex
Diatrizoate meglumine & sodium	Injection	Gastrografin	Squibb
Diatrizoate meglumine & sodium	Injection	Gastrovist	Berlex
Diatrizoate meglumine & sodium	Injection	Hypaque-76	Nycomed
Diatrizoate meglumine & sodium	Injection	Hypaque-M 75%	Nycomed
Diatrizoate meglumine & sodium	Injection	Hypaque-M 76%	Nycomed
Diatrizoate meglumine & sodium	Injection	MD-76	Mallinckrodt
Diatrizoate meglumine & sodium	Injection	MD-Gastroview	Mallinckrodt
Diatrizoate meglumine & sodium	Injection	Renografin-60	Squibb
Diatrizoate meglumine & sodium	Injection	Renografin-76	Squibb
Diatrizoate meglumine & sodium	Injection	Renovist	Squibb
Diatrizoate meglumine & sodium	Injection	Renovist II	Squibb
Diatrizoate sodium	Injection	Hypaque Oral (Canada)	Nycomed
Diatrizoate sodium	Injection	Hypaque Sodium 25%	Nycomed
Diatrizoate sodium	Injection	Hypaque Sodium 50%	Nycomed
Diatrizoate sodium	Injection	Hypaque Sodium Oral Powder	Nycomed
Diatrizoate sodium	Injection	Hypaque Sodium Oral Solution	Nycomed
Diatrizoate sodium	Injection	Urovist Sodium 300	Berlex
Ethiodized oil	Injection	Ethiodol	Savage
Iocetamic acid	Tablets	Cholebrine	Mallinckrodt
Iodamide meglumine	Injection	Renovue-65	Squibb
Iodipamide meglumine	Injection	Cholografin	Squibb
Iodixanol	Injection	Visipaque	Nycomed
Iohexol	Injection	Omnipaque	Nycomed
Iopamidol	Injection	Isovue-128	Squibb
Iopamidol	Injection	Isovue-200	Squibb

Generic Name	Dose Form	Trade Name	Manufacturer
Iopamidol	Injection	Isovue-300	Squibb
Iopamidol	Injection	Isovue-370	Squibb
Iopamidol	Injection	Isovue-M 200	Squibb
Iopamidol	Injection	Isovue-M 300	Squibb
Iopanoic acid	Tablet	Telepaque	Nycomed
Iopental		Imagopaque	Nycomed
Iopromide	Injection	Ultravist	Berlex
Iothalamate meglumine	Injection	Conray	Mallinckrodt
Iothalamate meglumine	Injection	Conray-30	Mallinckrodt
Iothalamate meglumine	Injection	Conray-43	Mallinckrodt
Iothalamate meglumine	Injection	Conray-60	Mallinckrodt
Iothalamate meglumine	Injection	Cysto-Conray	Mallinckrodt
Iothalamate meglumine	Injection	Cysto-Conray II	Mallinckrodt
Iothalamate meglumine & sodium	Injection	Vascoray	Mallinckrodt
Iothalamate sodium	Injection	Angio-Conray	Mallinckrodt
Iothalamate sodium	Injection	Conray-325	Mallinckrodt
Iothalamate sodium	Injection	Conray-400	Mallinckrodt
Ioversol	Injection	Optiray 160	Mallinckrodt
Ioversol	Injection	Optiray 240	Mallinckrodt
Ioversol	Injection	Optiray 320	Mallinckrodt
Ioversol	Injection	Optiray 350	Mallinckrodt
Ioxaglate meglumine & sodium	Injection	Hexabrix	Mallinckrodt
Ioxaglate meglumine & sodium	Injection	Hexabrix 200	Mallinckrodt
Ioxaglate meglumine & sodium	Injection	Hexabrix 320	Mallinckrodt
Ipodate calcium	Granules	Oragrafin	Squibb
Ipodate sodium	Capsules	Bilivist	Berlex
Ipodate sodium	Capsules	Oragrafin Sodi.	Squibb
Isosulfan blue	Injection	Lymphazurin	Hirsch Industries
Metrizamide	Powder for Inj	Amipaque	Nycomed
Polyvinyl chloride	Capsules	Sitzmarks	Konsyl Pharm
Propyliodone in peanut oil	Suspension	Dionosil Oily	Allen & Hanburys
Tyropanoate sodium	Capsules	Bilopaque	Nycomed
nd		Iopamiron	Berlex

nd = No data available.

Radio-Isotopes

Active Isotope	Generic Name	Dose Form or Packaging	Trade Name	Manufacturer
18-F	Fluorine F-18	Injection	nd	Medi-Physics
32-P	Chromic Phosphate P-32	Suspension	Phosphocol P32	Mallinckrodt
		Injection	Phosphotope	Squibb
		Oral Solution	Phosphotope	Squibb
32-P	Sodium Phosphate P-32	Capsules	nd	Mallinckrodt
		Oral Solution	nd	Mallinckrodt
51-Cr	Sodium Chromate Cr-51	Injection	Chromitope	Squibb
		Injection	nd	Mallinckrodt
57-Co	Cyanocobalamin Co-57	Capsules	nd	Mallinckrodt
		Kit	Rubratope-57	Squibb
57&58-Co	Cyanocobalamin Co-57 & Co-58	Kit	Dicopac Kit	Amersham
59-Fe	Ferrous Citrate Fe-59	Injection	nd	Mallinckrodt
60-Co	Cyanocobalamin Co-60	Capsules	Rubratope-60	Squibb
67-Ga	Gallium Citrate Ga-67	Injection	nd	DuPont-Merck
		Injection	nd	Mallinckrodt
		Injection	nd	Medi-Physics
		Injection	Neoscan	Medi-Physics
75-Se	Selenomethionine Se-75	Injection	Sethotope	Squibb
		Injection	nd	Mallinckrodt
		Injection	nd	Medi-Physics
81m-Kr	Krypton Kr-81m	Gas Generator	nd	Medi-Physics
82-Sr&Rb	Strontium Sr-82/Rubidium Rb-82	Generator	Cardiogen-82	Squibb
89-Sr	Strontium Chloride Sr-89	Injection	Metastron	Medi-Physics/ Amersham
99m-Tc	Technetium Tc-99m	Generator	nd	Cintichem
		Generator (fission)	nd	DuPont-Merck
		Generator (neutron)	nd	DuPont-Merck
		Generator	Ultra-TechneKow	Mallinckrodt
		Generator	Minitec II	Squibb
		Generator	Technetope II	Squibb
99m-Tc	Technetium-99m Albumin Aggegated	Kit	AN Stannous Ag.	Benedict Nuclear
		Kit	nd	CIS-US
		Kit	Pulmolite	DuPont-Merck
		Kit	TechneScan MAA	Mallinckrodt
		Kit	Lungaggregate Reagent	Medi-Physics
		Kit	nd	Merck
		Kit	Macrotec	Squibb
99m-Tc	Technetium-99m Albumin Colloid	Kit	Microlite	DuPont-Merck
99m-Tc	Technetium-99m Arcitumomab	Kit	CEA-Scan	Immuno-medics/ Mallinckrodt
99m-Tc	Technetium-99m Serum Albumin	Kit	nd	Medi-Physics

Active Isotope	Generic Name	Dose Form or Packaging	Trade Name	Manufacturer
99m-Tc	Technetium-99m Bicisate	Kit	Neurolite	DuPont-Merck
99m-Tc	Technetium-99m Disofenin	Kit	Hepatolite	DuPont-Merck
99m-Tc	Technetium-99m Etidronate	Kit		
		Kit	Tc-99m Diphos-phonate-Tin	Medi-Physics
		Kit	Tc-99m HEDSPA	Medi-Physics
		Kit	Stannous Diphosphonate	Medi-Physics
99m-Tc	Technetium-99m Exametazime	Kit	Ceretec	Amersham
99m-Tc	Technetium-99m Lidofenin	Kit	TechneScan HIDA	Merck
99m-Tc	Technetium-99m Mebrofenin	Kit	Choletec	Squibb
99m-Tc	Technetium-99m Medronate	Kit	Amer-Scan MDP	Amersham
		Kit	AN-MDP	CIS-US
		Kit	Osteolite	DuPont-Merck
		Kit	nd	Medi-Physics
		Kit	TechneScan MDP	Merck
		Kit	MDP-Squibb	Squibb
99m-Tc	Technetium-99m Mertiatide	Kit	TechneScan MAG3	Mallinckrodt
99m-Tc	Technetium-99m Oxidronate	Kit	Ostescan HDP	Mallinckrodt
99m-Tc	Technetium-99m Pentetate Sodium	Kit	AN-DTPA	CIS-US
		Kit	MPI DTPA Kit	Medi-Physics
		Kit	TechneScan DTPA	Merck
		Kit	Techneplex	Squibb
		Kit	Renotec-Iron	Squibb
			Ascorbate-DTPA	nd
99m-Tc	Tc-99m Pyro- & Trimeta- Phos-phates	Kit	AN-Pyrotec	CIS-US
		Kit	Pyrolite	DuPont-Merck
		Kit	TechneScan PYP	Mallinckrodt
		Kit	Tc-99m Poly-phosphate	Medi-Physics
		Kit	Phosphotec	Squibb
99m-Tc	Technetium-99m Red Blood Cell	Kit	RBC-Scan	Cadema Med.
		Kit	Ultratag	Mallinckrodt
99m-Tc	Technetium-99m Sestamibi	Kit	Cardiolite	DuPont-Merck
99m-Tc	Technetium-99m Sodium Gluceptate	Kit	Glucoscan	DuPont-Merck
		Kit	Technescan Gluceptate	Merck
99m-Tc	Technetium-99m Succimer	Kit	Tc-99m DMSA	Medi-Physics

Active Isotope	Generic Name	Dose Form or Packaging	Trade Name	Manufacturer
99m-Tc	Technetium-99m Sulfur Colloid	Injection	nd	CIS-US
		Injection	nd	Mallinckrodt
		Injection	nd	Medi-Physics
		Inj. & Kit	nd	Medi-Physics
		Kit	nd	CIS-US
		Kit	TSC	Medi-Physics
		Kit	TechneColl	Mallinckrodt
		Kit	Tesuloid	Squibb
99m-Tc	Technetium-99m Teboroxime	Kit	CardioTec	Squibb
99m-Tc	Sodium Pertechnetate Tc-99m	Injection	nd	CIS-US
		Injection	nd	Mallinckrodt
		Injection	nd	Medi-Physics
99m-Tc	Tc-99m Nofetumomab Merpentan	Kit	Verluma	NeoRx/ DuPont Merck
111-In	Indium-111 Capromab Pendetide	Kit	ProstaScint	Cytogen
111-In	Indium-111 Imciromab Pentetate	Kit	Myoscint	Centocor
111-In	Indium-111 Oxine	Solution	nd	Amersham
111-In	Indium-111 Oxyquinoline Sodium	Solution	nd	Amersham
111-In	Indium-111 Pentetate Disodium	Injection	In-111 DTPA	Medi-Physics
111-In	Indium-111 Pentetreotide	Injection	OctreoScan	Mallinckrodt
111-In	In-111 Satumomab Pentetide	Injection	OncoScint CR/OV	Cytogen
123-I	Sodium Iodide-123	Capsules	nd	Benedict Nuclear
		Capsules	nd	Mallinckrodt
		Capsules	nd	Medi-Physics
123-I	Iohippurate Sodium I-123	Injection	Nephroflow	Medi-Physics
123-I	Iofetamine HCl I-123	Injection	Spectamine	Medi-Physics
125-I	Iothalamate Sodium I-125	Injection	Glofil-125	Iso-Tex
125-I	Iodinated Albumin I-125	Injection	Jeanatope 125-I	Iso-Tex
		Injection	nd	Mallinckrodt
125-I	Iodinated Fibrinogen I-125	Injection	Ibrin	Amersham
127-Xe	Xenon Xe-127	Gas	nd	Mallinckrodt
131-I	Iodinated Albumin I-131	Injection	Megatope	Iso-Tex
131-I	Iodinated-131 Albumin Aggegated	Injection	Albumitope L-S	Squibb
131-I	Iodohippurate Sodium I-131	Injection	nd	CIS-US
		Injection	Hippuran	Mallinckrodt
		Injection	Hipputope	Squibb
131-I	Rose Bengal Sodium I-131	Injection	Robengatope	Squibb
131-I	Sodium Iodide I-131	Capsules	nd	CIS-US
		Capsules	nd	Mallinckrodt
		Capsules	nd	Squibb
		Capsules	nd	Syncor

Active Isotope	Generic Name	Dose Form or Packaging	Trade Name	Manufacturer
		Oral Solution	nd	CIS-US
		Oral Solution	nd	Mallinckrodt
		Oral Solution	nd	Squibb
		Oral Solution	nd	Syncor
133-Xe	Xenon Xe-133	Injection	nd	DuPont-Merck
		Gas	nd	DuPont-Merck
		Gas	nd	General Electric
		Gas	nd	Mallinckrodt
		Gas	nd	Medi-Physics
		Kit (V.S.S.)	nd	Medi-Physics
197-Hg	Chlormerodrin Hg-197	Injection	nd	Squibb
198-Au	Gold Au-198	Injection	Aureotope	Squibb
201-Tl	Thallous Chloride Tl-201	Injection	nd	DuPont-Merck
		Injection	nd	Mallinckrodt
		Injection	nd	Medi-Physics
		Injection	nd	Squibb

nd = No data available.

Agents for Imaging

Agents for MRI Imaging				
Active Isotope	Generic Name	Dose Form	Trade Name	Manufacturer
	Gadodiamide & caldiamide sodium	Injection	Omniscan	Sanofi Ny
	Gadopentetate dimeglumine	Injection	Magnevist	Berlex
	Gadoteridol & calteridol calcium	Injection	ProHance	Squibb
	Perflubron	Liquid	Imagent GI	Alliance
	Ferumoxides (investigational)		Feridex	Nycomed
Agents for PET Imaging				
13-N	Nitrogen	nd	nd	nd
15-O	Oxygen	nd	nd	nd
18-F	Fludeoxyglucose [2-fluoro(F-18)-2-deoxyglucose]	nd	nd	nd
82-Rb	Rubidium	nd	nd	nd
Agents for Ultrasonic Imaging				
	Perfluorodecalin & Perfluorotripropylamine		Fluosol-DA	nd
	Investigational		Levovist	Berlex
	Investigational		Cavisomes	Berlex

nd = No data available.

Pharmaceutical Company Labeler Code Index

LISTED IN NUMERICAL ORDER

00002
Eli Lilly and Co.

00003
Apothecon
Braccho Diagnostics
Bristol-Myers Squibb
ConvaTec
Westwood Squibb Pharmaceuticals

00004
Roche Laboratories

00005
ESI Lederle Generics
Lederle Laboratories

00006
Merck & Co.

00007
SmithKline Beecham
   Pharmaceuticals

00008
Wyeth-Ayerst Laboratories

00009
Pharmacia & Upjohn

00011
Becton Dickinson Microbiology
   Systems

00013
Pharmacia & Upjohn

00014
Searle

00015
Apothecon

00016
Pharmacia & Upjohn

00017
Wampole Laboratories

00019
Mallinckrodt Medical, Inc.

00021
Schwarz Pharma

00023
Allergan Herbert
Allergan, Inc.

00024
Sanofi Winthrop Pharmaceuticals

00025
Searle

00026
Bayer Corporation (Biological
   Division and Pharmaceutical
   Division)

00028
Novartis

00029
SmithKline Beecham
   Pharmaceuticals

00031
Whitehall Robins Laboratories
Wyeth-Ayerst

00032
Solvay

00033
Roche Laboratories
Syntex Laboratories

00034
Purdue Frederick Co.

00037
Wallace Laboratories

00039
Hoechst-Marion Roussel

00041
Oral-B Laboratories, Inc.

00043
Sandoz Consumer

00044
Knoll Laboratories
Knoll Pharmaceuticals

00045
McNeil Consumer Products Co.
McNeil Pharmaceutical
Ortho McNeil Corp.

00047
Warner Chilcott Laboratories
Watson Laboratories

00048
Knoll Laboratories
Knoll Pharmaceuticals

00049
Roerig

00052
Organon, Inc.

00053
Centeon

00054
Roxane Laboratories, Inc.

00056
Du Pont Pharma

00062
Advanced Care Products
Ortho McNeil Corp.

00065
Alcon Laboratories, Inc.

00066
Dermik Laboratories, Inc.

00067
Novartis

00068
Hoechst-Marion Roussel

00069
Pfizer US Pharmaceutical Group

00070
Arcola Laboratories

00071
Parke-Davis
Warner Lambert Consumer Health
   Products

00072
Westwood Squibb Pharmaceuticals

00074
Abbott Diagnostics
Abbott Hospital Products
Abbott Laboratories
Ross Laboratories

00075
Rhone-Poulenc Rorer
   Pharmaceuticals, Inc.

00076
Star Pharmaceuticals, Inc.

00077
PBH Wesley Jessen

00078
Sandoz Pharmaceuticals

00081
Glaxo Wellcome
Warner Lambert Consumer Health
   Products

00083
Novartis

00085
Key Pharmaceuticals
Schering-Plough Corp.
Schering Plough Healthcare
   Products

00086
Carnrick Laboratories, Inc.

00087
Bristol-Myers Squibb
Mead Johnson Nutritionals

00088
Hoechst-Marion Roussel

00089
3M Personal Healthcare
    Products
3M Pharmaceutical

00091
Schwarz Pharma

00093
Lemmon Co.
Teva Pharmaceuticals USA

00094
Du Pont Merck Pharmaceutical

00095
ECR Pharmaceuticals

00096
Person and Covey, Inc.

00108
SmithKline Beecham
    Pharmaceuticals

00116
Xttrium Laboratories, Inc.

00118
Bayer Corporation (Allergy
    Division)

00121
Pharmaceutical Associates, Inc.

00122
Rexall Group

00127
Ulmer Pharmacal Co.

00128
SmithKline Beecham
    Pharmaceuticals

00131
Central Pharmaceuticals, Inc.
Schwarz Pharma

00132
C. B. Fleet, Inc.

00137
Johnson & Johnson

00140
Roche Laboratories

00143
West-Ward, Inc.

00145
Stiefel Laboratories, Inc.

00147
Camall, Inc.

00149
Procter & Gamble Pharm.

00150
Murray Drug Corp.

00152
Gray Pharmaceutical Co.

00154
Blair Laboratories

00161
Bayer Corp. (Biological and
    Pharmaceutical Div.)

00163
ICN Pharmaceuticals, Inc.
Zeneca Pharmaceuticals

00164
Carter Products

00165
Blaine, Inc.

00168
E. Fougera and Co.

00169
Novo/Nordisk Pharm., Inc.

00172
Zenith Laboratories, Inc.

00173
Allen & Hanburys
Glaxo Wellcome

00178
Mission Pharmacal Co.

00182
Goldline Laboratories, Inc.

00185
Eon Labs Manufacturing, Inc.

00186
Astra USA, Inc.

00187
ICN Pharmaceuticals, Inc.
Zeneca Pharmaceuticals

00192
Bayer Corp. (Biological and
    Pharmaceutical Div.)

00193
Bayer Corp. (Diagnostic Division)

00196
Houba, Inc.

00205
Immunex Corp.

00209
Marsam Pharmaceuticals, Inc.

00212
Sandoz Nutrition Corp.

00217
Dunhall Pharmaceuticals, Inc.

00222
Boyle and Co. Pharm.

00223
Consolidated Midland Corp.

00224
Konsyl Pharmaceuticals

00225
B. F. Ascher and Co.

00228
Purepac Pharmaceutical Co.

00234
Schmid Products Co.

00245
Upsher-Smith Labs, Inc.

00252
Jones Medical Industries

00254
Gambro, Inc.

00256
Fleming & Co.

00258
Forest Pharmaceuticals, Inc.
Inwood Laboratories

00259
Mayrand, Inc.

00263
Rystan, Inc.

00264
McGaw, Inc.

00268
Center Laboratories

00273
Young Dental

00274
Scherer Laboratories, Inc.

00275
Arco Pharmaceuticals, Inc.

00276
Misemer Pharmaceuticals, Inc.

00277
Laser, Inc.

00281
Savage Laboratories

00283
Beutlich, Inc.

00288
Fluoritab Corp.

00295
Denison Laboratories, Inc.

00298
Vortech Pharmaceuticals

00299
Galderma Laboratories, Inc.

00300
Tap Pharmaceuticals

00304
J.J. Balan, Inc.

00310
Zeneca Pharmaceuticals

00314
Hyrex Pharmaceuticals

00316
Del-Ray Laboratory, Inc.

00317
Whorton Pharmaceuticals, Inc.

00327
Guardian Laboratories

00332
Biocraft Laboratories, Inc.
Lemmon Co.
Teva Pharmaceuticals USA

00346
Ciba Vision Ophthalmics

00348
Medtech Laboratories, Inc.

00349
Parmed Pharmaceuticals, Inc.

00362
Novocol Chemical Mfr. Co.

00364
Schein Pharmaceutical, Inc.

00372
Scot-Tussin Pharmacal, Inc.

00374
Lyne Laboratories

00378
Mylan Pharmaceuticals

00386
Gebauer Co.

00394
Mericon Industries, Inc.

00395
Humco Holding Group, Inc.

00396
Milex Products, Inc.

00398
C & M Pharmacal, Inc.

00402
Steris Laboratories, Inc.

00406
Mallinckrodt Chemical

00407
Nycomed Inc.

00418
Taylor Pharmaceuticals

00421
Fielding Co.

00426
Morton Grove Pharmaceuticals

00433
Research Industries Corp.

00436
Century Pharmaceuticals, Inc.

00451
Muro Pharmaceutical, Inc.

00454
Lexis Laboratories

00456, see 00258 Forest

00463
C. O. Truxton, Inc.

00466
Macsil, Inc.
Forest Pharmaceutical, Inc.

00469
Fujisawa USA, Inc.

00472
Alpharma

00482
Kenwood Laboratories

00485
Edwards Pharmaceuticals, Inc.

00486
Beach Pharmaceuticals

00487
Nephron Pharmaceuticals Corp.

00494
Foy Laboratories

00496
Ferndale Laboratories, Inc.

00501
Warner Lambert Consumer Health
    Products

00514
Dow B. Hickam, Inc.

00516
Glenwood, Inc.

00517
American Regent

05128
Zila Pharmaceuticals, Inc.

00521
Chesebrough-Pond's, USA

00524
Knoll Laboratories
Knoll Pharmaceuticals

00527
Lannett, Inc.

00535
Forest Pharmaceuticals, Inc.

00536
Rugby Labs, Inc.
Eon Labs Manufacturing, Inc.

00537
Spencer Mead, Inc.

00539
American Urologicals, Inc.

00548
I.M.S., Ltd.

00551
Seatrace Pharmaceuticals

00555
Barr Laboratories, Inc.

00556
H.R. Cenci Labs, Inc.

00563
Bock Pharmacal Co.

00573
Spencer Mead, Inc.
Whitehall Robins Laboratories

00574
Paddock Laboratories

00575
Baker Norton Pharmaceuticals

00576
Medical Products Panamericana

00585
Medeva Pharmaceuticals

00586
Heather Drug, Inc.

00588
Keene Pharmaceuticals, Inc.

00590
DuPont Pharma

00597
Boehringer Ingelheim, Inc.

00598
Health for Life Brands, Inc.

00603
Qualitest Products, Inc.

00615
Vangard Labs, Inc.

00619
Walker Pharmacal Co.

00641
Elkins-Sinn, Inc.

00642
Everett Laboratories, Inc.

00659
Circle Pharmaceuticals, Inc.

00663
Pfizer US Pharmaceutical Group

00665
International Laboratories

00677
Circa Pharmaceuticals, Inc
United Research Laboratories

00682
Marnel Pharmaceuticals, Inc.
Mikart, Inc.

00684
Primedics Laboratories

00686
Raway Pharmacal, Inc.

00689
Jones Medical

00703
Gensia Laboratories, LTD.

00713
G & W Laboratories

00725
Circa Pharmaceuticals, Inc.

00729
Fidelity Halsom

00731
Alto Pharmaceuticals, Inc.

00741
Walker, Corp. and, Inc.

00744
Daywell Laboratories Corp.

00766
SmithKline Beecham Consumer
   Healthcare

00777
Dista Products Co.

00781
Geneva Pharmaceuticals

00785
Forest Pharmaceuticals

00813
Pharmics, Inc.

00814
Interstate Drug Exchange

00832
Morton Grove Pharmaceuticals
Rosemont Pharmaceutical Corp.

00837
Columbia Laboratories, Inc.

00839
H.L. Moore Drug Exchange, Inc.

00879
Halsey Drug Co.

00884
Pedinol Pharmacal, Inc.

00904
Major Pharmaceuticals

00905
SCS Pharmaceuticals

00917
Wesley Pharmacal, Inc.

00918
General Medical Corp.

00927
Pfeiffer Co.

00938
Davis and Geck

00944
Baxter Hyland

00961
Cook-Waite Laboratories, Inc.

00978
SmithKline Diagnostics

00998
Alcon Laboratories, Inc.
PolyMedica Pharmaceuticals

01020
Cumberland Packing Corp.

05128
Zila Pharmaceuticals, Inc.

05745
Nastech Pharmaceutical, Inc.

05973
Nabi

08026
Smith & Nephew United

08884
Sherwood Medical

10019
Ohmeda Pharmaceuticals

10038
Ambix Laboratories, Inc.

10106
Mallinckrodt-Baker

10116
Bartor Pharmacal Co.

10118
Norstar Consumer Products

10119
Bausch & Lomb Personal
   Products Division

10157
Blistex, Inc.

10158
Block Drug, Inc.

10160
Bluco Inc./Med. Discnt. Outlet

10223
Cetylite Industries, Inc.

10310
Del Pharmaceuticals, Inc.

10331
E. E. Dickinson Co.

10337
Doak Dermatologics

10356
Beiersdorf, Inc.

10432
Freeda Vitamins, Inc.

10481
Gordon Laboratories

10486
C. S. Dent & Co. Division

10651
Lavoptik, Inc.

10706
Manne

10712
Marlyn, Inc.

10742
Mentholatum, Inc.

10797
Oakhurst Co.

10812
Neutrogena Corp.

10865
Parthenon, Inc.

10888
Advanced Nutritional Technology

10952
Recsei Laboratories

10956
Reese Pharmaceutical, Inc.

10961
Requa, Inc.

10974
Pegasus Medical, Inc.

11012
Schaffer Laboratories

11086
Summers Laboratories, Inc.

11089
McGregor Pharmaceuticals, Inc.

11290
Thompson Medical Co.

11370
Warner Lambert Co.

11414
Baker Norton Pharmaceuticals

11428
Wonderful Dream Salve Corp.

11444
W. F. Young, Inc.

11509
Combe, Inc.

11584
International Ethical Labs

11704
Survival Technology, Inc.

11793
Pasteur-Mérieux-Connaught

11808
ION Laboratories, Inc.

11845
Mason Distributors, Inc.

11940
Medco Lab, Inc.

11980
Allergan America

12071
Richie Pharmacal, Inc.

12120
Wisconsin Pharmacal Co.

12136
Bird Corp.

12165
Graham Field

12225
Quality Formulations, Inc.

12463
Jones Medical

12496
Reckitt & Colman

12622
Olin Corp.

12758
Mason Pharmaceuticals, Inc.

12843
Bayer Corp. (Consumer Division)

12934
Nion Corp.

12939
Marlop Pharmaceuticals, Inc.

13723
Dr. Nordyke Footcare Products

14362
Mass. Public Health Bio. Lab.

16500
Bayer Corp. (Consumer Div)

16837
J & J Merck Consumer Pharm.

17022
Veratex Corp.

17156
MediPhysics, Inc., Amersham
  Healthcare

17204
Miller Pharmacal Group, Inc.

17314
Alza Corp.

17478
Akorn, Inc.

17808
Himmel Pharmaceuticals, Inc.

18393
Roche Laboratories
Syntex Laboratories

18686
InnoVisions, Inc.

19200
Reckitt & Coleman

19458
Eckerd Drug Co.

19810
Bristol-Myers Products

21406
Columbia Laboratories, Inc.

21659
Pharmaceutical Labs, Inc.

22200
Mennen Co.

22840
Greer Laboratories, Inc.

23317
NMC Laboratories

23558
Lee Pharmaceuticals

23731
Cytosol Laboratories

23900
Procter & Gamble Co.

24208
Bausch & Lomb Pharmaceuticals

25077
Hudson Corp.

25332
Legere Pharmaceuticals, Inc.

25358
Donell DerMedex

25866
Vicks Pharmacy Products

28105
Hill Dermaceuticals, Inc.

28851
Kendall Health Care Products

30103
Randob Laboratories, Ltd.

30727
Merit Pharmaceuticals

31280
Becton Dickinson & Co.

31600
Kiwi Brands, Inc.

31795
Fibertone Co.

33130
Continental Quest Research

33984
Solgar, Inc.

34044
Continental Consumer Products

34567
Milex Products, Inc.

34999
Nutraloric

37000
Procter & Gamble Co.

38083
Campbell Laboratories

38130
Econo Med Pharmaceuticals

38137
Spectrum Chemical Mfg. Corp.

38245
Copley Pharmaceutical, Inc.

38697
ALK Laboratories

39506
Somerset Pharmaceuticals

39769
SoloPak Pharmaceuticals, Inc.

39822
Pharma Tek, Inc.

41383
AKPharma, Inc.
Lactaid, Inc.

41701
Stolle

41785
Unimed

42987
Roche Laboratories
Syntex Laboratories

44087
Serono Laboratories, Inc.

44184
Bajamar Chemical, Inc.

44437
Bolan Pharmaceutical, Inc.

45334
Pharmaceutical Specialties, Inc.

45565
Med-Derm Pharmaceuticals

45802
Clay-Park Labs, Inc.

45809
Shionogi USA

46287
Carolina Medical Products

46500
Rydelle Laboratories

46672
Mikart, Inc.

47144
Polymer Technology Corp.

47992
Holles Laboratories, Inc.

48017
Hermal Pharmaceutical Labs

48028
Aplicare Inc.

48532
Delmont Laboratories, Inc.

48558
Arther, Inc.

48663
Unitek Corp.

48723
Apothecus, Inc.

49072
McGuff, Inc.

49158
Thames Pharmacal, Inc.

49281
Pasteur-Mérieux-Connaught

49447
Chattem Consumer Products

49483
Time-Cap Labs, Inc.

49502
Dey Laboratories, Inc.

49669
Alpha Therapeutic Corp.

49731
Sherman Pharmaceuticals, Inc.

49884
Par Pharmaceuticals

49938
Jacobus Pharmaceutical Co.

50111
Sidmak Laboratories, Inc.

50185
McHenry Laboratories, Inc.

50242
Genentech, Inc.

50272
General Generics, Inc.

50289
Birchwood Laboratories, Inc.

50361
Pasteur-Mérieux-Connaught

50383
Health Care Products

50419
Berlex Laboratories, Inc.

50458
Janssen Pharmaceutical, Inc.

50474
Whitby Pharmaceuticals, Inc.

50486
Blairex Labs, Inc.

50520
Optimox Corp.

50673
Hirsch Industries, Inc.

50694
Seres Laboratories

50744
Dermol Pharmaceuticals, Inc.

50752
Creighton Products Corp.

50893
Westport Pharmaceuticals, Inc.

50914
Iso Tex Diagnostics, Inc.

50924
Boehringer Mannheim Diags.

50930
Parnell Pharmaceuticals, Inc.

50962
Xactdose, Inc.

51079
UDL Laboratories, Inc.

51081
Nutripharm Laboratories, Inc.

51201
American Dermal Corp.

51244
I.C.P. Pharmaceuticals

51285
Duramed Pharmaceuticals

51301
Great Southern Laboratories

51318
Stellar Pharmacal Corp.

51353
Sanitube Co.

51432
Harber Pharmaceutical Co.

51479
Dura Pharmaceuticals

51641
Alra Laboratories, Inc.

51655
Pharmaceutical Corp.

51662
Healthfirst Corp.

51672
Taro Pharmaceuticals USA, Inc.

51687
Fischer Pharmaceuticals, Inc.

51801
Nomax, Inc.

51875
Royce Laboratories, Inc.

51944
Ocumed, Inc.

51991
Breckenridge Pharmaceutical, Inc.

52041
Dayton Laboratories, Inc.

52152
Amide Pharmaceuticals, Inc.

52189
Invamed, Inc.

52238
Optopics Laboratories, Corp.

52268
Braintree Laboratories, Inc.

52311
Biosearch Medical Products

52489
Chemi-Tech Laboratories

52544
Watson Laboratories

52555
Martec Pharmaceutical, Inc.

52584
General Injectables & Vaccines

52604
Jones Medical

52747
US Pharmaceutical Corp.

52761
GenDerm Corp.

52836
Milance Laboratories, Inc.

53014
Adams Laboratories

53020
Trinity Technologies, Inc.

53118
Millgood Laboratories, Inc.

53124
Lederle-Praxis Biologicals

53159
Palisades Pharmaceuticals, Inc.

53169
Boehringer Mannheim Corp.
Monarch Pharmaceuticals

53191
Bio-Tech

53258
VHA Supply Co.

53335
Tyson & Associates, Inc.

53385
Standard Drug Co.

53489
Mutual Pharmaceutical, Inc.

53905
Chiron Therapeutics

53926
Amsco Scientific

53978
Med-Pro, Inc.

53983
Natren, Inc.

54022
Vitaline Corp.

54092
Roberts Pharmaceuticals

54129
Immuno U.S., Inc.

54198
Liquipharm

54323
Flanders, Inc.

54391
R & D Laboratories, Inc.

54396
Gynex Pharmaceuticals, Inc.

54429
Chase Laboratories

54482
Sigma-Tau Pharmaceuticals

54569
Allscrips

54627
ValMed, Inc.

54686
Ethitek Pharmaceuticals

54765
GynoPharma Laboratories

54799
Cynacon/OCuSOFT

54807
R.I.D., Inc.

54838
Silarx Pharmaceuticals, Inc.

54891
Vision Pharmaceuticals, Inc.

54921
IPR Pharmaceuticals, Inc.

54964
Murdock, Madaus, Schwabe

55298
3M Personal Healthcare Products

55299
Kingswood Laboratories, Inc.

55326
3M Personal Healthcare Products

55390
Bedford Laboratories

55422
Pharmakon Laboratories, Inc.

55425
Dal-Med Pharmaceuticals

55499
Numark Laboratories, Inc.

55505
Kramer Laboratories, Inc.

55513
Amgen, Inc.

55515
Oclassen Pharmaceuticals, Inc.

55516
Dyna Pharm, Inc.

55559
Calgon Vestal Laboratories

55566
Ferring Laboratories, Inc.

55688
Speywood Pharmaceuticals, Inc.

55806
Effcon Labs, Inc.

55953
Novopharm USA, Inc.

55994
Dakryon Pharmaceuticals

56091
Johnson & Johnson Medical

56146
Nexstar

57267
Summit Pharmaceuticals

57317
Fujisawa USA, Inc.

57480
Medirex, Inc.

57506
American Drug Industries, Inc.

57664
Caraco Pharmaceutical Labs

57665
Enzon, Inc.

57706
Storz Ophthalmics

57782
Bausch & Lomb Pharmaceuticals

57844
Gate Pharmaceuticals

58174
Baker Cummins Dermatologicals

58177
Ethex Corp.

58178
US Bioscience

58197
Pharmacel Laboratory, Inc.

58223
Kirkman Sales, Inc.

58281
Medtronic

58337
Berna Products Corp.

58406
Immunex Corp.

58407
Huckaby Pharmacal, Inc.

58468
Genzyme Corp.

58521
Richwood Pharmaceutical, Inc.

58573
Hogil Pharmaceutical Corp.

58607
ME Pharmaceuticals, Inc.

58869
Dartmouth Pharmaceuticals

58887
Novartis

58914
Scandipharm, Inc.

58980
Stratus Pharmaceuticals, Inc.

59010
ECR Pharmaceuticals

59012
Pratt Pharmaceuticals

59016
Niche Pharmaceuticals, Inc.

59046
Caprice-Greystoke

59075
Athena Neurosciences, Inc.
Eli Lilly and Co.

59081
Lafayette Pharmaceuticals, Inc.

59148
Otsuka America Pharmaceutical

59196
WE Pharmaceuticals, Inc.

59229
Horus Therapeutics, Inc.

59310
Wakefield Pharmaceuticals, Inc.

59366
Glades Pharmaceuticals

59417
Lotus Biochemical

59426
CooperVision

59512
Healthline Laboratories, Inc.

59527
BioDevelopment Corp.

59591
West Point Pharma

59630
Horizon Pharmaceutical Corp.

59640
UBI Corp.

59676
Ortho Biotech, Inc.

59702
Atley Pharmaceuticals, Inc.

59911
ESI Lederle Generics

59930
Warrick Pharmaceuticals, Corp.

60077
Young Dental

60432
Morton Grove Pharmaceuticals

60574
Medimmune, Inc.

60575
Respa Pharmaceuticals, Inc.

60793
King Pharmaceuticals Inc.

60799
Liposome Co.

60951
Endo Laboratories

61113
Astra Merck

61563
Medisan

61646
Iomed

62592
Ucyclyd Pharma, Inc.

64855
Young Again Products

70501
Neutrogena Corp.

71114
Circa Pharmaceuticals

72363
Brimms, Inc.

72559
NCI Medical Foods

72959
Alva Laboratories

74300
Pfizer US Pharmaceutical Group

74312
NBTY, Inc.

74684
Goody's Manufacturing Corp.

75137
Medtech Laboratories

76660
Procter & Gamble

79511
Triton Consumer Products, Inc.

83926
Tec Laboratories, Inc.

87900
Menley & James Labs, Inc.

88395
J. R. Carlson Laboratories

89223
Stockhausen, Inc.

89709
Amcon Laboratories

90605
Amcon Laboratories

93312
Trask Industries, Inc.

97692
S.G. Labs, Inc.

99207
Medicis Dermatologicals, Inc.

99766
Faulding USA

Pharmaceutical Manufacturer and Drug Distributor Listing

LISTED IN ALPHABETICAL ORDER

00089, 55298, 55326
3M Personal Healthcare
  Products
3M Center
Building 275-5W-05
St. Paul, MN 55133
612-733-1110

00089
3M Pharmaceutical
3M Center
Building 275-3E-09
St. Paul, MN 55133
612-736-4930

12463
Abana Pharmaceuticals, Inc.
See Jones Medical

00074
Abbott Diagnostics
Customer Support Center
Dept. 94P
Abbott Park, IL 60064
800-323-9100

00074
Abbott Hospital Products
1 Abbott Park Road
Abbott Park, IL 60064-3500
847-937-6100

00074
Abbott Laboratories
1 Abbott Park Road
Abbott Park, IL 60064-3500
847-937-6100

Able Laboratories, Inc.
6 Hollywood Ct.
South Plainfield, NJ 07080
908-754-2253

Academic Pharmaceuticals, Inc.
25720 Saunders Road North
Lake Forest, IL 60045

Acme United Corp.
75 Kings Highway Cutoff
Fairfield, CT 06430
203-332-7330

53014
Adams Laboratories
14801 Sovereign Road
Ft. Worth, TX 76155-2645
817-545-7791

Adolphs
75 Merritt Blvd.
Trumbull, CT 06611
203-381-3500

Adria Laboratories
See Pharmacia & Upjohn

00062
Advanced Care Products
Route 202
P.O. Box 610
Raritan, NJ 08869
908-218-8625

10888
Advanced Nutritional
  Technology
P.O. Box 3225
Elizabeth, NJ 07207
201-354-2740

Advanced Polymer Systems
3697 Haven Avenue
Redwood City, CA 94063
415-366-2626

Advanced Vision Research
7 Alfred Street,
Suite 330
Woburn, MA 01801
617-932-8327

Agouron Pharmaceuticals
10350 North Torrey Pines
La Jolla, CA 92037-1020
619-622-3000

A.H. Robins Consumer
  Products
See Wyeth-Ayerst

00031
A.H. Robins, Inc.
See Wyeth-Ayerst

17478
Akorn, Inc.
100 Akorn Drive
Abita Springs, LA 70420
504-893-9300

41383
AKPharma, Inc.
P.O. Box 111
Pleasantville, NJ 08232
609-645-5100

A.L. Labs
One Executive Drive
P.O. Box 1399
Ft. Lee, NJ 07024
201-947-7774

00065, 00998
Alcon Laboratories, Inc.
6201 South Freeway
Ft. Worth, TX 76134
817-293-0450

ALK Laboratories, Inc.
27 Village Lane
Walllingford, CT 06492
203-949-2727

38697
ALK Laboratories
2840 Eighth Street
Berkeley, CA 94710-2707
510-843-6846

00173
Allen & Hanburys
See Glaxo Wellcome

Allercreme
See Carme, Inc.

11980
Allergan America
2525 DuPont Drive
Irvine, CA 92715-9534
800-433-8871

00023
Allergan Inc.
2525 DuPont Drive
Irvine, CA 92715-9534
800-433-8871

00023
Allergan, Inc.
2525 DuPont Drive
Irvine, CA 92715-9534
800-433-8871

Allermed
7203 Convoy Ct.
San Diego, CA 92111
619-292-1060

Alliance Pharmaceuticals
3040 Science Park Road
San Diego, CA 92121
619-558-4300

54569
Allscrips
1033 Butterfield Road
Vernon Hills, IL 60061
708-680-3515

Alpha 1 Biomedicals, Inc.
6903 Rockledge Drive
Bethesda, MD 20817
301-564-4400

49669
Alpha Therapeutic Corp.
5555 Valley Blvd.
Los Angeles, CA 90032
213-225-2221

00472
Alpharma
333 Cassell Drive
Suite 3500
Baltimore, MD 21224
410-558-7250

Alpharma USPd
7205 Windsor Blvd.
Baltimore, MD 21244-2654
800-638-9096

51641
Alra Laboratories, Inc.
3850 Clearview Court
Gurnee, IL 60031
708-244-9440

Altana Incorporated
60 Baylis Road
Melville, NY 11747
516-454-7677

00731
Alto Pharmaceuticals, Inc.
P.O. Box 1910
Land O'Lakes, FL 34639-1910
813-949-7464

72959
Alva Laboratories
6625 Avondale Ave.
Chicago, IL 60631
312-792-0200

17314
Alza Corp.
950 Page Mill Road
Palo Alto, CA 94303-0802
415-494-5000

10038
Ambix Laboratories, Inc.
210 Orchard Street
East Rutherford, NJ 07073
201-939-2200

89709, 90605
Amcon Laboratories
40 N. Rock Hill Road
St. Louis, MO 63119
314-961-5758

Americal Pharmaceutical, Inc.
See Akorn, Inc.

51201
American Dermal Corp.
51 Apple Tree Lane
P.O. Box 900
Plumsteadville, PA 18949-0900
610-454-8000

57506
American Drug Industries, Inc.
5810 S. Perry Ave.
Chicago, IL 60621
312-667-7070

American Lecithin Company
115 Hurley Road, Unit 2B
Oxford, CT 06478
800-364-4416

00517
American Regent
1 Luitpold Drive
Shirley, NY 11967
516-924-4000

00539
American Urologicals, Inc.
7881 Hollywood Blvd.
Suite 4
Pembroke Pines, FL 33024
305-438-5070

55513
Amgen, Inc.
1840 Dehavilland Drive
Thousand Oaks, CA 91320-1789
805-499-5725

52152
Amide Pharmaceuticals, Inc.
101 E. Main Street
Little Falls, NJ 07424
201-890-1440

53926
Amsco Scientific
1002 Lufkin Road
P.O. Box 747
Apex, NC 27502
800-388-5155

Amswiss Scientific, Inc.
2170 Broadway
Suite 1200
New York, NY 10024

Anaquest
See Ohmeda Pharmaceuticals

Andrew Jergens
2535 Spring Grove
Cincinnati, OH 45214
513-421-1400

Andrulis Research Corp.
11800 Baltimore Ave.
Beltsville, MD 20705
301-419-2400

Anthra Pharmaceuticals, Inc.
19 Carson Road
Princeton, NJ 08540

Antibodies, Inc.
P.O. Box 1560
Davis, CA 95617
916-758-4400

48028
Aplicare Inc.
P.O. Box 237
Prichard, WV 25555
304-486-5656

Apotex Critical Care, Inc.
1776 Broadway
Suite 1900
New York, NY 10019
800-700-3092

Apothecary Products, Inc.
11531 Rupp Drive
Burnsville, MN 55337
612-890-1940

00003, 00015
Apothecon
P.O. Box 4500
Princeton, NJ 08543-4500
800-321-1335

48723
Apothecus, Inc.
20 Audrye Avenue
Oyster Bay, NY 11771
516-624-8200

Applied Biotech
10237 Flanders Ct.
San Diego, CA 92121
619-587-6771

Applied Genetics
205 Buffalo Ave.
Freeport, NY 11520
516-868-9026

Applied Medical Research
1600 Hayes Street
Nashville, TN 37203
615-327-0676

Approved Drug
See Health for Life Brands, Inc.

00275
Arco Pharmaceuticals, Inc.
90 Orville Drive
Bohemia, NY 11716
516-567-9500

00070
Arcola Laboratories
500 Arcola Road
Collegeville, PA 19426
610-454-8000

Argus Pharmaceuticals, Inc.
3400 Research Forest Drive
The Woodlands, TX 77381

Armour Pharmaceutical
See Centeon

48558
Arther, Inc.
P.O. Box 1455
W. Caldwell, NJ 07007
201-226-5288

61113
Astra Merck
725 Chesterbrook Blvd.
Wayne, PA 19087-5677
800-236-9933

00186
Astra USA, Inc.
50 Otis Street
Westborough, MA 01581
508-366-1100

59075
Athena Neurosciences, Inc.
800 Gateway Blvd.
South San Francisco, CA 94080
415-877-0900

59702
Atley Pharmaceuticals, Inc.
340 S. Richardson Road
Suite 1
Ashland, VA 23005
804-550-1979

Autoimmune, Inc.
128 Spring Street
Lexington, MA 02173
617-860-0710

Axion Pharmaceuticals
395 Oyster Point Blvd.
Suite 405
South San Francisco, CA 94080

00225
B. F. Ascher and Co.
15501 W. 109th St.
Lenexa, KS 66219
913-888-1880

44184
Bajamar Chemical, Inc.
9609 Dielman Rock Island
St. Louis, MO 63132
314-997-3414

58174
Baker Cummins
  Dermatologicals
50 Northwest 176 Street
Miami, FL 33169
800-842-6704

00575, 11414
Baker Norton Pharmaceuticals
8800 N.W. 36th Street
Miami, FL 33178-2404
305-590-2200

00304
J.J. Balan, Inc.
5725 Foster Ave.
Brooklyn, NY 11234
718-251-8663

00555
Barr Laboratories, Inc.
2 Quaker Road
Pomona, NY 01970
914-362-1100

10116
Bartor Pharmacal Co.
70 High Street
Rye, NY 10580
914-967-4219

58887
Basel Pharmaceuticals
See Novartis

10119
Bausch & Lomb Personal
  Products Division
1400 N. Goodman Street
P.O. Box 450
Rochester, NY 14692-0450
716-338-6000

24208, 57782
Bausch & Lomb
  Pharmaceuticals
8500 Hidden River Pkwy.
Tampa, FL 33637
813-975-7700

Baxter Healthcare
550 North Brand Blvd.
Glendale, CA 91203
818-956-3200

00944
Baxter Hyland
550 North Brand Blvd.
Glendale, CA 91203
818-956-3200

00118
Bayer Corp. (Allergy Div.)
P.O. Box 3145
Spokane, WA 99220
509-489-5656

00026, 00161, 00192
Bayer Corp. (Biological and
  Pharmaceutical Div.)
400 Morgan Lane
West Haven, CT 06516
203-937-2000

12843, 16500
Bayer Corp. (Consumer Div.)
P.O. Box 5967
Parsippany, NJ 07054
800-331-4536

00193
Bayer Corp. (Diagnostic Div.)
P.O. Box 3100
Elkhart, IN 46515-3100
800-248-2637

BDI Pharmaceuticals, Inc.
P.O. Box 78610
Indianapolis, IN 46278-0610
317-228-5008

00486
Beach Pharmaceuticals
P.O. Box 128
Conestee, SC 29636
803-277-7282

31280
Becton Dickinson & Co.
One Becton Drive
Franklin Lakes, NJ 07417-1881
201-847-6800

00011
Becton Dickinson Microbiology
  Systems
250 Schilling Circle
Cockeysville, MD 21031
410-771-0100

55390
Bedford Laboratories
300 Northfield Road
Bedford, OH 44146
216-232-3320

Behringwerke Aktiengesellschaft
500 Arcola Road
P.O. Box 1200
Collegeville, PA 19426-0107

10356
Beiersdorf, Inc.
P.O. Box 5529
S. Norwalk, CT 06856-5529
203-853-8008 956

50419
Berlex Laboratories, Inc.
300 Fairfield Road
Wayne, NJ 07470-2095
201-694-4100

58337
Berna Products Corp.
4216 Ponce De Leon Blvd.
Coral Gables, FL 33146
305-443-2900

Best Generics
See Goldline Laboratories, Inc.

00283
Beutlich, Inc.
1541 Shields Dr.
Waukegan, IL 60085
708-473-1100

Biocare International, Inc.
2643 Grand Avenue
Bellmore, NY 11710
516-781-5800

00332
Biocraft Laboratories, Inc.
See Teva Pharmaceuticals

Biocryst Pharmaceuticals, Inc.
2190 Parkway Lake Drive
Birmingham, AL 35244

59527
BioDevelopment Corp.
8180 Greensboro Drive
Suite 1000
McLean, VA 22102
703-506-0290

Biofilm, Inc.
3121 Scott Street
Vista, CA 92083-8323
619-727-9030

Biogen
14 Cambridge Center
Cambridge, MA 02142
617-679-2000

BioGenex Laboratories
4600 Norris Canyon Road
Suite 400
San Ramon, CA 94583
510-275-0550

Bioline Labs, Inc.
See Zenith Goldline

Biomedical Frontiers, Inc.
1095 10th Ave. S.E.
Minneapolis, MN 55414
612-378-0228

Biomerica, Inc.
1533 Monrovia Ave.
Newport Beach, CA 92663
714-645-2111

Biomune Systems, Inc.
40 East South Temple
Suite 310
Salt Lake City, UT 84111

Biopure Corp.
68 Harrison Ave.
Boston, MA 02111

52311
Biosearch Medical Products
P.O. Box 1700
Somerville, NJ 08876
908-722-5000

53191
Bio-Tech
P.O. Box 1992
Fayetteville, AR 72702
501-443-9148

Bio-Technology General Corp.
70 Wood Ave. South
Iselin, NJ 08830
908-632-8800

BIRA Corp.
2525 Quicksilver
McDonald, PA 15057
412-796-1820

50289
Birchwood Laboratories, Inc.
7900 Fuller Road
Eden Prairie, MN 53344
800-328-6156

12136
Bird Corp.
1100 Bird Center Drive
Palm Springs, CA 92262
619-778-7200

00165
Blaine, Inc.
1465 Jamike Lane
Erlanger, KY 41018-1878
606-283-9437

00154
Blair Laboratories
100 Connecticut Ave.
Norwalk, CT 06850-3590
203-853-0123

50486
Blairex Labs, Inc.
P.O. Box 2127
Columbus, IN 47202-2127
812-378-1864

10157
Blistex, Inc.
1800 Swift Drive
Oak Brook, IL 60521
708-571-2870

10158
Block Drug, Inc.
257 Cornelison Ave.
Jersey City, NJ 07302
201-434-3000

10160
Bluco Inc./Med. Discnt. Outlet
14849 W. McNichols
Detroit, MI 48235
313-273-0322

00563
Bock Pharmacal Co.
P.O. Box 419056
St. Louis, MO 63141-9056
314-579-0770

00597
Boehringer Ingelheim, Inc.
900 Ridgebury Road
Ridgefield, CT 06877
203-798-9988

53169
**Boehringer Mannheim
 Corp.**
101 Orchard Ridge Drive
Gaithersburg, MD 20878
800-621-3784

50924
Boehringer Mannheim Diags.
9115 Hague Road
P.O. Box 50100
Indianapolis, IN 46250-0100
800-428-5074

44437
Bolan Pharmaceutical, Inc.
P.O. Box 230
Hurst, TX 76053
817-268-6110

Boots Pharmaceuticals, Inc.
See Knoll Laboratories

00222
Boyle and Co. Pharm.
1613 Chelsea Rd.
San Marino, CA 91108
818-441-0284

00003
Bracco Diagnostics
P.O. Box 5225
Princeton, NJ 08543
609-897-4200

Bradley Pharmaceutical
See Kenwood Laboratories

52268
Braintree Laboratories, Inc.
60 Columbian
P.O. Box 361
Braintree, MA 02184
617-843-2202

51991
Breckenridge Pharmaceutical, Inc.
P.O. Box 206
Boca Raton, FL 33429
407-367-8512

72363
Brimms, Inc.
425 Fillmore Ave.
Tonawanda, NY 14150
716-694-7100

Bristol Laboratories
See Bristol-Myers Squibb

Bristol-Myers Oncology
P.O. Box 4500
Princeton, NJ 08543
609-897-2000

19810
Bristol-Myers Products
345 Park Ave. 4th Floor
New York, NY 10154
800-468-7746

00003, 00087
Bristol-Myers Squibb
P.O. Box 4000
Princeton, NJ 08543-4000
609-252-4000

Britannia Pharmaceuticals
Forum Hs Brighton Road Redhill
Surrey, UK RH 1 6YS

Burroughs Wellcome Co.
See GlaxoWellcome

00398
C & M Pharmacal, Inc.
1721 Maple Lane
Hazel Park, MI 48030-1215
313-548-7846

00132
C. B. Fleet, Inc.
4615 Murray Place
Lynchburg, VA 24506
804-528-4000

00463
C. O. Truxton, Inc.
P.O. Box 1594
Camden, NJ 08101
609-365-4118

10486
C. S. Dent & Co. Division
317 E. Eighth Street
Cincinnati, OH 45202
513-241-1677

55559
Calgon Vestal Laboratories
P.O. Box 147
St. Louis, MO 63166-0147
314-535-1810

**California Department
   Health Service**
2151 Berkeley Way
Berkeley, CA 94704

00147
Camall, Inc.
P.O. Box 307
Romeo, MI 48065-0307
313-752-9683

Cambridge Neuroscience, Inc.
1 Kendall Square
Building 700
Cambridge, MA 02139
617-225-0600

38083
Campbell Laboratories
P.O. Box 639
Deerfield Beach, FL 33443
305-570-9834

Can-Am Care Corp.
Cimetra Industrial Park
Chazy, NY 12921
800-461-7448

Cangene Corp.
104 Chancellor Matheson Road
Winnipeg, R3T 2N2
204-989-6850

Capmed USA
P.O. Box 14
Bryn Mawr, PA 19010

59046
Caprice-Greystoke
1259 Activity Drive
Vista, CA 92083
619-598-9300

57664
Caraco Pharmaceutical Labs
1150 Elijah McCoy Drive
Detroit, MI 48202
313-871-8400

Care Technologies, Inc.
55 Holly Hill Lane
Greenwich, CT 06830

Carme, Inc.
84 Galli
Novato, CA 94949
415-382-4000

Carnation
800 North Brand Blvd.
Glendale, CA 91203
800-628-2229

00086
Carnrick Laboratories, Inc.
65 Horse Hill Road
Cedar Knolls, NJ 07927
201-267-2670

46287
Carolina Medical Products
P.O. Box 147
Farmville, NC 27828
919-753-7111

Carrington Labs
1300 E. Rochelle Blvd.
Irving, TX 75062
214-518-1300

00164
Carter Products
Half Acre Road
P.O. Box 1001
Cranbury, NJ 08512-0181
609-655-6000

Cavitation-Control Technology
55 Knollwood Road
Farmington, CT 06032
203-673-0507

Celgene Corp.
7 Powder Horn Drive
Warren, NJ 07059
908-271-1001

Cell Pathways, Inc.
1700 Broadway
Suite 2000
Denver, CO 80290

Cell Technology
1668 Valtec Lane
Boulder, CO 80301
303-790-0587

Cellegy Pharmaceuticals, Inc.
371 Bel Marin Keys
Suite 210
Novato, CA 94949

Celtrix Pharmaceuticals, Inc.
3055 Patrick Henry Drive
Santa Clara, CA 95054

00053
Centeon
1020 First Avenue
King of Prussia, PA 19406-1310
800-683-1288

00268
Center Laboratories
35 Channel Drive
Port Washington, NY 11050
516-767-1800

Centers for Disease Control
1600 Clifton Road
Mail Stop D-09
Atlanta, GA 30333
404-639-3670

Centocor, Inc.
200 Great Valley Pkwy.
Malvern, PA 19355
610-651-6000

00131
Central Pharmaceuticals, Inc.
See Schwarz Pharma

00436
Century Pharmaceuticals, Inc.
10377 Hague Road
Indianapolis, IN 46256-3399
317-849-4210

Cephalon, Inc.
145 Brandywine Pkwy.
West Chester, PA 19380
215-344-0200

00173
Cerenex Pharmaceuticals
See Glaxo Wellcome

10223
Cetylite Industries, Inc.
9051 River Road
P.O. Box 90006
Pennsauken, NJ 08110
609-665-6111

54429
Chase Laboratories
280 Chestnut Street
Newark, NJ 07105-1598
201-589-8181

49447
Chattem Consumer Products
1715 W. 38th Street
Chattanooga, TN 37409
615-821-4571

Chembiomed, Ltd.
P.O. Box 8050
Edmonton, AB T6H4NP

52489
Chemi-Tech Laboratories
74-80 Marine Street
Farmingdale, NY 11735

00521
Chesebrough-Pond's, USA
33 Benedict Place
Greenwich, CT 06830
203-661-2000

Chiesi Pharmaceuticals, Inc.
150 Danbury Road
Ridgefield, CT 06877

53905
Chiron Therapeutics
4560 Horton Street
Emeryville, CA 94608
800-244-7668

Chiron Vision
500 Iolab Drive
Claremont, CA 91711
909-624-2020

Chugai-Upjohn, Inc.
6133 North River Road
Suite 800
Rosemont, IL 60018

00067, 00083
Ciba Self-Medication, Inc.
See Novartis

00346
Ciba Vision Ophthalmics
11460 Johns Creek Pkwy.
Duluth, GA 30136
404-418-4101

00083
Ciba-Geigy Pharmaceuticals
See Novartis

00677, 00725, 71114
Circa Pharmaceuticals, Inc.
33 Ralph Ave.
Copiague, NY 11726-0030
516-842-8383

00659
Circle Pharmaceuticals, Inc.
6320 B Rucker Road
Indianapolis, IN 46220
317-475-1921

City Chemical Corp.
132 W. 22nd Street
New York, NY 10011
201-653-6900

45802
Clay-Park Labs, Inc.
1700 Bathgate Ave.
Bronyx, NY 10457
212-901-2800

Clintec Nutrition
Three Pkwy. North
Suite 500
Deerfield, IL 60015
708-317-2800

Cocensys, Inc.
213 Technology Drive
Irvine, CA 92718
714-453-0131

Colgate Oral Pharmaceuticals
1 Colgate Way
Canton, MA 02021
617-821-2880

Collagen Corp.
2500 Faber Place
Palo Alto, CA 94303
415-856-0200

00837, 21406
Columbia Laboratories, Inc.
2665 South Bayshore Drive
Miami, FL 33133
305-860-1670

11509
Combe, Inc.
1101 Westchester Ave.
White Plains, NY 10604
914-694-5454

11793, 49281, 50361
Connaught Labs
See Pasteur-Mérieux-Connaught

00223
Consolidated Midland Corp.
20 Main St.
Brewster, NY 10509
914-279-6108

34044
Continental Consumer
  Products
770 Forest
Suite B
Birmingham, MI 48009
800-542-5903

33130
Continental Quest Research
220 W. Carmel Drive
Carmel, IN 46032
800-451-5773

00003
ConvaTec
P.O. Box 5254
Princeton, NJ 08543-5254
908-359-9200

00961
Cook-Waite Laboratories, Inc.
90 Park Ave.
New York, NY 10016
212-907-2000

Cooper Biomedical, Inc.
One Technology Court
Malvern, PA 19355
215-219-6300

Cooper Development Co.
455 East Middlefield Road
Mountain View, CA 94043
415-969-9030

59426
CooperVision
10 Faraday
Irvine, CA 92618
714-597-8130

38245
Copley Pharmaceutical, Inc.
25 John Road
Canton, MA 02021
617-821-6111

Cord Labs
See Geneva Pharmaceuticals

Coulter Corp.
11800 S.W. 147 Ave.
P.O. Box 169015
Miami, FL 33116
305-380-3800

50752
Creighton Products Corp.
59 Route 10
East Hanover, NJ 07936-1080
201-503-6099

CTRC Research Foundation
11812 Becket Street
Potomac, MD 20854

01020
Cumberland Packing Corp.
35 Old Ridgefield Road
P.O. Box 7688
Willton, CT 06897
203-762-7227

55326
Curatek Pharmaceuticals
See 3M Pharmaceuticals

Cutter Biologicals
See Bayer Corp. (Biological and
  Pharmaceutical Div.)

Cyclin Pharmaceuticals Inc.
429 Gammon Place
Madison, Wi 53715
608-833-8462

54799
Cynacon/OCuSOFT
P.O. Box 429
Richmond, TX 77406-0429
800-233-5469

Cytel Corp.
3525 John Hopkins Court
San Diego, CA 92121
619-552-3000

Cytogen
600 College Road East
Princeton, NJ 08540
609-987-8200

23731
Cytosol Laboratories
55 Messina Drive
Braintree, MA 02184

CytRx
150 Technology Pkwy.
Norcross, GA 30092
404-368-9500

55994
Dakryon Pharmaceuticals
2579 S. Loop
Suite 8
Lubbock, TX 79423-1400
806-745-2872

55425
Dal-Med Pharmaceuticals
5701 N. Pine Island Road
Tamarac, Fl 33321
800-543-9151

Danbury Pharmacal
See Schein Pharmaceutical, Inc.

00689
Daniels Pharmaceuticals, Inc.
See Jones Medical

Dapat Pharmaceuticals, Inc.
5040 Linbar Drive,
Suite 102
Nashville, TN 37211
615-833-2616

Darby Pharmaceuticals, Inc.
100 Banks Ave.
Rockville Centre, NY 11570

58869
Dartmouth Pharmaceuticals
19 Whaler's Way
North Dartmouth, MA 02747
508-636-5553

00938
Davis and Geck
One Cyanamid Plaza
Wayne, NJ 07470
201-831-2000

52041
Dayton Laboratories, Inc.
3307 NW 74th Ave.
Miami, FL 33122
305-594-0988

00744
Daywell Laboratories Corp.
78 Unquowa Place
Fairfield, CT 06430
203-255-3154

Degussa Corp.
65 Challenger Road
Ridgefield Park, NJ 07660
201-641-6100

10310
Del Pharmaceuticals, Inc.
163 East Bethpage
Plainview, NY 11803
516-293-7070

48532
Delmont Laboratories, Inc.
P.O. Box 269
Swarthmore, PA 19081
215-543-3365

00316
Del-Ray Laboratory, Inc.
22 20th Ave. N.W.
Birmingham, AL 35215
205-853-8247

00295
Denison Laboratories, Inc.
60 Dunnell Lane
P.O. Box 1305
Pawtucket, RI 02862
401-723-5500

00066
Dermik Laboratories, Inc.
500 Arcola Road
P.O. Box 1200
Collegeville, PA 19426
610-454-8000

50744
Dermol Pharmaceuticals, Inc.
3807 Roswell Road
Marietta, GA 30062
404-977-7779

49502
Dey Laboratories, Inc.
2751 Napa Valley Corporate Dr.
Napa, CA 94558
707-224-3200

**Discovery Experimental &
Development, Inc.**
29949 SR 54 West
Wesley Chapel, FL 33543
813-973-7200

00777
Dista Products Co.
Lilly Corp. Center
Indianapolis, IN 46285
317-276-4000

10337
Doak Dermatologics
383 Route 46 West
Fairfield, NJ 07004-2402
201-882-1505

25358
Donell DerMedex
342 Madison Ave.
Suite 1422
New York, NY 10173
212-697-3800

00514
Dow B. Hickam, Inc.
P.O. Box 2006
Sugarland, TX 77487
713-240-1000

13723
Dr. Nordyke Footcare Products
1650 Palma Drive
Suite 102
Ventura, CA 93003
805-650-8333

00094
Du Pont Merck Pharmaceutical
4301 Lancaster Pike
Wilmington, DE 19805
302-892-7050

00056, 00590
Du Pont Pharma
P.O. Box 800723
Wilmington, DE 19880
800-474-2762

00217
Dunhall Pharmaceuticals, Inc.
P.O. Box 100
Gravette, AR 72736
501-787-5232

51479
Dura Pharmaceuticals
5880 Pacific Center Blvd.
San Diego, CA 92121-4202
619-457-2553

51285
Duramed Pharmaceuticals
5040 Lester Road
Cincinnati, OH 45213
513-731-9900

55516
Dyna Pharm, Inc.
P.O. Box 2141
Del Mar, CA 92014-2141
619-792-9523

10331
E. E. Dickinson Co.
2 Enterprise Drive
Shelton, CT 06484
203-929-1197

00168
E. Fougera and Co.
60 Baylis Road
Melville, NY 11747
516-454-6996

Eagle Vision, Inc.
6263 Poplar Ave.
Suite 650
Memphis, TN 38119
901-767-3937

Eastman Kodak Co.
10 Indigo Creek Drive
Rochester, NY 14650-0862
800-526-8811

Eaton Medical Corp.
2288 Dunn Ave.
Memphis, TN 38114
901-744-8024

19458
Eckerd Drug Co.
P.O. Box 4689
Clearwater, FL 34618
813-397-7461

38130
Econo Med Pharmaceuticals
4305 Sartin Road
Burlington, NC 27217-7522
919-226-1091

00095, 59010
ECR Pharmaceuticals
3981 Deep Rock Road
Richmond, VA 23233
804-527-1950

00485
Edwards Pharmaceuticals, Inc.
111 Mulberry Street
Ripley, MS 38663
601-837-8182

55806
Effcon Labs, Inc.
1800 Sandy Plains Pkwy.
Marietta, GA 30066
404-428-7011

Elan Corp.
1300 Gould Drive
Gainesville, GA 30504
404-534-8239

Elder
See Zeneca

00002, 59075
Eli Lilly and Co.
Lilly Corp. Center
Indianapolis, IN 46285
317-276-2000

00641
Elkins-Sinn, Inc.
See Wyeth Ayerst

EM Industries, Inc.
5 Skyline Drive
Hawthorne, NY 10532
914-592-4660

60951
Endo Laboratories
P.O. Box 80390
Wilmington, DE 19880
800-462-4467

57665
Enzon, Inc.
40 Kingsbridge Road
Piscataway, NJ 08854-3998
908-980-4500

00185, 00536
Eon Labs Manufacturing, Inc.
227-15 North Conduit Ave.
Laurelton, NY 11413
718-276-8600

Epitope Inc.
8505 SW Creekside Place
Beaverton, OR 97008
503-641-6115

E.R. Squibb & Sons, Inc.
See Bristol-Myers Squibb

Escalon Ophthalmics, Inc.
182 Tamarack Circle
Skillman, NJ 08558
609-497-9141

00005, 59911
ESI Lederle Generics
P.O. Box 8299
Philadelphia, PA 19101
610-688-4400

58177
Ethex Corp.
10888 Metro Court
St. Louis, MO 63043-2413
314-567-3307

Ethicon, Inc.
Route 22 West
P.O. Box 151
Somerville, NJ 08876-0151
908-218-0707

54686
Ethitek Pharmaceuticals
7701 North Austin
Skokie, IL 60077
708-675-6611

00642
Everett Laboratories, Inc.
71 Glenwood Place
East Orange, NJ 07017
201-674-8455

Evreka
600 Montgomery Street
San Francisco, CA 94111
415-627-2040

Falcon Ophthalmics, Inc.
6201 S. Freeway
Fort Worth, TX 76134
800-343-2133

Farmacon, Inc.
90 Grove Street
Suite 109
Ridgefield, CT 06877-4118
203-431-9989

99766
Faulding USA
200 Elmora Ave.
Elizabeth, NJ 07207
800-526-6978

00496
Ferndale Laboratories, Inc.
780 W. Eight Mile Road
Ferndale, MI 48220-1218
313-548-0900

55566
Ferring Laboratories, Inc.
400 Rella Blvd.
Suite 201
Suffern, NY 10901
914-368-7900

31795
Fibertone Co.
14851 N. Scottsdale Road
Scottsdale, AZ 85254
800-462-7596

00729
Fidelity Halsom
1330 Farr Drive at Stanley
Dayton, OH 45404
800-356-3065

Fidia Pharmaceutical
1401 I Street N.W.
Washington, DC 20005
202-371-9898

00421
Fielding Co.
94 Weldon Pkwy.
Maryland Heights, MO 63043
314-567-5462

51687
Fischer Pharmaceuticals, Inc.
165 Gibraltar Court
Sunnyvale, CA 94089
408-747-1760

Fiske Industries
339 N. Main Street
New City, NY 10956
914-634-5099

Fisons Consumer Health
See Ciba Self-Medication, Inc.

00585
Fisons Corp.
See Medeva Pharmaceuticals

54323
Flanders, Inc.
P.O. Box 39143
Charleston, SC 29407-9143
803-571-3363

00256
Fleming & Co.
1600 Fenpark Drive
Fenton, MO 63026-2918
314-343-8200

00288
Fluoritab Corp.
P.O. Box 507
Temperance, MI 48182-0507
313-847-3985

00258, 00456, 00535, 00785
Forest Pharmaceutical, Inc.
13622 Lakefront Drive
St. Louis, MO 63045
314-344-8870

00494
Foy Laboratories
906 Penn Ave.
Wyomissing, PA 19610
215-678-9460

Free Radical Sciences, Inc.
245 First Street
Cambridge, MA 02142
617-374-1200

10432
Freeda Vitamins, Inc.
36 E. 41st Street
New York, NY 10017-6203
212-685-4980

Fuisz Technologies, Ltd.
3810 Concorde Pkwy.
Suite 100
Chantilly, VA 22021
703-803-3260

00469, 57317
Fujisawa USA, Inc.
3 Parkway North Center
Deerfield, IL 60015-2548
708-317-0600

00713
G & W Laboratories
111 Coolidge Street
South Plainfield, NJ 07080
908-753-2000

Galagen, Inc.
4001 Lexington Ave. North
Arden Hills, MN 55126-2998
612-481-2105

00299
Galderma Laboratories, Inc.
P.O. Box 331329
Ft. Worth, TX 76163
817-263-2600

00254
Gambro, Inc.
1185 Oak Street
Lakewood, CO 80215
800-525-2623

57844
Gate Pharmaceuticals
650 Cathill Road
Sellersville, PA 18960
800-292-4283

00386
Gebauer Co.
9410 St. Catherine Ave.
Cleveland, OH 44104
216-271-5252

00028
Geigy Pharmaceuticals
See Novartis

Gencon
6116 N. Central Expy. 200
Dallas, TX 75206
214-373-4665

52761
GenDerm Corp.
600 Knightsbridge Pkwy.
Lincolnshire, IL 60069-3657
708-634-7373

50242
Genentech, Inc.
460 Point San Bruno Blvd.
South San Francisco, CA 94080
415-225-1000

50272
General Generics, Inc.
P.O. Box 510
Oxford, MS 38655
601-234-0130

52584
General Injectables & Vaccines
U.S. Hwy. 52
Bastian, VA 24314
703-688-4121

00918
General Medical Corp.
8741 Landmark Road
Richmond, VA 23261
804-264-7500

Genetic Therapy, Inc.
938 Copper Road
Gaithersburg, MD 20878
301-590-2626

00781
Geneva Pharmaceuticals
2599 W. Midway Blvd.
P.O. Box 469
Broomfield, CO 80038-0469
800-525-8747

Gen-King
See Kinray

00703
Gensia Laboratories, LTD.
19 Hughes
Irvine, CA 92718-1902
800-331-0124

58468
Genzyme Corp.
One Kendall Square
Cambridge, MA 02139
617-252-7500

Geriatric Pharmaceutical Corp.
See Roberts Pharmaceuticals

Gilead Sciences, Inc.
353 Lakeside Drive
Forsten City, CA 94404

59366
Glades Pharmaceuticals
255 Alhambra Center
Suite 1000
Coral Gables, FL 33134
800-452-3371

00081, 00173
GlaxoWellcome
Five Moore Drive
Research Triangle Pk., NC 27709
919-248-2100

00516
Glenwood, Inc.
83 N. Summit Street
Tenafly, NJ 07670
201-569-0050

Global Source
3001 N. 29th Ave.
Hollywood, FL 33020
305-921-0006

Glycomed, Inc.
860 Atlantic Ave.
Alameda, CA 94501
510-523-5555

00182
Goldline Laboratories, Inc.
See Zenith Goldline Pharmaceuticals

74684
Goody's Manufacturing Corp.
436 Salt Street
Winston Salem, NC 27108
910-723-1831

10481
Gordon Laboratories
6801 Ludlow Street
Upper Darby, PA 19082-1694
215-734-2011

12165
Graham Field
400 Rabro Drive East
Hauppauge, NY 11788
516-582-5900

00152
Gray Pharmaceutical Co.
100 Connecticut Ave.
Norwalk, CT 06856
203-853-0123

51301
Great Southern Laboratories
10863 Rockley Road
Houston, TX 77099
713-530-3077

Green Turtle Bay Vitamin Co.
P.O. Box 642
Summit, NJ 07902
908-277-2240

8225
Greenstone
Moors Bridge Road
Portage, MI 49002
800-447-3360

22840
Greer Laboratories, Inc.
P.O. Box 800
Lenoir, NC 28645-0800
704-754-5327

00327
Guardian Laboratories
230 Marcus Blvd.
Hauppauge, NY 11788
516-273-0900

54396
Gynex Pharmaceuticals, Inc.
1175 Corporate Woods Pkwy.
Vernon Hills, IL 60061
708-913-1144

54765
GynoPharma Laboratories
50 Division Street
Somerville, NJ 08876
908-725-3100

00879
Halsey Drug Co.
1827 Pacific Street
Brooklyn, NY 11233
718-467-7500

**Hannan Ophthalmic Marketing
  Services, Inc.**
163 Meetinghouse Road
Duxbury, MA 02332

51432
Harber Pharmaceutical Co.
350 Meadowlands Pkwy.
Secaucus, NJ 07094
201-348-3700

HDC Corporation
2109 O'Toole Ave.
San Jose, CA 95131
408-954-1909

Health & Medical Techniques
See Graham Field

50383
Health Care Products
369 Bayview Ave.
Amityville, NY 11701
516-789-8455

00598
Health for Life Brands, Inc.
1643 E. Genesee Street
Syracuse, NY 13210
315-478-6303

51662
Healthfirst Corp.
22316 70th Ave. W.
Mountlake Terrace, WA 98043
206-771-5733

59512
Healthline Laboratories, Inc.
835 Potts Ave.
Green Bay, WI 54304
414-497-3322

00586
Heather Drug, Inc.
1 Fellowship Road
Cherry Hill, NJ 08003
609-424-3663

Helena Laboratories
P.O. Box 752
Beaumont, TX 77704-0752
409-842-3714

HEM Research
1617 John F. Kennedy Blvd.
Philadelphia, PA 19103
215-988-0080

Hemacare Corp.
4954 Van Nuys Blvd.
Sherman Oaks, CA 91403
818-986-3883

Herald Pharmacal Inc.
6503 Warwick Rd.
Richmond, VA 23225
804-524-3112

Herbert Laboratories
See Allergan Inc.

48017
Hermal Pharmaceutical Labs
163 Delaware Ave.
Delmar, NY 12054
518-475-0175

28105
Hill Dermaceuticals, Inc.
P.O. Box 149283
Orlando, FL 32814-9283
407-896-8280

17808
Himmel Pharmaceuticals, Inc.
P.O. Box 5479
Lake Worth, FL 33466-5479
407-585-0070

50673
Hirsch Industries, Inc.
4912 West Broad Street
Richmond, VA 23230-0964
804-355-4500

Hiscia
CH-4144, Arlesheim Kirshweg
Switzerland
4106172-2323

00839
H.L. Moore Drug Exchange, Inc.
389 John Downey Drive
New Britain, CT 06050
203-826-3600

00039, 00068, 00088
Hoechst-Marion Roussel
P.O. Box 9627
Kansas City, MO 64134
908-231-2000

58573
Hogil Pharmaceutical Corp.
1 Byram Brook Place
Armonk, NY 10504
914-273-9666

47992
Holles Laboratories, Inc.
30 Forest Notch
Cohasset, MA 02025-1198
617-383-0741

Hollister-Stier
See Bayer Corp. (Allergy Div.)

Home Diagnostics, Inc. (HDI)
51 James Way
Eatontown, NJ 07724
908-542-7788

Hope Pharmaceuticals
2961 W. MacArthur Blvd.
Santa Ana, CA 92704
714-556-4673

59630
Horizon Pharmaceutical Corp.
1125 Northmeadow Pkwy.
Roswell, GA 30076
404-442-9707

59229
Horus Therapeutics, Inc.
2320 Brighton-Henrietta Town
Rochester, NY 14623
716-292-4820

00196
Houba, Inc.
P.O. Box 190
Culver, IN 46511
219-842-3305

00556
H.R. Cenci Labs, Inc.
1420 E. Street
P.O. Box 12524
Fresno, CA 93778-2524
209-237-3346

58407
Huckaby Pharmacal, Inc.
104 E. Main Street
LaGrange, KY 40031
502-222-4700

25077
Hudson Corp.
90 Orville Drive
Bohemia, NY 11716
516-567-9500

00395
Humco Holding Group, Inc.
P.O. Box 2550
Texarkana, TX 75504
903-793-3174

Hybritech
P.O. Box 269006
San Diego, CA 92196-9006
619-455-6700

Hyland Therapeutics
See Baxter Hyland

Hynson, Westcott & Dunning
See Becton Dickinson Microbiology
Systems

00314
Hyrex Pharmaceuticals
P.O. Box 18385
Memphis, TN 38181-0385
901-794-9050

Iatric Corp.
2330 S. Industrial Park Drive
Tempe, AZ 85282-1893
602-966-7248

ICI Pharmaceuticals
See Zeneca Pharmaceuticals

00163, 00187
ICN Pharmaceuticals, Inc.
See Zeneca Pharmaceuticals

51244
I.C.P. Pharmaceuticals
P.O. Box 294
Cudahy, WI 53110
414-521-4647

IDEC Pharmaceuticals
11099 N. Torrey Pines Road #160
La Jolla, CA 92037
619-458-0600

Immucell Corp.
56 Evergreen Drive
Portland, ME 04103
207-878-2770

00205, 58406
Immunex Corp.
51 University Street
Seattle, WA 98101
206-587-0430

Immuno Clinical Research Corp.
155 East 56th Street
New York, NY 10022
212-759-3521

54129
Immuno U.S., Inc.
1200 Parkdale Road
Rochester, MI 48307-1744
313-652-7872

Immunobiology Research Inst.
Route 22 East
P.O. Box 999
Annandale, NJ 08801-0999
908-730-1700

ImmunoGen
148 Sidney Street
Cambridge, MA 02139
617-661-9312

Immunomedics
300 American Road
Morris Plains, NJ 07950
201-605-8200

Immunotherapeutics
3505 Riverview Circle
Morehead, MN 56560
701-232-9575

Imreg
144 Elk Place
Suite 1400
New Orleans, LA 70112
504-523-2875

00548
I.M.S., Ltd.
1886 Santa Anita Ave.
South El Monte, CA 91733
818-913-4660

Infusaid, Inc.
1400 Providence Highway
Norwood, MA 02062
617-769-8330

18686
InnoVisions, Inc.
6065 Frantz Road
Suite 202
Dublin, OH 43017
614-766-5477

Interchem Corp.
120 Route 17 North
Suite 115
Paramus, NJ 07652

Interfalk U.S., Inc.
25 Margaret
Plattsburgh, NY 12901

Interferon Sciences
783 Jersey Ave.
New Brunswick, NJ 08901
908-249-3250

11584
International Ethical Labs
Reparto Metropolitano
Rio Piedras, PR 00921
809-765-3510

00665
International Laboratories
901 Sawyer Road
Marietta, GA 30062
404-578-5583

Interneuron Pharmaceuticals
1 Ledgemont Center
99 Hayden Ave.
Lexington, MA 02173
617-861-8444

Interpro
P.O. Box 1823
Haverhill, MA 01831
508-373-2438

00814
Interstate Drug Exchange
1500 New Horizons Blvd.
Amityville, NY 11701-1130
516-957-8300

Intramed
102 Tremont Way
Augusta, GA 30907

52189
Invamed, Inc.
2400 Route 130N
Dayton, NJ 08810
908-274-1040

Inveresk Research
4470 Redwood Hwy.
San Rafael, CA 94903
415-491-6460

00258
Inwood Laboratories
300 Prospect Street
Inwood, NY 11696
516-371-1155

Iolab Pharmaceuticals
See Ciba Vision Ophthalmics

61646
Iomed
7425 Pebble Drive
Fort Worth, TX 76118
817-589-7257

11808
ION Laboratories, Inc.
7431 Pebble Drive
Ft. Worth, TX 76118
817-589-7257

IOP, Inc.
3100 Airway Ave.
Suite 106
Costa Mesa, CA 92626
714-549-1185

54921
IPR Pharmaceuticals, Inc.
P.O. Box 6000
Carolina, PR 00984
800-477-6385

50914
Iso Tex Diagnostics, Inc.
P.O. Box 909
Friendswood, TX 77546
713-482-1231

16837
J & J Merck Consumer Pharm.
Camp Hill Road
Ft. Washington, PA 19034
215-233-7000

88395
J. R. Carlson Laboratories
15 College Drive
Arlington Heights, IL 60004-1985
708-255-1600

49938
Jacobus Pharmaceutical Co.
37 Cleveland Lane
Princeton, NJ 08540
609-921-7447

50458
Janssen Pharmaceutical, Inc.
P.O. Box 200
Titusville, NJ 08560-0200
609-730-2000

JMI-Canton Pharmaceuticals
See Jones Medical Industries

00137
Johnson & Johnson
Grandview Road
Skillman, NJ 08558-9418
908-524-0400

56091
Johnson & Johnson Medical
P.O. Box 130
Arlington, TX 76004-0130
800-433-5009

00252, 52604, 00689, 12463
Jones Medical Industries
P.O. Box 46903
St. Louis, MO 63146-6903
314-576-6100

10106
J.T. Baker, Inc.
See Mallinckrodt-Baker

KabiVitrum, Inc.
See Pharmacia & Upjohn

Kanetta
90 Park Ave.
New York, NY 10016
212-907-2690

00588
Keene Pharmaceuticals, Inc.
P.O. Box 7
Keene, TX 76059-0007
817-645-8083

28851
Kendall Health Care Products
15 Hampshire Street
Mansfield, MA 02048
508-261-8000

Kendall-McGaw Labs, Inc.
See McGaw, Inc.

00482
Kenwood Laboratories
383 Rt. 46 W.
Fairfield, NJ 07006-2402
201-882-1505

00085
Key Pharmaceuticals
2000 Galloping Hill Road
Kenilworth, NJ 07033
908-298-4000

60793
King Pharmaceuticals Inc.
501 Fifth Street
Bristol, TN 37620
615-989-6232

55299
Kingswood Laboratories, Inc.
10375 Hague Road
Indianapolis, IN 46256
317-849-9513

Kinray
152-35 10th Ave.
Whitestone, NY 11357
718-767-1234

58223
Kirkman Sales, Inc.
P.O. Box 1009
Wilsonville, OR 97070-1009
503-694-1600

31600
Kiwi Brands, Inc.
447 Old Swede Road
Douglassville, PA 19518-1239
215-385-9322

KLI Corp.
1119 Third Ave. S.W.
Carmel, IN 46032
317-846-7452

00044, 00048, 00524
Knoll Laboratories
3000 Continental Drive North
Mt. Olive, NJ 07828-1234
201-426-2600

00044, 00048, 00524
Knoll Pharmaceuticals
3000 Continental Drive North
Mt. Olive, NJ 07828-1234
201-331-7633

Kodak Dental
343 State Street
Rochester, NY 14650

00224
Konsyl Pharmaceuticals
4200 South Hulen
Suite 513
Ft. Worth, TX 76109
817-763-8011

55505
Kramer Laboratories, Inc.
8778 S.W. 8th Street
Miami, FL 33174-9990
305-223-1287

La Haye Laboratories, Inc.
2205 152nd Ave. N.E.
Redmond, WA 98052
206-644-2020

Lacrimedics, Inc.
9008 Newby St.
Rosemead, CA 91770

41383
Lactaid, Inc.
7050 Camp Hill Road
Ft. Washington, PA 19034
215-233-7000

59081
Lafayette Pharmaceuticals, Inc.
P.O. Box 4499
Lafayette, IN 47903-4499
317-447-3129

Lake Pharmaceutical, Inc.
625 Forest Edge Dr.
Vernon Hills, IL 60061
708-793-0230

00527
Lannett, Inc.
9000 State Road
Philadelphia, PA 19136
215-333-9000

00277
Laser, Inc.
2200 W. 97th Place
P.O. Box 905
Crown Point, IN 46307
219-663-1165

10651
Lavoptik, Inc.
661 Western Ave.
St. Paul, MN 55103
612-489-1351

00005
Lederle Laboratories
North Middletown Road
Pearl River, NY 10965-1299
914-732-5000

53124
Lederle-Praxis Biologicals
North Middletown Road
Pearl River, NY 10965
914-272-7000

23558
Lee Pharmaceuticals
1444 Santa Anita Blvd.
South Elmonte, CA 91733
800-950-5337

Leeming
See Pfizer US Pharmaceutical Group

25332
Legere Pharmaceuticals, Inc.
7326 E. Evans Road
Scottsdale, AZ 85260
602-991-4033

19200
Lehn & Fink
See Reckitt & Coleman

Leiner Health Products
1845 W. 205th Street
Torrance, CA 90501
310-835-8400

Leiras Pharmaceuticals, Inc.
2345 Waukegan Road
Suite N-135
Bonnockburn, IL 60015

00093, 00332
Lemmon Co.
See Teva Pharmaceuticals

Lenti-Chemico Pharmaceuticals
500 Frank W. Burr Blvd.
Teaneck, NJ 07666
201-836-1196

00454
Lexis Laboratories
P.O. Box 202887
Austin, TX 78720
512-328-8484

Lifescan
1000 Gibraltar
Milpitas, CA 95035-6312
408-263-9789

Ligand Pharmaceuticals, Inc.
9393 Towne Centre Drive
San Diego, CA 92121
619-535-3900

00002, 59075
Eli Lilly and Co.
Lilly Corp. Center
Indianapolis, IN 46285
317-276-2000

Lincoln Diagnostics
P.O. Box 1128
Decatur, IL 62525
217-877-2531

60799
Liposome Co.
One Research Way
Princeton, NJ 08540
609-452-7060

54198
Liquipharm
10716 McCune Avenue
Los Angeles, Ca 90034
310-558-3344

Loch Pharmaceuticals
See Bedford Laboratories

00273
Lorvic Corp.
See Young Dental

59417
Lotus Biochemical
7335 Lee Highway
P.O. Box 3586
Radford, VA 24143-3586
703-633-3500

LTR Pharmaceuticals, Inc.
145 Sakonnet Blvd.
Narragansett, RI 02882

LuChem Pharmaceuticals, Inc.
See H.N. Norton Co.

00374
Lyne Laboratories
260 Tosca Drive
Stoughton, MA 02072
508-583-8700

00466
Macsil, Inc.
P.O. Box 29276
Philadelphia, PA 19125-0976
215-739-7300

00904
Major Pharmaceuticals
1640 W. Fulton
Chicago, IL 60612
312-666-9600

10106
Mallinckrodt-Baker
222 Red School Lane
Phillipsburg, NJ 08865
908-859-2151

00406
Mallinckrodt Chemical
16305 Swingley Ridge Drive
Chesterfield, MO 63017
314-530-2058

00019
Mallinckrodt Medical, Inc.
675 McDonnell Blvd.
P.O. Box 5840
St. Louis, MO 63134
314-895-2000

10706
Manne
P.O. Box 825
Johns Island, SC 29457
800-517-0228

Marlin Industries
P.O. Box 560
Grover City, CA 93483-0560
805-473-2743

12939
Marlop Pharmaceuticals, Inc.
5704 Mosholu Ave.
P.O. Box 536
Bronx, NY 10471
800-345-7192

10712
Marlyn, Inc.
14851 N. Scottsdale Road
Scottsdale, AZ 85254
800-462-7596

00682
Marnel Pharmaceuticals, Inc.
206 Luke Drive
Lafayette, LA 70506
318-232-1396

00209
Marsam Pharmaceuticals, Inc.
P.O. Box 1022
Cherry Hill, NJ 08034
609-424-5600

52555
Martec Pharmaceutical, Inc.
P.O. Box 33510
Kansas City, MO 64120-3510
816-241-4144

11845
Mason Distributors, Inc.
5105 N.W. 159th Street
Hialeah, FL 33014-6370
305-624-5557

12758
Mason Pharmaceuticals, Inc.
4425 Jamboree
Suite 250
Newport Beach, CA 92660
714-851-6860

14362
Mass. Public Health Bio. Lab.
305 South Street
Jamaica Plains, MA 02130
617-522-3700

Matrix Laboratories
1430 O'Brian Drive
Suite G
Menlo Park, CA 94025
415-326-6100

00259
Mayrand, Inc.
915 Bridge Street
Winston Salem, NC 27101
910-765-4252

00264
McGaw, Inc.
P.O. Box 19791
Irvine, CA 92713-9791
714-660-2000

11089
McGregor Pharmaceuticals, Inc.
8420 Ulmenton Road
Suite 305
Largo, FL 34641
813-530-4361

49072
McGuff, Inc.
3617 W. MacArthur Blvd.
Suite 507
Santa Ana, CA 92704
800-854-7220

50185
McHenry Laboratories, Inc.
118 N. Wells, Lee Building
Edna, TX 77957
512-782-5438

00045
McNeil Consumer Products Co.
Camp Hill Road
Mail Stop 278
Ft. Washington, PA 19034-2292
215-233-7000

MCR American Pharmaceuticals
120 Summit Parkway,
Suite 101
Birmingham, AL 35209
205-942-6415

58607
ME Pharmaceuticals, Inc.
2800 Southeast Pkwy.
Richmond, IN 47375
800-637-4276

Mead Johnson Laboratories
See Bristol-Myers Squibb

00087
Mead Johnson Nutritionals
2404 Pennsylvania Street
Evansville, IN 47721
812-426-6000

Mead Johnson Oncology
See Bristol-Myers Oncology

Mead Johnson Pharmaceuticals
See Bristol-Myers Squibb

**Medac GmbH c/o Princeton
    Regulatory Assoc.**
65 South Main Street
Pennington, NJ 08534
609-951-9596

Medarex
1545 Rte. 22E
P.O. Box 953
Annandale, NJ 08801
908-713-6001

MedChem
232 W. Cummings Park
Woburn, MA 01801
800-451-4716

Medclone, Inc.
2435 Military Avenue
Los Angeles, CA 90064

11940
Medco Lab, Inc.
P.O. Box 864
Sioux City, IA 51102-0864
712-255-8770

Medco Research, Inc.
P.O. Box 13886
Research Triangle Park, NC 27709
919-549-8117

45565
Med-Derm Pharmaceuticals
P.O. Box 5193
Kingsport, TN 37663
615-477-3991

Medea Research Laboratories
200 Wilson Street
Port Jefferson, NY 11776
516-331-7718

00585
Medeva Pharmaceuticals
755 Jefferson Road
Rochester, NY 14623-0000
888-963-3382

Medi Aid Corp.
8250 S. Akron Street
Suite 205
Englewood, CO 80155
303-790-1655

00576
Medical Products Panamericana
647 West Flagler Street
Miami, FL 33130
305-545-6524

99207
Medicis Dermatologicals, Inc.
100 East 42nd Street, 15th Floor
New York, NY 10017-5613
212-599-2000

60574
Medimmune, Inc.
35 West Watkins Mill Road
Gaithersburg, MD 20878
301-417-0770

Medimorphics
245 East 6th Street
St. Paul, MN 55101
612-224-2800

17156
**MediPhysics, Inc., Amersham
    Healthcare**
2636 S. Clearbrook Drive
Arlington Heights, Il 60005
800-322-6334

Medi-Plex Pharm., Inc.
See ECR Pharmaceuticals

57480
Medirex, Inc.
20 Chapin Road
Pine Brook, NJ 07058
201-227-4774

61563
Medisan
400 Lanidex Plaza
Parsippany, NJ 07054
201-515-5300

MediSense, Inc.
266 Second Street
Waltham, MA 02154

53978
Med-Pro, Inc.
210 E. 4th Street
Lexington, NB 68850
308-324-4571

00348, 75137
Medtech Laboratories, Inc.
3510 N. Lake Creek
P.O. Box 1108
Jackson, WY 83011-1108
307-733-1680

58281
Medtronic
800 53rd Ave. N.E.
Minneapolis, Mn 55421
612-572-5000

87900
Menley & James Labs, Inc.
100 Tournament Drive
Horsham, PA 19044
215-441-6500

22200
Mennen Co.
Hanover Ave.
Morristown, NJ 07962-1928
201-631-9000

10742
Mentholatum, Inc.
1360 Niagara Street
Buffalo, NY 14213
716-882-7660

00006
Merck & Co.
P.O. Box 4
West Point, PA 19486
215-652-5000

00394
Mericon Industries, Inc.
8819 N. Pioneer Road
Peoria, IL 61615
309-693-2150

Merieux Institute, Inc.
See Pasteur-Mérieux-Connaught

30727
Merit Pharmaceuticals
2611 San Fernando Road
Los Angeles, CA 90065
213-227-4831

Michigan Department of Health
P.O. Box 30035
Lansing, MI 48909
517-335-8000

00682, 46672
Mikart, Inc.
2090 Marietta Blvd. N.W.
Atlanta, GA 30318
404-351-1125

52836
Milance Laboratories, Inc.
P.O. Box 368
Millington, NJ 07946
908-580-1591

Miles, Inc.
See Bayer Corp. (Consumer Div.)

Miles, Inc.
See Bayer Corp. (Diagnostic Div.)

00396, 34567
Milex Products, Inc.
5915 Northwest Hwy.
Chicago, IL 60631-1032
312-631-6484

17204
Miller Pharmacal Group, Inc.
350 Randy Road, Unit #2
Carol Stream, IL 60188
630-871-9557

53118
Millgood Laboratories, Inc.
250 D Arizona Ave.
P.O. Box 170159
Atlanta, GA 30317
404-377-6538

00276
Misemer Pharmaceuticals, Inc.
4553 S. Campbell
Springfield, MO 65810-5918
417-881-0660

00178
Mission Pharmacal Co.
P.O. Box 786099
San Antonio, TX 78278-6099
800-531-3333

53169
Monarch Pharmaceuticals
355 Beecham Street
Bristol, TN 37620
800-776-3637

Montgomery Medical Ventures
600 Montgomery Street
San Francisco, CA 94111

00426, 00832, 60432
Morton Grove Pharmaceuticals
6451 West Main Street
Morton Grove, IL 60053
708-967-5600

Morton Salt
100 N. Riverside Plaza
Chicago, IL 60606-1597
312-807-2000

MSD
See Merck & Co.

Mt. Vernon Foods, Inc.
13246 Wooster Road
Mt. Vernon, OH 43050
800-932-5525

54964
Murdock, Madaus, Schwabe
1400 Mountain Springs Pkwy.
Springvale, UT 84663
801-489-1500

00451
Muro Pharmaceutical, Inc.
890 East Street
Tewksbury, MA 01876-9987
508-851-5981

00150
Murray Drug Corp.
415 S. 4th Street
Murray, KY 42071
502-753-6654

53489
Mutual Pharmaceutical, Inc.
1100 Orthodox Street
Philadelphia, PA 19124
215-288-6500

00378
Mylan Pharmaceuticals
P.O. Box 4310
Morgantown, WV 26505
304-599-2595

05973
Nabi
5800 Park of Commerce Blvd.
  Northwest
Boca Raton, FL 33487
305-625-5303

05745
Nastech Pharmaceutical, Inc.
129 Oser Ave.
Hauppauge, NY 11788
516-273-0101

National Patent Medical
P.O. Box 419
Dayville, CT 06241
800-243-1172

53983
Natren, Inc.
3105 Willow Lane
Westlake Village, CA 91361

Natures Bounty, Inc.
See NBTY, Inc.

74312
NBTY, Inc.
105 Orville Drive
Bohemia, NY 11716
516-567-9500

72559
NCI Medical Foods
5801 Ayala Ave.
Irwindale, CA 91706
818-812-3393

Neorx Corp.
410 West Harrison
Seattle, WA 98119
206-281-7001

00487
Nephron Pharmaceuticals Corp.
4121 S.W. 34th Street
Orlando, FL 32811-6458
407-246-1389

Nephro-Tech, Inc.
P.O. Box 14703
Lenexa, KS 66285
913-894-6646

NeuroGenesis/Matrix Tech., Inc.
100 Louisiana
Suite 600
Houston, TX 77002
800-345-8912

10812, 70501
Neutrogena Corp.
5760 W. 96th Street
Los Angeles, CA 90045-5595
310-642-1150

Neutron Technology Corp.
877 Main Street
Boise, ID 83702
208-345-3460

New World Trading Corp.
P.O. Box 952
DeBary, FL 32713
407-668-7520

Newport Pharmaceuticals
140 Columbia
Laguna Hills, CA 92656-1459
714-362-1330

56146
Nexstar
2860 Wilderness Place
Boulder, CO 80301
303-444-5893

59016
Niche Pharmaceuticals, Inc.
200 N. Oak Street
P.O. Box 449
Roanoke, TX 76262
807-491-2770

12934
Nion Corp.
15501 First Street
Irwindale, CA 91706
818-969-1932

23317
NMC Laboratories
70-36 83rd Street
Glendale, NY 11385
718-326-1500

51801
Nomax, Inc.
40 North Rock Hill Road
St. Louis, MO 63119
314-961-2500

Norcliff Thayer
See SmithKline Beecham Consumer
  Healthcare

10118
Norstar Consumer Products
206 Pegasus Ave.
Northvale, NJ 07647
201-784-8155

North American Biologicals, Inc.
16500 N.W. 15th Ave.
Miami, FL 33169
305-625-5303

Novaferon Labs
2658 Patton Road
Roseville, MN 55713

00028, 00067, 00083, 58887
Novartis
556 Morris Ave.
Summit, NJ 07901
908-277-5000

Noven
11960 S.W. 144th Street
Miami, FL 33186
305-253-5099

00362
Novocol Chemical Mfr. Co.
P.O. Box 11926
Wilmington, DE 19850
302-328-1102

00169
Novo/Nordisk Pharm., Inc.
100 Overlook Center
Suite 200
Princeton, NJ 08540
800-727-6500

55953
Novopharm USA, Inc.
165 E. Commerce
Suite 100
Schaumberg, IL 60173-5326
708-882-4200

NPDC-AS101, Inc.
783 Jersey Avenue
New Brunswick, NJ 08901
716-636-9096

55499
Numark Laboratories, Inc.
P.O. Box 6321
Edison, NJ 08818
800-338-8079

34999
Nutraloric
350 N. Lantana, Unit G1
Camarillo, CA 93010
805-388-2811

NutraMax
9 Blackburn Drive
Gloucester, MA 01930
508-283-1800

Nutricia, Inc.
See Mt. Vernon Foods, Inc.

51081
Nutripharm Laboratories, Inc.
Salem Industrial Park
Building 5
Lebanon, NJ 08833
908-534-6267

00407
Nycomed Inc.
101 Carnegie Center
Princeton, NJ 08540-6231
609-514-6438

10797
Oakhurst Co.
3000 Hempstead Turnpike
Levittown, NY 11756
516-731-5380

55515
Oclassen Pharmaceuticals, Inc.
100 Pelican Way
San Rafael, CA 94901
415-258-4500

O'Connor, Inc.
See Columbia Laboratories, Inc.

51944
Ocumed, Inc.
119 Harrison Ave.
Roseland, NJ 07068
201-226-2330

Ohm Laboratories, Inc.
P.O. Box 7397
N. Brunswick, NJ 08902
908-297-3030

10019
Ohmeda Pharmaceuticals
110 Allen Road
Liberty Corner, NJ 07938
908-647-9200

12622
Olin Corp.
120 Long Ridge Road
Stamford, CT 06904-1355
203-356-2000

Omex International, Inc.
6001 Savoy
Suite 110
Houston, TX 77036
713-975-8325

Oncotherapeutics, Inc.
1002 East Park Blvd.
Cranbury, NJ 08512
609-655-5300

ONY, Inc.
1576 Sweet Home Road
Amherst, NY 14228
716-636-9096

Ophidian Pharmaceuticals, Inc.
2800 S. Fish Hatchery Road
Madison, WI 53711
608-271-0878

O.P.R. Development, LP
1501 Wakarusa Drive
Lawrence, KS 66047
913-749-0034

Optikem International, Inc.
2172 S. Jason Street
Denver, CO 80223
303-936-1137

50520
Optimox Corp.
2720 Monterey
Suite 406
Torrance, CA 90503
310-618-9370

52238
Optopics Laboratories, Corp.
32 Main Street
P.O. Box 210
Fairton, NJ 08320-0210
508-283-1800

00041
Oral-B Laboratories, Inc.
1 Lagoon Drive
Redwood City, CA 94065
415-961-8130

00052
Organon, Inc.
375 Mt. Pleasant Ave.
West Orange, NJ 07052
201-325-4500

Organon Teknika Corp.
100 Akzo Ave.
Durham, NC 27704
919-620-2000

Orion Diagnostica
71 Veronica Ave.
P.O. Box 218
Somerset, NJ 08875-0218
908-246-3366

Orphan Medical
13911 Ridgedale Drive
Minnetonka, MN 55305
612-513-6900

59676
Ortho Biotech, Inc.
700 US Hwy. 202
P.O. Box 670
Raritan, NJ 08869-0670
800-325-7504

00062
Ortho McNeil Pharmaceutical
Route 202
P.O. Box 600
Raritan, NJ 08869
908-218-6000

59148
Otsuka America
  Pharmaceutical
2440 Research Blvd.
Rockville, MD 98101
206-682-5300

Owen/Galderma
See Galderma Laboratories, Inc.

Oxis International
6040 N. Cutter Circle
Suite 317
Portland, OR 97212
503-283-3911

00574
Paddock Laboratories
3940 Quebec Avenue
North Minneapolis, MN 55427
612-546-4676

53159
Palisades Pharmaceuticals, Inc.
64 N. Summit Street
Tenafly, NJ 07670
201-569-8502

Pan America Labs
P.O. Box 8950
Mandeville, LA 70470-8950
504-893-4097

49884
Par Pharmaceuticals
One Ram Ridge Road
Spring Valley, NY 10977
914-425-7100

00071
Parke-Davis
201 Tabor Road
Morris Plains, NJ 07950
800-223-0432

00349
Parmed Pharmaceuticals, Inc.
4220 Hyde Park Blvd.
Niagara Falls, NY 14305
716-284-5666

50930
Parnell Pharmaceuticals, Inc.
Larkspur Landing Circle
Larkspur, CA 94939
415-461-4900

10865
Parthenon, Inc.
3311 W. 2400 South
Salt Lake City, UT 84119
801-972-5184

00418
Pasadena Research Labs
See Taylor Pharmaceuticals

11793, 49281, 50361
Pasteur-Mérieux-Connaught Labs
Route 611
P.O. Box 187
Swiftwater, PA 18370-0187
717-839-7187

00077
PBH Wesley Jessen
7976 Engineer Road
San Diego, CA 92111
619-614-7600

Pediatric Pharmaceuticals
718 Bradford Ave.
Westfield, NJ 07090
908-225-0989

00884
Pedinol Pharmacal, Inc.
30 Banfi Plaza North
Farmingdale, NY 11735
516-293-9500

10974
Pegasus Medical, Inc.
1 Technology Drive
Building 1C
Suite 525
Irvine, CA 92718-2325
714-753-9055

Pennex Pharmaceutical, Inc.
See Morton Grove
  Pharmaceuticals

Permeable Technologies, Inc.
712 Ginesi Drive
Morganville, NJ 07751
908-972-8585

00096
Person and Covey, Inc.
616 Allen Ave.
P.O. Box 25018
Glendale, CA 91221-5018
818-240-1030

00927
Pfeiffer Co.
43-45 N. Washington
P.O. Box 100
Wilkes-Barre, PA 18701
717-826-9000

Pfipharmecs
See Pfizer US Pharmaceutical Group

00069, 00663, 74300
Pfizer US Pharmaceutical Group
235 E. 42nd Street
New York, NY 10017-5755
800-438-1985

39822
Pharma Tek, Inc.
P.O. Box 1920
Huntington, NY 11743-0568
516-757-5522

58197
Pharmacel Laboratory, Inc.
203 South Coolidge Ave.
Tampa, FL 33609
813-289-2750

00121
Pharmaceutical Associates, Inc.
P.O. Box 128
Conestee, SC 29636
803-277-7282

Pharmaceutical Basics, Inc.
See Rosemont Pharmaceutical

51655
Pharmaceutical Corp.
12348 Hancock Street
Carmel, IN 46032
317-573-8000

21659
Pharmaceutical Labs, Inc.
1229 W. Corporate Drive
Arlington, TX 76006
817-633-1461

45334
Pharmaceutical Specialties, Inc.
P.O. Box 6298
Rochester, MN 55903
507-288-8500

Pharmachemie USA, Inc.
P.O. Box 145
Oradell, NJ 07049
201-265-1942

00013, 00016
Pharmacia & Upjohn
P.O. Box 16529
Columbus, OH 43216-6529
614-764-8100

PharmaControl
661 Palisade Ave.
P.O. Box 931
Englewood Cliffs, NJ 07632
201-567-9004

Pharmafair
See Bausch & Lomb
  Pharmaceuticals

55422
Pharmakon Laboratories, Inc.
6050 Jet Port Industrial Blvd.
Tampa, FL 33634
813-886-3216

Pharmaquest Corp.
See Inveresk Research

Pharmatec
County Road 2054
P.O. Box 730
Alachua, FL 32615
904-462-1210

Pharmavene, Inc.
35 West Watkins Mill Road
Gaithersburg, MD 20878
301-417-0033

Pharmedic Co.
28101 Ballard Road
Suite F
Lake Forest, IL 60045
708-549-8600

00813
Pharmics, Inc.
P.O. Box 27554
Salt Lake City, UT 84127
801-972-4138

Plexus Pharmaceuticals, Inc.
8122 Datapoint Drive
Suite 600
San Antonio, TX 78229

Plough, Inc.
See Schering-Plough Healthcare
  Products

00998
PolyMedica Pharmaceuticals
2 Constitution Way
Woburn, MA 01801
617-933-2020

47144
Polymer Technology Corp.
100 Research Drive
Wilmington, MA 01887
800-343-1445

**Polymer Technology
International**
1595 N.W. Gilman Blvd.
Suite 17
Issaquah, WA 98027
206-391-2650

Porton Product Limited
See Speywood Pharmaceuticals, Inc.

Poythress
See ECR Pharmaceuticals

59012
Pratt Pharmaceuticals
235 E. 42nd Street
New York, NY 10017-5755
800-438-1985

Precision-Cosmet
500 Iolab Drive
Claremont, CA 91711
800-423-1871

Premier, Inc.
See Advanced Polymer Systems

00684
Primedics Laboratories
15524 S. Broadway
Gardenia, CA 90248
213-770-3005

Princeton Pharm. Products
See Bristol-Myers Squibb

23900, 37000, 76660
Procter & Gamble Co.
1 Procter & Gamble Plaza
Cincinnati, OH 45202
513-983-1100

00149
Procter & Gamble Pharm.
P.O. Box 191
Norwich, NY 13815-0191
607-335-2111

00034
Purdue Frederick Co.
100 Connecticut Ave.
Norwalk, CT 06850-3590
203-853-0123

00228
Purepac Pharmaceutical Co.
200 Elmora Ave.
Elizabeth, NJ 07207
908-527-9100

QLT Phototherapeutics, Inc.
401 North Middletown Road
Pearl River, NY 10965

00603
Qualitest Products, Inc.
1236 Jordan Road
Huntsville, AL 35811
205-859-4011

12225
Quality Formulations, Inc.
P.O. Box 827
Zachary, LA 70791-0827
504-654-6880

Quidel Corp.
10165 McKellar Court
San Diego, CA 92121
619-552-1100

54391
R & D Laboratories, Inc.
4640 Admiralty Way,
Suite 710
Marina Del Rey, CA 90292
310-305-8053

R & R Registrations
P.O. Box 262079
San Diego, CA 92196-2069
619-586-0751

00196
Rachelle Laboratories, Inc.
See Houba Inc.

30103
Randob Laboratories, Ltd.
P.O. Box 440
Cornwall, NY 12518
914-699-3131

00686
Raway Pharmacal, Inc.
15 Granit Road
Accord, NY 12404-0047
914-626-8133

12496, 19200
Reckitt & Colman
1901 Huguenot Road
Suite 110
Richmond, VA 23235
804-379-1090

10952
Recsei Laboratories
330 S. Kellogg
Building M
Goleta, CA 93117-3875
805-964-2912

48028
Redi-Products Labs, Inc.
See Aplicare Inc.

00021
Reed & Carnrick
See Schwarz Pharma

10956
Reese Pharmaceutical Inc.
10617 Frank Ave.
Cleveland, OH 44106
216-231-6441

Regeneron Pharmaceuticals
777 Old Saw Mill River Road
Tarrytown, NY 10591-6707
914-347-7000

Reid Rowell
See Solvay

Remel, Inc.
12076 Santa Fe Drive
Lenexa, KS 66215

10961
Requa, Inc.
1 Seneca Place
P.O. Box 4008
Greenwich, CT 06830
203-869-2445

00433
Research Industries Corp.
6864 S. 300 West
Midvale, UT 84047
801-562-0200

**Research Triangle
Pharmaceuticals**
4364 S. Alston Ave.
Durham, NC 27713
919-544-4029

60575
Respa Pharmaceuticals, Inc.
P.O. Box 88222
Carol Stream, IL 60188
708-462-9986

00122
Rexall Group
4031 N.E. 12th Terrace
Ft. Lauderdale, FL 33334
800-255-7399

Rexar Pharmaceuticals
See Richwood Pharmaceutical

RH Pharmaceuticals, Inc.
See Cangene Corp.

**Rhone-Poulenc Rorer Consumer,
Inc.**
See Novartis

00075
**Rhone-Poulenc Rorer
Pharmaceuticals, Inc.**
500 Arcola Road
P.O. Box 1200
Collegeville, PA 19426
610-454-8000

Ribi Immunochem Research
553 Old Corvallis Road
Hamilton, MT 59840-3131
406-363-6214

Richardson-Vicks, Inc.
See Procter & Gamble Co.

12071
Richie Pharmacal, Inc.
197 State Ave.
P.O. Box 460
Glasgow, KY 42141
800-626-0250

58521
Richwood Pharmaceutical, Inc.
P.O. Box 6497
Florence, KY 41022
800-974-4700

54807
R.I.D., Inc.
609 North Mednik Avenue
Los Angeles, CA 90022-1320
213-268-0635

54092
Roberts Pharmaceuticals
4 Industrial Way West
Eatontown, NJ 07724
908-389-1182

**A.H. Robins Consumer
   Products**
See Wyeth-Ayerst

00031
A.H. Robins, Inc.
See Wyeth-Ayerst

Roche Diagnostic Systems, Inc.
1080 U.S. Highway 202
Somerville, NJ 08876-3771
908-253-7200

00004, 00033, 00140, 18393, 42987
Roche Laboratories
340 Kingsland Street
Nutley, NJ 07110-1199
800-526-6367

00049
Roerig
See Pfizer

00832
Rosemont Pharmaceutical Corp.
301 South Cherokee Street
Denver, CO 80223
303-733-7207

00074
Ross Laboratories
6480 Busch Blvd.
Columbus, OH 43229
614-624-3333

00054
Roxane Laboratories, Inc.
P.O. Box 16532
Columbus, OH 43216-6532
614-276-4000

51875
Royce Laboratories, Inc.
16600 N.W. 54 Ave.
Miami, FL 33014
305-624-1500

00536
Rugby Labs, Inc.
898 Orlando Ave.
West Hempstead, NY 11552
516-536-8565

Russ Pharmaceuticals
See UCB Pharmaceuticals

46500
Rydelle Laboratories
1525 Howe Street
Racine, WI 53403-5011
414-631-2000

00263
Rystan, Inc.
P.O. Box 214
Little Falls, NJ 07424-0214
201-256-3737

00043
Sandoz Consumer
59 Route 10
East Hanover, NJ 07936
201-503-7500

00212
Sandoz Nutrition Corp.
5320 W. 23rd Street
Minneapolis, MN 55440
800-999-9978

00078
Sandoz Pharmaceuticals
59 Route 10
East Hanover, NJ 07936
201-503-7500

51353
Sanitube Co.
19 Concord Street
S. Norwalk, CT 06854
203-853-7856

00024
**Sanofi Winthrop
   Pharmaceuticals**
90 Park Ave.
New York, NY 10016
800-446-6267

00281
Savage Laboratories
60 Baylis Road
Melville, NY 11747-2006
800-231-0206

**Scandinavian Natural Health &
   Beauty Products**
13 N. 7th St.
Perkasie, PA 18944
215-453-2505

58914
Scandipharm, Inc.
22 Inverness Center Pkwy.
Suite 310
Birmingham, AL 35242
800-950-8085

11012
Schaffer Laboratories
1058 North Allen Ave.
Pasadena, CA 91104
818-798-8644

00364
Schein Pharmaceutical, Inc.
100 Campus Drive
Florham Park, NJ 07932
914-278-3724

00274
Scherer Laboratories, Inc.
16200 N. Dallas Pkwy.
Suite 165
Dallas, TX 75248
800-858-9888

00085
Schering-Plough Corp.
2000 Galloping Hill Road
Kenilworth, NJ 07033-0530
908-298-4000

00085
**Schering-Plough Healthcare
   Products**
110 Allen Road
Liberty Corner, NJ 07938
908-298-4000

Schiapparelli Searle
See SCS Pharmaceuticals

Schiff Products
P.O. Box 26708
Salt Lake City, UT 84126
801-975-1166

00234
Schmid Products Co.
P.O. Box 4703
Sarasota, FL 34230-4703
800-827-0987

Scholl, Inc.
See Schering-Plough Healthcare
 Products

00021, 00091, 00131
Schwarz Pharma
5600 W. County Line
Mequon, WI 53092
800-558-5114

Scios Nova, Inc.
2450 Bayshore Pkwy.
Mountain View, CA 94043
415-966-1550

00372
Scot-Tussin Pharmacal, Inc.
50 Clemence Street
P.O. Box 8217
Cranston, RI 02920-0217
800-638-7268

00905
SCS Pharmaceuticals
P.O. Box 5110
Chicago, IL 60680
800-323-1603

00014, 00025
Searle
Box 5110
Chicago, IL 60680-5110
847-982-7000

00551
Seatrace Pharmaceuticals
P.O. Box 363
Gadsden, AL 35902-0363
205-442-5023

Sequus Pharmaceuticals, Inc.
960 Hamilton Court
Menlo Park, CA 94025
415-833-7207

50694
Seres Laboratories
3331 Industrial Drive
P.O. Box 470
Santa Rosa, CA 95401
707-526-4526

44087
Serono Laboratories, Inc.
100 Longwater Circle
Norwell, MA 02061
617-982-9000

97692
S.G. Labs, Inc.
500 North Broadway
Jericho, NY 11753
516-822-2900

49731
Sherman Pharmaceuticals, Inc.
P.O. Box 1377
Mandeville, LA 70470-1377
504-893-0007

08884
Sherwood Medical
1915 Olive Street
St. Louis, MO 63103
314-621-7788

45809
Shionogi USA
3848 Carson Street
Suite 206
Torrance, CA 90503
310-540-1161

50111
Sidmak Laboratories, Inc.
P.O. Box 371
East Hanover, NJ 07936
201-386-5566

54482
Sigma-Tau Pharmaceuticals, Inc.
800 S. Frederick Avenue
Gaithersburg, MD 20877-4150
301-948-1041

54838
Silarx Pharmaceuticals, Inc.
19 West Street
Spring Valley, NY 10977
914-352-4020

08026
Smith & Nephew United
11775 Starkey Road
Largo, FL 34643
800-876-1261

00766
**SmithKline Beecham Consumer
 Healthcare**
1500 Littleton
Parsippany, NJ 07054-3884
201-631-8700

00007, 00029, 00108, 00128
**SmithKline Beecham
 Pharmaceuticals**
One Franklin Plaza,
P.O. Box 7929
Philadelphia, PA 19103
215-751-4000

00978
SmithKline Diagnostics
225 Baypoint Pkwy.
San Jose, CA 95134-1622
800-877-6242

Sola/Barnes-Hind
See Pilkington Barnes Hind

33984
Solgar, Inc.
410 Ocean Ave.
Lynbrook, NY 11563
516-599-2442

39769
SoloPak Pharmaceuticals, Inc.
1845 Tonne Road
Elk Grove Village, IL 60007-5125
847-806-0080

00032
Solvay Pharmaceuticals
901 Sawyer Road
Marietta, GA 30062-2224
770-578-9000

39506
Somerset Pharmaceuticals
5215 West Laurel Street
Tampa, FL 33607
813-223-7677

Sparta Pharmaceuticals
P.O. Box 13288
Research Triangle Park, NC 27709
919-361-3461

Spectra Pharmaceuticals
See Cooper Pharmaceuticals

38137
Spectrum Chemical Mfg. Corp.
14422 S. San Pedro Street
Gardena, CA 90248-9985
800-772-8786

00537
Spencer Mead, Inc.
100 Banks Ave.
Rockville Center, NY 11570
800-645-3737

55688
Speywood Pharmaceuticals, Inc.
27 Maple Street
Milford, MA 01757-2658
508-478-8900

Sphinx Pharmaceutical Corp.
P.O. Box 52330
Durham, NC 27717
919-489-0909

Squibb Diagnostic Division
See Bracco Diagnostics

Stanback Co.
P.O. Box 1669
Salisbury, NC 28145-1669
704-633-9231

53385
Standard Drug Co.
P.O. Box 710
Riverton, IL 62561
217-629-9884

00076
Star Pharmaceuticals, Inc.
1990 N.W. 44th Street
Pompano Beach, FL 33064-1278
305-971-9704

51318
Stellar Pharmacal Corp.
1990 N.W. 44th Street
Pompano Beach, FL 33064
800-845-7827

00402
Steris Laboratories, Inc.
620 N. 51st Ave.
Phoenix, AZ 85043
602-278-1400

Sterling Health
See Bayer Corp. (Consumer Div.)

Sterling Winthrop
See Sanofi Winthrop
  Pharmaceuticals

00145
Stiefel Laboratories, Inc.
255 Alhambra Circle
Coral Gables, FL 33134
800-327-3858

89223
Stockhausen, Inc.
2408 Doyle Street
Greensboro, NC 27406
800-334-0242

41701
Stolle
6954 Cornell Road
Cincinnati, OH 45242
513-489-4235

57706
Storz Ophthalmics
3365 Tree Court Industrial
St. Louis, MO 63122-6694
314-225- 5051

58980
Stratus Pharmaceuticals, Inc.
P.O. Box 4632
Miami, FL 33265
800-442-7882

Stuart Pharmaceuticals
See Zeneca Pharmaceuticals

Sublingual Products International
See Pharmaceutical Labs, Inc.

11086
Summers Laboratories, Inc.
103 G.P. Clement Drive
Collegeville, PA 19426
610-454-1471

57267
Summit Pharmaceuticals
556 Morris Ave.
Summit, NJ 07901
908-277-5000

11704
Survival Technology, Inc.
2275 Research Blvd.
Rockville, MD 20850
301-926-1800

Syncom Pharmaceuticals, Inc.
155 Passaic Ave.
Fairfield, NJ 07004

Synergen, Inc.
1885 33rd Street
Boulder, CO 80301
303-938-6200

00033, 18393, 42987
Syntex Laboratories
3401 Hillview Ave.
Palo Alto, CA 94304
415-855-5050

Syntex-Synergen Neuroscience
1885 33rd Street
Boulder, CO 80301
303-442-1926

Syva Co.
929 Queensbridge
St. Louis, MO 63021
314-391-5374

Tag Pharmaceuticals
P.O. Box 904
Sellersville, PA 18960
215-723-5544

Tambrands, Inc.
777 Westchester Ave.
White Plains, NY 10604
914-696-6060

Tanning Research Labs, Inc.
1190 U.S. 1 North
Ormond Beach, FL 32174
904-677-9559

00300
Tap Pharmaceuticals
2355 Waukegan Road
Deerfield, IL 60015
800-621-1020

51672
Taro Pharmaceuticals USA, Inc.
Six Skyline Drive
Hawthorne, NY 10532-9998
914-345-9001

00418
Taylor Pharmaceuticals
P.O. Box 5136
San Clemente, CA 92674-5136
714-492-4030

83926
Tec Laboratories, Inc.
615 Water Ave. S.E.
P.O. Box 1958
Albany, OR 97321-0512
503-926-4577

Telluride Pharm. Corp.
146 Flanders Drive
Hillsborough, NJ 08876-4656
908-359-1375

00093, 00332
Teva Pharmaceuticals USA
650 Cathill Road
Sellersville, PA 18960

49158
Thames Pharmacal, Inc.
2100 Fifth Ave.
Ronkonkoma, NY 11779-6906
516-737-1155

Therakos, Inc.
201 Brandywine Pkwy.
West Chester, PA 19380
610-430-7900

Therapeutic Antibodies, Inc.
1500 21st Ave.
Suite 310
Nashville, TN 37212
615-327-1027

11290
Thompson Medical Co.
222 Lakeview Ave.
West Palm Beach, FL 33401
407-820-9900

T/I Pharmaceuticals, Inc.
See Fischer Pharmaceuticals

49483
Time-Cap Labs, Inc.
7 Michael Avenue
Farmingdale, NY 11735
516-753-9090

TNI Pharmaceuticals
5105 N. Pearl Street
Schiller Park, IL 60176
708-678-3067

93312
Trask Industries, Inc.
163 Farrell Street
Somerset, NJ 08873
908-214-9267

Triage Pharmaceuticals
See Health for Life Brands, Inc.

Triangle Labs, Inc.
1000 Robins Road
Lynchburg, VA 24504-3558
804-845-7073

53020
Trinity Technologies, Inc.
28510 Hayes
Roseville, MI 48066
313-778-5630

79511
Triton Consumer Products, Inc.
561 West Golf
Arlington Heights, IL 60005
708-228-7650

Tsumura Medical
1000 Valley Park Drive
Shakopee, MN 55379
612-496-4700

Tweezerman
55 Sea Cliff Ave.
Glen Cove, NY 11542-3695
516-676-7772

53335
Tyson & Associates, Inc.
12832 Chadron Ave.
Hawthorne, CA 90250-5525
310-675-1080

UAD Laboratories, Inc.
See Forest Pharmaceutical, Inc.

59640
UBI Corp.
2920 N.W. Boca Raton Blvd.
Boca Raton, FL 33431
407-367-1252

UCB Pharmaceuticals, Inc.
P.O. Box 4410
Hampton, VA 23664-0410
804-851-4618

62592
Ucyclyd Pharma, Inc.
10819 Gilroy Road,
Suite 100
Hunt Valley, MD 21031
410-584-0001

51079
UDL Laboratories, Inc.
P.O. Box 10319
Rockford, IL 61131-3019
815-282-1201

Ueno Fine Chemicals Industry
31 Koraibashi
Osaka 541, Japan
06-203-0761

00127
Ulmer Pharmacal Co.
2440 Fernbrook Lane
Plymouth, MN 55447-9987
612-559-0601

41785
Unimed
2150 E. Lake Cook Road
Buffalo Grove, IL 60089
800-541-3492

00677
United Research Laboratories
3600 Marshall Lane
P.O. Box 8546
Bensalem, PA 19020-8546
215-638-2626

48663
Unitek Corp.
2724 South Peck Road
Monrovia, CA 91016
818-445-7960

Univax Biologics
12280 Wilkins Ave.
Rockville, MD 20852
301-770-3099

00009
Upjohn Co.
See Pharmacia & Upjohn

00245
Upsher-Smith Labs, Inc.
14905 23rd Ave. N.
Minneapolis, MN 55447
612-473-4412

58178
US Bioscience
100 Front Street
Suite 400
West Conshohocken, PA 19428
800-447-3969

US Packaging Corp. Medical
506 Clay Street
LaPorte, IN 46350
219-362-9782

52747
US Pharmaceutical Corp.
2401-C Mellon Court
Decatur, GA 30035
(770) 987-4745

54627
ValMed, Inc.
203 Southwest Cutoff
Northboro, MA 01532
800-477-0487

00615
Vangard Labs, Inc.
P.O. Box 1268
Glasgow, KY 42142-1268
502-651-6188

17022
Veratex Corp.
1304 E. Maple Road
P.O. Box 4031
Troy, MI 48007
810-619-0800

Vertex Pharmaceuticals, Inc.
40 Allston Street
Cambridge, MA 02139-4211
617-576-3111

53258
VHA Supply Co.
300 Decker Drive
P.O. Box 160909
Irving, TX 75016
214-650-4444

23900
Vicks Health Care Products
See Procter & Gamble Co

25866
Vicks Pharmacy Products
One Far Mill Crossing
Shelton, CT 06484
203-929-2500

Vintage Pharmaceuticals, Inc.
3241 Woodpark Blvd.
Charlotte, NC 28256
704-596-0516

Viratek
3300 Hyland Ave.
Costa Mesa, CA 92627
714-540-1866

54891
Vision Pharmaceuticals, Inc.
P.O. Box 400
Mitchell, SD 57301-0400
605-996-3356

54022
Vitaline Corp.
385 Williamson Way
Ashland, OR 97520
503-482-9231

Vita-Rx Corp.
P.O. Box 8229
Columbus, GA 31908
706-568-1881

00298
Vortech Pharmaceuticals
6851 Chase Road
Dearborn, MI 48126
313-584-4088

11444
W. F. Young, Inc.
111 Lyman Street
Springfield, MA 01102
413-737-0201

59310
Wakefield Pharmaceuticals, Inc.
1050 Cambridge Square
Suite C
Alpharetta, GA 30201
404-664-1661

00741
Walker, Corp. and, Inc.
P.O. Box 1320
Syracuse, NY 13201
315-463-4511

00619
Walker Pharmacal Co.
4200 Laclede Ave.
St. Louis, MO 63108
314-533-9600

00037
Wallace Laboratories
Halfacre Road
Cranbury, NJ 08512
609-655-6000

00017
Wampole Laboratories
Half Acre Road
P.O. Box 1001
Cranbury, NJ 08515-0181
609-655-6000

00047
Warner Chilcott Laboratories
182 Tabor Road
Morris Plains, NJ 07950
800-521-8813

00071, 00081, 00501, 11370
**Warner Lambert Consumer Health
  Products**
201 Tabor Road
Morris Plains, NJ 07950
201-540-2000

59930
Warrick Pharmaceuticals, Corp.
1095 Morris Ave.
Union, NJ 07083
908-629-3600

00047, 52544
Watson Laboratories
311 Bonnie Circle Drive
Corona, CA 91720
909-270-1400

59196
WE Pharmaceuticals, Inc.
P.O. Box 1142
Ramona, CA 92065
619-788-9155

Wendt Laboratories
P.O. Box 128
Belle Plaine, MN 56011
800-328-5890

00917
Wesley Pharmacal, Inc.
114 Railroad Drive
Ivyland, PA 18974
215-953-1680

59591
West Point Pharma
P.O. Box 4
West Point, PA 19486-0004
212-652-2121

50893
Westport Pharmaceuticals, Inc.
1 Turkey Hill Road S.
Westport, CT 06880
203-226-0622

00143
West-Ward, Inc.
465 Industrial Way W.
Eatontown, NJ 07724
908-542-1191

00003, 00072
**Westwood Squibb
  Pharmaceuticals**
100 Forest Ave.
Buffalo, NY 14213
716-887-3400

50474
Whitby Pharmaceuticals, Inc.
See UCB Pharmaceuticals, Inc.

00031, 00573
Whitehall Robins Laboratories
Five Giralda Farms
Madison, NJ 07940-0871
201-660-5500

00317
Whorton Pharmaceuticals, Inc.
4202 Gary Ave.
Fairfield, AL 35064
205-786-2584

Willen Pharmaceuticals
See Baker Norton
  Pharmaceuticals

Winthrop Consumer
See Bayer Corp. (Consumer Div.)

Winthrop Pharmaceuticals
See Sanofi Winthrop
  Pharmaceuticals

12120
Wisconsin Pharmacal Co.
1 Repel Road
Jackson, WI 53037
414-677-4121

11428
Wonderful Dream Salve Corp.
18546 Old Homestead
Harper Woods, MI 48225
313-521-4233

Woodward Laboratories, Inc.
10357 Los Alamitos Blvd.
Los Alamitos, CA 90720
310-598-0800

WTD, Inc.
8819 N. Pioneer Road
Peoria, IL 61615
309-693-2150

00008, 00031
Wyeth-Ayerst Laboratories
P.O. Box 8299
Philadelphia, PA 19101
610-688-4400

50962
Xactdose, Inc.
722 Progressive Lane
South Beloit, IL 61080
815-624-8523

Xoma
2910 Seventh Street
Berkeley, CA 94710
510-644-1170

00116
Xttrium Laboratories, Inc.
415 West Pershing Road
Chicago, IL 60609
312-268-5800

64855
Young Again Products
43 Randolph Road
Suite 125
Silver Spring, MD 20904
301-622-1073

00273, 60077
Young Dental
13705 Shoreline Court E.
Earth City, MO 63045
314-344-0010

Young Pharmaceutical
1840 Berlin Turnpike
Wethersfield, CT 06109
203-529-7919

00163, 00187, 00310
Zeneca Pharmaceuticals
1800 Concord Pike
Wilmington, DE 19897
302-886-3000

00172
Zenith Goldline Pharmaceuticals
1900 W. Commercial Blvd.
Ft. Lauderdale, FL 33309
305-491-4002

05128
Zila Pharmaceuticals, Inc.
5227 N. 7th Street
Phoenix, AZ 85014-2817
602-266-6700

Zymogenetics, Inc.
1201 Eastlake Ave. E.
Seattle, WA 98102
206-547-8080

ISBN 1-57439-029-5

90000